PEDIATRIC ENDOCRINOLOGY

THIRD EDITION, REVISED AND EXPANDED

Compliments of

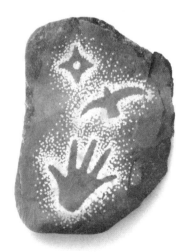

Pharmacia
&Upjohn

Clinical Pediatrics

Series Editor

Fima Lifshitz

Maimonides Medical Center
and State University of New York
Health Science Center at Brooklyn
Brooklyn, New York

Additional Volumes in Preparation

PEDIATRIC ENDOCRINOLOGY

THIRD EDITION, REVISED AND EXPANDED

EDITED BY

FIMA LIFSHITZ

**Maimonides Medical Center
and State University of New York Health Science Center at Brooklyn
Brooklyn, New York**

Marcel Dekker, Inc.

New York • Basel • Hong Kong

Library of Congress Cataloging-in-Publication Data

Pediatric endocrinology: a clinical guide / edited by Fima Lifshitz. — 3rd ed., rev. and
    expanded.
        p.   cm. — (Clinical pediatrics; v. 8)
    Includes bibliographical references and index.
    ISBN 0-8247-9369-2 (alk. paper)
    1. Pediatric endocrinology.   I. Lifshitz, Fima.   II. Series: Clinical pediatrics
(Marcel Dekker, Inc.); v. 8.
    [DNLM: 1. Endocrine Diseases—in infancy & childhood. 2. Endocrine
Diseases—physiopathology.   W1 CL761Y v.8 1996 / WS 330 P3713 1996]
RJ418.P43   1996
618.92'4—dc20
DNLM/DLC
for Library of Congress   95-35524
                                                                                    CIP

The publisher offers discounts on this book when ordered in bulk quantities. For more information, write to Special Sales/Professional
Marketing at the address below.

This book is printed on acid-free paper.

MARCEL DEKKER, INC.
270 Madison Avenue, New York, New York 10016

Current printing (last digit):
10 9 8 7 6 5 4 3 2

Printed in the United States of America

*To all those who helped in the creation, establishment,
and success of the Maimonides Children's Center*

About the Series

"Clinical Pediatrics" is a series of books designed to continuously update the knowledge of the practicing pediatrician in diverse areas of the specialty. Each volume in the series addresses rapidly developing topics that are changing the attitudes and treatment approaches of the clinician. The chapters comprising the volumes represent the state of the art on the various subjects from the vantage point of recognized experts in the field.

The books already published in this series are *Common Pediatric Disorders*, *Congenital Metabolic Diseases*, *Antimicrobial Therapy in Infants and Children*, *Food Allergy*, *Metabolic Bone Disease*, and *Pediatric Endocrinology*. The first edition of the latter book was published in 1985 and the second edition in 1990. This book has become the most sought after reference book in the field, making necessary an updated, third edition. This third edition of *Pediatric Endocrinology* is the eighth book in the "Clinical Pediatrics" series. It is an updated, improved, and greatly expanded version, which covers the field in a comprehensive manner to update clinicians on the numerous recent advances in pediatric endocrinology. The most frequent encounters by pediatricians are covered and reviewed in a practical, patient-oriented, yet scientific style, making it an invaluable resource for pediatricians and specialists alike.

These books serve as the foundation for the volumes that will follow, each complementing the other. Together, they will constitute a comprehensive review of the most recent developments in pediatrics.

Fima Lifshitz

Foreword

There is no greater challenge to the academician than writing a textbook that meets the needs of practitioners and academicians. Dr. Lifshitz met that challenge with the first edition of his textbook. It is no easy task to organize and publish a textbook, and it is an even more difficult task to organize and publish two additional editions, which Dr. Lifshitz has done, in an admirable manner. He states in his preface how these three books have come to pass, how the quality of the second surpassed that of the first, and how the quality of the third now markedly surpasses that of the second. The table of contents speaks for itself in respect to its broadness and completeness. You, the reader, will find the most up-to-date concepts in molecular biology, pathophysiology, and diagnosis and treatment of patients with growth disturbances, nutritional disorders, ambiguities of sexual differentiation, and various metabolic problems. Dr Lifshitz is the ideal person to have organized such a textbook because of his own multiple interests and accomplishments in the fields of growth, metabolism, and nutrition. National recognition of his expertise in all these areas has helped him organize this textbook in a way that those of us less broad in our knowledge and expertise could not. He is to be congratulated for accomplishing this work, and you are to be congratulated for seeking out this text for answers to your questions and search for knowledge. These observations and analyses are in addition to those I stated in the forewords to the previous two editions, to which you may wish to refer.

Robert M. Blizzard, M.D.
Professor of Pediatrics Emeritus
University of Virginia School of Medicine
Charlottesville, Virginia

Foreword

The study of endocrinology emerged as a specialty within the medical discipline of pediatrics over four decades ago, and, in the United States today, there are now over 600 practitioners who are board-certified pediatric endocrinologists. The field has broadened widely over the course of time: Originally concerned with physiological and anatomical topics as they related to sexual development, our understanding of endocrine science now encompasses a knowledge of molecular biology, biochemistry, and the genetic foundations of many varieties of endocrine disease. The modern pediatric endocrinologist must be part geneticist, part nutritionist, part gynecologist–urologist, and, as always, part auxologist.

The scope of this book is reflective of this growing field in pediatric endocrinology, offering a detailed guide for very specific problems in an age where pressure abounds to generalize. Dr. Fima Lifshitz, our colleague and the editor of this wonderful teaching tool, has assembled between these covers the foremost specialists in all areas of pediatric endocrinology. The end result, as I am sure you will agree, is a book that offers state-of-the-art information, techniques, and treatment options for pathophysiological disorders, and makes them accessible not only to endocrinologists but to all other pediatric specialists and general pediatricians as well.

I would like to congratulate our editor and friend, Fima Lifshitz, on possessing the forbearance necessary for an undertaking of this magnitude.

Maria I. New, M.D.
New York Hospital–Cornell Medical Center
New York, New York

ix

Preface to the Third Edition

That is a good book which is opened with expectation and closed in profit.

Amos Bronson Alcott

The third edition of the book *Pediatric Endocrinology* is the eighth volume in the "Clinical Pediatrics" series started in 1984. The aim of this series is to continuously update the knowledge of the practicing pediatrician in diverse areas of the specialty. With *Pediatric Endocrinology*, this goal is accomplished; every five years we have completed an updated, revised and expanded version. The first edition, published in 1985, included 33 contributors and contained 27 chapters; the second, more complete edition, included 57 contributors and 49 chapters. The growth process continued, culminating with this third edition, which constitutes a very comprehensive treatise in pediatric endocrinology, with 78 contributors, and 61 chapters with the most updated information in the field.

Updated material and increased size are not the only characteristics of the third edition. Unlike the previous editions, this book is fully inclusive, covering all aspects of the practice of pediatric endocrinology. Each chapter is written by recognized experts from all over the world. Every one of the 61 chapters provides the practicing pediatrician and the pediatric endocrinologist with an updated, comprehensive discussion addressing a clinical situation encountered in the practice of this specialty. Included are common and frequent problems faced daily, e.g., short stature, failure to thrive, menstrual abnormalities, vaginal bleeding, adrenal hyperplasia, hirsutism, hypothyroidism, diabetes mellitus, and obesity. More infrequent disorders, such as hypopituitarism, thyroid carcinoma, metabolic bone disorders, Mg alterations, hypoglycemia, and autoimmune endocrinopathies, are also covered. And there are new chapters addressing the most recent needs of pediatric endocrine practices, including psychosocial issues, treatment of short stature, Turner syndrome, and new advances in diabetes mellitus, as well as the endocrine aspects of patients with AIDS, long-term cancer survivors, eating disorders, and nontraditional inheritance of endocrine disorders.

As in the previous edition, this book was written with the needs of clinicians in mind, yet at a level fit for the subspecialist. Each chapter was conceptualized to enhance the knowledge of the practitioner and provide the reader with the necessary information to address and answer questions posed in the care of patients with endocrine and endocrine-related diseases. The answers and latest thoughts regarding each disease entity and group of alterations are contained here. From pathophysiology to treatment, readers will find the information necessary to care for their patients. The reviews are practical and provide the practicing physician with a succinct and clear understanding of the problem, with specific recommendations for diagnosis and treatment. The book is divided into six parts, each dealing with a specific area of childhood endocrinology: growth and growth disorders; sexual development abnormalities and adrenal disorders; thyroid; calcium and phosphorus; diabetes mellitus and hypoglycemia; and miscellaneous disorders. In addition, there is a chapter on laboratory aids and tolerance testing, and one with reference charts, figures, and tables supplying pertinent data, for easy reference. The third edition of *Pediatric Endocrinology* constitutes a clear and useful treatise in the field and is an excellent source for all those who care for children.

I am particularly grateful to all the contributors who have revised and updated their chapters and/or have provided new sections for this book. All of them made significant contributions, which combine to make this book a most valuable and necessary tool for pediatricians and pediatric endocrinologists alike. I am also very grateful to my assistant, Ms. Gladys G. Greenberg, whose help and contribution to this book shall not remain unrecognized. Her dedication and talent helped greatly in the realization of this book, and I thank her for it all.

Fima Lifshitz

Preface to the Second Edition

The essence of knowledge is, having it, to apply it; not having it, to confess your ignorance.

Confucius

Pediatric Endocrinology, the seventh volume in the "Clinical Pediatrics" series, focuses on current findings and concepts in the field. This volume is the second edition of what has become a very useful and successful book, published in 1985. The second edition has been greatly expanded and enhanced, and it now provides the practicing pediatrician with a review of the most relevant topics in pediatric endocrinology. The book is divided into six parts dealing with aspects of childhood endocrine disorders: growth and growth disorders, adrenals and sexual development; thyroid; calcium and phosphorus; diabetes mellitus and hypoglycemia; and other endocrine disorders. In addition, there is a chapter outlining the procedures of tolerance testing and supplying pertinent data and tables as an easy reference for the practitioner.

Each of the contributors of this book is an expert on his or her field. The authors convey the state of the art of each topic in a succinct and practical fashion, delving into the pathophysiological background of each disorder in order to make it clear and understandable to the practicing physician. This book contains pertinent practical information on a variety of problems with the most frequent complaints covered in great detail. The book constitutes a clear and useful reference source for all those who care for children.

Fima Lifshitz

Preface to the First Edition

Knowledge is to ignorance what the sun is to a morning fog.

O. A. Battista

Pediatric Endocrinology, the third volume in the "Clinical Pediatrics" series, focuses on current concepts in the field. It is not an all-inclusive treatise of pediatric endocrinology, but rather a review for the practicing pediatrician of some of the most relevant topics in this field. The book is divided into six parts dealing with aspects of childhood endocrine disorders, namely: growth, adrenals and sexual development, thyroid, calcium and phosphorus, diabetes mellitus and hypoglycemia, and other endocrine disorders. In addition, there is an appendix outlining the procedures of tolerance testing.

Each of the contributors of this book is an expert in his or her field. The authors convey the state of the art of each topic in a succinct and practical fashion, delving into the pathophysiological background of the topic in order to make it clear and understandable. The book also contains updated information that will be of considerable value to the pediatric endocrinologist.

Stimulation to pursue academic activities for continuous medical education has come from several sources, not the least being my close associates in the Division of Pediatric Endocrinology, Metabolism, and Nutrition. They have contributed with their writings and suggestions for the book, as well as assumed many responsibilities in order to allow me to pursue this endeavor.

Fima Lifshitz

Contents

SEXUAL DEVELOPMENT ABNORMALITIES AND ADRENAL DISORDERS

Contributors

Jose E. Abdenur, M.D. Assistant Professor, Human Genetics and Pediatrics, and Co-Director, Biochemical Genetics Laboratory, Mount Sinai School of Medicine, New York, New York

Ramin Alemzadeh, M.D. Assistant Professor, Department of Pediatrics, University of Tennessee Medical Center at Knoxville, Knoxville, Tennessee

David B. Allen, M.D. Professor of Pediatrics, and Director of Pediatric Endocrinology and Endocrinology Residency Training Program, University of Wisconsin School of Medicine, Madison, Wisconsin

Albert Altchek, M.D. Clinical Professor of Obstetrics, Gynecology, and Reproductive Science, and Chief of Pediatric and Adolescent Gynecology, Mount Sinai School of Medicine, New York, New York

Joseph N. Attie, M.D. Clinical Professor, Department of Surgery, Albert Einstein School of Medicine, Bronx, New York

Ronald R. Bainbridge, M.B.B.S. Associate Attending Neonatologist and Endocrinologist, Department of Pediatrics, Maimonides Medical Center, and Assistant Professor of Pediatrics, State University of New York Health Science Center at Brooklyn, Brooklyn, New York

Dorothy J. Becker, M.B., B.Ch., F.C.P.(P) Professor, Department of Pediatrics, Children's Hospital of Pittsburgh and University of Pittsburgh, Pittsburgh, Pennsylvania

Barry B. Bercu, M.D. Professor of Pediatrics, Pharmacology, and Therapeutics, Department of Pediatrics, University of South Florida College of Medicine, Tampa, Florida

Sandra L. Blethen, M.D., Ph.D. Associate Professor, Department of Pediatrics, School of Medicine, State University of New York at Stony Brook, Stony Brook, New York

Robert M. Blizzard, M.D. Professor of Pediatrics Emeritus, University of Virginia School of Medicine, Charlottesville, Virginia

Hans Henning Bode, M.D. Professor and Chairman, School of Pediatrics, University of New South Wales, Prince of Wales Children's Hospital, Sydney, New South Wales, Australia

Glenn D. Braunstein, M.D. Chairman of Medicine, Cedars-Sinai Medical Center, and Professor of Medicine, UCLA School of Medicine, Los Angeles, California

Stuart J. Brink, M.D. Director, Pediatric and Adolescent Diabetes and Endocrinology, Newton Wellesley Hospital, Newton, and Senior Physician, New England Diabetes and Endocrinology Center (NEDEC), Chestnut Hill, Massachusetts

Rosalind S. Brown, M.D., F.R.C.P.(C) Associate Professor of Pediatrics, and Director, Division of Pediatric Endocrinology/Diabetes, University of Massachusetts Medical School, Worcester, Massachusetts

Anamaria Bulatovic, M.D. Department of Pediatrics, Johns Hopkins Bayview Medical Center, Baltimore, Maryland

Salvador Castells, M.D. Professor, Department of Pediatrics, State University of New York Health Science Center at Brooklyn, Brooklyn, New York

Cecilia D. Cervantes, M.D. Assistant Professor, Department of Pediatrics, North Shore University Hospital, Manhasset, New York

Fred I. Chasalow, Ph.D. Director, Pediatric Endocrinology Laboratory, Department of Pediatrics, Maimonides Medical Center, Brooklyn, New York

Takeshi Chihara Instructor, Institute for Comprehensive Medical Science, Fujita Health University, Toyoake, Japan

Richard M. Cowett, M.D. Professor, Department of Pediatrics, Brown University School of Medicine and Women and Infants Hospital of Rhode Island, Providence, Rhode Island

Christopher Crawford Academic Research Specialist, Division of Pediatric Endocrinology, Department of Pediatrics, Cornell University Medical Center, New York, New York

John D. Crawford, M.D. Professor of Pediatrics Emeritus, Harvard Medical School, and Emeritus Chief, Pediatric Endocrine Metabolism Unit, Massachusetts General Hospital, Boston, Massachusetts

John S. Dallas, M.D. Assistant Professor, Department of Pediatrics, University of Texas Medical Branch, and Children's Hospital of Galveston, Galveston, Texas

Marco Danon, M.D. Chief, Division of Pediatric Endocrinology, Department of Pediatrics, Maimonides Medical Center, and Associate Professor, Department of Pediatrics, State University of New York Health Science Center at Brooklyn, Brooklyn, New York

Allan L. Drash, M.D. Professor of Pediatrics and Epidemiology, University of Pittsburgh, and Director of Research, Division of Endocrinology, Metabolism, and Diabetes Mellitus, Department of Pediatrics, Children's Hospital of Pittsburgh, Pittsburgh, Pennsylvania

Thomas P. Foley, Jr., M.D. Professor, Department of Pediatrics, University of Pittsburgh, and Professor and Director, Division of Endocrinology, Metabolism, and Diabetes Mellitus, Department of Pediatrics, Children's Hospital of Pittsburgh, Pittsburgh, Pennsylvania

Pavel F. Fort, M.D. Associate Professor of Clinical Pediatrics, Division of Pediatric Endocrinology and Metabolism, Department of Pediatrics, North Shore University Hospital, Manhasset, New York

Carol M. Foster, M.D. Associate Professor, Department of Pediatrics, University of Michigan Medical School, Ann Arbor, Michigan

S. Douglas Frasier, M.D. Professor of Pediatrics, UCLA School of Medicine, Los Angeles, California

Steven C. Friedman, M.D. Chief, Division of Pediatric Urology, Department of Urology, Maimonides Medical Center, Brooklyn, New York

Joseph M. Gertner, M.B., M.R.C.P. Professor, Department of Pediatrics, New York Hospital–Cornell University Medical Center, New York, New York

Lucia Ghizzoni, M.D. Department of Pediatrics, University of Parma, Parma, Italy

Lori J. Ginsberg, R.N., M.A. Nurse Coordinator, Division of Adolescent Medicine, Department of Pediatrics, North Shore University Hospital, Manhasset, New York

Judith G. Hall, M.D.   Professor and Head, Department of Pediatrics, British Columbia Children's Hospital, University of British Columbia, Vancouver, British Columbia, Canada

Alberto Hayek, M.D.   Professor, Department of Pediatrics, University of California at San Diego, La Jolla, California

Muhammad A. Jabbar, M.D.   Assistant Professor, Department of Pediatrics, Hurley Medical Center, Michigan State University, Flint, Michigan

Jean-Claude Job, M.D.   Professor Emeritus of Pediatrics, Faculté de Médecine Cochin, Paris, France

Ann J. Johanson, M.D.   Clinical Professor, Department of Pediatrics, University of Virginia School of Medicine, Charlottesville, Virginia

Winston W. K. Koo, M.B.B.S., F.R.A.C.P.   Associate Professor of Pediatrics, Obstetrics, and Gynecology, Department of Pediatrics, University of Tennessee at Memphis, Memphis, Tennessee

Roberto L. Lanes, M.D.   Pediatric Endocrinologist, Unidad de Endocrinologia Pediatrica, Hospital de Clinicas Caracas, Caracas, Venezuela

Peter A. Lee, M.D., Ph.D.   Professor, Department of Pediatrics, University of Pittsburgh and Children's Hospital of Pittsburgh, Pittsburgh, Pennsylvania

Lynne L. Levitsky, M.D.   Chief, Pediatric Endocrine Unit, and Associate Professor of Pediatrics, Children's Service, Massachusetts General Hospital, and Department of Pediatrics, Harvard Medical School, Boston, Massachusetts

Eric A. Lifshitz, M.D.   Clinical Instructor, Department of Psychiatry, UCLA Neuropsychiatric Institute, Los Angeles, California

Fima Lifshitz, M.D.   Chairman, Department of Pediatrics, Maimonides Medical Center, and Professor of Pediatrics, State University of New York Health Science Center at Brooklyn, Brooklyn, New York

Elena Lopez-Rangel, M.D., M.Sc.   Research Associate, Department of Pediatrics, British Columbia Children's Hospital, University of British Columbia, Vancouver, British Columbia, Canada

Claude J. Migeon, M.D.   Professor of Pediatrics, Johns Hopkins University School of Medicine, Baltimore, Maryland

Francis B. Mimouni, M.D.   Director, Division of Neonatology, Department of Pediatrics, Maimonides Medical Center, and Professor of Pediatrics, State University of New York Health Science Center at Brooklyn, Brooklyn, New York

John Money, Ph.D.   Professor Emeritus of Medical Psychology and of Pediatrics, Deparment of Psychiatry and Behavioral Sciences, Johns Hopkins University School of Medicine and Johns Hopkins Hospital, Baltimore, Maryland

Adib Moukarzel, M.D., Ph.D.   Director, Division of Pediatric Gastroenterology and Nutrition, Department of Pediatrics, Maimonides Medical Center, and Assistant Professor, Department of Pediatrics, State University of New York Health Science Center at Brooklyn, Brooklyn, New York

E. Kirk Neely, M.D.   Clinical Assistant Professor, Department of Pediatrics, Stanford University, Stanford, California

Maria I. New, M.D.   Chief, Division of Pediatric Endocrinology, and Professor and Chairman, Department of Pediatrics, New York Hospital–Cornell Medical Center, New York, New York

Yoshikazu Nishi, M.D.   Chairman, Department of Pediatrics, Hiroshima Red Cross Hospital, Hiroshima, Japan

Songya Pang, M.D.   Professor, Department of Pediatrics, College of Medicine, University of Illinois, Chicago, Illinois

Jaakko Perheentupa, M.D., D. Med. Sci.   Professor and Director, Department of Pediatrics, Children's Hospital, University of Helsinki, Helsinki, Finland

Gerald F. Powell, M.D.   Associate Professor of Pediatrics, University of Texas Medical Branch, Galveston, Texas

Robert Rapaport, M.D.   Associate Professor of Pediatrics, and Director, Division of Pediatric Endocrinology and Metabolism, University of Medicine and Dentistry–New Jersey Medical School and Children's Hospital of New Jersey, Newark, New Jersey

Raphael Rappaport, M.D.   Professor of Pediatrics, Pediatric Endocrinology Unit, Hôpital des Enfants Malades, Paris, France

Bridget F. Recker, R.N., Ed.M.   Clinical Coordinator, Department of Pediatrics, Maimonides Medical Center, Brooklyn, New York

David L. Rimoin, M.D., Ph.D.   Steven Spielberg Chairman of Pediatrics, Director, Ahmanson Pediatric Center, Director, Medical Genetics Birth Defect Center, Cedars-Sinai Medical Center, and Professor of Pediatrics and Medicine, UCLA School of Medicine, Los Angeles, California

Scott A. Rivkees, M.D.   Associate Professor of Pediatrics, Pediatric Endocrine Unit, Riley Hospital for Children, Indianapolis, Indiana

Alicia A. Romano, M.D.   Assistant Professor of Pediatrics, Division of Pediatric Endocrinology, New York Medical College, Valhalla, New York

Arlan L. Rosenbloom, M.D.   Professor, Department of Pediatrics, University of Florida College of Medicine, Gainesville, Florida

Ron G. Rosenfeld, M.D.   Professor and Chairman, Department of Pediatrics, and Physician-in-Chief, Doernbecher Memorial Hospital for Children, and Department of Pediatrics, Oregon Health Sciences University, Portland, Oregon

Max Salas, M.D.   Associate Professor, Department of Pediatrics, University of Medicine and Dentistry of New Jersey–Robert Wood Johnson Medical School, New Brunswick, New Jersey

David E. Sandberg, Ph.D.   Assistant Professor in Psychiatry and Pediatrics, Division of Child and Adolescent Psychiatry, Department of Psychoendocrinology, State University of New York at Buffalo and Children's Hospital of Buffalo, Buffalo, New York

Mordechai Shohat, M.D.   Director, Department of Medical Genetics, Beilinson Medical Center, Petah Tikva, Israel

Melanie M. Smith, M.N.S., R.D., C.S.   Chief Pediatric Nutritionist, Department of Pediatrics, Maimonides Medical Center, and Instructor in Pediatrics, State University of New York Health Science Center at Brooklyn, Brooklyn, New York

Phyllis W. Speiser, M.D.   Chief, Division of Pediatric Endocrinology, North Shore University Hospital, Manhasset, New York

Mark A. Sperling, M.D.   Vira I. Heinz Professor and Chairman, Department of Pediatrics, University of Pittsburgh and Children's Hospital of Pittsburgh, Pittsburgh, Pennsylvania

Susan E. Stred, M.D.   Assistant Professor, Pediatric Endocrine Center and Cell and Molecular Biology Program, State University of New York Health Science Center at Syracuse, Syracuse, New York

Omer Tarim, M.D.*   Pediatric Endocrinologist, Maimonides Medical Center, and Assistant Professor, State University of New York Health Science Center at Brooklyn, Brooklyn, New York

Elisabeth Thibaud   Consultant in Pediatric and Adolescent Gynecology, Department of Pediatric Endocrinology, Hôpital des Enfants Malades, Paris, France

Reginald C. Tsang, M.B.B.S.   Director, Division of Neonatology, University of Cincinnati, and Associate Chairman, Department of Pediatrics, Children's Hospital Medical Center, Cincinnati, Ohio

Raffaele Virdis, M.D.   Associate Professor, Department of Pediatrics, University of Parma, Parma, Italy

Mary L. Voorhess, M.D.   Professor Emeritus, Department of Pediatrics, State University of New York at Buffalo, and Division of Endocrinology, Children's Hospital of Buffalo, Buffalo, New York

Joseph B. Warshaw, M.D.   Professor and Chairman, Department of Pediatrics, Yale University School of Medicine, and Physician-in-Chief, Children's Hospital at Yale, New Haven, Connecticut

William E. Winter, M.D.   Associate Professor, Department of Pathology and Laboratory Medicine, Department of Pediatrics, and Department of Molecular Genetics and Microbiology, Medical Director, Clinical Chemistry Laboratory, and Section Chief, Clinical Chemistry Section, University of Florida College of Medicine, Gainesville, Florida

David Zangen, M.D.   Fellow in Pediatric Endocrinology, Massachusetts General Hospital and Harvard Medical School, Boston, Massachusetts

---

Present affiliation: Associate Professor of Pediatrics, ULUDAG University of Bursa, Turkey.

1
Short Stature

Fima Lifshitz
*Maimonides Medical Center and State University of New York Health Science Center at Brooklyn,
Brooklyn, New York*

Cecilia D. Cervantes
North Shore University Hospital, Manhasset, New York

I. THE GENERAL PROBLEM

One of the primary concerns of pediatricians is the appropriate growth of their patients. Parents and children also worry about "growth" as evidence of good health. Organic alterations, as discussed later, may alter the height and weight of a patient; these must be diagnosed and treated. There are other problems in being short, however, even when the body size is only mildly affected. Indeed, any person who is below average height (in the United States 5 feet 9 inches for men and 5 feet 5 inches for women) may also expect to have a number of psychosocial difficulties. Dwarfs have these problems to a greater degree, with various amounts of tolerance and rejection according to the different customs and beliefs of the locality in which they live. The psychosocial prejudice toward the small person transcends age, sex, race, creed, and financial status: all short people may be victims of discrimination. This seldom mentioned form of prejudice, like sexism or racism, is well established in this country and may be prevalent throughout the world. It has been called heightism. (The reader is referred to the book *The Height of Your Life*, by Ralph Keyes, for a very comprehensive and interesting review of this problem.) This book approaches heightism in a wry and humorous fashion. It highlights facts regarding height so basic to our relationships with others that we have ceased to think about them. It is from this book that the following comments have been extracted.

So pervasive is the bias against short people that no one notices it—no one, that is, except the short person. The English language illustrates this bias clearly. *Feisty* is the classic example, a word normally used in tandem with "little." *Distinguished*, by contrast, may not be synonymous with "tall" but rarely is used to refer to short persons. Other very important phrases remind us regularly of the importance of height: compare "looks up to" and "looks down upon." The question is always, How tall are you? instead of the neutral, What is your height? The song "Short People" by Randy Newman describes those below average in height have "grubby little fingers" and "dirty little minds" with "no reason to live." This song is a spoof of bigotry with a catchy tune, yet it made the hit parade. The composer meant it as a joke; of course, he is 5 feet 11 inches!

Height is one of the most important traits both parties try to match when it comes to selecting a personal relationship. In romantic matters, little men are "cut down to size." An ideal lover is never short, and at present both sexes seem to feel that in relationships the male should be taller than the female. Even Sandy Allen, who at 7 feet 7½ inches is certified by *The Guiness Book of World Records* as the tallest woman in the world, was quoted as saying, "I've got this old-fashioned idea, I will never marry anyone smaller than I am." She never married. Thus, the tall man seems to have all of womankind to choose from, whereas the short man appears to be limited to short women. Indeed, there may be more interreligious and interracial marriages than there are couples in which the man is shorter than the woman. Former Secretary of State Henry Kissinger was acknowledged as a truly unusual phenomenon because he married a taller woman.

Rewards for being tall in our society include money. Business, it seems, is interested in the short men mostly as customers for elevator shoes. The president of the Mutual Life Insurance Company surveyed its policy holders and found a nearly perfect correlation between body height and policy value. Several studies have pointed out that taller persons earn higher salaries. Corporate recruiters also tend to choose the taller of two equally qualified applicants. Even when he succeeds, despite the odds against him, the short person is often accused of being a "Little Napoleon."

Height is more than a mere statistic: for men it is a measure of manhood. Height brings acknowledgement, deference, and power. *Big* and *strong* are, from childhood, considered nearly the same word. The dominant figures in advertisements and legendary figures in the movies are usually represented by tall people. Height is equated with power to such a degree that it plays a very important role in politics. Most U.S. presidents have not been short; the shortest was Madison at 5 feet 4 inches. Only six other presidents were slightly below the present average height. Americans have usually favored the taller political candidate. As a matter of fact, the taller of the two major presidential candidates is usually sent to the White House. There have been only three exceptions. In 1924, Calvin Coolidge (5 feet 10 inches) defeated John Davis (5 feet 11 inches); in 1972, Nixon (6 feet) defeated McGovern (6 feet 1 inch); and in 1976 Carter (5 feet 6 inches) defeated Ford (6 feet 1 inch). Mr. Carter's political advisors recognized the problem of lack of height and insisted that both contestants appear of equal size during the presidential debates on television. His advisors requested that Mr. Carter stand on a stool behind the podium. The 1984 political contenders were both tall, but Ronald Reagan won over the slightly shorter Walter Mondale. The 1988 Democratic candidate Mike Dukakis (5 feet 7 1/2 inches) faced the public standing on a platform behind the podium so that he appeared of equal size to George Bush (6 feet 2 inches), his Republican opponent. Perhaps to improve his chances to win the presidency, he selected a tall running mate, Lloyd Bentsen, who is a bit over 6 feet tall—to no avail. Again, in 1992, the tallest candidate, Bill Clinton, was elected president, with a third-party very short candidate, Ross Perot, trailing way behind. The U.S. public again voted by the inch!

Although human esthetics and social tastes clearly favor tallness, nature shows no such preference. Anthropologists estimate that, for most of history, natural selection kept adult male heights within a range below our current averages. Supporting the natural selection process, infants' skeletons, which are abundant in old graveyards, are rather tall, in fact comparable to our present norms. Some experts think that these two phenomena are related. It seems that environmental problems were more detrimental to youngsters destined to be large, and only those destined to be small survived the rigors of malnutrition and disease. Ashley Montagu wrote, "At least in part the recent increase in overall size visible in the modern adult population is due to the fact that improved standards of food and medical care have allowed genetic combinations to survive which would have been selected against in ages past" (C. F. Brace and A. Montagu, *Human Evolution*).

II. THE MEDICAL PROBLEM

Pediatricians are often consulted by parents worried about short stature in their children. This term needs definition. "Short stature" has been defined as height below the third percentile; therefore, 3% of normal children would be classified as being short. "Dwarfism," the severe form of short stature, is defined as height below 3 standard deviations (SD) from the mean. The

population selected for reference is important when judgments are made about the shortness of an individual. A number of different reference charts have been used in this country in recent decades, each varying somewhat from others because of the representative population from whom the data were derived (e.g., predominantly rural children from Iowa versus Boston city children). The most common reference charts now in use are the National Center for Health Statistics growth charts (1). These are compiled from growth data gathered from many diverse population groups in the United States and are applicable to all racial groups.

Pediatricians know that most children with mild short stature eventually become average-sized adults; however, some children have serious growth disturbances that may prevent them from reaching normal adult size. The Newcastle study in England supported the need for an explanation of the cause of short stature in all children whose height falls below the third percentile (2). Almost half of the 5000 infants born in Newcastle in 1960 were measured for height at age 10. The height of 111 children fell below the third percentile: 16 were found to have previously unsuspected organic disease as a cause of short stature. These findings show that it is unusual for a "normal" child to have a height below the third percentile. It may also be inferred that in 10–15% of children who are short, a pathologic condition may be found to account for the short stature. Therefore, the cause of short stature should be investigated. At times the diagnosis is not simple and requires expert advice.

Growth-related disorders are also the most frequent problems encountered by pediatric endocrinologists in university hospitals. Pediatricians often seek consultation to help in the diagnosis and management of children with growth disturbances (Fig. 1). Even in a pediatric endocrine referral center, a large proportion of patients with short stature are healthy children. At times children are referred for short stature although they are of normal height. This is because of either poor, inaccurate measurements or the need of a pediatric endocrinologist in reassuring a patient or the family when the child is growing in the lower end of the normal range. In only a bit over one-third does an organic pathologic condition account for poor growth or short stature. In most instances of short stature a diagnosis is usually made, although in some patients, the cause of short stature may defy the differential diagnosis of numerous experts.

III. DIAGNOSIS OF SHORT STATURE

The different causes of short stature in children are listed in Table 1. This simplified classification distinguishes most forms of short stature into two main categories: short patients who are normal, and short patients who have an abnormality. These two basic concepts must be considered in the diagnosis of all short patients. It must be determined whether a child is normal but has constitutional growth delay and/or familial short stature. That is, one must distinguish between the short child who is healthy and growing normally and who will attain an adequate adult height and one whose shortness is of genetic

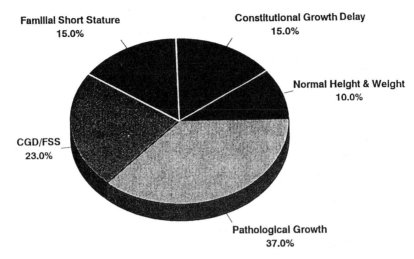

Figure 1 Patients referred because of short stature. Patients were referred to the Pediatric Endocrine Ambulatory Center at North Shore University Hospital from January 1973 through June 1991. Short stature was defined as a height below the third percentile for American standards. CGD/FSS = combination of constitutional growth delay and familial short stature.

origin, that is, a patient who is healthy and growing normally but is small, although within normal limits when allowance is made for his or her parents' heights. Most important, a clinician must determine whether a child is subject to pathologic causes of short stature or poor growth. These causes must be diagnosed to provide treatment and allow the patient to grow whenever possible.

Each of these possible categories of short stature denotes not only the cause but also the pathophysiologic process involved and the prognosis for final adult height. The specific applicable situation should be recognized by the physician before subjecting the patient to expensive and complicated investigations.

Other classifications to determine the different categories of short patients are used by pediatric endocrinologists. For example, in one review (3), familial or genetic short stature was referred to as "intrinsic shortness." Constitutional growth delay was called delayed growth, and all other disorders resulting in poor growth were called attenuated growth. Other authors have used the term "idiopathic short stature" to describe short individuals below the third percentile who have no demonstrable functional abnormality and whose parents are normal in height. However, these terms to classify short patients are unnecessary because the two categories proposed are inclusive and sufficient to understand and clarify growth problems. A specific diagnosis can usually be arrived at to define the patient's condition accurately.

A. Growth Patterns

The importance of obtaining previous growth and weight data for every patient with a growth problem cannot be over-emphasized (Fig. 2). Growth data can be plotted on standard growth charts devised by the National Center for Health Statistics. However, attention must be paid to the various growth patterns of specific patients, stages of development,

racial groups, or population types (4–7). For some conditions (Turner syndrome, achondroplasia, low birth weight, and Down syndrome), specific growth charts have been devised (see Chap. 61 for these charts) (8–13). Because growth is an active process, growth velocity charts are even more useful than standard growth charts in determining the normality of growth (14).

A record of consecutive accurate heights and weights over a considerable time span yields more important information than isolated measurements. Additionally, a child's growth should be evaluated over a period of time. It has been shown that growth is not a steady continuous process but occurs by episodic saltatory increments, and there may be a 3–60 day interval of no growth at all. Thus, a sound analysis of growth requires an observation period of at least 6 months before any definitie conclusions can be made about the growth pattern and before altering any mode of treatment (15).

There is also a significant scasonal variation in growth (16). Peak growth rates have been observed to occur in the summer and spring months, with a nadir in the fall and winter months. This pattern applies even to patients receiving growth hormone treatment. The best growth data are often obtainable from schools that measure children regularly once or twice a year. Often children may be seen erratically in physicians' offices for acute problems, and height may not be recorded. A serious growth problem may be overlooked for many years if no height and weight records are kept, or a patient may be referred and evaluated needlessly because of inaccurate measurements. About 10% of patients referred to our center because of short stature are found to be of normal height (see Fig. 1).

Children with abnormal growth velocity should be evaluated for possible pathologic conditions. In interpreting the patient's growth velocity, allowance must be made for age, puberty, and other factors. The fastest growth occurs in uterine life. Linear growth peaks around the fourth month of gestation, when it reaches 2.5 cm/week (130 cm/year). It then slows until

Table 1   Causes of Short Stature

I. Normal
   A. Constitutional growth delay
   B. Genetic-familial short stature
   C. Constitutional growth delay and familial short stature
II. Pathologic
   A. Nutritional
      1. Hypocaloric
      2. Chronic inflammatory bowel disease
      3. Malabsorption
      4. Celiac disease
      5. Zinc deficiency
   B. Endocrine
      1. Hypothyroidism
      2. Isolated growth hormone deficiency
      3. Hypopituitarism
      4. Excess cortisol
      5. Precocious puberty
   C. Chromosome defects
      1. Turner syndrome
      2. Down syndrome
   D. Low birth weight short stature (intrauterine growth retardation)
      1. Sporadic
      2. Characteristic appearance
         a. Russell-Silver syndrome
         b. De Lange syndrome
         c. Seckel bird-headed dwarfism
         d. Dubowitz syndrome
         e. Bloom syndrome
         f. Johanson-Blizzard syndrome
   E. Bone development disorders
      1. Achondroplasia
      2. Chondrodystrophies
      3. Other skeletal disorders
   F. Metabolic
      1. Mucopolysaccharidosis
      2. Other storage disorders
   G. Chronic illness
      1. Chronic renal disease
      2. Chronic liver disease
      3. Congenital heart disease
      4. Pulmonary (cystic fibrosis, bronchial asthma)
      5. Poorly controlled diabetes mellitus
      6. Chronic infections (including human immunodeficiency virus infection)
   H. Associated with birth defects or mental retardation
      1. Specific syndromes
      2. Nonspecific defects
   I. Psychosocial
   J. Chronic drug intake
      1. Glucocorticoids
      2. High-dose estrogens
      3. High-dose androgens
      4. Methylphenidate
      5. Dextroamphetamine

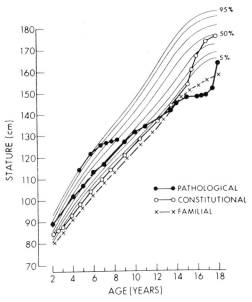

Figure 2 The growth patterns of three patients with short stature and one patient with pathological growth disorder who nevertheless was of normal height. The patient with pathological short stature received treatment at age 17 and attained catch-up growth.

birth. However, birth size and even size in the first 2 years may not correlate with childhood and adult height. In the first year of life, linear growth is still very fast: a total of approximately 25 cm is gained. However, the rate of growth declines rapidly over the first year, from 38 cm/year in the first 2 months to 28 cm/year at 4 months of age and 12 cm/year at 1 year of age. In the second year of life it is 10 cm/year, in the third through fourth years 7 cm/year, and in the fifth through sixth years 6 cm/year. From then on to puberty it is 5 cm/year (17,18). Guidelines for abnormal growth rates adjusted for chronologic age are fewer than 7 cm/year under age 4 years, fewer than 6 cm before age 6, and fewer than 4.5 cm from 6 years until puberty. For more precise growth velocity rates at various ages, specific charts should be consulted. Recent reference data have been published on expected weight and linear growth gains of children during the first 2 years of life. These are useful in screening for deviations from normal growth and may aid in early detection of failure to thrive or excessive weight gain during early life (19).

The second acceleration in height velocity takes place at puberty. Girls have their peak height velocity during early puberty and before menarche (Tanner stages II–III), during which time they grow at a mean velocity of 9 cm/year. Boys reach their peak height velocity during midpuberty (Tanner stages III–IV), during which time they grow at a mean rate of 10.3 cm/year. Boys' puberty growth spurt period is longer than girls' (17,18). Obese children have a faster rate of growth and reach puberty earlier than nonobese children. Their final height, however, may be slightly less than that of their nonobese peers (20). Boys are slightly taller than girls in the first 2 years of life. After this, until puberty, heights are

similar. For girls, skeletal age is more advanced for chronologic age than for boys.

An evaluation of the patient's pattern of growth is the most helpful clue in the differential diagnosis of short stature. The various growth patterns of patients with short stature are depicted in Figure 2. Patients with constitutional growth delay usually have a severe deceleration of growth within the first 2–3 years of life, with subsequent definition of a growth channel and normal growth increments paralleling the normal curve (see later). These patients usually do not have very severe short stature, although at times they may be below 3 SD from the mean, particularly when they have a concomitant familial short stature. They also have a delayed adolescent growth spurt that can result in an apparent deviation from their own growth curves at this time. Because of the bone age delay, however, they continue to grow after the average child has stopped growing and therefore may attain an appropriate adult height.

Patients with genetic or familial short stature grow at constant rates proportional to those in children of average height, and they enter puberty at an appropriate age. Their final height is consistent with parental height.

On the other hand, pathologic growth or short stature should always be considered in children who are very short and in those who do not grow well regardless of height. Any patient who falls behind in growth, across 2 major percentiles of the growth chart, should undergo a complete evaluation even when the height is not below the third percentile. This therefore includes patients with constitutional growth delay who are seen during the deceleration phase before 3 years of age. There is no other way to evaluate such patients at that time except by a thorough assessment to rule out disease. In contrast, there may be pathologic conditions without alterations in growth or in growth rate. For example, patients with hypopituitarism characteristically grow normally during the first few months of life, but they then reach a plateau and subsequent growth falls further and further behind. Patients with acquired hypothyroidism generally develop a plateau in their growth curves despite a progressive gain in weight. A similar growth pattern may be observed in Cushing syndrome or in children who are chronically taking pharmacologic doses of glucocorticoids for various conditions, such as chronic inflammatory bowel disease or bronchial asthma.

Other pathologic conditions of severe short stature do not alter the rate of growth of the patient (see Table 1). In the past, the term "primordial" or "ateliotic" dwarfism was used to define some of these patients. This term includes such conditions as intrauterine short stature, specific syndromes, and bone development disorders, generally referred to as bone dysplasias (Chaps. 7 and 10). Therefore, we prefer to specify the condition by the appropriate term instead of the broad category of primordial short stature. Children with short stature resulting from any of these conditions may or may not have a low birth weight and length. Those who are born small usually fail to exhibit catch-up growth during infancy. However, all grow at normal rates that parallel the normal curves. It is recommended that the growth rates of these patients be followed in growth charts specifically designed for each condition when available (5,9–11).

Usually, however, among pediatric endocrinologists and other physicians, growth patterns simply imply the assessment of the stature of the patient, with little consideration given to body weight progression. We now know that nutritional dwarfing may be a frequent cause of pathologic growth (see Chap. 8). These patients may be readily recognized by assessment of body weight progression throughout life. Children with nutritional causes of growth retardation usually demonstrate an initial fall in weight gain followed by a deceleration in growth rate (21,22). However, the nutritional growth-retarded patient is not necessarily underweight for height (23,24). Therefore, a record of previous weights is as essential as previous heights in the evaluation of a short child (see Chap. 8).

There are certain conditions in infancy in which weight progression does not necessarily affect growth. For example, in a recent study comparing the growth of breast-fed versus formula-fed infants during the first 18 months, the mean weight of breast-fed infants dropped from the median beginning at 6–8 months and was significantly lower than that of the formula-fed group between 6 and 18 months. However, length and head circumference were similar between the two groups (25). It has been suggested that breast-fed infants be plotted on a growth chart specific for their group, because they appear faltering when plotted on standard charts even if they are healthy and thriving.

Aside from body weight progression, attention must be given to the changes in body proportions during growth. The skeleton does not grow in a completely proportionate manner. At birth, the upper to lower body ratio is 1.7. As the legs grow, the ratio becomes 1.0 by 10 years of age. If growth plates close early, as in precocious puberty, the proportions are those of a child, with short limbs compared with the trunk. On the other hand, if growth is prolonged as in hypogonadism, the limbs are much longer compared with the trunk (26). Various types of tubular bone altrations are often found among short patients (see later). These categorize the patients into specific diagnostic categories and potential treatments.

Thus, aside from accurate measurement of height and weight, every child who presents with a growth problem should be evaluated for disproportionate limb shortening. Because this information helps to narrow the differential diagnosis, including ruling out skeletal dysplasia, a detailed anthropometric evaluation of a child's body segments is indispensable.

B. Anthropometric Measurements

Accurate weight measurements should be made on a regular hospital weighing scale. An infant should be stripped of clothes and diapers, and older children should wear a hospital gown or light clothing. These measures minimize inaccuracies resulting from variability in clothing weight, which varies with the different seasons of the year. Adherence to these rules is important if we are to take note of changes in weight over time.

Unfortunately, the most frequent method of measuring height, using a flip-up horizontal bar on a weighing scale, is subject to great errors caused by the child's slumping posture and considerable variation in the angle of the horizontal bar. Children should be measured standing upright and fully extended against a wall or firm vertical structure to which a properly mounted, accurate measuring device is attached. A steel tape measure, properly affixed to the wall, serves this purpose well and economically. The child stands shoeless, heels down, as erect as possible, and with the head directly forward. The back of the head, chest, gluteal area, and heels should touch the vertical surface. A firm object (e.g., a carpenter's angle) is then placed at a right angle over the top of the head and against the wall above the head. We utilize the Harpenden stadiometer (Holtain Limited, Crymych, Dyfed, U.K.), which determines height accurately (within 0.25 cm). Ross Laboratories and Genentech devised an inexpensive plastic instrument that they provide gratis; it is comparable in accuracy to the more expensive Harpenden stadiometer (27).

The arm span should be measured with the patient standing against a flat wall, the arms stretched out as far as possible, to create a 90° angle with the torso. The distance between the distal ends of both middle phalanges is measured to determine the arm span. Normally, the arm span is shorter than the height in boys under the age of 10–11 years and in girls under 11–14 years, after which the arm span becomes longer than the height, so that the average adult male has an arm span that is about 5.3 cm greater than his height and the adult female has an arm span 1.2 cm greater than her height (28). Conditions that adversely affect the vertebrae, may result in growth retardation and disproportionately long arms. Children with arm spans that are disproportionately longer than their heights should also be evaluated for scoliosis.

Determination of the upper to lower body segment ratio is also essential because skeletal dysplasias that result in growth problems are usually characterized by disproportionate shortening of the lower limbs or the spine. This can be done by measuring the distance between the upper border of the symphysis pubis and the floor in a patient who is standing against a flat wall in the proper position for height measurement. This measurement is difficult to obtain accurately because the superior border of the symphysis pubis is difficult to locate and palpate, particularly in some obese patients. Preferably, the sitting height can be measured to represent the upper segment, using a Harpenden sitting table (Holtain Limited). The patient is asked to sit on the table with the back of the knees touching the table edge. The vertical unit is then moved close to the patient's back and the patient positioned so that the entire back, including the back of the head, touches the vertical surface. The sitting height is indicated by a counter, and the sitting height to standing height ratio or relative sitting height is calculated and multiplied by 100. The normal absolute and relative sitting heights of the different ages and sexes are listed in Chapter 61.

Conditions that cause disproportionate limb shortening include achondroplasia, hypochondroplasia, and Turner syndrome. On the other hand, the trunk height may be disproportionately shorter than the limbs in scoliosis or in spondyloepiphyseal dysplasia.

The determination of rhizomelia should be made by accurate measurements of the proximal and distal segments of the limbs. This is important to assess for skeletal dysplasias, some of which may present clinically as short stature, without any other associated feature, such as mild hypochondroplasia (29–31) or short-limbed short stature of genetic or familial nature (32).

Disproportion between the upper arm and forearm length may be determined by measuring the shoulder-to-elbow (SE) length and the elbow-to-metacarpal length (EMC; Fig. 3) using an anthropometer. For SE length, the blades of the anthropometer are positioned from the midshoulder to the distal end of the humerus, with the elbow at a 90° angle and the upper arm next to the lateral side of the chest. To obtain the EMC length, the blades are positioned from the tip of the elbow to the distal end of the third metacarpal of the closed hand. Normally, the SE/EMC ratio is about unity. Rhizomelia is present if this ratio is lower than 0.98 (32).

Similarly, the presence of shortening of specific bones may lead to the diagnosis of certain syndromes, such as type E brachydactyly (33), Turner syndrome (34), or pseudo-pseudohypoparathyroidism (35). These patients may be seen by the physician because of short stature and must be distinguished from patients with other types of genetic or familial short stature in whom fifth metacarpal bone shortening has been observed to be very prevalent (32,36).

To detect fifth metacarpal shortening, a ruler is placed in front of the patient's fist. In most of the normal population the three knuckles of the third, fourth, and fifth fingers touch the ruler simultaneously. In brachymetacarpia V, however, there is a gap of 2 mm or more between the fifth knuckle and the edge of the ruler, as shown in Figure 4. This clinical observation has been confirmed radiologically (36). In Turner syndrome and pseudo-pseudohypoparathyroidism, fourth metacarpal shortening is frequent. This can be detected radiologically and clinically in a manner similar to that used to detect fifth metacarpal bone shortening (34,35). There is a gap between the fourth knuckle and the edge of the ruler, which touches the third and fifth knuckles simultaneously.

C. Physical and Dental Examinations

Aside from obtaining accurate anthropometric measurements, a detailed physical examination may help elucidate the cause of short stature or growth failure. Specific stigmata are present in common dysmorphology syndromes, such as Russell-Silver syndrome, William syndrome, Turner syndrome, and Prader-Willi syndrome. Signs of chronic illness should be looked for, such as pallor, dry skin, abnormal hair texture, splenomegaly, enamel hypoplasia, or dental caries.

An important part of the physical examination that may provide insight into a child's maturational development is evaluation of dental age. Tables 2 and 3 list the ages at which primary and secondary teeth are expected to erupt (37). Remember that there are wide variations in the time of eruption, which may be affected by local and environmental factors, such as the size of the jaw, position of the unerupted teeth, and the premature loss of deciduous teeth (38).

Children with growth hormone deficiency or untreated hypothyroidism usually have a significantly delayed dentition (39). Mild delays may occur in constitutional delay of growth and development.

D. Bone Maturation Patterns

The bone maturation pattern is also helpful in differentiating the type of short stature. The two most commonly used methods of assessing the maturation or skeletal age are the Greulich and Pyle (G-P) (40) and the Tanner-Whitehouse (TW$_2$-RUS) methods (41). The former method utilizes standards derived from U.S. children living in Cleveland; the latter was derived from British children (42). The G-P method of assessing bone age is usually done by comparing an x-ray film of the frontal view of the left hand and wrist with given

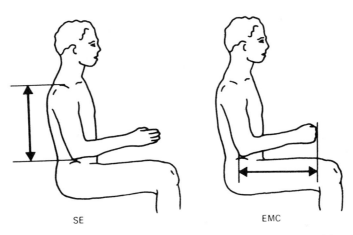

Figure 3 Measurement of shoulder-to-elbow length (SE) and elbow-to-end-of-third metacarpal length (EMC) is shown using an anthropometer. SE is the distance between the shoulder and the tip of the elbow, whereas EMC is the distance between the tip of the elbow and the distal end of the third metacarpal on a closed fist. (From Ref. 32.)

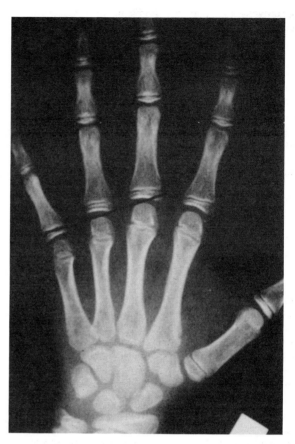

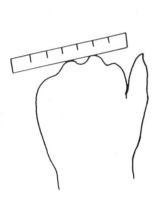

Figure 4 A straight ruler is applied against the distal ends of the third, fourth, and fifth metacarpals of a tightly closed fist. The clinical observation of brachymetacarpia V was confirmed radiologically when the fifth metacarpal bone failed to intercept a straight line connecting the distal ends of the third and fourth metacarpal bones by more than 2 mm (From Ref. 36.)

standards of the G-P atlas. The TW₂-RUS method is always done by assigning scores to each of the 20 hand bones, including the radius, ulna, carpals, metacarpals, and phalanges, depending on their stage of maturation. The total score determines the bone age. The advantage of the TW₂-RUS method over the G-P method is that it appears to be more objective. Moreover, it can differentiate bone age up to one-tenth of a year, whereas the G-P method gives only a rough approximation, with intervals of 6–12 months between standards. Thus, the TW₂-RUS method is more sensitive in following small changes in bone age, but it is more time consuming.

Table 2 Eruption of Primary Teeth

Tooth	Age (months)
Central incisor	6–9
Lateral incisor	7–10
Canine	16–20
First molar	12–16
Second molar	20–30

Table 3 Eruption of Secondary Teeth

Tooth	Age (years)
Maxilla	
Central incisor	7–8
Lateral incisor	8–9
Canine	11–12
First premolar	10–11
Second premolar	10–12
First molar	6–7
Second molar	12–13
Third molar	17–25
Mandible	
Central incisor	6–7
Lateral incisor	7–8
Canine	9–11
First premolar	10–12
Second premolar	11–12
First molar	6–7
Second molar	11–13
Third molar	17–25

Studies comparing the two methods of bone age determination in the same ethnic population among children aged 2–24 years suggest that the median G-P skeletal ages were similar to the chronologic ages of the children studied. In contrast, the TW$_2$-RUS skeletal ages were markedly greater than the corresponding chronologic ages, particularly from 6 to 9 years in boys and from 4 to 8 years in girls. The differences between these scales could be a result of real differences in the rates of skeletal maturation in the different populations. Studies were also done to determine whether there are significant differences among methods of evaluating skeletal age in relation to the group of bones studied. The results seem to suggest that when bone age is assessed by examining all bones (excluding the carpals), there is a high correlation with the bone age detected by measuring the maturation of all bones (43).

The bone growth in children with constitutionally delayed growth is slightly retarded (2 or at the most 3 years), and it is usually proportional to height. When adolescence begins and the growth spurt occurs, the bone age increases proportionally to height. The bone age in familial or genetic short stature is seldom retarded more than 1 year compared with chronologic age, and it usually follows a normal maturation pattern. In contrast, there may be a marked bone age delay in pathologic short stature, such as hypothyroidism, growth hormone deficiency, or chronic disease. The bone age may be even further behind than that expected for height. A short adolescent with sexual infantilism and a bone age maturation delay greater than 3 years is more likely to have pathologic short stature, such as that caused by hypopituitarism or hypothyroidism. The degree of delay may also reflect the length of time the patient has had the disease.

E. Methods of Adult Height Prediction

1. Target Height or Midparental Height

Another important parameter for the assessment of a short patient is the potential adult height that may be attained. It may help distinguish patients who are short but appropriate for family patterns from those who are short even for their own genetic potential. It may also be useful in distinguishing pathologic short stature from familial or genetic short stature or constitutional growth delay. If the predicted adult height falls within the range of the target height for the family, the patient most likely has familial short stature or constitutional growth delay whereas when the predicted adult height falls significantly below the target height range, further investigation for a pathologic process must be carried out.

A simple way of evaluating whether a child is within the normal limits of height for the family is to compare the stature of the patient with the midparental height in charts developed specially to assess the correlation coefficient of these variables (Fig. 5). This correlation coefficient changes little between ages 2 and 9 years. For this norm, a simple chart plotting the age in relation to parents' heights can be constructed with the usual percentile for the family stature. See Figure 5 for charts of three patients with different diagnoses. Patient A's height falls on the 3rd percentile, and his parents' heights have an

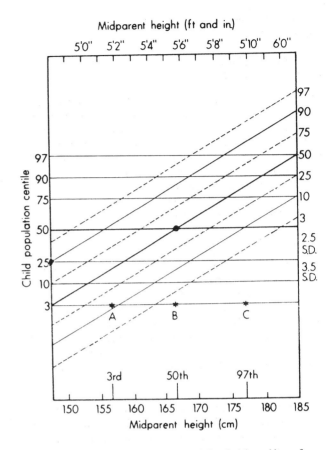

Figure 5 The Tanner standards for height of girls and boys from 2 to 9 years in relation to parents' height. (From Ref. 46.)

average of 157 cm. The position of this patient's stature in the chart is between the 10th and 25th percentiles. Thus, for the population at large, this patient would be small, but he would be appropriate for his immediate family. Therefore, this patient may have familial short stature. In contrast, patient B, who has the same height as patient A, has parents of average height (midparental height 167 cm). This means that patient B is actually very short for the family and requires further workup. Child C is a more extreme case: his parents are actually tall. Although this patient's height is equal to that of the other two patients, his stature falls more than 3 SD from the family norm.

The parents' height and that of other relatives should be *measured*, not guessed. Estimated height may differ significantly from actual measured height. In a number of patients, the diagnosis would be clear if the father's or mother's height were actually known instead of guessed.

Another way of estimating the appropriateness of a patient's height for his or her family is done by comparing the projected height with the target or midparental height. This can be obtained by adding 13 cm to the mother's height (if a boy's height is being considered) or subtracting 13 cm from the father's height (for a girl); this figure is averaged with the height of the other parent:

Target height for males = (father's height + mother's height + 13)÷2

Target height for females = (father's height − 13 + mother's height)÷2

The parents height and the target height obtained should be plotted into the 18 year line of the sex-appropriate growth chart. The projected height is determined by extrapolating the child's growth along his or her own channel to the anticipated adult height (44). If the projected or anticipated adult height is within the target or midparental height, ±5 cm, the child's height is appropriate for the family. If, on the other hand, the target and projected adult height differ by more than 5 cm, then a pathologic cause should be considered.

2. Predicted Adult Height

Currently, three popular methods are being used for calculating a child's predicted adult height. The Bayley-Pinneau method is most commonly used (45). It is based on the axiom that skeletal age correlates well with the proportion of adult height achieved by the child at the time of the x-ray study. After 9 years of age, the skeletal age correlates well (0.86) with the percentage of mature height eventually attained; height predictions after this age are more accurate than those calculated before age 9.

The second method used for predicting adult height is the Tanner-Whitehouse method, utilizing TW_2-RUS standards for calculating bone maturity (46). In addition to bone age, actual height, chronologic age, and parental heights, it also takes into consideration the occurrence of menarche in girls. For boys between 4 and 12 years of age, adult height can be predicted in 95% of cases to within 7 cm. For girls between 13 and 14 years, height can be predicted to within 6 cm. Height for girls between 4 and 11 years can be predicted to within 6 cm, for premenarcheal girls aged 12 and 13 years to within 5 and 4 cm, and for postmenarcheal girls aged 12 and 13 years to within 4 cm.

Last, the Roche-Wainer-Thissen (RWT) method of predicting adult height also incorporates a comprehensive system with attention given to the child's weight or nutritional status (47). Additionally, instead of standing height, the RWT method utilizes the recumbent length; the G-P standards are used to calculate the bone age. Regression techniques are used to estimate the weights of each of the following five predictor variables: recumbent length, weight, bone age, chronologic age, and parental heights. If only height is available, the recumbent length can be approximated with little loss of accuracy by adding 1.25 cm to the height.

One of the main sources of inaccuracy of adult height prediction is the inaccuracy of the bone age estimation. A small difference in bone age determination can lead to a great difference in height prediction, especially during the pubertal spurt (48). Height prediction, as such, is useful only in children with normal growth rates and has limited usefulness in children who are not growing at normal rates.

Comparability studies of the various methods of adult height prediction suggest that the RWT method is the most

accurate, but it involves the greatest amount of calculation. Its inaccuracy increases with age, and it therefore should not be used when more than half of the bones are adult (47,48). In general, height prediction methods differ with respect to their accuracy and their tendency to overestimate or underestimate adult height (48).

IV. CONSTITUTIONAL GROWTH DELAY

The most common cause of short stature and sexual infantilism in the adolescent is constitutionally delayed growth and sexual development. This constitutes a large proportion of the growth disorders seen by pediatric endocrinologists (Fig. 1). The total incidence in the population may even be higher, because pediatricians usually do not refer these patients to an endocrinologist. This entity is characterized by short stature as a variant of normal growth. These patients are the typical "slow growers" and "late bloomers," with a familial prevalence. Often it is recognized long before adolescence, when sexual development is not yet a concern.

The child with constitutional delay of growth and development typically is characterized by a retarded linear growth occurring during the first 3 years of life, followed by normal growth paralleling the normal curve throughout the rest of the prepubertal years and a catch-up growth or growth spurt after the usual expected time of pubertal spurt. Fathers usually report a similar pattern of growth and delayed puberty. Patients with constitutional growth delay usually follow a familial pattern of growth; growth delay is itself inherited from multiple genes from both sides of the family. There may be no short stature in the family, but there may be similar growth patterns. Usually it occurs in boys, only occasionally in girls. The diagnosis of constitutional growth delay in girls should be made only after eliminating other possibilities for pathologic growth patterns.

In a longitudinal study it was clearly shown that growth progression in constitutional growth delay patients slows within 3–6 months of life (49). Both height and weight gain decelerate, and infants destined to have constitutional growth delay downcross percentiles until age 2–3 years. Thereafter, they grow at a normal rate until adolescence. This type of deceleration is also seen in infants with familial short stature. However, body weight progression differs between the two types of infants. In constitutional growth delay patients body weight gain slows, whereas in familial short stature it does not. Thus, constitutional growth delay patients appear to fail to thrive with body weight deficits for length, whereas familial short stature infants maintain a normal or even an excess body weight for length. These growth patterns are maintained throughout childhood, but before puberty constitutional growth delay patients exhibit body weight gain and recover the body weight deficits for height before exhibiting sexual development (50). These data suggest that in constitutional growth delay there may be an association with suboptimal nutrition (Chap. 8). Of interest is that in developing countries suboptimal nutrition was also shown to produce a growth pattern similar to that of constitutional growth delay (50). In children with primary malnutrition, when the nutritional intake improved growth continued to progress at a lower percentile, as in constitutional growth delay. Once there was downregulation of the growth, the patients canalized their growth at a lower percentile.

There may also be an apparent deviation from the normal curve sometime between 10 and 14 years, but this may represent merely the difference between the prepubertal child with constitutional delay of growth and development and the average child already having a pubertal growth spurt. There is also a 2–4 year delay in skeletal maturation, a retarded sexual development, and a 60–90% chance of familial history of delayed growth and pubertal development (51). The mechanism of this phenomenon is still unclear. Some investigators consider it the result of a transient or partial growth hormone deficiency (52–54). Other groups believe that it is the result of permanently diminished growth hormone secretion (55). Some investigators think that the growth hormone alterations in these patients are caused by a deficiency of testosterone or estrogen, which are known to stimulate the production and secretion of growth hormone (56). In most patients with constitutional growth delay, however, there are no abnormalities in growth hormone secretion, nor are there any other detectable endocrine alterations (57).

Although children with constitutional delay attain a normal height during adulthood, they generally end up falling along the lower end of the normal height for the family (58). Studies have shown that in boys with untreated constitutional delay in growth and puberty, there was no significant difference between final and predicted adult height, but there was a significant difference between final height and measured midparental height. Thus, although these boys reach their predicted height, they were short for their families (59). This is probably the result of the lower peak height velocity attained by later maturers than normal or early maturers (60). Other factors may play a role: for example, the selection for presentation to the clinic probably accounts for the finding that children with constitutional growth delay do not, on the average, attain the average percentile of their parents as expected (58). This may indicate that only the smallest of the sibships come to the attention of the physician. Also, the possible effects of malnutrition in infancy on their growth percentile and of suboptimal nutriton on their ultimate height and bone density (59) must be considered (49,50). Based on various data available, it can be concluded that a child with constitutional delay of growth and puberty with a target or predicted height of 3 SD below the population mean is unlikely to reach the normal adult range of height (61).

Most patients with constitutional growth delay are also short for genetic reasons. Most of the children who have this type of short stature and who come to the attention of the pediatric endocrinologist have both constitutional growth delay and familial short stature (Fig. 1). If a child is destined to be an average-sized adult (50th percentile) but has a 2 year delay as a child, at age 10 he or she is at the population 5th percentile and, at 14 years, 5 cm below the general population's 5th percentile. Such patients may not come to the attention of the pediatric endocrinologist, especially because

one or both of the parents may remember that they were late bloomers and realize what is happening. If a patient is destined to reach only the 10th percentile as an adult and is 2 years late as a child, however, then at age 14 he or she is about 2–3 cm below the 3rd percentile, that is, more than 2 SD below the mean and therefore in the range of possible pathologic conditions (see Fig. 2).

The typical boy with this syndrome is otherwise healthy, 10 years of age, and with the height and bone age of an average 8 year old. At the age of 12 (2 years later), height age and bone age are appropriate for age 10 years. Linear and skeletal growth remain consistent, but delayed, until the body becomes 16 or 17. At that time his adolescent growth spurt takes place and secondary sexual characteristics appear. This condition is often difficult to diagnose when the patient is first seen unless measurements at various earlier ages are available, and follow-up height increments are assessed. The main concern with these patients is the psychologic aspect of both the short stature and the lack of secondary sexual characteristics. In severe cases there may be a defective self-image and social withdrawal.

Treatment of patients with constitutional delay of growth and development is controversial. Human growth hormone (hGH) is commercially available, and so the practicing physician is now under mounting pressure to prescribe hGH for short children who are not deficient in this hormone. The medical literature contains reports of improved growth with this treatment in "normal short children" who are experiencing a variety of mixtures of constitutional delay and familial short stature (3,62). There now is no definite evidence that even if such children transiently respond with improved growth rates to hGH treatment, or any growth-promoting agent for that matter, there will be any permanent beneficial effect on ultimate stature. For a complete review of the subject of growth hormone treatment of short children, the reader is referred to Chapter 5.

Although puberty eventually occurs spontaneously, treatment with testosterone in boys for a limited duration is recommended primarily for amelioration of the psychologic problems associated with delayed puberty (63). However, recent reports suggest that boys with untreated constitutional delay of growth and puberty may not reach their expected midparental height (59). Treatment is recommended only if the bone age is greater than 12 years. Before this age, there may be a risk of inappropriately advancing the bone age and thus compromising the eventual adult height (64). The recommended dose is 50 mg intramuscular testosterone enanthate or 17β-cypionate every month for 4–6 months. The 6 month course can be repeated if puberty does not progress spontaneously. Methyltestosterone is not recommended because of its potential toxicity to the liver.

The use of anabolic steroids has been utilized to stimulated growth as well as to promote sexual development (65–68). Ideally, this should promote both these objectives with minimal side effects and without danger of damage to the gonads or a decrease in the patient's final adult height. In addition, there seems to be a psychologic advantage to inducing puberty in patients who might otherwise have very delayed maturation. Treatment with these medications should be reserved for patients who have attained the psychologic development appropriate for puberty. Therapy may not be indicated in any patient with a chronologic age of under 12 years or a bone age under 10 years. One should always keep in mind that anabolic steroids given for short periods may accelerate growth and bone maturation but will not increase ultimate height (69). In fact, they may even prevent attainment of maximum height potential. Fluoroxymesterone is one anabolic compound that seems to be the best growth-promoting agent available. Long-term studies have shown that this drug causes accelerated growth without adversely causing rapid bone maturation or compromising adult height (65). For a comprehensive review of the effects of oxandrolone on growth, the reader is referred to an excellent article published elsewhere (69).

Aside from androgens and anabolic steroids, other pharmacologic agents that have been used in the treatment of these non–growth hormone-deficient children include propranolol, clonidine, and dopaminergic drugs, such as L-dopa (levodopa) and bromocriptine (70–75). Clonidine treatment of constitutional short stature improved the growth of some, but not all, patients treated, nor in placebo-controlled studies (71–73). Other drugs used include luteinizing hormone releasing hormone administration at physiologic intervals to stimulate testosterone production by means of pituitary gonadotropin secretion (64). However, these regimens are expensive and cumbersome. Although these drugs have been shown to increase growth hormone secretion, the growth-promoting effects are debatable. Also, long-term studies on their effect on the final height of children treated by such drugs are not promising (69,76).

The decision to use pharmacologic intervention must necessarily be based on the patient's emotional outlook and the severity of delay to prevent osteoporosis. Most children with constitutional delay of growth and development are able to cope with this condition, if they are properly reassured about their ultimate height and development. This diagnosis, by definition, presages eventual normal maturity and height without medical intervention. A good deal of caution is warranted when treating such a benign alteration, although the induction of more rapid maturation with medications is an immediate reward. A careful assessment of the nutritional intake is recommended with particular attention to deficits in micronutrients, iron, and calcium. If deficits are uncovered, nutritional therapy is recommended.

V. FAMILIAL SHORT STATURE

Familial short stature has also been defined as genetic short stature. These patients are short throughout life and are short as adults, but characteristically they grow at normal rates in their own percentile (see Fig. 2); however, their height is within normal limits when allowance is made for parental heights (77). The growth of these patients in infancy reveals that they changed growth channels sometime between 6 and 18 months of age (50). After 2–3 years of age growth assumes a steady channel below the 5th percentile. This is because a child's size at birth is mostly determined by maternal factors.

After 6 months, the genetic influence predominates, and therefore a child who was born of average size may now shift to lower channels because his or her parents are of short stature. In contrast to patients with constitutional growth delay, these infants gain weight at a steady rate, do not exhibit weight deficits for height, and have no bone age delay (50).

The bone age of patients with familial short stature is consistent with their chronologic age, although usually there is a component of constitutional delay in growth and development (see Fig. 1). The diagnosis of familial short stature is made when the child's height is normal, when allowance is made for parental heights or the predicted adult height falls within the target range for the family.

Recently, tubular bone alterations were described as significantly more prevalent in familial short stature children and adults than in the normal height population (32). These tubular bone alterations include fifth metacarpal bone shortening (brachymetacarpia V, Figs. 3 and 4), rhizomelia, and disproportionate shortening of the arms and lower limbs. Most children and adults with familial short stature had two to four types of tubular bone alterations, whereas most individuals with normal stature had either none or only one type of tubular bone defect. Interestingly, a direct linear relationship was observed between the degree of shortening of the fifth and first metacarpal bones, but not of the other metacarpal bones (36).

These findings suggest that, in familial short stature, there is an inherited defect in endochondral ossification, the major process involved in tubular bone elongation and increase in stature. This defect may result not only in overall decrease in stature but also in disproportionate limb shortening.

Some patients thought to have familial short stature may suffer from a heterogeneous group of conditions manifesting only as short stature, minor tubular bone alterations, and disproportionate limb shortening, with no other stigmata. For example, patients with type E brachydactyly have no other skeletal abnormalities but short stature and metacarpal and metatarsal shortening (33). Hypochondroplasia, particularly when mild, may manifest only with a slight, disproportionate limb shortening and brachydactyly (30,31). Unless careful observations and measurements of the different body segments are made, these patients can be underdiagnosed as plain and simple familial short stature. In these cases, a detailed radiologic study and segregation analysis of the family members must be done.

Although it is important to consider the parents' heights in evaluating a child's short stature, it should be remembered that a parent's stature is not necessarily familial or genetic. Stature also depends on a multitude of environmental factors that may have affected a parent's growth, including food limitation, drugs, and illness (78). Thus, considering the heights of the parents' siblings and parents, as well as obtaining a medical history on the parents, is also important before making a diagnosis of simple familial short stature.

VI. PATHOLOGIC SHORT STATURE

Pathologic short stature is the least frequently occurring but most serious cause of short stature. Pathologic short stature should be suspected in children who do not grow normally, with a growth velocity of less than 4.5 cm/year after 6 years of age, and in those with marked short stature (see Table 1). Bone maturation is usually quite delayed, often behind that expected for height. These patients usually fail to develop sexually, and the prognosis for ultimate height is dependent on the specific diagnosis. Pathologic short stature has accounted for over one-third of the short patients referred to our center (see Fig. 1). This incidence is high compared with the general population (2) but appropriate for a referral center.

It is essential to recognize these patients. A precise diagnosis must be established for early treatment. Often the only evidence of disease is the growth abnormality. The disturbances found to account for the short stature in these children may vary. In our center, the causes are most often nutritional, endocrine, or metabolic disturbances. Undoubtedly, other disturbances known to interfere with growth in children, such as renal or cardiac, predominate in other subspecialty centers. We do not discuss the specific pathologic causes of short stature in detail here because they are reviewed in other chapters of this book.

Conditions worth noting here are occult celiac disease and chronic inflammatory bowel disease. Several investigators have reported that short stature may be the only manifestation of these diseases (79). Recently, mild to moderate zinc deficiency was also demonstrated in a group of otherwise healthy children with idiopathic short stature (80). For further details of growth retardation, in these conditions, see Chapter 8.

In addition to organic causes of pathologic growth, it is important to recognize intrauterine growth retardation (IUGR), with failure to catch up, as a cause of short stature. Intrauterine growth retardation occurs in a heterogeneous group of patients who fail to grow in utero (see Chap. 7). Although most small-for-date children may grow and develop normally and attain normal stature as adults, some do not exhibit "catch-up" growth and remain short throughout life. About 10% of our patients displayed IUGR. There may have been no concomitant family history or congenital anomalies. Many of these occurrences may result from injuries occurring in utero (81), for example maternal alcoholism and the use of tobacco. In some patients the characteristic appearance leads to a specific diagnosis (5). Aside from the absence of catch-up growth, these children with IUGR may have early puberty and be unusually short as adults (82).

Frequently, the presenting problem is "lack of appetite" or "poor feeding." Indeed, the diagnosis of failure to thrive is often made in patients with IUGR. Although growing normally, they may be subjected to unnecessary diagnostic and therapeutic studies. One such patient was evaluated twice for failure to thrive, and forced feedings were advised and enforced to increment weight gain and growth, to no avail. A cursory examination of the anthropometric measurements of this patient ruled out the diagnosis of failure to thrive (Fig. 6). He more than tripled his birth weight by 1 year of age and quadrupled it by 2 years. Similarly, his length remained proportional to weight throughout. Failure to thrive cannot be considered when birth weight is tripled within the first year

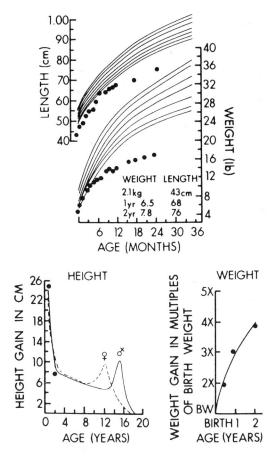

Figure 6 (Top) Growth pattern of a patient with intrauterine growth retardation is shown in upper figure. The growth velocity plotted against normal standards are shown in lower figures. Note that this patient did not have failure to thrive nor was it suspected because he was growing at a normal velocity.

of life, because this rate of growth occurs in normal children. When children start with a tremendous deficit, however, they may be expected to remain proportionally small thereafter (see Chap. 7).

It is also important to remember that low birth weight, preterm infants have different patterns of growth than term infants during the first 3 years of life, even with plotting corrected for gestational age (83). Although there has been a controversy regarding the potential for preterm low birth weight infants to catch up to the typical growth patterns for normal birth weight term infants of the same age, recent long-term data seem to show no compensatory growth in a large cohort through 36 months of corrected gestational age in weight or head circumference. The head circumference of the largest preterm infants seem to be moving away from the pattern of term infant growth, and the head growth of the smallest preterm infants seems to proceed even more slowly. For length, there seems to be some rebound growth noted during the first year of life, but this is followed by a stabilization in growth pattern with little further catch-up to term infant size regardless of birth weight (see Chap. 7). Therapy with hGH or dopaminergic drugs may be of value in these patients (see Chap. 5) (75,84).

There may be other causes of short stature (see Table 1). Individuals with Turner syndrome have sex chromosome abnormalities and often present because of short stature. The karyotype could be either pure 45,XO or a variety of mosaicism. In the latter case, the girl may present only as short stature with or without delayed puberty, with none of the dysmorphic features of Turner syndrome (see Chap. 19). The pathogenesis of the short stature is unclear, but recent studies suggest a functional abnormality of the hypothalamic-pituitary axis. During an overnight study of their nocturnal growth hormone secretion patters, children with Turner syndrome had a significantly decreased number and frequency of peaks compared with normal children. Moreover, their responses to acute growth hormone releasing hormone (GHRH) stimulation are lower. This abnormal growth hormone neuroregulation is thought to be caused by the absence of gonadal steroids (85).

Human growth hormone, anabolic steroids, and low-dose estrogen therapy, alone or in combination, have been recommended for increasing these patients' heights (Chapts. 5 and 19) (69,86–92).

The most common autosomal abnormality is Down syndrome, which is also the most common malformation in humans; it occurs with an incidence of 1:600. These children follow a typical growth pattern and have obvious dysmorphic features. The average adult female height is about 57 inches, and the average adult male is about 61 inches. They have a tendency to be overweight beginning in late infancy and throughout the remainder of the growing years (10). Growth and weight gain are affected by a concomitant congenital heart defect. The underlying cause of short stature remains unexplained, however. Low circulating levels of insulin-like growth factor I (IGF-I) and diminished provoked and spontaneous growth hormone secretion have been reported in some patients (93,94). However, most of the studies performed on Down syndrome patients in regard to hGH secretion were done without consideration of obesity, which is a known cause of decreased growth hormone secretion (95). Thus, caution is encouraged in interpreting the results of growth hormone testing in these patients and thereby justifying treatment with growth hormone. Growth hormone treatment of a small number of patients with Down syndrome has resulted in an accelerated average short-term linear growth and an increase in head circumference. However, it is recommended that careful and cautious evaluation of the safety, efficacy, and ethical ramifications of growth hormone treatment of children with Down syndrome be undertaken before embarking on this form of intervention (96).

Short stature associated with congenital anomalies is also seen with bone diseases classified as skeletal development disorders that result in disproportionate short stature (Chap. 10). The primary error may affect either the cartilaginous or the bone-forming stage of bone development. More than 250 different types of bone dysplasia are known, but the cause of most of these is unknown. The classification

is therefore based largely on morphologic criteria rather than metabolic or molecular (97). This disproportion seen in many skeletal dysplasias may have therapeutic implications because some bones grow better than others. Therefore, growth-promoting agents may accentuate the disparity among the various bones.

There is a group of conditions that are characterized by severe short stature and typical dysmorphic features. This group of conditions is occasionally referred to as primordial dwarfism because no specific etiology for the short stature is defined and no skeletal dysplasia is identifiable. Short stature is prenatal in onset, these children are born small for gestational age, and skeletal age is retarded (98).

The most notable among the causes of primordial dwarfism is Russell-Silver syndrome, described independently by Silver in 1953 and Russell in 1954. Skeletal asymmetry is a distinct feature of this disorder, as well clinodactyly of the fifth finger and small triangular face with downturning of the corners of the mouth. Café au lait spots are usually present (98).

De Lange syndrome typically is characterized by mental retardation, microbrachycephaly, bushy eyebrows and synophrys, and long, curly eyelashes. Patients have a small nose, anteverted nostrils, high arched palate, micrognathia, hirsutism, delayed dentition, micromelia, phocomelia and/or oligodactyly, hypospadias, undescended testes, and hypoplastic external genitals (98). There may or may not be associated endocrinopathies (99).

Bloom syndrome is characterized by mild microcephaly with dolichocephaly, malar hypoplasia, and facial telangiectatic erythema. There may be a mild mental deficiency and immunoglobulin deficiency. Death is usually caused by a lymphoreticular malignancy (98).

Johanson-Blizzard syndrome is characterized by varying degrees of intellectual impairment. Clinical characteristics include hypoplastic or aplastic alae nasi, hypoplastic deciduous teeth, and absent permanent teeth. They may have cryptochoridism, micropenis, imperforate anus, hy-dronephrosis, septate or double vagina, primary hypothyroidism, and/or pancreatic insufficiency (98).

Seckel syndrome is characterized by microcephaly, mental deficiency, premature synostosis, receding forehead, prominent nose, micrognathia, low set, malformed ears, relatively large eyes with downslanting palpebral fissures, clinodactyly of the fifth finger, and dislocation of the radial head and/or hips. These patients are referred to as bird-headed dwarfs because of the disproportionately large nose size in comparison with the mandible and face (98).

Finally, William syndrome is characterized by varying degrees of mental retardation, medial eyebrow flare, short palpebral fissures, depressed nasal bridge, epicanthal folds, periorbital fullness of subcutaneous tissues, blue eyes, anteverted nares, long philtrum, and prominent lips with open mouth. Nails are hypoplastic, and there may be cardiovascular anomalies, including supraalveolar aortic stenosis, pulmonary artery stenosis, ventricular or atrial septal defects. There may also be renal artery stenosis, hypertension, and hypoplasia of the aorta (98).

VII. LABORATORY AIDS IN DIFFERENTIATING SHORT STATURE

Any patient who falls below the third percentile in height and has decreased growth rates (falling across the major percentiles) should receive a complete diagnostic evaluation. Because there are multiple causes of short stature and growth retardation, laboratory investigation should be geared toward confirming or ruling out the differential diagnoses based on information obtained from history and physical examination: history of chronic illness, drug intake, mid-parental and target height, birth size, growth pattern, nutritional state, pubertal stage, body segment proportions, bone age, and predicted adult height. The following simple laboratory screening tests should be performed: urinalysis, urine metabolic screening, complete blood count, sedimentation rate, venous blood gases, liver and kidney function tests, and antigliadin antibodies. A karyotype and luteinizing hormone and follicle stimulating levels are imperative in every girl with short stature even in the absence of the stigmata of Turner syndrome. Children who demonstrate skeletal abnormalities on radiograph or physical examination deserve evaluation for both organic and inorganic metabolic bone disease, such as mucopolysaccharidosis, mucolipidosis, and gangliosidosis (100). Endocrine causes can be determined by evaluating thyroid function and assessing the hypothalamic-pituitary axis (Chaps. 2 and 60). Evaluating the sella turcica on a lateral skull x-ray may be helpful in screening for pituitary tumors, and so is a visual field test. Finally, a thorough nutritional assessment should be made if there is a growth pattern of nutritional dwarfing or eating disorders. If zinc deficiency is suspected, a zinc clearance test should be performed and treatment instituted as indicated (80).

A number of tests to assess growth hormone status have been devised using insulin, L-dopa, arginine, clonidine, and other agents, because growth hormone is secreted at intervals, so random growth hormone measurements are useless. Pituitary function may be evaluated comprehensively using a combined hormonal stimulation test (101). This utilizes sequentially administered insulin or arginine or L-dopa, thyrotropin releasing hormone, and gonadotropin releasing hormone. In addition, deficiency of growth hormone releasing hormone may be ruled out by giving human pituitary GHRH and evaluating the patient's growth hormone response. Additionally, neurosecretory growth hormone dysfunction can be determined by performing an overnight growth hormone study and assessing growth hormone pulsatile secretions under physiologic conditions, such as sleep (see Chap. 4). In the last test, a child may demonstrate a normal growth hormone response to pharmacologic stimuli but may not be able to secrete growth hormone under physiologic conditions (102). There is no completely reliable test for diagnosing or excluding growth hormone deficiency in short children (Chap. 2). IGF-I and IGF binding protein 3 levels are reportedly decreased in growth hormone deficiency and may help in interpreting the results of provocative or physiologic tests for growth hor-

mone deficiency (103). Finally, in children with pathologic growth with normal or increased growth hormone levels, the growth hormone resistance syndromes should be ruled out. Measuring levels of growth hormone binding protein or IGF binding proteins may help differentiate the different conditions, as well as IGF levels and their response to exogenous growth hormone administration (104–106). Details of the foregoing tests and procedures are described in Chapter 60.

VIII. FINAL CONSIDERATIONS

Short children and their parents face a number of specific psychologic problems (Chap. 11). These problems are frequently associated with the developmental stage of the child's life. The parents frequently have difficulty in accepting the child's height and in treating the child according to age level. By 7 or 8 years of age the child usually has become acutely aware of his or her dwarfism. The teenage years are much more difficult for the dwarf than for the child of normal height. The problems of short stature are often compounded by lack of sexual development and withdrawal from heterosexual social activities or by other transition periods, such as moving to a new school or community. Despite these developmental problems, the short individual frequently makes an adequate adjustment to life as an adult (see Chap. 11).

Other issues transcend the purely developmental aspects of short stature, such as the general personality mechanisms of the small child and his or her parents. Of importance are the school achievements of such children and the specific techniques they develop in coping more effectively with their environment. One of the most important problems of short people is being treated in an infantile manner, appropriate for their size, but not for their age. Some short people respond to being treated as a younger child by behaving immaturely (Peter Pan reaction). Others rebel against being pampered and sometimes develop various neurotic and psychosomatic symptoms, including denial, withdrawal, phobias, and compensatory fantasies. Still others find a more satisfactory solution in the reaction of "mascotism."

Frankness (diplomatic rather than brutal) is desirable in counseling short and dwarfed people about their situation in life. They are then able to plan the future realistically, to discuss the taboos that beset them, and to perfect techniques in dealing with silly comments about their size and age. Emotional problems may cause a certain type of dwarfism, but definite answers still cannot be given to this issue. Short stature is not typically associated with intellectual defect. Dwarfed people may expect to be employed and, under some circumstances, to graduate from college. Short people can meet one another by joining such organizations as Little People of America, P.O. Box 622, San Bruno, CA 94006 or the Human Growth Foundation, Inc., 4607 Davidson Drive, Cherry Lane, MD 20815. They may legitimately hope for romance, marriage, and a successful sex life.

REFERENCES

1. Hamill PVV, Drizd TA, Johnson CL, Reed RB, Roche AF, Moore WM. Physical growth: National Center for Health Statistics percentiles. Am J Clin Nutr 1979; 32:607–629.
2. Lacey KA, Parkin JM. Causes of short stature. A community study of children in Newcastle-upon-Tyne. Lancet 1974; 1:42–45.
3. Rudman D, Kutner MH, Blackstone RD, Cushman RA, Bain RP, Patterson JH. Children with normal variance short stature: treatment with human growth hormone for six months. N Engl J Med 1981; 305:123–131.
4. Tanner JM, Whitehouse RH, Marubini E, Resele L. The adolescent growth spurt of the boys and girls of the Harpenden Growth Study. Ann Hum Biol 1976; 3:109–126.
5. Tanner JM, Lejarraga H, Cameron N. The natural history of Silver-Russell syndrome: a longitudinal study of 35 cases. Pediatr Res 1975; 9:611–623.
6. Taranger J, Bruning B, Claesson I, et al. Skeletal development from birth to 7 years. In: Taranger J, ed. The Somatic Development of Children in a Swedish Urban Community. Acta Paediatr Scand (Suppl) 1967; 258:98–108.
7. Tuddenham RD, Snyder MM. Physical growth of California boys and girls from birth to eighteen years. Univ Calif Publ Child Dev 1954; 1:183–364.
8. Horton WA, Rotter JI, Rimoin DL. Standard growth curve for achondroplasia. J Pediatr 1978; 93:435–438.
9. Babson SG, Benda GI. Growth graphs for the clinical assessment of infants of varying gestational age. J Pediatr 1976; 89:814–820.
10. Cronk C, Crocker AC, Pueschel SM, et al. Growth charts for children with Down syndrome: 1 month to 18 years of age. Pediatrics 1988; 81:102–110.
11. Lyon AJ, Preece MA, Grant DB. Growth curve for girls with Turner syndrome. Arch Dis Child 1985; 60:932–935.
12. Horton WA, Hall JG, Scott CI. Growth curves for diastrophic dysplasia, spondyloepiphyseal dysplasia and pseudoachondroplasia. Am J Dis Clin Child 1982; 136:316–319.
13. Witt DR, Keena BA, Hall JG, Allanson JE. Growth curves for height in Noonan syndrome. Clin Genet 1986; 30:150–153.
14. Brook GGD, Hindmarsh PC, Healy MJR. A better way to detect growth failure. BMJ 1986; 293:1186.
15. Lampl M, Veldhuis JD, Johnson ML. Saltation and stasis: a model of human growth. Science 1992; 258:801–803.
16. Tiwary C. Seasonal and latitudinal effects on growth in patients on Protropin growth hormone in the U.S. and Canada. Genentech National Cooperative Growth Study Summary Report 15, June 1993.
17. Tanner JM, Whitehouse RH, Takaishi M. Standards from birth to maturity for height, weight, height velocity and weight velocity in British children. Arch Dis Child 1966; 41:613–616.
18. Tanner JM, Whitehouse RH. Clinical longitudinal standard for height, weight, height velocity, weight velocity and stages of puberty. Arch Dis Child 1976; 51:170–171.
19. Guo S, Roche AF, Fomon SJ, et al. Reference data on gains in weight and length during the first two years of life. J Pediatr 1991; 119:355–362.
20. Merritt J, Russel S. Obesity. Curr Prob Pediatr 1982; 12:18.
21. Publiese MT, Lifshitz F, Grad G, Fort P, Marks-Katz M. Fear of obesity: a cause of short stature and delayed puberty. N Engl J Med 1983; 309:513–518.
22. Lifshitz F, Moses N, Cervantes C, Ginsberg L. Nutritional dwarfing in adolescents. Semin Adol Med 1987; 3:255–266.
23. Desai ID, Garcia-Tavares ML, Dutra De Oliveira BS, et al. Anthropometric and cycloergometric assessment of the nutri-

tional status of the children of agricultural migrant workers in southern Brazil. Am J Clin Nutr 1981; 34:1934–1935.
24. Trowbridge FL, Marks JS, Lopez de Romana G, Madrid S, Boutton TW, Klein PD. Body composition of Peruvian children with short stature and high weight-for-height. II. Implications for the interpretation of weight-for-height as an indicator of nutritional status. Am J Clin Nutr 1987; 46:411–418.
25. Dewey KG, Heinig MJ, Nommsen LA, Peerson JM, Lönnerdal B. Growth of breast-fed and formula-fed infants from 0 to 18 months: the DARLING study. Pediatrics 1992; 89:1035–1041.
26. Pritchett JW. Practical Bone Growth. Seattle: James W. Pritchett, 1993:35–36.
27. Roche AF, Guo S, Baumgartner RN, Falls RA. The measurement of stature. Am J Clin Nutr 1988; 47:922.
28. Wilkins L. The Diagnosis and Treatment of Endocrine Disorders in Children and Adolescence. Springfield, IL: Charles C. Thomas, 1966:33.
29. Bailey JA. Disproportionate Short Stature: Diagnosis and Management. Philadelphia: W.B. Saunders. 1973.
30. Scott CI Jr. The genetics of short stature. In: Steinberg AG, Bearn AG, eds. Progress in Medical Genetics. New York: Grune & Stratton, 1974.
31. Kozlowski K. Hypochondroplasia. Pol Przegl Radiol (Warsaw) 1965; 19:450–459.
32. Cervantes C, Lifshitz F. Tubular bone alterations in familial short stature. Hum Biol 1988; 60:151–165.
33. Bell J. Brachydactyly and symphalangism. In: Penrose LS, ed. Treasury of Human Inheritance. London: Cambridge University Press, 1951.
34. Archibald RM, Finby N, DeVito F. Endocrine significance of short metacarpals. J Clin Endocrinol Metab 1959; 19:1312–1322.
35. Van der Werf Ten Bosch JJ. The syndrome of brachymetacarpal dwarfism ("pseudopseudohypoparathyroidism") with and without gonadal dysgenesis. Lancet 1959; 1:69–71.
36. Cervantes CD, Lifshitz F, Levenbrown J. Radiologic anthropometry of the hand in patients with familial short stature. Pediatr Radiol 1988; 18:210–214.
37. Stewart RE, Horton WA, Eteson DJ. General concepts of growth and development. In: Stewart RE, Barber TK, Troutman KC, Wei SHY, eds. Pediatric Dentistry: Scientific Foundations and Clinical Practice. St. Louis: C.V. Mosby, 1982:3–34.
38. Duterloo HS. An Atlas of Dentition in Childhood. London: Wolfe Publishing, 1991:93–96.
39. Blizzard RM. The practitioner's dilemmas about growth and short stature. Pediatric rounds: growth, nutrition, development. June 1992; 1:2–5.
40. Greulich WW, Pyle SI. Radiographic Atlas of Skeletal Development of the Hand and Wrist. Stanford, CA: Stanford University Press, 1950.
41. Tanner JM, Whitehouse RH, Cameron N, Marshall WA, Healy MJR, Goldstein H. Assessment of Skeletal Maturity and Prediction of Adult Height (TW$_2$ Method). London: Academic Press, 1983.
42. Roche AF, Davila GH, Leyman SL. A comparison between Greulich-Pyle and Tanner-Whitehouse assessment of skeletal maturity. Radiology 1971; 98:273–280.
43. Roche AF, Johnson JM. A comparison between methods of calculating skeletal age (Greulich-Pyle). Am J Phys Anthropol 1966; 30:221–229.
44. Kaplan SA. Growth and growth hormone: Disorders of the anterior pituitary. In: Kaplan SA, ed. Clinical Pediatric and Adolescent Endocrinology. Philadelphia: W.B. Saunders, 1982.

45. Bayley N, Pinneau SR. Tables for predicting adult height from skeletal age: revised for use with the Greulich-Pyle hand standard. J Pediatr 1952; 40:423–441.

46. Tanner JM, Whitehouse RH, Marshall WA, Carter BS. Prediction of adult height from height, bone age, and occurrence of menarche, at ages 4 to 16, with allowance for midparent height. Arch Dis Child 1975; 50:14–26.

47. Roche AF, Wainer H, Thissen D. The RWT method for the prediction of adult stature. Pediatrics 1975; 56:1026–1033.

48. Lenko HL. Prediction of adult height with various methods in Finnish children. Acta Pediatr Scand 1979; 68:85–92.

49. Horner JM, Thorsson AV, Hinz RL. 6 month deceleration patterns in children with constitutional short stature: an aid to diagnosis; Pediatrics 1978; 62:529–534.

50. Vaquero-Solans C, Lifshitz F. Body weight progression and nutritional status of patients with familial short stature with and without constitutional delay in growth. Am J Dis Child 1991; 146:296–302.

51. Bierich JR. Constitutional delay of growth and development. Growth Genet Horm 1987; 3:9–12.

52. Gourmelen M, Pham-Huu-Trung MT, Girard F. Transient partial hGH deficiency in prepubertal children with delay of growth. Pediatr Res 1979; 13:221–224.

53. Kastrup KW, Andersen H, Eskildsen PC, Jacobsen BB, Krabbe S, Petersen KE. Combined test of hypothalmic-pituitary function in growth-retarded children treated with growth hormone. Acta Paediatr Scand (Suppl) 1979; 227:9–13.

54. Clayton PE, Shalet SM, Price DA. Endocrine manipulation of constitutional delay in growth and puberty. J Endocrinol 1988; 116:321–323.

55. Bierich JR, Brogmann G, Schippert R. Assessment of sleep-associated HGH secretion in normal children and in endocrine disorders. Pediatr Res 1985; 19:609.

56. Link K, Blizzard RM, Evans WS, Kaiser DL, Parker MW, Rogol AD. The effect of androgens on the pulsatile release and the twenty-four-hour mean concentration of growth hormone in peripubertal males. J Clin Endocrinol Metab 1986; 62:159–164.

57. Abdenur JE, Publiese MT, Cervantes C, Fort P, Lifshitz F. Alterations in spontaneous growth hormone secretion and the response to GH-releasing hormone in children with nonorganic nutritional dwarfing. J Clin Endocrinol Metab 1992; 75:930–934.

58. Preece MA, Greco L, Savage MD, Cameron N, Tanner JM. The auxology of growth delay. Pediatrics 1981; 15:76.

59. Crowne EC, Shalet SM, Wallace WHB, Eminson DM, Price DA. Final height in boys with untreated constitutional delay in growth and puberty. Arch Dis Child 1990; 65:1109–1112.

60. Hägg U, Taranger J. Pubertal growth and maturity pattern in early and late maturers. Swed Dent J 1992; 16:199–209.

61. Ranke MB, Aronson AS. Adult height in children with constitutional short stature. Acta Paediatr Scand (Suppl) 1989; 362:27–31.

62. Von Vliet G, Styne PN, Kaplan SL, Grumbach MM. Growth hormone treatment for short stature in children. N Engl J Med 1983; 309:1016–1023.

63. Rosenfeld RG, Northcraft GB, Hintz RL. A prospective, randomized study of testosterone treatment of constitutional delay of growth and development in male adolescents. Pediatrics 1982; 69:681–687.

64. Lee PA, St. L. O'Dea L. Primary and secondary testicular insufficiency. Pediatr Clin North Am 1990; 37:1359–1385.

65. Strickland AL. Long-term results of treatment with low-dose fluoxymesterone in constitutional delay of growth and puberty and in genetic short stature. Pediatrics 1993; 91:716–720.

66. Bettmann HK, Goldman HS, Abramowics M, Sobel EH. Oxandrolone treatment of short stature, effect on predicted matrix adult height. J. Pediat 1971; 79:1018–1023.

67. Buyukgebiz A, Hindmarsh PC, Stanhope R, Preece MA, Brook CGD. Long term outcome of oxandrolone treatment in boys with constitutional delay of growth and puberty. J Pediatr 1990; 117:588–591.

68. Blethen SL, Gaines S, Welden V. Comparison of predicted and adult heights in short boys: effects of androgen therapy. Pediatr Res. 1984; 18:467–469.

69. Blizzard RM, Hindmarsh PC, Stanhope R. Oxandrolone therapy: 25 years experience. Growth Genet Horm 1991; 4(1):1–6.

70. Chihara K, Kodama H, Kaji H, et al. Augmentation by propranolol of growth hormone-releasing hormone-(1–44)-NH2-induced growth hormone release in normal short and normal children. J Clin Endocrinol Metab 1985; 61:229–233.

71. Pintor C, Cella SG, Loche S, et al. Clonidine treatment for short stature. Lancet 1987; 1:1226–1230.

72. Allen DB. Effects of nightly clonidine administration on growth velocity in short children without growth hormone deficiency: a double-blind, placebo-controlled study. J Pediatr 1993; 122:32–36.

73. Pescovitz OH, Tan E. Lack of benefit of clonidine treatment for short stature: a clonidine therapy of non-growth hormone deficient patients: double-blind, placebo trial. Lancet 1988; 2:874–877.

74. Lanes R, Insausti A, Carrillo E, Perez I. Effect of prolonged L-dopa therapy on the linear growth and the growth hormone and somatomedin concentration of healthy short children. International Symposium on Growth. Growth: Basic and Clinical Aspects, June 14–18, 1987.

75. Huseman C. Growth enhancement by dopaminergic therapy in children with intrauterine growth retardation. J Clin Endocrinol Metab 1985; 61:514–519.

76. Martin MM, Martin ALA, Mossman KL. Testosterone treatment of constitutional delay of growth and development: effect of dose on predicted vs definitive height. Acta Enderimol 1981: 279 (Suppl); 147–153.

77. Tanner JM, Goldstein H, Whitehouse RH. Standards of children's height at ages 2 to 9 years allowing for height of parents. Arch Dis Child 1970; 45:755.

78. Gebhardt-Henrich SG. Heritability of growth curve parameters and heritability of final size: a simulation study. Growth Dev Aging 1992; 56:23–34.

79. Ashkenazi A. Occult celiac disease: a common cause of short stature. Growth Genet Horm 1989; 5(2):1–4.

80. Nakammra T, Nishiyama S, Futagoishi-Suginohara Y, Matsuda I, Higashi A. Mild to moderate zinc deficien- cy in short children: effect of zinc supplementation on linear growth velocity. J Pediatr 1993; 123:65–69.

81. Miller H. Prenatal factors affecting intrauterine growth retardation. Clin Perinatol 1985; 12:307–318.

82. Arisaka G, Arisaka M, Kiyokawa N, Shimizu T, Nakayama Y, Yabuta K. Intrauterine growth retardation and early adolescent growth spurt in two sisters. Clin Pediatr (Phila) 1986; 25:559–561.

83. Casey PH, Kraemer HC, Bernbaum J, Yogman MW, Sells JC. Growth status and growth rates of a varied sample of low birth weight, preterm infants: a longitudinal cohort from birth to 3 years of age. J Pediatr 1991; 119:599–605.

84. Moore KC, Donaldson DL, Ideus PL, Gifford RA, Moore WV. Clinical diagnoses of children with extremely short stature and their response to growth hormone. J Pediatr 1993; 122:687–692.

85. Bermasconi S, Ghizzoni L, Volta C, Morano M, Giovanelli G. Spontaneous growth hormone secretion in Turner's syndrome. J Pediatr Endocrinol 1992; 5(12):101–105.

86. Tzagouris M. Response to long-term administration of human growth hormone in Turner's syndrome. JAMA 1969; 210: 2373–2376.

87. Tanner JM, Whitehouse RH, Hughes PCR, Vince FP. Effect of human growth hormone treatment for 1 to 7 years on growth of 100 children with growth hormone deficiency, low birth weight, inherited smallness, Turner's syndrome and other complaints. Arch Dis Child 1971; 46:745–756.

88. Raiti S, Moore WV, Van Vliet G, Kaplan SL. Growth-stimulating effects of human growth hormone therapy in patients with Turner syndrome. J Pediatr 1986; 109:944–949.

89. Rosenfeld RG, Hintz RL, Johanson AJ, et al. Methionyl human growth hormone and oxandrolone in Turner syndrome: preliminary results of a prospective randomized trial. J Pediatr 1986; 109:936–943.

90. Rose JL, Long IM, Skerda M, et al. Effect of low doses of estradiol on 6-month growth rates and predicted height in patients with Turner's syndrome. J Pediatr 1986; 109:950–953.

91. Sybert VP. Adult height in Turner syndrome with and without androgen therapy. J Pediatr 1984; 104:365–369.

92. Rosenfeld RG, Frane J, Attie KM, et al. Six-year results of a randomized, prospective trial of human growth hormone and oxandrolone in Turner syndrome. J Pediatr 1992; 121:49–55.

93. Anneren G, Gustavson K-H, Sara VR, Tunemo T. Growth retardation in Down syndrome in relation to insulin-like growth factors and growth hormone. Am J Med Genet (Suppl) 1990; 7:59–62.

94. Torrado C, Bastian W, Wisniewski KE, Castells S. Treatment of children with Down syndrome and growth retardation with recombinant human growth hormone. J Pediatr 1991; 119: 478–483.

95. Lifshitz F. Commentary. Growth Genet Horm 1993; 9(2): 1011.

96. Allen DB, Frasier SD, Foley TP Jr, Pescovitz OH. Growth hormone for children with Down syndrome. A commentary from the Lawson Wilkins Pediatric Endocrine Society Board of Directors and Drug and Therapeutics Committee. J Pediatr 1993; 123:742–743.

97. Spranger J. Classification of skeletal dysplasias. Acta Paediatr Scand (Suppl) 1991; 377:138–142.

98. Jones KL. Smith's Recognizable Patterns of Human Malformation, 4th ed. Philadelphia: W.B. Saunders, 1988.

99. Schwartz ID, Schwartz KJ, Kouseff BG, Bercu BB, Root AW. Endocrinopathies in Cornelia de Lange syndrome. J Pediatr 1990; 117:920–922.

100. Cervantes C, Lifshitz F. Skeletal dysplasias with primary abnormalities in carbohydrate, lipid, and amino acid metabolism. In: Castells S, ed. Metabolic Bone Diseases in Children. New York: Marcel Dekker, pp 329–379.

101. Pugliese M, Lifshitz F, Fort P, Cervantes C, Recker B, Ginsberg L. Pituitary function assessment in short stature by a combined hormonal stimulation test. Am J Dis Child 1987; 141:556–561.

102. Spilliotis BE, August GP, Hung W, Sonis W, Mendelson W, Bercu BB. Growth hormone neurosecretory dysfunction—a treatable cause for short stature. JAMA 1984; 25: 2223–2330.

103. Smith WJ, Nam TJ, Underwood LE, Busby WH, Celnicker A, Clemmons DR. Use of insulin-like growth factor-binding protein-2 (IGFBP-2), IGFBP-3, and IGF-I for assessing growth hormone status in short children. J Clin Endocrinol Metab 1993; 77:1294–1299.

104. Kowarski AA, Ben-Galim E, Weldon VV, Daughaday WH. Growth failure with normal serum RIA-GH and low somatomedin activity: somatomedin restoration and growth acceleration after exogenous GH. J Clin Endocrinol Metab 1978; 47:461–464.

105. Baumann G. Diagnostic implications of growth hormone binding proteins. J Pediatr Endocrinol 1992; 5(1–2):31–35.

106. Savage MO, Blum WF, Ranke MB, Clinical features and endocrine status in patients with growth hormone insensitivity. J Clin Endocrinol Metab 1993; 77:1465–1471.

2

Hypopituitarism

Sandra L. Blethen

*School of Medicine, State University of New York at Stony Brook,
Stony Brook, New York*

I. INTRODUCTION

The pituitary gland is located at the base of the brain. In the adult, it is composed of the anterior pituitary (adenohypophysis) and the posterior pituitary (neurohypophysis). The former is an ectodermal structure arising from the pharynx as Rathke's pouch. The latter is composed of neural tissue that descends from the floor of the third ventricle.

The anterior pituitary synthesizes and secretes the following hormones: growth hormone (GH), the gonadotropins, luteinizing hormone (LH), follicle stimulating hormone (FSH), adrenocorticotropic hormone (ACTH), thyroid stimulating hormone (TSH), and prolactin. Production of anterior pituitary hormones is regulated by hypothalamic factors that are transported to the pituitary via the portal veins of the pituitary stalk (1,2). Thus, any damage to the pituitary stalk or the hypothalamus is followed by anterior pituitary dysfunction. Indeed, much of what we call hypopituitarism is really a reflection of hypothalamic dysfunction (3,4).

The posterior pituitary does not synthesize hormones. It consists of axons with cell bodies located in the supraoptic and paraventricular nuclei of the hypothalamus. The posterior pituitary hormones arginine vasopressin (or antidiuretic hormone, ADH) and oxytocin are synthesized in the hypothalamus, transported along the neurohypophyseal tract of the pituitary stalk, stored in the posterior pituitary, and released in response to neurohypophyseal stimuli.

The clinical presentations of pituitary dysfunction vary with the age of the patient and the specific hormones that are deficient. Documentation of a deficiency in one pituitary hormone requires evaluation of the others. In this chapter, I describe different clinical situations that should prompt an evaluation of the hypothalamic-pituitary axis. Although testing for specific hormone deficits is found in other chapters devoted to those hormones, a brief outline of an appropriate diagnostic evaluation is given here. Strategies for treatment,

long-term follow-up, and specific syndromes known to be associated with pituitary dysfunction are discussed.

II. PRESENTING SIGNS AND SYMPTOMS

The signs and symptoms of hypopituitarism can be nonspecific in the newborn. Even if congenital hypopituitarism is not recognized in the immediate postnatal period, a careful history taken later in childhood may indicate the presence of symptoms at that time.

A. Hypopituitarism in the Newborn

Disease in the newborn usually presents with one or more of a limited number of signs and symptoms. For this reason, a high index of suspicion is necessary to make an accurate diagnosis in a timely fashion.

1. Hypoglycemia

The signs of hypoglycemia in a newborn are themselves nonspecific and include the following: apnea, cyanosis, pallor, lethargy, jitteriness, and seizures. In most nurseries, measurement of capillary blood glucose levels at the bedside with glucose oxidase strips is a part of the routine evaluation of an infant with any of these signs (Chap. 49). If hypoglycemia is found, a confirming sample (preferably collected in a tube containing sodium fluoride to inhibit erythrocyte glycolysis while the tube is awaiting processing) should be obtained. Serum insulin, GH, and cortisol levels should be obtained simultaneously with the confirming glucose. GH should be greater than 10 μg/L; cortisol, greater than 550 nmol/L (20 μg/dl). The ratio of insulin (μU/ml) to glucose (mg/dl) should be less than 0.4.

In newborn infants during the first week of life, serum GH levels are higher than later in life (5), so that a low (less than 10 μg/L) random GH obtained during this time is also indicative of GH deficiency when it would not be so in an older child.

Because glucagon increases glucose levels in an infant with hypoglycemia secondary to hyperinsulinemia (one of the major diagnoses that should be considered in the hypoglycemic newborn), a glucagon stimulation test has much to recommend it as a means of diagnosing GH deficiency in infants. A dose of 0.03 mg/kg of glucagon is given intramuscularly with glucose measurements at 15 and 30 minutes and concomitant glucose and GH levels at 60, 90, 120, and 180 minutes postglucagon (6). Serum cortisol should be greater than 550 nmol/L (20 µg/dl) 180 minutes after glucagon.

If additional testing is necessary to confirm the diagnosis of GH deficiency in the hypoglycemic infant, an arginine stimulation test (although requiring venous access) is a safe and reliable means of inducing GH secretion (6). L-arginine (0.5 mg/kg, maximum 30 g) is given as an intravenous infusion over 30 minutes. Serum for GH determination is obtained at 20 minute intervals for 120 minutes.

Most infants with hypopituitarism presenting as hypoglycemia have multiple pituitary hormone deficiencies (7,8). Therefore, the evaluation of such an infant should include thyroid function testing and gonadotropin measurements, as well as the GH and cortisol measurements already described.

2. Hyperbilirubinemia

Clinically apparent jaundice is seen in about 60% of full-term infants during the first week of life. Typically, physiologic jaundice appears on the second or third day of life and resolves by the end of the first week. The differential diagnosis of prolonged jaundice in the newborn infant is extensive and includes hemolysis, hemorrhage, polycythemia, sepsis, congenital infections, inborn errors of metabolism, hypothyroidism, and hypopituitarism.

In an infant with hypothyroidism secondary to deficiencies of TSH or of thyrotropin releasing hormone, the hyperbilirubinemia is caused by increased levels of unconjugated (indirect) bilirubin. However, an increase in *conjugated* bilirubin levels (direct hyperbilirubinemia) can be seen in infants with GH or ACTH deficiencies (9–11).

3. Turbulent Neonatal Course

A review of the medical history of infants with hypopituitarism often reveals numerous evaluations for sepsis, unexplained apnea, hypotension, or temperature instability (12, 13). Such problems are common in the small preterm infant, but their presence in a full-term baby should prompt consideration of a diagnosis of hypopituitarism. This is particularly true if hypoglycemia is present or if physical examination reveals the presence of one or more of the physical characteristics known to be associated with hypopituitarism (see later).

4. Hyponatremia

Low serum sodium not associated with hypovolemia and unresponsive to fluid restriction and infusion of hypertonic saline can been seen in infants with untreated hypopituitarism.

In contrast to the hyponatremia seen with the salt-losing crisis of congenital adrenal hyperplasia caused by a deficiency of 21-hydroxylase, serum potassium is normal or low (Chap. 21). The hyponatremia of hypopituitarism responds to physiologic replacement doses of glucocorticoids (8,14). In adults with untreated hypopituitarism and hyponatremia, serum levels of ADH are inappropriately elevated relative to serum osmolality (15). When patients with hyponatremia secondary to hypopituitarism were reevaluated after glucocorticoid replacement, the relation between ADH levels and osmolality was normal. Thus, although the ADH secretion in these patients may be "inappropriate" for their sodium level, it is a reflection of their ACTH deficiency.

5. Physical Findings in Hypopituitarism

Although infants with hypopituitarism usually have normal birth weights and body proportions (7,12,16–18), certain physical characteristics, if present, should suggest a diagnosis of hypopituitarism.

The association between the presence of a *micropenis* and hypopituitarism is well described (8,19). The phallus is formed during the first trimester under the influence of androgens synthesized in the fetal testes. At this time, androgen synthesis is independent of pituitary gonadotropins. However, growth of the penis during the second and third trimesters requires pituitary LH. Thus, a male infant who is gonadotropin deficient has a small but normally formed phallus. The presence of hypoglycemia, jaundice, or unexplained deteriorations in clinical well-being in an infant with a small penis is definitely an indication for a complete evaluation of pituitary function. In fact, most boys with hypopituitarism who are diagnosed in the first 2 years of life are recognized because of underdeveloped genitalia (7,8). Because testosterone and gonadotropin levels are higher after birth than they are in childhood (20), measurement of random testosterone, LH, and FSH should be sufficient to evaluate the hypothalamic-pituitary-gonadal axis in the newborn.

An underdeveloped clitoris can be a sign of hypopituitarism in girls. Data on normal clitoral length as a function of gestational age are available (21).

The association of optic nerve hypoplasia with hypopituitarism and absence of the septum pellucidum ("septooptic dysplasia" or de Morsier syndrome) was first described by Hoyt et al. (22). However, not all features of this syndrome are present in all cases. In a study of 45 individuals with optic nerve hypoplasia ascertained through a New York State registry of the blind, Acer (23) found 12 with midline structural defects on computed tomographic (CT) scan. Of these, 6 had hypopituitarism. Because pituitary hormone studies were not done on the remaining 33 subjects with normal CT scans, the incidence of hypopituitarism in those with optic nerve hypoplasia and an intact septum pellucidum was not reported. Other authors have described cases of hypopituitarism with optic nerve hypoplasia and an intact septum pellucidum (24). Because of the high mortality associated with hypoglycemia and hypopituitarism, the true incidence of hypopituitarism in patients with optic nerve hypoplasia may be underestimated. For this reason, the presence of clinically significant nystagmus should prompt an evaluation of pituitary function in addition to the ophthalmologic examination and brain imaging studies (magnetic resonance imaging or CT scan) that are typically performed.

Because the anterior pituitary is derived from midline structures, it is not surprising that defective embryologic development of these structures is associated with defective development of the pituitary gland itself. Any child with a midline defect should be considered at risk for pituitary hormone deficiencies and should be evaluated accordingly. Specific development defects associated with hypopituitarism are described later (Sec. II.B.7).

B. Hypopituitarism Presenting in Infancy and Childhood

Any of the manifestations of pituitary hormone deficiency seen in the newborn period can also be found in older infants and children, but the frequency of different presenting complaints is different.

1. Hypoglycemia

Particularly if not evaluated thoroughly in the newborn period, hypoglycemia can be a presenting sign of hypopituitarism in older infants (Chap. 50). The evaluation of hypoglycemia in an infant or child is most efficiently conducted if serum is obtained at the time of hypoglycemia ("critical sample"). In a child with failure to thrive, short stature, or slow growth, documented hypoglycemia is a definite indication for complete evaluation of hypothalamic-pituitary function.

2. Growth Failure

Whether pituitary GH is a major determinant of human growth in utero is unclear. Most infants with congenital GH deficiency have a normal birth weight (12,25), but children with total GH deficiency caused by mutations of the GH gene often have intrauterine growth retardation (Chap. 3) (18,26–29).

In contrast, the important role of GH in determining childhood growth (30,31) is well documented. Therefore, in older infants and children, growth failure is the major presenting complaint in hypopituitarism.

Growth failure may be present for some time before it is recognized. In the best circumstances, the child's primary care physician has made regular measurements of length (or height) and plotted them on appropriate charts, such as those complied from data from the National Center for Health Statistics (32), and the child is referred for evaluation when a substantial deviation from the normal growth pattern is observed. In other cases, the parents may recognize growth failure when the child enters school, and they note a marked discrepancy between his or her height and that of the classmates. A younger sibling who begins to approach the child's height (particularly a younger *sister*) often prompts parental concern. A child who is growing normally should need larger sizes of clothing yearly, and growth failure may be signaled by the failure to outgrow clothing regularly (Chap. 1).

Bone growth and ossification are regulated by GH, thyroxine, and the sex hormones (33). During growth, cartilage is produced by chrondrocytes in the epiphyseal growth plate. Subsequently, there is calcium deposition. As calcification of the cartilage matrix proceeds, the chondrocytes stop dividing, degenerate, and become part of the metaphyseal zone (33). In normal children, these processes occur in different bones at different times. If there is a lack of GH and/or the other hormones involved in this process, this is reflected in the pace of bone maturation. Clinically, this is recognized when the bone age (BA) of a child is determined by comparing an x-ray film of his or her hand to published standards. Typically, the BA of a GH-deficient child is less than the height age. An indication of delayed skeletal maturation can also be given by dental development, for example, age when the first tooth erupted and the number of primary and secondary teeth.

3. Diabetes Insipidus

Most older children and adults who develop acquired diabetes insipidus can recognize the symptoms of polydipsia and polyuria. In many cases, they can give an accurate indication of the time of onset of symptoms. In contrast, in infancy, the signs of diabetes insipidus may be nonspecific. They include irritability and unexplained fever. The diagnosis of diabetes insipidus is made when the serum osmolarity exceeds 285 m Osmol and the urine osmolarity is less than the serum osmolarity. Central diabetes insipidus caused by lack of ADH can then be differentiated from nephrogenic diabetes insipidus (as a result of end-organ resistance to ADH) by giving vasopressin or the long-acting vasopressin analog, desmopressin, and measuring urine specific gravity and osmolality. In central diabetes insipidus, these increase after vasopressin; in nephrogenic diabetes insipidus, they do not (Chap. 5).

4. Disorders of Pubertal Development

Gonadotropin deficiency may present in infancy with microgenitalia. Acquired gonadotropin deficiency or milder degrees of gonadotropin deficiency present as delayed or absent puberty. Because gonadal steroids affect growth both directly and via an effect on GH secretion (33), the adolescent with gonadotropin deficiency does not grow as rapidly as his or her age mates (34,35). Unlike the child with both GH and gonadotropin deficiency, the child with gonadotropin deficiency alone responds to sex hormone replacement therapy with growth that is normal for age (Chap. 18).

In Kallman syndrome, hypogonadotropic hypogonadism occurs with anosmia (or hyposmia). Family studies indicate that Kallman syndrome can be inherited in an autosomal dominant, autosomal recessive, or X-linked manner. In the X-linked form, which is the most common, the gene for Kallman syndrome has been mapped to the distal part of the short arm (Xp22.3) (36). Patients with X-linked Kallman syndrome may also have other problems, such as mirror movements, abnormal visual-spatial attention, high-arched or cleft palate, and unilateral renal aplasia; secretion of other pituitary hormones remains intact. A candidate gene has been mapped to the Xp22.3 region. On the basis of its deduced amino acid sequence, it is postulated to be an extracellular matrix protein that may have a role in neuronal migration (37).

5. Visual and Neurologic Complaints

If optic nerve hypoplasia has not been recognized in infancy, it may present in childhood as diminished visual acuity (38). The same evaluation of pituitary function recommended in infancy is suggested for children in whom the diagnosis has been delayed. In addition, once a child has been diagnosed as having optic nerve hypoplasia, careful follow-up, particularly of linear growth, should be maintained and a reevaluation of GH secretion and other pituitary hormones undertaken if there is growth deceleration. Although the association between hypopituitarism and "septooptic dysplasia" is well described, absence of the septum pellucidum is of little significance in the long-term prognosis of these children (39). Hypopituitarism and other brain abnormalities are more important in determining outcome. For this reason (38,39), another designation for this condition may be desirable.

Although growth failure and other signs of hypopituitarism are often present in children who are diagnosed as having a craniopharyngioma or other tumors in the region of the hypothalamus, most come to medical attention because of headaches, visual disturbances, and other neurologic complaints (Table 1) (40–44). If possible, a preoperative evaluation of pituitary function should be undertaken, and postoperative endocrine evaluation and follow-up are mandatory.

6. History of Breech Delivery

A number of authors (13,45) have noted the correlation between a complicated perinatal course, including breech delivery, and the later development of pituitary hormone deficiencies. A history of a breech delivery is more common in children with multiple pituitary hormone deficiencies, but it is also more common in children with brain anomalies (46). Whether breech delivery is the cause of hypopituitarism or a reflection of an underlying neuroendocrine abnormality is not clear. However, the fact that many of the males with hypopituitarism have a microphallus (8,19,47) suggests that, at least in some cases, hypopituitarism is of prenatal origin: lack of gonadotropins in utero would lead to decreased fetal testosterone synthesis and poor phallic growth.

7. Developmental Defects

Pituitary hormone deficiencies have been reported in association with congenital malformation syndromes, some of which are inherited (48). The associations between optic nerve hypoplasia and hypopituitarism and anosmia and gonadotropin deficiency have been described. Other malformation syndromes are discussed here.

Anencephaly is the most severe form of brain malformation. There is complete absence of the hypothalmus and a variable degree of pituitary hypoplasia (48).

The holoprosencephalies are associated with defective cleavage of the forebrain. In some cases, chromosomal abnormalities are present; in others, the condition appears to be inherited, with variable expression ranging from the presence of a single central incisor to more severe manifestations (49,50). Because of this association, a child presenting with growth failure and a single central incisor should have a complete evaluation of pituitary function. If hypopituitarism is found, magnetic resonance imaging (MRI) of the brain should be done; other family members should have a careful physical examination looking for a single central incisor and other signs of holoprosencephaly because this condition may be inherited in an autosomal dominant manner (49). The association of cleft lip and palate with hypopituitarism may be an example of a mild form of holoprosencephaly (48).

Destruction of the anterior pituitary with interstitial inflammation and fibrosis has been described at autopsy in up to 50% of infants with congenital syphilis (51). Two cases of congenital syphilis in small for gestational age, preterm infants with severe, symptomatic hypoglycemia caused by GH and ACTH deficiencies were recently described (52). Because the incidence of congenital syphilis is increasing, this association should be kept in mind in the infant with congenital syphilis who is having seizures, apnea, and bradycardia in association with hypoglycemia.

Autosomal dominant inheritance of isolated GH deficiency in Rieger syndrome (malformation of the iris and dental hypoplasia) has been described (53). The finding of primary empty sella in a patient with Rieger syndrome suggests that this association is the result of a common developmental defect (54).

Hypopituitarism has also been associated with other physical anomalies, such as Pallister-Hall syndrome, which consists of postaxial polydactyly, hypothalamic hamarto-blastoma, imperforate anus, abnormal external genitalia in males (micropenis, cryptorchidism, and testicular hypoplasia), and characteristic facies, including a broad, flat nasal bridge, dysplastic teeth, low-set or malformed ears, upward-slanting palpebral fissures, and abnormalities of the palate (55–58). Hypopituitarism, when present, is caused by aplasia or dysplasia of the pituitary gland. Some cases of Pallister-Hall syndrome are associated with an unbalanced chromosome translocation (58); others appear to be the result of an autosomal dominant pattern of inheritance (57).

8. Characteristic Facies and Body Habitus

In addition to the specific syndromes and physical anomalies associated with hypopituitarism already described, children with severe hypopituitarism often have characteristic facial features and body habitus. Because growth of the skull is dependent on brain growth and is less subject to hormonal regulation than that of the lower face and the axial skeleton, these children often appear to have large heads compared with the rest of their bodies. In fact, I have seen several youngsters in whom CT scans were done to evaluate their "large heads" when plotting head circumference and height on the appropriate growth charts showed that head growth was appropriate for age but statural growth was severely retarded.

Delayed skeletal maturation can be reflected in delayed dental development. Older children with long-standing hypopituitarism may not only have delayed dentition but also experience severe wearing down of the primary teeth.

Children with GH deficiency also tend to have a characteristic pattern of fat deposition with truncal obesity (59,60). Treatment with GH decreases the fraction of body weight that is fat and increases lean body mass. There is also a redistribution of fat from central to peripheral depots.

III. DIAGNOSTIC EVALUATION

The evaluation of a child with a complaint of short stature is outlined elsewhere in this book (Chap. 1). Briefly, it should begin with a history, including a perinatal history inquiring about the presence of any of the signs of hypopituitarism in the newborn described earlier, a review of growth data, medical history, and family history, including heights, pattern of growth and pubertal development, and significant illnesses. If data are available, growth charts of height, weight, and head circumference should be constructed.

The physical examination should include measurements of body proportions, a careful notation of dysmorphic features, a funduscopic (ophthalmoscopic) examination, and examination of the external genitalia.

A. Evaluation of Hormone Deficits

In a child with hypoglycemia, low GH levels, if measured when hypoglycemia is confirmed, are diagnostic of GH deficiency. If samples obtained at this time are not available or if the presenting complaint is short stature, GH secretion can be evaluated by pharmacologic testing or studies of spontaneous GH secretion (Chap. 4) (6). In the past, when supplies of GH were limited, the diagnosis of GH deficiency was thought to be capable of rigorous definition. As supplies, first of pituitary GH and later of GH prepared by recombinant DNA technology increased, it became clear that there were children who did not meet rigorous criteria for GH deficiency but responded to exogenous GH with an increase in growth rate (Chap. 4). The question then arises, What is the purpose of testing for GH deficiency? If it is decided that such testing serves a purpose, the next question is, how best to define the GH deficient state. To quote two British pediatric endocrinologists, "tests of growth hormone secretion are currently in a mess" (61).

In Australia, where GH is provided through a single governmental agency, a clinical trial to determine whether GH testing is necessary for selecting children to receive GH treatment is nearing completion (62). In this study, certain groups of children, such as girls with Turner syndrome and children with a history of brain irradiation or a craniopharyngioma, are treated when there is substantial growth deceleration without testing GH secretory capacity. Children with severe short stature and a growth rate less than the 25th percentile for age are tested for GH deficiency, but the results of these tests are *not* used to determine access to GH. The decision to treat with GH is based solely on height and growth rate criteria. If the child's growth rate increases significantly with treatment, GH is continued. If the increase in growth

after 6 months is not satisfactory according to preestablished criteria, the dose of GH is increased. If this increased dose does not result in a substantial increase in growth, treatment is discontinued. The reasoning for this study is as follows: GH testing is expensive and has the potential for adverse effects (particularly the so-called gold standard insulin tolerance test, in which seizures, aspiration, and respiratory arrest have occurred). Because GH secretion is a major determinant of childhood growth rates (30,31,63,64), growth is an excellent bioassay for GH secretion and function. If this hypothesis is confirmed, the Australian government plans to discontinue GH testing as a requirement for GH treatment.

In contrast to this approach, studies indicate the severity of GH insufficiency is a major predictor of the response to exogenous GH (65), and children with severe GH deficiency typically have the best response to GH treatment (66). The problem lies in our desire to establish firm "cutoff values" or limits to define GH insufficiency when clearly there are other factors, such as nutrition (Chap. 8), that affect growth. One group has even suggested that a hypocaloric diet be given for 3 days before GH testing to improve the diagnostic rigor of the procedure (67). In any case, there is a substantial overlap between the GH values (whether in response to pharmacologic agents or spontaneously secreted) between tall, normally growing, and short children (not to mention the interassay variability in GH assays, which is discussed in Chaps. 4, 5, and 6), to indicate that there can be no single value of GH that indicates that a given child will not respond to exogenous GH with improved growth. It is my belief that GH testing provides additional information that is useful in evaluating a child with growth failure but that the decision to treat such a child with GH must be based on both auxologic and hormonal criteria. My (strictly personal) opinion is that selecting children for GH treatment is akin to the decision-making process in civil law, in which one looks at the preponderance of the evidence rather than looking for GH deficiency "beyond a reasonable doubt."

I approach the child referred for short stature as follows: screen children with heights less than 5th percentile (or less than 5th percentile for midparental height) or growth deceleration (if past growth records are available) for treatable causes of short stature, including measurements of thyroid function and insulin-like growth factor I (Chap. 1). In children with severe short stature (height less than 1st percentile), a low insulin-like growth factor I, or marked growth deceleration (height crossing more than one isopleth), I then test the GH response to a pharmacologic agent, such as clonidine, L-dopa (levodopa), or, in infants, glucagon. In youngsters in whom the maximum GH is less than 10 μg/L, a second pharmacologic test is done. I consider a child who failed to attain a GH greater than 10 μg/L on both tests to have "classic" GH deficiency and evaluate for the presence of other pituitary hormone deficiencies before beginning GH treatment. I continue to follow the other youngsters (less severe short stature or a GH greater than 10 μg/L on provocative testing). If one of these children continues to grow poorly (growth less than 25th percentile) for a year or more, I consider this child for GH treatment. Because I have seen children who had "normal" GH responses when tested at one time who continued to grow poorly and were found to be "GH deficient" when retested, I might repeat a GH test at this time, more for the purpose of documenting pituitary function than for making a decision regarding GH treatment.

Another reason to test GH secretion in children with growth failure is that GH is usually the first of the anterior pituitary hormones to become deficient when there is an ongoing organic process, and such a process may not be recognized if an endocrine evaluation is not done. Given the availability of sophisticated neuroimaging techniques (see later), this may no longer be the case. Whether a magnetic resonance imaging study of the head can substitute for a dynamic endocrine evaluation is a question that deserves further study. Certainly, I would not treat a child with short stature of unknown etiology with GH without either documenting normal anterior pituitary hormone reserves or doing MRI to study hypothalamic-pituitary anatomy.

Because ACTH is rapidly degraded by proteolytic enzymes in serum and samples require careful, specialized handling and because ACTH assays have only recently become commercially available, the evaluation of ACTH secretion has usually been based on measurement of cortisol and its metabolites. A spontaneous cortisol (or one obtained following spontaneous or insulin-induced hypoglycemia) greater than 550 nmol/L (or 20 μg/dl) is usually taken as indicating that adrenal function is satisfactory.

In addition to its role in the acute adrenal release of cortisol, ACTH is required for adrenal growth and maintenance. Therefore, the cortisol response to exogenous ACTH is blunted in long-standing hypopituitarism, and measurement of the cortisol response to injected synthetic ACTH (cosyntropin) can indicate the presence of ACTH deficiency (68). Because this test has minimal side effects (occasional brief nausea or unease), it is a safe way to evaluate the pituitary-adrenal axis in children in whom normal spontaneous cortisol levels have not been documented. Insulin-induced hypoglycemia has been regarded as the gold standard for evaluating both GH and ACTH secretion (69), but the symptoms and risks of hypoglycemia, particularly in a child with hypopituitarism, have made this test less popular than it was in the past. Studies in adults with pituitary dysfunction indicate that an integrated 2 h cortisol response to ACTH greater than 40.6 μmol $\times$ minute/dl (1450 μg $\times$ minute/dl) with samples taken for cortisol determination at times 0, 30, 60, and 120 minutes following a bolus of 250 μg synthetic ACTH is associated with a stable clinical course in patients with subnormal responses to metyrapone (70). Because patients with multiple pituitary hormone deficiencies should probably receive additional glucocorticoid replacement for general anesthesia, febrile illnesses, and other stresses in any case, the cortisol response to ACTH may indicate those children who can be spared the growth-attenuating effects of chronic glucocorticoids.

A low thyroxine (T$_4$) coupled with a normal TSH can be caused by either an abnormality of thyroid hormone binding proteins (particularly thyroxine binding globulin) or central hypothyroidism. In the former case, free thyroxine (either measured directly or as indicated by the free thyroxine index) is normal. In the latter case, free thyroxine is low.

The ability to evaluate the pituitary-gonadal axis depends on the patient's age. In early infancy (up to age 4–6 months), there is spontaneous secretion of LH and FSH in amounts that are easily measured by standard radioimmunoassay (20). Testosterone and estradiol levels are substantially higher than they will be until midpuberty. At this time, random levels of gonadotropin and sex hormones are informative regarding gonadal function. Later in infancy (up to age 4 years), spontaneous gonadotropin secretion declines, but the LH and FSH responses to gonadotropin releasing hormone are retained (71). During childhood, the activity of the hypothalamic-pituitary-gonadal axis is muted, and the ability to evaluate its functional integrity is limited. In a child with no other pituitary hormone deficits, the differential diagnosis between delayed puberty and hypogonadotropic hypogonadism is very difficult to sort out. When the age of normal puberty is reached (particularly the BA), then low spontaneous levels of LH and FSH coupled with low testosterone and estradiol levels in a child with known pituitary hormone deficiencies are indicative of gonadotropin deficiency.

B. Neuroimaging

Before the development of sophisticated neuroimaging techniques, most pediatric endocrinologists obtained a lateral skull film to look for suprasellar calcifications or an enlarged sella turcica as an indication of the presence of a craniopharyngioma or other mass lesion. The development of computed tomography and MRI techniques has made the plain skull film obsolete. More importantly, MRI findings have provided insights into the cause of "idiopathic" hypopituitarism.

A number of brain MRI studies of children with both multiple pituitary hormone deficiencies and isolated GH deficiency (4,8,72–76) have documented the presence of anatomic abnormalities in the hypothalamic-pituitary region and elsewhere. The abnormalities found have included the following: pituitary hypoplasia, absence of the pituitary stalk, and an ectopic posterior pituitary. In a study of 37 patients with idiopathic hypopituitarism, Maghnie et al. (47) found that 22 (12 with multiple pituitary hormone deficiencies and 10 with isolated GH deficiency) had anterior pituitary hypoplasia accompanied by pituitary stalk agenesis and an ectopic posterior pituitary lobe. The 15 patients who had only anterior pituitary hypoplasia all had isolated GH deficiency. In the group with stalk agenesis, a history of vaginal delivery from a breech presentation was associated with multiple pituitary hormone deficiencies (12 of 12). The three patients in this group who had a history of breech presentation with delivery by cesarean section had only isolated GH deficiency. These authors suggested that maldevelopment of hypothalamic-pituitary anatomy during the intrauterine period was associated with an increased risk of a breech presentation and that vaginal delivery from the breech presentation then resulted in multiple pituitary hormone deficits. A second conclusion from MRI studies of children with isolated GH deficiency is that the presence of an ectopic posterior pituitary may be an indication of risk of future development of other anterior pituitary hormone deficits (47,74).

MRI studies may be of particular help in the evaluation of children with acquired central diabetes insipidus. Surgical removal of a tumor in the hypothalamic-pituitary region is the most common cause of acquired central diabetes insipidus. In the patient lacking such a history (or a history of significant head trauma, which can also cause diabetes insipidus), a careful search for hypothalamic neoplasms and infiltrative and inflammatory processes must be undertaken. If no such lesions are found, careful, long-term follow-up, including repeat MRI studies, should be undertaken because the endocrine manifestations of these processes often precede their appearance on MRI. The presence of a thickened or enlarged pituitary stalk may be the first sign of Langerhans cell histiocytosis (77–82).

In a comparison of MRI and CT in children with idiopathic hypopituitarism (both isolated GH deficiency and multiple pituitary hormone deficits), Maghnie et al. (83) came to the conclusion that MRI was better than CT scanning for identifying anatomic abnormalities in the pituitary, pituitary stalk, and brain. Because neuroimaging studies, particularly MRI, are expensive, the question arises as to which children should have these studies. Certainly the child with acquired pituitary deficiencies of known etiology (e.g., after central nervous system, CNS, radiation) does not need such studies. In children with idiopathic pituitary hormone deficits, they serve several functions: first, to identify the child whose hypopituitarism is caused by a CNS tumor or infiltrative process; second, to provide insight into the etiology of "idiopathic" hypopituitarism; and third, in children with isolated GH deficiency, to identify those children who may be at risk for developing additional pituitary hormone deficits (see Sec. V). If the institution of GH therapy on height and growth rate criteria alone becomes the norm, then an MRI of the head before instituting GH may be the only way to identify youngsters with organic hypopituitarism. At present, the data that would allow a cost-benefit analysis of this question and provide guidelines are lacking. My inclination is to obtain such studies in any child with a pronounced growth deceleration, multiple hormone deficits, diabetes insipidus, or neurologic findings in addition to growth failure who does not have a history suggesting a cause for the hypopituitarism.

IV. SPECIFIC SYNDROMES ASSOCIATED WITH HYPOPITUITARISM

A. Congenital

Congenital syndromes of hypopituitarism can be divided into those known to be inherited and those that appear to represent sporadic developmental defects. The latter may also have a genetic component that has not been recognized.

Autosomal recessive isolated GH deficiency caused by deletions in the pituitary GH gene is described elsewhere in this book (Chap. 3). Recent applications of the techniques of molecular biology to other families with inherited multiple pituitary hormone deficiencies have identified mutations in the gene encoding the pituitary transcription factor Pit-1.

These mutations, which are also inherited in an autosomal recessive manner, result in GH, TSH, and prolactin deficiencies (84–86). A similar mutation is responsible for GH, TSH, and prolactin deficiencies in the Snell dwarf mouse (87).

In addition to the autosomal recessive forms of hypopituitarism, sex-linked forms have been identified. Two families in which X-linked hypogammaglobulinemia occurred in association with isolated GH deficiency have been reported (88,89). X-linked panhypopituitarism with variable hormone deficiencies has been described in several families, but at present the molecular basis of this syndrome is unknown (48,90–92).

The growth failure in Fanconi syndrome (autosomal recessive inheritance) can be ascribed to both intrauterine growth retardation and GH deficiency (93). The mechanism responsible for GH deficiency in Fanconi syndrome is unknown.

Autosomal dominant multiple malformation syndromes associated with hypopituitarism and Reiger and Pallister-Hall syndromes have already been described.

B. Acquired Forms of Hypopituitarism

Any injury to the hypothalamus or pituitary can result in hypopituitarism.

1. Tumors and Their Treatment

Tumors of the sella turcica, suprasellar, and pineal regions can result in endocrine abnormalities for several reasons. Growth of the tumor mass can destroy functional endocrine tissue, the tumor itself may secrete hormonally active substances, and finally, surgery and radiation used to treat the tumor can damage hypothalamic or pituitary tissue.

In children and adolescents, craniopharyngioma is probably the most common central nervous system tumor causing pituitary dysfunction (44). Craniopharyngiomas are benign tumors that arise from remnants of Rathke's pouch. Most craniopharyngiomas, particularly in children, have calcification that can be identified on CT scan, and the majority are cystic (43). Although visual and neurologic complaints are the most common reason for evaluation, many children with craniopharyngiomas have evidence of growth failure on presentation (Table 1). Even if pituitary hormone deficiencies are not present before surgery, most patients develop panhypopituitarism postoperatively (40,42,43). Damage to the satiety center of the hypothalamus, either by the tumor itself or as a result of aggressive tumor resection, can result in severe obesity. Some of the children with this syndrome exhibit normal or accelerated growth postoperatively even though they are GH deficient (40–42). Such growth is not always sustained, however (42), and all children with craniopharyngiomas should have close endocrinologic follow-up with institution of appropriate hormone replacement.

Pituitary adenomas are uncommon in children (94,95). Further, patients under 20 years of age account for less than 5% of cases of pituitary adenomas (94). Functional tumors—

Table 1 Presenting Complaints in Children with a Craniopharyngioma

| First author | Thomsett et al. | Bucher et al. | Blethen | Tomita et al. | Rivarola et al. |
Reference	40	41	42	43	44
Number of patients	42	19	23	27	22
Complaint					
Visual	15	4	15	15	19
Neurologic	21	12	10	21	13
Short stature	3	1	3	7	5
Short stature present[a]	14	3	9	No report	5
Diabetes insipidus	1	2	2	1	4
Precocious puberty	0	0	1	2	0

[a]Children in whom evidence of growth failure was present although the child was not referred for a growth problem.

prolactinoma 85%, corticotropinoma 10%, and somatotropinoma 3%—account for most. These tumors give rise to specific syndromes depending on the hormone produced in excess. These are described in Chapter 58.

2. Cranial Irradiation

Pituitary dysfunction, particularly GH deficiency, is a well-recognized complication of cranial radiation (Chap. 4). Initially, all children treated for neoplastic disease have growth failure caused by a combination of the illness itself and the side effects of radiation and chemotherapy (96). Long-term studies indicate a second phase of growth failure in children who have received cranial or cranial-spinal radiation (96–102). This is caused by GH deficiency. The onset of GH deficiency depends on the dose of radiation received, higher doses leading to an earlier onset of growth failure and GH deficiency (100,101). In children who receive lower doses of cranial radiation, the GH response to pharmacologic testing may be preserved but spontaneous GH secretion is lost (103). Younger age at the time of radiation seems to be associated with an earlier onset of GH deficiency (102). Cranial radiation can lead to precocious puberty, which in turn masks growth failure as a result of GH deficiency and shortens the time available for growth (102). Such children, if identified in time, may benefit from combined treatment with GH and a gonadotropin releasing hormone antagonist (104). All children who have received cranial radiation should be carefully followed for the appearance of growth deceleration and inappropriately early puberty so that appropriate hormonal interventions can be instituted. Many would treat a child with a history of cranial radiation and growth deceleration, without other obvious cause, as GH deficient, and manage them accordingly without GH testing (62,103). Because spinal radiation has an additional adverse effect on adult height (inhibiting vertebral growth), children who have received combined cranial-spinal radiation have a particularly poor prognosis with respect to adult height and deserve particularly close follow-up (105). In young children who receive cranial radiation, stunting of head growth is also found. Although poor head growth correlates with the presence of GH deficiency, it is not corrected with GH treatment (106).

3. Trauma

Severe head trauma (associated with prolonged loss of consciousness and skull fracture) that damages the pituitary stalk and infundibulum can result in the development of diabetes insipidus (107,108). The diabetes insipidus can be transient or permanent. Because the signs of diabetes insipidus are so dramatic, this diagnosis is rarely missed. However, follow-up studies indicate that anterior pituitary hormone deficiencies are not uncommon in these patients. In one study, 50% of patients with posttraumatic diabetes insipidus had GH deficiency (107). TSH, ACTH, and gonadotropin deficiencies were also noted. As mentioned, TSH and/or ACTH deficiency can mask the signs of diabetes insipidus. For this reason, all patients with posttraumatic diabetes insipidus should have a complete evaluation of anterior pituitary function even (especially) if the diabetes insipidus remits when high-dose glucocorticoid therapy is discontinued. Less severe head trauma even without neurologic sequelae can also lead to pituitary hormone deficiencies if there is damage to the pituitary stalk (109).

4. Infiltrative, Autoimmune, and Metabolic

Destruction of the hypothalamus, pituitary stalk, or the pituitary itself can result from a variety of processes. Langerhans cell histiocytosis can present as diabetes insipidus. On MRI, a thickened pituitary stalk may be the only abnormal finding (77–81,110). Such patients should be followed closely for the development of additional pituitary deficits and other manifestations of histiocytosis. Recently, a patient with isolated diabetes insipidus and no anterior pituitary hormone deficits who eventually developed skin manifestations of another rare histiocytic disorder, xanthoma disseminatum, was described (111).

Lymphocytic hypophysitis can also cause hypopituitarism. It most commonly is described in adult women in late pregnancy or the postpartum period (112). However, it has also been described in males (113). Many patients have a history of other autoimmune endocrinopathies, and antibodies to ADH-producing cells have been demonstrated in some patients (114). Because antibodies to ADH-secreting cells are also found in patients with demonstrated Langerhans cell histiocytosis, the relationship of the antibodies to these two entities is unclear (115). Disseminated tuberculosis and sarcoidosis can also be associated with hypopituitarism. Most (95%) patients with hypothalamic and/or pituitary sarcoidosis have evidence of systemic or other central nervous system manifestations of their disease in addition to pituitary hormone deficiencies. Gonadotropin and GH deficiency are the most common endocrine abnormalities, but all combinations of hypothalamic and pituitary dysfunction are possible. Although corticosteroids are indicated for neurosarcoidosis, recovery of pituitary function with steroid treatment has not been reported (116).

Hemochromatosis is characterized by iron deposition in various tissues. It can be idiopathic, but in children it often results from multiple blood transfusions used to treat hemoglobinopathies, such as thalassemia major. Although treatment with the chelating agent deferoxamine has been instituted in an attempt to prevent or delay the complications of transfusion therapy, iron deposition in the endocrine glands can lead to hormone deficiency. Studies on patients with idiopathic and transfusion-related hemochromatosis indicate that both hypothalamic and pituitary dysfunction are common, in addition to syndromes of primary glandular failure, such as diabetes mellitus (117–121). Gonadotropin deficiency seems to be the most common deficit (120,121), but GH deficiency is also found. Children with hemoglobinopathies who are receiving intensive transfusion therapy should receive careful monitoring of growth and pubertal development, and endocrine evaluation should be undertaken at the first sign of growth failure. Intensive chelation therapy may have the potential to prevent the development of some endocrine deficiencies but, as currently practiced, does not do so (120).

Cerebral edema is one of the most devastating complications of the treatment of diabetic ketoacidosis in children. Those children who survive this insult may develop hypopituitarism as a consequence (122–124).

The hypothalamic-pituitary axis functions in a carefully regulated manner. Any disturbance of the anatomy of this region, by trauma, hypoxia, ionizing radiation, infections, infiltrative processes, or hypoxia, can result in deficiencies of function. Careful follow-up of children subjected to these insults and a high index of suspicion of their adverse effects should allow appropriate evaluations to be conducted in a timely fashion.

V. TREATMENT OF HYPOPITUITARISM

A. Strategies for Hormone Replacement

The replacement doses of L-thyroxine, cortisol, or other glucocorticoids, GH, gonadotropins, and ADH are given in Chapters 18 and 52. The specifics of GH treatment are discussed in detail in Chapter 5. Here, I discuss some of the interactions of different hormones and develop strategies for introducing the different replacement hormones. In the child with multiple pituitary hormone deficiencies who needs glucocorticoid replacement, there are three major points to be kept in mind.

1. Effect of Glucocorticoids on Growth

Glucocorticoids have long been known as potent growth inhibitors (125–127). These effects are most apparent in children receiving pharmacologic doses of glucorticoids, but even doses that are considered to represent replacement of normal daily cortisol production can decrease the growth response to GH (126,127). In part this may be because previous estimates of normal cortisol production were, in fact, overestimates (128,129). Because of this growth suppressive effect, the doses of hydrocortisone (cortisol) given to children with idiopathic hypopituitarism should be kept as low as possible. A dose of 10 mg/m^2 of oral hydrocortisone per day is reasonable. An increased dose (up to 100 mg/m^2/day) should be given for stress, such as febrile illness or surgery.

2. Replacement of L-Thyroxine in Patients with Possible ACTH Deficiency

Because L-thyroxine affects the metabolic disposal of glucocorticoids (130), a patient who has both TSH and ACTH deficiency may not manifest signs of adrenal insufficiency while hypothyroid. Institution of replacement therapy with L-thyroxine in such a patient may precipitate an addisonian crisis. Therefore, thyroxine replacement in patients suspected of having multiple pituitary hormone deficiencies should be delayed until either (1) normal adrenal reserve is documented or (2) glucorticoid replacement has been instituted.

3. Effect of ACTH and TSH Deficiencies in Patients with Central Diabetes Insipidus

Thyroxine and cortisol both affect the ability of the kidneys to excrete free water (131). In a patient with acquired central diabetes insipidus and unrecognized anterior pituitary hormone deficiencies, the diabetes insipidus may appear to be remitting as serum levels of T$_4$ and cortisol decline. Serum sodium and potassium decrease during this process, but institution of replacement therapy with thyroxine and cortisol results in the reappearance of polyuria.

4. Treatment of ADH Deficiency

Details of the management of central diabetes insipidus are discussed in Chapter 5. Desmopressin acetate (DDAVP) is a synthetic analog of arginine vasopressin and can be given intranasally or by subcutaneous or intravenous injection. Nasal insufflation is the preferred method of administration, but parental administration is useful when there is nasal blockage, for example following transsphenoidal surgery with nasal packing. The parenteral dose is 0.1–0.2 that of the intranasal dose.

5. Timing of Sex Hormone Replacement in Gonadotropin-Deficient Patients

The specifics of sex hormone replacement are discussed in Chapter 18. Here, I discuss the question of the timing of induced puberty in the patient with hypopituitarism. The issues are these: the desire of a child for sexual maturity at a time when peers are developing versus the effect of sex hormones in accelerating bone maturation and, eventually, epiphyseal closure and cessation of linear growth. In a study of 137 Japanese children with GH deficiency (108 isolated and 29 with gonadotropin deficiency as well), Hibi et al. (132) found that spontaneous puberty had an adverse effect on adult height. They attributed this to the fact that spontaneous puberty occurred at a younger chronological age (CA), BA, and shorter height (Ht) compared with when puberty was induced (CA 14.5 ± 1.9 versus 19.8 ± 1.8 years, BA 12.2 ± 2.0 versus 13.8 ± 0.7 years, Ht 136.7 ± 8.9 versus 156.5 ± 8.3 cm; all $p < 0.01$). A collaborative study undertaken by Belgian pediatric endocrinologists also showed that height at the onset of puberty was an important determinant of adult height (133).

If GH treatment has been instituted at an early age, there has been sufficient catch-up growth, and the child's height is appropriate for genetic background, then psychosocial considerations and CA can be the factors determining the timing of sex hormone replacement. In the more usual case in which there is still a substantial height deficit, the question of timing becomes more difficult. For boys, a BA of 13 years or no change in BA for 1 year has been suggested as a criterion for beginning adrogen replacement (134). For girls, these same authors suggested that estrogen replacement begin when the BA is between 11.5 and 12.5 years or the growth rate < 3 cm/year (134). Although the data (132,133) suggest that delaying the onset of puberty as long as possible improves adult height, there are adverse physical as well as psychologic consequences of doing this. Because GH accelerates long bone growth over that of the vertebrae, the body proportions of children with both GH and gonadotropin deficiency in whom puberty was induced at an older age are abnormal (134). In this group of patients, leg length was normal (mean standard deviation score + 0.2) but sitting height was very subnormal (mean standard deviation score −3.0). Taken together, these data indicate the importance of early diagnosis and treatment of GH deficiency so that height is in the normal range when the age of onset of normal puberty is reached.

B. Follow-up of the Patient with Hypopituitarism

In the past, the patient with (presumed) isolated GH deficiency was followed until GH treatment was no longer indicated because of epiphyseal fusion, patient's desire to discontinue injections, or the reluctance of third-party payers to continue treatment. It now appears that some patients initially diagnosed as having isolated GH deficiency may present later in life with evidence of other anterior pituitary hormone deficits. For this reason, continued follow-up of pituitary function is essential throughout life (135–137). Such follow-up should include yearly evaluation of thyroid (T$_4$ level), adrenal (a.m. cortisol and possibly dynamic testing of adrenal reserve), and gonadal function (testosterone in males and menstrual history and estradiol levels in females). In patients who have had MRI studies of the brain, abnormalities of the pituitary stalk may identify those patients most at risk for developing additional hormone deficits (47,74,137). In view of studies showing an impaired cardiovascular response to stress in patients with multiple pituitary hormone deficiencies, lifelong hormone replacement is definitely indicated (138).

The pituitary continues to synthesize and secrete GH after linear growth is complete. Until recently, limitations of GH supply resulted in treatment being reserved for those children capable of increasing their stature. Evidence is now accumulating that GH deficiency in adults is accompanied by muscle atrophy, increased risk of cardiovascular events, and a generalized loss of energy (139,140). A number of clinical trials of GH treatment in GH-deficient adults are currently in progress, and it is possible that in the future GH treatment will not cease when adult height is reached (Chap. 5) (141,142).

REFERENCES

1. Frohman LA, Jansson JO. Growth hormone-releasing hormone. Endocr Rev 1986; 7:223–253.
2. Schwanzel-Fukuda M, Jorgenson KL, Berger HT, Weesner GD, Pfaff DW. Biology of normal luteinizing hormone-releasing hormone neurons during and after their migration from olfactory placode. Endocr Rev 1992; 13:623–634.
3. Schriock EA, Lustig R, Rosenthal SM, Kaplan SL, Grumbach MM. Effect of growth hormone (GH) releasing hormone (GRH) on plasma GH in relation to magnitude and duration of GH deficiency in 26 children and adults with isolated GH deficiency or multiple pituitary hormone deficiencies: evidence for hypothalamic GRH deficiency. J Clin Endocrinol Meta 1984; 58:1043–1049.
4. Maghnie M, Triulzi F, Larizza D, et al. Hypothalamic-pituitary dysfunction in growth hormone-deficient patients with pituitary abnormalities. J Clin Endocrinol Metab 1991; 73:79–83.
5. De Zegher F, Devileger H, Veldhuis JD. Properties of growth hormone and prolactin secretion by the human newborn on the day of birth. J Clin Endocrinol Metab 1993; 76:1177–1181.
6. Frasier SD. A review of growth hormone stimulation tests in children. Pediatrics 1974; 53:929–937.
7. Herber SM, Milner RDG. Growth hormone deficiency presenting under age 2 years. Arch Dis Child 1984; 59:557–560.
8. Brown RS, Bhatia V, Hayes E. An apparent cluster of congenital hypopituitarism in central Massachusetts: magnetic resonance imaging and hormonal studies. J Clin Endocrinol Metab 1991; 72:12–18.
9. Copeland KC, Franks RC, Ramamurthy R. Neonatal hyperbilirubinemia and hypoglycemia in congenital hypopituitarism. Clin Pediatr (Phila) 1981; 20:536–526.
10. Kaufaman FR, Costin G, Thomas DW, Sinatra FR, Roe TF, Neustein HB. Neonatal cholestasis and hypopituitarism. Arch Dis Child 1985; 60:787–789.
11. Leblanc A, Odievre M, Hadchouel M, Gendrei D, Chaussain JL, Rappaport R. Neonatal cholestasis and hypoglycemia: possible role of cortisol deficiency. J Pediatr 1981; 99:577–580.

12. Gluckman PD, Gunn AJ, Wray A, et al. Congenital idiopathic growth hormone deficiency associated with prenatal and early postnatal growth failure. J Pediatr 1992; 121:920–923.
13. Craft WH, Underwood LE, Van Wyk JJ. High incidence of perinatal insult in children with idiopathic hypopituitarism. J Pediatr 1980; 96:397–402.
14. McQueen MC, Copeland KC. Congenital hypopituitarism with free water intolerance and lack of thymic involution. Early recognition of clinical presentation. Clin Pediatr (Phila) 1989; 28:579–580.
15. Oelker W. Hyponatremia and inappropriate secretion of vasopressin (antidiuretic hormone) in patients with hypopituitarism. N Engl J Med 1989; 321:492–496.
16. Albertsson-Wikland K, Niklasson A, Karlberg P. Birth data for patients who later develop growth hormone deficiency: preliminary analysis of a national register. Acta Paediatr Scand (Suppl) 1990; 370:115–120.
17. Karlberg J, Albertsson-Wikland K. Infancy growth pattern related to growth hormone deficiency. Acta Paediatr Scand 1988; 77:385–391.
18. Goossens M, Brauner R, Czernichow P, Duquesnoy R, Rappaport R. Isolated growth hormone (GH) deficiency type I-A associated with a double deletion in the human GH gene cluster. J Clin Endocrinol Metab 1986; 62:712–716.
19. Lovinger RD, Kaplan SL, Grumbach MM. Congenital hypopituitarism associated with neonatal hypoglycemia and microphallus: four cases secondary to hypothalamic hormone deficiencies. J Pediatr 1975; 87:1171–1181.
20. De Zegher R, Devlieger H, Veldhuis JD. Pulsatile and sexually dimorphic secretion of luteinizing hormone in the human infant on the day of birth. Pediatr Res 1992; 32:605–607.
21. Sane K, Pescovitz OH. The clitoral index: a determination of clitoral size in normal girls and in girls with abnormal sexual development. J Pediatr 1992; 120:264–266.
22. Hoyt WF, Kaplan SL, Grumbach MM, Glaser JS. Septo-optic dysplasia and pituitary dwarfism. Lancet 1970; 1:893–894.
23. Acer TE. Optic nerve hypoplasia: septo-optic-pituitary dysplasia syndrome. Trans Am Ophthalmol Soc 1981; 79:425–457.
24. LaFranchi SH, Hanna CE. The clinical spectrum of optic nerve hypoplasia, hypopituitarism, and absent septum pellucidum. Pediatr Res 1981; 15:510.
25. Wit JM, van Unen H. Growth of infants with neonatal growth hormone deficiency. Arch Dis Child 1992; 67:920–924.
26. Illig R, Prader A, Ferrandez M, Zachman M. Hereditary prenatal growth hormone deficiency with increased tendency to growth hormone antibody formation A-type of isolated growth hormone deficiency. Acta Pediatr Scand (Suppl) 1971; 60:607.
27. Rivarola MA, Phillips JA III, Migeon CJ, Heinrich JJ, Hjelle BJ. Phenotypic heterogeneity in familial isolated growth hormone deficiency type I-A. J Clin Endocrinol Metab 1984; 59:34–40.
28. Laron Z, Kelijman M, Pertzelan A, Keret R, Shoffner IM, Parks JS. Human growth hormone gene deletion without antibody formation or growth arrest during treatment: a new disease entity? Isr J Med Sci 1985; 21:999–1006.
29. Nishi Y, Masuda H, Nishimura S, et al. Isolated human growth hormone deficiency due to the hGH-I gene deletion with (type I-A) and without (the Israeli type) hGH antibody formation during hGH therapy. Acta Endocrinol (Copenh) 1990; 122:267–271.
30. Karlberg J. On the construction of the infancy-childhood-puberty growth standard. Acta Paediatr Scand (Suppl) 1989; 356:26–37.
31. Tse WY, Hindmarsh PC, Brook CGD. The infancy-childhood-puberty model of growth:clinical aspects. Acta Paediatr Scand (Suppl) 1989; 356:38–43.
32. Tanner JM, Davies PSW. Clinical longitudinal standards for height and height velocity for North American children. J Pediatr 1985; 107:317–327.
33. Ohlsson C, Isgaadr J, Tornell J, Nilsson A, Isalsson OGP, Lindahl A. Endocrine regulation of longitudinal bone growth. Acta Paediatr (Suppl) 1993; 391:33–40.
34. Kerrigan JR, Rogol AD. The impact of gonadal steroid hormone action on growth hormone secretion during childhood and adolescence. Endocr Rev 1992; 13:281–298.
35. Van der Werff ten Bosch JJ, Bot A. Some skeletal dimensions of males with isolated gonadotropin deficiency. Neth J Med 1992; 41:259–263.
36. Ballabio A, Sebastio G, Carrozzo R, et al. Deletions of the steroid sulfatase gene in classical X-linked ichthyosis and X-linked ichthyosis associated with Kallman syndrome. Hum Genet 1987; 77:338–341.
37. Petit C. Molecular basis of the X-chromosome-linked Kallman's syndrome. Trends Endocrinol Metab 1993; 4:8–13.
38. Blethen SL, Weldon VV. Hypopituitarism and septooptic "dysplasia" in first cousins. Am J Med Genet 1985; 21:123–129.
39. Brodsky MC, Glasier CM. Optic nerve hypoplasia: clinical significance of associated central nervous system abnormalities on magnetic resonance imaging. Arch Ophthalmol 1993; 111:66–74.
40. Thomsett MJ, Conte FA, Kaplan SL, Grumbach MM. Endocrine and neurologic outcome in childhood craniopharyngioma: review of effect of treatment in 42 patients. J Pediatr 1980; 97:728–735.
41. Bucher H, Zapf J, Torresani T, Prader A, Froesch ER, Illig R. Insulin-like growth factors I and II, prolactin, and insulin in 19 growth hormone-deficient children with excessive, normal or decreased growth following removal of a craniopharyngioma. N Engl J Med 1983; 309:1142–1146.
42. Blethen SL. Growth in children with a craniopharyngioma. Pediatrician 1987; 14:242–245.
43. Tomita T, McLone DG. Radical resections of childhood craniopharyngiomas. Pediatr Neurosurg 1993; 19:6–14.
44. Rivarola MA, Mendilaharzu H, Warman M, et al. Endocrine disorders in 66 suprasellar and pineal tumors of patients of prepubertal and pubertal ages. Horm Res 1992; 37:1–6.
45. Rona RJ, Tanner JM. Aetiology of idiopathic growth hormone deficiency in England and Wales. Arch Dis Child 1977; 52:197–208.
46. Cruikshank DP. Breech presentation. Clin Obstet Gynecol 1986; 29:255–263.
47. Maghnie M, Larizza D, Triulzi F, Sampaolo P, Scotti G, Severi F. Hypopituitarism and stalk agenesis: a congenital syndrome worsened by breech delivery? Horm Res 1991; 35:104–108.
48. Rimoin DL. Hereditary forms of growth hormone deficiency and resistance. Birth Defects 1976; 12:15–29.
49. Berry SA, Pierpont ME, Gorlin RJ. Single central incisor in familial holoprosencephaly. J Pediatr 1984; 104:877–880.
50. Rappaport EB, Ulstrom RA, Gorlin RJ, Lucky AW, Colle E, Miser J. Solitary maxillary central incisor and short stature. J Pediatr 1977; 91:924–9.
51. Berger S, Edberg S, David G. Infectious disease in the sella turcica. Rev Infect Dis 1886; 129:747–755.
52. Daaboul JJ, Kartchner W, Jones KL. Neonatal hypoglycemia caused by hypopituitarism in infants with congenital syphilis. J Pediatr 1993; 123:983–985.
53. Sadeghi-Nejad A, Senior B. Autosomal dominant transmission

of isolated growth hormone deficiency in iris-dental dysplasia (Rieger's syndrome). J Pediatr 1974; 85:644–648.

54. Kleinmann RE, Kazarian EL, Raptopoulos V, Braverman LE. Primary empty sella and Rieger's anomaly of the anterior chamer of the eye: a familial syndrome. N Engl J Med 1981; 90–93.

55. Hall JG, Pallister PD, Clarren SK, et al. Congenital hypothalamic hamartoblastoma, hypopituitarism imperforate anus, and post axial polydactly. Am J Med Genet 1980; 7:47–74.

56. Culler FL, Jones KL. Hypopituitarism in association with postaxial polydactyly. J Pediatr 1984; 104:881–883.

57. Topf KF, Kletter GB, Kelch RP, Brunberg JA, Biesecher LG. Autosomal dominant transmission of the Pallister-Hall syndrome. J Pediatr 1993; 123:943–946.

58. Kuller JA, Cox VA, Schonberg SA, Golabi M. Pallister-Hall syndrome associated with an unbalanced chromosome translocation. Am J Med Genet 1992; 43:647–650.

59. Brasel J, Wright JC, Wilkkens L, Blizzard RM. An evaluation of seventy-five patients with hypopituitarism beginning in childhood. Am J Med 1965; 38:484–498.

60. Wabitsch M, Heinze E. Body fat in GH-deficient children and the effect of treatment. Horm Res 1993; 40:5–9.

61. Brook CGD, Hindmarsh PC. Tests for growth hormone secretion. Arch Dis Child 1991; 66:85–87.

62. Silink M. Alternative methods of diagnosis of growth hormone deficiency. J Pediatr Endocrinol 1992; 5:43–52.

63. Hindmarsh PC, Smith PJ, Brook CGD, Matthews DR. The relationship between height velocity and 24 hour growth hormone secretion in children. Clin Endocrinol (Oxf) 1987; 27:581–591.

64. Albertsson-Wikland K, Rosberg S. Analysis of 24-hour growth hormone profiles in children: relation to growth. J Clin Endocrinol Metab 1987; 67:493–500.

65. Blethen SL, Compton P, Lippe BM, et al. Factors predicting the response to growth hormone (GH) therapy in prepubertal children with GH deficiency. J Clin Endocrinol Metab 1993; 76:574–579.

66. Moore KC, Donaldson DL, Ideus PL, Gifford RA, Moore WV. Clinical diagnoses of children with extremely short stature and their response to growth hormone. J Pediatr 1993; 122:687–692.

67. Maghnie M, Valtorta A, Moretta A, et al. Diagnosing growth hormone deficiency: the value of short term hypocaloric diet. J Clin Endocrinol Metab 1993; 77:1372–1378.

68. May ME, Carey RM. Rapid adrenocorticotropic hormone test in practice: a retrospective study. Am J Med 1985; 79:679–684.

69. Borst GC, Michenfelder HJ, O'Brien JT. Discordant cortisol response to exogenous ACTH and insulin-induced hypoglycemia in patients with pituitary disease. N Engl J Med 1982; 306:1462–1464.

70. Beyer HS, Bantle JP, Mariash CN, et al. Use of the dexamethasone adrenocorticotropin test to assess the requirement for continued glucocorticoid replacement therapy after pituitary surgery. J Clin Endocrinol Metab 1985; 60:1012–1018.

71. Conte FA, Grumbach MM, Kaplan SL, Reiter EO. Correlation of luteinizing hormone-releasing factor-induced luteinizing hormone and follicle-stimulating hormone release from infancy to 19 years with the changing pattern of gonadotropin secretion in agonadal patients: relation to the restraint of puberty. J Clin Endocrinol Metab 1980; 50:163–168.

72. Kaufman BA, Kaufman B, Mapstone TB. Pituitary stalk agenesis: magnetic resonance imaging of "ectopic posterior lobe" with surgical correlation. Pediatr Neurosci 1988; 14: 140–144.

73. Root AW, Martinez CR, Muroff LR. Subhypothalamic high-intensity signals identified by magnetic resonance imaging in children with idiopathic anterior hypopituitarism: evidence suggestive of and "ectopic" posterior pituitary gland. Am J Dis Child 1989; 143:366–367.

74. Pellini C, diNatale B, De Angelis R, et al. Growth hormone deficiency in children: role of magnetic resonance imaging in assessing aetiopathogenesis and prognosis in idiopathic hypopituitarism. Eur J Pediatr 1990; 149:536–541.

75. Christophe C, Van Vliet G, Dooms G, et al. Panhypopituitarism without diabetes insipidus: magnetic resonance imaging of pituitary stalk transection. Eur J Pediatr 1990; 149:235–236.

76. Marwaha R, Menon PSN, Jena A, Rant C, Sethi AK, Sapra ML. Hypothalamo-pituitary axis by magnetic resonance imaging in isolated growth hormone deficiency patients born by normal delivery. J Clin Endocrinol Metab 1992; 74:654–659.

77. Maghnie M, Villa A, Arico M, et al. Correlation between magnetic resonance imaging of posterior pituitary and neurohypophyseal function in children with diabetes insipidus. J Clin Endocrinol Metab 1992; 74:795–800.

78. Dunger DB, Broadbent V, Yeoman E. The frequency and natural history of diabetes insipidus in children with Langerhans-cell histiocytosis. N Engl J Med 1989; 321:1157–1162.

79. Tien RD, Newton TH, McDermott MW, Dillon WP, Kucharczyk J. Thickened pituitary stalk on MR images in patients with diabetes insipidus and Langerhans cell histiocytosis. Am J Neuro Radiol 1990; 11:703–708.

80. Rosenfield NS, Abrahams J, Komp D. Brain MR in patients with Langerhans cell histiocytosis: findings and enhancement with GdTPA. Pediatr Radiol 1990; 20:433–436.

81. O'Sullivan RM, Sheehan M, Poskitt KJ, Graeb DA, Chu AC, Joplin GF. Langerhans cell histiocytosis of hypothalamus and optic chiasm: CT and MR studies. J Comput Assist Tomogr 1991; 15:52–55.

82. Stanhope R, Preece MA, Grant DB, Brook CGD. Is diabetes insipidus during childhood ever idiopathic? Br J Hosp Med 1989; 41:490–491.

83. Maghnie M, Trializ F, Larizza D, et al. Hypothalamic-pituitary dwarfism: comparison between MR imaging and CT findings. Pediatr Radiol 1990; 20:229–235.

84. Tatsumi K, Notomi T, Mizuno Y, Miyai K. Combined deficiencies of growth hormone, prolactin, and thyrotropin caused by a nonsense mutation in the et *Pit*1 gene. J Endocrinol Invest 1992; 15(Suppl. 4):67.

85. Radovick S, Nations M, Du Y, Berg LA, Weintraub BD, Wondisford FE. A mutation in the POU-homeodo- main of Pit-1 responsible for combined pituitary hormone deficiency. Science 1992; 257:1115–1118.

86. Pfaffle RW, DiMattia GE, Parks JS, et al. Mutation of the POU-specific domain of Pit-1 and hypopituitarism without pituitary hypoplasia. Science 1992; 257:118–1121.

87. Li S, Crenshaw EB, Rawson EJ, Simmons DM, Swanson LW, Rosenfeld MG. Dwarf locus mutants lacking three pituitary cell types result from mutations in the POU-domain gene *pit*-1. Nature 1990; 347:528–533.

88. Fleisher TA, White RM, Broder S, et al. X-linked hypogammaglobulinemia and isolated growth hormone deficiency. N Engl J Med 1980; 302:1429–1234.

89. Monafo V, Maghnie M, Terracciano L, et al. X-linked agammaglobulinemia and isolated growth hormone deficiency. Acta Paediatr Scand 1991; 80:563–566.

90. Zipf WB, Kelch RP, Bacon GE. Variable X-linked recessive hypopituitarism with evidence of gonadotropin deficiency in two pre-pubertal males. Clin Genet 1977; 11:249–254.

91. Schimke RN, Spaulding JJ, Hollowell JG. X-linked congenital panhypopituitarism. Birth Defects 1971; 7:21–23.

92. Phelan PD, Connelly J, Martin FIR, Wettenhall NB. X-linked recessive hypopituitarism. Birth Defects 1971; 7:24–27.

93. Nordan UZ, Humbert JR, MacGillivray MH, Fitzpatrick JE. Fanconi's anemia with growth hormone deficiency. Am J Dis Child 1979; 133:291–293.

94. Faglia G. Epidemiology and pathogenesis of pituitary ademonas. Acta Endocrinol (Copenh) 1993; 129(Suppl. 1):1–5.

95. Haddad SF, Vanglider JC, Menezes AH. Pediatric pituitary tumors. Neurosurgery 1991; 29:509–514.

96. Schriock EA, Schell MJ, Carter M, Hustu O, Ochs J. Abnormal growth patterns and adult short stature in 115 long-term survivors of childhood leukemia. J Clin Oncol 1991; 9:400–405.

97. Katz JA, Pollock BH, Jacaruso D, Morad A. Final attained height in patients successfully treated for childhood acute lymphoblastic leukemia. J Pediatr 1993; 123:546–552.

98. Sklar C, Mertens A, Walter A, et al. Final height after treatment for childhood acute lymphoblastic leukemia: comparison of no cranial irradiation with 1800 and 2400 centigrays of cranial irradiation. J Pediatr 1993; 123:59–64.

99. Willi SM, Cooke K, Goldwein J, et al. Growth in children after bone marrow transplantation for advanced neuroblastoma compared with growth after transplantation for leukemia or aplastic anemia. J Pediatr 1992; 120:726–732.

100. Costin G. Effects of low-dose cranial radiation on growth hormone secretory dynamics and hypothalamic-pituitary function. Am J Dis Child 1988; 142:847–852.

101. Clayton PE, Shalet SM. Dose dependency of time of onset of radiation-induced growth hormone deficiency. J Pediatr 1991; 118:226–228.

102. Rappaport R, Brauner R. Growth and endocrine disorders secondary to cranial irradiation. Pediatr Res 1989; 25:561–567.

103. Albertsson-Wikland K, Lannering B, Marky I, Mellander L, Wannholt U. A longitudinal study on growth and spontaneous growth hormone (GH) secretion in children with irradiated brain tumors. Acta Paediatr Scand 1987; 76:966–973.

104. Cara JF, Kreiter ML, Rosenfield RL. Height prognosis of children with true precocious puberty and growth hormone deficiency: effect of combination therapy with gonadotropin releasing hormone agonist and growth hormone. J Pediatr 1992; 120:709–715.

105. Shalet SM, Gibson B, Swindell R, Pearson D. Effect of spinal irradiation on growth. Arch Dis Child 1987; 62:461–464.

106. Clayton PE, Shalet SM, Price DA, Surtees RAH, Pearson D. The role of growth hormone in stunted head growth after cranial irradiation. Pediatr Res 1987; 22:402–404.

107. Barreca T, Perrie C, Sannia A, Magnani G, Rolandi E. Evaluation of anterior pituitary function in patients with posttraumatic diabetes insipidus. J Clin Endocrinol Metab 1980; 51:1279–1282.

108. Notman DD, Mortek MA, Moses AM. Permanent diabetes insipidus following head trauma: observations on ten patients and an approach to diagnosis. J Trauma 1980; 20:599–602.

109. Yamanaka C, Monoi T, Fujisawa I, et al. Acquired growth hormone deficiency due to pituitary stalk transection after head trauma in childhood. Eur J Pediatr 1993; 152:99–101.

110. Schmitt S, Wichmann W, Martin E, Zachmann M, Schoenle EJ. Pituitary stalk thickening with diabetes insipidus preceding typical manifestations of Langerhans cell histiocytosis in children. Eur J Pediatr 1993; 152:399–401.

111. O'Dell WD, Doggett RS. Xanthoma disseminatum, a rare cause of diabetes insipidus. J Clin Endocrinol Metab 1993; 76:777–780.

112. Bevan JS, Othman S, Lazarus JH, Parkes AB, Hall R. Reversible adrenocortitropin deficiency due to probable autoimmune hypophysitis in a woman with postpartum thyroiditis. J Clin Endocrinol Metab 1992; 74:548–552.

113. Guay AT, Agnello V, Tronic BC, Gresham DG, Freidberg SR. Lymphocytic hypophysitis in a man. J Clin Endocrinol Metab 1987; 64:631–634.

114. Pestell RG, Best JD, Alford FP. Lymphocytic hypophysitis. The clinical spectrum of the disorder and evidence for an autoimmune pathogenesis. Clin Endocrinol (Oxf) 1990; 33:457–466.

115. Scherbaum WA, Bottazzo GF, Czernichow P, Wass JAH, Doniach D. Role of autoimmunity in central diabetes insipidus. Front Horm Res 1985; 13:232–239.

116. Freda PU, Silverberg SJ, Kalmon KD, Wardlaw SL. Hypothalamic-pituitary sarcoidosis. Trends Endocrinol Metab 1992; 2:321–325.

117. Charbonnel B, Chupin M, Legrand A, Guillon J. Pituitary function in idiopathic hemochromatosis: hormonal study in 36 male patients. Acta Endocrinol (Copenh) 1981; 98:178–183.

118. Williams TCC, Frohman LA. Hypothalamic dysfunction associated with hemochromatosis. Ann Intern Med 1985; 103:550–551.

119. Vannasaeng S, Fucharoen S, Pootrakul P, Ploybutr S, Yansukon P. Pituitary function in thalassemic patients and the effect of chelation therapy. Acta Endocrinol (Copenh) 1991; 124:23–30.

120. Oerter KE, Kamp GA, Munson PJ, Nienhuis AW, Cassorla FG, Manasco PK. Multiple hormone deficiencies in children with hemochromatosis. J Clin Endocrinol Metab 1993; 76:357–361.

121. Duranteau L, Chanson P, Blumberg-Tick J, et al. Non-responsiveness of serum gonadotropins and testosterone to pulsatile GnRH in hemochromatosis suggesting a pituitary defect. Acta Endocrinol (Copenh) 1993; 128:351–354.

122. Tubiana-Rufi N, Thizon-deGaulle I, Czernichow P. Hypothalamopituitary deficiency and precocious puberty following hyperhydration in diabetic ketoacidosis. Horm Res 1992; 37:60–63.

123. Lufkin EJ, Reagan TJ, Doan DH, Yanagihara T. Acute cerebral dysfunction in diabetic ketoacidosis: survival followed by panhypopituitarism. Metabolism 1977; 26:363–369.

124. Keller RJ, Wolfsdorf JI. Isolated growth hormone deficiency after cerebral edema complicating diabetic ketoacidosis. N Engl J Med 1987; 316:857–859.

125. Blodgett FM, Burgin L, Iezzoni D, Gribetz D, Talbot NB. Effects of prolonged cortisone therapy on the statural growth, skeletal maturation and metabolic status of children. N Engl J Med 1956; 254:636–641.

126. Soyka LF, Crawford JD. Antagonism by cortisone of the linear growth induced in hypopituitary patients and hypophysectomized rats by human growth hormone. J Clin Endocrinol 1965; 25:469–475.

127. Van den Brande JL, Van Wyk JJ, French FS, Strickland AM, Radcliffe WB. Advancement of skeletal age of hypopituitary children treated with thyroid hormone plus cortisone. J Pediatr 1973; 82:22–27.

128. Esteban NV, Loughlin T, Yergey AL, et al. Daily cortisol production rate in man determined by stable isotope/dilution mass spectrometry. J Clin Endocrinol Metab 1991; 71:39–45.

129. Kerrigan JR, Veldhuis JD, Layo SA, Iranmanesh A, Rogol AD. Estimation of daily cortisol production and clearance ratios in normal pubertal males by deconvolution analysis. J Clin Endocrinol Metab 1993; 76:1505–1510.

130. Hellman L, Bradlow HL, Zumoff B, Gallagher TF. The influence of thyroid hormone on hydrocortisone production and metabolism. J Clin Endocrinol Metab 1961; 21:1231–1247.

131. Slessor A. Studies concerning the mechanism of water reten-

tion in Addison's disease and in hypopituitarism. J Clin Endocrinol Metab 1951; 11:700–723.

132. Hibi I, Tanaka T, Committee for treatment of growth hormone deficient children. Final height of patients with idiopathic growth hormone deficiency after long-term growth hormone treatment. Acta Endocrinol (Copenh) 1989; 120:409–415.

133. Bourguignon JP, Vandeweghe M, Vanderschueren-Lodeweyckx M, et al. Pubertal growth and final height in hypopituitary boys: a minor role of bone age at onset of puberty. J Clin Endocrinol Metab 1986; 63:376–382; Eur J Pediatr 1981; 137:155.

134. Burns EC, Tanner JM, Preece MA, Cameron N. Growth hormone treatment in children with craniopharyngioma: final growth status. Clin Endocrinol (Oxf) 1981; 14:587–595.

135. Hanna CE, LaFranchi SH. Evolving hypopituitarism in children with central nervous system lesions. Pediatrics 1983; 72:65–70.

136. Crowe EC, Shalet SM. Adult panhypopituitarism presenting as idiopathic growth hormone deficiency in childhood. Acta Paediatr Scand 1991; 80:255–258.

137. Hasegawa Y, Hasegawa T, Yokoyama T, Kotoh S, Tsuchiya Y. Gradual progress of ACTH deficiency in a child with panhypopituitarism associated with pituitary stalk transection. Endocrinol Jpn 1992; 39:165–167.

138. Stabler B, Turner JR, Girdier SS, Light KC, Underwood LE. Reactivity to stress and psychological adjustment in adults with pituitary insufficiency. Clin Endocrinol (Oxf) 1992; 36:467–473.

139. Björk S, Jönsson B, Westphal O, Levin JE. Quality of life of adults with growth hormone deficiency: a controlled study. Acta Paediatr Scand (Suppl) 1989; 356:55–59.

140. Cuneo RC, Salomon F, McGauley GA, Sonksen PH. The growth hormone deficiency syndrome in adults. Clin Endocrinol (Oxf) 1992; 37:387–397.

141. Salomon F, Cuneo RC, Hesp R, Sonksen PH. The effects of treatment with recombinant human growth hormone on body composition and metabolism in adults with growth hormone deficiency. N Engl J Med 1989; 321:1797–1803.

142. Whitehead HM, Boreham C, McIlrath EM, et al. Growth hormone treatment of adults with growth hormone deficiency: results of a 13-month placebo controlled cross-over study. Clin Endocrinol (Oxf) 1992; 36:45.

3

Hereditary Growth Hormone Deficiency and Growth Hormone Insensitivity Syndrome

Yoshikazu Nishi

Hiroshima Red Cross Hospital,
Hiroshima, Japan

I. BIOSYNTHESIS

Recent advances in recombinant DNA technology have enabled characterization of the sequence and organization of the human growth hormone (hGH) gene and hGH gene cluster. With a molecular mass of 22,000 D (22 kD), hGH consists of a single polypeptide chain of 191 amino acid residues and has two disulfide bridges (1,2). This hormone accounts for approximately 90% of pituitary hGH content. The hGH gene cluster contains genes coding for hGH and human chorionic somatomammotropic hormone (CSH, also known as placental lactogen), together with related genes that do not code for familial hormones (1,2). hGH and CSH have 85% amino acid homology and 92–98% homology between their mRNA coding sequences (1,2). The hGH gene cluster is mapped in chromosome 17q22–24 (1,2). Its cluster has five very similar genes in the order 5′ hGH-1, CSHP-1, CSH-1, hGH-2, and CSH-2 3′, encompassing a distance of around 50 kilobase pairs. hGH-1 encodes the known protein sequence, whereas the other locus (hGH-2) encodes a protein that differs by 13 amino acids (1,2). hGH-1 and hGH-2 genes are termed the hGH-N gene (N for normal) and hGH-V gene (V for variant), respectively. The hGH-1 gene is solely responsible for coding pituitary hGH. CSHP-1 is a pseudogene (an inactive gene) (1,2).

II. GROWTH HORMONE, GROWTH HORMONE RECEPTOR, AND INSULIN-LIKE GROWTH FACTOR I ABNORMALITIES

Growth hormone (GH), GH receptor, and insulin-like growth factor I (IGF-I) abnormalities result in slow growth that can be classified into four major categories: decreased hGH secretion, defective hGH action (structurally abnormal hGH or defective hGH receptor), defective IGF-I (somatomedin C) generation, and impaired response of cartilage to IGF-I.

Although most cases of decreased hGH secretion are caused by birth trauma, hereditary single-gene disorders and embryologic defects have also been identified as causes. Phillips et al. distinguished six distinct groups based on the mode of inheritance, other hormone deficiencies, and status of hGH genes (2,3).

In this chapter, the hereditary growth hormone deficiency syndromes and growth hormone insensitivity syndromes are reviewed (Tables 1, 2, and 3).

III. HEREDITARY GROWTH HORMONE DEFICIENCY

A. Isolated Growth Hormone Deficiency Type 1A

Illig et al. (4) described the clinical characteristics of patients with isolated hGH deficiency (IGHD) type 1A: (1) familial incidence; (2) short body length and early growth retardation resulting in extreme short stature in adulthood; (3) typical facies with large, vaulted forehead and small nose with retracted bridge (Fig. 1); (4) strong anabolic action of an initial course of hGH; and (5) early appearance of anti-hGH antibodies followed by arrest of growth after an initial, short growth spurt. However, some patients have no anti-hGH antibodies during hGH therapy (5,6). There is phenotypic heterogeneity in IGHD type 1A. This facial appearance is not specific in IGHD type 1A, because it also occurs in other hereditary hGH deficiencies, in Laron syndrome, and in Pit-1 gene abnormalities.

Examination of DNA after digestion with restriction endonuclease shows that patients with IGHD type 1A have deletion of the hGH-1 gene (3). Examination of DNA after *Bam*HI digestion showed deletion of the 3.8 kilobase (kb) fragment that normally contains the hGH-1 gene (Fig. 2). The amount of hybridization seen for the 3.8 kb fragment in DNA from parents was intermediate between that seen in DNA from

Table 1 Genetic Disorders with Human Growth Hormone Deficiency

	Inheritance	Endogenous hGH	Response to hGH
Isolated hGH deficiency			
1A	Autosomal recessive	Absent	Temporally
1B	Autosomal recessive	Decreased	Present
2	Autosomal dominant	Decreased	Present
3	X-linked recessive	Decreased	Present
Panhypopituitary short stature (hGH + LH, FSH, TSH, and/or ACTH deficiency)			
1	Autosomal recessive	Decreased	Present
2	X-linked recessive	Decreased	Present
Pit-1 gene abnormality	Autosomal recessive or autosomal dominant (in some cases)	Decreased	Present
"Bioinactive" GH	?	Inactive	Present
Potent circulating human growth factor	?	Decreased	?
IGF-I resistance	?	Normal or increased	Absent
Growth without growth hormone: "invisible" hGH syndrome	?	Active?	?
Familial short stature with very high levels of GH binding protein	?	Free hGH: low?	?

Source: Refs. 25, 81, and 82.

the control subjects and DNA from patients, indicating that the parents are heterozygous for the hGH-1 deletion (3,7). To determine whether the deletion were of the same size in different families, DNA samples were cleaved with *Hind*III digestion. The hGH-1 gene is contained in a 26 kb fragment. Patients have a 19.3, 19.0, or 18.4 kb fragment, replacing the 26 kb fragment seen in control subjects. This implies that they have deletions of approximately 6.7 kb (26–19.3 kb), 7.0 kb (26–19.0 kb), or 7.6 kb (26–18.4 kb) DNA, which includes their hGH-1 genes. It has been reported that most (70–80%) IGHD type 1A patients have the 6.7 kb deletion, and the remainder (20–30%) have the 7.6 or 7.0 kb deletion (8). The polymerase chain reaction (PCR) amplification technique provides an alternative to Southern blotting in the

Table 2 Growth Hormone Insensitivity Syndrome

Primary GH insensitivity syndromes (Laron syndrome; hereditary/congenital defects)
  GH receptor deficiency (encompassing quantitative and qualitative defects in the GH receptor)
  Abnormalities of GH signal transduction (postreceptor defects)
  Primary defect of synthesis of insulin-like growth factor I
  Pygmies
Secondary GH insensitivity syndromes (acquired conditions; sometimes transitory)
  Circulating antibodies to GH that inhibit GH action
    Isolated GH deficiency type 1A with poor response to GH treatment as a result of anti-GH antibodies
  Antibodies to the GH receptor
  GH insensitivity caused by malnutrition
  GH insensitivity caused by liver disease
  GH insensitivity associated with elevated GH binding protein in Alagille syndrome (54)
  Other conditions that cause GH insensitivity

Source: From Reference 35, supplemented.

Table 3 Embryologic Defects

Pituitary aplasia, congenital absence of the pituitary gland, congenital hypopituitarism
Holoprosencephaly
Septooptic dysplasia (de Morsier syndrome)
Cleft lip and/or palate
Solitary central maxillary incisor
Transsphenoidal meningoencephalocele
Rieger syndrome (iridogonioidysgenesis with somatic anomalies)
Empty sella syndrome
Ectrodactyly-ectodermal dysplasia-clefting syndrome
Fanconi anemia

detection of hGH-1 gene deletions (8). Digestion patterns of the PCR products with restriction endonucleases *Bgl*I, *Hae*II, or *Sma*I showed characteristic differences for each of the three deletion sizes (6.7, 7.0, and 7.6 kb) (8).

Italian and western Spanish subjects have a deletion of the hGH-1 gene and the CSH gene (9). French siblings have a double deletion in the hGH/CSH gene cluster, which could have been generated by homologous crossing over between two different chromosomes, one bearing deletions of the hGH-1 gene and one bearing deletions of DNA containing CSH-1, hGH-2, and CSH-2 sequences (10). In a Turkish family, a total of approximately 45 kb DNA, encompassing hGH-1, CSHP-1, CSH-1, and hGH-2 genes, was deleted (11).

Individuals with IGHD type 1A have a prenatal hGH deficiency that causes a lack of immune tolerance to exogenous hGH. Although the development of anti-hGH antibodies causes arrest of response to hGH treatment, several patients continued to grow even though they had antibodies (Fig. 3). Interestingly, the majority of subjects with larger (~7.6 kb) gene deletions responded well to hGH treatment without the formation of high titers of anti-hGH antibodies, suggesting that subjects with a small gene deletion of approximately 6.7 kb may be more prone to developing anti-hGH antibodies, which inhibit the response to hGH treatment (12). The different antibody responses are known to occur between siblings in different families. Two Italian siblings, in whom the gene deletion was 7.6 kb, containing the hGH-1 gene as well as the CSHP-1 gene, showed different responses to hGH; one female patient showed a good response to hGH injections despite high titers of anti-hGH antibodies, but the other male patient showed a fairly good response, with lower antibody titers (9). One of three Argentinian siblings, in whom the gene deletion was 6.7

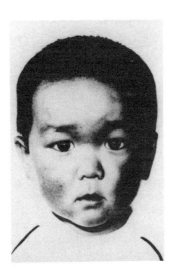

Figure 1 The characteristic face of IGHD type 1A; large, vaulted forehead and small nose with retracted bridge of our case at the age of 7 years.

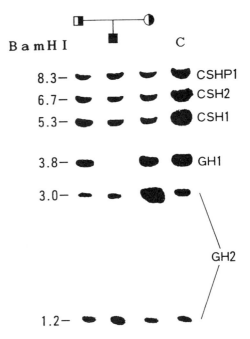

Figure 2 Autoradiogram patterns of DNA of IGHD type 1A from our Japanese boy, his parents, and control (C) after digestion with *Bam*HI restriction endonuclease. Fragment sizes in kilobases on the left.

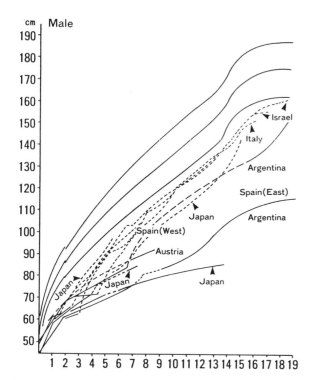

Figure 3 Growth curves of male patients with IGHD type 1A in various pedigrees. Solid lines indicate growth without therapy, and dotted lines show growth during hGH treatment. (Data from Refs. 6–10, 14, and 81.)

kb, continued to grow despite having a high titer of anti-hGH antibodies (13). Therefore, the role of anti-hGH antibodies as sole determinants of impaired growth response during continued hGH administration is equivocal. One could theorize that qualitative differences existed between the antibodies, permitting continued growth response in some, but not in other, persons. These differences must also be a result of factors other than hGH-1 gene deletion. Before hormone therapy, these factors may have included gene products from other loci that modify growth. During hGH therapy, these factors could be gene products, such as histocompatibility antigens (HLA), which could modify the qualitative or quantitative immune response (13).

Four Jewish siblings with a 7.6 kb deletion in four different families and two Japanese siblings with a 7.6 kb deletion in one family with the absence of anti-hGH antibodies showed a better response to hGH therapy (5,6). There are several possible explanations for divergence among patients with hGH-1 gene deletions. One possibility is that, despite similarity at the level of restriction endonuclease analysis, the deletions may differ in the antenatal production of peptides related to hGH, and thus differ in the induction of immune tolerance. The hGH-1 gene deletions may not necessarily result in antibody formation; rather, it may be a predisposing factor to produce antibody. Factors other than hGH-1 gene deletion can be surmised: HLA, complement, deficiency in the immune response gene, or an additional protective factor (6).

The Japanese family showed that parents had a limited response of hGH levels after various stimulation tests (7). This gene dosage effect has also been observed in the parents of the Argentinian and Austrian families (13,14). The subnormal response of hGH to provocative stimuli in heterozygotes does not seem to impair adult height significantly. Their parents did not have any anti-hGH antibodies and were capable of generating IGF-I normally.

Some patients with IGHD caused by point mutations in the hGH-1 genes have been reported. The hGH-1 sequence analysis of an affected patient from a consanguineous Turkish family had a G-A transition in codon 20 of the hGH-1 signal peptide. This substitution converts a TGG (tryptophan) to a TGA (stop) codon in exon 2 and generates a new *AluI* recognition site. Although two patients developed anti-hGH antibodies, one patient continued to respond to hGH treatment (15). In the Saudi family, a G-C transversion was found that alters the first base of the donor splice site of intron 4 in the hGH-1 genes. This substitution should perturb mRNA splicing, resulting in an altered protein product that should be unstable or bioinactive. Three affected patients responded well to hGH treatment and did not produce anti-hGH antibodies, suggesting the hGH proteins may be released that protect against the immune response to exogenous hGH (15). Two affected siblings were reported to be compound heterozygotes for a 6.7 kb deletion and a deletion of a C at position 371, causing a frameshift defect in the signal peptide coding region (16). Igarashi et al. (17) reported a compound heterozygote of a 6.7 kb deletion and a 2 bp deletion in exon 3 in the Japanese family.

The prevalence of IGHD type 1A has been reported. Using Southern blot analysis, Parks et al. (18) found that 5 (38%) of 13 Asian Jews with severe IGHD (height < –4 standard deviations, SD, score) had hGH-1 gene deletions. Kamijo et al. (12) and Vnencak-Jones et al. (19) reported that 3 (12%) of 26 Chinese subjects with severe IGHD had hGH-1 deletions using a polymerase chain reaction amplification method. Mullis et al. (20) observed a prevalence of an hGH-1 gene deletion in 3 (9%) of 32 North European, 3 (14%) of 22 Mediterranean, and 4 (17%) of 24 Turkish cases with IGHD (height < –4.5 SD score) using the PCR amplification method and Southern blotting. All affected families were consanguineous. In contrast, Mullis et al. (21) found no hGH-1 or GHRH gene deletions among 53 British children with a milder form of IGHD. Mullis and Brickell (22) reported the use of PCR to analyze chorionic villus DNA from fetuses with parents heterozygous for a 6.7 kb hGH-1 gene deletion. The PCR amplification method provides a real alternative to Southern blotting for identification and screening for hGH-1 gene deletions, because Southern blotting is slow, time consuming, and laborious compared with PCR analysis.

To date, there has been no way to treat these patients, and the attained height of the reported cases is rather poor. Hauffa et al. (23) observed that a patient with hGH-1 gene deletion (6.7 kb deletion) and anti-hGH antibodies for pituitary hGH responded well to methionyl hGH with decreased anti-hGH antibodies. The prospect of synthetic IGF-I offers a new aspect of treatment. Biosynthesis of the recombinant IGF-I has made possible the initiation of clinical trials. Our patient with IGHD type 1A with a 6.7 kb deletion with high titers of anti-hGH antibodies and poor growth during hGH therapy showed a good response of growth to IGF-I therapy for 2 years with decreased anti-hGH antibodies (24). IGF-I has a potential usefulness in the treatment of IGHD type 1A with poor response to hGH therapy as a result of high titers of anti-hGH antibodies.

Only a few families have been reported to have IGHD type 1A, but some cases may have gone unrecognized, especially when a single child in a family is affected. The search for a hGH-1 gene deletion should not be limited to patients with anti-hGH antibody formation and subnormal responses. When the technique of gene analysis becomes more generally available, it is probable that the recognition of this disorder will increase. Furthermore, gene analysis can also differentiate this disorder from other genetic types of IGHD in which the hGH-1 gene sequence is grossly normal.

B. Isolated Growth Hormone Deficiency Type 1B

Isolated hGH deficiency type 1B has an autosomal recessive mode of inheritance and is characterized by low but detectable levels of immunoassayable hGH after provocative stimuli, whereas hGH secretion is absent in IGHD type 1A.

Phillips et al. (25,26) studied DNA from individuals belonging to 12 different families in which two siblings were affected with IGHD type 1B. *Mps*I, *Bgl*II, and *Hinc*II restriction fragment length polymorphisms (RFLP) were used in linkage analysis of these families. Subjects in 7 families were discordant or differed in polymorphic restriction sites inherited from their parents and had inherited different hGH gene alleles from one or both parents. Subjects in 3 families were uninformative; those in 2 families inherited the same alleles from both parents. Because RFLP are very close to the hGH-1 locus, they should be reliable markers in which parental hGH-1 genes are inherited. The observed discordance between RFLP in at least 7 of 12 sibling pairs indicates that most of the mutation(s) causing IGHD type 1B phenotype segregate independently of the hGH gene cluster (25,26).

Patients with IGHD type 1B are considered to have isolated growth hormone releasing hormone (GHRH) deficiency based on the lack of adequate hGH responses to pharmacologic stimuli to hGH release and the large and brisk responses to GHRH injection (27). The lesion in this disorder appears to be in the hypothalamus and could be related to a lack of GHRH or a biologically inactive GHRH (25). These data suggest that the mutations causing IGHD type 1B affect a nonlinked locus (possibly one important for GHRH production or release or, alternatively, important for development of somatotropic cell function, rather than the hGH-1 gene) (25,26). The exact difference between type 1A and type 1B has not been determined. Recently, Phillips et al. (82) reclassified patients with splicing mutations from the Saudi family as having IGHD type 1B because of the nature of their hGH gene defects and their failure to produce anti-hGH antibodies in response to treatment with endogenous hGH. Both of these conditions imply that some hGH, although defective, is being made.

C. Isolated Growth Hormone Deficiency Type 2

Isolated hGH deficiency type 2 has an autosomal dominant inheritance. Affected subjects in the different families showed growth retardation, which responded well to exogenous hGH. A T-C transition of base 6 of the donor splice site of intron 3 was identified in a Turkish family with IGHD type 2 (28). The mutant hGH gene was transfected into cultured mammalian, and the hGH mRNA transcripts were analyzed by direct sequencing of their corresponding cDNAs. The mutation was found to destroy the donor splice site of intron 3, causing the donor splice site of intron 2 to be used in conjunction with the acceptor site of intron 3. This results in the splicing out or skipping of exon 3 and the loss of amino acids 32–71 from the corresponding mature hGH protein products. The mechanism by which the mutant hGH allele inactivates the normal hGH allele has not been proven but may involve the formation of a hGH dimer or disruption of normal intracellular protein transport (28).

Interestingly, Ohzeki et al. (29) reported a boy with hGH deficiency and IgM hyperimmunodeficiency in a Japanese family. The mode of transmission appears to be autosomal dominant. It is not known whether the two disorders are coincidental events.

D. Isolated Growth Hormone Deficiency Type 3

Isolated hGH deficiency type 3 has an X-linked recessive mode of inheritance. Some patients with IGHD type 3 have agammaglobulinemia, but others do not. Fleisher et al. (30) reported two brothers and two maternal uncles with hGH deficiency and hypogammaglobulinemia (deficient IgG, IgA, IgM, and IgE). The hGH-1 gene was normal. This disorder is considered to affect steps proximal to the hGH-1 gene or, alternatively, cellular development of the pituitary gland (25). Conley et al. (31) suggested that the combination of X-linked agammaglobulinemia and hGH deficiency may be caused by a small, contiguous, gene deletion syndrome involving the gene for X-linked agammaglobulinemia or an allelic variant of the gene for typical X-linked agammaglobulinemia. It is not known whether an allelic variant of the gene for typical X-linked agammaglobulinemia could code for a gene affecting transcription, translation, processing, or secretion of hGH. Interestingly, some subjects of IGHD have interstitial deletion of Xp22.3 or duplication of Xq13.3–q21.2, suggesting that multiple loci may cause IGHD type 3 (32,33).

Tang and Kemp (34) reported a boy with a combined defect in humoral and cellular immunity associated with IGHD whose immune defect was inherited in an X-linked recessive pattern.

The important point is that the poor growth of these children should not be attributed to growth retardation caused by infection, but the possibility of hGH deficiency per se should be contemplated.

E. Panhypopituitary Short Stature

Familial panhypopituitary short stature is associated with a deficiency of hGH and of one or more other pituitary hormones (luteinizing hormone, follicle stimulating hormone, adrenocorticotropic hormone, ACTH, and thyroid stimulating hormone, TSH) as well. Although almost all cases are sporadic, several kindreds have been reported. They are divided into two types by their modes of inheritance: type 1 is associated with autosomal recessive inheritance and type 2 with an X-linked recessive mode of inheritance. The clinical features depend on which of the trophic hormones is deficient. The most frequently associated hormonal deficiency is that of gonadotropin, followed in order of frequency by ACTH and TSH deficiency. There is both interfamilial and intrafamilial variability in the associated hormone deficiencies in both types: in certain families one individual may lack all the trophic hormones, whereas another may lack only hGH and gonadotropin. GHRH infusion tests showed a decreased release of hGH in these patients, indicating that the hypothalamus is the probable site of the basic defect, but a primary pituitary defect with varying severity cannot be excluded (27).

IV. GROWTH HORMONE INSENSITIVITY SYNDROME AND GROWTH HORMONE RESISTANCE

Classification of hGH insensitivity syndrome is proposed (Table 2) (35). To fill the definition of hGH insensitivity, affected patients must have adequate or inappropriately elevated serum hGH concentrations accompanied by low serum concentrations of IGF-I. Additionally, affected patients must have insensitivity to exogenous hGH.

A. Laron Syndrome, a GH Receptor Defect

Laron syndrome is a familial disorder with an autosomal recessive mode of inheritance, characterized by normal to high levels of circulating immunoreactive hGH, very low levels of circulating IGF-I, and unresponsiveness to exogenous hGH administration (36). The general appearance of patients with this disease is identical to that of patients with IGHD type 1A and pit-1 gene abnormalities [marked growth retardation; obesity; facial anomalies, such as frontal bossing, saddle nose, and small chin; small hands and feet; high-pitched voice, and small male genitalia (36)]. Puberty is delayed mainly in males, but full sexual development and reproductive capacity are attained. The largest cohorts described so far are from Israel, Asian Jewish, and Arab patients and from patients in Ecuador of Spanish and possibly Jewish descent. Isolated patients have also been reported, for example, in European countries, among black Americans, and in Japan. There is clinical heterogeneity between Ecuadorean and Israeli patients with this syndrome. Blue sclerae and limited elbow extension are noted in Ecuadorean patients, whereas they are not noted in Israeli patients (37). In contrast to the Israeli patients and others reported, the Ecuadorean patients are highly intelligent, with some exceptions (37). The Ecuadorean population also differed in that those patients coming from Loja province had a markedly skewed sex ratio (19 females and 2 males), but those from El Oro province had a normal sex distribution (14 females and 12 males). The phenotypic similarity between the El Oro and Loja patients

indicates that this abnormal sex distribution is not a direct result of Laron syndrome (37).

The human GH receptor gene is localized to the proximal short arm of chromosome 5. It spans at least 87 kb and includes nine exons (exons 2–10) that encode the hGH receptor and several additional exons in the 5'-untranslated region. Exon 2 encodes a secretion signal sequence; exons 3–7 the extracellular domain; exon 8 a transmembrane domain; and exons 9 and 10 the intracellular domain (38). The extracellular domain of the hGH receptor is normally found in serum as GH binding protein (GHBP), which is absent in Laron syndrome (38). However, families with Laron syndrome and normal circulating GHBP were recently reported, indicating a defect in the transmembrane or intracellular domain of the hGH receptor (39).

The cloning of the hGH receptor has enabled the investigation of the receptors in patients with Laron syndrome. Several types of receptor defects have been reported. Godowski et al. (40) found loss of exons 3, 5, and 6 and retention of exon 4 of the extracellular domain of the hGH receptor in two of seven Israeli patients of Iranian origin. Amselem et al. (41) reported a "serine" substitution to phenylalanine at position 96 in the extracellular domain. This alteration did not diminish the ability of the receptor to bind hGH but appeared to prevent normal trafficking of the molecule to the cell surface. Two different stop codon mutations were reported by Amselem et al. (42). A cysteine (TGC) to stop codon (TGA) mutation was detected at codon 38 in exon 4, and an arginine (CGA) to stop codon (TGA) mutation was found at codon 43 in exon 4 of Laron syndrome. Within this region, CpG dinucleotides seem to act as "hot spots" for the occurrence of mutations. Kou et al. (43) found amino acid substitutions in the intracellular part of the hGH receptor in a patient with Laron syndrome. At the second position of codon 422, a G to T transversion changes a cysteine residue to phenylalanine, whereas at the first nucleotide of codon 561 an alteration from C to A leads to the substitution of threonine for proline. Berg et al. (44) identified a substitution of G for A at the third position of codon 180, which is 24 nucleotides from the 3' end of exon 6 in Ecuadorean patients with this syndrome. This mutation does not cause an amino acid substitution, but it produces a consensus 5' splice sequence within exon 6 that results in the deletion of eight amino acids as a result of abnormal splicing of the 3' end of exon 6.

IGF-I treatment in Laron syndrome has been reported. Laron et al. (45) observed a dramatic growth-promoting effect of IGF-I on the body, limbs, and head circumference in five patients with Laron syndrome aged 3–14 years during 6–12 months of therapy. Heinrichs et al. (46) treated two patients with Laron syndrome aged 8.4 and 6.8 years using IGF-I subcutaneous injection, twice a day during 17 months. Increased linear growth velocity and bone mineralization, as well as increased bone maturation without remarkable adverse events, were observed. After 1 year of IGF-I therapy, growth response could no longer be observed in these two cases. Further studies are required to evaluate the efficacy of long-term IGF-I therapy on adult height and body proportions and the optimal effective dosage and safety of IGF-I in a large number of Laron syndrome cases.

B. Pygmies

African Pygmies have normal plasma levels of immunoreactive hGH, low levels of plasma GHBP activity, and peripheral unresponsiveness to hGH administration. Provocative hGH responses in Pygmies to arginine and insulin-induced hypoglycemia, however, are increased compared with normal (47). Merimee et al. (47) made the following observations. Prepubertal Pygmy children and normal children do not differ in linear growth or in serum concentrations of IGF-I and IGF-II. Adolescent Pygmies have lower levels of IGF-I than are found in control adolescents. In Pygmies, the serum levels of GHBP were less than normal in each age group. This difference was most marked in adolescents and adults, but it was also significant in children (48). Moreover, there was a marked acceleration of growth in control adolescents, but such an acceleration was absent or blunted in Pygmies (47). Baumann et al. (49) found that Pygmies have low levels of high-affinity GHBP in their plasma, which may indicate a reduced number of hGH receptors in their tissues. These findings suggest that the short stature of adult Pygmies is primarily caused by a failure of growth to accelerate during puberty, that IGF-I is the principal factor responsible for normal pubertal growth, and that partial hGH receptor deficiency, reduced hGH receptor number, and a defect in regulation of the hGH receptor gene, not a defect in the hGH receptor gene itself, may be responsible for their hGH resistance and short stature (47–49). Recent studies of Pygmy tissue have shown a normal sequence of hGH receptor gene, including its 3' and 5' extensions (48). It has also been postulated that a defect in promotor activity for the hGH receptor gene occurs in Pygmies (48). The study of allele frequencies of IGF-I gene failed to demonstrate any difference between Pygmy and non-Pygmy that suggest that this gene is involved in short stature (50). Geffner et al. (51) observed that the Pygmy T cell line showed no clonal responsiveness following stimulation with physiologic concentrations of IGF-I or any concentration of hGH, but it responded normally to insulin. IGF-I binding studies showed no binding to the Pygmy T cell line, with normal binding to control cells. These data suggest that the primary abnormality in the Pygmy is likely to be a genetic defect in IGF-I responsiveness associated with diminished IGF-I binding. These findings may explain both the short stature and hGH resistance of African Pygmies (51).

C. Mountain Ok People of Papua New Guinea

The height of the Mountain Ok people of Papua New Guinea generally falls below the fifth percentile of U.S. people from infancy to adulthood. Adult height is about 152 cm in males and 146 cm in females. These subjects have no major abnormalities of pubertal development. The possibility of nutritional deficits for short stature could be largely excluded because of normal serum levels of albumin and prealbumin (52). Serum concentrations of hGH, IGF-I, and IGF-II in Mountain Ok people were not different from those in controls (52). The high-affinity serum GHBP was decreased to 50% compared with sera of normal control subjects (53).

D. GH Insensitivity Associated with Elevated GHBP in Alagille Syndrome

Alagille syndrome is an autosomal dominant inherited disease with chronic intrahepatic cholestasis associated with a paucity of intralobular bile ducts in variable association with characteristic cardiac, skeletal, ocular, and facial features. Growth retardation occurs in approximately 50% of patients with Alagille syndrome and has been attributed to malnutrition. Recently, Bucuvalas et al. (54) reported that children with this syndrome, short stature, and decreased linear growth rate had low circulating IGF-I levels and elevated serum concentrations of hGH and GHBP. hGH insensitivity was demonstrated by no change in urinary Ca excretion, nitrogen metabolism, or circulating IGF-I levels after the administration of hGH. The growth disturbances and metabolic defects may be caused in part by failure to increase IGF-I concentrations in response to hGH. Growth-retarded children with this syndrome may benefit from IGF-I treatment.

V. ABNORMALITY OF PIT-1 GENE

Pit-1/GHF-1 (designated Pit-1 in humans for pituitary-specific factor 1), a member of the family of the POU domain DNA binding factors, is a pituitary-specific transcription factor that binds to and transactivates promoters of both hGH and prolactin genes (54). Pit-1 has a relatively minor role in transcription of the TSH-β gene. Pit-1 is also required for the differentiation, proliferation, and survival of anterior pituitary cells, somatotropes, lactotropes, and thyrotropes (55). Abnormalities in the Pit-1 gene were observed in congenital Snell and Jackson dwarf mice in which GH-, prolactin-, and TSH-producing cells were extremely hypoplastic (55).

In humans with congenital complete hGH and prolactin and complete or partial TSH deficiency, Pit-1 gene mutations were reported. The clinical features resemble those of IGHD type 1A and Laron syndrome. Magnetic resonance imaging (MRI) revealed a normal to small anterior lobe (56). Tatsumi et al. (56) reported a nonsense mutation at codon 172 in exon 4; a C to T transversion changed CGA encoding arginine to TGA encoding a nonsense or translational termination signal. In the case reported by Radovick et al. (57), the patient proved to be heterozygous for a single-base substitution in codon 271. This T for C substitution changed CGG encoding arginine to TGG encoding tryptophan. Pfäffle et al. (58) reported patients with a C for G substitution in codon 158 that changed GCA coding alanine to CCA encoding proline of exon 4. Ohta et al. (59) reported three Japanese children with Pit-1 gene mutations. In case 1, a single A for G transition that changed amino acid 143 from arginine to glycine was observed. In case 2, a T for C transition in one allele that changed amino acid 271 from arginine to tryptophan was observed. The patient was a heterozygote for the mutant allele and a normal allele similar to Radovick's case. In case 3, a T for C transition in one allele changed amino acid 24 from proline to leucine in exon 1. The patient was heterozygous for the mutant allele and a normal allele. This mutant Pit-1 may bind DNA normally but may act as a dominant inhibitor of Pit-1 action.

VI. BIOINACTIVE GROWTH HORMONE

There are at least two groups of patients with short stature but normal plasma radioimmunoactive hGH (60–63). Most of the patients reported are in one group. They show the following: plasma IGF-I is low, the ratio of radioreceptor-assayable to radioimmunoassayable hGH is low, and the response to exogenous hGH is good. This type of disorder is considered to be caused by the absence of or a low level of bioactivity of hGH, presumably because of abnormal structure. The defect is associated with a lack of generation of growth factors (60–64). Only three of these patients had a normal radioreceptor assay for hGH. Two of them were described by Rudman et al. (61) and showed a good response to treatment with hGH. A third patient, reported by Frazer et al. (62), did not respond to treatment. Valenta et al. (64) described a male patient with short stature who fits the first type of disorder of bioinactive hGH. His immunoassayable hGH was normal, but his radioreceptor-assayable and bioassayable hGH activities were low, and the response to hGH therapy was good. His plasma IGF-I was normal, however, which differentiated his case from the patients in the first group. The short stature of this patient was considered to be caused by the abnormal structure of his endogenous hGH. However, there is no clear evidence of inheritance and no definitive elucidation of specific molecular defects has been reported.

There is a group of a few patients with bioinactive hGH who demonstrate normal plasma hGH, IGF-I levels, and radioreceptor-assayable to radioimmunoassayable hGH ratio. In these patients the response to exogenous hGH is poor. In this type of disease the defect is apparently at the level of the target tissue (60,61). However, receptor assays reflect receptor binding but not subsequent cellular events leading to growth promotion. A questionable bioactivity of hGH also exists, because IGF-I is responsive to its action with normal levels.

Because neither radioreceptor assay nor bioassay of hGH is widely available and they are hampered by several difficulties, few children with this presumptive diagnosis have been reported. So far, a specific molecular defect has not been described.

VII. A POTENT CIRCULATING HUMAN GROWTH FACTOR

Geffner et al. (65) described a boy with hGH deficiency and early growth delay whose growth velocity spontaneously increased to supranormal levels despite continued absence of hGH. Both his radioimmunoassayable and radioreceptor-assayable hGH levels were low, IGF-I levels measured by radioimmunoassay (RIA) were low or low normal, and in vitro IGF-I bioactivity measured by bioassay was normal. Moreover, when the patient's serum was incubated with erythroid progenitor cells from the blood of a normal person and a Laron syndrome case, the proliferation of normal erythroid progenitors was almost double that obtained with physiologic concentrations of hGH or control sera. Laron erythroid progenitors, which were completely resistant to added hGH, also responded strongly to the patient's serum. These findings suggest that his growth is independent of hGH and other known growth factors and that there is a potent circulating human growth factor. There is no clear evidence of inheritance, however, and definitive proof of this factor is still lacking.

VIII. SHORT STATURE WITH IGF-I RESISTANCE

Heath-Monning et al. (66) reported a young girl with normal serum hGH responses to provocative stimuli and high normal to elevated IGF-I levels whose fibroblasts were insensitive to IGF-I. Other patients with possible IGF-I resistance were reported by Lanes et al. (67) and Bierich et al. (68). However, there is no clear evidence of inheritance. To substantiate a presumptive diagnosis of IGF-I resistance, biochemical studies of IGF-I action at the cellular level should be made.

IX. GROWTH WITHOUT GROWTH HORMONE: THE "INVISIBLE" hGH SYNDROME

Bistritzer et al. (69) described four nonobese boys who had normal linear growth despite apparent hGH deficiency as diagnosed by RIA measurements of hGH in provocation tests and 24 h integrated hGH concentration test. All four patients had normal hGH concentrations as measured with IM-9 cell radioreceptor assay (RRA). The RRA/RIA ratio of these four patients is significantly higher than that of the controls. These patients secrete a molecule with normal hGH receptor binding and bioactivity that is "invisible" to the standard hGH RIA. The variant hGH is possibly expressed from the hGH-2 gene or a mutant allele (69). However, definitive proof of this syndrome is still lacking.

X. FAMILIAL SHORT STATURE WITH VERY HIGH LEVELS OF GHBP

Rieu et al. (70) reported a familial syndrome of short stature associated with partial hGH resistance and very high levels of GH binding protein. In three individuals of the same family with growth failure, high circulating GH levels, both basal and stimulated, were found. Plasma IGF-1 levels were either normal or in the low normal range. GH binding activity was extremely elevated in the plasma of the three subjects, with very high maximum binding capacity (30- to 110-fold higher than that of normal adult plasma) and normal binding affinity. The cause and the exact consequences of the very high level of plasma GHBP, resulting in a low proportion of free circulating hGH, remain to be clarified. The short stature and the partial hGH resistance are probably related to high GHBP levels.

XI. EMBRYOLOGIC DEFECTS

A. Pituitary Aplasia, Congenital Absence of the Pituitary Gland, and Congenital Hypopituitarism

Complete absence of the anterior pituitary gland results in severe neonatal hGH deficiency, adrenal insufficiency, and hypothyroidism. Posterior pituitary tissue may be present or absent. Clinical features are early lethargy, hypoglycemia, seizure, cyanosis, jaundice, circulatory collapse, and small phallus (25,71). Several sibling pairs and an increased frequency of consanguinity suggest autosomal recessive inheritance (71). If untreated, patients usually die during the neonatal period. Therefore, it is important to make a diagnosis of adrenal insufficiency and to evaluate pituitary function at that time. Some cases may have gone unrecognized.

Brown et al. (72) evaluated five patients with congenital hypopituitarism by magnetic resonance imaging. All patients lacked a demonstrable pituitary stalk, and an ectopic bright spot, probably representing posterior tissue, was found. The height of the anterior pituitary remnant on MRI varied from undetectable to 4 mm. The significant correlation between the size and function of the anterior pituitary gland and the size of the ectopic posterior pituitary remnant suggests that the fetal pituitary gland secretes a factor necessary for the growth and descent of the neuroepithelium to form the infundibulum and posterior pituitary gland. Some cases of idiopathic hypopituitarism have a similar prenatal onset.

B. Holoprosencephaly

Holoprosencephaly is an embryologic anomaly of the brain in which there is interference with the midline cleavage of the forebrain. It is characterized by absence of olfactory bulbs and tracts, cleft lip, microophthalmia, and cyclopia. Severe mental and motor defects are usually present. Anomalies of the pituitary gland, ranging from malformation of the gland to its complete absence, result in IGHD or panhypopituitary short stature (25,71,73). Occasionally, this disorder occurs with trisomy 13, 13q, 18p, and triploidy (73). Cases are usually sporadic, but families with either autosomal dominant or autosomal recessive modes of inheritance have been reported (73).

C. Septooptic Dysplasia (De Morsier Syndrome) and Midline Craniocerebral and Midfacial Anomalies

This disorder is characterized by optic nerve hypoplasia with or without abnormalities of the septum pellucidum and corpus callosum. Pituitary insufficiency, varying from IGHD to panhypopituitarism, including diabetes insipidus, occurs in 60% of the cases. The defect is considered to reside in the hypothalamus (73). This disorder should be considered in any child with hGH deficiency who has nystagmus or abnormalities of the optic disc. There is no evidence for a mendelian basis for this disorder.

Other midline craniocerebral and midfacial anomalies associated with occasional hypothalamic-pituitary dysfunc-

tion are cleft lip or palate, or a combination (74), solitary central maxillary incisor (75), and transsphenoidal meningoencephalocele (76). Therefore, hypothalamic-pituitary function should be carefully evaluated in all patients with these conditions.

D. Rieger Syndrome: Iridogoniodysgenesis with Somatic Anomalies

Rieger syndrome is an autosomal dominant disorder associated with iris dysplasia, hypoplasia of the teeth, occasional optic atrophy, and hGH deficiency (71,73). Other ocular features are microcornea with opacity and glaucoma. Dysgenesis of the neural crest may result in ocular, dental, and hypothalamic abnormalities (71,73).

E. Empty Sella Syndrome

Empty sella syndrome is characterized by the radiologic appearance of a sella turcica that is partially or completely filled with cerebrospinal fluid (CSF). Primary empty sella syndrome results from an incompetent or incomplete sella diaphragma and increased cerebrospinal fluid pressure, which allows herniation of the subarachnoid space into the sella from above (77). Secondary empty sella results from pituitary surgery, radiation, or infarction, which allows herniation of the subarachnoid space to fill the empty sella (77). Primary empty sella in children in whom the sella is of normal size may be associated with (1) intrinsic pituitary hypoplasia, (2) unrecognized pituitary insult, (3) dysfunction of the hypothalamus or higher centers, resulting in decreased pituitary growth, or (4) herniation of CSF through an incompetent sella diaphragma, which occurs rapidly before sellar remodeling can occur.

The frequency of primary empty sella in children with hypothalamic-pituitary dysfunction, short stature, delayed puberty, and/or precocious puberty has been reported as 1–58% (78). Endocrine abnormalities were described in nearly all children; visual abnormalities were noted in only 6%. The most common endocrine abnormality in association with primary empty sella syndrome in childhood is hGH deficiency, isolated or associated with other pituitary hormone deficiencies (78). It is possible that many cases have gone unrecognized. One family has been reported in which empty sella syndrome was transmitted as an autosomal dominant trait in association with Rieger syndrome.

F. Ectrodactyly-Ectodermal Dysplasia-Clefting Syndrome

This syndrome is characterized by ectrodactyly of the hands and feet (from syndactyly to cleft hands and cleft feet), ectodermal dysplasia (thin, blond, and dry hair) and hypoplasia of the dental enamel, and cleft lip and/or palate (73,79). Urinary tract anomalies or absence of the septum pellucidum has been reported (73,79). The IGHD is probably secondary to developmental hypothalamic defects. Cases are frequently sporadic (probably new mutation), but families with an autosomal dominant mode of inheritance have been reported (73).

G. Fanconi Anemia

Fanconi anemia is characterized by anemia, leukopenia, thrombocytopenia, upper limb malformations, skin hyperpigmentation, malformations of the heart and kidney, and occasional hGH deficiency. This syndrome has an autosomal recessive mode of inheritance (73). The existence of at least two separate loci, homozygosity at either of which can result in Fanconi syndrome, was indicated by the complementation in cell hybrid studies by Zakrzewski and Sperling (80).

XII. SUMMARY

There are six single-gene disorders associated with hGH deficiency. These disorders are divided into six distinct groups based on mode of inheritance and associated with hormone deficiencies. Recently, a variety of molecular defects have been detected that causes these disorders. The classification is summarized as follows by type and mode of inheritance:

Isolated growth hormone deficiency: type 1A, autosomal recessive with absent hGH; type 1B, autosomal recessive with diminished hGH; type 2, autosomal dominant with diminished hGH; type 3, X-linked recessive with diminished hGH.
Panhypopituitary short stature: type 1, autosomal recessive with diminished hGH and other pituitary hormones; type 2, X-linked recessive with diminished hGH and other pituitary hormones.

Isolated hGH deficiency type 1A is caused by deletion of the hGH structural (hGH-1) gene. Some patients with IGHD caused by point mutations in the hGH-1 genes have been described, and compound heterozygotes have been reported. Several types of hGH receptor gene defects have also been found in Laron syndrome. Pit-1 gene abnormalities have also been reported. Further studies are needed to clarify the role of the hGH gene, hGH receptor gene, or pit-1 gene in genetic disorders with hGH deficiency or hGH insensitivity syndrome.

REFERENCES

1. Chen EY, Liao YC, Smith DH, Barrera-Saldana HA, Gelinas RE, Seeburg PH. The human growth hormone locus: nucleotide sequence, biology, and evolution. Genomics 1989; 4:479–497.
2. Phillips JA III. Inherited defects in growth hormone synthesis and action. In: Scriber CR, Beaudet AL, Sly WS, Valle D, eds. The Metabolic Basis of Inherited Disease, 6th ed. New York: McGraw-Hill Information Services, 1989:1965–1983.
3. Phillips JA III, Hjelle BL, Seeburg PU, Zackmann M. Molecular basis for familial isolated growth hormone deficiency. Proc Natl Acad Sci USA 1981; 78:6372–6375.
4. Illig R, Prader A, Ferrandez M, Zachman M. Hereditary prenatal growth hormone deficiency with increased tendency to growth hormone antibody formation. A type of isolated growth hormone deficiency. Acta Paediatr Scand (Suppl) 1971; 60:607.
5. Nishi Y, Masuda H, Nishimura S, et al. Isolated human growth hormone deficiency due to the hGH-I gene deletion with (type 1A) and without (the Israeli-type) hGH antibody formation during hGH therapy. Acta Endocrinol (Copenh) 1990; 122:267–271.
6. Laron Z, Kelijman M, Pertzelan A, Keret R, Shoffner JM, Parks JS. Human growth hormone gene deletion without antibody formation or growth arrest during treatment—a new disease entity? Isr J Med Sci 1985; 21:999–1006.
7. Nishi Y, Aihara K, Usui T, Phillips JA III, Mallonee RL, Migeon CJ. Isolated growth hormone deficiency type 1A in a Japanese family. J Pediatr 1984; 104:885–889.
8. Vnencak-Jones CL, Phillips JA III, Chen EY, Seeburg PH. Molecular basis of human growth hormone gene deletions. Proc Natl Acad Sci USA 1988; 85:5615–5619.
9. Braga S, Phillips JA III, Joss E, Schwarz H, Zuppinger K. Familial growth hormone deficiency resulting from a 7.6 kb deletion within the growth hormone gene cluster. Am J Med Genet 1986; 25:443–452.
10. Goossens M, Brauner R, Czernichow P, Duquesnog P, Rappaport R. Isolated growth hormone (GH) deficiency type 1A associated with a double deletion in the human GH gene cluster. J Clin Endocrinol Metab 1986; 62:712–716.
11. Akinci A, Kanaka C, Eblé A, Akar N, Vidinlisan S, Mullis PE. Isolated growth hormone (GH) deficiency type IA associated with a 45-kilobase gene deletion within the human GH gene cluster. J Clin Endocrinol Metab 1992; 75:437–441.
12. Kamijo T, Phillips JA III. Detection of molecular heterogeneity in GH-1 gene deletions by analysis of polymerase chain reaction amplification products. J Clin Endocrinol Metab 1992; 75:786–789.
13. Rivarola MA, Phillips JA III, Migeon CJ, Heinrich JJ, Hjelle BL. Phenotypic heterogeneity in familial isolated growth hormone deficiency type 1-A. J Clin Endocrinol Metab 1984; 59:34–40.
14. Frisch H, Phillips JA III. Growth hormone deficiency due to GH-N gene deletion in an Austrian family. Acta Endocrinol (Copenh) (Suppl) 1986; 27:107–112.
15. Cogan JD, Phillips JA III, Sakati N, Frisch H, Schober E, Milner RDG. Heterogenous growth hormone (GH) gene mutations in familial GH deficiency. J Clin Endocrinol Metab 1993; 76:1124–1128.
16. Duquesnoy P, Amselem S, Gourmelen M, Le Bouc Y, Goossens M. A frame shift mutation causing isolated growth hormone deficiency type 1A. Am J Hum Genet 1990; 47: A110.
17. Igarashi Y, Ogawa M, Kamijo T, et al. A new mutation causing inherited growth hormone deficiency: a compound heterozygote of a 6.7 kb deletion and a two base deletion in the third exon of the GH-1 gene. Hum Mol Genet 1993; 2:1073–1074.
18. Parks JS, Meacham LR, McKean MC, Keret R, Josefsberg Z, Laron Z. Growth hormone (GH) gene deletion is the most common cause of severe GH deficiency among oriental Jewish children. Pediatr Res 1989; 25:90A.
19. Vnencak-Jones CL, Phillips JA III, De-Fen W. Use of polymerase chain reaction in detection of growth hormone gene deletions. J Clin Endocrinol Metab 1990; 70:1550–1553.
20. Mullis PE, Akinci A, Kanaka CH, Eblé A, Brook CGD. Prevalence of human growth hormone-1 gene deletions among patients with isolated growth hormone deficiency from different populations. Pediatr Res 1992; 31:532–534.
21. Mullis P, Patel M, Brickell PM, Brook CGD. Isolated growth

hormone deficiency: analysis of the growth hormone (GH)-releasing hormone gene and the GH gene cluster. J Clin Endocrinol Metab 1990; 70:187–191.

22. Mullis PE, Brickell PM. The use of the polymerase chain reaction in prenatal diagnosis of growth hormone gene deletions. Clin Endocrinol (Oxf) 1992; 37:89–95.

23. Hauffa BP, Illig R, Torresani T, Stolecke H, Phillips JA III. Discordant immune and growth response in pituitary and biosynthetic growth hormone in siblings with isolated growth hormone deficiency type IA. Acta Endocrinol (Copenh) 1989; 121:609–614.

24. Nishi Y, Hamamoto K, Kajiyama M, et al. Treatment of isolated growth hormone deficiency type IA due to GH-I gene deletion with recombinant human insulin-like growth factor I. Acta Paediatr 1993; 82:983–986.

25. Phillips JA III. Regulation and defects in expression of growth hormone genes. In: Isaksson O, Binder C, Hall K, Hökfelt B, eds. Growth Hormone. Basic and Clinical Aspects. International Congress Series. Amsterdam: Excerpta Medica, 1987: 11–27.

26. Phillips JA III, Parks JS, Hjelle BL, et al. Genetic analysis of familial isolated growth hormone deficiency type I. J Clin Invest 1982; 70:489–495.

27. Rogol AD, Blizzard RM, Foley TP Jr, et al. Growth hormone releasing hormone and growth hormone: genetic studies in familial growth hormone deficiency. Pediatr Res 1985; 19: 489–492.

28. Cogan JD, Phillips JA III, Sakati NA, Schenkman SS, Milner D. Molecular basis of autosomal recessive and autosomal dominant inheritance in familial GH deficiency. Program and Abstract, Endocrine Society, 1993:376.

29. Ohzeki T, Hanaki K, Motozumi H, et al. Immunodeficiency with increased immunoglobulin M associated with growth hormone insufficiency. Acta Paediatr 1993; 82:620–623.

30. Fleisher TA, White RM, Broder S. X-linked hypogammaglobulinemia and isolated growth hormone deficiency. N Engl J Med 1980; 302:1429–1434.

31. Conley ME, Burks AW, Herrod HG, Puck JM. Molecular analysis of X-linked aggammaglobulinemia with growth hormone deficiency. J Pediatr 1991; 119:392–397.

32. Ogata T, Petit C, Rappold G, Matsuo N, Matsumoto T, Goodfellow P. Chromosomal localization of a pseudoautosomal growth gene(s). J Med Genet 1992; 29:624–628.

33. Yokoyama Y, Narahara K, Tsuji K, et al. Growth hormone deficiency and empty sella syndrome in a boy with dup(X)-(q13.3 → q21.2). Am J Med Genet 1992; 42:660–664.

34. Tang MLK, Kemp AS. Growth hormone deficiency and combined immunodeficiency. Arch Dis Child 1993; 68:231–232.

35. Laron Z, Blum W, Chatelain P, et al. Classification of growth hormone insensitivity syndrome. J Pediatr 1993; 122:241.

36. Laron Z. Laron-type dwarfism (hereditary somatomedin deficiency), A review. Ergeb Inn Med Kinderheilkd 1984; 51:117–150.

37. Guevara-Aguirre J, Rosenbloom AL, Vaccarello MA, et al. Growth hormone receptor deficiency (Laron syndrome): clinical and genetic characteristics. Acta Paediatr 1991; 377:96–103.

38. Phillips JA III. Molecular biology of growth hormone receptor dysfunction. Acta Paediatr (Suppl) 1992; 383:127–131.

39. Buchanan CR, Maheshwari HG, Norman MR, Morrell DJ, Preece MA. Laron-type dwarfism with apparent- ly normal high affinity serum growth hormone-binding protein. Clin Endocrinol (Oxf) 1991; 35:179–185.

40. Godowski PJ, Leung DW, Meacham LR, et al. Characterization of the human·growth hormone receptor gene and demonstration of a partial gene deletion in two patients with

Laron-type dwarfism. Proc Natl Acad Sci USA 1989; 86: 8083–8087.

41. Amselem S, Duquesnoy P, Attree O, et al. Laron dwarfism and mutations of the growth hormone-receptor gene. N Engl J Med 1989; 321:989–995.

42. Amselem S, Sobrier ML, Duquesnoy P, et al. Recurrent nonsense mutation in the growth hormone receptor from patients with Laron dwarfism. J Clin Invest 1991; 87:1098–1102.

43. Kou K, Lajara R, Rotwein P. Amino acid substitutions in the intracellular part of the growth hormone receptor in a patient with the Laron syndrome. J Clin Endocrinol Metab 1993; 76:54–59.

44. Berg MA, Guevara-Aguirre J, Rosenbloom AL, Rosenfeld RG, Francke U. Mutation creating a new splice site in the growth hormone receptor genes of 37 Ecuadorean patients with Laron syndrome. Hum Mutat 1992; 1:24–34.

45. Laron A, Anin S, Klinger B. Long-term IGF-I treatment of children with Laron syndrome. In: Laron Z, Parks JS, eds. Lessons from Laron syndrome (LS) 1966–1992. Pediatr Adol Endocrinol 1993; 24:226–236.

46. Heinrichs C, Vis HL, Bergmann P, Wilton P, Bourguignon JP. Effects of 17 months treatment using recombinant insulin-like growth factor-I in two children with growth hormone insensitivity (Laron) syndrome. Clin Endocrinol (Oxf) 1993; 38:647–651.

47. Merimee TJ. Similarities and dissimilarities between Pygmies and Laron-type dwarfs. In: Laron Z, Parks JS, eds. Lessons from Laron syndrome (LS) 1966–1992. Pediatr Adol Endocrinol 1993; 24:266–281.

48. Merimee TJ, Baumann G, Daughaday W. Growth hormone-binding protein. II. Studies in Pygmies and normal statured subjects. J Clin Endocrinol Metab 1990; 71:1183–1188.

49. Baumann G, Shaw MA, Merimee TJ. Low levels of high-affinity growth hormone-binding protein in African Pygmies. N Engl J Med 1989; 320:1705–1709.

50. Bowcock A, Sartorelli V. Polymorphism and mapping of the IGF1 gene, and absence of association with stature among African Pygmies. Huma Genet 1990; 85:349–354.

51. Geffner ME, Bailey RC, Bersch N, Vera JC, Golde DW. Insulin-like growth factor-I unresponsiveness in an efe Pygmy. Biochem Biophys Res Commun 1993; 193:1216–1223.

52. Schwarz J, Brumbach RC, Chiu M. Short stature, growth hormone, insulin-like growth factors, and serum proteins in the Mountain Ok people of Papua New Guinea. J Clin Endocrinol Metab 1987; 65:901–905.

53. Baumann G, Shaw MA, Brumbaugh RC, Schwartz J. Short stature and decreased serum growth hormone-binding protein in the Mountain Ok people of Papua New Guinea. J Clin Endocrinol Metab 1991; 72:1346–1349.

54. Bucuvalas JC, Horn JA, Carlsson L, Balistreri WF, Chernausek SD. Growth hormone insensitivity associated with elevated circulating growth hormone-binding protein in children with Alagille syndrome and short stature. J Clin Endocrinol Metab 1993; 76:1477–1482.

55. Parks JS, Kinoshita E, Pfäffle RW. Pit-1 and hypopituitarism. Trends Endocrinol Metab 1993; 4:81–85.

56. Tatsumi K, Miyai K, Notomi T, et al. Cretinism with combined hormone deficiency caused by a mutation in the pit1 gene. Nature Genet 1992; 1:56–58.

57. Radovick S, Nations M, Du Y, Berg LA, Weintraub BD, Wondisford FE. A mutation in the POU-homeodomain of pit-1 responsible for combined pituitary hormone deficiency. Science 1992; 257:1115–1158.

58. Pfäffle RW, DiMattia GE, Parks JS, et al. Mutation of the POU-specific domain of Pit-1 and hypopituitarism without pituitary hypoplasia. Science 1992; 257:1118–1121.

59. Ohta K, Nobukuni Y, Mitsubuchi H, et al. Mutations in the pit-1 gene in children with combined pituitary hormone deficiency. Biochem Biophys Res Commun 1992; 189:851–855.

60. Rudman D, Kunter MH, Blackston RD, Jansen RD, Patterson JH. Normal variant short stature: subclassification based on responses to exogenous growth hormone. J Clin Endocrinol Metab 1979; 49:92–99.

61. Rudman D, Kunter MH, Blackston RD, Cushman RA, Bain RP, Patterson JH. Children with normal-variant short stature: treatment with human growth hormone for six months. N Engl J Med 1981; 305:123–131.

62. Frazer T, Gavin JR, Daughaday WH, Hillman RE, Weldon VV. Growth hormone-dependent growth failure. J Pediatr 1982; 191:12–15.

63. Bright GM, Rogol AD, Johanson AJ, Blizzard RM. Short stature associated with normal growth hormone and decreased somatomedin C concentrations: response to exogenous growth hormone. Pediatrics 1983; 71:576–580.

64. Valenta LJ, Sigel MB, Lesniak MA, et al. Pituitary dwarfism in a patient with circulating abnormal growth hormone polymers. N Engl J Med 1985; 312:214–217.

65. Geffner ME, Lippe BM, Bersch N, et al. Growth without growth hormone: evidence for a potent circulating human growth factor. Lancet 1986; 1:343–346.

66. Heath-Moning E, Wohltmann HJ, Mills-Dunlap B, Daughaday WH. Measurement of insulin-like growth factor I (IGF-I) responsiveness of fibroblasts of children with short stature: identification of a patient with IGF-I resistance. J Clin Endocrinol Metab 1987; 64:501–507.

67. Lanes R, Plotnick LP, Spencer EM, Daughaday WH, Kowarski AA. Dwarfism associated with normal serum growth hormone and increased bioassayable, receptorassayable, and immunoassayable somatomedin. J. Clin Endocrinol Metab 1980; 50:485–488.

68. Bierich JR, Moeller H, Ranke MB, Rosenfeld RG. Pseudopituitary dwarfism due to resistance to somatomedin: a new syndrome. Eur J Pediatr 1984; 142:186–188.

69. Bistritzer T, Chalew SA, Lovchik JC, Kowarski AA. Growth without growth hormone: the "invisible" GH syndrome. Lancet 1988; 8581:321–323.

70. Rieu M, Bouc YL, Villares SM, Postel-Vinay MC. Familial short stature with very high levels of growth hormone binding protein. J Clin Endocrinol Metabl 1993; 76:857–860.

71. Rimon DL. Hereditary forms of growth hormone deficiency and resistance. Birth Defects 1976; 12:15–29.

72. Brown RS, Bhatia V, Hayes E. An apparent cluster of congenital hypopituitarism in central Massachusetts: magnetic resonance imaging and hormonal studies. J Clin Endocrinol Metab 1991; 72:12–18.

73. McKusick VA. Mendelian Inheritance in Man, 7th ed. Baltimore: Johns Hopkins University Press, 1986.

74. Rudman D, Davis T, Priest JH, et al. Prevalence of growth hormone deficiency in children with cleft lip or palate. J Pediatr 1978; 93:378–382.

75. Rappaport EB, Ulstrom RA, Gorlin RJ, Lucky AW, Colle E, Miser J. Solitary maxillary central incisor and short stature. J Pediatr 1977; 91:924–928.

76. Nishi Y, Muraki K, Sakoda K, Gen M, Uozumi T, Usui T. Hypopituitarism associated with transsphenoidal meningoencephalocele. Eur J Pediatr 1982; 139:81–84.

77. Shulman DI, Martinez CR, Bercu BB, Root AW. Hypothalamic-pituitary dysfunction in primary empty sella syndrome in childhood. J Pediatr 1986; 108:540–544.

78. Rapaport R, Logrono R. Primary empty sella syndrome in childhood: association with precocious puberty. Clin Pediatr (Phila) 1991; 30:466–471.

79. Knudtson J, Aarskog D. Growth hormone deficiency associated with ectrodactyly-ectodermal dysplasia-clefting syndrome and isolated absent septum pellucidum. Pediatrics 1987; 79:410–412.

80. Zakrzewski S, Sperling K. Analysis of heterogeneity in Fanconi's anemia patients of different ethnic origin. Hum Genet 1982; 56:321–323.

81. Phillips JA III, Ferrandez A, Frisch H, Illig R, Zuppinger K. Defects of growth hormone genes. Clinical syndromes. In: Raiti S, Tolman RA, eds. Growth Hormone. Basic and Clinical Aspects. New York: Plenum Press, 1986:211–226.

82. Phillips JA III, Cogan JD. Genetic basis of endocrine desease 6. Molecular basis of familial human growth hormone deficiency. J Clin Endocrinol Metab 1994; 78:11–16.

4

Disorders of Growth Hormone Neurosecretion

Barry B. Bercu
University of South Florida College of Medicine,
Tampa, Florida

I. INTRODUCTION

Over 35 years ago purified crude extracts of human growth hormone (hGH) from human cadavers were first used to stimulate growth in children with GH deficiency (1). As a result of the commercial production of hGH using recombinant DNA technology, pediatrics has entered a new era when hGH is no longer in limited supply. The timing of this major biotechnological advancement corresponds to the explosion of scientific information in the area of the neuroendocrine regulation of GH secretion. In this chapter, we review for the clinical practitioner the GH secretory dynamics in health and disease.

II. HUMAN GROWTH HORMONE: BIOCHEMISTRY AND PHYSIOLOGY

The pituitary somatotroph secretes a family of monomers and oligomers of hGH, 75% as a single-chain polypeptide (191 amino acids with two intrachain disulfide bridges, molecular weight 22,000). Of the net pituitary gland weight, 4–10% is hGH, that is, 5–11 mg/gland (Chap. 5). Another molecular form of hGH has a molecular weight of 20,000. This molecule retains the growth-promoting activity but not the diabetogenic action of the native GH molecule (2–6). Recent studies have demonstrated the specific diabetogenic fragment to be hGH (44–191) (7). High circulating levels of this fragment have caused diabetes mellitus in patients with gigantism or acromegaly (Bercu and Sinha, unpublished observations).

GH synthesis by the somatotroph is genetically controlled by the GH-N gene, one of a five-gene GH complex located on the long arm of chromosome 17. The GH-V gene is also present in the pituitary but is incapable of directing the somatotroph to synthesize GH. On the other hand, the GH-V gene is also located in the placenta, where it may play an important role in the growth of this organ (8–10). GH release by the somatotroph occurs by exocytosis. In adults, approximately 500 μg GH is secreted daily. Although GH circulates mainly in an unbound form in plasma, approximately 25% is complexed with a specific high-affinity, low-capacity GH binding protein. This GH binding protein is a fragment of the GH receptor (11,12). Approximately 20–25 minutes is the disappearance half-life of GH from the circulation. Recent studies have shown that the GH binding protein has three domains: intracellular, transmembrane, and extracellular (13). Each GH molecule dimerizes with two GH binding proteins for its cellular function. Extracellular binding protein acts as a reservoir in regulating GH secretory dynamics (14).

Under physiologic conditions, the anterior pituitary gland secretes approximately eight discrete peaks of GH each day, with very low basal levels between episodic pulses (15). Approximately 50% or more of the daily production of GH in children and young adults occurs during the early nighttime hours that follow the onset of deep sleep. Shifts in sleep-onset GH pulses occur with sleep advancement, sleep delay, or reversal. Daytime naps, interruptions in sleep, or forced fragmentation of sleep produces increases in GH secretion after sleep onset. "Jet lag" also causes disruptions in pulsatile GH secretion (16). In addition, GH secretion is stimulated by exercise, emotional stress, high-protein meals, rapid onset of hypoglycemia, and prolonged fasting. On the other hand, it is suppressed by elevated glucose levels in healthy nondiabetic subjects, hypothyroidism, obesity, and excess glucocorticoids. GH levels have also been found to change during periprandial periods (17).

Not yet elucidated is the exact mechanism of GH action. The extracellular domain of the GH receptor dimerizes with a single GH molecule (13). This then triggers the cAMP response typical of polypeptide hormones. In general terms, GH has anabolic effects, antagonizes the action of insulin, and possesses lipolytic activity. There are direct influences of GH on isolated extraskeletal tissues (e.g., hepatocytes, adipocytes, heart muscle, diaphragm, and hematopoietic cells) and on perfused organs (liver). In addition, GH plays an important role in the physiologic regulation of carbohydrate, fat, protein, and mineral metabolism.

The most widely accepted hypothesis (somatomedin hypothesis) (18–20) of GH action states that GH indirectly regulates linear growth via its ability to stimulate the production of growth factors (somatomedins), which in turn cause bone growth. There is also evidence of a direct GH effect on the growth plate (21). Somatomedin C (SmC) or insulin-like growth factor I (IGF-I) is the main GH-dependent growth factor that stimulates linear growth in children. GH also regulates IGF binding protein 3 (IGF BP-3). IGF BP-3, a glycoprotein, is one of six binding proteins and is the major high-affinity circulating and extracellular carrier or resevior for IGF-I and thus influences the amount of free IGF-1 available for cellular action (22,23). SmC/IGF-I is also involved in negative feedback of GH secretion. IFG-II, which may be important in fetal growth, is another somatomedin molecule in circulation but is not regulated by GH secretion (24,25).

A. Regulation of GH Secretion

Pituitary GH secretion is complex and under the dual regulatory control of two hypothalamic neurohormones, GH releasing hormone (GHRH, 44 amino acids) and GH inhibiting hormone (somatostatin or SRIH, 14 amino acids). Figure 1 illustrates the central and peripheral factors that influence GH secretion. GH secretion is inhibited by SmC/IGF-I and by GH itself; both work directly at the pituitary level and indirectly at hypothalamic regulatory centers by suppressing GHRH release and stimulating SRIH production.

GHRH and somatostatin are further regulated by neuro-

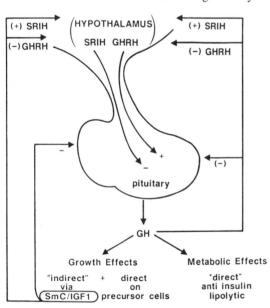

Figure 1 Hypothalamic-pituitary-peripheral interaction. SRIH, somatostatin; GHRH, growth hormone releasing hormone; SmC/IGF-I, somatomedin C/insulin-like growth factor I. (From Ref. 26.)

transmitters and possibly other neuropeptides (Fig. 2). The pharmacologic evidence for neurotransmitter secretory influences of GH secretion is summarized in part in Table 1 and reviewed elsewhere (27,28). In addition, corticotropin releasing hormone and thyrotropin releasing hormone also have effects in pharmacologic doses. Thyroid hormones, corticosteroids, calcitonin, and prostaglandins represent other circulating substances that influence GH secretion in pharmacologic studies.

Sex steroids also play a role in influencing growth rate, as exemplified by the adolescent growth spurt. Testosterone-deficient males grow normally until adolescence. Two-thirds of pubertal growth is independent of GH secretion (29). GH secretion is responsible for growth of the vertebral bodies and androgen mostly for leg length. Estrogens are stimulatory to GH secretion and inhibitory to skeletal growth. Estrogen and androgen receptors are present in the amygdala and hypothalamic areas involved in neuroregulation of GH secretion (30). Endogenous sex steroids influence GH secretion, also suggested by the increase in spontaneous GH secretion during normal (31,32) and precocious puberty (33). For a recent comprehensive review, the reader is referred to Reference 34.

B. Etiology of GH Deficiency

Growth hormone deficiency may result from dysfunction at the following sites: (1) higher brain centers (neurotransmitter defects)—lack of stimulators or excess of inhibitors; (2) neuropeptide defects in the hypothalamus—lack of GHRH or excess of somatostatin; (3) somatotroph in pituitary—lack of synthesis or secretion of GH or secretion of biologically inactive abnormal GH molecule; (4) receptor defects at various levels, including receptors of neurotransmitters, GHRH, and GH. Table 2 summarizes some causes of GH deficiency and GH resistance (site of defect is not specified).

1. Classic GH Deficiency

Patients with GH deficiency have a variety of presentations dependent on etiology, age at onset, and severity of the disorder. Idiopathic GH deficiency is more common than organic GH deficiency (disease as a result of tumor, trauma, embryologic defect, radiation therapy, and other causes; Chap. 2). Hereditary or congenital GH deficiency should be considered in infants in the following clinical settings: hypoglycemia, males with micropenis, and infants with midline facial defects (Chaps. 2 and 3). Characteristically, infants with congenital GH deficiency have normal birth length and weight and grow normally for 3–6 months, but linear growth rates decelerate thereafter. Growth rates in affected children after 3 years of age are almost always less than 4 or 5 cm/year. These patients have normal body proportions for chronologic age. As a general rule, children with GH deficiency are overweight for height. Skeletal age in the prepubertal hypopituitary patient is always delayed. The degree of bone age delay is usually proportional to that of height age. In addition, closure of the anterior fontanelle is usually very delayed.

During early infancy and childhood, children with congenital GH deficiency may have episodes of fasting hypoglycemia and convulsions. By 5 years of age, the tendency to fast-

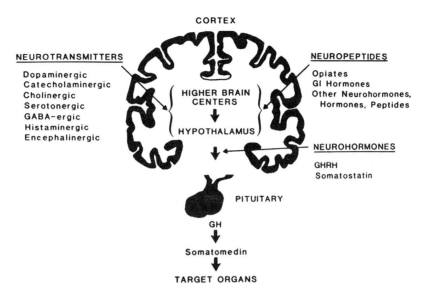

Figure 2 Neurotransmitters, neuropeptides, and neurohormones that regulate GH secretion. GH stimulates somatomedin C/insulin-like growth factor I from the liver. GABA, γ-aminobutyric acid. (From Ref. 27.)

ing hypoglycemia usually disappears; however, it may reappear if severe illnesses prevent oral intake for prolonged periods. Aside from the problems of hypoglycemia and seizures during the early childhood years, children with idiopathic GH deficiency are generally healthy and have normal intelligence. Their problems are more frequently emotional because these children often perceived to be much younger than their chronological age and are treated accordingly.

GH-deficient boys who have microphallus and hypoplastic testes are likely also to have partial or complete gonadotropin deficiency. The gonadotropin status usually cannot be accurately assessed until the adolescent years. Androgen treatment in small doses should be prescribed during infancy and early childhood to bring penis size into the normal range for age (Chap. 20). Testicular growth and enhanced virilization occur with appropriate medical therapy during the adolescent years. Puberty is often delayed in children with isolated idiopathic GH deficiency who begin hGH treatment late in childhood. This is in contrast to those children in whom treatment is initiated early. Hypopituitarism of organic origin (e.g., birth trauma and embryologic brain defects) carries a high risk of multiple hypothalamic-pituitary hormone deficiencies. The specific hereditary growth hormone syndromes are reviewed elsewhere, in Chapter 3.

Children with acquired GH deficiency have growth curves different from those of subjects with congenital GH deficiency. During childhood, children with acquired GH deficiency grow normally for a variable number of years and then cease to grow after GH deficiency develops or is severe enough to influence growth.

2. GH Neurosecretory Dysfunction: Experimental and Clinical Evidence

As noted earlier, GHRH and SRIH are regulated by neurotransmitters to varying degrees. Defects in the neuroregula-

tory control of GH secretion can result in decreased or disordered GH secretion. Ultimately, these abnormalities can be expressed as poor growth velocity and short stature.

For many years, the definition of GH deficiency was based on blunted provocative GH testing in the appropriate clinical setting (poor growth velocity and delayed skeletal age). It was suspected that some children may have abnormalities in GH secretion that were missed by standard provocative testing. Such a subgroup of children with a treatable cause of short stature are those with GH neurosecretory dysfunction (GHND), significantly short children with one or more normal GH provocative tests, poor growth velocity, and delayed skeletal age; Table 3). This observation results from a series of studies summarized briefly here.

Growth velocity is frequently diminished as a consequence of cranial radiation (Chap. 57). Classic GH deficiency results from high-dose cranial radiation therapy involving the hypothalamic-pituitary area (35,36). Smaller doses of cranial radiation cause variable results in conventional provocative GH tests (36–47). Clinical (41,42) and animal (47) studies were done in parallel by our group. A defect in endogenous neurosecretion of GH occurs in leukemic children who received prophylactic cranial radiation (41,42), whereas these children frequently have normal GH secretion after conventional GH testing. These studies can be summarized as follows: (1) a correlation of anatomic (leukoencephalopathy demonstrated with computed axial tomography of brain) abnormalities to endogenous GH secretion, and (2) a lack of correlation of endogenous GH secretion with provocative GH testing.

Using the monkey model, the question of cranial radiation damage without confounding chemotherapy was addressed (47). Arginine and levodopa readily stimulated GH secretion in central nervous system (CNS)-irradiated monkeys, whereas insulin did not unless the dose was doubled.

Table 1 Factors Regulating Growth Hormone Secretion

Stimulatory	Inhibitory
Physiologic	
Sleep	Psychologic stress
Exercise	↑ Fatty acids
Physical stress	↑ Glucose
↑ Amino acids	
↓ Glucose	
Pharmacologic	
Insulin-induced hypoglycemia	Glucocorticoids
Adrenocorticotropic hormone	Progesterone?
MSH	Melatonin?
Estradiol	
Vasopressin	
Galanin	
Gastrointestinal and hypothalamic hormones (motilin, vasoactive intestinal peptide, peptide histidine, isoleucine amino, glucagon, gastrin releasing peptide, secretin, gastrin inhibiting peptide, bombesin, cholecystokinin)	
Serotonin precursors (5-hydroxytryptamine)	Serotonin antagonists (methysergide)
Dopamine agonists (levodopa)	Dopamine antagonists (phenothiazines)
β-Adrenergic antagonists (propranolol)	β-Adrenergic agonists (isoproterenol)
α-Adrenergic agonists (clonidine)	α-Adrenergic antagonists (phentolamine)
Cholinergic agonists (methylcholine)	Cholinergic antagonists (imipramine)
γ-Aminobutyric acid (GABA) agonists	
Pathologic	
Starvation	Hypothyroidism
Protein deprivation	Obesity

The 24 h spontaneous endogenous GH secretion was dramatically reduced (Fig. 3). These studies were later confirmed in CNS-irradiated human leukemic patients (Fig. 4). We speculate that this reduced spontaneous GH secretion may cause the lack of catch-up growth frequently seen in leukemic children after cessation of all chemotherapy and while in remission. Destructive lesions in the arcuate and ventromedial nuclei of monkey (site of GHRH release in the monkey hypothalamus) abolish pulsatile GH secretion (Spiliotis, Mishkin, and Bercu, unpublished data).

We have extended our neurosecretory studies in CNS-radiated children (48). As previously described, spontaneous 24 h GH secretory pulsatile secretion is significantly reduced in a group of children who received CNS radiation for various reasons (1.8 ± 0.2 versus 3.9 μg/L, irradiated versus control, mean ± standard error of the mean, SEM) (48). Following GHRH stimulation in both normal and GH-deficient children, GH secretory response is variable; this is also the case for irradiated children. Because growing evidence suggests that somatostatin plays a greater role in the regulation of GH secretion than previously thought (49), one can speculate that damage to somatostatinergic neuronal fibers was greater in the two children with greater than normal GH secretory responses; this is demonstrated best in the patient shown in Figure 5 (50). Both standard provocative stimuli, which are, in fact, regulated by neurotransmitters and other neurotransmitter stimuli, were overall blunted in their GH secretory responses (Table 4).

The dramatic decrease in spontaneous but not provocative GH secretion in CNS-irradiated monkeys and children led us to consider that disorders of GH neurosecretion, other than classic GH deficiency, may be an etiology of pathologic short stature in nonirradiated children. We have termed the disorder in this subgroup of short stature children, growth hormone neurosecretory dysfunction (Fig. 6).

The hypothesis for different defects in the regulation of GH secretion as the basis for GHND is supported by the complexity of the CNS-hypothalamic-pituitary system. Dis-

Table 2 Causes of Growth Hormone Deficiency or Defective Growth Hormone Action

Congenital GH deficiency	Inflammatory diseases
Decreased GH secretion	Viral encephalitis
Idiopathic	Bacteria, group B streptococcal meningitis,
Hereditary—autosomal recessive or dominant	others
Embryologic defects—aplasia, hypoplasia,	Fungal
ectopia, anencephaly, arrhinencephaly, sep-	Granulomatous (tuberculosis, syphilis,
tooptic dysplasia, midline facial dysplasia,	sarcoidosis)
empty sella syndrome, miscellaneous	Unknown etiology
syndromes	GH resistance
Biologically inactive GH	Laron dwarfism
Neurosecretory defects	Pygmy
Acquired GH deficiency	Autoimmunity—lymphocytic hypophysitis
Idiopathic	Irradiation—CNS radiation for brain tumors,
Neurosecretory defects	leukemia
CNS tumors: Craniopharyngioma, dysgermi-	Vascular lesions—aneurysms, pituitary vessels,
noma, optic glioma, hamartoma	infarction
Trauma	Hematologic disorders—hemochromatosis, sickle
Perinatal insult (breech delivery, hypoxemia,	cell disease, thalassemia
asphyxia, difficult forceps delivery, intracra-	Histiocytosis
nial hemorrhage, precipitous or prolonged	Transient defects in hGH secretion or action,
delivery, twin pregnancy), child abuse,	peripuberty (secretion), primary hypothyroid-
accidental trauma	ism (secretion, action), psychosocial stress
	(secretion, action), malnutrition (action), glu-
	cocorticoid excess (?), drug use

Source: From Reference 26.

Table 3 Criteria for Diagnosis of Growth Hormone Neurosecretory Dysfunction

Height ≤ first percentile
Growth velocity ≤ 4 cm/year (prepubertal)
Bone age ≥ 2 years behind chronologic age
Abnormal 24 h GH secretory pattern
Normal provocative tests (peak GH ≥ 10 ng/ml)
Increased growth after exogenous hGH

ruption at any level, including neurotransmitter dysfunction, GHRH decrease, and/or somatostatin increase, could result in abnormalities in GH secretion, poor linear growth, and short stature (51).

Using GHRH as a biochemical pharmacologic probe demonstrated that most children with classic GH deficiency have a hypothalamic rather than a pituitary defect (52–54). These and other data suggest that many children with classic GH deficiency actually have defects in neurosecretion, as has been speculated for GHND children. In fact, there is overlap between classic GH deficiency and GHND. Part of this may be a result of how many and which provocative tests are used to make the diagnosis. In addition, the timing of GHRH stimulation relative to the endogenous GH pulse affects the GH secretory response (55,56).

To determine the diagnostic value of GHRH in assessing GH secretion in biochemical GH-deficient and GH-sufficient children, a GHRH bolus was administered to four groups of prepubertal children ($n = 85$): group I, classic GH deficiency; group II, biochemical GH deficiency and normal growth velocity; group III, biochemical GH sufficiency and poor growth velocity; and group IV, biochemical GH sufficiency and normal growth velocity. Briefly, these data suggest that GHRH-stimulated GH release is least in children with biochemical GH insufficiency, with and without poor growth velocity, and greater in children with biochemical GH sufficiency (Fig. 7) (56).

Another variable in the GH response to GHRH is likely related to the timing of bolus injection of exogenous GHRH and the pituitary release of GH. We arbitrarily defined the pulse, based retrospectively on GHRH pretreatment blood samples, as follows: upslope, downslope, and trough (56). We demonstrated variability in GH response following a standard GHRH challenge in normal short-statured children (Fig. 8). We believe that this same observation may apply to the interpretation of other provocative tests, although this has not been specifically examined. Thus, for these and other reasons, the diagnosis of GH-deficient states must be interpreted in the total context, which includes biochemical and anthropometric data and clinical observations.

GHRH challenge testing in classic GH deficiency (52, 56), GHND (53,54), and CNS-irradiated children (57,58) further suggests disordered control of GH secretion in these types of growth hormone-deficient states. Indeed, chronic

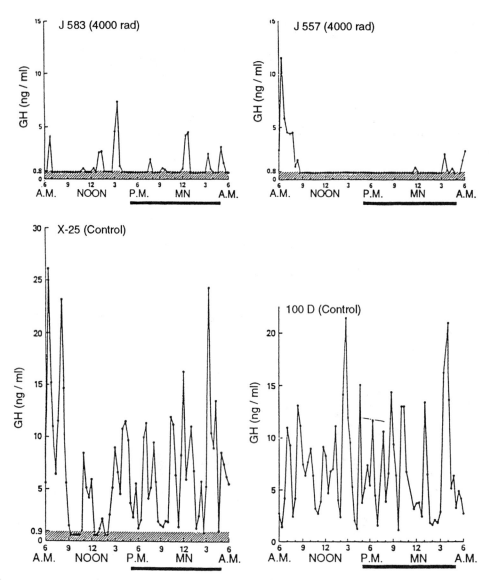

Figure 3 GH secretory pattern during a 24 h period in two primates treated with cranial radiation (4000 rad, top) and two normal controls (bottom). The study was performed 1 year after treatment. There was a decrease in the number (frequency) and amplitude of secretory spikes in the animals that received radiation. The shaded area represents the detection limit of the assay. The dark period was from 1700 to 0500 h (solid line). (From Ref. 47.)

GHRH administration has accelerated growth velocity in classic GH-deficient children (59,60). Of interest, children who fit the definition of GHND may increase their growth velocity for a sustained period of time (1 year) following a brief GHRH treatment interval (as little as 2 months) (61). GHRH challenge testing has been used in metabolic disorders, such as diabetes (62,63), and in other endocrine disorders, including acromegaly (64), hypothyroidism (65), and constitutional delay of growth and adolescent development (66). Body composition and nutritional status also affect GHRH testing results (67,68).

Somatostatin is a potent inhibitor of all known stimuli for GH release. Indirect evidence suggests its physiologic role

in the neuroregulation of GH is also important compared with GHRH. Our group has also used somatostatin infusion inhibition to demonstrate residual adenomatous pituitary tissue in a patient after surgery for her gigantism (unpublished data).

There is a spectrum of GH secretory abnormalities from absolute deficiency to more subtle deficiency states. Within this spectrum is a heterogeneous group including absolute and lesser degrees of classic GH deficiency and GHND (15,69), which may also be considered a GH deficiency state. Indeed, we have demonstrated an increased incidence of perinatal complications in children with GHND (70), as was observed previously in classic GH deficiency. Additional studies are

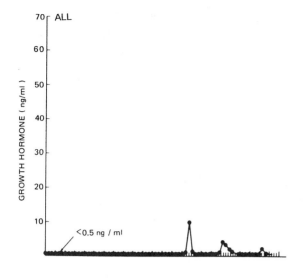

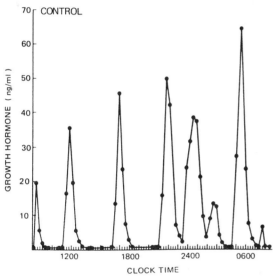

Figure 4 Spontaneous pulsatile growth hormone secretion in a representative patient with acute lymphoblastic leukemia (ALL) who received preventive therapy to the central nervous system with 2400 rad and in a control patient. (From Ref. 45.)

necessary to determine clearly the normal range for endogenous GH secretion because of the limited published data on normal-stature control subjects. (Indeed, the same statement could apply to peak GH responses to provocative testing in children). There are recent studies showing overlap with normal-stature prepubertal controls (71,72). Moreover, it is important to emphasize differences in assays in different laboratories (73). Clinicians should use caution when interpreting other investigators' published control data. Excess body fat decreases spontaneous and provocative GH secretion, so interpretation of results must take this information into account (68,74). This discussion, of course, does not take into account many of the factors, known and unknown, involved in growth.

In addition to classic GH deficiency and GHND as disorders of GH neurosecretion the list would be incomplete without mention of neuropsychiatric and metabolic disorders (Table 5).

SmC/IGF-I concentration correlates weakly with mean 24 h GH concentration ($r = 0.34$; Fig. 9) (54). Although normal spontaneous GH secretion and SmC/IGF-I concentrations have been demonstrated in many short control children, short children as a group have decreased endogenous GH secretion (75,76). In contrast, tall girls as a group have increased spontaneous GH secretion (76), very tall children and adults have increased SmC/IGF-I concentrations (77), and short children decreased levels (78) compared with age-matched control groups.

III. DIAGNOSIS OF GH NEUROSECRETORY DYSFUNCTION

Children with normal short stature must be distinguished from those with pathologic short stature to avoid unnecessary and expensive tests. Use of tests to diagnose GH deficiency should be considered in children with (1) abnormal linear growth rate for age, (2) subnormal height (>2 standard deviations, SD, below mean for age), (3) delayed bone age, (4) no organic disease that would cause growth failure, or (5) normal body proportions. Guidelines for abnormal growth rates adjusted for chronologic age are less than 7 cm/year before age 3 years, less than 4.5–5.0 cm/year from age 3 years, and less than 5.5–6.0 cm/year during pubertal years.

The diagnostic testing used to determine GH deficiency is classified as either pharmacologic (use of provocative agents) or physiologic (measurement of spontaneous endogenous GH secretion). We suggest that the provocative and/or spontaneous GH secretory data must be interpreted in the context of the clinical setting, that is, short stature, poor growth velocity, delayed bone age, and so on. It is critical to emphasize the term "context of the clinical setting." There are examples of children with either or even both decreased spontaneous and provocative GH secretion who are growing at a normal growth velocity. After eliminating other factors (e.g., precocious puberty in a CNS-irradiated child), the terms "classic GH deficiency" and "GHND" should not be based solely on biochemical laboratory criteria.

Spontaneous secretory studies are done by measuring discrete blood samples every 20 or 30 minutes for 24 or for 12 h at night. Another method, integrated concentration of GH, requires use of a continuous blood withdrawal system and removal of samples at 20 or 30 minute intervals (79). These two methods were compared in a small normal patient population, and the results were comparable (80). It is also helpful to assess other parameters of pulsatile secretion, including number and size of pulses and mean pulse amplitude, because it is possible that mean GH secretion is normal and the pulsatile pattern abnormal, suggestive of a neurosecretory defect (15,50,54). As a group, short children secrete less spontaneous GH (75,80) and taller stature children secrete more GH (80). A recent report suggests that prepubertal males

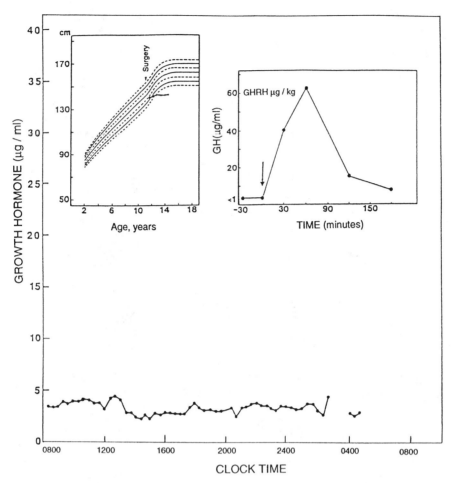

Figure 5   Growth hormone concentrations over 20 h, growth chart (vertical inset), and growth hormone response to growth hormone releasing hormone injection (horizontal inset). Mean growth hormone concentration over 20 h was 3.3 μg/L. (From Ref. 50.)

Table 4   Peak GH (μg/L) after Provocative Testing[a]

Stimulus	Irradiated	Control	p Value
GHRH	21.4 ± 5.0 (12)	38.1 ± 6.8 (22)	NS
Arginine	6.4 ± 1.2 (16)	14.7 ± 1.9 (29)	<0.005
Insulin	6.0 ± 0.9 (16)	14.7 ± 1.5 (38)	<0.001
L-dopa (dopaminergic)	4.9 ± 1.1 (15)	10.1 ± 1.6 (24)	<0.005
Clonidine (α-adrenergic)	6.0 ± 1.1 (17)	21.2 ± 2.0 (34)	<0.001
Propranolol (β-adrenergic)	3.9 ± 1.1 (12)	11.3 ± 1.5 (6)	<0.01
Cholinergic	7.2 ± 2.8 (11)	14.5 ± 3.4 (5)	<0.05
L-tryptophan (serotonergic)[b]	3.6 ± 0.8 (12)	22.3 ± 12.4 (6)	NS
Valproic acid (GABAergic)	3.4 ± 0.8 (10)	11.3 ± 3.8 (6)	<0.05

[a]GH, growth hormone; GHRH, growth hormone releasing hormone; NS, not significant. Values are mean ± SEM. Parentheses indicate number tested in each group. Statistical analyses by Mann-Whitney U test.

[b]L-tryptophan stimulation test did not reach statistical significance; there was an extremely variable response in the control group.

Source: From Reference 48.

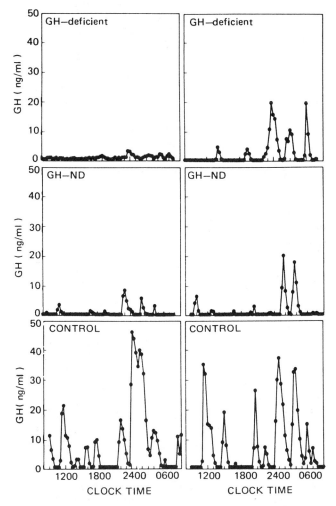

Figure 6 Representative 24 h GH secretory patterns in GH-deficient GHND (GH neurosecretory dysfunction), and control in lower left panel is Tanner stage I; control in right panel is Tanner stage IV. Note that a child with classic GH deficiency (upper right) had three GH pulses greater than 10 μg/ml and two above 20 ng/ml. This child had a mean spontaneous 24 h GH concentration less than that in two other children with GHND. By definition, the patients with GHND had two or more GH normal provocative tests (peak GH ≥ 10 ng/ml), unlike classic GH-deficient children (two or more GH provocative tests < 10 ng/ml). The GHND children had a linear growth response to exogenous GH similar to that in the classic GH-deficient subjects. (From Ref. 15.)

with constitutional delay of growth have altered reduced GH secretory dynamics (81). In addition, body composition and nutritional status affect interpretation of spontaneous GH secretory measurements (67,68,82–4).

In a report it was proposed that spontaneous GH secretion was not as sensitive as provocative testing in diagnosing GH deficiency states (71). In another study, using the same stimulation tests (insulin hypoglycemia-arginine tolerance test and L-dopa) 2 of 20 (10%) nonhypopituitary short children

had peak GH responses ≤ 7.0 μg/L and 4 of 20 (20%) had peak GH responses < 10 μg/ml, evidence that false positive results may occur despite using two or more stimulation tests of GH secretion (85). In these and other studies using provocative testing, normal-stature children were not compared and thus "short control" children have been the basis for almost all control data. Other investigators emphasize the overlap of peak GH secretion after insulin hypoglycemia (86).

Our interest in examining spontaneous GH secretion and describing GH neurosecretory dysfunction as part of the spectrum of GH deficiency (15,27,28,54,69) results from the observations of many investigators (79,85–101) who demonstrated that provocative testing using an arbitrary GH peak cutoff of 7 or 10 μg/L did not identify all children in whom there is acceleration in growth velocity after exogenous GH therapy. We recognize that spontaneous GH secretory studies are not practical in many clinical settings, but they offer a valuable research tool for assessment of "unprovoked" spontaneous GH secretion and its regulatory factors. The diagnosis of "GH deficiency" is difficult, but to exclude studies of spontaneous GH secretion in the appropriate patient in the pertinent clinical situation is premature. At the present time, pediatric endocrinologists in Australia are using height and growth velocity criteria alone to determine who should receive GH therapy. Our approach is to continue detailed provocative and spontaneous GH secretory testing and to apply the biochemical (and anatomic) results in the context of the clinical circumstances for the individual child. The cost of the treatment for even 1 year still far exceeds the cost of a detailed biochemical workup.

GH secretion is only part of the complex process of growth. Included in this process are the known influences of sex steroids and fuel and energy metabolism. In the end, it cannot be overemphasized that these tests must be analyzed in the context of the clinical setting.

IV. THERAPEUTIC OPTIONS

GHRH or a long-acting GHRH analog preparation still represents an experimental approach in the treatment of GH deficiency in certain children. In a recent limited study following a brief course of GHRH, children with decreased spontaneous GH secretion (who fit the definition of GHND) continued to grow after exogenous GHRH treatment (61). These limited observations in a small group of children suggest improved neuroregulation of GH secretion resulting from this temporary therapeutic manuever. In the future, this treatment may have specific application, as may recombinant DNA-prepared SmC/IGF-I. See Chapter 5 for recent reports on the successful administration of IGF-I in GH receptor deficiency syndrome. Drugs that effect neurotransmitter secretion (dopaminergic agonists, such as L-dopa and bromoergocriptine, and α-adrenergic drugs, such as clonidine) offer little promise for the future and are not recommended except as part of research protocols with long-term end points. It is interesting to speculate that neurotransmitter "replacement in pharmacologic" therapy might be more effective when used

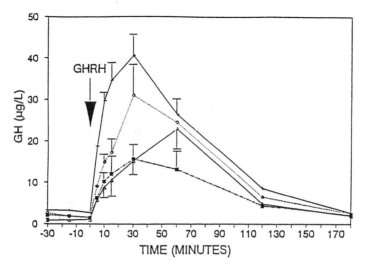

Figure 7 GH responses over time following GHRH administration in children with classic GH deficiency (group I, dashed line), biochemical GH deficiency and normal growth velocity (group II, solid line with triangle), biochemical GH sufficiency and subnormal growth velocity (group III, solid line with plus sign), and GH sufficiency and normal growth velocity (group IV, dotted line). Data are presented as mean ± SEM. (From Ref. 56.)

in a combination or "polypharmacy" approach. In general, we avoid using oxandrolone, a synthetic androgen, in the treatment of short stature because of concern about occasional inappropriate advancement of bone age. However, some pediatric endocrinologists use oxandrolone in the therapy of Turner syndrome and constitutional short stature. In Turner syndrome oxandrolone was used recently in combination with GH; both GH alone and in combination with oxandrolone impact positively on final height (102).

Both dopaminergic and α-adrenergic agonists stimulate growth velocity in classic GH deficiency (103,104) and intrauterine growth retardation (105). Clonidine, an α-adrenergic agonist, appears to have a growth-promoting benefit in

constitutional delay of growth and adolescent development and short stature (106,107), although a recent placebo control study did not support this conclusion (108).

Among the most exciting discoveries in this area is the development of new compounds that augment GH secretion; this includes drugs that are orally active. Several new compounds that stimulate growth hormone secretion have been identified recently, including growth hormone releasing peptide (GHRP-6), a synthetic enkephalin analog (His-D-Trp-Ala-Trp-D-Phe-Lys-NH₂) that stimulates GH secretion in a dose-dependent manner without an effect on other anterior pituitary hormones in vivo and in vitro (109,110). A recent study of nine children with short stature, slow growth, and

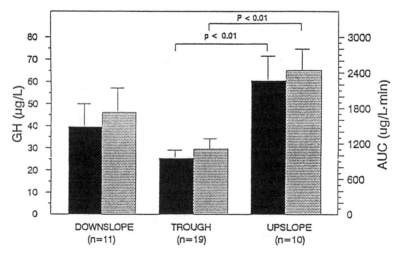

Figure 8 Peak GH response (C_{max}, solid bar), and area under the curve (AUC, stippled bar) after GHRH administration in children with normal GH secretion by standard GH provocative testing. AUC and C_{max} are significantly reduced during the trough compared with the upslope interval ($p < 0.01$). (From Ref. 56.)

Table 5 Disorders of Growth Hormone Neurosecretory Function

GH deficiency states (organic and functional)
    Classic GH deficiency
    GH neurosecretory dysfunction
Other pathologic states
    Neurologic disorders
    Cranial irradiation[a]
    CNS trauma[a]
    Huntington chorea
    Parkinson disease
    Shy-Drager syndrome
    Sleep disturbance disorders
    Nonorganic nutritional dwarfing
    Neuropsychiatric disorders
    Apallic syndrome
    Anorexia nervosa
    Manic depression
    Psychotic depression
    Psychosocial dwarfism
Metabolic disorders
    Diabetes mellitus
    Obesity
    Kidney failure
    Liver failure

[a]May be associated with decreased GH secretion; therefore, they can also be classified in the first subgroup.
Source: Adapted from Reference 27.

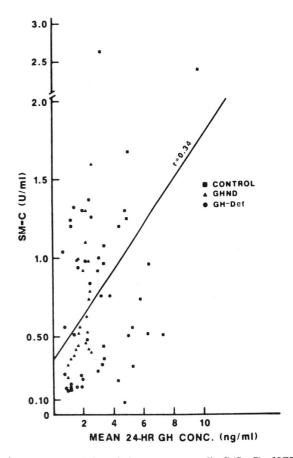

Figure 9 Correlation of plasma somatomedin C (SmC) of IGF-I and mean 24 h GH concentration in GH-deficient, GHND, and control children. The SmC/IGF-I concentration represents the mean of two samples (0900 and 2100 h). (From Ref. 54.)

delayed bone age treated with recombinant human GH therapy were investigated for their GH response to the oral administration of GHRP-6 (300 μg/kg). Of the nine children with classic GH deficiency, five had small or absent increases in serum GH concentration compared with four children with normal or nearly normal GH responses to provocative stimuli (111). Further safety and efficacy studies, along with evaluation of GH response to a multiple oral dosing regimen, remain before this peptide or other peptides (GHRP-1 and GHRP-2) may be considered for possible clinical use in the treatment of growth retardation (109). The nonpeptidyl compound L-692,429 is a very recent addition to the growing list of GH releasing compounds (112). L-692,429 has significant bioavailability as an oral agent and is significantly more potent than GHRP-6; it stimulates GH secretion similarly to GHRP-6 (112,113).

After thorough evaluation of the apparently healthy prepubertal child with significant short stature (≤3 SD below mean height for age), delayed bone age, slow growth velocity, and normal provocative and 24 h endogenous GH secretion, should hGH be administered? Our approach now is to offer a 6 month therapeutic trial of exogenous GH. A growth velocity increase of at least 2 cm/year over the pretreatment rate can be considered a satisfactory response and indication for longer treatment. If the reader is interested in a detailed analysis of GH replacement therapy, see Reference 108 and

Chapter 5. To determine whether to treat with GH, the clinician must carefully consider the risk-benefit ratio. Although the risks appear low, the reader is referred to recent discussions of this issue (114–116). Until more information is available, we must consider inadequate growth velocity, not short stature alone, the critical element in making the decision to treat. This must be considered in the context of the recent oral summary presentation of a questionnaire organized by Dr. H. Guyda at the combined Meeting of The Lawson Williams Pediatric Endocrine Society and European Society for Pediatric Endocrinology, San Francisco, CA, 1993. In a review of 50 pediatric endocrine clinics throughout the world, children who had normal GH secretion did not appear to receive long-term ultimate benefit from exogenous GH therapy. Further studies are necessary before definite conclusions can be reached.

ACKNOWLEDGMENT

I thank Ms. Becky Rains for her competent secretarial assistance.

REFERENCES

1. Raben MS. Treatment of a pituitary dwarf with human growth hormone. J Clin Endocrinol 1958; 18: 901–903.
2. Lewis UJ, Singh RNP, Tutweller GF, Sigel MB, Van der Laan EF, Van der Laan WP. Human growth hormone: a complex of proteins. Recent Prog Horm Res 1980; 36:477–508.
3. Chawla RK, Parks JS, Rudman D. Structural variants of human growth hormone: biochemical, genetic and clinical aspects. Annu Rev Med 1983; 34:519–547.
4. Baumann G, MacCart JC, Amburn K. The molecular nature of circulating growth hormone in normal and acromegalic man: evidence for a principal and minor monomeric forms. J Clin Endocrinol Metab 1983; 56:946–952.
5. Markoff E, Lee DW, Culler FL, Jones KL, Lewis UJ. Release of the 22,000 and the 20,000-dalton variants of growth hormone in vivo and in vitro by human anterior pituitary cells. J Clin Endocrinol Metab 1986; 62:664–669.
6. Stolar MW, Amburn K, Baumann G. Plasma "big" and "big-big" growth hormone (GH) in man: an oliogo-meric series composed of structurally diverse GH monomers. J Clin Endocrinol Metab 1984; 59:212–218.
7. Lewis UJ, Lewis LJ, Salem NR, Galosy SS, Krivi GG. A recombinant-DNA-derived modification of human growth hormone (hGH 44–191) with enhanced diabetogenic activity. Mol Cell Endocrinol 1991; 78:45–54.
8. Parks JS. Organization and function of human growth hormone genes cluster, In: Raiti S, Tolman RA, eds. Human Growth Hormone. New York: Plenum Publishing, 1986:199–209.
9. Frankenne F, Rentier-Delrue F, Scippo ML, Hennen G. Expression of the growth hormone variant gene in human placenta. J Clin Endocrinol Metab 1987; 64:635.
10. Hennen G, Frankenne F, Closset J, Gomez F, Pirens G, El Khayat N. A human placental GH: increasing levels during second half of pregnancy with pituitary GH suppression as revealed by monoclonal antibody radioimmunoassay. Int J Fertil 1985; 30:27.
11. Baumann G, Stoler MW, Ambrum K, Barsano CP, DeVries BC. A specific growth hormone binding protein in human plasma: initial characterization. J Clin Endocrinol Metab 1986; 62:134.
12. Baumann G, Shaw MA, Winter RJ. Absence of the plasma growth hormone-binding protein in Laron dwarfism. J Clin Endocrinol Metab 1987; 65:814.
13. Cunningham BC, Ultsch M, DeVos AM, Mulkerrin MG, Clauser KR, Wells JA. Dimerization of the extracellular domain of the human growth hormone receptor by a single hormone molecule. Science 1991; 254:821–825.
14. Martha PM, Rogol AD, Blizzard RM, Shaw MA, Baumann G. Growth hormone-binding protein activity is inversely related to 24-hour growth hormone release in normal boys. J Clin Endocrinol Metab 1991; 73:175–181.
15. Spiliotis B, August G, Hung W, Sonis W, Mendelson W, Bercu BB. Growth hormone neurosecretory dysfunction: a treatable cause of short stature. JAMA, 1984; 251:2223–2230.
16. Golstein J, Cauter EV, Desir D, et al. Effects of "jet lag" on hormonal patterns. IV. Time shifts increase growth hormone release. J Clin Endocrinol Metab 1983; 56:433–440.
17. Quabbe H-J. Hypothalamic control of GH secretion: pathophysiology and clinical implications. Acta Neurochir (Wien) 1985; 75:60–71.
18. Phillips LS, Vassilopoulou-Sellin R. Somatomedins. N Engl J Med 1980; 302:371.
19. Van Wyk J, Underwood LE. Relation between growth hormone and somatomedin. Annu Rev Med 1975; 26:427.
20. Daughaday WH, Garland JT. The sulfation factor hypothesis: recent observations. In: Pecile A, Mueller EE, eds. Growth and Growth Hormone. Amsterdam: Excerpta Medica, 1972:168–179.
21. Issaksson OGP, Isgaard J, Nilsson A, Lindahl A. Direction action of GH. In: Bercu BB, ed. Growth Hormone: Basic and Clinical Aspects. New York: Plenum Press, 1988:199–211.
22. Baxter RC. Physiological roles of the IGF binding proteins. In: Spencer EM, ed. Modern Concepts of Insulin-like Growth Factors. New York: Elsevier, 1991:371–380.
23. Smith WJ, Nan TJ, Underwood LE, Busby WH, Celnicker A, Clemmons DR. Use of insulin-like growth factor-binding protein-2 (IGFBP-2), IGFBP-3 and IGF-1 for assessing growth hormone status in short children. J Clin Endocrinol Metab 1993; 77:1294–1299.
24. Underwood LE, Van Wyk J. Normal and aberrant growth. In: Wilson JD, Oster DW, eds. Williams Textbook of Endocrinology. Philadelphia: W.B. Saunders, 1079–1138.
25. Zapf J, Walter H, Froesch ER. Radioimmunological determination of insulin-like growth factors I and II in normal subjects and in patients with growth disorders and extra-pancreatic tumor hypoglycemia. J Clin Invest 1981; 68:1321–1330.
26. Bercu BB, MacGillivray MH. Diagnosis and management of disorders of growth hormone secretion. Endocrine Science 1988.
27. Bercu BB, Diamond F. A determinant of stature: regulation of growth hormone secretion. In: Barness L, ed. Advances in Pediatrics, Chicago: Yearbook Medical Publishers, 1986:331–380.
28. Bercu BB, Diamond F. Growth hormone neurosecretory dysfunction. Clin Endocrinol Metab 1986; 15:537–590.
29. Tanner JM, Whitehouse RH, Hughes PCR, Carter BS. Relative importance of growth hormone and sex steroids for the growth at puberty of trunk length, limb length, and muscle width in growth hormone-deficient children. J Pediatr 1976; 89:1000–1008.
30. Agnati LF, Fuxe K, Kuonen D, et al. Effects of estrogen and progesterone on central alpha and beta adrenergic receptors in ovariectomized rats: evidence for gonadal steroid receptor. In: Fuxe K, Gustafsson JA, Wetterberg L, eds. Steroid Hormone Regulation of the Brain. Oxford: Pergamon Press, 1981:237.
31. Mauras N, Blizzard RM, Link K, Johnson ML, Rogol AD, Veldhuis JD. Augmentation of growth hormone secretion during puberty: evidence for a pulse amplitude-modulated phenomenon. J Clin Endocrinol Metab 1987; 64:596–601.
32. Zadik Z, Chalew SA, McCarter J Jr, Meistas M, Kowarski AA. The influence of age on the 24-hour integrated concentration of growth hormone in normal individuals. J Clin Endocrinol Metab 1985; 60:513–516.
33. Ross JL, Pescovitz OH, Barnes K, Loriaux DL, Cutler GB Jr. Growth hormone secretory dynamics in children with precocious puberty. J Pediatr 1987; 110:369–372.
34. Kerrigan JR, Rogol AD. The impact of gonadol steroid hormone action on growth hormone secretion during childhood and adolescence. Endocr Rev 1992; 13:281–298.
35. Richards GE, Wara WM, Grumbach MM, et al. Delayed onset of hypopituitarism: sequelae of therapeutic irradiation of central nervous system, eye and middle ear tumors. J Pediatr 1976; 89:553.
36. Shalet SM. Disorders of the endocrine system due to radiation and cytotoxic chemotherapy. Clin Endocrinol (Oxf) 1983; 18:637–659.
37. Shalet SM, Beardwell CG, Morris-Jones PH, Pearson D. Growth hormone deficiency after treatment of acute leukemia in children. Arch Dis Child 1976; 51:489–493.
38. Shalet SM, Beardwell CG, Pearson D, Morris-Jones PH. The

effect of varying doses of cerebral irradiation on growth hormone production in childhood. Clin Endocrinol (Oxf) 1976; 5:287–290.

39. Dacou-Vaitekakis C, Xypolyta A, Haidas ST, et al. Irradiation of the head: immediate effect on growth hormone secretion in children. J Clin Endocrinol Metab 1977; 44:791–794.

40. Swift PGF, Kearney PJ, Dalton RG, et al. Growth hormonal status of children treated for acute lymphoblastic leukemia. Arch Dis Child 1978; 53:890–894.

41. Oliff A, Bode U, Bercu BB, DiChiro G, Graves V, Poplack DG. Hypothalamic-pituitary dysfunction following CNS prophylaxis in acute lymphocytic leukemia: correlation with CT scan abnormalities. Med Pediatr Oncol 1979; 7:141–151.

42. Bode U, Oliff A, Bercu BB, DiChiro G, Glaubiger D, Poplack D. Absence of CT brain scan abnormalities with less intensive CNS prophylaxis. Am J Pediatr Hematol Oncol 1980; 2:21–24.

43. Romche CA, Zipf WB, Miser A, et al. Evaluation of growth hormone release and human growth hormone treatment in children with cranial irradiation-associated short stature. J Pediatr 1984; 104:177–181.

44. Dickinson WP, Berry DH, Dickinson L, et al. Differential effects of cranial radiation on growth hormone response to arginine and insulin infusion. J Pediatr 1978; 92:754–757.

45. Blatt J, Bercu BB, Gillin JC, Mendelson WB, Poplack D. Reduced pulsatile growth hormone secretion in children after therapy for acute lymphoblastic leukemia. J Pediatr 1984; 104:182–186.

46. Muhlendahl KEV, Gadner H, Riehm H, et al. Endocrine function after antineoplastic therapy in 22 children with acute lymphoblastic leukemia. Helv Paediatr Acta 1976; 31:463–471.

47. Chrousos GP, Poplack D, Brown T, O'Neill D, Schwade JG, Bercu BB. Effects of cranial radiation on hypothalamic-adenopypophyseal function: abnormal growth hormone secretory dynamics. J Clin Endocrinol Metab 1982; 54:1135–1139.

48. Jorgensen EV, Schwartz ID, Hvizdala E, et al. Neurotransmitter control of growth hormone secretion in children after cranial radiation therapy. J Pediatr Endocrinol 1993; 6:131–142.

49. Tannenbaum GS. Interrelationship of somatostatin and growth hormone-releasing hormone in the genesis of the rhythmic secretion of growth hormone. Acta Paediatr Scand 1990; 367:76–80.

50. Shulman DI, Bercu BB. The evaluation of impaired growth hormone secretion: provocative testing vs endogenous 24 hour growth hormone profile. Acta Paediatr Scand (Suppl) 1987; 337:61–71.

51. Bercu BB, Diamond FB. Regulation of growth hormone secretion: relevance to the pediatrician. Pediatrician 1987; 14:94–108.

52. Hizuka N, Takoano K, Shizume K, Hirose N, Ling ND. Plasma growth hormone responses to repetitive administrations of growth hormone releasing factor in patients with pituitary dwarfism. Endocrinol Jpn 1984; 31:697–704.

53. Chalew SA, Armour KM, Levin PA, Thorner MO, Kowarski AA. Growth hormone (GH) response to GH-releasing hormone in children with subnormal integrated concentrations of GH. J Clin Endocrinol Metab 1986; 62:1110–1115.

54. Bercu BB. Growth hormone neurosecretory dysfunction: update. In: Bercu BB, ed. Basic and Clinical Aspects of Growth Hormone. New York: Plenum Press, 1988:119–141.

55. Devesa J, Lima L, Lois N, et al. Reasons for the variability in growth hormone (GH) responses to GHRH challenge: the endogenous hypothalamic-somatotroph rhythm (HSR). Clin Endocrinol (Oxf) 1989; 30:367–377.

56. Cho KH, Yang SW, Hu C-S, Bercu BB. Growth hormone (GH) response to growth hormone-releasing hormone (GHRH) varies with intrinsic growth hormone secretory rhythm in children: can somatostatin pretreatment reduce this variability? J Pediatr Endocrinol 1992; 3:155–165.

57. Ahmed SR, Shalet SM. Hypothalamic growth hormone releasing factor deficiency following cranial irradiation. Clin Endocrinol (Oxf) 1984; 21:483–488.

58. Lustig RH, Schriock EA, Kaplan SL, Grumbach MM. Effect of growth hormone release in children with radiation-induced growth hormone deficiency. Pediatrics 1985; 76:274–279.

59. Thorner MO, Reschke J, Chitwood J, et al. Acceleration of growth in two children treated with human growth hormone-releasing factor. N Engl J Med 1985; 312:4–9.

60. Gelato MC, Ross JL, Malozowski S, et al. Effects of pulsatile growth administration of growth hormone (GH)-releasing hormone on short term linear in children with GH deficiency. J Clin Endocrinol Metab 1985; 61:444–450.

61. Lifshitz F, Lanes R, Pugliese M, et al. Sustained improvement in growth velocity and recovery from suboptimal growth hormone (GH) secretion after treatment with human pituitary GH-releasing hormone-(1–44)-NH$_2$. J Clin Endocrinol Metab 1992; 75:1255–1260.

62. Press M, Tamborlane MV, Thorner MO, et al. Pituitary response to growth hormone-releasing factor in diabetes: failure of glucose-mediated suppression. Diabetes 1984; 33:804–806.

63. Richards NT, Wood SM, Christofides ND, Bhuttacharji S-C, Bloom SR. Impaired growth hormone response to human pancreatic growth hormone releasing factor [GRF(1–44)] in type 2 (non-insulin-dependent) diabetes. Diabetologia 1984; 27:529–534.

64. Schulte HM, Benker G, Windeck R, Olbricht T, Reinwein D. Failure to respond to growth hormone releasing hormone (GHRH) in acromegaly due to GHRH secreting pancreatic tumor: dynamics of multiple endocrine testing. J Clin Endocrinol Metab 1985; 61:585–587.

65. Williams T, Maxon H, Thorner MO, Frohman LA. Blunted growth hormone (GH) response to GH-releasing hormone in hypothyroidism resolves in the euthyroid state. J Clin Endocrinol Metab 1985; 61:454–456.

66. Pintor C, Puggioni R, Fanni V, et al. Growth-hormone releasing factor and clonidine in children with constitutional growth delay: evidence for defective pituitary reserve. J Endocrinol Invest 1984; 7:253–256.

67. Abdenur JE, Pugliese MT, Cevantes C, Fort P, Liftshitz F. Alterations in spontaneous growth hormone (GH) secretion and the response to GH-releasing hormone in children with nonorganic nutritional dwarfing. J Clin Endocrinol Metab 1992; 75:930–934.

68. Abdenur JE, Solans C, Smith M, Carman C, Pugliese M, Lifshitz F. Body composition and spontaneous growth hormone secretion in normal in short stature children. J Clin Endocrinol Metab 1994; 78:277–282.

69. Bercu BB, Shulman D, Root AW, Spiliotis BE. Growth hormone provocative testing frequently does not reflect endogenous growth hormone secretion. J Clin Endocrinol Metab 1986; 63:709–716.

70. Bercu BB, Shulman DI, Root AW. High incidence of prenatal and perinatal complications associated with growth hormone neurosectory dysfunction (GHND) (abstract). Pediatr Res 1987; 21:244A.

71. Rose SR, Ross JL, Uriarte M, Barnes KM, Cassorla FG, Cutler GB. The advantage of measuring stimulated as compared with spontaneous growth hormone levels in the diagnosis

of growth hormone levels in the diagnosis of growth hormone deficiency. N Engl J Med 1988; 319:201–207.

72. Lin T-H, Kirkland RT, Sherman BM, Kirkland JL. Growth hormone testing in short children and their response to growth hormone therapy. J Pediatr 1989; 115:57–63; 23:280A (abstract).

73. Reiter EO, Morris AH, MacGillivray MH, Weber D. Variable estimates of serum GH concentrations by different radioassay systems. J Clin Endocrinol Metab 1987; 66:68.

74. Bercu BB, Shulman DI, Root AW. Obesity decreases endogenous growth hormone (GH) secretion in children with normal growth velocities (abstract). Pediatr Res 1988; 23:272A.

75. Zadik Z, Chalew SA, Raiti S, Kowarski AA. Do short children secrete insufficient growth hormone? Pediatrics 1985; 76:355–360.

76. Albertsson-Wikland K, Isaksson O, Rosberg S, Westphal O. Secretory pattern of growth hormone in children of different growth rates. Acta Endocrinol (Copenh) (Suppl) 1983; 103:72.

77. Gourmelen M, LeBouc Y, Girard F, Binoux M. Serum levels of insulin-like growth factor (IGF) and IGF binding protein in constitutionally tall children and adolescents. J Clin Endocrinol Metab 1984; 59:1197–1203.

78. Cacciari E, Cicognani A, Pirazzoli P, et al. Differences in somatomedin-C between short-normal subjects and those of normal height. J Pediatr 1985; 106:891–894.

79. Plotnick LP, Van Meter QL, Kowarski AA. Human growth hormone treatment of children with growth failure and normal growth hormone levels by immunoassay. Pediatrics 1983; 71:324–327.

80. Albertsson-Wikland K, Rosberg B. Analyses of 24-hour growth hormone profiles in children: relation to growth. J Clin Endocrinol Metab 1988; 67:493–500.

81. Kerrigan JR, Martha PM, Veldhuis JD, Blizzard RM, Rogol AD. Altered growth hormone secretory dynamics in prepubertal males with constitutional delay of growth. Pediatr Res 1993; 33:278–283.

82. Jorgensen EV, Shulman DI, Diamond FB, Root AW, Bercu BB. Spontaneous growth hormone secretion in children with normal and abnormal growth. In: Bercu BB, Walker RF, eds. Basic and Clinical Aspects of Growth Hormone II. New York: Springer-Verlag, pp. 286–298, 1994.

83. Iranmanesh A, Lizarralde G, Veldhuis JD. Age and relative adiposity are specific negative determinants of the frequency and amplitude of growth hormone (GH) secretory burses and the half-life of endogenous GH in healthy men. J Clin Endocrinol Metab 1994; 73:1081–1088.

84. Martha PM Jr, Gorman KM, Blizzard RM, Rogol AD, Veldhuis JD. Endogenous growth hormone secretion and clearance rates in normal boys, as determined by deconvolution analysis: relationship to age, pubertal status, and body mass. J Clin Endocrinol Metab 1994; 74:336–344.

85. Root AW, Russ RD. Effect of L-dihydroxyphenylalanine upon serum growth hormone concentrations in children and adolescents. J Pediatr 1973; 81:808–813.

86. Hindmarsh P, Smith PJ, Brook GD, Matthews DR. The relationship between height velocity and growth hormone secretion in short prepubertal children. Clin Endocrinol (Oxf) 1987; 27:581–591.

87. Van Vliet G, Styne DM, Kaplan SL, Grumbach MM. Growth hormone treatment for short stature. N Engl J Med 1983; 309:1016–1022.

88. Tanner JM, Whitehouse RH, Hughes PCR, Vince FP. Effect of human growth hormone treatment for 1 to 7 years on growth of 100 children, with growth hormone deficiency, low birth weight, inherited smallness, Turner's syndrome and other complaints. Arch Dis Child 1971; 46:745–782.

89. Schaff-Blass E, Burstein S, Rosenfield RL. Advances in diagnosis and treatment of short stature with special reference to the role of growth hormones. J Pediatr 1984; 104:801–813.

90. Rudman D, Kitner MH, Blackston RD, Cushman RA, Baine RP, Patterson JH. Children with normal variant short stature: treatment with human growth hormone for six months. N Engl J Med 1981; 305:123–131.

91. Valenta JJ, Sigel MB, Lesniak MA, et al. Pituitary dwarfism in a patient with. N Engl J Med 1985; 312:214–217.

92. Frazer TE, Gavin VR, Daughaday WH, Hillman RE, Wheldon VV. Growth hormone-dependent growth failure. J Pediatr 1982; 101:12–15.

93. Grunt JA, Howard CP, Daughaday WH. Comparison of growth and somatomedin C responses following growth hormone treatment in children with small for date short stature, significant idiopathic short stature and hypopituitarism. Acta Endocrinol (Copenh) 1984; 106:168–174.

94. Tokuhiro E, Dean HJ, Friesen HG, Rudman D. Comparison study of growth serum human growth measurements woth NB2 lymphoma cell bioassay, IM-9 receptor modulation assay and radioimmunoassay in children with disorders of growth. J Clin Endocrinol Metab 1984; 58:549–554.

95. Rudman D, Kutner MH, Goldsmith MA, et al. Further observations on four subgroups of normal variant short stature. J Clin Endocrinol Metab 1980; 52:1378–1384.

96. Lanes P, Plotnik LP, Spencer ME, Daughday WE, Kowarski AA. Dwarfism associated with normal serum growth hormone and increased bioassayable, receptorassayable and immunoassayable somatomedin. J Clin Endocrinol Metab 1980; 50:485–488.

97. Lenko HL, Leisti S, Perheentupa J. The efficacy of growth hormone in different types of growth failures: analysis of 101 cases. Eur J Pediatr 1982; 138:241–249s.

98. Hayek A, Peake GT. Growth and somatomedin-C responses to growth hormone in dwarfed children. J Pediatr 1981; 99:868–872.

99. Gertner JM, Genel M, Gianfredi SP, et al. Prospective clinical trial of human growth hormone in short children without growth hormone deficiency. J Pediatr 1984; 104:172–176.

100. Blethen SL, Chasalow FI. Use of a two-site immunoradiometric assay for growth hormone (GH) in identifying children with GH dependent growth failure. J Clin Endocrinol Metab 1983; 57:1031–1035.

101. Kaplan SL. Improvement in growth rate and mean predicted height during long-term treatment with growth hormone in children with non-growth hormone deficient short stature. In: Bercu BB, ed. Basic and Clinical Aspects of Growth Hormone. New York: Plenum Press, 1988:285–288.

102. Rosenfeld RG, Frand J, Attie KM, et al. Six-year results of a randomized, prospective trial of human growth hormone and oxandrolone in Turner syndrome. J Pediatr 1992; 121:49–55.

103. Huseman GA, Hassing JM. Evidence of dopaminergic stimulation of growth velocity in some hypopituitary children. J Clin Endocrinol Metab 1984; 58:419–425.

104. Pintor C, Cella SG, Corda R, et al. Clonidine accelerates growth in children with impaired growth hormone secretion. Lancet 1985; 1:1482–1483.

105. Huseman CA. Growth enhancement by dopamineric therapy in children with intrauterine growth retardation. J Clin Endocrinol Metab 1985; 61:514–519.

106. Pintor C, Locke S, Corda R, et al. Clonidine treatment for short stature. Lancet 1987; 1:1226–1229.

107. Castro-Magana M, Angulo M, Fuentes B, Castelar ME, Canas A, Espinoza B. Effect of prolonged clonidine administration on growth hormone concentrations and rate of linear growth

in children with constitutional growth delay. J Pediatr 1986; 109:784–787.

108. Pescovitz OH, Tan E. Lack of benefit of clonidine treatment for short stature in a clonidine therapy of non-growth hormone deficient. Double-blind, placebo-controlled trial. Lancet 1988; 2:874–877.

109. Bowers CY. GH releasing peptides-structure and kinetics. J Pediatr Endocrinol 1993; 6:21–31.

110. Bowers CY, Sartor AO, Reynolds GA, Badger TM. On the actions of the growth hormone-releasing hexapeptide, GHRP. Endocrinology 1991; 128:2027–2035.

111. Bowers CY, Alster DK, Frentz JM. The growth hormone-releasing activity of a synthetic hexapeptide in normal men and short statured children after oral administration. J Clin Endocrinol Metab 1992; 74:292–298.

112. Smith RG, Cheng K, Schoen WR, et al. A nonpeptidyl growth hormone secretagogue. Science 1993; 260:1640–1643.

113. Cheng K, Chan WW, Butler B, et al. Stimulation of growth hormone release from rat pituitary cells by L-692, 492, a novel non-peptidyl GH secretagogue. Endocrinology 1993; 132: 2729–2731.

114. Jorgensen JOL. Human growth hormone replacement therapy: pharmacological and clinical aspects. Endocr Rev 1991; 12:189–207.

115. Ritzen EM, Czernichow P, Preece M, Ranke M, Wit JM. European Society for Pediatric Endocrinology and the Lawson Wilkins Pediatric Endocrine Society. Safety of human growth hormone therapy. Human pituitary growth hormone and Creutzfeldt-Jakob disease. Does growth hormone increase the risk of malignancies? Horm Res 1993; 39:92–101.

116. Fradkin JE, Mills JL, Schonberg LB, et al. Risk of leukemia after treatment with pituitary growth hormone. JAMA 1993; 270:2829–2832.

5

Growth Hormone Treatment

David B. Allen
University of Wisconsin School of Medicine, Madison, Wisconsin

Ann J. Johanson and Robert M. Blizzard
University of Virginia School of Medicine, Charlottesville, Virginia

I. INTRODUCTION

Human growth hormone (hGH) was first used more than 30 years ago to stimulate growth in a child with hypopituitarism (1). Subsequently, a limited supply of pituitary glands from which hGH could be extracted and purified required that hGH therapy be restricted to children with the most severe and unequivocal GH deficiency. Strict, arbitrary laboratory criteria were established to identify patients likely to derive the greatest benefit from scarce GH. Delays in diagnosis and treatment, interruptions in therapy, and dosage restrictions were common during this time. Consequently, although hGH accelerated growth of these individuals, adult statures were usually less than average (2–4).

In 1985, the first case of Creutzfeld-Jakob disease (CJD) in patients who had received hGH was recognized; investigation disclosed that pituitary glands from which the hGH was derived were contaminated with subviral particles. Distribution of pituitary-derived hGH was stopped. Subsequently, in the United States, CJD was diagnosed in seven recipients of GH distributed by the National Hormone and Pituitary Program (5,6). Fortuitously, 192 amino acid biosynthetic hGH, first tested in the United States in 1981, was approved by the U.S. Food and Drug Administration in 1985 (7) and a second 191 amino acid biosynthetic hGH was approved in 1987. The production of hGH by biologic systems (*Escherichia coli* and, more recently, mammalian cells) (8) transplanted with the hGH gene yields a virtually unlimited supply of hGH.

Biosynthetic hGH therapy eliminated the risk of CJD and offered children with severe GH deficiency an opportunity for optimal treatment. Children with milder forms of inadequate GH secretion, previously excluded from hGH, could be treated. The increased availability of recombinant DNA-derived hGH has also allowed investigations of its growth-promoting effects in poorly growing children who do not fit traditional definitions of growth hormone deficiency, many of whom were previously believed to be unresponsive to GH treatment. In addition, the metabolic effects of hGH apart from linear growth promotion are now being studied extensively and may soon lead to new indications for hGH therapy.

The abundance of hGH has added complexity to decisions about the treatment of statural disorders. Human growth hormone *augmentation* therapy has now been added to hGH *replacement* therapy, thus expanding the traditional boundaries of endocrinologic endeavors, in which missing hormones are replaced and excessive hormone production suppressed. The advantages conferred by increased height in the social, economic, professional, and political realms of Western society are well documented. Concern about the social and psychological harm of short stature, and hope for effective therapy, has resulted in increased referrals for growth-promoting therapy. However, data confirming that stature per se is a primary determinant of psychologic health is limited, although some have reported a higher frequency of underachievement, behavior problems, and reduced social competency in short-statured children (9). Neuroendocrine dysfunction (e.g., classic growth hormone deficiency), rather than stature itself, may correlate most closely with psychologic and scholastic impairment (10). The physiologic benefits of hGH supplementation to children with severe GH deficiency appear obvious, but data confirming the efficacy of hGH therapy in improving the quality of life of non–GH-deficient recipients are scarce.

For many children, hGH treatment is appropriate after the cause of growth impairment, the concerns of patients and parents, and likelihood of success have been assessed. For most short children, however, efforts to build self-esteem through parental support, judicious selection of activities, and counseling are more effective than injectable hGH therapy. The decision to institute long-term hGH therapy should include both careful physical and psychologic evaluation, to determine whether the degree of disability and likelihood of therapeutic benefit justify investment of the required emotional and monetary resources. Although experience has shown that side effects appear minimal, other possible effects remain unknown. Unexpected benefits may also be found.

The spectrum of disorders for which hGH has been prescribed and the number of children receiving treatment (Fig. 1) has increased dramatically in the past several years. In this chapter, we review aspects of hGH treatment for classic GH deficiency, including recent information on nongrowth metabolic effects of hGH for adult GH-deficient individuals. Treatment of various short-stature conditions and catabolic disorders with hGH is also considered, reflecting the recent proliferation of investigations of the metabolic and growth-promoting effects of hGH in non–hGH-deficient individuals. Possible risks and ethical issues related to hGH therapy are also addressed.

II. GROWTH HORMONE PHYSIOLOGY

Human growth hormone is secreted by the anterior pituitary gland throughout life under the primary influence of stimulatory growth hormone releasing hormone (GHRH) and inhibitory somatostatin (SS). Both regulatory peptides are synthesized in and released from the hypothalamus. The cyclic pulsatile secretion of GH most likely results from the dominant effect of SS, which produces troughs that are interspersed with peaks of GH resulting from GHRH stimulation. Both GH and insulin-like growth factor I (IGF-I) exert positive feedback on SS secretion, and GH exerts negative feedback on GHRH secretion. Modulation of this system occurs through neurotransmitter, hormonal, and metabolic

substrate influences. Growth hormone is released in response to sleep, exercise, and relative hypoglycemia. Sleep-associated pulses of hGH release usually occur in the first 30–60 minutes of sleep and can occur at any time of day when individuals reach stages 3 and 4 of slow-wave sleep (11). Vigorous exercise for 15–20 minutes provokes a significant hGH surge in 90% of normal children (12). Because surges in hGH are more prolonged in physically unfit than in fit individuals performing comparable work, exercise-induced hGH release appears more related to physical stress than to exercise per se. Psychologic stress, such as venipuncture or general alarm, also produces hGH elevations (13). Rises in hGH occur with the postprandial decline in blood glucose concentration, and hGH secretory surges occur more often in the hours preceding meals than those following meals (14).

Human growth hormone is synthesized and stored in acidophils of the pituitary gland and accounts for as much as 8% of pituitary weight (15). About 80% of secreted hGH has a 191 amino acid sequence and molecular weight of 22 kD; the other 20% is approximately 20 kD and is produced by alternate gene splicing, which deletes amino acids 32–46 from the RNA (16). Human growth hormone is found in pituitary gland and plasma as monomers, dimers, and oligomers. Many other variants of hGH, including proteolytically cleaved, N-acetylated, and deamidated forms, may also be found as either physiologic variants or products of the extraction process (17). Because hGH is species specific, animal GH other than that from primates is ineffective in humans. Circulating hGH binding protein (GHBP) complexes about 50% of hGH and probably acts as a modulator of release and distribution to tissues (18). GHBP shows immunologic identity with the extracellular domain of the GH receptor, and concentrations of GHBP are low in patients with GH receptor deficiency (19). The regulation of GHBP remains uncertain; gonadal steroids, such as estrogen, increase GHBP activity, but hGH secretory status appears to play a minor role (20).

Serum hGH concentrations are high in full-term and

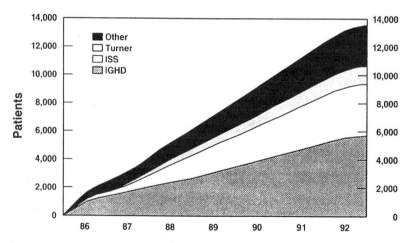

Figure 1 Growth in numbers of children in various diagnostic categories treated with hGH. (With permission, the National Cooperative Growth Study, Genentech, Inc.)

premature infants during the first 24 h of life, averaging 50–60 ng/ml (21) and resulting from both enhanced frequency and amplitude of pulses (22). In full-term, but not in premature infants, hGH levels fall after 48 h. Thereafter, growth hormone concentrations reflect pulsatile secretion, which occurs more often and with higher peaks during infancy, diminishes during childhood, and is lowest in late prepubertal childhood and in adults. Spontaneous puberty in boys or androgen treatment of prepubertal boys results in significant increases in hGH release (23,24). This sex hormone-induced augmentation of growth hormone secretion is primarily an amplitude-modulated phenomenon, although more frequent GH peaks occur (25). Interestingly, however, the effect of testosterone on pubertal growth may be largely independent of changes in circulating hGH (26). Stimulation of the somatotropic axis by testosterone is partly dependent upon its aromatization to estradiol (27); hGH levels in adult women are higher than those in men and rise in men when they are given estrogens (28).

The very short half-life (less than 20 minutes) of circulating hGH requires that blood sampling be carried out at frequent intervals to identify peaks. Studies of children indicate that both normal and short stature are associated with a broad range of hGH secretion patterns (29). Whereas it was previously thought that a bimodal distribution of hGH secretion discretely separated normal from abnormal, it now appears that (with the rare exception of complete GH deficiency secondary to GH gene deletion or abnormalities of expression) a continuum of "inadequate" hGH secretion likely spans classic and partially GH-deficient children, children with delayed growth and puberty, and other poorly growing children who pass provocative tests but still secrete less hGH than their peers. An asymptotic relationship between growth velocity and spontaneous GH secretion has been postulated for short children (Fig. 2) (30). This spectrum of hGH insufficiency, in which there are varying degrees of abnormal GH secretion (31), creates an enormous difficulty in interpreting tests of hGH secretion, to the extent that in such countries as Australia the selection of patients for hGH therapy is based solely upon anthropometric grounds rather than pharmacologic or physiologic tests of GH secretion.

III. GROWTH HORMONE EFFECTS

The objective of hGH therapy traditionally has been to increase the growth rate and adult height of short-statured GH-deficient children. The effectiveness of this therapy has been assessed through achievement of normal growth velocity and height. Linear growth promotion remains the focus of hGH therapy, but additional metabolic effects of hGH are being actively investigated for their potential clinical application. The major indirect actions of hGH are anabolic and growth promoting, mediated by insulin-like growth factors (principally IGF-I), and include cell proliferation and protein synthesis in both skeletal and nonskeletal tissues.

The IGFs are a family of peptides with molecular weight similar to that of insulin that have insulin-like activity (32,33).

Circulating IGFs are produced primarily by the liver in response to hGH stimulation and circulate bound to larger carrier proteins with molecular weight 28–150 kD. Because most organs synthesize IGFs (34), their action may occur within their cells of synthesis (autocrine), on cells in the immediate area (paracrine), and at distant sites (endocrine). The direct actions of hGH are those on lipid and fat metabolism, synergistic with cortisol and opposite to the actions of insulin and IGFs.

The most apparent metabolic effect of hGH is stimulation of linear growth in children before epiphyseal fusion. The relative roles of hGH and IGF-I in stimulating bone growth may be most accurately described by a "dual-effect" model of hGH action, in which hGH stimulates cartilage precursor cells first to differentiate and subsequently to produce, and become responsive to, the autocrine and paracrine mitogenic effects of IGF-I (35). The wide distribution of receptors for IGF-I (36), and the fact that blood levels of IGFs are higher than in any tissue, suggests that the endocrine function may also be important. However, administration of IGF-I to hypophysectomized rats does not promote growth equivalent to that of hGH (37). IGF-I also participates in negative feedback regulation of hGH secretion by stimulating hypothalamic somatostatin secretion (38) and by inhibiting the action of GHRH (39).

IGF-I is measured by radioimmunoassay, and its level correlates with the clinical state of hGH deficiency, sufficiency, or excess. Serum IGF-I levels are low in utero and in infancy, increase with age in both boys and girls, reach maximum values during puberty (earlier and higher in girls than boys), and decline to adult values as adolescence is completed (40). Although often used as part of the assessment of hypopituitarism, IGF-I levels do not exclusively reflect hGH production and are very age dependent. Concentrations of IGF-I correlate more closely with bone age and puberty (41) than with chronologic age (Fig. 3). Hypothyroidism, malnutrition, poorly controlled diabetes, and chronic disease may diminish secretion of IGF-I. Thus, a low serum IGF-I level is consistent with, but not diagnostic of, hGH deficiency. The normally low levels of IGF-I in infants and young children preclude its diagnostic utility for classic GH deficiency in this age group. Given these limitations, the use of IGF-I as a screening test for hGH status is of little diagnostic value but offers supportive information.

Other metabolic effects of hGH can be described as anabolic, lipolytic, and diabetogenic (Fig. 4). Growth hormone-induced growth acceleration is facilitated by concomitant enhancement of protein synthesis in bone, cartilage, skeletal muscles, the erythropoietic system, and other major organs. Administration of hGH produces positive nitrogen balance, increased amino acid transport into cells, increased intracellular RNA, and decreased urea production and blood urea nitrogen levels. The metabolic efficacy of total parenteral nutrition is also enhanced by hGH (42). A high normal or mildly elevated blood urea nitrogen level and low serum phosphorus and alkaline phosphatase level are usually observed in hGH deficiency (13) and reverse with GH treatment. Effects on mineral metabolism include increased intestinal

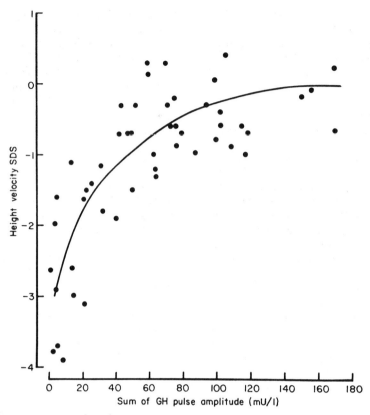

Figure 2 Relationship between height-velocity SDS for chronologic age and the sum of hGH pulse amplitudes. [With permission, Ref. 30, Hindmarsh P, Smith PJ, Brook CGD, Matthews DR. Clin Endocrinol (Oxf) 1987; 27:581–591.]

calcium absorption and urinary calcium excretion and reduced urinary phosphate excretion (43). Bone density and levels of osteocalcin, procollagen type I, and 1,25-dihydroxyvitamin D are reduced in hGH-deficient children and increase with long-term hGH therapy (44).

Growth hormone promotes site-specific free fatty acid release from adipose tissue, and GH-deficient children tend to demonstrate increased, predominantly abdominal, subcutaneous fat, which lessens and becomes more peripheral during therapy with exogenous hGH (45). Non–GH-deficient children also display a reduction in overall body fat during hGH therapy (46). The mechanism by which hGH reduces adipocyte size in vivo remains unclear, but in vitro studies suggest that hGH increases the basal rate of lipolysis and depresses reesterification of free fatty acids (47).

The effects of hGH on carbohydrate metabolism are complex. Intravenous administration of hGH causes an acute fall in blood glucose, most likely reflecting enhanced transport of glucose into adipose and skeletal muscle cells. In a child with hGH deficiency, insulin secretion is diminished, related in part to pancreatic islet cell hypoplasia. Glucose tolerance tests may reveal impaired ability to dispose of a carbohydrate load. However, hypoglycemia is common in such patients because of heightened sensitivity to insulin and may be a significant clinical problem. Administration of hGH reduces sensitivity to insulin, thereby correcting hypoglyce-

mia, and increases insulin secretion. The combined effects of hGH on both the release of and response to insulin create states of altered carbohydrate intolerance in situations of either hGH deficiency or excess.

IV. CLASSIC GROWTH HORMONE DEFICIENCY

The classic form of growth hormone deficiency is characterized by marked growth retardation, diminished growth velocity, delayed skeletal maturation, absence of other explanations for growth retardation, and subnormal secretion of hGH, both physiologic and in response to provocative stimuli. Genetic (e.g., altered hGH or GHRH gene), anatomic or congenital (e.g., midline cranial defects, septooptic dysplasia, or vascular malformations), and acquired abnormalities of the hypothalamus and pituitary (e.g., craniopharyngioma, glioma, or histiocytosis) are identifiable in many affected children. Evaluation of pituitary gland anatomy using magnetic resonance imaging has revealed a spectrum of more subtle morphologic abnormalities associated with the diagnosis of hGH deficiency (48). Irradiation or chemotherapy for malignancies and traumatic brain injury also cause organic hypopituitarism and account for an increasing incidence of hGH deficiency as survival of these individuals improves. Despite this growing list of etiologies, most children with hGH

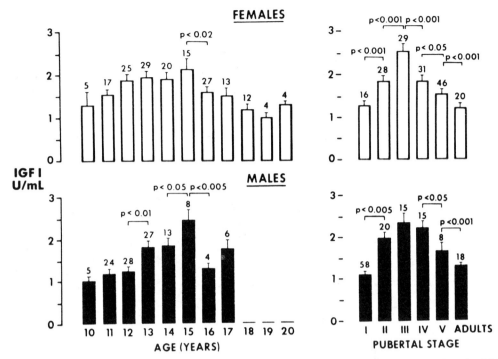

Figure 3 Serum IGF-I levels in females and males stratified by age and pubertal stage. (With permission, Grumbach MM, Styne DM. Puberty: ontogeny, neuroendocrinology, physiology, and disorders. In: Wilson JD, Foster DW, eds. Textbook of Endocrinology. Philadelphia: W.B. Saunders, 1992:1149.)

deficiency are still designated *idiopathic*, often because of apparently defective hypothalamic regulation of hGH release, rather than inability to synthesize hGH. It is likely that further improvement in imaging techniques will reveal additional organic lesions contributing to this dysfunction.

Idiopathic hGH deficiency usually occurs sporadically but may be familial (49). Its frequency has been reported to be from 1:4000 children to 1:60,000 (50,51). Although the latter figure is similar to the treated population in the United States before 1985, the true incidence of classic hGH deficiency is probably in the range of 1:10,000. These estimates are complicated by the fact that, with the exceptions of hGH gene deletion and severe pituitary or hypothalamic dysfunction, hGH deficiency is partial, rather than complete. The incidence of hGH deficiency is likely to rise during the 1990s because of prolonged survival of children who have received radiation therapy for malignancies.

Currently, arbitrary laboratory criteria provide a technical distinction between hGH deficiency and hGH sufficiency, even though it is generally accepted that there is no meaningful physiologic distinction between children whose provoked hGH levels fall slightly above or below laboratory threshold values. Evidence is accumulating to support the notion that hGH deficiency is not a distinct entity but rather a spectrum of disorders of hGH pulsatility. A continuum of hGH secretion may span essential absence of hGH, partial hGH deficiency, and a spectrum of "normal" hGH secretion (Fig. 5). Some investigators have found significant correlations between spontaneous hGH secretion and statural growth rates

(52); others have not (53). The blurring of what was once thought to be a clear distinction between hGH deficiency and sufficiency has combined with the luxury of available, expensive hGH to create new opportunities, uncertainties, and controversies in hGH therapy.

Profoundly hGH-deficient infants and young children may present initially with hypoglycemia. This may be associated with adrenocorticotropic hormone (ACTH) deficiency and hypocortisolism, but hypoglycemia often persists despite glucocorticoid replacement. Prompt administration of hGH is necessary to prevent the neurologic sequelae of persistent or recurrent hypoglycemia. Microphallus occurring in the newborn with hGH deficiency most often is associated with gonadotropin deficiency. Because hGH is largely responsible for phallic growth after the first few months of life, (untreated) isolated hGH-deficient males may display poor phallic growth during early childhood. This problem can be effectively treated with hGH and very small doses of androgen (54). Growth velocity may be mildly or severely impaired, depending upon the degree of hGH deficiency and/or presence of accompanying hormone deficiencies. Bone age (55) is usually delayed in hGH deficiency but is often less delayed than height age (age for which the child's height is average). Bone age is less delayed in isolated hGH deficiency than with multiple trophic hormone deficiencies. "Catch-up growth," a period of supranormal growth velocity often observed particularly during early hGH treatment, is accompanied by skeletal maturation proportional to growth achieved, leading to the *appearance* of accelerated bone age advancement.

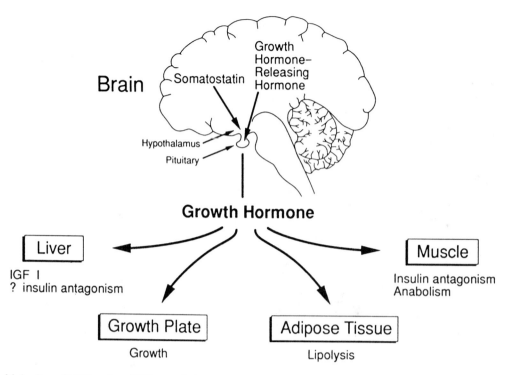

Figure 4 Multiple sites of hGH action. (With permission, Thorner MO, Vance ML, Horvath E, Kovacs K. The anterior pituitary. In: Wilson JD, Foster DW, eds. Textbook of Endocrinology. Philadelphia: W.B. Saunders, 1992:234.)

At least half the children with hGH deficiency were described in 1968 as having an isolated hormonal defect (56). This proportion has steadily risen as more children with partial or neurosecretory hGH deficiency have been recognized and diagnosed. A rise in hGH secretion and increase in growth velocity observed following pulsatile GHRH administration in many of these patients indicates that deficient the hypothalamic regulation of pituitary hGH secretion is the etiology of hGH deficiency in many patients with isolated hGH deficiency (57). However, hGH deficiency is often accompanied by deficiencies of other anterior pituitary hormones—adrenocroticotropic hormone, thyroid stimulating hormone (TSH), luteinizing hormone (LH), and follicle stimulating hormone (FSH)—and posterior pituitary antidiuretic hormone (ADH, synthesized in hypothalamic nuclei; see Chaps. 2 and 3). Hypopituitarism, the deficient production or release of one or more hormones from the pituitary, may be primary or secondary to hypothalamic dysfunction. When deficiencies other than hGH occur, they are, in decreasing order of frequency, LH and FSH, TSH, and ACTH (58).

Antidiuretic hormone deficiency, manifested as diabetes insipidus, usually occurs in acquired hGH deficiency (e.g., craniopharyngioma and surgical trauma). In contrast to anterior pituitary hormones, ADH is synthesized in the hypothalamus and transported to and stored for release in the posterior pituitary, which is embryologically distinct from the anterior pituitary. Consequently, deficiency of ADH is practically never seen with idiopathic hypopituitarism (59). On the other hand, extensive surgery for pituitary tumors usually results in ADH deficiency (if it was not present before) and variable but usually progressive loss of secretion of other pituitary hormones (60). A combination of less extensive surgery and irradiation, or irradiation alone, has been recommended as a more moderate approach to treatment of such patients (61). However, the gradual development of impaired hGH secretion is also observed in many children who receive cranial irradiation for neoplasms of the central nervous system (62). With radiation of the hypothalamic-pituitary axis, hGH is the first hormone to be affected, and the degree of hormonal deficit is related to the radiation dose (63). In one study, 5 years following 3.75–42.5 Gy radiation therapy, all patients were hGH deficient (Fig. 6); gonadotropin, ACTH, and TSH were deficient in 91, 77, and 42% of patients, respectively (64).

Timing of the onset of puberty normally is related most closely to a child's reaching a state of maturation (rather than chronologic age), corresponding to a bone age of 10–11 for girls and 12–13 for boys. Late recognition and treatment of hGH deficiency often results in delayed bone age and pubertal development. In addition, late diagnosis of hGH deficiency may not allow sufficient treatment time for height age to catch up to bone age before puberty; these children may experience rapid pubertal development without an adequate pubertal increment in height, resulting in adult short stature. The advent of LH releasing hormone agonist therapy, which can slow or stop pubertal advancement, may offer an effective means of "reclaiming" the time required for sufficient growth (65), but further controlled studies are needed to evaluate the

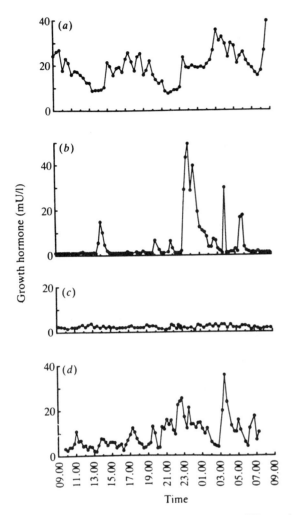

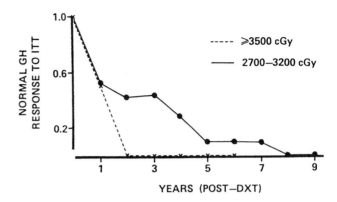

Figure 6 Incidence of GH deficiency in children receiving either 27–32 or 35 Gy cranial irradiation for a brain tumor in relation to the time from irradiation. (With permission from Littley MD. Radiation and the hypothalamic-pituitary axis. In: Radiation Injury to the Nervous System. New York: Raven Press, 1991:311.)

Figure 5 Four serum profiles of 24 h endogenous GH secretion from four 6-year-old boys. (a) Child with pituitary gigantism growing 7 cm/year. (b) Normal tall boy growing 7 cm/year. (c) Boy with GH deficiency growing 3 cm/year. (d) Boy with dysfunctional GH secretion growing 4 cm/year (note lack of return to baseline values between pulses). (Reprinted with permission from Brook CGD, Hindmarsh PC, Stanhope R. J Endocrinol 1988; 119:179–184.)

efficacy of this treatment. A preferable option is prompt recognition of hGH deficiency and optimization of hGH dosage and schedule, which facilitate both the achievement of normal prepubertal height and entrance into puberty at a more appropriate chronologic age.

V. TREATMENT OF GROWTH HORMONE DEFICIENCY

For over 30 years, the diagnosis of hGH deficiency was based on the analysis of serum hGH levels following at least two provocative stimuli. The limited amount of available pituitary-extracted hGH dictated that few short children could be

treated. Criteria were established by national committees of the National Pituitary Agency (which later became the National Hormone and Pituitary Program, NHPP) to ensure that the most severely affected hGH-deficient children would receive hGH treatment. Thus, only very short, very slowly growing children who had very low hGH levels on stimulation tests (66) qualified for hGH therapy, and these children were treated only until a height within −2 to −2.5 standard deviations (SD) of normal adult height was reached. This meticulous rationing of scarce hGH to the most severely affected children maximized the overal benefit that could be derived from this therapy.

Improved pituitary collection and extraction strategies increased the availability of hGH during the 1970s, and as a result, the criteria for treatment were relaxed. Whereas stimulated levels of hGH less than 3–5 ng/dl were originally considered sufficiently subnormal to indicate hGH deficiency, the threshold hGH level required for this diagnosis gradually rose to 7 ng/dl, then 10 ng/dl, and, in some clinics, 12 ng/dl. Currently, children with levels in the higher subnormal range (and children with normal stimulated hGH levels but low spontaneous hGH secretion) are now designated as having "partial" hGH deficiency.

Interpretation of tests for hGH is also complicated by laboratory variation: whereas the NHPP originally provided uniform material standards, and methodology for hGH testing, later commercialization of hGH assay methods created enormous variation in laboratory values for hGH in a single blood sample (63). Today, expanding definitions of partial hGH deficiency variations in hGH assays and unlimited hGH availability have transformed the historically clearly defined and tightly regulated practice of diagnosing and treating hGH deficiency into a rapidly evolving and controversial endeavor.

Growth failure caused by severe hGH deficiency is a universally accepted therapeutic indication for hGH treatment. Treatment of growth failure as a result of partial hGH deficiency, defined by subnormal stimulated hGH levels, has also become standard practice (68,69). However, it is now widely recognized that children with partial or subtle defects in the secretion of hGH are difficult to identify, and no individual assessment of hGH secretion or hGH-associated biochemical findings unerringly detects such subjects (70). A single provocative test for hGH (a necessary but not sufficient criterion for these diagnoses) appears to lack both specificity and sensitivity in identifying hGH insufficiency. In as many as 20% of children of normal stature, stimulated hGH levels may be <7 ng/ml (71). Specificity may be increased by performance of a second provocative test. On the other hand, a normal hGH response to provocative stimuli does not guarantee sufficient spontaneous hGH to maintain normal growth (72).

Attempts to define milder forms of hGH through frequent blood sampling and analysis of spontaneous hGH secretory pattern have led to the development of elaborate mathematical techniques for their interpretation. Children with subnormal hGH secretion following cranial irradiation, who may pass provocative hGH testing, may be identified solely by this frequent sampling method. [Over time, classic hGH deficiency develops in many of these patients (73).] However, determination of spontaneous hGH secretion requires considerable time, expense, and technical help and is complicated by technical difficulties, disturbed daily and nighttime routines of the patients, and lack of reproducibility (74,75). Current methods have been criticized for their inability to discriminate normal children from short, hGH-reponsive children, and even from classic hGH-deficient children. In summary, measurement and analysis of spontaneous hGH secretion are sometimes helpful in identifying hGH-sufficient subjects but add little in most instances to provocative tests in the identification of the hGH-deficient child. With either test, the notion of a discrete cutoff level of hGH secretion

that reliably distinguishes hGH deficiency from normal is historical and has limited relevance to current practice in pediatric endocrinology. The diagnosis of mild forms of hGH insufficiency depends primarily upon clinical perception; laboratory tests of hGH secretion provide ancillary information that helps to confirm or disprove the clinical diagnosis.

Various studies of time of initiation, dosage, and frequencies of hGH administration have advanced progress toward optimal treatment of hGH deficiency during childhood. Subcutaneous hGH administration is currently preferred while intranasal (76) and possibly long-acting preparations are being developed. Because growth before puberty is a major determinant of final adult height, early initiation of hGH treatment allows more complete normalization of height before puberty and an improved final height prognosis (Fig. 7) (77). There can be a temptation to defer injection therapy in young children to minimize discomfort and inconvenience, but the available evidence strongly supports early recognition, referral, diagnosis, and treatment of severely hGH-deficient patients as an important step toward optimizing their growth potential.

Increasing the dose of hGH improves growth rate; a dose-response equation derived from treatment of children of all ages with various degrees of hGH deficiency reveals a logarithmic relationship between hGH dose and growth rate for thrice weekly doses ranging from 0.015 to 0.1 mg/kg (Fig. 8) (78). The variation around the mean of each of these growth rate points is great, attesting to the poorly understood contribution of factors other than hGH levels to the normal linear growth process. Clinical studies of somatrem (methionyl hGH) in hGH-deficient children revealed that first-year growth rates improved from 8.5 cm/year using 0.05 mg/kg three times per week to 10.5 cm/year using 0.1 mg/kg three times per week (79). Recent studies implementing daily hGH

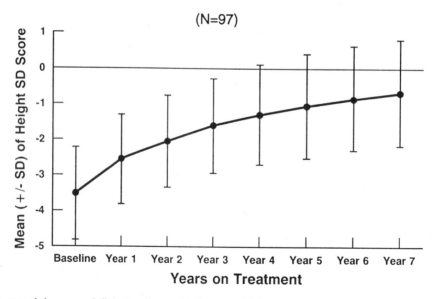

Figure 7 Long-term growth hormone-deficient patients with 7 years of follow-up: mean height standardized by age and sex. (With permission from the National Cooperative Growth Study, Genentech, Inc.)

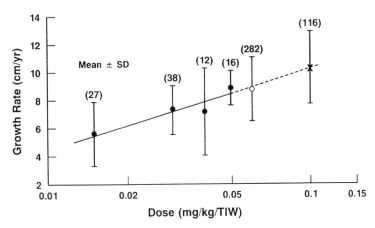

Figure 8 Growth hormone dose-response curve: naive growth hormone-deficient patients during the first 12 months of therapy. (With permission, Ref. 78, Frasier D, Costin G, Lippe BM, Aceto T, Bunge PF. J Clin Endocrinol Metab 1981; 53:1213–1217; and from the National Cooperative Growth Study, Genentech, Inc.)

injections have confirmed the relationship between growth rate and dose (80). Younger age, greater delay in height age and bone age, and greater severity of hGH deficiency based upon provocative testing each correlates with improved response to hGH therapy. The serum IGF-I response to hGH is also dose dependent, continuing to rise as hGH is administered in doses above currently prescribed levels (81). Trials of increased hGH dosage are currently underway, but it remains unclear to what extent higher doses of hGH improve growth or increase adverse effects. Current dosage recommendations for hGH range from 0.18 to 0.3 mg/kg/week.

Increased frequency of hGH administration improves growth rate, providing further evidence that the "pulsing" message of hGH to its target cells, in addition to adequacy of hGH levels, enhances linear growth. When the same weekly dose is given in daily injections rather than three times per week, an improvement in first-year growth rate of about 1.5 cm/year is observed (82). Nocturnal administration, which more closely mimics physiologic hGH secretion, may also add to efficacy (83), although this is not consistently observed. Regardless of the regimen chosen, the effect of hGH wanes with time, and the first year of treatment usually produces the greatest growth increment. Following this early phase of rapid growth, short-term increased replacement doses of hGH have been shown to produce renewed catch-up growth without adverse metabolic effects (84). Seasonal variations in growth rate during hGH therapy, with peaks in the summer and nadirs in the winter (North American population), have also been described (85).

Children from whom craniopharyngioma has been removed frequently experience growth acceleration in the absence of measurable hGH, a phenomenon that is unexplained but may be attributable to the postoperative hyperinsulinemia (86). Polyphagia and significant weight gain are usually also observed. Supplementation with hGH is not required while normal growth velocity is maintained. Avoidance of excessive cortisol replacement therapy is extremely important in these individuals. This growth pattern may persist for 1–2 years, allowing attainment of normal adult stature without hGH therapy.

The distinct augmentation of hGH pulsations (87) and increased production rates that occur during normal puberty raise the question of whether hGH replacement doses also should be increased during puberty. Insufficient dose and frequency of hGH administration have been shown to permit epiphyseal closure in hGH-deficient adolescents before adequate catch-up growth, thereby reducing expected adult height (88). In one recent study, doubling the dose of hGH during puberty did not significantly change growth rate but tended to advance pubertal maturation (89). Thus, the most effective frequency and dose of hGH therapy during puberty are yet to be determined.

Children treated with hGH may experience transient or persistent declines in serum thyroxine (T_4) levels; in approximately 25%, T_4 levels become abnormally low and impair response to hGH (68). Thyroid function tests should be monitored periodically (especially early) during hGH therapy to ensure detection of secondary T_4 deficiency and prevent this treatable cause of a poor response to hGH. Cortisol supplementation may also impair the growth response to hGH; as little as 7.5–10 mg/day of hydrocortisone may be growth suppressive in a school-age child. Thus, when ACTH deficiency has been documented, the dosage of daily cortisol replacement therapy should be reduced to a level sufficient to prevent symptoms of fatigue and lack of energy. In prepubertal children, these replacement levels are quite low, and some children with idiopathic hypopituitarism, even with evidence for ACTH deficiency, do not need cortisone replacement in the absence of illness or stress.

Testosterone or other anabolic agents enhance the growth velocity of a prepubertal hGH-deficient child taking hGH, but they (except for boys with microphallus) should not be given if the bone age is less than 9 years, and then in very low doses initially. Treatment for the purpose of virilization in a boy who is gonadotropin deficient should be initiated with low dosage (e.g., 50 mg intramuscular testosterone enanthate per month or 2.5 mg oxandrolone orally four times per day) to prevent accelerated epiphyseal maturation. Doses can be gradually increased to adult replacement levels (e.g., 200–300 mg testosterone enanthate every month) over the next several years. Oxandrolone in low dosages has also been useful in accelerating growth rate in girls. It is unknown whether estrogens have an accelerating effect on the growth resulting from hGH therapy; however, they have a potent effect on bone age acceleration in Turner syndrome patients.

With early diagnosis, careful attention to accompanying hormonal deficiencies, and progressive dose adjustments, children with hGH deficiency reach normal adult height (65). Bone age advances with hGH treatment, but usually no more than height age. Linear growth often accelerates faster than bone age following initiation of hGH therapy, leading to increases in predicted final height. During spontaneous puberty or sex hormone replacement therapy, however, undue acceleration in bone age maturation may limit ultimate stature. Even with successful long-term hGH therapy, correction of disabling short stature does not consistently normalize the psychosocial outcome for adults with hGH deficiency (90). Psychosocial counseling, which increases both therapeutic compliance during childhood and social outcome during adulthood (91), should be a consistent adjunct to parenteral hGH administration.

VI. CAUSES OF SHORT STATURE OTHER THAN hGH DEFICIENCY THAT MAY RESPOND TO GROWTH HORMONE TREATMENT

For every short child who has impaired hGH secretion, many more are short for other reasons. Parental concerns about the disadvantages of their child's short stature are legitimized by a "heightist" premise in the modern United States: to be tall is good, and to be short is to be stigmatized (92). The preponderance of white males in the hGH-treated population suggests that these social pressures give rise to ascertainment of short-statured patients biased by sex, race, and socioeconomic status (93). Stigmatization based upon height begins

in childhood. Feelings of incompetence and low self-esteem may arise from the short child's struggle with stature, although these problems may depend as much on the projection of parental perceptions of their child's vulnerability and immaturity as on short stature per se (94). Future studies investigating improvement in quality of life, as well as improved statural growth, of non–GH-deficient children treated with hGH will be of paramount importance.

Since the previous edition of this text, the medical literature has been replete with reports of non–hGH-deficient children treated with hGH, and numerous studies continue to investigate new indications for hGH (Table 1). Many extraordinarily short children have overlapping diagnostic conditions (e.g., familial short stature and constitutional growth delay), which complicates interpreting the response of a specific condition to hGH therapy. The discussion here reviews specific disorders that have undergone investigational trials to date.

A. Familial Short Stature (FSS) or Constitutional Growth Delay (CGD)

The prospect that hGH therapy may accelerate growth and increase adult height of markedly short but otherwise healthy children has generated great interest and debate. Serum hGH concentrations are usually normal in these children; however, children with severe CGD may demonstrate temporary failure to secrete hGH in response to stimuli, which normalizes with pubertal progression or induction (95,96). The finding that 10–15% of adults diagnosed as hGH deficient during childhood have normal hGH levels later suggests that this phenomenon is more common than generally recognized. Thus, repeat provocative testing for hGH following short-term sex hormone treatment is advisable before considering a commitment to hGH therapy for most nearly pubertal patients who fit the clinical criteria for CGD.

Administration of hGH at dosages used to treat hGH deficiency increases growth velocity in the majority of these children throughout at least 3 years of treatment. A controlled

Table 1 Statural Disorders and Metabolic Conditions for Which hGH Treatment Has Been Investigated

Familial short stature	Catabolic states
Constitutional delayed growth	Glucocorticoid-dependent disorders
Intrauterine growth retardation:	(renal transplant, asthma)
Russell-Silver syndrome	Postoperative wound healing
Turner syndrome	Burns
Skeletal dysplasia	Regenerative or reparative states
Hypochondroplasia	Fractures
Achondroplasia	Peripheral nerve damage
Spondyloepiphyseal dysplasia	Neural tube defects
Multiple epiphyseal dysplasia	Spina bifida
Vitamin D-resistant rickets	Myelomeningocele
Miscellaneous syndromes	Chronic illness
Noonan syndrome	Chronic renal failure
Prader-Willi syndrome	Cystic fibrosis
Down syndrome	Aging
Growth hormone deficiency in adults	

study reported that mean growth velocity increased during the first year, from 5.3 to 7.4 cm/year, and height SD score increased by 0.63 in hGH-treated children versus no change in velocity or SD score for untreated children (97). Growth rates declined during each successive year of therapy and, in one study, approximated pretreatment growth velocity by the fourth year (98). In a more recent study, however, daily hGH therapy during years 2 and 3 sustained growth rates of 7.6 and 7.2 cm/year, respectively, compared with the baseline growth rate of 4.6 cm/year (99). Short, non–hGH-deficient children who demonstrate sustained acceleration of growth rate on hGH therapy have attained prepubertal heights that are closer to but do not exceed their genetic height potential (100). In each of these studies, no clinical (e.g., pretreatment growth rate) or biochemical determinants (e.g., overnight endogenous hGH secretion) reliably predicted the individual response to hGH therapy. Some investigators report that the year 1 growth response to hGH is the best predictor of growth in subsequent years, suggesting that a clinical trial of hGH and periodic assessment of ongoing hGH responsiveness are necessary to identify individuals who will derive significant benefit from treatment.

Information regarding the efficacy of hGH in improving the final height of children with FSS or CGD is limited.

Short-term acceleration of growth rate is unlikely to increase final height, because a transient period of slowed growth frequently follows cessation of hGH therapy. Similarly, hGH treatment that improves growth might not improve ultimate stature if it induces an earlier onset or faster tempo of puberty. Because height at onset of puberty is a more important determinant of adult height than pubertal growth (because prepubertal growth normally contributes 85% of final height), the most effective hGH therapy will require substantial growth acceleration before puberty. Increases in standardized Bayley-Pinneau predictions of adult height have been consistently reported during prepubertal hGH therapy, but these gains do not improve substantially during treatment of pubertal subjects (Fig. 9) (99). Onset of puberty appears to occur at the expected time in hGH-treated children with FSS or CGD, but an accelerated tempo of puberty has been noted in boys (101). This possible decrement in height acquired during puberty probably accounts for reports of actual final heights of hGH-treated children, which fall short of earlier more optimistic height predictions (102). Thus, it remains unclear whether administration of hGH at currently recommended doses to non–hGH-deficient individuals during puberty is beneficial or detrimental to overall pubertal growth. Alternative strategies include administration of a high dose of hGH

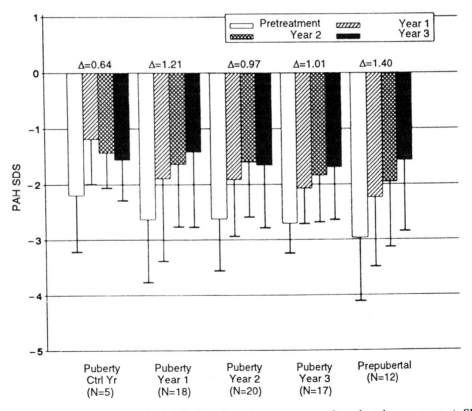

Figure 9 Bayley-Pinneau–predicted adult height (PAH) SDS for each treatment year by pubertal group mean ± SD. The change in PAH (delta) from before treatment to year 3 of treatment is shown for the pubertal groups based on year of treatment in which subjects entered puberty. Although overall gains were significant in each group ($p < 0.05$), there were no statistical differences among groups. (Reprinted with permission from Ref. 000, Hopwood N, et al. J Pediatr 1990; 123:215–222.)

for 2 years before puberty to achieve normalization of adolescent height, precluding the need for hGH therapy during puberty (103). Only after long-term studies reveal the final heights of hGH-treated individuals with FSS or CGD, and these results are compared with the costs and potential risks, can the value of this therapy be assessed.

B. Turner Syndrome (TS)

Between 95 and 100% of girls with TS experience growth failure, and the untreated mean final height of these patients is 143 cm (104). Growth curves specific for TS have been developed by European investigators, and North American patients closely match these data (105). An individual's height percentiles on this TS curve do not change from childhood to adulthood if they remain untreated. During childhood, average growth velocity is 4.44 cm for each year of bone age advancement. The lower final height results from the combined effects of a lack of a pubertal growth spurt (caused by ovarian failure to produce estrogens), abnormalities in growth plate cartilage (106), and a possible resistance to the action of hGH. Studies clearly show that TS patients do not have classic hGH deficiency, although endogenous hGH levels (107,108) and urinary hGH levels (109) are below normal after the age of 8 years. Estrogen administration, which increases hGH secretion, and oxandrolone, which accelerates growth through an apparent direct effect on growing cartilage, can accelerate growth rates in TS patients but have not been shown to increase final height.

With the exception of hGH-deficient children, girls with TS have received the longest trials of hGH therapy (up to 10 years). A multicenter prospective randomized trial of hGH, alone and in combination with oxandrolone, was begun in 1983 and now provides data on 62 patients who have received 3–6 years of hGH therapy. During the first year, growth rates increased from 3–4 to 6–8 cm/year. A hGH dose of 125% of that given to growth hormone-deficient patients or the addition of oxandrolone were both associated with higher growth rates (110). Similar results with short-term hGH treatment have been reported by others (111,112). During subsequent years of treatment, growth rates declined but remained higher than those of untreated girls. Of 17 girls receiving hGH alone, 14 equaled or exceeded their original projected adult heights, and 41 of 45 girls receiving combined oxandrolone-hGH therapy have done so (see Chap. 19). The mean height of 30 girls who completed therapy is 151.9 cm, a gain of 8.1 cm over the expected average height without treatment (113). These results suggest that an adult height above the lower limit of normal for U.S. women (150 cm) is now an attainable goal for many girls with this syndrome. Although still considered experimental in the United States, there is a growing consensus that hGH therapy is warranted for girls with TS whose height falls below the third percentile.

Adverse effects of hGH therapy in TS patients have been minimal. Osteopenia is more prevalent in TS, but bone mineral status is not impaired (and may be improved) in hGH-treated adolescents with TS (114). Autoantibodies to endocrine organs also occur in TS with increased frequency; hGH therapy does not alter immune function in TS (115). Glucose tolerance is of particular interest given the increased incidence of diabetes mellitus in adults with TS and the diabetogenic action of hGH. Frequency of impaired glucose tolerance is increased in children with TS over normal. Investigations to date have revealed no significant change in glucose tolerance tests or levels of glycosylated hemoglobin during hGH therapy (116). However, obese patients or patients with high insulin concentrations before start of hGH therapy may be at greater risk for deterioration (117). Elevations in plasma insulin concentrations are more frequent when hGH therapy is combined with oxandrolone, which may also impair glucose tolerance by induction of insulin resistance (117).

C. Intrauterine Growth Retardation (IUGR)

For some children with IUGR, the pattern of growth continues to be abnormal from intrauterine life to full maturity. Included in this group are children with dysmorphic features compatible with Russell-Silver syndrome. Even though bone age is often delayed early in childhood, the adolescent growth spurt usually occurs early and is reduced in magnitude (118). Although a minority of these children display subnormal spontaneous or provoked hGH concentrations, the results of these tests do not predict their responsiveness to hGH.

In a study reported more than 20 years ago, approximately 50% of prepubertal children with IUGR responded to twice or thrice weekly hGH injections with significant growth acceleration (119). Recent studies of daily administration of hGH reveal consistent increases in short-term growth velocity (e.g., from 6.7 to 10.4 cm/year) (120); greater increments in growth velocity have been achieved with higher hGH doses (121). Prolonged (3 years) hGH treatment of children with IUGR sustains an accelerated growth rate but has not increased height for bone age score, pointing to an unaltered final height outcome (122). Whether these children derive substantial psychologic benefits from a more rapid tempo of growth during childhood (even without enhanced final stature) remains uncertain. It is noted that the difficulty of accurately assessing bone age maturation in dysmorphic syndromes, such as Russell-Silver syndrome, may reduced the validity of predicted heights. Therefore, continuation of these clinical trials until final height is required to determine the efficacy of hGH for IUGR. Given the accelerated tempo of puberty in these patients, administration of gonadotrophic releasing hormone analog to permit a longer period of growth may be indicated for severely height-disabled individuals with IUGR.

D. Chronic Renal Failure (CRF)

Poor nutrition, anemia, and chronic metabolic acidosis contribute to the growth failure characteristic of CRF. In addition, elevated fasting hGH levels, exaggerated responses to provocative stimuli, depressed serum IGF-I levels, and increased levels of IGF-I binding protein suggest resistance to the action of hGH (123). Pharmacologic doses of hGH are able to overcome these growth-retarding influences in some patients with CRF. These salient effects may reflect metabolic effects of hGH (e.g., enhanced renal acid excretion) (124) in addition to its direct growth-promoting effect. A recent randomized double-blind placebo-controlled study of 125 prepubertal growth-retarded children with CRF revealed first-year (10.7 ± 3.1 cm/year) and second-year (7.8 ± 2.1 cm/year) growth rates in the hGH-treated group; these growth rates were significantly greater than those seen in the placebo group in the first (6.5 ± 2.6 cm/year) and second (5.5 ± 1.9 cm/year) years of study. Improved final height potential was suggested by an increment in height age that exceeded that of bone age (125). In general, responsiveness to hGH appears to be inversely related to the degree of renal function impairment and metabolic compromise. Multicenter trials continue to determine the effect of hGH on long-term growth of children with CRF.

Growth hormone excess produces hyperfiltration and increases glomerular sclerosis in the setting of uremia (126), raising a theoretical concern that hGH treatment of children with CRF could accelerate deterioration in renal function. However, current information suggests no adverse effect of hGH therapy on glomerular filtration rate (GFR); loss of GFR is unchanged during the first year of hGH treatment compared with the year before treatment (125,127). Reports of accelerated rises in serum creatinine may reflect increased body size and creatinine production without a commensurate increase in GFR (128). Thus, growth itself, rather than hGH, may place additional metabolic demands upon compromised but stable renal function. Hyperinsulinemia, often present before hGH therapy as a result of uremic insulin resistance, may remain stable (129) or worsen (127) during hGH therapy. However, glucose homeostasis, assessed by oral glucose tolerance testing and glycosylated hemoglobin levels, has remained stable.

E. Skeletal Dysplasias

Numerous forms of skeletal dysplasia may cause significant growth retardation. Detailed descriptions of clinical and radiologic features and inheritance patterns belie a lack of understanding of the basic pathophysiology for most of these disorders. Patients with achondroplasia demonstrate normal secretion of hGH, IGF-I levels, and IGF-I receptor activity (130) and do not appear to respond favorably to hGH, even when higher than conventional doses are used (131).

A short-term study of hGH therapy in children with hypochondroplasia showed an increase in first-year growth rate, which was proportionally distributed between limb and spine growth (132). Variation in response to hGH with regard to rate and proportionality of growth has also been reported and may be related to defects in the IGF-I gene in some patients (133). Growth response to hGH is generally less than that observed in children treated for classic hGH deficiency and declines after initial acceleration (132). Thus, at best, only modest improvement in adult height can be expected from currently used regimens of hGH therapy. Preliminary trials of hGH therapy for spondyloepiphyseal dysplasia and multiple epiphyseal dysplasia are in progress.

F. Glucocorticoid-Treated Children

Treatment of many chronic disorders (e.g., juvenile rheumatoid arthritis, asthma, renal transplantation, and inflammatory bowel disease), which themselves may lead to growth failure, includes glucocorticoid therapy. Glucocorticoids (GC) impede linear growth through several mechanisms, including promoting protein catabolism, inhibiting collagen synthesis, impairing the action of IGF-I, and suppressing endogenous hGH secretion through augmentation of hypothalamic somatostatin tone (134). These patients, who may demonstrate iatrogenic hGH insufficiency comparable to "neurosecretory dysfunction" (135), could be considered logical candidates to benefit from both the growth-promoting and anabolic effects of hGH therapy.

Early studies implementing relatively low dose and infrequent administration of hGH demonstrated marginal and inconsistent beneficial effects (136). Recent investigations of daily hGH therapy for children with stable GC-treated illness (137) or postrenal transplantation (138) show more consistent resumption of normal growth velocity during 1–3 years of treatment. Biochemical markers of growth (e.g., type I procollagen levels) are also normalized by hGH administration (137). Responsiveness to hGH appears greatest in those on moderate-dose GC regimens with stable, nonarthritic underlying disease. Reversal of GC-mediated protein catabolism (139) by hGH is an additional potential benefit requiring further study in the clinical setting.

A particular concern is that GC-induced insulin resistance could be exacerbated by hGH. Current doses of hGH do not appear to cause deterioration in carbohydrate metabolism, although some obese or pubertal patients or patients on high-dose glucocorticoid therapy have shown (reversible) increases in hyperinsulinemia and postprandial blood glucose levels (137). For these few patients, the risk of temporarily compromised glucose metabolism is unknown and must be balanced against the severity of growth disturbance. Increased doses of hGH, required either to sustain prolonged growth acceleration or to overcome larger doses of GC, may be more consistently detrimental to glucose homeostasis. Thus, hGH treatment of GC-dependent children, many of whom fit the criteria for "classic" hGH deficiency based upon provocative testing, should be carefully monitored and conducted within a treatment protocol.

G. Other Syndromes and Defects Associated with Short Stature

Short stature is a component of more than 100 syndromes. Subnormal secretion of hGH has been reported in some children with Down syndrome (140) and Prader-Willi syndrome (141). Preliminary treatment trials of these children show short-term responses to hGH similar to those of Russell-Silver syndrome and Turner syndrome. Anecdotal improvements in weight control have been reported in children with Prader-Willi syndrome. Short stature is also a common problem in children with neural tube defects, such as spina bifida or myelomeningocele, who may have spinal and/or lower abnormalities. Secretion of hGH is normal unless accompanying hydrocephalus impairs hypothalamic-pituitary function. In a small group of patients with neural tube defects, brief courses of hGH therapy increased annual growth velocity from 1.7 to 7.9 cm (142).

The expansion of hGH therapy into populations affected by mental disability or with limited ambulatory capability raises complex ethical questions by focusing attention on the expectation that successful hGH therapy ought to improve the quality of life, rather than merely the height, of treated individuals (143). For each of these groups of patients, analysis of larger, longer prospective trials, conducted within an hGH investigational protocol, are needed before recommendations about efficacy can be made. When this information is available, treatment decisions can be made for individual patients (rather than diagnostic groups) based upon degree of disability and likelihood of long-term enhancement of quality of life.

H. Adults with GH Deficiency and the Elderly

The increased availability of hGH has invigorated the option of extending hGH replacement therapy into adulthood. The function of hGH during normal adult life is unknown, but recent evidence suggests that lack of hGH leads to contraction of lean body mass and water, expansion of fat mass, and diminution of bone mineral content. Adults with hypopituitarism are known to have decreased life expectancy. Placebo-

controlled studies of hGH therapy in adults with complete hGH deficiency have revealed a marked increase in muscle mass, decrease in fat mass (Fig. 10) (144,145), and improvements in exercise performance (146). Subjective improvements in quality of life indicators, such as vigor, ambition, and sense of well-being, are also reported (145, 147).

The adverse effects of fluid retention (e.g., edema and carpal tunnel syndrome) occur frequently but reverse with dose reduction or continuation of the same dose. Appropriate replacement doses for adults may be approximately one-half those traditionally used for hGH-deficient children (145). Costs remain a formidable barrier, but a consensus is growing that the beneficial effects of hGH for hGH-deficient adults are of sufficient magnitude to warrant treatment. Should this become a reality, future allocation of hGH to adult patients will be complicated by diagnostic ambiguities as the relatively large number of today's children with the diagnosis of partial hGH deficiency reach adulthood.

The normal decline in the activity of the hGH-IGF-I axis that occurs with advancing age appears to contribute to the decrease in lean body mass, increase in adipose tissue mass, and, possibly, loss of energy. Administration of hGH to non–hGH-deficient men over 60 years old caused significant increases in lean body mass, bone density, and skin thickness, with concomitant reductions in fat mass (148). Following hGH therapy, deterioration in these parameters resumed in an age-appropriate fashion. The implications of such therapy are

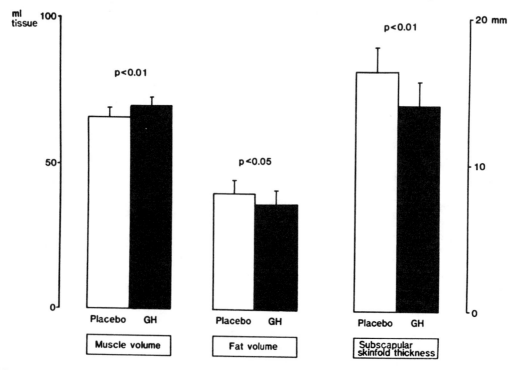

Figure 10 Mean ± standard error of the mean values of muscle and fat tissue volume and subscapular skinfold thickness at the end of the placebo and GH treatment period in adults. Muscle and fat volume are expressed in milliliters and measured by computed tomographic scan of a 0.8 cm cross-sectional slice of the midthigh region. (Reprinted with permission from Ref. 150, Jorgensen PH, Andreassen TT. Horm Metabol Res 1988; 20:490–493.)

enticing, but the risk-benefit ratio and cost effectiveness of hGH therapy in the general aging but healthy population are far from being established. Administration of hGH has also been used by younger adults in conjunction with heavy resistance exercise training in an effort to maximize skeletal muscle protein anabolism and strength. However, in a placebo-controlled study of young normal men, resistance training supplemented with hGH did not further enhance muscle anabolism and function (149). These results suggest that the increased fat-free mass seen with hGH supplementation was probably caused by an increase in lean tissue other than skeletal muscle.

I. Catabolic States

The well-documented anabolic effects of hGH have long stimulated interest in its possible ability to modify the course of catabolic, regenerative, or reparative states. The availability of recombinant DNA hGH has facilitated such investigations. Animal studies suggest that tissue mechanical strength and collagen formation are increased by pretreatment with hGH (150). The results of clinical studies, however, have been conflicting. Nitrogen balance is generally improved by hGH in postoperative patients even under hypocaloric conditions (151). Growth hormone also improves the efficiency of parenteral nutrient utilization in patients requiring total parenteral nutrition (13). These effects of hGH therapy have created interest in its use as ancillary therapy for chronic illnesses characterized by poor nutrition (e.g., cystic fibrosis and regional ileitis). Preliminary studies suggest that hGH treatment can reduce healing time for burns and speed acceptance of burn grafts (152). Savings in the costs of hospitalization could be expected to outweigh the cost of the drug. However, a placebo-controlled trial in normal adults showed that full-thickness wound healing was significantly *delayed* by hGH therapy (153). Growth hormone may also partially reverse nitrogen wasting in obese humans made catabolic by dietary restriction (154). During the next decade, we can look forward to considerable new knowledge about the anabolic effects of hGH in these and related settings.

VII. ADVERSE EFFECTS OF hGH TREATMENT

Recombinant biosynthetic hGH preparations are highly purified and free of contaminants (Table 2). The possibility of viral transmission through hGH has been essentially eliminated. However, surveillance of patients who received pituitary-derived hGH for development of Creutzfeldt-Jakob remains important. Antigenicity of hGH preparations is also low (155), although hGH antibodies can be detected in 10–30% of treated children. With rare exceptions (less than 0.1%), these antibodies do not impede the biologic effects of hGH.

As mentioned, hypothyroidism may develop in as many as 25% of hGH-deficient children treated with hGH. Declines in serum T_4 levels may reflect increased peripheral conversion of T_4 to triiodothyronine (156). An increased frequency of

slipped capital femoral epiphysis has been reported during treatment with hGH (157), although the precise contribution of hGH to this complication is unclear. Edema and sodium retention may occur early in the course of hGH therapy (particularly in older, heavier children and adolescents), attributable to an antinatriuretic effect on the renal tubule of hGH, IGF-I, or insulin. This effect abates with continued therapy. Pseudotumor cerebri has been reported rarely during hGH therapy; most instances have occurred in patients with other risk factors for this condition. Cessation of hGH therapy has reversed the symptoms in reported cases, and some patients experience spontaneous resolution of symptoms despite continued hGH treatment (158). Resumption of hGH treatment has been successfully accomplished with reinitiation at a lower dose and gradual return to the initial dose.

Until recently, hGH was used almost exclusively as replacement therapy for hGH deficiency. Other potential adverse effects of hGH therapy may be induced in non–GH-deficient (and GH-deficient) children by pharmacologic hGH augmentation therapy. Current recommendations for hGH dosage, derived largely from growth response data, are in excess of calculated estimates of normal hGH production in a child. The finding of IGF-I levels in hGH-treated girls with Turner syndrome that approach those found in acromegaly (159) supports the presence of a relative hGH excess. Anecdotal reports of the development of acromegaloid features (e.g., large hands and feet) during higher than conventional dose hGH therapy have appeared. In short non–GH-deficient children and in Turner syndrome patients, hGH therapy frequently increases insulin production but does not impair glucose disposal (160). Thus, normal levels of blood glucose and glycosylated hemoglobin may indicate compensated rather than normal carbohydrate metabolism. Persistent hyperinsulinemia is associated with the development of atherosclerosis and hypertension, but it is far from clear whether (temporarily) elevated insulin levels coincident with hGH therapy lead to harmful consequences. Only careful long-term evaluation of individuals during and after hGH therapy will resolve this issue.

Perhaps the greatest concern regarding hGH therapy is the theoretical possibility that hGH could facilitate the devel-

Table 2 Potential Side Effects of Human Growth Hormone Treatment

Physiologic replacement doses
  Growth attenuation from antibody formation
  Hypothyroidism
  Slipped femoral capital epiphysis
  Possible increased risk of leukemia
Pharmacologic doses
  Hyperinsulinism
  Possible glucose intolerance
  Salt and water retention
  Pseudotumor cerebri
  Acromegaloid features

opment of cancers. Growth hormone is mitogenic, and there is evidence in animals of a cause-and-effect relation between supraphysiologic doses of hGH and the development of leukemia (161). In 1988, a cluster of leukemia cases occurred in Japan among hGH-treated, hGH-deficient children (162). A recent survey of U.S. and Canada patients revealed a total of nine cases of leukemia among children exposed to hGH therapy. All but three had additional risk factors for malignancy, including previous radiation or chemotherapy or surgery for brain tumors without radiation (163). Similar findings were reported in an extended follow-up study of 6284 recipients of pituitary-derived hGH; the relative risk of leukemia in recipients of hGH was 2.6 (90% confidence interval 1.2–5.2). Of six subjects five had antecedent cranial tumors as the cause of hGH deficiency, and four had received radiotherapy (164). In both studies, if patients with these additional risk factors for neoplasia are subtracted, hGH-treated children do not differ from the general population with regard to risk for leukemia. Nevertheless, a widely quoted conclusion is that there may be a slight (less than twofold) increased risk of leukemia in children treated with hGH (165). In the United States, any increased risk appears to be confined to children who have received treatment for brain tumors. Current information also suggests that hGH therapy does not increase the risk of brain tumor recurrence and that abnormalities on computed tomography are not a contraindication to treatment with hGH (166).

In summary, a decade of experience with recombinant hGH has proven this therapy to be remarkably safe when used in conventional substitution doses for hGH deficiency. Higher dose therapy for other causes of growth retardation also appear to be safe, but surveillance of its metabolic effects is indicated. There appear to be very few medical contraindications to hGH therapy. Nevertheless, the experience of transmission of Creutzfeldt-Jakob via pituitary GH is a poignant reminder that a farsighted view must be taken of the potential ramifications of long-term hormonal therapy.

VIII. ETHICAL ISSUES OF hGH TREATMENT

The limited availability of hGH once provided a barrier to expanding its use beyond children who were unequivocally hGH deficient. Today, the increased supply of hGH has been matched by increased demand; more than twice as many children received hGH therapy in 1990 than in 1986, at an average annual cost per child of more than $10,000. Relaxed diagnostic criteria have obliterated any clear boundary between hGH deficiency and sufficiency, allowing many partially affected children access to treatment. Future goals of hGH therapy appear likely to shift further toward supplementing and enhancing individuals' well-being rather than merely returning them to some physiologic baseline. Careful longitudinal studies, many already in progress, are required to determine the efficacy of hGH in accomplishing these goals.

But what *can* be done with hGH is not necessarily what *should* be done. Ethical justification of these goals, not merely the efficacy of hGH therapy in accomplishing them, also

deserves careful scrutiny. New uses of hGH raise complex philosophic, psychologic, and economic as well as medical questions that physician-scientists alone cannot answer (167). Even if hGH is shown effectively to increase the growth of non–hGH-deficient children and even if treatment can be accomplished without toxicity, additional considerations are needed to responsibly balance expected benefit with issues of resource allocation and fairness.

The widespread distribution of hGH has been partially deterred by high drug costs. Paradoxically, although the source of hGH is no longer limited, the resources with which to pay for it are becoming increasingly so. Prescribing hGH requires a difficult and often uncomfortable balancing of the responsible use of medical resources with an obligation to do the best for each individual patient. But is taller really better for each patient (168)? Concern about psychologic harm is invoked as a primary rationale for treating short stature, yet data confirming the efficacy of hGH therapy in alleviating the psychosocial consequences of short stature are scarce. If the ultimate goal of hGH therapy is not tall stature, but, rather, an improved quality of life, documentation of psychosocial impairment caused by stature before therapy and improvement following hGH therapy ought to play an important role in the initiation of hGH therapy and evaluation of its efficacy (169). To date, however, growth rate and final adult height remain the measures by which therapeutic success is judged.

Responsiveness to hGH, described earlier in many groups of short-statured individuals, is a necessary but not sufficient indication for treatment. Because of enormous expense and concerns that such widespread access would not ameliorate the disadvantages of short stature, it seems appropriate to restrict access within this group based upon the presence of significant functional or psychologic disability related to stature and the likelihood of improvement with treatment (Fig. 11). Most short children do not satisfy these additional criteria. Children with severe hGH deficiency are likely to be both more disabled and more responsive than non–hGH-deficient children, justifying their preferential treatment. Is it justified to restrict access of others to hGH based on the laboratory diagnosis of hGH deficiency? Some have argued that equally short children share a similar disability, regardless of whether stimulated hGH levels fall just above or just below an arbitrary threshold. If both are hGH responsive and truly disabled by height, there appears to be little ethical justification for treating only the child with lower hGH test results (170).

Alleviating the disability of short stature, rather than normalization of hGH levels, has traditionally been the primary goal of hGH therapy. Determining an appropriate end point for hGH therapy remains controversial. Attainment of genetic potential for height, a realistic possibility with optimal diagnosis and treatment, remains a goal for many. Consistent adherence to the goal of alleviating disabling short stature, on the other hand, implies that hGH therapy be discontinued when *each* treated child reaches an adult height no longer considered a disability. No policy regarding hGH therapy will ever eliminate the first percentile, but the second strategy has as its goal bringing children into the *normal opportunity range for*

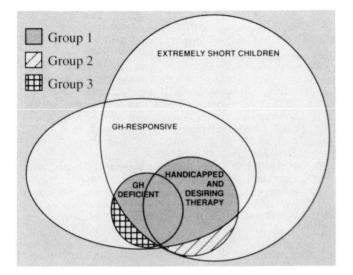

Figure 11 Proposal for allocation of growth hormone to children. Equitable but restricted entitlement to GH therapy based upon preferential allocation to children disabled by height who demonstrate GH responsiveness (group 1): children unresponsive to GH (group 2) or GH responsive but not sufficiently disabled by small stature (group 3, including GH-deficient children who have achieved nonhandicapping adult stature) would not receive public or privately subsidized therapy. (Reprinted with permission from Ref. 167, Allen DB. Growth hormone therapy for the disability of short stature. Growth Genet Horm 1992; 8:1–77.)

height without further enhancing those who have achieved a height within the normal adult distribution. By adhering to the *treatment* of disabling short stature and resisting the *enhancement* of normal stature, physicians treating children with hGH would minimize their contribution to society's heightist perception that to be taller is to be better (171).

REFERENCES

1. Raben MS. Treatment of a pituitary dwarf with human growth hormone (letter). J Clin Endocrinol 1958; 18:901.
2. Burns EC, Tanner JM, Preece MA, Cameron N. Final height and pubertal development in 55 children with idiopathic growth hormone deficiency, treated for between 2 and 15 years with human growth hormone. Eur J Pediatr 1981; 137:155–164.
3. Bundak R, Hindmarsh PC, Smith PJ, Brook CGD. Long term auxologic effects for human growth hormone. J Pediatr 1988; 112:875–879.
4. Joss E, Juppinger K, Schwarz HP, Roten G. Final height of patients with pituitary growth failure and changes in growth variables after long-term hormonal therapy. Pediatr Res 1983; 17:676–679.
5. Fradkin JE, Schonberger LB, Mills JL, et al. Creutzfeldt-Jakob disease in pituitary growth hormone recipients in the United States. JAMA 1991; 265:880–884.
6. Underwood LE, Fisher DA, Frasier SD, et al. Degenerative neurologic disease in patients formerly treated with human growth hormone—report of the Committee on Growth Hormone Use of the Lawson Wilkins Pediatric Endocrine Society, May 1985. J Pediatr 1985; 107:10.
7. Goeddel DV, Heyneker JL, Hozumi T, et al. Direct expression in *Escherichia coli* of a DNA sequence coding for human growth hormone. Nature 1979; 281:544.
8. Frasier SD, Rudlin CR, Zeisel HJ, et al. Effect of somatotropin of mammalian cell origin in growth hormone deficiency. Am J Dis Child 1992; 146:582–587.
9. Stabler B, Clopper RR, Siegel PT, Stoppani C, Compton PG, Underwood LE, National Cooperative Growth Study. Academic achievement and psychological adjustment in short children. J Dev Behav Pediatr 1993; (in press).
10. Stabler B, Siegel PT, Clopper RR. Growth hormone deficiency in children has psychological and educational comorbidity. Clin Pediatr (Phila) 1991; 30(3):156–160.
11. Sassin JF, Parker DC, Mace JW, Gorlin WR, Johnson LC, Rossman LG. Human growth hormone release: relation to slow-wave sleep and sleep-waking cycles. Science 1969; 165:513–515.
12. Johanson AJ, Morris GL. A single growth hormone determination to rule out growth hormone deficiency. Pediatrics 1977; 59:467–468.
13. Root A. Human Pituitary Growth Hormone. Springfield, IL: Charles C. Thomas, 1972.
14. Hunter WM, Rigal WM. The diurnal pattern of plasma growth hormone concentration in children and adolescents. J Endocrinol 1966; 34:147–153.
15. Martin JB. Neural regulation of growth hormone secretion. Medical progress report. N Engl J Med 1973; 228:1384.
16. Bauman G, Winter RJ, Shawn M. Circulating molecular variants of growth hormone in childhood. Pediatr Res 1987; 22:21.
17. Bauman G. Heterogenicity of growth hormone. In: Bercu B, ed. Basic and Clinical Aspects of Growth Hormone. New York: Plenum, 1988:13.
18. Leung DW, Spencer SA, Cachianes G, et al. Growth hormone receptor and serum binding protein: purification, cloning and expression. Nature 1987; 330:537–543.
19. Guevara-Aguirre J, Rosenbloom AL, Fielder PJ, Diamond FB, Rosenfeld RG. Growth hormone receptor deficiency in Ecuador: clinical and biochemical phenotype in two populations. J Clin Endocrinol Metab 1993; 76:417–423.
20. Ho KKY, Valiontis E, Waters MJ, Rajkovic IA. Regulation of growth hormone binding protein in man: comparison of gel chromatography and immunoprecipitation methods. J Clin Endocrinol Metab 1993; 76:302–308.
21. Cornblath M, Parker ML, Reisner SH, Forbes AE, Daughaday WH. Secretion and metabolism of growth hormone in premature and full-term infants. J Clin Endocrinol 1965; 25:209–218.
22. Miller MD, Esparza A, Wright NM, et al. Spontaneous growth hormone release in term infants: changes during the first four days of life. J Clin Endocrinol Metab 1993; 76:1058–1062.
23. Martha PM, Rogol AD, Veldhuis JD, Kerrigan JR, Goodman DW, Blizzard RM. Alterations in the pulsatile properties of circulating growth hormone concentrations during puberty in boys. J Clin Endocrinol Metab 1989; 69:563–570.
24. Martin LG, Clark JW, Conner TB. Growth hormone secretion enhanced by androgens. J Clin Endocrinol 1968; 28:425–428.
25. Kerrigan JR, Rogol AD. The impact of gonadal steroid hormone action on growth hormone secretion during childhood and adolescence. Endocr Rev 1992; 13:281– .
26. Keenan BS, Richards GE, Ponder SW, Dallas JS, Nagamani M, Smith ER. Androgen-stimulated pubertal growth: the effects of testosterone and dihydrotestosterone on growth hormone and insulin-like growth factor-1 in the treatment of short stature and delayed puberty. J Clin Endocrinol Metab 1993; 76:996–1001.

27. Weissberger AJ, Ho KKY. Activation of the somatotropic axis by testosterone in adult males: evidence for the role of aromatization. J Clin Endocrinol Metab 1993; 76:1407–1412.

28. Frantz AG, Rabkin MT. Effect of estrogen and sex difference on secretion of human growth hormone. J Clin Endocrinol 1965; 25:1470–1480.

29. Albertsson-Wiklund K, Rosberg S. Analysis of 24-hour growth hormone profiles in children: relationship to growth. J Clin Endocrinol Metab 1988; 67:493–500.

30. Hindmarsh P, Smith PJ, Brook CGD, Matthews DR. The relationship between height velocity and growth hormone secretion in short prepubertal children. Clin Endocrinol (Oxf) 1987; 27:581–591.

31. Brook CGD, Hindmarsh PC, Stanhope RJ. Endocrinology 1988; 119:179–184.

32. Phillips LS, Vassilopoulou-Sellin R. Somatomedins. Part 1. N Engl J Med 1980; 302:371.

33. Van Wyk JJ, Underwood LE. Relation between growth hormone and somatomedin. Annu Rev Med 1975; 26:427.

34. D'Ercole AJ, Stiles AD, Underwood LE. Tissue concentrations of somatomedin C: Further evidence for multiple sites of synthesis and paracrine or autocrine mechanisms of action. Proc Natl Acad Sci USA 1984; 81:935–939.

35. Isaksson OGP, Lindahl A, Nilsson A, Isgaard J. Mechanism of the stimulatory effect of growth hormone on longitudinal bone growth. Endocr Rev 1987; 8(4):426–438.

36. Rechler MM, Nilsson A, Lindahl A, Jonsson J-O, Isaksson O. Effects of local administration of GH and IGF-1 on longitudinal bone growth in rats. Am J Physiol 1986; 250: E367–372.

37. Guler HP, Zapf J, Scheiwiller E, et al. Recombinant human insulin-like growth factor I stimulates growth and has distinct effects on organ size in hypophysectomized rats. Proc Natl Acad Sci USA 1988; 85:4889–4893.

38. Berelowitz M, Szabo M, Frohman LA. Somatomedin-C mediates growth hormone negative feedback by effects on both the hypothalamus and the pituitary. Science 1981; 212:1279–1281.

39. Yamashita S, Melmed A. Insulin-like growth factor I action on rat anterior pituitary cells: suppression of growth hormone secretion and messenger ribonucleic acid levels. Endocrinology 1986; 118:176–182.

40. Bala RM, Lopatka J, Leung A, et al. Serum immunoreactive somatomedin levels in normal adults, pregnant women at term, children at various ages, and children with constitutionally delayed growth. J Clin Endocrinol Metab 1981; 52:508–512.

41. Rubin KR, Lichtenfels JM, Ratzan SK. Relationship of somatomedin-C concentration to bone age in boys with constitutional growth delay. Am J Dis Child 1986; 140:555–558.

42. Ziegler TR, Rombeau JL, Young LS, et al. Recombinant human growth hormone enhances the metabolic efficacy of parenteral nutrition: a double-blind randomized controlled study. J Clin Endocrinol Metab 1992; 74(4):865–873.

43. Chipman JJ, Zerwekh J, Nicar M, Marks J, Pak CJC. Effect of growth hormone administration: reciprocal changes in serum 1-alpha,25-dihydroxyvitamin D and calcium metabolism. J Clin Endocrinol Metab 1980; 51:321–324.

44. Saggese G, Baroncelli BI, Bertelloni S, Cinquanta L, DiNero G. Effects of long-term treatment with growth hormone on bone and mineral metabolism in children with growth hormone deficiency. J Pediatr 1993; 122:37–45.

45. Zachmann M, Fernandez F, Tassinari D, Thakker R, Prader A. Anthropometric measurements in patients with growth hormone deficiency before treatment with human growth hormone. Eur J Pediatr 1980; 133:277.

46. Walker, JM, Bond SA, Voss LD, Bets PR, Wootton SA,

47. Goodman HM, Grichting G. Growth hormone and lipolysis: a reevaluation. Endocrinology 1983; 113:1697.

48. Argyropoulou M, Perignon F, Brauner R, Brunelle F. Magnetic resonance imaging in the diagnosis of growth hormone deficiency. J Pediatr 1992; 120:886–891.

49. Rimoin DL, Merimee TJ, McKusick VA. Growth hormone deficiency in man: an isolated, recessively inherited defect. Science 1966; 152:1635.

50. Vimpani CV, et al. Prevalence of severe growth hormone deficiency. BMJ 1977; 2:427.

51. Pankin JM. Incidence of growth hormone deficiency. Arch Dis Child 1974; 49:905.

52. Stanhope R. Is growth hormone deficiency a discrete entity? Against the notion. In: Allen DB, ed. Access to Treatment with Human Growth Hormone: Medical, Ethical, and Social Issues. Growth Genet Horm 1992; 8(Suppl 1):6–9.

53. Veldhuis JD, Blizzard RM, Rogol AD, Martha PM, Kirkland JL, Sherman BM. Properties of spontaneous growth hormone secretory bursts and half-life of endogenous growth hormone in boys with idiopathic short stature. J Clin Endocrinol Metab 1992; 74:766–773.

54. Lovinger RD, Kaplan SL, Grumbach MM. Congenital hypopituitarism associated with neonatal hypoglycemia and microphallus. J Pediatr 1975; 87:1171.

55. Greulich W, Pyle SI. Radiographic Atlas of Skeletal Development of the Hand and Wrist, 2nd ed. Stanford, CA: Stanford University Press, 1959.

56. Goodman HG, Grumbach MM, Kaplan SL. Growth and growth hormone. II. A comparison of isolated growth hormone deficiency and multiple pituitary hormone deficiencies in 35 patients with idiopathic hypopituitary dwarfism. N Engl J Med 1968; 278:57.

57. Duck S, Schwarz HP, Costin G, et al. Subcutaneous growth hormone-releasing hormone therapy in growth hormone deficient children: first year of therapy. J Clin Endocrinol Metab 1992; 75:1115.

58. Brasel JA, Wright JC, Wilkins L, et al. An evaluation of 75 patients with hypopituitarism beginning in childhood. Am J Med 1965; 38:484.

59. Guyda H, Friesen H, Bailey JB, Leboeuf C, Beck JC. Medical Research Council of Canada therapeutic trial of human growth hormone: first 5 years of therapy. Can Med Assoc J 1975 112:1291–1309.

60. Thomsett MJ, Conte FA, Kaplan SL, et al. Endocrine and neurologic outcome in childhood craniopharyngioma. Review of effect of treatment in 42 patients. J Pediatr 1980; 97:728.

61. Jenkins JS, Gilbert CJ, Ang V. Hypothalamic-pituitary function in patients with craniopharyngiomas. J Clin Endocrinol Metab 1976; 43:394.

62. Blatt J, Bercu BB, Gillin JC, et al. Reduced pulsatile growth hormone secretion in children after therapy for acute lymphoblastic leukemia. J Pediatr 1984; 104:182–186.

63. Shalet SM. The effects of irradiation on endocrine function in children. Growth Genet Horm 1992; 8(3):7–11.

64. Littley MD. Radiation and the Hypothalamic-Pituitary Axis, Radiation Injury to the Nervous System. New York: Raven Press, 1991:311.

65. Bourguignon JP, Van Vliet B. Factors influencing final height in growth hormone treated patients. In: Frisch H, Thorner MO, eds. Hormonal Regulation of Growth. New York: Raven Press, 1989:261–271.

66. Frasier SD. A review of growth hormone stimulation tests in children. Pediatrics 1974; 53:929.

67. Celniker C, Chen B, Wert M Jr, Sherman BM. Variability in

Jackson AA. Treatment of short normal children with growth hormone—a cautionary tale? Lancet 1990; 336:1331.

the quantitation of circulating hormone using commercial immunoassays. J Clin Endocrinol Metab 1989; (in press).

68. Frasier SD. Human pituitary growth hormone (hGH) therapy in growth hormone deficiency. Endocr Rev 1983; 4:155–170.

69. Wit JM, Faber JAJ, Van den Brande JL. Growth response to human growth hormone treatment in children with partial and total growth hormone deficiency. Acta Paediatr Scand 1986; 75:767–773.

70. Root AW. Methods of assessing growth hormone secretion and determining growth hormone deficiency. In Allen DB, ed. Access to Treatment with Human Growth Hormone: Medical, Ethical, and Social Issues. Growth Genet Horm 1992; 8(Suppl 1):1–6.

71. Marin G, Barnes KM, Domene H. Failure of normal prepubertal children to respond to growth hormone stimulation tests. Endocrinology 1991; 128:82A.

72. Kaplan SA. Clinical Pediatric and Adolescent Endocrinology. Philadelphia: W.B. Saunders, 1982:36.

73. Brauner F, Rappaport R, Prevot C, et al. A prospective study of the development of growth hormone deficiency in children given cranial irradiation, and its relation to statural growth. J Clin Endocrinol Metab 1989; 68(2):346–351.

74. Rose SR, Ross JL, Uriarte M, Barnes KM, Cassorla FG, Cutler GB Jr. The advantage of measuring stimulated as compared with spontaneous growth hormone levels in the diagnosis of growth hormone deficiency. N Engl J Med 1988; 319:201–208.

75. Donaldson DL, Hollowell JG, Pan FP, Moore WV. Growth hormone profiles: significant variation on consecutive nights. Pediatr Res 1988; 23:276A (abstract 449).

76. Hedin L, Olsson B, Diczfalusy M, et al. Intranasal administration of human growth hormone in combination with a membrane permeation enhancer in patients with GH deficiency: a pharmacokinetic study. J Clin Endocrinol Metab 1993; 76:962–967.

77. Vanderschueren-Lodeweyckx M, Van den Broeck J, Wolter R, Malvaux P. Early initiation of growth hormone treatment: influence on final height. Acta Paediatr Scand (Suppl) 1987; 337:4–11.

78. Frasier SD, Costin G, Lippe BM, Aceto T, Bunge PF. A dose-response curve for human growth hormone. J Clin Endocrinol Metab 1981; 53:1213.

79. Kaplan SL, Underwood LE, August GP, et al. Clinical studies with recombinant-DNA, derived methionyl human growth hormone in growth hormone deficient children. Lancet 1986; 1:697–700.

80. Keizer-Schrama SMPF, Rikken B, Wynne HJ, et al. Dose-response study of biosynthetic human growth hormone (GH) in GH-deficient children: effects on auxological and biochemical parameters. J Clin Endocrinol Metab 1992; 74:898–905.

81. Jorgensen JOL, Flyvbjerg A, Lauritzen T, Alberti KGMM, Orskov H, Christiansen JS. Dose-response studies with biosynthetic human growth hormone (GH) in GH-deficient patients. J Clin Endocrinol Metab 1988; 67:36.

82. Sherman B, Frane J. Genentech National Cooperative Growth Study. Program of the Endocrine Society, 1988 (abstract 406).

83. Smith PJ, Hindmarsh PC, Brook CGD. Contribution of dose and frequency of administration to the therapeutic effect of growth hormone. Arch Dis Child 1988; 63:491–494.

84. Gertner JM, Tamborlane WV, Gianfredi SP, Genel M. Renewed catch-up growth with increase replacement doses of human growth hormone. J Pediatr 1987; 110(3):425–428.

85. Tiwary C. Seasonal and latitudinal effects on growth in patients on Protropin growth hormone in the US and Canada. Genentech National Cooperative Growth Study Summer Report 15, June 1993.

86. Costin G, Kogut MD, Phillips LS, Daughaday WH. Cranio-

pharyngioma: the role of insulin in promoting postoperative growth. J Clin Endocrinol Metab 1976; 42:370.

87. Mauras N, Blizzard RM, Link K. Augmentation of growth hormone secretion during puberty: evidence for a pulse amplitude modulated phenomenon. J Clin Endocrinol Metab 1987; 64:596–601.

88. Van der Werff ten Bosch JJ, Bot A. Growth of males with idiopathic hypopituitarism without growth hormone treatment. Clin Endocrinol (Oxf) 1990; 32:707–717.

89. Stanhope R, Uruena M, Hindmarsh P, Leiper AD, Brook CGD. Management of growth hormone deficiency through puberty. Acta Paediatr Scand 1991; 372:47–52.

90. Dean HJ. Demographic outcome of growth hormone deficient individuals. In: Holmes CS, ed. Psychoneuroendocrinology: Brain, Behavior, and Hormonal Interactions. New York, Springer-Verlag, 1990:79–91.

91. Bjork S, Jonsson B, Westphal O, Levin JE. Quality of life of adults with growth hormone deficiency: a controlled study. Acta Paediatr Scand (Suppl) 1989; 356:55–59.

92. Feldman SD. The presentation of shortness in everyday life: height and heightism in American society—toward a sociology of stature. In: Feldman SD, ed. Life-styles: Diversity in American Society. Boston: Little, Brown, 1975:437–452.

93. Lippe BM. Growth hormone treatment: does ascertainment bias determine treatment practices? In: Allen DB, ed. Access to Treatment with Human Growth Hormone: Medical, Ethical, and Social Issues. Growth Genet Horm 1992; 8(Suppl. 1):31–35.

94. Rotnem D, Benel M, Hintz RL, et al. Personality development in children with growth hormone deficiency. J Am Acad Child Psychiatry 1977; 16:412–426.

95. Penny R, Blizzard RM. The possible influence of puberty on the release of growth hormone in three males with apparent isolated growth hormone deficiency. J Clin Endocrinol 1972; 34:82–84.

96. Martin LG, Clark JW, Conner TB. Growth hormone secretion enhanced by androgens. J Clin Endocrinol Metab 1968; 28:425–428.

97. Hindmarsh PL, Brook CGD. Effect of growth hormone on short normal children. BMJ 1987; 295:573–577.

98. Albertsson-Wikland K. Growth hormone treatment in short children: short-term and long-term effects on growth. Acta Paediatr Scand (Suppl) 1988; 343:77–84.

99. Hopwood NJ, Hintz RL, Gertner JM, et al. Growth response of children with non-growth-hormone deficiency and marked short stature during three years of growth hormone therapy. J Pediatr 1993; 123:215–222.

100. Moore WV, Moore KC, Gifford R, Hollowell JG, Donaldson DL. Long-term treatment with growth hormone of children with short stature and normal growth hormone secretion. J Pediatr 1992; 120:702–708.

101. Attie KM, Hintz RL, Hopwood NJ, Johanson AJ, Genentech Collaborative Study Group. Growth hormone treatment of idiopathic short stature and its effect on the onset and tempo of puberty (abstract). Pediatr Res 1992; 31:72A.

102. Kaplan SL, Grumbach MM. Long-term treatment with growth hormone of children with non-growth hormone deficient short stature. In: Isaksson O, Binder C, Hall K, et al., eds. Growth Hormone: Basic and Clinical Aspects. Amsterdam: Excerpta Medica, 1987:197–204.

103. Lesage C, Walker M, Landier F, Chatelain P, Chaussain JL, Bougneres PF. Near normalization of adolescent height with growth hormone therapy in very short children without growth hormone deficiency. J Pediatr 1991; 119:29–34.

104. Lyon AL, Preece MA, Grant DB. Growth curve for girls with Turner syndrome. Arch Dis Child 1985; 60:932–935.

105. Lippe BM, Frane J, Attie K, Genentech National Collaborative Group Growth in Turner syndrome. Updating the United States experience (abstract). Proc 3rd Int Symp Turner Syndrome, 1992:32.

106. Rappaport R, Sauvion S. Possible mechanism for the growth retardation in Turner syndrome. Acta Paediatr Scand (Suppl) 1989; 356:82–86.

107. Ranke MG, Blum WF, Haug F, et al. Growth hormone somatomedin levels and growth regulation in Turner's syndrome. Acta Endocrinol (Copenh) 1987; 116:305–313.

108. Ross JL, Meyerson L, Loriauz DL, et al. Growth hormone secretory dynamics in Turner syndrome. J Pediatr 1985; 106:202–205.

109. Kohno H, Honda S. Low urinary growth hormone values in patients with Turner's syndrome. J Clin Endocrinol Metab 1992; 74:619–622.

110. Rosenfeld RG. Update on growth hormone therapy for Turner's syndrome. Acta Paediatr Scand (Suppl) 1989; 356:103–108.

111. Takano K, Shizume K, Hibi I. Turner' syndrome: treatment of 203 patients with recombinant human growth hormone for one year. Acta Endocrinol (Copenh) 1989; 120:559–568.

112. Lin TH, Kirkland JS, Kirkland RT. Growth hormone assessment and short term treatment with growth hormone in Turner syndrome. J Pediatr 1988; 112:919–921.

113. Rosenfeld RG, Frane J, Attie KM, et al. Six year results of a randomized prospective trial of human growth hormone and oxandrolone in Turner syndrome. J Pediatr 1992; 21:49–55.

114. Neely EK, Marcus R, Rosenfeld RG, Bachrach LK. Turner syndrome adolescents receiving growth hormone are not osteopenic. J Clin Endocrinol Metab 1993; 76:861–866.

115. Rongen-Weserlaken C, Rijkers GT, Scholtens EJ, et al. Immunologic studies in Turner syndrome before and during treatment with growth hormone. J Pediatr 1991; 119:268–272.

116. Stahnke N, Stubbe P, Keller E, et al. Effects and side effects of GH plus oxandrolone. In: Ranke MB, Rosenfeld RG, eds. Turner Syndrome: Growth Promoting Therapies. Amsterdam: Elsevier, 1991:241–249.

117. Haeusler G, Frisch H. Growth hormone treatment in Turner's syndrome: short and long-term effects on metabolic parameters. Clin Endocrinol (Oxf) 1992; 36:247–254.

118. Davies PSW, Valley R, Preece MA. Adolescent growth and pubertal progression in the Silver-Russell syndrome. Arch Dis Child 1988; 63:130–135.

119. Tanner JM, Whitehouse RH, Hughes PCR, Vince FP. Effect of human growth hormone treatment for 1 to 7 years on growth of 100 children with growth hormone deficiency, low birth weight, inherited smallness, Turner's syndrome and other complaints. Arch Dis Child 1971; 46:745–782.

120. Albertsson-Wikland K. Growth hormone secretion and growth hormone treatment in children with intrauterine growth retardation. Acta Paediatr Scand 1989; 349:35–41.

121. Stanhope R, Ackland F, Hamill G, Clayton J, Jones J, Preece MA. Physiological growth hormone secretion and response to growth hormone treatment in children with short stature and intrauterine growth retardation. Acta Paediatr Scand (Suppl) 1989; 349:47–52.

122. Stanhope R, Preece MA, Hamill, G. Does growth hormone treatment improve final height attainment of children with intrauterine growth retardation? Arch Dis Child 1991; 66:1180–1181.

123. Mehls O, Ritz E, Hunziker EB, Tonshoff B, Heinrich U. Role of growth hormone in growth failure of uremia: perspectives for application of recombinant growth hormone. Acta Paediatr Scand (Suppl) 1989; 343:118–126.

124. Allen DB, El-Hayek R, Friedman AL, Chobanian MC. Growth hormone stimulated urinary ammonia excretion in normal and 75% nephrectomized rats. Pediatr Res 1991; 29(4):2202.

125. Fine RN, Kohaut EC, Brown D, Perlman AJ. Growth following recombinant human growth hormone (rhGH) treatment in children with chronic renal failure (CRF): report of a multicenter randomized double-blind placebo-controlled study. J Pediatr (in press).

126. Allen DB, El-Hayek R, Friedman AL. Effects of prolonged growth hormone administration on growth, renal function, and renal histology in 75% nephrectomized rats. Pediatr Res 1992; 31:406–410.

127. Tonshoff B, Tonshoff C, Mehls O, et al. Growth hormone treatment in children with preterminal chronic renal failure: no adverse effect on glomerular filtration rate. Eur J Pediatr 1992; 151:601–607.

128. Andersson HC, Markello T, Schneider JA, Gahl WA. Effect of growth hormone treatment on serum creatinine concentration in patients with cystinosis and chronic renal disease. J Pediatr 1992; 120:716–720.

129. Koch VH, Lippe BM, Nelson PA, Boechat MI, Sherman BM, Fine RN. Accelerated growth after recombinant human growth hormone treatment of children with chronic renal failure. J Pediatr 1989; 115;365–371.

130. Rosenfeld RG, Hintz RL, Normal somatomedin and somatomedin receptors in achondroplastic dwarfism. Horm Metab Res 1980; 12:76–77.

131. Butenandt O. Growth hormone therapy is children with bone disease. Pediatr Adol Endocrinol 1987; 16:118–120.

132. Appan S, Laurent S, Chapman M, Hindmarsh PC, Brook CGD. Growth and growth hormone (GH) therapy in hypochondroplasia. Horm Res 1989; 31(Suppl. 1):170A.

133. Mullis PE, Patel MS, Brickell PM, Hindmarsh PC, Brook CGD. Growth characteristics and response to growth hormone therapy in patients with hypochondroplasia: genetic linkage of the insulin-like growth factor 1 gene at chromosome 12q23 to the disease in a subgroup of these patients. Clin Endocrinol (Oxf) 1991; 34:265–274.

134. Wehrenberg WB, Janowski BA, Piering AW, Culler F, Jones KL. Glucocorticoids: potent inhibitors and stimulators of growth hormone secretion. Endocrinology 1990; 126:3200–3203.

135. Spiliotis BE, August PA, Hung W, et al. Growth hormone neurosecretory dysfunction: a treatable cause of short stature. JAMA 1984; 251:2223–2230.

136. Butenandt O, Eder R, Clados-Kelch A. Growth hormone studies in patients with rheumatoid arthritis and Still syndrome. Verh Dtsch Ges Rheumatol 1976; 4:68–77.

137. Allen DB, Goldberg BD. Stimulation of collagen synthesis and linear growth by growth hormone in glucocorticoid-treated children. Pediatrics 1992; 89(3):416–421.

138. Van Dop CV, Jabs KL, Donohoue PA, Bock GH, Fivush BA, Harmon WE. Accelerated growth rates in children treated with growth hormone after renal transplantation. J Pediatr 1992; 120:244–250.

139. Horber FF, Haymond MW. Human growth hormone prevents the protein catabolic side effects of prednisone in humans. J Clin Invest 1990; 86:265–272.

140. Castells S, Torrado C, Bastian W, Wisniewski KE. Growth hormone deficiency in Down's syndrome children. J Intell Disability Res 1992; 36:29–43.

141. Angulo M, Castro-Magana M, Uy J. Pituitary evaluation and growth hormone treatment in Prader-Willi syndrome. J Pediatr Endocrinol 1991; 4:167–172.

142. Rotenstein D, Reigel DH, Flom LL. Growth hormone treatment accelerates growth of short children with neural tube defects. J Pediatr 1989; 115:417–420.

143. Allen DB, Pescowitz O, Frasier SD, Foley T. Growth hormone for children with Down syndrome. J Pediatr 1993; 123:742–743.

144. Salomon F, Cuneo RC, Hesp R, Sonksen PH. The effects of treatment with recombinant human growth hormone on body composition and metabolism in adults with growth hormone deficiency. N Engl J Med 1989; 321:1797–1803.

145. Bengtsson G, Eden S, Lonn L, et al. Treatment of adults with growth hormone deficiency with recombinant human GH. J Clin Endocrinol Metab 1993; 76:309–317.

146. Cuneo RC, Salomon R, Wiles CM, Hesp R, Sonksen PH. Growth hormone treatment in growth-hormone deficient adults. II. Effects on exercise performance. J Appl Physiol 1991; 70(2):695–700.

147. McGaulley GA. Quality of life assessment before and after growth hormone treatment in adults with growth hormone deficiency. Acta Paediatr Scand (Suppl) 1989; 356:70–72.

148. Rudman D, Feller AG, Hagraj HS, et al. Effects of growth hormone in men over 60 years old. N Engl J Med 1990; 323:1–6.

149. Yarasheski KE, Campbell JA, Smith K, Rennie MJ, Holloszy JO, Bier DM. Effect of growth hormone and resistance exercise on muscle growth in young men. Am J Physiol 1992; 262(25):E261–E267.

150. Jorgensen PH, Andreassen TT. The influence of biosynthetic human growth hormone on biomechanical properties and/or collagen formation in granulation tissue. Horm Metab Res 1988; 20:490–493.

151. Ponting GA, Halliday D, Teale JD, Sim AW. Postoperative positive nitrogen balance with intravenous hyponutrition and growth hormone. Lancet 1988; 1:438–439.

152. Herndon DN, Barrow RE, Kunkle KR, Broemeling L, Rutan RL. Effects of recombinant human growth hormone on donor site healing in severely burned children. Ann Surg 1990; 212:424–429.

153. Welsh K, Lamit M, Morhenn V. The effect of recombinant human growth hormone on wound healing in normal individuals. J Dermatol Surg Oncol 1991; 17:942–945.

154. Snyder DK, Clemmons DR, Underwood LE. Treatment of obese, diet-restricted subjects with growth hormone for 11 weeks: effects on anabolism, lipolysis, and body composition. J Clin Endocrinol Metab 1988; 67:54–61.

155. Buzi F, Buchanan C, Morrell DJ, Preece MA. Antigenicity and efficacy of authentic sequence recombinant human growth hormone (Somatropin): first year experience in the United Kingdom. Clin Endocrinol (Oxf) 1989; 30:531–538.

156. Sato T, Suzuki Y, Taketani T. Enhanced peripheral conversion of thyroxine to triiodothyronine during hGH therapy in GH deficient children. J Clin Endocrinol Metab 1977; 45:324–329.

157. Prassad B, Greig F, Bastian W, Castells S, Juan C, AvRuskin TW. Slipped capital femoral epiphysis during treatment with recombinant growth hormone for isolated partial growth hormone deficiency. J Pediatr 1990; 116:397–399.

158. Otten BJ, Rotteveel JJ, Cruysberg JRM. Pseudotumor cerebri following treatment with growth hormone. Horm Res 1992; 37(Suppl. 4):16.

159. Van Vliet G. Use of growth hormone in the management of growth disorders. In: Sizonenko PC, Aubert M, eds. Developmental Endocrinology. New York: Raven Press, 1990:195–202.

160. Walker J, Chaussain JL, Bougneres PF. Growth hormone treatment of children with short stature increases insulin secretion but does not impair glucose disposal. J Clin Endocrinol Metab 1989; 69:253–258.

161. Estrov Z, Meir R, Barak Y, Zaizov R, Zadik Z. Human growth hormone and insulin-like growth factor-1 enhance the proliferation of human leukemic cells. J Clin Oncol 1991; 9:394–399.

162. Watanabe S, Tsunematsu Y, Fujimoto J, Komiyama A. Leukemia in patients treated with growth hormone. Lancet 1988; 2:1159.

163. Lawson Wilkins Pediatric Endocrine Society. Addendum to Minutes of the Drug and Therapeutics Committee, Washington, DC, July 1991.

164. Fradkin JE, Mills JL, Schonberger LB, et al. Risk of leukemia after treatment with pituitary growth hormone. JAMA 1993; 270:2829–2832.

165. Fisher DA, Job J-C, Preece M, et al. Leukemia in patients treated with growth hormone. Lancet 1988; 1:1159–1160.

166. Ogilvy-Stuart AL, Ryder WDJ, Battamaneni HR, Clayton PE, Shalet SM. Growth hormone and tumour recurrence. BMJ 1992; 304:1601–1605.

167. Allen DB, ed. Access to Treatment with Human Growth Hormone: Medical, Ethical, and Social Issues. Growth Genet Horm 1992; 8(Suppl. 1):1–77.

168. Diekema DS. Is taller really better? Growth hormone therapy in short children. Perspect Biol Med 1990; 34:109–123.

169. Stabler B, Underwood LE. Growth hormone for short children. Lancet 1991; 337:1298.

170. Allen DB, Fost NC. Growth hormone for short stature: panacea or Pandora's box? J Pediatr 1990; 117:16–21.

171. Allen DB. Determining who needs growth hormone. Med Ethics Pediatrician 1991; 6:6–7.

6

Syndromes of Psychosocial Short Stature

Robert M. Blizzard
University of Virginia School of Medicine, Charlottesville, Virginia

Anamaria Bulatovic
Johns Hopkins Bayview Medical Center, Baltimore, Maryland

I. INTRODUCTION

Psychosocial short stature (PSS) consists of several syndromes characterized by growth failure and/or delayed puberty and occurs in infancy, childhood, and adolescence in association with psychologic harassment or emotional deprivation and for which there is no other explanation (1–18). The occurrence of PSS syndromes covers all socioeconomic groups, although the syndromes occur more frequently in the lower than in the upper economic groups. In this chapter the various types of PSS are defined, the historical aspects as they occurred chronologically related, and the diversity of the clinical picture presented. The pathophysiology is considered, and the diagnostic and therapeutic considerations are discussed.

II. TYPES OF PSYCHOSOCIAL SHORT STATURE

At least three subtypes of psychosocial short stature have been recognized (Table 1).

The first (type I) occurs in infants and children 2 years of age or younger. These infants usually have failure to thrive (nutritional deficiency), as well as short stature, and were very adequately described by Kreiger, Whitten, and colleagues (3–7). There is no evidence that these children have a hormonal disturbance, such as growth hormone (GH) deficiency, and they usually recover when sufficient calories are given. Their parents do not usually blatantly reject the child. The mothers characteristically have multiple children or responsibilities. They are usually disorganized, and the children do not receive the food or the attention they need, but the attention they receive apparently is usually adequate for infants to again grow, if they are given adequate calories. Nevertheless, growth in some may be inadequate without further psychosocial interventions, as reported by Bithoney et al. (8–10) (Chap. 9).

Type II PSS has been called transient hypopituitarism, reversible hyposomatotropism, emotional deprivation, maternal deprivation, psychosomatic dwarfism, abuse dwarfism, and the "garbage can" syndrome (1,2,11–18). The term PSS is preferable to definitions that include the presence or absence of growth hormone, the presence or absence of overt psychologic abuse, or emotional deprivation. This type occurs characteristically in children 3 years of age and older. There is a greater psychologic component, and GH may or may not be demonstrable in their serum of these patients after stimulation with pharmacologic agents, such as arginine or insulin, which cause the release of growth hormone from the pituitary into the serum. Other abnormalities indicating adrenocorticotropic hormone (ACTH), thyroid stimulating hormone, and gonadotropin deficiency may be noted; however, GH deficiency is the most common (19–23) endocrine aberrancy. The parents in this group usually reject their children and abuse them psychologically. The fathers and/or mothers are frequently chronic alcoholics (1,2). Occasionally type I patients are observed to advance into type II, which is not surprising.

The third (type III) was described by Boulton et al. (24), who studied seven children aged 3.6–11.6 years diagnosed with PSS, who did not have the bizarre signs and symptoms discussed by Powell et al. (1,2), who secreted growth hormone when tested, who were significantly depressed and/or had a disorder of attachment often dating from infancy, and who in contrast to previously reported patients had a significant increase in growth when given growth hormone. A lesser response was obtained with a placebo. The authors emphasized that this group did not show lack of discrimination in relationships, nor did they display the self-destructive behavior, pain agnosia, or bizarre eating and sleeping disorders seen in many type II patients. In addition, the parents

Table 1 Characteristics of Various PSS Syndromes

Type	Age of Onset	Failure to Thrive	Bizarre Behavior (Table 2)	Depression	GH Secretion	Parental Rejection	GH Responsiveness
I	Infancy	Usually	No	Often	Normal	No; see text	?
II	≥3 years	Some and some overweight	Usual	Very often	Decreased or absent often	Usual	Minimal at doses used
III	Infancy or later	Not usual	Not usual	Yes	Normal	Concern, not rejection	Significant at dose used

were not indifferent and rejecting, as are those with PSS type II. The parents also had insight into the problem, which was not characteristic of the parents of patients who were previously reported, and several felt guilty and/or had depression.

III. CHRONOLOGIC AND HISTORICAL DESCRIPTION

The chronologic history of PSS has been amply reviewed by Gardner (16) and by Green (25). Gardner relates that King Frederick II in Sicily took responsibility for children who died of lack of communication and attention. King Frederick was interested in learning the innate language of humans, and consequently, he isolated infants to learn what language they would speak spontaneously. These children did not grow and allegedly died because of lack of communication and attention. Obviously, King Frederick's experiment was unsuccessful, and he was not able to answer the question he asked, but his experience indicated a role for human interaction in proper childhood development.

The death of infants in foundling homes was described subsequently in Spain in the mideighteenth century. Such deaths also were subsequently described in England and other countries. For example, James Knox at the Johns Hopkins Institution described deaths of infants in the foundling homes in Baltimore in the year 1915 (26).

In 1947, Talbot and Sobel described patients with short stature they believed was caused by emotional disturbances. They postulated that these children could have a transient deficiency of growth hormone (27). The techniques to confirm their hypothesis were not yet available.

A classic example of the role of love and attention in influencing the somatic development of children was presented in a report by Widdowson in 1951 (28). She reported two German orphanages run by two women of different personalities. The data are shown in Figure 1. The children in group B were under the scrutiny of an unpleasant and dominating woman who rendered no loving tender care. The infants in group A were under the tutelage of a woman whose characteristics were the opposite: she gave loving care to the children for whom she was responsible. The intermediate group portrayed in Figure 1 included children who were the

favorites of the unkind supervisor in orphanage B. They grew better than most of the children who did not receive favorable attention from this matron. The diets were equivalent in both institutions. At the time portrayed by the vertical line in Figure 1, the supervisor of orphanage B moved to orphanage A. Children in orphanage A were given extra calories at this time. Those children in orphanage B who had not grown normally began to grow rapidly when given loving attention. The reverse occurred in orphanage A, probably as a result of the absence of attention. The favorites of the headmistress continued to do better than those she rejected. These observations demonstrated how loving care and attention are important to normal growth in many children.

Following this report, others, including Spitz, examined infants in foundling homes in the United States and Canada. Infants who did not receive attention showed evidence of anxiety, sadness, and retarded physical development, and more than one-third died, despite adequate food and meticulous care. Infants aged 7–12 months were reported to be most susceptible. Even those who survived were physically retarded (29,30).

Gardner and his collaborators, in 1955, began to report children who had been adversely treated and had failed to grow. These children were almost uniformly underweight for height, and many investigators believed that malnutrition was the causative factor. Gardner and his colleagues took these observations one step further and recognized that factors other than inadequate nutrition often were responsible (15,16,31–32).

In 1967, Powell et al. published the definitive study of the role of psychologic factors in the growth of children (1,2). These authors revealed how emotional deprivation could result in transient growth hormone deficiency. The case history of the proband is presented here because of its characteristics and historical importance.

A 7-year-old boy, with a height age (HA) of 3 years and a bone age of 3.5 years, was underweight for height. The mother gave a history compatible with steatorrhea. Initially it was believed that this child had malabsorption because of a protuberant abdomen and a history of steatorrhea, but this could not be documented while the patient was in the hospital.

The results of a metyrapone test indicated that the patient had limited corticotropin (ACTH) reserve. On the basis of this test, the delayed height and bone ages, and the absence

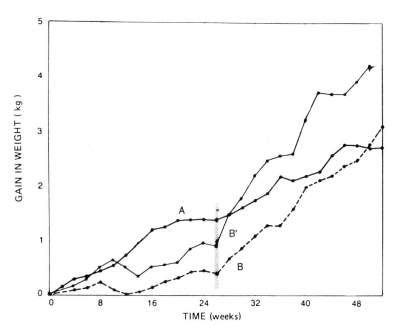

Figure 1 For six months the orphans in each home received nothing but basic rations, yet the children in orphanage A, supervised by a kindly matron, gained more weight than most of those in orphanage B, whose matron was a stern disciplinarian. An exception was a group (B') of favorites of the stern matron at B; they did better than their companions. After six months the matron at B was transferred to A and brought her favorites with her. Simultaneously the children at A were given extra rations, whereas the children at B remained on the same basic diet. (The transition is indicated by the vertical gray line.) Relieved of the stern matron's discipline, the children at B began to show a sharp increase in weight; those at A showed a weight gain that averaged somewhat less than during the preceding six months in spite of the larger ration. Again matron's favorites were an exception: their weight gain was greatest of any. (From Ref. 8, Gardner, L. I. *Deprivation dwarfism.* Copyright © 1972 by Scientific American, Inc.)

of other cause, the probable diagnosis was hypopituitarism. The child was placed in a foster home, and the responsible parties were advised to have the patient return in 12 months for follow-up. Upon return, the child had grown 17.5 cm in 1 year.

This boy had been reared in a home environment in which he was rejected by both mother and father. There was no evidence of physical abuse. The mother was pleased to relinquish his care to others. In retrospect, it was learned that he had raided garbage cans and drank water from the toilet bowl. These symptoms disappeared in the foster environment.

Many more cases of children 3 years of age and older were quickly recognized and reported after this syndrome (type II PSS) was brought to light. A majority, but not all, of the patients have had detectable endocrine abnormalities, GH deficiency being the most common aberrancy (20–24).

IV. CLINICAL MANIFESTATIONS OF PATIENTS WITH PSS

Infants and young children with failure to thrive (FTT), who do not have an organic etiology for their failure to thrive, should be suspected of having type I or early type III PSS. Infants with type I PSS often have mothers who are overburdened with life's problems and/or are immature and disorga-

nized. These characteristics prevent them from fulfilling either the emotional or nutritional needs of their infants or very young children. A number of maternal factors, such as low maternal responsiveness, communication, and encouragement for their infants, have been identified. These interfere with effective development and appropriate attachment. Vietze et al. (34) reported that the diagnosis of nonorganic failure to thrive is often associated with a low overall response by the mothers to their offspring, compared with that observed by mothers whose children thrive. These mothers demonstrated fewer verbal and physical contacts with their infants. A study using home observation by assessment of general maternal interactional behavior, including sensitivity, accessibility, acceptance, cooperation, delight, and their emotional expression, showed that mothers of nonorganic failure to thrive infants scored lower in all categories of interactional behaviors than mothers of normal infants. In another study (9), the mothers of FTT infants were reported to have extreme social isolation, lack of extended family, and a greater number of children than mothers of unaffected children.

The most overt signs and symptoms, as observed in the first 13 patients with type II PSS studied by Powell et al. (1,2), are given in Table 2. Some of these signs and symptoms are present in most but not all patients of type II. Signs of pain agnosia and depression also are frequent (18,35). In older patients, these bizarre symptoms and signs may have been

Table 2 Symptoms and Signs in the First 13 Patients Recognized in our Clinic with Type II Psychosocial Short Stature[a]

Symptom	Number
Polydipsia	13
Polyphagia	13
Stole food	12
Ate from garbage cans	11
Retarded speech	11
Played alone	9
Temper tantrums	9
Enuresis	9
Shy	9
Steatorrhea	8
Drank from toilet bowl	6
Prowled at night	7
Encopresis	6
Gorging and vomiting	8

[a]Not all patients have these symptoms and signs when seen.

present during childhood but may be absent later in childhood, when the child comes to the pediatric endocrinologist because of short stature and delayed puberty. An example of such a case is a 15.3-year-old girl who was seen because of short stature (height 136 cm, HA 9.5 years). She was sexually infantile and had a history of little growth for the past few years. The family history revealed that she was one of seven siblings and that she had been rejected by her mother and father. She particularly hated her father and refused to relate to male physicians in the clinic or hospital. Polyphagia, polydipsia, eating from the dog's dish, and drinking from puddles were part of her history at 7 and 8 years of age.

Laboratory testing revealed a bone age of 10. The results of the metyrapone test were abnormal, indicting limited ACTH production, as was the GH test secondary to both insulin and arginine stimulation. The serum thyroxine determination result was normal.

The patient was observed in the hospital for 1 month; she grew 2.5 cm and advanced from stage I to stage II of breast development. At this time, retesting with arginine and insulin revealed normal release of GH from the pituitary. When removed from the adverse environment, she grew more than 10 cm in the next 16 months. Simultaneously, development of both breasts and sexual hair advanced to Tanner stage III.

This patient exemplifies that the psychosocial short stature of type II may be present at adolescent age, that the usual signs and symptoms may have been present only at an earlier age in such patients, and that probing into the history may be necessary to elicit these. Such probing indicated that this was a patient with psychosocial short stature instead of idiopathic GH deficiency of the usual type.

Although most patients with type II PSS are passive and shy, an occasional patient is particularly aggressive. Such was a 3.5-year-old boy who was admitted to the hospital because of growth retardation (height 83.8 cm, HA 1.5 years). He was a smiling hyperactive child who had cataracts bilaterally and an enlarged liver. The endocrinologists were asked to evaluate him because of his short stature.

Psychosocial short stature was not suspected until the mother failed to come to see her son for 2 weeks. When she did, they passed each other in the hall without speaking. This prompted further observation of the maternal-child relationship, which strongly indicated that the mother rejected her son.

This boy was very aggressive, in contrast to most patients with psychosocial short stature. He wished to be surrounded by nurses, but he was aggressive toward the physicians and persisted in pinching and poking them. When stimulated with arginine and insulin to determine whether GH was released, he did not secrete significant GH into his serum.

The patient was removed from the home and grew approximately 15 cm in the next 12 months. The cataracts were determined to be congenital and of undetermined cause. The hepatomegaly was determined to be secondary to *Toxocara*. Eosinophilia was also present.

This patient exemplifies that all patients with type II PSS do not fit the same mold of shyness. This boy was exactly the opposite of most children with psychosocial short stature, and he did not have the other usual signs and symptoms of polyphagia, polydipsia, or drinking from the toilet bowl. Other variants are recorded by us elsewhere (36).

Patients with type III PSS were not described to have the bizarre symptomatology noted in type II patients, and the parents were not indifferent or rejecting as are the parents of patients with type II PSS. Boulton et al. described (24) and subsequently commented about (37) seven children 3.6–11.6 years of age with bone ages of 2–9.5 years with the diagnosis of psychosocial growth failure. Of these, six had a disorder of attachment for the parents, dating from infancy, with recurrent depression in three. The seventh child had reactive depression from current family stress.

In addition to differing from type II patients in having primarily an attachment and/or depressive disorder instead of the bizarre symptomatology intermittently and frequently found in type II patients, these patients released significant GH with arginine and insulin and during the collection of integrated concentrations of GH overnight. Also, these patients responded favorably to GH injections by growing at very accelerated rates (a growth velocity of 4.66 standard deviations, SD, $\pm$ 1.88 standard error of the mean, SEM, in contrast to the pretreatment growth SD velocity of -2.32 SD $\pm$ 0.122 SEM). Type II patients respond poorly to GH therapy (38,39).

The parents and their parental attitudes toward the children and problem differed from those of type II children in that the parents of type III PSS patients had insight into their problem and several felt guilty and/or had depression and readily accepted guidance and help for their children and themselves. Psychiatric assistance seemed to be readily accepted and was probably beneficial.

Table 3 Growth Measurements of 10 Patients with Type II Psychosocial Short Stature

Patient (Sex)	Chronological Age (Years)	Height Age (Years)	Bone Age (Years)	Weight × 100 (Weight for Age, %)
1 (M)	7.8	4.5	4.0	7
2 (M)	11.5	5.3	6.0	6
3 (M)	7.1	3.0	4.0	12
4 (F)	5.1	2.8	5.0	2
5 (F)	7.1	4.0	6.0	0
6 (M)	4.4	2.0	2.0	0
7 (M)	6.9	3.5	3.5	−6
8 (M)	5.1	2.0	2.5	−13
9 (M)	3.9	1.2	2.5	−20
10 (M)	5.8	3.0	4.0	−23

Patients with type I PSS characteristically have failure to thrive, are underweight for height, and have growth deficiency. Patients with type II and type III PSS may or may not be underweight for height.

The growth measurements in 10 sequential patients with type II PSS observed in the clinic are listed in Table 3. The height and bone ages of these patients were approximately half those expected for chronologic age. Many were not underweight for height, although 40% were. Only 20% of the group were significantly underweight. The growth pattern in Figure 2 is that of 1 patient who had significant PSS, who had been evaluated adequately before the diagnosis was made, and who had never been underweight for height. In fact, the converse was true: the patient was of greater weight than usual for height.

In the study by Ferholt et al. (18) of 10 patients who probably had type II PSS, all were at least 2 standard deviations below the mean height for age. Growth failure in 3 began in the second year of life or before, for 4 it began in

the third year, and for the remaining 3 children, in the sixth and seventh years.

V. PSYCHODYNAMICS

In 1985, Ferholt and coworkers (18) reported a psychodynamic study of psychosomatic short stature that classified this syndrome as one of depression, personality disorder, and impaired growth. An intensive longitudinal psychiatric study of 10 very short children, whose severe growth failure was reversed when the interpersonal environment was improved, was reported. Marked depression, personality disorders with narcissistic features, and a spectrum of eating disorders were present. The behavioral abnormalities and overt depression were almost immediately relieved by removing the children from their homes. This observation added much to our understanding of the psychiatric component of PSS. These authors noted that the growth failure was associated with overt depression, and the shortness of stature was directly proportional to the extent of social withdrawal and to a prolonged history of marked inactivity. During episodes of overt depression the growth rates were nil. The marked inactivity and withdrawal occurred almost exclusively at home, not at school. Admission to the hospital or removal from the adverse environment quickly reversed the depression (18), at least superficially, although experienced observers easily detected an underlying sadness. Often these patients had uncamouflaged suicidal fantasies.

Green et al. (40,41) published two excellent extensive reviews of the psychodynamics of PSS patients. Money et al. (42,43) extended our understanding of the complexity and variance of the principal participants (parents and child) when they reported that PSS occurs in association with Munchausen syndrome by proxy. In these instances, the mothers were seeking atonement of sins and guilt by way of sacrificing their children. Addiction to abuse by many of these patients also was noted by Money et al. (42). They found that these patients frequently precipitate abuse on themselves to gain attention

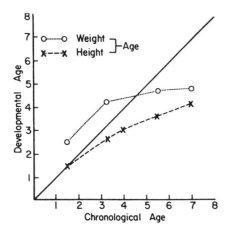

Figure 2 The growth curve of a patient with PSS type II. The weight was always greater than the average for height. Therefore, there was no evidence, for caloric deficiency.

from parents or keepers. The combination created a vigorous cycle of confrontation and further rejection by the parents.

The difference in psychodynamics for patients and their parents with type II and III PSS has been described. However, there is overlap in that patients in both groups have been described as depressed. Even in failure to thrive of nonorganic etiology in infancy, recent work has prompted the suggestion that the behavior attributes of children contribute significantly to the cycle (Chap. 9).

VI. PATHOPHYSIOLOGY

Because patients with type II PSS often have growth hormone deficiency, investigators have repeatedly asked whether patients with this type of PSS have short stature of endocrine origin or whether these patients have a nutritional deficiency that could be caloric or of a specific substrate, or whether both endocrine and nutritional factors could play roles (Chap. 8).

Nutritional causes are suspected because some patients are underweight for height and have protuberant abdomens and a history compatible with malabsorption. Hopwood and Becker described 35 PSS children; 20% had malodorous stools (44). Only 20% of the 35 were believed to have decreased food intake. Studies by Parra failed to demonstrate evidence of steatorrhea (Table 4) even in those who were symptomatic (45). Normal serum carotene levels were found in 94%, as well as normal xylose tolerance. Fecal fat was normal in six of seven. Results from examinations of jejunal biopsy specimens were normal in the five who were biopsied. These five also had normal "disaccharidase" activity.

Regardless of these data, a history of steatorrhea is often present in patients with type II PSS, as noted earlier. There is the possibility that malabsorption occurs while the patient is home but that it disappears when the patient is admitted to the hospital. The incompatibility of the history of steatorrhea with the physical and laboratory findings for malabsorption remains an enigma, although transient elevation of somatostatin or somatostatin activity could explain this finding.

Nutritional factors were not characteristic in the seven patients with type III PSS reported by Boulton et al. (24,37).

All except one of these patients were at or above the 45th percentile when weight was plotted for height. Gastrointestinal symptoms have not been described in type III patients, but so few patients have been described to date that these may be described subsequently for patients in this group.

The results of a study of type II patients made by Thompson et al. are presented in Table 5. Corticotropin secretion, as determined indirectly by metyrapone testing, was abnormal in 80% of those tested. Thyroid function, as determined by ^{131}I uptake, was abnormal in 36%. Growth hormone testing was abnormal in 54% (20). It was further demonstrated by Parra that many patients with psychosocial short stature failed to release GH, with arginine stimulation similar to that in patients with true idiopathic GH deficiency (45). Data are summarized in Figures 3 and 4. However, Green et al. in 1984 (41) reviewed the data available at that time and concurred that the finding of GH in significant levels after pharmacologic testing for GH release does not exclude the diagnosis. Patients with type III PSS have been reported to have normal growth hormone secretion (24).

The data regarding integrated concentrations of GH in type II patients are very limited. Howse et al. (46), in 1977, studied 3 children with PSS by drawing blood continuously over a 5 h period of sleep at night and correlated these levels with sleep electroencephalograms (EEGs). All 3 showed lower peak GH values, lower 5 hour mean GH values, and subnormal GH responses to insulin-induced hypoglycemia compared with a group of normal short children. We have studied 3 siblings, ages 4.5, 6.5, and 7.8 years, whose integrated concentrations of GH were <0.5, 0.9, and 0.8 ng/ml, respectively. These values are abnormally low for the chronologic ages (Chap. 3). In 1994, Albanese et al. studied spontaneous GH secretion over 18 h in 11 patients with type II PSS (47) over a 3 week period following diagnosis and hospitalization and separation from family. On the first day of admission, spontaneous GH secretion demonstrated a spectrum of abnormalities in the pattern of basal values, pulse frequency, and pulse amplitude. Such GH insufficiency showed reversibility during the 3 weeks in the hospital. Indeed, there was a significant increase in GH secretion that

Table 4 Gastrointestinal Data from Patients Admitted with Type II Psychosocial Short Stature and History of Steatorrhea

Test	Results		
	Normal	Abnormal	Total
Carotene	18	1	19
Xylose absorption	8	0	8
Fecal fat	6	1	7
Jejunal biopsy	5	0	5
Microscopic	5	0	5
Disaccharidase activity	5	0	5

Table 5 Endocrine Studies 2–3 Days After Admission in 25 Patients with Type II Psychosocial Short Stature

Test	Results		
	Normal	Abnormal	Total
Metyrapone	5	20	25
Thyroxine	21	4	25
^{131}I	14	8	22
Growth hormone			
Insulin tolerance test	8	9	17
Arginine tolerance test	5	9	14
Both	5	6	11

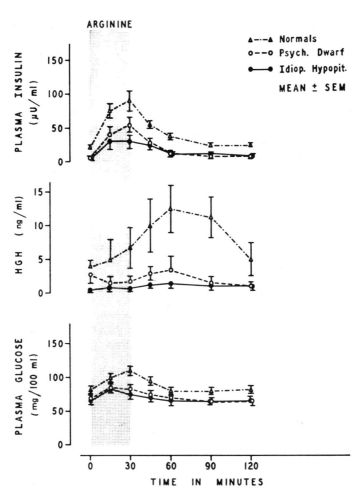

Figure 3 The concentration of insulin, growth hormone, and glucose after arginine stimulation of 11 growth hormone-deficient patients, 11 patients with Type II psychosocial short stature, and 11 normal controls.

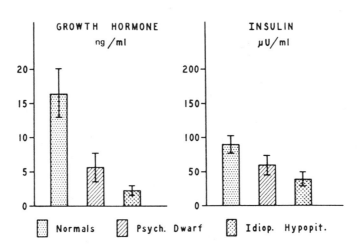

Figure 4 The peak values of insulin and growth hormone in the same groups as in Figure 3.

was amplitude modulated without any significant modification in pulse frequency.

Of considerable interest is the clinical observation of sleep disturbances, such as roaming and restlessness, as reported initially by Wolff and Money (48). At least two studies (40,49) have documented by use of EEG recording that a gross deficit of stage IV sleep and a decreased slow-wave sleep (stages III and IV) are found at the time of diagnosis in type II PSS patients. These changes reverse to normal within a brief period after the patients are removed from the adverse environment. The alterations in GH described earlier can be associated with the sleep disorders prevalent in these patients.

In the limited number of type II PSS patients whose somatomedin C (SmC) or insulin-like growth factor I (IGF-I) levels have been reported, the values were low during the period of growth failure (25,40,41). In 9 of 12 such patients included in a summary by Green, normalization of SmC levels occurred once the patient was removed from the adverse home environment. These rises were consistent with increased growth rates. The SmC levels as reported in seven type III patients were normal and were not affected by GH therapy.

The biochemical control of the endocrine and gastrointestinal systems deserves further consideration. Absolute or relative excess of somatostatin could account for the decrease in GH and thyroxine secretion and for the steatorrhea. These findings occur in the somatostatinoma syndrome (50).

As fascinating as all the previous observations is the one made by multiple authors, that the administration of GH to type II patients who remain in their adverse environment produces minimal or no growth response and induces only a minimal rise in SmC or IGF-I. At least nine such patients have now been tested in this manner (38–40,51). Therefore, in at least some patients, there appears to be a dual defect with the GH axis: decreased GH secretion and a decreased response to exogenous GH. Type III patients have been found to respond to GH treatment (24,37), although the dose used in the patients with type III PSS was a pharmacologic dose (1.2 units/kg/week) versus the doses (approximately 0.3 units/kg/week) used in the type II patients (38,39).

Animal models have also been useful in studying PSS. Miller et al. (52) described hyperphagia and polydipsia in socially isolated monkeys, and Schanberg et al. (53) found that restricting preweanling rat pups from active tactile interaction with their mothers produced specific abnormalities in at least three biochemical processes involving growth. The first was an immediate and significant decrease in tissue ornithine decarboxylase (ODC) in all tissues, including brain; second, a decrease in GH levels; and third, decreased peripheral sensitivity to GH. When exogenous GH was given to the pups, tissue ODC was unresponsive. Green (25) points out that although one obviously cannot generalize that data observed in the rat pups apply to children, marked similarities of physiologic responses to abnormal mothering gives additional support to the concept that an adverse psychosocial environment rapidly causes GH dysfunction and growth retardation.

In summary, endocrine dysfunction occurs frequently in children with type II psychosocial short stature, although not

in patients with types I and III. Endocrine dysfunction and growth inhibition are quickly reversible when the patient is removed from the adverse environment. These children characteristically have a reversal of the inability to release GH within a matter of 1 or 2 days after they are taken out of the adverse environment. Nutritional factors may also play a role in some patients with type II PSS (8), but with the limited data available (24,37), malnutrition is not a major contributor to the growth retardation of patients with type III PSS. An excess of endorphins could account for the pain agnosia and also suppression of gonadotropins that occur in teenagers with type II PSS.

VII. PROGNOSIS

The prognosis for growth is good or excellent if the patient's adverse environment can be altered significantly and early. Characteristic growth curves for patients with type II PSS are shown in Figure 5. It is the impression of many investigators that if type II children are not removed from their adverse environment until their early teens, it is unlikely they will reach their genetic height potential, although finite data are unavailable (54).

Growth also occurs rapidly in the skull (55), sometimes so rapidly that on x-ray films the sutures appear to be split. Radiologists who are unaware of the history have misdiagnosed this phenomenon.

The endocrine abnormalities, when present, often disappear within 2 or 3 days of admission to the hospital. The aberrancies of sleep and the EEG patterns that accompany these are restored to normal; the pain agnosia, when present, also disappears (35).

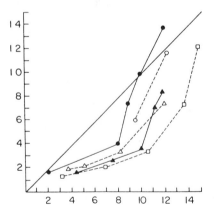

Figure 5 The growth curves of five patients with psychosocial short stature type II. The curve of the first patient (solid circles) resembles that observed for the first case described earlier. The prediagnosis growth rates are represented by solid lines, and the growth rates when the adverse environments were changed are represented by dotted lines. The third and fourth patients (triangles) are siblings: the fourth is the younger and, when he was removed from the home, his height soon surpassed that of his older brother.

The prognosis for intelligence in type II patients is guarded (56,57). If these patients are removed from the adverse environment at an early age and placed in an intellectually stimulating environment, they appear to have the capability eventually to function within normal limits. If the patients are removed from the adverse environment later in childhood (during the school years), they do not attain intellectual capability in the normal range.

Money et al. (56,57) demonstrated that children rescued before 5.5 years of age advanced their intelligence quotient (IQ) from 71 ± 21 to 104 ± 11, whereas those rescued after 5.5 years advanced from 63 ± 15 to only 78 ± 16. Each group had the same amount of time for catch-up. Annecillo and Money cited a girl of 3.8 years with an IQ of 36 who was rescued and who at age 13.7 years had an IQ of 120 (54).

The prognosis for the emotional stability of these children as adults is poor, particularly for those whose condition is diagnosed late in childhood. When they reach adulthood, these patients often abuse their children psychologically. Money and associates demonstrated that these children's parents had been psychologically abused. Early removal from the adverse environment into an emotionally stable environment is essential if the child is to have any chance to develop into an emotionally stable adult. The same guarded prognosis applies for healthy parenting.

Boulton et al. (24,37) were guardedly optimistic in predicting the outcome for type III patients because the parents of these individuals had greater insight into the problems of their children than did parents of children with PSS type II.

VIII. DIAGNOSTIC AND THERAPEUTIC CONSIDERATIONS

The failure to find an organic cause of growth retardation in any patient makes a psychologic cause probable. Physicians, nurses, and teachers who see children who are short and have no explanation for the limited stature must be aware of the frequency with which this syndrome occurs. Psychologic causes for growth inhibition occur in patients between early infancy and late adolescence, although there are at least the three types, referred to previously. Also, it is important to realize that the home environments of these patients may be very diverse. Its occurrence spans *all* socioeconomic groups.

The preceding case histories further elaborate upon the variability of the syndrome. This variability must be recognized if the syndrome is to be diagnosed in accord with the frequency of occurrence.

Unfortunately, the only treatment for type II patients is to change the child's psychologic environment. Often this means the geographic environment as well. Parents of infants with type I and apparently type III PSS are more open to education for parenting than are parents of type II children. Most of the parents of children with type II do not have the emotional constitution to alter their attitudes toward their children. Consequently, removel from the home is frequently necessary. Recently, Wolff and associates have had some success, in a few instances, when the parent(s) were treated in the home (58).

Unfortunately, many state laws do not make it easy to remove patients who are psychologically but not physically abused from the home. It is not within the scope of this chapter to suggest legislation or specific approaches. However, we encourage a team approach among social services, physicians, nurses, and legal authorities. Albanese et al. (47) suggested that evidence to support removal from the home may be difficult to achieve; however, documentation of reversibility of GH secretion during short-term hospitalization may provide evidence justifying a longer term separation on a legal basis.

Treatment of type III PSS needs to be directed toward improving the patients' depression and stressed psychologic relationships between the children and parents. Although these patients are reported to respond to GH therapy with increased growth, GH therapy should be considered only as adjunctive therapy if it is considered at all.

IX. FUTURE RESEARCH

Psychosocial short stature is of at least three types and represents fascinating biologic phenomena. There remain many unanswered questions, and the syndrome challenges us from the aspects of diagnosis, cause, and treatment.

Many questions that remain unanswered concerning this PSS syndrome include the following: (1) Why do some children treated in this manner respond with growth failure but others do not? (2) What is the biochemical mechanism that inhibits GH release and, sometimes, the release of other trophic hormones in type II PSS? Other questions that are pertinent to our understanding of PSS include the following: (1) What happens in the gastrointestinal tract so that a history that is strongly suggestive of steatorrhea in patients with type II PSS is frequently obtained, but evidence for steatorrhea is not found when the patient is admitted to the hospital? (2) How do we effectively treat patients and parents of these patients so they may stop or reverse the process?

REFERENCES

1. Powell GF, Brasel JA, Blizzard RM. Emotional deprivation and growth retardation simulating idiopathic hypopituitarism. I. Clinical evaluation of the syndrome. N Engl J Med 1967; 276:1271–1278.
2. Powell GJ, Brasel JA, Raiti S, Blizzard RM. Emotional deprivation and growth retardation simulating idiopathic hypopituitarism. II. Endocrinologic evaluation of the syndrome. N Engl J Med 1967; 276:1279–1283.
3. Krieger I. Food restriction as a form of child abuse in 10 cases of psychosocial deprivation dwarfism. Clin Pediatr (Phila) 1974; 13:127–133.
4. Krieger I, Mellinger RC. Pituitary function in the deprivation syndrome. J Pediatr 1971; 79:216–225.
5. Whitten C, Fischoff J. Evidence that growth failure from maternal deprivation is secondary to undereating. JAMA 1969; 209:1675–1682.
6. Krieger I. Endocrines and nutrition in psychosocial deprivation in the USA: comparison with growth failure due to malnutri-

tion on an organic basis. In: Gardner LI, Amacher P, eds. Endocrine Aspects of Malnutrition: Marasmus, Kwashirkor and Psychosocial Deprivation. Kroc Foundation, CA: Santa Ynez, 1973:129–162.

7. Krieger I, Whitten CF. Energy metabolism in infants with growth failure due to maternal deprivation, under-nutrition, or causes unknown. J Pediatr 1969; 75:374–379.

8. Bithoney WG, McJunkin J, Michalek J, Egan H, Snyder J, Munier A. Prospective evaluation of weight gain in both nonorganic and organic failure-to-thrive children: an outpatient trial of a multi-disciplinary team intervention strategy. Dev Behav Pediatr 1989; 10(1):27–31.

9. Bithoney WG, Newberger EH. Child and family attributes of failure-to-thrive. Dev Behav Pediatr 1987; 8(1):32–36.

10. Bithoney WG, Dubowitz H, Egan H. Failure to thrive/growth deficiency. Pediatr Rev 1992; 13(12):453–459.

11. Money J. The syndrome of abuse dwarfism (psychosocial dwarfism or reversible hyposomatotropism). Am J Dis Child 1977; 131:508–513.

12. Bakwin J. Emotional deprivation in infants. J Pediatr 1949; 35:512–521.

13. Silver J, Finklestein M. Deprivation dwarfism. J Pediatr 1967; 70:317–324.

14. Blodgett F. Growth retardation related to maternal deprivation. In: Solnit A, Provence S, eds. Modern Perspectives in Child Development. New York: International Universities Press, 1963:83–93.

15. Patton R, Gardner I. Influence of family environment on growth: the syndrome of maternal deprivation. Pediatrics 1962; 30:957–962.

16. Gardner LI. Deprivation dwarfism. Sci Am 1972; 227:76–82.

17. Money J, Wolff G. Late puberty, retarded growth and reversible hyposomatotropinism (psychosocial dwarfism). Adolescence 1974; 9:121–134.

18. Ferholt JB, Rotem DL, Genel M, et al. A psychodynamic study of psychosomatic dwarfism: a syndrome of depression, personality disorder and impaired growth. Am Acad Child Psychiatry 1985; 24:1:49– 57.

19. Langer G, Heinze G, Reim B, Matussek N. Reduced growth hormone responses to amphetamines in "endogenous" depressive patients. Arch Gen Psychiatry 1976; 33:1471–1475.

20. Thompson RG, Parra A, Schultz RB, Blizzard RM. Endocrine evaluation in patients with psychosocial dwarfism (abstract). Am Fed Clin Res 1969; 17:592.

21. Imura H, Yoshimi T, Ike Rubo K. Growth hormone secretion in a patient with deprivation dwarfism. Endocrinol Jpn 1971; 18:301–304.

22. Frisch H, Granditsch G, Wurst E. Psychosocial dwarfism and reversible growth hormone deficiency (German with English abstract). Wien Klin Wochenschr 1979; 91:726–731.

23. Neufeld ND. Endocrine abnormalities associated with deprivation dwarfism and anorexia nervosa. Pediatr Clin North Am 1979; 26:199–203.

24. Boulton TJC, Smith R, Single T. Psychosocial growth failure: a positive response to growth hormone and placebo. Acta Paediatr 1992; 81:322–325.

25. Green WH. Psychosocial dwarfism: psychological and etiological considerations. Adv Clin Child Psychol 1986; 9:245–278.

26. Bakwin H. Loneliness in infants. Am J Dis Child 1942; 62:30–40.

27. Talbot NB, Sobel EH, Burke BS, Lindemann E, Kaufman SB. Dwarfism in healthy children, its possible relation to emotional, nutritional, and endocrine disturbances. N Engl J Med 1947; 236:783–793.

28. Widdowson EM. Mental contentment and physical growth. Lancet 1951; 1:1316–1318.

29. Spitz R. Hospitalism, an inquiry into the genesis of psychiatric conditions in early childhood. Psychoanal Study Child 1945; 1:53–74.

30. Spitz R. Hospitalism, a follow-up report. Psychoanal Study Child 1946; 2:113–117.

31. Gardner LI, Amacher P, eds. Endocrine Aspects of Malnutrition: Marasmus, Kwashiorkor and Psychosocial Deprivation. Santa Ynez, CA: Kroc Foundation, 1973.

32. Patton RG, Gardner LI. Deprivation dwarfism (psychosocial deprivation); disordered family environment as cause of so-called idiopathic hypopituitarism. In: Gardner LI, ed. Endocrine and Genetic Diseases of Childhood and Adolescence, 2nd ed. Philadelphia: W.B. Saunders, 1975.

33. Gardner LI. The endocrinology of abuse dwarfism. Am J Dis Child 1977; 131:505–507.

34. Vietze PM, Falsey S, O'Connor S, et al. Newborn behavioral and interactional characteristics of nonorganic failure-to-thrive infants. In: Field TM, Goldberg S, Stern D, Sostek AM, eds. High Risk Infants and Children. New York: Academic Press, 1980:5–24.

35. Money J, Wolff G, Annecillo C. Pain agnosia and self-injury in the syndrome of reversible somatotropin deficiency (psychosocial dwarfism). J Autism Child Schizophr 1972; 2:127–139.

36. Blizzard RM, Bulatovic A. Psychosocial short stature: a syndrome with many variables. In: Bierich J, ed. Baillieres' Clinical Endocrinology and Metabolism, Vol. 6, No. 3. Philadelphia: W.B. Saunders, (Bailliere Tindall Limited), 1992.

37. Boulton TJC. Letter to the editor. Growth Genet Horm 1992; 9(1):4–5.

38. Tanner JH. Resistance to exogenous human growth hormone in psychosocial short stature (emotional deprivation). J Pediatr 1973; 82:171–172.

39. Frazier SD, Rallison O. Growth retardation and emotional deprivation: relative resistance to treatment with human growth hormone. J Pediatr 1972; 80:603–609.

40. Green WH, Deutsch SI, Campbell M. Psychosocial dwarfism, infantile autism, and attention deficit disorder. In: Nemeroff CB, Loosen PT, eds. Handbook of Psychoneuroendocrinology. New York: Guildford Press, 1987.

41. Green WH, Campbell M, David R. Psychosocial dwarfism: a critical review of the evidence. J Am Acad Child Psychiatry 1984; 23:39–48.

42. Money J, Annecillo C, Hutchinson JW. Forensic and family psychiatry in abuse dwarfism: Munchausen's syndrome by proxy, atonement, and addiction to abuse. J Sex Marital Ther 1985; 11:30–40.

43. Money J. Munchausen's syndrome by proxy: update. J Pediatr Psychol 1986; 11:583–584.

44. Hopwood NJ, Becker DJ. Psychosocial dwarfism: Detection, evaluation and management. In: Franklin AW, ed. Child Abuse and Neglect, Vol 3. London: Pergamon, 1979:439–447.

45. Parra A. Discussion of psychosocial dwarfism. In: Gardner LI, Amacher P, eds. Endocrine Aspects of Malnutrition: Marasmus, Kwashiorkor and Psychosocial Deprivation. Santa Ynez, CA: Kroc Foundation, 1973:155.

46. Howse PM, Rayner PHW, Williams JM, et al. Nyctohemeral secretion of growth hormone in normal children of short stature and in children with hypopituitarism and intrauterine growth retardation. Clin Endocrinol (Oxf) 1977; 6:347–359.

47. Albanese A, Hamill G, Jones J, et al. Reversibility of physiological growth hormone secretion in children with psychosocial dwarfism. Clin Endocrinol (Oxf) 1994; 40:687–692.

48. Wolff G, Money J. Relationship between sleep and growth in

patients with reversible somatotropin deficiency (psychosocial dwarfism). Psychol Med 1973; 3:18–27.

49. Taylor BJ, Brooke CGD. Sleep EEG in growth disorders. Arch Dis Child 1986; 61:754–760.

50. Krejs GJ, Orci L, Conon JM, et al. Somatostatinoma syndrome. N Engl J Med 1979; 301:285–292.

51. Sarr M, Job JC, Chaussain JL, Galse B. The diagnosis of psychosocial deprivation dwarfism: a critical study. Arch Fr Pediatr 1987; 44:331–338.

52. Miller RE, Mirsky IA, Caul WF, Sakata T. Hyperphagia and polydipsia in socially isolated rhesus monkeys. Science 1969; 165:1027–1028.

53. Schanberg SM, Evoniuk G, Kuhn CM. Tactile and nutritional aspects of maternal care: specific regulators of neuroendocrine function and cellular development. Proc Soc Exp Biol Med 1984; 175:135–146.

54. Annecillo C, Money J. Abuse of psychosocial dwarfism: an update. Growth Genet Horm. 1985; 1(4):1–4.

55. Reinhart JB, Drash AL. Psychosocial dwarfism: environmentally induced recovery. Psychosom Med 1969; 31:165–171.

56. Money J, Annecillo C, Kelley JF. Growth of intelligence: failure and catch-up associated respectively with abuse and rescue in the syndrome of abuse dwarfism. Psychoneuroendocrinology 1983; 8:309–319.

57. Money J, Annecillo C, Kelley JF. Abuse-dwarfism syndrome: after rescue, statural and intellectual catch-up growth correlate. J Clin Child Psychol 1983; 12:279–283.

58. Wolff G, Ehrich JHH. Psychosozialer Minderwuchs. In: Steinhausen HC, ed. Psychosomatische storungen und Krankheiton bei Kindern und Jugendlichen. Kohlhammer, Stuttgart, Germany 1981:58–75.

7

Intrauterine Growth Retardation

Joseph B. Warshaw

Yale University School of Medicine and Children's Hospital at Yale,
New Haven, Connecticut

I. INTRODUCTION

Intrauterine growth retardation or, preferably, intrauterine growth restriction (IUGR), represents a final common pathway by which diverse genetic and environmental influences result in low birth weight for gestational age. There has been some confusion about definitions of IUGR, which has been defined most commonly as a birth weight of less than the 10th percentile for gestational age. This likely results in an overestimation of IUGR because it is unlikely that 10% of all births in a given population have a pathologic restriction of growth. More than 10% of infants in areas with endemic malnutrition may have IUGR as well, but nourished middle class infants in the 5th to 10th percentile may be absolutely normal. Small infants in whom there is no evidence that adverse genetic or environmental influences are limiting to growth should be spared the IUGR label, which connotes pathology, and should be defined as small for gestational age (SGA). Further refinements of these definitions include the following: (1) "small for gestational age" should be applied to all infants < 10th percentile; and (2) "intrauterine growth restriction" generally should be reserved for infants < 3rd percentile, in recognition of the fact that some infants with growth restriction fall out of this range if an insult occurs late in gestation. Thus, although all IUGR infants are also SGA, not all SGA infants are IUGR.

The confusion is amplified further by differences in 10th percentile birth weights at each gestational age that have been used to define IUGR in different published studies. Differences in published standards of growth have likely been influenced by racial composition, socioeconomic status of the population studied, and elevation above sea level when the standards were developed (1–4). The commonly used Lubchenko grids (1), developed in Denver at about 5000 feet above sea level, may underestimate IUGR when these charts are used at sea level. What is necessary for an effective comparison between populations is the adoption of a single standard for fetal growth, for example, the standards developed by Brenner et al. based on 30,772 deliveries made at 21–44 weeks gestation in Cleveland (3).

II. INFLUENCES ON FETAL GROWTH

Fetal growth is ultimately controlled by the genetic endowment but is subject to diverse influences, summarized in Table 1.

The most obvious genetic influences on growth are seen in newborns with aneuploid chromosomal defects, including trisomy 18 and trisomy 13. Newborns with Turner syndrome are also characteristically small at birth.

Male infants are larger than females at birth, but this confers no survival advantage because infant mortality is greater in males. Size at birth differs greatly between different racial and ethnic groups; for example, the mean birth weight of populations in New Guinea is 2400 g compared with 3880 g in Native American populations (5). These weight differences likely reflect variations in maternal size, nutrition, and genetic factors.

Fetal endocrine status is of obvious importance for normal maturation and growth, but only insulin among the classic hormones has an apparent major influence on somatic growth and size at birth. The metabolic influences of insulin on fetal growth occur primarily in the last trimester, when there is rapid accumulation of adipose tissue. Insulin regulates fetal lipogenic activity and has a permissive effect on hepatic glycogen deposition and protein synthesis. A clinical example of the importance of insulin to fetal growth is the profound IUGR observed in infants with pancreatic agenesis or in those with an abnormal insulin receptor, as in the "leprauchan" syndrome (6). Such infants may exhibit little growth during the last trimester. Conversely, there can be a striking macrosomia in hyperinsulinemic infants of diabetic mothers who have increased adipose tissue and hepatic glycogen levels. Some of these effects of insulin are outlined in Table 2.

Table 1 Genetic, Hormonal, and Environmental Influences on Fetal Growth

Genetic and fetal factors
    Species, race, gender
    Congenital anomalies
    Chromosomal disorders
    Fetal hormones
    Growth factors
Maternal uterine environment
    Uterine and placental anatomy
    Uteroplacental function
    Human placental lactogen
    Substrate fluxes and transfer
    Uterine blood flow
    Maternal systemic disease
Macroenvironment
    Infectious agents
    Diet and nutrition
    Social and emotional stress
    Drugs and smoking
    Teratogens and toxins
    Altitude and temperature
    Ionizing radiation

Other classic hormones, including thyroxine, glucocorticosteroids, and sex hormones, have important influences on specific organ development or on functional and metabolic adaptation but have little influence on somatic growth. For example, thyroid hormones are important for central nervous system and skeletal maturation. Glucocorticoids modulate lung maturation and are of importance to the development of the surfactant system, and androgens are critical for sex differentiation.

Pituitary growth hormone itself is not a powerful determinant of fetal growth. However, in a recent report of 52 patients with idiopathic growth hormone deficiency, Gluckman et al. (7) reported a small decrease in birth length relative to weight in the growth hormone-deficient group. Over 60% of the males had microphallus, and among this group the effect on growth became far more significant during the first months of life.

The greater density of receptors for placental lactogen (HPL) in fetal ovine liver compared with receptors for growth hormone (8) suggests a role for HPL in fetal growth. This may account for a relatively small effect of growth hormone deficiency on size at birth. That HPL has a role in modulating

Table 2 Metabolic Effects of Insulin

Increases	Decreases
Lipogenesis	Lipolysis
Glycogenesis	Glycolysis
Protein synthesis	Gluconeogenesis

fetal growth is further supported by studies showing that maternal nutritional state influences the density of HPL receptors in fetal liver. In the ovine fetus, maternal starvation reduces the number of HPL receptors in fetal liver and may therefore play a role in the fetal growth restriction that accompanies maternal starvation (9).

Peptide growth factors play an important role in modulating fetal growth and maturation. These include the insulin-like growth factors (IGF-I and IGF-II), which in the fetus appear to be regulated independently of growth hormone. IGF-I influences the terminal differentiation of a number of tissues, including brain astrocytes, neural outgrowth, and myogenesis. Even though many of the influences of IGF-I appear to be local, serum concentrations of IGF-I correlate with birth weight (10). Both IGF-I and IGF-II are complexed to binding proteins that modulate their biologic activity. The IGFs and their binding proteins are regulated in a reciprocal direction by maternal starvation. Growth retardation in fetal rats caused by maternal starvation has been associated with the decreased expression of IGF-I and IGF-II and with the increased expression of IGF binding proteins in liver of the fetuses (11). Fetal rats with growth restriction induced by uterine artery ligation showed increased levels of IGF binding proteins and decreased IGF-II expression in placenta (12). Increased binding protein (IGF) likely decreases the bioavailability of the IGF. Bernstein et al. (13) reported a decrease in fetal plasma and placental and hepatic tissue IGF concentrations in nutritionally deprived, growth-retarded fetal rats. These studies, as well as older data showing a correlation between IGF levels and birth weight, suggest an important role for IGF in fetal growth regulation.

Epidermal growth factor (EGF) and transforming growth factor α, which may be its fetal form, influence growth and differentiation of a variety of epithelial cells, including those in lung and gut. Receptors for EGF are present throughout development and are increased in number in the placenta and lung of fetuses with growth restriction induced by uterine artery ligation (14). This suggests a role for EGF in fetal growth retardation. Additional evidence for an effect of EGF on somatic growth is the observation that exogenous EGF administered to rats less than 2 weeks of age decreases growth. This effect of EGF has been related to the suppression of IGF-I concentrations in growth-restricted fetuses (15).

Maternal constraint of fetal growth is an adaptation that may occur under conditions of decreased nutrient supply or when fetal growth is inappropriate for maternal size. The latter may involve changes in growth factor or hormonal signaling. Mice selected for high plasma IGF-I concentrations were not only larger but produced litters with heavier fetuses than mice selected for low IGF-I concentrations (16). Maternal constraints on fetal growth are also illustrated by the classic study of Walton and Hammond (17) showing that foals born to Shetland ponies bred to male Shire reflect maternal size at birth. Shire mares bred with Shetland males had offspring with a size typical of foals born to Shire mares.

Maternal constraints on fetal growth may be multigenerational. The adverse effect of maternal malnutrition on fetal growth may take several generations to correct after reinstitution of normal nutrition (18), which emphasizes the importance of maternal factors and the intrauterine milieu. For example, mothers who were IUGR themselves have an increased risk of having IUGR offspring (19).

III. CLINICAL PICTURE OF IUGR

The pattern of growth of the infant with IUGR often reflects the underlying condition that has resulted in growth restriction. The terms proportional and disproportionate have been used to distinguish newborns with decreased growth potential from those with restricted growth as a result of fetal malnutrition. Newborns with decreased growth potential caused by such conditions as chromosomal disorders, congenital infections, or exposure to environmental toxins are more likely to have body proportions that are proportional or symmetric; that is, the head, length, and weight generally follow similar percentile grids, or the head is small relative to the body. Obstetric monitoring of the fetus with decreased growth potential characteristically demonstrates decreased body growth, including that of the head, from midgestation or earlier. Fetuses with decreased growth potential are at high risk for having major malformations or congenital infection and are also at risk for poor neurobehavioral outcomes.

Newborns with fetal malnutrition caused by maternal malnutrition or decreased uteroplacental blood flow may have weight reduced out of proportion to length or head circumference. These infants, who exhibit a sparing of head growth during late gestation, are disproportionate, with the head circumference and length closer to the expected percentiles for gestational age than those for weight. Conditions in which fetal nutrition is compromised include multiple pregnancies and the smaller of twins, in which arteriovenous communications in the chorionic plate limit blood flow to one twin. IUGR is also seen in infants born at high altitudes or to mothers with cyanotic congenital heart disease, presumably because of decreased oxygen availability. Nutritional constraints on growth are unusual before 24–25 weeks of gestation; in most cases, only after that time does restriction in blood supply to the fetus result in IUGR. During the last trimester there is deposition of the storage fuels, glycogen and lipid, and the fetus quadruples in size. In mild to moderate degrees of IUGR, head growth may proceed along normal percentile grids, with a decrease in body fat and restriction in length and weight (disproportionate growth). When followed by serial fetal ultrasound, these infants may exhibit an increase in the head to abdominal circumference ratio. This sparing of head growth is thought to result from circulatory changes in the fetus that favor a redistribution of blood flow to the heart and brain. It is likely that the changes in blood flow that characterize the hemodynamic response to fetal nutrient restriction are also modulated by endocrine mechanisms. The mechanisms for head "sparing" are unclear but may relate to factors in the brain itself or be influenced by such factors as increases in the circulating levels of arginine vasopressin (20), which may contribute to decreased splanchnic blood flow and an

increase blood flow to the brain. Vasoactive prostaglandins are also likely to be important in modulating blood flow to the fetus and the hemodynamic changes that result in brain sparing. There may be exceptions to this general pattern, as with extreme nutritional restriction to the fetus with class D diabetes or other conditions that result in severely decreased uterine blood flow in which head growth becomes compromised.

Infants with either proportional or disproportionate IUGR should be evaluated carefully for conditions causing hydrocephalus or microcephaly, which may also confound the measurements. Figure 1 summarizes the classification of IUGR. The importance of environmental exposures, such as cigarette smoking, cannot be overestimated. In the developed countries of the world, cigarette smoking is the single greatest determinant of low birth weight (21,22).

The pattern of postnatal growth is also important to record and follow. A slow rate of postnatal growth may be seen in such conditions as genetic disorders, congenital infections, and the fetal alcohol syndrome. Infants with growth retardation secondary to fetal malnutrition often exhibit rapid growth when adequate nutrients are provided in the postnatal period; this is a good prognostic finding, even though these infants may stay relatively small throughout childhood. About 30% of nutritionally induced IUGR newborns are still below the third percentile at 2 years of age.

IV. MANAGEMENT OF IUGR

Management of IUGR should begin with recognition of the problem during pregnancy. This includes consideration of the options of cesarean section versus vaginal delivery. If biophysical data obtained during fetal monitoring show fetal distress, cesarean section may be the preferred mode of delivery. Decreased maternal weight gain and fundal growth should alert the caregiver to the likelihood of fetal growth retardation. Ultrasonography can then confirm the diagnosis by monitoring such parameters of fetal growth as the biparietal diameter or, as noted earlier, the relationship of head size to body size.

Strategies to treat fetal growth retardation have included therapies to decrease the platelet aggregation and abnormalities in uteroplacental circulation seen in toxemia of pregnancy (23,24).

Maternal parenteral nutritional supplementation is controversial. An adverse influence was observed when short-term administration of glucose to normal patients before delivery resulted in a significant increase in lactic acid and a fall in pH (25). This response is not surprising and is consistent with studies by Phillips et al. (26) showing that glucose infusion into fetal sheep resulted in increased oxygen consumption and lactate production, suggesting that increased substrate delivery can contribute to fetal hypoxemia under conditions of fetal oxygen deficiency. Similar mechanisms may contribute to the risk for sudden death in hyperglycemic fetuses of diabetic mothers. When the fetus is "adapted" to a decreased nutrient supply, there may be a potential risk to

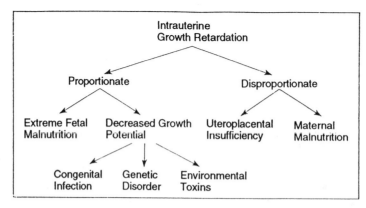

Figure 1 Classification of intrauterine growth retardation.

increasing nutritional intake without a corresponding increase in fetal oxygenation.

Important problems of the infant with IUGR secondary to intrauterine malnutrition are summarized in Table 3. Appropriate management can prevent may of these complications (Table 4). If there is birth asphyxia, support measures should be instituted immediately, including the establishment of an effective airway and the management of meconium if present.

Tracheal suction before the first breath if meconium is present at the level of the cords greatly reduced problems associated with meconium aspiration. Meconium aspiration is rarely seen in infants of less than 35 weeks gestation; therefore, in those infants, hypoxia per se is the major problem. An estimate of the degree of acidosis can be obtained from the cord blood pH. Hyaline membrane disease is generally less of a problem in infants with disproportionate IUGR because of the accelerated lung maturation commonly seen in these infants. Some asphyxiated newborns exhibit significant right-to-left cardiac shunting, making systemic oxygenation difficult to achieve. This is a consequence of chronic intrauterine hypoxia, which results in abnormal thickening of the smooth muscle of small pulmonary arterioles, thereby reducing pulmonary blood flow and increasing right-to-left blood flow at the atrial level or through the ductus arteriosus. Diagnosis of persistent pulmonary hypertension is confirmed by measuring the disparity between preductal (right radial) and postductal (umbilical arterial) PO_2. Nitric oxide therapy holds the greatest promise for treatment of persistent pulmonary hypertension and should largely supplant tolazoline and extracorporeal membrane oxygenation as therapeutic interventions.

Apgar scores should be assigned in the delivery room, and the infant should be dried rapidly and warmed to prevent hypothermia. As soon as the infant is stable, measurements should be taken and plotted on standard growth grids. Accurate measurements determine whether an IUGR newborn follows the disproportionate or proportional pattern. Measurements include the standard growth parameters of weight, height, and head circumference. The ponderal index, (weight in grams $\times$ 100) (length in cm^3), has also been used to identify infants with decreased weight relative to length; however, applications of standard measurements of length, weight, and head circumference to standard growth grids are generally more useful.

A careful assessment of gestational age should be done in all infants with IUGR. The examination most commonly used is a modification of a scale developed by Dubowitz et al. (27) that includes physical signs involving skin color and texture, hair, breast size, plantar creases, ear form and firmness, external genitalia, and neuromuscular assessment, which measures tone, posture, and reflexes. Scores are assigned for these measures, a total score being used to assign gestational age. This examination can be completed in about 10 minutes and has a predictive error or ± 2 weeks in infants weighing more than 1000 g. It is most accurate when performed within the first 6 h of life and by two observers.

Newborns with IUGR secondary to fetal malnutrition (e.g., those with disproportionate IUGR, with the head and length generally in higher percentiles than the weight) fre-

Table 3 Problems of the IUGR Newborn

Birth asphyxia	Hypothermia
Meconium aspiration	Hypoglycemia
Persistent fetal circulation	Hypocalcemia
Necrotizing enterocolitis	Polycythemia

Table 4 Management of the IUGR Infant

Gestational age assessment and careful history for drugs, other toxins
Prevent hypothermia
Check central hematocrit
Monitor blood sugar with first 45 minutes
Evaluate for congenital infections and congenital malformations
Chromosomal and genetic evaluation as indicated
Careful follow-up

quently appear scrawny as a result of their marked decrease in subcutaneous fat. They have an alert appearance and have higher Dubowitz ratings than premature infants with similar weights.

Infants should be examined for genetic causes of IUGR, including the presence of congenital malformations. They should also be evaluated for any stigmata of congenital infection. The examination should include weighing and examining the placenta to determine whether there are structural or vascular abnormalities contributing to IUGR.

Many of the problems of IUGR newborns relate to their markedly decreased metabolic reserves. There is a risk of perinatal asphyxia when oxygen and metabolic demands exceed the oxygen provided by the uteroplacental circulation. This underscores the need for careful biophysical monitoring of the at-risk fetus to alert the obstetrician to the presence of uteroplacental insufficiency. Hypoglycemia is found frequently in the immediate postnatal period. Hypothermia may increase both oxygen and glucose requirements. Blood glucose should be measured, and a central hematocrit should be performed to detect polycythemia. Hypoglycemia and polycythemia are primarily problems of nutritionally growth-retarded newborns. Those with IUGR secondary to congenital infection, genetic disorders, or environmental insults are less likely to experience these complications (Chap. 48).

Hypoglycemia is best treated by early recognition and prevention. All infants with IUGR should be tested with Dextrostix within the first 30–45 minutes of life. These infants are at risk for hypoglycemia because of decreased fuel stores secondary to their fetal malnourished state, decreased gluconeogenesis, and an increase in the peripheral use of glucose caused by polycythemia and cold stress. The best treatment for hypoglycemia is prevention by early feeding.

Hypocalcemia may also occur in the IUGR newborn, generally in association with neonatal stress. Only rarely do these infants require parenteral calcium, and this should be given with constant monitoring and with good venous access to avoid skin sloughing (Chap. 32).

Hyperviscosity secondary to polycythemia in infants with IUGR can result in venous thrombosis and central nervous system injury and can also contribute to hypoglycemia. Polycythemia results from increased erythropoietin levels secondary to relative fetal hypoxia. Because blood viscosity sharply increases when the central hematocrit exceeds 65%, partial exchange transfusion should be considered in IUGR infants when the hematocrit exceeds this level. There is some controversy concerning whether partial exchange transfusion should be done in asymptomatic polycythemic infants. However, infants treated with partial exchange transfusion appear to have fewer neurologic problems than those not transfused (28). The symptoms of polycythemia include respiratory distress, plethora, cardiac failure, and neurologic signs, including jitteriness and seizures. Partial exchange transfusion is done using normal saline or 5% salt-poor albumin to replace blood that is removed. This is preferable to plasma because of the high viscosity of adult fibrinogen in plasma. The formula used to calculate the amount of blood to be withdrawn (V) in a partial exchange transfusion is as follows: $V =$ estimated blood volume $\times$ [(actual hematocrit—the desired hematocrit)/the actual hematocrit].

V. NEWBORN OUTCOME

The most important aspect of IUGR is neurodevelopmental outcome, and this in large part reflects etiology. Infants with IUGR secondary to environmental insult or decreased growth potential generally have outcomes that are poor and reflect the underlying neuropathology of conditions caused by the environmental or genetic insult. Infants with IUGR with major genetic or chromosomal disorders—trisomy 18 or trisomy 13, for example—have virtually a 100% incidence of severe handicap and death, whereas outcome in those with congenital infection appears to be more variable (29). More than 75% of infants with congenital rubella infection have neurodevelopmental problems requiring special education. They may also have learning deficits and disturbances associated with hearing loss or blindness. Infants with cytomegalovirus infection may have only minor or no sequelae, whereas those who present with microcephaly or significant growth retardation are likely to have poor outcomes, with handicap rates generally exceeding 50%. It is important to test for hearing loss in all infants diagnosed with cytomegalovirus disease. Those infants who are at risk for neurodevelopmental delay should be identified early and be given the opportunity to be enrolled in stimulation and social enrichment programs.

When evaluating the outcome of newborns exposed to pharmacologic agents, it may be difficult to dissociate the effect of the primary disease state from that of the medication. It is clear, however, that many drugs are associated with poor outcomes. The fetal alcohol syndrome, for example, is associated with slow postnatal growth and poor developmental outcome. Prenatal cocaine exposure has been associated with IUGR and microcephaly. Exposures to therapeutic agents, such as phenytoin, warfarin sodium, and narcotics, may result in IUGR, slow postnatal growth, and a spectrum of developmental disabilities. Infants with these conditions require thorough and thoughtful evaluation, including appropriate counseling with the family.

Infants in whom brain growth has been spared may have more favorable neurodevelopmental outcomes even though there may be long-term consequences on growth. Even those infants in whom there has been a decrease in intrauterine brain growth may show significant postnatal catch-up. In a group of IUGR infants studied by Fitzhardinge and Inwood (30), acceleration of growth began shortly after birth but was limited to the first 9 months of age. Approximately 30% of IUGR infants were below the fifth percentile for height and weight by 2 years of age. Outcome is more difficult to predict in IUGR preterm infants, who appear to have a higher incidence of handicap than that of the general population. IUGR low birth weight infants at 3 years of age had lower weight and height than appropriate for gestational age-, weight-, or gestation-matched controls (31). That growth differences persist is further suggested by studies showing that IUGR infants continue to be underweight for height at 7 years of age (32) and that the smaller of twins, when weight differences were greater than 25%, had reduced height, head circumference, and intelligence quotient (IQ) compared with their normal siblings (33). In a group of IUGR infants followed for 13–19 years of age, significant deficits in height and weight were found, even after adjustment for differences in socioeconomic status and parental height (34). Children from higher social classes appear to score better on standard IQ tests and school achievement evaluations. Thus, although outlook for most infants with nutritional IUGR is favorable if the postnatal environment is adequate, there appears to be some increased risk for school problems and learning diability (35). Other studies have shown normal outcomes in IUGR. In a group of males weighing below the 2% at birth and matched with controls of the same social class, there were no differences in intelligence or school achievement (36).

Because IUGR infants are at risk for short stature, they have been considered candidates for treatment with human growth hormone (hGH, Chap. 5). This has been controversial, however, and has met with only limited success, likely because of the heterogeneity of the children treated (37). Blizzard's group reported a favorable response to hGH treatment, achieving up to twice the pretreatment growth velocity (38). However, the final height attained by these patients was not studied. In a recent study, a group of 25 children with a history of IUGR were treated with hGH for 4 years beginning at a median age of 6 years. This trial failed to demonstrate any differences in growth between IUGR and control infants (39). In a crossover study of hGH treatment of children with IUGR, Lanes et al. (40) reported that hGH had a sustained positive effect on increasing growth rates in children with IUGR, although the magnitude of the effect appeared to decrease with continued treatment. The variability in response to hGH treatment reported was likely caused by different etiologies of IUGR. As mentioned, growth hormone deficiency may contribute to IUGR (41). Similar to older children, IUGR patients with GH deficiency may respond to hGH therapy more than those who are not GH deficient. Treatment of IUGR newborns with hGH must be considered experimental and should not be used routinely until validated by larger clinical trials.

There are a number of recently reported longer term consequences of IUGR, including cardiovascular disease in later life (42,43). There is a reported increased risk of hypertension, coronary artery disease, and stroke, as well as a reported increased risk for glucose intolerance (44). These adult consequences of low newborn weight may result from the fetal adaptations to an adverse intrauterine environment that cause a permanent change in the structure and physiology of different organs. This phenomenon, termed programming, emphasizes the need for careful evaluation and long-term follow-up of IUGR infants.

In summary, IUGR is a final common pathway for diverse genetic and environmental influences on the developing fetus. Adverse environmental and genetic influences on fetal growth may result in permanent injury, but infants with low birth weight resulting from inadequate nutrient supply have a great potential for "catch-up" if they receive normal postnatal nutrition and social support.

REFERENCES

1. Lubchenko LO, Hansman C, Dressler, et al. Intrauterine growth as estimated from live born birth weight data at 24–42 weeks of gestation. Pediatrics 1963; 32:793–800.
2. Usher R, McLean F. Intrauterine growth of live born caucasian infants at sea level: standards obtained from measurements in 7 dimensions of infants born between 25 and 44. Pediatrics 1969; 74:901–910.
3. Brenner WE, Edelman DA, Hendricks CH. A standard for fetal growth for the United States of America. Am J Obstet Gynecol 1976; 126:55–564.
4. Sloan CT, Lorenz RP. Importance of locally derived birth weight normograms. J Reprod Med 1991; 36:598–602.
5. Meredith HV. Body weight at birth of viable human infants: a worldwide comparative treatise. Hum Biol 1970; 42:217–264.
6. Krook A, Brueton L, O'Rahilly S. Homozygous nonsense mutation in the insulin receptor gene in infant with leprechanism. Lancet 1993; 342:227–228.
7. Gluckman PD, Gunn AJ, Wray A, et al. Congenital idiopathic growth hormone deficiency associated with prenatal and early postnatal growth failure. International Board of the Kabi Pharmacia International Growth Study. Pediatrics 1992; 121(6):920–923.
8. Freemark M, Comer M, Mularoni T, Dercole J, Grandis A, Kokacki, L. Placental lactogen receptors in maternal sheep liver: effects of fasting and refeeding. Am J Physiol 1990; 258:E338–E346.
9. Freemark M, Comer M, Mularoni T, D'Ercole AJ, Granois A, Kodack L. Nutritional regulation of the placental lactogen receptor in fetal liver: implications for fetal metabolism and growth. Endocrinology 1989; 125:1504–1512.
10. Verhaeghe J, Van Bree R, Van Herck E, Laureys J, Bouillon R, Van Assche FA. C-peptide, insulin-like growth factors I and II, and insulin-like growth factor binding protein-1 in umbilical cord serum: correlations with birth weight. Am J Obstet Gynecol 1993; 169(1):89–97.
11. Straus DS, Ooi GT, Orlowski CC, Rechle MM. Expression of the genes for insulin-like growth factor-I (IGF-I) IGF-II and IGF-binding proteins-1 and 2 in fetal rat under conditions of intrauterine growth retardation caused by fasting. Endocrinology 1991; 128:518–525.
12. Price WA, Rong L, Stiles AD, D'Ercole J. Changes in IGF-I and II, IGF binding protein and IGF receptor transcript abundance after uterine artery ligation. Pediatr Res 1992; 32:291–295.
13. Bernstein IM, DeSourza MM, Copeland C. Insulin-like growth factor I in substrate deprived, growth-retarded fetal rats. Pediatr Res 1991; 30:154–157.
14. Lawrence S, Warshaw JB. Increased binding of epidermal growth factor to placental membranes in IUGR fetal rats. Pediatr Res 1989; 25:214–218.
15. Chernausek SD, Dickson BA, Smith EP, Hoath SB. Suppression of insulin-like growth factor induced growth retardation. Am J Physiol 1991; 260:E416–E421.
16. Kroonsberg C, McCutcheon SN, Siddiqui RA, et al. Reproductive performance and fetal growth in female mice from lines divergently selected on the basis of plasma IGF-1 concentrations. J Reprod Fertil 1989; 87:349–353.
17. Walton A, Hammond J. The maternal effects on growth and

conformation in Shire horse-Shetland pony crosses. Proc R Soc Lond [Biol] 1938; 124:311–335.

18. Stewart RJC, Pierce RF, Sheppard HG. Twelve generations of marginal protein deficiency. Br J Nutr 1975; 33:233–253.

19. Klebanoff MA, Meirik O, Berendes HW. Second generation consequences of small-for-dates birth. Pediatrics 1989; 84:343–347.

20. De Vane GW, Porter JC. An apparent stress-induced release of arginine vasopressin by human neonates. J Clin Endocrinol Metab 1980; 51:1412–1416.

21. Kramer MS. Intrauterine growth and gestational duration determinants. Pediatrics 1987; 80(4):502–511.

22. Stein ZA, Susser M. Intrauterine growth retardation: epidemiological issues and public health significance. Semin Perinatol 1984; 8:5–14.

23. Uzan S, Beaufils M, Breart G, Brazen B. Prevention of fetal growth retardation with low-dose aspirin: findings of the EPREDA trial. Lancet 1991; 337:1427–1431.

24. Battaglia C, Artini PG, D'Ambrogio G, Galli PA, Segne A, Genazzani AR. Maternal hyperoxygenation in the treatment of intrauterine growth retardation. Am J Obstet Gynecol 1992; 167:430–435.

25. Nicolini V, Hubinont C, Santolaya J, Fisk NM, Kodeck CN. Effects of fetal intravenous glucose challenge in normal and growth retarded fetuses. Horm Metab Res 1990; 22:426–430.

26. Phillips AF, Porte PJ, Stabinsky S, Rosenkrantz TS, Raye JR. Effects of chronic fetal hyperglycemic upon oxygen consumption in the ovine uterus and conceptus. J Clin Invest 1984; 74:279–286.

27. Dubowitz LM, Dubowitz V, Goldberg C. Clinical assessment of gestational age in the newborn infant. J Pediatr 1970; 77:1–10.

28. Black VD, Lubchenko LO, Luckey DW, et al. Developmental and neurological sequelae of neonatal hyperviscosity syndrome. Pediatrics 1982; 69P:426–431.

29. Allen MC. Development outcome and followup of the small for gestational age infant. Semin Perinatol 1984; 8:123–156.

30. Fitzhardinge PM, Inwood G. Acta Pediatr Scand 1989; 27–33.

31. Sung IK, Vohr B, Oh W. Growth and neurodevelopmental outcome of very low birth weight infants with intrauterine growth retardation: comparison with control subjects matched by birth weight and gestational age. J Pediatr 1993; 123(4):618–624.

32. Walther FJ. Growth and development of term disproportionate small-for-gestational age infants at the age of 7 years. Early Hum Dev 1988; 18(1):1–11.

33. Henrichsen L, Skinhoj K, Andersen GE. Delayed growth and reduced intelligence in 9–17 year old intrauterine growth retarded children compared with their monozygous co-twins. Acta Paediatr Scand 1986; 75(1):31–35.

34. Westwood M, Kramer MS, Nunz D, Lovett JM, Watters GV. Growth and development of fullterm nonasphyxiated small-for-gestational age newborns: follow-up through adolescence. Pediatrics 1983; 72:376.

35. Low JA, Handley-Derry MH, Burcke SO, et al. Association of intrauterine fetal growth retardation and learning deficits at age 9 to 11 years. Am J Obstet Gynecol 1992; 167:1499–1505.

36. Hawdon JM, Hey E, Kolvin I, Fundudis T. Born too small—is outcome still affected? Dev Med Child Neurol 1990; 32(11):943–953.

37. Tanner JM, Whitehouse RH, Hughes PCR, Vince FP. Effect of human growth treatment for 1 to 7 years on growth of 100 children, with growth hormone deficiency, low birthweight, inherited smallness, Turner's syndrome, and other complaints. Arch Dis Child 1971; 46:745–780.

38. Foley TP, Thompson RG, Shaw M, Baghdassarian A, Nissley SP, Blizzard RM. Growth responses to human growth hormone in patients with intrauterine growth retardation. J Pediatr 1974; 84(5):635–641.

39. Albanese A, Stanhope R. Growth and metabolic data following growth hormone treatment of children with intrauterine growth retardation. Horm Res 1993; 39(1-2):8–12.

40. Lanes N, Plotnick LP, Lee PA. Sustained effect of human growth hormone therapy on children with intrauterine growth retardation. Pediatrics 1979; 63(5):731–735.

41. Gluckman PD, Gunn AJ, Wray A, et al. Congenital idiopathic growth hormone deficiency associated with prenatal and early postnatal growth failure. J Pediatr 1992; 121:920–923.

42. Barker DJP, Gluckman PD, Godfrey KM, Harding JE, Owens JA, Robinson JS. Fetal nutrition and cardiovascular disease in adult life. Lancet 1993; 341:935–941.

43. Williams S, St. George IM, Silva PN. Intrauterine growth retardation and blood pressure at age seven and eighteen. J Clin Epidermiol 1992; 45:1257–1263.

44. Phipps K, Barker DJ, Hales CN, Fall CH, Osmond C, Clark PM. Fetal growth and impaired glucose tolerance in men and women. Diabetologia 1993; 36(3):225–228.

8

Nutritional Growth Retardation

Fima Lifshitz, Omer Tarim,* and Melanie M. Smith
Maimonides Medical Center and State University of New York Health Science Center at Brooklyn, Brooklyn, New York

I. INTRODUCTION

The single most important cause of growth retardation worldwide is poverty-related malnutrition (1). When suboptimal nutrition is continued for prolonged periods of time, stunting of growth occurs as the main clinical picture (2,3). However, nutritional dwarfing (ND), as found in a pediatric endocrine practice in the United States, is usually not the result of poverty-related malnutrition. Nutritional growth retardation and delayed sexual development among suburban upper middle class adolescents is most often a result of self-restrictive nutrient intake (4,5). Also, poor growth and inadequate nutrition have been found in such systemic problems as chronic inflammatory bowel disease (CIBD) and celiac disease (CD) (6,7).

Children with nutritional growth retardation are generally referred to the pediatric endocrinologist because of short stature or delayed puberty. Therefore, pediatricians and pediatric endocrinologists need to recognize nutritional dwarfing and become familiar with its etiology and treatment. This chapter reviews the diagnostic criteria, pathophysiology, and etiology of ND, as well as the treatment of patients with nutritional growth retardation.

II. DIAGNOSIS OF NUTRITIONAL DWARFING

Pediatric endocrinologists usually follow linear growth patterns accurately in the assessment of patients with short stature, but little consideration is given to body weight progression. Indeed, some growth charts used by pediatric endocrinologists feature height percentiles, growth velocity, and Tanner stages but do not depict current or previous weights (Serono Laboratories, Inc., Randolph, MA). Although the importance of evaluating the pattern of stature increments throughout life in the differential diagnosis of short stature cannot be overemphasized (Chap. 1), the assessment of the progression of body weight is equally relevant. Figure 1 illustrates this point. This 15-year-old male patient was referred to the endocrine clinic with short stature of unknown etiology. He was healthy in all other respects, and the only presenting symptom was deteriorating linear growth. On examination, both his height of 146.9 cm and weight of 37.6 kg were below the fifth percentile. No body weight deficit for height was evident, and sexual development was delayed (Tanner stage I). The initial measurements provided by the referring pediatrician indicated a decreasing growth rate with appropriate weight gain that was progressing just below the fifth percentile (Fig. 1a). This type of growth pattern usually denotes an endocrine disorder (Chap. 1).

However, after additional growth data were obtained and all height and weight records were compiled, a typical picture of nutritionally related growth retardation emerged (Fig. 1b). At 12 years of age, his weight gain ceased, which subsequently resulted in deceleration of linear growth and pubertal delay. Review of his nutritional intake showed that he was consuming only approximately 60% of his estimated energy needs based on age and sex. He was an athletic boy who described a desire to remain slim and avoid obesity, a syndrome that is discussed later in greater detail.

A. Anthropometric Parameters

1. Nutritional Dwarfing

The Wellcome Trust classification distinguishes ND from other types of malnutrition characterized by wasting and stunting (8). The anthropometric criteria for ND stipulate low weight for age with minimal deficit in weight for height. By these criteria, it may be difficult to differentiate ND children from those who have familial short stature, or constitutional growth delay, or who are constitutionally thin. Cross-sectional data in these normal children may also demonstrate weights below the mean for age. Only the longitudinal progression of body weight and height can more clearly reveal ND (9), which may occur even when there is weight for height

---

*Present affiliation: Associate Professor of Pediatrics, ULUDAG University of Bursa, Turkey

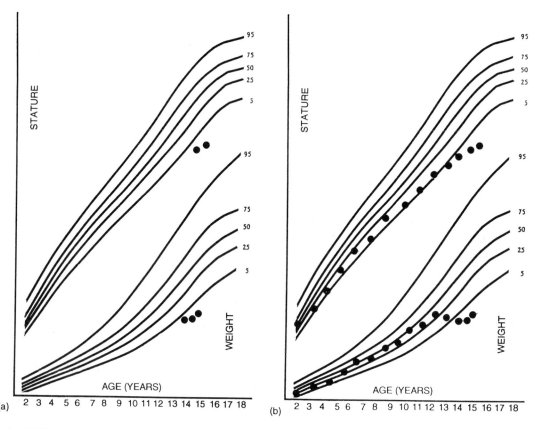

Figure 1   (a) The patient was referred because of short stature. Initially, the heights and weights depicted were the only available data. Signs of sexual development were absent. (b) Complete growth data for the patient, who began dieting at 12 years of age. (With permission from Semin Adoles Med 1987; 3.)

excess (10). In nutritional growth retardation, there is a deteriorating linear growth and/or delayed sexual development that is associated with inadequate weight gain (Fig. 2a and b) (5,6,9). This pattern of growth is seen in organic forms of ND, as in chronic inflammatory bowel disease (10), or in nonorganic forms, that is, ingestion of restrictive diets (11). Furthermore, although concern is heightened when weight or height measurements fall below the fifth percentile, deterioration across percentiles of weight and height may also indicate nutritional growth retardation (12) even when height and weight are above the fifth percentile (13). With nutritional rehabilitation, catch-up growth is usually achieved (14).

Indeed, the analysis of body weight progression may be the most important clue to diagnosis of suboptimal nutrition in patients with short stature (Fig. 2a and b). The calculation of theoretical weights and heights based on previous growth percentiles may be used to compare current anthropometric indices quantitatively with previously established patterns of weight and height progression (Fig. 2a). *Theoretical weight* is defined as the weight the patient should have had at the time of the examination, if the patient had continued to gain weight along the previously established percentile during the premorbid growth period (9). Body weight for height deficits are not common in ND, but there is often a body weight

deficit for theoretical weight (Fig. 2a and b). In contrast, short patients without ND, such as those with constitutional growth delay, continue to gain weight along established percentiles and the body weight at the time of assessment is equal to the theoretical body weight (Fig. 2c).

2.   *Normal Variations in Growth*

The growth patterns of nutritional dwarfing must also be distinguished from normal variations in growth that may occur as a result of variations in frame size, infant feeding practices, or constitutional factors resembling nutritional growth retardation.

a.   Variations in Frame Size.   Most normal children exhibit minimal deficits or excesses in body weight in proportion to height and grow along established percentiles (12). These constitutional variations in body weight are usually within one or two major percentiles of the height; they represent variations in frame size and do not necessarily reflect over- or undernutrition. The body weight and height increments of a child with constitutional thinness are depicted in Figure 3. Although his body weight was two major percentile lines below the height percentile, representing more than 20% body weight deficit for height, the adolescent grew

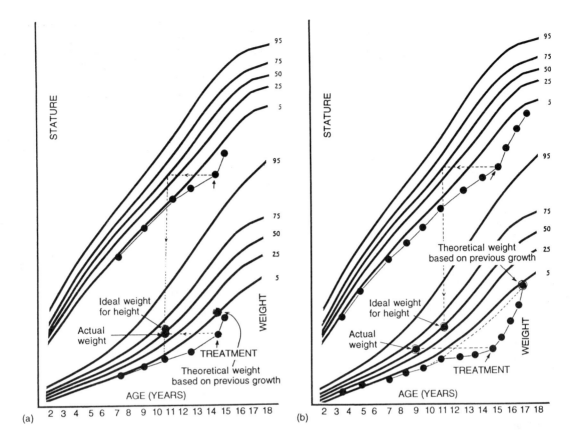

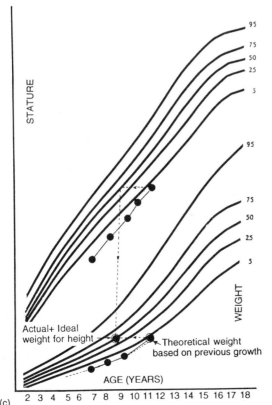

Figure 2 Growth pattern of nutritional dwarfing (a and b) compared with constitutional growth delay (c). The patient depicted in a shows that body weight gain and height progression decreased after 10 years of age. Extrapolated weight after age 14 years revealed a body weight deficit based on previous growth percentile. However, there was no body weight deficit for height; with nutritional rehabilitation, there was recovery in weight gain and catch-up growth. The patient shown in b demonstrates that there is a body weight deficit for height, but the deficit for theoretical weight is more marked. In contrast, c shows a patient who does not have nutritional dwarfing. This patient, with constitutional growth delay, shows a body weight gain consistently along the lower percentile, with no deviation in growth. Note that there was no body weight deficit for height or for theoretical weight based on previous growth. (Figure 2b was published in Lifshitz F, ed. Childhood Nutrition. Boca Raton, FL: CRC Press, 1995; 143–157.)

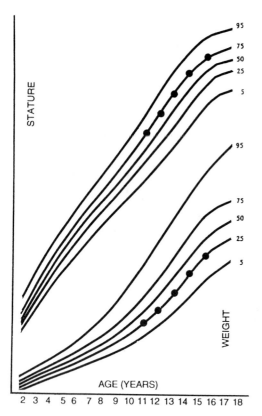

STATURE

95
75
50
25
5

95

75
50
25
5

WEIGHT

AGE (YEARS)

2 3   4   5   6   7   8   9 10 11 12 13 14 15 16 17 18

Figure 3 Constitutional underweight for height. Note the constant progression of both height and weight in the same percentiles for at least 4 years. Even though there is body weight deficit for height, there cannot be malnutrition because there must be a positive balance for growth to occur.

normally. A body weight deficit for height that remains constant and permits normal growth to proceed along a set percentile cannot be construed as abnormal. In contrast, a fall in growth associated with a poor rate of weight gain may indicate ND, even without an appreciable body weight deficit for height (Figs. 1b and 2a).

b. Breast-feeding and Growth. Growth rates of breast-fed infants have been shown to decelerate compared with those of formula-fed infants after the first 2–3 months of life (15). The differences between breast-fed and formula-fed infants were predominantly in weight, not length gain, both energy and protein intakes being lower in breast-fed infants (16). Although growth differences between groups are related to dietary intake, no disadvantagous effects on morbidity or mortality have been demonstrated (17).

Furthermore, growth charts are based on data derived primarily from formula-fed infants. Data have been published on weight and length gain of breast-fed infants enrolled in growth studies in Iowa between 1965 and 1987 (15). However, the breast-fed infants were allowed up to 8 ounces formula per day, and solid foods were allowed after 1 month of age. Therefore, additional data are necessary to construct

appropriate growth charts for infants exclusively breast-fed for the first 4–6 months and extensively breast-fed for the remainder of the first year. Long-term differences in growth status attributable to breast-feeding have not been reported in well-nourished populations.

The cause-effect relationship between breast-feeding and slower growth may not be purely nutritional. For example, prolonged breast-feeding may be more prevalent among poorer, less educated women. Thus, reasons including economic necessity and traditional norms, as well as access to better health care, which may improve health by preventing and treating disease, may also play a role. Furthermore, in a longitudinal study it was shown that weights of the infants were heaviest just before weaning, implying that mothers delayed weaning their children, which implies reverse causality (18).

Thus, the pediatrician who is following an exclusively breast-fed infant who slows in weight gain should consider all the possibilities (19). First, the adequacy of the infant's intake should be evaluated by assessing the frequency and duration of feedings. Milk production may be reduced with severe maternal restriction in caloric and protein intakes (20,21) and unusual feeding practices, such as the use of high-fiber grains and low-fat foods (22) or strict vegetarian diets (23). Although the composition of milk produced by a lactating woman does not seem to be altered despite restricted protein and energy intakes, rare cases of specific nutrient deficiencies, such as chloride, have been reported to cause failure to thrive in breast-fed infants (24). Additionally, lack of maternal support by the family or physician, insufficient knowledge about breast-feeding techniques (25), or inappropriate feeding routines (26,27) may also lead to inadequate milk supply. Other factors associated with a decrease in milk production, such as mastitis, birth control pills, resumption of menses, pregnancy, returning to work, or a poor suck because of various anatomic or functional causes affecting the infant, should also be considered. After excluding these factors and assuring an adequate milk supply, slower weight gain and linear growth should not be a concern and breast-feeding should continue. The multiple advantages of human milk are reviewed elsewhere, and the introduction of supplemental feedings, which may interfere with breast-feeding, should not be added unless there is a medical indication.

However, the prevalence of failure to thrive in breast-fed infants is reported to be as high as 22% (18,19), and any weight loss in a breast-fed baby warrants evaluation and intervention when necessary (Chap. 9).

c. Constitutional Growth Delay. The most common cause of short stature and sexual infantilism in the adolescent is constitutional growth delay (CGD). These patients are typically "slow growers" and "late bloomers" (Chap. 1). They usually exhibit a severe deceleration of growth within the first 2 years of life, with subsequent definition of a growth channel and normal growth increments paralleling the normal curve until adolescence, when a growth spurt occurs. Because of a delayed adolescent growth spurt, however, there may also be an apparent deviation from their own growth curves at this time. The delayed bone age and puberty permit growth after the average child has stopped growing. Thus, CGD patients may attain an appropriate adult height for the family.

However, we found significant differences between the growth of patients with CGD and those with familial short stature (FSS). The weight/length (W/L) ratio profiles and weight/height (W/H) ratio profiles from 4 months to 12 years of age differed among these two types of short stature (28). After 4 months of age, the W/L ratio of the patients with CGD was significantly lower than that of the FSS population. A weight deficit for length was also noted by month 6 of life in the CGD population. The difference became more noticeable by 18 months of age. In addition, nutritional parameters, such as mean creatinine-height index, retinol binding protein, serum iron, and transferrin saturation values, were lower among young CGD patients. These data suggested that suboptimal nutrition early in life contributes to the course of CGD. The deterioration in growth and weight progression that occurs in infancy could be the result of a nutritional insult. After an adaptive readjustment, these children resume normal growth rates and maintain appropriate weight gain increments later in life. Slowing the growth rate without other functional alterations may be an advantageous adaptation to limited food intake (29).

In a study of men with a history of CGD, bone mineral density was found significantly lower in comparison with men with normal growth and pubertal development. It was demonstrated that the timing of puberty remained a significant determinant of bone density after accounting for the effects of age, body mass index, exercise, alcohol intake, calcium intake, and serum testosterone. It was hypothesized that the timing of puberty is an important determinant of peak bone mineral density in males (30). However, the reverse could also be true. Although the effect of calcium intake seemed to be accounted for, a deficiency of calcium intake throughout childhood could have led to decreased bone mineral density, which in turn was associated with constitutional delay of growth and pubertal development.

Other studies also showed that children who had primary protein-calorie malnutrition in the first year of life had downregulation in their growth (31). Thereafter, with improved nutrition, they resumed growing at normal rates but, like CGD patients, rechanneled their growth percentiles at a lower level than that before the nutritional insult. They also had significant delays in sexual maturation and short stature in comparison with the control group until puberty. However, their growth rate during adolescence was equal to or better than that of the comparison group. This pattern of growth and sexual development among patients with primary malnutrition strikingly resembles the pattern in CGD patients. Thus, we believe that CGD represents an adaptation to suboptimal nutrition in infancy leading to readjustment of growth to a lower percentile until puberty. Patients diagnosed as CGD may have had subtle nutritional deficiencies in early life. Unless specifically looked for, these cannot be detected (28). Therefore, a workup for nutritional deficiencies is advisable during the deceleration phase of weight gain and height progression in the infancy and early childhood of patients with CGD (Chap. 1).

B. Biochemical Parameters

Patients with nutritional growth retardation do not appear to be wasted, and biochemical parameters of nutritional status, including serum levels of retinol binding protein, prealbumin, albumin, transferrin, and triiodothyronine (T_3) levels, do not distinguish ND patients from those with familial or constitutional short stature (Fig. 4a and b) (32). Similarly, other indices of malnutrition, such as the urinary creatine-height index or urinary nitrogen/creatinine ratio, do not usually reflect abnormalities (Fig. 4c). The reason is that ND patients have adapted to their suboptimal nutritional intake and they maintain homeostasis by decreasing growth, thereby reaching an equilibrium with preservation of all their nutritional markers (see later).

We also showed that insulin-like growth factor I (IGF-I) levels could not distinguish ND patients from familial constitutional short-stature children (Fig. 4a) (32). This is in contrast to other studies, which measured IGF levels and their binding proteins (IGFBP) in fasting and varying levels of nutritional intake both in rodents and in humans (33–42). These studies showed that IGF-I is reduced in children with protein-calorie malnutrition, in fasted rats, and in rats chronically deprived of nutrients. Reductions in IGF-I concentrations were observed in fasted volunteers (37). However, the degree of nutritional insufficiency in ND is not as severe as that observed in protein-calorie malnutrition or fasting. The amount of nutrient restriction in ND may impair growth by altering other cellular mechanisms without affecting the serum IGF-I levels. Because the energy restriction is mild and ND children consume sufficient dietary protein, IGF-I concentrations may be preserved within a range appropriate for bone age development. Likewise, studies in rats showed IGF-I concentrations to be maintained within normal ranges or to improve rapidly when diets containing 15% protein and 90% of the total energy requirements were consumed (43,44).

Similarly, serum IGF BP-3 concentrations are decreased in prolonged fasting and/or protein deficiency states (40). However, alterations in IGF PB-3 levels in more subtle forms of suboptimal nutrition like that observed in ND have not yet been studied (Table 1).

On the other hand, we reported that ND patients show decreased activity of erythrocyte Na^+, K^+-ATPase compared with familial short-stature children (32). This enzyme is involved with the active transport of sugars and amino acids and with cellular thermogenesis. It normally accounts for approximately one-third of the basal energy requirements (45). A diminished energy intake lowers the basal metabolic rate (46) and decreases Na, K-ATPase activity (47). Thus, it may be a good marker of ND. We have expanded our initial studies with increased numbers of patients, and the data continue to suggest that erythrocyte Na^+, K^+-ATPase activity is significantly reduced in patients with ND in comparison with that in children with familial short stature (Fig. 5). Furthermore, Na, K-ATPase activity was positively correlated with incremental body weight gain. The enzyme concentrations did not differ significantly with regard to sex, chronologic age, bone age, or pubertal status.

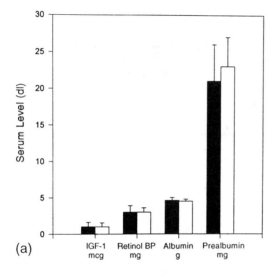

(a)

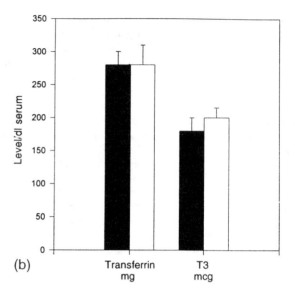

(b)

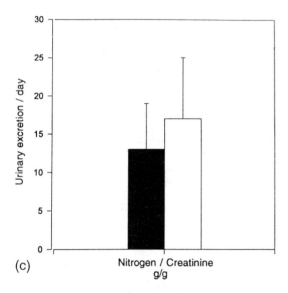

(c)

Figure 4 Comparison of common biochemical parameters in patients with nutritional growth retardation and in those with familial or constitutional short stature. (a) IGF-1, retinol binding protein, albumin, and prealbumin. (b) Transferrin and T_3. (c) Urinary nitrogen/creatinine excretion. None of the parameters was significantly different between the two groups to distinguish nutritional growth retardation from familial or constitutional short stature. Solid bar, nutritional short stature; open bar, familial/constitutional short stature.

Because anthropometric parameters may be lacking or inaccurate and biochemical markers may not be sufficient to detect ND, a more sensitive test is required for diagnosis. Erythrocyte Na^+, K^+-ATPase activity may offer such a diagnostic tool. To date, however, this assay has not been widely available for clinical purposes, it is cumbersome, and it can be applied only on a research basis.

III. PATHOPHYSIOLOGY

Patients with nutritional growth retardation have reached an equilibrium between their genetic growth potential and their nutritional intake because growth deceleration is the adaptive response to suboptimal nutrition (29,48). Diminished growth brings the nutrient demands into balance with the nutritional intake without adversely affecting biochemical or func-

tional homeostatic measures. Of course, there are limits to these adaptive possibilities. If nutritional deprivation becomes more severe, acute malnutrition may be superimposed on the chronic short stature. In such patients, malnutrition would be reflected by altered anthropometric measurements, such as weight and skinfold thickness or biochemical indices.

It has been known for many years that a diminished energy intake leads to a reduced metabolic rate even before there is a loss of body weight. The rate of protein synthesis may decrease in response to a reduction in energy intake, because this process is energy expensive and accounts for 10–15% of the basal metabolic rate (49,50). Protein catabolism is also sensitive to energy deprivation. Reduction in dietary energy sources may lead to an increased nitrogen flux in which protein breakdown is accelerated to provide energy (51). Nitrogen retention markedly increases during nutritional

Table 1 Endocrine Alterations in Different Types of Malnutrition[a]

Condition studied	Hormone	Direction of change	References
Acute fasting in adult human	GH pulse frequency	↑	146
	24 h integrated concentration	↑	
	Maximum pulse amplitude	↑	
Protein-calorie malnutrition in infants	Suppression by glucose	—	147
	GH response to arginine	—	148, 149
	GH clearance	N	150
ND	Mean overnight GH secretion		58
	Prepubertal	N	
	Pubertal	↓	
	GH response to GHRH		
	Prepubertal	↑	
	Pubertal	N	
Normal short children	Spontaneous GH secretion	Inversely correlated with adiposity	58
Protein-calorie malnutrition in children	IGF-I	↓	33–36, 42, 151–155
	IGF-II	↓	149
Anorexia nervosa in adolescents	IGF-I	↓	154, 155
Fasting in adults (after 72 h)	IGF BP-3	↓	40
Anorexia nervosa in adolescents	IGF BP-1	↓	41
	IGF BP-2	↓	
Acute fasting in adults	TSH	↓	156, 157
	TSH response to TRH	↓	
Adolescents with growth failure caused by fear of obesity	TSH response to TRH	Delayed but normal amplitude	155
Anorexia nervosa and ND	TSH response to TRH	N or delayed	151, 155, 158
Acute and chronic malnutrition in rats and children	T_3	↓	157, 159
	rT_3	↑	
Malnutrition and anorexia nervosa in children	24 h urine free cortisol	↑	151, 152, 160, 161
	P.M. free and total plasma cortisol	↑	
	Cortisol suppression after dexamethasone	Inadequate	
Protein-calorie malnutrition in children	Fasting blood glucose	↓	149, 162
	Glucose disposal	Delayed	
	Insulin release	Diminished	
Protein-calorie malnutrition in children and adults	Hypothalamopituitary and direct gonadal	Suppression	151, 152 161, 163

[a]TSH, thyroid-stimulating hormone; TRH, thyrotropin-releasing hormone; ↑: increased; ↓: decreased; N: normal.

rehabilitation of malnourished children (50,52). In addition, nutritional recovery normalizes the excretion of amino acids (51) and increases the rate of protein synthesis (53). In ND, the result of the altered rates of protein turnover and nitrogen retention may be the cessation of normal growth as an adaptive response to the decreased intake.

In addition to suboptimal energy intake, various mineral and vitamin deficiencies have been implicated in the etiology of nutritional growth retardation. The minerals implicated to cause specific deficiency syndromes and play a role in growth retardation include iron, calcium, phosphate, copper, chromium, and zinc (see later) (54). Zinc deficiency is a well-known cause of ND that responds to zinc supplementation with increased growth (55). We have also reported a high

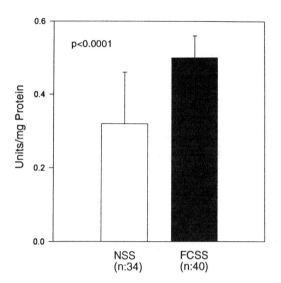

Figure 5 Erythrocyte Na$^+$, K$^+$-ATPase activity in nutritional short stature (NSS) and in familial or constitutional short stature (FCSS) patients. The enzyme activity was significantly reduced in patients with nutritional short stature. This data is modified from the data published elsewhere (41). It includes an expanded number of patients studied, NSS from 20 to 34 and FCSS from 32 to 40.

frequency of iron deficiency without anemia in ND patients who responded to iron therapy with improved growth (5).

However, it remains controversial whether decreased body size is an advantageous adaptation to a limited food supply or whether adverse health and functional impairments result (29,48). It has been demonstrated that physical activity is decreased with a 20% decrease in energy consumption (56), but other functional impairments are more difficult to assess. Regardless, the decreased growth velocity constitutes a functional compromise per se, which should be detected and treated as early as possible.

IV. ENDOCRINE ADAPTATION

The changes in the endocrine system in response to undernutrition are adaptive in nature and largely revert to the "normal" state after nutritional status is improved (57). Undernutrition may involve single or multiple micronutrient deficiencies, and thus any one or a combination of deficits could be the primary problem leading to the endocrine alterations. A detailed description of the hormonal alterations in malnutrition has been published elsewhere (57). In Table 1, we summarize the major endocrine changes associated with protein and energy deficiencies.

However, it must be remembered that most studies have been conducted in severely malnourished patients, which may not accurately reflect more subtle forms of suboptimal nutrition leading to ND. For example, although circulating growth hormone (GH) levels are increased in severe malnutrition, we

have shown that pubertal ND children show decreased overnight growth hormone secretion (Fig. 6) and prepubertal subjects have an increased growth hormone response to growth hormone-releasing hormone (GHRH) stimulation. Interestingly, body composition is a significant determinant of spontaneous growth hormone secretion. In normal children with short stature, the degree of adiposity modifies spontaneous growth hormone secretion and alters the amplitude of growth hormone pulses in puberty and the number of pulses in prepubertal children (58). These results indicate that interpretation of spontaneous growth hormone secretion must take into account the body composition and nutritional status of the patient (Chap. 4). Indeed, ND may be easily confused with growth hormone deficiency or neurosecretory dysfunction if the deterioration in weight progression is overlooked. An example of such an error is illustrated in Figure 7. This 10 year, 4 month girl was seen by a pediatric endocrinologist and was diagnosed to have neurosecretory GH deficiency. She was exhibiting deteriorating growth, and her height dropped below the fifth percentile. She did not have any secondary sexual development. After GH testing, the pediatric endocrinologist recommended GH treatment. However, a second opinion was sought. During the later evaluation, two facts emerged. The first was that weight progression had almost ceased since age 6 and preceded the deceleration in height. The second was that the child had been given a low-fat, low-cholesterol diet because of hypercholesterolemia and familial risks and consequences of hypercholesterolemia. Her grandmother died suddenly at

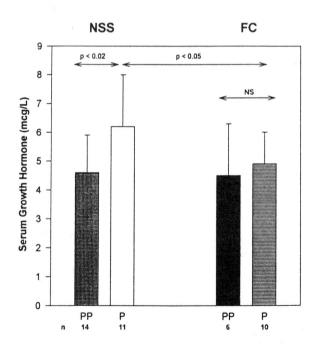

Figure 6 Mean overnight GH levels achieved by patients with NSS and FC short stature. The pubertal patients with NSS were not able to increase their spontaneous growth hormone secretion, contrary to the patients in FC group, who showed a marked increase in their mean overnight growth hormone levels. (With permission from Clin Endocrinol Metab 1992; 75(3):930–934.)

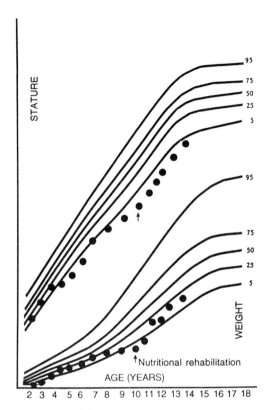

Figure 7 Nutritional dwarfing or growth hormone deficiency. The patient was diagnosed to have GH deficiency at age 10 years because of poor growth. However, because of inadequate weight gain associated with decreased growth increments, therapeutic trial with an adequate diet was tried in lieu of growth hormone. Note the catch-up growth after the initiation of nutritional rehabilitation.

age 49 years because of a heart attack when the patient was 6 years of age. During the examination, the dietary intake was found to be inadequate in terms of energy and other nutrients, as we have described elsewhere for patients with nutritional growth retardation undergoing treatment for hypercholesterol-emia (59). The patient was given nutritional rehabilitation. Her dietary intake was modified to provide all the necessary nutrients for growth, and GH was not recommended despite biochemical evidence of GH deficiency. With an appropriate intake, weight gain and height progression improved and catch-up growth was demonstrated.

Obviously, the preferable course of action, as in the patient shown in Figure 7, should be to replace the nutritional deficits and achieve a reasonable weight gain before considering growth hormone treatment. Nutritional rehabilitation should be less expensive and more acceptable for ND patients than GH.

V. ETIOLOGY

Suboptimal nutrition that leads to ND may be a result of organic or nonorganic causes (Table 2). Various pathologic

Table 2 Etiology of Nutritional Growth Retardation

Organic
  Chronic inflammatory bowel disease (CIBD)
  Celiac disease (CD)
  Mineral deficiencies
  Postgastoenteritis
  Developmental delay
  Chronic infection
  Human immunodeficiency virus (HIV)
  Cardiac disease
  Cystic fibrosis
  Cleft palate

Nonorganic
  Dieting in children
  Fear of obesity
  Cholesterol concern
  Hypercholesterolemia
  Treatment of obesity
  Parental health beliefs
  Nonorganic failure to thrive
  Psychosocial

conditions that lead to decreased nutritional intake or malabsorption may cause ND (60). Crohn's disease, celiac disease, and cystic fibrosis are some of the relatively more common pathologies. Crohn's disease may present with growth retardation that may precede weight loss (61). The primary presentation in the so-called occult type of celiac disease is short stature (62–65). The nutritional consequences of these diseases depend on the severity and duration of the problem before diagnosis and intervention. Therefore, a workup is necessary to rule out these diseases when there is an impairment in weight gain or height progression. Recently, the acquired immunodeficiency syndrome and human immunodeficiency virus (HIV) infection were also shown to be associated with short stature and poor growth that preceded any other manifestation of disease (Chap. 55) (66). These patients did not have body weight deficits for height or wasting and were therefore not considered to have nutritional growth retardation. However, the growth data in HIV-infected patients clearly indicate ND because body weight progression failed to proceed at appropriate rates even before any other symptom of the disease was apparent (66). In the most recent study by Gertner et al. (67), there was a failure to assess body weight progression and therefore the diagnosis of ND was missed. It is very likely that anorexia and decreased intake of nutrients lead to suboptimal nutrition in HIV-infected patients and cause ND even before other signs and symptoms of the disease become apparent.

However, ND in otherwise healthy children is usually because of nonorganic causes that reflect an adaptive response to voluntary reduction in food intake (4,5,11). Furthermore, inappropriate eating behaviors, dissatisfaction with body weight and appearance, and unhealthy approaches toward weight control may cause ND among well-to-do populations (see later).

A. Organic Nutritional Dwarfing

1. Chronic Inflammatory Bowel Disease

Impaired linear growth, retarded skeletal maturation, and delayed sexual development are estimated to occur in 5–10% of pediatric patients with ulcerative colitis and 25% of patients with Crohn's disease (68,69). Growth failure may be the first indication of chronic inflammatory bowel disease and may precede disease-related symptoms (61). Therefore, the diagnosis of CIBD should always be considered in children who cease to grow adequately, even in the absence of gastrointestinal complaints.

Although the pathogenesis is influenced by age at onset, duration of disease, disease activity, and medication, undernutrition is now recognized as the primary factor in growth failure in Crohn's disease (10). Multifactorial nutritional alterations include (1) decreased nutrient intake, (2) impaired absorption of nutrients, (3) specific nutrient deficiencies, and (4) enhanced protein losses through the gastrointestinal tract.

Decreased energy intake in children with CIBD has been associated with anorexia and the early satiety and discomfort that accompany eating. The total daily caloric intake of CIBD patients usually is not above the recommended dietary allowance (RDA) for height age (61). Multiple studies have documented catch-up growth when adequate energy is provided (61,68,69). Various forms of nutritional support (parenteral, elemental, or complex diet) have been employed, but it remains controversial whether the type of nutritional supplement can decrease disease activity (70–72).

In addition to energy and protein deficits, other nutritional alterations may affect growth in patients with CIBD. Iron deficiency, particularly when there is blood loss through the stools, may compound anorexia and poor growth (73). These patients also may have magnesium deficiency (74).

The potential contributing role of zinc deficiency in growth failure in CIBD has gained considerable attention. It has been shown that large enteric losses of zinc occur in CIBD patients who have diarrhea and small bowel disease (75). In addition, zinc absorption may be reduced (76,77). In contrast, Nakamura et al. (78) have shown that zinc clearance rather than absorption correlated with the clinical severity of Crohn's disease. Comparison of oral versus parenteral administration of zinc showed that zinc absorption was intact regardless of whether the disease was active or inactive. Hypozincemia was presumably related to an accelerated turnover rather than to a malabsorption of zinc. Other studies have demonstrated that circulating serum zinc levels are correlated with the presence or absence of hypoalbuminemia and that there are zinc deficits in CIBD patients as shown by oral zinc loads (77). Hypozincemia preceding any other alteration may also occur in some patients with short stature and decreased growth rates who eventually manifest CIBD (73). Zinc supplementation without additional medical therapy increased growth velocity in some CIBD patients (69,77). However, prospective studies remain to be done to ascertain the therapeutic effects of zinc replacement in CIBD.

The most commonly observed laboratory finding in active CIBD is protein-losing enteropathy (79,80). Successful therapeutic nutritional intervention, whether by elemental diet (69) or total parenteral nutrition (TPN) (81), is usually followed by normalization of enteric protein losses. Despite the observed protein-losing enteropathy, most studies of nitrogen balance demonstrate a positive balance in growth-impaired patients before therapeutic intervention (6,82,83). Protein synthesis and catabolism were different in CIBD patients than in healthy control children, although lean body and muscle mass were reduced by 30–35% in comparison with controls (83). Also, in children with CIBD, basal metabolic rates (6) and energy expenditure, calculated from stable isotope methods with doubly labeled water, are not greater than expected for age, sex, and height (82).

It is often assumed that intestinal malabsorption and the resulting loss of nutrients could explain the nutritional deficits and the growth failure of patients with CIBD. However, a wide range of absorptive dysfunction and protein-losing enteropathy can occur in children with CIBD (83). When groups of severely growth-impaired children have been studied to determine the prevalence of steatorrhea, impaired d-xylose, or impaired vitamin B_{12} absorption, only a few patients present alterations (6,80,81). Although the stool mineral concentrations of zinc, calcium, magnesium, and phosphorus were higher in teenagers with CIBD than healthy controls, balance studies of nitrogen, calcium, and phosphorus were not different from those of age-matched controls (80).

The nutritional dwarfing of these patients is evident even though they seem well adapted to decreased nutrient intake (61). Often the dietary intake is not reduced beyond that needed to maintain body weight and height at a level below that expected for age, but it is insufficient to permit normal growth. These patients may not be underweight, and only by use of stable isotope measurements may malnutrition be discerned. These well-adapted Crohn's disease patients slow their growth as an adaptive response to decreased nutrient availability (3,83).

Therefore, nutrition rehabilitation is essential for the treatment of CIBD patients. This may reverse the growth retardation and may even improve the disease itself (81,84). Nutritional support has been used successfully by a variety of methods, formulas, and means of administration. Long-term TPN at home and intermittent elemental enteral feedings given for 1 month every 4 months were shown to be sufficient to allow tripling of the growth rate during a year of nutritional therapy for CIBD patients (69,81).

The mechanism whereby nutritional rehabilitation results in improved growth appears to go beyond the provision of calories. The enteral or parenteral feedings provide all nutrients, not only calories, and usually eliminate food intake. Additionally, the patients receive supplements with vitamins and minerals, such as vitamin K, folic acid, and elemental iron. Any one or all of these nutrients could contribute to the patient's improvement. Also, the effect of "bowel rest" while receiving therapeutic infusions of monomeric enteral feedings or TPN may play a role in reducing antigen load and improving the disease activity (72). This could lead to a reduced steroid dosage for treatment, thereby allowing more growth. There may also be decreased energy needs by reduction in the hypermetabolic effects of the diseased bowel and by alleviating the anorexia of the patient. The food ingested would therefore be increased and yield better results. At a cellular level, there may be improved osteoclastic function, which is regulated by hormones, and a decrease in somatomedin, which limits energy expenditure for growth.

Some gastroenterologists now combine low-dose prednisone therapy with nasogastric infusion of monomeric feedings to determine whether prolonged remission in disease activity can be achieved (71). Alternate-day steroid treatment in low dosages may also alleviate the plateau effect in growth that is frequently observed when the elemental or chemically defined formula infusions are replaced by food (85).

However, it is clear that nutritional rehabilitation of Crohn's disease patients is essential. Nutritional rehabilitation should be attempted even before growth failure occurs, although this is not an easy task. The complications of parenteral nutrition are well described and are not repeated here. The unpalatability of oral supplements over extended periods usually results in intake being less than recommended. Also, food consumption may decrease when nasogastric infusions are used. Moreover, highly motivated compliant patients are required for long-term acceptance of nutritional support. The provision of all the necessary nutrients for growth should be attempted throughout the treatment of these patients. Surgery for the correction of the growth problem of Crohn's disease should be contemplated only when appropriate nutritional therapy fails.

2. Celiac Disease

Growth failure in association with gastrointestinal symptoms is common in children with active celiac disease. For example, in two studies, 36 and 55% of patients with CD were below the third percentile for height and 40 and 60% were below the same percentile for weight (86,87). In another study, it was reported that failure to thrive was present in 14 of 52 children with celiac disease at the time of diagnosis (88). However, several investigators have reported short stature as the sole manifestation of celiac disease (7,62–65). These asymptomatic patients were considered to have occult celiac disease.

The prevalance of asymptomatic CD is highly variable. It was reported to be 1.8, 5, and 8% in some studies (7,63,64), whereas in others it was higher, 24 and 48% (62,65). This may be a result of geographic differences in the prevalence of the disease and/or the level of suspicion in recognizing patients with short stature as the sole manifestation of the disease without intestinal malabsorption.

The incidence of CD in the western New York area, estimated by serum IgA-endomysial antibody, has been reported to be 1:7752. This calculation was based on the high sensitivity and specificity of IgA-EmA in correlation with histologic changes observed in CD (89).

The recognition of occult CD is dependent on the alertness of the clinician to consider CD as a cause of short stature. Many asymptomatic CD patients have a history of diarrhea at an early age or have microcytic anemia. They may also have some other alterations when studied (e.g., increased stool fat, antigliadin, and antiendomysial antibodies, low serum folate levels, and low serum ferritin levels) that point toward the possibility of CD (90–92) as the cause of short stature.

The xylose absorption test and serum antigliadin antibody panel may be used in screening for celiac disease (93). The xylose test has been reported to be sensitive (93%) but not specific (47%) for CD. The sensitivity of IgG antigliadin antibody (AGA) was 100% and that of IgA AGA was 53%. On the other hand, IgA AGA was more specific (93%) than IgG AGA (58%) (93). Although these methods may be used for screening purposes, they are not diagnostic. CD patients may have no other alterations except for short stature and an abnormal intestinal mucosa (2,62,65,89). Therefore, a small bowel biopsy is the "gold standard" for the diagnosis of CD. This should be performed in every short child showing ND from unidentified causes. A history of diarrhea during the first year of life and/or the presence of iron deficiency anemia in a short patient should also warrant a small bowel biopsy. It is also important to exclude CD in short-stature patients without endocrine cause in the United States. Asymptomatic CD presenting as short stature is less common than idiopathic growth hormone deficiency. In the United States, the prevalence of growth hormone deficiency is approximately 1:3500 (94) compared with the prevalence of 1:7752 for CD in western New York (90). In other parts of the world, however, CD is more common. The diagnosis of CD should be confirmed by documentation of catch-up growth in weight and height after institution of a gluten-free diet, the only treatment available for the treatment of the disease. Long-term studies of children with CD suggest that those who do not comply with the diet have significantly lower mean heights and weights and greater abnormality of the intestinal mucosa than those who are compliant.

3. Mineral Deficiencies

Regardless of etiology, ND patients may present multiple nutritional deficiencies that contribute to growth failure (95). There may be generalized malnutrition with multiple macro- and micronutrient deficits, or there may be more specific nutritional alterations. For example, individual mineral deficiencies, such as zinc and iron, may influence food intake and adversely affect growth (5,54,96). All aspects of nutritional status—energy and macronutrient and micronutrient balance—must be considered in ND. The importance of some of these deficiencies in nutritional short-stature patients is discussed next.

There are two types of mineral and other nutrient deficiencies, which differ in their response to the deficiency (97). Type I, "classic" deficiency, is characterized by a reduced tissue concentration of the particular nutrient. Additionally, the nutrient's primary function is not related to growth. The subject first presents with specific clinical signs of nutrient deficiency, and growth failure occurs later. Nutrient deficiencies in this group include selenium, iodine, iron, copper, calcium, manganese, thiamine, riboflavin, ascorbic acid, retinol, tocopherol, cobalamin, vitamin K, and vitamin D (97).

In contrast, type II deficiency is characterized by a primary cessation of growth. Tissue concentrations of the nutrient are not reduced, and no specific signs or symptoms are observed. Following a profound and prolonged deficiency, specific signs may appear long after growth ceases. The nutrients in this group are zinc, threonine, lysine, potassium, sodium, phosphorus, sulfur, magnesium, nitrogen, essential carbon skeletons of amino acids, and energy (97). ND may result from the lack of a specific single nutrient but is more likely to occur when there is a combination of nutrient deficiencies.

Mineral deficiencies in children may be caused by two different mechanisms: increased losses that lead to a negative mineral balance or an insufficient positive mineral balance in which the available nutrients do not meet the needs of a growing organism but are not associated with abnormal losses of endogenous mineral. The two mechanisms may lead to different physiologic manifestations because the losses of endogenous minerals may impair vital functions, whereas with an insufficient positive balance, cellular function may continue with the mineral already present. Moreover, the manifestations of mineral deficiencies in a growing organism may be more severe and may be quite different from the clinical picture seen in an adult (98,99).

A variety of diseases may lead to mineral deficiencies and poor growth or short stature. Often, the only evidence of disease may be the growth abnormality. For example, growth retardation may be the most prominent sign of familial hypophosphatemia (100). Similarly, poor growth may precede the development of any specific sign or symptom of the disease, for example CIBD. Mineral deficiencies associated with short stature could also be the consequence of iatrogenic manipulations, as with steroids or other drugs (101), or the result of specific inborn errors of metabolism, which could affect the absorption or excretion of specific minerals (102, 103). Different pathogenic processes may lead to one or several mineral deficiencies in each or any one of these groups of patients.

In humans, specific deficiency syndromes that lead to growth retardation have been identified for iron, calcium, phosphate, copper, and chromium (54,96). Under special circumstances, manganese, selenium, molybdenum, and cobalt deficiencies were also reported to induce growth failure in children (see later). We have found that the dietary intakes of children with nutritional growth retardation often provide insufficient minerals for growth and may thereby contribute to their short stature (95). The mineral deficits may also play a role in the anorexia that often characterizes these disorders. For example, we have shown that iron deficiency, even in the absence of anemia, is relatively frequent among adolescents with nutritional growth retardation (5). Nutritional rehabilitation of these patients is often facilitated by iron supplementation.

However, the diagnostic criteria to define mineral deficiencies in children is not precise. Gross deficits in dietary intakes or losses were evident in most reports. On the other hand, serum levels may be decreased or urinary excretion altered without evidence of deficiency of these minerals. For example, there may be hypozincemia without evidence of total zinc deficiency (104), and urinary zinc excretion may be increased despite low blood levels of this ion (101). Low concentrations of zinc in human hair have also been described in association with zinc deficiency, but these measurements are most unreliable (105).

Nakamura et al. defined methods of studying zinc kinetics that appear to be more reliable than random serum or tissue levels (78,106). These methods involve serial measurements of serum zinc levels after oral or intravenous administration to assess its exponential decline over time.

Milder manifestations of zinc deficiency associated with growth disorders in children have been studied (96). Hambidge et al. described 10 children with poor appetite, decreased taste acuity, short stature, and decreased hair zinc levels; all improved after zinc supplementation (107). Other studies also reported zinc deficits as possible cause of growth retardation and retarded bone age (108), and zinc deficit was implicated in the etiology of failure to thrive and pica (109). Hypozincemia was also reported to occur in asymptomatic short-stature patients who eventually developed CIBD (54). Furthermore, zinc as a supplement to infant formulas has been associated with an accelerated weight gain in normal, healthy children (110).

In addition to its anorectic effect, hypozincemia may cause hormonal alterations that may lead to growth retardation. In rats, zinc deficiency was associated with a significant decrease in the activity of IGF-I (111), lower serum concentrations of GH and testosterone, and higher serum luteinizing hormone and follicle-stimulating hormone levels (112). Although these results were not confirmed in humans (113), hypopituitarism and delayed growth (96,114,115) have been associated with zinc deficiency. The severity and duration of the deficiency may be important in determining its endocrine consequences.

Zinc and other mineral supplements are often employed in the treatment of short stature (108). Many studies have shown improved growth velocity with replacement therapy in zinc-deficient short children (116,117). However, treatment should be reserved for documented deficiency states. Zinc therapy is not without adverse consequences. Side effects include nausea, vomiting, abdominal pain, and diarrhea. Acute intoxication, resulting from the ingestion of excess zinc from food or beverages stored in galvanized containers, may produce fever, nausea, vomiting, diarrhea, seizures, and even death. Inhalation of zinc oxide fumes produces severe pneumonitis. Chronic toxicity with this mineral has been accompanied by anemia and poor growth (118). Treatment with zinc may also produce low serum histidine levels, copper deficiency, and hypercholesterolemia (119). It may also interfere with the absorption of other cations and elements in the diet. Zinc has also been shown to be a carcinogen under experimental conditions and to reduce immunity (120).

Manganese, cobalt, molybdenum, selenium, silicon, nickel, tin, lead, cadmium, and even arsenic are other trace elements of established nutritional importance that have not yet made an impact on the assessment of growth problems in children. Manganese plays an essential role in mucopolysaccharide synthesis, and its deficiency in young birds causes a variety of skeletal abnormalities with stunted growth (121). Manganese deficiency in humans produced weight loss, dermatitis, retarded growth of hair and nails, changes in hair color from black to red, and elevated serum cholesterol levels (122). Silicon deficiency in animals also causes depressed levels of collagen, leading to growth retardation and skeletal deformities (123).

The effects of selenium deficiency in animals (124), in malnourished children (125), and in patients maintained on prolonged TPN (126) have been described. Severe selenium deficiency has also been associated with cardiomyopathy, Keshan disease (127). Molybdenum deficiency was described in Crohn's disease treated with long-term TPN (128), and cobalt deficiency was described in a Scottish child, living in a cobalt-deficient area, who had marked geophagia (129). Lead and fluoride deficiencies are also associated with growth retardation and other abnormalities (125,130).

Because of the increased use of elemental diets or prolonged TPN in children with various diseases, the pediatric endocrinologist will encounter more problems arising from deficiencies of these minerals in the future. Further research will be necessary before the deficiency of these minerals can be accurately diagnosed and their role in the growth of children evaluated.

B. Nonorganic Nutritional Dwarfing

The prevalence of nonorganic ND leading to malnutrition and poor growth in affluent communities is unknown. Only those patients whose height is markedly impaired have been recognized thus far. However, suboptimal nutritional intake may result in a fall in height within the normal percentiles that may elude medical attention. In a survey of 1017 high school students from a middle-class parochial school, a high incidence of low-weight students was reported. Over 25% of these students weighed less than 90% of their ideal body weight for height, but only 1.8% of these high school students had growth patterns suggestive of ND (12).

In a pediatric endocrine clinic in a referral center located in the same geographic area as the high school just mentioned, we detected over 300 patients with ND. The most common causes of nutritional alterations that resulted in ND and delayed sexual development among adolescents referred to us were nonorganic. This group accounted for 73% of the patients with ND.

There were patients in whom a specific fear or health belief was identified as the cause of the poor nutritional intake leading to short stature (4,5,11,32,131). A fear of obesity or a fear of hypercholesterolemia was specifically verbalized by some. However, most patients with nonorganic ND caused by dieting expressed preoccupations that involved similar issues of body weight and cholesterol and concern with a "healthy" dietary intake. They avoided excess dietary fat and cholesterol and "junk food" (11). Regardless of the reason for the inadequate nutritional intake, the result in these children was short stature.

These patients with inadequate dietary intake appeared to be free of severe psychopathology. They did not meet the inclusion criteria for severe eating disorders (Chap. 59), namely, anorexia nervosa or bulimia nervosa. Moreover, in a controlled, double-blind, prospective study, we demonstrated that these children did not have behavioral or psychosocial deviations and did not differ from a group of normal or short-stature children (132). Thus, we concluded that the dietary habits that led to ND were a result of the prevalence of current health beliefs and preoccupation with slimness, weight control, and the search for longevity through the intake of idealized diets (4,5,11,32,60,133–139).

There is a high prevalence of extreme measures taken by high school students to avoid obesity throughout the country (135–137). They often diet, have inappropriate eating habits, and purging behaviors. These data indicate just how powerful and important it is for adolescents to achieve an ideal slim and trim figure. Young persons, even when they are not overweight, diet to avoid obesity at a time when they are still growing and developing (5,131,137). Regardless of their physical needs, they strive to reach a thin ideal, consequently developing nutritional short stature (5,11). In addition to growth retardation, other potential medical complications may be associated with excessive dieting, binging, and purging that include electrolyte disturbances, dental enamel erosion, acute gastric dilation, esophagitis, enlargement of the parotid gland, aspiration pneumonitis, and pancreatitis (Chap. 59).

However, it must be kept in mind that the population at large is also quite concerned about cholesterol and preoccupied with diets to lower cholesterol levels (140). These concerns are also prevalent among children (95). The medical profession and the American Academy of Pediatrics have also recommended a low-fat–low-cholesterol diet for the population at large (141) in an effort to prevent adult-onset diseases. However, there are potential harmful consequences of feeding children with adult diets (142) and low-fat–low-cholesterol intake may lead to nutritional short stature (5,11) and nutrient deficits (5,95).

Careful assessment of weight and height progression will clearly identify these children who are not gaining weight and growing appropriately (4,5,60,131). An awareness by health care providers and by pediatric endocrinologists of the prevailing eating attitudes and behaviors among adolescents in the population of the area in which they practice may help detect the adolescent at risk for more serious problems. Simple tests and questionnaires may help identify the patient with eating disorders (138). The 24 h dietary recall may identify short-stature patients with inappropriate dietary intake.

Patients with obesity constitute another group of children who often diet. Although these children do not come to the pediatric endocrinologist because of poor growth, when it occurs there may be great concerns about their health. A variety of endocrine disorders may affect obese children who do not grow well (Chap. 52). Diet-related growth failure may be uncovered by a careful history, thereby eliminating other concerns (Fig. 8).

Weight loss is associated with a negative balance that does not allow growth in height even if the child is obese (143). Therefore, during the treatment of obesity in children, allowances must always be made to maintain a balance between the needs of a patient to lose weight and the nutritional requirements that allow growth in height (Chap. 52).

In general, obese children are above average in height for their age and sex. The growth rate in obese children is faster and the age of puberty is earlier compared with nonobese children (11). Therefore, some physicians tolerate a slowing of the growth rate during treatment of obesity. This

decrease has been reported to bring children more in line with the heights of the parents (144). However, the final height may be slightly less than that of their nonobese peers (145). If there is a drastic decrease in the height velocity of an obese child, the individual should be reevaluated and the daily caloric and nutrient intake reassessed. To allow catch-up growth to take place, a new program, perhaps with different short-term goals (e.g., decreased rate of weight loss or weight maintenance), should be considered.

VI. TREATMENT

Nutritional rehabilitation for ND requires providing the patient with adequate caloric and nutrient intake for the resto-

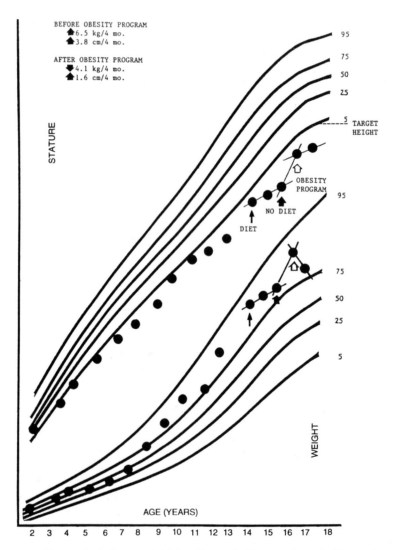

Figure 8 The patient began a self-prescribed diet at age 13 (small arrow). He grew 5 cm in 22 months and was able to reduce his weight gain, crossing one major percentile line (6 kg in same period). He discontinued his attempt at dieting (large arrow) for 4 months and demonstrated accelerated weight gain and linear growth. When enrolled in the obesity program (large open arrow), this patient was very successful at losing weight (4.1 kg/4 m), but consequently a deceleration in linear growth (1.6 cm/4 m) was observed.

ration of previous growth patterns. Initially, estimation of energy requirements should be based on the age- and gender-specific RDA using the patient's theoretical weight. Adequate intake of protein usually accompanies sufficient caloric intake, but care should be taken that micronutrient intakes meet the RDA. If biochemical tests reveal specific deficiencies, such as iron or zinc, these nutrients should be supplemented. Some patients may not be willing or able to consume a completely balanced diet and may require a multivitamin and mineral supplement.

A careful diet history can elucidate food preferences and eating patterns that can be used to devise an appropriate dietary plan. Our experience has been to offer general dietary suggestions rather than to prescribe a specific diet. Frequent follow-up visits provide an opportunity to revise and update dietary recommendations and to obtain weight and height measurements. Although the appropriate diet can be easily determined, successful intervention requires a change in dietary patterns and possibly health beliefs as well. Increasing the caloric density of the child's diet often involves raising the dietary fat content to at least 30–35% of calories. The increase in fat consumption may concern both the child and the parent, especially in patients who fail to grow because of dieting. The assurance that an appropriate nutritional intake will result in normal growth, without producing obesity, is necessary supportive therapy. This is of particular concern in the initial stages of the treatment, when weight increases rapidly, whereas no noticeable effect on height is observed.

REFERENCES

1. Torun B, Viteri FE. Protein energy malnutrition. In: Shils ME, Young VR, eds. Modern Nutrition in Health and Disease, 7th ed. Philadelphia: Lea & Febiger, 1988:746–773.
2. Nikens PR. Stature reduction as an adaptive response to food production in Mesoamerica. J Archaeol Sci 1976; 3:21–41.
3. Stin WA. Evolutionary implications of changing nutritional patterns in human populations. Am Anthropol 1971; 73:1019–1030.
4. Lifshitz F. Nutrition and growth. In: Paige DM, ed. Clinical Nutrition. Nutrition and Growth Supplement 4. St. Louis: C.V. Mosby, 1985:40–47.
5. Lifshitz F, Moses N, Cervantes C, et al. Nutritional dwarfing in adolescence. Semin Adolesc Med 1987; 3(4):255–256.
6. Kelts DG, Grand RJ, Shen G, et al. Nutritional basis of growth failure in children and adolescents with Crohn's disease. 1979; 76:720–727.
7. Stenhammar L, Fallstrom SP, Hansson G, et al. Coeliac disease in children of short stature without gastrointestinal symptoms. Eur J Pediatr 1986; 145:185–186.
8. Keller W, Fillmore CM. Prevalence of protein-energy malnutrition. World Health Stat Q 1983; 36:129–167.
9. Lifshitz F, Moses N. Nutritional growth retardation. In: Lifshitz F, ed. Pediatric Endocrinology. New York: Marcel Dekker, 1991:111–133.
10. Kirschner BS. Nutritional consequences of inflammatory bowel disease on growth. J Am Coll Nutr 1988; 7:301–308.
11. Lifshitz F, Tarim O. Nutritional dwarfing. Curr Probl Pediatr 1993; 23:322–336.
12. Pugliese M, Recker B, Lifshitz F. A survey to determine the prevalence of abnormal growth patterns in adolescence. J Adolesc Health Care 1988; 9:181–187.
13. Towbridge FL, Marks JS, DeRomana GL, et al. Body composition of Peruvian children with short stature and high weight for height: implication for the interpretation for weight-for-height as an indicator of nutritional status. Am J Clin Nutr 1987; 46:411–418.
14. Pugliese MT, Lifshitz F, Grad G, et al. Fear of obesity: a cause of short stature and delayed puberty. N Engl J Med 1983; 309:513–518.
15. Dewey KG, Heinig MJ, Nommesen LA, Peerson JM, Lonnderal B. Growth patterns of breastfed and formula-fed infants from 0–18 months: the DARLING study. Pediatrics 1992; 89:1035–1041.
16. Dewey KG, Heinig MJ, Nommesen LA, Peerson JM, Lonnderal B. Adequacy of energy intake among breastfed infants in the DARLING study: relationships to growth velocity, morbidity, and activity levels. J Pediatr 1991; 119:538–547.
17. Heinig MJ, Nommsen LA, Peerson JM, Lonnerdal B, Dewey KG. Energy and protein intakes of breastfed and formula-fed infants during the first year of life and their association with growth velocity: the DARLING study. Am J Clin Nutr 1993; 58:152–161.
18. Briend A, Bari A. Breast-feeding improves survival, but not nutritional status of 12–35 months old children in rural Banladesh. Eur L Clin Nutr 1989; 43:603–608.
19. O'Connor PA. Failure to thrive with breast feeding. Clin Pediatr (Phila) 1978; 17:833–835.
20. Whichelow MJ, King BE, Taylor S. Breast feeding in relation to maternal eating habits and weight change. Int J Obes 1979; 3:93–94.
21. Whichelow MJ. Calorie requirements for successful breast feeding. Arch Dis Child 1975; 50:669.
22. Motil KJ, Sheng HP, Montandon CM. Case report: failure to thrive in a breast-fed infant is associated with maternal dietary protein and energy restriction. J Am Coll Nutr 1994; 13:2:203–208.
23. Sklar R. Nutritional vitamin B_{12} deficiency in a breast-fed infant of a vegan-diet mother. Clin Pediatr (Phila) 1986; 25:219–221.
24. Lifshitz F, Moses Finch N, Ziffer Lifshitz J. Breast-feeding and lactation. In: Lifshitz F, ed. Children's Nutrition. Boston: Jones and Bartlett, 1991:160–185.
25. Neifert MR, Seacat JM. Contemporary breast-feeding management. Clin Perinatol 1985; 12:319–342.
26. Woolridge MW, Fisher C. Colic, "overfeeding," and symptoms of lactose malabsorption in the breast-fed baby: a possible artifact of feed management? Lancet 1988; 2:382–384.
27. Habbick BF, Gerrard JW. Failure to thrive in the contented breast-fed baby. Can Med Assoc J 1984; 131:765–768.
28. Solans CV, Lifshitz F. Body weight progression and nutritional status of patients with familial short stature with and without constitutional delay in growth. Am J Dis Child 1992; 146:296–302.
29. Montage A, Brace C. Human Evolution, 2nd ed. New York: Macmillan, 1977.
30. Finkelstein JS, Neer RM, Beverly MK, et al. Osteopenia in men with a history of delayed puberty. N Engl J Med 1992; 326:600–604.
31. Galler JR, Ramsey F, Solimano G. A follow-up study of the effects of early malnutrition on subsequent development. I. Physical growth and sexual maturation during adolescence. Pediatr Res 1985; 19:6:518–523.
32. Lifshitz F, Friedman S, Smith MM, et al. Nutritional dwarfing: a growth abnormality associated with reduced erythrocyte Na^{+}, K^{+} ATPase activity. Am J Clin Nutr 1991; 54:1–7.
33. Clemmons DR, Underwood LE. Nutritional regulation of IGF-I and IGF binding proteins. Annu Rev Nutr 1991; 11:393–412.

34. Thissen JP, Underwood IE, Maiter D, et al. Failure of IGF-I infusion to promote growth in protein-restricted rats despite normalization of serum IGF-I concentrations. Endocrinology 1991; 128:885–890.

35. Clemmons DR, Thissen JP, Maes M, et al. Insulin-like growth factor-I (IGF-I) infusion into hypophysectomized or protein-deprived rats induces specific IGF binding proteins in serum. Endocrinology 1989; 125:2967–2972.

36. Clemmons DR, Underwood LE, Dickerson RN, et al. Use of somatomedin-C, insulin-like growth factor I measurements to monitor the response to nutritional repletion in malnourished patients. Am J Clin Nutr 1985; 41:192–198.

37. Merimee TJ, Zapf J, Froesch ER. Insulin-like growth factors in the fed and fasted states. J Clin Endocrinol Metab 1982; 55:999.

38. Underwood LE, Thissen JP, Moats-Staats BM, et al. Nutritional regulation of IGF-I and postnatal growth. In: Spencer EM, ed. Modern Concepts of Insulin-Like Growth Factors. New York: Elsevier. 1991:37–47.

39. Donhue SP, Phillips LS. Response of IGF-I to nutritional support in malnourished hospital patients: a possible of short-term changes in nutritional status. Am J Clin Nutr 1989; 50:962–969.

40. Ranke MB, Blum WF, Frisch H. The acid-stable subunit of insulin-like growth factor binding protein (IGFBP-3) in disorders of growth. In: Drop SLS, Hintz RL, eds. Insulin-like Growth Factor Binding Proteins. Amsterdam: Excerpta Medica, 1989:103–113.

41. Guler HP, Zapf J, Schmid C, et al. Insulin-like growth factors I & II in healthy man. Estimations of half-lives and production rates. Acta Endocrinol (Copenh) 1989; 121:753.

42. Phillips LS, Unterman TG. Somatomedin activity in disorders of nutrition and metabolism. Clin Endocrinol Metab 1984; 13:145–189.

43. Phillips LS, Young HS. Nutrition and somatomedin. I. Effect of fasting and refeeding on serum somatomedin activity and cartilage growth activity in rats. Endocrinology 1976; 99:304–314.

44. Phillips LS, Orawski AT, Belosky DC. Somatomedin and nutrition. IV. Regulation of somatomedin activity and growth cartilage activity by quantity and composition of diet in rats. Endocrinology 1978; 103:121–124.

45. Golden MHN, Jackson AA. Chronic severe undernutrition. In: Olson RE, Broquist HP, Chichester CO, Darby WJ, Kolbye AC Jr, Stalvey RM, eds. Present Knowledge in Nutrition. Washington, DC: Nutrition Foundation, 1984:57–67.

46. Byung PY. Update on food restriction and aging. Rev Biol Res Aging 1985; 2:435–443.

47. Patrick J, Golden MHV. Leukocyte electrolytes and sodium transport in protein energy malnutrition. Am J Clin Nutr 1977; 30:1478–1481.

48. Beaton GH. The significance of adaptation in the definition of nutrient requirements and for nutrition policy. In: Baxter with, Waterlow K, eds. Nutritional Adaptation in Man. London: John Libley, 1985:219–232.

49. Poehlman F, Melby CL, Badylak SF. Resting metabolic rate and post-prandial thermogenesis in highly trained and un-trained males. Am J Clin Nutr 1988; 47:793–798.

50. Waterlow JC, Golder M, Picou D. Protein turnover in man. Am J Clin Nutr 1977; 30:1333–1339.

51. Read WW, McLaren DS, Tchalian M, et al. Studies with ^{15}N-labelled ammonia and urea in the malnourished child. J Clin Invest 1969; 48:1143–1149.

52. Waterlow JC, Golden MH, Garlick PJ. Protein turnover in man measured with ^{15}N-Comparison of end products and dose regimens. Am J Physiol 1978; 235(2):E165-E174.

53. Golden M, Waterlow JC, Pilou D. The relationship between dietary intake, weight change, nitrogen balance, and protein turnover in man. Am J Clin Nutr 1977; 30:1345–1348.

54. Lifshitz F, Nishi Y. Mineral deficiencies during growth. In: Anast C, DeLuca H, eds. Pediatric Diseases Related to Calcium. New York: Elsevier North-Holland, 1980:305–322.

55. Prasad AS. Zinc in growth and development and spectrum of human zinc deficiency. J Am Coll Nutr 1988; 7:377–384.

56. Viteri FE, Torun B. Nutrition, physical activity and growth. In: Ritzer M, Apsia A, Hall K, eds. The Biology of Normal Human Growth. New York: Raven Press, 1981: 269–273.

57. Lifshitz F, Brasel JA. Nutrition and Endocrine Disease. In: Kappy MS, Blizzard RM, Migeon C, eds. Wilkins Diagnosis and Treatment of Endocrine Disorders in Childhood and Adolescence. Springfield, IL: Charles C. Thomas, 1994:535–573.

58. Abdenur JE, Pugliese MT, Cervantes C, et al. Alterations in spontaneous growth hormone secretion and the response to growth hormone releasing hormone in children with nonorganic nutritional dwarfing. J Clin Endocrinol Metab 1992; 75(3):930–934.

59. Lifshitz F, Moses N. Growth failure: a complication of dietary treatment of hypercholesterolemia. Am J Dis Child 1989; 143:537–542.

60. Alemzadeh R, Pugliese M, Lifshitz F. Disorders of puberty. In: Friedman SB, Fisher M, Shonberg SK, eds. Comprehensive Adolescent Health Care. St. Louis, MO: Quality Medical Publishing, 1992:187–205.

61. Kanof ME, Lake AM, Bayless TM. Decreased height velocity in children and adolescents before diagnosis of Crohn's disease. Gastroenterology 1988; 95:1523–1527.

62. Groll A, Candy DCA, Preece MA, et al. Short stature as the primary manifestation of coeliac disease. Lancet 1980; 21: 1097–1099.

63. Verkasalo M, Kuitunen P, Leisti S, et al. Growth failure from symptomless celiac disease. A study of 14 patients. Helv Paediatr Acta 1978; 33:489–495.

64. Cacciari E, Salardi S, Volta U, et al. Can antigliadin antibody detect symptomless coeliac disease in children with short stature? Lancet 1985; 1:1469–1471.

65. Rosenback Y, Dinari G, Zahavi I, et al. Short stature as the major manifestation of celiac disease in older children. Clin Pediatr (Phila) 1986; 25:13–16.

66. Brettler DB, Forsberg A, Bolivar E, et al. Growth failure as a prognostic indicator for progression to acquired immunodeficiency syndrome in children with hemophilia. J Pediatr 1990; 117:4:584–588.

67. Gertner JM, Kaufman FR, Donfield SM, et al. Delayed somatic growth and pubertal development in human immunodeficiency virus-infected hemophiliac boys: Hemophilia Growth and Development Study. J Pediatr 1994; 124(6):896–902.

68. Kirschner BS, Sutton MM. Somatomedin C levels in growth impaired children and adolescents with chronic inflammatory bowel disease. Gastroenterology 1986; 91:830–836.

69. Belli DC, Seidman E, Bouthillier L, et al. Chronic intermittent elemental diet improves growth failure in children with Crohn's disease. Gastroenterology 1988; 94:603–610.

70. Seidman E, LeLeiko N, Ament M, et al. Nutritional issues in pediatric inflammatory disease. J Pediatr Gastroenterol Nutr 1991; 12:424–438.

71. Lindor KD, Fleming CR, Burnes JU, Neslon JK, Ilstrup DM. A randomized prospective trial comparing a defined formula diet, corticosteroids, and a define formula diet plus corticosteroids in active Crohn's disease. Mayo Clin Proc 1992; 67:328–333.

72. Logan RFA, Gillon J, Ferrington C, et al. Reduction of gastrointestinal protein loss by elemental diet in Crohn's disease of the small bowel. Gut 1981; 22:383–387.

73. Daum F, Aiges HW. Inflammatory bowel disease in children. In: Lifshitz F, ed. Clinical Disorders in Pediatric Gastroenterology and Nutrition. New York: Marcel Dekker, 1980:145–168.

74. La Sala MA, Lifshitz F, Silverberg M, et al. Magnesium metabolism studies in children with inflammatory disease of the bowel. J Pediatr Res Gastroenterol Nutr 1985; 4:75–81.

75. Wolman SL, Anderson H, Marliss EB, et al. Zinc in total parenteral nutrition: requirements and metabolic effects. Gastroenterology 1979; 76:458–467.

76. Stumiolo GC, Molokhia MM, Shields R, et al. Zinc absorption in Crohn's disease. Gut 1980; 21:387–391.

77. Nishi Y, Lifshitz F, Bayne MA, et al. Zinc status and its relation to growth retardation in children with chronic inflammatory bowel disease. Am J Clin Nutr 1980; 33:2613–2621.

78. Nakamura T, Higashi A, Takano S, Akagi M, Matsuda I. Zinc clearance correlates with clinical severity of Crohn's disease. Dig Dis Sci 1988; 33(12):1520–1524.

79. Kirschner BS, Voinchet O, Rosenberg IH. Growth retardation in children with inflammatory bowel disease. Gastroenterology 1978; 75:504–511.

80. Beeken W. Absorptive defects in young people with regional enteritis. Pediatrics 1973; 52:69–74.

81. Strobel CT, Byrne WJ, Ament ME. Home parenteral nutrition in children with Crohn's disease: an effective management alternative. Gastroenterology 1979; 77:272–279.

82. Kirschner BS, Schoeller DA, Sutton MM. Measurement of energy expenditure (EE) in adolescents with Crohn's disease (CD) using doubly-labelled water. (abstract). Gastroenterology 1984; 86:1136.

83. Motil KJ, Grand RJ, Maletskos CJ, et al. The effect of disease, drug and diet on whole body protein metabolism in adolescents with Crohn's disease and growth failure. J Pediatr 1982; 101:345–351.

84. Morin CL, Roulet M, Roy CC, et al. Continuous elemental enteral alimentation in children with Crohn's disease and growth failure. Gastroenterology 1980; 79:1205–1210.

85. Whittington PR, Barnes V, Bayless TM. Medical management of Crohn's disease in adolescence. Gastroenterology 1977; 72:1338–1344.

86. Hamilton JR, Lynch MJ, Reilly BJ. Active coeliac disease in childhood. Q J Med 1969; 38:135–158.

87. Young WF, Pringle EM. 110 children with coeliac disease. Arch Dis Child 1971; 46:421–436.

88. Walker-Smith JA. Celiac Disease. In: Walker WA, Durie PR, Hamilton JR, Walker-Smith JA, Watkins JB, eds. Pediatric Gastrointestinal Disease. Philadelphia: B.C. Decker, 1991: 700–715.

89. Rossi TM, Albini CH, Kumar V. Incidence of celiac disease identified by the presence of serum endomysial antibodies in children with chronic diarrhea, short stature, or insulin-dependent diabetes mellitus. J Pediatr 1993; 123:262–264.

90. Ashkenazi A, Branski D. Pathogenesis of celiac disease. Part I. Immunol Allergy Pract 1988; 10:227–234.

91. Ashkenazi A, Branski D. Pathogenesis of celiac disease. Part 2. Immunol Allergy Pract 1988; 10:268–277.

92. Ashkenazi A, Branski D. Pathogenesis of celiac disease. Part 3. Immunol Allergy Pract 1988; 10:315–323.

93. Rich EJ, Christie DL. Anti-gliadin antibody panel and xylose absorption test in screening for celiac disease. J Pediatr Gastroenterol Nutr 1990; 10:174–178.

94. Lindsay R, Feldkamp M, Harris D, et al. Utah Growth Study: growth standards and the prevalence of growth hormone deficiency. J Pediatr 1994; 125:29–35.

95. Lifshitz F, Moses N. Nutritional dwarfing: growth, dieting and fear of obesity. J Am Coll Nutr 1988; 7:368–376.

96. Prasad AS. Zinc in growth and development and spectrum of human zinc deficiency. J Am Coll Nutr 1988; 7:377–384.

97. Golden MHN. The nature of nutritional deficiency in relation to growth failure and poverty. Acta Pediatr Scand Suppl 1991; 374:95–109.

98. Lifshitz F, Harrison HC, Bull EC, et al. Citrate metabolism and the mechanism of renal calcification induced by magnesium depletion. Metabolism 1967; 16:345–357.

99. Walser M. Magnesium metabolism. In: Rev Physiol Biochem Exp Pharmacol. Springer-Verlag, Berlin Heidelberg-New York, 1967; 218.

100. Harrison HE, Harrison HC, Lifshitz F, et al. Growth disturbance in hereditary hyophosphatemia. Am J Dis Child 1966; 112:290–297.

101. Henkin RI. On the role of adrenocorticosteroids in the control of zinc and copper metabolism. In: Hoekstra WG, Suttie JW, Ganther NE, Mertz WE, eds. Trace Element Metabolism in Animals, Vol. 2. Baltimore: University Park Press, 1974:647–651.

102. Skyberg D, Stromme JH, Nesbakken R, Harnaes K. Neonatal hypomagnesemia with selective malabsorption of magnesium: a clinical entity. Scand J Clin Lab Invest 1968; 21:355–363.

103. Booth B, Johnson A. Hypomagnesemia due to renal tubular defect in reabsorption of magnesium. J Pediatr 1974; 84:350–354.

104. Henkin RI, Smith FR. Zinc and copper metabolism in acute viral hepatitis. Am J Med Sci 1972; 264:401–409.

105. Hambidge KM. Hair analysis: worthless for vitamins, limited for minerals. Am J Clin Nutr 1982; 36:943–949.

106. Nakamura T, Higashi A, Nishitama S, Fujimoto S, Matsuda I. Kinetics of zinc status in children with IDDM. Diabetes Care 1991; 14:553–557.

107. Hambidge KM, Hambidge C, Jacobs M, et al. Low levels of zinc in hair, anorexia, poor growth, and hypozincemia in children. Pediatr Res 1972; 6:868–874.

108. Ghavami-Maibodi SZ, Collipp PJ, Castro-Magana M, et al. Effect of oral zinc supplements on growth hormonal levels, and zinc in healthy short children. Ann Nutr Metab 1983; 27:214–219.

109. Hambidge KM, Silverman A. Pica with rapid improvement after dietary zinc supplementation. Arch Dis Child 1973; 48:567–568.

110. Walravens PA, Hambidge KM. Growth of infants fed a zinc supplemented formula. Am J Clin Nutr 1976; 29:1114–1121.

111. Cossack ZT. Somatomedin-C in zinc deficiency. Experientia 1984; 40:498–500.

112. Root AW, Duckett G, Sweetland M, Reiter EO. Effects of zinc deficiency upon pituitary function in sexually mature and immature male rats. J Nutr 1979; 109:958–964.

113. Fons C, Brun JF, Fussellier M, Cassanas G, Bardet L, Orsetti A. Serum zinc and somatic growth in children with growth retardation. Biol Trace Elem Res 1992; 32:399–404.

114. Nishi Y, Hatano S, Aihara K, Fujie A, Kihara M. Transient partial growth hormone defiociency due to zinc deficiency. J Am Coll Nutr 1989; 8(2):93–97.

115. Prasad AS, Halsted JA, Nadimi M. Syndrome of iron deficiency anemia, hepatosplenomegaly, hypogonadism, dwarfism and geophagia. Am J Med 1961; 31:532–546.

116. Walravens PA, Krebs NF, Hambidge KM. Linear growth of low income preschool children receiving a zinc supplement. Am J Clin Nutr 1983; 38:195–201.

117. Nakamura T, Nishiyama S, Futagoishi-Suginohara Y, Matsuda I, Higashi A. Mild to moderate zinc deficiency in short children: effect of zinc supplementation on linear growth velocity. J Pediatr 1993; 123:65–69.

118. Underwood EJ. Trace Elements in Human and Animal Nutrition, 3rd ed. New York: Academic Press, 1971:208–252.

119. Klevay IM. Hypercholesterolemia in rats produced by an increase in the ratio of zinc to copper ingested. Am J Clin Nutr 1973; 26:1060–1068.

120. Chandra RK. Nutrition and Immunology. New York: Alan R. Liss, 1986.

121. Leach RM Jr, Meunster AM, Wien EM. Studies on the role of manganese in bone formation. II. Effect upon chrondroitin sulfate synthesis in chick epiphyseal cartilage. Arch Biochem Biophys 1969; 133:22–28.

122. Doisy EA. Micronutrient controls on biosynthesis of clotting proteins and cholesterol. In: Hemphill DD, ed. Trace Substances in Environmental Health. Vol. VI. Columbia, MO: University of Missouri Press, 1972:193–199.

123. Carlisle EM. A silicon requirement for normal skull formation in chicks. J Nutr 1980; 110:352–359.

124. Ewan RC. Effect of selenium on rat growth, growth hormone, and diet utilization. J Nutr 1976; 106(5):702–709.

125. Linder MC. Nutrition and metabolism of the trace elements. In: Linder MC, ed. Nutritional Biochemistry and Metabolism: With Clinical Applications. New York: Elsevier, 1985:151–197.

126. Van Rij AM, Thomson CD, McKenzie JM, et al. Selenium deficiency in total parenteral nutrition. Am J Clin Nutr 1979; 32:2076–2086.

127. Keshan Disease Research Group. Epidemiologic studies on the etiologic relationship of selenium and Keshan disease. Clin Med J 1979; 92:477–482.

128. Abumrad NN. Molybdenum. Is it an essential trace metal? Bull NY Acad Med 1985; 60:163–171.

129. Shuttleworth VS, Cameron RS, Alderman G, et al. A case of cobalt deficiency in a child presenting as "earth eating." Practitioner 1961; 186:760–764.

130. Kirchgebner M, Reichlmayr-Lais AM. Lead deficiency and its effects on growth and metabolism. In: Howell JM, Gawthorne JM, White CL, eds. Trace Element Metabolism in Man and Animals (TEMA-4). Canberra: Australian Academy of Science, 1982:390–393.

131. Pugliese MT, Weyman-Daum M, Moses N, et al. Parental health beliefs as a cause of non-organic failure to thrive. Pediatrics 1987; 8:179–182.

132. Sandberg DE, Smith MM, Fornari V, et al. Nutritional dwarfing: is it a consequence of disturbed psychosocial functioning? Pediatrics 1991; 88(5):926–933.

133. Health and Public Policy Committee, American College of Physicians. Eating disorders: anorexia nervosa and bulimia. Ann Intern Med 1986; 105:790–794.

134. Smith NJ. Excessive weight loss and food aversion in athletes simulating anorexia nervosa. Pediatrics 1980; 66(1):139–142.

135. Storz NS, Greene WJ. Body weight, body image, and perception of fad diets in adolescent girls. J Nutr Ed 1983; 15:15–18.

136. Killen JD, Taylor CB, Telch MJ, et al. Self-induced vomiting and laxative and diuretic use among teenagers: precursors of the binge-purge syndrome. JAMA 1986; 255:1447–1449.

137. Moses N, Banilivy M, Lifshitz F. Fear of obesity among adolescent females. Pediatrics 1989; 83:393–398.

138. Garner DM, Garfunkel PE, The eating attitudes test: an index of the symptoms of anorexia nervosa. Psychol Med 1979; 9:273–279.

139. U.S. Department of Health and Human Services. Lipid Research Clinics Population Studies Data Book, Vol. I. The Prevalence Study. National Institutes of Health Publication No. 80-1527.

140. Consensus Conference. Lowering blood cholesterol to prevent heart disease. JAMA 1985; 253:2080–2086.

141. American Academy of Pediatrics, Committee of Nutrition. Prudent life-style for children: dietary fat and cholesterol. Pediatrics 1986; 78:521–525.

142. Tarim O, Newman TB, Lifshitz F. Cholesterol screening and dietary intervention for prevention of adult onset cardiovascular disease. In: Lifshitz F, ed. Childhood Nutrition. Boca Raton, FL: CRC Press 1995; 13–20.

143. Dietz WH, Hartung R. Changes in height velocity of obese preadolescents during weight reduction. Am J Dis Child 1985; 139:704–708.

144. Epstein LH, Rena RW. Long-term effects of family based treatment of childhood obesity. J Consult Clin Psychiatry 1987; 1:91–95.

145. Merrit RJ. Obesity. Curr Probl Pediatr 1982; 12:1–58.

146. Ho KY, Veldhuis JD, Johnson ML, et al. Fasting enhances growth hormone secretion and amplifies the complex rhythms of growth hormone secretion in man. J Clin Invest 1988; 81:968.

147. Pimstone BL, Barbezat G, Hansen JDL, et al. Growth hormone and protein-calorie malnutrition: impaired suppression during induced hyperglycemia. Lancet 1967; 2(530):1333–1334.

148. Beas F, Contreras I, Maccioni A, et al. Growth hormone in infant malnutrition: the arginine test in marasmus and kwashiorkor. Br J Nutr 1971; 26:169.

149. Soliman AT, Hassan AEHI, Aref MK, et al. Serum insulin-like growth factors I and II concentrations and growth hormone and insulin responses to arginine infusion in children with protein-energy malnutrition before and after nutritional rehabilitation. Pediatr Res 1986; 20(11):1122–1130.

150. Pimstone BL, Becker D, Kronheim S. Disappearance of plasma growth hormone in acromegaly and protein-calori malnutrition after somatostatin. J Clin Endocrinol Metab 1975; 40:168.

151. Becker DJ. The endocrine responses to protein calorie malnutrition. Ann Rev Nutr 1983; 3:187–212.

152. Brown PI, Brasel JA. Endocrine changes in the malnourished child. In: Suskind RM, Winter-Susking L. eds. The malnourished child. Nestle Nutrition Workshop Series, Vol 19, Raven Press, New York: 1990:213–228.

153. Clemmons DR, Klibanski A, Underwood LE, et al. Reduction of plasma immunoreactive somatomedin-C during fasting in humans. J Clin Endocrinol Metab 1981; 53:1247–1250.

154. Rappaport R, Prevot C, Czernichow P. Somatomedin activity and growth hormone secretion. I. Changes related to body weight in anorexia nervosa. Acta Pediatr Scand 1980; 69(1):37–41.

155. Pugliese M, Lifshitz F, Fort P, et al. Pituitary-hypothalmic response in adolescents with growth failuredue to fear of obesity. J Am Coll Nutri 1987; 6(2):113–120.

156. Komaki G, Tamai H, Kiyohara K, et al. Changes in the hypothalamic-pituitary-thyroid axis during acute starvation in non-obese patients. Endocrinol Japan 1986; 33(3):303–308.

157. Danforth E Jr, Burger AG. The impact on nutrition on thyroid hormone physiology and action. Annu Rev Nutr 1989; 9:201–207.

158. de Rosa G, Della Casa S, Corsello SM, et al. Thyroid function in altered nutritional state. Exp Clin Endocrinol 1983; 82(2):173–177.

159. Burman KD, Lukes Y, Wright FD, et al. Reduction in hepatic triiodothyronine binding capacity induced by fasting. Endocrinol 1977; 101:1331.

160. Jaya Rao KS. Endocrines in protein energy malnutrition. Wld Rev Nutr Diet. 1982; 39:53–84.

161. Pugliese MT. Endocrine function adaptations in undernutrition. Wld Rev Nutr Diet. 1990; 62:186–211.

162. Heard CRC. The effects of protein energy malnutrition on blood glucose homeostasis. World Rev Nutr Diet 1978; 30:107.

163. Van der Spuy ZM. Nutrition and reproduction. Clin Obstet Gynecol 1985; 12(3):579–604.

9
Failure to Thrive

Gerald F. Powell
University of Texas Medical Branch,
Galveston, Texas

I. INTRODUCTION

Failure to thrive (FTT) is a common problem of infancy, accounting for 1–5% of pediatric tertiary hospital admissions (1,2). Even larger numbers of FTT infants are managed as outpatients (3). "Failure to thrive," a term usually restricted to infants, is a sign or symptom, not a diagnosis or a disease state. The causes of FTT are many, and determination of the specific cause can be time consuming, expensive, and frustrating. Use of the term FTT usually implies that the cause is not immediately apparent.

Nonorganic failure to thrive (NOFTT) is a subset or type of FTT. Among other terms designating this subtype are maternal deprivation, emotional deprivation, sensory deprivation, and feeding disorder of infancy. However, *nonorganic* is the preferred adjective, because it does not imply a specific etiology but merely suggests that the cause is primarily external to the infant. This subtype accounts for 15–58% of FTT infants; the percentage varies from institution to institution (4,5).

The primary focus of this chapter is on the relationship of nutrition, hormones, and behavior to poor weight gain in NOFTT infants. Diagnosis and treatment of NOFTT are covered briefly, but social and legal aspects of this disorder are not covered. Psychosocial dwarfism in older children (6), which has some etiologic factors similar to those of NOFTT in infants, is covered elsewhere in this book.

II. DEFINITION

A lack of consensus among investigators has prevented the formulation of a single definition of FTT. Common to the many definitions is a weight below the fifth percentile on the growth chart or an abnormally low rate of weight gain. With most infants, the term FTT, is applied clinically when actual weight is perceptibly lower than the expected weight for measured length. A low rate of length gain is often not included as part of the definition, probably because longitudinal growth data are usually not available at the time the infant is first seen: The infant frequently is labeled as failing to thrive when only one length or weight measurement has been obtained. Additionally, undernutrition during infancy mainly seems to affect weight gain; linear growth may deteriorate only if malnutrition persists over a longer period. Although most FTT infants are developmentally delayed, delay is generally not included as part of the definition.

The definition of FTT with reference to growth should include one or more of the following:

1. Length or weight, or both, below the fifth percentile
2. Length or weight transversing percentiles in a downward deviation (i.e., length or weight rate not paralleling one of the percentile lines on the growth chart)
3. Measured weight less than 90% of the expected weight for measured length
4. Actual weight loss regardless of length

Caution must be used in applying the definition without longitudinal data because growth is a rate phenomenon. The use of a single length or weight measurement below the fifth percentile would wrongly include in the FTT category premature infants, infants with intrauterine growth retardation, and some normally small infants.

III. CATEGORIES OF CAUSES

There are many causes of FTT during infancy and childhood. Failure to thrive because of causes that are intrinsic to the infant is called organic failure to thrive (OFTT); that from causes extrinsic to the infant is called nonorganic failure to thrive (NOFTT). Examples of intrinsic causes of FTT are certain congenital heart defects and cystic fibrosis. Extrinsic factors, such as inadequate nutritional intake and deprived social environment, may define nonorganic causes of FTT. In many infants a combination of organic and nonorganic factors operates simultaneously. Most NOFTT results from a combination of nutritional and socioenvironmental factors. Physiologically, all failure to thrive is organic in the sense that these infants are underweight for length. Only the causes of FTT can be categorized as organic or nonorganic. Use of the term "nonorganic" to describe a cause must be distinguished from the incorrect use of the term to describe a pathophysiologic mechanism.

The pathophysiologic mechanism for nonorganic causes of FTT has been much debated in the literature and remains confused, primarily because some investigators have focused on behavioral abnormalities, whereas others have focused on growth or nutritional abnormalities. Although FTT is defined as a growth problem, the subset, NOFTT, is more than a growth problem: it is a syndrome consisting of a low rate of weight or length gain, or both, delayed development, abnormal behavior, and distorted caretaker-infant interaction (7,8). This chapter focuses on the causes of poor weight gain in the NOFTT syndrome, although interactions between behavioral and physiologic phenomena are also considered.

IV. DEFINITION OF NONORGANIC FAILURE TO THRIVE

Several criteria can be used in defining NOFTT. To be classified as NOFTT, the infant must not have an organic disorder as the primary underlying or root cause for FTT. However, an organic disorder, such as a small atrial septal defect, not directly causing the FTT, may be present. A deprived social and nutritional history is compatible with a nonorganic cause of poor weight gain, but such a history may or may not be forthcoming during initial examination. Development is usually delayed, and abnormal behaviors are usually present. However, proof of a nonorganic cause is established by catch-up growth and development in response to appropriate treatment. This important response criterion requires that treatment be initiated before certainty of the correct diagnosis of NOFTT. Complicating evaluation is that infants with OFTT may also come from deprived social environments and may gain weight in the hospital (9).

V. CLINICAL DESCRIPTION OF NONORGANIC FAILURE TO THRIVE

Symptoms and signs of NOFTT form a spectrum or continuum that is complex, and the expression of symptoms and signs ranges from mild to severe. Symptoms and signs vary with age and developmental level at time of onset of the failure to thrive. They may also vary with the underlying environmental cause or causes.

The average age of a NOFTT patient on initial medical presentation is 11 months (10). More than half of the infants are boys (2,11). Lack of weight gain is the most common presenting complaint of FTT. Other common problems are intermittent vomiting, diarrhea, and frequent upper respira-

tory infections (8). Vomiting is generally mild, but it may be severe when rumination is present. Diarrhea may also be present, but it is usually mild or intermittent. Developmental delay is a less frequent presenting complaint.

The major clinical presentation of deteriorating growth in patients with NOFTT varies with differences in the rate of weight gain and linear growth and the degree of wasting. The degree of wasting varies from mild to severe (10). Weight is usually more severely affected than length, especially in infants below 1 year of age. This accounts for the thin appearance of these infants. The more wasted infants have thin chests and prominent abdomens, with hanging skin folds under the arms and wasted buttocks. These features of wasting are indistinguishable from those of OFTT and do not clinically differentiate between NOFTT and OFTT.

The behavior of the infants with FTT may strongly suggest a nonorganic cause. In the more common clinical presentation of NOFTT, a general depression in gross motor activity is usual, as is decreased facial muscle activity, resulting in an expressionless face (2). Several gaze abnormalities can be present. Some infants have a wide-eyed stare, but most have some degree of gaze avoidance. Vocalization and socialization are most frequently and severely delayed. These behaviors are similar to those seen in adults with major depression (12). The younger infant's fists are often clenched, and there may be obsessive hand or thumb sucking. The infants usually do not cuddle and may actually push away from the caregiver instead of folding into the contour of this person, as normal infants do. Rumination may also be present (2,14). Infantile posturing is also common (15). Table 1 lists clinical features in young infants with NOFTT. Older infants with NOFTT, 16–24 months of age, may have fewer abnormal behaviors. The OFTT infants may also have abnormal behaviors, although they have fewer episodes of abnormal behavior than NOFTT infants, and their behaviors are less intense (2). Therefore, behavior alone does not distinguish NOFTT from OFTT.

A subtype of NOFTT, *infantile anorexia nervosa* (IAN), has a different behavioral presentation from the more common presentation of NOFTT described earlier (12,16,17). The onset of failure to thrive for IAN infants is usually 12–24

Table 1 Clinical Features of Young Infants with Nonorganic Failure to Thrive

Small for age
Thin
Wide-eyed expression or gaze aversion
Expressionless face
Decreased vocalization
Decreased gross motor activity
Decreased response to social stimuli
Lack of cuddling
Infantile posturing
Preoccupation with sucking
Clenched fists

months. IAN infants are often active rather than depressed in motor activity. Smiling and vocalization and other developmental milestones may be nearly normal, and they often are interested in exploring their environment. Common to IAN infants is refusal to eat or a very selective eating pattern. They frequently carry a bottle around with them. The infants are in control of feeding situations rather than the mother, and there is much dyadic conflict.

VI. CAUSES OF NONORGANIC FAILURE TO THRIVE

The syndrome of NOFTT probably results from multiple interacting causal factors. Inadequate nutrition (nature) and decreased or distorted social stimulation (nurture) contribute to the poor weight gain, delayed development, and abnormal behavior. There have been several hypothesis on the role of nature and nurture. One hypothesis postulates that lack of weight gain is a result of decreased caloric intake or endocrine factors related to starvation. Another hypothesis considers lack of weight gain to be caused by psychologic factors, mediated through decreased intestinal absorption, decreased utilization of calories, or abnormal endocrine function. The exact role of these factors and how they interact is undetermined (see Chap. 6). Both the macroenvironment (i.e., major factors within the home, such as the number of people in the home who are the caregivers) and the microenvironment (i.e., quality of caregiver-infant interpersonal interaction), play a role. More recent research efforts have been directed toward understanding these environmental factors (18–21). The role of the macroenvironment is illustrated in Figure 1. The microenvironment is considered in Section VIII. C.

VII. ETIOLOGY OF POOR WEIGHT GAIN

A. Undernutrition

Acute *undernutrition*, defined as a weight less than that expected for actual length, is present in most NOFTT infants. In a study that included all FTT infants admitted to the hospital during 1 year, 17 NOFTT and 17 OFTT infants had actual weights that were respectively 80.0 and 86.2% of expected for actual length (10). These differences in mean weights between groups of NOFTT and OFTT infants are not statistically significant. When anthropometric indices on individual NOFTT infants from all U.S. studies were grouped for degree of malnutrition, only 7% of infants had severe wasting (10), as defined by a weight-length (WT/LT) ratio of less than 70% of the expected, according to the Waterlow classification of malnutrition (22). Of NOFTT infants, 40% have a mild (80–89% WT/LT) and 31% a moderate (70–79% WT/LT) decrease in weight for actual length. Of NOFTT infants, 20% are equally delayed in length and weight but have abnormally slow rates of gain.

Two-thirds of NOFTT infants gain weight in the hospital (4,7,23,24). Several studies have demonstrated catch-up growth when normal caloric intake is achieved (25,26).

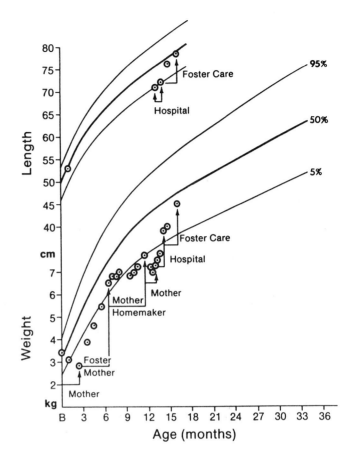

Figure 1 Macroenvironment of an NOFTT infant. This female infant lost weight in the first $2^{1/2}$ months of life while living at home with her mother. When placed in a foster home for the next 4 months, there was a dramatic weight gain. The infant was returned to her mother, and over the next 5 months, a homemaker came into the home every weekday and supervised feeding. Presumably intake was adequate, but it was not accurately measured. The rate of weight gain slowed. When the homemaker stopped coming there was dramatic weight loss. With hospitalization and later foster placement, there was again a rapid increase in weight and length. This case illustrates weight changes as a function of environment, but it does not identify the underlying mechanism. It is not fully understood how multiple factors interact or what is the final common pathway for poor weight gain.

However, weight gain is influenced not only by caloric intake, but also by nutritional status. The NOFTT infants whose ideal body weight-length ratio for age, was greater than 80% did not have a significant correlation between caloric intake and weight gain (27). Neither malabsorption nor increased caloric requirements have been demonstrated in NOFTT, and basal metabolic rate is normal in these patients (26,28). The quality of the caregiver-infant interpersonal interaction accounting for the poor appetite in infants with IAN may not change during hospitalization, accounting for lack of weight gain in infants in this NOFTT subtype.

Calorie intake may be lost through vomiting or diarrhea, and decreased intake is often associated with frequent infections. However, neither form of decreased intake has been documented in NOFTT infants. Although vomiting is mild in most instances, some mothers have electively restricted intake to decrease vomiting. Some infants have apparent anorexia in the hospital, but most infants eat normally.

Undereating is the most likely cause of the decreased weight in NOFTT, based on (1) anthropometric indices (7,23,25); (2) the Whitten et al. study of caloric intake (23); (3) that most of the infants gain weight in the hospital when provided adequate food (4,7,23,24); and (4) the lack of evidence for abnormal losses or abnormal metabolism. However, although undereating is suspected, actual intake has been poorly studied, and the reason for undereating is unclear. Determination of the reason for decreased intake is necessary if the situation is to be reversed.

If one assumes that decreased caloric intake is the cause for lack of weight gain, the question becomes, why are insufficient amounts of food consumed at home? Although food is in short supply in some homes, unavailability is not the usual problem in the United States. Assuming that sufficient food is available, are these infants simply not offered enough? Does the infant not signal hunger or satiety? If offered sufficient food, does the infant have a poor appetite or refuse food? Is the feeding environment not conducive to a good appetite? Do the infants not ingest or retain enough food? These are not trivial questions. Despite conjecture that inadequate food intake is the cause of the poor weight gain, in few NOFTT infants have accurate determinations been made to show a lower food intake before hospitalization (23).

Food refusal and food selection occur in infants with the IAN subtype. Behavior and development in IAN infants are different from those in most NOFTT infants, as is their attachment to their mothers (16). Pugliese et al. (29) have identified parents who deliberately restricted nutrition to their infants, based on health practices currently in vogue and recommended for adults by the medical community. In a study of 19 NOFTT subjects, 12–60 months of age, Pollitt reported a smaller caloric intake (as measured by calculations based on dietary recall) than in a normally growing group (30). Over 50% of the mothers of these 19 infants retrospectively reported having difficulties feeding their children during the first 12 months (31).

In addition to caloric undernutrition, NOFTT infants may be deficient in vitamins and minerals. Iron deficiency during infancy has been associated with anorexia, irritability, and lack of interest in surroundings (32). Therefore, underlying specific nutrient deficiencies may exacerbate the condition of NOFTT. Zinc supplementation of failure to thrive infants has been shown to be associated with increased weight gain (33).

B. Endocrine Factors

There has been debate about whether the lack of weight gain in NOFTT infants is secondary to undernutrition alone or is attributable to hormonal factors independent of nutrition. This debate arose because of (1) early studies reporting adequate caloric intake in infants (34,35); (2) a tendency to equate psychosocial dwarfism in older children with NOFTT infants; and (3) extrapolation of hormonal data from severely malnourished infants to NOFTT infants. Caloric intake was not accurately measured in these early studies of institutionalized infants. Psychosocial dwarfism, although similar to NOFTT, has distinctive characteristics suggestive of a different pathophysiologic cause of the growth problem. Extrapolation of data from severely malnourished infants may be unwarranted, because most NOFTT infants are not severely malnourished.

In fact, hormone status in NOFTT infants has received little study. Fasting and peak growth hormone values were normal in 13 of 14 NOFTT infants under 2 years of age in whom growth hormone was measured (36–38). An additional 3 infants had fasting and peak growth hormone evaluations (39), but the data are not clearly presented. At least 2 of these 3 infants had low fasting growth hormone on hospital admission. The generally normal growth hormone in NOFTT contrasts with the decreased growth hormone observed in many children with psychosocial dwarfism (40,41). Somatomedin levels have not been reported in NOFTT infants, but they are low in malnutrition and return to normal on nutritional recovery (39). The low thyroxine (T_4) levels reported in four infants with NOFTT are probably related to the undernutrition (42). Although not confined to NOFTT infants, sick infants have been shown to have high plasma somatostatin levels, which may be related to slow weight gain and may inhibit growth hormone (43). Of the circulating somatostatin, 90% is derived from the stomach. Gastrointestinal hormones may also play a role in the metabolism of ingested food, but these have not been studied in NOFTT. If such hormonal mechanisms contribute to poor weight gain in NOFTT infants, abnormal behavior may initiate the mechanism.

C. Behavior

Infant behavior may contribute to poor weight gain. Delayed motor, language, and social development are well recognized in NOFTT (7,8). However, there is more than merely delayed development. Infants with NOFTT behave in an unusual manner, and there is decreased spontaneous and interactive behavior (2,14,19,44). Developmentally, the NOFTT infant is capable of motor activity, vocalization, and smiling but electively does not perform these activities and may deliberately engage in avoidance of eye contact. Obsessive thumb sucking and rumination are additional, although less frequent, abnormal behaviors.

Although apathy and decreased motor activity are recognized behaviors in malnourished infants, many of the aforementioned behaviors are not attributable to malnutrition alone. In a recent study (2), NOFTT infants were shown to have a significantly more frequent association of specific behaviors than OFTT infants of equivalent nutritional status. Furthermore, the intensity of the most frequent behaviors was greater in NOFTT than OFTT infants. One interpretation of these results is that the behavioral abnormalities of the NOFTT infants could discourage social interaction. These behaviors may be interpreted by the mother as a personal rejection. If the infant demands feeding, the mother may not recognize the hunger signals, or if signals are recognized, she may be less likely to respond to them because of the infant's apathy. FTT infants express a less positive effect in feeding and nonfeeding situations and more negative effect in feeding than normally growing infants (21,44). They are also more fussy, demanding, and unsociable and less task oriented and persistent (19).

Many mothers of NOFTT infants are depressed or have other psychopathology (45–47). Most come from lower socioeconomic groups and are under multiple stresses (46,48–50). Mothers may not be knowledgeable about nutritional needs or have the emotional strength or motivation to interpret or meet the needs of the infant. It is known that NOFTT mothers engage less often in mutual gaze, and they interact with their infants less than control dyads (51). Additionally, mothers of NOFTT infants have less adaptive social interactional behavior, less positive affective behavior, and more arbitrary termination of feedings (18). They also express more negative emotions during play interaction (19).

There have been few studies examining the relationships between mother-infant interaction and feeding. Cravioto and DiLicardie identified lower scores in quantity and quality of socioemotional stimulation that are antecedent to clinical malnutrition (52). Pollitt (53) found less mother-child interaction in a growth-retarded group compared with a group with normal height and weight. The mean age of these children was 37 months. Within the growth-retarded group, the mother-child interaction measure was the only independent variable in the study that correlated significantly with both height and weight measures. The better nourished children had more frequent and more positive contact with the mother. Abnormal mother-infant interaction has been observed in NOFTT (51,53), but decreased caloric intake as a result of this interaction has not been documented.

Investigations of family influences on NOFTT with respect to food availability, allocation, dysfunctional feeding, and caregiving were recently reviewed (54). NOFTT family functioning is different from that of controls, but the mechanism whereby the physical growth and psychosocial development of infants is affected is not clear (55).

Rosenn et al. (56) reported that those NOFTT infants who subsequently gained weight had an accompanying positive change in behavior, and the weight gain was not necessarily correlated with the time of greatest caloric intake. With use of a behavior scale modified from Rosenn's, Goldstein and Field (57) noted an increase in positive affect across hospitalization only for infants who gained weight, suggesting that positive affect is related to weight gain. Thus, there appears to be a relationship between behavior and nutritional state, but the nature of this relationship is not clear. These studies do not clarify the crucial question of whether behavior affects nutrition and thus growth, or whether behavior also affects growth through hormonal mechanisms independently of nutrition.

Recently, Field et al. reported greater weight gain in premature infants given tactile kinesthetic stimulation com-pared with a nonstimulated control group receiving the same number of calories (58). In a replication of this study, the treated infants averaged a 21% greater weight gain per day and were discharged 5 days earlier (59). These data suggest stimulation factors in addition to nutrition may be important in weight gain. The underlying mechanism for this difference in weight gain is unknown. Lack of such factors may contribute to NOFTT.

VIII. DIAGNOSIS AND EVALUATION OF NONORGANIC FAILURE TO THRIVE

The diagnosis of NOFTT always demands a very careful history and physical examination, but a positive diagnosis of a nonorganic etiology can be made only retrospectively. Catch-up growth and development and decreased abnormal behavior must occur in response to intervention to confirm a diagnosis of NOFTT. A nonorganic etiology can be suspected from a compatible history, growth data showing intermittent improvement, and lack of demonstration of organic disease on physical and laboratory examination. The diagnosis of NOFTT should be made by inclusion of positive findings, not merely by exclusion of organic disease. Organic disease may be present concomitantly but should not account solely for the poor weight gain. Obviously, any suspected organic disease must be further evaluated and confirmed.

Initial history should include time of onset of the poor weight gain and an estimation of the caloric intake per kg body weight. The type of milk and other foods and liquids, the amounts ingested with each feeding, and the number of feedings, as well as who feeds the infant, should also be determined. The infant's appetite and hunger signals, length of feeding time, and signals of satiety should also be elicited. All forms of caloric intake and their amounts should be determined, with specific questions about the timing and amount of intake of juices and other sugar sources. Excess juice consumption is a contributing factor in NOFTT (60). It is very important to determine if appetite is present because therapy is much easier if appetite is present. Infants without an appetite or with food refusal may have IAN if the other behavioral characteristics of this NOFTT subtype are present. Lack of appetite may suggest milk allergy or other medical conditions mentioned later. A history of caloric losses, as with vomiting and/or diarrhea, should be sought. Social history should include maternal and environmental stresses and support systems and identification of other caregivers, as well as characteristics of the physical environment.

Infant behaviors are of great help in suggesting an underlying nonorganic cause. The infant should be carefully observed for the behaviors described earlier in both feeding and nonfeeding situations, including play both with the mother and with strangers. Infants with IAN are often indifferent to their mother's presence as they explore their environment. They are capable of vocalization but may not vocalize.

Mother-infant interaction should be observed with particular attention to what the mother does in response to the infant's communication efforts. Does the mother bring the infant to a socially alert state? Mother should be observed for evidence of depression, anxiety, and stress, as well as for her interest in caring for the infant. The infant should be observed being fed by the mother. Feeding by the examiner is also very informative, particularly with regard to establishing the presence of oral motor problems.

A group of conditions associated with poor growth or weight gain despite apparently adequate intake (Table 2) must be distinguished from NOFTT. These conditions can usually be diagnosed or suggested by careful examination and the laboratory tests suggested later. Medical conditions associated with a poor appetite include chronic infection, acidosis, elevated ammonia or amino acids, and an elevated blood urea nitrogen.

Because confirmation of the initial diagnosis is based on a growth and behavioral response to treatment, initial and repeated anthropometric measurements and behavioral evaluations must be obtained with great care to demonstrate later that increased growth and behavioral change have occurred with treatment. For infants of about 6 months of age, a weight gain of 0.045 g/day can be considered catch-up growth, three times the usual weight gain in this weight and age group. An increase in length is technically more difficult to demonstrate during a short hospitalization. Sutures may split as rapid brain growth exceeds growth of the skull (61). There should also be a demonstrable improvement in developmental status and a decrease in abnormal behavior patterns.

There are no laboratory tests that confirm NOFTT. However, laboratory evaluation is necessary to evaluate the presence and degree of biochemical complications of malnutrition and to rule out suspected organic disease. Determinations of blood gas levels and concentrations of electrolytes, glucose, blood urea nitrogen, total serum protein, and albumin, as well as a complete blood count, are a necessary minimum for evaluation of the malnutrition. These tests, along with a urinalysis and urine culture, are also helpful in detecting the presence of acidosis, urinary tract infection, and decreased renal function. On the other hand, "shotgunning"

Table 2 Conditions with Poor Weight Gain and Apparently Adequate Caloric Intake That Must Be Distinguished from Nonorganic Failure to Thrive

Various syndromes
Central nervous system damage
Malabsorption
Chronic "hidden" infection
Anemia
Large left-to-right shunt
Heart failure
Renal failure
Acidosis of any cause
Hyper- or hypothyroidism
Adrenal hyperplasia with salt loss

for organic disease with laboratory tests is rarely helpful (5,62). Laboratory evaluation for suspected organic disease and treatment of nonorganic problems should proceed immediately and simultaneously.

Hospitalization may not be necessary for the mildly malnourished infants if a nonorganic cause is likely and caretaker compliance is probable. If attempts at outpatient management are not successful after 2–4 weeks, and in those cases in whom accurate intake and weight gain are otherwise impossible to obtain or evaluate, admission to the hospital is usually necessary. Hospitalization is generally necessary for treatment of the moderately to severely malnourished infant and may also be necessary for behavioral therapy.

IX. TREATMENT

Like the clinical picture of NOFTT, treatment is also multifaceted and can be divided into immediate and long-term treatment of the infant, the mother and environment, and mother-infant interaction. Treatment of the infant includes nutritional, development, and behavioral therapy, as well as treatment for complicating factors, such as infection and anemia. Treatment of the mother-environment requires identification and modification of environmental stresses and improvement of support systems. Improvement of mother-infant interaction is needed if initial success during hospitalization is to be maintained in the home. This comprehensive approach to treatment is best accomplished through a team, usually consisting of a physician, nurse, dietitian, social worker, and developmental therapist (63,64).

A. Nutritional Therapy

Initial treatment of malnutrition is most easily accomplished through formula alone, feeding the young infant about 140 kcal (kg/day). Most infants under 1 year of age do not have difficulty taking this amount of formula. The giving of formula alone allows easy calculation of caloric intake and estimation of losses through vomiting. Nurses or trained therapists should feed the infant initially to allow identification of a feeding problem and to assure that intake is adequate. Except in the most severe malnutrition, tube feeding is rarely indicated. If tube feeding is under consideration because the infant refuses to eat for the mother, placement of the infant in foster care is probably indicated, particularly if treatment for IAN is unsuccessful. Vomiting is rarely a problem, because most infants with a history of vomiting cease vomiting soon after hospitalization. Continued gastroesophageal reflux may require thickened feedings and placing the infant in a semiupright position after feeding. Infants with rumination require considerable therapeutic attention, which is beyond the scope of this chapter.

Observation of mother-infant feeding and nonfeeding interaction is a necessary part of the evaluation. For example, does the mother relax the infant, yet gently encourage feeding, or does she passively feed the infant in a disinterested fashion? In nonfeeding interactions, does she offer a warm and pleasant smile and voice? Does she socially reward the infant for its responses?

Once it is known that the infant does not have a problem feeding and when intake is adequate, mother may again feed the infant under observation. Presumably, by this time rapport has been established with the mother, maternal stresses identified, and some social intervention has begun. Education of the mother concerning the infant's nutritional needs is an essential part of therapy.

B. Developmental Therapy

The goal in developmental therapy is to promote normal patterns of motor, language, personal-social, and adaptive behavior (64). To obtain a baseline, the developmental therapist formally identifies areas of delay by using assessment instruments, such as the Bayley Scales of Infant Development. Of equal importance is clinical assessment of the quality of movement and interactive behaviors. Developmental delay in NOFTT infants differs from that in neurologically damaged infants in that the delay is functional. The infant with NOFTT has the capacity to move and respond. There is a paucity in motor activity, and there may be gaps in developmental sequence or abnormal compensation for normal motor patterns. The therapist aids the NOFTT infant in developing normal patterns of movement, rather than compensating for problems in motor tone or inability.

Therapy is adjusted to the infant's level of performance. Positioning and social stimuli, such as play, as well as interaction modalities with toys, are used to motivate the infant. One example of encouraging a more normal movement pattern in an infant with strong extension might be to facilitate rolling over from the supine to prone by positioning the infant on its side to encourage antigravity or volitional flexion. Social stimuli as outlined in the next section should be used simultaneously to encourage normal developmental skills.

C. Behavioral Therapy

The goal in behavioral therapy with those infants with the behavioral characteristics of infantile depression is to change the infant's abnormal behaviors to positive, spontaneous, and interactive behaviors (64). This goal is based on the concept that the infant's behavior contributes to the problem. Although spontaneous behaviors cannot be induced, the infants become spontaneously active once their interactive behaviors improve. Thus, behavioral interventions are directed toward improving social responsiveness through social interaction (64).

Mutual eye contact must be established to induce social responsiveness. If gaze avoidance is present, eye contact can be established from about 6 feet away. Maintenance of eye contact may require the therapist to move repeatedly into the infant's line of vision. Together, a warm smile and vocalization are repeatedly used as stimuli. The infant is very carefully monitored for the slightest response, which is immediately and consistently reinforced by the therapist. A slight smile

involving the corners of the mouth is usually the first response, followed by increased motor activity. Vocalization is usually the last response to return. With improvement, the infant's response time to stimuli decreases and intensity of response increases. The intensity, frequency, and quality of the therapist's social stimuli and responses are determined by the infant. The therapist's exaggerated smiles and vocalizations are effective as stimuli and reinforcers. This is only a brief description of a comprehensive and intensive behavioral program.

Therapy sessions are most effective if offered in the morning after feeding, when the infant is neither tired nor hungry. Sessions are offered daily by the same therapists for about 30 minutes. Nutritional, developmental, and behavioral progress is monitored daily.

After the infant develops consistent social responsiveness with the therapist, the mother is reintroduced to the infant. The therapist models the technique, explaining it as he or she goes along, observes the mother interacting, and reinforces the mother's efforts. Success is measured by observing the infant's improved social responsiveness to the mother's efforts.

Therapy for the IAN subtype involves education of the mothers, particularly with regard to normal independent development of the infant and the management of the expression of this independence during feeding. The IAN subtype results from control issues, which often are displayed in nonfeeding situations as well. The control issue in general must be handled.

The purpose of hospitalization is to establish the correct cause of the failure to thrive and to initiate therapy. Once this has been accomplished, discharge can be considered. However, there should be some indication that the relational or environmental conditions that initiated or maintained the problem have improved. If there is little hope of improvement in the relational or home environment, placement in a foster home may be necessary.

Continued treatment after discharge is necessary. Enrollment in an infant stimulation program is suggested. The infant must be followed at intervals for a long time. Growth, development, and social behavior must be carefully and continually monitored. Therapy with regard to the mother involves identification and alleviation of her stresses, as well as education and demonstration of more appropriate interaction with her infant.

X. OUTCOME

There are few systematic long-term studies of growth and development in NOFTT infants. In Shaheen and coworkers' 15 month follow-up study (4), 22% in infants remained below the third percentile in weight, whereas 26% were below the third percentile in height. Glaser et al. followed 40 children for an average of 41 months (65): 42% remained below the third percentile for height or weight. Mitchell et al. (3) followed 30 cases for 3–6 years. Failure to thrive subjects were lighter but not shorter than controls; that is, height caught up, but weight remained low. Most NOFTT children improved in weight and height but remained short and thin. No intervention beyond the initial intervention was carried out in any of these studies.

The longest follow-up study of growth (14 years) was reported by Oates and colleagues (66), who found a difference between former failure to thrive and control children when the relationship between the height ages and weight ages of the children was compared with their chronologic ages. Of 14 children who had suffered from failure to thrive, in contrast to 1 child in the comparison group of 14 children, 6 were 1 year or more below the chronologic age for height and also for weight ($p < 0.04$).

There are more follow-up studies of development than studies of growth. Developmental studies have been mostly short term, and few have included interventions. In general, NOFTT infants continue to do poorly developmentally, despite improved weight gain. In a study by Singer (67), even after extended hospitalization, NOFTT infants manifested persistent intellectual delays at 3 year follow-up, despite maintenance of weight gains achieved during early hospitalization. In a follow-up study, these same children, as preschoolers, demonstrated deficits in behavioral organization and ego control. Their parents reported a higher level of behavioral symptoms (68). In a 13 year follow-up study by Oates and Yu (24), former NOFTT children were significantly behind in language development, reading age, and verbal intelligence with reference to their comparison group. They also scored lower than the comparison group on a social maturity rating.

Although delayed development is often attributed to early malnutrition, continued exposure to an adverse environment probably plays a major role.

XI. SUMMARY AND CONCLUSION

Nonorganic failure to thrive can be diagnosed and treated, yet many questions remain unanswered for this common problem of infancy. Despite the logistic difficulties, further studies are needed to assess whether inadequate intake occurs at home and, if so, why? Factors contributing to inadequate intake must be defined. The relationship of undernutrition and social factors to the infant's later social and cognitive development must be determined.

If, indeed, one-third of infants do not gain weight while receiving adequate caloric intake, the reasons for this phenomenon must be identified. The interaction of gastrointestinal hormones with social stimuli and nutrition may account for this lack of weight gain.

Interventions must be comprehensive and long term, and they must focus on improving nutrition and mother-infant interaction, in addition to other socioenvironmental factors. These interventions must be studied with appropriate design and controls. Although much has been written about NOFTT, much remains to be done if this problem is to be correctly diagnosed, effectively treated, and, it is hoped, prevented.

REFERENCES

1. English PC. Failure to thrive without organic reason. Pediatr Ann 1978; 7:774–781.
2. Powell GF, Low JF, Speers MA. Behavior as a diagnostic aid in failure-to-thrive. J Dev Behav Pediatr 1987; 8:18–24.
3. Mitchell WG, Gorrell RW, Greenberg RA. Failure to thrive: a study in a primary care setting, epidemiology and follow-up. Pediatrics 1980; 65:971–977.
4. Shaheen E, Alexander D, Truskowsky M, Barbero GJ. Failure to thrive—a retrospective profile. Clin Pediatr (Phila) 1968; 7:255–261.
5. Sills RH. Failure to thrive, the role of clinical and laboratory evaluation. Am J Dis Child 1978; 132:967–969.
6. Powell GF, Brasel JA, Blizzard RM. Emotional deprivation and growth retardation simulating idiopathic hypopituitarism. I. Clinical evaluation of the syndrome. N Engl J Med 1967; 276:1271–1278.
7. Leonard MF, Rhymes JP, Solnit AJ. Failure to thrive in infants. A family problem. Am J Dis Child 1966; 111:600–612.
8. Barbero GJ, Shaheen E. Environmental failure to thrive: a clinical view. J Pediatr 1967; 71:639–644.
9. Bithoney WG, McJunkin J, Michalek J, Egan H, Snyder J, Munier A. Prospective evaluation of weight gain in both nonorganic and organic failure to thrive children: an outpatient trial of a multidisciplinary team intervention strategy. J Dev Behav Pediatr 1989; 10:27–31.
10. Powell GF. Nonorganic failure to thrive in infancy: an update on nutrition, behavior and growth. J Am Coll Nutr 1988; 7:345–353.
11. Herman-Staab B. Antecedents of nonorganic failure to thrive. Pediatr Nurs 1992; 18:579–584.
12. Chatoor I, Egan J. Nonorganic failure to thrive and dwarfism due to food refusal: a separation disorder. J Am Acad Child Psychiatry 1983; 22:294–301.
13. Powell GF, Bettes BA. Infantile depression, nonorganic failure to thrive, and DSM-III-R: a different perspective. Child Psychiatry Hum Dev 1992; 22:185–198.
14. Powell GF, Low J. Behavior in nonorganic failure to thrive. J Dev Behav Pediatr 1983; 4:26–33.
15. Krieger I, Sargent DA. A postural sign in the sensory deprivation syndrome in infants. J Pediatr 1967; 70:332–339.
16. Chatoor I, Egan J, Getson P, Menvielle E, O'Donnell R. Mother-infant interactions in infantile anorexia nervosa. J Am Acad Child Adol Psychiatry 1988; 27:535–540.
17. Chatoor I. Infantile anorexia nervosa: a developmental disorder or separation and individuation. J Am Acad Psychoanal 1989; 17:43–64.
18. Drotar D, Eckerle D, Satola J, Pallotta J, Wyatt B. Maternal interactional behavior with nonorganic failure-to-thrive infants: a case comparison study. Child Abuse Negl 1990; 14:41–51.
19. Wolke D, Skuse D, Mathisen B. Behavioral style in failure-to-thrive infants: a preliminary communication. J Pediatr Psychol 1990; 15:237–254.
20. Ward MJ, Kessler DB, Altman SC. Infant-mother attachment in children with failure to thrive. Infant Mental Health J 1993; 14:208–220.
21. Lobo ML, Barnard KE, Coombs JB. Failure to thrive: a parent-infant interaction perspective. J Pediatr Nurs 1992; 7:251–261.
22. Waterlow JC. Classification and definition of protein-calorie malnutrition. B Med J 1972; 3:566–569.
23. Whitten CF, Pettit MG, Fischhoff J. Evidence that growth

failure from maternal deprivation is secondary to undereating. JAMA 1969; 209:1675–1682.

24. Oates RK, Yu JS. Children with non-organic failure to thrive, a community problem. Med J Aust 1971; 2:199–203.

25. Krieger I. The energy metabolism in infants with growth failure due to maternal deprivation, undernutrition, or causes unknown. Metabolic rate calculated from the insensible loss of weight. Pediatrics 1966; 38:63–76.

26. Ellerstein NS, Ostrov BE. Growth patterns in children hospitalized because of caloric-deprivation failure to thrive. Am J Dis Child 1985; 139:164–166.

27. Bell LS, Woolston JL. The relationship of weight gain and caloric intake in infants with organic and nonorganic failure to thrive syndrome. J Am Acad Child Psychiatry 1985; 24:447–452.

28. Krieger I, Chen YC. Calorie requirements for weight gain in infants with growth failure due to maternal deprivation, undernutrition and congenital heart disease. A correlation analysis. Pediatrics 1969; 44:647–654.

29. Pugliese MT, Weyman-Daum M, Moses N, Lifshitz F. Parental health beliefs as a cause of nonorganic failure to thrive. Pediatrics 1987; 80:175–182.

30. Pollitt E, Eichler A. Behavioral disturbances among failure-to-thrive children. Am J Dis Child 1976; 130:24–29.

31. Pollitt E, Eichler AW, Chan CK. Psychosocial development and behavior of mothers of failure-to-thrive children. Am J Orthopsychiatry 1975; 45:525–537.

32. Oski FA. Nutritional anemias of infancy. In: Lifshitz F, ed. Pediatric Nutrition. New York: Marcel Dekker, 1982:123–138.

33. Walravens PA, Hambridge KM, Koepfer DM. Zinc supplementation in infants with a nutritional pattern of failure to thrive: a double-blind, controlled study. Pediatrics 1989; 83:532–538.

34. Bakwin H. Loneliness in infants. Am J Dis Child 1942; 63:30–40.

35. Spitz RA. Hospitalism, an inquiry into the genesis of psychiatric conditions in early childhood. Psychoanal Study Child 1945; 1:53–74.

36. Kaplan SL, Abrams CAL, Bell JJ, Conte FA, Grumbach MM. Growth and growth hormone. I. Changes in serum level of growth hormone following hypoglycemia in 134 children with growth retardation. Pediatr Res 1968; 2:43–63.

37. Krieger I, Mellinger RC. Pituitary function in the deprivation syndrome. J Pediatr 1971; 79:216–225.

38. Guilhaume A, Benoit O, Gourmelen M, Richardet JM. Relationship between sleep stage IV deficit and reversible HGH deficiency in psychosocial dwarfism. Pediatr Res 1982; 16:299–303.

39. Van Den Brande JL, Van Buul S, Heinrich U, Van Roon F, Zurcher T, Van Steirtegem AC. Further observations on plasma somatomedin activity in children. In: Luft R, Hall K, eds. Advances in Metabolic Disorders, Vol. 8, Somatomedins and Some Other Growth Factors. New York: Academic Press, 1975:171–181.

40. Powell GF, Brasel JA, Raiti S, Blizzard RM. Emotional deprivation and growth retardation simulating idiopathic hypopituitarism. II. Endocrinologic evaluation of the syndrome. N Engl J Med 1967; 276:1279–1283.

41. Hopwood NJ, Becker DJ. Psychosocial dwarfism: detection, evaluation and management. Child Abuse Negl 1979; 3:439–447.

42. Krieger I, Good MH. Adrenocortical and thyroid function in the deprivation syndrome. Am J Dis Child 1970; 120:95–102.

43. Uvnas-Moberg K, Widstrom AM, Marchini G, Winberg J. Release of GI hormones in mother and infant by sensory stimulation. Acta Paediatr Scand 1987; 76:851–860.

44. Polan HJ, Leon A, Kaplan MD, Kessler DB, Stern DN, Ward MJ. Disturbances in affect expression in failure-to-thrive. J Am Acad Child Adol Psychiatry 1991; 30:897–903.

45. Evans SL, Reinhart JB, Succop RA. Failure to thrive. A study of 45 children and their families. J Am Acad Child Psychiatry 1972; 11:440–457.

46. Singer LT, Song LY, Hill BP, Jaffe AC. Stress and depression in mothers of failure to thrive children. J Pediatr Psychol 1990; 15:711–720.

47. Polan HJ, Kaplan MD, Kessler DB, et al. Psychopathology in mothers of children with failure to thrive. Infant Mental Health J 1991; 12:55–64.

48. Casey PH, Bradley R, Wortham B. Social and nonsocial home environments of infants with nonorganic failure to thrive. Pediatrics 1984; 73:348–353.

49. Altemeier WA, O'Connor SM, Sherrod KB, Vietze PM. Prospective study of antecedents for nonorganic failure to thrive. J Pediatr 1985; 106:360–365.

50. Bithoney WG, Newberger EH. Child and family attributes of failure to thrive. J Dev Behav Pediatr 1987; 8:32–36.

51. Berkowitz CD, Senter SA. Characteristics of mother-infant interactions in nonorganic failure to thrive. J Fam Pract 1987; 25:377–381.

52. Cravioto J, DeLicardie ER. Microenvironmental factors in severe protein-energy malnutrition. In: Scrimshaw NS, Behars M, eds. Nutrition and Agricultural Development: Significance and Potential for the Tropics. New York: Plenum Press, 1976.

53. Pollitt E. Failure to thrive: socioeconomic, dietary intake and mother-child interaction data. Fed Proc 1975; 34:1593–1597.

54. Drotar D. The family context of nonorganic failure to thrive. Am J Orthopsychiatry 1991; 61:23–34.

55. Drotar D, Eckerle D. The family environment in nonorganic failure to thrive: a controlled study. J Pediatr Psychol 1989; 14:245–257.

56. Rosenn DW, Loeb LS, Jura MB. Differentiation of organic from nonorganic failure to thrive syndrome in infancy. Pediatrics 1980; 66:698–704.

57. Goldstein S, Field T. Affective behavior and weight changes among hospitalized failure-to-thrive infants. Infant Mental Health J 1985; 6:187–194.

58. Field TM, Schanberg SM, Scafidi F, et al. Tactile/kinesthetic stimulation effects on preterm neonates. Pediatrics 1986; 77:654–658.

59. Scafidi FA, Field TM, Schanberg SM, et al. Massage stimulates growth in preterm infants: a replication. Infant Behav Dev 1990; 13:167–188.

60. Smith MM, Lifshitz F. Excess juice consumption as a contributing factor in nonorganic failure to thrive. Pediatrics 1994; 93:438–443.

61. Pearl M, Finkelstein J, Berman MR. Temporary widening of cranial sutures during recovery from failure to thrive. Clin Pediatr (Phila) 1972; 11:427–430.

62. Berwick DM, Levy JC, Kleinerman R. Failure to thrive: diagnostic yield of hospitalization. Arch Dis Child 1982; 57:347–351.

63. Bithoney WG, McJunkin J, Michalek J, Snyder J, Egan H, Epstein D. The effect of a multidisciplinary team approach on weight gain in nonorganic failure to thrive children. J Dev Behav Pediatr 1991; 12:254–258.

64. Hunter JG, Powell GF. Failure to thrive. In: Semmler CJ, Hunter JG, eds. Early Occupational Therapy Intervention, Neonates to Three Years. Gaithersburg, MD: Aspen Publishers, 1990:185–196.

65. Glaser HH, Heagarty MC, Bullard DM Jr, Pivchik EC. Physical and psychological development of children with early failure to thrive. J Pediatr 1968; 73:690–698.

66. Oates RK, Peacock A, Forrest D. Long-term effects of nonorganic failure to thrive. Pediatrics 1985; 75:36–40.

67. Singer L. Long-term hospitalization of failure to thrive infants: developmental outcome at three years. Child Abuse Negl 1986; 10:479–486.

68. Drotar D, Sturm L. Personality development, problem solving, and behavior problems among preschool children with early histories of nonorganic failure to thrive: a controlled study. J Dev Behav Pediatr 1992; 13:266–273.

10

The Skeletal Dysplasias

Mordechai Shohat
Beilinson Medical Center, Petah Tikva, Israel

David L. Rimoin
Cedars-Sinai Medical Center and UCLA School of Medicine, Los Angeles, California

I. INTRODUCTION

The human skeletal dysplasias are a heterogeneous group of disorders that result in disproportionate short stature. Although individually rare, these developmental defects of the skeleton cause a significant proportion of the cases of moderate to severe short stature.

Before 1970, the diagnosis for most patients with disproportionate shortening of the limbs was "achondroplasia," and those with short trunks were thought to have "Morquio syndrome." The understanding and appreciation of the heterogeneity within the skeletal dysplasias led to a systematic description of over 100 different forms, which have been primarily classified on the basis of clinical and radiographic changes. With the recent explosion of knowledge in the biochemistry and molecular biology of connective tissue, rapid progress should occur in the delineation of the basic defect in these disorders. It is important to make a specific diagnosis in each case so that an accurate prognosis can be given and proper genetic counseling provided. Furthermore, each of these disorders is associated with a variety of skeletal or nonskeletal complications, which an accurate diagnosis allows one to anticipate, treat promptly, or prevent.

II. DIFFERENTIATION OF THE SKELETAL DYSPLASIAS

The current nomenclature for these disorders is confusing. The specific name for a given condition usually describes the skeletal segment involved (e.g., the epiphyseal dysplasias and the metaphyseal dysplasias), or use a Greek term [e.g., thanatophoric (death bringing) dysplasia, metatropic (changing dysplasia), and diastrophic (twisted) dysplasia]. Some

disorders are eponyms (e.g., Kniest dysplasia and Ellis Van Creveld syndrome). Occasionally, the name attempts to describe the pathogenesis (osteogenesis imperfecta), but usually inacurately (e.g., achondroplasia and achondrogenesis).

The extent of the heterogeneity in these disorders and the variety of methods used for their classification have resulted in further confusion. Clinical classifications have divided the skeletal dysplasias into those with short-limbed dwarfism and those with short-trunk dwarfism. Age of onset of the disease and associated clinical abnormalities have also been used in subdividing these disorders. Still other disorders have been classified on the basis of their apparent mode of inheritance, for example the dominant and X-linked varieties of spondyloepiphyseal dysplasia.

The most widely used method for differentiating the skeletal dysplasias has been the detection of skeletal radiographic abnormalities. Radiographic classifications are based on the different parts of the long bones that are abnormal (epiphyses, metaphyses, or diaphyses; Figs. 1 and 2). Thus, there are epiphyseal and metaphyseal dysplasias that can be further divided depending on whether the spine is also involved (spondyloepiphyseal dysplasias and spondylometaphyseal dysplasias). Furthermore, each of these classes can be divided into several distinct disorders based on a variety of other clinical and radiographic differences.

As the morphology, pathogenesis, and especially the basic biochemical and molecular defect in each of these disorders are unraveled, this nomenclature is being changed to refer to the specific pathogenetic or metabolic defect. The etiologic or pathogenetic nomenclature is now being used for certain skeletal dysplasias, such as the mucopolysaccharidoses, mucolipidoses, and disorders of mineralization (e.g., β-glucuronidase deficiency, fucosidosis, and hypophosphatasia).

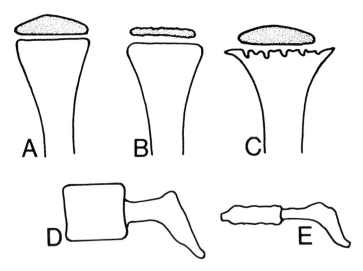

Figure 1 Classification of chondrodysplasias based on radiologic involvement of long bones (A–C) and vertebrae (D and E).

Involvement	Disease category
A + D	Normal
B + D	Epiphyseal dysplasia
C + D	Metaphyseal dysplasia
B + E	Spondyloepiphyseal dysplasia
B + C + E	Spondyloepimetaphyseal dysplasia

A. International Classification and Nomenclature

In an attempt to develop a uniform nomenclature for these syndromes, an international nomenclature and classification for the skeletal dysplasias were proposed in 1969 and updated in 1977, 1983, and 1991. The term "dwarfism" has been replaced by "dysplasia." The international classification divides the skeletal dysplasias into five major groups:

1. Osteochondrodysplasias: abnormalities of cartilage or bone growth and development
2. Dysostoses: malformation of individual bones, singly or in combination (does not reflect a generalized disorder of the skeleton)
3. Idiopathic osteolyses: a group of disorders associated with multifocal resorption of bone
4. Skeletal disorders associated with chromosomal aberrations
5. Skeletal disorders associated with primary metabolic disorders

In the differential diagnosis of short stature, osteochondrodysplasias are of major importance. These are a complex group of diseases that are caused by primary abnormalities of cartilage or of bone growth or development. This group is divided into the following:

1. Defects of growth of tubular bones or spine, or both (further referred to as chondrodysplasias)
2. Abnormalities in the amount, density, and remodeling of bone (includes disorders with a decrease or increase in bone and disorders of mineralization and mineral metabolism)
3. Disorders involving disorganized development of cartilage and fibrous connective tissue

The Fourth International Nomenclature committee, which met in Germany in 1991, not only updated the nomenclature with the addition of a number of newly described syndromes but also completely revised the organization of these disorders into a clinically and pathogenetically based classification (Table 1). Thus, disorders that share clinical, radiographic, or morphologic features, suggesting that they fall into a family of disorders that share common pathogenetic mechanisms, were grouped together. This classification will certainly undergo constant revision as the basic defect in each of these disorders is discovered.

III. DIAGNOSIS AND ASSESSMENT

The diagnosis of skeletal dysplasias is based on the clinical, radiographic, pathologic, and, in some instances, biochemical and molecular studies. Table 1 summarizes the clinical, genetic, and radiographic features of the common chondrodysplasias. Abnormalities in the amount, density, and remodeling of bone are described in Table 2.

A. History

An accurate medical and family history may be of major importance in arriving at a diagnosis. A complete family history, details of stillborn children, and parental consanguin-

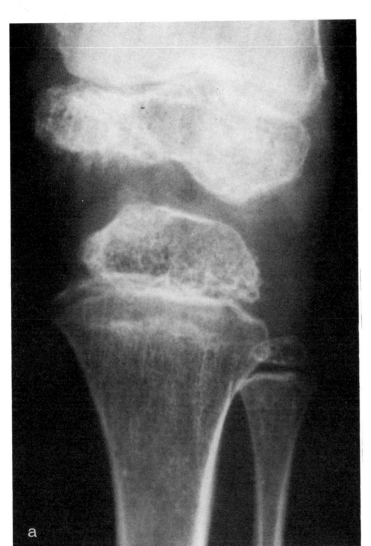

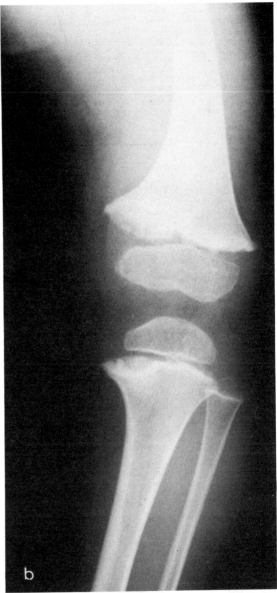

Figure 2 Radiographs of knee (a–c) and spine (d) from patients with a variety of chondrodysplasias. (a) Epiphyseal dysplasia: note the small irregular epiphyses and normal metaphyses from a patient with spondyloepiphyseal dysplasia congenita; (b) metaphyseal dysplasia: note the irregular and widened metaphyses with normal epiphyses from a patient with metaphyseal dysplasia, type Schmid; (c) epimetaphyseal dysplasia: note the abnormal epiphyses and metaphyses from a patient with spondyloepimetaphyseal dysplasia, type Strudwick; (d) platyspondyly: note the flat and irregular vertebrae from a patient with spondylometaphyseal dysplasia, type Kozlowski.

ity should be obtained. Parents should always be closely examined, looking for evidence of a dysplasia in a partially expressed form. Because each of the skeletal dysplasias most frequently appears as a sporadic case in the family, an isolated instance of a skeletal dysplasia in a family cannot provide information on the mode of inheritance of the particular disorder. However, the type of familial aggregation, when it occurs, can be helpful. For example, if two dwarfed siblings are born to normal parents, then achondroplasia, which is an

autosomal dominant trait, is unlikely, and one should suspect an autosomal recessive disorder. If two achondroplastic parents produce a severely affected offspring, it is most likely homozygous achondroplasia rather than thanatophoric dysplasia. However, different modes of inheritance have been observed in disorders that resemble each other clinically, such as the X-linked and certain autosomal forms of spondyloepiphyseal dysplasia. On the other hand, in some dominant disorders, a high incidence of gonodal mosaicism has been

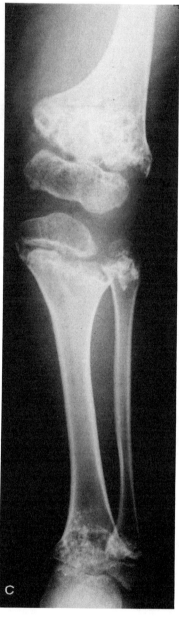

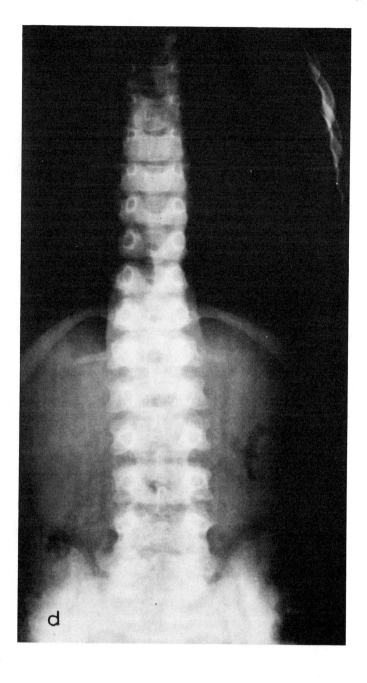

Figure 2   *(Continued)*

shown to account for recurrent cases in the same family. For example, in osteogenesis imperfecta type II, gonadal mosaicism may result in a recurrence risk of 6%.

Because the skeletal dysplasias become apparent at various ages, it is helpful to obtain accurate measurements from infancy onward and, especially, to know whether the shortening was evident at birth. Although in certain disorders marked variability in expression is seen with both prenatal and postnatal onset of the disease in the same family (e.g., osteogenesis imperfecta type I), this information may help limit the diagnosis to a small number of disorders. Thus, a child who was

normal until 2 years of age and then developed disproportionate short-limbed dwarfism is more likely to have pseudoachondroplasia or multiple epiphyseal dysplasia than achondroplasia or spondyloepiphyseal dysplasia congenita. In some disorders, growth may be normal for several years. For instance, in the X-linked form of spondyloepiphyseal dysplasia tarda, growth retardation is not apparent until between 5 and 10 years of age. Relative body proportions may change with age in some disorders, such as metatropic dysplasia, in which only the limbs are short at birth; because of progressive kyphoscoliosis, such patients become short-trunked dwarfs during childhood.

Table 1 Clinical, Genetic, and Radiographic Features in the Common Chondrodysplasias

Dysplasias	Clinical Features[a]	Radiologic Features
Achondroplasia group (the disorders in this group have similar radiographic changes but range from severe neonatally lethal thanatophoric dysplasia through achondroplasia to mild hypochondroplasia.		
Achondroplasia	AD; 80% represent new mutation; the most common skeletal dysplasia (1 : 25,000 births); rhizomelic shortening of limbs (recognizable at birth); final height averages 135 cm in men and 125 cm in women, with wide variability; hands are short and broad, wedge-shaped gap between third and fourth fingers (trident); lumbar gibbus in infancy usually replaced by prominant lumbar lordosis; limbs with skin folds in children; the mean head circumference follows a curve above the 97th percentile for normal individuals; specific curves are valuable to recognize hydrocephalus; prominant frontal bossing, hypoplasia of maxilla, mandibular prognathism; hypotonia is frequent during infancy; mental development is normal; except for patients with severe complications or sudden infant death, life span is normal; recurrent otitis media and chronic serous otitis are common and lead to conductive hearing loss in adults; overgrowth of fibula and joint laxity cause progressive genu varum; nerve root compression and signal claudication are common complications in adults; (FGFR3 mutation)	Large calvariua, short base of skull, small foramen magnum (computed tomographic scan norms are available); ribs are short, cupped anteriorly; decreased lumbosacral interpedicular distance, squared off ilia, small sacrosciatic notches; limbs are short and broad; oval radiolucency in proximal femur and humerus in infancy: overgrowth of fibula
Hypochondroplasia	AD; recognized from 2 to 3 years of age; short-limbed (rhizomelic) short stature; there is wide variability in severity and much overlap in appearance with achondroplasia; this type of skeletal dysplasia is probably very common and easily undiagnosed in mildly short individuals; head is normal; patients are stocky and muscular; hands and feet are short and broad; mild genu varum and mild lumbar lordosis; mild mental retardation has been reported in some cases	"Mild achondroplastic changes": skull normal or mildly enlarged; ribs are normal or slightly flaired; distal lumbosacral interpedicular narrowing; long bones; rhizomelia; short wide bones; elongated fibula; prominent deltoid tubercles
Thanatophoric dysplasia	AD; the most common lethal type; markedly short limbs; large bulging forehead ± cloverleaf skull; prominent eyes; small, narrowed, pear-shaped thorax; ±congenital heart and CNS defects (FGFR3 mutation)	The long bones are short and bowed; metaphyseal flaring with medial spikes; severe platyspondyly; the vertebrae are hypoplastic, U shaped on AP view; cupped and short ribs; large calvaria

Table 1 (*Continued*)

Dysplasias	Clinical Features[a]	Radiologic Features
Achondrogenesis group (a distinct lethal type of skeletal dysplasia)		
Achondrogenesis type IA and type IB	AR; lethal; very short limbs; short and barrel-shaped chest; extremely soft skull; round or oval face; types are classified according to radiologic and morphologic appearance	Characterized by poor ossification of the spine, more extreme shortening of femora and other long bones; long bones have concave ends and spurs in the middle shaft; type IA (Houston-Harris) is differentiated from type IB (Fraccaro) by the lack of rib fractures, appearance of the long bone, and cartilage histology
Metatropic dysplasia group		
Metatropic dysplasia	AD and AR; normal to long in length at birth, short limbed in infancy, becoming short trunked later with progressive kyphoscoliosis; prominent joints; tail-like sacral appendage, large head with ventriculomegaly may be present; C1–2 subluxation is frequent and requires surgical fusion; severe cases die in infancy of RDS	Extreme platyspondyly with flattening of vertebrae and relatively large intervertebral spaces; long bones: irregularly expanded metaphyses giving barbell-like appearance; flattened and irregular epiphyses; short and broad tubular bones in hands; marked flaring of iliac crests (halberd appearance)
Short rib dysplasia group (conditions in this group form a spectrum of disorders and probably represent different mutations of the same gene)		
Short-rib polydactyly syndrome (I, II, III)	AR; lethal, hydropic appearance, narrow thorax, severe RDS, polydactyly; in type I (Saldino Noonan) high frequency of cloacal abnormalities and postaxial polydactyly; type III is probably the mild end of type I disease; type II (Majewski) has high frequency of cleft lip and palate, multiple internal anomalies, and pre- and postaxial polydactyly	Extremely short horizontal ribs; the pelvis is small and hypoplastic in type I, whereas in II the pelvis is normal; in type I the long bones are very short with metaphyseal spurs; in type II the long bones have a more rounded appearance, especially the middle segment
Asphyxiating thoracic dysplasia (ATD) (Jeune)	AR; long narrow thorax and RDS with variable severity; ±postaxial polydactyly; progressive nephropathy; cystic changes in kidney, liver, and pancreas	Ribs are short, cupped anteriorly; square short ilia; flat acetabulum with spurs at ends (trident appearance).
Chondroectodermal dysplasia (Ellis Van Creveld)	AR; narrowed thorax, short limbs, and polydactyly; often with congenital cardiac anomalies (ASD, single atrium, PDA) and ectodermal abnormalities; hypoplastic nails, natal teeth, multiple frenula, cleft lip and palate, epispadias	Ribs and pelvis are similar to ATD; acromesomelic shortening of limbs; hamate-capitate fusion.
Atelosteogenesis and diastrophic dysplasia group (characterized by hypoplastic humeri or femora, absence of ossification several bones, or ossification of what should remain cartilage)		
Otopalatodigital syndrome type II	X-linked; characterized by distinct facies, short and broad distal segments of thumbs and toes; proportional short stature and sometimes mental retardation; facies have prominent forehead, flat nasal root, flattening of the midface and small jaw; ±hearing defect (conductive); dislocation of radial heads and/or hips may be present	Small illia; hypoplastic distal radius results in dislocations; wide lumbar interpedicular distance; small mandible; radiographic changes may not become apparent until later in infancy.

Dysplasias	Clinical Features[a]	Radiologic Features
Diastrophic dysplasia	AR; acute swelling of pinnea of ears in infancy; cauliflower ears; laryngomalacia; short limbed (rhizomelic), severe clubfeet, joint contractures, proximally placed abducted thumb; progressive scoliosis; there is wide variability in expression even within the same family; gene was mapped to chromosome 5q31–q34 (sulfate transporter)	Hypoplasia of epiphyses and flaring metaphyses in long bones; extracarpal bones; short and wide metacarpals and phalanges; lumbar interpedicular narrowing; C2/C3 dislocation; peritracheal, ear pinnae, and precocious costal cartilage ossification
Kniest-Stickler dysplasia group		
Kniest dysplasia	AD; short trunk, progressive kyphoscoliosis: joint limitation; face is flat and round; myopia and cleft palate are common; Swiss cheese cartilage; Kniest syndrome must be differentiated from Weissenbacher-Zweymuller syndrome, an AR condition characterized by only mild short stature and by improvement in the clinical and roentgenographic findings with age, and from Rolland-Desbuquois syndrome, an AR condition having many features in common with Kniest dysplasia but showing more severe vertebral segmentation defects; type II collagen abnormalities were recently shown to cause dysplasia	Coronal clefts in flattened vertebrae, small ilia, increased acetabular angles; barbell-like femora as a result of broad metaphyses, delayed ossification of femoral heads, cloud effect in epiphyseal region; squared-off metacarpals and phalanges
Stickler syndrome	AD; marfanoid habitus, myopia, retinal detachment, conductive hearing loss, hyperextension of joints, may lead to joint pains and morning stiffness; cleft palate and mandibular hypoplasia; recently cosegregation with the type II collagen gene was demonstrated in some families, whereas in others segregation was discordant	Mild epiphyseal dysplasia (especially proximal femur and distal tibia), degenerative arthrosis (hips), wedging of thoracic vertebra, and Schmorl's disease of spine
Spondyloepiphyseal dysplasia congenita group (all the disorders in this group share defects in type II collagen secondary to mutations in the COL2A1 gene on chromosome 12q 13.1).		
Spondyloepiphyseal dysplasia (SED) Congenita (Spranger-Wiedeman)	AD; evident at birth; variable severity; rhizomelic shortening of limbs, but these appear long relative to trunk; hands and feet are normal in size; clubfeet; neck is extremely short; it is important to rule out C1/C2 subluxation, which may lead to dislocation; broad barrel chest, lordosis; severe myopia, joint laxity, cleft palate, genu valgum or varum, waddling gait; the basic defect is in type II collagen	Platyspondyly and epiphyseal dysplasia; delayed ossification of ephiphyseal centers and the epiphyses appear irregular, fragmented, and flattened (especially femoral); coxa vara; vertebrae are ovoid in childhood but later become flat, irregular, with narrowed disk space; odontoid hypoplasia with C1/C2 subluxation
achondrogenesis II (Langer-Saldino) hypochondrogenesis)	AD; lethal; very short limbs; short and barrel-shaped chest; extremely soft skull; round or oval face; lack of type II and type I collagen is found in achondrogenesis type II	In contrast to achondrogenesis type I, the long bones are straighter, relatively longer with cupping of their ends, with milder cases known as hypochondrogenesis
Other spondyloepiphyseal- (meta)physeal dysplasias group		
SED tarda	X-linked recessive, short stature develops in midchildhood; short limbs and short trunk; mild to severe kyphoscoliosis; large chest capacity; hands and feet are normal in size; early onset osteoarthritis in back and hips	Flat vertebrae with hump-shaped centra; hypoplastic iliac wings; epiphyseal hypoplasia of large bones; premature osteoarthrosis of hips

Table 1 (*Continued*)

Dysplasias	Clinical Features[a]	Radiologic Features
Spondyloepimetaphyseal dysplasias AD (SEMD, Strudwick type)	Resembles SED congenitia at birth; SEMD is distinguished from SED by radiologic evidence of metaphyseal changes; Strudwick type is characterized by specific radiologic changes such as peripheral "popcornlike" ossification of the femoral epiphyses, pectus carinatum, and genu valgum; type II collagen abnormalities have been documented	Delayed epiphyseal ossification, clubbed shaped femora (first year), metaphyseal changes (>3 years), multiple epiphyseal centers in femoral heads, greater involvement of fibula and ulna than tibia and radius; platyspondyly; pear-shaped vertebrae; C1/C2 subluxation
Dyggve-Melchior-Clausen dysplasia	AR; short trunk, short stature with barrel chest, lumbar lordosis, restricted joint mobility, and waddling gait; mental retardation in most cases	Changes similar to those in SED; anterior beaking of vertebral bodies; a fine lace-like ossification above the iliac crest and irregular small carpal and metacarpal bones
Pseudoachondroplastic dysplasia	AD; short limb, short stature usually not apparent until 2–3 years; in some patients the limb shortening is predominantly rhizomelic, in others mesomelic; hyperlaxity of joints is associated with severe varus or valgus or as a combined ("windswept") deformity; the facies are characteristically attractive; gene was recently mapped to the pericentromeric region of chromosome 19	Epiphyses and metaphyses of the tubular bones are involved, with platyspondyly and anterior tonguing of the vertebral bodies; acetabular irregularity, hypoplastic ischium and pubis; striking hand involvement with shortening of tubular bones, irregular metaphyses, and small round epiphyses
Spondylometaphyseal dysplasia group (association of vertebral changes along with metaphyseal abnormalities in the long bones		
Spondylometaphyseal dysplasia (SMD) Kozlowski type	AD; growth retardation is usually apparent after 1–2 years; short trunk short stature and waddling gait develop; pectus carinatum, kyphoscoliosis, and precocious osteoarthritis; numerous other less well defined types of SMD have been described	Platyspondyly and general metaphyseal irregularities in the tubular bones; "open staircase" appearance to vertebrae on AP films; marked retardation of carpal ossification
Epiphyseal dysplasia group		
Multiple epiphyseal dysplasias (Fairbanks and Ribbing types)	AD; mild short stature; pain and stiffness in knees, hips, and ankles; waddling gait is common in severe Fairbanks type; osteoarthropathy of hips in mild Ribbing type	Characterized by flattened, fragmented, or irregular epiphyses (all areas, including hands and feet in Fairbanks; primarily the hips in Ribbing); earliest features may be delay in epiphyseal ossification; no metaphyseal or vertebral changes are seen; Schmorl's nodes are common
Chondrodysplasia punctata group (stippled epiphyses)		
Chondrodysplasia punctata (punctate epiphyseal dysplasia)	Several dysplasias (AR, rhyzomelic type; XLD Conradi-Hunerman, and XLR forms); laryngomalacia and upper airway obstruction; limbs are proximally shortened in the rhizomelic type and asymmetrically shortened in the XLD types; cataract, ichthyosis, and contractures are common; rhizomelic type is caused by a peroxisomal defect. The gene for Conardi-Hunerman was mapped to Xq-28, and the XLR type to Xpter-p22.32	Stippled calcification of epiphyses, periarticular tissues, and growth plate zones; stippling of laryngeal cartilage; coronal clefts of vertebrae

Dysplasias	Clinical Features[a]	Radiologic Features
Metaphyseal dysplasia group		
Metaphyseal dysplasias		All types are characterized by metaphyseal in-
Jansen	AD; severe short stature; recognizable in early infancy; rhizometic shortening, severe leg bowing, mandibular hypoplasia; joints are large with contractures; arms less affected than legs	volvement; all metaphyses including hands and feet are severely affected but improve with age
Schmid	AD; mild to moderate short stature (130–160 cm) and bowing of legs; enlarged wrists and flaring of rib cage; coxa vara	Most prominent changes are in hips, shoulders, knee, ankles, and wrists
McKusick type (cartilage-hair hypoplasia)	AR; severe to moderate postnatal growth deficiency, short broad hands and loose joints; genu varum; fine, light, sparse hair and light complexion; increased susceptibility to severe varicella infection	Knees especially are involved, in contrast to Schmid; proximal femoral metaphyses are very mildly involved; fibula is long relative to tibia; ribs are short with anterior cupping
Others	[Combination of metaphyseal abnormalities and immune deficiency can also be found in Schwachman syndrome (AR), associated with pancreatic insufficiency and chronic neutropenia; metaphyseal chondrodysplasia— thymic alymphopenia syndrome (AR); and adenosine deaminase deficiency (AR)]	
Mesomelic dysplasia group	Heterogeneous group characterized predominantly by shortening of the middle segments of the limbs	In all types, the bones of the forearm and legs are disproportionately shortened
Dyschondrosteosis	AD, the common type; mesomelic short stature (mild to moderate); Madelung deformity of the wrist	Hypoplasia of the distal ulna; ±radial head dislocation (Madelung deformity)
Langer type	AR, rare, respresents the homozygote (double-dose) form of dyschondrosteosis; severe short stature, mandibular hypoplasia	Limb bones are short and thick; hypoplastic fibula and distal ulna
Robinow	AD; flat facial profile, mesomelic shortening, and genital hypoplasia; hypoplastic mandible and hypertelorism, flat nose, and hypoplastic nails	Madelung deformity; posterior osseous fusion of vertebra; hemivertebrae
Nievergelt type	AD; brachydactyly and clubfeet	Rhomboid-shaped radius, ulna, tibia, fibula; radioulna and tarsal synostosis
Rheinhardt	AD; radial bowing of hands and lateral bowing of legs	Short radius and ulna; hypoplasia of distal ulna and proximal fibula
Acromelic and acromesomelic dysplasia group (shortening of the limbs, primarily affecting the hands and feet)		
Acromesomelic dysplasia	AR; several distinct skeletal dysplasias characterized by disproportionate shortening, predominantly affecting forearms, hands, feet, and legs; recognizable at birth; trunk slightly shortened	Mild epiphyseal ossification delay; brachydactyly with cone epiphyses; hypoplasia of iliac base and irregular acetabulum; wedging of vertebrae in adults
Trichorhinophalangeal (TRP) dysplasia	AD; mild disproportionate short stature, sparse hair, pear-shaped nose, medial accentuation of the eyebrows; short stubby hands; multiple joint contractures; severe genu valgum or varum; recently small chromosomal deletion in 8q24.12 was shown to be the cause for all types; the previously entitled TRP type I contains smaller deletion than in the previous type 2	Numerous phalangeal cone-shaped epiphyses of the hands; Legg-Perthes–like changes occasionally occur in the hips

Table 1 (*Continued*)

Dysplasias	Clinical Features[a]	Radiologic Features
Pseudohypoparathyroidism (several types): AD (A.R?, XLD?), mild short stature, marked short IV metacarpal in hand (±feet); ±hypocalcemia, ±parathyroid hormone unresponsiveness; short IV metacarpals		
Dysplasia with significant membranous bone involvement		
Cleidocranial dysplasia	AD; variable expressivity; large prominent forehead, wide persistent open fontanelles, drooping shoulders, narrow chest, abnormal dentition, coxa vara and joint laxity, short and squared fingers; proportionate short stature may occur	Varying degree of hypoplasia of membranous bones; absent or hypoplastic clavicles, narrowed and high pelvis; delayed closure of the anterior fontanelle with wormian bones are characteristic
Bent-bone dysplasia group		
Campomelic dysplasia	AR; bending of long bones; cutaneous dimples at the site of bend; large head, flat face; sex reversal (females 47 XY) in phenotypic females is common; some with severe RDS because of small thorax, hypoplastic tracheal rings, and other anomalies; various short-limb types have been described (kyphomelic dysplasia) (Sox 9 mutations on 17q)	Slender bent femur and tibia; enlarged dolichocephalic skull with shallow orbits; pelvis is tall and narrow; hypoplastic ischiopubic rami
Multiple dislocations with dysplasia group		
Larsen syndrome	AD (AR?); marked hyperlaxity and multiple dislocations (especially hips, knees, elbows) are characteristic; prominent forehead, low nasal bridge, hypertelorism, and cleft uvula are common features; disproportionate short stature; the associated skeletal abnormalities and craniofacial features help to distinguish Larsen syndrome from Ehlers-Danlos syndrome (especially type III, VII), and otopalatodigital syndrome	Multiple joint dislocations with secondary epiphyseal deformities; supernumerary carpal and tarsal ossification centers develop; premature fusion of the epiphyses and shaft of the first distal phalanges

[a]AR, autosomal recessive; AD, autosomal dominant; RDS, respiratory distress syndrome; XLR, X-linked recessive; XLD, X-linked dominant; XLR, X-linked recessive; ASD, atrial septal defect; PDA, patent ductus arteriosus; CNS, central nervous system; AP, anterioposterior.

B. Physical Examination

A detailed physical examination may disclose the correct diagnosis or point to the likely diagnostic category. It is essential to determine whether the shortening is proportional. In general, patients with disproportionate short stature have skeletal dysplasias, whereas those with relatively normal body proportions have endocrine, nutritional, prenatal, or other nonskeletal defects. There are exceptions to these rules: cretinism can lead to disproportionate short stature, and a variety of skeletal dysplasias, such as osteogenesis imperfecta and hypophosphatasia, may result in normal body proportions.

A disproportionate body habitus may not be readily apparent on casual physical examination. Measurements that are essential for determining whether an abnormally short individual is disproportionate include the following:

1. Upper/lower segment ratio (U/L ratio): Although sitting height is a more accurate measure of the head and trunk length, it requires special equipment for consistent accuracy. U/L segment ratio, on the other hand, provides a fairly accurate measure of body proportions and can be easily obtained. The lower segment measure is taken from the symphysis pubis to the floor at the inside of the heel, and the upper segment is obtained by subtracting the lower segment value from the total height. McKusick has published standard U/L curves for both white and black

Table 2 Conditions Associated with Abnormal Amount, Density, and/or Remodeling of Bone

Disorder	Clinical features	Radiologic features	Inheritance[a]
Decreased bone density group			
Osteogenesis imperfecta (share defect in collagen type I as a result of mutations in either COL2A1 gene or COL1A2 gene)			
Type 1	Excessive bone fragility, blue sclerae, conductive hearing loss in adolescence, hyperlaxity of ligaments, nonprogressive aortic root dilatation (12%), most have late-onset short stature, some families with opalescent teeth	General osteopenia (especially vertebral bodies), angulation at site of previous fractures, wormian bones in skull	
Type 2	Lethal, low birth weight and short birth length, soft skull, beaking of the nose, hypotelorism, short and deformed limbs, thin and fragile skin; prenatal diagnosis by ultrasound and molecular genetic studies	Extreme beading of ribs, crumpled appearance of long (femora), diffuse osteopenia of skull	Most are AD; gonadal mosaicism
Type 3	Nonlethal severe bone fragility leading to progressive deformity and marked short stature, sclerae may be blue at birth but become less blue with age, most with opalescent dentin, cardiorespiratory complications may lead to death	General osteopenia and marked deformity of bones; fractures may be present at birth, bowed long bones, progressive platyspondyly (codfish vertebra) and kyphoscoliosis, wormian bones in skull	AR and AD
Type 4	As type 1 but with white sclerae (may be blue at birth), less hearing abnormality, some families with opalescent teeth	Osteopenia, variability in severity and age of onset of fractures, multiple wormian bones of skull	AD
Disorders of mineralization			
Hyperphosphatesemia with osteoectasia	Onset 2–3 years, progressive painful skeletal deformity, fractures, short stature, large skull; elevation of alkaline phosphatase	Dense areas interspersed wih lucent areas, generalized demineralization (juvenile Paget's disease)	AR
Hypophosphatasia			
Congenital lethal	Disproportionate short stature at birth, bowing deformity, thin skull vault, death from respiratory distress; low serum alkaline phosphatase	Generalized poor ossification, thin ribs, hypoplastic vertebrae, splayed and frayed metaphyses	AR
Tarda	Milder, onset in childhood, bowing of legs, premature loss of teeth; reduced serum alkaline phosphatase, elevated phosphoethanolamine in the urine	As in congenital type but milder changes	AD
Hypophosphatemic rickets	X-linked hypophosphatemic rickets; bowing of legs and short stature, late dentition; low serum phosphate	Radiographic changes are those of rickets	X-linked dominant

Table 2 (*Continued*)

Disorder	Clinical features	Radiologic features	Inheritance[a]
Pseudo vitamin D deficiency rickets (VDD)			
Type 1	Defective 1α-hydroxylation of 25-hydroxyvitamin D	As in rickets	AR
Type 2	Impaired target organ responsiveness to vitamin D	As in rickets	AR?
Increased bone volume or density			
Osteopetrosis			
Precocious form	Onset in early infancy, failure to thrive, malignant hypocalcemia, anemia, thrombocytopenia, hepatosplenomegaly, optic atrophy leading to blindness, impaired bone resorption as a result of defect in maturation of osteoclasts; early bone marrow transplantation may be successful	Generalized hyperostosis at birth, "bone in bone" appearance (vertebrae), crowded marrow cavity, dense base of skull	AR
Tarda	Onset in chilhood; may go undetected until adulthood; excessive fractures, mild craniofacial disproportion, mild anemia, osteonecrosis of bones (especially mandible) may develop; a distinct form with renal tubular acidoses and mental retardation has been found to be caused by a deficiency of carbonic anhydrase type 2; chromosome location: 8q22	Generalized increased density, defective metaphyseal modeling, dense base of skull	AD or AR
Pycnodysostosis	Short-limb, short stature from infancy; wide anterior fontanelle, large cranium with open fontanelle, small chin, short hands and feet, increased fractures, sclerae may be blue	General hyperostosis, hypoplasia of distal phalanges in hands, wide sutures, and wormian bones	AR
Dysosteosclerosis	Postnatal onset of short stature, severe hypodontia and early loss of teeth, fractures, visual and hearing loss	General hyperostosis, platyspondyly	AR
Osteopoikilosis	Commonly asymptomatic, joint pains	Numerous small osteodense foci in epiphyses and carpal centers or tubular bones	AD
Craniotubular dysplasias Craniometaphyseal dysplasia	Broad osseous prominence of nasal root, bony encroachment on cranial foramina and nasal passages	Hyperostosis of skull, mandible, nasal and maxillary bones; lack of modeling of metaphyses of long bones (Ehrlenmeyer flask appearance)	AD and AR
Diaphyseal dysplasia (Camurati Engelmann)	Failure to thrive and fatigability, onset at age 4–10 years, progressive increased pain in the legs, encroachment on cranial nerves; syndactyly, enamel hypoplasia	Symmetric fusiform enlargement of the diaphyses, normal metaphyses and epiphyses, sclerosis of anterior base of skull	AD

Disorder	Clinical features	Radiologic features	Inheritance[a]
Craniodiaphyseal dysplasia	Flattening of nasal root in early infancy, with increasing hypertelorism, marked encroachment of cranial nerves in foramina, normal stature	Massive hyperostosis and sclerosis of the skull and face with widened shafts of tubular bones	AR
Endosteal hyperostosis and sclerosteosis	Progressive mandibular enlargement from childhood; in adults sclerotic encroachment of optic and acoustic nerves	Marked accretion of osseous tissue at the endosteal surface, fusion between carpal bones	AR and AD
Tubular stenosis (medullary stenosis)	Hypocalcemia, delayed closure of fontanelle, and early-onset myopia	Narrowing of medullary cavity caused by widening diaphyseal cortex	AD
Pachydermoperiostosis	Progressive thickening of the skin, clubbing of fingers, easy fatigability, joint pain, blepharitis, sensory hearing loss	Subperiosteal thickening of tubular bones	AD
Frontometaphyseal dysplasia	Pronounced supraorbital ridge	Prominent frontum, ±large frontal sinuses; no hyperostosis of rest of skull; mild metaphyseal changes in long bones	X-linked dominant
Osteodysplasty (Melnick-Needles)	Abnormal gait and bowing of extremities, dislocation of hip, delayed closure of fontanelle, usually normal stature, exophthalmos, protruding cheeks, micrognathia, incurving of the distal segment of the thumbs	Uneven thickening of cortex bones, metaphyseal modeling defect, wavy ribs, narrowed iliac wings	AD (AR rare)

[a]AR, autosomal recessive; AD, autosomal dominant.

Americans that are quite useful for rapid assessment of proportion (1). For example, a white infant has an upper/lower segment ratio of approximately 1.7; it reaches 1.0 at approximately 7–10 years and then falls to an average U/L of 0.95 as an adult. Blacks, on the other hand, have relatively long limbs and reach a U/L of approximately 0.85 as adults.

2. Arm span: Another index of limb versus trunk length, this measurement usually falls within a few centimeters of total height.

These measurements must be obtained before the possibility of a mild skeletal dysplasia, such as hypochondroplasia or multiple epiphyseal dysplasia, can be excluded. Short-limbed dwarfs have an abnormally high U/L ratio and an arm span that is considerably shorter than the height.

If a child has short-limbed dwarfism, it is important to determine whether all segments of the limb are equally shortened or whether the shortening primarily affects the proximal (rhizomelic), middle (mesomelic), or distal (acromelic) segment (Fig. 3).

The presence or absence of extraskeletal manifestations may be helpful in making a diagnosis. During the examination, attention should be given to the head size, facial appearance, and specific physical findings, such as myopia, cleft palate, clubfoot, hearing, joint laxity, and bone deformity. In the older child or adult, the complications associated with specific disorders may provide additional information for making the diag-

nosis. For example, spinal stenosis with spinal cord claudication is characteristic of achondroplasia; odontoid hypoplasia and C1/C2 subluxation are frequently found in Morquio sydrome, spondyloepiphyseal dysplasia, and metatropic dysplasia; and fibular overgrowth (and genu varum) is seen in achondroplasia and cartilage hair hypoplasia.

C. Skeletal Radiographs

A full series of skeletal views is usually required. These views include anteroposterior (AP), lateral, and Towne views of the skull, AP and lateral views of the spine, and AP views of the pelvis and extremities, with separate views of hands and feet. Lateral views of the foot are particularly helpful in identifying punctate calcifications of the calcaneus, which may be a clue to the diagnosis of the milder forms of chondrodysplasia punctata, confirming the delayed ossification of the calcaneus and talus in newborns with spondyloepiphyseal dysplasia congenita, and in delineating the double ossification centers of the calcaneus in the Larsen syndrome.

Attention should be paid to the specific parts of the skeleton that are involved (spine, limbs, pelvis, and skull) and, within each, where the abnormality is located (epiphysis, metaphysis, diaphysis, or combination). Because the skeletal radiographic features in many of these disorders change with age, reviewing radiographs taken at different ages is helpful. Moreover, epiphyseal closure, which occurs after puberty,

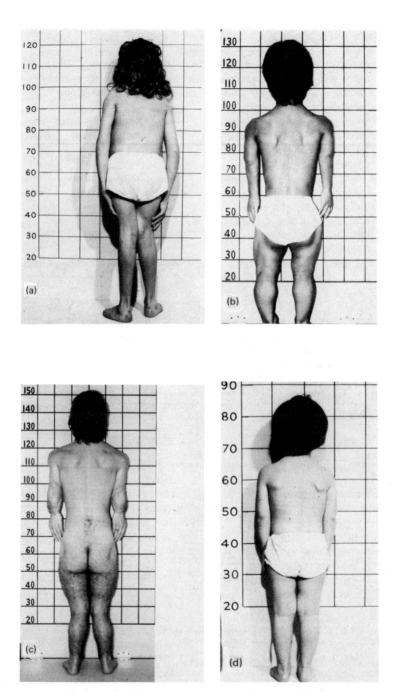

Figure 3 Different forms of disproportionate dwarfism. (a) Short-trunk dwarfism in a girl with Dyggve-Melchior-Clausen syndrome; (b) short-limb dwarfism of the rhizomelic type in a boy with achondroplasia; (c) short-limb dwarfism of the mesomelic type in a boy with mesomelic dysplasia, Langer type; (d) short-limb dwarfism of the acromelic type in a girl with peripheral dysostosis.

frequently obliterates the specific abnormalities that would have permitted a specific diagnosis to be made had the films been taken before puberty. Nevertheless, skeletal radiographs alone are often sufficient to make the diagnosis because the classification of these disorders has been based primarily on their radiographic features. In many instances, however, only

the general type of dysplasia, such as a spondyloepiphyseal dysplasia, can be recognized, but the specific entity cannot be identified on radiographic grounds alone.

Apart from the changes in the epiphyses, diaphyses, and metaphyses, some radiographic features characterize certain disorders:

"Dumbell-shaped" femur in the newborn period: metatropic dysplasia and Kniest dysplasia.

Bending of long bones (campomelia): common in campomelic dysplasia, kyphomelic dysplasias, osteogenesis imperfecta, congenital hypophosphatasia, and thanatophoric dysplasia.

Calcified projections or spikes on lateral borders of the metaphyses of the femur: thanatophoric dysplasia, achondrogenesis, and short-rib polydactyly syndrome type I/III.

Fractures of long bones in the newborn: osteogenesis imperfecta, congenital osteopetrosis, and severe hypophosphatasia. In the older individual, fractures may also be seen in a variety of osteopetrotic syndromes, including dysosteosclerosis and pyknodysostosis.

Marked delay in epiphyseal center ossification: spondyloepiphyseal dysplasia (SED) congenita, Kniest dysplasia, and other SED and multiple epiphyseal dysplasias.

Stippled epiphyses: the chondrodysplasia punctatas, cerebrohepatorenal syndrome, warfarin-related embryopathy, and, occasionally, with chromosomal trisomy, lysosomal storage diseases, diphenylhydantoin-induced embryopathy, the Smith-Lemli-Opitz syndrome, and congenital infections.

Severely shortened ribs: short-rib polydactyly syndromes, asphyxiating thoracic dysplasia, chondroectodermal dysplasia, thanatophoric dysplasias, and metatropic dysplasia.

Decreased ossification of the vertebral bodies: most severe in the achondrogenesis syndromes.

Severe platyspondyly: metatropic dysplasia, thanatophoric dysplasia (U shaped in thoracic spine and inverted U shape in the lumbar spine), osteogenesis imperfecta type II, congenital hypophosphatasia, Morquio syndrome, spondylometaphyseal dysplasia, brachyolmia, and others.

Coronal clefts of the vertebra: Kniest dysplasia, Rolland-Desbuquois syndrome, Weisenbach-Zweymuller syndrome, short-rib polydactyly syndrome type 1, chondrodysplasia punctata, and atelosteogenesis.

Oval translucent appearance of the proximal femora and humeri in infants: achondroplasia.

These examples are representative of only a few of the many typical radiographic features seen in the skeletal dysplasias (see Table 1). Furthermore, many other radiographic differences within what is now considered a given skeletal dysplasia may be found as the complete heterogeneity of this group of disorders is delineated by the morphologic and biochemical studies.

D. Microscopic Evaluation

Histologic examination of the chondroosseous tissue can be useful in making an accurate diagnosis of several specific skeletal disorders, especially the lethal neonatal types. In certain other conditions the pathologic examination is useful in ruling out a diagnosis. (A protocol for the collection of skeletal tissues can be found in Sec. V.)

On morphologic grounds, the chondrodysplasias can be broadly divided into the following disorders:

1. Minimal or no qualitative abnormality in endochondral ossification: Achondroplasia and hypochondroplasia (in which abnormalities in the height and arrangement of proliferative columns, particularly in the center of the large growth plates, are the only changes).

2. Abnormalities mainly in cellular morphology: Large chondrocytes, containing prominent inclusions; for example, achondrogenesis IA, pseudoachondroplasia, and certain SEDs; sparse matrix with collagen rings around the chondrocytes as in achondrogenesis IB, suggesting a metabolic defect leading to reduced synthesis of a matrix component. Dilatation of the chondrocyte rough endoplasmic reticulum (RER): the SEDs, pseudoachondroplasia, spondylometaphyseal dysplasia, autosomal recessive type of multiple epiphyseal dysplasia, and Kniest dysplasia (in the latter there are also special matrix abnormalities). Thus dilatation of the RER is not a diagnostic finding, although it suggests defective synthesis or abnormal processing of the matrix proteins in these conditions.

3. Abnormalities in matrix morphology: Areas of cell degeneration with wide collagen fibrils, scar formation, and intracartilaginous ossification: diastrophic dysplasia. "Swiss-cheese" appearance of cartilage: Kniest dysplasia. Large lacunae containing numerous chondrocytes: Dyggve-Melchior-Clausen syndrome. Areas of dystrophic ossification, fibrous dysplasia, and fat deposition in the reserve zone cartilage of the matrix: chondrodysplasia punctata. Wide interwoven connective septa in epiphyseal cartilage and basal zone: fibrochondrogenesis.

4. Abnormalities primarily localized to the area of chondroosseous transformation: Reduced and disorganized columnization: thanatophoric dysplasia, short-rib polydactyly syndromes. Broad matrix septa surrounding clusters of hypertrophic cells: the metaphyseal dysplasias.

E. Biochemical Studies

Great progress has been made in recent years in our knowledge about the biochemical defect involved in certain of the skeletal dysplasias. These findings may help us understand the basic biology of the normal bone and provide us with new means for prenatal diagnosis.

Biochemical studies are still of diagnostic value in only a few of the skeletal dysplasias. Until recently, the basic defect had been uncovered only in the mucopolysaccharidoses, mucolipidoses, and certain of the mineralization defects, such as hypophosphatasia, hypophosphatemic rickets, and vitamin D dependency rickets.

Various structural abnormalities in collagen have been demonstrated in different skeletal dysplasias: mutations (or deletion) along the α_1- and α_2-procollagen genes have been demonstrated in all four types of osteogenesis imperfecta, whereas mutations along the type II collagen gene may result in achondrogenesis II—hypochondrogenesis, the SEDs, Kniest dysplasia, SEMD-Strudwick-type cases, and at least some Stickler syndrome cases. Defects in type X collagen have been described in the Schmid type of metaphyseal dysplasia. Pseudo-achondroplasia has been mapped to the pericentromeric region of chromosome 19, diastrophic dysplasia to 5q31–34 (sulfate transportor defect), cartilage hair hypoplasia (metaphyseal chondrodysplasia, type McKusick) to chromosome 9, trichorhinophalangeal dysplasia to 8q24, and campomelic dysplasia to 17q (box 9 gene mutation). Impaired cell division appears to cause the metaphyseal dysplasia in adenosine deaminase deficiency and mutations in the fibroblast growth factor receptor 3 gene in achondroplasia and thanatophoric dysplasia.

The rapid increase in our knowledge of the basic biology and technology of collagen and proteoglycan chemistry should pave the way for an exciting era in the detection of the basic defect in many of the skeletal dysplasias.

IV. MANAGEMENT

Effective management requires (1) precise diagnosis, (2) prompt recognition of specific skeletal and nonskeletal complications, (3) appropriate orthopedic and rehabilitative care, (4) emotional support and psychosocial counseling, and (5) genetic counseling. There is no specific cure for any of these conditions. The effects of recombinant human growth hormone (hGH) in the skeletal dysplasias are now being studied, but it is unlikely to do much more than increase height by several inches. The use of androgenic hormones has given no evidence of sustained growth and no gains that outweigh its potential side effects.

Orthopedic management aims at maximizing mobility and correcting deformity; if deformities in the lower limbs are left uncorrected beyond puberty, early onset of osteoarthritis may lead to mechanically unsound joints. Early recognition of spinal deformity and its early treatment with bracing or surgical intervention may reduce morbidity (from scoliosis) in adult life.

Recently, new leg-lengthening techniques have been developed in Europe, with encouraging results. The safety of these methods still needs careful study.

Prenatal diagnosis is now available for many of the skeletal dysplasias. Ultrasound femoral length examination at 18 weeks gestation may be used as a reliable test in many severe dysplasias, such as the type II osteogenesis imperfectas, thanatophoric dysplasia, achondrogenesis, and so forth. An atlas of normal skeletal radiography throughout fetal life was recently published, along with examples of numerous dysplasias, which can serve as a reference guide to the diagnosis of these disorders in affected fetuses (2). New

molecular genetic techniques may be used for early prenatal diagnosis in those conditions in which linkage to a marker gene is known or, more directly, when the exact DNA abnormality is known.

V. COLLECTION OF SKELETAL TISSUES

A variety of histologic, histochemical, immunohistochemical, ultrastructural, and biochemical studies of chondroosseous tissue and skin can be performed. Specimens can be sent to one of the laboratories that specialize in processing and interpreting tissue from the skeletal dysplasias [e.g., International Skeletal Dysplasia Registry, Cedars-Sinai Medical Center, 444 South San Vicente, Suite 1001, Los Angeles, CA 90048, (310) 855-2211]. The following handling of tissues is recommended.

A. Site of Biopsy

The iliac crest is recommended for biopsy. An iliac crest biopsy should be wedge shaped, including cartilage, growth plate, and bone, approximately 2 cm wide at the surface.

B   Site of Autopsy

It is desirable to collect specimens of costochondral junction (both bone and cartilage), chest plate, iliac crest, whole long bones, and a block of vertebrae.

C.   Specimens for Morphologic Studies

The specimens for morphologic analysis should be placed in formalin for histology and thin slices of cartilage placed in glutaraldehyde for electron microscope studies.

D.   Specimens for Biochemical Studies

At autopsy, it is ideal to obtain the chest plate (sternum plus costal cartilages) with several costochondral junctions attached, a portion of iliac crest containing cartilage and bone, and a long bone (including epiphyseal cartilages) frozen for biochemical studies. Before freezing, a slice of growth plate can be cut from the center of the block for morphologic studies without impairing the usefulness of the specimen for biochemical studies. These specimens should be wrapped in aluminum foil and frozen immediately in liquid nitrogen or on dry ice, stored at −20 to −70°C, and shipped on dry ice. Pieces of cartilage can be shipped in tissue culture medium for chondrocyte culture. In addition, skin samples in tissue culture medium should be sent for fibroblast culture.

E.   Transport of Specimens to the Laboratory

Specimens for histologic, histochemical, and electron microscope (EM) studies can be shipped in a well-sealed sturdy container at room temperature, labeled appropriately. Histology and EM specimens fixed in formaldehyde or glutaraldehyde should be stored at 4°C until shipped. These specimens should then be shipped at room temperature as quickly as possible or with an ice pack (keep away from dry ice). Cartilage and skin for culture should be shipped at room temperature.

Deep-frozen specimens should be shipped on dry ice with instructions to refrigerate during transit. It is important to ship histology and culture specimens in a separate container so that they are not frozen during transit.

ACKNOWLEDGMENTS

The authors thank Dr. Ralph Lachman and Helen Gruber for their help and Sheilah Levin and Eli Spear for the preparation of this paper. This work was supported in part by U.S. Public Health Service National Institutes of Health Program Project Grant HD-22657.

REFERENCES

1. Rimoin DL, Lachman RS. Genetic disorders of the osseous skeleton. In: Beighton P, ed. McKusick's Heritable Disorders of Connective Tissue. St. Louis: C. V. Mosby, 1992:557.
2. Ornoy A, Borochowitz Z, Lachman R, Rimoin DL. Atlas of Fetal Skeletal Radiology. Chicago: Year Book Medical Publishers, 1988.

11

Short Stature: Intellectual and Behavioral Aspects

David E. Sandberg
State University of New York at Buffalo and Children's Hospital of Buffalo, Buffalo, New York

I. INTRODUCTION

Recent developments in clinical diagnosis and biotechnology have modified our concepts of growth hormone (GH) deficiency and the clinical management of growth failure in children with short stature (SS). GH therapy is no longer restricted to those children meeting the "classic criteria" of GH deficiency (GHD) but has been extended to children with non-GHD growth problems (1–3). Some endocrinologists have suggested that the ultimate test of GHD is an increased growth velocity in response to a therapeutic trial (4). This approach potentially opens the door for large numbers of short, non-GHD children to be treated in the future. The advent of recombinant DNA technology now provides an inexhaustible supply of GH. This technological development, along with a better understanding of the complex pathophysiology of growth disorders, has dramatically changed the long-standing policy of providing GH only to those individuals with pathologic growth associated with classic GHD.

Providing GH therapy to non-GHD short children is not without controversy (5–8), and the practice is currently receiving considerable attention (9–11). In the summer of 1992, the National Institutes of Health temporarily suspended clinical trials of GH therapy in GH-sufficient children in response to a petition by the Foundation on Economic Trends, a watchdog organization (12). The estimated annual cost of $20,000 for a 30 kg child (9) has also added intensity to the "treat or not to treat" debate.

One of the justifications for providing GH therapy to children and adolescents with SS is to improve the presumed poor academic achievement and disturbed psychosocial adjustment thought to occur as a consequence of the predictable effects of SS on social interactions (13). A role for specific cognitive weaknesses in particular patient groups (for example, GHD) has also been examined (14). The majority of studies indicating problems of psychosocial adjustment have been restricted to

patient groups with either hypopituitarism (e.g., Refs. 15–19), a chondrodystrophy (20,21), or a chromosomal anomaly (22). These heterogeneous diagnostic categories share the common feature of SS, but each is associated with unique features that may serve as a barrier to healthy psychosocial adjustment and educational advancement. It is unclear whether these findings can be generalized to non-GHD children with SS who are currently being evaluated by pediatric endocrinologists, a portion of whom will go on to receive GH therapy.

One objective of this chapter is to familiarize the reader with aspects of the older literature, as well as to present some of the most recent studies on the educational and psychosocial aspects of SS. The studies selected assess the intellectual and behavioral adaptation of both endocrine clinic-referred and community samples of children and adolescents with SS. Special emphasis is given to two primary domains of functioning: intellectual and educational performance and problems of behavioral and emotional functioning.

An additional objective is to describe a clinical service and research program at Children's Hospital of Buffalo. This program involves the routine psychosocial and educational screening of all children and adolescents referred to a regional endocrinology clinic for evaluation and possible treatment of SS. Findings from this ongoing survey are presented, along with a discussion of their relevance for the debate regarding the appropriateness of GH therapy in cases of nongrowth hormone-deficient SS.

II. INTELLECTUAL AND ACADEMIC FUNCTIONING

A. Clinic-Referred Samples

Table 1 summarizes intellectual and academic functioning findings from selected studies of clinically referred samples of children and adolescents with SS arising from a variety of conditions. Pollitt and Money (16) reported that intelligence

Table 1 Selected Studies of Intellectual Functioning and Academic Achievement in Clinic-Referred Samples of Children and Adolescents with SS[a]

Study	N (Age range, years)	Diagnosis	General intelligence	Specific cognitive deficits	Academic achievement	Comments
16	15 (3–15)	Panhypopituitary (n = 5) IGHD (n = 3) Primordial (n = 2) Turner syndrome (n = 1) Undiagnosed (n = 4)	>5 years old (n = 13) FSIQ = 102.9 ± 16.3 <5 years old (n = 2) FSIQ = 48.0 ± 8.0	No effect	"Average or below average"	Diagnostically heterogeneous Sample selected for positive psycho- logic adjustment Nonstandardized measures of aca- demic achievement No control subjects
23	29 (3–38)	IGHD (n = 15) MPHD (n = 14)	Normal IQ distribution IGHD > MPHD (after controlling for SES)	No effect	Not assessed	No control subjects
25	11 (4–18)	IGHD (n = 4) Panhypopituitary (n = 4) IGHD and other serious medical problem (n = 3)	FSIQ = 88.2 ± 17.2	Visual-motor integration ↓	Commensurate with IQ Grade retention in 45%	Diagnostically heterogeneous Sampling bias?; disproportionate number of low SES cases No control subjects
14	42 (6–16)	IGHD (n = 28) MPHD (n = 14)	VIQ = 93.9 ± 18.3 PIQ = 94.0 ± 16.3 VIQ/PIQ differences higher in IGHD	VIQ-PIQ difference ↑ Visual-motor integration ↓ (26% of sample)	Arithmetic ↓ Reading (no effect)	No control subjects
26	166 (5–16)	IGHD (n = 86) ISS (n = 80)	IGHD IQ = 111.0 ± 14.9 ISS IQ = 110.3 ± 17.3	Not assessed	Average range and no group differences Achievement lower than IQ	Potential sampling bias No control subjects
30	47 (6–16)	IGHD (n = 14) MPHD (n = 2) Turner syndrome (n = 10) CGD (n = 21)	(see Academic achievement)	Not assessed	5 of 16 GHD retained a grade VIQ retained < nonretained PIQ retained < nonretained	Diagnostically heterogeneous No control subjects
29	116 (18–38)	GHD Idiopathic GHD (n = 85) Craniopharygioma (n = 16) Familial IGHD (n = 6) Postirradiation (n = 4) Posttraumatic (n = 3) Chromophobe adenoma (n = 1) Histiocytosis X (n = 1)	Not assessed	Not assessed	Same or higher than parents and similar to siblings	Utilizes sibling comparison group

[a]CGD, constituional growth delay; FSIQ, full-scale IQ; IGHD, isolated growth hormone deficiency; ISS, idiopathic short stature; MPHD, multiple pituitary hormone deficiency; PIQ, performance IQ; SES, socioeconomic status; VIQ, verbal IQ.

quotients (IQs) of 13 of 15 patients who had not yet received GH therapy fell in the average range. The 2 youngest GHD children in this series (3 and 4 years old) received IQ scores that fell in the moderately mentally retarded range. Significant differences between the verbal and performance portions of the IQ test were not detected, nor were there significant differences between factor scores that are based upon the grouping of IQ subtests. Despite average intelligence in the school-age portion of the sample, the children were rated by school officials and/or parents as "average or below average" in school achievement. The authors attributed academic weaknesses to emotional problems stemming from these children's "search for approval" rather than being from intellectual deficits intrinsic to their medical conditions.

In a larger study restricted to individuals with idiopathic GHD, a normal IQ distribution and absence of deficits in specific mental abilities were once again reported (23). The investigators also compared the performance of individuals with isolated GHD with those who had multiple pituitary hormone deficiencies in an attempt to detect IQ differences between diagnostic subgroups of patients. After controlling for socioeconomic background factors, significantly more isolated GHD than multiple hormone-deficient patients showed higher IQs. This finding suggests that additional hormone deficiencies associated with GHD (and/or factors that were responsible for the condition, such as subtle abnormalities in brain function) may contribute to lower IQs. A similar difference between isolated GHD and multiple hormone-deficient patients has been reported by other investigators (14,24).

In contrast to the studies just cited, other reports have suggested that GHD is associated with specific cognitive deficits. Abbott et al. (25) reported in a study of patients with varied forms of pituitary insufficiency, all of which included GHD, that visual-motor integration skills were significantly below average and lower than expected based upon scores of global intelligence. Academic achievement, however, was commensurate with intelligence. Grade retention in 5 of 11 children was attributable to absenteeism related to serious illnesses and hospitalization. An additional 5 children performed at or above average in school.

In a more recent study by Siegel and Hopwood (14) of children with pituitary insufficiency, the difference between the verbal and performance subtests of an intelligence test was significantly higher than for the test's standardization sample. Further, 11 of 42 hypopituitary children (26%) showed significant visual-motor integration deficits on the Bender-Gestalt test.

Virtually all these studies suffer from the weaknesses of small sample size, diagnostic heterogeneity of the study population, and absence of a control or comparison group. A collateral research protocol of the National Cooperative Growth Study (NCGS) (26) addresses the first two problems. The purpose of this research, involving 166 children and adolescents with heights below the third percentile, was to describe both the learning and behavioral profiles of short children before initiating GH therapy. Subjects were enrolled from 27 centers participating in the NCGS, and they fell into two diagnostic groups: 86 subjects (GHD group) were diagnosed as GHD as determined by a peak stimulated GH level < 10 ng/ml. The second group (idiopathic SS group, ISS) comprised 80 subjects who tested GH sufficient. Patients with additional pituitary hormone deficiencies and/or other diagnoses were excluded.

General intelligence was estimated with an IQ screening test and academic achievement by standardized assessment. Mean IQs for the GHD and ISS groups were in the high average range and did not differ significantly by diagnosis. Academic achievement subtest scores fell in the average range, and these also did not differ by diagnosis. However, achievement scores were significantly lower than IQ scores for both diagnostic groups. The authors interpret this finding as implying that both GHD and ISS children and adolescents show academic "underachievement." Thus, response to GH stimulation tests does not predict intellectual functioning or academic achievement: both GHD and GH-sufficient groups perform similarly. This study appears to rule out GH (at least as assessed by provocative testing of the pituitary) as mediating academic underachievement observed in this population.

Because no details are provided by the authors concerning the recruitment procedures employed in this behavioral component of the NCGS, it is unclear to what extent the findings are representative of all children and adolescents being followed (2331 cases recruited from 112 centers in the United States) (27). If those children with the greatest academic difficulties were more likely to be enrolled into the research protocol, then this factor alone could account for the apparent association between SS and academic underachievement as measured by the Child Behavior Checklist (CBCL).

Holmes et al. (28) reported that 5 of 16 (31%) children (ages 6–16 years) with GHD (isolated and multiple pituitary hormone deficits combined) had repeated a grade. Retention typically occurred in the primary school years, kindergarten to grade 3. Those who were retained (a combined group of children with GHD and other diagnoses responsible for SS) had lower verbal (mean 94) and performance (mean 92) IQ scores than those with the same diagnoses who had never been held back (means 105 and 107 for verbal and performance IQs, respectively). This finding was replicated by Siegel and Hopwood (14). Thus, it appears that when children with GHD (as well as other conditions associated with SS) perform poorly academically and are retained, they are more likely to represent that subgroup with lower intellectual potential, in general.

Reporting on a study of GHD adults who had been treated with GH, Dean et al. (29), in the only controlled study of its type, interviewed 116 GHD patients concerning various aspects of life adjustment, including educational status. In general, the level of educational attainment (i.e., last grade or degree completed) of the GHD group was the same or higher than that of parents and similar to that of siblings. This finding contrasts with other reports (14,30) and suggests that GHD is less of a predictor of *ultimate* level of educational attainment than it is of achievement during the early years of schooling.

Another syndrome that has been extensively studied from the standpoint of intellectual functioning and academic achievement is Turner syndrome (TS). All evidence points to the conclusion that global intelligence in this condition is normal. Nevertheless, TS is associated with a specific pattern of cognitive strengths and weaknesses. It has occasionally been the practice to group individuals with TS together with other conditions that share SS as a common feature (e.g., Refs. 16, 28, and 30) in the discussion of the intellectual functioning in patient groups with SS. This practice can be misleading because it obscures the fact that features other than SS may be even more important in accounting for the learning and psychosocial difficulties observed in this group. For this reason, TS is not discussed in this chapter. Instead, the reader is referred to recent review articles (31,32).

Although there are exceptions (e.g., Refs. 16 and 26), it is important to note that many GHD patients are already receiving GH replacement therapy at the time of the psychometric assessment. For instance, Meyer-Bahlburg et al. (23) reported that IQ was not significantly correlated with age at onset or length of GH treatment. Also, there was no significant difference between patients who were receiving GH treatment at the time of testing and those who were not. Abbott et al. (25) also failed to detect changes in IQ from pretest (i.e., before initiating GH replacement therapy) to posttest occurring approximately 1 year into the course of treatment. Performance scores on certain tests actually declined 1 year after treatment had begun. Thus, GH treatment in childhood and adolescence does not seem positively to influence intelligence. These findings appear to undermine the rationale of providing GH therapy to improve intellectual functioning directly (33), at least when treatment is initiated beyond the infancy stage. There remains the possibility, however, that academic achievement (if not cognitive functioning itself) is indirectly facilitated via GH-induced improvements in relative height, psychologic well-being, and psychosocial adjustment of the child or adolescent with SS. This assumes, of course, that children and adolescents with SS are experiencing, as a group, significant problems of academic and psychosocial adjustment before receiving GH therapy and that poor academic achievement is attributable to SS-related psychosocial difficulties. The Stabler et al. study (26) does not support this possibility: of the 30 children identified as having problems of academic achievement, only 4 (13%) showed behavioral adjustment problems. The issue of the psychosocial adaptation of youth with SS is addressed in detail in the following section.

There are two additional reports from preliminary studies that leave open the possibility that GH replacement in GHD individuals enhances certain aspects of cognitive performance. Smith et al. (34) found in a double-blind, placebo-controlled study that children (ages 8.7–14.1 years) showing higher blood levels of GH after an injection of GH administered 12 h earlier showed enhanced performance on tasks assessing various aspects of attention. The relationship between GH levels and performance on psychometric tests was not simple, however. The group showing higher blood levels of GH after an injection of GH also outperformed those with lower levels under the placebo conditions as well. Thus, the investigators did not attribute the superior performance in the group with the higher GH levels to the injections received during the experiment. Complicated speculation regarding the differential metabolism of GH in the two groups was adopted to explain the pattern of findings.

In a second, nonblinded study conducted in adults (ages 22–26 years) with multiple pituitary hormone deficiencies who had received GH therapy in childhood, investigators reported a statistically significant improvement in a memory function test when subjects were receiving GH compared with baseline (35). Although differences in the predicted direction (i.e., improved cognitive performance) were noted on the majority of measures across five separate cognitive tasks, these differences did not achieve statistical significance. These two studies suggest a potential cognitive benefit of GH therapy, but the data at this time are much too preliminary for them to be of any utility regarding issues of clinical management of individuals with GHD.

B. Community Samples

Studies of medically unselected (and presumably healthy) community samples potentially elucidate the role of stature in influencing different aspects of intellectual and educational performance. It is within the context of these population-based studies that investigations of the specific medical conditions reviewed earlier must be evaluated. Findings from these studies are summarized in Table 2.

In a study of middle-childhood boys, Weinberg et al. (36) reported that height correlated significantly with two standardized measures of intelligence after statistically controlling for family socioeconomic status. Neither subject's height nor other physical measures significantly correlated with reading proficiency. Subject's head circumference served as an even stronger predictor of IQ scores. The authors pointed out that socioeconomic status of the family easily accounted for the greatest amount of variance in IQ scores (38%). Adding in six physical variables (only one of which was the subject's height) caused the multiple correlation to increase by only 5%. This study illustrates how findings can achieve statistical significance (i.e., $p < 0.05$) and still be small in terms of "clinical" significance.

In a study of seventh grade students (boys and girls) attending regular classes, Richards et al. (37) failed to detect a significant correlation between student's height and grade point average. The same held true for performance on academic achievement tests. Contrasting the academic performance of the tallest (height ≥ 1 standard deviation, SD) and the shortest (height ≤ 1 SD) children also failed to detect significant differences for either boys or girls. Although limited by the small numbers of such cases, these authors were unable to demonstrate a relationship between height and school performance even when restricting data analyses to children above and below 1.5, 2, or 2.5 SD from the mean for height norms.

In the largest study of its type and the only one conducted on a national probability sample of the U.S. population,

Table 2 Relationship Between Stature, Intellectual Functioning, and Academic Functioning in Community Samples[a]

Study	N (Age range, years)	Sample origin	Relation between stature and dependent measure	Comments
36	334 (8–9)	School (United States)	WISC $r = 0.14$ PPVT $r = 0.20$ Reading: no effect	Socioeconomic status far stronger predictor of intellectual functioning than anthropometric indices. Six anthropometric measures accounted for 5% of variance in IQ scores (SES accounted for 38%) Head circumference measures are stronger predictors than stature: WISC, $r = 0.21$; PPVT, $r = 0.30$
37	481 (seventh grade)	School (United States)	GPA: no effect Iowa Achievement Test: no effect Sort Form Test of Academic Aptitude: no effect	
38	Cycle II: 7, 119 (6–11) Cycle III: 6, 768 (12–17) 2, 177 (studied at 8–11 and again 2–5 years later)	General population (United States)	WISC/WRAT: height accounts for approximately 2% of variance after controlling for demographic variables. No correlation between change in height Z score from childhood to adolescence and WISC or WRAT scores No sex differences	
39	Same as 38	General population (United States)	Children and adolescents with SS (≤ 1.5 SD) received lower "school adjustment" scores than individuals of average (within 1.5 SD) and tall stature (≥ 1.5 SD) Proportion of variance accounted for by height classification was small (0.4–0.7%) No sex differences Changes in height Z from childhood to adolescence unrelated to school adjustment Relationship between height Z and school performance maintained when SS defined as -2 and -3 SD below norms	
40	141 (7–9)	School (United Kingdom)	No IQ difference between SS ($<$3rd percentile) pupils and average stature (10th–90th percentile) pupils "Reading" and "number" scale scores on academic ability test lower in SS group. Statistically controlling for SES differences between SS and average-stature children reduces academic performance differences	Covariation between stature and SES is emphasized, replicating findings from independent studies (47,48)

[a]GPA, grade point average; PPVT, Peabody Picture Vocabulary Test; WISC, Wechsler Intelligence Scale for Children; WRAT, Wide Range Achievement Test.

Wilson et al. (38) assessed the relationship between stature and two measures of intellectual functioning. The data for this study come from cycles II and III of the National Health Examination Survey (NHES) conducted by the National Center for Health Statistics during the 1960s. Cycle II (1963–1965) involved the assessment of 7119 children 6–11 years of age. Cycle III (1966–1970) comprised 6768 adoles-

cents 12–17 years of age. A longitudinal component was incorporated into the design of the study so that 2177 children 8–11 years of age who were first evaluated during cycle II were subsequently reevaluated 2–5 years later during cycle III. Using stepwise multiple linear regression to control statistically for potentially confounding subject and family background characteristics, subject's standardized height (Z)

scores contributed significantly to the prediction of IQ and academic achievement. The percentage of variance accounted for, however, was very small (approximately 2%). An additional finding of considerable interest was that a significant correlation could not be detected between change in subject's relative height from cycle II to cycle III and change in either set of tests.

In an attempt to explain the statistically significant correlation between subject's height and intelligence, Wilson et al. (38) speculate that both variables covary with another factor, such as subtle intrauterine damage or postnatal malnutrition. The finding that measures of intelligence did not covary with increases in relative height across time suggested to the authors that the processes that contribute to the relationship between height, IQ, and school performance must occur relatively early in childhood.

Using the same NHES database, Vance et al. (39) further investigated the relation between subject's height and measures of academic achievement. The variable subject's height was trichotomized as "short of stature" (≤1.5 SD from the population mean), "average" (within 1.5 SD of mean), and "tall" (≥1.5 SD from mean). Statistical analyses controlling for background variables revealed that the short group in both cycles II and III received statistically lower scores on a school adjustment scale. The proportion of variance in school adjustment accounted for by the subject's height classification was very small (0.4 and 0.7% in cycles II and III, respectively) and did not differ by subject's sex. These investigators also found, similar to the Wilson et al. study (38), that change in subject's relative height from childhood to adolescence was not statistically related to school adjustment. Supplementary analyses by these authors (40), in which short of stature was defined as –1 SD, –2 SD, and –3 SD from the population mean, yielded the same pattern of findings.

The absence of a relationship between increased relative height and measures of intellectual functioning further weakens one of the implicit justifications of providing GH therapy to children or adolescents with SS. First, studies reviewed earlier in this chapter do not provide support for the hypothesis that GH therapy in clinic-referred populations directly or indirectly improves intellectual functioning or academic achievement. Second, results from the aforementioned epidemiologic studies (38,39) suggest that increments in relative height (in this case brought about through normal developmental processes) are also not related to improvements in either of these domains.

In the ongoing Wessex Growth Study of the scholastic and psychosocial sequelae of SS in a school-based sample being conducted in the United Kingdom, schoolchildren with SS (i.e., heights < 3rd percentile for norms) are being evaluated longitudinally and performance is being contrasted with a matched comparison group of classmates who are of average stature (10th–90th percentiles) (41). At the time of the first study report, the children were between 7 and 9 years old. The SS group received comparable scores on a measure of intelligence. Despite this similarity, the SS group received lower scores than the control group on measures of academic attainment. Thus, the SS group appeared to be showing "underachievement" relative to the average-statured group. This discrepancy was partially resolved when the socioeconomic background of the children was taken into consideration; under these circumstances, the differences between the SS and control groups were attenuated, although not entirely eliminated.

In conclusion, it appears that height is related to measures of intellectual functioning and academic achievement in the general population: shorter children tend to have lower IQs and show poorer academic achievement relative to taller children. Such findings must be interpreted very cautiously. Most important to keep in mind is that although such effects are statistically reliable (i.e., the findings are replicable with independent samples), the demonstrated effect sizes are rather small and are partially attributable to socioeconomic factors that covary with stature in the general population (38,41).

III. BEHAVIORAL AND EMOTIONAL FUNCTIONING

In the second edition of this text, Meyer-Bahlburg (13) reviewed the behavioral and educational problems associated with various SS conditions. His analysis suggested that the difficulties encountered by children and adolescents with SS develop as a consequence of the predictable effects of SS on everyday social interactions and the chronic adjustments that typically develop as a result. The social effects and consequences are summarized in Table 3.

The research and clinical data supporting the idea that these processes and behavioral sequelae occur suffer from many of the same weaknesses as those studies that have been used to imply that SS is associated with significant intellectual and/or academic problems. This is because both domains of functioning are commonly assessed within the same study.

Table 3 Common Social Experiences Associated with Short Stature and Potential Maladaptive Adjustment

Reaction of parents, peers
Infantilizing
Overprotection
Demands low for age
Stigmatization
Teasing
Avoidance
Rejection
Potential long-term maladaptation
Social retardation
Peer relationship problems
Withdrawal from peer group
Lack of assertiveness
Dependence on parents
Poor self-image
Depression

Source: Adapted from Ref. 13.

Thus, as in the studies of intellectual functioning, investigations of the behavioral adaptation of children and adolescents with SS tend to be restricted to highly selected patient groups. As noted earlier, individuals with these conditions (e.g., hypopituitarism, chondrodystrophies, chromosomal variations, and constitutionally delayed puberty) experience syndrome-specific sequelae as well as more general consequences that flow from the shared psychosocial experience related to SS.

More recent investigations provide information on the full range of SS patients, both clinic referred and nonreferred. Patient groups not previously studied (e.g., GH sufficient with poor growth velocity) are included, and sample sizes are typically larger than in previous clinic-based studies on SS. Also, investigators have placed greater attention on potential subject selection factors that can result in a systematic biasing of findings. Together, these studies possibly provide a "cleaner" picture of the psychosocial impact of SS than have earlier investigations.

A. Clinic-Referred Samples

The study of GHD and idiopathic SS children by Stabler et al. (26), described earlier, included a component concerned with patients' social competencies and behavioral and emotional functioning. Compared with the nonclinical sample used in the standardization of the parent-reported Child Behavior Checklist, the GHD group received significantly lower "school" and "total social competency" scores. The ISS group, in contrast, could not be differentiated from the comparison group in terms of social or academic competencies. In the domain of behavioral and emotional functioning, parents of subjects in both the GHD and ISS groups reported significantly more problems in their children than parents of the nonclinical standardization sample.

The authors interpreted these differences as representing a "high frequency of behavior problems" in both SS groups. A different interpretation is that the 1983 CBCL nonclinical norms, which were used for comparison, are not a suitable substitute for an independent control group for such a study. First, the CBCL nonclinical samples (42) adopted by Stabler et al. for comparison to the SS samples were recruited from a geographically limited area within the United States (Washington, D.C., Maryland, and northern Virginia). Children participating in the NCGS study, in contrast, were recruited from across the country. Other studies of community (i.e., psychiatrically unselected) samples conducted at different locations within the United States have demonstrated that children can receive scores on the CBCL that are indicative of both poorer social competencies and increased behavior disturbance compared with the CBCL nonclinical standardization norms (43–44).

Second, the CBCL nonclinical norms may be an excessively stringent criterion against which the mental health of children and adolescents with SS should be gauged. The standardization procedures for the CBCL called for exclusion from the "nonclinical" (i.e., normative) sample frame all individuals who had received mental health services or special

remedial school classes within the preceding 12 months. Excluding such cases from the GHD and ISS samples would potentially minimize or even eliminate any differences between the clinical and nonclinical samples. Such a methodologic approach is obviously flawed because a major goal of such behavioral studies of SS groups is to ascertain the prevalence of psychosocial problems, and any procedure that *a priori* excludes those cases who may be experiencing the greatest difficulties is of dubious validity. This reasoning points to the critical need for controlled studies to be conducted in which clinically nonreferred children and adolescents with SS are compared to children with average stature without imposing *a priori* exclusion criteria related to psychosocial functioning or utilization of mental health or special educational services.

In a recent study taking a very different approach, Zimet and colleagues (45) assessed several domains of adult psychologic functioning in 31 individuals who as short children (during the 1970s) were referred for endocrinologic evaluation but were not eligible for GH therapy because they were found to be GH sufficient or did not otherwise meet eligibility requirements for GH therapy. Standardized heights at the time of initial endocrine evaluation (2–16 years) ranged from –3.7 to –0.2 SD (mean –2.15 SD) and from –3.1 to 1.1 SD (mean –1.56 SD) at the time of the study (18–33 years). The sample comprised the following diagnostic groups: familial SS (13%), constitutional growth delay (16%), mixed familial SS and constitutional growth delay (19%), idiopathic SS (23%), primordial SS (3%), glucocorticoid excess (3%), greater than fifth percentile for standing height (13%), and definitive diagnosis not possible because the child was adopted (10%).

The assessment protocol included standardized measures: emotional adjustment, including distress, restraint, and defensiveness; self-esteem; and perceived social support. Compared to nonclinical norms for these instruments, the clinical sample was different in only limited respects. For example, on a measure of psychologic adjustment, the Weinberger Adjustment Inventory (WAI), the clinical sample scored higher on the restraint and repressive-defensiveness scales but were not different on the distress or denial of distress scales. The measure of social support also did not differentiate the clinical group from several normative samples. Correlational analyses of the relationship between subject's child height (i.e., at the time of endocrine evaluation) and adult height (i.e., at the time of the study) and the psychosocial measures produced mixed findings. Relatively few achieved statistical significance: taller child height was correlated with more *negative* self-statements regarding intellectual competence and taller adult height predicted *lower* distress scores but *higher* restraint, denial of distress, and repressive-defensiveness scores on the WAI. Taller adult stature was also associated with more positive self-perceptions of the sense of humor and global self-worth on the Adult Self Perception Profile. Adult height did not correlate significantly with any scales of the social support measure.

The authors interpreted these findings as providing only modest support for the contention that children with non-GHD SS go on to experience significant problems of psychosocial adjustment in adulthood. They conclude that these findings "bring into question an often stated justification for GH treatment with non-GHD short children; that short stature in childhood, if left untreated, will lead to poor psychosocial adjustment in adulthood" (45).

This conclusion must be accepted very tentatively because of the significant methodologic problems noted by the authors. First, the participation rate was quite poor. Of the 181 non-GHD children who were originally evaluated and eligible for inclusion in the study, protocols were completed by only 31 (17%). The possibility that selection bias in subject recruitment led to an unrepresentative picture of the adult psychosocial functioning of this SS group must therefore be seriously considered. Second, the study relied on the use of nonclinical norms associated with the various instruments instead of recruiting its own control group. These limitations notwithstanding, the design of this study is creative and well deserving of replication with a more complete sample and appropriate control and comparison groups.

B. Community Samples

Vance et al. (39) extended their secondary analyses of the NHES database beyond academic achievement (see earlier discussion for details) to consider such psychosocial variables as peer relations and aggression (cycle II, 6–11 years) and immaturity and anxiety (cycle III, 12–17 years). These dependent variables were all assessed through parent-completed questionnaires. In statistical analyses that controlled for subject and family background variables, subject's height was unrelated to these measures. Furthermore, the longitudinal component of this study (described earlier) also did not reveal a relationship between changes in relative height from childhood to adolescence and scores on the psychosocial variables. Although the authors' original set of analyses defined SS as ≤ 1.5 SD from the population mean, further analyses demonstrated the generalizability of these relationships when SS was defined as –1 SD, –2, or –3 SD from the population mean (40). It thus appears that children and adolescents with SS in the general population, as a group, function similarly to individuals with average or tall stature. The authors conclude that GH therapy for non-GHD youths based upon the justification of improving their psychosocial status may be unwarranted.

The longitudinal Wessex Growth Study compares the psychosocial functioning of schoolchildren with SS (i.e., heights < 3rd percentile for norms) with a matched group of classmates of average stature (10th–90th percentiles) (46). The research protocol includes a self-report measure of self-esteem and a teacher-reported behavior rating scale. No statistically significant differences were detected on the self-esteem measure or in teacher ratings of problems. As in intellectual functioning and academic achievement (see earlier), whatever differences were detected were diminished or eliminated by statistically controlling for the socioeconomic background of the subjects. To ensure that severity of the SS was not a factor contributing to the negative findings, data from the 18 shortest children with a height ≤ 2.5 SD were examined separately. Once again, differences between the short and average-stature children did not achieve statistical significance on any of the psychometric measures.

Voss and Mulligan (46) point out that identification of SS in the general population may be related to social deprivation. This underscores the importance of statistically controlling for this variable in all data analyses. This observation was made previously (47,48). They also note that any conclusions concerning the adaptive functioning of short nonreferred children must be restricted to the developmental stage assessed (ages 7–9 years). The longitudinal aspect of this study will provide data in time to address whether the academic and social challenges of advancing years are associated with increased symptomatology in this group.

IV. THE PSYCHOSOCIAL SCREENING PROJECT: AN ONGOING SURVEY

The Psychosocial Screening Project refers to a clinical service provided to all new patients receiving a growth evaluation for SS through the Division of Pediatric Endocrinology at Children's Hospital of Buffalo. Based upon clinical reports that children and adolescents with SS show increased problems of academic and psychosocial adjustment, we set out to identify those individuals who were already experiencing difficulties and to provide preventive information to families in which the child or adolescent was currently adapting well. Approximately 200 new patients each year have undergone the psychosocial screening evaluation since its inception in late 1989.

At the time of their initial visit to endocrinology, all patients (8 years and older) referred with a chief complaint of short stature and an accompanying parent complete paper-and-pencil questionnaires selected to characterize the individual's psychosocial profile. The protocol is completed during waiting intervals between physician examinations or while waiting for blood tests or a bone-age x-ray. Feedback from the evaluation and any indicated recommendations are provided to the family 2 weeks after the endocrine clinic visit. A summary of the psychosocial screening report is filed in the endocrine chart, and a copy is forwarded to the referring primary care physician. This behavioral assessment, which occurs at the point of entry to the growth clinic, provides clinicians, both medical and mental health, with information that can enhance the clinical management of SS, whether or not an endocrinologic intervention is indicated. The screening evaluation also serves to inform families of common psychosocial sequelae of SS and of the counseling and psychoeducational services available to them through the psychoendocrinology program.

The clinical service that involves the *routine* evaluation of large numbers of short individuals also provides an important research opportunity. We are in the position to learn not only about the individual case referred by professionals or family members to mental health professionals during a time of crisis but also about short children in the aggregate whose growth problems are related to a wide range of etiologies.

A. Preliminary Screening Findings

A total of 288 patients met the age and height criteria, but 10% (30 cases) were excluded according to a priori criteria (i.e., marked physical and/or intellectual impairments; see Ref. 49 for details). The 258 patients described here were between 4 and 18 years old, with a height ≤ fifth percentile for age and sex norms. There were 180 boys (mean ± SD age = 11.4 ± 3.5) and 78 girls (mean ± SD age = 10.4 ± 3.5). The 2.3:1 boy-girl ratio is commonly observed in clinically referred samples and is thought to represent the enhanced significance attributed to the stature of males. The sample was predominantly white (87%). Mean parental educational attainment fell above the rating for partial college (at least 1 year) or specialized training but below that for standard college or university graduation. The majority of the children (72.4%) were living in intact homes with both parents present.

Of the SS sample 54% was classified as having normal variant SS (i.e., genetic SS, 15.5%; constitutional growth delay, 13.6%; transient prepubertal growth deceleration, 1.6%; or a combination of these, 23.3%). A variety of conditions accounted for the pathologic growth observed in the rest of the sample: GHD (14.4%); "idiopathic growth failure" (defined as a height ≤ fifth percentile with pathologic growth velocity (≤5 cm/year) but a normal GH peak (≥10 ng/ml) to a provocative test, 7.8%); undernutrition (4.7%); intrauterine growth retardation (1.9%); skeletal dysplasia (0.8%); chromosomal anomaly (0.8%); chronic disease (0.8%); dysmorphic syndrome (0.4%); and hypothyroidism (0.4%). A conclusive diagnosis could not be established for 35 children (13.6%). The mean ± SD standardized height for the boys and girls, combined, was –2.3 ± 0.5 SD, with a range of –4.0 to –1.6 SD.

Data are provided here from only three methods used in the screening: the Issues Related to Growth Problem and Height (IRGPH, a questionnaire developed specifically for the screening), the CBCL (50), and Youth Self-Report (YSR) (51). Because not all of the questionnaires used in the protocol were introduced simultaneously, the number of cases for whom data are available varies by method. Also, scheduling difficulties within the clinic resulted in some patients and parents not fully completing the assessment protocol.

The IRGPH was designed to collect information from both the parent and guardian and the child concerning factors the clinical research literature on short stature and our own clinical experience suggest are important in modulating the psychosocial impact of short stature. A combination of open- and closed-ended questions was utilized. The child version is suitable for administration to children 8 years and older. The present analysis is restricted to portions of multicomponent items concerning ongoing stigmatization and juvenilization related to short stature and whether there was a younger sibling in the home who is taller than the patient being evaluated. The items concerning juvenilization and the presence in the home of a younger, taller sibling were added to the IRGPH after the rest of the protocol was already in use. Thus, data for these items are not available for the total

sample. The CBCL and YSR have been used as broad-range psychosocial screening instruments in several of the studies reviewed earlier in this chapter.

1. Short Stature-Related Experiences

A total of 207 parents (145 boys and 62 girls) provided responses to the IRGPH item, Does your child currently report teasing that is related to his/her height? Approximately one-half of the parents of both boys (59.3%) and girls (56.5%) reported that their son or daughter currently experiences teasing related to SS. The mean frequency of teasing experienced (rated on an eight-point scale) was 3.8 (±1.9) and 3.3 (±1.6) for the boys and girls, respectively, which falls between the verbal anchors of two to three times per month (3) and once per week (4).

The parallel item from the patient version of the questionnaire (Does anyone tease you these days because you are shorter than most children your age?) was completed by 156 patients 8 years and older (116 boys and 40 girls). A higher proportion of patients than parents reported experiencing teasing: 61.2% of the boys and 65% of the girls. Further, they reported that the teasing occurred more frequently than reported by the parents: 6.0 ±2.0 or four to six times per week for the boys and 4.9 ±2.6 or close to the verbal anchor or two to three times per week (5) for the girls.

A total of 142 parents (of 102 boys and 40 girls) answered the question, Do you think that people treat your child as if he/she were younger than his/her age? The majority (72.5% for boys and 75.0% for girls) answered affirmatively. The parallel item from the patient version (Do you think that people treat you as if you are younger than your age?) was completed by 112 subjects (85 boys and 27 girls): 52.9 and 48.1% of the boys and girls, respectively, answered this item affirmatively.

The finding that the majority of clinic-referred short children are teased because of their height and that there is a tendency on the part of others to treat them as if they are younger is not surprising and replicates earlier reports (13). Consequently, SS might be considered a chronic psychosocial stressor that places the individual at heightened risk for the development of emotional and behavioral disturbance. This assumption was examined using the parent-reported CBCL and self-reported YSR.

2. Social Competencies and Behavior Problems: SS Boys

The CBCL comprises 20 social competency items that are grouped into three scales: activities, social, and school. The 118 behavior problem items are grouped into eight or nine (boys and girls ages 4–11 years only) factor-analytically derived "narrow-band" scales. Factor analyses of the narrow-band scales yield two "broad-band" behavior syndrome scales (internalizing and externalizing) that reflect the distinction between fearful, inhibited, and overcontrolled behavior versus aggressive, antisocial, and undercontrolled behavior.

SS boys (ages 4–11 and 12–18 years) received generally lower social competency scores than the CBCL nonclinical (i.e., normative) samples (Tables 4 and 5). The SS samples

Table 4 Direction of Differences in CBCL Scale Scores Between 4- to 11-Year-Old SS Boys and Girls and the CBCL Nonclinical Samples[a]

	Boys		Girls	
Variable	SS ($n = 83$) versus normals ($n = 582$)	p (two-tailed)	SS ($n = 50$) versus normals ($n = 619$)	p (two-tailed)
Social competencies[b]				
Activities	↓[c]	<0.001	—	NS
Social	↓	<0.001	—	NS
School	↓	<0.001	↓	<0.001
Total competence	↓	<0.001	—	NS
Behavior problems				
Withdrawn	↑	<0.05	—	NS
Somatic complaints	↑	<0.001	↑	<0.05
Anxious or depressed	—	NS	—	NS
Social problems	↑	<0.001	↑	<0.001
Thought problems	—	NS	—	NS
Attention problems	↑	<0.05	—	NS
Delinquent behavior	↑	<0.05	—	NS
Aggressive behavior	—	NS	—	NS
Sex problems	—	NS	—	NS
Internalizing	↑	<0.01	—	NS
Externalizing	—	NS	—	NS
Total problems	↑	<0.01	—	NS

[a]SS = short stature; NS = not significant.

[b]N vary slightly for social competency data because these scales are not computed for ages 4–5 years.

[c]SS group received significantly ($p < 0.05$) higher (↑) or lower (↓) scale score or were not significantly ($p \geq 0.05$) different (—) from the CBCL nonclinical sample. p Values are associated with t tests for independent samples.

(4–11 and 12–18 year age groups) also received significantly higher scores (indicating more problems) on 7 of 12 narrow- and broad-band behavior problem scales. For both age groups, the SS sample consistently received higher behavior problem scores on narrow-band scales, with factor loadings on the internalizing scale (i.e., withdrawn, somatic complaints, and anxious or depressed). Scores on the externalizing scale did not differentiate the SS and CBCL nonclinical samples.

Because the CBCL nonclinical samples comprise only children and adolescents who had *not* received mental health services in the past 12 months (see earlier discussion), this comparison group is biased toward mental health and, therefore, possibly too stringent a standard by which to gauge the psychosocial functioning of the SS sample. To determine whether this difference in the exclusion criteria for the two samples was responsible for the impression of greater adjustment problems in the male SS group, the clinic sample was compared to an unselected school sample that had been recruited for a separate study (43). Because the earlier study was restricted to children 6–10 years, this was the age range used for comparison with the SS group. As expected, a direct comparison of these groups (without *a priori* exclusion of cases who had mental health contacts in the past year) greatly minimized the differences previously observed when the SS sample was compared with the CBCL nonclinical sample. This was particularly true for the behavior problems scales of the CBCL, in which only 2 of 12 scale score comparisons achieved statistical significance (52).

When the SS boys were compared to norms for a psychiatric-referred sample (50), marked differences were observed, but in the *opposite* direction: SS boys were described as more socially competent and as showing fewer behavior problems, except the 12–18 year group, who continued to receive higher mean somatic complaints scores.

The SS boys' (ages 11–18 years only) own reports of their overall social competencies on the YSR corroborated their parent's reports (i.e., indicating reduced social competencies relative to the YSR nonclinical sample), although the particular scales showing effects by self-report were different from those by parent report. In marked contrast, the SS boys' own reports of behavior problems did not differentiate them from the nonclinical sample on any of the scales. Contrary to expectations, the SS group scored significantly lower (indicating fewer problems) on the withdrawn scale.

3. Social Competencies and Behavior Problems: SS Girls

Compared with the SS boys, relatively limited differences between the SS girls and CBCL nonclinical samples were

Table 5 Direction of Differences in CBCL Scale Scores Between 12- to 17-Year-Old SS Boys and Girls and the CBCL Nonclinical Samples[a]

	Boys		Girls	
	SS ($n = 93$) versus	p	SS ($n = 28$) versus	p
Variable	normals ($n = 450$)	(two-tailed)	normals ($n = 459$)	(two-tailed)
Social competencies				
Activities	—[b]	NS	—	NS
Social	↓	<0.001	—	NS
School	↓	<0.01	↓	<0.01
Total competence	↓	<0.01	—	NS
Behavior problems				
Withdrawn	↑	<0.01	—	NS
Somatic complaints	↑	<0.001	—	NS
Anxious or depressed	↑	<0.001	—	NS
Social problems	↑	<0.001	—	NS
Thought problems	—	NS	—	NS
Attention problems	—	NS	—	NS
Delinquent behavior	—	NS	—	NS
Aggressive behavior	↑	<0.05	—	NS
Internalizing	↑	<0.001	—	NS
Externalizing	—	NS	—	NS
Total problems	↑	<0.001	—	NS

[a]SS = short stature; NS = not significant.
[b]SS group received significantly ($p < 0.05$) higher (↑) or lower (↓) scale score or were not significantly ($p \geq 0.05$) different (—) from the CBCL nonclinical sample. p Values are associated with t tests for independent samples.

observed for the social competency scales. The school scale for both age groups was the only scale found to be significantly lower than norms (Tables 4 and 5). The relatively weak effect of SS in girls was also observed on the behavior problem scales. The 4- to 11-year-old SS girls received significantly higher behavior problem scores on only 2 of 12 scales (somatic complaints and social problems). The 12- to 18-year-old SS group was statistically indistinguishable from the nonclinical sample on all of the behavior problem scales.

The SS girls' own reports corroborated the parent reports: there were no statistically significant differences between the SS and nonclinical samples in the direction of poorer social competencies or greater behavior disturbance. On the contrary, the SS girls reported significantly *fewer* behavior problems classified specifically as "delinquent behavior" and globally as "externalizing."

4. Height Deficit and Psychosocial Function

Patients' heights at the time of the psychosocial screening extended from –4.0 to –1.6 SD (range 2.4 SD). Increased height deficits were not predictive of lower social competencies or increased behavior disturbance on any of the measures as assessed by multiple-regression analyses in which demographic background variables were statistically controlled. The opposite was true: relatively *taller* children within the SS group received higher scores (i.e., indicating more problems)

on the CBCL somatic complaints (incremental $R^2 = 0.021$; $p = 0.02$) and internalizing (incremental $R^2 = 0.015$; $p = 0.04$) scales.

5. Influence of Younger, Taller Sibling on Psychosocial Functioning

Multiple-regression analyses were also used to ascertain the influence on the SS child (boys and girls combined) of having a younger, taller sibling. SS children and adolescents with a younger, taller sibling received significantly ($p < 0.05$) lower scores on the social and total competence scales and higher scores on all behavior problem scales. The percentage of unique variance in CBCL social competency scores accounted for by this social contextual variable ranged from 2.8% (total social competencies) to 3.3% (social) after statistically controlling for demographic variables and subject's height. For the behavior problem scales, the percentage of variance in scale scores accounted for ranged from 1.9% (somatic complaints) to 8.2% (withdrawn).

B. Summary of Screening Findings

These findings both confirm and challenge earlier findings on the topic of the psychosocial functioning of children and adolescents with SS. Stigmatization and juvenilization are common psychosocial sequelae in clinic-referred boys and girls with SS. SS boys are somewhat less socially competent and have more behavioral or emotional problems than boys of comparable age in the nonclinical sample. When we contrasted our SS patients with a psychiatrically unselected school sample of our own (52), the differences were greatly diminished. The SS girls were comparable in psychosocial functioning to both the CBCL nonclinical norms and our own school-based sample.

When the SS boys were compared with the CBCL clinical (i.e., psychiatric-referred) sample, marked differences (in the direction of better psychosocial adjustment) were observed. Furthermore, the magnitude of the differences in scale scores between the SS samples and CBCL psychiatric norms were larger than the parallel differences between the SS and CBCL nonclinical samples. Thus, an elevation in symptomatology observed in the SS group (boys in particular), does not imply the presence of disturbance of a magnitude observed in children who are being evaluated for mental health problems.

The anecdotal impression that short boys are more troubled by their stature than short girls received some empirical support. Supplementary analyses focusing on possible sex-related variation in behavioral adaptation to SS did not reveal statistically significant differences in the proportions of 4- to 11-year-old male and female SS subjects receiving either social competency or behavior problem scores that placed them in the borderline clinical or clinical range according to parent report on the CBCL. For the 12- to 18-year-old SS group, however, a significantly higher percentage of boys than girls received clinically elevated scores on the scales (withdrawn and somatic complaints) labeled "internalizing" within the CBCL categorization scheme. There was no significant difference for the older group in the proportion of cases receiving clinically elevated social competency scores. The findings from the present study suggest that clinic-referred boys with SS, but not girls, are those showing increased problems of behavioral adjustment, and these appear to be rather mild in nature.

The present finding that degree of height deficit was unrelated to psychosocial adjustment was unexpected based upon the behavioral clinical literature regarding SS, but not without precedent. As mentioned earlier in the context of population-based studies of the psychosocial aspects of SS, Vance et al. (39,40) found only very subtle (although statistically significant) differences between children that could be accounted for by their height.

The observation that children referred for SS who have younger but taller siblings show poorer social competencies and increased behavior problems suggests that these children are not impervious to all negative psychosocial sequlae of their SS. Although the magnitude of the effect of this family contextual variable was quite small (1.9–8.2% of unique variance accounted for on the various CBCL scales), this finding points out that relative height alone may be less important than other individual and family background factors in accounting for variability in day-to-day functioning.

V. CONCLUDING REMARKS

Findings from the Psychosocial Screening Project and those of others (39–41,46) give the impression that short children and adolescents, both referred and nonreferred, are functioning relatively well and certainly better than one would have expected based upon earlier clinic-based studies of SS. A reconciliation of these apparent discrepant findings may rest in methodologic differences between the current survey and earlier clinic-based reports. First, earlier studies have typically been restricted to highly selected patient groups (see earlier), whereas all children referred for evaluation of SS, including those with normal variant SS, were included in the present series. Future analyses will contrast diagnostic subgroups of patients. It is expected that if there were large numbers of children with particular diagnoses, such as Turner syndrome, hypopituitarism, or psychosocial SS, a direct comparison with the normal variant SS group (statistically controlling for height differences) would probably yield some of the syndrome-specific differences noted by others (22,25, 53,54). Second, because earlier studies have provided scant details regarding the formation of the study group, it is possible that it has been the poorer functioning individuals who end up being recruited. Because the data presented here derive from a clinical service that is a routine component of the growth evaluation, this path to potential selection bias is effectively neutralized.

In conclusion, if clinically significant behavioral or emotional problems are detected among referred children with SS, then factors other than relative height may serve as crucial determinants of how the individual functions psychosocially. For instance, such factors as the particular underlying medical condition or the presence of family background circumstances that sensitize the individual to his or her SS may provide far greater explanatory power of the variability in psychosocial functioning.

Finally, because stature by itself does not appear to be predictive of behavioral outcomes, GH therapy should not be initiated with the objective of improving assumed psychosocial disturbance in SS children. At this time, the strongest indication for GH therapy should remain evidence of an underlying disease state. Nevertheless, there will likely be individual cases in whom SS is associated with significant psychosocial morbidity and who may benefit from GH therapy. The psychosocial screening methodology described in this report serves as a practical means of systematically identifying such "at-risk" cases.

ACKNOWLEDGMENTS

This work was supported in part by a grant from the Human Growth Foundation. The author is greatly indebted to the Children's Growth Foundation (Buffalo) for its support of the Psychosocial Screening Project described in this chapter and the other clinical services provided by the psychoendocrinology program. Thanks are owed to the following research assistants for their help in supporting various aspects of the Psychosocial Screening Project: Limor Azizy, Christopher

Barrick, Amy Brook, Angelique Fusco, Patricia Michael, Kassia Pryzstal, David Romanowski, Jennifer Stern, and Patricia Tolsma. Special thanks to Margaret H. MacGillivray, Mary L. Voorhess, and Tom Mazur for facilitating the development and continued support of the Psychosocial Screening Project. The collaborative research efforts of Susana P. Campos are greatly appreciated. Thanks also to William Tallmadge, Caroline Fung, and Patricia Michael for assistance in preparing the manuscript.

REFERENCES

1. Gertner JM, Genel M, Gianfredi SP, Hintz RL, Rosenfeld RG, Tamborlane WV. Prospective clinical trial of human growth hormone in short children without growth hormone deficiency. J Pediatr 1984; 104(2):172–176.

2. Genentech Collaborative Study Group. Idiopathic short stature: results of a one-year controlled study of human growth hormone treatment. J Pediatr 1989; 115(5):713–719.

3. Wit JM, Fokker MH, de Munick Keizer-Schrama SMPF, et al. Effects of two years of methionyl growth hormone therapy in two dosage regimens in prepubertal children with short stature, subnormal growth rate, and normal growth hormone response to secretogogues. J Pediatr 1989; 115(5):720–725.

4. Allen DB, Fost NC. Growth hormone therapy for short stature: panacea or Pandora's box? J Pediatr 1990; 117:16–21.

5. Bercu BB. Growth hormone treatment and the short child: to treat or not to treat? J Pediatr 1987; 10:991–995.

6. Grumbach M. Growth hormone therapy and the short end of the stick. N Engl J Med 1988; 319:238–240.

7. Ritzen EM, Albertsson-Wikland K, eds. Growth hormone treatment of short stature. State of the art in 1989. Acta Pediatr Scand 1989; 362(Suppl):1–60.

8. Lippe B, Frasier SD. How should we test growth hormone deficiency, and who should we treat? J Pediatr 1989; 115:585–587.

9. Lantos J, Siegler M, Cuttler L. Ethical issues in growth hormone therapy. JAMA 1989; 261:1020–1024.

10. Allen DB, Fost N, Blizzard RM, eds. Access to treatment with human growth hormone: medical, ethical, and social issues. Growth Genet Horm 1992; 8(Suppl 1):1–77.

11. Hopwood N, Hintz RL, Gertner JM, et al. Growth response of children with non-growth-hormone-deficiency and marked short stature during three years of growth hormone therapy. J Pediatr 1993; 123:215–222.

12. Stone R. NIH to size up growth hormone trials. Science 1992; 257:739.

13. Meyer-Bahlburg HFL. Short stature: psychological issues. In: Lifshitz F, ed. Pediatric Endocrinology. A Clinical Guide, 2nd ed. New York: Marcel Dekker, 1990:173–196.

14. Siegel PT, Hopwood NJ. The relationship of academic achievement and the intellectual functioning and affective conditions of hypopituitary children. In: Stabler B, Underwood LE, eds. Slow Grows the Child: Psychosocial Aspects of Growth Delay. Hillsdale, NJ: Erlbaum, 1986:57–71.

15. Kusalic M, Fortin C. Growth hormone treatment in hypopituitary dwarfs: longitudinal psychological effects. Can Psychiatric Assoc J 1975; 20:325–331.

16. Pollitt E, Money J. Studies in the psychology of dwarfism. I. Intelligence quotient and school achievement. J Pediatr 1964; 64:415–421.

17. Money J, Pollitt E. Studies in the psychology of dwarfism. II. Personality maturation and response to growth hormone treatment in hypopituitary dwarrfs. J Pediatr 1966; 68:381–390.

18. Rotnem D, Genel M, Hintz RL, Cohen DJ. Personality development in children with growth hormone deficiency. J Am Acad Child Psychiatry 1977; 16:412–426.

19. Rotnem D, Cohen DJ, Hintz R, Genel M. Psychological sequelae of relative "treatment failure" for children receiving growth hormone replacement. J Am Acad Child Psychiatry 1979; 18:505–520.

20. Drash PW, Greenberg NE, Money J. Intelligence and personality in four syndromes of dwarfism. In: Gardner LI, ed. Endocrine and Genetic Diseases of Childhood. Philadelphia: W. B. Saunders, 1969:1014–1022.

21. Weinberg MS. The problems of midgets and dwarfs and organizational remedies: a study of the Little People of America. J Health Social Behav 1968; 9:65–71.

22. Downey J, Ehrhardt AA, Gruen R, Bell JJ, Morishima A. Psychopathology and social functioning in women with Turner syndrome. J Nerv Ment Dis 1989; 177:191–201.

23. Meyer-Bahlburg HFL, Feinman JA, MacGillivray MH, Aceto T Jr. Growth hormone deficiency, brain development, and intelligence. Am J Dis Child 1978; 132:565–572.

24. Galatzer A, Aran O, Beit-Halachmi N, et al. The impact of long-term therapy by a multidisciplinary team on the education, occupation and marital status of growth hormone deficient patients after termination of therapy. Clin Endocrinol (Oxf) 1987; 27:191–196.

25. Abbott D, Rotnem D, Genel M, Cohen DJ. Cognitive and emotional functioning in hypopituitary short-statured children. Schizophr Bull 1982; 8:310–319.

26. Stabler B, Clopper RR, Siegel PT, Stoppani C, Compton PG, Underwood LE. Academic achievement and psychological adjustment in short children. J Dev Behav Pediatr 1994; 15:1–6.

27. August GP, Lippe BM, Blethen SL, et al. Growth hormone treatment in the United States: demographic and diagnostic features of 2331 children. J Pediatr 1990; 116:899–903.

28. Holmes CS, Thompson RG, Hayford JT. Factors related to grade retention in children with short stature. Child Care Health Dev 1984; 10:199–210.

29. Dean HJ, McTaggert TL, Fish DG, Friesen HG. The educational, vocational, and marital status of growth hormone-deficient adults treated with growth hormone during childhood. Am J Dis Child 1985; 139:1105–1110.

30. Holmes CS, Karlsson JA, Thompson RG. Longitudinal evaluation of behavior patterns in children with short stature. In: Stabler B, Underwood LE, eds. Slow Grows the Child: Psychosocial Aspects of Growth Delay. Hillsdale, NJ: Erlbaum, 1986:1–12.

31. Rovet JF. The cognitive and neuropsychological characteristics of females with Turner syndrome. In: Berch DB, Berger BG, eds. Sex chromosome abnormalities and human behavior. Boulder, CO: Westview, 1990:38–77.

32. Rovet JF. The psychoeducational characteristics of children with Turner syndrome. J Learn Disabil 1993; 26:333–341.

33. Laron Z, Galatzer A. Effect of hGH on head circumference and IQ in isolated growth hormone deficiency. Early Hum Dev 1981; 5:211–214.

34. Smith MO, Shaywitz SE, Shaywitz BA, Gertner JM, Raskin LA, Gelwan EM. Exogenous growth hormone levels predict attentional performance: a preliminary report. J Dev Behav Pediatr 1985; 6:273–278.

35. Almqvist O, Thorén M, Sääf M, Eriksson O. Effects of growth hormone substitution on mental performance in adults with growth hormone deficiency: a pilot study. Psychoneuroendocrinology 1986; 11:347–352.

36. Weinberg WA, Dietz SG, Penick EC, McAlister WH. Intelligence, reading achievement, physical size, and social class. J Pediatr 1974; 85:482–489.

37. Richards GE, Marshall RN, Kreuser IL. Effect of stature on school performance. J Pediatr 1985; 106:841–842.

38. Wilson DM, Hammer LD, Duncan PM, et al. Growth and intellectual development. Pediatrics 1986; 78:646–650.

39. Vance MD, Ingersoll G, Golden M. Short stature and psychosocial risk in a non-clinical sample. Paper presented at the Biennial Meeting of the Society for Research in Child Development, Seattle WA, 1991.

40. Vance, MD. Short stature and psychosocial risks in a nonclinical sample. Proceedings of the Fourth North Coast Conference of the Society of Pediatric Psychology, Amherst, NY, 1992.

41. Voss LD, Bailey BJR, Mulligan J, Wilkin TJ, Betts PR. Short stature and school performance—the Wessex Growth Study. Acta Pediatr Scand 1991; 377(Suppl):29–31.

42. Achenbach T, Edelbrock C. Manual for the Child Behavior Checklist and Revised Child Behavior Profile. Burlington, VT: University of Vermont Department of Psychiatry, 1983.

43. Sandberg DE, Meyer-Bahlburg, HFL, Yager, TJ. The Child Behavior Checklist nonclinical standardization samples: should they be utilized as norms? J Am Acad Child Adolesc Psychiatry 1991; 30:124–134.

44. Costello EJ, Edelbrock C, Costello AJ, Dulcan MK, Burns BJ, Brent D. Psychopathology in pediatric primary care: the new hidden morbidity. Pediatrics 1988; 82:415–424.

45. Zimet G, Cutler M, Owens R, Dahms W, Litvene M, Cuttler L. Psychosocial functioning of adults who were short as children. Paper presented at the Growth, Stature and Adaptation Symposium, Chapel Hill, NC, 1993.

46. Voss LD, Mulligan J. The short "normal" child in school: self-esteem, behavior and school performance before puberty (the Wessex Growth Study). Paper presented at the Growth, Stature and Adaptation Symposium, Chapel Hill, NC, 1993.

47. Campani GV, Vimpani AI, Lidgard GP, Cameron E, Farquhar JW. Prevalence of severe growth hormone deficiency. BMJ 1977; 2:427–430.

48. Lacey KA, Parkin JM. The normal short child. Community study of children in Newcastle-upon-Tyne. Arch Dis Child 1974; 49:417–424.

49. Sandberg DE, Brook AE, Campos SP. Short stature: a psychosocial burden requiring growth hormone therapy? Pediatrics 1994; 94:832–840.

50. Achenbach T. Manual for the Child Behavior Checklist/4-18 and 1991 Profile. Burlington, VT: University of Vermont Department of Psychiatry, 1991.

51. Achenbach TM. Manual for the Youth Self-Report and 1991 Profile. Burlington, VT: University of Vermont Department of Psychiatry, 1991.

52. Sandberg DE, Brook AE, Campos SP. Short stature in middle childhood: a survey of psychosocial functioning in a clinic-referred sample. Paper presented at the Growth, Stature and Adaptation Symposium, Chapel Hill, NC, 1993.

53. Clopper RR, Meyer WJ III, Udvarhelyi GB, et al. Postsurgical IQ and behavioral data on twenty patients with a history of childhood craniopharyngioma. Psychoneuroendocrinology 1977; 2:365–372.

54. Blizzard RM, Bulatovic A. Psychosocial short stature: a syndrome with many variables. Ballieres Clin Endocrinol Metab 1992; 6:687–712.

12

Tall Stature and Excessive Growth Syndromes

S. Douglas Frasier
UCLA School of Medicine,
Los Angeles, California

I. INTRODUCTION

Tall stature and excessive growth are relatively rare concerns in pediatric and pediatric endocrine practice. Nevertheless, an important group of pathologic conditions and variants in the pattern of normal growth and development are first brought to the physician's attention by these complaints. The causes of excessive growth that are important in children and adolescents are shown in Table 1. This presentation considers growth hormone excess, the nonendocrine disorders listed in Table 1, and constitutional tall stature. Disorders of sexual maturation are discussed elsewhere in this volume.

II. GROWTH HORMONE EXCESS

As recently reviewed (1) and is exemplified by several single case reports (2–9), growth hormone excess, although rare, must be considered a cause of tall stature and rapid growth in all patients with these symptoms.

A. Etiology and Pathogenesis

Excessive growth hormone secretion is generally associated with a functioning pituitary adenoma. These tumors usually take up the eosin present in standard stains and are classified as eosinophilic adenomas. However, the tumor may be chromophobic and not take any stain. In these instances, the final diagnosis may depend on electron microscopy. If growth hormone excess is present, the pituitary tumor contains typical growth hormone secretory granules. Occasionally, the tumor secretes excess prolactin in addition to growth hormone (10,11) and prolactin secretory granules are also demonstrated. A growth hormone-secreting pituitary adenoma is usually present as an isolated abnormality, but associations occur with McCune-Albright syndrome (12–14) and tuberous sclerosis (15).

As with all functioning endocrine tumors, the specific pathogenesis of growth hormone-secreting adenomas is not completely understood. In some patients, the excess secretion of GH may be caused by unrestrained stimulation of the somatotrophs by growth hormone-releasing hormone (16). Impaired somatostatin (somatotropin release inhibiting factor) secretion is also a theoretical etiologic consideration. Various mutations in the gene for the α subunit of the stimulatory G protein, which increases cyclic AMP formation, have been demonstrated in growth hormone-secreting pituitary adenomas (17–19). These putative oncogenes may cause somatotropin hyperplasia and the development of an adenoma through the unrestrained production of cyclic AMP, which leads to an increase in both cell growth and cell function. A specific constitutive G protein α gene mutation leading to the substitution of histidine or cysteine for arginine at position 201 has been demonstrated in patients with McCune-Albright syndrome and pituitary adenoma (20).

B. Clinical Manifestations

Growth hormone excess leads to either gigantism or acromegaly, depending on whether the epiphyses are open or closed. Typically, gigantism is produced in young children and acromegaly is seen in adults. The adolescent who still has open epiphyses shows a mixed picture of rapid growth and acromegalic features—acromegalic gigantism (Fig. 1).

Young patients with excess growth hormone secretion both are tall and grow at a rate that is greater than normal for their age. Their growth curve progressively deviates from normal. When growth hormone excess begins during adolescence, there is enlargement of the lower jaw, hands, and feet in addition to the rapid increase in height.

Rarely, this clinical picture may be imitated by the syndrome of pseudoacromegaly or acromegaloidism in which growth hormone secretion is normal but other non–growth hormone-dependent growth factors may be present in excess (21).

Table 1 Causes of Tall Stature and Excessive Growth

I. Endocrine disorders
    A. Growth hormone excess
    B. Disorders of sexual maturation
        1. Precocious puberty
        2. Virilization
        3. Feminization
        4. Hypogonadism
II. Nonendocrine disorders
    A. Cerebral gigantism (Sotos syndrome)
    B. Klinefelter syndrome
    C. XYY males
    D. Marfan syndrome
    E. Homocystinuria
III. Normal variants: constitutional tall stature

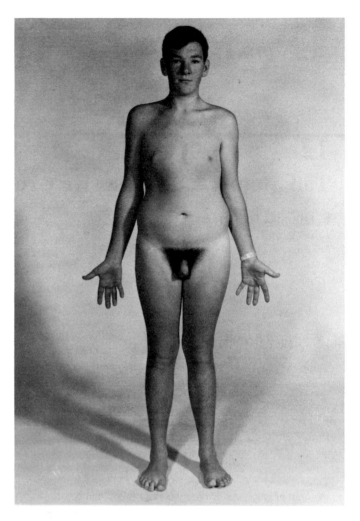

Figure 1 A 17-year-6-month-old boy with growth hormone excess caused by a pituitary adenoma. Height was 193 cm, and weight was 108.3 kg. (Previously published in Frasier SD, Pediatric Endocrinology. New York: Grune and Stratton, 1980.)

Expanding adenomas may interfere with the secretion of one or more pituitary trophic hormones. Thus, a growth hormone-secreting adenoma may be associated with gonadotropin deficiency leading to delayed or arrested puberty and, less often, adrenocorticotropic hormone and/or thyroid-stimulating hormone deficiency. When there is combined growth hormone excess and gonadotropin deficiency, patients may show both excessive growth and eunuchoid body proportions.

Impaired vision and visual field abnormalities may accompany growth hormone excess. The characteristic abnormality is bitemporal homonymous hemianopsia ("tunnel vision") because of midline compression of the optic chiasm. However, a wide variety of visual field defects may be produced depending on the size and location of the tumor. Expanding intrasellar tumors may also lead to increased intracranial pressure and/or symptoms of hypothalamic dysfunction.

C. Diagnosis

The clinical diagnosis of growth hormone (GH) excess is confirmed by demonstrating an elevated serum concentration of growth hormone that is not suppressed by raising the concentration of blood glucose during performance of a standard glucose tolerance test. The administration of glucose by mouth in a dose of 1.75 g/kg, up to a maximum of 100 g, raises the blood glucose concentration to a level that suppresses the serum GH concentration to less than 5 ng/ml in normal persons. The lowest concentration of GH is seen between 60 and 120 minutes after the ingestion of glucose. Failure to suppress the serum concentration of GH supports the diagnosis of growth hormone excess as a result of hypothalamic or pituitary dysfunction (3). Confirmation of the diagnosis is also aided by demonstrating an elevated serum somatomedin C (insulin-like growth factor type I, IGF-I) concentration (22). The level of growth hormone activity may be better correlated with the somatomedin C concentration than with the concentration of growth hormone after glucose suppression.

In at least 25% of patients there is glucose intolerance and hyperinsulinism. There are also failure to increase the serum concentration of growth hormone above the already elevated levels in response to hypoglycemia and relative resistance to the hypoglycemic effects of exogenous insulin.

When growth hormone excess is confirmed, the possibility of pituitary trophic hormone deficiencies should be investigated by performing standard tests of pituitary function.

Complete neuroradiologic studies aimed at demonstrating the size and location of the pituitary adenoma are essential in planning therapy. Recommended studies include skull films, cone-down views of the sella turcica, sellar polytomography, computed tomography (CT), and magnetic resonance imaging (MRI). Of these, MRI is the preferred technology.

D. Treatment

Treatment is directed at eliminating excess growth hormone secretion (23). In the past this has meant destruction of the tumor, and a number of ablative techniques have been employed. Radiation from an external source is least effective. Transsphenoidal microsurgery appears to offer the best possibility of complete removal of the tumor with preservation of remaining pituitary function. This technique is particularly useful when small tumors without extrasellar extension are the source of the excess GH secretion (24). When the tumor is too large for this approach, a craniotomy with direct visualization and removal of the tumor must be performed.

Recent interest has focused on pharmacologic management of growth hormone excess with the dopamine receptor agonist, bromocriptine, or with a long-acting analog of somatostatin, octreotide. Bromocriptine inhibits the secretion of both growth hormone and prolactin through direct effects on the pituitary. There is also evidence indicating an inhibitory effect on cell growth leading to a decrease in the size of some pituitary tumors. This agent has been used successfully in several children with growth hormone excess (25,26). In these patients, excess growth hormone secretion was partially inhibited and associated excess prolactin secretion was abolished. There was significant clinical improvement even though the suppression of GH secretion was incomplete. Between 10 and 20 mg/day of bromocriptine was therapeutic, and no significant side effects were observed.

Somatostatin is the potent inhibitor of growth hormone secretion that was initially isolated from the hypothalamus. It is present in a variety of tissues and has a generalized inhibitory activity, particularly on the secretion of insulin. Although native somatostatin inhibits GH secretion in acromegaly, its effect is very short-lived and variable effects on glucose metabolism are induced by somatostatin administration. Octreotide, which may be given every 6–8 h and which has relatively little effect on insulin secretion, has been found to be useful in the management of GH excess. This agent has now been administered to pediatric patients with growth hormone-producing tumors (8,27,28). Effective doses were 50–100 μg given every 6–8 h. Side effects have been minimal, and both growth hormone secretion and pituitary tumor size have decreased significantly in response to octreotide administration.

E. Prognosis

The rarity of growth hormone excess and the very recent application of transsphenoidal surgery and medical suppression of growth hormone secretion make generalizations regarding the prognosis of GH excess in children and adolescents difficult. However, a report from Manchester, England (29) describes the serious physical and psychologic disability observed in 10 untreated or partially treated patients. Marked skeletal deformity and psychologic problems were common. More aggressive therapy and current methods of management may improve this poor outcome.

III. CEREBRAL GIGANTISM: SOTOS SYNDROME

Cerebral gigantism is a clinical syndrome of rapid growth in infancy, dysmorphic features, and a nonprogressive neurologic disorder first described by Sotos and others in 1964 (30). Since this initial description, over 100 patients have been reported in numerous case reports and in several reviews (31–33).

A. Etiology and Pathogenesis

The underlying cause(s) of cerebral gigantism are not understood. Most instances of this syndrome are sporadic, but there have been reports of familial occurrence and dominant inheritance has been suggested in at least four families (34,35). In addition, there have been reports of the syndrome in first cousins, siblings in a highly inbred family, and monozygotic twins (32), suggesting the possibility of recessive inheritance. One report identified fragile X chromosomes in two affected patients (36), but this appears to be a fortuitous association. These data clearly suggest genetic heterogeneity as well as clinical heterogeneity in cerebral gigantism and make a single etiology unlikely.

The constellation of abnormalities suggests hypothalamic dysfunction, but no specific neuropathologic lesions have been identified (37). Extensive investigation has not shown any consistent abnormality of growth hormone secretion or somatomedin concentration. Although it is possible that other abnormal growth factors are present, they have not yet been identified.

B. Clinical Manifestations

The major clinical manifestations of cerebral gigantism are shown in Table 2 (31). Patients are often large at birth in terms of both weight and length (33), and growth is rapid during the first year. By 1 year of age most patients are above the 97th percentile height for age and sex. Growth velocity also exceeds the 97th percentile. Rapid growth continues for the first 3–4 years (Fig. 2). Body proportions are abnormal, arm span exceeding height by as much as 5 cm. This

Table 2 Cerebral Gigantism: Clinical Manifestations (%)

Gigantism	100
Rapid growth in infancy	100
Prominent forehead	96
High-arched palate	96
Hyperteleorism	91
Long head	84
Pointed chin	83
Developmental retardation	83
Advanced bone age	74
Impaired fine motor control	52
Neonatal irritability	44
Feeding problems	44

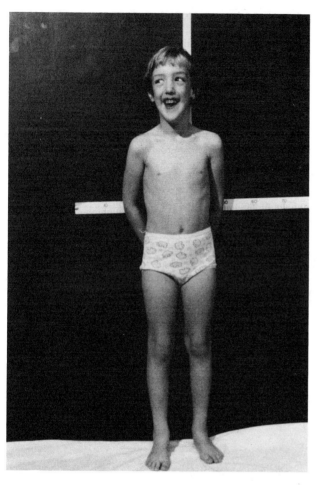

Figure 2 A 4 year 9 month old girl with cerebral gigantism. Height was 55.7 cm (height age 11 years 9 months), and weight was 33.7 kg (weight age 10 years, 10 months). Developmental level was 3 to 3 years, 6 months. (Courtesy of Juan F. Sotos, MD, Children's Hospital, Columbus, Ohio.)

difference is normally negative up to age 12 and exceeds 2 cm only in males older than 13 or 14 years (31).

Fine motor control is impaired in infancy and early childhood, and developmental milestones are delayed. Intellectual impairment is mild to moderate, with median IQ score between 70 and 75 (31,38). The neonatal period is characterized by irritability and feeding problems in addition to large size.

The bone age is generally advanced between 1 and 2 years. Mildly dilated cerebral ventricles are present in the majority of patients when they are studied by pneumoencephalography or CT scanning.

C. Diagnosis

The diagnosis depends on the characteristic clinical picture. There are no definitive physical findings and no specific laboratory results.

D. Treatment

Treatment is directed at improving the level of motor and intellectual function, as is the case with any child who manifests developmental delay and intellectual handicap. Modification of ultimate height might be considered under very unusual circumstances (see later).

E. Prognosis

The prognosis for normal adult intellectual function is poor even in the best of circumstances. Few patients have been followed to final height, but predicted height exceeds 200 cm (6 feet 6 inches) in many of them. Concern has been expressed that patients with cerebral gigantism may be particularly susceptible to the development of tumors (33,39). This may represent another facet of growth without proper control that may be the basic mechanism underlying this and other overgrowth syndromes.

IV. KLINEFELTER SYNDROME

Klinefelter syndrome is a relatively common abnormality in phenotypic males occurring in between 1:500 and 1:1000 live males births (40,41). It may present in a variety of different ways, but tall stature is a frequent finding in both children and adolescents (Chap. 18).

A. Etiology and Pathogenesis

Klinefelter syndrome is caused by an abnormality in chromosome number in which two or more X chromosomes are present in male patients. By far the most usual abnormal karyotype is 47, XXY. Mosaic karyotypes, however, such as XY/XXY, have also been described, as have other aneuploid karyotypes, such as 48, XXXY or 49, XXXXY. The presence of one or more extra X chromosomes is associated with testicular failure, which results in infertility and impaired testosterone production. The testes show hyalinization and fibrosis of the seminiferous tubules, with histologically intact interstitial cells.

B. Clinical Manifestations

Klinefelter syndrome is infrequently diagnosed in prepubertal children. Several clinical clues point to this diagnosis, however, which should lead to appropriate laboratory evaluation (40). Prepubertal boys with an extra X chromosome are often tall for their age. Body proportions are often abnormal, with relatively long legs reflected in a low upper/lower segment ratio. Patients tend to be thin and underweight for height and age. Genital abnormalities, such as small phallus, hypospadias, and cryptorchidism, may be present. The testes are often normal in size before puberty, but they are abnormally small (<2 ml in volume) in a few patients. The major means of finding Klinefelter syndrome before puberty is studying boys with mental retardation or school and/or behavior difficulties.

Learning and psychologic problems are common in this group of children.

Adolescent patients with Klinefelter syndrome are usually taller than expected for their age and have eunuchoid proportions, with a long arm span and long leg length. The latter leads to a diminished upper/lower body segment ratio (42).

The testes are disproportionately small for the level of pubertal development. Testicular development begins with the onset of puberty but regresses by midadolescence, and testicular volume rarely exceeds 2–3 ml. Testicular length is generally below 2.0 cm. The testes are usually firm and show diminished sensitivity to pressure. Androgen function is initially preserved, and almost all boys enter puberty. Penile development and the development of public hair are generally satisfactory. However, oligospermia or aspermia are uniformly present. Adolescent development may be delayed, and impotence or other problems with sexual function may develop (42–44).

Gynecomastia is common. This begins as simple adolescent breast enlargement but is often marked and persistent. It is frequently the reason for seeking medical advice and is very distressing to most patients.

As a group, patients with Klinefelter syndrome have lower than expected verbal intelligence quotient scores and a significant increase in learning, behavioral, and psychosocial problems (45,46).

C. Diagnosis

The clinical picture of tall stature, gynecomastia, and small testes in a male with adequate secondary sex characteristics is often diagnostic. The clinical diagnosis of Klinefelter syndrome is confirmed by the demonstration of one or more extra X chromosomes in the karyotype. Primary gonadal failure is reflected in elevated serum concentrations of pituitary gonadotropins. Although both luteinizing hormone and follicle-stimulating hormone (FSH) are elevated, the major increase is in FSH (43,44). Testosterone concentrations are variable but usually in the low normal adult male range (43). Average concentrations are clearly below those seen in normal adolescent boys (42).

D. Treatment

The administration of testosterone may be helpful when adolescent development is delayed or when sexual function is impaired. Full replacement therapy with 200–400 mg long-acting, intramuscular testosterone every 3 or 4 weeks should be given to restore serum testosterone concentrations to the normal range. Gynecomastia may require surgical therapy with simple mammoplasty using a circumareolar incision.

E. Prognosis

Some patients function quite normally, but impaired intellectual function and psychosocial difficulties persist in a signif-

icant number. Sexual function may be impaired, and fertility is not restored by any currently available therapy.

V. THE XYY SYNDROME

The presence of an extra Y chromosome also predisposes to tall stature (45,47). Males with the XYY syndrome are relatively common in the general population. Newborn screening studies indicate an incidence of between 1:500 and 1:1000 live male births (41). Although there is no uniform phenotypic expression of this abnormal karyotype, the incidence is mugh higher when males whose height exceeds 183 cm (72 inches) are screened.

In addition to tall structure, there appear to be few phenotypic expressions of the XYY syndrome. Those that have been described include severe acne, hypospadias and/or cryptorchidism, radioulnar synostosis, and mild or moderate mental retardation (45,46,48,49). The finding of an XYY karyotype in a newborn does not necessarily predict intellectual function or behavior. Generalizations cannot be made regarding the correlation between karyotype and behavioral phenotype (45,46).

VI. MARFAN SYNDROME

Marfan syndrome is a heritable disorder of connective tissue in which tall stature is one of a spectrum of abnormalities that lead to significant morbidity and early mortality.

A. Etiology and Pathogenesis

Marfan syndrome is an autosomal dominant disorder. In 65–75% of patients one parent is affected, and sporadic new mutations account for 25–35% of patients. There is a 50% recurrence risk in the offspring of affected individuals. The degree of expression and severity of clinical features may vary from family to family, but involvement in a particular individual cannot be predicted from knowledge of the family history.

Marfan syndrome is caused by mutations in the fibrillin gene (50,51), located on chromosome 15 (52). The affected gene product, fibrillin, a 350 kD glycoprotein, is a structural component of a microfibril, the elastin-associated microfibril, found in the extracellular matrix of connective tissue. Patients with Marfan syndrome have a deficiency of elastin-associated microfibrils that leads to the clinical manifestations of this disorder (53).

B. Clinical Manifestations

A complex constellation of abnormalities characterize Marfan syndrome. As shown in Table 3, the skeletal, ocular, and cardiovascular systems are involved (54,55).

Height is increased, and body proportions are abnormal. Both arm and leg length are greater than normal, so that arm span is significantly greater than height and the upper/lower segment ratio is diminished. *Arachnodactyly*, long fingers and

Table 3 Marfan Syndrome: Clinical Manifestations

Skeletal
    Tall stature
    Long, thin extremities
    Long fingers (arachnodactyly)
    Loose joints
    Scoliosis
    Pectus deformity

Ocular
    Flat cornea
    Dislocated lens
    Myopia
    Retinal detachment

Cardiovascular
    Diffuse aortic aneurysm
    Dissecting aortic aneurysm
    Mitral regurgitation

toes, is seen in the majority of patients. There is often a pectus excavatum chest deformity, and scoliosis is common. The joints are hyperextensible and lax.

Ocular abnormalities are extremely common. The cornea is flat, and congenital subluxation of the lens with upward displacement is frequently present. The ability to accommodate is retained. Refractive errors, particularly myopia, are present in many patients. Retinal detachment is a common complication.

The shortened life span of patients with Marfan syndrome is a result of its cardiovascular manifestations. The combination of physical examination and echocardiography shows some abnormality in almost all patients. Both aortic and mitral regurgitation are present. Aortic root dilatation is seen relatively early when sophisticated diagnostic tools are employed. Aortic regurgitation, dissection, and rupture are major life-threatening complications (56).

C. Diagnosis

The characteristic familial, musculoskeletal, ocular, and cardiovascular manifestations of Marfan syndrome are usually diagnostic. Specific molecular diagnosis, although possible, is not yet generally available. Careful measurements including assessment of body proportions, ocular examination, including slit lamp evaluation, and cardiovascular studies, including echocardiography, should allow the clinician to make the correct diagnosis once it is considered a possibility.

D. Treatment

There is no specific treatment, although several approaches may reduce the morbidity and perhaps even the mortality of patients with Marfan syndrome (55). Early recognition and correction of a refractive error prevent the amblyopia that

often limits vision. Prevention or correction of scoliosis and repair of the pectus deformity may be very helpful.

When significant aortic regurgitation is noted, an aortic valve prosthesis may be utilized. Progressive aortic dilatation may be managed by graft placement. Attempts have been made to limit progression of aortic dilatation by administering propranolol or some other β-adrenergic blocking agent. Theoretically this decreases left ventricular ejection impulse and protects the aortic root from a maximal exposure to left ventricular pressure. It remains to be seen whether such a therapy is effective.

E. Prognosis

The life expectancy of patients with Marfan syndrome is about half that in the general population. Half of affected males are dead by age 40–45, and half of affected females die by age 50–55. In over 95% of patients death is a result of cardiovascular complications (56).

VII. HOMOCYSTINURIA

Homocystinuria caused by a deficiency of cystathionine β-synthase is an unusual disorder of amino acid metabolism (57) in which the phenotype has a significant resemblance to Marfan syndrome. It also carries a significant morbidity and mortality (58–60).

A. Etiology and Pathogenesis

Cystathionine β-synthase deficiency is inherited as an autosomal recessive inborn metabolic error. The recurrence rate is 25% for each pregnancy when both parents are carriers. This enzyme is active in the pathway through which methionine is converted to cystine. It catalyzes the metabolic step at which homocystine and serine combine to form cystathionine. When the enzyme is deficient, homocystine and methionine accumulate in plasma and homocystinuria is seen. The plasma concentrations of cystathionine and cystine are markedly reduced. There is a significant quantitive and, probably, qualitative heterogeneity in the enyme deficiency. The most clear example of this is the dichotomy between patients in whom the administration of pyridoxine (vitamin B_6) leads to correction of the medical abnormality and those in whom it does not. There is apparent segregation of these two types of abnormality among affected families (59,60).

B. Clinical Manifestations

The clinical manifestations of homocystinuria are shown in Table 4. In addition to tall stature and marfanoid habitus, patients with homocystinuria show abnormalities that involve multiple organ systems. The eye, the nervous system, the skeleton, and the vascular system are all affected. Patients are usually normal at birth, and the clinical manifestations come to the physician's attention in the first few years of life.

Mental retardation is very frequent and is often the presenting abnormality. The original patients were found by

Table 4 Homocystinuria: Clinical Manifestations

Tall stature
Marfanoid habitus
Mental retardation
Dislocated lens
Osteoporosis
Thrombosis

screening a population of retarded children for aminoaciduria. Convulsions are seen in 10–20% of patients.

The optic lens is dislocated in the majority of patients. Displacement is usually downward, and the eyes lose their ability to accommodate. There are marked myopia and astigmatism. Osteoporosis, scoliosis, and vertebral collapse may be seen.

Thromboembolic phenomena, especially in the postoperative period, are life-threatening complications. Both arterial and venous occlusion are seen, and sudden death may result. Heterozygotes develop premature thrombotic disease affecting the coronary, cerebral, and peripheral arteries (61).

C. Diagnosis

Cystathionine β-synthase deficiency may be suspected on the basis of homocystinuria and elevated plasma concentrations of homocystine and methionine. Plasma cystine concentrations are low. Confirmation depends on demonstrating deficiency of cystathionine β-synthase in liver biopsy, cultured phytohemagglutinin-stimulated lymphocytes, or skin fibroblasts.

D. Treatment

Dietary methionine is restricted, and dietary cystine is supplemented. Special synthetic diets that are virtually methionine free are generally used.

All patients should be given a trial of therapy with pyridoxine. Patients should not be considered pyridoxine unresponsive until 500–1000 mg pyridoxine each day for 3–4 weeks is shown to be ineffective. Responsive patients can usually be managed with 150–250 mg pyridoxine daily.

E. Prognosis

Methionine restriction ameliorates mental retardation when it is begun after diagnosis on the basis of newborn screening. When patients are not diagnosed in the newborn period, a significant number are mentally retarded and have other complications by age 15. The prognosis also depends significantly on whether the patient is pyridoxine responsive (59). Lens dislocation, osteoporosis, and late thromboembolic phenomenon are less frequent in B$_6$-responsive patients. However, there is an increase in mortality as a result of thromboembolism in both responsive and nonresponsive pa-

tients. Almost 25% of nonresponsive patients and 5% of responsive patients die by age 30.

VIII. BECKWITH-WIEDEMANN SYNDROME

Beckwith-Wiedemann syndrome (BWS) (62,63), which is also termed exomphalos-macroglossia-gigantism syndrome, is generally recognized in the neonatal period on the basis of a characteristic phenotype, which includes somatic overgrowth and hypoglycemia.

A. Etiology and Pathogenesis

Beckwith-Wiedemann syndrome is a genetically determined set of phenotypic features in which there are abnormalities of a region of the short arm of chromosome 11, 11p15.5 (64,65). This disorder is an example of chromosomal imprinting in which the abnormality is derived from only the male or female parent. In BWS the abnormality is paternal (66–68), and affected patients show either trisomy for this region, the duplication arising in the father, or paternal disomy for this region, with loss of the maternal chromosome contribution. The specific gene or genes that are duplicated have not yet been determined, but the IGF-II gene is the putative candidate. The IGF-II gene or some other growth promoter appears to be the probable cause of the characteristic phenotype of this disorder.

B. Clinical Manifestations

The typical clinical appearance of patients with Beckwith-Wiedemann syndrome (Table 5) includes macroglossia, umbilical abnormalities, such as ompholocele, umbilical hernia, and diastasis recti, cranofacial anomalies, such as midface hypoplasia, prominent occiput, flat nasal bridge, and high-arched palate, increased birth weight and postnatal gigantism, earlobe anomalies that include groves, pits, and notches, enlarged liver, kidneys, and other organs, facial flame nevus, and hyperinsulinemic hypoglycemia. A significant number of patients have somatic assymetry, which may be associated with the development of various cancers, particularly neph-

Table 5 Beckwith-Wiedemann Syndrome: Major Clinical Manifestations (%)

Macroglossia	95
Craniofacial anomalies	80
Visceromegaly	80
Umbilical anomalies	75
Earlobe anomalies	70
Increased birth weight	60
Postnatal gigantism	60
Facial flame nevus	60
Hypoglycemia	55
Cardiac defects	35

roblastoma (Wilms' tumor), adrenocortical carcinoma, hepatoblastoma, and rhabdomyosarcoma (69,70).

Hypoglycemia, if it is present, usually occurs in the first few days of life. It is extremely important to recognize and manage this feature of BWS as soon as possible to prevent subsequent brain damage, developmental delay, and microcephaly, which may result from an unrecognized chronic low blood glucose concentration. Blood glucose should be monitored frequently during the first 72 h of life in all neonates showing the clinical features of this disorder (Chap. 49).

C. Diagnosis

As with other dysmorphic syndromes, the diagnosis of BWS depends on a characteristic clinical picture rather than on any specific diagnostic test. Demonstration of the underlying genetic abnormalities requires extremely sophisticated methodology that is beyond the scope of a standard clinical or genetics laboratory. The major features (Table 5) should be present before a diagnosis of BWS is assigned to an individual patient.

D. Treatment

Treatment is directed at specific features of this syndrome. Surgical repair of umbilical abnormalities is sometimes necessary. Management of associated cardiac anomalies depends on the nature of the defect and on whether cardiac failure is present. Associated tumors require specific management plans.

Because the pathogenesis of the neonatal hypoglycemia of BWS is hyperinsulinism, treatment is directed at reducing the excess insulin secretion. A number of agents, such as glucocorticoids, Susphrine®, and zinc glucagon, have been employed, but most effective medical management has been with diazoxide. Subtotal pancreatectomy is reserved for patients who are not made normoglycemic with diazoxide therapy.

E. Prognosis

There is a very high mortality rate in infancy among BWS patients, 20–25% dying by age 1 year (62). The causes of death are not well documented, but associated heart disease and unrecognized hypoglycemia are significant contributors. Very little information is available regarding patients with Beckwith-Wiedemann syndrome beyond infancy. Patients generally continue to grow excessively, and the majority remain above the 95th percentile for height and weight through adolescence. Intellectual function is variable, and delayed development is often seen when hypoglycemia has been recognized late or when its management has been suboptimal. When malignancies develop in BWS patients, the prognosis becomes that of the associated cancer.

IX. HEMIHYPERTROPHY

Hemihypertrophy, or asymmetric overgrowth, is of particular significance because of its association with malignancy. By far the most common associated cancer is Wilms' tumor (71). Other tumors that develop in patients with hemihypertrophy are adrenocortical carcinoma and adenoma, rhabdomyosarcoma, and hepatoblastoma. These cancers are the same as those noted in patients with Beckwith-Wiedemann syndrome. As in BWS, abnormalities of chromosome 11 at the 11p15.5 site are found in these tumors (66,72). By far the most significant aspect of hemihypertrophy is not the overgrowth itself but the development of malignancy. All such patients require close follow-up to discover these tumors at the earliest possible time.

X. CONSTITUTIONAL TALL STATURE

Constitutional tall structure is a variant of the normal pattern of childhood growth and development. Its incidence varies with the sociocultural definition of normal and the level of parental concern regarding height. In the past, pediatric endocrinologists were often asked to see tall girls whose tall mothers were concerned about their daughters finding suitable dance partners and husbands. A great deal of the initial concern over the patient's height reflected whatever problems her mother may have had as a tall adolescent and young adult. She anticipated that her daughter would have similar difficulties. As the role of women in U.S. society has expanded and as it has become first permitted and then fashionable for girls to be athletic and to concentrate on physical training, the frequency of this complaint has declined significantly. It has always been extremely unusual for American families to consider that their sons were too tall.

A. Etiology and Pathogenesis

The growth pattern of patients with constitutional tall stature follows that of one or both parents who are also tall. Thus, genetic and familial factors appear to play the most important role in etiology and pathogenesis.

Endocrinologic studies of tall children have yielded variable results. An increased serum concentration of growth hormone in response to both glucose loading (73,74) and the administration of thyrotropin-releasing hormone (74) has been demonstrated, and similar observations have been made in normal pubertal children (75). This apparent paradoxic growth hormone response may be a phenomenon of normal adolescence (75,76) and have no significance relative to tall structure.

B. Clinical Manifestations

Patient with constitutional tall structure are between 2 and 4 standard deviations above the average height for their age. Length is normal at birth, and tall stature is evident by age 3 or 4 years. Growth velocity is accelerated in early childhood but slows after 4 or 5 years of age, when the growth curve is parrallel to the normal curve (77). Body proportions are normal. There is the same variability in the timing of adolescent development as in children of average height, and the age of onset of puberty tends to follow the pattern characteristic of the patient's family.

C. Diagnosis

The diagnosis is generally clear from the family history, record of growth, and physical examination. Specific laboratory studies of endocrine function are rarely indicated. Bone age determination as part of the initial evaluation is essential so that the most accurate prediction of adult height can be given to the patient and the patient's family. The bone age shows the same variability as that in the general population of children. Advanced bone age is not associated with constitutional tall stature in the same way that delayed bone age is associated with constitutional short stature.

D. Treatment

Management of tall children and adolescents remains among the more controversial topics in pediatric endocrinology. Generally, therapy has been aimed at inducing incomplete precocious puberty and accelerating the rate of development of secondary sex characteristics through the pharmacologic administration of gonadal steroids. Theoretically, the acceleration of epiphyseal maturation that accompanies gonadal steroid administration should lead to early closure of the epiphyses. Somatomedin generation may also be inhibited by pharmacologic doses of estrogen (78).

A large number of reports have appeared describing the administration of estrogens in tall girls. A variety of preparations and dose schedules have been employed. These include injectable estradiol valerate (79,80), implanted estradiol pellets (81), and oral stilbestrol, 3 mg/day (82), diethylstibestrol, 5 mg/day (83), ethinyl estradiol, 0.1 mg/day (84), 0.25 mg/day (83), 0.3 mg/day (84,85), or 0.5 mg/day (84,86), and conjugated estrogens, 2.5–10.0 mg/day (78,87, 88). There is general agreement that a favorable effect on ultimate height results from such pharmacologic therapy (89). The overall average decrease in ultimate height has varied from 3.5 to 7.3 cm, and much greater effects have been claimed in selected patients. Most investigators believe that the effects are greatest when therapy is begun at a bone age below 12–13 years and/or a chronologic age below 11–12 years. The exact age at which estrogen treatment should be started and the predicted mature height that would serve as an indication for treatment remain in question.

Short-term side effects of estrogen administration include nausea, weight gain, pigmentation, leg cramps, and transient hypertension (78–88). There may be the induction of hyperlipidemia, glucose intolerance, or cholelithiasis. Thromboembolism is a potential hazard (90). During treatment, the gonadotropin response to gonadotropin-releasing hormone is uniformly suppressed (78,91). Menstrual function generally returns promptly after discontinuing estrogen administration, however, and fertility has been normal in treated patients. The overall late effects of pharmacologic estrogen administration on gonadal function and both genital tract and breast neoplasia are unknown.

There remains considerable disagreement regarding whether the benefits of the effect on ultimate height outweigh the risks of high-dose estrogen administration in young girls. I believe that too much is unknown with regard to the late effects of such therapy on reproductive function and the development of neoplasms of the breast and female genital tract. In my opinion, the potential risks outweigh the benefits. Girls with the Marfan syndrome and the potential development of scoliosis may be a special case (92). The difficulties a patient's tall stature present to her and, more often, to her mother can usually be dealt with through sympathetic support. Occasionally, more intensive individual or family psychotherapy is necessary.

Although tall stature has not been a complaint among adolescent boys in the United States, it has been a sufficient cause of concern in Europe to lead to gonadal steroid therapy (85,93). The administration of a long-acting intramuscular testosterone preparation, 500 mg every 2 or 3 weeks (mean dose 500 mg/m^2/month) has produced a significant reduction in predicted mature height. Long-term gonadal function was normal in treated boys. The same questions regarding benefits and risks, as well as the same psychologic considerations, apply to the treatment of tall boys as to tall girls.

Bromocriptine has also been used to treat tall patients. If growth hormone secretion were suppressed in tall adolescents while pubertal epiphyseal maturation progressed at a normal rate, ultimate height might be reduced. There are conflicting reports of the efficacy of bromocriptine in limiting adult height. An initial report suggested a significant effect (94), but subsequent studies have reported equivocal (95) or negative (96) results.

Recently octreotide was used in small groups of tall children to inhibit growth hormone secretion and growth velocity (97,98). Preliminary results suggest a role for this agent in the management of tall stature, but a great deal of additional data must accumulate before the administration of somatostatin analogs can be considered other than experimental therapy.

E. Prognosis

The long-term prognosis for mature height in a patient with constitutional tall stature is consistent with the height attained by the rest of the family. An accurate prognosis for ultimate height obtained as part of the initial evaluation often indicates that the patient will not be nearly as tall as the parents fear. In these instances, the prognosis becomes part of the supportive therapy given to the family.

ACKNOWLEDGMENT

Ms. Adrianna Gonzales provided invaluable and expert secretarial assistance.

REFERENCES

1. Daughaday WH. Pituitary gigantism. Endocrinol Metab Clin North Am 1992; 21:633–647.
2. Lopis S, Rubenstein AH. Measurements of serum growth

hormone and insulin in gigantism. J Clin Endocrinol Metab 1967; 28:393–398.

3. Frasier SD, Kogut MD. Adolescent acromegaly: studies of growth-hormone and insulin metabolism. J Pediatr 1968; 71:832–839.

4. Spence HJ, Trias EP, Raiti S. Acromegaly in a 9½ year old boy. Am J Dis Child 1972; 123:504–506.

5. AvRuskin TW, Sau K, Tang S, Juan C. Childhood acromegaly: successful therapy with conventional radiation and effects of chlorpromazine on growth hormone and prolactin secretion. J Clin Endocrinol Metabb 1973; 37:380–388.

6. Haigler ED Jr, Hershman JM, Meador CK. Pituitary gigantism. Arch Intern Med 1973; 132:588–594.

7. Blumberg DL, Sklar CA, David R, Rothenberg S, Bell J. Acromegaly in an infant. Pediatrics 1989; 83:998–1002.

8. Gelber SJ, Heffez DS, Donohoue PA. Pituitary gigantism caused by growth hormone excess from infancy. J Pediatr 1992; 120:931–934.

9. Lu PW, Silink M, Johnston I, Cowell CT, Jimenez M. Pituitary gigantism. Arch Dis Child 1992; 67:1039–41.

10. Guyda H, Robert F, Colle E, Hardy J. Histologic, ultrastructural, and hormonal characterization of a pituitary tumor secreting both hGH and prolactin. J Clin Endocrinol Metab 1973; 36:531–547.

11. Moran A, Asa SL, Kovacs K, et al. Gigantism due to pituitary mammosomatotroph hyperplasia. N Engl J Med 1990; 323: 322–327.

12. Joishy SK, Morrow LB. McCune-Albright syndrome associated with a functioning pituitary chromophobe adenoma. J Pediatr 1976; 89:73–75.

13. Lightner ES, Penny R, Frasier SD. Pituitary adenoma in McCune-Albright syndrome: follow-up information. J Pediatr 1976; 89:159.

14. Nakagawa H, Nagasaka A, Sugiura T, et al. Gigantism associated with McCune-Albright's syndrome. Horm Metab Res 1985; 17:522–527.

15. Hoffman WH, Perrin JCS, Halac E, Galla RR, England BG. Acromegalic gigantism and tuberous sclerosis. J Pediatr 1978; 93:478–480.

16. Zimmerman D, Young WF Jr, Ebersold MJ, et al. Congenital gigantism due to growth hormone releasing hormone excess and pituitary hyperplasia with adenomatous transformation. J Clin Endocrinol Metab 1993; 76:216–222.

17. Landis CA, Masters SB, Spada A, Pace AM, Bourne HR, Vallar L. GTPase inhibiting mutations activate the α chain of G$_s$ and stimulate adenylyl cyclase in human pituitary tumours. Nature 1989; 340:692–696.

18. Lyons J, Landis CA, Harsh G, et al. Two G protein oncogenes in human endocrine tumors. Science 1990; 249: 655–659.

19. Melmed S. Acromegaly. N Engl J Med 1990; 322:966–976.

20. Weinstein LS, Shenker A, Gejman PV, Merino MJ, Friedman E, Spiegel AM. Activating mutations of the stimulatory G protein in the McCune-Albright syndrome. N Engl J Med 1991; 325:1688–1695.

21. Ashcraft NW, Hartzband PI, Van Herle AJ, Bersch N, Golde DW. A unique growth factor in patients with acromegaloidism. J Clin Endocrinol Metab 1983; 57:272–276.

22. Clemmons DR, Van Wyk JJ, Ridgway EC, Kliman B, Kjellberg RN, Underwood LE. Evaluation of acromegaly by radioimmunoassay of somatomedin-C. N Engl J Med 1979; 301:1138–1142.

23. Frohman LA. Clinical review: therapeutic options in acromegaly. J Clin Endocrinol Metabl 1991; 72:1175–1181.

24. Arafah BM, Rodkey JS, Kaufman B, Velasco M, Manni A, Pearson OH. Transsphenoidal microsurgery in the treatment

of acromegaly and gigantism. J Clin Endocrinol Metabl 1980; 50:578–585.

25. Lightner S, Winter SD. Treatment of juvenile acromegaly with bromocriptine. J Pediatr 1981; 98:494–496.

26. Ritzen EM, Wettrell G, Davies G, Grant DB. Management of pituitary gigantism: the role of bromocriptine and radiotherapy. Acta Paediatr Scand 1985; 74:807–814.

27. Geffner ME, Nagel RA, Dietrich RB, Kaplan SA. Treatment of acromegaly with a somatostatin analog in a patient with McCune-Albright syndrome. J Pediatr 1987; 111:740–743.

28. Barkan AL, Kelch RP, Hopwood NJ, Beitins IZ. Treatment of acromegaly with the long-acting somatostatin analog SMS 201–995. J Clin Endocrinol Metab 1988; 66:16–23.

29. Whitehead EM, Shalet SM, Davies D, Enoch BA, Price DA, Beardwell CG. Pituitary gigantism: a disabling condition. Clin Endocrinol (Oxf) 1982; 17:271–277.

30. Sotos JF, Dodge PR, Muirhead D, Crawford JD, Talbot NB. Cerebral gigantism in childhood: a syndrome of excessively rapid growth with acromegalic features and a nonprogressive neurologic disorder. N Engl J Med 1964; 271:109–116.

31. Jaeken J, Van Der Scheren-Lodeweyckx M, Eeckels R. Cerebral gigantism syndrome. A report of 4 cases and review of the literature. Z Kinderheilk 1972; 112:332–346.

32. Sotos JF. Cerebral gigantism. Am J Dis Child 1977; 131:625–627.

33. Wit JM, Beemer FA, Barth PG, et al. Cerebral gigantism (Sotos syndrome). Compiled data of 22 cases. Analysis of clinical features, growth and plasma somatomedine. Eur. J Pediatr 1985; 144:131–140.

34. Zonana J, Sotos JF, Romshe CA, Fisher DA, Elders MJ, Rimoin DL. Dominant inheritance of cerebral gigantism. J Pediatr 1977; 91:251–256.

35. Winship IM. Sotos syndrome—autosomal dominant inheritance substantiated. Clin Genet 1985; 28:243–246.

36. Beemer FA, Veenema H, de Pater JM. Cerebral gigantism (Sotos syndrome) in two patients with fra(X) chromosomes. Am J Med Genet 1986; 23:221–226.

37. Whitaker MD, Scheithauer BW, Hayles AB, Okazaki H. The hypothalamus and pituitary in cerebral gigantism: a clinicopathologic and immunocytochemical study. Am J Dis Child 1985; 139:679–682.

38. Rutter SC, Cole TRP. Psychological characteristics of Sotos syndrome. Dev Med Child Neurol 1991; 33:898–902.

39. Hersh JH, Cole TRP, Bloom AS, Bertolone SJ, Hughes HE. Risk of malignancy in Sotos syndrome. J Pediatr 1992; 120:572–574.

40. Caldwell PD, Smith DW. The XXY (Klinefelter's) syndrome in childhood: detection and treatment. J Pediatr 1972; 80:250–258.

41. Nielsen J, Wohlert M. Chromosome abnormalities found among 34,910 newborn children: results from a 13 year incidence study in Arhus, Denmark. Hum Genet 1991; 87:81–83.

42. Ratcliffe SG, Bancroft J, Axworthy D, McLaren W. Klinefelter's syndrome in adolescence. Arch Dis Child 1982; 57:6–12.

43. Ratcliffe SG. The sexual development of boys with the chromosome constitution 47,XXY (Klinefelter's syndrome). Clin Endocrinol Metab 1982; 11:703–716.

44. Salbenblatt JA, Bender BG, Puck MH, Robinson A, Faiman C, Winter JSD. Pituitary-gonadal function in Klinefelter syndrome before and during puberty. Pediatr Res 1985; 19:82–86.

45. Ratcliffe SG, Butler GE, Jones M. Edinburgh study of growth and development of children with sex chromosome abnormalities. IV. Birth Defects 1991; 26:1–44.

46. Walzer S, Bashir AS, Silbert AR. Cognitive and behavioral factors in the learning disabilities of 47,XXY and 47,XYY boys. Birth Defects 1991; 26:45–58.

47. Ratcliffe SG, Pan H, McKie M. Growth during puberty in the XYY boy. Ann Hum Biol 1992; 19:579–587.

48. Court Brown WM. Males with an XYY sex chromosome complement. J Med Genet 1968; 5:341–359.

49. Valentine GH, McClelland MA, Sergovich FR. The growth and development of four XYY infants. Pediatrics 1971; 48:583–594.

50. Dietz HC, Cutting GR, Pyeritz RE, et al. Marfan syndrome caused by a recurrent de novo missense mutation in the fibrillin gene. Nature 1991; 352:337–339.

51. Dietz HC, Pyeritz RE, Puffenberger EG, et al. Marfan phenotype variability in a family segregating a missense mutation in the epidermal growth factor-like motif of the fibrillin gene. J Clin Invest 1992; 89:1674–1680.

52. Kainulainen K, Pulkkinen L, Savolainen A, Kaitila I, Peltonen L. Location on chromosome 15 of the gene defect causing Marfan syndrome. N Engl J Med 1990; 323:935–939.

53. Milewicz DM, Pyeritz RE, Crawford ES, Byers PH. Marfan syndrome: defective synthesis, secretion, and extracellular matrix formation of fibrillin by cultured dermal fibroblasts. J Clin Invest 1992; 89:79–86.

54. Pyeritz RE, McKusick VA. The Marfan syndrome: diagnosis and management. N Engl J Med 1979; 14:772–777.

55. Pyeritz RE. The Marfan syndrome. Am Fam Physician 1986; 34:83–94.

56. Roberts WC, Honig HS. The spectrum of cardiovascular disease in the Marfan syndrome: a clinico-morphologic study of 18 necropsy patients and comparison to 151 previously reported necropsy patients. Am Heart J 1981; 104:115–135.

57. Carson NAJ, Cusworth DC, Dent CE, Field MB, Neill DW, Westall RG. Homocystinuria: a new inborn error of metabolism associated with mental deficiency. Arch Dis Child 1963; 38:425–436.

58. Mudd SH, Levy HL. Disorders of transsulfuration. In: Stanbury JB, Wyngaarden JB, Fredickson DS, Goldstein JL, Brown MS, eds. The Metabolic Basis of Inherited Disease, 5th ed. New York: McGraw-Hill, 1983:522–559.

59. Mudd SH, Skovby F, Levy HL, et al. The natural history of homocystinura due to cystathionine β-synthase deficiency. Am J Hum Genet 1985; 37:1–31.

60. Skovby F. Homocystinuria: clinical, biochemical and genetic aspects of cystathionine β-synthase and its deficiency in man. Acta Paediatr Scan Suppl 1985; 321:1–21.

61. Rodgers GM, Chandler WL. Laboratory and clinical aspects of inherited thrombotic disorders. Am J Hematol 1992; 41:113–122.

62. Pettenati MJ, Haines JL, Higgins RR, Wappner RS, Palmer CG, Weaver DD. Wiedemann-Beckwith syndrome: presentation of clinical and cytogenetic data on 22 new cases and review of the literature. Hum Genet 1986; 74:143–154.

63. Engstrom W, Lindham S, Schofield P. Beckwith-Wiedemann syndrome. Eur J Pediatr 1988; 147:450–457.

64. Koufos A, Grundy P, Morgan K, et al. Familial Beckwith-Wiedemann syndrome and a second Wilms tumor locus both map to 11p15.5. Am J Hum Genet 1989; 44:711–719.

65. Ping AJ, Reeve AE, Law DJ, Young MR, Boehnke M, Feinberg AP. Genetic linkage of Beckwith-Wiedemann syndrome to 11p15. Am J Hum Genet 1989; 44:720–723.

66. Little M, Van Heyningen V, Hastie N. Dads and disomy and disease. Nature 1991; 351:609–610.

67. Henry I, Bonaiti-Pellie C, Chehensssssssse V, et al. Uniparental paternal disomy in a genetic cancer-predisposing syndrome. Nature 1991; 351:665–667.

68. Viljoen D, Ramesar R. Evidence for paternal imprinting in familial Beckwith-Wiedemann syndrome. J Med Genet 1992; 29:221–225.

69. Wiedemann HR. Tumours and hemihypertrophy associated with Beckwith-Wiedemann syndrome. Eur J Pediatr 1983; 141:129.

70. Sotelo-Avila C, Gonzalez-Crussi F, Fowler JW. Complete and incomplete forms of Beckwith-Wiedemann syndrome: their oncogenic potential. J Pediatr 1980; 96:47–50.

71. Fraumeni JR Jr, Geiser CF, Manning MD. Wilms' tumor and congenital hemihypertrophy: report of five new cases and review of literature. Pediatrics 1967; 40:886–899.

72. Stalens JP, Maton P, Gosseye S, Clapuyt P, Ninane J. Hemihypertrophy, bilateral Wilms' tumor, and clear-cell adenocarcinoma of the uterine cervix in a young girl. Med Pediatr Oncol 1993; 21:671–675.

73. Pieters GFFM, Smals AGH, Kloppenborg PWC. Defective suppression of growth hormone after oral glucose loading in adolescence. J Clin Endocrinol Metab 1980; 51:265–270.

74. Evain-Brion D, Garnier P, Schimpff RM, Chaussain JL, Job JC. Growth hormone response to thyrotropin-releasing hormone and oral glucose-loading tests in tall children and adolescents. J Clin Endocrinol Metab 1983; 56:429–432.

75. Eiholzer U, Torresani T, Bucher H, Prader A, Illig R. Paradoxical rise of growth hormone after oral glucose load in tall girls: a physiological finding in puberty? Pediatr Res 1985; 19:633.

76. Hindmarsh PC, Stanhope R, Kendall BE, Brook CGD. Tall stature: a clinical, endocrinological and radiological study. Clin Endocrinol (Oxf) 1986; 25:223–231.

77. Dickerman Z, Loewinger J, Laron Z. The pattern of growth in children with constitutional tall stature from birth to age 9 years. Acta Paediatr Scand 1984; 73:530–536.

78. Bierich JR. Estrogen treatment of girls with constitutional tall stature. Pediatrics 1968; 62:1196–1201.

79. Whitelaw MJ. Experiences in treating excessive height in girls with cyclic oestradiol valerate: a ten year survey. Acta Endocrinol (Copenh) 1967; 54:473–484.

80. Andersen H, Jacobsen BB, Kastrup KW, et al. Treatment of girls with excessive height prediction. Acta Paediatr Scand 1980; 59:293–297.

81. Colle ML, Alperin H, Greenblatt RB. The tall girl: prediction of mature height and management. Arch Dis Child 1977; 52:118–120.

82. Wettenhall HNB, Cahill C, Roche AF. Tall girls: a survey of 15 years of management and treatment. J Pediatr 1975; 86:602–610.

83. Crawford JD. Treatment of tall girls with estrogen. Pediatrics 1968; 62:1189–1197.

84. Gruters A, Heidemann P, Schluter H, Stubbe P, Weber B, Helge H. Effect of different oestrogen doses on final height reduction in girls with constitutional tall statue. Eur J Pediatr 1989; 149:11–13.

85. Prader A, Zachmann M. Treatment of excessively tall girls and boys with sex hormones. Pediatrics 1978; 62: 1202–1210.

86. Kuhn N, Blunck W, Stanhnke N, Wiebel J, Willig RP. Estrogen treatment in tall girls. Acta Paediatr Scand 1977; 66:161–167.

87. Frasier SD, Smith FG Jr. Effect of estrogens on mature height in tall girls: a controlled study. J Clin Endocrinol Metab 1968; 28:416–419.

88. Schoen EJ, Solomon IL, Warner O, Wingerd J. Estrogen treatment of tall girls. Am J Dis Child 1973; 125:71–74.

89. Sorgo W, Scholler K, Heinze F, Heinze E, Teller WM. Critical analysis of height reduction in estrogen-treated tall girls. Eur J Pediatr 1984; 142:260–265.

90. Werder EA, Waibel P, Sege D, Flury R. Severe thrombosis during oestrogen treatment for tall stature. Eur J Pediatr 1990; 149:389–390.

91. Hanker JP, Schellong G, Schneider HPG. The functional state of the hypothamo-pituitary axis after high-dose estrogen therapy in excessively tall girls. Acta Endocrinol (Copenh) 1979; 91:19–29.

92. Skovby F, McKusick VA. Estrogen treatment of tall stature in girls with the Marfan syndrome. Birth Defects 1977; 13:155–161.

93. Zachmann M, Ferrandez A, Murset G, Gnehm HE, Prader A. Testosterone treatment of excessively tall boys. J Pediatr 1976; 88:116–123.

94. Evain-Brion D, Garnier P, Blanco-Garcia M, Job J. Studies in constitutionally tall adolescents. II. Effects of bromocriptine on growth hormone secretion and adult height prediction. J Clin Endocrinol Metab 1984; 58:1022–1026.

95. Schwarz HP, Joss EE, Zuppinger KA. Bromocriptine treatment in adolescent boys with familial tall stature: a pair-matched controlled study. J Clin Endocrinol Metab 1987; 65:136–140.

96. Schoenle EJ, Theintz G, Torresani T, Prader A, Illig R, Sizonenko PC. Lack of bromocriptine-induced reduction of predicted height in tall adolescents. J Clin Endocrinol Metab 1987; 65:355–358.

97. Hindmarsh PC, Pringle PJ, di Silvio L, Brook CGD. A preliminary report on the role of somatostatin analogue (SMS 201-995) in the management of children with tall stature. Clin Endocrinol (Oxf) 1990; 32:83–91.

98. Tauber MT, Tauber JP, Vigoni F, Harris AG, Rochicchioli P. Effect of the long-acting somatostatin analogue SMS 201-995 on growth rate and reduction of predicted adult height in ten tall adolescents. Acta Paediatr Scand 1990; 79:176–181.

13

Disorders of Puberty

Peter A. Lee
University of Pittsburgh and Children's Hospital of Pittsburgh,
Pittsburgh, Pennsylvania

I. NORMAL PUBERTY

A. Definition and Mechanism

Puberty is the period during which sexual maturity is completed, resulting in the capacity for reproduction. It involves growth and maturation of the primary sexual characteristics (gonads and genitals) and the appearance of secondary sexual characteristics (sexual hair, female breast development, and voice change). During puberty, menstruation begins and spermarche (the onset of emission of sperm) occurs. The changes of puberty are caused by increased stimulation from heightened sex steroid secretion, primarily estrogen (as estradiol) in females and testosterone in males. Increased gonadal activity occurs as the result of increased stimulation by the pituitary gonadotropins luteinizing hormone (LH) and follicle-stimulating hormone (FSH). The increased sex hormone production by the testes results from increased LH stimulation; FSH stimulates primarily maturation of spermatogonia. In the female, both LH and FSH are necessary for hormonogenesis and FSH plays a larger role in the maturation of ova.

The physiologic secretion pattern of gonadotropins is a periodic intermittent release, more dramatically apparent for LH whether using traditional immunoassays or more sensitive assays (1–5). Before puberty, the amplitude of release is low and occurs infrequently. The onset of pubertal hormonal changes is first evident in dramatic episodes of LH release of short duration that first occur during sleep. With maturity, this release occurs regularly throughout the day (6). The intermittent release of gonadotropin is reflective of the episodic release of gonadotropin-releasing hormone (GnRH), also called luteinizing hormone-releasing hormone, from the hypothalamus (7). Currently, the understanding of the onset of puberty is that the pituitary and gonad are ready and capable of full function at any age after a relatively short period of priming or upregulation. During childhood this system is down-regulated because GnRH secretion is minimal. Puberty begins when the episodic secretion of GnRH is enhanced. The mechanisms by which this occurs are incompletely understood, but they appear to involve the stimulatory and inhibitory influences of such neurotransmitters as acetylcholine, catecholamines, γ-aminobutyric acid, opioid peptides, prostaglandins, and serotonin.

Negative-feedback mechanisms of hypothalamic-pituitary gonadotropin-gonadal control are operative from fetal life onward (8). A change in the sensitivity of this feedback is inadequate to explain the changes in fetal, neonatal, childhood, and pubertal physiology. Overriding central nervous system (CNS) control appears to be the necessary component. Episodic release is present in the neonatal period and childhood, although total gonadotropin secretion is diminished in childhood (9). Mean LH and FSH levels are low in childhood, FSH levels being relatively higher than LH levels, particularly in girls (3,5,9). At any age, the pituitary gland is capable of response to GnRH stimulation. The response pattern of childhood is relatively diminished and similar to that present among some hypogonadotropic adults. With the onset of puberty, the mean LH and FSH levels increase, with a relatively greater rise in the LH levels. For any single patient, however, baseline values may overlap; hence, levels of pubertal individuals may be within the prepubertal range, and vice versa. The response of LH to exogenous GnRH stimulation becomes more pronounced with pubertal maturity (9,10). Therefore, GnRH stimulation may be useful in differentiating a pubertal from a prepubertal response. The incremental rise in FSH after GnRH stimulation is less indicative of pubertal maturation (9–11). It is already clearly evident in prepubertal children, particularly girls, and may not increase discernibly with puberty.

Synchronized episodic increased gonadotropin stimulation sets into motion all that is necessary for full development and ovulation or spermatogenesis (8,9). By the end of puberty, episodic release of gonadotropins is characteristic of the waking hours as well as those of sleep and, in the female, varies predictably during different phases of the menstrual cycle.

Serum bioactive LH levels generally rise as expected during pubertal development, but FSH changes little or not at all. In girls before puberty, bioactive FSH are relatively elevated, as are immunoactive levels, but bioactive LH is low. During puberty, bioactive FSH increases modestly but LH shows the expected greater rise (12). Among boys, the rise in bioactive LH is relatively greater than the rise in immunoactive levels, but serum bioactive FSH levels do not change significantly (13).

B. Normal Female Development

Milestones of female puberty include thelarche (the onset of pubertal breast development) and menarche (the onset of menstrual periods). "Pubarche" is a term used to signify the onset of sexual hair development, commonly considered to result from an increase in adrenarche (pubertal elevation of androgen secretion), although androgen production by the ovaries also occurs with the increased steroidogenesis during puberty.

The most common first evidence of puberty in girls is thelarche (Fig. 1), although it may occasionally be preceded by pubarche (pubic hair development) (14). The mean age for the onset of puberty in girls is about 11 years, with a range from 8 to 13 or 14 years (Fig. 1) (14). The duration of pubertal development is usually 3–3 1/2 years, but it may occur within 2 years or take as long as 5–6 years (14). Mean LH, FSH, and estradiol levels have significantly increased before physical changes begin (15), but because of fluctuation within and between individuals, this rise may not be discernible in individual instances. The rise in estradiol signifies that gonadarche has occurred; the estrogen-stimulated development that follows includes breast, genital, and uterine maturation and fat distribution in the typical female contours (16). Breast growth, which may begin asymmetrically, progresses throughout puberty and may be classified into five Tanner stages (Table 1) (17). Pubic hair growth, which begins within about 6 months of breast development, can also be staged to follow progression (Table 1). This and other androgen-caused changes, such as axillary hair, apocrine gland development (body odor), and acne, are caused by increased androgen secretion from both adrenal and ovarian sources.

Adrenarche, which is characterized by a relatively increased adrenal androgen production in relation to other adrenal corticosteroids, precedes the pubertal rise in gonadotropins and gonadarche. It can be detected as young as age 6 or 7 in girls by an increase in circulating levels of dehydroepiandrosterone (DHA) and DHA sulfate (DHAS) (18). The cause of adrenarche is unknown: no stimulating factor has been identified.

The pubertal growth spurt in girls occurs during the first half of puberty, usually detectable at the time of the appearance of the first signs of puberty (Fig. 1). During puberty, girls experience an increase in body fat content and fat-free mass (19). The average girl experiences menarche 2 years after the onset of pubertal breast growth, but there is considerable variation. The pace of pubertal development correlates with the level of sex steroids during early puberty (16). The magnitude of sex steroid exposure before menarche also relates to the amount of statural growth after menarche, those with greater exposure being close to final height at menarche. The average girl grows 4–6 cm after menarche, although growth after menarche varies considerably. Those with relatively early menarche may grow as much as 10 cm, whereas those with a more prolonged estrogen stimulation time before the onset of menses may grow fewer than 4 cm. Generally, earlier menses is correlated with shorter adult height. Commonly, adolescent girls have irregular menses for a year or longer after menarche; although some always menstruate regularly, others have irregular periods for years.

C. Normal Male Development

Although pubic hair growth is the first evidence of puberty that is usually noticed, increased testicular size is the first physical evidence of puberty among boys (20). A testis is pubertal sized if the longest axis is 2.5 cm or more in length. This occurs, on the average, by 11.5–12 years and may occur normally as early as 9.5 years (14). Pubertal development in males can be gauged by Tanner staging (Table 1) of genital size and pubic hair (Fig. 2) (14). Stage 1 is prepubertal and stage 5 adult for all staging.

During puberty, there is a progressive evaluation of circulating levels of LH, FSH, and testosterone indicative of a continuing upregulation of secretion of the hypothalamic-pituitary-testicular axis (1,2,4,21). The increased gonadotropin secretion results from increased episodic GnRH secretion. Other hormonal changes include a progressive elevation of

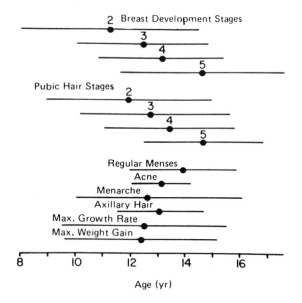

Figure 1 Mean ages (dots) and ranges (horizontal lines) of onset of pubertal development in girls.

Table 1 Staging of Pubertal Development (Tanner)

Staging	Pubic hair staging	Concomitant changes	Prader orchidometer (ml)
Girls: breast			
1 Prepubertal, papilla elevation	No pigmented hair		
2 Budding; larger areolae; palpable and visible elevated contour	Pigmented hair, mainly labial	Accelerated growth rate	
3 Enlargement of the breast and areola	Coarser, spread of pigmented hair over mons	Peak growth rate, thicker vaginal mucosa, axillary hair	
4 Secondary mound of areola and papilla	Adult type but smaller area	Menarche (stage 3 or 4) Decelerated growth rate	
5 Mature	Adult distribution		
Boys: genital size		Concomitant changes	
1 Prepubertal	No pigmented hair	Long testis axis <2.5 cm	1, 2, 3
2 Early testicular, penile, and scrotal growth	Minimal pigmented hair at base of penis	Early voice changes; testes length 2.5–3.3 cm	3, 4, 5, 6, 8
3 Increased penile length and width; scrotal and testes growth	Dark, coarse, curly hair extends midline above penis	Light hair on upper lip, acne, maximal growth, testes length 3.3–4.0 cm	10, 12, 15
4 Increased penis size including breadth; pigmented scrotum	Considerable, but less than adult distribution	Early sideburns; testes 4.0–4.5 cm	15, 20
5 Adult size and shape	Adult distribution, spread to medial thighs or beyond	Beard growth; testes >4.5 cm	25

steroids of adrenal or testicular origin: estrone, estradiol, androstenedione, 17-hydroxyprogesterone, DHA, and DHAS (21,22). The rise in the last two signifies adrenarche and precedes the onset of the gonadotropin and testosterone rise and the beginning of Tanner stage 2 (18). Müllerian inhibiting hormone has an inverse relationship to testosterone: levels progressively fall throughout puberty (23,24).

During midpuberty, the period when testosterone levels are rapidly rising (14,21,25), the peak of the pubertal growth spurt, voice change, and the onset of axillary hair growth occur (Fig. 2). Testosterone produces a progressive increase in total-body bone mineral content and lean body mass and a progressive decrease in body fat (19,26). The onset of acne (14) and gynecomastia (27) are also midpubertal events. Gynecomastia, palpable or visible breast tissue, occurs in at least two-thirds of boys sometime during puberty. It begins before testosterone levels have reached the adult range and, in most, persists for 18–24 months. If the quantity of breast tissue is considerable and regression is not apparent after 2 years, plastic surgical excision should be offered (see Chap. 14). Facial hair growth begins about 3 years after the onset of pubic hair growth. The thickness and distribution of the

beard, chest, abdominal, and pubic hair may progress for years after puberty and vary considerably among adult men. These correlate more with familial or genetic factors than with hormonal levels.

In contrast to girls, the period of accelerated growth occurs during midpuberty rather than generally concomitant with the onset (14,25). Peak growth velocity is generally at 14–15 years of age and during Tanner stages 3 and 4. Onset of spermarche (first evidence of completed spermatogenesis, usually first observable by the presence of sperm in urine, particularly the first morning void), is usually at Tanner stage 3 based on pubic hair or genital development and occurs sometime in year 13. It occurs after considerable testosterone stimulation but before adult levels are reached (25,28).

II. PRECOCIOUS PUBERTY

A. Classification

When pubertal development occurs too early, the condition is, by definition, precocious puberty. On the basis of the early

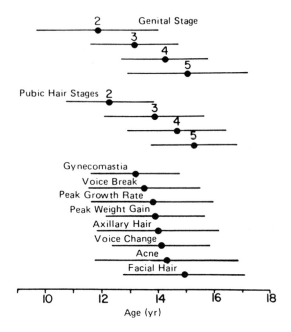

Figure 2 Mean ages (dots) and ranges (horizontal lines) of various pubertal changes in boys.

limits of age for the normal onset of pubertal changes, puberty before age 8 years in girls and 91/2 in boys is precocious (14). Early pubertal development is classified as physiologically normal but early (GnRH driven) or GnRH independent (Table 2). GnRH-driven or central (true) precocious puberty results from early onset of pubertal hypothalamic-pituitary-gonadal activity; it is (true) physiologic gonadotropin stimulation emanating from the GnRH secretion of (central) CNS-hypothalamic origin. In central precocious puberty, in contrast to peripheral or precocious pseudopuberty, the sex steroid stimulating the physical changes of puberty is not produced as a result of physiologic pituitary gonadotropin secretion. The source of sex steroid may be exogenous or endogenous, gonadal or extragonadal. The hormone may be autonomously produced and is independent of gonadotropin stimulation or control.

The terminology "complete" or "incomplete" sexual precocity has been used with different meanings. Central precocious puberty has been called complete and peripheral incomplete, but the more common designation has used *complete* for any form of precocious puberty; *incomplete* designates some partial early pubertal development, such as thelarche or pubarche. Because of the confusion with this terminology, the latter changes are more appropriately called partial development or variations of normal. Further classification can be used to differentiate *isosexual precocity*, early pubertal development appropriate for sex (e.g., development of female characteristics in females), from *contrasexual* or *heterosexual precocity*, early development inappropriate for sex or appropriate for opposite sex (e.g.,

estrogen effects with breast development in boys and excessive androgen stimulation with clitoromegaly in girls). Such abnormal development is clearly in a different category from precocious puberty and should be considered a hyperandrogenic state in females and as feminizing conditions in males.

B. Girls

1. Central Precocious Puberty

Central precocious puberty is diagnosed if the development of physical pubertal changes and laboratory testing are consistent with the progressive changes of normal puberty. The majority of girls and about half of boys who present with precocious puberty have the central form (29). Such premature activation of the hypothalamic-pituitary axis is also about five times more common in girls than in boys, although in contrast to males, in most instances among females no underlying pathology is demonstrable. Precocious puberty may be associated with no anatomic changes or changes within the CNS that disrupt the restraint typical of childhood. A more frequent association with this form of precocious puberty has become patients surviving CNS tumors who have received radiation and chemotherapy. Associated abnormalities with central precocious puberty in girls are listed in Table 2.

Girls with central precocious puberty have thelarche, accelerated growth and skeletal maturation, and hormone levels and responses consistent with gonadarche. Basal and GnRH-stimulated gonadotropin levels are within the pubertal range; LH responses increase to a greater degree with pubertal onset and are hence more useful in diagnosing central precocious puberty. Patients who present with early puberty progress at very different rates (30). Some patients develop and grow rapidly, with clear diminution of adult height potential; others, being tall for age, continue to grow along the same percentile without accelerated skeletal maturation rates (Fig. 3). A more frequently diagnosed CNS congenital malformation since the availability of better imaging techniques is the GnRH-secreting hypothalamic hamartoma (31–33). This apparently redundant CNS tissue containing GnRH neurons is independent of CNS inhibitory influences and functions as an ectopic hypothalamus episodically secreting GnRH. The loss of such episodic release after complete removal of a pedunculated hamartoma was early evidence that the pulse generator itself resides within the network of communicating GnRH-secreting neurons (31).

2. Peripheral Precocious Puberty

Precocious pseudopuberty in girls results from excessive estrogen stimulation for age from ovarian, adrenal cortical, or exogenous source. Pseudopuberty is relatively rare in girls (Table 2).

a. McCune-Albright Syndrome. The McCune-Albright syndrome, which occurs in females far more frequently than in males, includes a unique form of peripheral precocious puberty in which there is an activating missense

Table 2 Differential Diagnosis of Precocious Puberty

Central (GnRH driven)
  Idiopathic (sporadic or familial)
  Central nervous system abnormalities
    Acquired (abscess, chemotherapy, granulomas, inflammation, radiation, surgical, trauma)
    Congenital anomalies (arachnoid cysts, hydrocephalus, hypothalamic hamartomas, septo-optic
      dysplasia, suprasellar cyst
    Tumors (LH-secreting adenoma, astrocytoma, glioma (may be associated with neurofibroma-
      tosis), craniopharyngiomas, ependymomas
    Secondary to chronic exposure to sex steroids (causes of peripheral puberty; CVAH, GIP,
      tumors)
    Reversible forms: space-occupying or pressure-associated lesions (abscess, hydrocephalus)
Peripheral (GnRH independent)
  Genetic disorders (mutations)
    Congenital virilizing adrenal hyperplasia (CVAH), males
    Gonadotropin-independent puberty (GIP), males
    McCune-Albright syndrome
  Tumors
    Adrenal sex steroid secreting (adenoma, carcinoma)
    Gonadotropin-producing (choriocarcinoma, chorioepithelioma, dysgerminoma, hepatoblastoma,
      hepatoma, teratoma)
    Ovarian (granulosa cell, may be associated with Peutz-Jeghers syndrome); granulosa, theca cell
    Testicular (Leydig cell)
  Limited or reversible forms
    Chronic primary hypothyroidism
    CVAH
    Exogenous sex steroid or gonadotropins
    Ovarian cysts
Variants of normal development
  Premature pubarche (secondary to premature adrenarche)
  Premature thelarche

mutation in the gene for the α subunit of G_s, the G protein that stimulates cyclic adenosine monophosphate formation (34). Abnormalities in this syndrome consist of multicentic localized osseous lesions called polycystic fibrous dysplasia, melanotic cutaneous macules called café au lait spots, and endocrinopathy (35). The endocrinopathies may include sexual precocity (Fig. 4), hyperthyroidism, hyperadrenocorticism, pituitary gigantism or acromegaly, and hypophosphatemia. The mutation has been found in variable abundance in affected tissues, a finding consistent with a mosaic distribution of aberrant cells from a somatic cell mutation (34) and also compatible with variable expression and exacerbations and remissions of disease activity characteristic of this syndrome. The excessive endocrine function appears to be caused by autonomous excessive hormone production, as if trophic hormone stimulation were present; female patients with sexual precocity secrete increased ovarian estrogen without gona dotropin stimulation. It appears that mechanisms usually stimulated by the trophic hormones are activated as a result of this mutation. Because ovarian estrogen secretion in patients with the McCune-Albright syndrome is not gonado tropin driven, such secretion is not suppressed by GnRH analog therapy. Thus, other therapy is indicated (see Sec. II.E).

As with other entities of peripheral precocious puberty, skeletal age and biologic maturity become advanced, and eventually, mature hypothalamic-pituitary control of ovarian function commences, even at an early age. After hypothalamic-pituitary maturation, ovarian function is under the usual control mechanisms and GnRH analogs may have a place in therapy for early puberty. Eventually these patients ovulate, and true menstrual cycling, and pregnancy may occur (35).

b. Ovarian Cysts. Ovarian cysts, readily identified by sonography, may occur with central precocious puberty (36), as part of the normal ovarian development of childhood (37), secondary to intermittent unsustained gonadotropin stimulation, and in the McCune-Albright syndrome. An isolated follicular cyst may be present with apparent autonomous estrogen production, presenting with the finding of peripheral precocious puberty. Such cysts are usually self-limiting; estrogen levels falling as the cyst spontaneously regresses. Such a drop in estrogen levels may be accompanied by withdrawal bleeding. Initial treatment of an isolated follicular cyst should be conservative, with careful monitoring and without surgical intervention, unless a surgical emergency,

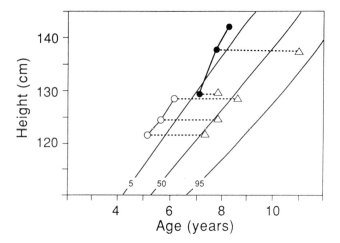

Figure 3 Growth chart for girls showing percentile of height for age. The solid circles represent height for age for a girl presenting with central precocious puberty; the connected triangles depict height for bone age. Note that although growth rate is accelerated, bone age has accelerated considerably more in the same time period, resulting in a decrease in projected adult height. In contrast, the patient whose heights are depicted with Tanner stage 2 breast and pubic hair development, did not have an acceleration in growth rate or bone maturity. Although she was tall for age with early pubertal development, she did not have a decreased adult height potential.

such as torsion, is likely. Follow-up sonography and estrogen levels after 1–4 months usually show regression.

c. Chronic Primary Hypothyroidism. Although hypothyroidism is usually accompanied by growth, skeletal, and pubertal delay, a few patients with thyroid gland failure and elevated thyroid-stimulating hormone (TSH) levels have evidence of advanced pubertal development (38). Marked pituitary enlargement may occur in this syndrome (39). An excessive secretion of the α subunit accompanies the TSH hypersecretion. The excess of the α subunit, as newer assays suggest, may activate gonadotropin receptors. Alternatively, there may be excessive production of FSH and LH as well as prolactin. Patients present with breast development that may be accompanied by galactorrhea. Treatment of the hypothyroidism with appropriate thyroid replacement results in negative feedback suppression of the TSH and a concomitant drop in the levels of other hormones. Pubertal changes regress, and no other therapy is necessary.

3. Diagnostic Evaluation

The approach to the assessment of the girl with early pubertal development is outlined in Table 3. A diagnostic workup sufficient to discern the underlying etiology is necessary so that appropriate treatment can be given.

A complete history should be taken, emphasizing the points noted in Table 3 and with careful consideration of any possible exposure to exogenous hormone, previous or current CNS abnormalities or symptoms, pubertal history of other

family members, and height and growth rates. Physical examination should include careful height, weight, span, and upper/lower body segment ratio. Pubertal staging should be done with inspection of the genitalia for pubertal maturation and visualization of the vaginal mucosa.

Visual inspection should be adequate to assess the effect of estrogen stimulation upon the vaginal mucosa and to avoid traumatizing the patient. If the patient is positioned prone with knees drawn up and legs spread, the introitus can be visualized without touching the vulva but by gently spreading the labia. A glistening red appearance is consistent with a thin, non–estrogen-stimulated mucosa, whereas a pink mucosa with a mucous covering indicative of a thicker, more cornified mucosa and mucous secretion is suggestive of concomitant estrogen stimulation. However, irritation or infection can also result in the latter appearance. A bimanual abdominal-rectal examination may be traumatizing and usually can be avoided if an adequate abdominal pelvic ultrasound study is done.

A determination of plasma estradiol is indicated as well as a GnRH stimulation test to determine whether gonadotropin responses are consistent with pubertal pituitary gonadotropin secretion. The LH response is more helpful in demonstrating a pubertal pattern characteristic of central precocious puberty, and patients with peripheral precocious puberty are expected to have a prepubertal or suppressed response. Interpretation of GnRH responses requires that the normal prepubertal response be known for the assays used. Figure 5 shows the range of responses in 12 prepubertal girls. The FSH range is wide, and most pubertal patients do not have a response outside this range; hence FSH responses are seldom discriminatory. On the other hand, the low responses of both LH and FSH, which are normal for prepubertal individuals, demonstrates why it may not be possible to separate a suppressed from a prepubertal response.

If the patient is menstruating regularly, progesterone during the second half of the cycle may indicate a luteal phase and verify ovulation. Other laboratory testing may involve thyroid function tests, including TSH to rule out primary hypothyroidism and plasma DHA, DHAS, or urinary 17-ketosteroid levels to determine whether adrenarche has occurred or excessive adrenal androgen secretion should be ruled out. A skeletal maturity (bone age) roentgenogram should be obtained to estimate the extent of excessive stimulation and remaining growth potential. Pelvic sonography should be done in all patients to determine whether ovaries and uterus are enlarged for age but appropriate for stage of puberty (consistent with central precocious puberty); unilateral or asymmetric ovarian enlargement may be indicative of a tumor or cysts.

All young girls (less than 5 years) with central precocious puberty in whom the etiology is not already explained should have computed tomography (CT) or magnetic resonance imaging (MRI) of the CNS, particularly the hypothalamic region, looking for unapparent lesions (Table 2) even if the neurologic examination is normal. Lesions are unlikely to be demonstrated among girls aged 6–8 years, so the need for such a study should be determined for each patient individu-

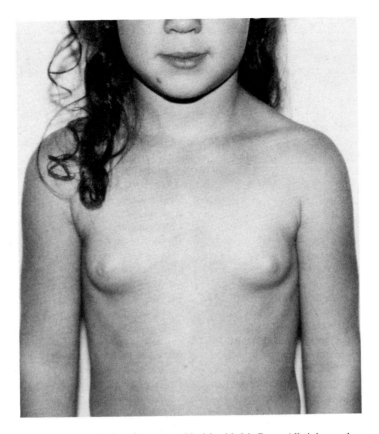

Figure 4   Premature breast development (stage 3) in a four-year-old girl with McCune–Albright syndrome.

ally. An electroencephalogram is not generally indicated, even though abnormalities have been reported in central precocious puberty.

C. Boys

1. Central Precocious Puberty

The causes of early pubertal development among boys are outlined in Table 2. In contrast with girls, although central precocity is less frequent, a larger percentage of boys with central precocity have CNS lesions than the idiopathic variety. Therefore, the CNS assessment of boys with early puberty, usually including an MRI scan, should be emphasized unless the cause is already explained. The CNS disorders may include hamartomas (Fig. 6), which are congenital malformations rather than tumors and rarely have neurologic consequences. Puberty in patients with these tumors may be suppressed using GnRH analogs (see Sec. II.E), or if the patient is very young and the tumor pedunculated, surgical excision may be considered (31,32). Other tumors, including astrocytomas, craniopharyngiomas, ependymomas, germinomas, and gliomas, that may be associated with central precocious puberty require the indicated treatment to obliterate them or attempt to control their growth.

As among girls, a more common recent cause of central precocity is previous CNS radiation therapy, with or without chemotherapy (Chap. 56). As the cure rate of malignancies rises, this late sequela can be expected to be identified with increasing frequency, not infrequently in conjunction with growth hormone deficiency. Other poorly understood CNS-related causes include trauma, surgery, inflammation, and severe neurologic-mental deficits of congenital or acquired origin. Precocity related to hydrocephalus, brain abscesses, or granulomas may be related to pressure changes and, in some instances, is reversible when pressure is decreased.

In either sex, central precocity may be secondary to prolonged sex steroid exposure associated with peripheral precocious puberty. Boys may develop central precocious puberty as a consequence of a prolonged hyperandrogenic state in inadequately treated congenital virilizing adrenal hyperplasia (40). Patients with this disorder may initially have peripheral precocity but later develop central early puberty after prolonged excessive androgen stimulation. After appropriate treatment of their adrenal hyperplasia, these individuals have a persistence of pubertal development with hormonal, including pubertal, response to GnRH stimulation and physical evidence of early maturation of the hypothalamic-pituitary axis. If this occurs, it is among patients who have advance in biologic maturation evidenced by bone age maturation to or beyond 12.5 years.

Central precocity in males is characterized not only by pubertal testosterone levels and basal and GnRH-stimulated

Table 3 Criteria to Plan Diagnostic Evaluation of Premature Pubertal Development

	Girls	Both sexes	Boys
A Clinical findings of precocious puberty	Breast development Genital maturation Accelerated linear growth ± Sexual hair ± Menstruation		Genital development with testicular growth Sexual hair Accelerated linear growth Increased muscle mass
		Assess the following depending upon particular situation:	
		History Exposure to exogenous hormones CNS trauma, anomalies, or infection CNS symptoms Familial history of age of pubertal onset Growth pattern and rates Physical examination	Familial forms usually involve males
	Tanner breast and pubic hair stage Clitoral size Rectal-abdominal bimanual examination Inspect for galactorrhea, estrogenized vaginal mucosa	Pubertal maturational staging (Tanner) Body proportions (upper/lower segment ratios) Body and skeletal symmetry Acne and skin pigmentation Fundoscopic and visual field examinations Thyroid examination Evidence of thyroid dysfunction Neurologic examination Laboratory evaluation Serum or plasma assessment	Tanner genital size and pubic hair stages Penis size Stretched length Description of width Testicular examination Size: long axis or volume Symmetry Consistency
	Estradiol	LH, FSH Thyroid function tests DHA or DHAS	Testosterone hCG
	Increased LH response	GnRH stimulation Radiologic assessment Skeletal age MRI of hypothalamic region (if "peripheral" causes excluded)	Increased LH and FSH rise
	Abdominal-pelvic sonography	Other	Testicular sonography
	Vaginal cytology		Morning void for sperm

gonadotropin levels but also by full physical pubertal development, including testicular growth. The forms of peripheral precocious puberty in which androgen production is autonomous generally do not present with symmetric testicular size consistent with stage of pubertal development.

2. Peripheral Precocious Puberty

The most common cause of peripheral precocious puberty in boys is endogenous androgen excess in undiagnosed or inadequately treated congenital adrenal hyperplasia (CAH) caused by 21-hydroxylase deficiency. Precocity in boys results not only from adrenal hyperplasia but also from the inappropriate presence of androgen from endogenous or exogenous sources or, rarely, from Leydig cell testosterone secreted after stimulation by abnormal gonadotropin production. Unusual causes include 11-hydroxylase deficiency CAH and tumors that secrete excess androgen, such as Leydig cell tumors and adrenocortical androgen-secreting tumors. Chorionic gonadotropin-secreting tumors, such as teratomas, em-

		History	
B Clinical findings of premature thelarche	Breast development without growth acceleration or other pubertal findings	Exposure to gonadotropins or estrogen	(see Table 5 for contrasexual development)
		Growth pattern	
		Physical examination: thorough examination (see earlier)	
		Laboratory examination Serum LH, FSH, estradiol Skeletal age x-ray **Pelvic sonography**	
		Follow-up Reassess growth rate, pubertal progression after 2–6 months Repeat sonography if follicular cysts	
C Clinical findings of adrenarche	Sexual hair (pubic or axillary) without growth acceleration or other pubertal changes (Table 5)	History Exposure to androgens Growth pattern	
		Physical examination Laboratory examination Plasma DHA or DHAS Skeletal age x-ray Follow-up: reassess growth rate and pubertal progression in 3–6 months	

bryonal tumors, hepatoblastomas, and CNS germinomas, cause peripheral precocity among males, although it is not clear whether hCG excess alone can cause precocity among females.

a. Familial Gonadotropin-Independent Puberty. An unique entity of male gonadotropin-independent precocity occurs in which gonadal steroidogenesis and spermatogenesis proceed even though gonadotropin stimulation is age appropriately low or suppressed (41,42). Gonadotropin levels, episodic release, and responses to exogenous GnRH are all prepubertal, but testosterone production and levels reach the adult male range. Pubertal development is full, including testicular growth. Fathers with this condition transmit it to all their sons; inheritance is consistent with an autosomal dominant but male-limited pattern. Family history may include males in each generation who were affected with early puberty.

A mutation of the LH receptor involving a single base change has been found among affected individuals (43). The mutant receptor has been demonstrated to increase cyclic AMP production, providing evidence that the autonomous Leydig cell activity is the result of a constitutively activated LH receptor. It has not yet been fully explained why this mutation is not expressed in females unless the LH effects of the mutation are insufficient for ovarian steroidogenesis without FSH (tumors secreting human chorionic gonadotropin, hCG, have not been shown to cause precocity in females); in the male, not

only is Leydig cell steroidogenesis activated, but spermatogenesis is sufficient to produce mature forms and considerable seminiferous tubular growth without FSH. Eventually, a pubertal hypothalamic-pituitary-testicular axis can be demonstrated among affected males, with normal fertility and adult height that may be foreshortened. This is a form of peripheral precocious puberty that may be followed by central precocity.

Gonadotropin-independent precocity may be misdiagnosed as idiopathic central sexual precocity because patients present with physical findings of complete puberty, including bilateral testicular enlargement. Testosterone levels are pubertal or adult, and other laboratory screening tests may be consistent with idiopathic puberty. GnRH stimulation testing is indicated not only to diagnose central precocity but as part of the assessment for this entity. There is a prepubertal gonadotropin response to GnRH, unless presentation and evaluation are sufficiently delayed after pubertal onset that secondary hypothalamic maturation has occurred. Lack of suppression of testosterone with an GnRH analog is characteristic of this entity (44). Even after maturation of the hypothalamic-pituitary axis has occurred, GnRH analog treatment results in suppression of the LH and FSH response to exogenous GnRH, but testosterone levels are not suppressed. Although GnRH analog administration is useful in confirming the diagnosis of testotoxicosis, it cannot be used alone to treat the combined peripheral-central pubertal condition because pubertal levels of testosterone persist.

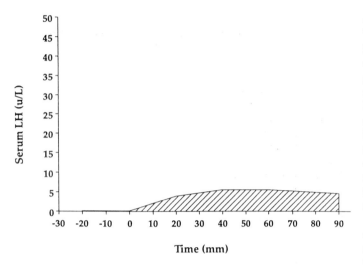

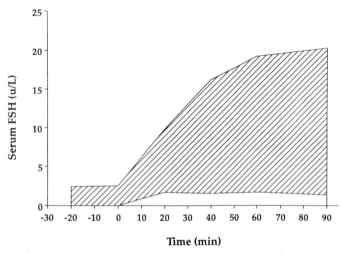

Figure 5 Range of serum LH and FSH responses to GnRH stimulation in 12 prepubertal females showing the wide variation in response, especially FSH. Actual units vary depending upon the gonadotropin assay used, but pubertal individuals have an LH response greater than the prepubertal response, although the height of the FSH response cannot be expected to be greater. The initial rise in FSH may be more brisk, so that values within the first 40 minutes may be somewhat greater than the prepubertal range, and maximum incremental rise does not differ. Therefore, to verify central precocious puberty, a rise in LH above the prepubertal range should be demonstrated.

b. Chronic Primary Hyperthyroidism. Rarely, prepubertal-aged boys with chronic primary hyperthyroidism present with testicular enlargement. Testicular enlargement may be the result of increased prolactin, α subunit, or FSH stimulation (45). Hyperprolactemia and galactorrhea may be present. Gonadotropin and prolactin levels fall and testicular size decreases when TSH levels are suppressed by thyroid replacement therapy.

3. Assessment

The evaluation of males with early puberty should be guided by the important aspects of history, physical examination, and laboratory assessment outlined in Table 3. A history of growth patterns and pubertal progression can provide clues concerning etiology. Tanner staging and testicular size should be verified. Generally, prepubertal-sized testes (less than 2.0 cm in the longitudinal axis) suggest a cause other than pubertal hypothalamic-pituitary gonadotropin function; pubertal-sized testes (longer than 2.5 cm) suggest central precocious puberty (Fig. 7). Asymmetrically enlargement or unilateral enlargement suggests a Leydig cell tumor or hyperplasia adrenal rest tissue. The latter is seen in inadequately treated CAH and may also be bilateral.

Gonadotropin response to GnRH stimulation should be documented, with particular attention to whether the LH response is within the prepubertal or pubertal range. Testosterone levels above the prepubertal range verify the early pubertal status, but such levels do not differentiate the source or stimulation of such hormone production. Skeletal age should be documented to judge androgen-stimulated advanced maturity and remaining growth potential. Because of the high incidence of CNS lesions in male sexual precocity, MRI or CT scans should be done unless the cause is otherwise explained.

D. Natural History

The natural history of central sexual precocity is outlined in Figure 8. This condition involves all phases of pubertal development; thus, not only is there early sexual development, including spermatogenesis, but also a premature pubertal growth acceleration. If untreated, this early pubertal development leads to premature attainment of adult sexual and reproductive capabilities. The increased sex steroid levels stimulate bone growth and maturation. However, the untimely stimulation may result in less total increase in height for the degree of skeletal maturity. Because of this premature growth spurt and skeletal maturation, children with precocity are likely to be tall for age during childhood. However, if their skeletal maturity becomes relatively more advanced than their stature (for example, a 5 year old with the mean height for a 7 year old but a skeletal age of 10 years), projected adult height is less than genetic potential would suggest. Because of the disproportionately advanced bone age, it is expected that such children will complete growth at a younger age and that they will be shorter as adults than they would have been if puberty and its growth spurt had occurred during the usual adolescent years. Therefore, the indications for treatment are not only to stop or cause regression of pubertal characteristics but also to attempt to increase adult height if the tempo of puberty is such that adult height is or is expected to be compromised.

The tall stature for age, as well as the advanced pubertal development, may cause social and psychologic adjustment problems. Early menarche may add to this, especially for very young girls for whom practical aspects of care are difficult. Psychosocial concerns are an indication for counseling, in

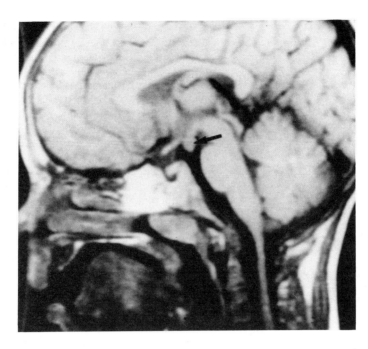

Figure 6 A hypothalamic hamartoma associated with episodic gonadotropin-releasing hormone secretion in a young boy with central precocious puberty. The arrow points to the hamartoma.

addition to consideration of medical treatment to suppress excessive growth rate and pubertal advancement.

Whether or not the precocity is treated medically, the patient and parents need to understand what is happening. If puberty is idiopathic, they should understand that normal things are happening, but at an early age. Discussion of pubertal development with the patient should include age-appropriate sex education. Psychosexual development is generally commensurate with age, not physical maturity, and hence inappropriate sexual behavior is seldom a problem. In contrast with being sexually aggressive, patients may be naive and misinterpret sexual advances by older individuals. Girls and, to a lesser extent, boys are potential victims of sexual encounters with older persons who would take advantage of their child-like concept of, and vulnerability to, intimacy. Both boys and girls may be potentially fertile, but once they recognize that they are more mature, they tend to avoid incidents of childhood sex play. Children with early puberty share interests with age peers. Even though boys experience frequent erections and masturbation and may have the capacity for ejaculation, they are not an increased threat of potential sexual aggression.

E. Therapy

If there is an underlying cause resulting in early puberty, medical therapy involves treatment of this cause if possible. A treatable underlying cause is infrequently present. In some of these, such as malignant tumors, the underlying disease is a considerably greater threat to the patient's well-being than the early puberty. Examples of treatment for underlying

conditions include surgery and radiation or chemotherapy for CNS, ectopic gonadotropin-producing, gonadal, or adrenal tumors. Adrenal suppression is indicated in CAH, thyroid replacement in primary hypothyroidism, and cessation of administration of inappropriate steroid or gonadotropin treatments in those instances. If the underlying treatment is completely successful and central pubertal maturation has not occurred, progression of pubertal development should cease and some regression may follow. In patients with autonomous gonadal steroid production, such as those with the McCune-Albright syndrome or male familial gonadotropin-independent puberty, various treatment agents are used (46,47). In the former instance, medroxyprogesterone has been used (48), although efficacy has not been established. Testolactone may be effective (47). Ketoconazole to inhibit androgen production (49), testolactone to block androgen action, and spironolactone via several effects (46) have been used alone or in combination with variable effectiveness in gonadotropin-independent precocity. Patients so treated should be carefully monitored for pubertal development, testosterone levels, and side effects of the agent(s) used. As mentioned, GnRH analogs are indicated if a secondary central component is present.

Among patients with central puberty, idiopathic or otherwise, marked by a pubertal pattern of gonadotropin response to GnRH stimulation, gonadotropin production can be stopped with GnRH analogs (50–53). If therapy is indicated to stop the progression of puberty or menses and to preclude or attempt to reclaim compromised growth potential, GnRH analog therapy is the treatment of choice. The GnRH analogs contain amino acid substitutions of the nat-

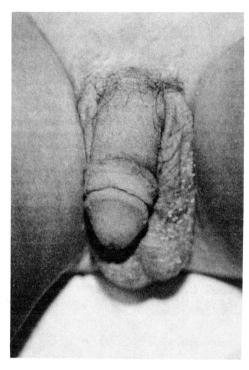

Figure 7 Genitalia of a 25-month-old boy with sexual precocity associated with a hypothalamic hamartoma. Tanner stage 2 pubic hair, Tanner stage 3 genital development and enlarged testes for age are evident.

urally occurring decapeptide that prolong the duration of effectiveness (Table 4). The basis for this treatment is the interference with the episodic secretion of gonadotropins by overriding the episodic release of GnRH with continual high levels of GnRH analog. Although the initial response to GnRH analog treatment is gonadotropin release, the long-term effect of persistent adequate dosing is downregulation of responsiveness; GnRH receptor numbers decrease, and gonadotropin responses are suppressed. The result of such treatment is first a fall in circulating gonadotropins, followed by a return of sex steroids to prepubertal levels. Adequacy of suppression should be monitored by the demonstration of the lack of gonadotropin response to exogenous GnRH stimulation.

GnRH analogs have been developed for suppression using depot injections, short-acting injections, and nasal spray. The effectiveness of treatment is monitored by clinical indices and hormonal testing, including GnRH stimulation. Hormonal secretion should revert to a prepubertal level, and physical development should cease or regress. An effective dosage is reached when the LH and FSH response to exogenous GnRH is obliterated. In boys, a fall in plasma testosterone to a prepubertal range is indicative of adequate dosage, whereas in girls estradiol levels are less helpful because of fluctuating and low levels that are present in the pubertal state. Treatment can be initiated after baseline studies, including GnRH stimulation, verify the pubertal

status. Repeat hormone determinations should be done at 1 to 2 months after beginning treatment to verify that suppression is complete. If not, and if the recommended dosage is being appropriately administered, the per kilogram dose should be increased. Once suppression is verified, patients should be monitored at 3–6 month intervals, with GnRH testing at 6–12 month intervals and skeletal age x-ray films taken at least annually.

The hormonal suppression that follows GnRH analog treatment results in a deceleration of the puberty growth rate and a cessation of pubertal development. In female patients, breasts stop growing and may regress, the vaginal mucosa becomes nonestrogenized, and menses cease. In boys, genital, including testicular, growth ceases and regression may occur. Growth rates and skeletal maturity decelerates. Projected final adult heights may increase among those with compromised predictions before beginning therapy. Also, patients begun on therapy early in the course of precocity may avoid the compromised height that might otherwise have occurred without treatment.

Long-term data are available only for the initial patients treated, who tend to have been older (53–55). Following discontinuation, gonadotropin levels and responses promptly return to pubertal, as does progression of pubertal development. Menarche among most occurs within 2 years, but for some a considerably longer period has been observed (55). Ovulation and pregnancy have been documented. Data concerning adult heights indicate that this surpasses pretreatment height predictions but fails to reach target heights calculated by sex-adjusted midparental heights. The need for complete suppression has been demonstrated (56): growth velocity and bone maturation have been shown to be higher among patients with more phases of incomplete suppression compared with a completely suppressed group.

The purpose of treatment should be carefully considered before therapy is begun. If physical pubertal development is minimal, treatment can delay these changes until an age-appropriate time. If menses has not begun, treatment can prevent it, although withdrawal bleeding may occur within the first 2 weeks of initiating treatment. Although growth rate and skeletal maturation can be slowed unless skeletal age is advancing faster than concomitant growth, the precocious puberty may be proceeding at a pace that does not compromise height. In such a situation, treatment should not be prescribed in the context of improving height. The actual effect of reversing the tall child–short adult phenomenon can only be anticipated if treatment is begun before height is excessive. If a pubertal growth spurt has already occurred, only a small percentage of growth potential remains; hence treatment may not be expected to affect ultimate height dramatically.

F. Partial Pubertal Development: Variants of Normal

1. Premature Thelarche: Girls

Premature thelarche (isolated premature breast development) commonly occurs during two age periods. Significant breast

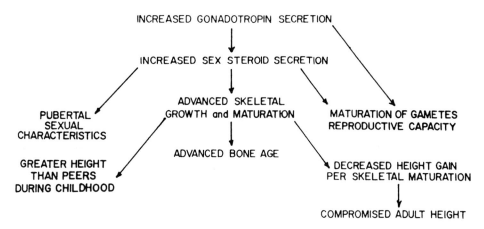

Figure 8 Schematic representation of the natural history of early pubertal development. (Used by permission, Year Book Medical Publishers.)

tissue is most commonly noted during the first 2 years of life. In most instances, the history suggests that this is a persistence or increase in the palpable breast tissue present at birth caused by a persistence of infant gonadotropin physiology. Ovarian hormone production is greater during infancy than later childhood, and breast growth may occur because of increased stimulation or extraresponsive breast tissue. Such breast growth almost always regresses before 24 months of age.

The second period when isolated breast growth may be noted is after age 6 years. As in normal puberty, when breast development is first noticed it may be asymmetric or unilateral. It may be caused by temporarily increased ovarian steroid secretion or by breast tissue that is very sensitive to low pubertal circulating estrogen levels, or both. However, if breast development is not accompanied by other evidence of puberty, limited workup is indicated (see Table 3[B]). Estrogen levels, height, and bone age may be normal or slightly advanced for age. Rarely, an ovarian follicular cyst may be identified but does not persist. Because the condition is benign and may regress, treatment can be limited to education and counseling. Because there may be episodes of greater gonadotropin secretion during childhood in girls, however, it may be difficult to ascertain where along the continuum from premature thelarche and central precocity a given patient lies. Occasionally, what initially

appears to be isolated breast development may actually be the first sign of what will eventually become manifest central precocity; thus, careful follow-up examination should be done.

2. Premature Pubarche
Premature pubarche, the early development of sexual hair, is the result of premature adrenarche, an early onset of the increase in adrenal androgen production. Adrenarche usually precedes pubertal maturation of the gonad, is independent at gonadarche (57), is not accompanied by a mature response to GnRH stimulation (58), and is not suppressed by GnRH analog therapy (59). Premature pubarche is more common in girls than boys and is rare before 6 years of age. The early pubic hair may be an isolated finding or be accompanied by mild acne, oily skin, onset of adult-type body odor, and axillary hair. If there are no other associated findings or pathologic conditions, minimal workup is required (Table 3[C]). Documentation of the status of adrenarche can be confirmed by demonstrating that serum or plasma levels of DHA or DHAS are above the prepubertal range. Height and skeletal age may be normal or transiently advanced (60). Growth and subsequent pubertal development should be expected to occur normally. The degree of advancement should be followed; abnormal progression, excessive viriliza-

Table 4 Gonadotropin-Releasing Hormone Analogs (GnRHa)

Analog	Trade name	Manufacturer	Formulation
Buserelin	—	Hoechst	—
Goserelin	Zoladex	Zeneca	Subcutaneous (SC) depot implant[a]
Histrelin	Supprelin	Roberts	SC injection[b]
Leuprolide	Lupron depot	TAP	IM depot[b] and SC injection
Nafarelin	Synarel	Syntex	Nasal spray[b]
Tryptorelin	—	Lederle	—

[a]Not appropriate for precocious puberty.
[b]Approved for precocious puberty before 1994.

tion, or elevated DHA and DHAS levels may indicate pathologic causes of excessive androgen.

III. CONTRASEXUAL PUBERTAL DEVELOPMENT

Contrasexual pubertal development during childhood or puberty is the development of sexual characteristics inappropriate for the sex of the individual (i.e., feminization among boys and virilization among girls). Causes among girls include the differential of androgen excess and, for boys, estrogen excess.

A. Girls

Although premature development of sexual hair (premature pubarche) in girls is not uncommon, excessive virilization of the prepubertal girl is rare and may present with the development not only of sexual hair, oily skin, and acne but also clitoromegaly and hirsutism. Etiologies are listed in Table 5. Generally, the degree of virilization with adrenal hyperplasia or adrenal and ovarian tumors is much more marked than with adrenarche. Mild forms of adrenal hyperplasia may present as premature adrenarche. Thus, if bone age, growth rate, or degree of virilization is more than slightly excessive, adrenal steroid metabolites should be measured. Androgen levels, measured as plasma androstenedione, DHA, DHAS, or testosterone, and urinary 17-ketosteroids are within the pubertal range in adrenarche but above normal ranges in adrenal hyperplasia and dramatically elevated with adrenal tumors. 17-Hydroxyprogesterone levels are elevated in 21-hydroxylase deficiency adrenal hyperplasia. Corticotropin (adrenocorticotropic hormone) stimulation testing with measurement of adrenal steroid intermediate metabolites may be useful in identifying these mild forms (61). In the presence of persistently elevated levels of androgens, adrenal suppression should be attempted to differentiate adrenal hyperplasia from adrenal tumors or ovarian sources. Although adrenal hyperplasia is uncommon among patients presenting with early

pubarche without clear excessive virilization, there may be an increased incidence of ovarian hyperandrogenism (62).

B. Boys

Gynecomastia, either unilateral or bilateral, in a pubertal boy is usually a variation of normal puberty (Chap. 14) (25). The most common pathologic cause of gynecomastia is hypogonadism, particularly Klinefelter syndrome. Gynecomastia caused by abnormal estrogen production (Table 5) is rare, but it should be ruled out in a prepubertal boy or at any age when the degree or progression is troublesome. Plasma estrogen levels or total urinary estrogen levels are elevated if there is a persistent source of abnormal endogenous estrogen. Appropriate plasma and urinary levels, an otherwise normal history and physical examination, and a negative history of contact with estrogen-containing medicine or cosmetics are sufficient to delay further workup with follow-up to watch for progression of gynecomastia.

IV. DELAYED PUBERTY

A. Definition and General Approach

If the initial physical changes of puberty are not present by age 13 years in girls or age 14 in boys, evaluation should be considered for possible causes of lack of pubertal development. An abnormality may be present if pubertal development has begun but does not progress appropriately. Therefore, evaluation may also be indicated if more than 5 years has elapsed between the first signs of puberty and menarche in girls or completion of genital growth in boys. The aim of the assessment is to determine whether the delay or lack of development is a result of a lag in normal pubertal maturation of the hypothalamic-pituitary-gonadal axis or represents an underlying abnormality (Table 6; see also Chap. 18).

If patients have no pertinent findings on medical history, a delay in the onset of puberty is likely to be so-called

Table 5   Causes of Contrasexual Pubertal Development, Prepubertal or Pubertal Onset

Virilization in girls
   Adrenal sources of androgen excess: adenoma, carcinoma, virilizing adrenal hyperplasia
   Exogenous androgen
   Idiopathic hirsutism
   Ovarian sources of androgen excess: arrhenoblastoma, teratoma, polycystic ovarian syndrome
Feminization in boys
   Adolescent, pubertal, or idiopathic gynecomastia
   Drugs (amphetamines, antineoplastics, gonadotropin, isoniazid, ketoconazole, marijuana, sex
      steroids, tricyclic antidepressants, others)
   Neoplasms (adrenal or testicular steroid-producing tumors, teratomas)
   Primary hypogonadal conditions
      Congenital (anorchia, dysgenetic testes, enzyme biosynthetic defects, Klinefelter syndrome,
         partial androgen insensitivity syndrome)
      Acquired (cryptorchidism, infection, radiation, torsion, trauma)
   Systemic illness: hepatic, renal, recovery from malnutrition

constitutional delay of puberty. Such patients are healthy but generally have a history of delayed growth and development throughout childhood, including short stature but a relatively normal growth rate.

The initial approach to patients of both sexes with delayed or lack of progression of puberty is to determine gonadotropin status (Table 6) and skeletal age. Skeletal age or bone age is determined by radiographic analysis of the ossification centers of the hands and wrists. The extent of ossification is compared with the average for age and sex. If bone age is less than biologic age of the onset of puberty (10.5–11 years for girls and 12.5–13 for boys), it is impossible to determine whether gonadotropin secretion is delayed and immature or defective. In either situation, gonadotropin levels, both before and after GnRH stimulation, are within the prepubertal range, although as patients grow older assessment may show persistence of a decreased response in deficient patients. Persistently low gonadotropin secretion over time suggests a deficiency at the hypothalamic or pituitary level, whereas a progressive rise is consistent with normal but delayed puberty. If bone age, an index of biologic age, is at or beyond the age of puberty, gonadotropin (LH and FSH) levels should be elevated if gonadal failure is present because of lack of negative feedback by sex steroids. Excessive responses of LH and FSH to acute GnRH stimulation also reflect this phenomenon.

B. Boys

1. Assessment

Most boys who present with normal but underdeveloped genitalia and delayed pubertal development have constitutional delay and eventually have normal testicular function. Many of these patients present with a history of short stature. A plot of previous heights for age on a growth curve indicates low normal growth rates (Chap. 1). The delay in biologic maturity is evident by skeletal maturation. Such patients have immature body proportions (a greater upper/lower ratio than usual for age or usually short legs for height) and descended testes that are prepubertal in size and consistency. Primary

Table 6 Etiologies of Delay or Lack of Pubertal Development

Hypergonadotropic states (primary gonadal failure)
  Chromosomal, genetic disorders, and syndromes: androgen enzymatic synthesis defects, complete and partial androgen insensitivity syndrome, 46, XX males, 47, XYY syndromes, galactosemia, Klinefelter syndrome (47, XXY), mixed 45, X/46, XY gonadal dysgenesis, multiple X-Y syndromes, multiple Y syndromes, myotonic dystrophy, Noonan syndrome, pure 46, XY gonadal dysgenesis, 5α-reductase deficiency, resistant ovary syndrome, Turner syndrome, vanishing testes syndrome
  Acquired: autoimmune, chemotherapy, infectious (coxsackie, mumps), irradiation, surgical, torsion, traumatic
Hypogonadotropic states (hypothalamic-pituitary defect or lag)
  Hypothalamic-pituitary deficiencies
    Gonadotropin deficiency
      LH only (fertile eunuch syndrome)
      LH and FSH
        Acquired [autoimmune, cranial irradiation, granulomatous disease, hemosiderosis (thalassemia), sickle cell disease]
        Congenital, genetic, syndromes [Alstrom syndrome, Borjenson-Forssman-Lehmann syndrome, CHARGE syndrome, idiopathic Kallmann syndrome, Laurence-Moon-Bardet-Biedl syndrome, multiple lentigines syndrome, Prader-Willi syndrome, prosencephalon defects (associated with central incisor syndrome, cleft-lip palate, midfacial cleft), septooptic dysplasia]
    Endocrinopathies (may include gonadotropin deficiency): hypopituitarism [idiopathic or secondary to empty sella syndrome, inflammation, pituitary dysgenesis, radiation, Rathke pouch cysts, surgery, trauma, tumors (craniopharyngioma, pituitary adenomas, prolactinomas)]
  Delayed or deferred function
    Constitutional delay of growth and/or puberty
    Chronic illness [cardiac, gastrointestinal (regional enteritis), hematologic (sickle cell disease), malignancy, pulmonary (cystic fibrosis), renal]
    Drug abuse
    Excessive energy expenditure, exercise
    Exogenous obesity
    Endocrinopathies: diabetes mellitus, growth hormone deficiency, glucocorticoid excess, hyperprolactinemia, hypothyroidism
    Malnutrition
    Psychiatric illness (anorexia nervosa, psychosocial dwarfism)

hypogonadism (testicular failure) and hypergonadotropism are very unlikely in such a patient (Chap. 18).

Gonadotropin are usually low for age in delayed puberty, as in gonadotropin deficiency. It usually is not possible at presentation at ages 13–16 years to determine definitely which patients have a temporary delay of gonadotropin secretion and which have a permanent deficiency unless there is a concomitant finding associated with hypogonadotropism, such as anosmia. The range of LH and FSH responses to GnRH stimulation in individuals with an immature prepubertal hypothalamus overlap with the response range in those with permanent defect of the hypothalamus and pituitary, even though the latter group has a mean response that is less.

The initial workup should involve an evaluation aimed at the differential diagnosis listed in Table 6. The history should include a review of rates of weight and height gain, testicular descent, any other evidence suggestive of gonadal endocrinopathy, including associated hypopituitarism, hypothyroidism, adrenal insufficiency, diabetes insipidus, or midline facial malformations. Current or prior illnesses and their treatment, including irradiation, surgery, chemotherapy, or glucocorticoid therapy, should be considered. A family history of pubertal delay, hypogonadism, or infertility should be sought. Evidence of craniofacial-CNS midline defects, including anosmia or hyposmia, are important and suggestive of Kallmann syndrome, a unique hypogonadotropic syndrome with concomitant defects in the sense of smell (63,64). Physical examination must include careful documentation of height, weight, pubertal stage (Table 1), and upper/lower (U/L) segment ratios. This ratio is determined by subtracting, from standing height (U), the vertical distance from the pubic symphysis to the floor (L) or by subtracting the sitting height (U) from standing height (L). A ratio higher than normal suggests immaturity and delay, whereas a ratio lower than normal is suggestive of a defect or prolonged delay. In general, a ratio of less than unity (0.88 in blacks) results from excessive leg (long-bone) growth characteristic of hypogonadism. Such eunuchoid ratios are often abnormal in instances of primary hypogonadism, such as Klinefelter syndrome. Testicular location (scrotal, inguinal, or nonpalpable), size, and consistency are important. A testis less than 2.0 cm along the longitudinal axis is prepubertal in size; if longer than 2.5 cm, there has been some pubertal growth. A testes in a pubertal-aged boy of 1.0 cm or less, particularly if unusually firm or soft, is suggestive of a hypogonadal state. A careful neurologic examination should be done, including assessment of fundi, visual fields, and sense of smell.

Laboratory evaluation should include, at least, measurement of plasma or serum LH and FSH levels. A skeletal x-ray for bone age is indicated to document biologic age and time of expected pubertal maturation, because puberty in girls should start when bone age is 10–11 years and in boys at about 12.5 years. Assessment of growth hormone secretion and thyroid function may be indicated if growth rate is subnormal, although growth rates slow just before the onset of puberty in normal boys. Various studies may be indicated to rule out CNS, renal, or gastrointestinal disease and may include blood and urinary pH, urinary specific gravity,

sedimentation rates, blood urea nitrogen, creatinine, and MRI of the head. If testes are small and firm or if there is other evidence suggestive of Klinefelter syndrome, a karyotype is indicated. The GnRH stimulation test is usually not helpful in the diagnosis of gonadal failure, because although excessive responses indicate testicular failure, in most instances patients also have elevated basal gonadotropin levels. The response in patients with hypogonadotropism is variable and may be indistinguishable from normal responses. A human chorionic gonadotropin stimulation test is indicated if testes are nonpalpable or a testicular defect is suspected and the gonadotropin levels are not elevated. A rise in circulating testosterone levels to higher than 300 ng/dl after 5 days of stimulation demonstrates adequate Leydig cell function. Many hCG regimens are used (Chap. 18). A dosage of 3000 units/m^2 per injection for 5 days of stimulation is adequate, with the following limits. The maximum stimulation should be limited to a total of 3000 units per injection, or 15,000 units for the treatment period. A minimum of 5000 units should be given during the treatment period. Within these total dosage limits, the drug may be administered two or three times a week. A blood sample for the testosterone should be obtained within 1 day of the last injection.

2. Elevated Gonadotropin: Primary Hypogonadism and Testicular Failure

The initial laboratory testing identifies patients with elevated gonadotropin if bone age is over 12.5 years. This indicates failure of the testes to produce adequate sex steroids to suppress the maturing hypothalamic-pituitary axis. The possible conditions of primary testicular failure listed in Table 6 should be a guide to further evaluation. A karyotype is indicated in boys who have small testes and hypergonadotropism. If there is a documented history of destruction of normal testes (e.g., torsion or radiation), a karyotype determination is unnecessary.

Patients with primary hypogonadism and their parents should be informed about therapeutic possibilities. Such boys should be counseled appropriately for their level of understanding. The counseling should be based on an understanding of the two basic functions of the testes: male hormone and sperm production.

Patients can be assured that the hormone can be replaced and that they will develop physically into normal men at the appropriate age. They also need to know that they will be able to function sexually, the same as any other man. They also need to understand, however, that their children may be by adoption or by some other way available to men who have a problem producing sperm, including sperm donation. They should have the choice, which most select, to have prosthetic testes placed in the scrotum. Prosthetic testes come in a graded series of sizes, from juvenile to adult. If the condition is discovered before pubertal hormonal stimulation is appropriate, a decision must be made about whether to implant smaller testes temporarily. Although having an empty scrotum may have psychologic effects during boyhood, the advantage of placing prostheses that must later be replaced by larger prostheses needs to be weighed. It may be wiser to delay the implant until it is appropriate to place organs of adult size, thereby avoiding repeated surgical procedure. Usually the knowledge that testes will be implanted during early to midpubertal development is psychologically satisfying. Adult-sized testes can be inserted as soon as there is enough pubertal scrotal growth to accommodate them. One should be sure that the patient and his parents understand that the prostheses are, on the one hand, for cosmetic or appearance purposes only, but, on the other, that they look and feel so normal that no one can tell.

Hormonal replacement should begin at the usual age of the onset of puberty, 12.5–13 years, or as soon thereafter as the need is recognized. Occasionally there are reasons to delay treatment, including general growth failure, short stature, and emotional or psychologic immaturity. The initial dosage may vary depending on the rapidity of pubertal development desired based on the age, social and intellectual maturation, and psychologic needs of the patient (see Sec. IV.B.4). Although early treatment with androgens accelerates bone age and may ultimately decrease adult height, if replacement therapy is given at the age of usual pubertal development, it does not have a detrimental effect on adult height (65).

3. Low Gonadotropin

If gonadotropin levels are low (Table 6), if there are no organic or associated conditions of pituitary malfunction, and if there is no other cause to account for delayed maturation, it usually is not possible to determine whether gonadotropin deficiency or simply delayed maturation exists (Chap. 18). Gonadotropin, particularly LH, responses to GnRH stimulation may be helpful if a clear pubertal response is present. Although, as a group, patients with gonadotropin deficiency have poorer responses than those with constitutional delay, only rarely are the responses so minimal they indicate a definite diagnosis of hypogonadotropism. A rise consistent with a pubertal response may be discernible before clinical evidence of the onset of puberty, suggesting constitutional delay. Also, the demonstration of episodic LH release with 10–20 minute sampling during sleep, the normal physiology of the prepubertal state (66), suggests normal developmental potential and therefore constitutional delay. Patients with Kallmann syndrome may have occasional pulses but nocturnal augmentation has not been demonstrated. However, the lack of demonstration of such episodic release may be a prepubertal pattern, nonrepresentative sampling, or a hypogonadotropic state and is not diagnostic.

When pubertal delay occurs with low gonadotropin levels, hormonal stimulation can be begun, even if delay cannot yet be differentiated from deficiency. Short-term treatment with testosterone (Fig. 9) is appropriate if age and psychosocial development indicate a need for physical pubertal maturation. Such exposure to androgens at a biologic age (bone age) of 12–13 years or older has no detrimental effects upon those with either constitutional delay or hypogonadotropic hypogonadism (65). Subsequent development in the former is normal, and spermatogenesis in response to exogenous gonadotropin stimulation in the latter is no different between those previously treated with testosterone and those not (67).

When a diagnosis is not yet possible, androgen treatment can be testosterone (enanthate or cypionate) given for a first treatment course of no longer than 4–6 months. The dosage can range from 50 to 100 mg intramuscularly (IM) every 4 weeks. Higher dosages may result in a too rapid stimulation, with dramatic reddening and sensitivity in the genital area and frequent erections. After the initial months of stimulation, no treatment should be given for at least 2 months so that basal testosterone levels can be measured to determine endogenous androgen production. If testosterone levels are clearly within the pubertal range (>100 ng/dl), this suggests a diagnosis of constitutional delay. Further treatment is not indicated at this point, but such patients should be followed at intervals of 6 months or longer to assess progression of puberty and testosterone levels. Once values reach the adult male range (>300 ng/dl), normal hypothalamic-pituitary-testicular function has been documented.

If testosterone levels are still low, more time, which may include a second course of testosterone treatment, is necessary to determine whether gonadotropin deficiency exists. When this diagnosis is made based on persistently low LH, FSH, and testosterone levels, physical pubertal development should be completed and maintained with testosterone replacement therapy. All males with hypogonadotropism should be informed that spermatogenesis and fertility may be possible after exogenously extracted (hCG and hCG plus human menopausal gonadotropin [hMG]) (68) or biosynthetic gonadotropin therapy. Similar results are expected after exogenous GnRH-stimulated pituitary gonadotropin release (69). Patients should understand that only a portion of patients so treated respond with adequate spermatogenesis. Response is predicted by initial testis size (68). However, the response to gonadotropin stimulation is not adversely affected by prior exogenous androgens (67). Because of expense and injection schedules, such treatment is not indicated until fertility is desired. Testosterone replacement is the treatment of choice until that time.

4. Therapy

Full replacement of androgen to attain and maintain an adult male state physically and sexually requires parenteral testosterone. Traditionally this has been given as a depot injection of testosterone enanthate or cypionate. The full adult replacement is a dosage of no more than 100 mg/week. It should be given at intervals of 2 weeks (200 mg) or 3 weeks (300 mg). Injections of 400 mg every 4 weeks are not recommended because they result in supraphysiologic levels for 7–10 days and then during the fourth week the levels are subnormal. Transdermal scrotal patches may become a substitute for this mode of therapy. The dosage of initial therapy depends upon the age and maturity of the patient and the rapidity of pubertal development desired. The usual starting dosage for intramuscular injections ranges from 50 to 100 mg every 4 weeks; higher dosages are sometimes used. The higher dosages stimulate more rapid development and can achieve considerable development within 4–6 months. The lower dosages stimulate pubertal changes at more of a natural pace.

Dosages can be gradually titered upward after full-re-

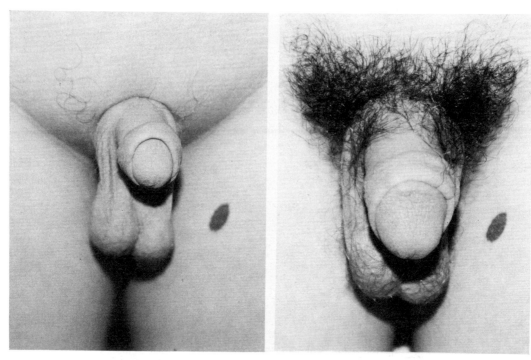

Figure 9 Genitalia of a male with delayed puberty before (left) and after (right) five monthly injections of 200 mg of testosterone enanthate IM. Pubertal development was Tanner 2 before the injections and skeletal age was 12-1/2 years at 14-8/12 years of age. After the injections at 15-2/12 years pubertal development progressed to Tanner 4. A subsequent endogenous testosterone level of 192 ng/dl verified a diagnosis of constitutional delay of puberty.

placement dosages after 3–4 years. Often patients learn to give their own injections into the thigh, keeping their medications at home. It is often important to reassure them that no one can tell that they require injections and that their physical development (except testicular, of course) and sexual function can be expected to be normal. If accessary sexual glands are appropriately formed, ejaculation, semen volume, and semen appearance are normal.

Other forms of androgen replacement are usually inadequate to produce full androgen stimulation. In situations in which the beginning of pubertal growth and development is required, mild oral androgens can be given. Oxandrolone causes somatic growth acceleration and the onset of penile, scrotal, and pubic hair growth. Therefore, it may be useful in such instances as constitutional pubertal delay in which the beginning of pubertal development is of psychosocial benefit. To achieve this effect, the dosage should be 0.25 mg/kg per day. Less than 0.1 mg/kg per day produces little, if any, virilization. The dosage should not exceed 10 mg daily. Buccal or oral oxandrolone, fluoxymesterone, and methyltestosterone tablets do not provide full replacement, however, and have limited usefulness. In addition, oral replacement of methyltestosterone is associated with malignant hepatocellular changes. Aqueous testosterone injections would have to be given daily or more often.

Some hypogonadotropic hypogonadal males have the potential for spermatogenesis and testosterone production if appropriately stimulated with gonadotropin or GnRH. Because of the expense and frequency of administration, such therapy is generally reserved for adult men at the time they desire paternity.

C. Girls

1. Assessment

Onset delay of pubertal development is a less common complaint among girls than among boys and is more likely to have an underlying pathologic cause. Delay is usually considered present if development of breasts and pubic hair has not begun by age 13 years or menarche by 15.5–16 years. Also, lack of completion of pubertal development to Tanner stage 5 within 4 years is considered delay. Categorization of patients as having elevated or low gonadotropin levels (Table 6) should be done initially, together with documentation of skeletal age (bone age x-ray). A GnRH stimulation test and periodic sleep-related blood sampling for gonadotropins may be indicated if basal gonadotropin levels are not diagnostic. Initial assessment should include a careful history, looking for evidence of chronic illness (e.g., occult Crohn's disease), endocrinopathy, prior illnesses and therapy, sense of smell, and a family history of lack of puberty or infertility (Kallmann syndrome). The physical examination should concentrate on body proportions, breast and genital development, neurologic examination, and possible evidence of Turner syndrome.

Laboratory evaluation should generally be similar to that for boys, although hCG testing is not indicated because hCG alone appears not to stimulate precocious puberty in girls.

2. Elevated Gonadotropins

If elevated gonadotropin levels are found and there is not ample evidence to explain the hypergonadotropic state, such as surgery, radiation, and chemotherapy, a karyotype evaluation should be done. This can verify Turner syndrome (70) if stigmata are present or can identify a variant or mosaic of Turner syndrome with subtle or no stigmata. A karyotype also identifies the very rare entity, pure gonadal dysgenesis, with a 46, XY karyotype, a condition with female genital differentiation caused by the complete lack of testicular development or function. Rarely, pure ovarian agenesis with a 46, XX karyotype also occurs (Chap. 19).

If the hypergonadotropic state is not explained by history and karyotype, the presence of antiovarian antibodies to rule out autoimmune disease and steroid intermediate metabolites to rule out enzyme deficiency can be measured. Although most enzyme deficiencies will have appeared earlier with other complaints, those that block estrogen synthesis include 17-hydroxylase-17,20-desmolase deficiency (elevated progesterone, pregnenolone 17-hydroxyprogesterone, and 17-hydroxypregnenolone levels) and desmolase deficiency (all steroids are low).

3. Low Gonadotropin Levels

If gonadotropin levels are low, the search for the cause is also an attempt to determine whether the hypogonadotropism represents a permanent hypothalamic-pituitary defect. If there is an underlying chronic illness, if there has been prolonged pharmacologic glucocorticoid therapy, or if there is excessive emotional stress, unusual physical activity, or an inadequate nutritional state, the hypogonadotropism is likely a secondary and potentially reversible condition. If the underlying problem can be adequately treated, normal gonadotropin secretion should follow. Treatment with estrogen while the underlying problem persists is usually not followed by much response. Idiopathic hypogonadotropism is less common in females than in males, although Kallmann syndrome occurs in both sexes, sometimes within the same family.

In an attempt to differentiate patients with a permanent defect from those with delayed or temporary hypogonadotropism, GnRH-stimulated or sleep-related periodic gonadotropin levels can be measured, although such testing is often not helpful except in the older adolescent patient. Persistence of low basal or GnRH-stimulated LH and FSH levels and lack of demonstration of episodic secretion in a patient without an underlying cause, or the finding of such levels in a patient in late-teenage years with a bone age over 11–12 years, is indicative of a defect of gonadotropin secretion.

As outlined for boys, skeletal maturation should be documented and followed with periodic bone-age x-ray films at intervals no more frequently than every 6 months. This should be done whether or not sex steroid treatment is used.

4. Treatment

Replacement therapy for girls should eventually consist of cyclic estrogen-progesterone therapy. However, initial therapy for young pubertal-aged patients can be daily low-dosage estrogen therapy for 6 to at most 12 months. If breakthrough bleeding occurs during this time, cyclic medication should be initiated. The lowest available estrogen dosage preparation (such as 0.3 mg Premarin or 0.02 mg ethinyl estradiol daily or the 0.05 mg transdermal patch applied once or twice a week) is appropriate for initial treatment. Cyclic estrogen-progesterone therapy can be given by administering low-estrogen birth control pills. Alternatively, a daily estrogen regimen or the transdermal form can be used for the first 3 weeks (21 days) of the calendar month, regardless of the length of the month, with progesterone added for the last 10 of the 21 days (days 12–21). With this regimen the patient is easily aware, based on the actual date, of what pills she should take. From day 22 until the end of the month, no matter how many days in the month, she should take no medication. On the first of the month, even if her period has not stopped, she should begin estrogen again. The dosage of estrogen can be varied, gauged to the rapidity and adequacy of pubertal development. Ethinyl estradiol (0.02–0.10 mg/day), conjugated estrogen (0.3–1.25 mg/day), or transdermal treatment to deliver 0.05 or 0.1 mg daily can be used. Once full pubertal development has been reached, the estrogen dosage should be the minimum that maintains normal menstrual flow and prevents calcium bone loss, equivalent to 0.625 mg conjugated estrogen. Progesterone in this regimen can be given as medroxyprogesterone (5 or 10 mg/day) or norethindrone (5 mg/day).

It should be recognized that spontaneous menstruation may occur with Turner syndrome; replacement therapy may not be needed in all patients, and some may be fertile (71). In addition, patients with Turner syndrome and others with ovarian failure but normal müllerian duct differentiation are candidates for in vitro fertilization using donated ova (72).

REFERENCES

1. Dunkel L, Alfthan H, Stenman U, Tapanainen P, Perheentupa J. Pulsatile secretion of LH and FSH in prepubertal and early pubertal boys revealed by ultrasensitive time-resolved immunofluorometric assays. Pediatr Res 1990; 27:215–219.
2. Goji K, Tanikaze S. Comparison between spontaneous gonadotropin concentration profiles and gonadotropin response to low-dose gonadotropin-releasing hormone in prepubertal and early pubertal boys and patients with hypogonadotropic hypogonadism: assessment by using ultrasensitive, time-resolved immunofluorometric assay. Pediatr Res 1992; 31:535–539.
3. Apter D, Bützow TL, Laughlin GA, Yen SSC. Gonadotropin-releasing hormone pulse generator activity during pubertal transition in girls: pulsatile and diurnal patterns of circulating gonadotropins. J Clin Endocrinol Metab 1993; 76:940–949.
4. Kletter GB, Padmanabhan V, Foster CM, Brown MB, Kelch RP, Beitins IZ. Luteinizing hormone pulse characteristics in early pubertal boys are the same whether measured by radioimmuno- or immunofluorometric assay. J Clin Endocrinol Metab 1993; 76:1173–1176.

5. Goji K. Twenty-four-hour concentration profiles of gonadotropin and estradiol (E_2) in prepubertal and early pubertal girls: the diurnal rise of E_2 is opposite the nocturnal rise of gonadotropin. J Clin Endocrinol Metab 1993; 77:1629–1635.

6. Delemarre-Van De Waal HA, Wennink JMB, Odink RJH. Gonadotropin and growth hormone secretion throughout puberty. Acta Paediatr Scand 1991; 372:26–31.

7. Knobil E. The neuroendocrine control of the menstrual cycle. Recent Prog Horm Res 1980; 36:53–88.

8. Lee PA. Pubertal neuroendocrine maturation: early differentiation and stages of development. Adolesc Pediatr Gynecol 1988; 1:3–12.

9. Lee PA. Neuroendocrine maturation and puberty. In: Lavery JP, Sanfilippo JS, eds. Pediatric and Adolescent Obstetrics and Gynecology. New York: Springer-Verlag, 1985:12–26.

10. Dickerman A, Prager-Levin R, Laron Z. Response of plasma LH and FSH to synthetic LHRH in children at various pubertal stages. Am J Dis Child 1976; 130:634–638.

11. Lee PA. Advances in the management of precocious puberty. Clin Pediatr (Phila) 1994; 33:54–61.

12. Kasa-Vubu JZ, Padmanaghan V, Kletter GB, et al. Serum bioactive luteinizing and follicle-stimulating hormone concentrations in girls increase during puberty. Pediatr Res 1993; 34:829–833.

13. Kletter GB, Padmanabhan V, Brown MB, Reiter EO, Sizonenko PC, Beitins IZ. Serum bioactive gonadotropins during male puberty: a longitudinal study. J Clin Endocrinol Metab 1993; 76:432–438.

14. Lee PA. Normal ages of pubertal events among American males and females. J Adolesc Health Care 1980; 1:26–29.

15. Lee PA, Zenakis T, Winer J, Matsenbaugh S. Puberty in girls: correlation of serum levels of gonadotropins, prolactin, androgens, estrogens and progestins with physical change. J Clin Endocrinol Metab 1976; 43:775–784.

16. DeRidder CM, Thijssen JHH, Bruning PF, Van Den Brande JL, Zonderland ML, Erich WBM. Body fat mass, body fat distribution, and pubertal development: a longitudinal study of physical and hormonal sexual maturation of girls. J Clin Endocrinol Metab 1992; 75:442–446.

17. Tanner JM. Growth at Adolescence, 11th ed. Oxford: Blackwell Scientific, 1962.

18. DePeretti E, Forest MG. Unconjugated dehydroepiandrosterone plasma levels in normal subjects from birth to adolescence in humans: the use of a sensitive radio-immunoassay. J Clin Endocrinol Metab 1976; 43:982–991.

19. Rico H, Revilla M, Villa LF, Hernandez ER, Alvarez de Buergo M, Villa M. Body composition in children and Tanner's stages. A study with dual-energy x-ray absorptiometry. Metabolism 1993; 42:967–970.

20. Winter JSD, Faiman C. Pituitary-gonadal relations in male children and adolescents. Pediatr Res 1972; 6:126–135.

21. Lee PA, Migeon CJ. Puberty in boys: correlation of plasma levels of gonadotropins (LH, FSH), androgens (testosterone, androstenedione, dehydroepiandrosterone, and its sulfate), estrogens (estrone and estradiol) and progestins (progesterone, 17-hydroxyprogesterone). J Clin Endocrinol Metab 1975; 41:556–562.

22. Richards RJ, Svec F, Bao W, Srinivasan SR, Berenson GS. Steroid hormones during puberty: racial (black-white) differences in andorstenedione and estradiol—the Bogalusa Heart Study. J Clin Endocrinol Metab 1992; 75:624–631.

23. Baker ML, Hutson JM. Serum levels of mullerian inhibiting substance in boys throughout puberty and in the first two years of life. J Clin Endocrinol Metab 1993; 76:245–247.

24. Rey R, Lordereau-Richard I, Carel JC, et al. Anti-Müllerian hormone and testosterone serum levels are inversely related during normal and precocious pubertal development. J Clin Endocrinol Metab 1993; 77:1220–1226.

25. Nielson CT, Skakkabak NE, Darling JA, et al. Longitudinal study of testosterone and leuteinizing hormone (LH) in relation to spermarche, pubic hair, height and sitting height in normal boys. Acta Endocrinol (Copenh) Suppl 1986; 279:98–106.

26. Forbes GB, Porta CR, Herr BE, Griggs RC. Sequence of changes in body composition induced by testosterone and reversal of changes after drug is stopped. JAMA 1992; 267:397–399.

27. Lee PA. The relationship of concentrations of serum hormones to pubertal gynecomastia. J Pediatr 1975; 89:212–215.

28. Hirsch M, Lunenfeld B, Modan M, Ovadia J, Shemesh J. Spermarche—the age of onset of sperm emission. Sex Active Teenagers 1988; 2:34–38.

29. Pescovitz OH, Comite F, Hench K, et al. The NIH experience with precocious puberty: diagnostic subgroups and response to short-term luteinizing hormone releasing hormone analogue therapy. J Pediatr 1986; 108:47–54.

30. Kreiter M, Burstein S, Rosenfield RL, et al. Preserving adult height potential in girls with idiopathic true precocious puberty. J Pediatr 1990; 117:364–370.

31. Price RA, Lee PA, Albright AL, Ronnekleiv OK, Gutai JP. Treatment of sexual precocity by removal of a luteinizing hormone-releasing hormone secretion hamartoma. JAMA 1984; 251:2247–2249.

32. Starceski PJ, Lee PA, Albright AL, Migeon CJ. Hypothalamic hamartomas and sexual precocity. Evaluation of treatment options. Am J Dis Child 1990; 144:225–228.

33. Mahachoklertwattana P, Kaplan SL, Grumbach MM. The luteinizing hormone-releasing hormone-secreting hypothalamic hamartoma is a congenital malformation: natural history. J Clin Endocrinol Metab 1993; 77:118–124.

34. Shenker A, Weinstein LS, Moran A, et al. Severe endocrine and nonendocrine manifestations of the McCune-Albright syndrome associated with activating mutations of stimulatory G protein G_s. J Pediatr 1993; 123:509–518.

35. Lee PA, VanDop C, Migeon CJ. McCune-Albright syndrome: long-term followup. JAMA 1986; 256:2980–2984.

36. Stanhope R, Adams J, Jacobs HS, Brook CG. Ovarian ultrasound assessment in normal children, idiopathic precocious puberty, and during low dose pulsatile gonadotropin releasing hormone treatment of hypogonadotropic hypogonadism. Arch Dis Child 1985; 60:116–119.

37. Cohen HL, Eisenberg P, Mandel F, Haller JO. Ovarian cysts are common in premenarchal girls: a sonographic study of 101 children 2–12 years old. AJR 1992; 159:89–91.

38. Lee PA, Blizzard RM. Serum gonadotropins in hypothyroid girls with and without sexual precocity. Johns Hopkins Med J 1974; 135:55–60.

39. Atchison JA, Lee PA, Albright AL. Reversible suprasellar pituitary mass secondary to hypothyroidism. JAMA 1989; 262:3175–3177.

40. Pescovitz OH, Comite F, Cassorla F, et al. True precocious puberty complicating congenital adrenal hyperplasia: treatment with a luteinizing hormone-releasing hormone analog. J Clin Endocrinol Metab 1984; 58:857–861.

41. Rosenthal SM, Grumbach MM, Kaplan SL. Gonadotropin independent familial sexual precocity with premature Leydig and germinal cell maturation (familial testotoxicosis): effects of a potent luteinizing hormone-releasing factor agonist and medroxyprogesterone acetate therapy in four cases. J Clin Endocrinol Metab 1983; 57:571–579.

42. Boepple PA, Frisch LS, Wierman ME, Hoffman WH, Crowley WF Jr. The natural history of autonomous gonadal function, adrenarche, and central puberty in gonadotropin-in-

dependent precocious puberty. J Clin Endocrinol Metab 1992; 75:1550–1555.

43. Shenker A, Laue L, Kosugi S, Merendino JJ Jr, Minegishi T, Cutler GB Jr. A constitutively activating mutation of the luteinizing hormone receptor in familial male precocious puberty. Nature 1993; 365:652–654.

44. Pescovitz OH, Comite F, Hench K, et al. The NIH experience with precocious puberty: diagnostic subgroups and response to short term luteinizing hormone releasing hormone analogue therapy. J Pediatr 1986; 108:47–54.

45. Pringle PJ, Stanhope R, Hindmarch P, Brook CG. Abnormal pubertal development in primary hypothyroidism. Clin Endocrinol (Oxf) 1988; 28:479–486.

46. Lau L, Jones J, Barnes DM, Cutler GB Jr. Treatment of familial male precocious puberty with spironolactone, testolactone, and deslorelin. J Clin Endocrinol Metab 1993; 76:151–155.

47. Feuillan PP, Jones J, Cutler GB Jr. Long term testolactone therapy for precocious puberty in girls with the McCune-Albright syndrome. J Clin Endocrinol Metab 1993; 77:647–651.

48. Lee PA. Medroxyprogesterone therapy for sexual precocity in girls. Am J Dis Child 1981; 135:443–445.

49. Holland FJ, Kirsch SE, Selby R. Gonadotropin-independent precocious puberty ("testotoxicosis"): influence of maturational status on response to ketoconazole. J Clin Endocrinol Metab 1986; 64:328–333.

50. Lee PA, Page JG, Leuprolide Study Group. The effects of leuprolide in the treatment of central precocious puberty. J Pediatr 1989; 114:321–324.

51. Parker KL, Lee PA. Depot leuprolide acetate for treatment of precocious puberty. J Clin Endocrinol Metab 1989; 69:689–691.

52. Parker KL, Baens-Bailon RG, Lee PA. Depot leuprolide acetate dosage for sexual precocity. J Clin Endocrinol Metab 1991; 73:50–52.

53. Clemons RD, Kappy MS, Stuart TE, Perelman AH, Hoekstra FT. Long-term effectiveness of depot gonadotropin-releasing hormone analogue in the treatment of children with central precocious puberty. Am J Dis Child 1993; 147:653–657.

54. Oerter KE, Manasco P, Barnes KM, Jones J, Hill S, Cutler GB Jr. Adult height in precocious puberty after long-term treatment with deslorelin. J Clin Endocrinol Metab 1991; 73:1235–1240.

55. Jay N, Mansfield MJ, Blizzard RM, et al. Ovulation and menstrual function of adolescent girls with central precocious puberty after therapy with gonadotropin-releasing hormone agonists. J Clin Endocrinol Metab 1992; 75:890–894.

56. Partsch CJ, Hümmelink R, Peter M, et al., German-Dutch Precocious Puberty Study Group. Comparison of complete and incomplete suppression of pituitary-gonadal activity in girls with central precocious puberty: influence on growth and predicted final height. Horm Res 1993; 39:111–117.

57. Sklar CA, Kaplan SL, Grumbach MM. Evidence for dissociation between adrenarche and gonadarche: studies in patients with idiopathic precocious puberty, gonadal dysgenesis, isolated gonadotropin deficiency, and constitutionally delayed growth and adolescence. J Clin Endocrinol Metab 1980; 51:548–556.

58. Lee PA, Gareis FJ, Gonadotropin and sex steroid response to luteinizing hormone-releasing hormone in patients with premature adrenarche. J Clin Endocrinol Metab 1967; 43:195–197.

59. Wierman ME, Beardsworth DE, Crawford JD, et al. Adrenarche and skeletal maturation during luteinizing hormone releasing hormone analogue suppression of gonadarche. J Clin Invest 1986; 77:121–126.

60. Ibanez L, Virdis R, Potau N, et al. Natural history of premature pubarche: an auxological study. J Clin Endocrinol Metab 1992; 74:254–257.

61. Siegel SF, Finegold DN, Urban MD, McVie R, Lee PA. Premature pubarche: etiological heterogeneity. J Clin Endocrinol Metab 1992; 74:239–247.

62. Ibanez L, Potau N, Virdis R, et al. Postpubertal outcome in girls diagnosed of premature pubarche during childhood: increased frequency of functional ovarian hyperandrogenism. J Clin Endocrinol Metab 1993; 76:1599–1603.

63. Hermanhussen M, Sippell WG. Heterogeneity of Kallmann's syndrome. Clin Genet 1985; 28:106–111.

64. Franco B, Guioli S, Pragliola A, et al. A gene deleted in Kallmann's syndrome shares homology with neural cell adhesion and axonal path-finding molecules. Nature 1991; 353:529–536.

65. Zachmann M, Studer S, Prader A. Short-term testosterone treatment at bone age of 12 to 13 years does not reduce adult height in boys with constitutional delay of growth and adolescence. Helv Paediatr Acta 1987; 42:21–28.

66. Wu FCW, Butler GE, Kelnar CJH, Stirling HF, Huhtaniemi I. Patterns of pulsatile luteinizing hormone and follicle-stimulating hormone secretion in prepubertal (midchildhood) boys and girls and patients with idiopathic hypogonadotropic hypogonadism (Kallmann's syndrome): a study using an ultrasensitive time-resolved immunofluorometric assay. J Clin Endocrinol Metab 1991; 72:1229–1237.

67. Ley SB, Leonard JM. Male hypogonadotropic hypogonadism; factors influencing response to human chorionic gonadotropin and human menopausal gonadotropin, including prior exogenous androgens. J Clin Endocrinol Metab 1985; 61:746–752.

68. Burris AS, Rodbard HW, Winters SJ, Sherins RJ. Gonadotropin therapy in men with isolated hypogonadotropic hypogonadism: the response to human chorionic gonadotropin is predicted by initial testis size. J Clin Endocrinol Metab 1988; 66:1144–1151.

69. Hoffman AR, Crowley WF Jr. Induction of puberty in men by long-term pulsatile administration of low-dose gonadotropin-releasing hormone. N Engl J Med 1982; 307:1237–1241.

70. Saenger P. The current status of diagnosis and therapeutic intervention in Turner's syndrome. J Clin Endocrinol Metab 1993; 77:297–301.

71. Kaneko N, Kawagoe S, Hizoi M. Turner's syndrome—review of the literature with reference to a successful pregnancy outcome. Gynecol Obstet Invest 1990; 29:81–87.

72. Navot D, Laufer N, Kopolovic J, et al. Artificially induced endometrial cycles and the establishment of pregnancies in the absence of ovaries. N Engl J Med 1986; 314:806–811.

14

Pubertal Gynecomastia

Glenn D. Braunstein

Cedars-Sinai Medical Center and UCLA School of Medicine,
Los Angeles, California

I. INTRODUCTION

Gynecomastia is a benign condition of males in which the glandular components of the breast proliferate, resulting in a concentric enlargement of one or both breasts (Fig. 1). Clinical gynecomastia in children and adolescents may be detected when the diameter of the glandular tissue exceeds 0.5 cm. Gynecomastia is an extraordinarily common clinical condition with three well-defined time periods of occurrence: the neonatal period, during puberty, and in older adults. This chapter concentrates on gynecomastia occurring during late childhood and puberty, and readers are referred to several reviews for a discussion of adult gynecomastia (1–3).

II. PREVALENCE OF PUBERTAL GYNECOMASTIA

Table 1 presents the results of several studies that have examined the prevalence of pubertal gynecomastia (4–10). As is clearly apparent, there is a wide variation between studies, the prevalence figures ranging from 4 to 69%. Some of this variation is a result of the clinical definition of gynecomastia used in the studies, and some of the variation can be accounted for by the distribuion of the ages of the patients studied. This can be appreciated from the data shown in Figure 2, which depicts the prevalence of gynecomastia by age from four population studies of large numbers of male adolescents (4,5,8,11). As can be seen, pubertal gynecomastia has an onset between the ages of 10 and 12 years, with a peak occurrence between ages 13 and 14, when Tanner stage 3–5 is reached. After a duration that is rarely longer than 18 months there is involution, which is complete by ages 16–17. Thus, the prevalence is heavily dependent upon the age at which the subjects are examined.

III. NORMAL BREAST DEVELOPMENT

There appears to be no inherent differences between the breast tissue of males and females with regard to their sensitivity to sex steroid hormones. At birth, 60–90% of neonates demonstrate breast enlargement caused by proliferation of the glandular tissue from the transplacental transfer of estrogens from the maternal-placental-fetal unit (11,12). Indeed, a small amount of fluid may be expressed from the nipples ("witches' milk") because of the effect of lactogenic hormones, as well as the decrease in estrogen levels that occurs following birth. Although the breast enlargement may last as long as 6 months, it usually remits within a period of 2–3 weeks. Breast tissue undergoes involution and does not develop further until the time of puberty.

In males, the relative imbalance between estrogen and testosterone levels during puberty (*see later*) leads to pubertal gynecomastia, which in most boys is transient, with resolution when adult androgen-estrogen ratios are achieved, usually by age 17. In females, the large amounts of estrogens that are produced by the pubertal ovaries brings about marked proliferation of the ductal and periductal tissues and, following the institution of ovulatory menstrual cycles with luteal-phase progesterone production, there is further differentiation into terminal acini. Thus, it is the hormonal milieu, not the presence of sexual dimorphism in the breast tissue, that determines the growth and development of breast tissue.

IV. NORMAL SEX STEROID HORMONE PRODUCTION AND METABOLISM

The three steroid-producing tissues are the maternal-placental-fetal unit during pregnancy, the adrenals, and the testes (Fig. 3). The placenta transforms adrenal steroid hormones, such as dehydroepiandrosterone and dehydropiandrosterone sulfate, from both the maternal and fetal compartments to estrone and estradiol, some of which enters the fetus and binds to target tissues, including the breasts. As noted earlier, this stimulation is responsible for the presence of breast enlargement in newborns.

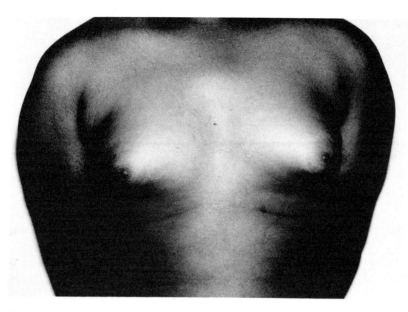

Figure 1 Concentric enlargement of both breasts in a 17-year-old male with persistent pubertal gynecomastia.

The majority of circulating estrogen in adolescent boys and men is derived from extraglandular conversion of androgens secreted by the testes and adrenals. Approximately 95% of the circulating testosterone is secreted by the testes. This is taken up by extragonadal tissues, including liver, skin, fat, muscle, kidney, and bone, in which aromatization to estradiol through an aromatase enzyme takes place. In addition, estrone and estradiol are intraconverted through the enzyme 17-ketosteroid reductase in peripheral tissues (3). The estradiol formed in extragonadal tissues then enters the blood, where it combines with estradiol that is directly secreted by the testes, the latter source accounting for approximately 15% of the circulating estradiol concentration. The major estrogen precursor secreted by the adrenal glands is androstenedione, which also enters extragonadal tissues, where it is converted by the same aromatase enzyme system to estrone. The estrone formed directly by aromatization or derived from estradiol through the 17-ketosteroid reductase enzyme system then enters the blood.

In the circulation, the majority of the androgens and estrogens are bound to sex hormone binding globulin (SHBG), which has a greater affinity for androgens than for estrogens. The sex hormones that are not bound to SHBG exist in either a free or unbound state or are weakly bound to albumin. The free and weakly bound hormones are able to diffuse into the target cells, where they bind with appropriate cytoplasmic receptors. Estrone and estradiol bind with an estrogen receptor, and testosterone binds to an androgen receptor. In some target

Table 1 Prevalence of Pubertal Gynecomastia

Author	Group studied	Criteria	Age range	Total N	Gynecomastia N	Gynecomastia %
Nydick et al. (4)	Boy Scouts	~0.5 cm$^+$	10 −16¹	1865	722	38.7
Neyzi et al. (5)	Turkish schoolboys	Firm, subareolar tissue	9 −17	993	70	7.0
Lee (6)	U.S. schoolboys	Firm, subareolar disk	Pubertal boys	29	20	69
Fara et al. (7)	Italian schoolboys	≥0.5 cm	11 −14	681	228	33.4
Harlan et al. (8)	U.S. youths	≥1 cm	12 −17	3522	147	4.2
Moore et al. (9)	Normal Swiss volunteers	≥0.5 cm	8.5−17.5	135	30	22.2
Biro et al. (10)	U.S. schoolboys	Palpable glandular tissue	10 −15	377	183	48.5

Source: Braunstein GD. N Engl J Med 1993; 328:490–495.

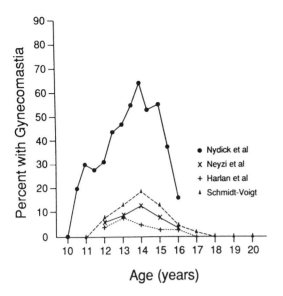

Figure 2 Prevalence of gynecomastia in adolescent males at various chronologic ages. Data derived from four population studies (4,5,8,11).

cells, testosterone undergoes metabolic conversion to dihydrotestosterone through the same enzyme, 5α-reductase, and the dihydrotestosterone binds to the androgen receptor. Once the estrogen or androgen receptors are occupied, they are translocated into the nucleus, where the DNA binding domain binds to the hormone-responsive element of the hormone-responsive genes, which results in initiation of transcription, ultimately resulting in hormone action (13).

V. PATHOGENESIS OF GYNECOMASTIA

Gynecomastia results from an imbalance between estrogen and androgen action (14). An absolute or relative increase in estrogen levels, hypersensitivity of breast tissue to normal concentrations of estrogens, or a decrease in the production, circulating concentrations, or action of free androgen may result in gynecomastia (Table 2). In many instances, there are multiple pathophysiologic mechanisms that result in the imbalance between free estrogen or free androgen levels or action in patients who present with gynecomastia.

VI. CONDITIONS ASSOCIATED WITH GYNECOMASTIA

Although the list of conditions associated with gynecomastia is large (see Ref. 1), the clinically relevant situations in which gynecomastia is seen in the pubertal and peripubertal age groups are listed in Table 3 and are discussed here.

A. Pubertal Gynecomastia

The etiology of pubertal gynecomastia has not been clearly defined. A number of studies have found no differences in the serum concentrations of testosterone, estradiol, estrone, luteinizing hormone, or follicle-stimulating hormone (6,8,15, 16). Therefore, it has been hypothesized that such studies missed the peaks of excessive estrogen production, which may occur at the beginning of the gynecomastia, or that gynecomastia is the result of the rate of change in estrogen and androgen production during puberty or hypersensitivity of the breast tissue to estrogens. Indeed, there are data to

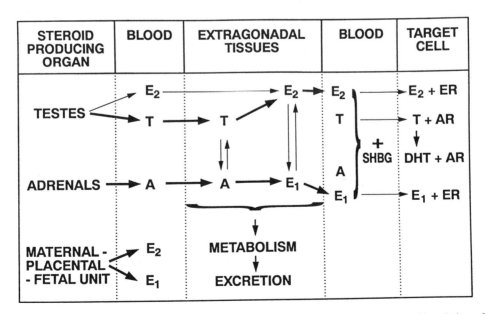

Figure 3 Sites of production and metabolism of sex steroid hormones in males. See text for details. Abbreviations: E_2, estradiol; T, testosterone; A, androstenedione; E_1, estrone; SHBG, sex hormone binding globulin; ER, estrogen receptor; AR, androgen receptor; DHT, dihydrotestosterone.

Table 2 Pathophysiologic Mechanisms in the Genesis of Gynecomastia

Absolute increase in free estrogens
  Direct secretion from
    Maternal-placental-fetal unit
    Testes
    Adrenal
  Extraglandular aromatization of precursors
  Displacement from SHBG
  Decreased metabolism
  Exogenous estrogen administration
Decreased endogenous free androgens
  Decreased secretion
  Increased metabolism
  Increased binding to SHBG
Relative increase in free estrogen to free androgen ratio
Androgen insensitivity
  Congenital defects in androgen receptor structure
    and function
  Displacement of androgens from androgen receptor
Other
  Estrogen-like effect of drugs
  Enhanced sensitivity of breast tissue?

Source: Braunstein GD. N Engl J Med 1993; 328:490–495.

Table 3 Pathologic Conditions Associated with Adolescent Gynecomastia

Neoplasms
  Testicular
    Leydig cell tumor
    Sertoli cell (sex cord) tumor
    Germ cell tumor
  Adrenal
Gonadal dysfunction
  Primary hypogonadism
  Secondary hypogonadism
  Enzymatic defects of testosterone production
  True hermaphroditism
Androgen insensitivity syndromes
Hyperthyroidism
Excessive extraglandular aromatase activity
Drugs
  Androgens and anabolic steroids
  Estrogens
  Human chorionic gonadotropin
  Ketoconazole
  Marijuana
  Amphetamines?

support each of these hypotheses. Lee (6) studied 29 peripubertal and pubertal males, 20 of whom developed pubertal gynecomastia. These workers found that there was a significant increase in estradiol concentrations with the onset of gynecomastia compared with the prior samples, and the mean serum estradiol concentrations were higher in the patients with gynecomastia than in control patients at the same stage of puberty. In addition to the transient increase in estradiol concentrations at the onset of puberty, there are ample opportunities during puberty for a relative imbalance in the concentrations of estrone and estradiol to testosterone. La-Franchi et al. (17) noted that 6 of 16 boys with pubertal gynecomastia had elevated serum estradiol concentrations and that 11 of the 16 had high estradiol-testosterone ratios for the stage of puberty that returned toward normal as puberty progressed. During puberty, the serum concentrations of testosterone increase 30-fold, the estradiol concentrations increase 3-fold, and the serum estradiol concentrations in pubertal males reach adult levels before the testosterone concentration peak (9,16,18). An interesting study was carried out by Large and Anderson (19), who investigated the 24 h profile of circulating androstenedione, testosterone, estrone, and estradiol in pubertal males and noted that there were wide fluctuations in estradiol throughout the day and that boys with gynecomastia tended to have an absolute increase in the 24 h concentration of estradiol relative to testosterone. Part of this increase may be a result of enhanced intraconversion of adrenal androgens to estrogens, as suggested by the studies of Moore and colleagues (9), who noted that the ratio of dehydroepiandrosterone sulfate to estrone and

estradiol was lower in patients with pubertal gynecomastia at the onset than in individuals without pubertal gynecomastia. An increase in the aromatization of androgen precursors to androgens in the breast tissue itself may also be of pathogenetic importance in the onset of gynecomastia, because aromatase activity has been found to be increased in public skin fibroblasts from patients with isolated gynecomastia, including some with pubertal gynecomastia (20). Finally, the breast tissue of males who develop pubertal gynecomastia may be inherently more sensitive to normal circulating levels of estrogen than the breast tissue of boys who do not develop gynecomastia. Support for this concept comes from an observation that patients with protracted neonatal gynecomastia are more likely to develop pubertal gynecomastia than those who do not have excessive neonatal gynecomastia (12).

B. Pathologic Conditions Associated with Gynecomastia During Peripubertal and Pubertal Age Ranges

1. Testicular Neoplasms

Leydig cell tumors account for less than 2% of all testicular tumors, and 20–30% of affected patients have gynecomastia. About 10% of the tumors are malignant, with a median survival of 4 years. There is a bimodal age distribution, with peaks at 6–10 years, generally presenting with virilization, and 26–35 years, presenting with an isolated testicular mass in association with gynecomastia, impotence, and loss of libido (21). The tumors both directly secrete estradiol and exhibit increased aromatization (22,23). Testosterone production is reduced because of the intratesticular inhibitory effects of estradiol on testosterone biosynthesis and from the estradiol inhibition of gonadotropin secretion, which in turn leads to a secondary hypogonadism. Injections of human chorionic gonadotropin (hCG) result in a prolonged rise in estradiol, which can be helpful diagnostically, especially in conjunction with an undetectable serum hCG concentration and unilateral testicular enlargement (24). Nonpalpable tumors may be detected through testicular echograms (24). Sertoli cell tumors of the testes are derived from the primitive gonadal stromal cells, which also may differentiate into Leydig cells. Therefore, it is not surprising that some of these tumors may also secrete estrogens (25).

Of all testicular neoplasms 95% are germ cell tumors, and these are the most common neoplasms in males between the age of 15 and 35. From 2.5 to 6% exhibit gynecomastia at the time of presentation (26). The gynecomastia is associated with a marked elevation in serum human chorionic gonadotropin levels and correlates with the presence of foci of choriocarcinona or trophoblast giant cells. These patients exhibit normal or low serum testosterone levels and elevated serum and urine estrogen concentrations. There is a Leydig cell dysfunction in the face of chronic elevations of hCG, because the exogenous administration of hCG to these patients does not lead to a further rise in testosterone (27). The high circulating endogenous hCG leads to an inhibition of the cytochrome P_{-450} c17 enzyme mediating 17,20-lyase and 17α-hydroxylase activities, as well as stimulating interstitial aromatase activity (28,29). The trophoblast tumor cells also contain aromatase, converting androgen precursors to estrone and estradiol. The presence of gynecomastia in this setting is a poor prognostic sign (26). In contrast, the onset of gynecomastia following effective surgery, chemotherapy, and/or radiation therapy, which occurs in approximately 15% of patients, does not affect predicted survival. Cytotoxic chemotherapy or radiation therapy damage to the remaining testicle leads to primary hypogonadism, which often spontaneously resolves in 4–12 months (26,30). In this situation, the serum hCG is undetectable. The pathogenesis of the gynecomastia seen with extragonadal germ cell tumors is the same as with testicular germ cell tumors.

2. Feminizing Adrenal Cortical Tumors

Adrenal cortical neoplasms are rare tumors during adolescence. In a series of 52 patients reviewed by Gabrilove and coworkers (31), 3 presented between the ages of 14, and 20 and all had gynecomastia. In general, approximately three-quarters of feminizing adrenal cortical tumors are malignant, metastisizing to the liver, lung, and lymph nodes, with a median survival of 1½ years. Of all patients, 98% have gynecomastia, 58% exhibit a palpable tumor, and approximately half have evidence of testicular atrophy. Laboratory studies reveal an increase in urinary 17-ketosteroid excretion, increased serum levels of 17-hydroxyprogesterone and estradiol, and decreased concentrations of total and free testosterone. Luteinizing hormone and follicle-stimulating hormone levels are generally normal or low. The pathogenesis of the gynecomastia in these patients is through overproduction of estrogens by the tumors, as well as possibly increased peripheral aromatization of estrogen precursors of adrenal origin.

3. Gonadal Dysfunction and Androgen Insensitivity Syndromes

These topics are covered in detail elsewhere in this book. However, several comments regarding the pathophysiology of gynecomastia with these conditions are in order.

Patients who have primary hypogonadism from congenital abnormalities, such as Klinefelter syndrome, or enzymatic defects in the biosynthesis of testosterone or who have acquired testicular abnormalities from infection, chemotherapy, or injury commonly exhibit gynecomastia. Each of these conditions is associated with a decrease in the testosterone production rate and decreased concentrations of circulating testosterone. The loss of appropriate negative feedback at the level of the hypothalamus and pituitary results in an elevation of serum luteinizing hormone, which in turn stimulates interstitial cell aromatase activity and enhances estradiol secretion. The increase in estradiol production also inhibits the cytochrome P_{-450} c17 enzyme activities in the testes, further reducing the production of testosterone (29). Because adrenal estrogen precursors continue to be produced and aromatize to estrogens in extragonadal tissues, the net result is an imbalance between free estradiol and estrone concentrations relative to free testosterone. In patients who are agonadal or who have secondary hypogonadism with low concentrations of luteinizing hormone, which results in a low testosterone production rate, the continued production of adrenal estrogen precursors ultimately results in a similar imbalance.

True hermaphrodites have both testicular and ovarian tissue and may develop gynecomastia from the secretion of estrogens directly by the ovarian component. In addition, the elevated estrogen levels may suppress cytochrome P_{-450} c17 enzyme activities in the testes, leading to a reduction in testosterone production.

Patients with the androgen insensitivity syndrome caused by the absence of or defects in the androgen receptors exhibit gynecomastia through two mechanisms. The decreased inhibition of pituitary luteinizing hormone secretion because of the androgen insensitivity at the pituitary and hypothalamic areas leads to an elevation of luteinizing hormone concentrations, which in turn results in the excess secretion of androgens from the testes. The elevated serum testosterone is converted into estradiol through extraglandular aromatization, raising the estradiol concentrations. However, the major pathophysiologic mechanism for gynecomastia in these syndromes is related to the unopposed estrogen action at the breast tissue level. Because androgens are unable to act and thereby counteract some of the effects of estrogen (32), these patients exhibit exuberant stimulation of the breast glandular tissue.

4. Hyperthyroidism

Gynecomastia has been noted in between 25 and 40% of males with hyperthyroidism from Graves' disease (33,34). Although most of the studies defining the pathophysiology of hyperthyroidism-induced gynecomastia have been carried out in older males, it is likely that the pathogenesis of hyperthyroidism-associated gynecomastia in adolescence is the same. Hyperthyroidism induces the liver to increase its production of SHBG. This in turn results in increased binding of testosterone, leading to a slight decrease in free testosterone as well as an increase in luteinizing hormone. Because estradiol also binds to SHBG, one anticipates that there would be a balanced reduction in free testosterone to free estradiol levels. However, testosterone is bound more avidly by the protein than estradiol. Thus, the free testosterone level is actually relatively lower than the free estradiol level when SHBG is increased. In addition, hyperthyroidism is associated with increased aromatization of androstenedione to estrone and testosterone to estradiol in extraglandular tissues (35,36). The combination of overproduction of estrogens and decreased free androgen levels is sufficient to bring about stimulation of breast growth.

5. Excessive Extraglandular Aromatase Activity

Extraglandular aromatization of estrogen precursors is increased in several clinical settings (Table 4). Hemsell and colleagues (37) described an 8-year-old boy who developed severe feminization with gynecomastia and accelerated growth in bone maturation caused by a 50-fold increase in the extraglandular conversion of plasma androstenedione to estrone in extrahepatic sites. These authors hypothesized that the heterosexual precocity was caused by a failure of the fetal aromatase and sulfokinase activities to regress following birth (37). Subsequently, Berkovitz et al. (38) described five males in two generations of a family with a similar defect, suggesting that this condition can occur in a familial setting as an X-linked recessive or a sex-limited autosomal dominant trait.

6. Drugs

A multitude of drugs have been associated with gynecomastia. The clinically important agents in the adolescent age group are listed in Table 3. Androgens and anabolic steroids paradoxically produce gynecomastia, possibly from enhanced

Table 4   Clinical Situations In Which Extraglandular Aromatization of Estrogen Precursors Is Increased

Aging
Obesity
Hyperthyroidism
Liver disease
Testicular feminization
17-Ketosteroid reductase deficiency
Congenital adrenal hyperplasia
Sertoli cell or sex cord tumors
Trophoblastic tumors
Klinefelter syndrome
Drugs: Spironolactone
Idiopathic: Persistence of fetal aromatase

conversion of testosterone to estradiol in peripheral tissues. In addition, the suppression of pituitary gonadotropins with the resulting decrease in endogenous testosterone production with unabated estrogen precursor production by the adrenal glands may be of pathophysiologic importance. Several surveys have shown that between 5 and 10% of male high school students admit to having taken anabolic steroids to improve athletic performance, treat sport injuries, or improve physical appearance (39). Therefore, the use of these drugs in adolescents with persistent pubertal gynecomastia should be suspected.

Another illicit drug consumed by adolescents and associated with gynecomastia is marijuana. Although it was initially thought that the pharmacologically active component of marijuana, tetrahydrocannabinol, interacts with the intracellular steroid hormone receptors, this has been proven not to be the case (40). Rather, it appears that the phytoestrogens present in some marijuana preparation are the ingredients that interact with the estrogen receptors and stimulate breast growth (41). Amphetamine abuse has also been associated with gynecomastia and an increase in estrone, although the pathophysiologic mechanism for this has not been defined (42).

Although estrogens are not used therapeutically in peripubertal or pubertal males, inadvertent estrogen ingestion is a well-documented cause of gynecomastia. Estrogen contamination of the clothes of male workers in a pharmaceutical plant that produced contraceptives resulted in breast enlargement in the workers' children (43). Contamination of other drugs with estrogens has also been described as a cause of gynecomastia in children (44), as has accidental exposure to estrogen-containing hair creams (45). Outbreaks of breast enlargement in children in Bahrain who drank milk from a cow that had received estrogen injections and an outbreak of gynecomastia in Italian schoolchildren following the ingestion of poultry or veal suspected of having been treated with estrogens have also been reported (7,46).

hCG injections to treat cryptorchidism may also be associated with gynecomastia through stimulation of estradiol secretion from enhanced interstitial cell aromatase activity, which in turn leads to an inhibition of the cytochrome P_{-450} c17 enzyme activity (28,29). This is generally not seen unless there has been prolonged use of hCG injections for this purpose. hCG injections are also used by athletes to prevent the testicular atrophy that accompanies anabolic steroid abuse.

The antifungal agent ketoconazole decreases testosterone synthesis as well as displaces estradiol from SHBG, raising the free estradiol level and increasing the estradiol-testosterone ratio (47,48). The incidence of this adverse effect is directly related to the dosage and is seen in as many as 20% of patients treated with doses in the range of 800–1200 mg/day (48).

VII. DIAGNOSIS

The condition that must be differentiated from gynecomastia is pseudogynecomastia, which is breast enlargement as a result of fat accumulation rather than an increase in the glandular component. With the patient laying supine with his hands locked together underneath the back of his head, the examiner should place his or her thumb and forefinger at opposite ends of the breast and slowly bring them together. In patients with pseudogynecomastia there is no resistance until the thumb and forefinger meet, but in patients with true gynecomastia there is a firm or rubbery disk of tissue that extends concentrically outward from beneath the nipple (49). Often patients with pubertal gynecomastia complain of pain in the breasts and exhibit tenderness during examination; those with pseudogynecomastia do not. Other conditions may present as breast masses. These include neurofibromas, lymphangiomas, hematomas, lipomas, and dermoid cysts. These conditions are rare, unilateral, and often eccentric in position rather then concentric to and beneath the areolar area. Breast carcinoma is not a consideration in this age group.

A pubertal or adolescent male presenting with gynecomastia should be questioned about the use of anabolic steroids, hCG, marijuana, and amphetamines. He should also undergo a careful physical examination, with particular attention to signs of feminization, such as spider hemangiomata or palmar erythema, examination of the abdomen for adrenal masses, careful examination of the external genitalia for ambiguities or abnormalities that might be suggestive of prenatal androgen insufficiency, and a careful examination of the testicles for size and consistency as well as the presence of masses. If the history does not reveal drug use and there are no abnormalities on physical examination, then the patient should be reassured that the gynecomastia is a normal concomitant of puberty and that it will resolve within the next 12–18 months. The patient should be reexamined in 6 months.

If the gynecomastia persists or worsens during the period of observation, then measurement of serum concentrations of hCG, estradiol, and luteinizing hormone should be performed. If the hCG concentration is elevated, then a testicular ultrasound should be carried out to determine whether a germ cell tumor of the testicle is present. If the ultrasound is negative, then other radiographic studies, including a chest x-ray, should be performed, looking for an extragonadal germ cell tumor. An elevation in the serum estradiol concentration should be followed by ultrasound of the testicles to detect a Leydig or Sertoli cell tumor. If this is negative, then computed tomography or, magnetic resonance imaging of the adrenal glands should be carried out to diagnose the presence of an adrenal neoplasm. In the face of elevated estradiol, if neither the testicles nor the adrenal glands appear abnormal, then the possibility exists that the patient has increased extraglandular aromatase activity. Measurement of serum estrone in this setting may be helpful because the estrone levels are relatively higher than estradiol concentrations in the idiopathic excessive extraglandular aromatase activity syndrome. Finally, if the luteinizing hormone level is elevated, the patient may have primary hypogonadism and must be evaluated for Klinefelter syndrome and other conditions associated with testicular damage.

VIII. THERAPY

The majority of patients with pubertal gynecomastia require no specific therapy other than reassurance that this is a normal manifestation of pubertal development and that they are not "turning into a girl." They should also be reassured that complete spontaneous regression is the rule for the vast majority of boys (see Fig. 2). If this explanation does not relieve the anxiety or the adolescent is extremely emotionally distraught, then psychotherapy and/or medical therapy should be considered.

Medical therapy for gynecomastia is indicated for boys who are so mortified because of their breast enlargement that they refuse to interact socially with their peers. Therapy is also indicated in boys who have extreme breast pain and tenderness. Several different drugs have been used to treat gynecomastia. However, it is difficult to evaluate the results of the studies critically, for several reasons. First, pubertal gynecomastia has a high spontaneous remission rate, and therefore, the number of boys needed to show a significant difference between those treated with the active agents and those treated with a placebo would be quite large. Second, many of these studies have included patients with gynecomastia from various causes, not pubertal gynecomastia alone. Third, the potential responsiveness of the breast tissue to pharmacologic agents is highly dependent upon the duration of gynecomastia. Histologic studies have shown that gynecomastia begins with an active or florid stage characterized by ductal proliferation with hyperplasia of the epithelial lining and an increase in the periductal connective tissue and vasculature, as well as periductal edema. The florid stage predominates during the first 6 months after the onset of gynecomastia. After 12 months of gynecomastia, the epithelium returns to a resting stage, the ducts dilate, and hyalinization and fibrosis take place in the stroma. Between 6 and 12 months there is an intermediate stage (50–53). The time when medical therapy is most likely to be efficacious is during the proliferative phase; little effect is anticipated once hyalinization and fibrosis have taken place.

Three types of medical therapies have been tried: androgens, antiestrogens, and an aromatase inhibitor. Because gynecomastia results from an imbalance between estrogen and androgen effects on the breast tissue, androgen therapy seems to be a logical means for treating gynecomastia. Although testosterone has been used, it does not appear to be any more effective than placebo alone and has the potential for actually increasing gynecomastia through aromatization of the testosterone. To circumvent this, both percutaneous and injectable forms of dihydrotestosterone, an androgen that is not aromatized to estrogens, have been tried. Percutaneous dihydrotestosterone was used in 40 males, including 37 adolescents, in whom gynecomastia was present for more than 18 months (54). Of the 40 patients 10 had complete disappearance of the gynecomastia, 19 of the 40 had partial disappearance and 11 of the 40 demonstrated no change over a period of 4–20 weeks. The investigators noted that breast tenderness remitted first, followed by softening of the breast glandular tissue and then a reduction in the volume of the breast size in those individuals who responded. In another study, injections of dihydrotestosterone heptonate were used in 4 males with pubertal gynecomastia (55). During a 16 week period of injections, all had improvement in the gynecomastia, which did not recur following discontinuation of therapy. Neither of these studies were placebo controlled or blinded, and therefore it is difficult to interpret the results. Another androgenic steroid, danazol, has been used in a small number of patients in an unblinded fashion, with improvement noted in approximately three-quarters of the pubertal boys treated (56,57). The side effects of weight gain, edema, acne, and gastrointestinal distress limit the usefulness of this drug.

The two antiestrogens that have been used are clomiphene citrate and tamoxifen. In one study that used clomiphene, 28 adolescent boys who had gynecomastia for more than 2 years were treated with 100 mg/day for 6 months, and 60% of the patients noted a decrease in the size of the breast tissue (58). In another study, 12 boys received 50 mg/day, and only 5 were found to have a greater than 20% reduction in the size of the breast tissue. Most were not satisfied with the results (59). In another uncontrolled study, 19 patients received 50 mg/day of clomiphene citrate, which was switched to 50 mg every other day after response was obtained (60). Over 8 weeks, 18 of the 19 had a decrease in the breast size, with the maximum response noted between 4 and 8 weeks. However, less than half of the patients were satisfied with their response. Tamoxifen has been studied in several groups of patients with gynecomastia of various causes and has been found to be effective in decreasing breast size and pain with doses of 10 mg twice per day, and it has been free of side effects when used up to 3 months at this dose (61–63).

The aromatase inhibitor testolactone has been used safely at a dose of 450 mg/day for up to 6 months in 22 patients with pubertal gynecomastia (64). As a group there was improvement, but unfortunately the study was not blinded or controlled and patient satisfaction was not noted. Testolactone would certainly be the therapy of choice in individuals who have documented excessive extraglandular aromatase activity.

Finally, surgical removal of the breast glandular tissue and subglandular adipose tissue through a periareolar incision should be strongly considered in boys who have had persistent pubertal gynecomastia and have completed or nearly completed puberty. Surgical removal before this time carries a risk of recurrence of gynecomastia if the relative androgen-estrogen imbalance has not been resolved.

REFERENCES

1. Braunstein GD. Gynecomastia. N Engl J Med 1993; 328:490–495.
2. Carlson HE. Gynecomastia: pathogenesis and therapy. Endocrinologist 1991; 1:337–342.
3. Wilson JD, Aiman J, MacDonald PC. The pathogenesis of gynecomastia. Adv Intern Med 1980; 29:1–32.
4. Nydick M, Bustos J, Dale JH Jr. Rawson RW. Gynecomastia in adolescent boys. JAMA 1961; 178:449–454.
5. Neyzi O, Alp H, Yalcindag A, Yakacikli S, Orphon A. Sexual maturation in Turkish boys. Ann Hum Bio 1975; 2:251–259.
6. Lee PA. The relationship of concentrations of serum hormones to pubertal gynecomastia. J Pediatr 1975; 86:212–215.
7. Fara GM, DelCorvo G, Bernuzzi S, et al. Epidemic of breast enlargment in an Italian school. Lancet 1979; 2:295–297.
8. Harlan WR, Grillo GP, Cornoni-Huntley J, Leaverton PE. Secondary sex characteristics of boys 12 to 17 years of age: the U.S. Health Examination Survey. J Pediatr 1979; 95:293–297.
9. Moore DC, Schlaepfer LV, Paunier L, Sizonenko PC. Hormonal changes during puberty. V. Transient pubertal gynecomastia: abnormal androgen-estrogen ratios. J Clin Endocrinol Metab 1984; 58:492–499.
10. Biro FM, Lucky AW, Huster GA, Morrison JA. Hormonal studies and physical maturation in adolescent gynecomastia. J Pediatr 1990; 116:450–455.
11. Schmidt-Voigt J. Brustdrüenschwellungen bei männlichen Jugendlichen des Pubertätsalter (Pubertätsmakromastie). Z Kinderheilkd 1941; 62:590–606.
12. Hall PF. Gynaecomastia. Glebe: Australasian Medical Publishing, 1959.
13. Lazar MA. Steroid and thyroid hormone receptors. Endocrinol Clin North Am 1991; 20:681–695.
14. Edmondson HA, Glass SJ, Soll SN. Gynecomastia associated with cirrhosis of the liver. Proc Soc Exp Biol Med 1939; 42:97–99.
15. Knorr D, Bidlingmaier Gynaecomastia in male adolescents. Clin Endocrinol Metab 1975; 4:157–171.
16. Bidlingmaier F, Knorr D. Plasma testosterone and estrogens in pubertal gynecomastia. Z Kinderheilkd 1973; 115:89–94.
17. LaFranchi SH, Parlow AF, Lippe BM, Coytupa J, Kaplan S. Pubertal gynecomastia and transient elevation of serum estradiol level. Am J Dis Child 1975; 129:927–931.
18. Nuttall FQ. Gynecomastia as a physical finding in normal men. J Clin Endocrinol Metab 1979; 48:338–340.
19. Large DM, Anderson DC. Twenty-four-hour profiles of circulating androgens and estrogens in male puberty with and without gynecomastia. Clin Endocrinol (Oxf) 1979; 11:505–521.
20. Bulard J, Mowszowicz I, Schaison G. Increased aromatase activity in public skin fibroblasts from patients with isolated gynecomastia. J Clin Endocrinol Metab 1987; 64:618–623.
21. Gabrilove JL, Nicolis GL, Mitty HA, Sohval AR. Feminizing interstitial cell tumor of the testis: personal observations and a review of the literature. Cancer 1975; 35:1184–1202.
22. Bercovici J-P, Tater D, Khoury S, Charles J-F, Floch J, Leroy J-P. Leydig cell tumor with gynecomastia: hormonal effects of an estrogen-producing tumor. J Clin Endocrinol Metab 1981; 53:1291–1296.
23. Bercovici J-P, Nahoul K, Ducasse M, Tater D, Kerlan V, Scholler R. Leydig cell tumor with gynecomastia: further studies—the recovery after unilateral orchidectomy. J Clin Endocrinol Metab 1985; 61:957–962.
24. Kuhn JM, Mahoudeau JA, Billaud L, et al. Evaluation of diagnostic criteria for leydig cell tumours in adult men revealed by gynaecomastia. Clin Endocrinol (Oxf) 1987; 26:407–416.
25. Gabrilove JL, Freiberg EK, Leiter E, Nicolis GL. Feminizing and nonfeminizing sertoli cell tumors. J Urol 1980; 124:757–767.
26. Tseng A Jr, Horning SJ, Freiha FS, Resser KJ, Hannigan JF, Torti FM. Gynecomastia in testicular cancer patients. Prognostic and therapeutic implications. Cancer 1985; 56:2534–2538.
27. Fox H, Reeve NL. Endocrine effects of testicular neoplasms. Invest Cell Pathol 1979; 2:63–73.
28. Forest MG, Lecoq A, Saez JM. Kinetics of human chorionic

gonadotropin-induced steroidogenic response of the human testis. II. Plasma 17α-hydroxyprogesterone, Δ4-androstenedione, estrone, and 17β-estradiol: evidence for the action of human chorionic gonadotropin on intermediate enzymes implicated in steroid biosynthesis. J Clin Endocrinol Metab 1979; 49:284–291.

29. Jones TM, Fang VS, Landau RL, Rosenfield R. Direct inhibition of Leydig cell function by estradiol. J Clin Endocrinol Metab 1978; 47:1368–1373.

30. Turner AR, Morrish DW, Berry J, MacDonald RN. Gynecomastia after cytotoxic therapy for metastatic testicular cancer. Arch Intern Med 1982; 142:896–897.

31. Gabrilove JL, Sharma DC, Wotiz HH, Dorfman RI. Feminizing adrenocortical tumors in the male. A review of 52 cases including a case report. Medicine (Baltimore) 1965; 44:37–79.

32. Rochefort H, Garcia M. The estrogenic and antiestrogenic activities of androgens in female target tissues. Pharmacol Ther 1984; 23:193–216.

33. Chopra IJ, Tulchinsky D. Status of estrogen-androgen balance in hyperthyroid men with Graves' disease. J Clin Endocrinol Metab 1974; 38:269–277.

34. Ashkar FS, Smoak WM III, Gilson AJ, Miller R. Gynecomastia and mastoplasia in Graves' disease. Metabolism 1970; 19:946–951.

35. Bercovici J-P, Mauvais-Jarvis P. Hyperthyroidism and gynecomastia: metabolic studies. J Clin Endocrinol Metab 1972; 35:671–677.

36. Olivo J, Gordon GG, Rafii F, Southren AL. Estrogen metabolism in hyperthyroidism and in cirrhosis of the liver. Steroids 1975; 26:47–56.

37. Hemsell DL, Edman CD, Marks JF, Siiteri PK, MacDonald PC. Massive extraglandular aromatization of plasma androstenedione resulting in feminization of a prepubertal boy. J Clin Invest 1977; 60:455–464.

38. Berkovitz GD, Guerami A, Brown TR, MacDonald PC, Migeon CJ. Familial gynecomastia with increased extraglandular aromatization of plasma carbon 19-steroids. J Clin Invest 1985; 75:1763–1769.

39. Yesalis CE. Incidence of anabolic steriod use: a discussion of methological issues. In: Yesalis CE, ed. Anabolic Steroids in Sport and Exercise. Champaign: Human Kinetics Publishers, 1993:49–69.

40. Smith RG, Besch NF, Besch PK, Smith CG. Inhibition of gonadotropin by Δ⁹-tetrahydrocannabinol: mediation by steroid receptors. Science 1979; 204:325–327.

41. Sauer MA, Rifka SM, Hawks RL, Cutler GB Jr, Loriaux DL. Marijuana: interaction with the estrogen receptor. J Pharmacol Exp Ther 1983; 224:404–407.

42. Bridgman JF, Buckler JMH. Drug-induced gynaecomastia. BMJ 1974; 2:520–521.

43. Landrigan PJ, Harrington JM. Gynecomastia. N Eng J Med 1981; 304:234–235.

44. Weber WW, Grossman M, Thom JV, Sax J, Chan JJ, Duffy MP. Drug contamination with diethylstibestrol. Outbreak of precocious puberty due to contaminated isonicotinic acid hydrazide (INH). N Engl J Med 1963; 268:411–415.

45. Edidin DV, Levistky LL. Prepubertal gynecomastia associated with estrogen-containing hair cream. Am J Dis Child 1982; 136:587–588.

46. Kimball AM, Hamadeh R, Mahmood RAH, et al. Gynaecomastia among children in Bahrain. Lancet 1981; 1:671–672.

47. Grosso DS, Boyden TW, Pamenter RW, Johnson DG, Stevens DA, Galgiani JN. Ketoconazole inhibition of testicular secretion of testosterone and displacement of steroid hormones from serum transport proteins. Antimicrob Agents Chemother 1983; 23:207–212.

48. Pont A, Goldman ES, Sugar AM, Siiteri PK, Stevens DA. Ketoconazole-induced increase in estradiol-testosterone ratio. Probable explanation for gynecomastia. Arch Intern Med 1985; 145:1429–1431.

49. Braunstein GD. Diagnosis and treatment of gynecomastia. Hosp Pract 1993; 28:37–46.

50. Nicolis GL, Modlinger RS, Gabrilove JL. A study of the histopathology of human gynecomastia. J Clin Endocrinol Metab 1971; 32:173–178.

51. Williams MJ. Gynecomastia. Its incidence, recognition and host characterization in 447 autopsy cases. Am J Med 1963; 34:103–112.

52. Bannayan GA, Hajdu SI. Gynecomastia: clinicopathologic study of 351 cases. Am J Clin Pathol 1972; 57:431–437.

53. Andersen JA, Gram JB. Gynecomasty. Histological aspects in a surgical material. Acta Path Microbiol Immunol Scand 1982; 90:185–190.

54. Kuhn J-M, Roca R, Laudat M-H, Rieu M, Luton J-P, Bricaire H. Studies on the treatment of idiopathic gynaecomastia with percutaneous dihydrotestosterone. Clin Endocrinol (Oxf) 1983; 19:513–520.

55. Eberle AJ, Sparrow J, Keenan BS. Treatment of persistent pubertal gynecomastia with dihydrotestosterone heptanoate. J Pediatr 1986; 109:144–149.

56. Buckle R. Studies on the treatment of gynaecomastia with danazol (danol). J Int Med Res 1977; 5(Suppl 3):114–123.

57. Beck W, Stubbe P. Endocrinological studies of the hypothalamo-pituitary gonadal axis during danazol treatment in pubertal boys with marked gynecomastia. Horm Metab Res 1982; 14:653–657.

58. LeRoith D, Sobel R, Glick SM. The effect of clomiphene citrate on pubertal gynecomastia. Acta Endocrinol (Copenh) 1980; 95:177–180.

59. Plourde PV, Kulin HE, Santner SJ. Clomiphene in the treatment of adolescent gynecomastia. Clinical and endocrine studies. Am J Dis Child 1983; 137:1080–1082.

60. Stepanas AV, Burnet RB, Harding PE, Wise PH. Clomiphene in the treatment of pubertal-adolescent gynecomastia: a preliminary report. J Pediatr 1977; 90:651–653.

61. Hooper PD. Puberty gynaecomastia. J R Coll Gen Pract 1985; 35:142.

62. Parker LN, Gray DR, Lai MK, Levin ER. Treatment of gynecomastia with tamoxifen: a double-blind crossover study. Metabolism 1986; 35:705–708.

63. Alagaratnam TT. Treating puberty gynaecomastia. J R Coll Gen Pract 1987; 37:178.

64. Zachmann M, Eiholzer U, Muritano M, Werder EA, Manella B. Treatment of pubertal gynaecomastia with testolactone. Acta Endocrinol (Copenh) Suppl 1986; 279:218–226.

15

Nonendocrine Vaginal Bleeding

Albert Altchek
*Mount Sinai School of Medicine,
New York, New York*

I. INTRODUCTION

A. General Considerations

The vast majority of abnormal bleeding in children is a result of local causes, not precocious puberty or other endocrine causes.

Unfortunately, there have been reports from distinguished authorities indicating that the leading cause of bleeding is precocious puberty (for example, Ref. 1). Clearly such reports are a result of case selection bias.

Such distorting of the relative incidence of precocious puberty causing bleeding, combined with the training and interests of pediatricians, causes an immediate reaction to assume that the first thing to rule out if there is bleeding is precocious puberty. Thus it is essential that pediatric endocrinologists recognize and diagnose patients with nonendocrine vaginal bleeding to avoid misdirected investigation that may involve radiation exposure; be wasteful of resources and funds; be prolonged; be stressful to the child, parents, and pediatrician; and delay discovery of the statistically probable local, nonendocrine cause of the bleeding.

Because menstruation may be considered physiologic in children age 10 or over, bleeding in girls under age 10 is considered abnormal (1). Ideally, in all cases of vaginal bleeding local nonendocrine causes should be ruled out (Chap. 13).

Even if the presumptive diagnosis is precocious puberty, there should be consideration of the possibility of a nonendocrine, local cause of bleeding. It may even be possible that there is a local cause of bleeding together with precocious puberty. If this occurs, then the bleeding pattern and the lack of response to precocious puberty therapy cause great confusion. Gynecologic investigation is relatively brief and inexpensive and, except for the possible need for general anesthesia for vaginoscopy, relatively without danger.

B. Differences Between Endocrine and Nonendocrine Bleeding

Usually with true, constitutional precocious puberty, there is a similarity to the normal puberty sequence of events except that they occur at an earlier age. Therefore, by the time the child has her first episode of vaginal bleeding, she has already had breast development, public and axillary hair, and other physical signs of puberty. In addition, the vaginal cytology smear (or urine cytology) shows an estrogenic effect, with superficial and intermediate cells.

By contrast, the child with a local, nonendocrine cause of bleeding does not have the physical changes of puberty, and the vaginal cytology shows an anestrogenic maturation index with mostly parabasal cells, with few if any superficial or intermediate cells. In addition, a local bleeding site is present. Furthermore, the history may give positive clues, such as trauma, symptoms of vulvovaginitis, dysuria, scratching, the presence of a vaginal or vulvar mass, or pain on defecation.

C. Endocrine Bleeding Posing as Nonendocrine Bleeding

Infrequently, an endocrine cause may pose as a local cause because of an absence of physical signs of puberty when bleeding starts as an apparently isolated phenomenon. However, the vaginal smear cytology is usually estrogenic because the vaginal mucosa is the most estrogen sensitive tissue.

1. The newborn may have physiologic vaginal (uterine estrogen withdrawal bleeding) bleeding and discharge (from the estrogenic vagina).
2. The first clinical sign of McCune-Albright syndrome is often vaginal bleeding. The diagnosis requires the characteristic café au lait pigmentation and radiologic bone disease. Eventually secondary sexual development occurs (Chap. 13).

3. Estrogen-secreting ovarian neoplasms, such as gran-ulosa cell tumors, even though small, may also cause bleeding before physical signs of puberty. They may be palpable on rectal examination and can be imaged by ultrasound (Chap. 57).

4. Patients with isolated premature menarche may have isolated or recurrent vaginal bleeding without other signs of precocious puberty (2). Sleep luteinizing hormone (LH) may show pulsations; however, fol-licle-stimulating hormone (FSH) responds more than LH after LH-releasing hormone stimulation, as in prepuberty. There may be transient elevation of estradiol and a later return of LH to a prepubertal pattern. This entity is usually benign and self-limit-ing and is thought to be the result of a partial, transient activation of true precocious puberty. Care-ful evaluation and follow-up are required.

5. Prepubertal vaginal bleeding without signs of pre-cocious puberty may be infrequently caused by prolonged, untreated hypothyroidism. In these pa-tients, there may be breast enlargement, galactor-rhea, hyperprolactinemia, enlarged sella turcica, ovarian follicular cysts, elevated gonadotropins (mainly FSH), and an estrogenic vaginal smear. There is no androgen excess or pubarche and no pubertal growth spurt. There is a delayed bone age (Chap. 27) (3).

6. Accidental estrogen ingestion may also set off vaginal bleeding without puberty development.

7. Sometimes, precocious puberty caused by a central nervous system lesion may have bleeding before secondary sexual development (1). Brain imaging is necessary for diagnosis.

II. ETIOLOGY OF LOCAL NONENDOCRINE BLEEDING

A. Causes

The local causes of nonhormonal vaginal bleeding in the child are listed in Table 1. These conditions can also cause abnormal bleeding in the adolescent. The vast majority of adolescent abnormal bleeding is caused by anovulatory dys-functional uterine bleeding because half of all adolescents do not ovulate at menarche (Chap. 16).

B. Incidence and Prevalence

There are no reliable data on the incidence and causes of local bleeding in the child because of case selection factors and age group bias. Adolescent statistics may also reflect pregnancy and its complications (miscarriage, abortion, or ectopic preg-nancy), sexually transmitted disease, misuse of oral contra-ceptives, voluntary sexual activity, and rape.

Among 1300 Viennese children, average age 7.6 years, seen in elective clinic visits for gynecologic problems, the most frequent conditions were vulvovaginitis (43%), "patho-logic vaginal bleeding" (13%), vulva disorders (7%), and

suspicion of foreign body (5%) (4). In adolescents, most of the bleeding was anovulatory dysfunctional bleeding.

Emergency rooms tend to report trauma and urethral prolapse as bleeding causes because of the acute and severe presentations. Private pediatric offices and clinics acquire cases with less dramatic bleeding and tend not to report them.

A London referral hospital reported that among 52 girls 10 years of age and under with vaginal bleeding, 28 had a local lesion, of which 11 had malignant vaginal tumors. These included 8 rhabdomyosarcomas, 2 clear cell adenocarcino-mas, and 1 endodermal sinus tumor. Bleeding from vulvar lesions included lichen sclerosus, warts, and cavernous he-mangioma, as well as urethral prolapse, trauma, and vulvo-vaginitis. Precocious puberty occurred in 11 children: constitutional in 2, granulosa cell tumor of the ovary in 3, and premature menarche in 6. In 13 cases, no cause for bleeding was found (5). I believe that the high incidence of malignancy and precocious puberty and the absence of foreign bodies in the vagina were a result of case selection. The lack of a cause for bleeding may have been a result of a severe vaginitis that cleared by the time of vaginoscopy. In their precocious puberty cases (only 2 of 11 were constitutional), most had bleeding without other signs of secondary sexual development and with normal bone age. Isolated bleeding as the first sign of puberty was also found in another select series (1).

There have been several recent reviews of vaginal bleeding in children (6–11). There is general agreement that the most frequent causes of local vaginal bleeding include trauma, vulvovaginitis (especially vaginitis), vulvar lesions, vaginal foreign bodies, and urethral prolapse.

Malignant conditions of the vagina are very rare but may present initially as unexplained vaginal bleeding (even only staining for a few days) in an otherwise healthy child. With early discovery, local resection, and contemporary chemo-therapy, the dismal prognosis of 30 years ago has been removed from about 85% fatality to apparent cure.

Trauma may result from sexual abuse, which may also be part of general mistreatment of the child. The suspicion of abuse requires reporting to legal authorities. Ideally, sexual abuse should not be overlooked (even though there may not be definite physical findings), and sexual abuse should not be misdiagnosed in conditions that simulate its physical findings (such as lichen sclerosus with bleeding, laceration-like fissures, and ecchymoses).

III. SEVERE VAGINAL INFECTIONS AS A CAUSE OF LOCAL NONENDOCRINE BLEEDING

A. Vulvovaginitis

Vulvovaginitis is the leading gynecologic problem of the child, which can cause bleeding. The child is susceptible to infection because of a vulva which

1. lacks the thick adult labial pads and pubic hair
2. has delicate skin
3. is close to the anus.

Table 1 Nonhormonal Causes of Bleeding

I. Severe, usually specific, infections of the vagina, with secondary vulvitis
   A. Group A β-hemolytic streptococcus
   B. *Candida*
   C. *Neisseria gonorrhoeae*
   D. *Chlamydia*
   E. *Gardnerella* (bacterial vaginosis)
   F. *Trichomonas vaginalis*
   G. Rare (geographic endemic) *Shigella*, schistosomiasis, amebiasis
   H. Pinworm infestation
II. Trauma
   A. Management of bleeding
   B. Types of injury
   C. Suspicion of sexual abuse
III. Foreign body in the vagina
   A. Rolled-up wads of toilet tissue
   B. "Arrowhead" narrow plastic bottle caps
   C. Trapped pinworms
IV. Vulva lesions
   A. Severe nonspecific vulvitis with secondary vaginitis, scratching
   B. Skin lesions
      1. General skin disease, seborrheic, atopic, psoriasis, candidiasis
      2. Hemangioma
      3. Condylomata acuminata
      4. Lichen sclerosus
      5. Diaper rash
      6. Ulcers: herpetic, syphilis, chancroid
      7. Systemic infection: chicken pox
      8. Local infection: bacterial, tinea
      9. Allergic-irritant: contact
      10. Scabies
V. Prolapse of urethra, hematuria, prolapse of bladder, rhabdomyosarcoma, prolapse of ureterocele
VI. Anal fissure, pinworms, perianal dermatitis, condyloma acuminatum, hemorrhoid caused by pelvic cavernous hemangioma, laceration.
VII. Hymen polyps
VIII. Malignant tumors of the vagina
   A. Rhabdomyosarcoma
   B. Midline germ cell endodermal sinus tumor
   C. Clear cell adenocarcinoma
IX. Rare coagulation defect (in association with skin and mucous membrane bleeding)

The child is also susceptible because of a vaginal mucosa which

1. is anestrogenic and thin (about 6 cells thick rather than the approximately 5 times thicker adult)
2. lacks glycogen (and Lactobacilli) and therefore is of neutral pH rather than the adult acid pH
3. might lack immune globulin of the adult.

In addition, children tend to have poor local hygiene.

Most vulvovaginitis is primary vulvitis with secondary vaginitis set off by an episode of poor hygiene.

Primary vaginitis is less common and more deserving of investigation. A culture of the vagina above the hymen is required for diagnosis.

B. Group A β-Hemolytic Streptococcus Vaginitis

Group A β-hemolytic streptococcus is the most frequent cause of a specific vaginal infection causing bleeding, although bleeding does not occur in every case. Q-tip culturing often provokes bleeding. On vaginoscopy, there is a severe inflammation of the upper posterior vaginal wall and fornix with extensive petechial hemorrhages in the anestrogenic atrophic mucosa. Blood comes from a broad area. A single bleeding site cannot be visualized. Although vaginoscopy is recommended, a positive culture with cure after 10 days of antibiotic therapy (similar to a pharyngitis) and observation is a reasonable alternative.

Group A β-hemolytic streptococcus (GAHS) has been

reported in 18% of girls who were cultured for clinical vulvovaginitis (actually vaginitis). The incidence is higher in the age group up to 9 years, as opposed to the 10–14 year age group. The younger child is expected to have streptococcal vaginitis; the older child, because of an estrogenic thicker vaginal wall, is resistant. It is also increased in the winter months, when streptococcal pharyngitis is increased. The organism is probably transmitted from the pharynx to the vagina (12). This suggests that GAHS is more commonly associated with vulvovaginitis than previously thought. It could indicate a true increase in frequency or better recognition by more liberal use of cultures.

C. Candida Vaginitis

Candida may cause a vaginitis with a cottage cheese discharge, a vulvitis with severe excoriation, a perianal dermatitis, a diaper rash, and a secondary infection of any vulvar lesion. The diagnosis is made by inspection, scraping, culture, or microscopic potassium hydroxide wet mount smear.

D. Sexually Transmitted Disease

Any sexually transmitted disease raises the question of sexual molestation (gonorrhea, chlamydia, trichomonads, *Gardnerella*, condyloma, etc.), although it is possible that all of these can be acquired without molestation at the time of vaginal delivery, from a caretaker, or close physical contact with the mother. Trichomonads prefer the estrogenic vagina and tend to be found in the newborn and older child.

E. Unusual Infections

There are rare severe vaginal infections usually associated with geographic endemic areas which can cause bleeding.

Recurrent vaginal bleeding and bloody discharge may be due to *Shigella* causing a distal localized intense vaginitis. It originates from a previous enteric infection and there may or may not be a residual positive stool culture. Sometimes, prolonged treatment may be required. Contacts should be cultured even if asymptomatic. In the United States, these cases are infrequent. Patients often come from Indian reservations in the Southwest and usually have *Shigella flexneri*. In Peru, the usual cause is *Shigella sonnei* (13). Other rare causes include *Schistosomiasis* and *Amoebiasis* (14).

IV. TRAUMA AS A CAUSE OF LOCAL NONENDOCRINE BLEEDING

The physician is faced with two problems: the specific injury (and treatment) and the question of sexual abuse and, with it, sexually transmitted disease.

A. Management of Bleeding

When the child is first seen by the pediatrician, there is the tendency to watch and wait with the hope that the bleeding will spontaneously stop. Unfortunately, if there is persistent

active bleeding several hours may be lost, with significant blood loss. A cold compress should be applied to the vulva for about 10 minutes. If significant bleeding persists, the child should be taken to the operating room for meticulous hemostasis, suturing of lacerations, and reconstruction using fine absorbable nonreactive sutures. The integrity of the bladder and rectum is checked by having the child void, catheterization, and rectal examination. Vaginal lacerations and possible transvaginal peritoneal injury are checked and consideration given to blunt abdominal trauma. Despite fecal contamination, immediate repair of fresh rectal tears gives good results. Antibiotics and tetanus prevention should be considered.

Bleeding as a result of trauma often causes external bleeding. Occasionally, blunt trauma from a fall may result in a deep pelvic hematoma that a number of days later ruptures laterally into the vagina, resulting in the vaginal discharge of old blood.

Most bleeding from trauma is not dangerous. There is often a hematoma of the anterior labia majora.

Genital injury gives rise to anxiety: the little girl is disturbed by pain and bleeding, her parents are worried about serious damage, and the physician is concerned about possible sexual abuse.

Accidental injury is more common than molestation. With the former, there is prompt reporting by the patient and her mother, a clear history, and findings consistent with the history (15).

B. Types of Injury

A prospective 33 month study from the accident and emergency department of the Royal Liverpool Children's Hospital revealed 87 girls with genital injuries (15). Of these, 82 had a clear clinical history. Most of the injuries (74) were straddle or falling onto hard objects, which compresses the vulvar soft tissue against the public ramus bone. This resulted in asymmetric bruising (sometimes severe), abrasion, and (usually superficial) lacerations anteriorly between the labia majora and minora. There may be unilateral medial thigh scraping. With the usual straddle accident, one foot slips and the child falls forward and to one side. Accidents occurred on bicycles, falling on small toys, climbing on furniture, falling astride a fence or bathtub wall, on play or sport apparatus, and from kicking. There were 5 girls with vaginal-penetrating injuries caused by railing spikes, sticks, and a bath tap. These injuries were severe and required examination under anesthesia and suturing. There were tears of the posterior vestibule and posterior vaginal wall. Stretch injuries ("splits") occurred in 3 cases, with superficial tears in the perineum and fourchette, especially in those with labial adhesions; 2 girls had self-inflicted scratch injuries. Of the 87 girls with genital injuries, 80 were considered accidental. Sexual abuse was alleged by only 3 of the 7 girls with suspicion of abuse (15).

C. Sexual Abuse

Suspicion of sexual abuse is raised by an absent or vague history and a delay in presentation in cases of injury to the hymen, (severe) posterior fourchette, perineum, or posterior vaginal wall and failure to have a return visit. The posterior fourchette is distal to the hymen in the vestibule. The gynecologic perineum is between the vagina and anus (the anatomic perineum includes the entire vulva) (15). With sexual abuse, there may be sexually transmitted disease.

V. FOREIGN BODIES IN THE VAGINA AS A CAUSE OF LOCAL NONENDOCRINE BLEEDING

Foreign bodies in the vagina tend to cause a persistent, foul, bloody vaginal discharge. This is a primary vaginitis and secondary vulvitis. The usual material is rolled-up wads of toilet tissue. These are almost always multiple and of different ages. X-rays usually do not detect them because most foreign bodies are not radiopaque. Also, these wads cannot be detected by rectal examination or ultrasound. Levator muscle action causes these wads to be pulled to the upper posterior vagina, and thus they are usually not visualized by inspection of the vulva. Vaginal cultures may yield any or all of the colon bacteria.

Another frequent foreign body is the hard plastic, narrow bottle cap with an "arrowhead" configuration. It may cause trauma on insertion. It can be palpated on rectal examination.

Almost any small object has been found in the vagina, including rolled-up pieces of cloth and green peas. Rarely, trapped pinworms may be lost on their return migration from the rectum.

The object is usually inserted by the child herself, who forgets or does not wish to remember because she knows that it is not proper. I believe that the child pushes her finger rolled up with toilet tissue into the vagina because of itching, and the tissue remains. Thus, there is usually no history of insertion.

Rolled-up wads of toilet tissue tend to reaccumulate, probably because of a habit formation.

On discovery, there is an emotional melodrama as the mother berates the child.

Sometimes, the foul odor results in the child being isolated, with secondary physiologic reactions developed before the diagnosis is discovered.

VI. VULVAR LESIONS AS A CAUSE OF LOCAL NONENDOCRINE BLEEDING

A. Trauma

Because of (1) play, abrasions, scratching, and binding clothing combined with (2) an unprotected vulva with delicate skin, children often get nonspecific abrasions, excoriations, and nonspecific infections of the vulva. These may bleed spontaneously or after rubbing.

B. Skin Disease

1. Condyloma Acuminatum

The incidence of childhood condyloma acuminatum is progressively increasing. It is readily diagnosed by inspection. Scratching or other trauma readily provokes bleeding. The lesions have a characteristic dry, warty, hard, pointed appearance on the skin of the labium majus, perineum, and perianal areas. At the vaginal introitus with mucosa, the lesions are soft, bulky, and rounded, containing 1 mm clear granuloma-like areas suggestive of tapioca pudding. Personal observation suggests that children with sensitive skin (seborrheic or atopic dermatitis) are more susceptible (see Fig. 1).

The presence of vulvar and perianal condyloma acuminatum requires that sexual molestation be ruled out because this is a sexually transmitted disease. Nevertheless, it is possible that in most children anogenital warts are acquired by nonsexual transmission. The sources may be the mother's birth canal, caretakers by direct contact, washcloths, and general body cutaneous verruca vulgaris (16).

In the differential diagnosis of genital verrucous lesions is Darier disease (keratosis follicularis), an autosomal dominant acantholytic disorder that may also result from a spontaneous mutation. Initially it resembles a chronic diaper rash or candidiasis, and later, painful infected masses develop (17). A biopsy is necessary for the diagnosis.

2. Symmetric Fissures

Seborrheic and atopic dermatitis are frequent childhood skin diseases occurring in over 5% of all children. Although not generally recognized, I find a high incidence of vulvar involvement and a frequently underestimated cause of chronic vulvovaginitis. The reason is that the usual diagnosis is made from the vaginal culture and the vulva is overlooked. Both these conditions have characteristic general signs, such as fissures and crusts behind the ears, a prominent lower eyelid fold (Dennie's lines and Morgan's folds), keratosis pilaris of the outer arms, and eczema of the elbow creases. There may be some overlap between these two conditions on purely clinical grounds. Both have a similar, transient subacute appearance of the vulva, with symmetric fissures between the labia minora and majora and in the midline perineum. There may also be fissures in the midline anterior to the clitoris, radial in the perianal area, and in the midline posterior to the anus (see Fig. 2). When deep, the fissures can bleed. They may be confused with sexual molestation; however, the fine precise symmetric lesions and the general body distribution confirm the diagnosis.

Lichen sclerosus et atrophicus, now referred to as lichen sclerosus, in its advanced form has fissures in a similar distribution; however, they are coarser and chronic and bleed more readily (see Fig. 3). They are often misdiagnosed as sexual molestation. A biopsy confirms the lesion. It begins as white, flat papules that coalesce into atrophic "cigarette paper" plaques in the anogenital region. The skin becomes thin and fragile, with upper dermal edema and collagen homogenization. It is easily traumatized, causing purpura and bleeding. Mothers may report "blood blisters" after the child goes on long

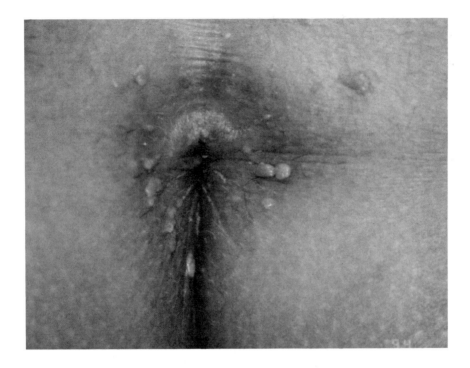

(a)

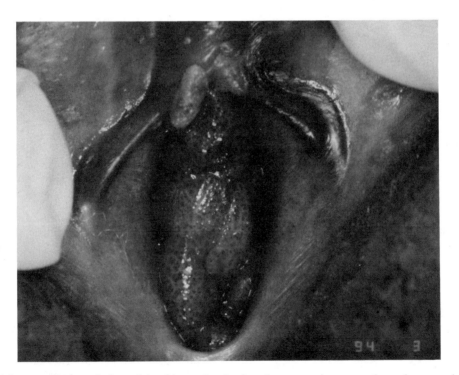

(b)

Figure 1   (a) Condylomata acuminata lesions of the skin are dry, hard, and warty, as is seen on the perineum and perianal areas. In this case, they are less pointed because of previous podophyllin (podophyllun resin) therapy (b). The lesions of the introitus and periurethral areas (mucosa) are soft and bulky and resemble tapioca pudding.

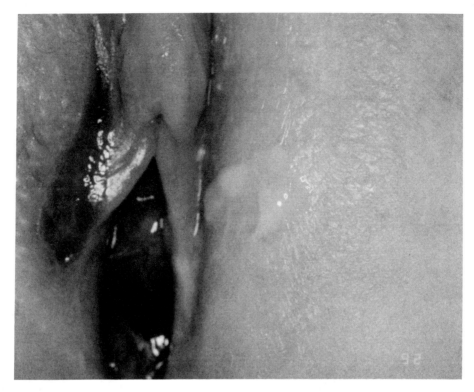

Figure 2 Fissure that caused bleeding on the child's right side between the labia minus and majus.

bicycle rides. A biopsy confirms the diagnosis. Whereas in adults topical 2% testosterone in petrolatum has been recommended, topical 1% progesterone may help in children (18).

3. Psoriasis

Psoriasis is not unusual in children. If it first appears on the vulva, it is frustrating because the local heat, humidity, and rubbing modify the typical appearance and it resists therapy. If it appears on the vulva after general body involvement is present, then the diagnosis is simple. Abrasion and chafing can cause bleeding.

4. Diaper Rash, Allergies, and Contact

The usual diaper rash is an irritant dermatitis related to chemical and bacterial action of the urine and stool. It usually starts on the convex surfaces of the vulva closer to the diaper.

Diaper area rashes also may be caused by candidiasis, atopic eczema dermatitis, seborrheic dermatitis, and psoriasis, and, less often, by dermatophyte fungi or histiocytosis. The last may represent a serious systemic illness and presents as deep intertriginous fissures with severe seborrheic-like dermatitis that resists treatment.

The usual seborrheic dermatitis begins in the intertriginous creases but is less severe and responds to treatment.

The child's sensitive skin is easily irritated by contact or allergic reactions to perfumes, dyes, bubble bath, hot water, excessive soap, and so on.

5. Hemangiomas

As many as 10% of all infants have hemangiomas. They may grow rapidly in the early months. Slow spontaneous regression usually starts at 6–10 months of age. Vulvar lesions are easy to visualize. Scratching or trauma may cause recurrent bleeding. Vaginal hemangiomas require vaginoscopy for identification. Rare, deep pelvic cavernous hemangiomas may have vulvar extensions, bladder extensions (causing hematuria), and rectal extensions (causing large hemorrhoids). Uncomplicated hemangiomas are observed. Complications are traditionally treated with oral or intralesional glucocorticosteroids (19). Dry ice sticks have also been used. There are two new modality treatments that seem to be relatively safe and effective and are being evaluated. They are the vascular-specific pulsed dye laser and interferon-α2a (20).

Aside from the hemangiomas, the other vascular birthmark is the vascular malformation. It persists throughout life, may involve complex combined vascular malformations, requires evaluation, and is rare (21,22).

The rare giant hemangioma, which may present as a subcutaneous soft mass, may have a dangerous consumption coagulopathy and thrombocytopenia (Kasabach-Merritt syndrome). Those that do not respond to conventional therapy may respond to systemic subcutaneous interferon-α (23).

There are extremely rare, rapidly growing, congenital hemangiopericytomas that simulate hemangiomas but spontaneously ulcerate with severe bleeding (24).

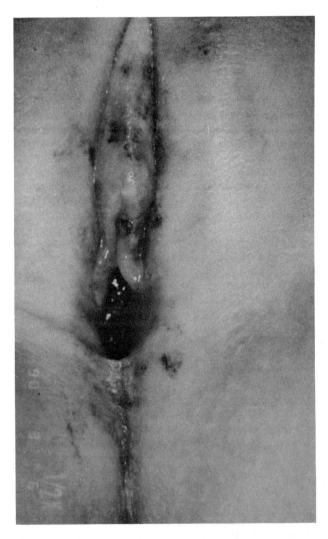

Figure 3 Lichen sclerosus of the vulva. There are chronic coarse deep fissures that readily bleed and white skin. The trauma of bicycle riding can cause ecchymoses.

6. *Vulvar Infections*

Vulvar candidiasis can cause severe pruritic erythematous lesions with sharp irregular borders and satellite lesions. It suggests diabetes or immune deficiency.

Staphylococcus and streptococcus can cause vulvar and buttock pustules and brawny induration (erysipelas).

Tinea skin infections cause elevated circular lesions.

The chicken pox (varicella) lesions are also present on the vulva, where they are readily infected with bacteria and therefore persist.

The most common vulvar ulcers are caused by herpes. Figure 4 shows multiple confluent vulvar ulcers covered with a white exudate of colon-type bacteria. Bacterial culture of itself is misleading. The syphilis lesion may be a primary chancre, secondary congenital condyloma lata, or generalized macular rash. Chancroid ulcers are shaggy and painful and

simulate herpetic ulcers. Tumor chemotherapy can cause vulvar ulcers (25).

In refugee situations with enforced closeness, scabies spreads rapidly and causes intense genital itching. Pediculosis publis occurs in the older child.

There are many rare vulvar lesions.

Chronic bullous dermatosis of childhood has subepidermal blisters with the deposition of IgA in a linear pattern along the basement membrane. It may also develop in other areas besides the genitalia, such as the trunk, extremities, and oral and tracheal mucosa (26).

Crohn's disease of the vulva may occur as a direct extension of this granulomatous intestinal disease as ulcerations and fistulas or separately ("metastatic"). Histologically, the latter is a sterile, noncaseating, nonspecific granuloma.

Granular cell tumors are slow-growing solitary nodules or plaques with a smooth or hyperkeratotic hyperpigmented verrucous surface that may be confused with squamous cell carcinoma or condyloma (27).

VII. PROLAPSE OF THE URETHRA AS A CAUSE OF LOCAL NONENDOCRINE BLEEDING

In some emergency rooms, urethral prolapse is the leading cause of vaginal bleeding. It presents as acute bleeding with pain and urinary symptoms. On inspection, there is a friable, shaggy, necrotic, bleeding mass suggestive of a malignancy. The diagnosis can be confirmed by passing a urethral catheter. The predisposing factors are an increase in intraabdominal pressure and trauma. Management options include conservative therapy (sitz baths and topical estrogen cream), ligation over a Foley indwelling catheter, and excision under general anesthesia. The last gives the best results (28). Milder cases with conservative therapy tend to remain in a subacute condition (see Fig. 5).

The differential diagnosis includes hematuria (from bladder or urethral hemangioma), prolapse of ureterocele, and bladder rhabdomyosarcoma.

VIII. ANAL LESIONS AS A CAUSE OF LOCAL NONENDOCRINE BLEEDING

A. Fissures

The most common anal lesion causing bleeding is the fissure. It may cause spontaneous bleeding, blood covering the stool, pain, and fear of bowel movement. The usual cause (which is not generally recognized) is seborrheic or atopic dermatitis, in which there are the characteristic, symmetric, interlabial vulvar fissures, midline perineal fissures, and perianal radial fissures. There is often an anterior edematous skin tag.

B. Perianal Dermatitis

Perianal dermatitis on culture usually reveals *Candida*, but *Streptococcus* group A and *Staphylococcus aureus* (29), as well as all the colon bacteria, may be present. A single

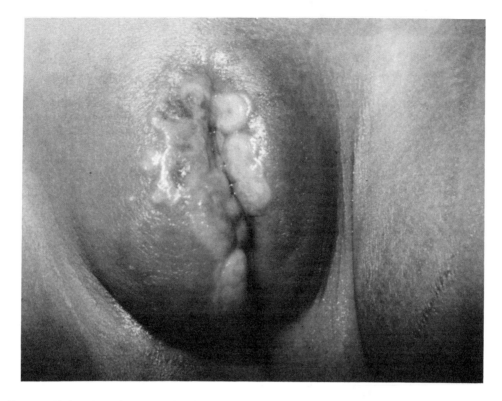

Figure 4   Confluent multiple vulvar ulcers caused by herpes, covered by a white exudate of colon-type bacteria.

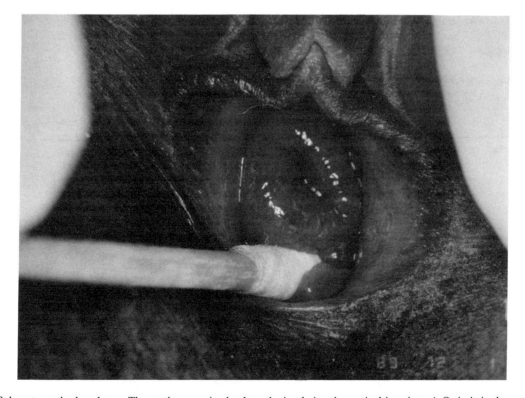

Figure 5   Subacute urethral prolapse. The urethra remained enlarged, simulating the vaginal introitus. A Q-tip is in the actual vagina.

infecting organism may be predominant and the presumptive cause, but the condition, especially if recurrent, may be caused by the predisposing fissures of seborrheic and atopic dermatitis with secondary infection.

C. Pinworm

Pinworm infestation is common in children. About 20% of cases are significantly symptomatic, usually with nocturnal itching and sometimes with abdominal pain. Scratching tears the skin and encourages reinfection. Nocturnal itching may also be the result of blankets that cause an increase in heat and moisture in atopic dermatitis.

D. Condylomata Acuminata

Condylomata acuminata are often perianal in distribution. Their presence requires consideration of molestation. Even without molestation, it occurs in this area especially in children with atopic dermatitis, who are particularly susceptible.

E. Hemorrhoids and Trauma

True hemorrhoids are unusual in children and suggest a large pelvic cavernous hemangioma.

Trauma may be a result of molestation, foreign bodies,

or an innocent accident. Prompt evaluation and reconstruction if needed usually result in healing despite contamination.

IX. POLYPS OF THE HYMEN AS A CAUSE OF LOCAL NONENDOCRINE BLEEDING

It is not unusual to find a prominent, fleshy hymen in the newborn, often with a polypoid posterior lip as a result of maternal estrogen. After a week, these recede, with absence of estrogen. Occasionally, there are true polyps that persist and may tear and bleed. Figure 6 shows large true polyps in a 1-week-old child. Even small polyps may persist. Polyps of the hymen are usually benign.

X. MALIGNANT TUMORS OF THE VAGINA AS A CAUSE OF NONENDOCRINE BLEEDING

A. Rhabdomyosarcoma

Malignant vaginal tumors are rare but potentially fatal. The victims when first seen always look in deceivingly perfect health. The most common is rhabdomyosarcoma, which gynecologists call sarcoma botryoides. About 30 years ago, it was generally fatal within 2 years, and the only survivors were those who were discovered early and had pelvic exenteration. In recent years, with early discovery, local resection,

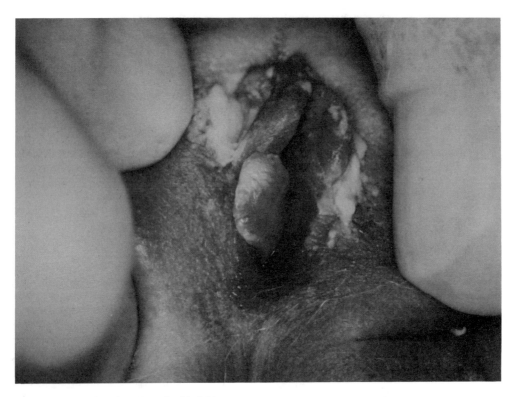

Figure 6 Large true hymen polyps in a 1-week-old child.

and contemporary chemotherapy, the prognosis has been reversed, with the expectation of a cure in 85%. The tumor originates in the submucosal mesenchyme of the vagina and initially presents as a protruding polypoid mass and bleeding. Because the tumor surface is normal mucosa, even experienced physicians are misled. In addition, superficial biopsies may be misleading, because aside from the normal surface mucosa, a deep section is necessary: the pathologic diagnosis requires more than one cell type and the dermis layer. The tumor usually develops in the upper anterior vaginal wall. The important fact is that although polyps of the hymen are usually benign, polyps that originate above the hymen are considered malignant until proven otherwise. Figure 7 shows a 6-year-old girl (most are younger) who had staining for 3 days and a normal hymen. Vaginoscopy revealed a polypoid tumor. On straining, a polyp protruded with a normal vaginal mucosal surface whose origin was above the hymen. Early small rhabdomyosarcoma polypoid masses do not prolapse on straining, and this is not a reliable test. Resection of the polyp showed it to be a rhabdomyosarcoma. If the frozen section confirms the diagnosis, then it is advisable to perform cystoscopy with the same anesthesia to detect possible bladder invasion.

Large vaginal rhabdomyosarcomas may suddenly protrude out of the vagina in grape-like clusters, sometimes after straining at stool. Figure 8 shows such an 11-month-old child.

Part of the tumor has become necrotic because of a vascular disturbance. Despite the size, the child was cured.

B. Germ Cell Tumors

Endodermal (yolk sac) germ cell tumors are very malignant, midline body neoplasms. They tend to develop in the upper vagina and cause bleeding but usually do not prolapse to the introitus. In the past 10 years, with contemporary chemotherapy, the previous usually fatal outcome has been reversed.

C. Adenocarcinoma

Clear cell adenocarcinoma (CCA) has been associated with female fetal exposure to maternal ingestion of diethylstilbesterol (DES) (30). Despite this discovery in 1971 and the discontinuation of DES for pregnant women, this cancer still occurs, although at a reduced rate. It is a cause of vaginal bleeding, and the tumor usually is not visible at the vulva.

DES is the first discovered, hormonal transplacental carcinogen. If given in the first trimester to a pregnant woman with a female fetus, DES can cause a CCA of the vagina or cervix at a delayed time, usually at or just after puberty.

DES became popular in the 1940s because it was the first synthetic, inexpensive oral estrogen. It is nonsteroidal.

There were 547 cases of CCA reported as of 1989. In

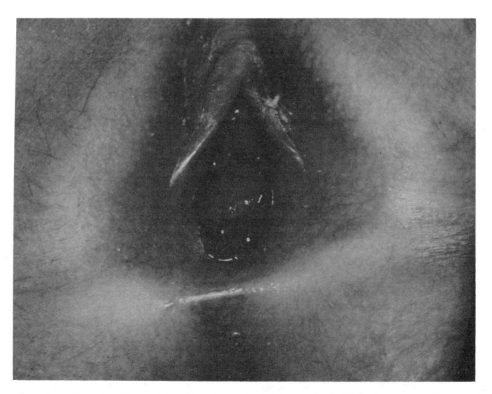

Figure 7 Vaginoscopy showed a polyp. On straining, the polyp protruded as seen here. The surface mucosa is normal vaginal mucosa. Under the normal mucosa of the apparently benign polyp is the very malignant mesenchymal rhabdomyosarcoma. Any vaginal polyp that originates above the hymen is considered malignant until proven otherwise.

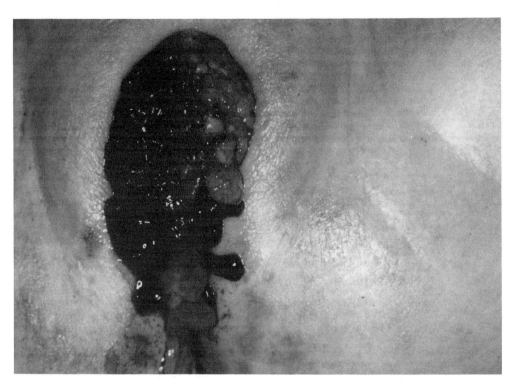

Figure 8 Large vaginal rhabdomyosarcoma protruding from the vagina. The grape-like cluster ("sarcoma botryoides") is noted. Part of the tumor is necrotic because of vascular disturbance.

about one-quarter of the cases, there was no history of hormonal exposure. The age range at discovery was 7–34.4 years, with 91% between 15 and 27 and a median age of 19.0. This suggests a stimulation effect of puberty, especially because of a sharp, dramatic rise at age 14.

Before the use of DES, CCA was very rare and tended to occur in older women.

DES was used to treat women with a history of repeated spontaneous abortion. Such women tend to have affected children more than women on DES without pregnancy losses.

About 60% of CCA are vaginal, usually in the anterior upper third. The remainder are on the ectocervix (portio). They are unifocal. CCA is fatal if untreated.

The risk of developing CCA in a DES-exposed female is 1 in 1000.

Benign changes are much more frequent, about 35% having vaginal adenosis (glandular, endocervical-type epithelium). About 25% have cervix structural abnormalities with cervical hoods, ridges, collars, pseudopolyps, or vaginal septa. All the benign changes occur more frequently with higher doses of DES and with earlier use in pregnancy.

In early embryonic life, the paired müllerian (paramesonephric) ducts (with glandular, columnar, endocervical-type epithelium) form and fuse at about 8 weeks at the urogenital sinus, forming a tubercle or vaginal plate. The latter then grows cephalad as a solid core of squamous epithelium into the fused ducts. Later, the solid core canalizes to become the

vagina. Usually, the separation of the two types of epithelium is at the external os of the cervix.

DES, or any stilbene-type estrogen, prevents normal development of the genital epithelium. It can also cause abnormal proliferation of the adjacent connective tissue, resulting in gross structural abnormalities.

DES is considered an incomplete carcinogen, and there may be other unknown predisposing factors.

The benign and malignant changes are not found with steroidal estrogen exposure.

DES-exposed males do not have an increased risk of cancer. There are conflicting reports of possible benign anatomic and seminal abnormalities (30).

Personal speculation is that because DES is still used to fatten chickens and cows for slaughter, this may be a continuing source of ingestion because it can be stored in animal fat.

A very rare cause of vaginal malignancy is mesonephric duct remnant carcinoma.

XI. COAGULATION DEFECTS AS A CAUSE OF LOCAL NONHORMONAL BLEEDING

Symptomatic coagulation defects are an unusual cause, and any vaginal bleeding is part of the overall body tendency to bleed.

The most common congenital hemostatic abnormality in

children is von Willebrand disease. It is not limited to one ethnic group. The prevalence is 1.3% when the diagnosis is based on a personal history of bleeding, decreased von Willebrand factor activity, and a positive family history. The true incidence is probably higher, especially with blood group O. Because screening tests are not reliable, it is recommended that von Willebrand factor activity be measured in children with mucosal bleeding. Affected children tend to have easy bruising, epistaxis, prolonged bleeding after trauma, and oral bleeding. Adolescents tend to have menorrhagia (31).

With Glanzmann's thrombasthenia the initial bleeding occurs before 5 years of age. The frequent presentations include epistaxis, gingival bleeding, posttraumatic bruises, menorrhagia (often requiring transfusions), and gastrointestinal and postoperative bleeding (32).

Rarely there may be severe acute onset of a general tendency to bleed because of hypoprothrombinemia associated with a lupus anticoagulant (33).

Other coagulation defects may be associated with viral infections, leukemia, or collagen vascular disease.

XII. EVALUATION

A. History

It is important to obtain a reliable history from the mother, the child's caretaker, and if possible from the child herself. Some suggestions follow.

The bleeding history is detailed: onset, color (bright red or brownish red, mixed with discharge), odor, amount, and continuation—course, pain, and association with scratching, wiping, urination, bowel movement, and tight clothing.

Inquiry is made about vulvovaginitis symptoms: vulvar itching, burning, and pain; vaginal discharge; rubbing; use of bubble baths, perfumed soaps, or deodorants; or use of tights, leotards, and ballet outfits. Dysuria caused by vulvitis is vulvar dysuria with external pain, a reluctance to void, a distended bladder, and occasionally acute urinary retention. Dysuria caused by cystitis-urethritis causes deep pain, frequency, urgency, and bladder spasms.

Has there been recent antibiotic or hormonal therapy or respiratory or skin infection? Does the child have allergies or general chronic skin disturbances, such as atopic or seborrheic dermatitis, eczema, or psoriasis? Does she have diabetes, chronic illnesses (kidney, hepatic, or intestinal), or immunodeficiency defect? Is there a coagulation disturbance?

Was there an acute trauma, such as falling from a play device or from standing on a chair? Could the child have been molested (even by an adult male relative) and have been threatened if she reveals it? Is she left without supervision?

Was the pregnancy uneventful? Did the mother take any unusual medications?

The family history includes the health of siblings and such illnesses as diabetes; atopic dermatitis, allergies, asthma, and eczema; bleeding disorders; immunodeficiency states; and malignancies.

B. Physical Examination

Before examination, as an educational device, I indicate to the child in the presence of the mother that only mothers and doctors are allowed to examine, look at, or touch children's "private parts." The mother is kept in the room to reassure the child. Try to communicate in a friendly fashion with the child to help her relax and create a nonthreatening environment.

The panties are inspected for blood and discharge.

The physical examination begins with a general examination.

1. Are there signs of precocious puberty? Is there mammary tissue on palpation, or do the breasts seem enlarged because the child is chubby?
2. Does the child seem irritable? Does she scratch herself generally? Is there white dermatographism? Are there signs of general skin disease, especially seborrheic or atopic dermatitis characterized by erythematous fissures behind the ears with flaking; scalp margins and paranasal erythematous greasy scales; pityriasis alba of the face; prominent lower eyelid skin folds (Morgan's folds) with white edematous edges; keratosis pilaris of the outer arms and thighs, eczema of the elbows, wrists, and popliteal space; and ichthyosis of the legs? Are there signs of psoriasis or chicken pox? Are there skin infections? Is there pharyngitis, rhinitis, or cough? Is there adenopathy (cervical, axillary, or inguinal), abdominal masses, or ecchymosis?

The frequent local nonhormonal bleeding areas that require attention in the physical examination are listed in Table 2.

As a minimum, the vulva must be visualized. Further office testing must be individualized in accord with the reaction of the child, source of bleeding, experience of the physician, appearance of the vulva, history, and perceived seriousness.

The child may be placed in small stirrups in dorsal lithotomy position or in frog leg position on the examination table or in the lap of the mother, who sits on the table. A good cold light is necessary.

The labia majora are gently held apart and downward to permit adequate inspection. Sometimes, the child's hands can be used by the examiner as retractors to reduce anxiety. Careful inspection requires a trained eye. One method is to start anteriorly and proceed posteriorly, viewing the mons publis; presence of hair; erythematous fissures in the midline anterior to the clitoris, then between the labia majora and minora symmetrically, in the midline perineum (between vagina and rectum), radially around the anus, and in the midline posterior to the anus; the clitoris; the urethra; the hymen and its orifice; the vestibule (just outside the hymen); the posterior fourchette; the perineum; the perianal area; and the groin and the adjacent buttocks. Very often the distal vagina can be visualized.

If the site and cause of the bleeding can be identified by

Table 2 Frequent Causes of Nonhormonal Bleeding According to Site

    I. Urethra: prolapse urethra (necrotic, sloughing)
   II. Anus: deep fissure (pain, skin tag edema)
  III. Vulva (inspection with good light and gentle retraction)
      A. Trauma
      B. Skin disease and lesions
      C. Fissures (associated with seborrheic and atopic dermatitis and lichen sclerosus)
      D. General ecchymoses (coagulation defect)
      E. Hymen polyp
  IV. Inspection of distal vagina
      A. Vaginal discharge
      B. Vaginal bleeding
   V. Vaginal bleeding
      A. Severe streptococcus A vaginitis (usually upper vagina)
      B. Foreign body (usually multiple rolled-up wads of toilet tissue causing a foul, bloody discharge)
      C. Rhabdomyosarcoma (rare but very malignant, with only drops of blood)

visualizing the exposed vulva, then the examination may be discontinued. If these are not apparent, then further investigation is needed and examination under anesthesia may be required to avoid anxiety, thrashing, and resistance by the child.

Placing a Q-tip in the vagina may show blood and indicate the vaginal source of bleeding. Another device is an eye or medicine dropper. Vaginal secretion may be tested for Papanicolaou cytology, bacterial culture, Gram stain, gonorrhea culture, *Chlamydia* culture, saline wet mount (for motile trichomonads, white blood cells, lactobacilli, "clue" cells of *Gardnerella* bacterial vaginosis), and 10% potassium hydroxide wet mount for *Candida*. Cytology is not reliable to rule out a vaginal malignancy. Cytologic maturation index (MI) is helpful in evaluating estrogen activity. The usual anestrogenic prepubertal child has an MI of 0% superficial, 0% intermediate, and 100% parabasal cells. Superficial vaginal cells are large, flat, and polygonal with a small pyknotic nucleus and are indicative of the presence of estrogen. In England and Canada, laboratories often reverse the MI sequence and report parabasal, intermediate, and superficial vaginal cells. The newborn has a temporary estrogenic smear of superficial vaginal epithelial cells because of in utero maternal estrogen exposure.

Although not as reliable as an early morning swab, a clear cellophane type of perianal swab may be made to check for microscopic pinworm ova and to show the mother how to do it at home in the early morning.

Bimanual rectal examination usually cannot detect toilet tissue wads in the vagina but can detect a hard vaginal foreign object, a normal cervix, a firm vaginal tumor mass, and the lower pole of an ovarian neoplasm (the infant's ovary is pelvic). It might "milk out" vaginal discharge or bleeding.

With a cooperative older child, the "knee-chest" position may result in a ballooning out of the vagina to permit visualization of the distal two-thirds of the vagina with a hand-held light (see Fig. 9).

If the bleeding source is not apparent from visualization

of the exposed vulva and distal vagina or if a Q-tip inserted into the vagina produces bleeding, then *vaginoscopy* is appropriate. There may be a specific severe infection (streptococcus A), a foreign body (rolled-up wads of toilet tissue), or a malignant and potentially fatal neoplasm. Vaginoscopy is done generally for the suspicion of significant trauma, foreign body, neoplasm, congenital anomaly, or persistent vaginitis.

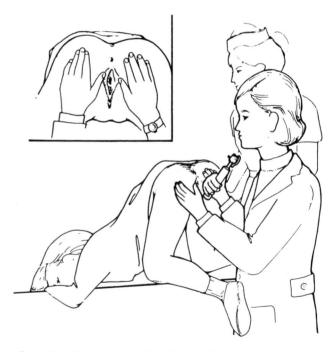

Figure 9 Knee-chest position for visualizing the vagina in the cooperative older child using a hand-held light. (Reproduced with permission from Emans SJ. Section 11. Gynecology. In: Avery ME, First LR, eds. Pediatric Medicine. Baltimore: Williams & Wilkins, 1989:652.)

Unfortunately, no standard vaginoscope is in use. The vaginoscope instruments that have been used include a simple tube with obturator; a Cameron-Miller tube with obturator, distal light bulb, magnifying glass; a fiberoptic Storz instrument; a hysteroscope; a cystoscope; or a miniature bivalve speculum. Miniature alligator forceps to remove foreign bodies, and long microsurgical instruments should be available for biopsy and local excision of tumors. Experience is required for operative procedures.

Sometimes observation vaginoscopy can be done as an office procedure; however, operative vaginoscopy is best done in an operating room with general anesthesia by an expert pediatric anesthesiologist.

If there is an expectation of a malignant vaginal tumor, then a frozen section is considered and cystoscopy with biopsy may be done with the same anesthesia to check for spread.

Abdominal and pelvic *ultrasound* are considered for the suspicion of a vaginal neoplasm, large or rigid foreign body, and congenital anomaly (therefore the kidneys require imaging). Rolled-up wads of toilet tissue and small vaginal malignant neoplasms may not be able to be imaged.

X-rays are avoided if possible.

XIII. CONCLUSION

Vaginal bleeding is unusual in children. It creates great anxiety in the child and her parents. The vast majority of bleeding is caused by local, nonhormonal causes. Bleeding requires prompt investigation to determine the site, cause, and management.

The special concerns include precocious puberty, sexual molestation, and malignancy.

If required for the diagnosis of blood coming from the vagina from a site that cannot be visualized externally, vaginoscopy under general anesthesia (if necessary) is appropriate.

REFERENCES

1. Heller ME, Savage MO, Dewhurst J. Vaginal bleeding in childhood: a review of 51 patients. Br J Obstet Gynaecol 1978; 85:721–725.
2. Saggese G, Ghirri P, DelVecchio A, Papini A, Pardi D. Gonadotropin pulsatile secretion in girls with premature menarche. Horm Res 1990; 33:5–10.
3. Rakover Y, Weiner E, Shalev E, Luboshitsky R. Vaginal bleeding: presenting symptom of acquired primary hypothyroidism in a seven year old girl. J Pediatr Endocrinol 1993; 6:197–200.
4. Grunberger W. Diagnose und therapie bei gynakologisch erkrankten madchen. Wien Klin Wochenschr 1987; 99:763–767.
5. Hill NC, Oppenheimer LW, Morton KE. The aetiology of vaginal bleeding in children: a 20 year review. Br J Obstet Gynaecol 1989; 96:467–470.
6. Altchek A. Vaginal discharges. In: Stockman JA III, ed. Difficult Diagnosis in Pediatrics. Philadelphia: W.B. Saunders, 1990:383–389.
7. Emans SJH, Goldstein DP. Pediatric and adolescent gynecol-

ogy. In: Vulvovaginal Problems in the Prepubertal Child, 3rd ed. Boston: Little, Brown, 1990:67–93.
8. Fishman A, Paldi E. Vaginal bleeding in premenarchal girls: a review. Obstet Gynecol Surv 1991; 46:457–460.
9. Pokorny SF. Prepubertal vulvovaginopathies. Obstet Gynecol Clin North Am 1992; 19:39–58.
10. Wilson MD. Vaginal discharge and vaginal bleeding in childhood. In: Carpenter SEK, Rock JA, eds. Pediatric and Adolescent Gynecology. New York: Raven Press, 1992:139–151.
11. Muram D, Sanfilippo JS, Hertweck SP. Vaginal bleeding in childhood and menstrual disorders in adolescence. In: Sanfilippo JS, Muram D, Lee PA, Dewhurst J, eds. Pediatric and Adolescent Gynecology. Philadelphia: W.B. Saunders, 1994: 222–232.
12. Dhar V, Roker K, Adhami MZ, Mckenzie S. Streptococcal vulvovaginitis in girls. Pediatr Dermatol 1993; 10:366–367.
13. Yanovski JA, Nelson LM, Willis ED, Cutler GB Jr. Repeated childhood vaginal bleeding is not always precocious puberty. Pediatrics 1992; 89:149–151.
14. Magana-Garcia M, Arista-Viveros A. Cutaneous amebiasis in children. Pediatr Dermatol 1993; 10:352–355.
15. Pierce AM, Robson WJ. Genital injury in girls—accidental or not? Pediatr Surg Int 1993; 8:239–243.
16. Obalek S, Misiewicz J, Jablonska S, Favre M, Orth G. Childhood condyloma acuminatum: association with genital and cutaneous human papillomaviruses. Pediatr Dermatol 1993; 10:101–106.
17. Salopek TG, Krol A, Jimbo K. Case report of Darier disease localized to the vulva in a 5 year old girl. Pediatr Dermatol 1993; 10:146–148.
18. Serrano G, Millan F, Fortea JM, Grau M, Aliaga A. Topical progesterone as treatment of choice in genital lichen sclerosis et atrophicus in children (correspondence). Pediatr Dermatol 1993; 10:201.
19. Cook CL, Sanfilippo JS, Verdi GD, Pietsch JP. Capillary hemangioma of the vagina and urethra in a child: response to short term steroid therapy. Obstet Gynecol 1989; 73:883–885.
20. Morelli JG. On the treatment of hemangiomas (commentary). Pediatr Dermatol 1993; 10:84.
21. Pehr K, Moroz B. Cutis marmorata telangiectatica congenita: long term follow-up, review of the literature, and report of a case in conjunction with congenital hypothyroidism. Pediatr Dermatol 1993; 10:6–11.
22. Enjolras O, Mulliken JB. The current management of vascular birthmarks. Pediatr Dermatol 1993; 10:311–333.
23. Hatley RM, Sabio H, Howell CG, Flickinger F, Parrish RA. Successful management of an infant with a giant hemangioma of the retroperitoneum and Kasabach-Merritt syndrome with alpha-interferon. J Pediatr Surg 1993; 28:1356–1359.
24. Resnick SD, Lacey S, Jones G. Hemorrhagic complications in a rapidly growing, congenital hemangiopericytoma. Pediatr Dermatol 1993; 10:267–270.
25. Muram D, Gold SS. Vulvar ulcerations in girls with myelocytic leukemia. South Med J 1993; 86:293–294.
26. Hruza LL, Mallory SB, Fitzgibbons J, Mallory GB. Linear IgA bullous dermatosis in a neonate. Pediatr Dermatol 1993; 10:171–176.
27. Guenther L, Shum D. Granular cell tumor of the vulva. Pediatr Dermatol 1993; 10:153–155.
28. Fernandes ET, Dekermacher S, Sabadin MA, Vaz F. Urethral prolapse in children. Urology 1993; 41:240–242.
29. Montemarano AD, James WD. *Staphylococcus aureus* as a

cause of perianal dermatitis. Pediatr Dermatol 1993; 10:259–262.

30. Herbst AL, Anderson D. Clear cell adenocarcinoma of cervix and vagina and DES-related abnormalities. In: Coppleson M, Monaghan JM, Morrow CP, Tattersall MHN, eds. Gynecologic Oncology. Fundamental Principles and Clinical Practice, 2nd ed., Vol. 1. New York: Churchill Livingstone, 1992:523–533.

31. Werner EJ, Broxson EH, Tucker EL, Giroux DS, Shults J, Abshire TC. Prevalence of von Willebrand disease in children: a multi-ethnic study. J Pediatr 1993; 123:893–898.

32. Agarwal MB, Agarwal UM, Viswanathan C, Bhave AA, Billa V. Glanzmann's thrombasthenia. Indian Pediatr 1992; 29:837–841.

33. Bernini JC, Buchanan GR, Ashcraft J. Hypoprothrombinemia and severe hemorrhage associated with a lupus anticoagulant. J Pediatr 1993; 123:937–939.

16
Adolescent Menstrual Abnormalities

Carol M. Foster

University of Michigan Medical School,
Ann Arbor, Michigan

I. INTRODUCTION

The pubertal transition is a period of marked hormonal change that results in the development of secondary sexual characteristics and attainment of the ability to reproduce. Changes occur in central nervous system function that permit maturation of the hypothalamic-pituitary axis, which result in increased sex steroid production leading to breast development, pubic hair growth, and menses. A thorough understanding of the physiology of pubertal maturation, including its normal timing and tempo, and of the hormonal events underlying puberty and the menstrual cycle is essential in assessment of adolescent menstrual disorders (Chapter 13). Our understanding of the physiology of puberty is evolving rapidly. Hormone radioimmunoassays in use for many years are now giving way to ultrasensitive and precise immunoassays (1,2) and bioassays for both peptide hormones, such as gonadotropins and steroid hormones. The biology of the activin, inhibin, and follistatin, peptides produced in the gonads and elsewhere, is now being elucidated. The role these peptides play in reproduction is as yet unknown but is undergoing active investigation (3–6). These advances, the availability of hypothalamic-releasing peptides for study of gonadotropin release, and inferences made from animal studies are altering traditional views of how pubertal maturation occurs and how menstrual cycles and ovulation are regulated.

II. NORMAL GROWTH AND DEVELOPMENT

Sexual development is a continuous process beginning in the fetus and extending throughout childhood and adolescence until reproductive competence is achieved in adulthood. Sexual development can be more readily understood when divided into four stages: (1) fetal differentiation; (2) early infancy and childhood; (3) puberty; and (4) adulthood.

A. Fetal Development

Sexual differentiation of the gonad is determined genetically (Chapter 20). Fetal ovarian development is apparent by the tenth week (7), when primordial germ cells are already beginning to divide. Six to seven million oogenia are formed by the 20th week (8,9). The fetal hypothalamic-pituitary axis also develops at this time and becomes remarkably active, secreting both luteinizing hormone (LH) and follicle-stimulating hormone (FSH) under the control of hypothalamic gonadotropin releasing peptide (GnRH) (10,11). GnRH secretion increases, as do LH and FSH secretion, and peaks around 20 weeks of gestation when LH pulses can be detected at intervals occurring about every 2 h. LH concentrations achieved during this time exceed those seen in puberty and adulthood. The pituitary gonadotropins advance some oogenia into meiotic prophase and result in subsequent investment of the oocytes with a layer of granulosa cells to form the first primordial follicles. The increase in sex steroids, and perhaps in gonadal peptides, is thought to produce a decrease in GnRH and gonadotropin secretion, demonstrating the development of hypothalamic sensitivity to ovarian negative feedback (11). As gonadotropin secretion declines, ovarian germ cells also decline to approximately 2 million. From the seventh month of gestation and onward throughout reproduction life, primordial follicles undergo maturation to graafian follicles. The development of granulosa cells and thecal differentiation in the follicles result in estrogen secretion. Follicles also undergo atresia. The hypothalamic-pituitary axis becomes increasingly sensitive to negative feedback regulation, so there is a decline in GnRH and gonadotropin secretion as fetal maturation occurs (9,11).

B. Early Infancy and Childhood

With the separation of the fetus from placental steroids and human chorionic gonadotropin (hCG) at birth, there is often a brief increase of serum gonadotropin concentrations increasing to near-castrate levels by 3 months of age (12,13). Estradiol is also produced from maturing antral follicles. Feedback sensitivity to these steroids and perhaps to other gonadal peptides inhibits gonadotropin secretion. By 2–4 years of age, the hypothalamic-pituitary gonadal axis is relatively quiescent and will remain so until pubertal maturation begins (14). The cause for this quiescent phase is the subject of debate. While the hypothalamic-pituitary gonadal axis becomes exquisitely sensitive to the negative feedback effects of any gonadal steroids produced, the childhood decline in gonadotropins may be related to intrinsic central nervous system changes, since girls with ovarian dysgenesis also have a remarkable decline in gonadotropin secretion despite their inability to synthesize estradiol in the concentrations seen in normal girls (15,16). Recent animal studies suggest the restraint of the hypothalamic-pituitary axis may be under control of inhibitory tone produced by GABA-secreting neurons (17). Whatever the cause, low-amplitude, infrequent gonadotropin pulses occur during childhood until the onset of puberty (1,18,19).

C. Puberty

The hormonal or central nervous system changes responsible for the onset of puberty are not known (Chapter 13). The primary determinants of the timing of puberty are probably genetic, but nutrition, physical health, and psychological factors can influence both the onset of and the rate of progression through puberty (20–22). Pubertal maturation is usually preceded for 2–3 years by an increase in adrenal androgens such as dehydroepiandrosterone sulfate (23). The control of adrenal maturation is also not understood, and although this maturation could be important to the subsequent apparent decrease in sensitivity of the hypothalamic-pituitary axis to negative feedback from gonadal steroids, a role for adrenal androgens in pubertal development has not been found (24). At the same time that the adrenals are maturing, body weight and fat content are increasing. Although metabolic rate and body fat content cannot be the only signals for the initiation of puberty, heavy children usually mature relatively early while thin children mature relatively late, compared to children with an average body habitus (25).

Whatever the cause for this maturation, puberty is heralded by an increase in the amplitude and frequency of the episodic secretion of LH resulting in an increase in mean serum LH concentration (26–28). The increase in LH secretion first occurs at night, coincident with the onset of sleep (Fig. 1). The increase in LH is followed about 6 hr later by an increase in plasma estradiol concentration (29). Both LH and FSH concentrations increase as puberty progresses, and their increase is paralleled by an increase in plasma estradiol concentration (Fig. 2) (30). The increase in gonadotropins and sex steroids is associated with physical changes, including an increase in height and weight, breast development, and pubic hair growth. Ninety-five percent of girls have onset of breast development between 8 and 12 years, and the onset of pubic hair growth occurs closely around the time of breast

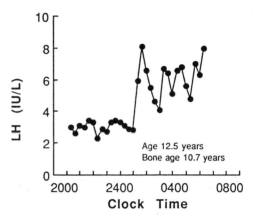

Figure 1 LH concentrations in an early pubertal girl. LH was measured in blood obtained every 20 min from 20:00 to 08:00 hr in a 12.5-year-old girl with constitutional delay of growth and adolescence. LH concentrations fluctuated episodically and the amplitude and frequency of these episodic fluctuations increased coincident with the onset of sleep. An increase in LH concentration, pulse frequency, and pulse amplitude is characteristic of girls in early to midpuberty reflecting an increase in GnRH pulse frequency and amplitude.

development (Fig. 3) (31,32). Pubic hair growth and development of acne are the result of an increase in circulating testosterone concentration produced from both ovarian and adrenal sources. An increase in growth rate occurs in early puberty and reaches a peak shortly before the onset of menses, which occurs in late puberty (32).

D. Adult Stage and the Menstrual Cycle

The mean age for menarche in American girls is 12.8 ± 1.2 years (SD) (33). In midpuberty, there is sufficient estradiol

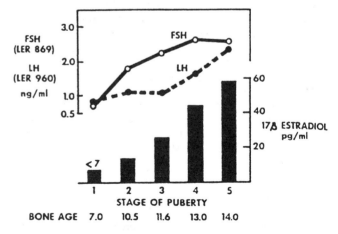

Figure 2 Hormonal concentrations with advancing puberty. The standard used for follicle-stimulating hormone (FSH) was LER 869 and for luteinizing hormone (LH), LER 960. (From Ref. 30.)

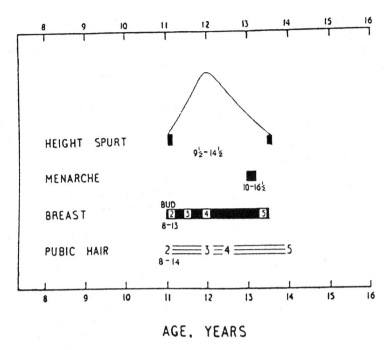

AGE, YEARS

Figure 3 Stages of sexual development are represented within the bars. The range of ages when some of the changes occur is indicated by the numbers below the bars. (From Taner JM. Growth at Adolescence, ed 2. Oxford: Blackwell, 1962.)

in response to gonadotropin stimulation of the ovary to permit the development of an endometrial lining that will shed after estradiol withdrawal. The hallmark of adult development in girls, however, is the development of positive estrogen feedback on the hypothalamus, producing an LH surge that initiates ovulation and cyclical episodes of menses (34,35). This feedback loop requires 6–18 months to develop after the onset of estrogen withdrawal bleeding (36,37). Positive feedback requires that ovarian follicles can, under FSH priming, secrete sufficient estradiol to maintain a critical concentration in the circulation; that the pituitary gland is sensitive to GnRH and contains sufficient LH to support an LH surge; and that the GnRH neurons in the hypothalamus can produce or release sufficient GnRH into the portal circulation to produce an LH surge (34,35). The hormone patterns of estradiol, LH, and FSH that culminate in an LH surge and the subsequent increase in progesterone character-istic of a normal menstrual cycle are diagrammed in Figure 4. Studies of hormone patterns, progesterone secretion, and basal body temperature suggest that 50–60% of cycles in the first 2 years after menarche in most girls are anovulatory. Five years after menarche, the percentage of cycles that are anovulatory decreases to less than 20% (38). Once cycles are ovulatory, adult reproductive status has been achieved.

III. MENSTRUAL DISORDERS

Irregular menstrual periods occur commonly during adoles-cence. The focus of this discussion are those entities that should be recognized as pathological so as to be differentiated

from normal variations in pubertal development. These dis-orders include primary and secondary amenorrhea, oligomen-orrhea, dysfunctional uterine bleeding, essential dysmenor-rhea, and premenstrual syndrome.

A. Primary Amenorrhea

Primary amenorrhea is defined as the absence of onset of menstruation by the age of 16 years. In general, menses can be expected to occur 2.3 ± 1.0 (SD) years after onset of breast development (32). Ninety-five percent of all girls have onset of menses by 16 years of age and 98% by 18 years of age. Evaluation is guided by a careful history and physical examination taking into consideration whether the adolescent has delayed or normal development of secondary sexual characteristics, and whether there is evidence of virilization. A plasma FSH concentration is also useful in determining whether there is a primary disorder of the ovary resulting in ovarian failure (elevated FSH) or whether the disorder is likely to involve the hypothalamic pituitary axis (low or normal FSH) (Chapter 3–18). The differential considerations for the girl with primary amenorrhea are outlined in Table 1.

1. Primary Amenorrhea in Association with Normal or Decreased FSH Concentrations and Otherwise Normal Pubertal Development

Girls who have normal development of secondary sexual characteristics but absence of menses may have anatomical abnormalities of the genital tract that can be congenital or acquired. Radiation to the pelvis may result in endometrial atrophy. Labial aglutination may occur as a result of infection

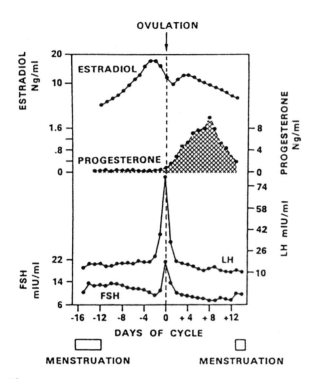

Figure 4 Hormonal changes in a normal adult menstrual cycle. (From Hung W, August GP, Glasgow AM, eds. Ovary in Pediatric Endocrinology. New York: Medical Examination Publishing Co., 1978.)

and obstruct menstrual flow (39). Aplasia of the vaginal hymen or vaginal webs may result in absent menses (40). Uterine agenesis may occur from severe abnormalities of müllerian differentiation such as the Mayer-Rokitansky-Kuster-Hauser syndrome of müllerian agenesis. In other cases involving errors of müllerian differentiation, the uterus may not fuse normally leaving a blind uterine horn. Accumulation of menstrual blood behind on obstruction to uterine outflow may lead to cyclical pain. Some disorders of intersex may allow breast development despite absent development of müllerian structures. Phenotypical female adolescents with a 46,XY karyotype and complete androgen resistance will produce estradiol sufficient for normal breast development but will have had in utero müllerian regression with absent uterus and a blind vaginal pouch (41,42). These girls will have minimal sexual hair. Those with partial androgen resistance may have some degree of virilization with clitoral enlargement and sexual hair growth. Serum FSH is usually normal but may be slightly increased. In contrast, LH concentrations are usually increased, and testosterone concentrations are in the adult male range.

2. Primary Amenorrhea in the Girl with Delayed Adolescent Development and Elevated FSH

Girls with primary amenorrhea and delayed or absent pubertal development may have primary hypogonadism, as indicated by an elevated plasma FSH concentration (Chapter 13–18).

The differential diagnosis of these primary ovarian disorders may include both congenital and acquired conditions. An association with short stature should alert the physician to consider gonadal dysgenesis on the basis of karyotypic disorders of the X chromosome including 45,XO, 46,XX/45,XO mosaicism or other disorders including isochromosome and ring abnormalities of the X chromosome (43). These girls often, but not always, exhibit phenotypic features characteristic of Turner syndrome, including nail dysplasia, webbed neck, foreshortening of the fourth and fifth metacarpals, midfacial hypoplasia, and cubitus valgus deformity. Other congenital disorders of differentiation resulting in gonadal dysgenesis are associated with 46,XX and 46,XY karyotypes (44,45). These individuals are phenotypic girls with normal stature and sexual infantilism (Chapter 19).

Congenital disorders resulting in hypergonadotropic hypogonadism also include those disorders that prevent steroid synthesis or prevent gonadotropins from producing intracellular signals in the ovaries. The steroid synthesis disorders include the forms of congenital adrenal hyperplasia that do not allow estradiol synthesis (e.g., 17α-hydroxylase deficiency) (46). These disorders are quite rare and are usually associated with a lack of cortisol production. Gonadotropins may not be able to produce a signal to the ovaries in conditions where there is a defect in the gonadotropin receptor–adenylate cyclase complex such as may occur in Albright's hereditary osteodystrophy (pseudohypoparathyroidism) (47) or in other forms of the resistant ovary syndrome (48).

Acquired causes of ovarian failure include autoimmune oophoritis, which may occur in isolation or in association with other autoimmune disorders including hypoparathyroidism, adrenal insufficiency, thyroiditis, and pernicious anemia (49,50). Trauma involving both ovaries, surgical bilateral oophorectomy, or invasion of the ovaries by neoplasms all may result in acquired ovarian failure. Radiation of the pelvis with or without chemotherapy for treatment of pelvic neoplasms may also result in ovarian failure although more commonly such treatment destroys the germ cells without impairing the ovarian steroid production underlying the development of secondary sexual characteristics (51–53). Galactosemia, an inborn error of metabolism of galactose, is associated with primary ovarian failure (54). Girls with galactosemia are usually, but not always, detected by newborn screening. Those who are discovered later in life usually give a history of avoidance of galactose-containing foods such as milk.

3. Primary Amenorrhea and Delayed Pubertal Development in Association with Decreased Serum FSH

The most common cause of delayed adolescence in girls is constitutional delay of growth and adolescence (Chapter 13). This disorder is associated with short stature, delay in bone development (delayed bone age), and height and growth velocity appropriate for bone age. Frequently, these girls are slender, and all have normal body proportions (55). This pattern of development is frequently associated with a family history of adolescent delay in a parent. If pubertal development has begun and the girl has a delayed bone age, a height

Table 1 Causes of Amenorrhea

I. Abnormal genital structure
   A. Aplasia
      1. Hymenal
      2. Vaginal
      3. Müllerian structures
      4. Intersex disorders associated with normal female external genitalia
   B. Intersex disorders associated with ambiguous genitalia and virilization at puberty
   C. Acquired
      1. Radiation
      2. Infection
II. Hypogonadism with low gonadotropins
   A. Constitutional delay in growth and development
   B. Hypogonadotropic hypogonadism
      1. Congenital absence of GnRH
         a. Isolated
         b. Combined with anosmia (Kallman syndrome)
         c. Associated with other syndromes (Bartlett-Biedl, Prader-Willi, Friedreich's ataxia)
      2. Acquired
         a. Postencephalitis
         b. Trauma
         c. Tumors (craniopharyngioma, glioma, pinealoma, histiocytosis)
III. Hypogonadism with elevated gonadotropism
   A. Congenital ovarian disorders
      1. Gonadal dysgenesis (45,X; XO/XX; "pure" XY)
      2. 17α-hydroxylase deficiency
   B. Acquired ovarian disorders
      1. Oophoritis
         a. Isolated
         b. Associated with other autoimmune disorders (hypoparathyroidism, thyroiditis, adrenal insufficiency, pernicious anemia)
      2. Trauma
      3. Neoplasms
      4. Oophorectomy
      5. Radiation
      6. Galactosemia
IV. Primary amenorrhea associated with virilization
   A. Congenital disorders
      1. True hermaphroditism
      2. Congenital virilizing adrenal hyperplasia
   B. Acquired
      1. Polycystic ovary syndrome
      2. Hyperthecosis
      3. Functioning ovarian tumors
      4. Adrenal tumors

age appropriate for the bone age, and a growth velocity of 5 cm per year in association with a positive family history, it is usually sufficient to reassure the girl that her development will proceed normally.

Constitutional delay of growth and adolescence must be differentiated from other disorders associated with short stature and adolescent delay, including growth hormone deficiency (Chapter 1). In general, children with isolated growth hormone deficiency will have a subnormal growth rate and may have increased truncal adiposity, since growth hormone is lipolytic. These children may have depressed serum insulin-like growth factor-I (IGF-I) and/or decreased IGFBP-3 (56,57), and their growth hormone response to provocative stimuli will be subnormal (58,59). Isolated growth hormone deficiency is associated with normal sensitivity of the pituitary to GnRH (60). The delay in adolescent development seen with growth hormone deficiency may be related to the decreased serum concentrations of IGF-I, which is known to be an important mediator of ovarian steroid synthesis and differentiation (61–63).

Congenital absence of GnRH in isolation or in association with anosmia (Kallman syndrome) is also associated with delayed adolescent development. The disorder is 5–7 times more common in males than in females, and most cases are the result of an X-linked mutation. Autosomal dominant and recessive forms of the disorder have also been reported (64). The diagnosis is difficult to make, but in general, skeletal development is not delayed and short stature is not a prominent feature (64,65). Testing with GnRH usually reveals an absent or prepubertal gonadotropin response (65). GnRH deficiency may occur in asociation with the absence of other pituitary hormones including growth hormone, ACTH, and thyroid stimulating hormone, as the result of congenital disorders of hypothalamic pituitary development or from acquired disorders such as neoplastic invasion.

Careful history taking may direct investigation toward acquired causes of GnRH deficiency. A history of trauma or encephalitis or the presence of visual and neurological symptoms suggestive of an intracranial neoplasm or craniopharyngeoma (66,67) will direct the need for neuroimaging studies. A GnRH stimulation test will also demonstrate a prepubertal or absent gonadotropin response, if delayed adolescence is related to these acquired disorders. Chronic illnesses, dieting, exercise, and anorexia may be associated with acquired absence of GnRH secretion and should be ruled out by history (68–72). Endocrinopathies such as hypo- or hyperthyroidism (72,73), hypercortisolism from Cushing's disease or syndrome (68,72,74), and uncontrolled diabetes mellitus (75,76) can be excluded by appropriate tests.

Some syndromes are associated with hypogonadotropism and sexual infantilism or delayed adolescence. The Prader-Willi syndrome is characterized by infantile hypotonia and feeding difficulties, short stature, massive obesity with onset in early childhood, small hands and feet, mental retardation, emotional disturbances, characteristic facies with almond-shaped eyes, and hypogonadism associated with hypothalamic dysfunction (77). About 60% of individuals have a deletion in the long arm of chromosome 15 (78). The Laurence-Moon and Bardet-Biedl syndromes are autosomal recessive syndromes of obesity, mental retardation, and retinitis pigmentosa with or without polydactyly associated with hypogonadotropic hypogonadism and occasionally with primary gonadal failure (79).

4. Primary Amenorrhea Associated with Virilization

Elevations of androgens and estrogens may be seen in girls with hirsutism and/or virilization (Chapter 17). These steroids may provide sufficient negative feedback in the hypothalamus and pituitary to inhibit gonadotropin secretion and delay puberty and the onset of menses (80). Hirsutism and virilization may be seen in some intersex disorders associated with abnormalities of müllerian development including true hermaphroditism. Elevation of 17-hydroxyprogesterone and androstenedione as well as testosterone will be seen in congenital virilizing adrenal hyperplasia due to 21-hydroxylase or 11-hydroxylase deficiency severe enough to delay adolescent

development while producing virilization. Abnormal values can be suppressed by treatment with dexamethasone. Adrenal and ovarian tumors may also serve as a source of androgen secretion. In the absence of an enzyme disorder, a careful investigation of the adrenals and ovaries by imaging studies is warranted to determine the source of the excess androgen secretion. Polycystic ovarian syndrome may also cause primary amenorrhea if the disorder is severe. This disorder is more often associated with secondary amenorrhea and is discussed later.

5. Management

Rational therapy of primary amenorrhea relies on identification of the underlying disorder. While girls with constitutional delay of growth and adolescence can be treated with reassurance, those with functional hypogonadotropic hypogonadism require elimination of the underlying cause such as dieting, stress, or excessive exercise. Those individuals with congenital or acquired hypogonadism resulting in insufficient estradiol production, whether the disorder stems from dysfunction of the hypothalamus, pituitary, or ovary, will need estrogen replacement. Conjugated estrogen in doses of 0.3 mg daily or ethinyl estradiol at doses of 5–20 µg daily given orally can be used to induce pubertal development. Development should be observed within 6 months of onset of therapy (81). The replacement therapy can be increased as necessary to achieve sexual maturation over 1–2 years. Once adequate sexual development has been achieved, cycling to achieve monthly shedding of the endometrium should be begun. Estrogens are given on days 1–21 of the cycle and a progestin such as 5 mg of medroxyprogesterone acetate is given on days 15–21 of each month. Following a 7–10-day withdrawal period when no hormones are given, the cycle is then reinstituted the following month. Some girls prefer taking a fixed combination low-dose oral contraceptives such as Lo-Ovral to maintain their sexual development. Fertility issues may be addressed as each girl or family desires. Girls with hypogonadotropic hypogonadism may be counseled that ovulation can be induced by pulsed administration of GnRH (82). For those girls with primary ovarian failure, adoption has served as the main means of acquiring a child. With the advancement of reproductive technologies, it may be possible to conceive using a donor cycle and in vitro fertilization techniques with proper hormonal replacement.

B. Secondary Amenorrhea

Menses may be irregular in the years following the first episode of vaginal bleeding. Intervals of 12 months during the first year after onset of menses and 6 months in the second postmenarchal year may occur normally (38,83,84). Secondary amenorrhea is defined as the cessation of menses for at least 6 months during the third postmenarchal year. Many of the causes of primary amenorrhea are also causes of secondary amenorrhea. The most common causes in adolescence are stress, excessive exercise, dieting, which may be strenuous or to the extreme of anorexia nervosa, pregnancy, and polycystic ovarian disease. Central nervous system pathology, ovarian or adrenal tumors, and ovarian failure may also occur after the onset of menses, resulting in secondary amenorrhea.

Disorders that increase plasma androgen concentrations may produce primary amenorrhea but more often are associated with postpubertal development of virilization and secondary amenorrhea. These disorders include polycystic ovary syndrome, late-onset congenital adrenal hyperplasia, hyperprolactinemia, and acromegaly, or they may be idiopathic (85). Polycystic ovary syndrome is the most common of these disorders. Its cause is poorly understood, but there appears to be functional ovarian production of excess androgen in association with a relative increase in plasma LH and a decrease in plasma FSH (86). Polycystic ovary syndrome is strikingly associated with obesity, insulin resistance, and glucose intolerance (87,88). Reduction of plasma insulin concentration decreases serum testosterone in women with obesity and polycystic ovary syndrome, suggesting a causal role for insulin in producing hyperandrogenism (89).

Hyperprolactinemia produces both primary and secondary amenorrhea that is often associated with galactorrhea (90). Some girls may develop hyperandrogenism with a clinical picture similar to those with polycystic ovary syndrome and chronic anovulation, although hyperprolactinemia may also cause irregular menses with cycles. Hyperprolactinemia may result from prolactinomas or other hypothalamic or pituitary tumors, acromegaly, and hypercortisolism, or from hypothalamic dysfunction. Treatment involves removal of the underlying cause, surgery, or bromocriptine for microadenomas.

1. Evaluation

Since many teens are sexually active, pregnancy must be excluded by sensitive history taking or by laboratory determination. A careful history obtained after rapport is established with the patient will help define the amount of exercise and stress and nutritional status. Symptoms of chronic illness, endocrine disorders, and neurological disorders should be elucidated. During the physical examination, the degree of breast and pubic hair maturation and the presence of galactorrhea should be assessed. Inspection for evidence of virilization, including acne, hirsutism, and evidence of clitoromegaly, should be performed. A neurological examination including evaluation of visual fields should also be performed. A gynecological examination or a rectoabdominal examination is necessary to assess ovarian size and contour. Determination of plasma LH, FSH, and prolactin is often useful. Imaging studies of the head can be performed if neurological symptoms are present. If virilization is present, measurement of testosterone, free testosterone, dehydroepiandrosterone-sulfate (DHEA-S), or adrenal androgens may be needed. Ovarian ultrasonography may be warranted if polycystic ovarian disorder or an ovarian tumor is suspected. Additional studies as dictated by the history and physical examination may be performed.

2. Management

Treatment of secondary amenorrhea, like treatment of primary amenorrhea, is directed by the underlying cause. For secondary amenorrhea resulting from stress, exercise, or dieting, a change in life-style is required. This may, in many cases, require referral to a mental health professional. The advisability of estrogen treatment is controversial for those unable to modify their life-styles or stress levels. Estrogen therapy will further suppress the hypothalamic-pituitary axis, and it is not known whether the institution of estrogen therapy will predispose to future menstrual disorders. The absence of adequate estrogen in young women may predispose to development of postmenopausal osteoporosis (91,92), although a cause-effect relationship has not been definitely proven. If the association between estrogen and preservation of bone mass is proven, then estrogen therapy may prove to have benefits in those with chronic anovulation and hypogonadism. If estrogen therapy is instituted, periodic treatment with a progestin to allow withdrawal bleeding, as described for primary amenorrhea, will be required.

3. Treatment

Treatment of secondary amenorrhea due to polycystic ovarian disease is symptomatic. Weight reduction is to be encouraged in girls with obesity. This may reduce androgen concentrations and allow menses. The main goal of therapy, however, is to prevent the progression of hirsutism. Once excessive hair growth has occurred, it will not regress. Hair then must be shaved or bleached and may be permanently removed by electrolysis. Prevention of further hair growth and development of male-pattern baldness can be accomplished by treatment with combination estrogen-progestin treatment. Combination pills employing progestins with minimal androgen side effects should be selected. Obese patients require relatively more estrogen (1/50 formulation) than nonobese girls to prevent breakthrough bleeding. Estrogen therapy decreases free testosterone concentrations by reducing gonadotropin secretion, thereby decreasing ovarian stimulation, by increasing sex hormone-binding globulin. There may also be a modest reduction in production of DHEAS (85). If estrogen-progestin combination pills are not tolerated, long-acting agonist analogs of GnRH may be employed to reduce gonadotropin secretion (93). Long-term therapy with GnRH agonist analogs may suppress plasma sex steroids to an extent where bone mineralization and osteoporosis become a concern. Spironolactone, which interferes with androgen receptor-binding target sites such as the hair follicle, may also serve as an alternative therapy for hirsutism (94). High doses of 50–100 mg given twice daily are required, and side effects such as hyperkalemia and hypotension may limit their use.

Treatment of anovulation not associated with polycystic ovarian disease may be accomplished with periodic oral progestin therapy in the girl with adequate estrogen. A 5-day oral course of 10 mg medroxyprogesterone acetate or 5 mg Norlutin daily can serve as a test of adequate estrogen exposure. Following withdrawal of the progestin, an episode of menses should occur if estrogen has allowed an adequate endometrium to develop. Treatment for 5 days every other month for 6 months is often sufficient to establish a normal cycle.

C. Oligomenorrhea

Oligomenorrhea is defined as menstrual bleeding that occurs at intervals of more than 6 weeks but less than 1 year. Since anovulatory cycles occur commonly during the first 2 years after menarche, oligomenorrhea is often observed in adolescent girls (95). This is related to either an inadequate LH surge during each cycle or insufficient progesterone secretion in the corpus luteum to allow a normal withdrawal bleed at the termination of the cycle. Since the problem is self-limited as the hypothalamic-pituitary axis matures, reassurance is usually sufficient. Continued oligomenorrhea more than 2 years after menarche requires an investigation as outlined for secondary amenorrhea.

D. Abnormal Bleeding

The duration of menstrual flow is normally 4–6 days with the loss of 25–60 ml of blood (96). Bleeding that exceeds this amount is excessive. The most common cause for abnormal bleeding is dysfunctional uterine bleeding that is not attributable to genital tract pathology and is related to anovulatory cycles (97). The diagnosis of dysfunctional uterine bleeding is made by exclusion (98). In girls who are sexually active, pregnancy must be considered. Threatened, incomplete, or spontaneous abortion, ectopic pregnancy, and molar pregnancy may all be associated with abnormal bleeding. Blood-clotting abnormalities, particularly von Willebrand's disease, idiopathic thrombocytopenic purpura, and leukemia, must also be considered. Rarely, an intrauterine myoma or polyp or tumors of the vagina or cervix may also cause bleeding. Patients with infections of the genitourinary tract or who have trauma or vaginal foreign bodies may also experience abnormal bleeding.

1. Evaluation

The absence of cramping and symptoms of bloating and breast tenderness with bleeding suggest that ovulation has not occurred and point to a diagnosis of anovulatory dysfunctional uterine bleeding. A blood count and clotting studies should be performed to determine whether a blood dyscrasia is present and whether anemia has occurred from the blood loss. An hCG level should be obtained to exclude pregnancy as a cause.

2. Management

Most anovulatory bleeding in adolescents is self-limited. Should anemia be present, an iron supplement can be provided. If the episodes are severe, the bleeding can be terminated by administration of combination estrogen-progestin pills given 3–4 times daily until the bleeding stops, and then daily for 21 days followed by withdrawal, which will be followed by a heavy episode of menstrual bleeding (99). Alternatively, 2.5 mg Premarin may be given every 6 h until the bleeding stops. Then 2.5 mg of Premarin can be given daily in combination with 20 mg of medroxyprogesterone acetate for 5 days. A withdrawal bleed will occur following the termination of hormone therapy. Continued monthly cycles with combination pills or 1.25 mg Premarin on days 1–21 of the cycle and a progestin on days 15–21 of the cycle may be needed for several months until the hypothalamic-pituitary axis matures sufficiently to support regular menses. An iron supplement can be given to replete diminished iron stores. Severe bleeding associated with profound anemia and orthostatic hypotension may occur. This bleeding requires hospitalization and blood transfusion. Estrogen-progestin combination pills can be given orally every 6 h until the bleeding ceases or Premarin can be given IV at a dose of 25 mg every 6 hr. This should be followed with 10 mg of medroxyprogesterone acetate daily for 5 days and then a withdrawal bleed. Dilatation and curettage is usually not needed in an adolescent. Adolescents with severe episodes of dysfunctional uterine bleeding often have abnormal function of the hypothalamic-pituitary-gonadal axis. They may need indefinite follow-up and should be warned that menstrual problems and infertility may occur in the future (100).

E. Dysmenorrhea

Essential dysmenorrhea is menstrual pain not associated with recognized pelvic pathology. It is the most common of all gynecological disorders. About 50% of all adolescent girls experience dysmenorrhea and 10% cannot attend classes regularly (101). Other causes of dysmenorrhea should be excluded, including pain from endometriosis, endometrial polyps, adenomyosis, submucous or intramural fibroids, cervical stenosis, or pelvic inflammatory disease. Intractable pelvic pain and dysmenorrhea in adolescents is most often associated with endometriosis (102). Uterine hypoplasia and retroflexion are not associated with pain (103).

Essential dysmenorrhea is associated with ovulatory cycles. The painful cramps are associated with uterine contractions. The pain is sharp and colicky with localization to the suprapubic area and may radiate to the back and thighs. Gastrointestinal symptoms of nausea, vomiting, and diarrhea, palpitations, flushing, dizziness, and headache are associated with dysmenorrhea. Since similar symptoms occur after administration of prostaglandins, these substances have been implicated as the cause of essential dysmenorrhea. Menstrual sloughing releases lyzosomal enzymes, which then release phospholipids from cell membranes. The release of phospholipids results in increased local prostaglandin synthesis, which in turn causes myometrial contractions, vasoconstriction, ischemia, and pain (104,105). Progesterone, produced during ovulatory cycles, increases the synthesis of the prostaglandins (106). Girls with anovulatory cycles have lower prostaglandin levels and essentially no dysmenorrhea (101, 106).

Girls with dysmenorrhea have been treated with a multitude of simple, but generally ineffective, measures, including genital hygiene, exercise, heat, vitamins, and psychotherapy. A more rational approach to therapy is based on the recognition that prostaglandins are likely to play a pivotal role in the pathogenesis of dysmenorrhea. These girls benefit from treatment with inhibitors of prostaglandin synthetase as shown in Table 2 (101). Medication should be started at the time of

Table 2 Doses of Oral Prostaglandin Synthetase Inhibitors for Dysmenorrhea

Drug	Dose	Relief (%)	Side effects
Ibuprofen	400 mg q4–6 hr	80	Gastrointestinal
Naproxen	500 mg, then 250 q6–8hr	100	Gastrointestinal
Indomethacin	25–50 mg q3–4hr	63–100%	Headache
Mefenamic acid	500 mg q3–4hr	89	Gastrointestinal
Meclofenamate	100 mg q8hr	90	Gastrointestinal

Source: Adapted from Ref. 101.

the appearance of menstrual flow. Teens should be reassured that their menses are normal. Those girls with severe pain related to endometriosis may achieve relief with oral contraceptives, danazol, or GnRH agonists (107).

F. Premenstrual Syndrome

The premenstrual syndrome is a complex disorder that occurs in a cyclical pattern with onset of symptoms preceding the onset of menses. A prerequisite for the diagnosis is the absence of symptoms during the follicular phase of the cycle (108). Many women experience symptoms of breast tenderness, abdominal bloating, constipation, edema, fatigue, food cravings, and mood swings prior to the onset of menses, but in premenstrual syndrome, these symptoms are heightened, resulting in anxiety, restlessness, and irritability that may interfere with daily life activities in as many as 5–10% of women (109,110). The incidence in adolescence is not clear, but 89% of girls in one survey reported at least one severe symptom (111).

The criteria for establishing a diagnosis of premenstrual syndrome have been controversial. There are legal, social, and political ramifications of recognition of this disorder. It is difficult to separate those who have another psychiatric disorder from those with premenstrual syndrome, so strict diagnostic criteria must be used (112). Because of the difficulty in establishing diagnostic criteria, the underlying basis for the disorder has yet to be elucidated. The fact that the disorder remits after surgical hysterectomy and oophorectomy (113) or medical oophorectomy (114) provides evidence that there is a premenstrual disorder that is separate from depressive or other known psychiatric illness. Current hypotheses for the pathogenesis of the disorder include psychosomatic influences, endogenous opioid withdrawal, and serotonin dysfunction (115–117).

Therapy for the disorder includes treatment with progesterone and vitamin B_6, although there is no evidence that this therapy is effective (108). Remarkable improvement in symptoms can be achieved by performing a medical oophorectomy using GnRH agonist therapy (114). Estrogen and progestins have been provided to prevent bone loss without redevelopment of symptoms (117). Further research is required, how-

ever, to characterize this disorder and determine appropriate treatment strategies.

IV. SUMMARY

A thorough understanding of the events and hormonal changes that accompany puberty can be successfully utilized to diagnose adolescent menstrual disorders. It is important to recognize the normal maturational events that take place within the hypothalamic-pituitary axis and within the ovary, to design rational therapy for adolescent disorders. An understanding of the timing of development of negative and positive feedback control of estradiol on hypothalamic-pituitary function can guide the timing of interventions. Extensive research has shown the prudence of reassurance and nonintervention in some disorders while dictating rational therapy in others, such as use of prostaglandins to treat dysmenorrhea. Continued efforts to better understand the pathogenesis of many adolescent disorders, such as polycystic ovary syndrome and premenstrual syndrome, will continue to be needed to advance the health and well-being of adolescent girls.

REFERENCES

1. Wu FC, Butler GE, Kelnar CJ, Stirling HF, Huhtaniemi I. Patterns of pulsatile luteinizing hormone and follicle-stimulating hormone secretion in prepubertal (midchildhood) boys and girls and patients with idiopathic hypogonadotropic hypogonadism (Kallmann's syndrome): a study using an ultrasensitive time-resolved immunofluorometric assay. J Clin Endocrinol Metab 1991; 72:1229–1237.
2. Kletter GB, Padmanabhan V, Foster CM, et al. Luteinizing hormone pulse characteristics in early pubertal boys are the same whether measured by radioimmuno- or immunofluorometric assay. J Clin Endocrinol Metab 1991; 72:1229–1237.
3. Ying SY. Inhibins, activins, and follistatins: gonadal proteins modulating the secretion of follicle-stimulating hormone. Endocr Rev 1988; 9:267–293.
4. Risbriger GP, Robertson DM, de Kretser DM. Current perspectives of inhibin biology. Acta Endocrinol (Copenh) 1990; 122:673–682.
5. Mather JP, Woodruff TK, Krummen LA. Paracrine regulation of reproductive function by inhibin and activin. Proc Soc Exp Biol Med 1992; 201:1–15.
6. Meriggiola MC, Dahl KD, Mather JP, Bremmer WJ. Follistatin decreases activin-stimulated FSH secretion with no effect on GnRH-stimulated FSH secretion in prepubertal male monkeys. Endocrinology 1994; 134:1967–1970.
7. Gillman J. The development of the gonads in man, with a consideration of the whole fetal endocrines and the histogenesis of ovarian tumors. Contrib Embryol Carnegie Inst Wash 1948; 32:67–80.
8. Wartenberg H. Development of the early human ovary and the role of the menophrose in the differentiation of the cortex. Anat Embryol 1982; 165:253–280.
9. Carr BR. Disorders of the ovary and female reproductive tract. In: Wilson JD, Foster DW, eds. Williams Textbook of Endocrinology. Philadelphia: WB Saunders. 1992:733–798.
10. Faiman C, Winter JSD, Reyes FI. Patterns of gonadotropins and gonadal steroids throughout life. Clin Obstet Gynecol 1976; 3:467–483.

11. Kaplan SL, Grumbach MM, Aubert ML. The ontogenesis of pituitary hormones and hypothalamic factors in the human fetus: maturation of the central nervous system regulation of anterior pituitary function. Recent Prog Horm Res 1976; 32:161–243.

12. Plant TM. Pulsatile luteinizing hormone secretion in the neonatal male rhesus monkey (Macaca mulatta). J Endocrinol 1982; 93:71–74.

13. Waldhauser F, Weissenbacher G, Frisch H, Pollak A. Pulsatile secretion of gonadotropins in early infancy. Eur J Pediatr 1981; 137:71–74.

14. Marshall JC, Kelch RP. Gonadotropin-releasing hormone: role of pulsatile secretion in the regulation of reproduction. N Engl J Med 1986; 315:1459–1468.

15. Conte FA, Grumbach MM, Kaplan SL. A diphasic pattern of gonadotropin secretion in patients with the syndrome of gonadal dysgenesis. J Clin Endocrinol Metab 1975; 40:670–674.

16. Foster CM, Borondy M, Markovs ME, Hopwood NJ, Kletter GB, Beitins IZ. Growth hormone bioactivity in girls with Turner's syndrome: correlation with insulin-like growth factor I. Pediatr Res 1994; 35:218–222.

17. Mitsushima D, Hei DL, Terasawa E. Gamma-aminobutyric acid is an inhibitory neurotransmitter restricting the release of luteinizing hormone-releasing hormone before the onset of puberty. Proc Natl Acad Sci USA 1994; 91:395–399.

18. Penny R, Olambiwonnu NO, Frasier SD. Episodic fluctuations of serum gonadotropins in pre- and post-pubertal girls and boys. J Clin Endocrinol Metab 1977; 45:307–311.

19. Jakacki RI, Kelch RP, Sauder SE, Lloyd JS, Hopwood NJ, Marshall JC. Pulsatile secretion of luteinizing hormone in children. J Clin Endocrinol Metab 1982; 55:453–458.

20. Warren MP. The effects of exercise on pubertal progression and reproductive function in girls. J Clin Endocrinol Metab 1980; 51:1150–1157.

21. Frisch RE, McArthur JW. Menstrual cycles: fatness as a determinant of the minimum weight for height necessary for their maintenance or onset. Science 1974; 185:949–951.

22. Eisenstein TD, Gerson MJ. Psychosocial growth retardation in adolescence. A reversible condition secondary to severe stress. J Adolesc Health Care 1988; 9:436–440.

23. Lashansky G, Saenger P, Fishman K, et al. Normative data for adrenal steroidogenesis in a healthy pediatric population: age- and sex-steroid changes after adrenocorticotropin stimulation. J Clin Endocrinol Metab 1991; 73:674–686.

24. Cutler GB Jr, Loriaux DL. Andrenarche and its relationship to the onset of puberty. Fed Proc 1980; 39:2384–2390.

25. Heald FP. Juvenile obesity. In: Winick M, ed. Childhood Obesity III. New York: Wiley, 1975:81–88.

26. Oerter E, Uriarte M, Rose SR, Barnes KM, Cutler GB, Jr. Gonadotropin secretory dynamics during puberty in normal girls and boys. J Clin Endocrinol Metab 1990; 71:1251–1258.

27. Apter D, Cacciatore B, Alfthan H, Stenman H. Serum luteinizing hormone concentrations increase 100-fold in females from 7 years of age to adulthood, as measured by time-resolved immunofluorometric assay. J Clin Endocrinol Metab. 1989; 68:53–57.

28. Apter D, Butzow TL, Laughlin GA, Yen SSC. Gonadotropin-releasing hormone pulse generator activity during pubertal transition in girls: pulsatile and diurnal patterns of circulating gonadotropins. J Clin Endocrinol Metab 1993; 76:940–949.

29. Goji K. Twenty-four-hour concentration profiles of gonadotropin and estradiol (E2) in prepubertal and early pubertal girls: the diurnal rise of E2 is opposite the nocturnal rise of gonadotropin. J Clin Endocrinol Metab 1993; 77:1629–1635.

30. Grumbach MM. Onset of puberty. In: Berenberg SR, ed.

31. Grumbach MM, Styne DM. Puberty: Ontogeny, neuroendocrinology, physiology, and disorders. In: Wilson JD, Foster DW, eds. Williams Textbook of Endocrinology. Philadelphia: WB Saunders, 1992:1139–1221.

32. Marshall WA, Tanner JM. Variations in pattern of pubertal changes in girls. Arch Dis Child 1969; 44:291–303.

33. MacMahen B. Age at menarche. In: National Health Survey. DHEW Publication No. (HRA) 74-1615, Series II, No. 133 Washington, DC: Government Printing Office, 1973:1.

34. Fillcori M, Butler JP, Crowley WE. Neuroendocrine regulation of the corpus luteum in the human. J Clin Invest 1984; 73:1638–1647.

35. Liu JH, Yen SSC. Induction of midcycle gonadotropin surge by ovarian steroids in women: a critical evaluation. J Clin Endocrinol Metab 1983; 57:797–802.

36. Apter D, Raisanen I, Ylostalo P, et al. Follicular growth in relation to serum hormone patterns in adolescence compared with adult menstrual cycles. Fertil Steril 1987; 47:82–88.

37. Frasier IS, Michie EA, Wide L, et al. Pituitary gonadotropin and ovarian function in adolescent dysfunctional uterine bleeding. J Clin Endocrinol Metab 1973; 37:407–414.

38. Apter D, Vihko R. Serum pregnenolene, progesterone. 17-hydroxyprogesterone, testosterone, and 5α-dihydro-testosterone during female puberty. J Clin Endocrinol Metab 1977; 45:1039–1048.

39. Capraro VJ, Greenbarg H. Adhesions of the labia minora. A study of 50 patients. Obstet Gynecol 1972; 39:65–69.

40. Soules MR. Adolescent amenorrhea. Pediatr Clin North Am 1987; 43:1083–1103.

41. Griffin JE, Wilson JD. The syndromes of androgen resistance. N Engl J Med 1980; 302:198–209.

42. Madden JD, Walsh PC, MacDonald PC, et al. Clinical and endocrinologic characterization of a patient with the syndrome of incomplete testicular feminization. J Clin Endocrinol Metab 1973; 41:751–760.

43. Rosenfeld RG, Grumbach MM, eds. Turner Syndrome. New York: Marcel Dekker, 1990:1–512.

44. Levinson G, Zarate A, Guzman-Toledano R, et al. An XX female with sexual infantilism, absent gonads, and lack of müllerian ducts. J Med Genet 1976; 13:68–69.

45. Simpson JL. Gonadal dysgenesis and abnormalities of the human sex chromosomes: current status of phenotypic-karyotypic correlations. Birth Defects 1975; 11:23–59.

46. McDonough PG. Molecular biology in reproductive endocrinology. In: Yen SSC, Jaffe RB, eds. Reproductive Endocrinology. Philadelphia: WB Saunders, 1991:25–64.

47. Aurbach GD, Marx SJ, Spiegel AM. Parathyroid hormone, calcitenia, and the calciferols. In: Wilson JD, Foster DW, eds. Williams Textbook of Endocrinology. Philadelphia: WB Saunders, 1992:1397–1517.

48. Evers JLH, Rolland R. The gonadotropin resistant ovary syndrome: a curable disease? Clin Endocrinol 1981; 14:99–103.

49. Lucky AW, Rebar RW, Blizzard RM, et al. Pubertal progression in the presence of elevated serum gonadotropins in girls with multiple endocrine deficiencies. J Clin Endocrinol Metab 1977; 45:673–678.

50. Fotsiou F, Botta ZZO GF, Doniach D. Immunofluorscence studies on auto-antibodies to steroid producing cells, and to the germline cells in endocrine disease and infertility. Clin Exp Immunol 1980; 39:97–111.

51. Barrett A, Nicholls J, Gibson B. Late effects of total body irradiation. Radiother Oncol 1987; 9:131–135.

52. Perrone L, Sinisi AA, Sicuranza R, et al. Prepubertal endo-

crine followup in subjects with Wilms' tumor. Med Pediatr Oncol 1988; 16:255–258.

53. Nicosia SV, Matus Ridley M, Meadows AT. Gonadal effects of cancer therapy in girls. Cancer 1985; 55:2364–2372.

54. Kaufman FR, Kogut MD, Donnell GN, et al. Hypergonadotropic hypogonadism in female patients with galactosemia. N Engl J Med 1981; 304:994–998.

55. Prader A. Delayed adolescence. Clin Endocrinol Metab 1975; 4:143–155.

56. Furlannetto RW, Underwood LE, Van Wyk JJ, D'Ercole AJ. Estimation of somatomedin-C levels in normals and patients with pituitary disease by radioimmunoassay. J Clin Invest 1977; 60:648–657.

57. White RM, Nissley SP, Moses AC, Rechler MM, Johnsonbaugh RE. The growth hormone dependence of a somatomedin-binding protein in human serum. J Clin Endocrinol Metab 1981; 53:49–57.

58. Lanes R, Hurtado E. Oral clonidine—an effective growth hormone-releasing agent in prepubertal subjects. J Pediatr 1982; 100:710–714.

59. Raiti S, Davis WT, Blizzard RM. A comparison of the effects of insulin hypoglycemia and arginine infusion of release of human growth hormone. Lancet 1967; 1:321–323.

60. Foster CM, Hopwood NJ, Beitins IZ, et al. Evaluation of gonadotropin responses to synthetic gonadotropin-releasing hormone in girls with idiopathic hypopituitarism. J Pediatr 1992; 121:528–532.

61. Adashi EY, Resnick CE, D'Ercole AJ, et al. Insulin-like growth factors as intra ovarian regulators of granulosa cell growth and function. Endocr Rev 1985; 6:400–420.

62. El-Roeiy A, Chen X, Roberts VJ, et al. Expression of insulin-like growth factor-I (IGF-I) and IGF-II and the IGF-I, IGF-II, and insulin receptor genes and localization of the gene products in the human ovary. J Clin Endocrinol Metab 1993; 77:1411–1418.

63. Yeshimura Y, Iwahita M, Karube M, et al. Growth hormone stimulates follicular development by stimulation of ovarian production of insulin-like growth factor-I. Endocrinology 1994; 135:887–894.

64. Van Dop C, Burstein S, Conte FA, et al. Isolated gonadotropin deficiency in boys: clinical characteristics and growth. J Pediatr 1987; 111:684–692.

65. Job JC, Chaussain JL, Toublanc JE. Delayed puberty. In: Grumbach MM, Sizonenke PC, Aubert ML, eds. Control of the Onset of Puberty. Baltimore: Williams & Wilkins, 1990: 588–619.

66. Petito CK, DeGirolami U, Earle KM. Craniopharyngiomas, a clinical and pathological review. Cancer 1976; 37:1944–1952.

67. Banna M. Carniopharyngioma in children. J Pediatr 1973; 83:781–785.

68. Gold PW, Goodwin FK, Chrousos GP. Clinical and biochemical manifestations of depression. Relation to the neurobiology of stress. N Engl J Med 1988; 319:413–420.

69. Pugliese MT, Lifshitz F, Grad G. Fear of obesity. A cause of short stature and delayed puberty. N Engl J Med 1983; 309:513–518.

70. Biller MK, Federoff MJ, Koenig JL, et al. Abnormal cortisol secretion and responses to corticotropin-releasing hormone in women with hypothalamic amenorrhea. J Clin Endocrinol Metab 1990; 70:311–317.

71. Nelson MA, Dyment PG, Goldberg B, et al. Amenorrhea in adolescent athletics. Pediatrics 1989; 84:394.

72. Rosenfield RL. Puberty and its disorders in girls. Endocrinol Metab Clin North Am 1991; 20:15–42.

73. Burrow GN. The thyroid gland and reproduction. In: Yen SSC, Jaffe RB, eds. Reproductive Endocrinology. Philadelphia: WB Saunders, 1991:555–575.

74. Styne DM, Grumbach MM, Kaplan SL, et al. Treatment of Cushing disease in childhood and adolescence by transphenoidal microadenomectomy. N Engl J Med 1984; 310:889–893.

75. Ibrahim II, Sakr R, Ghaly IM, et al. Endocrine profiles in pediatric andrology. II. Insulin-dependent diabetic adolescents. Arch Androl 1983; 11:45–51.

76. Wise JE, Kolb EL, Sauder SE. Effect of glycemic control on growth velocity in children with IDDM. Diabetes Care 1992; 15:826–830.

77. Cassidy SB, Ledbetter DH. Prader-Willi syndrome. Neurol Clin 1989; 7:37–54.

78. Ledbetter DH, Mascarello JT, Riccardi VM. Chromosome 15 abnormalities and the Prader-Willi syndrome: a follow-up report of 40 cases. Am J Hum Genet 1982; 34:278–285.

79. Reinfrank RF, Nichols FL. Hypogonadotropic hypogonadism in the Laurence-Moon syndrome. J Clin Encrinol Metab 1964; 24:48–53.

80. Sultan C, Medlej IZ, Chevalier C, Lobaccaro JM. Management of the hyperandrogenism in adolescent girls. Horm Res 1991; 36:160–164.

81. Rosenfield RL. Diagnosis and management of delayed puberty. J Clin Endocrinol Metab 1990; 70:559–562.

82. Schoemaker J, Vankessel H, Simmons AH, et al. Induction of first cycles in primary hypothalamic amenorrhea with pulsatile luteinizing hormone-releasing hormone: a mirror of female pubertal development. Fertil Steril 1987; 48:204–212.

83. Metcalf MG, Mackenzie JA. Incidence of ovulation in young women. J Biosoc Sci 1980; 12:345–352.

84. Lemarchand-Beraud T, Zufferey MM, Reymond M. Maturation of the hypothalamic-pituitary ovarian axis in adolescent girls. J Clin Endocrinol Metab 1982; 54:241–246.

85. Ehrmann DA, Rosenfield RL. An endocrinologic approach to hirsutism. J Clin Endocrinol Metab 1990; 71:1–4.

86. Judd HL, McPherson RA, Rakoff JS, Yen SSC. Correlation of the effects of dexamethasone administration on urinary 17-ketosteroid and serum androgen levels in patients with hirsutism. Am J Obstet Gynecol 1977; 128:408–417.

87. Burghen GA, Givens JR, Kitabchi AE. Correlation of hyperandrogenism with hyperinsulinism in polycystic ovarian disease. J Clin Endocrinol Metab 1980; 50:113–116.

88. Dunaif A, Segal KR, Futterweit W, Dobrjansky A. Profound peripheral insulin resistance, independent of obesity, in polycystic ovary syndrome. Diabetes 1989; 38:1165–1174.

89. Nestler JE, Barlascini CO, Matt DW, et al. Suppression of serum insulin by diazoxide reduces serum testosterone levels in obese women with polycystic ovary syndrome. J Clin Endocrinol Metab 1989; 68:1027–1032.

90. Howlett TA, Wass JAH, Grossman A, et al. Prolactinomas presenting as primary amenorrhoea and delayed or arrested puberty: response to medical therapy. Clin Endocrinol 1989; 30:131–140.

91. Kritz-Silverstein D, Barrett-Connor E. Early menopause, number of reproductive years, and bone mineral density in postmenopausal women. Am J Public Health 1993; 83:983–988.

92. Young N, Formica C, Szmkler G, Seeman E. Bone density at weight-bearing and nonweight-bearing sites in ballet dancers: the effects of exercise, hypogonadism, and body weight. J Clin Endocrinol Metab 1994; 78:449–454.

93. Friedman AJ, Barbieri RL. Leuprolide acetate: applications in gynecology. Curr Probl Obstet Gynecol Surv 1989; 44(Suppl): 326–329.

94. Corvol P, Michaud A, Menard J, et al. Antiandrogenic effect

of spironolactones: mechanisms of action. Endrocrinology 1975; 97:52–58.

95. Wentz AC. Oligomenorrhea and secondary amenorrhea in the adolescent. Med Clin North Am 1975; 59:1385–1394.

96. Halberg L, Hogdahl AM, Nilsson L, et al. Menstrual blood loss—a population study: variations at different ages and attempts to define normality. Acta Obstet Gynecol Scand 1966; 45:320–351.

97. Bettendorf G, Leidenberger F. Amenorrhea and dysfunctional uterine bleeding in puberty. Clin Endocrinol Metab 1975; 4:89–106.

98. Hertweck SP. Dysfunctional uterine bleeding. Obstet Gynecol Clin North Am 1992; 19:129–148.

99. Beitins IZ. Menstrual abnormalities during adolescence. Primary Care 1981; 8:3–18.

100. Southam AL, Richart RM. The prognosis for adolescents with menstrual abnormalities. Am J Obstet Gynecol 1966; 94:637.

101. Ylikorkala O, Dawood MY. New concepts in dysmenorrhea. Am J Obstet Gynecol 1978; 130:833.

102. Goldstein DT, DeCholnoky C, Emans SJ. Adolescent endometriosis. J Adolesc Health Care 1980; 1:37–41.

103. Abraham GH. Primary dysmenorrhea. Clin Obstet Gynecol 1978; 21:139.

104. Neinstein LS. Menstrual problems in adolescents. Med Clin North Am 1990: 74:1181–1203.

105. Russell PT, Owens OM. Dysmenorrhea and other menstrual disorders. In: Bygdemam M, et al., eds. Prostoglandins and Their Inhibitors in Clinical Obstetrics and Gynecology. Norwell, MA: Kluwer Academic, 1986:315.

106. Dawood MY. Nonsteroidal anti-inflammatory drugs and changing attitudes toward dysmenorrhea. Am J Med 1988; 84(Suppl 51):23–29.

107. Strauss JF, Gurpide E. The endometrium: regulation and dysfunction. In: Yen SSC, Jaffe RB, eds. Reproductive Endocrinology. Philadelphia: WB Saunders, 1991:309–356.

108. Reid RL. Premenstrual syndrome. Am Assoc Clin Chem 1987; 5:1.

109. Chakmakjian ZH. A critical assessment of therapy for the premenstrual tension syndrome. J Reprod Med 1983; 28:532–538.

110. Robinson GE. Premenstrual syndrome: current knowledge and management. Can Med Assoc J 1989; 140:605–611.

111. Fisher M, Trieller K, Napolitano B. Premenstrual syndrome in adolescents. J Adolesc Health Care 1989; 10:369–375.

112. Mortola JF, Girton L, Beck L, Yen SSC. Depressive episodes in premenstrual syndromes. Am J Obstet Gynecol 1989; 161:1682–1687.

113. Casper RF, Hearn MT. The effect of hysterectomy and bilateral oophorectomy in women with severe premenstrual syndrome. Am J Obstet Gynecol 1990; 162:105–109.

114. Muse KN, Celel NS, Futtermen LA, Yen SSC. N Engl J Med 1984; 311:1345–1349.

115. Walker JM, Khachaturian H, Watson SJ. Some anatomical and physiological interactions among noradrenergic systems and opioid peptides. Front Clin Neurosci 1984; 2:74.

116. Fachinetti F, Martignoni E, Petraglia F, Sances MG, Nappi G, Genazzani AR. Premenstrual fall of plasma β-endorphin in patients with premenstrual syndrome. Fertil Steril 1987; 47:570.

117. Rapkin AJ, Edelmuth E, Chang LC, Reading AE, McGuire MT, Su T-P. Whole-blood serotonin in premenstrual syndrome. Obstet Gynecol 1987; 70:533.

118. Mortola JF, Girton L, Fischer U. Successful treatment of severe premenstrual syndrome by combined use of GnRH-agonist and estrogen/progestin. J Clin Endocrinol Metab 1991; 72:252A-252F.

17

Hirsutism and Polycystic Ovary Syndrome

Songya Pang

College of Medicine, University of Illinois,
Chicago, Illinois

I. INTRODUCTION

Skin and muscle are two major target tissues of androgens in postnatal life. Androgen excess symptoms in peripubertal and postpubertal females may thus include hirsutism, acne, and virilization or masculinization.

Hirsutism is clinically defined as excess body hair growth in women involving primarily areas of the face, chin, neck, midline chest and abdomen, upper and lower back, buttocks, and inner aspects of the thigh. In general, hirsutism by itself is a mild symptom of androgen overproduction or enhanced androgen metabolism in the skin tissue. Similarly, increased androgen activity in the sebaceous and apocrine glands may be associated with development of acne vulgaris. The androgen metabolic response of hair follicles and sebaceous glands of the skin do not behave identically and vary greatly between sites (1). This may be one of the reasons some adolescent girls and women develop only hirsutism, or acne, or both hirsutism and acne together as symptoms of androgen excess or enhanced androgen metabolic activity in the skin tissue.

Hypertrichosis is characterized by generalized increased fine body hair with no special preferential sites. This condition is generally not associated with androgen over-production. Either genetic or ethnic makeup in body hair growth may be a contributing factor in hypertrichosis. In some cases, however, hypertrichosis may be the early manifestation of mild androgen excess or may be induced by chronic ingestion of drugs that affect the metabolism of certain androgens.

Clinically, the more severe androgen excess symptoms involve both skin and muscle, as well as the reproductive system, and are termed virilization or masculinization. These include some or all of the following symptoms of hyperandrogenism: clitoral enlargement, masculine body habitus, temporal hair loss, voice changes, breast atrophy, and menstrual disorders (2). Virilization and masculinization are usually manifestations of significant pathology causing androgen overproduction in women. On the other hand, hirsutism may be defined as cutaneous virilism, as suggested by Shuster (3), and results from increased or normal androgen production in women who comprise a spectrum of clinical and biochemical features, frequently defying specific pathophysiologic classification. In addition, clinical expression of androgen excess symptoms does not always correlate with the degree of androgen production or circulating androgen levels. This suggests that androgen metabolic activity in the target tissue is in part governed by an as yet undefined and independent local mechanism that may play an important role in hirsutism.

Thus, this chapter discusses the physiology of androgen metabolism in women and disorders of androgen metabolism in regard to production, peripheral metabolism, and skin metabolic activity resulting in the manifestation of excess androgen symptoms in peripubertal and postpubertal females.

II. BIOACTIVITY OF ANDROGENS

"Androgenicity" is the term used to describe the bioactivity of a steroid that produces masculine characteristics. The bioactivity of androgens in a laboratory setup is measured either by determining an exogenous steroidal effect of a known quantity on the weight increase in the seminal vesicle or prostate of castrated male rats or mice or by measuring the growth of a cock's comb (4). The androgenicity determined by these methods provides its bioactivity only in relation to one end point.

Essentially all androgenic steroids are C_{19} steroid compounds, and the biopotency is dependent on the presence of a 17-oxygen function of a 17-hydroxyl group in its configuration (4). Naturally occurring C_{19} compounds that possess a 17-hydroxyl group are testosterone (T), 5α-dihydrotestosterone (DHT), and 5α-androstanediol (Fig. 1). T and DHT are almost equally biopotent androgens, based on the bioassay described earlier (Fig. 2) (5). 5α-Androstanediol is significantly less

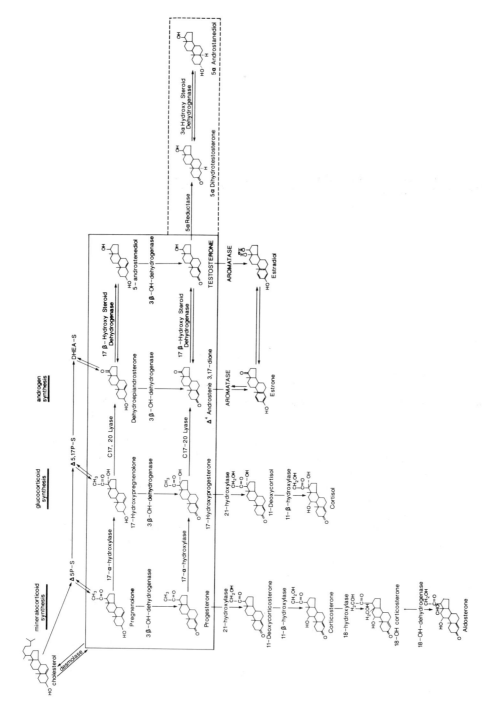

Figure 1 Steroid biosynthetic pathway. The pathway within the box occurs in both adrenal cortical and ovarian tissue. The pathway in the dotted box is intracellular metabolism.

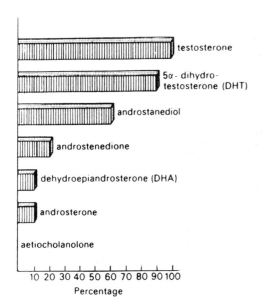

Figure 2 Androgen biopotency in relation to testosterone determined by bioassay. (Reproduced with permission of author and publisher, Sommerville IF, et al. In: Advances in Steroid Biochemistry and Pharmacology. New York: Academic Press, 1970:266.)

biopotent than T or DHT because it lacks a 3-oxo group in its configuration. T and DHT are the most important androgens, but other clinically significant androgens are androstenedione and dehydroepiandrosterone, which are 17-oxosteroids. These steroids by themselves have considerably reduced or smaller androgenic activity compared with T or DHT because of the lack of a 17-oxygen function and/or 3-oxo configuration (Fig. 2). Nevertheless, these weak androgens are important precursor steroids in androgen biosynthesis and bioaction. Other C_{19} steroids, such as 11β-hydroxyandrostenedione and androstenediol, circulate in the plasma of women. However, these steroids are clinically insignificant in androgenic activity because of their low concentration or lack of bioactivity (6).

III. ANDROGEN METABOLISM IN NORMAL WOMEN

Both adrenal cortical and ovarian tissue possess Δ^5 and Δ^4 steroidogenic pathways for androgen biosynthesis (Fig. 1). Thus the adrenal cortex and ovaries are important sources of androgens from an early peripubertal age. Androgens and other C_{19} steroids either are directly secreted by the glands or may arise by extraadrenal or extraovarian conversion of precursor steroids. The rate of androgen production generally influences the circulating levels of androgens.

A. Adrenal Androgen Secretion

A simplified schematic pathway for adrenal androgen biosynthesis is shown in Figure 1. Pregnenolone and progesterone

are metabolized to androgens through this pathway. The 17 side-chain cleavage of the 17α-hydroxypregnenolone (Δ5-17P) leads to the formation of dehydroepiandrosterone (DHEA). DHEA is converted to androstenedione (Δ4-A) by 3β-hydroxysteroid dehydrogenase activity, followed by an isomerase reaction, or can be converted to DHEA sulfate (DHEA-S) by sulfakinase activity. The major androgens secreted by the adrenals are DHEA, DHEA-S, and Δ4-A. The zona reticularis is very active in the 17 side-chain cleavage of Δ5-17P or 17α-hydroxyprogesterone (17-OHP) to form androgens. DHEA and DHEA-S are mainly the products of zona reticularis, Δ4-A and T are secreted by both zona reticularis and zona fasciculata (7–9). Under normal circumstances, smaller quantities of T and even smaller amounts of androstenediol are secreted by the adrenals (6). Secretion of all adrenal androgens gradually increases from midchildhood onward as the histologic development and hormonal biosynthesis of the zona reticularis mature. These then reach a plateau toward the late stages of pubertal maturation (10).

Corticoptropin (adrenocorticotropic hormone, ACTH) is the major trophic hormone for adrenal androgen biosynthesis and secretion (7). There are clinical situations, however, in which disparity in adrenal androgen and cortisol secretory patterns suggest the possibility for the existence of an additional trophic factor for adrenal androgen synthesis (11, 12). Despite descriptions of a pituitary substance other than ACTH capable of stimulating androgen secretion (13,14), the only pituitary substance that unequivocally regulates adrenal androgen secretion in human adrenal physiology remains ACTH. Under ACTH regulation, adrenal androgens are secreted synchronously with cortisol in both the episode of secretion and the circadian pattern (15,16). The circadian pattern of adrenal steroids in women is depicted in Figure 3. DHEA and Δ5-17P concentration are thus normally higher in early morning and decline gradually throughout the day (16). 17-OHP and Δ4-A concentrations in normal women also tend to be higher in the morning hours than thereafter because of the adrenal contribution (16). However, the circadian difference in 17-OHP levels is likely minimized during the luteal phase of the menstrual cycle, when ovarian 17-OHP production is increased. DHEA-S, on the other hand, shows very little circadian or episodic variation in plasma concentration because of the slow rate of clearance of the sulfate (16,17). Its plasma concentration is nearly 300–400 times greater than that of unconjugated DHEA because of high secretion by the adrenals and low clearance of this conjugate (16). DHEA, DHEA-S, and Δ4-A are further metabolized to etiocholanolone and androsterone. 11β-OH-androstenedione and a small amount of cortisol are metabolized to 11-oxy,17-oxysteroids. These metabolites of C_{19} steroids are generally excreted in the urine as 17-ketosteroids (17-oxosteroids).

The adrenal contribution of androgens in relation to overall androgen production and circulating concentration in women is depicted in Table 1 (18–24). Circulating DHEA and DHEA-S are directly from the adrenal secretion contribution. Approximately equal amounts of Δ4-A are secreted by the adrenals and ovaries from puberty onward. The androgens secreted by the adrenal cortex and ovaries undergo

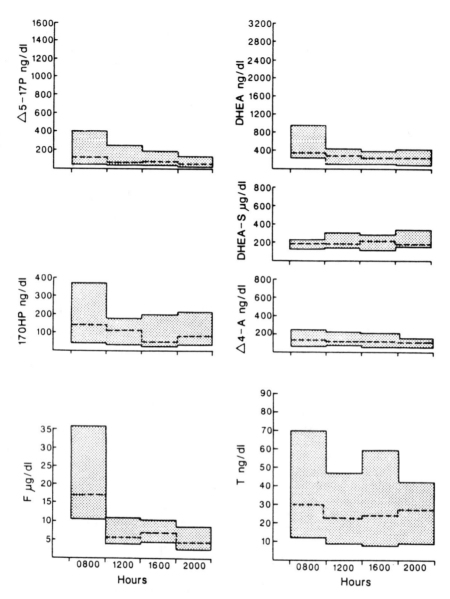

Figure 3 Circadian patterns of adrenal and gonadal steroids in normal women. (Modified from Pang S, et al. J Clin Endocrinol Metab 1985; 60:434.)

peripheral metabolism and contribute to the blood production rate of androgens. Under normal circumstances, the peripheral contribution to the blood production of DHEA, DHEA-S, and Δ4-A is small. The major source of T blood production in women is via peripheral conversion of Δ4-A (Table 1) (20,21). The blood production rate of Δ4-A is approximately 10–15 times that of T, and the rate of fraction of the blood Δ4-A pool conversion to the blood T pool is 5.6% (20,21). Therefore, approximately 60% of circulating T production is derived from the circulating Δ4-A. Consequently, the conditions associated with increased Δ4-A production simultaneously increase the blood production of T. With advancing age, from the fourth to sixth decades of life, adrenal androgen secretion normally declines (25,26) without significant

changes in cortisol. This event is independent of the menopausal event (27).

B. Ovarian Androgen Secretion

The principle sites of steroid synthesis in ovarian tissue are theca cells, the granulosa cells of the follicle, and the corpus luteum. The pathway involving the Δ5 and Δ4 steroid biosynthesis process in the ovarian cells is similar to that described for the adrenal cortex (Fig. 1). Ovarian androgen synthesis occurs mainly in the theca cells, stroma cells, and the corpus luteum under luteinizing hormone (LH) stimulation (28–30). The ovary further aromatizes the androgens to estrogen in the granulosa cell layers through follicle-stimulating hormone

Table 1 Contribution of C_{-19} Steroids in Normal Women by Adrenal and Ovarian Secretion and Peripheral Metabolism

	Gland	DHEA	DHEA-S	Δ4-A		T	
% Secretion	Adrenal	90	>99	40	−66	50	−66
	Ovary	10	<1	34	−60	34	−50
Secretion rate, mg/day	Adrenal + ovary	0.8– 8	5– 7.7	3	− 3.8	0.15– 0.35	
% Contribution in plasma concentration via production	Adrenal	67	90	36	−60	20	−26
	Peripheral[a]	25	10	<0.1		60	
	Ovary	8	0	30	−56	14	−20
Blood production rate, mg/day		6 −16	8–16	3.3– 3.4		0.23– 0.34	

[a]Extraadrenal and extragonadal source.

Source: Data were derived from References 18–24.

(FSH) stimulation. Estrogens are thus largely produced by the granulosa cells, regulated by FSH and estrogen. Progesterone is secreted largely from the granulosa cells of the late follicular and midcycle phase and by the corpus luteum derived from granulosa cells (28,29).

The major androgens secreted by the ovaries are Δ4-A and T (Table 1). The amount of androgen secreted by the ovary is far greater than the amount of estrogens produced. The ovarian source of androgen also increases gradually with the onset of gonadarche. Following menarche, ovarian androgen secretion appears to alter throughout the cycle. The secretion of T and Δ4-A into the ovarian vein is at its highest when estrogens are being maximally secreted. The variable production of androgen by the ovary on the contribution in plasma is to some extent masked by the adrenal source of androgens and by interconversion that occurs after secretion (31). Peripheral concentrations of Δ4-A and T levels are generally higher at midcycle because of the ovarian contribution (32,33), although others reported higher Δ4-A and T levels in the luteal phase of normal women (34). The ovarian contribution of androgens to the overall blood production rate and circulating androgen concentration in plasma pool is shown in Table 1. In general, the amount of ovarian Δ4-A and T secretion is similar to that of adrenal secretion, thereby contributing equally to the blood production and concentration of these androgens. In the periovulatory phase, 65% of increased blood production rate of Δ4-A is contributed by the increased secretion of the ovarian source of Δ4-A (6). The ovaries contribute very little to DHEA production and none to DHEA-S. With menopause, ovarian Δ4-A production declines (35) and, with aging, probably diminishes overall androgen secretion by the ovary (8).

C. Bioactive Androgens in Blood

The circulating sex steroid hormones are in part present in a protein-bound form and in part in a free form unbound to protein (Table 2). The specific binding proteins with a high affinity for sex steroids, such as testosterone and estradiol, are called sex hormone binding globulin (SHBG). Recent evidence suggests that the biologically active T includes both the free and albumin-bound fraction; SHBG-bound androgens are not readily available for bioaction (36). Approximately 1% of the circulating T and DHT in normal females is unbound (Table 2) (37). This unbound T freely diffuses into the target cells to bind to receptor of the target cell. At puberty, the SHBG concentration falls slightly in girls but a greater drop in concentration is noted in boys (31). SHBG concentration is decreased by the androgens and is increased by estrogen (38). Estrogen, by its action in increasing the concentration of SHBG, decreases biologically active free fractions of androgens (31). Thus a hyperandrogenic state further causes availability of the free bioactive form of T. The increased availability of free T or DHT to the target cells by the decrease in SHBG in the presence of normal circulating T levels has been proposed as one of the pathogenic mechanisms of hirsutism in women (39). The binding of DHEA and Δ4-A to SHBG in circulation is negligible (40).

IV. PHYSIOLOGY OF HAIR GROWTH AND SKIN ANDROGEN METABOLISM

Hair growth on the face, neck, trunk, and extremities is generally androgen dependent. Pubic and axillary hair growth are also androgen dependent. Androgen stimulation in these androgen-dependent areas usually promotes terminal hair growth that is thick, long, and dark.

The life cycle of hair follicles consists of three distinct and yet transitional periods (Fig. 4) (41). Basically, the active proliferative growth phase of the hair is called anagen. During anagen, formation of the hair by proliferation and pigmentation of cells occurs from an epidermal matrix of the hair bulb. The transitional or regressing stage of the hair, catagen,

Table 2 Total Protein-Bound Testosterone and Free Testosterone Concentration in a Representative Normal Adult Man and Woman

	Total plasma T (%)	SHBG-bound T (%)*	Albumin-bound T (%)*	Free T (%)[a]
Male, ng/dl	810	486	307	22
	(100%)	(60%)	(38%)	(2%)
Female, ng/dl	49	39	9.3	0.7
	(100%)	(80%)	(19%)	(1%)

[a]Percentage of total T concentration.

Source: Data were derived from References 31 and 40.

begins at the termination of anagen, followed by a resting stage, telogen (41). Generally, in males, the duration of anagen for the moustache is 4 months, and for thigh hair it is 2 months. In females, the duration of anagen for thigh hair is less than 1 month (42). The length of the hair is influenced by the length of the anagen phase, which is by comparison more important than the rate of hair growth. The longer thigh hair in men is thus attributed to the longer anagen period. The telogen phase of facial hair is approximately 2–3 months. The growth cycle of the moustache is therefore 6–7 months or more at the very least and is more than 3 months for thigh hair (43). Duration of the hair cycle differs, therefore, depending on location.

Androgens most likely prolong the growth of hair by lengthening the duration of anagen, as evidenced by a reduction in the length of hair by antiandrogen treatment in hirsute women (44). Androgen-dependent hair growth is influenced not only by the amount of androgen delivered to the target cells but also by the target cell response to the androgen. In some instances, the peripheral target cell response may even be more important in the manifestation of androgen excess symptoms because no correlation has been found between the rate of hair growth and circulating total, protein-bound, or free T (45).

Androgen bioaction at the cellular level involves the uptake of prehormone or active hormone and conversion to DHT, which binds to a specific receptor protein and then transfers to the nucleus (Fig. 5) (46). All skin structures, including epidermis, sweat and sebaceous glands, hair follicles, and dermis, possess 5α-reductase activity and 3β-hydroxysteroid dehydrogenase-Δ^{4-5}-isomerase and 17β-, 3β-, and 3α-hydroxysteroid dehydrogenase activities (Fig. 5) (47). Human skin thus has the capacity not only to convert T to DHT but also to convert the precursor weak androgens DHEA to Δ^5-androstenediol or to Δ4-A, which in turn is converted to T and eventually to DHT. DHT is then further reduced to 3α-androstanediol (3α-adiol) and its glucuronide (gluc; Fig. 5). The measurement of circulating concentrations of DHT does not reflect the metabolic activities of androgens in peripheral tissue because only a fraction of this peripherally

formed androgen escapes into circulation: most of it is further metabolized in situ (Fig. 5) (48,49). Glucuronidation is one of the effective disposal mechanisms in skin tissue (50). 3α-Adiol and its gluc have been reported to be good markers of peripheral skin androgen activity in view of the evidence that (1) it is produced exclusively at the extrasplanchic tissue (50); (2) there is no evidence at the present time that these hormones are secreted directly in considerable amounts by the adrenals or gonads (50); and (3) muscle does not contain 5α- or 3α-reductase activity (51). Circulating concentrations of serum 3α-adiol and its gluc were reported to be increased in hirsute women (52–54). Studies from our laboratory indicate that serum 3α-adiol gluc levels were significantly correlated with the degree of hirsutism in women with excess adrenal androgen production and idiopathic causes but not in women with excess ovarian androgen production (Fig. 6) (55). No correlation was found, however, between precursor or circulating androgen levels and the hirsutism scores (Fig. 6) (55). In addition, 3α-adiol gluc levels in hirsute females correlated significantly with circulating DS and DHEA levels (55). These findings suggest that in women 3α-adiol gluc may be the marker of metabolic activity of largely weak adrenal androgens in the skin tissue.

The androgen receptor binding capacity of genital skin from hirsute and normal women showed no differences (56). On the other hand, 5α-reductase activity of homogenate or fibroblast from pubic skin in hirsute women, with or without apparent excess androgen production, was greatly increased (57). Furthermore, the amount of DHEA converted to T by the skin of hirsute women was nearly eight times greater than that of normal women (58). This suggests that the abnormally high conversion of androgens by skin plays a major roll in the production of hirsutism. Normal androgen metabolism was found in isolated hairs from women with idiopathic hirsutism, however, suggesting a fundamental defect in the regulation of hair growth as a pathogen of this disorder (59). Additional studies by other investigators nevertheless support the concept that idiopathic hirsutism is primarily caused by an alteration in androgen metabolism in the target skin androgen-dependent structures (60).

V. HIRSUTISM AND POLYCYSTIC OVARY SYNDROME

A. Pathophysiology and Etiology of Hirsutism

The pathogenesis of hirsutism and other related increased androgen symptoms in women can be classified as follows: (1) increased glandular secretion of androgens or exogenous androgen administration; (2) increased extraglandular production of active androgens via increased peripheral conversion of precursor steroids; (3) increased availability of circulating bioactive androgens; and (4) primary or secondary increased sensitivity of target cells to androgen or increased androgenic biosynthetic enzymatic activity in the androgen-dependent skin structures. One or more of these pathogenetic mechanisms may play a role in hirsutism.

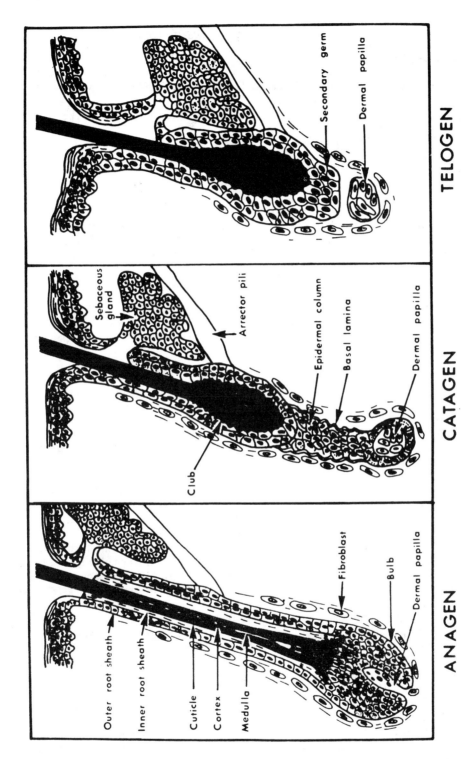

Figure 4 Human hair cycle. (Reproduced with permission of author and publisher, Ebling FJG. In: Clinics in Endocrinology and Metabolism. Philadelphia: W. B. Saunders 1986:319.)

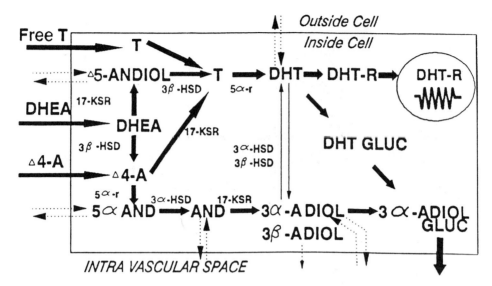

Figure 5 Conversion of androgens in skin tissue. DHT-R, DHT and its receptor complex; 5α AND, 5α-androstenedione; AND, androsterone; Δ5-ANDIOL, Δ^5 androstenediol; 3α-ADIOL, 3α-androstanediol; GLUC, glucuronide; 3βHSD, 3β-hydroxysteroid dehydrogenase, Δ$^{4-5}$-isomerase; 17-KSR, 17-ketosteroid reductase; 5α-r, 5α-reductase. (Reproduced with permission of author and publisher, Pang S, et al. J Clin Endocrinol Metab 1992; 75:243.)

Experience and observation reveal that generally hirsutism associated with virilism and menstrual disorder is primarily caused by unequivocal excess adrenal and/or ovarian androgen production. Hirsutism and menstrual disorder alone may result from moderately increased androgen production. Hirsutism and acne, alone or together, coupled with normal menses are frequently caused by mildly increased androgen production or normal androgen secretion in association with mechanisms 2, 3, or 4, as just described.

Clinically, the most easily distinguished excess androgen-producing lesions are those associated with classic manifestations of excess glucocorticoid hormone production (Cushing disease or Cushing syndrome) and those presenting with sudden onset and rapidly advancing androgen excess symptoms caused by adrenal or ovarian androgen-producing tumors (Table 3). These lesions, although rare, usually cause virilization and amenorrhea. The majority of hirsute women, however, present with either peripubertal or postpubertal onset of increased hair growth or acne, with or without menstrual dysfunction, and with no obvious clinical cause for increased androgen symptoms. The causes of clinically indistinguishable hirsutism are many, including those conditions associated with mild to moderately increased adrenal and/or ovarian sources of androgens (16,55,61–65), as well as other conditions associated with apparently normal androgen levels (Table 3). Recent studies of hirsutism have further defined some specific etiologies of adrenal and ovarian androgen excess production in women (Table 3).

1. Late-Onset Genetic Steroidogenic Enzyme Deficiencies

a. 21-Hydroxylase Deficiency. A partial or mild adrenal 21-hydroxylase deficiency is a well-defined cause of excess adrenal androgen secretion resulting in peripubertal or postpubertal onset of hirsutism and acne, with or without menstrual dysfunction (16,66–78). This entity has frequently been termed late-onset adrenal hyperplasia, attenuated congenital adrenal hyperplasia, or symptomatic form of nonclassic congenital adrenal hyperplasia and has been studied in great detail over the past two decades (66–78). The mild form of 21-hydroxylase deficiency may manifest excess androgen symptoms well before puberty, causing premature pubarche, acne, oily hair, and accelerated skeletal maturation in childhood (Chap. 21) (68,71).

The mild late-onset form of 21-hydroxylase deficiency results from a missense mutation in the 21-B gene as a result of a single base pair change in exon 1, 7, or 10 and a combined base pair change in exon 8/10 (79–84). These missense mutations appear to result from the microgene conversion of 21-B to a "21-A-like" gene. This mild 21-hydroxylase deficiency disorder has been reported in genetic linkage disequilibrium with HLA B14 in Ashkenazi Jews (68,73–75). A high frequency of this disorder reported in whites (individuals of mainly European descent) and Ashkenazi Jews, based on the family studies of the affected patients (74), must be verified by an adequate population screening. In hirsute females, varying frequencies (0–16%) of this disorder have been reported (16,70,78,85–90). The varying incidence in part appears to result from different hormonal criteria used for diagnosing mild 21-hydroxylase deficiency (85–90). Using an identical hormonal criterion, the author has diagnosed both a high frequency (13%) of mild 21-hydroxylase deficiency in hirsute females of largely physician referral cases (16) and a low frequency of the disorder (2%) in self-referral cases of hirsute females. The ethnic and racial makeup of hirsute females may be another factor for the varying incidence of

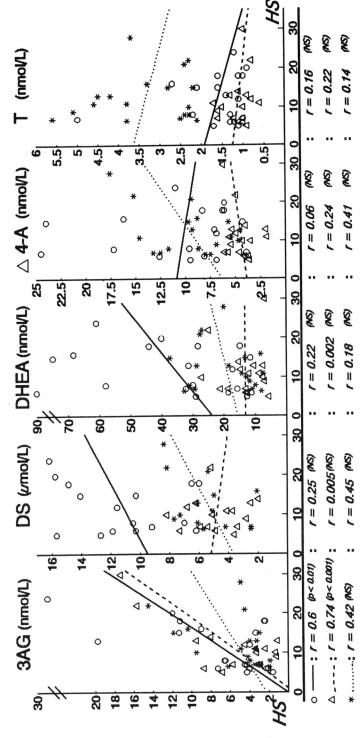

Figure 6 Correlations between serum 3α-Adiol ; Gluc and HS in each hirsutism group. Increased adrenal androgen group (circles); idiopathic cause (triangles); increased ovarian androgen group (asterisks); NS, not significant; HS, hirsutism score as based on a modified Ferriman and Gallwey method (18). Lines indicate the regression between hormone level and HS. To convert steroids, multiply DHEA by 28.6 (ng/dl), Δ⁴-A and T by 28.8 (ng/dl), and 3AG by 48.4 (ng/dl). (Reproduced with permission of author and publisher, Pang S, et al. J Clin Endocrinol Metab 1992; 75:243.)

Table 3 Causes of Excess Androgen Symptoms in Peripubertal and Postpubertal Females

Increased androgen production		
Adrenal	Ovarian	Other
Cushing syndrome, disease	Primary polycystic ovaries	Idiopathic hirsutism (normal
Androgen-producing adrenal	Stromal hyperthecosis	androgen production)
tumor (adenoma, carcinoma)	Secondary polycystic ovaries	Ingestion, injection of androgen
Late-onset genetic defects in	Androgen-producing ovarian	or androgenic substance
adrenal steroidogenesis	tumor (lipoma, luteoma, hilar	Hypothyroidism
21-Hydroxylase deficiency	cell tumor, stromal tumor)	Ingestion of nonsteroidal drug
3β-HSD deficiency	Hilar cell hyperplasia	Diazoxide
11β-Hydroxylase deficiency	Genetic defects in ovarian	Minoxidil
Isolated increased adrenal an-	steroidogenesis	Phenytoin
drogen-producing condition of	17-Ketosteroid reductase	
undefined etiology	deficiency	
Hyperprolactinemia	3β-HSD deficiency	
	aromatase deficiency	

the mild form of the disorder among various hirsute female populations because this mild form of the disorder was found more frequently in Ashkenazi Jews.

Characteristic hormonal abnormalities for the mild form of 21-hydroxylase deficiency in women are elevated circulating 17-hydroxyprogesterone and Δ4-A. Testosterone is also frequently mildly to moderately elevated. These adrenal sources of hormonal abnormalities can be more accurately detected by early morning blood sampling because of their circadian variations. Confirmative diagnosis of this condition, however, is made by evaluating the adrenal steroid response to exogenous ACTH stimulation regardless of time of day (16,68,85–89). ACTH-stimulated 17-OHP and androgen levels in normal and 21-hydroxylase-deficient hirsute females are depicted in Table 4 (55). The 17-OHP response to ACTH stimulation in these women was 3 standard deviations (SD) above the mean 17-OHP response of known carriers for 21-hydroxylase deficiency (16,55,68). All other steroid responses, including C_{19} steroid levels to ACTH stimulation, in these women overlapped with the steroid response of hirsute women with other causes (16,55,68). The moderately increased 17-OHP levels with or without ACTH stimulation, together with prompt suppression by exogenous glucocorticoid hormone administration, unequivocally confirm the diagnosis of mild form of 21-hydroxylase deficiency for patients of all ages.

Late-onset 11β-hydroxylase deficiency in women with hirsutism has also been reported (66). In the author's study of over 200 hirsute patients from two different populations, partial 11β-hydroxylase deficiency was not found. Thus, this disorder is an extremely rare cause of hirsutism in women.

b. 3β-Hydroxysteroid Dehydrogenase (3β-HSD) Deficiency. Early studies reported salt-losing symptoms in early life as the presenting signs of 3β-HSD deficiency (91).

However, the diagnosis of the non–salt-losing form of 3β-HSD deficiency may be delayed until later in life, when either premature pubic hair growth occurs during childhood or hirsutism occurs during puberty as symptom of a 3β-HSD defect (92–94). A partial adrenal 3β-HSD deficiency was first described in a woman with pubertal onset of hirsutism two decades ago (95). Thus, partial genetic 3β-HSD deficiency is a possible cause of pubertal or postpubertal hirsutism and polycystic ovaries in women (93,94). In the past decade, mild late-onset 3β-HSD deficiency was suspected in children with premature pubarche and in women with hirsutism if their ACTH-stimulated Δ^5 precursor steroids Δ5-17P and DHEA levels and Δ^5 precursor to Δ^4 product steroid ratios were greater than 2 SD above the age and pubertal stage-matched normal subject's mean value (16,86,87,89,90,96,97). However, questions remain regarding the validity of these hormonal criteria for diagnosing mild late-onset 3β-HSD deficiency disorder because of a lack of evidence that the subtle hormonal abnormalities were caused by a defect in the 3β-HSD gene. Recently, two types of human genes encoding 3β-HSD enzyme were characterized (98,99). The type I gene is primarily expressed in extraadrenal and extragonadal tissue, and the type II gene is primarily expressed in adrenal and gonadal tissue (98,99). Furthermore, mutation of the type II 3β-HSD gene has been identified in patients with the severe salt-wasting and non–salt-wasting forms of 3β-HSD deficiency (100–103). Molecular analysis of the type II 3β-HSD gene in several patients with Δ^5 precursor steroids and Δ^5 precursor to Δ^4 product steroid ratios greater than 2–8 SD above the normal mean value revealed no mutation in the type II 3β-HSD gene (104). Thus, a genuine mild late-onset 3β-HSD deficiency could not be verified unequivocally in these patients. Furthermore, DNA-proven obligate carriers for severe 3β-HSD deficiency did not demonstrate hormonal abnormalities upon ACTH stimulation (104). Therefore, the

Table 4 Mean ± SD Reference Baseline and ACTH-Stimulated Steroid Levels in Normal Females and Hirsute Females (HF) of Various Etiology and Hirsutism Scores (HS)[a]

| | Normal female (n = 28) | | ↑ Adrenal androgen HF | | | | ↑ Ovarian androgen | | Idiopathic HF | |
| | | | Undefined (n = 14) | | 21(OH)D (n = 5) | | HF (n = 18) | | (n = 17) | |
	Base	ACTH	Base	ACTH	Base	ACTH	Base	ACTH	Base	ACTH
DHEA	12 ± 7	45 ± 10	38 ± 26[b]	89 ± 33[b]	31 ± 2[b]	52 ± 15[c]	19 ± 10	32 ± 11	13 ± 6.4	40 ± 13
DS	5.2 ± 3	5.4 ± 2.2	11 ± 3.2[b]	12 ± 3[b]	7, 6, 7[d]	7, 5[d]	5.5 ± 2	5.7 ± 2.6	4.8 ± 1.8	5.1 ± 1.7
Δ4-A	4.7 ± 2.2	7.3 ± 2.0	9.3 ± 5.5[b]	11 ± 4.0[c]	12.4 ± 7[b]	19 ± 3.4[b]	9.4 ± 3.8[b]	12.5 ± 4.8[b]	4.5 ± 1.3	6.6 ± 2
T	1.0 ± 0.4	1.1 ± 0.3	1.4 ± 0.4	1.5 ± 0.4	2.3 ± 1.7[b]	3 ± 1.0[b]	3.3 ± 1.1[b]	4.0 ± 1.5[b]	1.1 ± 3.2	1.3 ± 0.3
Δ5-17P	3.0 ± 1.6	29 ± 11	11 ± 12[b]	46 ± 20[b]	6.2, 2.7[d]	25, 32[d]	5.6 ± 4.2	31 ± 11	2.8 ± 2.4	24 ± 13
17-OHP	2.8 ± 2.9	5.0 ± 2.3	3.6 ± 3.0	7.5 ± 6.1	15 ± 10[b]	185 ± 57[c]	4 ± 1.6	6.4 ± 3	2 ± 2	6 ± 5
S	0.6 ± 0.2	4.0 ± 1.8	0.6 ± 0.2	3.1 ± 0.9	1.8, 0.3[d]	4, 5.6[d]	1.3 ± 0.9	6 ± 3.3	0.6 ± 0.2	3.5 ± 1.3
F	0.3 ± 0.1	0.7 ± 0.2	0.4 ± 0.2	0.8 ± 0.2	0.3 ± 0.2	0.6 ± 0.2	0.4 ± 0.2	0.8 ± 0.4	0.4 ± 0.2	0.9 ± 0.5
HS	—		12 ± 6		12 ± 5		13 ± 6		12 ± 6	—

[a]All units nM except DS and F (μM). To convert: × 28.6 for DHEA (ng/dl); × 37 for DS and F (μg/dl); × 34.7 for S (ng/dl); × 28.8 for 4-A and T (ng/dl); × 33.3 for 17-OHP and Δ5-17P (ng/dl). Base: mean of −15 and 0 time. ACTH, 60 min after ACTH. The data do not represent the incidence of various causes of hirsutism. They provide only the reference values (55).

[b]$p < 0.01-0.0001$, significant difference from normal females.

[c]$p < 0.05$, significant difference from normal females.

[d]Individual values.

subtle findings of decreased adrenal 3β-HSD activity in hirsute females or in premature pubarche children were not a result of the heterozygote state for 3β-HSD deficiency. Thus, the hormonal criteria for mild late-onset 3β-HSD deficiency are not yet established. A hormonal criterion for this disorder analogous to that of mild late-onset 21-hydroxylase deficiency (i.e., precursor steroid response 8 SD above the normal general population mean) (105–107) appears acceptable for bona fide mild late-onset 3β-HSD deficiency.

On the other hand, to those hirsute females with only mildly increased Δ^5 precursor steroid levels and Δ^5 precursor to Δ^4 product steroid ratio (<8 SD above the normal mean) we now arbitrarily assign the diagnosis "mildly decreased adrenal 3β-HSD activity of unknown etiology." These hirsute women have clearly increased adrenal androgen secretion. In addition, in some women with this mildly decreased adrenal 3β-HSD activity of unknown etiology, clinical and/or hormonal findings of polycystic ovary syndrome may be present (16,97). It is now apparent that true mild late-onset 3β-HSD deficiency resulting from the type II 3β-HSD gene mutation is a rare disorder in hirsute females. The mildly decreased adrenal 3β-HSD activity of unknown etiology without the type II 3β-HSD gene mutation appears to be more frequent than true 3β-HSD deficiency in hirsute females, and its pathogenesis must be investigated.

Ovarian function and polycystic ovaries (PCO) in hirsute females with mild 21-hydroxylase and bona fide 3β-HSD deficiencies are discussed in Section V.B.

2. Isolated Increased Adrenal Androgen-Producing Condition of Undefined Etiology

In a study of over 125 hirsute females, approximately 10 patients demonstrated only elevated baseline or ACTH-stimulated levels of DHEA and or DHEA-S. A specific cause for increased adrenal androgen secretion was not found in these patients because they did not meet the criteria of any enzyme deficiency or decreased enzyme activity and had no hormonal or radiologic evidence of adrenal hyperplasia or adrenal tumor (55). This isolated increased adrenal androgen-producing condition was thus labeled undefined increased adrenal androgen producing condition (55). Our therapeutic approach to this condition is the same as for those women with bona fide adrenal 3β-HSD deficiency or decreased mild adrenal 3β-HSD activity.

3. Cushing Disease or Syndrome

Inappropriate ACTH secretion by a pituitary tumor or by a disturbed CRH-ACTH axis in the central nervous system (CNS; Cushing disease) and ectopic ACTH secretion by the malignant tumor often result in excess adrenal glucocorticoid and androgen secretion simultaneously. Autonomously functioning adrenal cortical tumor (adenoma and carcinoma) may also secrete increased amounts of cortisol and androgen (Cushing syndrome). Thus, patients with Cushing disease or syndrome manifest symptoms not only of glucocorticoid excess but of hirsutism or virilism as well. These conditions are rare causes of hirsutism and are usually clinically more easily recognizable because of the presence of cushingoid features and muscle-wasting signs. Biochemically abnormal cortisol and/or ACTH dynamics is apparent in these disorders. Classic hormonal abnormalities are non-suppressed or partially suppressible excess cortisol, DHEA, and DHEA-S levels by dexamethasone administration. Radiologic studies are also an essential part of the differential diagnosis of Cushing disease and/or syndrome (Chap. 22).

4. Adrenal Androgen-Producing Tumor

An androgen-producing tumor of the adrenal may be adenoma or carcinoma; however rare, it is a cause of virilism.

Generally, the supraphysiologic amount of androgen secreted by these tumors characteristically causes extremely elevated circulating DHEA and DHEA-S levels. Other androgens, such as Δ4-A and T, or progestational steroid levels may also be elevated by either direct secretion or peripheral conversion of DHEA and DHEA-S. Some androgen-producing tumors may also have the capacity to secrete cortisol, but the patient may not present with cushingoid features. Clinically these diseases are manifested by sudden onset; hormonal symptoms are rapidly progressive. In carcinomas, the metastasis to liver or ovarian tissue may occur, and metastatic tissue often secretes steroids inappropriately. Radiologic and hormonal evaluations are essential for the diagnosis; tumor tissue should be removed as soon as possible (Chap. 57).

5. Hyperprolactinemia

Elevated adrenal androgen levels (DHEA and DHEA-S) have been found in some hirsute women with high prolactin levels (108,109) and a normal metabolic clearance rate of these steroids (110). Increase plasma Δ4-A and cortisol response to ACTH stimulation and low SHBG in hirsute and hyperprolactinemic patients were also described (111). To date, the mechanism by which excess prolactin induces increased adrenal androgen levels has not been defined. Reduction in prolactin by bromocriptine did not lower circulating levels of androgens (112). This also suggests that high prolactin and adrenal androgen levels may be associated findings, rather than cause and effect. Enhanced androgen effect at the target tissue by a permissive action of prolactin was also described (113). The associated findings of PCO in some hyperprolactinemic women suggest an additional cause of hirsutism in the hyperprolactinemic state.

B. Pathophysiology and Etiology of Polycystic Ovary Syndrome

Clinically PCO is a syndrome in which the spectrum of hyperandrogenic symptoms and signs, including chronic anovulation (associated with irregular menses, amenorrhea, dysfunctional bleeding, or infertility) in the presence or absence of hirsutism, acne, and/or virilism and or obesity, is caused by excess androgen production of ovarian or extra-ovarian source (114–116). The morphologic changes of ovaries include bilaterally and symmetrically enlarged ovoid ovaries, but ovaries may be unilateral or normally shaped (117). An oyster-gray color and smooth glistening surface surrounding a thickened capsule in association with numerous small subcapsular cysts 2–15 mm in size and many ovary atretic follicles are characteristic morphologic findings of PCO (117). Approximately 70% of women with PCO in the United States were reported to be hirsute, and the remaining 30% of patients were not hirsute despite hyperandrogenism (116).

PCO appears to be caused by or associated with multifactorial conditions (Table 5) and has been found not uncommonly in conditions associated with primary causes of increased ovarian or adrenal androgen production. In excess adrenal androgen-producing conditions, such as 21-hydroxylase deficiency, 11β-hydroxylase deficiency, 3-HSD deficiency, adrenal androgen-producing tumor, and Cushing disease or syndrome or with exogenous administration of androgen, the proposed pathogenetic mechanism for PCO development is a direct adverse effect of androgen either affecting ovarian estrogen synthesis or altering gonadotropin secretion by increased free androgen or estrogen, thereby causing PCO changes (118–123). Impaired ovarian estradiol synthesis caused by ovarian 17-ketosteroid reductase deficiency (124), ovarian 3β-HSD deficiency (93,94), and, possibly, aromatase deficiency, will likely lead to PCO either as a result of the increased intraovarian androgen effect resulting from the enzyme deficiency or because of the increased gonadotropin effect via feedback regulation. PCO in ovarian androgen-producing tumor may be caused by either the direct effect of androgen on the process of ovarian estrogen synthesis or by altering gonadotropin secretion via excess androgen or free estrogen converted from excess androgen. It is not known

Table 5 Proven or Proposed Etiology of Polycystic Ovarian Disease

Ovarian	Adrenal	Other
Intraovarian defect in E₂ synthesis	Increased adrenal androgen production	Brain-hypothalamic in origin, leading to increased LH
17-Ketosteroid reductase deficiency	21-OH deficiency (congenital and late onset)	Dopamine deficiency
3β-HSD deficiency	3β-ol dehydrogenase deficiency (late onset)	Psychologic stress
Other steroidogenic enzyme deficiency: aromatase	1β-OH deficiency (congenital and late onset)	Increased free androgen, estrogen causing increased LH
Ovarian androgen-producing tumor	Adrenal tumor	Ovarian and adrenal source of excess androgens
Other pathology?	Cushing syndrome	Obesity?
	Extra-ovarian, adrenal	Insulin resistance, hyperinsulinemia
	Exogenous androgens	Heredity (?)
	Hyperprolactinemia	

whether excess androgen production in these adrenal and ovarian conditions alters some growth factor action in the modulation of gonadotropin on the ovarian function, thereby leading to the development of PCO.

A majority of the women with PCO, however, have no discernible cause of PCO and manifest increased ovarian androgen secretion. This hyperandrogenic cause of primary PCO is elaborated on further later. Several hypotheses have been proposed for the pathogenetic mechanism of PCO (123), including (1) dopamine deficiency in the CNS; supporting evidence for this is decreased LH response to LH-releasing hormone (LHRH) following a week of L-dopa (lerodopa) treatment in women with PCO; (2) psychologic stress leading to chronic anovulation; (3) decrease in SHBG by androgens or by obesity, resulting in increased peripheral free estrogen production, leading to increased LH and PCO; (4) excess insulin, resulting in increased ovarian androgen production in insulin resistance syndrome; and (5) genetic theory.

1. Ovarian Causes of Hirsutism

a. Primary PCO. In general, most women with primary PCO (nonadrenal and nonexogenous excess androgen induced) have normal onset of menarche, although infrequently primary amenorrhea or oligomenorrhea may be present from the beginning (114,125,126). Frequently a history of significant weight gain preceding menarche can be obtained in many primary PCO patients (127). Hirsutism is a frequent symptom in primary PCO and generally begins during the late pubertal stage following the menarche (127). Progressive manifestation of hirsutism and menstrual dysfunction correlated with the ovarian androgen production rate (114,128, 129). Some genetic factors may modify the effects of increased ovarian androgen secreted in some PCO women who are not hirsute (114). The clinical spectrum of primary PCO therefore ranges from no apparent symptoms, to anovulation and menstrual abnormalities without hirsutism, to mild hirsutism with no apparent menstrual abnormalities, to severe hirsutism and/or virilism and menstrual abnormalities and/or infertility (114,116,129).

Hormonal manifestations of primary PCO include a frequently increased ovarian source of Δ4-A and/or T production. Elevated basal levels of T and/or Δ4-A in the absence of elevated adrenal androgens (DHEA and DS) generally signify primary PCO. However, in some patients, combination of both increased ovarian T and/or Δ4-A production and increased adrenal androgen levels may be present simultaneously in the absence of any known enzyme defect in adrenal and/or ovarian biosynthesis. The increased ovarian androgen production in primary PCO is frequently associated with inappropriate gonadotropin secretory patterns, including elevated basal LH levels (116, 129, 130), elevated basal LH/FSH ratios, high LH amplitude (130,131), or hyperresponse of LH to LHRH stimulation (Fig. 7) (130). Nonbioactive gonadotropin measurement, such as radioimmunoassay, however, did not demonstrate abnormally elevated LH levels in approximately 25% of primary PCO patients (132).

The inappropriately elevated LH levels in the primary PCO patients were not related to an alteration in the negative feedback regulation between estradiol and LH secretion because estradiol infusion effectively suppressed elevated LH in these patients (130). In addition, the positive feedback mechanism of estrogen on LH release was apparently intact in PCO patients because the preovulatory elevation of estradiol via clomiphene citrate administration induced an LH surge in primary PCO patients (133). The pathogenesis of the inappropriate gonadotropin secretion in the primary PCO has not yet been clearly defined. Inappropriate gonadotropin secretion may arise as inappropriate feedback because of abnormal ovarian steroidogenesis or as a primary hypothalamic-pituitary defect, as elaborated earlier. The presence of both negative and positive feedback mechanisms of gonadotropin secretion in primary PCO patients led to the conclusion that anovulation in primary PCO is less likely to be caused by an intrinsic hypothalamic abnormality (130,134). Defective secretion of FSH may play a crucial role in the pathogenesis of PCO because FSH or clomiphene administration resulted in ovulation in primary PCO patients (130,134,135). An extraglandular source of estrogen (estrone) via the peripheral conversion of androstenedione is related to body weight and has been speculated to be of etiologic importance in the maintenance of chronic anovulation (134,136). A possible role of inhibin has also been speculated in PCO because inappropriate gonadotropin secretion is not fully explained by the effective feedback of estrogen on FSH and the feedback modulation of FSH may be inhibin dependent (134).

Hyperprolactinemia may also be found in primary PCO patients (137). The mechanism of altered reproductive function in hyperprolactinemic females is complex (137). Estrogen's stimulatory effect on the pituitary lactotropes has been speculated to cause hyperprolactinemia in patients with this disorder (137). Recently, dysregulation (increased activity) in P_{450} 17α-hydroxylase and 17,20-desmolase activity in ovarian steroidogenesis was proposed in PCO (138). The complex determinants in the hormonal regulation of ovarian (and adrenal) steroidogenesis make it difficult to postulate whether such dysregulation is the cause or effect of altered steroidogenesis.

b. Insulin Resistance in Primary PCO. A well-recognized and common etiologic factor of primary PCO is the varying degree of insulin resistance (139–141) and is not affected by changes in circulating androgen levels (142,143). Many studies suggest there is a strong relationship between hyperinsulinemia and ovarian hyperandrogenemia (116,139–144). Patients with insulin resistance may or may not be obese; however, obesity contributes to the problem by inducing a greater degree of insulin resistance and decreasing SHBG levels in women with PCO. The mechanism by which hyperinsulinemia in insulin resistance for carbohydrate metabolism, resulting in increased ovarian androgen production, has been the subject of investigation in the past decade. Altered insulin and insulin-like growth factor (IGF) may exert their effect on ovarian IGF-I receptors because insulin and IGF-I receptors are present in human ovaries. In vitro insulin or IGF-I in large doses stimulated ovarian stromal androgen production (144–146). Interaction between insulin/IGF-I and

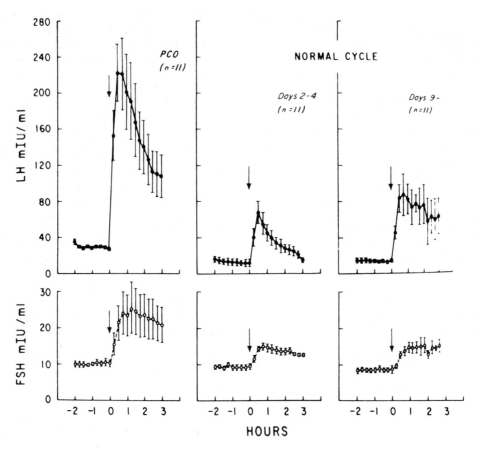

Figure 7   Comparison of LH and FSH response to LHRH administration (150 mg IV bolus at time 0) in primary PCO females versus normal females in the early and late follicular phases of the menstrual cycle (mean ± standard error of the mean). (Reproduced with permission of author and publisher, Rebar R, et al. J Clin Invest 1976; 57:1320.)

LH in the regulation of ovarian (stromal and thecal) androgen production must be further explained.

IGF-I also stimulates 5α-reductase activity, and hair growth is influenced by IGF-I (147). Serum IGF-I levels were reported to be normal, but IGF binding protein levels were decreased in primary PCO (148). Whether or how the effects of insulin and IGF-I play a role on hair growth directly in the insulin-resistant state also needs further investigation.

c. Genetic Causes of Insulin-Resistant Syndrome and Ovarian Stromal Hyperthecosis.   A severe degree of excess ovarian androgen production has been found in genetic disorders of severe insulin-resistant syndrome caused by a point mutation of the gene encoding insulin receptor function (149–152). These patients manifest HAIR-AN syndrome (hyperandrogenism, HA; insulin resistance, IR; and acanthosis nigricans, AN) and are usually virilized. Leprechaunism characterized by severe congenital growth retardation appears also to be caused by insulin receptor gene mutation (149) and the development of PCO, although severe cases do not survive long. Kahn type B insulin resistance syndrome caused by the presence of circulating antibodies for insulin receptors also causes HAIR-AN syndrome. AN is a dermatologic manifestation of severe hyperinsulinemia and hyperan-

drogenism. However, less than 30% of women with insulin resistance manifest AN (144). Patients with AN are therefore at high risk of HAIR-AN syndrome. In patients with HAIR-AN syndrome, ovarian histology almost always reveals marked stromal hyperthecosis, which results in severe excess ovarian androgen production (144).

d. Hyperthecosis of Stroma.   This condition is characterized by the nests of luteinized theca cells within the stroma of bilaterally enlarged ovaries (2,153,154). The thickened capsule without subcapsular cysts differentiates hyperthecosis from PCO (153,154), and excess androgen is produced by the theca cells. Patients with stromal hyperthecosis have progressive symptoms of androgen excess and are usually amenorrheic. Serum T levels are generally >150 ng/dl (2,144). This condition, however, is differentiated from most of the androgen-producing tumors clinically by the nature of slowly progressive symptoms and hormonally by the elevated basal and LHRH-stimulated LH levels.

In the author's experience of PCO syndrome in young hirsute females, more than 200 young hirsute females evaluated in the last decade, intrinsic primary PCO syndrome, defined by clinical presentation of hirsutism with (majority) or without (minority) apparent menstrual disorders and documented increased ovarian Δ-A and or T production in the absence of increased adrenal androgen secretion, was diagnosed in one-quarter to one-third (16,55). Primary ovarian hyperthecosis and HAIR-AN syndrome have been found in only a few patients. The baseline LH levels, LH/FSH ratios, and LH response to LHRH administration in the primary PCO patients were elevated or apparently appropriate despite increased ovarian androgen secretion. Generally, the increased ovarian source of Δ-A and or T in these patients was not significantly dexamethasone suppressible, but all other adrenal steroid levels were promptly suppressed. PCO associated with both increased ovarian and adrenal androgen secretion of undefined cause was found in about 5% of the patients. Menstrual disorder was observed in about one-half of patients with isolated increased adrenal androgen secretion without an enzyme defect. In these patients, despite clinical manifestation of PCO syndrome, the ovarian androgen secretion appeared normal. Menstrual disorder was also observed in many patients with "mildly decreased adrenal 3β-HSD activity" associated with increased adrenal androgen secretion, although ovarian androgen secretion was either normal or mildly increased in some cases. In mild 21-hydroxylase deficiency patients, menstrual disorders were present in about one-half, but most of these patients had normal ovarian androgen secretion despite menstrual problems. Previous studies demonstrated that the menstrual disorder in either 21-hydroxylase deficiency or "decreased adrenal 3β-HSD activity" patients (no longer 3β-HSD deficiency) had PCO by ultrasound, laparoscopy, or laparotomy study (16). Thus, PCO syndrome in patients with primarily increased adrenal androgen secretion was associated with both normal and mildly increased ovarian androgen production. However, in the poorly controlled severe classic virilizing form of congenital adrenal hyperplasia patients, classic PCO pathology findings and increased ovarian androgen production were demonstrated (118–122).

e. Genetic Defects in Ovarian Steroidogenesis.

i. Ovarian 17-Ketosteroid Reductase (17-KSR) Deficiency. The existence of 17-KSR, which converts the precursor hormone androstenedione to the product hormone T (and estrone to estradiol) in human adrenal and gonadal tissue, is well known. Furthermore, a genetic defect or deficiency of this enzyme in testicular tissue is a well-defined etiology of male pseudohermaphroditism as a result of insufficient T production beginning in early fetal life (155,156). This enzyme deficiency is probably transmitted as an auto- somal recessive trait (although X-linked recessive transmission cannot be totally excluded) (157). Thus, the chances of a genetic female inheriting this disorder is presumably the same as that of a genetic male.

We first described three female siblings whose hormonal studies indicated that ovarian 17-KSR deficiency was the likely cause of excess ovarian Δ4-A secretion beginning in puberty (124). This excess ovarian androgen secretion resulted in hirsutism, acne, clitoromegaly, amenorrhea, and apparent polycystic ovarian disease. Serum Δ4-A and T levels in these siblings were, beginning with the youngest,

336 and 49 ng/dl, respectively, 421 and 59 ng/dl in the middle sibling, and 871 and 114 ng/dl in the oldest sibling (124). The normal Δ4-A is 140 ± 56 ng/dl; normal T is 40 ± 22 ng/dl (124).

17-KSR deficiency in ovarian tissue in the index case was confirmed by the increased ovarian Δ4-A secretion (11.6 mg/day; normal 2.5–3.0 mg/day), together with a very low rate of ovarian T secretion (0.05 mg/day in the patient compared with the normal female 0.15 mg/day). The rate of ovarian Δ4-A secretion to ovarian T secretion was extremely high in this patient (patient ratio 232; normal ratio 12–24). The LH response to LHRH stimulation in the index patient was comparable to that seen in agonadal females; the FSH response was normal. These data further supported the evidence of a defect in intraovarian estrogen biosynthesis caused by the 17-KSR deficiency. The index patient demonstrated unequivocal findings of classic PCO on ultrasound study. We hypothesized that both increased LH stimulation and increased direct ovarian androgen secretion in this patient synergistically and adversely affected ovarian morphology, leading to the development of PCO in ovarian 17-KSR deficiency (124).

ii. Ovarian 3β-HSD Deficiency and Ovarian Aromatase Deficiency. 3β-HSD deficiency has been demonstrated in both adrenal and gonadal tissue in patients with severe 3β-HSD deficiency. To date, two females with proven severe non–salt-losing 3β-HSD deficiency CAH have demonstrated a defect in ovarian 3β-HSD, and both manifested hirsutism, menstrual disorders, and PCO (93,94). Thus, combined intraadrenal and intraovarian genetic 3β-HSD deficiency is a cause of ovarian dysfunction and PCO. In addition, hypothetically decreased intraovarian aromatase deficiency leads to a similar pathology and increased ovarian androgen production and PCO.

f. Ovarian Androgen-Producing Tumors. Clinically, the presentation of androgen-producing tumors by the ovary is similar to that of the androgen-producing tumor of the adrenals. Thus, in general, marked virilism occurs in short duration in women with ovarian androgen-producing tumors. However, there are exceptional cases whose symptomatology of excess androgen production by the ovarian tumor was slowly progressive and of long standing (158). Both clinically rapid and slowly progressive androgen-secreting ovarian tumors are associated with extremely high circulating levels of mainly Δ4-A and T regardless of the histopathologic classification of the tumors. Serum DHEA and DHEA-S may be mildly elevated or normal, except in metastasized adrenal carcinoma of the ovary. The tumorous androgen-producing cells arise from lipoid cells, hilus cells, Sertoli-Leydig cells, granulosa-theca cells, and stromal cells (Chap. 57).

2. Idiopathic Hirsutism

By strict definition, idiopathic hirsutism should be applied to those females presenting with hirsutism and/or acne and no other androgen excess symptoms or other clinical or hormonal causes of hirsutism. Thus, these women usually have normal circulating total androgen concentration either in the basal state or under dynamic test of adrenal or ovarian steroidogenic function. Further, these women usually have apparently normal ovarian function as evidenced by normal menses or normal reproductive function.

Several pathogenetic mechanisms have been speculated for idiopathic hirsutism. Increased intracellular conversion of precursor androgens to DHT by increased intracellular 5α-reductase activity was found in some women with idiopathic hirsutism (57,159). Further increased skin androgen metabolic activity has also been noted in those women with idiopathic hirsutism as evidenced by the increased circulating 3α-adiol gluc levels (Fig. 6) (52–55,160). Serum 3α-adiol gluc, however, largely reflects 5α-reductase activity (160) and peripheral adrenal androgen metabolism (55). Thus, the increased 5α-reductase activity in the skin of these women could be a causative factor in idiopathic hirsutism.

Another proposed theory for the mechanism of idiopathic hirsutism is the increased availability of bioactive androgens. That hirsutism corresponds better to the plasma free T than to the plasma total T is evidence that free T is a determinant factor in androgen action, and free T was elevated in number of hirsute women with normal total T concentration (42,161). Thus the decreased SHBG and increased free T or DHT may be etiologic factors in idiopathic hirsutism.

The third theory involves increased skin tissue sensitivity to the circulating androgen for idiopathic hirsutism. The increased skin 5α-reductase activity may enhance the effect of androgen at the target cells, but the androgen binding capacity at the receptor protein of the target cell shows no differences between normal and hirsute females (56).

In review, abnormalities found in some women with idiopathic hirsutism include increased skin androgen-metabolizing activity and/or increased bioactive free androgens. Whether these are primary abnormalities or are caused by enzyme and receptor protein regulation disorders secondary to the circulating androgen, particularly by an increase in the free component of androgen, remains to be elucidated. The mechanism of low SHBG and high free T in this disorder also remains to be elucidated.

3. Hirsutism Associated with Thyroid Disorder

Thyroid hormones increase the concentration of SHBG in plasma (18). Thus, the high testosterone levels observed in some patients with hyperthyroidism are a result of increased protein-bound testosterone levels, with no clinical androgen excess symptoms. On the other hand, hypothyroidism may be associated with hirsutism. Only three women with hirsutism have been found by the authors in the last 15 years to have hypothyroidism. These women had normal circulating total androgen levels. Thus hypothyroidism seems to be a condition rarely associated with hirsutism. To the best of our knowledge, no studies have been reported with regard to the androgen metabolism, SHBG, or free androgen concentration in hypothyroidism.

C. Clinical Assessment of Hirsutism

A detailed history and careful physical examination are essential in evaluating hirsute patients. History of puberty,

including adrenarche, thelarche, onset of hirsutism and its progression, menarche, and menstrual disorders should be obtained. A similar history should be taken of the family members as well. Evaluation of the severity and progression of terminal hair growth is an essential part of the physical examination in hirsute females. A detailed history of cosmetic care, in terms of frequency, method, and the last treatment date of depilation or shaving, is necessary to estimate the degree of hair growth in the native state.

The degree of hirsutism on various parts of the body should be examined, including face, chin, neck, chest, areolae, abdomen, pelvic area, upper and lower back, buttocks, inter-gluteal region, thighs, and other parts of the extremities. The best method to determine the degree of hirsutism was described by Ferriman and Gallwey (162). Their original scoring system included 14 areas of the body, using a total of 4 points for grading each area, with a total score of 44. Further modification of the charts and scoring system of Ferriman and Gallwey was described by Cooke and Goodal (111) and Hatch et al. (163). The scoring system modified by Cooke and Goodal identifies hirsute scores in 9 more hormonally sensitive areas and 2 less hormonally sensitive areas, with a total score of 36 (Fig. 8). We find that this modified scoring system is easy and more informative in evaluating the initial state and for follow-up of treated hirsute patients. Presence or absence and extent of acne, seborrhea, oily hair, masculine body habitus, and clitoral size should also be examined in all hirsute patients.

D. Differential Diagnosis

In the previous section, many of the specific clinical and hormonal abnormalities of each disorder were discussed. In this section, a general approach to the laboratory investigation for the diagnosis and differential diagnosis of hirsutism is described. The reference data for basal steroid levels in normal women and in hirsute women with various etiologies are depicted in Table 4.

In hirsutism associated with virilism and menstrual disorders, the dynamics of adrenal and ovarian steroidogenic function is usually warranted to determine the source of excess androgen production. Radiologic evaluation (ultrasonographic and/or computed tomography or magnetic resonance imaging of abdomen and pelvis) of adrenals and ovaries are also essential. The logical sequence of dynamic studies may include early morning basal hormonal study or circadian basal hormonal study followed by adrenal stimulation and suppression and ovarian suppression and stimulation contiguously. Suppression tests are generally more important than the stimulation test in evaluating excess androgen production. For adrenal stimulation, generally 0.25 mg ACTH is administered by intravenous (IV) bolus and various adrenal steroids and C_{19} steroids responses are examined 1 h following ACTH stimulation. The adrenal suppression test is performed by administering a pharmacologic dose of dexamethasone, 2 mg/day in four divided doses/day $\times$ 3–5 days. The key circulating adrenal steroids, including C_{19} androgens and urinary metabolites of C_{19} steroids, may be determined on

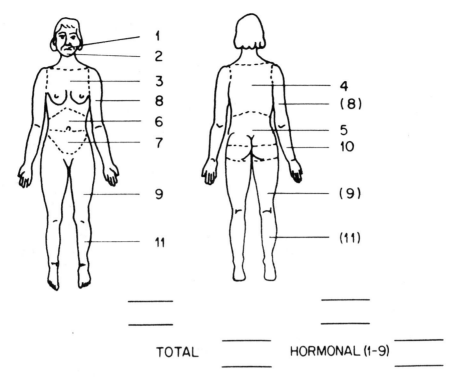

Figure 8 Modified Ferriman and Gallwey hirsutism scoring chart. (Reproduced with permission of authors and publishers, Cooke and Sawers, In: Androgens and Anti-androgen Therapy. New York: John Wiley and Sons, 1982:95.)

days 3–5 after dexamethasone administration. The adrenals are suppressed by dexamethasone, but ovarian suppression may be evaluated by administering a gonadotropin suppressant, such as synthetic estrogen (50–100 μg oral ethinyl estradiol twice per day), or a progestational compound, such as norethindrone acetate (10 mg orally three times per day) for 5–6 days. The ovarian stimulation test may be performed by administering human chorionic gonadotropin (hCG), 3000–5000 IU/day × 3 days, and the ovarian steroidal response should be examined from 2 to 24–48 h after the last dose of hCG. An LHRH stimulation test (100–150 μg IV bolus) or LHRH analog stimulation test has proven to be useful in the differential diagnosis of increased ovarian androgen production. These gonadotropin stimulation tests, however, must be performed before the ovarian suppression or ovarian stimulation test just described.

Very high basal DHEA (>1500 ng/dl) levels, DHEA-S (>500 μg/dl) levels, and urinary 17-ketosteroid levels, with or without moderately elevated Δ4-A and T levels, can be seen in adrenal tumors and in women with partial adrenal 3β-HSD deficiency (93,94), in the isolated increased adrenal androgen-producing condition of undefined etiology (55), or in mildly decreased adrenal 3β-HSD activity of unknown etiology (no longer 3β-HSD deficiency) (16,104). The basal Δ5-17P, however, is highly elevated in true 3β-HSD deficiency (93,94), and Δ5-17P may also be elevated in adrenal androgen-producing tumors and mildly elevated in mildly decreased adrenal 3β-HSD activity of unknown etiology

(16,104). With dexamethasone, in adrenal tumor, DHEA, DHEA-S, and other C_{19} steroids and their urinary metabolites may be only slightly or partially decreased. In adrenal 3β-HSD deficiency, mildly decreased adrenal 3β-HSD activity of unknown etiology, and isolated increased adrenal androgen-producing condition of unknown etiology, these steroid levels are promptly suppressed (55,93,94). Clinically, these patients rarely present with virilism. Occasionally patients with partial 21-hydroxylase deficiency present with virilism and menstrual disorder. In these patients, 17-OHP levels (>600 ng/dl) in the basal state, after ACTH stimulation (>2000 ng/dl), are unequivocally high. Serum DHEA and DHEA-S may be moderately elevated, but Δ4-A and T are also generally higher in the early morning hours. These steroidal abnormalities are quickly suppressed by dexamethasone administration.

Extremely high basal Δ4-A (>350 ng/dl) and T (>150–200 ng/dl) levels without concomitantly increased levels of DHEA and DHEA-S are usually seen in ovarian tumor, long-standing stromal hyperthecosis, and ovarian 17-KSR deficiency. These patients generally manifest virilism. The ovarian source of androgen is promptly suppressed in ovarian 17-KSR deficiency, whereas androgen secretion by the tumor may not change or may partially decrease. The LHRH stimulation test results in a LH hyperresponse in ovarian hyperthecosis and 17-KSR deficiency (124). In stromal hyperthecosis, suppression of androgens by administration of estrogen or progestational agents is not as good as in the patient with PCO; however, long-term (>3 month) LHRH analog treatment suppresses ovarian androgen secretion in these patients. The definitive differential diagnosis of these three conditions requires ovarian hormonal dynamic studies, radiologic evaluation, gynecologic examination, and possibly laparoscopic examination in some cases. Laparotomy may also have to be carried out if there is a high suspicion of tumorous lesions in the ovary.

In hirsute patients without virilism, androgen levels are generally not as high as in the patient with virilism, and hirsute patients with menstrual disorders have generally elevated ovarian and/or adrenal androgen levels. In this group of patients, hormonal evaluation of early morning blood sampling may include DHEA/DHEA-S, 17-OHP, Δ4-A, T, LH, FSH, prolactin, and thyroxine. In those patients with mildly to modestly elevated morning levels of DHEA/DHEA-S, 17-OHP, and Δ4-A or T simultaneously, the ACTH stimulation test differentiates partial 21-hydroxylase deficiency, mildly decreased adrenal 3β-HSD activity of unknown etiology, 3β-HSD deficiency, 11β-hydroxylase deficiency, isolated increased adrenal androgen-producing condition of undefined etiology, and PCO syndrome (Table 4). Pelvic ultrasound may be performed to look for both classic and other types of PCO (164–166) in those patients with proven increased androgen production by the adrenals and/or ovaries. The occurrence of menstrual disorders and PCO-like syndrome in all adrenal androgen-producing conditions was discussed earlier. The author's experience indicates that the response of LH to LHRH stimulation is variable in primary PCO and secondary PCO as a result of increased adrenal androgen production.

In those hirsute patients with normal menses, normal basal and ACTH-stimulated steroid levels, and normal pelvic sonogram findings, serum 3α-adiol gluc, serum free T, and SHBG measurements are useful in diagnosing idiopathic hirsutism.

E. Treatment

The specific and nonspecific therapy for the various cause of hirsutism described here are based on the author's experience and review of literature. The treatment of hirsute symptoms is most effective if aimed at correcting the primary pathology. This is not easily done in patients with PCO, ovarian hyperthecosis, or idiopathic hirsutism. Both specific and nonspecific therapies are discussed in each disorder.

1. Late Onset 21-Hydroxylase Deficiency, 3β-HSD Deficiency, Mildly Decreased Adrenal 3β-HSD Activity of Unknown Etiology, and Isolated Increased Adrenal Androgen-Producing Condition of Undefined Etiology

Suppression of excess adrenal androgen production in these conditions can be easily achieved by administration of a relatively low dose of glucocorticoid hormone. We have used prednisone in a dose of 2.5 mg twice per day, or 5 mg in the morning and 2.5 mg at night, or 0.25–0.375 mg dexamethasone at bedtime. The dose of glucocorticoid should be adjusted based on the clinical and hormonal response, as well

as other unwanted side effects of glucocorticoid, such as weight gain, striae, and cushingoid features. Use of 0.5 mg dexamethasone at bedtime caused mild cushingoid features in some women with late-onset adrenal hyperplasia within 4–8 weeks.

The aim of treatment is to reduce adrenal androgen secretion to a low normal level, not complete adrenal suppression, thereby minimizing the side effects. Our experience indicates that marginal to significant clinical improvement in hirsutism in a large number of women with the preceding increased adrenal androgen-producing conditions occurred within 8 months to 1 year of treatment. By the second year of treatment, a majority of the patients showed good improvement in hirsutism. In almost all cases, recovery of menses occurred in 2–3 months following adequate suppression of excess adrenal androgen secretion. Therapeutic monitoring of 21-hydroxylase deficiency requires periodic follow-up measurement of 17-OHP, Δ4-A, and T levels. Periodic measurement of DHEA, DHEA-S, Δ4-A, and T is necessary for monitoring 3β-HSD deficiency, mildly decreased adrenal 3β-HSD activity of unknown etiology, and isolated increased adrenal androgen-producing condition of undefined etiology. Ovarian function and the outcome of PCO in some women with these adrenal causes of excess androgen-producing conditions require follow-up.

2. Primary (Intrinsic) PCO

Primary PCO is a more difficult condition to treat successfully. There are often two specific problems in young women with primary PCO, hirsutism and menstrual disorders (amenorrhea or oligomenorrhea or dysfunctional bleeding). Currently acceptable and available medical treatment using hormonal preparations or drugs is not designed to attack both problems. By and large, most young hirsute women with PCO desire treatment for hirsutism. Oral contraceptives (OC) used in an attempt to decrease ovarian androgen secretion and to lower free T levels have been partially successful. Cyclic combined estrogen and progestin or OC therapy in primary PCO patients has an additional long-term benefit for the prevention of endometrial hyperplasia secondary to an unopposed effect of increased free estrogen in this disorder.

Spironolactone (50–200 mg/day) treatment alone was not generally useful in women with PCO. However, a combination of spironolactone and OC therapy generally improves hirsutism in PCO patients to a degree. Successful medical treatment for hirsutism is possible by the use of combined cyproterone acetate (an antiandrogenic agent) and sex hormone replacement therapy (167,168). A short- (6 month) or long-term (1 year) LHRH analog treatment in conjunction with OC therapy demonstrated a marked reduction in ovarian androgen secretion and a marked improvement in hirsutism in patients with primary PCO and ovarian hyperthecosis (169–171). No significant side effects of these combined therapies was noted in our experience; however, a recurrence of increased ovarian androgen secretion occurred 6 weeks to 2 months following discontinuation of the LHRH analog and OC therapy (171). Maintenance OC therapy alone continuously when the LHRH analog therapy has been discontinued prevented the progression of hirsutism in several PCO patients in the author's clinic. High doses (800–1200 mg/day) of ketoconazole have also been used in hirsute patients with decreased serum androgen levels. The therapeutic effect of ketoconazole on hirsutism was seen after 6 months of therapy (172). The use of clomiphene citrate (Clomid), LHRH, FSH, and bromocriptine has aided in the recovery of ovarian function. The medical treatment pertaining to infertility in primary PCO is not elaborated on in this chapter.

3. Idiopathic Hirsutism

In the treatment of idiopathic hirsutism, antiandrogen agents as well as a local or systemic 5α-reductase inhibitor may be more specific therapeutic agents. However, all these antiandrogenic agents entail a risk of a teratogenic effect in women of child-bearing age. Therefore, absolute contraceptive measures are a must in women during antiandrogenic therapy.

There are several antiandrogenic compounds (173), including such steroid compounds as spironolactone, cyproterone acetate, RU-2956, and medrogestone, and nonsteroid compounds, such as cimetidine, flutamide, Finasteride, and stilbestrol. Of these, the medically acceptable agents used in the management of hirsutism are spironolactone and cyproterone acetate; however, combined flutamide and OC therapy also demonstrated marked improvement in hirsutism in one patient without side effects (174).

High-dose spironolactone (200–400 mg/day) interferes with DHT binding to its receptor and forms inactive complexes at the nuclear level, minimizing the androgen effect on hair growth. Spironolactone treatment has variable results in hirsute females, and other cosmetic hair removal is often necessary. In our experience, this agent alone or with OC was more effective in women with so-called idiopathic hirsutism defined by normal androgen levels.

Cyproterone acetate is a synthetic steroid derivative of 17-OHP and has both anti-androgenic activity and antigonadotropic actions (175). This agent is effective not only in the treatment of idiopathic hirsutism but also in other causes of androgen excess because of its antiandrogenic properties and because it reduces androgen production via suppression of gonadotropin secretion (176). Overall, the combination of cyproterone acetate and estrogen therapy reduces the production, transport, metabolism, and action of androgens (175). Numerous European sources indicate successful treatment of hirsutism of various causes using this combination.

5α-Reductase inhibitor should theoretically be an effective agent in the treatment of hirsutism. The 5α-reductase isoenzyme type 1 predominates in peripheral tissue and the type 2 isoenzyme in reproductive systems. A variety of compounds are found to have 5α-reductase inhibitory activity in vivo, including Δ^4-androsten-3-one-17β-carboxylic acid (177) and (4R)-5,10-seco-19-norpregna-4,5-diene-3,10,20-trione (178), as well as Δ^4-azasteroidal inhibitor. To date, the clinical use of systemic 5α-reductase inhibitor is limited to prostate cancer. Further research is necessary to develop a safe agent for the treatment of hirsutism, with precautions against teratogenic sequelae in women of child-bearing age.

VI. SUMMARY

This chapter has presented a review of androgen metabolism and disorders of androgen metabolism in peripubertal and postpubertal females. Although advances have been made in the knowledge of androgen physiopathology and in the method of diagnosis of various causes of hirsutism and PCO over the years, the results of current therapy are still largely unsatisfactory. Further advances in defining both the specific etiology for PCO and idiopathic hirsutism would result in the development of more specific therapeutic agents for these conditions. Currently, a few new agents are being experimented with, and the search for better therapeutic regimens must continue.

The psychologic impact of hirsutism in adolescent females and women continues to be underestimated in medical practice. Special attention should be given to these females' emotional well-being, in addition to the medical therapy described.

ACKNOWLEDGMENTS

This study was supported in part by Grant No. RO1 HD24360 from the U.S. Public Health Service and by a biomedical research grant from the University of Illinois at Chicago College of Medicine.

REFERENCES

1. Ebling FJG. Hair follicles and associated glands as androgen targets in androgen metabolism in hirsute and normal females. In: Horton R, Lobo RA, eds. Clinics in Endocrinology and Metabolism. Philadelphia: W. B. Saunders, 1986:319–339.
2. Goebelsman U, Lobo RA. Androgen excess. In: Mischell DR, Davajan V, eds. Infertility, Contraception, and Reproductive Endocrinology. Oradell, NJ: Medical Economics, 1987:303–317.
3. Shuster S. The sebaceous glands and primary cutaneous virilism. In: Jeffcotes SL, ed. Androgens and Anti-androgen Therapy. Chichester: John Wiley & Sons, 1982:1–21.
4. Gower DB, Fotherby K. Biosynthesis of the androgens and oestrogens. In: Makin HLJ, ed. Biochemistry of Steroid Hormones. London: Blackwell Scientific, 1975:77–104.
5. Sommerville IF, Collins WP. Indices of androgen production in women. In: Briggs MH, ed. Advances in Steroid Biochemistry and Pharmacology. New York: Academic Press, 1970:267–307.
6. Longcope C. Adrenal and gonadal androgen secretion in normal females. In: Horton R, Lobo RA, eds. Clinics in Endocrinology and Metabolism. Philadelphia: W. B. Saunders, 1986:213–228.
7. Pang S, Levine LS, Legido A, New MI. Adrenal androgen response to metyrapone, ACTH and corticotropin releasing factor (CRF) stimulation in children with hypopituitarism. J Clin Endocrinol Metab 1987; 64:282–284.
8. Jones T, Griffith K. Ultramicrochemical studies on the sites of formation of dehydroepiandrosterone sulfate in the adrenal cortex of the guinea pig. J Endocrinol 1968; 42:559–565.
9. McKerns KW. Steroidogenesis and metabolism in the adrenal cortex. In: Steroid Hormones and Metabolism. New York: Appleton-Century-Crofts, 1969:9–30.

10. Korth-Schutz S, Levine LS, New MI. Serum androgens in normal, prepubertal and pubertal children and in children with precocious adrenarche. J Clin Endocrinol Metab 1976; 42: 117–124.

11. Zumoff BB, Walsh T, Katz JL, et al. Subnormal plasma dehydroxyandrosterone to cortisol ratio in anorexia nervosa: a second hormonal parameter of ontogenic regression. J Clin Endocrinol Metab 1983; 56:668–672.

12. Cutler GB, Davis SE, Johnsonbaugh RE, Louriaux DL. Dissociation of cortisol and adrenal androgen secretion in patients with secondary adrenal insufficiency. J Clin Endocrinol Metab 1979; 49:604–609.

13. Parker LN, Odell WD. Evidence for existence of cortical androgen stimulating hormone. Am J Physiol 1979; 236:616–620.

14. Parker LN, Lifrak ET, Odell WD. A 60,000 molecular weight human pituitary glycopeptide stimulates adrenal androgen secretion. Endocrinology 1983; 13:2092–2096.

15. Rosenfeld RS, Hellman H, Roffwarg H, Weitzman ED, Fukushima DK, Gallagher TF. Dehydroisoandrosterone is secreted episodically and synchronously with cortisol by normal men. J Clin Endocrinol Metab 1971; 33:87–92.

16. Pang S, Lerner A, Stoner E, Oberfield S, Engle I, New MI. Late-onset adrenal steroid 3β-hydroxysteroid dehydrogenase deficiency: a cause of hirsutism in pubertal and post pubertal women. J Clin Endocrinol Metab 1985; 60:428–439.

17. DeJong FH, Van Der Molen HJ. Determination of dehydroepiandrosterone and dehydroepiandrosterone-sulfate in human plasma using electron capture detection of 4-androstene-3,6,-17-trione after gas liquid chromatography. J Endocrinol 1972; 53:461–474.

18. James VHT, Goodal AM. Androgen production in women. In: Jeffcote SL, ed. Androgens and Anti-androgen Therapy. Chichester: John Wiley & Sons, 1982:23–40.

19. Jeffcoate SL, Brookes RV, Lemi NY, London DR, Prienty FFG, Spathes GS. Androgen production in hypogonadal men. J Endocrinol 1967; 37:401–411.

20. Bardin CW, Lipsett MB. Testosterone and androstenedione blood production rates in normal women and women with idiopathic hirsutism or polycystic ovaries. J Clin Invest 1967; 46:891–902.

21. Horton E, Tait JF. Androstenedione production and interconversion rates measured in peripheral blood and studies on the possible sites of its conversion to testosterone. J Clin Invest 1966; 45:301–313.

22. Lloyd CW, Lobotsky J, Baird DT, et al. Concentration of unconjugated estrogens, androgens and gestagens in ovarian and peripheral venous plasma of women: the normal menstrual cycle. N Engl J Med 1971; 32:155–166.

23. Nieschlag E, Loriaux DL, Ruder HJ, Zucker IR, Kirschner MA, Lipsett MB. The secretion of dehydroepiandrosterone and DHEA-S in man. J Endocrinol 1973; 57:123–134.

24. Vande Wiele R, McDonald P, Gurpide E, Lieberman S. Studies on the secretion and interconversion of the androgens. Rec Pro Horm Res 1963; 19:275–310.

25. Zumoff B, Rosenfeld RS, Stain GW, Levin J, Fukushima DK. Sex differences in twenty-four hour mean plasma concentration of dehydroepiandrosterone (DHEA) and dehydroepiandrosterone sulfate (DHEAS) and the DHEA to DHEAS ratio in normal adults. J Clin Endocrinol Metab 1980; 57:330-333.

26. Purifoy FE, Koopmans LH, Tatum RW. Steroid hormones and aging; free testosterone, testosterone, and androstenedione in normal females aged 20–87 years. Hum Biol 1980; 52:181–192.

27. Parker LN, Odell WD. Control of adrenal androgen secretion.

28. Fritz MA, Speroff L. The endocrinology of the menstrual cycle; the interaction of folliculogenesis and neuroendocrine mechanisms. Fertil Steril 1982; 38:509–529.

29. McNatty KP, Makris A, Degrazia C, Osathanondh R, Ryan KJ. Production of progesterone, androgens and estrogens by granulosa cells, thecal tissue and stromal tissue from human ovaries in vitro. J Clin Endocrinol Metab 1979; 49:687–700.

30. Rice BF, Hammerstein J, Savard K. Steroid hormone formation in the human ovary: androstenedione, progesterone and estradiol during the human menstrual cycle. Am J Obstet Gynecol 1974; 119:1026–1032.

31. Brooks RV. Androgens: physiology, and pathology In: Makin HLJ ed. Biochemistry of Steroid Hormones. Oxford: Blackwell Scientific, 1975:289–311.

32. Judd HL, Yen SSC. Serum androstenedione and testosterone levels during the menstrual cycle. J Clin Endocrinol Metab 1973; 36:475–481.

33. Abraham GE. Ovarian and adrenal contribution to peripubertal androgens during the menstrual cycle. J Clin Endocrinol Metab 1974; 39:340–346.

34. Aedo AR, Pederson PH, Pederson SC, Diczfalusy E. Ovarian steroid secretion in normally menstruating women. 1. The contribution of the developing follicles. Acta Endocrinol (Copenh) 1980; 95:212–221.

35. Judd HL, Judd GE, Lucas WE, Yen SSC. Endocrine function of the post menopausal ovary: concentration of androgens and estrogens in ovarian and peripheral vein blood. J Clin Endocrinol Metab 1974; 39:1020–1024.

36. Cumming DC, Wall SR. Non-sex hormone binding globulin-bound testosterone as a marker for hyperandrogenism. J Clin Endocrinol Metab 1985; 61:873–876.

37. Vermeulen A. The physical state of testosterone in plasma. In: James VHT, Seria MS, Martini L, eds. The Endocrine Function of the Human Testis. New York: Academic Press, 1973:157–170.

38. Burke CW, Anderson DC. Sex-hormone-binding-globulin is an oestrogen amplifier. Nature 1972; 240:38–40.

39. Pentti K, Niklas HS. Changing concepts of active androgens in blood. In: Horton R, Lobo RA, eds. Clinics in Endocrinology and Metabolism. Philadelphia: W. B. Saunders, 1986: 247–258.

40. Rosenfield RL, Maudelonde T, Moll GW. Biologic effects of hyperandrogenism in polycystic ovary syndrome. Semin Reprod Endocrinol 1984; 281–295.

41. Klingman AM. The human hair cycle. J Invest Dermatol 1959; 33:307–316.

42. Rosenfield RL. Pilosebaceous physiology in relation to hirsutism and acne. In: Horton R, Lobo RA eds. Clinics in Endocrinology and Metabolism. Philadelphia: W. B. Saunders, 1986:341–362.

43. Peereboom-Wynia JDR, Beck CH. The influence of cyproterone-acetate orally on the hair root state in women with idiopathic hirsutism. Arch Dermatol Res 1977; 260:137–142.

44. Ebling FJ, Cooke ID, Randall VA, et al. Einfluss Von cyproteronacetat auf die aktivitat der haarfouikel und talgdrüsen beim menschen. In: Hammerstein J, Lachnit-Fixon U, Neumann F, Plewig G, eds. Androgenisierungser Schlinungen bei der Frau. Amsterdam: Excerpta Medica, 1979:243–249.

45. Ebling FJG, Randall VA, Sawers RS. Interrelationship between body hair growth, sebum excretion and endocrine parameters. Prostate 1984; 5:347–348.

46. Fang S, Andersen KM, Liao S. Receptor proteins for androgens; on the role of specific proteins in the retention of

17β-hydroxy-5α-androstan-3-one by the rat ventral prostate in vivo and in vitro. J Biol Chem 1969; 244:6584–6595.

47. Hay JB, Hodgins MB. Distribution of androgen metabolizing enzymes in isolated tissues of human forehead and axillary skin. J Endocrinol 1978; 79:29–39.

48. Mauvais-Jarvis P, Kutten F, Mowszowicz I. Androgen metabolism in human skin: importance of dihydrotestosterone formation in normal and abnormal target cells. In: Molinatti GM, Martini L, James VHT, eds. Androgenization in Women. New York: Raven Press, 1983:47.

49. Toscano V, Petrangeli E, Admo MV, Foli S, Caiola S, Sciarra F. Simultaneous determination of 5α-reduced metabolites of testosterone in human plasma. J Steroid Biochem 1981; 14:574–572.

50. Moghissi E, Ablan F, Horton R. Origin of plasma androstanediol glucuronide in men. J Clin Endocrinol Metab 1984; 59:417–421.

51. Morimoto I, Edmiston A, Hawks D, Horton R. Studies on the origin of androstanediol and androstanediol glucuronide in young and elderly men. J Clin Endocrinol Metab 1981; 52:772–778.

52. Deslyper JP, Sayed A, Punjabi U, Verdonck L, Vermeulen A. Plasma 5α-androstane-3α,17β-diol and urinary 5α-androstane-3α,17β-diol glucuronide, parameters of peripheral androgen action: a comparative study. J Clin Endocrinol Metab 1982; 54:386–391.

53. Horton R, Hawks D, Lobo RA. 3α,17β-Androstanediol glucuronide in plasma. J Clin Invest 1982; 69:1203–1206.

54. Lobo RA, Goebelsmann U, Horton R. Evidence for the importance of peripheral tissue events in the development of hirsutism in polycystic ovary syndrome. J Clin Endocrinol Metab 1983; 57:393–397.

55. Pang S, Wang M, Jeffries S, Riddick L, Clark A, Estrada E. Normal and elevated 3α-androstanediol glucuronide concentrations in women with various causes of hirsutism and its correlation with degree of hirsutism and androgen levels. J Clin Endocrinol Metab 1992; 75:243–248.

56. Mowszowicz I, Melinatou E, Doukane A, et al. Androgen binding capacity and 5α-reductase activity in pubic skin fibroblast from hirsute patients. J Clin Endocrinol Metab 1983; 56:1209–1213.

57. Kuttenn F, Mowszowicz I, Schaison G, Mauvais-Jarvis P. Androgen production and skin metabolism in hirsutism. J Endocrinol 1977; 75:83–91.

58. Thomas JP, Oake RJ. Androgen metabolism in the skin of hirsute women. J Clin Endocrinol Metab 1974; 38:19–122.

59. Glickman SP, Rosenfield RL. Androgen metabolism by isolated hairs from women with idiopathic hirsutism is usually normal. J Invest Dermatol 1984; 82:62–66.

60. Mauvais-Jarvis P, Kuttenn F, Gauthier-Wright F. Testosterone 5α-reductase in human skin as an index of androgenicity. In: James VHT, Serio M, Giusti G, eds. The Endocrine Function of the Human Ovary. London: Academic Press, 1976:481–494.

61. Cruikshak DD, Chapler FK, Yannone ME. Differential adrenal and ovarian suppression. Obstet Gynecol 1971; 38:724–733.

62. Abraham GE, Manlimos. The role of the adrenal cortex in hirsutism. In: James VHT, Serio M, Giusti G, Martini L, eds. The Endocrine Function of the Human Adrenal Cortex. London: Academic Press, 1976: 325–355.

63. Kirshner A, Jacobs J. Combined ovarian and adrenal vein catheterization to determine the site(s) of androgen overproduction in hirsute women. J Clin Endocrinol Metab 1971; 33:199–209.

64. Stahl NL, Teeslink CR, Greenblatt RB. Ovarian adrenal and

65. Moltz L, Schwartz U. Gonadal and adrenal androgen secretion in hirsute females. In: Horton R, Lobo RA, eds. Clinics in Endocrinology and Metabolism. Philadelphia: W. B. Saunders, 1986:229–245.

66. Newmark S, Dluhy RG, Williams GH, Pochi P, Rose LI. Partial 11-β and 21-hydroxylase deficiencies in hirsute women. Am J Obstet Gynecol 1977; 127:594–598.

67. Brooks RV, Mattingly D, Mills IH, Prunty FIG. Postpubertal adrenal virilism with biochemical disturbance of the congenital type of adrenal hyperplasia. BMJ 1960; 1:1294–1298.

68. Kohn B, Levine LS, Pollack MS, et al. Late-onset steroid 21-hydroxylase deficiency: a variant of classical congenital adrenal hyperplasia. J Clin Endocrinol Metab 1982; 55:817–827.

69. DeWailly D, Vantyghem-Haudiquet MC, Sainsard C, et al. Clinical and biological phenotypes in late-onset 21-hydroxylase deficiency. J Clin Endocrinol Metab 1986; 63:418–423.

70. Kutten F, Couillin P, Girard F, et al. Late-onset adrenal hyperplasia in hirsutism. N Engl J Med 1985; 313:224–231.

71. Temeck JW, Pang S, Nelson C, New MI. Genetic defects of steroidogenesis in premature adrenarche. J Clin Endocrinol Metab 1987; 64:609–617.

72. Chrousos GP, Loriaux DL, Mann D, Cutler JR. Late-onset 21-hydroxylase deficiency is an allelic variant of congenital adrenal hyperplasia characterized by attenuated clinical expression and different HLA haplotype association. Horm Res 1982; 16:193–200.

73. Pollack MS, Levine LS, O'Neill GJ, et al. HLA linkage and B14,DR1,BfS haplotype association with the genes for late-onset and cryptic 21-hydroxylase deficiency. Am J Hum Genet 1981; 33:540–550.

74. Speiser PW, Dupont B, Rubinstein P, Piazza A, Kastelan A, New MI. High frequency of non-classical steroid 21-hydroxylase deficiency. Am J Hum Genet 1985; 37:650–667.

75. Laron Z, Pollack MS, Zamir R, et al. Late-onset 21-hydroxylase deficiency and HLA in the Ashkenazi population: new allele at the 21-hydroxylase locus. Hum Immunol 1980; 1:55–56.

76. Speiser PW, New MI, White PC. Molecular genetic analysis of non-classic steroid 21-hydroxylase deficiency associated with HLA-B14,DR1. N Engl J Med 1988; 319:19–23.

77. Garlepp MJ, Wilton AN, Dawkins RL, White PC. Rearrangement of 21-hydroxylase gene in disease associated MHC supratypes. Immunogenetics 1986; 23:100–105.

78. Child DF, Builock DE, Anderson DC. Adrenal steroidogenesis in hirsute women. Clin Endocrinol (Oxf) 1980; 12:595–601.

79. Helmberg A, Tusie-Luna MT, Tabarelli M, Kofler R, White PC. R339H and P453S: CYP21 mutations associated with nonclassic steroid 21-hydroxylase deficiency that are not apparent gene conversions. Mol Endocrinol 1992; 6:1318–1322.

80. Higashi Y, Tanae A, Inoue H, Hiromasa T, Fuji-Kuriyama Y. Aberrant splicing and missense mutations cause steroid 21-hydroxylase [P-450(C21)] deficiency in humans: possible gene conversion products. Proc Natl Acad Sci USA 1988; 85:7486–7490.

81. Owerbach D, Sherman L, Ballard AL, Azziz R. Pro 453 to Ser mutation in CYP21 is associated with nonclassic steroid 21-hydroxylase deficiency. Mol Endocrinol 1992; 6:1211–1215.

82. Speiser PW, New MI, White PC. Molecular genetic analysis of non-classic steroid 21-hydroxylase deficiency associated with HLA-B14,DR1. N Engl J Med 1988; 319:19–23.

peripheral testosterone levels in the polycystic ovary syndrome. Am J Obstet Gynecol 1973; 117:194–200.

83. Wu DA, Chung B. Mutations of P450c21 at Cys[428], Val[281], or Ser[268] result in complete, partial, or no loss of enzymatic activity. J Clin Invest 1991; 88:519–523.

84. White PC, New MI. Genetic basis of endocrine disease 2: congenital adrenal hyperplasia due to 21-hydroxylase deficiency. J Clin Endocrinol Metab 1992; 74:6–11.

85. Azziz R, Zacur HA. 21-Hydroxylase deficiency in female hyperandrogenism: screening and diagnosis. J Clin Endocrinol Metab 1989; 69:577–584.

86. Eldar-Geva T, Hurwitz A, Vecsei P, Palti Z, Milwidsky A, Rosler A. Secondary biosynthetic defects in women with late-onset congenital adrenal hyperplasia. N Engl J Med 1990; 323:855–863.

87. Siegel S, Finegold DN, Lanes R, Lee PA. ACTH stimulation tests and plasma dehydroepiandrosterone sulfate levels in women with hirsutism. N Engl J Med 1990; 323:849–854.

88. Killeen AA, Hanson NQ, Eklund R, Cairl CJ, Eckfeldt JH. Prevalence of nonclassical congenital adrenal hyperplasia among women self-referred for electrolytic treatment of hirsutism. Am J Med Genet 1992; 42:197–200.

89. Arnaout MA. Late-onset congenital adrenal hyperplasia in women with hirsutism. Eur J Clin Invest 1992; 22:651–658.

90. Hawkins LA, Chasalow FI, Blethen SL. The role of adrenocorticotropin testing in evaluating girls with premature adrenarche and hirsutism/oligomenorrhea. J Clin Endocrinol Metab 1992; 74:248–253.

91. Bongiovanni AM. Unusual steroid pattern in congenital adrenal hyperplasia: deficiency of 3β-hydroxysteroid dehydrogenase. J Clin Endocrinol Metab 1961; 21:860–862.

92. Pang S, Levine LS, Stoner E, Opitz JM, New MI. Non–salt-losing congenital adrenal hyperplasia due to 3β-hydroxysteroid dehydrogenase deficiency with normal glomerulosa function. J Clin Endocrinol Metab 1983; 56:808–818.

93. Chang YT, Kulin HE, Garibaldi L, Suriano MJ, Bracki K, Pang S. Hypothalamic-pituitary-gonadal axis function in pubertal male and female siblings with glucocorticoid treated nonsalt-wasting 3β-hydroxysteroid dehydrogenase deficiency congenital adrenal hyperplasia. J Clin Endocrinol Metab 1993; 77:1251–1257.

94. Rosenfield RL, Rich BH, Wolfsdorf JI, et al. Pubertal presentation of congenital Δ5-3β-hydroxysteroid dehydrogenase deficiency. J Clin Endocrinol Metab 1980; 51:345–353.

95. Axelrod LR, Goldzieher JW, Ross SD. Concurrent 3β-hydroxysteroid dehydrogenase deficiency in adrenal and sclerocystic ovary. Acta Endocrinol (Copenh) 1965; 48:392–412.

96. Bongiovanni AM. Acquired adrenal hyperplasia: with special reference to 3β-hydroxysteroid dehydrogenase. Fertil Steril 1981; 35:599–608.

97. Lobo RA, Goebelsman U. Evidence for reduced 3β-ol-hydroxysteroid dehydrogenase activity in some hirsute women thought to have polycystic ovary syndrome. J Clin Endocrinol Metab 1981; 53:394–400.

98. Lorence MC, Murray BA, Trant JM, Mason JI. Human 3β-hydroxysteroid dehydrogenase/$\Delta^{5->4}$ isomerase from placenta: expression in non-steroidogenic cells of a protein that catalyzes the dehydrogenation/isomerization of C21 and C19 steroids. Endocrinology 1990; 126:2493–2498.

99. Rhéaume E, Lachance Y, Zhao H, et al. Structure and expression of a new complementary DNA encoding the almost exclusive 3β-hydroxysteroid dehydrogenase/Δ^{5}-Δ^{4} isomerase in human adrenals and gonads. Mol Endocrinol 1991; 5:1147–1157.

100. Rhéaume E, Simard J, Morel Y, et al. Congenital adrenal hyperplasia due to point mutations in the type II 3β-hydroxysteroid dehydrogenase gene. Nat Gene 1992; 1:239–245.

101. Simard J, Rhéaume E, Sanchez R, et al. Molecular basis of congenital adrenal hyperplasia due to 3β-hydroxysteroid dehydrogenase deficiency. Mol Endocrinol 1993; 7:716–728.

102. Chang YT, Kappy MS, Iwamoto K, Wang J, Yang X, Pang S. Mutations in the type II 3β-hydroxysteroid dehydrogenase gene in a patient with classic salt-wasting 3β-HSD deficiency congenital adrenal hyperplasia. Pediatr Res 1993; 34:698–700.

103. Sanchez R, Rhéaume E, Laflamme N, Rosenfield RL, Labrie F, Simard J. Detection and functional characterization of the novel missense mutation Y254D in type II 3β-hydroxysteroid dehydrogenase (3βHSD) gene of a female patient with nons-alt-losing 3βHSD deficiency. J Clin Endocrinol Metab 1994; 78:561–567.

104. Chang YT, Zhang L, Mason I, et al. Redefining hormonal criteria for mild 3β-hydroxysteroid dehydrogenase (3β-HSD) deficiency (def) congenital adrenal hyperplasia (CAH) by molecular analysis of the type II 3β-HSD gene. Pediatr Res 1994; 35:96A.

105. Kohn B, Levine LS, Pollack MS, et al. Late-onset steroid 21-hydroxylase deficiency: a variant of classical congenital adrenal hyperplasia. J Clin Endocrinol Metab 1982; 55:817–827.

106. Levine LS, Dupont B, Lorenzen F, et al. Genetic and hormonal characterization of cryptic 21-hydroxylase deficiency. J Clin Endocrinol Metab 1981; 53:1193–1198.

107. New MI, Lorenzen AF, et al. Genotyping steroid 21-hydroxylase deficiency hormonal reference data. J Clin Endocrinol Metab 1983; 57:320–326.

108. Kandel FR, Rudd BT, Butt WR, Logan R, Loden DR. Androgen and cortisol response to ACTH stimulation in women with hyperprolactinemia. Clin Endocrinol (Oxf) 1980; 9:123–130.

109. Vermeulen A, Ando S. Prolactin and adrenal androgen secretion. Clin Endocrinol (Oxf) 1978; 8:295–303.

110. Belisle S, Menard J. Adrenal androgen production in hyperprolactinemic state. Fertil Steril 1986; 33:396–400.

111. Cooke ID, Sawers RS. Investigation of hirsutism and selection of patients for treatment. In: Jeffcoate SL, ed. Androgens and Anti-androgen Therapy. New York: John Wiley and Sons, 1982: 95–112.

112. Carter JM, Tyson JE, Warne GL, McNeilly AS, Faiman C, Friesen HG. Adrenalcortical function in hyperprolactinemic women. J Clin Endocrinol Metab 1977; 45:973–980.

113. Ebling FJ, Ebling E, Skinner J. The influence of pituitary hormones on the response of the sebaceous glands of the rat to testosterone. J Endocrinol 1969; 45:245–256.

114. Futterweit W. Clinical features of polycystic ovarian disease. In: Polycystic Ovarian Disease. New York: Springer-Verlag, 1984:83–95.

115. Coney P. Polycystic ovarian disease: current concepts of pathophysiology and therapy. Fertil Steril 1984; 42:667–682.

116. Lobo RA. Hirsutism in polycystic ovary syndrome: current concepts. Clin Obstet Gynecol 1991; 34:817–826.

117. Futterweit W. The pathologic anatomy of polycystic ovarian disease. In: Polycystic Ovarian Disease. New York: Springer-Verlag, 1984:41–46.

118. Pang S, Levine LS, New MI. Puberty in congenital adrenal hyperplasia. In: Grumbach MM, Sizonenko PC, Aubert ML, eds. Control of the Onset of Puberty. Baltimore: Williams and Wilkins, 1990:669–687.

119. Levine LS, Korth-Schutz S, Saenger P, Sweeney WJ III, Beling CG, New MI. Disordered puberty in treated congenital adrenal hyperplasia. In: Lee PA, et al., eds. Congenital Adrenal Hyperplasia. Baltimore: University Park Press, 1977: 511–526.

120. Sizonenko PC, Schindler AM, Kohlberg IJ, Paunier L. Gonadotropins, testosterone and oestrogen levels in relation

to ovarian morphology in 11β-hydroxylase deficiency. Acta Endocrinol (Copenh) 1972;71:539–550.

121. Bergman P, Siogren B, Hakansson B. Hypertensive form of congenital adrenocortical hyperplasia: analysis of a case with co-existing polycystic ovaries. Acta Endocrinol (Copenh) 1962; 40:555–564.

122. Abu-Haydar N, Laidlaw JC, Nusimovich B, Sturgis S. Hyperadrenocorticism and the Stein-Leventhal syndrome. Abstract of paper presented at 36th Annual Meeting of the Endocrine Society. J Clin Endocrinol Metab 1954; 14:766.

123. Lobo RA. Polycystic ovarian syndrome. In: Mishell DR Jr, Dacajan V, eds. Infertility, Contraception and Reproductive Endocrinology, 2nd ed. Oradell, NJ: Medical Economics Co., 1985:319–336.

124. Pang S, Softness B, Sweeney WJ III, New MI. Hirsutism, polycystic ovarian disease and ovarian 17-ketosteroid reductase deficiency. N Engl J Med 1987; 316:1295–1301.

125. Canales ES, Zarate A, Castelazo-Ayala. Primary amenorrhea associated with polycystic ovaries: endocrine, cytogenetic and therapeutic considerations. Obstet Gynecol 1971; 37:205–210.

126. Yen SSC, Chaney C, Judd HL. Functional aberrations of the hypothalamic-pituitary system in polycystic ovary syndrome: a consideration of the pathogenesis. In: James VHT, Serio M, Giusti G, eds. The Endocrine Function of the Human Ovary. New York: Academic Press, 1976:373–385.

127. Yen SSC. The polycystic ovary syndrome. Clin Endocrinol (Oxf) 1980; 12:177–207.

128. Kirschner MA, Zucker IR, Jespersen DL. Ovarian and adrenal vein catheterization studies in women with idiopathic hirsutism. In: James VHT, Serio M, Giusti G, eds. The Endocrine Function of the Human Ovary. New York: Academic Press, 1976:443–456.

129. Takai I, Taii S, Takakura K, Mori T. Three types of polycystic ovarian syndrome in relation to androgenic function. Fertil Steril 1990; 56:856–862.

130. Rebar R, Judd HL, Yen SSC, Rakoff J, Vadenberg G, Naftolin F. Characterization of the inappropriate gonadotropin secretion in polycystic ovarian syndrome. J Clin Invest 1976; 57:1320–1329.

131. Burger CW, Korsen T, van Kessel H, van Dop PA, Caron FJM, Schoemaker J. Pulsatile luteinizing hormone patterns in the follicular phase of the menstrual cycle, polycystic ovarian disease (PCOD) and non-PCOD secondary amenorrhea. J Clin Endocrinol Metab 1985; 61:1126–1132.

132. Lobo RA, Kletzky OA, Campeau JD, et al. Elevated bioactive luteinizing hormone in women in polycystic ovary syndrome. Fertil Steril 1983; 39:674.

133. Rebar RW. Gonadotropin secretion in polycystic ovarian disease. Semin Reprod Endocrinol 1984; 2:223.

134. Futterweit W. Pathophysiology of polycystic ovarian disease. In: Polycystic Ovarian Disease. New York: Springer-Verlag, 1984:49–82.

135. Schoemaker J, Wentz AC, Jones GS, et al. Stimulation of follicular growth with "pure" FSH in patients with anovulation and elevated LH levels. Obstet Gynecol 1978; 51:270–277.

136. Siiteri PK, MacDonald PC. Role of extraglandular estrogen in human endocrinology. In: Greep RO, Astwood EB, eds. Handbook of Physiology: Endocrinology, Vol. II, Sec. 7. Washington, DC: American Physiological Society, 1973:615–629.

137. Futterweit W. Hyperprolactinemia and polycystic ovarian disease. In: Polycystic Ovarian Disease. New York: Springer-Verlag, 1984:97–111.

138. Rosenfield RL, Barnes RB, Cara JF, et al. Dysregulation of cytochrome P450c17α as the cause of polycystic ovarian syndrome. Fertil Steril 1990; 53:785.

139. Shoupe D, Kumar DD, Lobo RA. Insulin resistance in polycystic ovarian syndrome. Am J Obstet Gynecol 1983; 147:588–592.

140. Stuart CA, Peters EJ, Prince MJ, Richards G, Cavallo A, Meyer WJI. Insulin resistance with acanthosis nigricans: the role of obesity and androgen excess. Metabolism 1986; 35:197–205.

141. Jialal I, Naiker P, Reddi K, Moodley J, Joubert SM. Evidence for insulin resistance in nonobese patients with polycystic ovarian disease. J Clin Endocrinol Metab 1987; 64:1066–1069.

142. Geffner ME, Kaplan SA, Bersch N, Golde DW, Landaw EM, Chang RJ. Persistence of insulin resistance in polycystic ovarian disease after inhibition of ovarian steroid secretion. Fertil Steril 1986; 45:327–333.

143. Dunaif A, Green G, Futterweit W, Doberjansky A. Suppression of hyperandrogenism does not improve peripheral or hepatic insulin resistance in the polycystic ovary syndrome. J Clin Endocrinol Metab 1990; 70:699–704.

144. Barbieri RL. Hyperandrogenic disorders. Clin Obstet Gynecol 1990; 33:640–654.

145. Barbieri RL, Makris A, Ryan KJ. Insulin stimulates androgen accumulation in incubations of human ovarian stroma and theca (abstract). Obstet Gynecol 1984; 64(Suppl):73.

146. Barbieri RL, Makris A, Randall RW, et al. Insulin stimulates androgen accumulation in incubations of ovarian stroma obtained from women with hyperandrogenism. J Clin Endocrinol Metab 1986; 62:904.

147. Pasupuleti V, Horton R. Insulin-like growth factor can alter steroid 5α-reductase activity and formation of dihydrotestosterone in skin fibroblast. Clin Res 1990; 39:2088.

148. Kiddy DS, Hamilton-Fairley D, Seppala M, et al. Diet-induced charges in sex hormone binding globulin and free testosterone in women with normal or polycystic ovaries: correlation with serum insulin and insulin-like growth factor-I. Clin Endocrinol. (Oxf) 1989; 31:757.

149. Kadawaki T, Berins C, Cama A, et al. Two mutant alleles of the insulin receptor gene in a patient with extreme insulin resistance. Science 1988; 240:787.

150. Yoshimas Y, Seino S, Whittaker J, et al. Insulin resistant diabetes due to a point mutation that prevents insulin proreceptor processing. Science 1988; 240:784.

151. Moller DE, Flier JS. Detection of an alternation in the insulin-receptor gene in a patient with insulin resistance, acanthosis nigricans and the polycystic ovary syndrome (type A insulin resistance). N Engl J Med 1988; 319:1526.

152. Kahn CR, White MF. The insulin receptor and the molecular mechanism of insulin action. J Clin Invest 1988; 82:1151.

153. Judd HL, Scully RE, Herbst AL, et al. Familial hyperthecosis; comparison of endocrinologic and histologic findings with polycystic ovarian disease. Am J Obstet Gynecol 1973; 117:976–982.

154. Behrman SJ, Scully RE. Case records of the Massachusetts General Hospital; infertility and irregular menses in a 27 year old woman. N Engl J Med 1972; 217:1192–1195.

155. Saez JM, de Peretti E, Morera AM, David M, Bertrand J. Familial male pseudohermaphroditism with gynecomastia due to a testicular 17-ketosteroid reductase defect. I. Studies in vivo. J Clin Endocrinol Metab 1971; 32:604–610.

156. Saez JM, Morera AM, de Peretti E, Bertrand J. Further in vivo studies in male pseudohermaphroditism with gynecomastia due to a testicular 17-ketosteroid reductase defect (compared to a case of testicular feminization). J Clin Endocrinol Metab 1972; 34:598–600.

157. Virdis R, Saenger P. 17β-Hydroxysteroid dehydrogenase

deficiency; pediatric and adolescent endocrinology. In: Laron Z, New MI, Levine LS, eds. Adrenal Disease in Childhood. Basel: Karger, 1984: 110–124.

158. Pang S, Leibel RL, Sweeney WJ III, New MI. Hirsutism due to gonadotropin-dependent androgen secreting lipoid cell ovarian tumor. In: 7th International Congress of Endocrinology. Amsterdam: Excerpta Medica, 1984:1254.

159. Wright F, Mowszowicz I, Mauvais-Jarvis P. Urinary 5α-androstane 3α, 17β-diol radioimmunoassay: a new clinical evaluation. J Clin Endocrinol Metab 1978; 47:850–854.

160. Horton R, Lobo RA. Peripheral androgens and the role of androstanediol glucuronide. In: Horton R, Lobo RA, eds. Clinics in Endocrinology and Metabolism. Philadelphia: W. B. Saunders, 1986:293–300.

161. Rosenfield RL, Moll CW Jr. The role of proteins in the distribution of plasma androgens and estradiol. In: Molinatti GM, Martini L, James VHT, eds. Androgenization in Women. New York: Raven Press, 1983:25.

162. Ferriman D, Gallwey JD. Clinical assessment of body hair growth in women. J Clin Endocrinol Metab 1961; 21:1440–1447.

163. Hatch R, Rosenfield RL, Kim MH, Tredway D. Hirsutism: implication, etiology, and management. Am J Obstet Gynecol 1981; 140:815–830.

164. Swanson M, Sauerbrei EE, Cooperberg PL. Medical implications of ultrasonically detected polycystic ovaries. J Clin Ultrasound 1981; 9:219–220.

165. Parisi L, Tramont M, Casciano S, Zurli A, Gazzarrini O. The role of ultrasound in the study of polycystic ovarian disease. J Clin Ultrasound 1982; 10:167–168.

166. Morley P, Barnett E. The ovarian mass. In: Saunders RC, James AE, eds. The Textbook of the Principle and Practice of Ultrasonography in Obstetrics and Gynecology. New York: Appleton-Century-Crofts, 1980:357–386.

167. Inaudi P, Dambrogio G, Massafra C, Facchini V, Genazzani AR. Impaired pregnenolone secretion after combined cyproterone acetate and ethinyl estradiol therapy in hirsute patients. Gynecol Obstet Invest. 1982; 14:106–120.

168. Jones DB, Ibraham I, Edward CR. Hair growth and androgen response in hirsute women treated with continuous cyproterone acetate and cyclinical ethinyl estradiol. Acta Endocrinol (Copenh) 1987; 116:497–501.

169. Mongioi A, Maugeri G, Macchi M, et al. Effects of gonadotrophin-releasing hormone analogue (GnRH-A) administration on serum gonadotrophin and steroid levels in patients with polycystic ovarian disease. Acta Endocrinol (Copenh) 1986; 111:228–234.

170. Andreyko JL, Monroe SE, Jaffe RB. Treatment of hirsutism with a gonadotropin-releasing hormone agonist (nafarelin). J Clin Endocrinol Metab 1986; 63:854–859.

171. Suriano MJ, Riddick L, Faries S, et al. (sponsor Pang S) Clinical, hormonal, and radiological studies in adolescent hirsute females with increased ovarian androgen production during and after long term LHRH analog (Lupron®) treatment. In: 75th Annual Endocrine Society Meeting, Program and Abstract, 1993: 396.

172. Martikainen H, Heikkinen J, Roukonen A, Kaupila A. Hormonal and clinical effects of ketoconazole on hirsute women. J Clin Endocrinol Metab 1988; 66:987–991.

173. Trembly RR. Treatment of hirsutism with spironolactone. In: Horton R, Lobo RA, eds. Clinics in Endocrinology and Metabolism. Philadelphia: W. B. Saunders, 1986:363–372.

174. Cusan., Belanger A, Tremblay RR, Manhes G, Labrie F. Treatment of hirsutism with the pure antiandrogen flutimide. J Am Acad Dermatol 1990; 23:464–469.

175. Miller JA, Jacobs HS. Treatment of hirsutism and acne with cyproterone acetate. In: Horton R, Lobo RA, eds. Clinics in Endocrinology and Metabolism. Philadelphia: W. B. Saunders, 1986:373–390.

176. Neumann F, Schleusener A. Pharmacology of cyproterone acetate with special reference to the skin. In: Vokaer R, Fanta D, eds. Proceedings of the Diane Symposium. Excerpta Medica: Brussels, 19–51.

177. Voigt W, Hsia SL. The antiandrogenic action of 4-androsten-3-one-17β-carboxylic acid and its methyl ester on hamster flank organ. Endocrinology 1980; 92:1216–1222.

178. Robaire B, Covey DF, Robinson CH, Ewing LL. Selective inhibition of rat epididymal steroid Δ4-5 reductase by conjugated allenic 3-oxo-5, 10-secosteroids, J Steroid Biochem 1977; 8:307–310.

18

Hypogonadism at Adolescence: Lack or Delay of Sexual Development?

Jean-Claude Job
Faculté de Médecine Cochin,
Paris, France

I. INTRODUCTION

Lack of sexual development at adolescence is not synonymous with hypogonadism (Chap. 13). The clinical situations described in this chapter cover the entire spectrum of cases in which adolescent sexual development is incomplete or is completely lacking beyond an age corresponding to the physiologic limit of 2 standard deviations above the average (1,2).

Hypogonadism at adolescence may result from primary gonadal defects; primary deficiency of the pituitary gonadotropic hormones follicle-stimulating hormone (FSH) and/or luteinizing hormone (LH); or genetic, nutritional, and various other factors that influence general and/or sexual maturation. Any one of these alterations may result in partial or complete lack of pubertal achievement (see Table 6 in Chap. 13).

From a practical point of view, there is a difference between primary gonadal failure, in which elevated gonadotropins allow an immediate and easy diagnosis, and hypogonadism, with low gonadotropin output, which makes the diagnosis uncertain and requires protracted follow-up in an often critical psychologic situation.

II. HYPERGONADOTROPIC HYPOGONADISM

Primary gonadal failure or dysgenesis is a common cause of complete or partial lack of sexual development in phenotypic girls. In contrast, it is uncommon in phenotypic males with absent or delayed puberty. Most adolescents in this group have elevated levels of LH and/or FSH in plasma and urine, which allow easy indirect recognition of the gonadal defect. Few patients demonstrate levels of gonadotropins that remain at the upper limit of the normal range after age 10 years: this elevation must then be confirmed by measurement of pituitary reserve using the gonadorelin (gonadotropin-releasing hormone and LH-releasing hormone, LHRH) test.

A. Phenotypic Females

1. Turner Syndrome

Turner syndrome is the main cause of primary hypogonadism with the female phenotype, as described in detail in Chapter 19. Diagnosis should be made before age 10 years to ensure proper management. The secondary female characteristics of adolescence are completely lacking in at least half of patients. In at least one-third of girls with Turner syndrome, partial breast development occurs at the usual age or a little later. Very seldom do girls with Turner syndrome reach Tanner's stage 5 or menstruate.

2. Noonan Syndrome

Turner syndrome must be distinguished from its dysmorphic copy, Noonan syndrome (3), because both are characterized by short stature with slow growth and similar external dysmorphic features. The peculiar characteristics of Noonan syndrome include mental impairment, pulmonic stenosis or atrial septal defect, and normal karyotype 46, XX in female cases and 46, XY in male cases. Partial hypogonadism is frequent in male patients with Noonan syndrome but rare in females. Most cases are sporadic, although a few familial cases have been reported (3).

3. Other Types of Primary Gonadal Dysgenesis in Phenotypic Females

Pure gonadal dysgenesis is a rare entity defined by the complete or nearly complete absence of ovaries in phenotypic girls with normal height and no dysmorphic features. Sexual development may be completely lacking. More often, these patients have some degree of breast development but remain amenorrheic during and after adolescence. Diagnosis is facilitated through demonstration of high levels of gonadotropins. Pelvic ultrasonography shows normal, small prepubertal uterus and fallopian tubes, without measurable ovaries. The dysgenetic gonads are streak gonads as in Turner syndrome or hypoplastic ovaries.

In most cases, the karyotype is normal female, 46, XX. The XX pure gonadal dysgenesis may be a familial disease transmitted as an autosomal recessive character (4). Familial cases strongly suggest the role of one or several autosomal genes on ovarian organization of primordial gonads. There are also sporadic or apparently sporadic cases.

Karyotype 46, XY is found in approximately one-fifth of cases, usually tall girls with large shoulders and female genitalia. Familial cases exist, suggesting either recessive inheritance, with both female and ambiguous individuals in the kindred, or dominant transmission (5). More cases appear as sporadic. Recent genetic studies have demonstrated microdeletions on either the Y (6) or the X (7) chromosome. XY gonadal dysgenesis carries the risk of gonadoblastoma and/or carcinoma in the gonadic rudiments. Thus castration is mandatory and should be performed before the end of adolescence.

Primary gonadal dysgenesis may be associated with other malformations, such as camptomelia (8), congenital deafness, Perrault syndrome (8,9), cleft lip (10), cerebellar ataxia and other neurologic abnormalities (11,12). Gonadal dysgenesis can also exist in autosomal anomalies, such as trisomy 13, trisomy 18 (8), and translocation 18 (13).

4. Acquired Ovarian Lesions

Pelvic exposure to radiation doses over 10 Gy involving the ovaries was frequent in the management of abdominopelvic tumors and lymphomas and, for a time, became a common cause of adolescent infantilism in girls (14). Advances in chemotherapy have largely replaced the use of radiation in recent years. Chemotherapy for leukemia or tumors during childhood may also damage the ovocytes (14). However, some compensation of ovarian function after puberty is possible (15). Under such conditions, partial hypogonadism may be suspected but not ascertained at adolescence.

Traumatic ovarian lesions may result from various accidents, but the main cause is bilateral torsion of the fallopian tubes during childhood. In these girls, the degree of ovarian atrophy can seldom be determined before midpuberty. Unilateral torsion leads to the recommendation of ovariopexy on the other side, because torsion of the second ovary, possibly caused by bilateral cysts, is a high risk, whereas ovariopexy is easy surgery. Bilateral recurring cysts or tumors of the ovaries rarely necessitate complete prepubertal castration.

Other acquired diseases may lead to ovarian insufficiency at adolescence. Juvenile autoimmune polyendocrinopathy, which may be associated with chronic moniliasis, involves the ovaries less often than the thyroid, parathyroid, or pancreatic islets (Chap. 1) (16). Infectious oophoritis from viral (mumps) or bacterial origin is seldom a cause of adolescent hypogonadism.

Congenital diseases are also causes of ovarian failure.

This was frequent in galactosemia when diagnosis and dietary treatment were not available at birth (17). Congenital adrenal hyperplasia (see Chap. 9) related to the rare recessive diseases 17-hydroxylase deficiency (Biglieri type, with hypertension and hypokalemia) and 17, 20-lyase deficiency present as complete infantilism with elevated plasma levels of progesterone and 17-hydroxyprogesterone because the defect involves sex steroid biosynthesis (18,19). Most patients are phenotypic females, with either 46, XX or XY karyotype. Affected XY subjects may also have ambiguous external genitalia.

Another rare congenital cause of female hypogonadism is the "resistant ovary" syndrome, resulting from abnormality of the FSH receptor. Differential diagnosis with gonadal dysgenesis needs biopsy. Resistance may be improved by estrogen therapy (20).

B. Phenotypic Males: Klinefelter Syndrome

Klinefelter syndrome, the most frequent cause of hypergonadotropic hypogonadism in phenotypic males (approximately 1:1000 in extended studies), does not delay the onset of sexual development. Puberty starts at the usual age, but with small testes. The secondary sex characteristics do not attain normal adult development. The persisting small testicular size provides speculation, but the diagnosis is confirmed by the presence of one or more extra X chromosomes in the karyotype. Tall stature with long legs and arms and poor muscular development are obvious at adolescence (Chap. 12). Gynecomastia is not constant and occurs later (Chap. 14).

School performance is usually poor, with an average verbal intelligence quotient 10–20 points below that of controls (21), without increased prevalence of psychopathology. Hormonal measurements at adolescence usually show high FSH levels, moderately elevated LH, and plasma testosterone in the low normal range. After years, gonadotropins increase and testosterone decreases, with an increasing estradiol-testosterone ratio.

The mechanism for an extra X chromosome may be nondisjunction of one X during meiosis of the gametes or early mitosis of the zygote. Recent studies have shown that half of cases result from meiotic nondisjunction in the spermatogonial meiosis and the other half from the same event in the meiosis occurring in the first step of ovocyte maturation (rarely during the second step) (22).

Variants with more than one extra gonosome usually have more severe genital and mental impairment. The most frequent have XXXY and XXYY karyotypes (23). The XXXXY variant is rare and has multiple malformations (24). Various mosaic versions of the X polygonosomia have been reported. XX human maleness with or without hypospadias may be considered another variant of Klinefelter syndrome. This has allowed important discoveries regarding the role of the Y chromosome and X-Y interchanges (25,26).

Other types of primary congenital testicular failure in otherwise normal males include anorchia, or the "vanishing testes syndrome," which features normal male genitalia but an empty scrotum at birth (27). It can be differentiated from abdominal cryptorchidism by the high levels of LH and/or FSH, their elevated response to the LHRH test, and, most importantly the lack of a testosterone response to a short stimulation test with human chorionic gonadotropin (hCG; Chap. 20).

LH resistance caused by an LH receptor abnormality has been reported as a cause of infantilism in a phenotypic male (28).

Acquired bilateral lesions of the testes that occur during childhood and may lead to hypogonadism at adolescence include bilateral testicular torsion, severe scrotal trauma, and unskilled surgery for cryptorchidism. The sequelae of orchitis during childhood (e.g., mumps) are exceptional causes of overt hypogonadism. Prepubertal testicular exposure to x-rays and/or to chemotherapies, such as cyclophosphamide or chlorambucil, affects germ and Sertoli cells more than Leydig cells and thus causes infertility with small testes rather than complete lack of puberty (29,30). However, early and incomplete puberty is possible after treatment for leukemia (15).

C. Gender-Ambiguous Patients

Congenital adrenal hyperplasia with 17α-hydroxylase and 17,20-lyase or 20,22-desmolase deficiency prevents testosterone biosynthesis and is a possible but extremely rare cause of hypogonadism in an ambiguous male (18).

Various malformative syndromes with ambiguous genitalia or simple hypospadias and a small penis show some degree of hypogonadism with elevated gonadotropins at adolescence. Variants of Turner syndrome, other chromosomal anomalies, and Noonan syndrome are included (Chaps. 19 and 20). Primary male hypogonadism has also been reported in the following syndromes: Alström (with retinitis); Bloom (with photosensitive erythema); CHARGE association (with choanal atresia and heart defect); Leopard (with lentiginosis); Louis-Bar (with ataxia and telangectasia); Rothmund-Thomson (with poikiloderma); Smith-Lemli-Opitz (with peculiar facies and failure to thrive); and Steinert syndrome (with myotonia) (8,31). Genetic investigation may show how gene deletions or mutations cause such associations.

Syndromes of congenital resistance to androgens include various types of hypogonadism (32) in a spectrum of ambiguous subjects (Chap. 20).

A distinctive group of male gonadal dysgenesis includes the syndromes associating male pseudohermaphroditism and hypogonadism with early chronic nephropathy and/or Wilms' tumor: syndromes of Drash or Denys-Drash, Frasier (33–36), and Wilms-aniridia-gonadoblastoma-retardation (WAGR) syndrome related to a 11p13 gene deletion.

Partial testicular dysgenesis, first described as "syndrome of rudimentary testes," is another distinctive group of males with hypospadias and/or micropenis, very small testes, and no detected cytogenetic abnormality (37). Some cases are familial, with intrakindred variability including various types of primary gonadal dysgenesis, possibly hermaphroditism (38,39).

Testicular unresponsiveness to LH results in the absence of Leydig cells, poorly masculinized or ambiguous external genitalia, and hypogonadism with a high output of LH at adolescence. The absence or defect of the LH receptor on Leydig cells has been demonstrated (28). Familial cases have been reported.

D. Treatment of Hypergonadotropic Hypogonadisms

Primary gonadal failure requires replacement therapy with gender-appropriate steroids. Treatment should begin when the bone age approaches 13 years in males and 10.5 years in females, provided that the patient has reached the corresponding height.

In males, long-acting testosterone derivates, such as enanthate, via intramuscular (IM) injection, offer the most appropriate replacement. A monthly dose of 100 mg during the first 2 years is generally sufficient to induce good development of the penis and sexual hair, to allow normal linear growth, and to improve the male appearance. From the third year, it should be increased to 200–300 mg/month, preferably divided into injections every 2–3 weeks. Later it should be adjusted to produce both testosterone levels in the normal adult range and satisfactory erections. Higher doses during the first year can provoke gynecomastia and acceleration of bone epiphyseal fusion. We have no experience with oral testosterone undecanoate (40) or with transcutaneous dihydrotestosterone, which require daily treatment and are less appropriate for hypogonadic adolescents. Psychologic support for these patients is extremely important and requires skilled doctors, nurses, and psychologists who can devote substantial time to both the patient and his family. For smallness of testes, implanting protheses after the 2–3 years required for appropriate development of the scrotum completes the management.

In females, replacement therapy consists of cyclic administration of estrogens. We preferably prescribe conjugated estrogens for 21–24 days per month at daily doses increasing from 0.3 mg in the first 6 months to 0.62 mg for 1 or 2 years and then to 1.25 mg per day. Oral ethinyl estradiol and 17β-estradiol, transcutaneous estradiol gel or patches, may also be used. From month 6, monthly administration of a progestagen, such as 10 mg/day of dydrogestone or 0.5 mg/day of demegestone from day 12 or 13 up to the end of each cycle, is mandatory. The development and consistency of the breast and the menses are the best guides for adjusting individual treatments. Follow-up of blood lipids and coagulability is required. Contraceptive pills, often requested by hypogonadic girls for convenience and other personal reasons, are not appropriate.

III. HYPOGONADOTROPIC HYPOGONADISM

Primary deficiency of the pituitary gonadotropins FSH and LH may be isolated, may be associated with other disturbances of anterior pituitary secretions, or may be secondary to various chronic diseases.

A. Multiple Pituitary Deficiencies or Disturbances

These are the most frequently seen in pediatric practice. Hypopituitarism resulting from such malformations as septo-optic dysplasia and other midline defects or various acquired neonatal and postnatal lesions of the pituitary, its stalk, and the suprahypophyseal hypothalamic zone, frequently associates both growth hormone (GH) and gonadotropin insufficiency, thus leading to short stature and hypogonadotropic hypogonadism (Chap. 2).

The absence of puberty at the usual age in GH-deficient adolescents does not preclude further spontaneous sexual development, however, because it can also be caused by a delay in body maturation. It is well known (41) that puberty in isolated idiopathic GH deficiency is delayed at least 2 years.

Interpretation of blood and urine gonadotropin measurements and the LHRH test may be difficult in GH-deficient patients until the bone age has reached 12.5–13 years in males and 10.5–11 years in females. Complete unresponsiveness to the acute LHRH test, which is highly characteristic of hypogonadotropism, was found in only one-quarter of children and adolescents with idiopathic GH deficiency in our series (42). In the other GH-deficient patients in this study, the response of one or both gonadotropins was in the normal prepubertal range, but it did not preclude further clinical evidence of gonadotropic deficiency.

Hyperprolactinemia, a well-known cause of hypogonadotropism in adults, is less frequent during adolescence (43), and galactorrhea is uncommon at this age. Headache is the first symptom in most cases. However, low gonadotropin levels in subjects with pubertal delay or hypogonadism at any age requires prolactin measurement and, if prolactin is elevated, appropriate neuroradiologic examination for an adenoma. Prolactinomas are more frequent in girls than in boys. The diagnosis of primary hyperprolactinemia, with or without detectable adenoma, requires specific treatment with bromocriptine and its derivatives.

B. Isolated Gonadotropic Deficiency

Isolated gonadotropic deficiency (IGD) was first described by Kallmann and colleagues (44) as a familial multisymptomatic disease. During adolescence, it is often difficult to distinguish IGD from constitutional delay of puberty (CDP) if familial history and/or associated features characteristic of Kallmann syndrome are not found. This stresses the importance of repeated extensive examination of the patient and recording the familial history in hypogonadic patients with low gonadotropin levels.

At adolescence, IGD is diagnosed much more often in males than in females, with a sex ratio of 5:1 in our series (42). This was higher than in the adult series, which included females referred for amenorrhea or anovulation following an apparently normal puberty.

1. Males

Our patients were referred and/or diagnosed at age 16–17 years for absence of puberty (42). Their height was in the normal range for age, with some degree of macroskelia, poor muscular development, and excess fat. The bone age was delayed by 1–6 years. Half had some pubic hair, but the penis was small, either in the normal prepubertal range in two-thirds of cases, or definitely small, below 3.5 cm length, in the remaining cases. A history of undescended testes, treated by chorionic gonadotropin and/or surgery, was reported by two-thirds of patients. More than 80% had very small testes, 2.1 ± 0.4 ml; occasional patients had a testicular size in the early pubertal range of 4–6 ml. Associated defects and familial history are detailed later.

All our IGD patients had blood FSH and LH levels in the prepubertal range or in the lower limit of the pubertal range. The acute test with LHRH, 0.1 mg/m^2 in a single-bolus intravenous injection, showed completely blunted FSH and LH responses in half of the patients and responses in the normal prepubertal range in the other half (42). Overt pulsatility and/or nocturnal peak of gonadotropins were rarely observed. Indirect evidence of IGD by measurement of Leydig cell secretion was more reliable. Plasma testosterone remained prepubertal, below 0.5 ng/ml, when bone age reached 12.5–13 years. The testosterone response to stimulation with three IM injections of hCG, 1500 IU/m^2 on alternate days, did not exceed 2 ng/ml in most patients. A close correlation between the LH peak after LHRH and the testosterone level after hCG ($r = 0.70$, $p < 0.001$) suggested that the ability of Leydig cells to secrete testosterone depends on previous stimulation by endogenous gonadotropin(s) (42).

The associated anomalies in patients and/or their relatives include anosmia and hyposmia, which are not often mentioned by the patients, nor are they easy to recognize. They may also have partial color blindness, congenital partial or complete deafness (44), cleftlip and cleft palate (44), unilateral renal agenesis (45), and various neurologic defects, such as mirror movements and pes cavus (46).

2. Females

IGD is seldom diagnosed at adolescence in girls, probably because they carry or express milder forms of the IGD genetic defect. Females with IGD are more often referred for primary infertility at adult age than for infantilism or primary amenorrhea at adolescence.

As in males, the body size and proportions are in the normal range, with a slight degree of macroskelia. There is usually a contrast between the pubic hair, which is present, and the absent or poor breast development.

The hormonal pattern regarding gonadotropins does not differ in female compared to male cases of IGD. Low estradiol measurements are not helpful for diagnosis. Pelvic ultrasonography showing normal prepubertal internal genitalia is more important in practice.

3. Pathophysiology

It was recently shown in animal models (47) that Kallmann syndrome results from a defect in migration of a discrete group of cells from the olfactory placode that give rise to the olfactory nerves. These cells migrate along the olfactory tract as a subpopulation that ends as specific LHRH cells in the hypothalamus. Immunocytochemistry in a human fetus from a Kallman's lineage has shown that the hypothalamic LHRH cells and olfactory nerves failed to reach their normal position and ended prematurely in the meninges (48). Other recent data confirm that hypogonadotropism in Kallman syndrome can be attributed to a failure of LHRH neurons to migrate into the brain (49,50).

The genetic heterogeneity of IGD has been hypothesized since 1973 (51) and confirmed by more recent reports (52,53). In fact, IGD without anosmia has been observed in kindreds born from normal, fertile, but consanguineous parents (42, 52). However, most pedigrees are of a dominant type (53). A few with an anosmic father suggest autosomal dominant transmission with variable expressivity (54,55). Most, being transmitted from mother or maternal lineage to children, with a strong male predominance, suggest X-linked inheritance.

Biochemical studies (56,57) have localized the gene responsible for the X-linked Kallman syndrome to the terminal part of the X chromosome short arm (locus Xp22.3). Complete deletions of the gene have been found in only a few patients. Extended deletions are probably rare.

4. Other Types of Isolated Gonadotropic Deficiency

Isolated LH deficiency or LH abnormality, known as syndrome of fertile eunuchoidism (58) with normal sense of smell, has been reported in male or ambiguous patients with an absence of secondary sex characteristics contrasting with normally sized testes. Treatment with LH-like chorionic gonadotropin hCG is indicated.

5. Hypogonadotropic Hypogonadism in Malformative Syndromes

Gonadotropic deficiency with overt hypogonadism at adolescence is a main component of Prader-Willi-Labhart syndrome. This disease is related to the lack of paternal chromosome 15. Its features include congenital hypotonia, growth retardation, obesity, and mental impairment (59,60). Hypogonadotropic hypogonadism is also found in Laurence-Moon-Bardet-Biedl syndrome, in which the main features are polydactyly, retinitis pigmentosa, obesity, and mental retardation (8,61). It may also be a part of other malformative syndromes, among which Biemond syndrome (with coloboma, polydactyly, and obesity) (31) and blepharophimosis syndrome (with short palpebral fissures) (8).

IV. OTHER TYPES OF HYPOGONADOTROPIC HYPOGONADISM OR DELAYED PUBERTY

The distinction between gonadotropic deficiency with normal olfaction and constitutional delay of puberty should be deferred until other causes known to inhibit or delay sexual development have been investigated and eliminated.

A. Delayed Puberty Secondary to Chronic Systemic Diseases

Nutritional and metabolic disturbances are the most frequent of these causes. Anorexia nervosa and/or such eating disorders as fear of obesity (62) are much more frequent in females than in males. Mild malnutrition is usually difficult to recognize (Chap. 60). Some of these patients present with digestive disturbances, either imaginary or related to inappropriate diet or hidden laxative abuse. The borderline weight-height ratio or body mass index may be the only means of suspecting malnutrition as the cause of pubertal delay. It can be very difficult to determine whether such thin girls are underfed or constitutionally slim persons. Body weight gain over time is the best index to recognize nutritional growth alterations, because weight gain may have ceased with growth stunting, without apparent deficit in the weight for height measurements of the child (Chap. 8).

The results of hormonal investigations in juvenile anorexia nervosa with delayed puberty vary according to the degree of undernutrition. The discharge of LH during sleep is usually lacking. Low plasma and urine levels of gonadotropins and sex steroids and low responses to LHRH and to clomiphene citrate are common in severe malnutrition (24).

Treatment of anorexia nervosa in adolescents is very difficult. Undernutrition may persist for years, and sexual characteristics do not develop. Therapy with steroids is useless. Whenever substantial weight gain is obtained, sexual development may not occur or recur for several months or years, despite repeated hormonal investigations showing substantial improvement (Chap. 60).

Malnutrition also exists as a consequence of the late forms of gluten intolerance (celiac disease), in which a gluten-free diet induces rapid sexual development and catch-up growth. Chronic intestinal diseases, particularly Crohn's disease, also have a delayed or absent sexual maturation (Chap. 8).

Intensive physical training in athletes, such as runners, swimmers, skaters, and ballet dancers, often delays or blocks sexual development. The prognosis is much more favorable than in anorexia, and regular follow-up may be sufficient.

Juvenile diabetes, when poorly controlled, may be associated with a delay in puberty and growth. No such delay occurs in well-controlled diabetics (Chaps. 41 and 43).

Almost all chronic organic and metabolic disturbances of childhood may cause a delay in puberty, usually associated with a similar delay in growth and bone maturation. Renal glomerular and tubular defects (63), including Bartter syndrome, and other long-term diseases such as hemoglobin defects and chronic anemias, hemosiderosis, respiratory insufficiency in patients with severe asthma or cystic fibrosis, and chronic hepatic and intestinal diseases, are causes of such a delay (42). These situations require only treatment of the primary disease. Treatment of hypogonadism, which is its consequence, is of no value in improving the situation of the patient.

Hypogonadotropic hypogonadism exists in adrenal diseases: as a consequence of hypercortisolism in Cushing's disease or Cushing syndrome; of hyperandrogenism in poorly controlled congenital virilizing adrenal hyperplasia (Chap. 21); or of associated disease in Prader's type congenital adrenal hypoplasia (64), which is an X-linked genetic disease affecting contiguous genes. In thyroid diseases, hypo- or hyperthyroidism can delay sexual development unless appropriately treated.

B. Lack of Puberty Without Detectable Cause: Simple Delay?

During adolescence, constitutional delay of puberty (CDP) or of growth and puberty is the most frequent cause of sexual immaturity (Chap. 1). It has the same male predominance as isolated gonadotropic deficiency and may be difficult to distinguish from this condition. Late puberty in the parents or other relatives may support the diagnosis of CDP but does not offer sufficient evidence.

Select clinical features facilitate the differential diagnosis between CDP and IGD. On average, CDP patients are shorter than IGD patients. The bone maturation is also retarded, but the ratio of height to bone age is not significantly different in either male or female CDP and IGD groups (42). The main differences are found in males: CDP boys have a normal prepubertal penis size, usually no history of cryptorchidism, and a testicular volume of at least 4 ml (25 × 15 mm).

The most significant hormonal measurement is basal serum testosterone in males, which is greater than 0.6 ng/ml in CDP patients when the bone age exceeds 12.5 years (42). A testicular stimulation test using chorionic gonadotropin is seldom useful at adolescence. Serum estradiol in females is meaningless. Assay of urinary gonadotropins may contribute to the diagnosis. Serum FSH and LH are not significantly different in CDP and IGD. Furthermore, the responses to the stimulation test using gonadoliberin LHRH overlap between the two groups, so that only the lack of response is of real diagnostic value (42).

A special type of delay in females is delayed menarche, defined as the absence of menstruation in adolescent girls who have reached complete breast development. These girls demonstrate normal adult genitalia on pelvic ultrasonography, no health or nutritional disturbances, and no detectable cause for hypogonadism. They later develop normal spontaneous cycles and need only reassurance and follow-up (65).

V. MANAGEMENT OF HYPOGONADOTROPIC HYPOGONADISM AND DELAYED PUBERTY

Treatment of obvious gonadotropic deficiency is difficult. In males, the question is whether sex steroids or gonadotropins, or both, should be prescribed. Testosterone may be used as in hypergonadotropic hypogonadism (see earlier). Less masculinization is obtained, however, and the size of the testes fails to increase. Addition of chorionic gonadotropin hCG, 200–3000 IU/week, or chorionic plus human menopausal gonadotropin (hMG), has not, in our experience, improved the results in adolescent patients. Thus, we reserve gonad-

otropins to induce fertility in adults, because their efficiency is not reduced by previous testosterone treatment.

In adolescent females with gonadotropic deficiency, treatment should also be limited to sex steroids, used in cyclic courses as in primary ovarian deficiencies (see earlier). The use of hMG and hCG at this age should be avoided because it requires close supervision and should be delayed until treatment for ovulation and fertility are indicated.

There have been numerous attempts to use LHRH and analogs in the treatment of primary gonadotropic deficiency (66–68). Despite various models of pulsatile administration, very few have been able to ensure the proper conditions of pubertal development in patients with infantilism. As gonadotropin treatment, LHRH should be reserved for attempts to induce fertility in patients who have reached a sufficient degree of sexual maturity.

Delayed puberty secondary to detectable nutritional, visceral, or other systemic causes needs only treatment of the primary disease. Very short courses of sex steroids may be offered if the spontaneous onset of sexual development does not occur at the appropriate time.

When simple constitutional delay is probable, careful follow-up with periodic control and reassurance may be sufficient for a time. However, beyond 2 or 3 standard deviations from the average age in other adolescents, the patient would feel deeply different from peers. At this time, sex steroids are useful for psychologic reasons and should be given as one or two courses of 6 months, with the hope of triggering the onset or progression of spontaneous puberty. Testosterone, 50 mg monthly, or oxandrolone, 1–2 mg daily, can be prescribed in boys and conjugated estradiol, 0.3 mg daily, to girls. Appropriate psychologic support and follow-up must be added to hormonal treatment.

REFERENCES

1. Marshall WA, Tanner JM. Variations in the pattern of pubertal changes in girls. Arch Dis Child 1969; 44:291–301.
2. Marshall WA, Tanner JM. Variations in the pattern of pubertal changes in boys. Arch Dis Child 1970; 45:13–21.
3. Mendez HMM, Opitz JM. Noonan syndrome: a review. Am J Hum Genet 1985; 21:493–506.
4. Vesely DL, Bower RH, Kohler PO, Char F. Familial ovarian dysgenesis in 46 XX females. Am J Med Sci 1980; 280:157–166.
5. Fechner PY, Marcantonio SM, Ogata T, et al. Report of a kindred with X-linked (or autosomal dominant sex-limited) 46 XY partial gonadal dysgenesis. J Clin Endocrinol Metab 1993; 76:1248–1253.
6. Blagovidow N, Page DC, Huff DE, et al. Ullrich Turner syndrome in a XY female fetus with deletion of the sex-determining portion of the Y chromosome. Am J Med Genet 1989; 34:159–162.
7. Scherer G, Shempp W, Baccichetti C, et al. Duplication of an Xp segment that includes the ZFX locus causes sex inversion in man. Hum Genet 1989; 81:291–294.
8. Jones KL. Smith's Recognizable Patterns of Human Malformation, 4th ed. Philadelphia: W. B. Saunders, 1988.
9. Pallister PD, Opitz JM. The Perrault syndrome: autosomal

recessive ovarian dysgenesis with facultative, non sex-limited sensorineural deafness. Am J Med Genet 1979; 4:239–246.

10. Nishi Y, Hamamoto K, Kajiyama M, Kawamura I. The Perrault syndrome: clinical report and review. Am J Med Genet 1988; 31:623–629.

11. Brosnan PG, Lewandovski RC, Toguri AG, et al. A new familial syndrome of 46, XY gonadal dysgenesis with anomalies of ectodermal and mesodermal structures. J Pediatr 1980; 97:586–590.

12. Skre H, Bassoe HH, Berg K, et al. Cerebellar ataxia and hypergonadotropic hypogonadism in two kindreds. Chance occurrence, pleiotropism, or linkage? Clin Genet 1976; 9:234–244.

13. Larizza D, Maraschio P, Maghnie M, Sampaolo P. Hypogonadism in a patient with balanced X/18 translocation and pituitary hormone deficiency. Eur J Pediatr 1993; 152:424–427.

14. Nicosia S, Matus Ridley M, Meadows AT. Gonadal effects of cancer therapy in girls. Cancer 1985; 55:2364–2372.

15. Quigley C, Cowell C, Jiminez M, et al. Normal or early development of puberty despite gonadal damage in children treated for acute lymphoblastic leukemia. N Engl J Med 1989; 321:143–151.

16. LaBarbera AR, Miller MM, Ober C, et al. Autoimmune etiology in premature ovarian failure. Am J Reprod Immunol Microbiol 1988; 16:115–122.

17. Kaufman FR, Xu YK, Ngo WG, et al. Gonadal function and ovarian galactose metabolism in classic galactosemia. Acta Endocrinol (Copenh) 1989; 120:129–133.

18. Yanase T, Simpson ER, Waterman FR. 17alpha-Hydroxylase/17,20-lyase deficiency: from clinical investigation to molecular definition. Endocr Rev 1991; 12:91–108.

19. Larrea F, Lisker R, Banuelos R, et al. Hypergonadotropic hypogonadism in an XX female subject due to 17–20 desmolase deficiency. Acta Endocrinol (Copenh) 1983; 103:400–405.

20. Evers JLH, Rolland R. The gonadotropin resistant ovary syndrome: a curable disease? Clin Endocrinol (Oxf) 1981; 14:99–103.

21. Graham JM Jr, Bashir AS, Stark RE, et al. Oral and written language abilities of XXY boys: implications for school guidance. Pediatrics 1988; 81:795–806.

22. Jacobs PA, Hassold TJ, Whittington E, et al. Klinefelter's syndrome: an analysis of the origin of the additional sex chromosome using molecular probes. Ann Hum Genet 1988; 52:93–109.

23. Stewart DA, Netley CT, Park E. Summary of clinical findings in children with 47 XXY, 47 XYY and 47 XXX karyotypes. Birth Defects 1982; 18:1–5.

24. Borghgraeff M, Fryns JP, Smeets E, et al. The 49 XXXXY syndrome. Clinical and psychologic follow-up data. Clin Genet 1988; 33:429–434.

25. Anderson M, Page DC, de la Chapelle A. Chromosome Y-specific DNA is transferred to the short arm of X chromosome in human XX males. Science 1986; 223:786–788.

26. Petit C, de la Chapelle A, Levilliers J, et al. An abnormal X-Y interchange accounts for most but not all cases of human XX maleness. Cell 1987; 49:595–602.

27. Lustig RH, Conte FA, Kogan BA, et al. Ontogeny of gonadal secretion in congenital anorchism; sexual dimorphism versus syndrome of gonadal dysgenesis and diagnostic considerations. J Urol 1987; 138:587–591.

28. David R, Yoon DJ, Landin L, et al. A syndrome of gonadotropin resistance possibly due to a luteinizing hormone receptor defect. J Clin Endocrinol Metab 1984; 59:156–160.

29. Matus Ridley M, Nicosia SV, Meadows AT. Gonadal effects of cancer therapy in boys. Cancer 1985; 55:2353–2363.

30. Bramswig JH, Heimes U, Heiermann E, et al. The effects of different cumulative doses of chemotherapy on testicular function. Cancer 1990; 65:1298–1302.

31. Buyse ML, ed. Birth Defects Encyclopedia. Cambridge, MA: Blackwell, 1990.

32. Hughes I, Evans B. Androgen insensitivity in forty-nine patients: classification based on clinical and androgen receptor phenotypes. Horm Res 1987; 28:25–29.

33. Drash A, Sherman F, Hartmann WH, et al. A syndrome of pseudohermaphroditism, Wilm's tumor, hypertension and degenerative renal disease. J Pediatr 1970; 76:585–593.

34. Friedman BL, Finlay JL. The Drash syndrome revisited. Diagnosis and follow-up. Am J Med Genet (Suppl) 1987; 3:293–296.

35. Pelletier J, Bruening W, Kashtan CE, et al. Germline mutations in the Wilm's tumor suppressor gene are associated with abnormal urogenital development in Denys-Drash syndrome. Cell 1991; 67:437–447.

36. Coppes MJ, Huff V, Pelletier J. Denys-Drash syndrome: relating a clinical disorder to genetic alterations in the tumor suppressor gene WT1. J Pediatr 1993; 123:673–678.

37. Acquafredda A, Vassal J, Job JC. Rudimentary testes syndrome revisited Pediatrics 1987; 80:209–214.

38. Bergada C, Cleveland WW, Jones HW Jr, et al. Variants of embryonic testicular dysgenesis: bilateral anorchia and the syndrome of rudimentary testes. Acta Endocrinol (Copenh) 1962; 40:521–536.

39. Josso N, Briard ML. Embryonic testicular regression syndrome: variable phenotypic expression in siblings. J Pediatr 1980; 97:200–204.

40. Butler GE, Sellar RE, Walker RF, et al. Oral testosterone undecanoate in the management of delayed puberty in boys: pharmacokinetics and effects on sexual maturation and growth. J Clin Endocrinol Metab 1992; 75:37–44.

41. Tanner JM, Whitehouse RH. A note on the bone age at which patients with true isolated growth hormone deficiency enter puberty. J Clin Endocrinol Metab 1975; 41:788–790.

42. Job JC, Chaussain JL, Toublanc JE. Delayed puberty. In: Grumbach MM, Sizonenko PC, Aubert ML, eds. Control of the Onset of Puberty. Baltimore: Williams & Wilkins, 1990: 588–613.

43. Patton ML, Woolf PD. Hyperprolactinemia and delayed puberty: a report of three cases and their response to therapy. Pediatrics 1983; 71:572–575.

44. Kallmann FJ, Schoenfeld WA, Barrera SE. The genetic aspects of primary eunuchoidism. Am J Ment Defic 1944; 48:203–236.

45. Wegenke JD, Uehling DT, Wear JB, et al. Familial Kallmann syndrome with unilateral renal aplasia. Clin Genet 1975; 7:368–381.

46. Schwankhaus JD, Currie J, Jaffe MJ, et al. Neurologic findings in men with isolated hypogonadotropic hypogonadism. Neurology 1989; 39:223–226.

47. Wray S, Grant P, Gainer H. Evidence that cells expressing luteinizing hormone-releasing hormone mRNA in the mouse are derived from progenitor cells in the olfactory placode. Proc Natl Acad Sci USA 1989; 86:1132–1136.

48. Bick D, Curry CJR, McGill JR, et al. Male infant with ichtyosis, Kallmann's syndrome, chondrodysplasia punctata and an Xp chromosome deletion Am J Med Genet 1989; 33:100–107.

49. Schwanzel-Fukuda M, Jorgenson KL, Bergen HT, et al. Biology of normal luteinizing hormone-releasing hormone neurons during and after their migration from olfactory placode. Endocr Rev 1992; 13:624–634.

50. Crowley WF, Jameson JL. Gonadotropin-releasing hormone

deficiency: perspectives from clinical investigation. Endocr Rev 1992; 13:635–640.

51. Santen RJ, Paulsen CA. Hypogonadotropic eunuchoidism. I. Clinical study of the mode of inheritance. J Clin Endocrinol Metab 1973; 36:47–54.

52. White BJ, Rogol AD, Brown KS, et al. The syndrome of anosmia with hypogonadotropic hypogonadismp: a genetic study of 18 new families and a review. Am J Med Genet 1983; 15:417–435.

53. Chaussain JL, Toublanc JE, Feingold J, et al. Mode of inheritance in familial cases of primary gonadotropic deficiency. Horm Res 1988; 29:202–206.

54. Merriam GR, Beitins IZ, Bode HH. Father-to-son transmission of hypogonadism with anosmia. Am J Dis Child 1977; 131:1216–1219.

55. Evain-Brion D, Gendrel D, Bozzola M, et al. Diagnosis of Kallmann's syndrome in early infancy. Acta Paediatr Scand 1982; 71:937–940.

56. Hardelin JP, Levilliers J, Young J, et al. Xp22.3 deletions in isolated familial Kallmann's syndrome. J Clin Endocrinol Metab 1993; 76:827–831.

57. Prager D, Braunstein GD. X-chromosome-linked Kallmann's syndrome: pathology at the molecular level (editorial). J Clin Endocrinol Metab 1993; 76:824–825.

58. Smals AGH, Kloppenborg PWC, Van Haelst UJG, et al. Fertile eunuch syndrome versus classic hypogonadotrophic hypogonadism. Acta Endocrinol (Copenh) 1978; 87:389–399.

59. Kauli R, Prager-Lewin R, Laron Z. Pubertal development in the Prader-Labhart-Willi syndrome. Acta Paediatr Scand 1978; 67:763–770.

60. Bray GA, Dahms WT, Swerdloff RS, et al. The Prader-Willi syndrome: a study of 40 patients and a review of the literature. Medicine (Baltimore) 1983; 62:59–80.

61. Perez-Palacio G, Uribe M, Scaglia H, et al. Pituitary and gonadal function with the Laurence-Moon-Bardet-Biedl syndrome. Acta Endocrinol (Copenh) 1977; 84:191–199.

62. Pugliese MT, Lifshitz F, Grad G, et al. Fear of obesity, a cause of short stature and delayed puberty. N Engl J Med 1983; 309:513–518.

63. Castellano M, Turconi AZ, Chaler E, et al. Hypothalamic-pituitary-gonadal function in prepubertal boys and girls with chronic renal failure. J Pediatr 1993; 122:46–51.

64. Hay ID, Smail PJ, Forsyth CC. Familial cytomegalic adrenocortical hypoplasia; an X-linked syndrome of pubertal failure. Arch Dis Child 1981; 56:715–721.

65. Blanco-Garcia M, Evain-Brion D, Toublanc JE, Job JC. L'aménorrhée primaire des adolescentes: fréquence du retard isolé d'apparition des règles Arch Fr Pediatr 1984; 41:377–382.

66. Hoffman AR, Crowley WF Jr. Induction of puberty in men by long-term pulsatile administration of low-dose gonadotropin-releasing hormone. N Engl J Med 1982; 307:1237–1241.

67. Santoro N, Filicori M, Crowley WF Jr. Hypogonadotropic disorders in men and women: diagnosis and therapy with pulsatile gonadotropin-releasing hormone. Endocr Rev 1986; 7:11–23.

68. Stanhope R, Pringle PJ, Brook CGD. The mechanism of the adolescent growth spurt induced by low dose pulsatile GnRH treatment. Clin Endocrinol (Oxf) 1988; 28:83–91.

19

Turner Syndrome

E. Kirk Neely
Stanford University, Stanford, California

Ron G. Rosenfeld
Doernbecher Memorial Hospital for Children and Oregon Health Sciences University, Portland, Oregon

I. INTRODUCTION

Humans need an intact X chromosome to survive. When the second sex chromosome, the X or the Y chromosome, is absent, a characteristic prenatal and postnatal phenotype results. These individuals are phenotypic females who usually have dysgenetic ovaries, short stature, and other typical but highly variable dysmorphic features (Fig. 1). Otto Ullrich first described the syndrome in a case report in the German literature in 1930, and University of Oklahoma Professor Henry Turner described seven patients with "infantilism, congenital webbed neck, and cubitus valgus" in 1938 (1). As a consequence, the syndrome associated with X chromosome loss is called Ullrich-Turner syndrome in Germany and Turner syndrome in most of the world. For simplicity, we use Turner syndrome (TS) here.

Turner likened the "osseous and sexual retardation" seen in his syndrome to the endocrine effects of hypopituitarism. He became, presumably, the first physician to use pharmacologically relevant agents in TS, administering injections of various pituitary extracts and estrogen-containing preparations to several of his patients. Rudimentary ovaries, or streak gonads, were identified in 1944 by Wilkins and Fleishman as the cause of the sexual infantilism (2), and the term 45, X gonadal dysgenesis is often used to identify TS (3). The recognizable infantile phenotype of lymphedema and neck folds was later described by Ullrich and is sometimes referred to as the Bonnevie-Ullrich syndrome (4). Other manifestations of the syndrome were cataloged during this period and termed collectively "Turner stigmata" (5,6).

Elucidation of the chromosomal basis of TS began with the discovery in 1954 that TS patients were sex chromatin negative (7). After new cytogenetic culture techniques allowed human chromosomes to be accurately counted, TS was

associated with X chromosome monosomy in 1959 by Ford et al. (8) in a prepubertal 14 year old with short stature and typical features. The development of routine cytogenetic analysis in the 1960s led to recognition of the diverse chromosomal complements associated with TS (6). Most patient series have reported approximately half of their TS patients to have a 45, X karyotype; the rest are caused by either mosaicisms or structural anomalies resulting in loss of major portions of the X chromosome, the most common being isochromosome (duplication) of the long arm (9–12). The relative proportions of karyotypes found in several large patient series over the past two decades are presented in Table 1.

II. FEATURES OF TURNER SYNDROME

A. Ascertainment Patterns

TS may be detected incidentally during prenatal diagnostic procedures for advanced maternal age, by classic features at birth, growth failure in childhood, failed puberty, or for miscellaneous reasons. Unlike trisomies or Klinefelter syndrome, the incidence of TS does not increase with maternal age (13); therefore, few children with TS are ascertained by prenatal diagnosis. TS may be detected by elevated α-fetoprotein levels in maternal serum. Approximately a third of TS patients are identified at birth by pterygium coli (webbed neck) or lymphedema of the hands and feet. Most of these infants have 45, X karyotypes (Fig. 2), because these physical findings, in contrast with other stigmata of TS, are more common in patients with complete X monosomy than in patients with mosaicism or structural abnormality of the X (6,9–11).

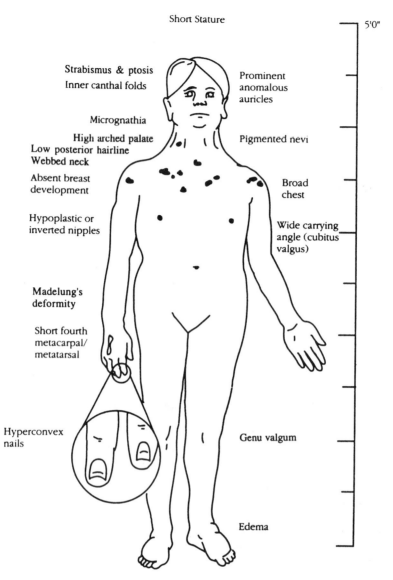

Figure 1   Features of Turner syndrome commonly visible on physical examination. (Modified from Ref. 101.)

TS is additionally suspected in many girls in mid-childhood, when growth failure results in a height noticeably below the normal range. Recognition of TS during childhood may have been enhanced in the last decade by availability of recombinant human growth hormone for treatment of short stature. Nevertheless, many patients are not recognized until pubertal failure or short stature in the teenage years leads to medical evaluation. Finally, the diagnosis may be made upon referral in adulthood for primary or secondary amenorrhea, infertility, or recurrent miscarriage. Patients are also occasionally detected on the basis of one of the less evident features of TS, such as facial or bony abnormalities, learning problems, strabismus, or otitis or hearing loss. It is likely that some patients, particularly those with mosaicism, have manifestations that are mild enough to escape detection altogether.

B.   Fetal Demise

X monosomy is the most commonly occurring sex chromosome anomaly, but the vast majority of Turner conceptuses are spontaneously aborted. It is probable that more than 1% of conceptions involve X chromosome loss, and up to 10% of spontaneously aborted fetuses have 45, X karyotypes (14). As a result, TS occurs with an incidence of only about 1 in 2500 live female births, which is less common than Klinefelter syndrome (approximately 1 in 800), or 45, XXX postnatally. Because the peak of fetal deaths occurs at 11–13 weeks of gestation, most 45, X fetuses are spontaneously aborted before the gestational age at which amniocentesis is routinely performed. A smaller proportion of fetuses is aborted in the second trimester, with autopsy findings of massive lymphedema and cystic nuchal hygroma (15).

Table 1 Percentages of Karyotypes in Four Large Series of Patients with Turner Syndrome

Karyotype	Palmer and Reichman (9)	Hall et al. (10)	Park et al. (11)	Held et al. (17)
45, X	58.2	55.0	61.2	20.7
46, XisoXq	7.3	5.5	6.0	5.7
Mosaicism (with 45, X)				
46, XX	8.2	13.4	11.2	17.2
46, XisoXq	11.8	4.7	7.8	12.6
46, XringX	5.5	3.9	1.7	3.5
46, XY	5.4	3.1	2.6	2.3
46, XXp⁻	0.9	0.8	2.6	2.3
46, XXq⁻	0	1.6	1.7	3.5
47, XXX and 46, XX/47, XXX	1.8	0.8	0.9	6.9
46, X + marker	0	0.8	0	18.4

Several investigators have contended that all fetuses with complete 45, X karyotypes are spontaneously aborted and, conversely, that all live-born individuals with TS are actually occult X chromosome mosaics, secondary to early mitotic errors (14,16). Aborted fetuses with X chromosome loss are indeed overwhelmingly 45, X, implying a relative fetoprotective effect of mosaicism. By employing rigorous techniques, Held et al. (17) have been able to document a higher level of mosaicism in live-born TS patients than has previously been reported, largely by the detection of small marker chromosomes in some cell populations (Table 1). Mosaicism may theoretically be present in multiple tissues without detectability in blood cells, and the presence of mosaicism in the trophoblast or in placental tissue may be all that is required

to avoid lethality. Nonetheless, obligate mosaicism in live-born TS remains only a theory (18).

C. Cardiac and Renal Anomalies

To detect cardiac malformations, echocardiography should be performed as soon as the diagnosis of TS is confirmed. In large patient series, coarctation of the aorta is reported in approximately 20% of patients (range 15–68%) and is more frequent in association with a 45, X karyotype (9–11). The advent of high-resolution echocardiography has revealed other anomalies with probable greater frequency in TS. Miller et al. (19) documented isolated bicuspid aortic valve in 34% of patients, in addition to bicuspid aortic valve with coarctation. Echocardiography has also demonstrated isolated aortic root dilation in approximately 10% of patients (20). These anomalies place TS patients at risk for catastrophic aortic dissection and aneurysmal rupture (21), as well as bacterial endocarditis and development of aortic stenosis. Mitral valve prolapse is also commonly reported. TS patients with significant cardiac anomalies should be referred to a cardiologist. It is not known whether follow-up echocardiography is helpful in TS patients without cardiac lesions on the initial examination. Patients should be routinely screened for hypertension, which may occur in the absence of a detectable anomaly.

In studies of second-trimester fetal pathology, a high frequency of heart vessel defects (juxtaductal coarctation, diminution of the ascending aorta, and dilated pulmonary arteries) has been noted in association with edema, nuchal cystic hygromas, and lymphatic aberrations at the base of the major vessels. This association suggests a causal link between lymphedema and cardiac anomalies (22). Cardiac anatomy is normal in many fetuses with severe edema as well, however, and the etiology of cardiac defects remains conjectural.

The etiology of renal abnormalities in TS is also unknown, and cardiac and renal anomalies usually occur inde-

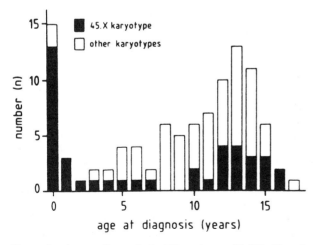

Figure 2 Age at diagnosis in 100 patients with TS. Note the greater percentage of patients with 45, X karyotype diagnosed in infancy. (From Ref. 102.)

pendently. Because dysmorphic renal structures can be adequately visualized by either ultrasonography or intravenous pyelography, a single-screening renal ultrasound is recommended for all patients at the time of diagnosis. Most renal anomalies are silent and do not become clinically significant. Renal abnormalities were documented in one-third of 141 patients with various karyotypes in the series of Lippe et al. (23). The most frequent abnormalities were double collecting systems (8%), horseshoe kidney (7%), and rotational abnormalities (6%). Abnormalities requiring urologic referral included ureteropelvic and ureterovesicle junction obstruction (6%) and absent kidney (3%). In this study, the incidence of renal dysmorphology in girls with 45, X karyotype was 45%, compared with 18% in other karyotypes combined, but this difference has not been found in other series.

D. Craniofacial and Skeletal Anomalies

The characteristic facial appearance in TS is comprised of epicanthal folds, ptosis, downslanting palpebral fissures, midfacial hypoplasia, small mandible, prominent ears, neck webbing, low hairline, and short neck. Many patients have a high arched palate, which may contribute to the feeding difficulties commonly encountered in infancy. Anatomic anomalies at the cranial base probably alter the angle of the eustachian tube, leading to the high incidence of otitis media; sinusitis and mastoiditis are also observed. The incidence of hearing loss in adults with TS may be as high as 30% and can be of either conductive or sensorineural origin. The small jaw and high palate are associated with orthodontic problems, such as crowding and malocclusion. Reconstructive surgery of the ears or neck is controversial because of the reported frequency of keloid formation.

Diverse bone abnormalities are found in TS, but they are usually documented only after the diagnosis has been made. The most common anomalies are short fourth metacarpal and cubitus valgus. Less frequent skeletal abnormalities include thinning of parietal bones, Madelung deformity of the wrist, pectus excavatum, premature fusion of the ossification centers of the sternum, "drumstick" appearance of the distal phalanges, decreased bitrochanteric breadth, android appearance of the pelvic inlet, genu valgum, and fusion of the tarsal bones. The common bone abnormalities appear to be seen equally in patients with 45, X monosomy, structural abnormality, and mosaicism. Cubitus valgus and Madelung's wrist deformity are easily seen on physical examination, and a short fourth metacarpal is documented on bone age films. Patients should be routinely evaluated for scoliosis, which may worsen as medical therapies are initiated. Congenital dislocation of the hip may be seen in more than 5% of infants with TS (24). Many investigators have documented short-leggedness and abnormal body segment ratios in TS, and patients tend to exhibit a short, square body habitus (25,26). The appearance of widely spaced nipples (shield chest) may be attributable to this phenomenon.

Osteopenia has been widely reported in TS and may be secondary to an underlying bone dysplasia. Bone mineral status is additionally concerning in TS, because ovarian failure, as well as reduced growth hormone (GH) secretion in adolescence, likely contributes to insufficient acquisition and maintenance of bone mass. Radiographic evidence of diminished bone mass includes a coarse trabecular pattern of vertebral and carpal bones and reduced metacarpal cortical thickness (27,28). Osteopenia has been reported employing computed tomographic scans in adults with TS, but absorptiometric methods are now utilized to determine bone mineral content (BMC) and density (BMD), the latter method compensating for the surface area of bones. In adults with TS, early limited studies documented a markedly reduced BMC, with less reduction in patients receiving estrogen replacement (29–31). However, measurements in TS may be artifactually low because both BMC and BMD are dependent upon body and bone size. The studies of osteopenia in children and adolescents with TS are even less convincing and have not effectively delineated when relative demineralization begins to occur (32–34). Our group has reported that adolescents with TS receiving growth hormone therapy exhibit normal bone mineral properties (35). Other investigators have reported an increase in biochemical markers of bone turnover at initiation of GH therapy. Thus, it is not clear whether bone density can be accurately interpreted in TS or whether early estrogen replacement or GH therapy is helpful for bone accretion or maintenance.

E. Gonadal Dysgenesis

Gonadal dysgenesis is one of the hallmarks of partial or complete X chromosome loss. In most 45, X individuals during childhood, the ovaries are already pale gonadal streaks consisting of normal fibrous stroma with greatly diminished numbers of primordial follicles. Histologic studies of the gonadal ridge have documented normal densities of primordial germ cells at up to 12 weeks of gestation, but in the early second trimester oocyte formation and folliculogenesis fail to occur normally and connective tissue proliferates instead. Oocytes undergo premature atresia in a highly variable manner that may be completed before birth or may continue into adolescence or adulthood. Massarano et al. have reported the ultrasound appearance of ovaries in 104 TS girls of variable age (36). The ovaries of two-thirds of the subjects were classified as streak gonads, and ovarian volumes in the remaining one-third of subjects were in the lower range of normal. Ovaries that were nearly normal in size were most easily detected in infants and toddlers or in girls of pubertal age, matching the pattern of gonadotropin stimulation (37). Prepubertal uterine volumes were in the normal range, consistent with the anatomically normal and hormonally responsive uterus (as well as vagina and external genitalia) found in patients with TS.

Ovarian failure is reflected in reduced steroid feedback on the hypothalamic-pituitary axis and marked elevations in serum follicle-stimulating hormone (FSH) and luteinizing hormone. Significantly elevated gonadotropin levels are clinically detectable from birth to approximately 4 years old but may fall to normal prepubertal levels in midchildhood before rising again to very high levels at the usual age of puberty

(37). The phenotypic manifestations of the declining numbers of functioning ovarian follicles constitute a spectrum from absence of any pubertal development in 70–80% of girls, to midpubertal failure in approximately 10–20%, to failure to progress to menses, secondary amenorrhea, or early menopause. Pregnancy occurs in an occasional TS patient, predominantly but not exclsively in those with mosaic karyotypes. In these cases, miscarriages are common and prenatal diagnosis may be advised because of the increased incidence of chromosomal anomalies in the offspring.

From a management point of view, it is important to remember that progressive follicular atresia results in two functional deficits, failure to secrete estrogen and progesterone, on the one hand, and loss of germ cells and infertility, on the other. For the pediatric endocrinologist, only the former requires medical intervention, as discussed in a later section. Nevertheless, families appreciate a frank discussion of the probable infertility and potential options, including adoption and assisted reproductive technologies.

F. Growth

The natural history of growth in TS is comprised of distinct phases in the evolution of short stature. Moderate intrauterine growth retardation results in birth weight and length that are below the mean but are usually overlooked; mean birth weight in TS is approximately 2800 g. Growth velocity in the first 3 years of life is relatively normal, but a progressive decline occurs during the remainder of childhood (Fig. 3). The 5th percentile of the normal female curve and the 95th percentile of the TS curve diverge at about 9 years of age. Growth failure becomes even more obvious in adolescence because of the absence of a pubertal growth spurt, and the height nadir in TS relative to normal females occurs at about 14 years of age. TS patients ordinarily continue to exhibit slow, consistent growth during late adolescence as a result of delayed bone maturation and epiphyseal fusion, with typical closure at 18–20 years. This delay affords some measure of catch-up growth and provides an opportunity for prolonged growth therapy.

Lyon et al. (38) combined the growth data of Ranke et al. (39) and other European studies to create growth standards for TS in the absence of hormonal therapy. The Lyon curve, as well as other growth standards, such as those of Naeraa and Nielsen (40), provide an important means of evaluating growth therapies. These standard curves permit an accurate projection of adult height on the basis of the current height, and a high degree of correlation has been demonstrated between first measured height in childhood and final adult height (41). Adult heights projected on the basis of standardized curves are as accurate as heights predicted from bone age, which may be difficult to interpret. The mean final height of the Lyon curve is 142.9 ± 7.3 cm, a figure close to the height reported for the combined European-U.S. experience over the last 20 years. It cannot be ignored that several studies have reported taller adult heights, however, most notably mean heights of approximately 147 cm in TS populations from Denmark and Seattle (40,42).

Resolution of discrepancies regarding untreated final heights is crucial for assessing the benefits of growth therapies, because published studies with human growth hormone have not utilized long-term control groups. Most investigators are convinced that a mean untreated adult height of 143 cm is a reasonably accurate assumption for the U.S. population, but interpretation of final height data is complicated by many factors, including karyotype, parental heights, ethnicity, spontaneous puberty, and earlier hormonal treatment with estrogens or androgens. There has probably been a secular trend toward increased adult height, although this may reflect previous underestimations of adult height because of ascertainment bias: TS was less likely to be diagnosed in more phenotypically normal patients. Patients with 45, X/46, XX karyotype have a greater mean final height, but the height effect of other mosaicisms is unclear. The influence of spontaneous puberty on adult height has also not been conclusively determined. In the minority of patients in whom it occurs, it is generally associated with a slight pubertal growth spurt. Massa et al. reported an increased adult height in patients with spontaneous puberty, but other studies have found no significant differences or even reduced height from endogenous puberty (43,44).

Etiology of growth failure in TS is essentially unknown, but it may be caused by the combined effects of a primary skeletal dysplasia, growth hormone secretory dysfunction, and estrogen deficiency. Pathologic bone development could represent either an intrinsic defect in ossification secondary to loss of critical genes on the X chromosome or, alternatively, another of the protean manifestations of intrauterine edema. Although increased bone resorption and defective osteoblast function have been reported and cartilage from TS patients has been noted to have narrowed growth zones (45), there has been no consistent histologic finding in the bones of patients with TS. Furthermore, most patients with Turner syndrome are not GH deficient as classically defined by provocative GH testing. Occasional patients exhibit frank growth hormone deficiency, and any girl whose growth velocity is below normal for TS (i.e., falling across TS percentiles) should be screened for GH deficiency and hypothyroidism.

On the other hand, evidence of diminished growth hormone secretion in adolescence is convincing. TS adolescents, but not younger children, have reduced mean 24 h GH levels, peak amplitudes, and peak frequencies compared with age-matched controls (46). Comparably, serum levels of insulin-like growth factor I (IGF-I) are generally in the normal range in childhood but fall to the low end of normal in adolescence (47). The failure in TS of the usual pubertal increase in GH secretion or IGF-I levels may be secondary to estrogen deficiency, a thesis supported by an increase in GH concentrations in response to low-dose estrogen therapy (48,49). However, spontaneous puberty does not appear to benefit final height. Growth failure is apparent in most girls with TS during childhood, before deficiencies in the GH/IGF axis are demonstrable, implying that an intrinsic bone defect, not an endocrine abnormality, is primarily responsible for short stature. It remains an irony that one of the fundamental,

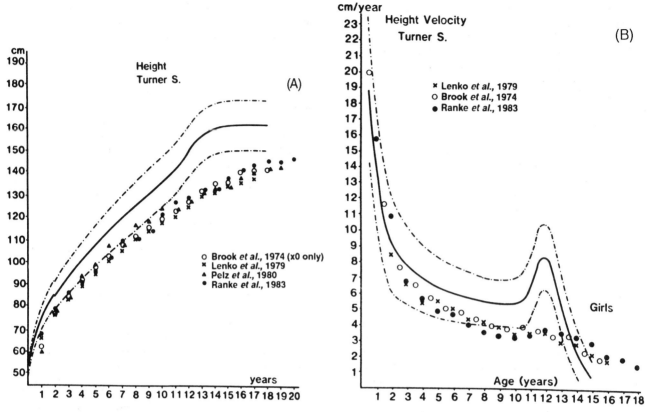

Figure 3 Mean height (A) and height velocity (B) in untreated European girls with Turner syndrome from four European studies, plotted on the growth curve for normal females. Note the steady decline in height velocity beginning in early childhood and the absence of a pubertal growth spurt. (From Ref. 39.)

treatable manifestations of TS has not been adequately explained.

G. Cognitive and Psychosocial Effects

It is essential to remember that individuals with TS are not mentally retarded, as was erroneously reported in some early studies. Later studies reported an increased incidence of retardation (full-scale intelligence quotient less than 80) only in patients with ring X karyotypes (50,51), and this has not been adequately confirmed. Modern psychologic investigations have revealed only specific impairments in cognitive functioning. The most commonly reported deficits relate to visual-spatial processing and visual memory, often reported as difficulties on tasks assessing spatial and numeric abilities (52,53). These deficits result in measurable reductions in performance IQ, in contrast with the normal verbal IQ, in a subset of TS children and adults. A cerebral lateralizing defect has been hypothesized as the lesion underlying cognitive impairment in TS, but more recently investigators have postulated a global problem involving attention, information processing, and visual memory, perhaps attributable to early alterations in brain function (54,55). Newer imaging studies have inconsistently documented abnormalities in

brain function in TS (56). Cognitive impairment seems to be unrelated to karyotype or to physical stigmata, except that deficits may be less frequent in 45, X/46, XX mosaicism.

Few studies have actually examined academic outcome in large numbers of subjects (57). Children with TS are not disruptive in the classroom setting and so may not be referred by the schools for evaluation. Nonetheless, it is crucial that patients with TS receive both psychologic and educational evaluation early in their school careers. Hearing evaluation, because of the high incidence of both conductive and sensorineural hearing loss, is very important as an adjunct measure to improve the social and academic skills of girls with TS. Girls may benefit from psychologic counseling at several times during childhood and adolescence. An increased incidence of anorexia, clinical depression, and social isolation has been reported (58). Life expectancy is reportedly diminished, but these studies predate the introduction of modern medical monitoring and therapies.

H. Autoimmunity

Several types of autoimmunity are found in increased incidence in TS, including inflammatory bowel disease, rheumatoid arthritis, and thyroid autoimmunity. Although glucose intolerance is present in 25–60% of adults with TS, frank diabetes occurs in only 5%, and this is type 2 insulin resistant diabetes. Estimates of prevalence in TS of specific thyroid autoantibodies range from 25 to 60% (59), in contrast to a 1–2% prevalence of thyroid autoimmunity in the general population. The frequency of thyroid autoimmunity is increased in patients of all karyotypes. The incidence of frank hypothyroidism is lower but increases with age, developing in 10–20% of TS patients. Individuals should be screened periodically for hypothyroidism, particularly if thyroid antibodies have been detected. There does not appear to be an increase in polyglandular autoimmunity associated with thyroid autoimmunity, because islet cell and adrenal antibodies are not elevated. The etiology of thyroid and other autoimmunities is not known. The presence of two cell lines may be contributory, and patients with long-arm isochromosomes seem to be even more prone to autoimmune disorders. Parents of patients with TS have a higher than expected incidence of thyroid autoimmunity. This has led to the speculation that familial thyroid autoimmunity is associated with nondisjunction or related chromosomal defects, but, on the other hand, it may paradoxically provide a protective effect against the lethality of X chromosome monosomy in utero (60).

III. SEARCH FOR THE GENETIC BASIS OF TS

The routine availability of TS karyotypes in the 1960s allowed initial attempts to correlate phenotypic manifestations with the variations in X chromosomal loss (61). In a well-known review of the early literature in 1965, Ferguson-Smith hypothesized that 45, X subjects demonstrated the "complete Turner syndrome" and that the short stature and stigmata of TS were attributable to monosomy of loci on the short arm (6). According to his review of data, 45, X patients exhibited a higher incidence of some features, including neck webbing, congenital lymphedema, and cardiac malformations, than patients with mosaicism or X structural abnormalities. Short stature was a universal feature when the short arm was missing, as in 45, X and karyotypes with long-arm isochromosomes. In contrast, normal stature occurred in 20% of 45, X/46, XX, 50% of 45, X/47, XXX, and 63% of long-arm deletions. Spontaneous pubertal development and menses, which occurred in only 8% of 45, X patients, were more likely in girls with 45, X/46, XX mosaicism (21%) and deletions of the short arm (25%). Large patient series since the 1960s have more or less corroborated these findings. Various studies have confirmed the lower incidence of common TS features in certain mosaics, although many features, such as bony abnormalities or pigmented nevi, seem to occur equally in X monosomy and mosaicisms.

Use of better banding techniques and X chromosome probes has provided a more detailed localization of X chromosome breakpoints. Simpson presented updated reviews of phenotype-karyotype correlations in the late 1970s (62). Location of the breakpoint correlates poorly with the resulting phenotype, and basically any feature of TS can be seen with a major deletion of either Xp or Xq. Nonetheless, there is a crude association of short-arm deletions with short stature and of long-arm deletions with ovarian dysgenesis. Therman and Susman more recently reviewed the literature on phenotypes of nonmosaic adults with X long- or short-arm terminal deletions (63). Short stature occurred in 43 and 88% of the Xq^- and Xp^- cases, respectively (Table 2). Turner stigmata were frequently associated with short-arm deletions, but their incidence in short-arm deletions was diminished in comparison with patients with complete X monosomy. Ovarian failure, including both primary and secondary amenorrhea, occurred in 93 and 65% of Xq^- and Xp^- karyotypes, respectively. Essentially the entire long arm is involved in ovarian development and maintenance: deletion breakpoints with apparently identical degrees of ovarian failure are scattered along the length of the long arm. Lymphedema and cardiovascular anomalies were rare in *both* short- and long-arm deletions, although lymphedema has resulted from the loss of the distal short arm of the Y in XY females.

Identification of the parental origin of the remaining X chromosome in TS has been undertaken to look for clues to the etiology of X monosomy and to evaluate whether genomic imprinting might explain the phenotytic variation seen with the 45, X karyotype. Sanger determined by assessment of Xg blood groups that the paternal X or Y was lost in 77% of cases (64). Restriction fragment length polymorphism analysis has verified that the remaining X in 45, X monosomy is maternal (X^m) approximately 80% of the time (65). However, there is no difference in the prevalence of maternally or paternally imprinted X in spontaneous abortuses (66), and early studies have not discerned any postnatal phenotypic

Table 2 Frequency (%) of Phenotypic Features in Adults with Complete X Monosomy (45, X), Short-Arm Deletion (46, XXp^-), or Long-Arm Delection (46, XXq^-)

Feature	45, X (n = 332)	46, XXp^- (n = 52)	46, XXq^- (n = 67)
Short stature	100	88	43
Gonadal dysgenesis	91	65	93
Short neck	77	38	21
Cubitus valgus	77	25	16
"Shield chest"	74	35	13
Low hairline	72	19	9
Delayed bone age	64	17	10
Pigmented nevi	64	27	19
Nail anomaly	57	8	7
Short metacarpal	55	29	12
Renal anomaly	44	8	6
Webbed neck	42	2	1
Hypertension	37	8	7
Cardiac anomaly	23	2	0
Thyroid disease	18	6	3

Source: Adapted from Reference 63.

distinctions in 45, X subjects on the basis of parental chromosomal origin (67).

A model to explain the Turner syndrome phenotype invokes halved expression of a gene or genes on the X chromosome; such a gene must have homologs on the X and the Y and must escape X inactivation. The second X is inactivated throughout all developmental phases and tissues, except in the oocyte and during initial zygotic cell divisions (68). Many genes that escape X inactivation have been identified in recent years, and regions of the distal short arm (including the pseudoautosomal region) and pericentromeric regions appear not to be inactivated. Page (69) has nominated both ZFX (a transcription factor) and RPS4X (a ribosomal subunit component) as candidate Turner genes, supported by observations that Zfx and Rps4, in contrast with the situation in humans, are X inactivated in mice, in which no prenatal lethality or phenotypic abnormality in XO is seen (70). However, other evidence argues against these genes as factors in TS (71). Despite the growing list of X chromosome genes that escape inactivation, in essence there has been little progress in elucidating the genetic basis of TS since phenotype-karyotype correlations were first drawn 30 years ago. The remarkable similarity in phenotypes resulting from loss of either the short or long arm, survivorship of only a small fraction of TS fetuses, incidence of coarctation and renal anomaly in only a minority of 45, X patients, and the occasional 45, X patient with normal ovaries are all mysteries.

IV. Y CHROMOSOME MOSAICISM

X chromosomal monosomy occurs in mosaicism with 46, XY cells in approximately 5% of patients with Turner syndrome. The phenotype associated with the 45, X/46, XY karyotype, ranging from female to male, provides an interesting story and a cautionary tale about ascertainment bias. The phenotype has historically been described predominantly as ambiguous genitalia and mixed gonadal dysgenesis (streak ovary with dysgenetic testicular elements and possible asymmetry of wolffian and müllerian structures). In an early review, 60% of cases exhibited ambiguous genitalia and mixed gonadal dysgenesis, 25% were phenotypic females with bilateral streak gonads and other features of TS, and the remaining 15% had the appearance of undervirilized males (72). Approximately two-thirds of 45, X/46, XY individuals diagnosed at birth are raised as females. In contrast, 90–95% of the cases diagnosed *prenatally* have been normal phenotypic males at birth, and features of TS have been rare (73,74). These data suggest that characteristics of TS are seen less commonly in 45, X/46, XY individuals than in comparable mosaicisms, such as 45, X/46, XX. Adequate longitudinal studies have not been performed, however, and the incidence of TS features and gonadal dysgenesis may be higher than expected from first reports of normal male external genitalia.

The incidence of gonadal malignancy in 45, X/46, XY mixed gonadal dysgenesis engenders considerable clinical discussion. In Scully's series of 30 cases of gonadoblastoma, 10 were associated with 45, X/46, XY mosaicism (75). The

risk of a patient with this karyotype developing gonadoblastoma or dysgerminoma has been estimated at 15–20% (62). Because this risk assessment was derived before recognition that the postnatal phenotype is usually normal, it is possibly overestimated for the 45, X/46, XY karyotype in general. Nevertheless, it seems prudent to assume that the risk of malignancy remains high in the phenotypic subgroups with either female (TS) or ambiguous genitalia. Prophylactic gonadectomy should be performed in TS patients with XY mosaicism, certainly before adolescence and preferably in early childhood. This recommendation has consequently raised the question of whether techniques other than routine cytogenetics should be utilized to detect Y material in TS. Southern blotting, in situ hybridization, or polymerase chain reaction with Y-specific primers definitely should be used to determine the origin of marker chromosomes or small rings (76). Analysis of cells from series of patients with TS has revealed an incidence of previously undetected Y material ranging from 0 to 15% (77), but the utility of these techniques as an adjunct to routine karyotyping is not yet clear.

V. MEDICAL THERAPIES (TABLE 3)

A. Growth Therapy: Androgens and Estrogens

Androgens were widely utilized for growth promotion in clinical trials in TS before the time that human growth hormone (hGH) became widely available. Most investigations of androgen therapy for short stature in TS have demonstrated short-term efficacy in stimulating growth. A number of studies have also reported modest increases in final or predicted adult height from androgen therapy (78,79). However, most of the early studies were flawed in being small, retrospective, uncontrolled, or controlled only by an estro-

Table 3 Management of Turner Syndrome in Childhood

Preventive measures
    Karyotype analysis: rule out Y material
    Renal ultrasound
    Echocardiography (may be repeated)
    Regular thyroid screening
    Hypertension monitoring
    Possible orthopedic referral (scoliosis)
    Ophthalmology (strabismus, others)
    Ear, nose, and throat (recurrent otitis)
    Audiologic evaluation
    Cognitive evaluation
    Psychologic counseling
    Support groups
Medical therapy
    Begin hGH therapy at height <fifth percentile
    Initiate estrogen at 12–15 years/cycle within 2 years

---

gen-treated group. Lenko et al. (80) analyzed growth and final height data in 76 girls treated with fluoxymesterone or conjugated estrogens and found that initial growth velocity was greatest when both were used, followed by the androgen and estrogen groups, but mean final heights were not distinguishable. In a retrospective analysis of 66 TS patients, Sybert (42) reported that the mean adult height of patients given either oxandrolone or fluoxymesterone (148 cm) did not differ significantly from the height of untreated patients (146.3 cm).

In contrast, a 3–5 cm increase in final height (relative to predicted heights) has been documented in three separate oxandrolone trials (81–83). In aggregate, these studies suggest that anabolic steroids accelerate growth over several years of treatment and may result in modest improvement of adult height, perhaps by as much as 3–5 cm. However, the final height data are not persuasive enough to consider androgens, which are quite inexpensive relative to hGH, as more than a secondary treatment option. Potential growth benefits must be weighed against potential androgenic side effects. Oxandrolone is available on a limited clinical research basis in the United States and has limited side effects at a dose of 0.0625 mg/kg-day. It can be added to an hGH regimen if growth rate falls below 4 cm/year or if initiation of growth therapy has been delayed to a relatively advanced age (>12 years old) in a patient in the lower half of the TS growth curve.

As with androgens, estrogen therapy in TS definitely results in growth acceleration. Most studies have failed to document any improvement in predicted or final adult height, however, and estrogen therapy fundamentally appears only to accelerate short-term growth while sacrificing duration of growth. Several studies have demonstrated that TS patients given full-dose estrogen replacement during early adolescence have final heights in the 140 cm range, possibly less than the expected mean height of 143 cm in TS (78). Investigators have therefore attempted to identify a reduced, nonfeminizing dose of estrogen that might be an effective long-term growth stimulant. It has been argued that estrogen has a biphasic effect upon skeletal growth, stimulating growth at low concentrations but inhibiting growth at higher dosages. In this vein, Ross et al. reported that a low dose of ethinyl estradiol (EE, 100 ng/kg-day) resulted in a 70% increase in growth rate in 16 Turner girls, ages 5–15 years, during 6 month crossover treatments (84). This result raised hopes that low-dose estrogen might be effective in preadolescent Turner girls in stimulating growth without skeletal advancement or feminization. The short-term growth stimulation from low-dose EE was confirmed in subsequent studies, but it did not occur without accompanying effects on bone. In a study by Martinez et al. (85) using 100 ng/kg-day of EE, growth velocity more than doubled but bone age advanced by 1.6 years per year and predicted height was unchanged. Similarly, growth rate increased from 4.2 to 7.9, 4.8, 2.8, and 1.8 cm/year during years 1–4 of treatment in 35 girls treated with a low dose of 17β-estradiol (86), but skeletal maturation was particularly rapid in the younger patients and no significant improvement in final height was observed.

Although the previous studies suggested that low-dose estrogen given alone provides a brief growth stimulation and may not adversely influence final height, no additional growth at all is observed when estrogen is added to hGH therapy. Vanderschueren-Lodeweyckx et al. (87) administered hGH alone or in combination with a very low dose of EE (25 ng/kg-day) to 40 Turner patients, and no significant differences in growth rates were found between the two groups. Nevertheless, increased skeletal maturation was noted in TS patients treated with hGH plus low-dose EE before 11 years of age. Mean "near final height" of 20 girls with BA > 13 years was 149.3 cm after 4 years of treatment, with no discernible differences between the hGH alone and hGH plus ethinyl estradiol groups (88). Similarly, studies by Ross et al. (89) failed to show that the combination of hGH and 50 ng/kg-day of EE was superior to hGH alone. Several studies in progress appear to confirm the acceleration of bone age during low-dose EE therapy (90), particularly in younger subjects. If these findings are substantiated, EE in combination with hGH may ironically have a deleterious effect upon final height because skeletal maturation is increased without benefit of an increase in growth velocity. Estrogen therapy is contraindicated in preadolescent patients and plays no role in growth therapy in TS, and as a corollary, the timing of initiating estrogen for feminization remains debatable.

B. Growth Therapy: Human Growth Hormone

Turner undertook the first documented administration of exogenous growth hormone in TS and was unsuccessful, presumably giving injections of bovine pituitary extract, because hGH was not available until the 1950s. In 1960, Escamilla et al. (91). administered hGH to a patient with TS, resulting in an increase in growth velocity from 3.8 to 7.5 cm/year over several months. Later trials of pituitary-derived hormone supported the efficacy of hGH in the treatment of short stature in TS. With the development of recombinant hGH in the 1980s, TS was the first group (after GH deficiency) in which clinical trials were initiated, largely because of the relative homogeneity of the population and the lengthy potential treatment period.

hGH trials in TS have universally demonstrated an increase in growth velocity, but long term treatment and final height data are just beginning to appear. In almost every study, hGH has augmented pretreatment growth velocity by 50–150% in the first year, depending upon dosing and whether hGH was used in combination with androgens. As in hGH treatment of GH deficiency (GHD) or idiopathic short stature, growth acceleration in girls with TS is sustainable but is most pronounced in the first year of therapy. Most early trials used three times per week dosing regimens, and virtually none of the trials has utilized a control group, except in the first year. Many of the early trials combined hGH with estrogens or androgens, which were previously established as short-term growth stimulants. The anabolic effects of oxandrolone had been observed in the absence of a marked increase in serum IGF-I levels, implying that the actions of growth hormone and androgens are additive. Nilsson et al. (92), using combination daily hGH and oxandrolone in

Swedish TS patients, reported an increase in growth velocity from 3.9 to 9.4 and 6.8 cm/year in the first 2 years of therapy. The increment in growth velocity was more pronounced in the combination group. In the Belgian experience using hGH alone, growth velocity increased from 4.0 cm/year at baseline to 7.4, 5.8, 5.0, and 3.7 cm/year in each of 4 years of therapy (93). In the German collaborative study, height velocities in the hGH-treated group were 4.0, 6.3, and 5.3 cm/year at baseline and in the first 2 years, respectively, and predicted adults heights increased by approximately 4 cm (94).

The first and most influential trial in TS began in the United States in 1983 (95). A total of 70 girls between 4.7 and 12.4 years of age, with normal provocative GH tests, were randomly assigned to a control group (no treatment), oxandrolone (0.125 mg/kg-day), hGH (0.125 mg/kg three times per week), or combination oxandrolone and hGH. After 12–20 months, all subjects except the hGH group were placed into the combination group at a reduced oxandrolone dose (because of virilization in 30% of subjects). After the third year of treatment, when trials in GHD had revealed a better response to daily hGH, subjects received hGH daily instead of three times per week. In subjects receiving hGH alone, growth velocity increased from 4.5 cm/year in the pretreatment period to 6.6 and 5.4 cm/year in the first and second years, respectively. Mean growth rates in the first 3 years in subjects started on hGH and oxandrolone (at the lower dose of 0.0625 mg/kg/day) were 8.3, 6.7, and 6.3 cm/year, and the first year growth rate with hGH and the higher oxandrolone dose was 10 cm/year. In the most recent report (95), 50 subjects had finished 5 years of therapy. Figure 4 presents the mean annual growth rate in comparison with the expected untreated growth rate calculated from the Lyon curve. By this method of presentation, it can be seen that growth rates of 5.2, 5.1, and 4.3 cm/year in years 4–6 of treatment with hGH alone are greater than expected, because of the progressive decline of growth velocity normally seen in untreated TS. A positive growth response has been sustained throughout the entire 6 years of treatment in both the hGH and combination groups.

The primary therapeutic objective of hGH therapy is augmentation of final height, which can be achieved if growth velocity increases without undue advance in skeletal age. Figure 4C expresses the U.S. study data as cumulative growth in comparison with untreated patients. Over 6 years, total growth of 19 cm without treatment was expected by projection on the Lyon curve, whereas subjects receiving hGH alone grew 31.2 cm, and those in the combination group grew 37.3 cm. The expected bone age (BA) advance in TS is approximately 0.8 years per year of chronologic age. hGH therapy for 6 years resulted in skeletal age advancement of 5.2 ± 1.4 years versus BA advance of 6.3 ± 1.6 years from combination therapy. Thus, preliminary results suggest that treatment with hGH alone slightly accelerates BA, but the long-term benefit is positive. In contrast, oxandrolone provides additional short-term growth benefit but offers minimal additional long-term benefit when combined with hGH in TS. The 6.2 cm excess in cumulative growth in the combination group may diminish as the study progresses.

At this point, 82% of subjects in the hGH group and 91% in the combination arms of the U.S. study have already exceeded projected adult heights, and many patients are still growing. Mean current height for the 30 patients who have terminated therapy is 151.9 ± 4.8 cm, as opposed to the initial mean projected height of 143.8 ± 6.0 cm. Mean chronologic age at enrollment for the U.S. study was 9.3 years, and mean skeletal age at entry was 8.0 years; these relatively advanced degrees of skeletal maturation may have limited the length of potential treatment.

The U.S. and international studies do not provide information regarding the appropriate time to initiate or terminate hGH therapy (96). Data are convincing that daily administration is preferable to less frequent dosing. This was suggested by the increase in growth rate in the U.S. study following a change from three times per week to daily dosing in year 3. Additionally, the Dutch group randomized 52 girls to 24 IU/m² per week, given either three or six times weekly (93). After 2 years, total height increment was 8.6 and 11.3 cm in the two groups, respectively. Although bone age advance was slightly greater with more frequent hGH dosing, change in height SDS for BA was still 0.4 SDS greater with the daily dosing regimen.

Some dosage data are also available and suggest that GH doses in excess of 0.05 mg/kg-day result in greater growth stimulation in the first year, possibly at the cost of diminished growth velocity in later years of therapy. Takano et al. reported the Japanese experience with different dosages in 46 children over 3 years (97). Growth rate in the group receiving the higher dose was significantly greater in the first year only; after 3 years, relative advances in BA were 2.5 and 2.9 years in the two groups, respectively. Thus, it is unclear whether final height would be significantly improved with higher doses of hGH.

Our current policy is to offer treatment with hGH alone, 0.05 mg/kg-day, as soon as a TS patient falls below the fifth percentile on the normal female growth curve, although we have not treated any girls under 2 years of age. We utilize this arbitrary percentile criterion on the unproven supposition that therapeutic response is most successful if therapy can be sustained over many years. The decision to begin therapy also depends upon the readiness of the family to undertake a regimen of daily injections, and so therapy is often delayed until the patient reaches school age. Possible side effects are always discussed (98,99). We do not routinely perform provocative growth hormone testing in girls with TS, because most subjects respond positively to hGH therapy despite adequate stimulated GH levels. The appropriate time to discontinue hGH has not been established; without any data to support more definitive criteria, we generally use a growth rate <2.5 cm/year together with a bone age >14 years.

Although pediatric endocrinologists are widely engaged in discussions regarding appropriate medical uses of hGH, a consensus has been reached that hGH therapy is beneficial for most, but possibly not all, girls with TS. Dissent from this view comes either from rejection of the 143 cm figure for untreated final height or from a broader ethical argument that a 8–10 cm height benefit does not justify the risk or

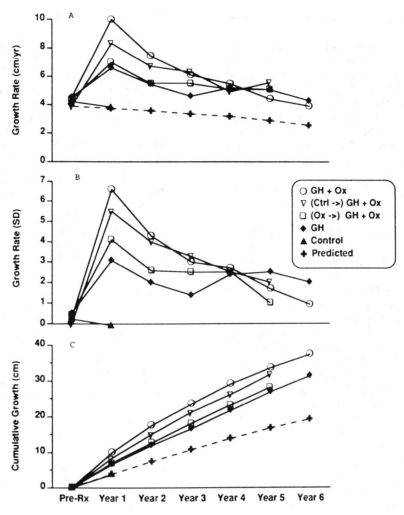

Figure 4 Annual growth for each U.S. Turner study group as indicated. (A) Growth velocity expressed as cm/year and compared with predicted untreated growth rate; (B) growth velocity standard deviation score (SDS); (C) cumulative growth as cm/year in excess of expected cumulative growth for untreated patients. (From Ref. 95.)

expense involved. In our opinion, TS patients and their families are generally eager for hGH therapy.

C. Estrogen Replacement

Most adolescents with TS have markedly elevated FSH values, indicating ovarian failure (37). As many as 20–30% of TS patients may exhibit breast budding, but few complete pubertal development and reach menarche spontaneously (9–11). Thus, estrogen replacement for secondary sexual development is required in most girls with TS. Ironically, many studies of estrogen use in TS have concentrated upon the objective of growth stimulation and have failed to provide detailed analysis of the feminizing effects. Consequently, the timing and dose of estrogen replacement are still controversial issues. The difficulty rests upon a general belief that physiologic estrogen replacement in early adolescence may diminish

final height, although this assumption relies upon older and poorly controlled studies.

Balancing the legitimate psychologic need to begin pubertal development against concerns about final height, our routine practice is to begin conjugated estrogens at the relatively advanced age of 13–15 years, when most growth has been completed. In our regimen, the initial dosage is 0.3 mg/day and is increased to 0.625 mg approximately 6 months later. After 1–2 years of therapy, estrogens are modified to days 1–26 only, and 5–10 mg medroxyprogesterone acetate is added on days 17–26, to induce menses and diminish the risk of endometrial hyperplasia or carcinoma. This estrogen replacement regimen may adversely influence skeletal maturation. In the first year following introduction of conjugated estrogens, the bone age of 12- to 15-year-old girls receiving this estrogen regimen advances approximately 50% faster than in girls on hGH alone (unpublished data), and younger girls are at greater risk of skeletal age acceleration. Nevertheless, there are no definitive data confirming a reduction in final height.

If estrogens are to be employed for feminization before final height has been achieved, the lowest effective dose should be used, to avoid accelerated epiphyseal fusion. Because some earlier studies of estrogen for growth stimulation suggested that low doses of estrogen, such as 100 ng/kg-day of ethinyl estradiol, could stimulate breast development without affecting predicted adult height (at least in girls with bone ages > 11 years), it has recently been thought possible to introduce low-dose estrogen at a more physiologically appropriate age, perhaps at 11–13 years of age. Of course, the mean bone age of 12- to 13-year-old females with TS is approximately 10–11 years, putting substantial future growth at risk if bone age accelerates unduly.

The Belgians have reported that the very low dose of ethinyl estradiol (25 ng/kg-day) added to hGH therapy resulted in breast budding in 9 of 20 recipients (87). Martinez et al. treated subjects with 100 ng/kg-day of ethinyl estradiol, and all progressed to Tanner 2 breast stage (85). The problem with very low doses of estrogens is that girls cannot be considered adequately feminized until reaching at least Tanner B3–4. We have undertaken a double-blind, multicenter trial of 0, 25, or 100 ng/kg-day of oral ethinyl estradiol in 12- to 15-year-old females with TS with Tanner breast stage 1 or 2, all of whom were already receiving a standardized dose of hGH as growth therapy (100). There was no significant advance in bone age using 25 ng/kg-day, and only about 20% of the girls achieved B3. On the other hand, B3 was reached in approximately 60% of subjects in the 100 ng/kg-day group, but BA advancement increased by about one-third without any improvement in height velocity. Thus, an effective feminizing dose will probably have skeletal effects, although some girls appear to be quite sensitive to the feminizing effects of low-dose estrogens.

As a result, no perfect dose of estrogen may be adequate to achieve feminization without inducing an acceleration of bone age, with its implicit (but not documented) reduction in adult height. The apparent estrogen-induced acceleration in skeletal age jeopardizes the primary objective of hGH therapy and has made practitioners reluctant to begin "early" estrogen replacement. On the other hand, the practice of delaying estrogen replacement until 15–18 years of age, in an effort to maximize growth, guarantees signficant delays in pubertal development, risks a lifelong diminution of bone mineral density, and potentially accentuates the social isolation and stigmatization of girls with TS. Thus, a prudent and sympathetic approach is to customize therapy according to the current height and psychologic needs of each patient but to delay estrogen therapy until bone age reaches approximately 11 years.

REFERENCES

1. Turner HH. A syndrome of infantilism, congenital webbed neck, and cubitus valgus. Endocrinology 1938; 23:566–574.
2. Wilkins L, Fleischmann W. Ovarian agenesis: pathology, association with clinical symptoms, and their bearing on the theories of sex differentiation. J Clin Endocrinol Metab 1944; 4:357–368.
3. Grumbach MM, Van Wyk JJ, Wilkins L. Chromosomal sex in gonadal dysgenesis: relationship to male pseudohermaphroditism and theories of human sex differentiation. J Clin Endocrinol Metab 1955; 15:1161–1193.
4. Ullrich P. Turner's syndrome and status Bonnevie-Ullrich. Am J Hum Genet 1949; 1:179–202.
5. Haddad HM, Wilkins L. Congenital anomalies associated with gonadal aplasia. Pediatrics 1959; 23:885.
6. Ferguson-Smith MA. Karyotype-phenotype correlations in gonadal dysgenesis and their bearing on the pathogenesis of malformations. J Med Genet 1965; 2:142–145.
7. Polani PE, Hunter WF, Lennox B. Chromosomal sex in Turner's syndrome with coarctation of the aorta. Lancet 1954; 2:120.
8. Ford CE, Miller OJ, Polani PE, de Almeida JC, Briggs JH. A sex chromosome anomaly in a case of gonadal dysgenesis (Turner's syndrome). Lancet 1959; 1:711–713.
9. Palmer CG, Reichman A. Chromosomal and clinical findings in 110 females with Turner syndrome. Hum Genet 1976; 35:35–42.
10. Hall JG, Sybert VP, Williamson RA, Fisher NL, Reed SD. Turner's syndrome. West J Med 1982; 137:32–44.
11. Park E, Bailey JD, Cowell CA. Growth and maturation of patients with Turner's syndrome. Pediatr Res 1983; 17:1–7.
12. Otto PG, Vianna-Morgante AM, Otto PA, et al. The Turner phenotype and the different types of human X isochromosome. Hum Genet 1981; 7:159–164.
13. Warburton D, Kline J, Stein Z, Susser M. Monosomy X: a chromosomal anomaly associated with young maternal age. Lancet 1980; 1:167.
14. Hook EB, Warburton D. The distribution of chromosomal genotypes associated with Turner's syndrome: livebirth prevalence rates and evidence for diminished fetal mortality and severity in genotypes associated with structural X abnormalities or mosaicism. Hum Genet 1983; 62:24–27.
15. Canki N, Warburton D, Byrne J. Morphological characteristics of monosomy X in spontaneous abortions. Ann Genet 1988; 31:4–13.
16. Hecht F, Macfarlane JP. Mosaicism in Turner's syndrome reflects the lethality of XO. Lancet 1969; 2:1197–1198.
17. Held KR, Kerber S, Kaminsky E, et al. Mosaicism in 45, X Turner syndrome: does survival in early pregnancy depend on the presence of two sex chromosomes? Hum Genet 1992; 88:288–294.
18. Burns JL, Hall JG, Powers E, Callis JB, Hoehn H. No evidence for chromosomal mosaicism in multiple tissues of 10 patients with 45, XO Turner syndrome. Clin Genet 1979; 15:22–28.
19. Miller MJ, Geffner ME, Lippe BM, et al. Echocardiography reveals a high incidence of bicuspid aortic valve in Turner syndrome. J Pediatr 1983; 102:47–50.
20. Allen DB, Hendrich A, Levy JM. Aortic dilation in Turner syndrome. J Pediatr 1986; 109:302–305.
21. Lin AE, Lippe BM, Geffner ME, et al. Aortic dilation, dissection, and rupture in patients with Turner syndrome. J Pediatr 1986; 109:820–822.
22. Clarke EB. Web neck and congenital heart defects: a pathogenic association in 45XO Turner syndrome? Teratology 1984; 29:355–361.
23. Lippe B, Geffner ME, Dietrich RB, Boechat MI, Kangarloo H. Renal malformations in patients with Turner syndrome: imaging in 141 patients. Pediatrics 1988; 82:852–856.
24. Hall JG. Turner syndrome. In: King RA, Rotter JI, Motulsky AG, eds. The Genetic Basis of Common Disorders. London: Oxford University Press, 1992:895–914.

25. Rongen-Westerlaken C, Rikken B, Vastrick P, et al. Body proportions in individuals with Turner syndrome. Eur J Pediatr 1993; 152:813–817.

26. Hughes PCR, Ribeiro J, Hughes IA. Body proportions in Turner syndrome. Arch Dis Child 1986; 61:506–507.

27. Lubin MB, Gruber HE, Rimoin DL, Lachman RS. Skeletal abnormalities in the Turner syndrome. In: Rosenfeld RG, Grumbach MM, eds. Turner Syndrome. New York: Marcel Dekker, 1990:281–300.

28. Barr DGO. Bone deficiency in Turner's syndrome measured by metacarpal dimensions. Arch Dis Child 1974; 49:821–822.

29. Smith MA, Wilson J, Price WH. Bone demineralization in patients with Turner's syndrome. J Med Genet 1982; 19:100–103.

30. Stepan JJ, Musilova J, Pacovsky V. Bone demineralization, biochemical indices of bone remodeling, and estrogen replacement therapy in adults with Turner's syndrome. J Bone Miner Res 1989; 4:193–198.

31. Naeraa RW, Brixen K, Hansen RM, et al. Skeletal size and bone mineral content in Turner's syndrome: relation to karyotype, estrogen treatment, physical fitness, and bone turnover. Calcif Tissue Int 1991; 49:77–83.

32. Kirkland RT, Lin T-H, LeBlanc AD, Kirkland JL, Evans HJ. Effects of hormonal therapy on bone mineral density in Turner syndrome. In: Rosenfeld RG, Grumbach MM, eds. Turner Syndrome. New York: Marcel Dekker, 1990:319–325.

33. Rubin KR. Osteoporosis. In: Rosenfeld RG, Grumbach MM, eds. Turner Syndrome. New York: Marcel Dekker, 1990:310–317.

34. Ross JL, Long LM, Feuillan P, Cassorla F, Cutler GB. Normal bone density of the wrist and spine and increased wrist fractures in girls with Turner's syndrome. J Clin Endocrinol Metab 1991; 73:355–359.

35. Neely, EK, Marcus R, Rosenfeld RG, Bachrach LK. Bone mineral apparent density is normal in adolescents with Turner syndrome. J Clin Endocrinol Metab 1993; 76:861–866.

36. Massarano AA, Adams JA, Preece MA, Brook CGD. Ovarian ultrasound appearances in Turner syndrome. J Pediatr 1989; 114:568–573.

37. Conte FH, Grumbach MM, Kaplan SL. A diphasic pattern of gonadotropin secretion in patients with the syndrome of gonadal dysgenesis. J Clin Endocrinol Metab 1975; 40:670–676.

38. Lyon AJ, Preece MA, Grant DB. Growth curve for girls with Turner syndrome. Arch Dis Child 1985; 60:932–935.

39. Ranke MB, Pfluger H, Rosendahl W, et al. Turner syndrome: spontaneous growth in 150 cases and review of the literature. Eur J Pediatr 1983; 141:81–88.

40. Naeraa RW, Nielsen J. Standards for growth and final height in Turner's syndrome. Acta Paediatr Scand 1990; 79:182–190.

41. Zachmann M, Sobradillo B, Frank M, Frisch H, Prader A. Bayley-Pinneau, Roche-Wainer-Thissen, and Tanner height predictions in normal children and in patients with various pathologic conditions. J Pediatr 1978; 93:749–755.

42. Sybert VP. Adult height in Turner syndrome with and without androgen therapy. J Pediatr 1984; 104:365–369.

43. Massa G, Vanderschueren-Lodeweyckx M, Malvaux P. Linear growth in patients with Turner syndrome: influence of spontaneous puberty and parental height. Eur J Pediatr 1990; 149:246–250.

44. Page LA. Final heights in 45, X Turner's syndrome with spontaneous sexual development. Review of European and American reports. J Pediatr Endocrinol 1993; 6:153–158.

45. Horton WA. Growth plate biology and the Turner syndrome. In: Rosenfeld RG, Grumbach MM, eds. Turner Syndrome. New York: Marcel Dekker, 1990:259–266.

46. Ross JL, Long LM, Loriaux DL, Cutler GB, Jr. Growth hormone secretory dynamics in Turner syndrome. J Pediatr 1985; 106:202–206.

47. Cuttler L, Van Vliet G, Conte FA, Kaplan SL, Grumbach MM. Somatomedin-C levels in children and adolescents with gonadal dysgenesis: differences from age-matched normal females and effect of chronic estrogen replacement. J Clin Endocrinol Metab 1985; 60:1087–1092.

48. Massarano AA, Brook CGD, Hindmarsh PC, et al. Growth hormone secretion in Turner's syndrome and influence of oxandrolone and ethinyl estradiol. Arch Dis Child 1989; 64:587–592.

49. Mauras N, Rogol AD, Veldhuis JD. Increased hGH production rate after low-dose estrogen therapy in prepubertal girls with Turner's syndrome. Pediatr Res 1990; 28:626–630.

50. Garron DA. Intelligence among persons with Turner's syndrome. Behav Genet 1977; 7:105–127.

51. Fryns JP, Kleczkowska A, Van Den Berghe H. High incidence of mental retardation in Turner syndrome patients with ring chromosome X formation. Genetic Couns 1990; 38:161–165.

52. Rovet J, Netley C. Processing deficits in Turner's syndrome. Dev Psychol 1982; 18:77–94.

53. Bender B, Puck M, Salbenblatt J, Robinson A. Cognitive development of unselected girls with complete and partial X monosomy. Pediatrics 1984; 73:175–182.

54. Gordon H, Galatzer A. Cerebral organization in patients with gonadal dysgenesis. Psychoneuroendocrinology 1980; 5:235–244.

55. McCauley E, Kay T, Ito J, Treder R. The Turner syndrome: cognitive deficits, affective discrimination, and behavior problems. Child Dev 1987; 58:464–473.

56. Murphy DG, DeCarli C, Daly E, et al. X-chromosome effects on female brain: a magnetic resonance imaging study of Turner's syndrome. Lancet 1993; 342:1197–1200.

57. Pennington BF, Bender B, Puck M, Salbenblatt J, Robinson A. Learning disabilities in children with sex chromosome anomalies. Child Dev 1982; 53:1182–1192.

58. Swillen A, Fryns JP, Kleczkowska A, Massa G, Vanderschueren-Lodeweyckx M, Van den Berghe H. Intelligence, behaviour and psychosocial development in Turner syndrome. A cross-sectional study of 50 pre-adolescent and adolescent girls (4–20 years). Genetic Couns 1993; 4:7–18.

59. Papendieck LG, Iorcansky S, Coco R, Rivarola MA, Bergada C. High incidence of thyroid disturbances in 49 children with Turner syndrome. J Pediatr 1987; 111:258–261.

60. Schatz R, Maclaren NK, Lippe BM. Autoimmunity in Turner syndrome. In: Rosenfeld RG and Grumbach MM, eds. Turner Syndrome. New York: Marcel Dekker, 1990:205–220.

61. Neely EK, Rosenfeld RG. Phenotypic correlates of X chromosome loss. In: Wachtel SS, ed. Molecular Genetics of Sex Determination. Orlando, FL: Academic Press, 1993:311–339.

62. Simpson JL. Gonadal dysgenesis and sex chromosome abnormalities: phenotypic-karyotypic correlations. In: Vallet HL, and Porter IH, eds. Genetic Mechanisms of Sexual Development. New York: Academic Press, 1979:365–405.

63. Therman E, Susman B. The similarity of phenotypic effects caused by Xp and Xq deletions in the human female: a hypothesis. Hum Genet 1990; 85:175–183.

64. Sanger R, Tippett P, Gavin J. Xg groups and sex abnormalities in people of Northern European ancestry. J Med Genet 1971; 8:417–426.

65. Hassold T, Kumlin E, Takeesu N, et al. Determination of the parenteral origin of sex chromosome monosomy using restriction fragment length polymorphisms. Am J Hum Genet 1985; 37:965–972.

66. Hassold T, Pettay D, Robinson A, Uchida I. Molecular studies

of parental origin and mosaicism in 45, X conceptuses. Hum Genet 1992; 89:647–652.

67. Mathur A, Stekol L, Schatz D, Maclaren NK, Scott ML, Lippe B. The parental origin of the single X chromosome in Turner syndrome: lack of correlation with parental age or clinical phenotype. Am J Hum Genet 1991; 48:682–686.

68. Lyon M. X inactivation. In: Wachtel SS, ed. Molecular Genetics of Sex Determination. Orlando, FL: Academic Press, 1993:123–142.

69. Fisher EMC, Beer-Romero P, Brown LG, et al. Homologous ribosomal protein genes on the human X and Y chromosomes: escape from X inactivation and possible implications for Turner syndrome. Cell 1990; 63:1205–1218.

70. Ashworth A, Rastan S, Lovell-Badge R, Kay G. X-chromosome inactivation may explain the difference in viability of XO humans and mice. Nature 1991; 351:406–408.

71. Just W, Geerkens C, Held KR, Vogel W. Expression of RPS4X in fibroblasts from patients with structural aberrations of the X chromosome. Hum Genet 1992; 89:240–242.

72. Hsu LYF. Prenatal diagnosis of 45, X/46, XY mosaicism—a review and update. Prenat Diagn 1989; 9:31–48.

73. Chang HJ, Clark RD, Bachman H. The phenotype of 45, X/46, XY mosaicism: an analysis of 92 prenatally diagnosed cases. Am J Hum Genet 1990; 46:156–168.

74. Wheeler M, Peakman D, Robinson A, et al. 45X/46XY mosaicism: contrast of prenatal and postnatal diagnosis. Am J Med Genet 1988; 29:565–571.

75. Scully RE. Gonadoblastoma: a review of 74 cases. Cancer 1970; 25:1340–1356.

76. Lindgren V, Chen C, Bryke CR, Lichter P, Page DC, Yang-Feng TL. Cytogenetic and molecular characterization of marker chromosomes in patients with mosaic 45, X karyotypes. Hum Genet 1992; 88:393–398.

77. Medlej R, Lobaccaro JM, Berta P, et al. Screening for Y-derived sex determining gene SRY in 40 patients with Turner syndrome. J Clin Endocrinol Metab 1992; 75:1289–1292.

78. Ranke MB, Rosenfeld RG, eds. Turner Syndrome: Growth Promoting Therapies. Amsterdam: Excerpta Medica, 1991.

79. Urban MD, Lee PA, Dorst JP, Plotnick LP, Migeon CJ. Oxandrolone therapy in patients with Turner syndrome. J Pediatr 1979; 94:823–827.

80. Lenko HL, Perheentupa J, Soderholm A. Growth in Turner's syndrome: spontaneous and fluoxymesterone stimulated. Acta Paediatr Scand Suppl 1979; 227:57–63.

81. Joss E, Zuppinger K. Oxandrolone in girls with Turner's syndrome. A pair-matched controlled study up to final height. Acta Paediatr Scand 1984; 73:674–679.

82. Naeraa RW, Nielsen J, Pedersen IL, Sorensen K. Effect of oxandrolone on growth and final height in Turner's syndrome. Acta Paediatr Scand 1990; 79:784–789.

83. Crock P, Werther GA, Wettenhall HNB. Oxandrolone increases final height in Turner syndrome. J Paediatr Child Health 1990; 26:221–224.

84. Ross JL, Long LM, Skerda M, et al. Effect of low doses of estradiol on 6-month growth rates and predicted height in patients with Turner syndrome. J Pediatr 1986; 109:950–953.

85. Martinez A, Heinrich JJ, Domene H, et al. Growth in Turner's syndrome: long-term treatment with low dose ethinyl estradiol. J Clin Endocrinol Metab 1987; 65:253–258.

86. Kastrup KW. Oestrogen therapy in Turner's syndrome. Acta Paediatr Scand Suppl 1988; 343:43–46.

87. Vanderschueren-Lodeweyckx M, Massa G, Maes M, et al. Growth-promoting effect of growth hormone and low-dose ethinyl estradiol in girls with Turner's syndrome. J Clin Endocrinol Metab 1990; 70:122–126.

88. Massa G, Vanderschueren-Lodeweyckx M. Growth promoting effect of growth hormone and low dose ethinyl estradiol in girls with Turner syndrome: 4 year results. In: Hibi I, Takano K, eds. Basic and Clinical Approach to Turner Syndrome. Amsterdam: Elsevier, 1993:327–332.

89. Ross JL, Cassorla F, Carpenter G, et al. The effect of short-term treatment with growth hormone and ethinyl estradiol on lower leg growth rate in girls with Turner's syndrome. J Clin Endocrinol Metab 1988; 67:515–518.

90. Hibi I, Takano K, eds. Basic and Clinical Approach to Turner Syndrome. Amsterdam: Elsevier, 1993.

91. Escamilla RF, Hutchings JJ, Deamer WC, Li CH. Clinical experiences with human growth hormone (LI) in pituitary infantilism and in gonadal dysgenesis. Acta Endocrinol Suppl (Copenh) 1960; 51:253A.

92. Nilsson KO. Swedish Paediatric Study Group for Growth Hormone Treatment. The Swedish Somatonorm Turner Trial: two-year results. Acta Paediatr Scand Suppl 1989; 356:160A.

93. Rongen-Westerlaken C, van Es A, Wit J-M, et al. Growth hormone therapy in Turner's syndrome. Am J Dis Child 1992; 146:817–820.

94. Stahnke N, Stubbe P, Keller E. Recombinant human growth hormone and oxandrolone in treatment of short stature in girls with Turner syndrome. Horm Res 1992; 37(Suppl 2):37–46.

95. Rosenfeld RG, Frane J, Attie KM, et al. Six year results of a randomized prospective trial of human growth hormone and oxandrolone in Turner syndrome. J Pediatr 1992; 121:49–55.

96. Price DA, Albertsson-Wikland K. Demography, auxology and response to recombinant human growth hormone treatment in girls with Turner's syndrome in the Kabi Pharmacia International Growth Study. Acta Paediatr Scand 1993; 82(Suppl 391):69–74.

97. Takano K, Shizume K, Hibi I. Treatment of 46 patients with Turner's syndrome with recombinant human growth hormone for three years: a multicentre study. Acta Endocrinol (Copenh) 1992; 126:292–302.

98. Hintz RL. Untoward events in patients treated with growth hormone in the USA. Horm Res (Suppl) 1992; 38:44–49.

99. Wilson DM, Frane JW, Sherman B, et al. Carbohydrate and lipid metabolism in Turner syndrome: effect of therapy with growth hormone, oxandrolone, and a combination of both. J Pediatr 1988; 112:210–217.

100. Neely EE, Rosenfeld RG, Gynex Cooperative Study Group. First year results of a randomized, placebo-controlled trial of low-dose ethinyl estradiol for feminization during growth hormone therapy for Turner syndrome. Pediatr Res 1993; 33:S89.

101. Rosenfeld RG. Turner syndrome: a guide for physicians. Wayzata, MN: Turner's syndrome Society, 1989.

102. Massa G, Vanderschueren-Lodweyckx M. Age and height at diagnosis in Turner syndrome: influence of parental height. Pediatrics 1991; 88:1148–1152.

20

Ambiguous Genitalia, Micropenis, Hypospadias, and Cryptorchidism

Marco Danon
Maimonides Medical Center and State University of New York Health Science Center at Brooklyn, Brooklyn, New York

Steven C. Friedman
Maimonides Medical Center, Brooklyn, New York

I. NORMAL SEX DETERMINATION AND SEX DIFFERENTIATION

Sex differentiation is a complex process by which the undifferentiated genitalia of the embryo evolve into male or female reproductive organs. This process comprises the following three events:

1. Differentiation of the bipotential gonad into testis or ovary
2. Differentiation of the wolffian ducts into epididymidis, vasa deferentia, and seminal vesicles, or differentiation of the müllerian ducts into uterus, fallopian tubes, and upper vagina
3. Development of the external genitalia into penis and scrotum or clitoris and labia

Sexual determination and differentiation are sequential processes starting with the establishment of genetic sex at conception, followed by gonadal determination in early embryogenesis. The main event in this process is the differentiation of the bipotential genital ridge into either a testis or an ovary. This sex determination event ultimately determines both the gonadal and phenotypic sex because male sex differentiation is regulated by testicular signals, whereas female sex differentiation occurs in the absence of fetal gonadal signals.

A. Testicular Development

From human chromosome analysis, evidence was obtained for the regulation of testicular gonadogenesis by a gene (or genes) on the Y chromosome. The short arm of the Y chromosome contains a gene (or genes) that controls testis determination and, therefore, maleness. This gene works in a dominant fashion and leads to differentiation of the bipotential gonad as a testis. There have been three hypotheses to explain testicular morphogenesis: (1) the H-Y antigen hypothesis, (2) the ZFY gene as the sex-determining locus, and (3) the SRY gene as control of male sex determination.

1. H-Y Antigen

An Y-linked antigen was thought to be the gene product initiating the sex determination event. This antigen, named H-Y, was recognized in experiments on inbred mice. It was observed that skin transplants from males were rejected, although transplants between same-sex pairs and from females to males were accepted. This was thought to be secondary to a histocompatibility antigen, coded by a Y-linked gene. H-Y is one of the so-called minor histocompatibility antigens. These antigens play a role in cellular rather than serologic immunity and are coded for by genes localized outside the major histocompatibility complex cluster of loci (1).

A technique was developed for assaying what appeared to be a serologic equivalent of H-Y. The simplicity of the serologic technique made it possible to identify this antigen as that responsible for transplantation rejection. In comparative studies on different species, the antigen appeared to be highly evolutionarily conserved. It was suggested that the H-Y antigen is the testis-determining factor (TDF) and, therefore, that the gene coding for it is the long-sought TDF (2). The serologic test for H-Y antigen provided a simple assay of genetic sex. However, problems with the assay surfaced. The techniques for serologic H-Y depended on subjective evaluations (e.g., of cytotoxicity as judged by trypan blue staining). Because of this and because the serologically detected H-Y is a "weak" antigen (hardly raising an antibody), the test did not distinguish well between male and female specimens.

Therefore, the assumptions that serologic and transplantation H-Y are identical, that H-Y is a single, male-specific molecule, and that it is identical with the testis-determining factor have all been questioned. Multiple studies in favor and against the H-Y antigen hypothesis have been published. The problems regarding the reproducibility and specificity of the H-Y antigen assay have led to the rejection by most investigators of a role for H-Y antigen in sex determination (3).

2. ZFY Gene

When the immunologic approach to identifying a primary sex-determining molecule was unsuccessful, the molecular genetic approach was intensified. The first success was reported from studies in patients with anomalous sex chromosomes (4). When XX males (normal male phenotype except for small testis and infertility) were investigated, they were found to have some Y chromosomal DNA. On the other hand, XY females are known to have microdeletion of the Y chromosome. These investigations identified 140 kB of DNA present in an XX male and absent in an X, Y:22 translocation female. This female's Y:22 translocation was a microdeletion of the TDF region of the Yp associated with a reciprocal translocation between Yq and autosome 22. Using information about the Y-specific DNA present in XX males and absent in this female made it possible to characterize TDF. TDF appeared to induce testicular differentiation by encoding a transcriptional regulatory protein called a "zinc finger protein," with multiple "finger" domains to facilitate its penetration into grooves of DNA or RNA.

Several investigations have cast doubts on the ZFY as the only sex-determining gene. The initial report on ZFY described some XX males who did not contain this sequence. Whether these were true XX males or XX hermaphrodites— the latter well known not to contain Y sequences—was not clarified. The ZFY hypothesis was therefore abandoned when this report and others demonstrated that it could not be TDF, and the search for TDF began again (5,6).

3. SRY Gene

The isolation of the sex-determining region of the Y (SRY), a single-copy gene, has fulfilled the criteria for TDF. Situated in the smallest Y chromosome region capable of sex reversal, it is expressed in the genital ridge during the appropriate time in embryonic development and it is deleted in some cases of human XY females. Furthermore, Sry (equivalent gene expressed in the mouse) can sex-reverse transgenic XX mice to males.

SRY belongs to a family of DNA binding proteins with an 80 amino acid sequence motif, resembling the same motif in high-mobility group (HMG) proteins called the HMG box. This family has two groups: those with a highly conserved HMG box and those including SRY, with a more divergent HMG box. Unlike the conserved HMG box proteins, the divergent HMG box proteins bind to specific DNA sequences implicated in transcriptional regulation. However, recent work suggests that these divergent HMG box proteins do not function as traditional transcription factors that directly increase transcription, but rather they bend or kink the DNA

(DNA bending proteins), possibly facilitating an interaction between proteins bound on either side that then alters transcription.

Evidence that SRY is the testis-determining gene (TDF) has been demonstrated by sex reversal in XX transgenic mice carrying the Sry transcript and the production of XY females by site-directed mutagenesis of the Sry gene. The Sry gene has been inserted into female mouse embryos and produced XX sex-reversed transgenic mice. It is possible that other genes on the short arm of the Y chromosome also play a role in male sex determination. It is also possible that autosomal genes are involved in the regulation of SRY expression, and others could be targets of SRY (7,8).

B. Ovarian Development

Two intact X chromosomes are required in the human for differentiation of the indifferent gonad into a normal ovary, in contrast to the mouse, in which a 45, X sex chromosome constitution allows the development of an ovary (although it leads to accelerated atresia of ovarian follicles). Females with 45, X chromosomes and those with deletions of the short arm (Xp) or long arm (Xq) of the X chromosome have ovarian development in utero, but the oocytes usually do not survive meiosis and folliculogenesis fails. This results in loss of germ cells, oocyte degeneration, and, secondarily, gonadal dysgenesis (streak gonads). Both X chromosomes appear to be active in the germ cell and oocyte from the onset of meiosis to ovulation. It has been suggested that genes controlling ovarian differentiation and function are located on both arms of the X chromosome. The viability of the germ cells and oocytes is also dependent on the genetic contribution of both X chromosomes. The familial 46, XX gonadal dysgenesis (an autosomal recessive trait condition) suggests that autosomal genes besides the genes on the X chromosomes are expressed through direct or indirect actions on the germ cell and are essential to ovarian development. It is therefore possible that a mutant autosomal gene contributes to a defect in the development of the ovary or in the synthesis or action of the putative meiosis-stimulating factor that leads to familial 46, XX gonadal dysgenesis (9).

II. ANATOMIC SEX DIFFERENTIATION OF THE REPRODUCTIVE TRACT

A. The Ambisexual Stage

The reproductive tract is anatomically the same until week 8 of gestation in male and female human fetuses, consisting of unipotential wolffian and müllerian ducts and bipotential external genital primordia (Figs. 1 and 2). Wolffian ducts, the primordia for the male sex organs, originally serve as excretory canals for the primitive kidney, the mesonephros, and are incorporated in the genital system when renal function is taken over by the metanephros, or definitive kidney. Müllerian, or paramesonephric ducts, the primordia for the female internal reproductive tract, originate from a cleft

FEMALE   INDIFFERENT STAGE   MALE

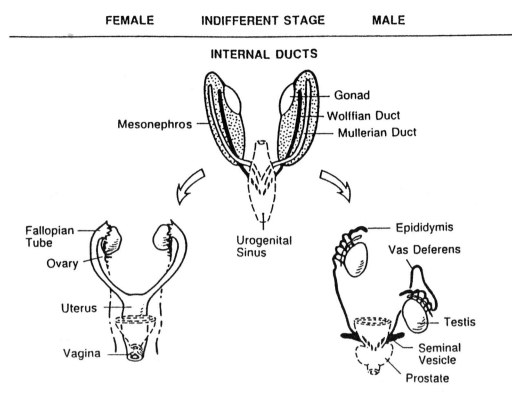

Figure 1 Phenotypic differentiation of internal ducts in male and female embryos.

lined by coelomic epithelium between the gonadal ridge and the mesonephros and grow parallel to the wolffian duct, then crossing it ventrally to join with the duct on the opposite side. By week 8, the paired ducts reach the dorsal wall of the urogenital sinus, where they cause an elevation, the müllerian tubercle. The müllerian tubercle separates the cranial vesicourethral canal from the caudal urogenital sinus. The fused tips of the müllerian ducts are separated from the dorsal wall of the urogenital sinus by a solid mass, the vaginal cord (Figs. 1 and 2).

The undifferentiated external genitalia includes the genital membrane, which closes the ventral part of the cloaca. The cloacal membrane within the folds becomes the urogenital and anal membrane at week 6 of gestation. By week 8 the cloaca is divided into an anterior urogenital sinus and a posterior anorectal canal. The genital tubercle is located ventrally, and the genital folds or labioscrotal swellings are located laterally (10).

B. Male Differentiation

Müllerian duct regression is the first event of somatic male differentiation. Testis-mediated müllerian regression begins at fetal week 8; müllerian ducts undergo regression only if exposed to testicular tissue before that date and cannot be rescued beyond that period when removed from testicular influence (11,12). The regression of the müllerian duct represents an unusual pattern of cell death: few cells actually die; instead,

they lose their polarity and orientation and cease to divide. The basement membrane dissolves, and a tight ring of connective tissue forms around the cells (13). In the human, müllerian ducts have nearly completely disappeared at 10 weeks.

The second aspect of internal male sex differentiation is the integraton of wolffian ducts in the genital system and their subsequent differentiation into epididymis, vas deferens, and seminal vesicles. Mucous epididymal secretion is demonstrable from 25 weeks of gestation.

Male orientation of the urogenital sinus is characterized by development of the prostate. Prostatic buds appear at approximately 10 weeks at the site of the müllerian tubercle and grow into solid branching cords. Maturation of the prostatic gland is accompanied by development of the prostatic utricle, the male remnant of the vaginal pouch. Two buds of epithelial cells, the sinoutricular bulbs, develop from the urogenital sinus close to the opening of the wolffian ducts and grow inward, fusing with the medial müllerian tubercle to form the sinoutricular cord, which makes contact with the caudal tip of the fused müllerian ducts and canalizes at 18 weeks to form the prostatic utricle (14).

Masculinization of the external genital organs begins in 9-week-old human fetuses by lengthening of the anogenital distance, followed by fusion of the labioscrotal folds and closure of the rims of the urethral groove, leading to the formation of a perineal and penile urethra. Penile organogenesis is completed at 11 weeks of gestation, but until week 16 penis and clitoris are more or less the same size (15).

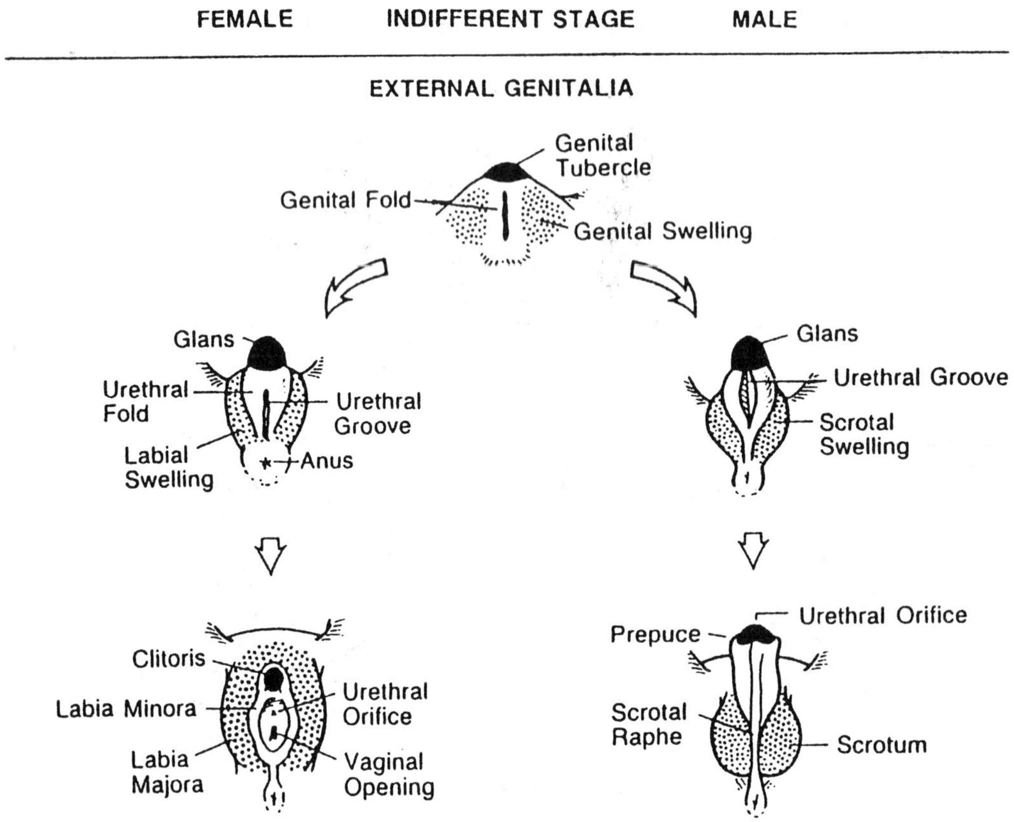

FEMALE   INDIFFERENT STAGE   MALE

EXTERNAL GENITALIA

Figure 2   Phenotypic differentiation of external genitalia in male and female embryos.

The testicular descent from its position around the kidney to its final location in the scrotum is a complex process that starts at week 12 of fetal age. Transabdominal movement brings the testis to the internal inguinal ring at midgestation, around 22 weeks. The actual passage of the testis through the inguinal canal into the scrotum does not occur until after week 28 and may be delayed until the immediate postnatal period. The mechanism of testicular descent is not fully understood and probably results from a combination of mechanical and humoral factors. Increase in intraabdominal pressure is certainly involved initially. The gubernaculum testis, a jelly-like structure extending from the caudal pole of the testis to the inguinal ring, precedes the testis into the inguinal canal and reaches the scrotum at 22 weeks (16). The gubernaculum is thought to have a critical role in testicular descent (17), but the testicular factors controlling its growth and differentiation are not completely recognized. Androgens are involved, mainly in the transinguinal part of the descent (18).

C.   Female Differentiation

Differentiation of the female genital tract is characterized by stabilization of the müllerian ducts and their differentiation into fallopian tubes and uterus. Wolffian ducts begin to degenerate at 10 weeks, and the remnants are incorporated into the wall of müllerian derivatives. In male pseudohermaphroditism associated with lack of regression of müllerian derivatives, the latter are attached to the male excretory ducts and the vas deferens is often embedded in the posterior uterine wall extending into the cervix (19). Mobilizable müllerian derivatives are pulled down in the inguinal canal by the descending testis, leading to what is known as the syndrome of hernia uteri inguinalis (20).

The developmental origin of the vagina remains controversial; the most likely embryologic hypothesis includes the müllerian, wolffian, and sinusal structures. The first stages of vaginal development are quite similar to those that in the male lead to the formation of the prostatic utricle. At 11 weeks, the vaginal primordium is formed by the caudal tip of the müllerian ducts and by outgrowths of the posterior sinusal wall, the sinovaginal bulbs laterally and the müllerian tubercle medially. At 15 weeks, these structures fuse to form the vaginal cord of plate, which acquires a lumen approximately halfway through prenatal life. The major difference between male and female organogenesis is in the downgrowth of the vaginal plate. Whereas in males the prostatic utricle, the male equivalent of the vagina, opens below the bladder neck, in females the vaginal cord proliferates and migrates down the urethra to acquire a separate opening on the perineum (Fig. 3). The process of feminization of the external

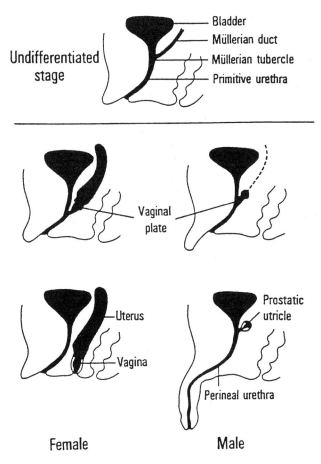

Figure 3 Sex differentiation of the urogenital sinus and external genitalia.

genitalia is simultaneously completed with follicular growth around week 26 of gestation, suggesting a role of the fetal ovaries in these events (21). Fetal exposure to diethylstilbestrol disturbs the normal migration of the female reproductive tract, and a significant percentage of the daughters of women who received the drug during pregnancy are at risk for adenocarcinoma of the vagina (22).

III. HORMONAL CONTROL OF SEX DIFFERENTIATION

A. The Jost Theory

Hormonal control of somatic sex differentiation was demonstrated by the experiments of Jost (23,24). When fetal rabbits were castrated very early, at the ambisexual stage of reproductive tract differentiation, all developed female somatic characteristics, regardless of the histologic nature of the fetal gonads. Fetal ovaries play no part in female sex differentiation, the key factor being the presence or absence of the fetal testis. The active part played by male-determining factors, as opposed to the constitutive nature of female

differentiation, is a general feature of sex differentiation that applies to the genital tract.

The male differentiation of the reproductive tract included two steps: müllerian regression and wolffian stabilization. Two testicular products were shown to be responsible for both steps, namely testosterone and müllerian inhibiting factor. Until that time, testosterone had been the only hormone known to be secreted by the testis. By inserting a testosterone crystal near the ovary of a developing rabbit at the ambisexual stage, it was shown that müllerian ducts were not influenced by androgen but regressed when exposed to a graft of testicular tissue. The testicular agent responsible for müllerian regression was termed müllerian inhibitor, now known as müllerian inhibiting substance (MIS) or antimüllerian hormone.

B. Müllerian Inhibiting Substance

MIS is a glycoprotein member of the transforming growth factor β (TGF-β) family, together with inhibin, activins, and various differentiation factors. Members of the TGF-β family are usually produced as large precursors, which require cleavage for expression of their biologic activity. Although MIS seemed to be an exception in this regard, the full-length molecule is cleaved by plasmin at a site located 109 amino acids away from the carboxyl terminus, generating a TGF-β-like carboxyl-terminal fragment that is thought to contain the biologically active site. Inhibin and activin, other members of the TGF-β family, are also produced by the fetal gonads of both sexes, but their physiologic significance remains to be elucidated (25,26).

The human MIS gene has been cloned and mapped to the short arm of chromosome 19. MIS is synthesized by Sertoli cells soon after testicular differentiation and is detectable in human serum until puberty. Serum MIS is a marker of testicular function in infancy; levels have been reported to be useful in the diagnosis and management of patients with a variety of intersex and gonadal abnormalities (27–29). Granulosa cells of the postnatal ovary also produce MIS, and elevated serum levels have been reported in a case of granulosa cell tumor (30).

Despite that MIS is produced by Sertoli cells until puberty and by postnatal granulosa cells and would therefore be expected to exert physiologic effects in both sexes after birth, this has not been confirmed. Lack of regression of uterus and tubes is the only aspect of sex differentiation constantly affected in the persistent müllerian duct syndrome (PMDS), as a result of MIS gene mutations. Incomplete testicular descent, commonly observed in this PMDS, could be caused by mechanical restraint of the testis by the uterus and tubes as well as a direct influence on testicular descent (31–33). The effect of MIS on ovarian function is controversial, but MIS has been reported to inhibit the progress of oocyte meiosis (34).

MIS is a masculinizing agent of the fetal female reproductive tract, as demonstrated in the freemartin condition. Freemartins are bovine females united to a male cotwin by placental anastomoses established very early in fetal development. At birth, these females have no internal reproductive tract and their ovaries are either reduced to fibrous streaks or masculinized. Proof that MIS is responsible for the ovarian abnormalities was obtained in organ culture and in transgenic mice expressing the MIS gene. MIS also sex-reverses the pattern of steroidogenesis in the fetal ovary by inhibiting aromatase activity. Despite the masculinizing effect on fetal ovaries, MIS is not required for testicular development, because mutations impairing MIS production do not affect testicular organogenesis (35–37).

C. Testosterone

Interstitial Leydig cells appear in the fetal testis between weeks 7 and 8 in the human fetus, coinciding with testosterone secretion. Serum and testicular testosterone concentrations increase to a peak of 300 ng/dl between 15 and 18 weeks, when they decrease, correlating with the histologic pattern of fetal Leydig cell development.

Gonadal steroidogenesis in both fetal testis and ovaries is initiated at similar times, each producing its own characteristic hormone. The rate-limiting enzyme for testosterone synthesis is 3β-hydroxysteroid dehydrogenase, which is approximately 50 times higher in the fetal testis than in the ovary at similar ages. In contrast to adult Leydig cells, in which the response to gonadotropic stimulation with increased androgen production is restrained by a refractory state, secondary to receptor down-regulation, fetal Leydig cells escape this desensitization, and therefore they maintain a high testosterone secretion during the several weeks required for completion of the male differentiation of the genital tract (38,39).

Human chorionic gonadotropin appears to control fetal gonadal steroidogenesis despite the initial lack of influence on the adenyl cyclase activity of fetal testicular homogenates. The testicular and serum levels of testosterone are closely correlated with human chorionic gonadotropin (hCG) concentration. hCG peaks at 12 weeks of fetal age. When hCG declines, in the third trimester, the hypothalamic-pituitary axis gains control over testicular function. Failure of this takeover is associated with hypoplastic male external genitalia. Micropenis is often observed in children with congenital hypopituitarism, and anencephalic infants have a significantly diminished population of Leydig cells.

D. Mechanism of Hormonal Action in the Reproductive Tract

The mechanism of action of MIS has not been elucidated, and its receptor is still unknown. The regression of the müllerian duct by MIS with the formation of a ring of connective tissue around the epithelial cells has suggested that the mesenchyme is the primary target tissue for MIS. It has been hypothesized that MIS acts by activating phosphotyrosyl protein phosphatase, thereby opposing epidermal growth factor-mediated membrane phosphorylation.

The mechanisms by which androgens masculinize the male fetus have been clearly elaborated. Testosterone is the gonadal steroid secreted by fetal testis in the circulation and enters cells by passive diffusion. The wolffian duct, which is adjacent to the fetal testis, also takes up testosterone by pinocytosis. This local source of androgen is important for wolffian duct development, which does not occur if testosterone is supplied only via the peripheral circulation, as in female pseudohermaphroditism as a result of adrenal hyperplasia.

At the intracellular level, testosterone is converted to dihydrotestosterone (DHT) by the enzyme 5α-reductase. The conversion of testosterone to DHT amplifies the androgenic signal through several mechanisms. DHT cannot be aromatized to estrogen, and thus its actions are purely androgenic. Furthermore, DHT binds to the androgen receptor with greater affinity and stability than does testosterone. Thus, those target tissues with 5α-reductase enzyme activity at the time of sex differentiation, such as the prostate, urogenital sinus, and external genitalia, generate DHT as the active androgen. Patients with 5α-reductase deficiency fail to virilize because the DHT is not synthesized. At high concentrations, however, testosterone interacts with the androgen receptor similarly to DHT. In contrast, the wolffian ducts do not form DHT before sex differentiation, but because they are exposed to high concentrations of testosterone, they virilize.

The enzyme 5α-reductase activity has two pH optima in cultured genital skin fibroblasts, one at pH 5.5 and another one near pH 8, corresponding to two distinct enzymes. The alkaline enzyme, human steroid 5α-reductase 1, has been cloned, and it has been mapped to the short arm of chromosome 5, band 15; however, the predominant enzyme in the prostate is the acid 5α-reductase 2. A deletion in the gene coding for the acid enzyme has been detected in intersex patients with 5α-reductase deficiency. It has been mapped to the short arm of chromosome 2, band 23 (40).

The gene coding for the androgen receptor has been cloned. It is localized to the q11–12 region of the X chromosome, and it belongs to the family of nuclear steroid receptors. Mutatons in the exon 2 and 3 code for the DNA region have been described in patients with the so-called receptor-positive form of androgen insensitivity, because binding of DHT is not affected. Most mutations occur in exons 4–8, which code for the steroid hormone binding domain. Deletions and point mutations in this region lead to "receptor-negative" androgen insensitivity (41).

E. Estrogens

Estrogen synthesis is detectable in the female human embryo just after 8 weeks. The rate-limiting enzyme is aromatase, which is higher in the fetal ovary than in the fetal testis. Estrogens are not required for normal female differentiation of the reproductive tract. However, estrogen receptors in female external genitalia suggest that maternal estrogen influences its development. Estrogens can interfere with male differentiation in various ways: prenatal estrogen treatment is associated with reproductive tract abnormalities in males, and estrogen blocks the effect of MIS on müllerian ducts. Local estradiol may be needed for completion of ovarian differentiation; it has been suggested that the masculinizing effect of MIS on fetal ovaries is linked to the capacity of MIS to decrease aromatase activity and, therefore, estrogen production (26,42).

F. Environmental Factors

Environmental factors modulate the expression of genetic potential and may be important determinants of both external and internal genitalia development in the fetus. These nongenetic factors include the uterine and maternal environments and the external influences that may affect the mother and, thus, impact the fetus. Environmental influences on fetal development include the intrauterine environment, determined largely by uterine blood flow, placental function, local uterine circulation, and placental and umbilical circulation. These factors determine the substrate necessary to support fetal development. Maternal nutritional deprivation may compromise fetal development. Intrauterine growth retardation is associated with diminished placental blood flow. Tobacco smoking is known to induce placental insufficiency and may affect fetal growth and development. Other environmental factors that may affect fetal growth and therefore organ development include the effects of altitude, radiation, and environmental toxins, as well as drugs or maternal addiction. The fetal alcohol syndrome has been associated with malformations of the sex organs, including absence or hypertrophy of the labia, clitoris, and vagina; hypoplastic or absent penis or scrotum; and intersex and unspecified genital anomalies (43). There is an expanding list of environmental factors that may lead to intrauterine organ maldevelopment and congenital malformations. These agents result in growth restriction by arresting cell replication during critical stages of development, causing patterns of malformations that may include the external genitalia.

IV. AMBIGUOUS GENITALIA

A newborn infant with ambiguous genitalia is an urgent problem that must be considered a "social emergency." New parents should be able to answer the question that is always asked, Is it a boy or a girl? The condition may not be life threatening, but mismanagement or delay in diagno-

sis and inappropriate gender assignment could induce lifetime repercussions for both family and patient. Recent advances in cytogenetics, immunogenetics, endocrinology, and experimental embryology have clarified the pathogenesis of these disorders and now allow the pediatric endocrinologist to manage these patients in an orderly fashion without being overwhelmed by the complexity of these conditions and the extent of the malformations.

Rapid and organized evaluation should be initiated immediately after birth to assign the appropriate gender, identify a possible life-threatening medical condition, and begin the required medical, surgical, and psychologic management. The following approach to the diagnostic evaluation is outlined, along with suggested management of these complex patients.

Four major diagnostic categories can cause gender confusion at birth: (1) female pseudohermaphroditism, (2) male pseudohermaphroditism, (3) true hermaphroditism, and (4) mixed gonadal dysgenesis (Table 1). Such criteria as gonadal symmetry, chromosomal analysis (fluorescent Y staining), and imaging can be determined in the first 48 h of life and together can allow close to 90% accuracy in diagnosis.

A. Female Pseudohermaphroditism

Female pseudohermaphroditism, comprising approximately one-third to one-half of patients with ambiguous genitalia, refers to an individual possessing ovaries with masculinized genitalia. Female pseudohermaphrodites have a 46, XX karyotype, normal müllerian duct structures (uterus, fallopian tubes, and upper vagina), and no wolffian duct structures (epididymidis, vasa deferentia, and seminal vesicles). Exposure of the female fetus to androgens results in the virilization of the external genitalia seen in these patients. The major cause of female pseudohermaphroditism is congenital adrenal hyperplasia (CAH) (44).

Female pseudohermaphroditism (Table 2) is the easiest of the sexual anomalies to understand: the ovaries and müllerian derivatives are normally developed, and the anatomic ambiguity is limited to the external genitalia. In the absence of testis, the tendency for the external genitalia is to feminize, unless a female fetus is exposed to androgens. The degree of fetal masculinization is determined by the stage of

Table 1 Ambiguous Genitalia in the Newborn: Differential Diagnosis

	Karyotype	Gonads	Genitalia
Female pseudohermaphroditism	46,XX	Symmetric (ovary and ovary)	Virilized female
Male pseudohermaphroditism	46,XY	Symmetric (testis and testis)	Incomplete masculinization
True hermaphroditism	46,XX (mosaics)	Asymmetric (testis and ovary)	Male, female, or ambiguous
Mixed gonadal dysgenesis	45,X/46,XY	Asymmetric (ovotestis and streak)	Ambiguous

Table 2 Classification of Female Pseudohermaphroditism

Fetal androgens: congenital adrenal hyperplasia caused by
    deficiency
    3β-Hydroxydehydrogenase
    P-450$_{c21}$ (21-hydroxylase)
        Type 1: partial, incomplete, or simple virilizing form
        Type 2: complete, salt-losing form
    P-450$_{c11}$ (11-hydroxylase)
Maternal androgens
    Iatrogenic: androgens, progestins
    Virilizing ovarian or adrenal tumor
    Luteoma of pregnancy
Congenital abnormalities
    Structural or teratogenic factor
    Idiopathic
Aromatase deficiency

differentiation at the time of exposure. Once the vagina has separated from the urogenital sinus (at fetal week 12), androgens cause only clitoral hypertrophy. Despite the severe masculinization of the external genitalia, the uterus and fallopian tubes are normal, because regression of the müllerian duct structures requires secretion of MIS by the fetal testis. The virilized genitalia usually indicates evidence of an androgenic influence during gestation. However, ambiguous genitalia, resembling those induced by androgens, can also be occasional feature of other, more generalized teratologic malformations.

The most frequent etiology of ambiguous genitalia in the newborn is congenital adrenal hyperplasia caused by steroid P- 450$_{c21}$ (21-hydroxylase) deficiency (Chap. 21). The differential diagnosis includes true hermaphroditism, in which case there is usually a 46, XX karyotype, but the gonads will be constituted of both ovarian and testicular tissue. Virilizing ovarian or adrenal tumors in the mother or drugs administered to the mother during pregnancy may masculinize the genitalia of the genetic female. Other causes of female pseudohermaphroditism have included maternal androgens, congenital abnormalities, and aromatase deficiency (45–47).

B. Male Pseudohermaphroditism

Male pseudohermaphrodites are individuals with testis but with female or ambiguous genitalia. They have a 46, XY karyotype and no müllerian duct structures (because of normal production of müllerian inhibiting substance by the testis). Inadequate androgen exposure during the first trimester results in absent or hypoplastic wolffian duct structures and undervirilization of the external genitalia. Testosterone biosynthetic defects, 5α-reductase deficiency, and androgen insensitivity syndromes are forms of male pseudohermaphroditism.

Male pseudohermaphroditism is incomplete masculinization of the external genitalia in an individual with a normal 46, XY karyotype (48). It is a heterogeneous condition in

which both gonads are exclusively testis but the genital ducts or external genitalia are incompletely masculinized, with various degrees of phenotypic characteristics of a female. The clinical spectrum ranges from individuals in whom the external genitalia are completely feminized to milder forms in phenotypic males with hypospadias, cryptorchidism, or minimal ambiguity of the external genitalia (Table 3).

Male pseudohermaphroditism in 46, XY individuals with relatively normal embryonic differentiation of the testis are the most common. In such patients, defective male development is secondary to failure of the fetal testis to overcome the inherent tendency toward feminization of the somatic sex structures. This failure originates either from a secretory failure of the testis during the fetal sex differentiation or failure of the target organs to androgen stimulation. Table 3 represents a classification of the several forms of male pseudohermaphroditism on the basis of etiology.

The capacity of the testes to virilize at puberty is frequently a reminder of their ability to masculinize the external genitalia in utero. The larger the development of the phallus in an infant, the greater is the likelihood that male secondary sexual characteristics will happen at the time of puberty. Patients with ambiguous genitalia have increased chances to remain eunuchoid, develop mild masculinization, or exhibit gynecomastia and other feminine secondary sexual characteristics. Those individuals with an external female phenotype usually either feminize or remain sexually infantile. However, individuals with partial androgen resistance and patients with 5α-reductase deficiency develop male sexual characteristics at puberty.

1. Enzyme Defects of Testosterone Biosynthesis

Five enzymatic defects in testosterone biosynthesis have been described, one at each of the enzymatic steps required for the conversion of cholesterol to testosterone. Three of the defects (P-450$_{scc}$, 3β-hydroxysteroid deficiency (3β-

Table 3 Classification of Male Pseudohermaphroditism

Inadequate testosterone production
    Testosterone biosynthetic defects
        P-450$_{scc}$ deficiency
        3β-HSD deficiency
        P-450$_{c17}$ deficiency
        P-450$_{c17}$ (17,20-lyase) deficiency
        17β-Hydroxysteroid oxidoreductase deficiency
    Leydig cell hypoplasia or agenesis
Peripheral unresponsiveness to androgens
    End-organ resistance
        Testicular feminization syndrome
        Partial androgen insensitivity
    5α-Reductase deficiency
Dysgenetic male pseudohermaphroditism
    Incomplete gonadal dysgenesis
    Hernia uteri inguinale
    Testicular regression syndrome

HSD), and $P-450_{c17}$ hydroxylase) involve enzymes affecting both glucocorticoid and gonadal steroid biosynthesis; the remaining two enzymes, 17,20-desmolase and 17-ketoreductase, are required for the formation of androgens only and therefore are clinically expressed by sexual ambiguity alone. The pattern of inheritance in each of these defects indicates an autosomal recessive mode of transmission (49).

The biochemical heterogeneity within each defect and the subsequent variability of the testosterone biosynthetic block make it impossible to distinguish these enzyme disorders based on the appearance of the external genitalia alone. The clinical presentation ranges from a normal female external genitalia to incomplete labioscrotal fusion and a clitoris-like phallus. Milder forms include hypospadias, chordee, or cryptorchidism. The testis may be situated within the labioscrotal folds, inguinal canals, or peritoneal cavity. The wolffian derivatives may present a normal development or may be hypoplastic, depending on the severity of the testosterone biosynthetic block. Müllerian structures are usually absent because the secretion of MIS by Sertoli cells is unaffected. Some of the specific presentations of each defect are outlined here.

a. $P-450_{scc}$ Deficiency (Cholesterol Side-Chain Cleavage Deficiency or Lipoid Adrenal Hyperplasia). The first step in gonadal and adrenal steroidogenesis is the conversion of cholesterol to pregnenolone, which involves three reactions: 20α-hydroxylation, 22-hydroxylation, and side-chain cleavage of cholesterol. A defect in the conversion of cholesterol to pregnenolone is the etiology of the condition known as congenital lipoid adrenal hyperplasia (CLAH). CLAH infants present very early in life with severe adrenal insufficiency and salt wasting. Affected 46, XY males present with female external genitalia and, in a few cases, with mild masculinization.

Cytochrome $P-450_{scc}$, a mitochondrial mixed-function oxidase, is involved in the conversion of cholesterol to pregnenolone. The $P-450_{scc}$ gene is located in the q23–q24 region of chromosome 15 (50,51). CLAH is suspected in any newborn male pseudohermaphrodite (or phenotypic female) with adrenal insufficiency. Laboratory confirmation is obtained with decreased serum and urinary levels of both adrenal and gonadal steroids, even after adrenocorticotropic hormone (ACTH) or hCG stimulation. ACTH levels are elevated. Hyponatremia, hyperkalemia, and metabolic acidosis indicate salt-wasting adrenal insufficiency. Computed tomography (CT) or magnetic resonance imaging (MRI) of the abdomen demonstrates large adrenal glands, secondary to the accumulation of cholesterol and cholesterol esters. The adrenal insufficiency in these patients is managed with glucocorticoid and mineralocorticoid therapy.

b. 3β-Hydroxysteroid Dehydrogenase Deficiency. 3β-Hydroxysteroid dehydrogenase catalyzes the conversion of 3β-hydroxy-Δ^5-steroids to 3-keto-Δ^4-steroids (pregnenolone, 17-hydroxypregnenolone, and dehydroepiandrosterone to progesterone, 17-OH-progesterone and androstenedione, respectively). Two genes encoding 3β-HSD include type I for placental and type II gene for adrenal and gonadal 3β-HSD.

A point mutation in the type II gene has been found in patients with classic 3β-HSD deficiency. A deficiency of 3β-HSD impairs both adrenal and gonadal steroidogenesis. Affected 46, XY individuals exhibit incomplete masculinization, with a small phallus, hypospadia, and partial fusion of the labioscrotal folds. The urogenital sinus leads to a blind vaginal pouch. The testes are palpated in the scrotum, and the wolffian structures are normal (52,53).

c. $P-450_{c17}$ (17-Hydroxylase) Deficiency. Affected 46, XY individuals exhibit a wide range of impaired masculinization depending on the severity of the biosynthetic defect. The external genitalia show a small phallus, hypospadia, and a blind vaginal pouch. The testes may be in the inguinal canal or in the labioscrotal folds. The wolffian duct derivatives are hypoplastic, and there are no müllerian structures. Clinical findings include hypertension with hypokalemic alkalosis secondary to the excess mineralocorticoids. At puberty, these genetic males undergo significant virilization and some develop gynecomastia.

d. $P-450_{c17}$ (17,20-Lyase) Deficiency. Genetic males with this deficiency present with various clinical variants: one is associated with an incomplete defect, with partial virilization and perineal hypospadias and a bifid scrotum, and a second one with a more complete defect, with a female phenotype but absence of uterus and an almost complete deficiency of testosterone and lack of pubertal virilization. In both variants, plasma androgens are low and do not increase on hCG stimulation. A single gene encoding cytochrome $P-450_{c17}$ controls both 17α-hydroxylase and 17,20-desmolase activities. Combined defects have been described regardless of the clinical phenotype (54).

e. 17β-Hydroxysteroid Dehydrogenase Deficiency. These genetic males present with female external genitalia and associated clitoromegaly and mild labioscrotal fusion. The testes are palpable in the labioscrotal folds. They are often misdiagnosed as testicular feminization and raised as females. They are diagnosed at puberty, when they develop breasts as well as virilization signs, such as acne, hirsutism, voice deepening, and amenorrhea, because they have no müllerian structures. They have elevated blood androstenedione and estrone, with low testosterone levels, and these alterations can be further magnified by hCG stimulation. Baseline luteinizing hormone (LH) and follicle stimulating hormone (FSH) levels are markedly elevated at puberty. It is an autosomal recessive condition (55).

f. Leydig Cell Hypoplasia. Hypoplasia or agenesis of the Leydig cells of the testis is a cause of male pseudohermaphroditism because of insufficient testosterone production. The inheritance pattern appears male limited and autosomal recessive. Affected 46, XY individuals have a female phenotype, with mild posterior labial fusion and a urogenital sinus present with an anterior urethra and a blind vaginal pouch. Wolffian duct structures are present but hypoplastic. These findings are caused by low levels of local testosterone production as well as insufficient circulating fetal levels in early gestation. Müllerian structures are absent because of normal secretion of MIS by the Sertoli cells, a further suggestion that Leydig cells are not required for this Sertoli cell function. Small testes are located in the inguinal canals or the abdomen.

The testicular tissue from postpubertal or hCG-stimulated prepubertal individuals have demonstrated absent or decreased Leydig cells, normal Sertoli cells, hyalinization of the seminiferous tubules, and incomplete spermatogenesis. A luteinizing hormone/hCG receptor defect has been suggested.

Leydig cell hypoplasia in affected 46, XY infants is associated with low basal testosterone levels and absent response to hCG stimulation. The low levels of testosterone precursors also demonstrate that there is no testosterone biosynthetic defect. The diagnosis is made by histologic examination of hCG-stimulated testis showing absence of Leydig cells with normal-appearing seminiferous tubules (56).

2. Peripheral Unresponsiveness to Androgens

A failure in the mechanism of action of androgens on their target cells can result in male pseudohermaphroditism. Two forms have been described: (1) end-organ resistance to androgenic hormones (androgen receptor defects) and (2) errors in testosterone metabolism by peripheral tissues (5α-reductase deficiency).

a. End-Organ Resistance to Androgens.

Several forms of androgen resistance have been identified. The phenotypes in 46, XY individuals with androgen resistance syndromes have ranged from subjects with normal female external genitalia through subjects with ambiguous genitalia to subjects with a normal male external genitalia but a small phallus. Both qualitative and quantitative defects in the androgen receptor have been described. The gene for the androgen receptor (AR) has been cloned and localized to Xq11–Xq12 (41).

The AR is a steroid receptor and a ligand-activated nuclear transcription factor, which on DNA binding induces transcription of specific target genes. The gene encoding the AR is situated in the q11–12 region in the human X chromosome. It encodes a receptor protein that mediates steroid binding, nuclear translocation, DNA binding, and transcriptional activation of target genes.

Two main defects in AR function have been described: (1) abnormalities of androgen binding, and (2) abnormalities of DNA binding. Defects in receptor androgen binding include reduced binding affinity, reduced levels of normal affinity binding, and qualitative abnormalities, such as thermolability of binding, increased ligand dissociation, or altered binding specificity. Receptor levels and androgen binding affinity correlate minimally with the degree of masculinization. In a family with the complete form of androgen insensitivity syndrome (AIS), affected siblings had normal androgen binding capacity and only a three- to fourfold decrease in androgen binding affinity in cultured genital skin fibroblasts (57,58).

The molecular defects in the etiology of androgen resistance can be described as (1) major structural abnormalities of the AR gene; (2) point mutations altering the AR

messenger RNA; and (3) point mutations that alter a single amino acid (59,60).

Structural abnormalities of the AR gene. Deletions of the AR gene have been present in individuals with complete AIS; however, deletions are uncommon, representing only about 10% of AR gene mutations. No deletion has been described in partial AIS. Complete deletion of the AR gene results in total absence of the AR protein.

Point mutations that alter receptor mRNA. Single-base changes have been described in various locations within the coding region of the AR gene that convert a codon for an amino acid into a premature termination codon. Such mutations result in the expression of a defective, truncated receptor or may destabilize the mRNA, causing reduced receptor protein production.

Single-base mutations that change a single amino acid. Point mutations that alter a single amino acid have been found in AR genes of subjects with both complete and partial AIS. About 50% of the mutations occurring in the AR gene are new mutations in each kindred, the remaining being recurrent mutations at a number of distinct sites.

The complete form of AIS was previously known as testicular feminization syndrome. It is an X-linked disorder in which affected males are phenotypic females and develop female secondary sexual characteristics at puberty but fail to menstruate. They are genetic males with the 46, XY karyotype, and they present with normal female external genitalia but with a blind vaginal pouch. They have absent müllerian structures, and their testes are situated in the labia, inguinal canal, or intraabdominally, as well as the hypoplastic wolffian derivatives. The testes appear as normal as prepubertal testes before puberty. After puberty, the seminiferous tubules become atrophic, with no spermatogenesis. The Leydig cells are hyperplastic and are found in clumps. The testes have a tendency to develop neoplasia, although the risk of malignancy is low before age 25, after which it increases significantly. The risk of malignancy in these individuals is slightly higher than that in normal men with cryptorchid testes.

AIS must be suspected in phenotypic females with an inguinal hernia and a gonadal mass in the inguinal region or in the labia discovered in the neonatal period, infancy, or childhood. It has been estimated that 1–2% of phenotypic females with inguinal hernias have androgen insensitivity. At puberty, female secondary sexual characteristics develop, including normal breasts and female body habitus but no menses. Pubic and axillary hairs are minimal and are absent in about one-third of patients. A minimal amount of pubic hair may be present. The clitoris is normal or small, the vagina is shallow and ends in a blind pouch, and the labia minora are underdeveloped. Wolffian duct derivatives are absent or hypoplastic; müllerian structures are absent because of the normal secretion of MIS by the fetal Sertoli cells.

A small percentage of patients have been described with various degrees of slight ambiguity of the external genitalia at birth (posterior fusion of the labioscrotal folds and minimal clitorimegaly). These individuals may show virilization at puberty, with mild pubic and axillary hairs as well as breast development. The latter group is considered a variant of complete AIS, and the term "incomplete AIS or incomplete testicular feminization" has also been used (48,59,61). Partial AIS comprises a heterogeneous group of 46, XY individuals. The external genitalia are predominantly male or ambiguous. The pattern of inheritance is consistent with an X-linked recessive trait. Previous literature reports by Lubs, Gilbert-Dreyfus, Reifenstein, and Rosewater described all various forms of partial androgen insensitivity (62). The variable degree of masculinization of affected males within and between kinships has ranged from micropenis and hypospadias to significant ambiguous genitalia. Infants are recognized at birth. They present as an apparent male with third-degree hypospadias (the urethral orifice located at the base of the phallus), a small penis, and, frequently, cryptorchidism. Müllerian duct derivatives are absent; in some patients wolffian duct derivatives are present but usually hypoplastic. At adolescence, pubic and axillary hairs and gynecomastia usually appear, with poorly developed male secondary sexual characteristics. The testes remain small and exhibit germinal cell arrest. Patients with partial androgen insensitivity demonstrate elevated concentrations of plasma LH and testosterone; the high LH concentrations are not suppressed by exogenous androgens. Estradiol and testosterone production rates are increased. Their degree of feminization at puberty, despite elevated estradiol secretion, is much less than in the complete form of androgen insensitivity.

b. Errors in Testosterone Metabolism. 5α-reductase is an enzyme that converts testosterone into dihydrotestosterone. The deficiency of 5α-reductase during the differentiation of the fetal external genitalia and urogenital sinus causes incomplete masculinization of these structures because of insufficient DHT production. The resulting genitalia are ambiguous and demonstrate clitoral-like phallus with hypospadias and chordee, a bifid scrotum, and persistent urogenital sinus on the perineum with a blind vaginal pouch. The testis, epididymides, vasa deferentia, and seminal vesicles are normally developed. The testes are found in the labioscrotal folds or inguinal canals. Müllerian structures are absent because MIS is produced by the Sertoli cells. The pattern of inheritance in 5α-reductase deficiency is autosomal recessive. Heterozygous males or homozygous females do not have clinical manifestations, but they have biochemical abnormalities (63).

Reduced 5α-reductase activity has been demonstrated in cultured genital skin fibroblasts from these patients. However, genetic heterogeneity of the enzyme has been suggested by differences in enzyme stability and affinity for testosterone. The hypothesis that this enzyme heterogeneity represents gene mutations is suggested by the isolation of two human cDNA clones for 5α-reductase. The 5α-reductase 1 encodes the alkaline enzyme present in normal prostate and has been mapped to 5p15. The other clone, 5α-reductase 2, encodes the major isozyme in genital tissue based on its acid pH

optimum and its presence in the major human prostate 5α-reductase enzyme. Molecular analyses of the 5α-reductase 2 genes in several kindreds have demonstrated different mutations, and it has been mapped to the 2p23 chromosome (64).

At puberty, a considerable degree of virilization occurs in the affected males as a result of increased testosterone, even though the DHT levels continue to be low. The body habitus becomes very muscular. The phallus enlarges up to 8 cm in length, and the labioscrotal folds become rugated and pigmented. The testes enlarge and descend into the labioscrotal folds. Acne, facial hair, and enlargement of the prostate do not occur, suggesting that these organs are dependent on DHT activity. Gynecomastia does not occur because the ratio of testosterone to estrogen is normal. In a study of affected individuals in the Dominican Republic kindred who initially were raised as females, 17 of 18 changed to male gender identity during puberty. It has therefore been hypothesized that testosterone exposure of the brain has a greater effect in determining male gender identity than sex of rearing. It is also possible that cultural factors may have had a significant influence in these individuals' decisions (65–67).

The diagnosis of 5α-reductase deficiency in infancy requires an elevated ratio of plasma testosterone to DHT after stimulation with hCG. In normal infants (2 weeks to 6 months), the hCG-stimulated ratio is 4.8 ± 2.2 (mean ± standard deviation). Affected infants have markedly increased ratios of testosterone to DHT in the 20–60 range. Diminished 5α-reductase activity in genital skin fibroblast cultures has been the most direct but invasive diagnostic method (68,69).

3. Dysgenetic Male Pseudohermaphroditism

Ambiguous development of the external genitalia occurs in individuals with XY karyotype and gonadal dysgenesis. Some patients have 45, X/46, XY mosaicism, similar to mixed gonadal dysgenesis. There are also patients with a familial form of 46, XY gonadal dysgenesis. These disorders may be considered abnormalities of gonadal differentiation, but their partial testicular determination exhibits the clinical phenotype of male pseudohermaphroditism. Therefore, these disorders must be considered in the differential diagnosis of ambiguous genitalia. The term "dysgenetic male pseudohermaphroditism" was suggested to designate patients presenting with bilateral dysgenetic gonadal development ranging from gonadal streaks to dysgenetic testis to normal appearing testis (70). The prevalence of malignancy in dysgenetic male pseudohermaphroditism is increased.

a. The 46, XY Incomplete Gonadal Dysgenesis. "46, XY partial gonadal dysgenesis" refers to individuals with partial testicular differentiation and a normal-appearing 46, XY karytoype. Other terms that have been applied to this condition include "dysgenetic male pseudohermaphroditism" and "46, X/46, XY mixed gonadal dysgenesis" by its different chromosomal constitution. However, both syndromes share similar clinical features. 46, XY partial gonadal dysgenesis has a normal amount of mutant SRY gene, whereas 45, X/46,

XY individuals have a decreased amount of normal SRY gene.

Individuals with 46, XY partial gonadal dysgenesis are diagnosed in the newborn period because of ambiguous genitalia. The degree of masculinization depends on the extent of testicular differentiation. The levels of testosterone vary from low to normal, but the response to hCG is blunted, indicating a dysgenetic gonad. A genitogram shows a utriculovaginal pouch. Patients have both wolffian and müllerian structures, indicating variable fetal müllerian inhibiting substance and testosterone production. Individuals with 46, XY partial gonadal dysgenesis may also present with the stigmata of Turner syndrome.

The diagnosis of 46, XY gonadal dysgenesis should be considered in a child with ambiguous genitalia, a 46, XY karyotype, and a subnormal plasma concentration of testosterone, without elevated levels of testosterone precursors. The presence of müllerian structures on genitourethrogram or sonogram increases the suspicion of this condition. The diagnosis is made by gonadal histology.

Because of the presence of uterus, a female sex rearing is preferred and the gonadal tissue and wolffian structures should be removed. It is recommended that laparotomy be performed as early as possible because of the increased risk of malignancy in the dysgenetic gonads and because gonadoblastoma has been reported in a child with 46, XY partial gonadal dysgenesis at 15 months. Even if the sex rearing is male, removal of dysgenetic gonads is recommended to prevent the occurrence of malignancy (71–73).

b. Hernia Uteri Inguinale (19,20). These individuals are also referred as having persistent müllerian duct syndrome. They are phenotypically normal 46, XY males who present at the time of surgery for unilateral or bilateral inguinal hernias and/or cryptorchidism in infancy or early childhood. Imaging studies have been useful in PMDS with bilateral cryptochidism (74). The usual finding at the time of the inguinal exploration is uterus inguinale, or retained müllerian duct structures in the inguinal hernia sac. The testes of these patients are usually normal, except for cryptorchidism consequences if discovered in adolescence or adulthood. Vasa deferentia are present, as well as epididymis, so fertility is likely if normal spermatogenesis occurs. Resection of the rudimentary uterus and tubes is indicated.

This condition is often familial, presenting as sex-limited autosomal recessive. However, there is evidence for both end-organ unresponsiveness to MIS despite normal production of the hormone and deficiency of the MIS, suggesting PMDS is a heterogeneous disorder (31,32).

c. Testicular Regression Syndrome. Patients with 46, XY karyotype without gonadal elements and variable differentiation of the genital ducts, urogenital sinus, and external genitalia have been referred as having fetal testicular regression or vanishing testis syndrome. Other terms to describe the spectrum of anomalies include true agonadism, bilateral anorchia, XY gonadal agenesis, and rudimentary testis syndrome. Sporadic and familial forms have led to speculation of autosomal or X-linked transmission, but the nature of the underlying defect is not known. The clinical features are related to the time of the embryonic testicular regression. The regression may occur at different stages of the male development in utero, and therefore the neonate may present as bilateral cryptorchidism with a normal male phenotype to various degrees of ambiguity of the external genitalia. The diagnosis is based on the absence of palpable gonads and lack of testicular response to hCG stimulation and is finally made by laparotomy (75,76).

C. True Hermaphroditism

True hermaphroditism represents a gonadal differentiation disorder in an individual with both ovarian and testicular tissue. The genitalia may be male, female, or ambiguous, depending on the amount of functioning testicular tissue. Patients with this disorder may have bilateral ovotestis, an ovary or testis on one side and an ovotestis on the other or an ovary on one side and a testis on the other. The ovarian tissue contains primordial follicles, and the testicular tissue contains seminiferous tubules and germ cells. The gonadal tissue of both sexes may be ovary and testis separately or combined in an ovotestis. The most common combination is an ovary on one side of the abdomen and a testis on the other. The second most common consists of an ovotestis and a contralateral ovary, followed by bilateral ovotestis (77).

Internally, a uterus is almost constantly present, but the development of müllerian and wolffian structures is variable and generally depends on the adjacent gonad. Usually, on the side of the testis, there is a vas, and with the ovary there is a tube. The external genitalia are usually ambiguous, but they may be either completely male or completely female.

True hermaphroditism has been described with many chromosomal patterns. The most common karyotype is 46, XX, occurring in about 60% of patients. In 13% of patients, 46, XX/46, XY chimerism has been described. The 46, XY true hermaphroditism occurs in 12% of patients. The remaining 15% were patients with mosaicism, such as 46, XY/47, XXY and 45, X/46, XY (78).

In patients with 46, XX/46, XY chimerism, the chromosomal abnormality is caused by mitotic or meiotic errors or chimerism from double fertilization or fusion of two normally fertilized ova. In patients with true hermaphroditism associated with 45, X/46, XY mosaicism, the abnormal gonadal determination is determined by the number of cells that contain a Y chromosome compared with those without a Y. Patients with 45, X/46, XY partial gonadal dysgenesis are said to represent a true hermaphroditism in utero.

The etiology of 46, XY true hermaphroditism is not clear. It is believed that the etiology of 46, XY true hermaphroditism is similar to the proposed mechanism for 46, XY partial gonadal dysgenesis. When testis differentiation is partial because of a mutation in a gene in the early stages of testis development, some areas of the gonadal ridge undergo testicular differentiation, whereas other areas undergo ovarian differentiation. Consequently, the primordial follicles in the ovarian tissue undergo involution because of the absence of two X chromosomes. As has been proposed, the phenotype is determined according to the timing of the ovarian involution: if follicles remain, the diagnosis is true hermaphroditism, but if the follicles have degenerated and only ovarian stroma remains, then it is diagnosed as gonadal dysgenesis. Therefore, the ovotestis and the dysgenetic gonad are likely to be different manifestations of a similar process (79,80).

The risk of gonadal tumor has been described in true hermaphroditism. It has been estimated that malignant gonadal tumors occur in 4% of patients with a 46, XX karyotype and 10% among patients with either 46, XY or 46, XX/46, XY. Gonadoblastoma, dysgerminoma, seminoma, and embryonal carcinoma have been the reported gonadal tumors (81,82).

The definite diagnosis of true hermaphroditism is made by gonadal biopsy. If the infant is raised as male, both ovarian gonadal tissue and the müllerian structures are removed. The testes are brought down into the scrotum. If the infant is raised as female, both wolffian structures and testicular gonadal tissue are removed. A biopsy of an intrascrotal gonad in a 46,XY subject with ambiguous genitalia is usually obtained to rule out an ovotestis. The testicular portion of an ovotestis is removed in patients with 46, XX true hermaphroditism raised as females to preserve ovarian function at puberty. The gonadal tissue is dissected at surgery to outline and remove the unwanted part of the gonad.

1. Syndromes of Testicular Differentiation with 46, XX Chromosomes

The syndromes characterized by testicular differentiation in individuals with a normal 46, XX chromosomes include 46, XX maleness and 46, XX true hermaphroditism. In the 46, XX maleness syndrome, testicular differentiation appears to be complete, whereas in 46, XX true hermaphroditism, testicular differentiation undergoes incomplete development of both ovarian and testicular tissue.

a. Syndrome of 46, XX Maleness. The syndrome 46, XX maleness is the development of testes in a patient with two X chromosomes but no Y chromosome. The majority have normal male external genitalia, and only 10% are described with hypospadias. A small number of individuals with 46, XX maleness are associated with cardiac anomalies. Virtually all 46, XX males are infertile.

The incidence of 46, XX maleness is 1 in 20,000 newborn males. Patients with this syndrome may present clinically with pubertal gynecomastia, delayed pubertal development, or gonadal dysfunction.

The clinical features are similar to those of Klinefelter syndrome: the penis and scrotum are normal, but the testicular size is decreased. The levels of LH and FSH in plasma are elevated, and plasma testosterone levels are low normal. The testicular histology is similar to that of Klinefelter syndrome: it is normal in prepubertal patients, but in adults, there is absence of spermatogonia, degeneration of seminiferous tubules, and Leydig cell hyperplasia.

b. Syndrome of 46, XX True Hermaphroditism. The syndrome is diagnosed when both testicular and ovarian tissue are demonstrated. The affected individual has an ovary on one side of the abdomen and a testis or ovotestis on the other. The external genitalia and development of the internal ducts depend on the extent of testicular development.

Mechanisms to explain testicular differentiation in individuals with 46, XX chromosomes include (1) translocation of some part of the Y chromosome, including the SRY gene, from paternal Y to the X chromosome; (2) an autosomal mutation allowing testicular differentiation in the absence of SRY; and (3) hidden mosaicism with a Y-carrying cell line (83–85).

2. Translocation of Some Part of the Y Chromosome from the paternal Y to the X Chromosome

Sex reversal in 46, XX subjects was thought to be secondary to the translocation of some Y genetic material to the X chromosome. The pseudoautosomal regions of X and Y chromosomes were pointed out as the regions at the end of the short arms of these two chromosomes, which are the site of X-Y pairing during male meiosis. It has been demonstrated that an obligatory crossing occurs between the X and Y pseudoautosomal regions. Because the SRY gene is so close to the pseudoautosomal region, an unequal crossover results in the translocation of SRY from the Y chromosome to the X chromosome.

DNA analysis from individuals with 46, XX maleness has demonstrated that two-thirds of XX males have the SRY gene in their genomes. The quantity of Y chromosome translocated to the X chromosome has ranged from most of the short arm of the Y chromosome to a small amount of genetic material next to the pseudoautosomal region.

Most individuals with 46, XX true hermaphroditism have absence of the SRY gene. However, the description of individuals with 46, XX true hermaphroditism and translocated SRY gene has originated controversy about incomplete testicular differentiation despite the presence of the SRY gene. The proposed mechanisms include (1) rearrangement of a mutaton of the SRY gene during translocation; (2) a diminished SRY gene expression caused by flanking sequences at the site of the translocation; (3) absence of Y sequences that are needed for SRY expression; and (4) timing and extent of X inactivation in the translocated X.

3. Autosomal Mutation Allowing Testicular Differentiation

Testicular differentiation in the absence of SRY occurs in individuals with 46, XX true hermaphroditism and in individuals with 46, XX maleness. Families with an inherited form of 46, XX maleness have an autosomal mode of inheritance, suggesting that one or more autosomal genes play a role in the etiology of 46, XX sex reversal. Both 46, XX maleness and 46, XX true hermaphroditism have been present in the same family, indicating a role of specific autosomal genes in the etiology of the two abnormalities.

4. A Hidden Mosaicism with a Y-Carrying Cell Line

This situation has been described as a Y-bearing cell line in the gonadal ridge at the time of the testicular differentiation. This explanation in 46, XX maleness does not rule out other possibilities for etiology.

D. Mixed Gonadal Dysgenesis (MGD)

Mixed gonadal dysgenesis is a gonadal differentiation disorder presenting with ambiguous genitalia. These individuals have at least one dysgenetic testis and no ovarian tissue or an ovotestis on one side and a streak ovary on the other. Subnormal production of testosterone by the dysgenetic testis may result in hypoplasia of wolffian duct structures and inadequate virilization of the external genitalia. The insufficient production of MIS allows the formation of a uterus and fallopian tubes. As in true hermaphroditism, asymmetric development of the internal ducts occurs when testicular tissue is present on only one side.

MGD is associated with mosaicism of two or more cell lines with different karyotypes, derived from a single zygote. MGD includes the syndromes associated with 45, X/46, XY, 45, X/47, XYY, 46, XX/47, XXY, and other karyotypes. The mosaicism is caused by a loss of the Y chromosome by nondisjunction. It is associated with an alteration of the Y chromosome, either rearrangement or deletion. The most common pattern is the 45, X/46, XY karyotype. Mixed gonadal dysgenesis represents the second most common intersexuality seen in the nursery.

Data from prenatal diagnosis have estimated the various clinical presentations in individuals with 45, X/46, XY mosaicism. When 76 cases of 45, X/46, XY mosaicism were studied, 90% had normal male external genitalia. In the remaining individuals with ambiguous genitalia, there were male phenotypes with hypospadias and female genitalia and mild clitoromegaly. The individuals with normal male genitalia had abnormal testicular histology in 27%, suggesting that although the majority of subjects with 45, X/46, XY mosaicism have normal male phenotypes, a number of them have gonadal dysfunction (86). The abnormal gonadal development in 45, X/46, XY individuals is related to the relative proportion of 45, X and 46, XY cells in the gonadal ridge. However, during a prenatal diagnosis study, there was no correlation between the percentage of 45, X cells in the cultured amniocytes and the presence of abnormal gonadal development (87).

Patients with 45, X/46, XY mosaicism present during infancy or at puberty with a wide range of phenotypes. The newborn has ambiguous genitalia, with asymmetry of the labioscrotal folds. There is an urogenital sinus opening that leads to a vagina. If this condition is not recognized at birth, patients are evaluated in endocrinology, urology, and gynecology clinics, where they consistently present with ambiguous genitalia. However, the majority of 45, X/46, XY individuals have a normal male phenotype, whereas others have a completely female phenotype with bilateral streak gonads. About 50% of these subjects have short stature, and Turner stigmata are present in about one-third. All patients with mixed gonadal dysgenesis have a rudimentary uterus and at least one fallopian tube, suggesting insufficient MIS secretion by dysgenetic gonads (88,89).

The management of subjects with 45, X/46, XY mosaicism and abnormal sexual differentiation depends upon the recommended sex of rearing. If the individual is raised as female, all gonadal tissue and wolffian structures should be removed. If the individual is raised as male, the intrascrotal testis or the abdominal testis is brought down into the scrotum, with removal of müllerian duct derivatives and the discordant streak gonad. However, careful examination and periodic sonogram examinations of the testis are important because of the increased risk of gonadal malignancy (90).

Two patterns of gonadal histology have been present in 45, X/46, XY individuals. One pattern consists of a streak gonad on one side of the abdomen and an ovotestis on the other side. This pattern is the classically referred as mixed gonadal dysgenesis. It is associated with müllerian structures on the side of the streak and wolffian structures on the ovotestis side. In the second pattern, the gonads may be bilateral ovotestis, bilateral dysgenesis testis, or a dysgenetic testis in association with a normal testis, classically referred as dysgenetic male pseudohermaphroditism.

Gonadal tumors occur in 30% of 45, X/46, XY individuals with abnormal sexual differentiation. This risk of malignancy increases with age. However, a gonadoblastoma in infancy has suggested an early intervention. Early removal of the gonads in MGD is considered in the neonatal period and will prevent the development of gonadoblastoma and dysgerminoma.

V. DIAGNOSTIC STEPS FOR AMBIGUOUS GENITALIA

When a child is born with ambiguous genitalia, a specialized care team should be convened. The situation is considered a pediatric emergency, not only for medical reasons but also because of the social implications. While the birth certificate is placed on hold, a rapid and organized evaluation is initiated to develop information about genetic, gonadal, and internal body sex. Here an approach is offered for the diagnostic evaluation and management of these infants.

A. Diagnostic Evaluation

1. History

A thorough family history is very important regarding perinatal or neonatal deaths, infertility, consanguinity, or questionable sex assignment at birth. Additional information includes family members with genital anomalies and inguinal hernias with prolapsed gonads. The patterns of inheritance in the various intersex disorders must be considered in the differential diagnosis.

A maternal history includes any abnormalities during pregnancy, especially during the first trimester. An androgen-secreting tumor in the mother can virilize a female fetus. Among drugs or hormones administered during pregnancy, hydantoin may induce incomplete masculinization by inhibiting the 5α-reductase enzyme and progesterone in the first trimester has been correlated with hypospadias in the male fetus. Androgen therapy for endometriosis may virilize the female fetus. Maternal alcohol intake has been associated with hypertrophy of the clitoris in females and hypoplastic penis in males.

2. Physical Examination

Ambiguity of the genitalia may have the same appearance in a virilized female or in an undermasculinized male. Thus, all the details in the physical examination should be emphasized. Findings during this examination may provide clues to the underlying pathology.

The physical examination should address such questions as whether the infant has dysmorphic features or a "chromosomal look." A good number of syndromes are associated with ambiguity of the genitalia. Intrauterine growth retardation may suggest a chromosomal abnormality. Abnormal body proportions may suggest an associated bone dysplasia syndrome. Abnormalities of external gentialia are common in infants with chromosome abnormalities. Stigmata, such as webbed neck and edematous hands and feet, may be present in mixed gonadal dysgenesis. Table 4 includes some of the conditions associated with genital ambiguity (91,92).

Asymmetry of the external genitalia is the hallmark of mixed gonadal dysgenesis as the testicular tissue on one side descends and the streak gonad does not. If palpable gonads are present, they are assessed for their position. Mobile, oval masses palpated below the inguinal ligament will prove to be testes, in keeping with "Federman's rule" that a gonad palpated below that ligament is a testis until proven otherwise, even if they are within the labia majora. Each gonad is evaluated for size, texture, and the presence of an epididymis.

The phallus length is measured along the dorsum of the stretched penis from the pubic ramus to the tip of the glans.

Table 4 Ambiguous Genitalia: Associated Syndromes

	Clinical Findings
Chromosomal Abnormalities	
Trisomy 13	Holoprosencephaly, polydactyly, cleft lip, hypospadias, cryptorchidism
Trisomy 18	Clenched hand, short sternum, malformed auricles, incomplete masculinization, virilized females
Triploidy	Prenatal growth failure, microphthalmia, congenital heart defects, hypospadias, micropenis, cryptorchidism
4p⁻	Supraorbital ridges, synophrys, large ears, incomplete masculinization
13q⁻	Microcephaly, colobomata, thumb hypoplasia, incomplete masculinization
Aniridia-Wilms	Microcephaly, ptosis, nystagmus, male pseudohermaphroditism
Syndromes	
Aarskog	Hypertelorism, brachydactyly, shawl scrotum, cryptorchidism
Camptomelic dwarfism	Flat facies, bowed tibiae, hypoplastic scapulae, male pseudohermaphroditism
Carpenter	Acrocephaly, polydactyly and syndactyly of feet, lateral displacement of inner canthi, hypogenitalism
CHARGE	Colobomata, heart defect, choanal atresia, retarded growth, genital hypoplasia, ear anomalies
Ellis-Van Creveld	Mesomelic dwarfism, polydactyly, cardiac anomalies, cryptorchidism
Fraser	Cryptophthalmos, defect of auricle, incomplete genitalia development: males with cryptorchidism and hypospadias, females with vaginal atresia
Meckel-Gruber	Encephalocele, polydactyly, renal cystic dysplasia, incomplete development of external genitalia
Opitz-Frias	Hypertelorism, hypospadias, bifid scrotum, cryptorchidism
Robinow	Flat facies profile, mesomelic dwarfism, hemivertebrae, small penis, clitoris, labia majora, cryptorchidism
Rieger	Iris dysplasia, maxillary hypoplasia, hypospadias
Smith-Lemli-Opitz	Anteverted nostrils, ptosis, toe syndactyly, hypospadias, cryptorchidism
VACTERL	Vertebral anomalies, anal atresia, tracheo-esophageal fistula, radial and renal dysplasia, bifid scrotum

Measurements for normal penile length in neonates and preterm infants are available (Chap. 61) (15). The degree of development of the corpora may be assessed by palpation of the shaft. Clitoral length should be assessed: premature infants may appear to have clitoromegaly because they have a larger clitoral breadth compared with body size.

The urogenital sinus opening is assessed by a careful look at the ventral area of the phallus for grooves and chordees. The urethral meatus may be at the tip of the phallus, along the shaft, or on the perineum. The presence of a vagina or vaginal pouch should be examined with a number 5 Hegar dilator to assess its depth. The vagina tends to be short in testicular feminization and long in mixed gonadal dysgenesis. The labioscrotal folds are examined for degree of fusion, development of rugae, and pigmentation. Posterior fusion may be the only finding in mild adrenal hyperplasia syndrome as well as the other extreme of the spectrum, with a penile urethra and empty rugated scrotum.

Genital hyperpigmentation in the congenital adrenal hyperplasia syndromes may be associated with increased pigmentation of the linea nigra from the umbilicus down the midline as well as the areolae. Some forms of congenital adrenal hyperplasia are associated with hypertension, so that blood pressure measurements should be noted.

3. Laboratory Evaluation

The most urgent investigations in patients with ambiguous genitalia include the chromosome analysis and the hormonal profile. Rapid karyotypes can be achieved on lymphocytes within 48 h on an emergency basis. Occasionally bone marrow chromosomes may be assessed in a few hours. When confronted with possible mosaicism, at least 50 cells must be counted.

Buccal smears to look for Barr chromatin bodies are often inaccurate and are not helpful in the newborn period. Examination of leukocytes by quinacrine staining of interphase for Y chromosome fluorescence may provide helpful results within a few hours if available.

With the initial blood sample for karyotyping, an aliquot is obtained for 17-hydroxyprogesterone. An increased level indicates a diagnosis of congenital adrenal hyperplasia, the most common cause of ambiguous genitalia. In the first few days of life, however, the levels may not be diagnostic and it should be repeated in 48 h. If the trend is upward, it leads to a diagnosis of CAH (P-450$_{c21}$ or 21-hydroxylase) deficiency. The presence of hyponatremia and hyperkalemia points to the CAH diagnosis.

Other adrenal steroid precursors may be indicated if CAH is a possibility. An increased level of 11-deoxycortisol indicates P-450$_{c11}$ (11β-hydroxylase) deficiency, and elevated dehydroepiandrosterone is present in 3β- hydroxysteroid dehydrogenase deficiency. Other evaluations may include serum testosterone levels before and after stimulation with human chorionic gonadotropin. This is particularly important for diagnosis of male pseudohermaphroditism because testosterone levels will not rise if there is a testosterone biosynthetic defect. hCG is usually given every other day for two doses intramuscularly, and blood samples are obtained, one at

baseline, a second before the second hCG injection, and a third blood sample 2 days later. A normal response is doubling the testosterone level from baseline to 48 h, the latter level being doubled on the third blood sample (Chap. 60). If the response is insufficient testosterone secretion, measurements of the different precursors of testosterone will indicate the level of the biosynthetic defect. If the testosterone response is normal, then the ratios of testosterone to dihydrotestosterone are estimated for diagnosis of 5α-reductase deficiency.

4. Imaging Studies

The pediatric radiologist's help should be enlisted to ascertain the nature of the pelvic organs and the size of the adrenals. A genitogram with retrograde injection of contrast media via the urogenital orifice should be performed to detect the presence of müllerian structures as well as to outline the anatomy of the urethra. Sonography is used to assess adequacy of the urinary tract. It may also detect müllerian structures and uterus behind the bladder, as well as ovaries. It can also identify undescended testes.

Magnetic resonance imaging may be helpful to delineate pelvic anatomy in infants with abnormal sexual differentiation (93). It may support the clinical picture in CAH by demonstrating normal ovaries and uterus. In male pseudohermaphroditism, MRI confirms the absent uterus and can demonstrate testicular location. However, because the immature testis and ovary have a similar appearance on MRI, gonadal characterization is ultimately a histologic diagnosis.

B. Management Considerations

It is important to remember that the laboratory requirements for gender assignment are the most promptly needed, but these are different from those that ultimately are needed for final diagnosis. For gender role selection, the primary criterion is the potential for future sexual and reproductive function, taking into consideration the cause of the disorder, the anatomic abnormalities, and the capabilities and limitations of reconstructive surgery. A newborn with female pseudohermaphroditism, even if severely virilized, should always be assigned the female sex. Male pseudohermaphrodites with complete or severe androgen resistance do not masculinize sufficiently for sexual function and should be given a female sex assignment. In other male pseudohermaphrodites, the sex of rearing depends upon the penile length at birth and its response to testosterone. If the full-term neonate stretched penile size is less than 1.9 cm, the individual should be given a female sex assignment. If a male assignment is being considered, the response of the phallic size to 25 mg testosterone enanthate or cypionate intramuscularly every 3 weeks for four doses must be assessed. If penile size does not reach the 2.5 cm range or above, a male sex assignment is not advisable. It is important for the pediatric surgeon to be involved in the diagnostic evaluation of these infants to plan the timing and techniques of the surgical reconstruction (90,94–96).

VI. MICROPENIS

Micropenis has been defined as a penile stretched length of less than $2\frac{1}{2}$ standard deviations below the mean for age or stage of sexual development (96). The standards for normal penile size have been provided by classic studies and are summarized in Figure 23 in Chapter 61. The penile length measurement should be made of the fully stretched rather than flaccid penis. A ruler should be pressed against the pubic ramus, depressing the suprapubic fat pad as completely as possible. The penis should be stretched by grasping the glans between the thumb and forefinger. The measurement is made along the dorsum to the tip of the glans without including the foreskin, if present.

Accurate examination and measurement are essential in determining whether micropenis is present. Micropenis must be differentiated from "hidden penis syndrome," which is one buried in excessive suprapubic fat, and from a penis held in marked chordee, which presents a downward bowing as a result of a congenital anomaly (97). Only very rarely is the entire penis absent in a condition named aphallia (98).

A. Etiologic Factors

The micropenis or incomplete masculinization of an XY individual may represent an end-organ defect resulting from unresponsiveness to androgen or from inadequate androgen production. Therefore, patients with micropenis may be classified into four major groups: (1) inadequate androgen production secondary to a hypothalamic or a pituitary disorder, leading to insufficient gonadotropin secretion and called hypogonadotropic hypogonadism (Table 5); (2) inadequate androgen production caused by a deficiency of any one of the enzymes necessary for testosterone synthesis, also called hypergonadotropic hypogonadism or primary gonadal disorder. This group of patients includes syndromes associated with primary gonadal failure, such as Klinefelter syndrome, other X polysomies, and Robinow syndrome (fetal facies and brachymesomelic dwarfism); other cases of primary hypogonad-

ism have included a variant of Laurence Moon-Biedl; (3) partial androgen insensitivity, when the mechanism of androgen action in target cells is defective (this group includes patients with partial androgen insensitivity syndrome associated with hypogenitalism); and (4) idiopathic micropenis with normal hypothalamic pituitary-gonadal function and appropriate virilization at puberty. Idiopathic micropenis is diagnosed if there is normal hypothalamic gonadal function, a normal penile size responsiveness to exogenous androgens, and normal masculinization at puberty. Environmental factors adversely influencing the intrauterine development of the penis without other sequelae may be considered the etiology in some cases.

B. Diagnostic Evaluation and Therapy

The workup of all patients with micropenis should be directed toward early diagnosis and therapy. The most important issue is whether the child will have sufficient penile growth to allow sexual function as an adult. Therefore, early evaluaton in the neonatal period is done so that gender change can be an option. In an infant with clearly diminished penile size of less than 1.9 cm and lack of adequate penile growth after treatment, sexual reassignment should be considered. Reassignment should be performed before 18 months of age because gender identity is clearly established by then (Chap. 23). The studies include karyotyping to rule out Klinefelter syndrome or variant forms of gonadal dysgenesis with a Y chromosome cell line. The syndromes associated with hypothalamic-pituitary insufficiency, such as growth hormone deficiency, should be ruled out or treated before hypoglycemia occurs. If indicated, cortisol levels and growth hormone following glucagon stimulation should be measured. Plasma FSH, LH, and testosterone levels, as well as the pituitary response to LH releasing hormone, will help to differentiate hypothalamic from pituitary deficiency. The testosterone response to hCG stimulation will differentiate primary from secondary testicular deficiency. The hCG may be given as 3000 units/m^2 per dose for two doses every other day, with the last testosterone sample taken on day 6 of the test. A normal testosterone response will be doubling the baseline on day 3 and redoubling on day 6. The hCG may also be given as 3000 U/m^2 body surface area per day, intramuscularly for 4 days after baseline plasma testosterone is determined. The response in testosterone at 4 day after the last injection is adequate when the level is above 200 ng/dl (Chap. 60).

An assessment should be made of the ability of the penis to respond to testosterone; testosterone cypionate or enanthate in oil, 25 mg intramuscularly, may be given every 3 weeks for 4 months (99,100). The side effects of this short course of testosterone therapy are minimal and include temporary accelerated growth velocity and bone age. A possible drawback of this androgen treatment is the imprinting on brain behavior in the infant who will be raised as female because of inadequate response. It is unclear whether this is indeed a factor in future psychosocial development. The response to this testosterone trial is considered a failure if the penis does

Table 5 Syndromes Associated with Micropenis and Hypogonadotropic Hypogonadism

Syndrome	Associated findings
Kallmann	Hyposmia, X-linked recessive
Prader-Willie	15q11–13 (deletion), perinatal hypotonia, obesity, short stature, small hands and feet, developmental delays
Rud	Hyposmia, congenital ichthyosis, developmental delays
Septooptic-dysplasia (de Morsier)	Hypopituitarism, absent septum pellucidum, hypoplastic optic disks
Laurence-Moon-Biedl (Laurence-Moon and Bardet-Biedl)	Short stature, retinal pigmentation, polydactyly, obesity, developmental delays

not increase in length. A lack of response is likely to represent androgen resistance and therefore possible failure to virilize at puberty. A diagnosis of partial androgen insensitivity is done if receptor assays of cultured genital fibroblasts demonstrate abnormal androgen binding and affinity of the steroid for the receptor (101).

VII. HYPOSPADIAS

Hypospadias is defined as abnormal anatomic location of the urethral meatus on the ventral aspect of the penis. It is a common anomaly of the genitourinary tract, with an estimated incidence of 8.2 in every 1000 male births.

The formation of the ventral foreskin of the penis is related to normal urethral development: failure of the urethra to reach the tip of the glans penis is accompanied by absence of the ventral foreskin. The absence of this foreskin causes an abnormal ventral curvature of the penis known as chordee. Hypospadias is frequently accompanied by chordee. If normal development of the urethra is arrested and the urethral folds fail to fuse, the meatus may be found anywhere along the course of the penis from the perineum to the glans.

Hypospadias are classified according to the anatomic site of the meatus, such as glandular; coronal; distal, middle, and proximal shaft; penoscrotal; scrotal; and perineal.

Uncomplicated hypospadias has been described in several generations of affected individuals. Once an affected child is present in a family, the recurrence risk for subsequent male siblings is up to 10%, suggesting a genetic factor, with a multifactorial mode of inheritance. Hypospadias may be associated with other anomalies and syndromes of human malformation, such as Smith-Lemli-Opitz syndrome (ptosis of eyelids, anteverted nostrils, and cryptorchidism) and cerebrohepatorenal syndrome (flat facies, hepatomegaly, and hydroureter).

Surgical reconstruction of hypospadias requires chordee correction when present. It is recommended that boys with hypospadias not be circumcised, because the foreskin may be used in the urethroplasty. If hypospadias is associated with micropenis, treatment with testosterone is done before surgery. Severe hypospadias, especially when associated with cryptorchidism, should be thoroughly studied as a patient with intersex disorder before embarking on a surgical reconstruction procedure.

VIII. CRYPTORCHIDISM

A. Definition and Anatomy

Cryptorchidism is defined as a developmental defect characterized by the failure of the testis to descend completely into the scrotum. Cryptorchidism represents one of the most common genital disorders of childhood. Cryptorchidism means "hidden testis" and refers to any testis that has not come to rest within the scrotal sac. The testicle originally develops within the abdominal cavity and therefore can be located anywhere within the abdomen, inguinal canal, or one of several ectopic locations. The majority of cases occur as isolated conditions, although there are a number of congenital disorders and syndromes of which cryptorchidism is a part. Undescended testes have been known to be associated with infertility and an increased risk of malignancy. Interest in the early treatment of undescended testis has sparked research into the migration of the testicle from the abdomen into the scrotum. Distinction between true cryptorchidism and the normal variation "retractile testis" is often difficult yet critical for both diagnostic and therapeutic reasons. Whereas cryptorchidism may be associated with chromosome abnormalities and malformation syndromes, retractile testis is a benign diagnosis, not associated with significant abnormalities. The majority of children with cryptorchidism referred to pediatric endocrinologists actually prove to have retractile testis, requiring no further evaluation. The retractile testis is an otherwise normal testis that has an active cremasteric reflex that retracts the testis into the groin. This testis can be "milked" into the dependent portion of the scrotum, where is should remain without tension. With growth, as the testis becomes larger and heavier, retraction becomes more difficult. Retractile testis usually are bilateral, can often be manipulated into the scrotum when the child assumes a squatting position, or may be seen in the scrotum during a hot bath. By contrast, cryptorchidism is usually 90% unilateral, with 55% more commonly right sided. A compensatory hypertrophy in the contralateral testicle frequently develops. Clues to a clinical diagnosis of true cryptorchidism include scrotal hypoplasia, testis palpable extremely high in the inguinal canals or not at all, and testis palpable in an ectopic location.

The infant with totally nonpalpable testes requires a more rapid and thorough evaluation than others with cryptorchidism. If hypospadias or genital skin hyperpigmentation is present, the absence of palpable testis should alert the pediatrician to the very distinct diagnosis of congenital adrenal hyperplasia or a chromosomal disorder.

The cryptorchid testis is usually located along the line of testicular descent, with 10% intraabdominal, 40% in the inguinal canal, and 25% just distal to the external ring. Another 25% may be located ectopically outside the normal pathway (superficial inguinal pouch, perineum, femoral canal, prepenile position, or contralateral scrotum). The cryptorchid testis may be absent or atrophic as a result of vascular impairment or injury with descent.

B. Embryology and Hormonal Aspects

Various factors play a role in the embryology of testicular descent. They include the gubernaculum, the epididymis, abdominal pressure, müllerian inhibiting substance, the genitofemoral nerve, and the hypothalamic-pituitary-testicular axis (102).

By week 6 of gestation, the primordial germ cells migrate to reach the genital ridges. By 7 weeks, the indifferent gonad differentiates into the fetal testis. During week 8 of gestation, the fetal testis secretes müllerian substance, causing regression of the müllerian ducts. At 10 weeks of gestation, the fetal testis produces testosterone, stimulating the wolffian duct to form the epididymis, vas deferens, and seminal vesicle. The external genitalia is masculinized between 10 and 12 weeks by testosterone conversion to dihydrotestosterone by the 5α-reductase enzyme. During week 5, the gubernaculum forms from the wolffian duct and extends from the abdominal wall to the genital swellings (scrotum). With the ascent of the kidney as a result of the elongation of the embryo, the testis stays anchored at the internal inguinal canal by the gubernaculum. In the third month, the processus vaginalis forms and gradually extends to the scrotum. The process of testicular descent remains dormant until the seventh month of gestation, when the gubernaculum increases in size, distending the inguinal canal and the scrotum. The testis then descends rapidly into the scrotum. The role of the gubernaculum in testicular descent has been debated. At present, the gubernaculum is said to function by either mechanical forces or hormonal response to androgens. Theories for the mechanical mechanism of the gubernaculum are as follows:

1. The gubernaculum's surrounding cremasteric muscle pulls the testicle into the scrotum.
2. The gubernacular regression and subsequent immobility serve to fix the testicle in position, with descent of the testicle caused by differential body growth.
3. The gubernaculum acts as a guide for the testicle, which is pushed into the scrotum by abdominal pressure.

Studies suggest that the gubernaculum is under androgen direction during testicular descent. Ligand binding assays in fetal rat and porcine gubernacular tissues demonstrated the presence of a gubernacular androgen receptor protein. Following descent, the gubernaculum persists as a fibrous band at the lower pole of the testis and the processus vaginalis obliterates before birth.

Undescended testicles occur commonly in patients with an abnormality of the hypothalamic-pituitary axis. This further correlates the role of androgen in descent of the testis. Anencephaly, pituitary aplasia, and Kallman syndrome are frequently noted to have cryptorchidism. In addition, disorders of testosterone production or insensitivity syndromes are commonly associated with cryptorchidism.

Testosterone induces testicular descent, but the descent appears regulated primarily by DHT. MIS may be involved in the initial phases of testicular descent. Support for this is based on the observation that in the persistent müllerian duct syndrome, in which there is a failure of müllerian regression, cryptorchidism is almost always present. In addition, the ovary, which does not produce MIS, never "descends" into the labia, even in congenital adrenal hyperplasia, in which severe virilization occurs (33,103).

C. Incidence and Classification

Cryptorchidism represents the most common genital abnormality in infancy. Approximately 4% of newborn males

have undescended testis. At 1 month, however, the incidence is 1.8% and by 1 year of age is only 0.8% (1 in 125 boys). The incidence is much higher in premature infants (1 in 3), and the lower the birth weight, the greater the incidence of cryptorchidism. Approximately 75% of males born with an undescended testis exhibit spontaneous descent during the first year of life. Subsequently, however, spontaneous descent is rare. Recognition of these statistics is important in determining the optimal age for treatment (104–106).

A variety of classifications of cryptorchid testis are used. Most are based on whether the testicle is palpable or nonpalpable. Certain assumptions must be made to understand the rationale for the following organization. If the testicle does not develop, müllerian structures will be present on that side. If the processus vaginalis does not form, the gubernaculum also will not form and the testicle will be intraabdominal. Testicular descent is complete by 9 months. Descent after 9 months of age is evidence of testicular retractility.

If the pituitary gland is normal, hCG does not result in descent of a true undescended testis. The same may be true for gonadotropin releasing hormone. Testicular retractility does not impair eventual fertility, because this is a normal variant. Retractile testis are most commonly palpated in the groin but can be moved to the base of the scrotum. The hemiscrotum is well developed. These are not truly undescended but withdrawal of the scrotal sac because of an active cremasteric reflex. The spermatic cord length is normal. Maturation and fertility are normal. These patients respond to hormonal manipulation. Ectopic testes have deviated from the path of normal migration. The most common site is the superficial inguinal pouch, but other sites include the perineum, the femoral canal, the base of the penis, or the opposite scrotum. The hemiscrotum is usually small and flat.

Truly undescended testicles are in the normal path of descent, either within the inguinal canal or just below the external ring by the scrotal inlet. A nonpalpable testicle may become palpable with increased abdominal pressure by sliding through the internal ring into the canal (gliding undescended testicle). Iatrogenic undescended testis occurs after groin surgery, in which the testicle has become trapped and pulled up out of the scrotum, the most common being herniorrhaphy. Only 20% of nonpalpable testes will be absent. The remainder will be in either the intraabdominal or intracanalicular position. If the testis never developed (absent testis), ipsilateral müllerian structures should be present. Usually, there is an atrophic testicle with blind-ending spermatic vessels and vas deferens on that side.

D. Implications of Cryptorchidism

The potential implications of cryptorchidism include testicular atrophy, malignancy, infertility, testicular torsion, and inguinal hernia. There may be psychologic factors as well.

Long-term follow-up has shown that testicular atrophy eventually results if the condition is untreated. This atrophy is often accompanied by contralateral testicular enlargement, but testicular insufficiency in adulthood may occur despite such compensatory hypertrophy (107). The risk of testicular malignancy in cryptorchid testis is increased. The risk of malignancy in the general population is 1 in approximately 45,000 males, but 10% of adult testicular tumors occur in men who have a history of cryptorchidism. The risk of tumor in a cryptorchid testis is approximately 20 times greater than in a normally descended testis. The location of the testis is also a factor in the development of malignancy; an intraabdominal testis is five times more likely to develop a malignancy than is an inguinal one (108).

Most studies indicate that bringing the testis down into the scrotum does not reduce the risk of subsequent malignancy. It has also been suggested that very early orchiopexy offers some protection against the later development of malignancy, but this requires more long-term follow-up. In any event, bringing the testis to a scrotal location allows easier examination by both the patient and the pediatrician. Self-examination of the scrotum is a skill that the patient with cryptorchidism should acquire early and perform monthly, beginning in adolescence.

The incidence of infertility is increased in cryptorchidism. Impaired fertility is 5% in the male population and rises to 40% in unilateral cryptorchidism and up to 70% in bilateral cryptorchidism. The intrascrotal temperature is between 1.5 and 2.5°C lower than that of the abdomen; the higher temperature to which an intraabdominal testis is exposed may severely retard normal germinal maturation.

Histologic studies have demonstrated normal morphology and spermatogonia content in most cryptorchid testis during first 2 years of life. By the beginning of the third year, however, cryptorchid testes have a statistically significant deterioration in number of germ cells, spermatogonia, and Leydig cells, which progresses with time. There is also an increase in interstitial fibrosis and collagenization in peritubular connective tissue after the second year of life in the cryptorchid testis.

There is indirect evidence that unilateral cryptorchidism affects the contralateral descended testis at an early age. Autoantibodies to the cryptorchid testis may be produced and can cause degenerative changes in the descended testis. There is a suggestion that improved fertility is obtained with early orchiopexia (before 2 years of age) (109).

The majority of boys with cryptorchidism do not have a clinical hernia but have a patent processus. At the time of the orchiopexy, the hernia must be repaired. Testicular torsion may result from the lack of adequate fixation of the testis and occurs most frequently in the postpubertal male. Sudden painful inguinal swelling in association with cryptorchidism can represent testicular torsion or clinical hernia with incarceration and indicates the need for urgent intervention.

E. Treatment

The therapeutic goals in treating cryptorchidism include (1) improve fertility, (2) allow the testis to be more accessible for physical examination and detection of malignancy, (3) correct, if present, an associated hernia, and (4) alleviate psychologic stress caused by the empty scrotum.

1. Hormonal Therapy

Because testicular descent is influenced by the hypothalamic-pituitary-gonadal axis, both human chorionic gonadotropin and gonadotropin releasing hormone (GnRH) have been used in cryptorchidism.

Various regimens of hCG administration have been recommended. They all have had variable success. Maximum stimulation may be obtained by as little as 100 units hCG per kg given every 5 days for 3–4 weeks (110). The World Health Organization recommends 250 IU twice a week for 5 weeks in males up to 1 year of age. From 1 to 5 years of age, 500 IU is given twice weekly for 5 weeks. Older boys are given 1000 IU twice weekly for 5 weeks (111). However, dosages and treatment schedules have varied from 100 to 4000 IU per injection given 2–3 days per week for 1–5 weeks.

Successful treatment of the true undescended testis with hCG has varied from 6 to 65% (112). On the other hand, hCG is quite useful when it is suspected that a testis is retractile. In these cases, hCG, 3000 $IU/m^2/week$, may be given intramuscularly three times per week for 4 weeks. The child is reexamined 1 week after the last injection. If the testis has "descended" into the scrotal sac, then it is probably retractile. The child should be reexamined 6 months following completion of hormonal therapy to reassess the location of the testis. If it has returned to an apparently undescended position, then a formal orchiopexy should be performed.

GnRH has been used intranasally at a dose of 1–1.2 mg daily for 4 weeks. It is simple and painless and without side effects. However, it appears no more effective than hCG or a placebo.

Most investigations conclude that hormonal therapy causes descent of those testes that ultimately would have descended without surgery. Hormone administration has been advised as a way of distinguishing testes destined to descend spontaneously from those requiring orchiopexy.

2. Surgical Therapy

The standard treatment for undescended testis is surgical when hormone therapy fails. The decision about the optimum time of orchiopexy depends on such factors as technical, psychologic, and risk of not operating early. Technically, successful orchiopexy can be performed early by experienced surgeons with good pediatric anesthesia. The optimal time to operate on a child is between birth and 6 months, when the infant is not aware of separation from his mother. Because the diagnosis of cryptorchidism is usually confirmed after 12 months, surgery at this age includes the mother staying with the child. The recommendation as proposed by the Action Committee on Surgery of the Genitalia is to perform orchiopexy at 12 months of age. Numerous studies have shown that 75% of testes will descend spontaneously by this age without further chance of descent thereafter. Anesthesia risk by this age is minimal with experienced pediatric anesthesiologists. It has been shown that testicular damage occurs by 2 years of age. Most orchiopexies can be performed as an ambulatory procedure. Ectopic testes and canalicular testes are brought into the scrotum by a small inguinal crease incision. The gubernaculum and cremasteric muscle are separated from the testicle, and the lateral Prentiss fibers are divided, thereby allowing the testis a more direct route into the scrotum. The testis is then fixed in place with a suture. There is a 90% incidence of inguinal hernia with undescended testis, which is repaired simultaneously. The success rate of this operation is reported to be over 95%.

Bilateral inguinal testis can be operated upon at the same setting. Nonpalpable undescended testis can now be located by laparoscopy to inspect the peritoneal cavity. Of nonpalpable testes, 20% are atrophic, and blind-ending spermatic vessels and vas deferens are noted intraabdominally. Numerous radiologic investigations have been performed, including sonograms, CT scans, venography of the spermatic vessels, and, most recently, MRI. These are all inaccurate and are not recommended. If at the time of laparoscopy the testicle is located, an orchiopexy can be performed at that time. Most testicles can be placed within the scrotal sac by one procedure. However, when the spermatic vessels are extremely short, a two-stage orchiopexy can be performed. The spermatic vessels are ligated or divided during the first stage, allowing collateral blood supply via the vasal artery to develop. Then, 4–6 months later, the testicle is brought into the scrotal sac and nourished with the vasal blood supply, with a success rate of 90%. In bilateral nonpalpable testis, hCG stimulation tests should be performed before laparoscopy to rule out testicular agenesis. Laparoscopy in children has been shown to be safe by the age of 1 year and can be done as an ambulatory procedure (113).

REFERENCES

1. Erickson RP, Blecher SR. Sex determination. In: Polin RA, Fox WW, eds. Fetal and Neonatal Physiology. Philadelphia: WB Saunders, 1992:1851–1853.
2. Wachtel SS, Koo GC, Boyse EA. Evolutionary conservation of H-Y ("male") antigen. Nature 1975; 254:270–272.
3. Goldberg E. H-Y antigen and sex determination. Philos Trans R Soc Lond (Biol) 1988; 32:72–81.
4. Page DC, Mosher R, Simpson EM, et al. The sex-determining region of the human Y chromosome encodes a finger protein. Cell 1987; 51:1091–1104.
5. Palmer MS, Sinclair AH, Berta P, et al. Genetic evidence that ZFY is not the testis-determining factor. Nature 1989; 342:937–939.
6. Moore CCD, Grumbach MM. Sex determination and gonadogenesis: a transcription cascade of sex chromosome and autosome genes. Semin Perinatol 1992; 16:266–278.
7. Grumbach MM, Conte FA. Disorders of sex differentiation. In: Wilson JD, Foster DW, eds. Williams Textbook of Endocrinology. Philadelphia: WB Saunders, 1992:853–951.
8. Hawkins JR. The SRY gene. Trends Endocrinol Metab 1993; 4:328–332.
9. Jirasek JE. Germ cells and the indifferent gonad (genital ridge). In: Polin RA, Fox WW, eds. Fetal and Neonatal Physiology. Philadelphia: WB Saunders, 1992:1854–1864.
10. Jirasek JE. Development of the Genital System and Male Pseudohermaphroditism. Baltimore: Johns Hopkins Press, 1971:121.
11. Josso N, Picard JY, Tran D. The anti-Mullerian hormone. Recent Prog Horm Res 1977; 33:117–160.
12. Taguchi O, Cunha GR, Lawrence WD, et al. Timing and irreversibility of müllerian duct inhibition in the embryonic reproductive tract of the human male. Dev Biol 1984; 106:394–398.
13. Trelstad RL, Hayashi A, Hayashi K, et al. The epithelial mesenchymal interface of the male rate müllerian duct: loss of basement membrane integrity and ductal regression. Dev Biol 1982; 92:27–40.
14. Glenister TW. The development of the utricle and of the so-called "middle" or "median" lobe of the human prostate. J Anat 1962; 96:443–445.
15. Feldman KW, Smith DW. Fetal phallic growth and penile standards for newborn male infants. J Pediatr 1975; 86:395–398.
16. Gier HT, Marion GB. Development of the mammalian testis and genital ducts. Biol Reprod 1969; 1:1–23.
17. Heyns CF. The gubernaculum during testicular descent in the human fetus. J Anat 1987; 153:93–112.
18. George FW. Developmental pattern of 5-alpha-reductase activity in the rat gubernaculum. Endocrinology 1989; 124:727–732.
19. Stallings MW, Rose AH, Auman GL, et al. Persistent müllerian duct structures in a male neonate. Pediatrics 1976; 57:568–569.
20. Guerrier D, Tran D, VanderWinden JM, et al. The persistent müllerian duct syndrome: A molecular approach. J Clin Endocrinol Metab 1989; 68:46–52.
21. Ammini AC, Pandey J, Vijyaraghavan M, Sabherwal U. Human female phenotypic development: role of fetal ovaries. J Clin Endocrinol Metab 1994; 79:604–608.
22. Herbst AI. Problems of prenatal DES-exposure. In: Herbst AI, Mishell DR, Stenchever MA, Droegemueller W, eds. Comprehensive Gynecology. St. Louis: Mosby Yearbook, 1992:179.
23. Jost A. Problems of fetal endocrinology: the gonadal and hypophyseal hormones. Recent Prog Horm Res 1953; 8:379–418.
24. Jost A, Vigier B, Prepin J, et al. Studies on sex differentiation in mammals. Recent Prog Horm Res 1973; 29:1–46.
25. Lee MM, Donahoe PK. Müllerian inhibiting substance: a gonadal hormone with multiple functions. Endocr Rev 1993; 14:152–164.
26. Josso N. Hormonal regulation of sexual differentiation. Semin Perinatol 1992; 16:279–288.
27. Miller WL. Immunoassays for human müllerian inhibitory factor (MIF)—new insights into the physiology of MIF. J Clin Endocrinol Metab 1990; 70:8–10.
28. Josso N, Boussin L, Knebelmann B, Nihoul-Fekete C, Picard JY. Anti-müllerian hormone and intersex states. Trends Endocrinol Metab 1991; 2:227–233.
29. Gustafson ML, Lee MM, Asmundson L, MacLaughlin DT, Donahoe PK. Müllerian inhibiting substance in the diagnosis and management of intersex and gonadal abnormalities. J Pediatr Surg 1993; 28:439–444.
30. Gustafson ML, Lee MM, Scully RE, et al. Müllerian inhibiting substance as a marker for ovarian sex-cord tumor. N Engl J Med 1992; 326:466–471.
31. Knebelmann B, Boussin L, Guerrier D, et al. Anti-müllerian hormone Bruxelles: a nonsense mutation associated with the persistent müllerian duct syndrome. Proc Natl Acad Sci USA 1991; 88:3767–3771.
32. Loeff DS, Imbeaud S, Reyes HM, Meller JL, Rosenthal IM. Surgical and genetic aspects of persistent müllerian duct syndrome. J Pediatr Surg 1994; 29:61–65.

33. Hutson JM, Donahoe PK. The hormonal control of testicular descent. Endocr Rev 1986; 7:270–283.

34. Takahashi M, Koide SS, Donahoe PK. Müllerian inhibiting substance as oocyte meiosis inhibitor. Mol Cell Endocrinol 1986; 47:225–234.

35. Vigier B, Watrin F, Magre S, et al. Purified bovine AMH induces a characteristic freemartin effect in fetal rat prospective ovaries exposed to it *in vitro*. Development 1987; 100:43–55.

36. Behringer RR, Cate RL, Froelick GJ, et al. Abnormal sexual development in transgenic mice chronically expressing mullerian inhibiting substance. Nature 1990; 345:167–170.

37. Di Clemente N, Ghaffari S, Pepinsky RB, et al. A quantitative and interspecific test for biological activity of anti-müllerian hormone: the fetal ovary aromatase assay. Development 1992; 114:721–727.

38. Pelliniemi LJ, Dym M. The fetal gonad and sexual differentiation. In: Tulchinsky D, Little AB, eds. Maternal-Fetal Endocrinology. Philadelphia: WB Saunders, 1994:297–320.

39. Gustafson ML, Donahoe PK. Male sexual determination: current concepts of male sexual differentiation. Annu Rev Med 1994; 45:505–524.

40. Jenkins EP, Andersson S, Imperato-McGinley J, Wilson JD, Russell DW. Genetic and pharmacological evidence for more than one human steroid 5-alpha-reductase. J Clin Invest 1992; 89:293–300.

41. French FS, Lubahn DB, Brown TR, et al. Molecular basis of androgen insensitivity. Recent Prog Horm Res 1990; 46:1–42.

42. Kalloo NB, Gearhart JP, Barrack ER. Sexually dimorphic expression of estrogen receptors, but not of androgen receptors in human fetal external genitalia. J Clin Endocrinol Metab 1993; 77:692–698.

43. Mills JL, Graubard BI. Is moderate drinking during pregnancy associated with an increased risk for malformations? Pediatrics 1987; 80:309–314.

44. Miller WL. Congenital adrenal hyperplasias. Endocrinol Metab Clin North Am 1991; 20:721–749.

45. Shozu M, Akasofu K, Harada T, Kubota Y. A new cause of female pseudohermaphroditism: placental aromatase deficiency. J Clin Endocrinol Metab 1991; 72:560–566.

46. Conte FA, Grumbach MM, Ito Y, Fisher CR, Simpson ER. A syndrome of female pseudohermaphroditism, hypergonadotropic hypogonadism, and multicystic ovaries associated with missense mutations in the gene encoding aromatase (P 450 arom). J Clin Endocrinol Metab 1994; 78:1287–1292.

47. New MI. Female pseudohermaphroditism. Semin Perinatol 1992; 16:299–318.

48. Kupfer SR, Quigley CA, French FS. Male pseudohermaphroditism. Semin Perinatol 1992; 16:319–331.

49. Mastroyannis C, Wallach EE. Male pseudohermaphroditism: inborn errors in testosterone biosynthesis. Semin Reprod Endocrinol 1987; 5:261–276.

50. Miller WL. Molecular biology of steroid hormone synthesis. Endocr Rev 1988; 9:295–318.

51. Sparkes RS, Klisak I, Miller WL. Regional mapping of genes encoding human steroidogenic enzymes: P450scc to 15q23-q24, adrenodoxin to 11q22, adrenodoxin reductase to 17q24-q25 and P450c17 to 10q24-q25. DNA Cell Biol 1991; 10:359–365.

52. Rheaume E, Simard J, Morel Y, et al. Congenital adrenal hyperplasia due to point mutations in the type 11 3β-hydroxysteroid dehydrogenase gene. Nature Genet 1992; 1:239–245.

53. Rheaume E, Sanchez R, Simard J, et al. Molecular basis of congenital adrenal hyperplasia in two siblings with classical non-salt losing 3β-hydroxysteroid dehydrogenase deficiency. J Clin Endocrinol Metab 1994; 79:1012–1018.

54. Yanase T, Simpson ER, Waterman MR. 17-Alpha- hydroxylase/17,20 lyase deficiency: from clinical investigation to molecular definition. Endocr Rev 1991; 12:91–108.

55. Rosler A, Belanger A, Labrie F. Mechanisms of androgen producton in male pseudohermaphroditism due to 17 β-hydroxysteroid dehydrogenase deficiency. J Clin Endocrinol Metab 1992; 75:773–778.

56. Martinez-Mora J, Saez JM, Toran M, et al. Male pseudohermaphroditism due to Leydig cell agenesis and absence of testicular LH receptors. Clin Endocrinol (Oxf) 1991; 34:485–491.

57. Keenan BS, Kirkland JL, Kirkland RT, et al. Male pseudohermaphroditism with partial androgen insensitivity. Pediatrics 1977; 59:224–231.

58. Gyorki S, Warne GL, Khalid BAK, et al. Defective nuclear accumulation of androgen receptors in disorders of sexual differentiation. J Clin Invest 1983; 72:819–825.

59. Quigley CA, Friedman KJ, Johnson A, et al. Complete deletion of the androgen receptor gene: definition of the null phenotype of the androgen insensitivity syndrome and determination of carrier status. J Clin Endocrinol Metab 1992; 74:928–934.

60. Griffin JE. Androgen resistance—the clinical and molecular spectrum. N Engl J Med 1992; 326:611–618.

61. Rutgers JL, Scully RE. The androgen insensitivity syndrome (testicular feminization): a clinicopathologic study of 43 cases. Int J Gynecol Pathol 1991; 10:126–144.

62. Griffin JE, Wilson JD. The syndromes of androgen resistance. N Engl J Med 1980; 302:198–209.

63. Fratianni CM, Imperato-McGinley J. The syndrome of 5α-reductase deficiency. Endocrinologist 1994; 4:302–314.

64. Wilson JD, Griffin JE, Russell DW. Steroid 5α-reductase 2 deficiency. Endocr Rev 1993; 14:577–593.

65. Imperato-McGinley J, Peterson RE, Gautier T, et al. Androgens and the evolution of male-gender identity among male pseudohermaphrodites with 5α-reductase deficiency. N Engl J Med 1979; 300:1233–1237.

66. Wilson JD. Sex hormones and sexual behavior. N Engl J Med 1979; 300:1269–1270.

67. Imperato-McGinley J, Miller M, Wilson JD, et al. A cluster of male pseudohermaphrodites with 5α-reductase deficiency in Papua New Guinea. Clin Endocrinol (Oxf) 1991; 34:293–298.

68. Imperato-McGinley J, Gautier T, Pichardo M, et al. The diagnosis of 5α-reductase deficiency in infancy. J Clin Endocrinol Metab 1986; 63:1313–1318.

69. Saenger P, Goldman AS, Levine LS, et al. Prepubertal diagnosis of 5α-reductase deficiency. J Clin Endocrinol Metab 1978; 46:627–634.

70. Federman DD. Abnormal Sexual Development. Philadelphia: WB Saunders, 1967:82.

71. Berkovitz GD. Abnormalities of gonadal determination and differentiation. Semin Perinatol 1992; 16:289–298.

72. Berkovitz GD, Fechner PY, Zacur HW, et al. Clinical and pathologic spectrum of 46,XY gonadal dysgenesis: its relevance to the understanding of sex differentiation. Medicine (Baltimore) 1991; 70:375–383.

73. Olsen MM, Caldamone AA, Jackson CL, et al. Gonadoblastoma in infancy: indications for early gonadectomy in 46,XY gonadal dysgenesis. J Pediatr Surg 1988; 23:270–271.

74. Adamsbaum C, Rolland Y, Josso N, Kalifa G. Radiological findings in three cases of persistent müllerian duct syndrome. Pediatr Radiol 1993; 23:55–56.

75. Josso N, Briard M-L. Embryonic testicular regression syndrome: variable phenotypic expression in siblings. J Pediatr 1980; 97:200–204.

76. Coulam CB. Testicular regression syndrome. Obstet Gynecol 1979; 53:44–49.

77. Berkovitz GD, Fechner PY, Zacur HW, et al. Clinical and pathological spectrum of 46, XY gonadal dysgenesis: its relevance to the understanding of sex differentiation. Medicine (Baltimore) 1991; 70:375–383.

78. Van Niekerk WA, Retief AE. The gonads of human true hermaphrodites. Hum Genet 1981; 58:117–122.

79. McKelvie J, Jaubert F, Nezelof C. True hermaphroditism. A primary germ cell disorder. Pediatr Pathol 1987; 7:31–41.

80. Tho SPT, Layman LC, Lanclos KD, Plouffe L, Byrd JR, McDonough PG. Absence of the testicular determining factor gene SRY in XX true hermaphrodites and presence of this locus in most subjects with gonadal dysgenesis caused by Y aneuploidy. Am J Obstet Gynecol 1992; 16:1794–1802.

81. Scully RE. Neoplasia associated with anomalous sexual development and abnormal sex chromosomes. Pediat adolesc endocr 1981; 8:203–217.

82. Ramani P, Yeung CK, Habeebu SS. Testicular intratubular germ cell neoplasia in children and adolescents with intersex. Am J Surg Pathol 1993; 17:1124–1133.

83. Fechner PY, Marcantonio SM, Jaswaney V, et al. The role of the sex-determining region Y gene in the etiology of 46, XX maleness. J Clin Endocrinol Metab 1993; 76:690–695.

84. Pereira ET, Cabral de Almeida JC, Gunha A, et al. Use of probes for ZFY, SRY and the Y pseudoautosomal boundary in XX males, XX true hermaphroditism, and an XY female. J Med Genet 1991; 28:591–595.

85. Berkovitz GD, Fechner PY, Marcantonio SM, et al. The role of the sex-determining region of the Y chromosome (SRY) in the etiology of 46, XX true hermaphroditism. Hum Genet 1992; 88:411–416.

86. Donahoe PK, Crawford JD, Hendren WH. Mixed gonadal dysgenesis, pathogenesis and management. J Pediatr Surg 1979; 14:287–300.

87. Chang HJ, Clark RD, Bachman H. The phenotype of 45, X/46, XY mosaicism: an analysis of 92 prenatally diagnosed cases. Am J Hum Genet 1990; 46:156–167.

88. Davidoff F, Federman DD. Mixed gonadal dysgenesis. Pediatrics 1973; 52:725–742.

89. Robboy SJ, Miller T, Donahoe PK, et al. Dysgenesis of testicular and streak gonads in the syndrome of mixed gonadal dysgenesis. Hum Pathol 1982; 13:700–716.

90. Donahoe PK, Powell DM, Lee MM. Clinical management of intersex abnormalities. Curr Probl Surg 1991; 28:513–579.

91. Buyse M, Feingold M. Syndromes associated with abnormal external genitalia. In: Vallet HL, Porter IH, eds. Genetic Mechanisms of Sexual Development. New York: Academic, 1979:425–435.

92. McGillivray BC. The newborn with ambiguous genitalia. Semin Perinatol 1992; 16:365–368.

93. Gambino J, Caldwell B, Dietrich R, Walot I, Kangarloo H. Congenital disorders of sexual differentiation: MR findings. Am J Roentgenol 1992; 158:363–367.

94. Meyers-Seifer CH, Charest NJ. Diagnosis and management of patients with ambiguous genitalia. Semin Perinatol 1992; 16:332–339.

95. Rock JA, Katz E. Ambiguous genitalia. Semin Reprod Endocrinol 1987; 5:327–329.

96. Lee PA, Mazur T, Danish R, et al. Micropenis. I. Criteria, etiologies and classification. Johns Hopkins Med J 1980; 146:156–163.

97. Bergeson PS, Hopkin RJ, Bailey RB, McGill LC, Piatt JP. The inconspicuous penis. Pediatrics 1993; 92:794–799.

98. Skoog SJ, Belman AB. Aphallia: its classification and management. J Urol 1989; 141:589.

99. Guthrie RD, Smith DW, Graham CB. Testosterone treatment for micropenis during childhood. J Pediatr 1973; 83:247–252.

100. Burstein S, Grumbach MM, Kaplan SL. Early determination of androgen responsiveness is important in the management of microphallus. Lancet 1979; 2:983–986.

101. Amrhein JA, Meyer WJ, Danish RK, Migeon CJ. Studies of androgen production and binding in 13 male pseudohermaphrodites and 13 males with micropenis. J Clin Endocrinol Metab 1977; 45:732–738.

102. Fonkalsrud EW, Mengel W. The Undescended Testis. Chicago: Yearbook Medical, 1981.

103. Elder JS. Cryptorchidism: isolated and associated with other genitourinary defects. Pediatr Clin North Am 1987; 34:1033–1053.

104. Frey HL, Rajfer J. Incidence of cryptorchidism. Urol Clin North Am 1982; 9:327–329.

105. Scorer GC, Farrington GH. Congenital Deformities of the Testis and Epididymis. New York: Appleton-Century-Crofts, 1971.

106. Berkowitz GS, Lapinsky RH, Dolgin SE, Gazella JG, Bodian CA, Holzman IR. Prevalence and natural history of cryptorchidism. Pediatrics 1993; 92:44–49.

107. Laron Z, Dickerman Z, Ritterman I, et al. Follow-up of boys with unilateral compensatory testicular hypertrophy. Fertil Steril 1980; 33:303.

108. Martin DC. Malignancy in the cryptorchid testis. Urol Clin North Am 1982; 9:37.

109. Hadziselimovic F. Cryptorchidism. In: Gillenwater JY, Grayhack JT, Howards SS, Duckett JW, eds. Adult and Pediatric Urology. St. Louis: Mosby Yearbook, 1991:2217–2228.

110. Forest MG, David M, Lecoq A, et al. Kinetics of the HCG-induced steroidogenic response of the human testis. III. Studies in children of the plasma levels of testosterone and HCG: rationale for testicular stimulation test. Pediatr Res 1980; 14:819.

111. Rabinowitz R, Hulbert WC. Cryptorchidism. Pediatr Rev 1994; 15:272–274.

112. Rajfer J, Handelsman DJ, Swerdloff RS, et al. Hormonal therapy of cryptochidism: a randomized, double-blind study comparing human chorionic gonadotropin and gonadotropin-releasing hormone. N Engl J Med 1986; 314:466.

113. Holcomb GW. Laparoscopic evaluation for a contralateral inguinal hernia or a nonpalpable testis. Pediatr Ann 1993; 22:678–684.

21
Update on Congenital Adrenal Hyperplasia

Maria I. New
New York Hospital–Cornell Medical Center, New York, New York

Lucia Ghizzoni
University of Parma,
Parma, Italy

Phyllis W. Speiser
North Shore University Hospital, Manhasset, New York

I. INTRODUCTION

Congenital adrenal hyperplasia (CAH) is a family of inherited disorders of adrenal steroidogenesis. Each disorder results from a deficiency of one of the several enzymes necessary for normal steroid synthesis. Since the earliest case of CAH documented in 1865 by the Neapolitan anatomist De Crecchio (1), numerous investigators have unraveled the mechanisms of adrenal steroid synthesis and the associated enzyme defects responsible for the clinical syndromes. This report includes recent advances in the investigation and understanding of these disorders.

II. PATHOPHYSIOLOGY

The adrenal gland synthesizes three main classes of hormones: mineralocorticoids, glucocorticoids, and sex steroids. Figure 1 shows a simplified scheme of the adrenal synthesis of these steroids from the cholesterol precursor molecule. Each enzymatic step is indicated.

The pituitary regulates adrenal steroidogenesis via adrenocorticotropic hormone (ACTH). ACTH stimulates steroid synthesis by acting on the adrenals to increase the conversion of cholesterol to pregnenolone, the principal substrate for the steroidogenic pathways. The central nervous system controls the secretion of ACTH, its diurnal variation, and its increase in stress via corticotropin-releasing factor (2,3). The hypothalamic-pituitary-adrenal feedback system is mediated through the circulating level of plasma cortisol; any condition that decreases cortisol secretion results in increased ACTH secretion. Cortisol therefore exerts a negative feedback effect on ACTH secretion.

An enzyme deficiency acts as a dam behind which steroid precursors accumulate. In congenital adrenal hyperplasia, an enzyme defect blocks cortisol synthesis, thus impairing cortisol-mediated negative feedback control of ACTH secretion (Fig. 2). Oversecretion of ACTH ensues, which stimulates excessive synthesis of the adrenal products of those pathways unimpaired by an enzyme deficiency and causes an accumulation of precursor molecules in pathways blocked by an enzyme deficiency.

The clinical symptoms of the different forms of congenital adrenal hyperplasia result from the particular hormones that are deficient and that are produced in excess. In the most common case, that of 21-hydroxylase deficiency, the aldosterone and cortisol pathways are blocked and the androgen pathway, which does not involve 21-hydroxylation, is overstimulated (Fig. 3). The characteristic virilization caused by 21-hydroxylase deficiency is caused by excessive secretion of adrenal androgens.

An enzymatic deficiency of 11β-hydroxylase also results in decreased cortisol synthesis with consequent overproduction of cortisol precursors and sex steroids, as seen in 21-hydroxylase deficiency. Thus, 11β-hydroxylase deficiency shares the clinical feature of virilization with the 21-hydroxylase disorder. An additional finding in many, but not all, patients with 11β-hydroxylase deficiency is hypertension. The hypertension is thought to derive from the excess accumulation of the aldosterone precursor, deoxycorticosterone (DOC), a steroid with salt-retaining activity.

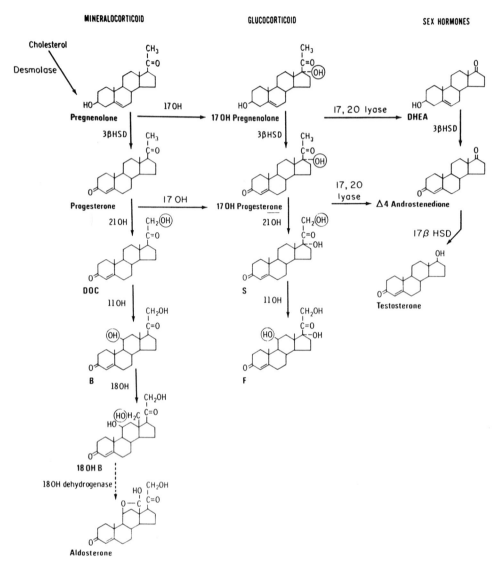

Figure 1 Simplified scheme for adrenal synthesis of the three main classes of adrenal hormones. Each hydroxylation step is indicated, and the newly added hydroxyl group is circled. DOC, deoxycorticosterone; B, corticosterone; S, 11-deoxycortisol; F, cortisol; DHEA, dehydroepiandrosterone; 3β-HSD, 3β-hydroxysteroid dehydrogenase; OH, hydroxylase (for enzymes). The 18-OH-dehydrogenase step is now known to be catalyzed by an isozyme closely related to the 11β-hydroxylase (11 OH) enzyme. (From Ref. 125, with permission.)

Disorders of adrenal steroidogenesis have also been described in association with deficiencies of the enzymes 3β-hydroxysteroid dehydrogenase, cholesterol desmolase, 18-hydroxylase, 18-dehydrogenase, and 17β-hydroxysteroid dehydrogenase. A summary of the biochemical features of these disorders is presented in Table 1.

III.   CLINICAL FEATURES

The most prominent clinical feature of 21- and 11β-hydroxylase deficiency is virilization. Because adrenocortical function begins in month 3 of gestation, a fetus with 21- or 11β-hydroxylase deficiency is exposed to oversecreted adrenal androgens at the critical time of sexual differentiation. In

a female fetus, the excessive adrenal androgens masculinize the external genitalia and female pseudohermaphroditism results. In rare cases, the masculinization is so profound that the urethra is penile (4). The internal genitalia (i.e., uterus and fallopian tubes), which arise from the müllerian ducts, are normal because the female fetus does not possess testes, the source of müllerian inhibiting factor. The female genital abnormalities are present only in the androgen-responsive external genitalia. Males with 21- or 11β-hydroxylase deficiency do not manifest genital abnormalities at birth.

The simple virilizing form of 21-hydroxylase deficiency is characterized by excess adrenal androgen secretion, which causes prenatal virilization of the genetic female and postnatal virilization of both boys and girls. The salt-wasting form, in

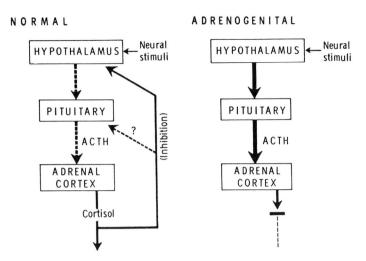

Figure 2 Regulation of cortisol secretion in normal subjects and in patients with congenital adrenal hyperplasia. (From Ref. 125, with permission.)

addition to the excess adrenal androgens, has an aldosterone deficiency that causes low serum sodium, high serum potassium, and vascular collapse. In the more severe salt-wasting form, both newborn boys and girls are subject to early, life-threatening, salt-wasting crises within the first few weeks of life.

The various clinical and biochemical features associated with the different forms of congenital adrenal hyperplasia are indicated in Table 1. Continued oversecretion of adrenal androgens as a result of untreated 21- or 11β-hydroxylase deficiency results in progressive penile or clitoral enlargement; advanced bone age and tall stature in early childhood with ultimate short stature caused by premature epiphyseal

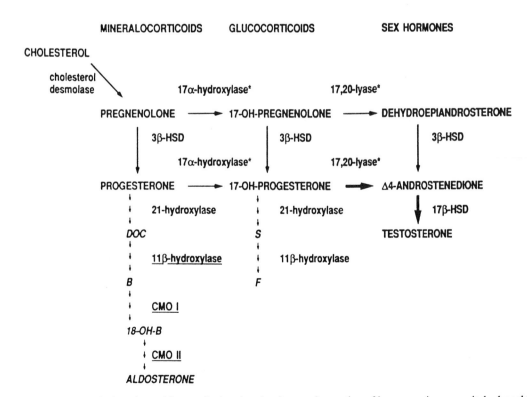

Figure 3 Simplified scheme of adrenal steroidogenesis showing the abnormal secretion of hormones in congenital adrenal hyperplasia resulting from 21-hydroxylase deficiency. For abbreviations, see Figure 1.

Table 1 Clinical and Laboratory Features of Various Disorders of Adrenal Steroidogenesis

Deficiency (syndrome)	Genital ambiguity	Postnatal virilization	Salt metabolism	Diagnostic hormones	Treatment
21-Hydroxylase					
Classic					
Salt-wasting (SW)	F	Yes	Salt wasting	17-hydroxyprogesterone[a] Δ^4-Androstenedione(Δ^4-A)	Hydrocortisone (HC), 15–20 mg/m^2/day orally (PO), and fludrocortisone acetate (9αFF), 0.05–0.2 mg/day PO
Simple virilizing	F	Yes	Normal (↑ renin)	17-OHP,[a] Δ^4-A	HC (same); addition of 9αFF (same) if ↑ renin
Nonclassic (symptomatic and asymptomatic)	No	Yes	Normal	17-OHP, Δ^4-A	HC, 10–15 mg/m^2/day or dexamethasone, 0.25–0.5 mg/day h.s., or prednisone 5–10 mg/day
3β-ol Dehydrogenase					
Classic	M ($\pm$F)	Yes	Salt wasting	17-OHP[a] Dehydroepiandrosterone (DHEA)	HC and 9αFF as for SW 21-Hydroxylase deficiency[b]
Nonclassic	No	Yes	Normal	17-OHP DHEA	HC as for nonclassic 21-hydroxylase deficiency
11β-Hydroxylase					
Classic (hypertensive CAH)	F	Yes	Salt retention	Deoxycorticosterone (DOC)[a] 11-Deoxycortisol (S)	HC, 15–20 mg/m^2/day
Nonclassic	No	Yes	Normal	S $\pm$ DOC	HC, dexamethasone, or prednisone as for nonclassic 21-hydroxylase deficiency
Corticosterone methyl oxidase type II	No	No	Salt wasting	18-Hydroxycorticosterone[a]	9αFF, 0.1–0.2 mg/day
17α-Hydroxylase	M	No	Salt retention	DOC[a] Corticosterone (B)	HC, 15–20 mg/m^2/day[b]
17,20-Lyase	M	No	Normal	None	HC, 15–20 mg/m^2/day
Cholesterol desmolase (lipoid hyperplasia)	M	No	Salt wasting	None	HC, 15–20 mg/m^2/day 9αFF, 0.05–0.2 mg/day[b]

[a]Increased in serum of affected patients before or after ACTH stimulation.
[b]With addition of sex steroid replacement at puberty.

closure; early appearance of facial, axillary, and pubic hair; and acne. In 11β-hydroxylase deficiency, as noted earlier, hypertension is frequently, although not necessarily, an additional finding. Girls with congenital adrenal hyperplasia who remain untreated do not develop breasts or menstruate and are further virilized. In untreated boys, the testes may remain small and there may be infertility, although some untreated men have been fertile (5).

IV. CLINICAL FORMS OF ADRENAL HYPERPLASIA CAUSED BY 21-HYDROXYLASE DEFICIENCY

Two major phenotypes are recognized in 21-hydroxylase deficiency: classic and nonclassic (late onset; Fig. 4). Within the latter class of patients are those who demonstrate the biochemical defect but lack any overt stigmata of hyperandrogenism. Table 2 delineates the differences between classic and nonclassic 21-hydroxylase deficiency.

A. Classic

Classic congenital adrenal hyperplasia is a well-known genetic disorder transmitted by an autosomal recessive gene. The biochemical and clinical abnormalities of this form of CAH are clearly present in patients both prenatally and postnatally. Progesterone, 17-OH-progesterone, androstenedione, and testosterone are secreted in excess, consequent to increased ACTH stimulation resulting from an inherited 21-hydroxylase deficiency that impairs cortisol synthesis (6–13). As expected, the urinary excretion of the metabolites of these steroids is also increased (14,15).

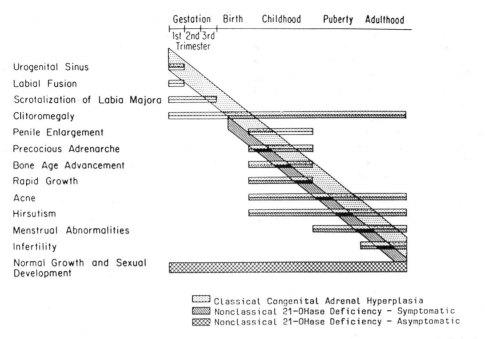

Figure 4 Clinical spectrum of HLA-linked steroid 21-hydroxylase deficiency. There is a wide spectrum of clinical presentation in 21-hydroxylase deficiency, ranging from prenatal virilization with labial fusion to precocious adrenarche, to pubertal or postpubertal virilization. During their lifetimes, patients may change from symptomatic to asymptomatic with 21-hydroxylase deficiency. (From New MI, Dupont B, Grumbach K, Levine LS. In: Stanbury JB, Wyngaarden JB, et al., eds. The Metabolic Basis of Inherited Disease, 5th ed. New York: McGraw-Hill, 1983:973–1000; with permission.)

Table 2 Comparison of Classic and Nonclassic 21-Hydroxylase Deficiency

Feature	Classic	Nonclassic
Disease frequency	1:12,000	1:100 all whites 1:30 Ashkenazi Jews
Prenatal virilization	Females	No
Postnatal virilization	Males and females	Variable
Salt wasting	60–75% of cases	No
17-Hydroxyprogesterone levels after ACTH challenge	Extreme elevation (>20,000 ng/dl)	Moderate elevation (2000–15,000 ng/dl)
Genotype of CYP21B	Severely affected allele/ severely affected allele	Mildly affected allele/ mildly affected allele; or severely affected allele/ mildly affected allele
Associated HLA haplotype	B47; DR7	B14; DR1
Mutation		
Simple virilizing	Ile^{-172} → Asn Intron 2, A → G	Val^{-281} → Leu Pro^{-30} → Leu
Salt wasting	Deletion Lg. conversion Intron 2, A → G Exon 3, -8 bp Codons 234–238 Gln^{-318} → end Arg^{-356} → Trp	Pro^{-453} → Ser

In genetic females with congenital 21-hydroxylase deficiency, the developing fetus is exposed to the excessive adrenal androgens, equivalent to the male fetal level, secreted by the hyperplastic adrenal cortex. External genitalia in the genetic female range from mildly ambiguous to completely virilized. The internal genitalia (uterus and fallopian tubes) are not affected by the excess androgens. Boys with 21-hydroxylase deficiency do not manifest genital abnormalities at birth. Postnatally, in untreated boys and girls, continued excessive androgen production results in rapid somatic growth, advanced epiphyseal maturation, progressive penile or clitoral enlargement, early appearance of facial, axillary, and pubic hair, and acne. Without treatment, early epiphyseal closure and short stature result (16).

In three-quarters of cases with classic 21-hydroxylase deficiency, salt wasting occurs, as defined by hyponatremia, hyperkalemia, inappropriate natriuresis, and low serum and urinary aldosterone with concomitantly high plasma renin activity. The increase in the proportion of salt-wasting cases in recent years may be attributed in part to enhanced ascertainment because of advancements in diagnostic capabilities, as well as increased survival because of the availability of exogenous mineralocorticoid supplements. Salt wasting results from inadequate secretion of salt-retaining steroids, especially aldosterone. In addition, hormonal precursors of 21-hydroxylase may act as mineralocorticoid antagonists in the marginally competent sodium-conserving mechanism of the immature newborn renal tubule (17–20). It has been observed that an aldosterone biosynthetic defect apparent in infancy may be ameliorated with age (21,22), and a spontaneous partial recovery from salt wasting in adulthood was recently described in a patient with severe salt wasting in infancy. This variation in the ability to produce mineralocorticoids may be attributable to another adrenal enzyme with 21-hydroxylase activity (23). Therefore, it is desirable to follow the sodium and mineralocorticoid requirements carefully by measuring plasma renin activity in patients who have been labeled neonatally as salt wasters.

Although it has been claimed that salt wasting correlates with severe virilism (24), it is important to recognize that the extent of virilism may be the same in simple virilizing and salt-wasting CAH. Thus, even a mildly virilized newborn with 21-hydroxylase deficiency should be observed carefully for signs of a potentially life-threatening crisis within the first few weeks of life.

B. Nonclassic 21-Hydroxylase Deficiency

An attenuated, late-onset form of adrenal hyperplasia was first suspected by gynecologists in clinical practice who used glucocorticoids for the treatment of women with physical signs of hyperandrogenism, including infertility (25,26). The first documentation of suppression of 21-hydroxylase precurors in the urine of such individuals after glucocorticoid therapy was by Baulieu and coworkers in 1957 (27). The precise diagnosis of a mild 21-hydroxylase defect was made possible when a radioimmunoassay for 17-hydroxyprogesterone (17-OHP) the direct precursor of the enzyme in the adrenal zona fasciculata, was developed (28). The autosomal

recessive mode of genetic transmission of the nonclassic form of 21-hydroxylase deficiency (NC21-OHD) became apparent through family studies of classic 21-OHD (29–31). The establishment of linkage to HLA (32,33) confirmed the existence of this disorder as an allele of classic 21-OHD (29,34). The HLA associations for nonclassic 21-OHD (32, 35,36) are distinct from those found in classic 21-OHD and differ according to ethnicity (33,37,38).

The clinical symptomatology of NC21-OHD is variable and may present at any age. NC21-OHD can result in premature development of pubic hair in children; to our knowledge, the youngest such patient was noted to have pubic hair at 6 months of age (30). In a review of 23 cases presenting to The New York Hospital–Cornell Medical Center for evaluation of premature pubarche, 7 children demonstrated a 17-OHP response to ACTH stimulation consistent with the diagnosis of nonclassic 21-hydroxylase deficiency, a prevalence of 30% in this preselected group of pediatric patients at high risk (39). Other investigators found 7 of 46 children (15%) with premature pubarche demonstrating an ACTH-stimulated 17-OHP response greater than that of obligate heterozygote carriers of the 21-hydroxylase deficiency gene (40). Elevated adrenal androgens promote the early fusion of epiphyseal growth plates, and it is common, but not universally found, that children with the disorder have advanced bone age and accelerated linear growth velocity and ultimately are shorter than the height that might be predicted based on midparental height and linear growth percentiles before the apparent onset of excess androgen secretion (41).

Severe cystic acne refractory to oral antibiotics and retinoic acid has been attributed to NC21-OHD. In one study of 31 young female patients with acne and/or hirsutism tested with low-dose ACTH stimulation after overnight dexamethasone suppression, no cases of 21-hydroxylase deficiency were found (42). In another study comparing the responses of 11 female patients with acne and 8 (female) control subjects to a 24 h infusion of ACTH, elevated urinary excretion of pregnanetriol in 6 patients was suggestive of a partial 21-hydroxylase deficiency (43).

Additionally, male pattern baldness in young women with this disorder has been noted as the sole presenting symptom. Severe androgenic alopecia in association with marked virilization has also been reported in an undiagnosed and therefore untreated 59-year-old woman with the simple virilizing form of the disease (44). Menarche may be normal or delayed, and secondary amenorrhea is a frequent occurrence. The syndrome of polycystic ovarian disease includes a subgroup of women with NC21-OHD. The pathophysiology of this phenomenon probably relates to adrenal sex steroid excess disrupting the usual cyclicity of gonadotropin release and/or the direct effects of adrenal androgens upon the ovary, leading ultimately to the formation of ovarian cysts, which then may autonomously produce androgens.

Retrospective analysis of the etiologies of hirsutism and oligomenorrhea revealed that 16 of 108 (14%) of young women presenting to this institution for endocrinologic evaluation of these complaints had nonclassic 21-hydroxylase deficiency (45). In other published series the prevalence of nonclassic

21-hydroxylase deficiency in hirsute, oligomenorrheic women ranges from 1.2% to 30% (46–52). The disparity in frequency of nonclassic 21-hydroxylase deficiency reported by different authors may be attributed to differences in the ethnic groups studied because the disease frequency is ethnic specific.

In boys, early beard growth, acne, and growth spurt may be detected. A highly reliable constellation of physical signs of adrenal (as opposed to testicular) androgen excess in boys is the presence of pubic hair, enlarged phallus, and relatively small testes. In men, signs of androgen excess are difficult to appreciate and may theoretically be manifest only by adrenal sex steroid-induced suppression of the hypothalamic-pituitary-gonadal axis, resulting in diminished fertility.

Oligospermia and subfertility have been reported in men with nonclassic 21-hydroxylase deficiency (53,54) and reversal of infertility with glucocorticoid treatment in three men (54–56).

The presence of 21-hydroxylase deficiency can be discovered during the evaluation of incidental adrenal masses (57). An increased incidence of adrenal incidentalomas has in fact been found in male and female patients with homozygous congenital adrenal hyperplasia (82%) and also in the heterozygote subjects (45%), probably arising from hyperplastic tissue areas and not requiring surgical intervention (58).

A subset of NC-21OHD individuals are overtly asymptomatic when detected (usually as part of a family study), but it is thought, based on longitudinal follow-up of such patients, that symptoms of hyperandrogenism may wax and wane with time. The gene defect in these so-called cryptic 21-hydroxylase-deficient subjects is the same as that found in symptomatic nonclassic patients.

V. PUBERTAL MATURATION IN CLASSIC CONGENITAL ADRENAL HYPERPLASIA

A. Onset of Puberty

In most patients treated satisfactorily from early life, the onset of puberty in both girls and boys with classic CAH occurs at the expected chronologic age (59–62). The pattern of gonadotropin response to luteinizing hormone-releasing hormone (LHRH) is appropriate for age in prepubertal and pubertal girls with well-controlled CAH (63,64). Physiologic secretion of gonadotropins, however, may not be entirely normal (65,66).

True precocious puberty may occur in some well-treated children with CAH, perhaps correlated with bone age. Another setting in which central puberty sometimes occurs in CAH is after initiation of glucocorticoid therapy, producing a sudden decrease in sex steroid levels and leading to hypothalamic activation. LHRH analogs may be employed as an adjunct to therapy with hydrocortisone in such children (67). Long-term data on final height in a small number of CAH patients suggest that LHRH analogs are not only effective in arresting the pubertal process but also improve final height (68).

In most untreated or poorly treated adolescent girls and in some adolescent boys, spontaneous true pubertal development does not occur until proper treatment is instituted (Table 3) (60,61,69–71). Studies suggest that excess adrenal androgens (aromatized to estrogens) inhibit the pubertal pattern of gonadotropin secretion by the hypothalamic-pituitary axis (70). The inhibition probably occurs via a negative feedback effect; whether it is primarily at the hypothalamus or pituitary is not known. This inhibition is reversible by suppression of the adrenal hormone production by glucocorticoid treatment.

Following gonadarche, in a majority of successfully treated patients, the milestones of further development of secondary sex characteristics in general appear to be normal (59,62), although a somewhat delayed sequence of pubertal events was present in girls (59).

B. Menstrual Disorders

Many patients with treated classic CAH have regular menses after menarche (60,61,72). However, expected age at menarche of treated CAH patients from various clinics, as shown

Table 3 Pubertal Disorders in 21-Hydroxylase Deficiency CAH

Puberty	Poorly treated or untreated classic CAH		Nonclassic: abnormal	Cryptic CAH: normal
	Abnormal	Normal		
Girls	No thelarche; no menarche; secondary amenorrhea or menstrual irregularity; cystic ovaries, anovulation, infertility	None reported	Precocious adrenarche, hirsutism, cystic acne; amenorrhea or menstrual irregularity; anovulation, infertility, cystic ovaries	No abnormalities
Boys	Small testes[a]	Normal testicular size	Precocious adrenarche	No abnormalities
	Decreased spermatogenesis	Spermatogenesis	Cystic acne	

[a]Adolescent males may have nodular testes as a result of adrenal rest tumor.

in Table 3, suggests that menarche was significantly delayed, especially when those patients who were not menstruating after 16 years of age were included (59–62,73). Menarche was not observed in untreated patients, only in patients who had received suppressive glucocorticoid treatment (59–61, 74).

Menstrual irregularity and secondary amenorrhea with or without hirsutism are not uncommon complications in postmenarchal girls (5,61,62,64,74–76). These menstrual abnormalities have been frequently found in patients with inadequately controlled disease (Table 1) (59,60,62,72,74,76). Several studies subsequently reported menarche or the normalization of the menstrual cycle following adequate suppression of adrenal sex steroids with long-acting and more potent glucocorticoid treatment (74,76,77). Delayed menarche or even primary amenorrhea may result from poor treatment or overtreatment. In poorly treated patients, the mechanism for delayed menarche may be interference by adrenal sex steroids in the cyclicity of the hypothalamic-pituitary-ovarian axis (59,60). The delayed menarche in patients who are overtreated may be related to the delay in bone age and general maturation known to occur with excessive glucocorticoid treatment (59).

Many treated women have had successful pregnancies with the delivery of a normal, healthy, full-term infant (60,78–80). A recent retrospective survey of fertility rates in a large group of women affected with 21-hydroxylase deficiency showed that simple virilizers were more likely than salt wasters to become pregnant and carry the pregnancy to term (81). Adequacy of glucocorticoid therapy is probably an important variable with respect to fertility outcome. Among all patients questioned, only 50% reported that the vaginal introitus was adequate for intercourse; 5% reported homosexual preference, and 38% had no sexual experience. Based on these data, it seems prudent to perform early surgical correction of clitoromegaly but to delay vaginoplasty until adolescence (when the patient can be expected to assume responsibility for vaginal dilatation and strict adherence to medical therapy).

The clinical observation of gonadal function as described earlier clearly suggests that excess adrenal sex steroid production is the major contributing factor to gonadal dysfunction, menstrual disorders, anovulation, and infertility in girls with classic CAH. The generally accepted theory is that the excessive adrenal androgens may disrupt gonadotropin secretion, leading ultimately to hypogonadism (62,65,70,74).

C. Male Reproductive Function

Several long-term studies indicate that in a majority of successfully treated male patients with CAH, pubertal development, normal testicular function, and normal spermatogenesis and fertility occur (5,61,62,82,83). However, complications of small testes and aspermia have been reported in some patients with inadequately controlled disease (5,61,71,72, 84). In contrast to this observation, some investigators have reported normal testicular maturation and normal spermatogenesis and fertility in patients who had never received

glucocorticoid treatment (5,69,83,85,86) or in those whose glucocorticoid therapy was discontinued for several years (5,83). Thus, male patients with CAH and excessive adrenal androgens may have either normal gonadal function or hypogonadism. The factors resulting in such a disparity in puberty among patients with the same disorder are not known. Some patients with normal gonadal function may have nonclassic rather than classic CAH (see later). Hormonal studies in untreated classic patients with normal sexual maturation have shown either normal or increased gonadotropin production (87) or concentrations (5,83) and follicle-stimulating hormone excretion (5,87). Of great interest is that in these male patients, excess adrenal sex steroids or their precursor steroids did not seem to affect gonadotropin secretion. Adrenal androgen levels in untreated boys with normal gonadal function did not appear to be lower than those in patients with gonadal dysfunction in poor control (5,61,84). This suggests that adrenal androgens alone have no effect on gonadotropin secretion via a negative feedback mechanism in male patients.

Another frequently reported complication in postpubertal boys with inadequate control of CAH is hyperplastic nodular testes. Almost all patients with such complications were found to have adenomatous adrenal rests within the testicular tissue, as indicated by the presence of specific 11β-hydroxylated steroids in the blood from gonadal veins (88). These tumors have been reported to be ACTH dependent and to regress following adequate steroid therapy (89–95).

VI. GENETICS

Studies of families carrying 21-hydroxylase deficiency have demonstrated that the disease locus is situated in the HLA major histocompatibility complex on the short arm of the sixth chromosome (96,97). Both classic and nonclassic 21-hydroxylase deficiency are inherited in a recessive manner as allelic variants. Characteristic combinations of HLA alleles, or haplotypes, are associated with different forms of 21-hydroxylase deficiency. Whereas HLA-Bw47;DR7 is observed at an increased frequency in the classic form of the disorder (98–100), HLA-B14;DR1 is associated with nonclassic 21-hydroxylase deficiency (32,33,35,36). These associations, combined with hormonal studies of families carrying both classic and nonclassic forms, suggest that classic 21-hydroxylase deficiency results from the presence of two severely affected alleles and that nonclassic 21-hydroxylase deficiency results from the presence of either two mild 21-hydroxylase deficiency alleles or one severe and one mild allele (101).

Based on estimates of its frequency among Ashkenazi Jews (3%) and all ethnic whites (individuals of mainly European descent) (1%) (37), it is apparent that nonclassic 21-hydroxylase deficiency is among the most frequent human autosomal recessive disorders. Molecular genetic studies have demonstrated that the gene encoding the cytochrome P_{450} enzyme specific for 21-hydroxylation (P_{450} c21) is located in the HLA complex between the genes encoding the transplantation antigens, HLA-B and HLA-DR. This gene, CYP21, and an inactive homolog or pseudogene, CYP21P, are immediately adjacent to the C4B and C4A genes encoding the fourth component of serum complement (102,103). The protein-encoding sequence of CYP21P is 98% homologous to that of CYP21, but it contains several deleterious mutations, three of which completely prevent the synthesis of a functional protein (104–106). In recent studies evaluating the phenotype-genotype relationship, a good correlation between the severity of clinical disease and the discrete mutations was observed (107,108). However, there are patients whose phenotype is different from that predicted by their mutations (108,109), the reason for which requires further investigation.

Approximately 25% of classic 21-hydroxylase deficiency alleles result from deletions of CYP21 (110–112). The remaining three-quarters of classic alleles are caused by smaller mutations in CYP21, some of which are de novo point mutations resulting in amino acid substitutions (107,113–115) that significantly disrupt synthesis of the protein. Nonclassic 21-OHD is associated with conservative (or mild) amino acid substitutions in highly conserved portions of the gene encoding the active 21-hydroxylase (116–118).

VII. EPIDEMIOLOGY

Screening studies indicate that the worldwide incidence of classic 21-OHD is 1:14,199 live births (119), of which approximately 75% are salt wasters. The frequency of non-classic 21-OHD is considerably higher; based on population genetic studies this allelic variant occurs in 1:100 persons in the general white population and in higher frequency among selected ethnic groups, most notably Ashkenazi Jews (37).

VIII. DIAGNOSIS

Congenital adrenal hyperplasia must be suspected in infants born with ambiguous genitalia. The physician is obliged to make the diagnosis as quickly as possible, to initiate therapy and to arrest the effects of the enzyme disorders. The diagnosis and a rational decision of sex assignment must rely on the determination of genetic sex, the hormonal determination of the specific deficient enzyme, and an assessment of the patient's potential for future sexual activity and fertility. Physicians are urged to recognize the physical findings of ambiguous genitalia characteristic of congenital adrenal hyperplasia in newborns and to refer such cases to appropriate clinics for full endocrine evaluation.

As indicated in Table 1, each form of congenital adrenal hyperplasia has its own unique hormonal profile, consisting of elevated levels of precursors and elevated or diminished levels of adrenal steroid products (12,13). Traditionally, laboratory tests have measured the urinary excretion of adrenal hormones or their urinary metabolites (e.g., 17-keto-steroids). Collection of 24 h urine excretion may be difficult, however, and the results in neonates may often be misleading (13). The development of simple and reliable radioimmuno-assays for circulating serum levels of adrenal steroids is a significant advance in the laboratory diagnostic technique

(12). The direct serum measurement of accumulated precursors and oversecreted adrenal steroids, such as 17-hydroxy-progesterone, Δ^4-androstenedione, and dehydroepiandroster-one, is now possible, and more exact hormonal profiles of the different forms of congenital adrenal hyperplasia have been established (Table 1).

A. Hormonal Standards for Genotyping 21-Hydroxylase Deficiency

In our experience, the best diagnostic test for genotyping for 21-hydroxylase deficiency has proven to be an ACTH (Cor-trosyn, 0.25 mg) stimulation test measuring the serum concentration of 17-OHP at 0 and 60 minutes after intravenous bolus ACTH administration (120). The nomogram (Fig. 5) provides hormonal standards for assignment of the 21-hydroxylase genotype; that is, patients whose hormonal values fall on the regression line within a defined group are assigned to this group. Because of the diurnal variation in 17-OHP, an early morning serum concentration of 17-OHP may be useful as a screening test for genotyping 21-OHD. In addition, early morning salivary 17-OHP has proven to be an excellent screening test for the nonclassic form (121). ACTH stimulation, however, remains the most definitive diagnostic test (52,122,123).

Diagnosis of 21-hydroxylase deficiency can also be made by microfilter paper radioimmunoassay for 17-hydroxypro-gesterone; this has been useful as a rapid screening test for congenital adrenal hyperplasia in newborns (11). This convenient test requires only 20 μl blood, obtained by heel prick and blotted on microfilter paper, to provide a reliable diagnostic measurement of 17-hydroxyprogesterone, a cortisol precursor that accumulates in elevated concentrations in 21-hydroxylase deficiency. Because of the simplicity of the test and the ease of transporting microfilter paper specimens through the mail, we have proposed that a congenital adrenal hyperplasia newborn screening program be instituted using the 17-hydroxyprogesterone microfilter paper radioimmuno-assay, similar to the existing screening programs for phenyl-ketonuria and hypothyroidism.

B. Prenatal Diagnosis and Prenatal Treatment

1. Prenatal Diagnosis

Since the report by Jeffcoate et al. (124) of the successful identification of an affected fetus by elevated concentrations of 17-ketosteroids and pregnanetriol in the amniotic fluid, several investigators have undertaken prenatal diagnosis for congenital adrenal hyperplasia by similar measurements of hormone levels in pregnancy (125,126). The most specific hormonal diagonostic test for 21-hydroxylase deficiency is amniotic fluid 17-OHP (28,127–130); Δ^4-androstenedione may be employed as an adjunctive diagnostic assay (129). It has been suggested that elevated amniotic fluid 21-deoxycort-isol may also be a marker for 21-hydroxylase deficiency (131). Amniotic fluid testosterone levels may not be outside the normal range in an affected male (129,132).

HLA genotyping of amniotic fluid cells is a possible

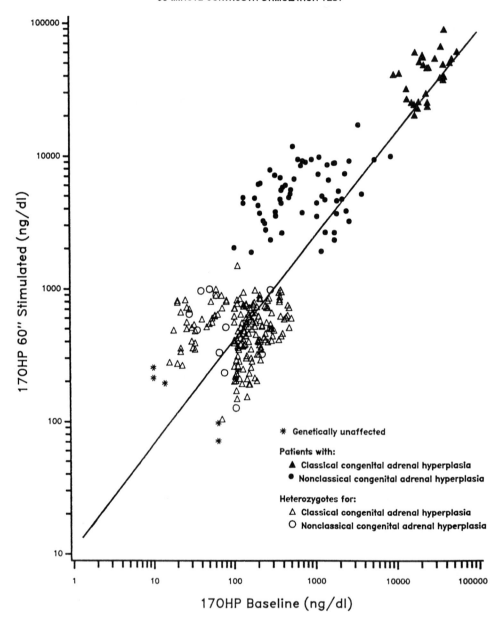

The data for this nomogram was collected between 1982 and 1991 at the Department of Pediatrics. The New York Hospital–Cornell Medical Center. New York. NY. 10021.

Figure 5 Nomogram relating baseline to ACTH-stimulated serum concentrations of 17-hydroxyprogesterone (17-OHP). The scales are logarithmic. A regression line for all data points is shown.

means of diagnosis but has now been superseded by direct molecular analysis of the 21-hydroxylase locus.

With the advent of chorionic villus sampling (CVS), evaluation of the fetus at risk is now possible in the first trimester at 8–11 weeks gestation. Because normative standards for hormonal levels measurable at this early stage

remain to be established, CVS diagnosis now depends on molecular typing for restriction fragment length polymorphisms (RFLPs) of the chromosome 6 loci, 21-hydroxylase gene, and HLA (133,134). In the 26 pregnancies followed at The New York Hospital in which a villous sample was obtained, the DNA diagnosis was correct in 24 cases.

Moreover, fetal diagnosis by CVS and molecular genetic analysis reduced the duration of unnecessary prenatal treatment in males and unaffected females.

The introduction of DNA amplification by polymerase chain reaction (PCR) has further hastened fetal diagnosis. The specific mutations responsible for the disease are directly assayed using PCR, which constitutes an improvement compared with analysis using the less specific RFLP markers. The procedure has the advantage of requiring small amounts of DNA, and because it is a direct assay of disease mutations, it is not subject to errors arising from recombination events. By this method, prenatal diagnosis of CAH was successful in all four cases reported thus far (135,136). An algorithm for the diagnostic management of potentially affected pregnancies is given in Figure 6.

2. Prenatal Treatment

Treatment with dexamethasone was recently employed in pregnancies at risk for 21-hydroxylase deficiency (134,137–139). In pregnancies at risk for 21-hydroxylase deficiency in which treatment was begun at 3–10 weeks gestation (0.5 mg dexamethasone orally twice daily), all had complete suppression of adrenocortical hormones at amniocentesis. Only when dexamethasone therapy was discontinued before amniotic fluid sampling were the amniotic fluid hormone levels elevated. Masculinization of genitalia was completely prevented in 1 of 3 affected female fetuses and partially prevented in another female. In the third case in which treatment failed, the mother had begun dexamethasone at 10 weeks and terminated therapy at 28 weeks. In 10 affected females followed at The New York Hospital whose mothers were treated with dexamethasone from week 4 of gestation until delivery, the virilization of the genitalia was significantly less than in the index case (140). No congenital malformations were found in any of the treated fetuses. The failure of one group of investigators to find evidence of suppression of the fetal pituitary-adrenal axis after acute administration of dexamethasone at midterm (141) is not necessarily reflective of the situation in which chronic therapy is begun in the first trimester. German investigators (138) also found high amniotic fluid 17-OHP levels in two pregnancies at risk for CAH treated with dexamethasone from weeks 10 to 17, although therapy was stopped 5 days before the amniocentesis. The latter group postulated increased metabolic clearance of dexamethasone or inadequate dosage.

The current recommendation is to treat the mother with a pregnancy at risk for 21-hydroxylase deficiency with dexamethasone in a dose of 0.5 mg three times daily as soon as pregnancy is recognized (142). The total daily dose should not exceed 20 μg/kg/day for the woman's prepregnancy weight.

Theoretically, institution of such therapy at 6–7 weeks of gestation, before onset of adrenal androgen secretion, would effectively suppress adrenal androgen production and allow normal separation of the vaginal and urethral orifices, in addition to preventing clitoromegaly. Obviously, if dexamethasone is to be administered at such an early date, treatment is blind to the status of the fetus. After HLA and/or

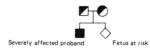

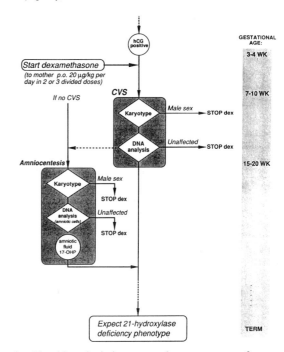

Figure 6 Algorithm depicting prenatal management of pregnancy in families at risk for a fetus affected with 21-hydroxylase deficiency. (Adapted from New MI, et al. In: Scriver CR, Beaudet WS, Sly WS, Vale D, eds. The Metabolic Basis of Inherited Disease, 6th ed. New York: McGraw-Hill, 1988:1881–1971, and from Ref. 134, with permission.)

DNA analysis by either chorionic villus sampling or amniocentesis, cessation of prenatal therapy may be considered if the fetus is male or an unaffected female.

To date, no fetus of a mother treated with dexamethasone in low doses has been found to have any congenital malformation. Specifically, no cases have been reported of cleft palate, placental degeneration, or fetal death, which have been observed in a rodent model of *in utero* exposure to high-dose glucocorticoids (143). In contrast, in a few cases, significant maternal side effects have been reported, including excessive weight gain, cushingoid facial features, severe striae resulting in permanent scarring, and hyperglycemic response to oral glucose administration (144). In The New York Hospital experience, maternal complications were observed in only 6 pregnancies of 67, and none of them were permanent (140). Therefore, we believe that prenatal treatment of fetuses at risk for CAH can be considered effective and safe.

IX. TREATMENT

In ambiguous genitalia caused by congenital adrenal hyperplasia, appropriate surgical repair may be made once a sex assignment has been made based on a reliable diagnosis of the underlying enzyme disorder. In female pseudohermaphroditism caused by 21- or 11β-hydroxylase deficiency, the aim of surgical repair should be to remove the redundant erectile tissue, preserve the sexually sensitive glans clitoris, and provide a normal vaginal orifice that functions adequately for menstruation, intromission, and delivery (145). Because of the normal internal genitalia in these patients, normal puberty, fertility, and childbearing are possible when there is early therapeutic intervention.

The aim of endocrine therapy is to replace the deficient hormones. In 21- and 11β-hydroxylase deficiencies, replacing cortisol both corrects the deficiency in cortisol secretion and suppresses ACTH overproduction. Proper replacement prevents excessive stimulation of the androgen pathway, preventing further virilization and allowing normal growth and a normal onset of puberty.

The recent demonstration of the importance of the renin-angiotensin system in congenital adrenal hyperplasia has made better therapeutic control of this condition possible. In addition to hypothalamic-pituitary regulation of adrenal steroidogenesis, the renin-angiotensin system exerts a primary influence on the adrenal secretion of aldosterone. The juxtaglomerular apparatus of the kidney secretes the enzyme renin in response to the state of electrolyte balance and plasma volume. Renin initiates a series of reactions that produce angiotensin II, a potent stimulator of aldosterone secretion (146).

Although aldosterone levels are not deficient in the simple virilizing form of 21-hydroxylase deficiency, plasma renin activity is commonly elevated in the simple virilizing as well as in the salt-wasting forms (147). Despite elevated plasma renin activity, it has not been customary to supplement conventional glucocorticoid replacement therapy with the administration of salt-retaining steroids in simple virilizing 21-hydroxylase deficiency. However, Rosler et al. have demonstrated that adding salt-retaining hormone to glucocorticoid therapy in patients with classic simple virilizing CAH with elevated plasma renin activity in fact improves the hormonal control of the disease (148). When plasma renin activity was normalized by the addition of 9α-fludrocortisone acetate, a salt-retaining steroid, the ACTH level also fell and excessive androgen secretion decreased. The addition of salt-retaining steroids to the therapeutic regimen often made possible a decrease in the glucocorticoid dosage. Normaliza-

tion of plasma renin activity also resulted in improved statural growth.

Steroid radioimmunoassay methods have been an asset not only for the initial diagnosis of congenital adrenal hyperplasia, but also for improved monitoring of hormonal control once therapy has been instituted. Studies indicate that serum 17-hydroxyprogesterone and Δ^4-androstenedione levels provide the most sensitive index of biochemical control. In girls and prepubertal boys (but not in newborn and pubertal boys), the serum testosterone level is also a useful index (12). The combined determination of plasma renin activity, 17-hydroxyprogesterone, and serum androgens, as well as the clinical assessment of growth and pubertal development, must all be considered in adjusting the dosage of glucocorticoid and salt-retaining steroid. Recently, 3α-androstenediol (3AG) has been proposed as a useful serum metabolic marker of integrated adrenal androgen secretion in CAH patients. However, whether serum 3AG determinations would be useful for therapeutic monitoring of CAH requires further long-term study (149). Both in our clinic and in others, combinations of hydrocortisone and 9α-fludrocortisone acetate have proven to be highly effective treatment modalities (150). Monitoring of plasma renin activity is also a useful index of hormonal control in other forms of congenital adrenal hyperplasia.

X. CONCLUSION

Abnormalities of sexual differentiation and development, often in combination with hypertension (as in 11β-hydroxylase deficiency) or severe salt wasting (associated with 21-hydroxylase and 3β-hydroxysteroid dehydrogenase deficiency), are clinical hallmarks of congenital adrenal hyperplasia. The pathophysiology can be traced to discrete, inherited defects in the adrenal enzyme system. Treatment of CAH is targeted to replace the hormones that are produced in insufficient quantity. With proper hormone replacement therapy, normal and healthy development may often be expected. Radioimmunoassay of serum and urinary steroid levels permits reliable diagnosis of the various forms of congenital adrenal hyperplasia. Prenatal diagnosis and therapy are possible in 21-hydroxylase deficiency.

The most common form of CAH, 21-hydroxylase deficiency, has served as a prototype for examination of the molecular genetic basis of phenotypic diversity. Similar studies in other enzymatic defects are now in progress.

REFERENCES

1. De Crecchio L. Sopra un caso di apparenze virile in una donna. Morgani 1951; 7:1865.
2. Ganong WF. The central nervous system and the synthesis and release of adrenocorticotrophic hormone. In: Nalbandov AV, ed. Advances in Neuroendocrinology. Urbana, IL: University of Illinois Press, 1963:92.
3. Guillemin R, Schally AV. Recent advances in the chemistry of neuroendocrine mediators originating in the central nervous system. In: Nalbandov AV, ed. Advances in Neuroendocrinology. Urbana, IL: University of Illinois Press, 1963:314.

4. Wilkins L. Adrenal disorders. II. Congenital virilizing adrenal hyperplasia. Arch Dis Child 1962; 37:231.

5. Prader A, Zachmann M, Illig R. Normal spermatogenesis in adult males with congenital adrenal hyperplasia after discontinuation of therapy. In: Lee PA, Plotnick LP, Kowarski AA, Migeon CJ, eds. Congenital Adrenal Hyperplasia. Baltimore: University Park Press, 1977:397.

6. Levine LS, New MI, Pitt P, Peterson RE. Androgen production in boys with sexual precocity and congenital adrenal hyperplasia. Metabolism 1972; 21:457.

7. Lippe BM, LaFranchi SH, Lavin N, Parlow A, Coyotupa J, Kaplan SA. Serum 17α-hydroxyprogesterone, progesterone, estradiol, and testosterone in the diagnosis and management of congenital adrenal hyperplasia. J Pediatr 1974; 85:782.

8. Janne O, Perheentupa J, Viinikka L, Vihko R. Plasma pregnenolone, progesterone, 17-hydroxyprogesterone, progesterone, estradiol, and testosterone in the diagnosis and management of congenital adrenal hyperplasia. Clin Endocrinol (Oxf) 1975; 4:39.

9. Solomon IL, Schoen EJ. Blood testosterone values in patients with congenital virilizing adrenal hyperplasia. J Clin Endocrinol Metab 1975; 40:355.

10. Hughes IA, Winter JSD. The application of a serum 17-OH-progesterone radioimmunoassay to the diagnosis and management of congenital adrenal hyperplasia. J Pediatr 1976; 88:766.

11. Pang S, Hotchkiss J, Drash AL, Levine LS, New MI. Microfilter paper method for 17α-hydroxyprogesterone radioimmunoassay: its application for rapid screening for congenital adrenal hyperplasia. J Clin Endocrinol Metab 1977; 45:1003.

12. Korth-Schutz S, Virdis R, Saenger P, Chow DM, Levine LS, New MI. Serum androgens as a continuing index of adequacy of treatment of congenital adrenal hyperplasia. J Clin Endocrinol Metab 1978; 46:452.

13. Pang S, Levine LS, Chow D, Faiman C, New MI. Serum androgen concentrations in neonates and young infants with congenital adrenal hyperplasia due to 21-hydroxylase deficiency. Clin Endocrinol (Oxf) 1979; 11:575.

14. Bongiovanni AM, Eberlein WR, Cara J. Studies on metabolism of adrenal steroids in adrenogenital syndrome. J Clin Endocrinol Metab 1954; 14:409.

15. Butler GC, Marrian GF. The isolation of pregnane-3,17,20-triol from the urine of women showing the adrenogenital syndrome. J Biol Chem 1937; 119:565.

16. New MI, Levine LS. Adrenal hyperplasia in intersex states. In: Laron Z, Tikva P, eds. Pediatric and Adolescent Endocrinology, Vol. 8. Basel: Karger, 1981:51.

17. Prader A, Spahr A, Neher R. Erhöhte Aldosteronausscheidung beim kongenitalen adrenogenitalen Syndrom. Schweiz Med Wochenschr 1955; 85:45.

18. Klein R. Evidence for and evidence against the existence of a salt-losing hormone. J Pediatr 1960; 57:452.

19. Kowarski AA, Finkelstein JW, Spaulding JS, Holman GS, Migeon CJ. Aldosterone secretion rate in congenital adrenal hyperplasia. A discussion of the theories on the pathogenesis of the salt-losing form of the syndrome. J Clin Invest 1965; 44:1505.

20. Kuhnle U, Land M, Ulick S. Evidence for the secretion of an antimineralocorticoid in congenital adrenal hyperplasia. J Clin Endocrinol Metab 1986; 62:934.

21. Stoner E, DiMartino J, Kuhnle U, Levine LS, Oberfield SE, New MI. Is salt wasting in congenital adrenal hyperplasia genetic? 1986; 24:9.

22. Luetscher JA. Studies of aldosterone in relation to water and electrolyte balance in man. Rec Prog Horm Res 1956; 12:175.

23. Speiser PW, Agdere L, Ueshiba H, White PC, New MI.

Aldosterone synthesis in salt-wasting congenital adrenal hyperplasia with complete absence of adrenal 21-hydroxylase. N Engl J Med 1991; 324:145–149.

24. Verkauf BS, Jones HW. Masculinization of the female genitalia in congenital adrenal hyperplasia: relationship to the salt-losing variety of the disease. South Med J 1970; 63:634.

25. Jones HW, Jones GES. The gynecological aspects of adrenal hyperplasia and allied disorders. Am J Obstet Gynecol 1954; 68:1330.

26. Jefferies WM, Weir WC, Weir DR, Prouty RL. The use of cortisone and related steroids in infertility. Fertil Steril 1958; 9:145.

27. Decourt MJ, Jayle MF, Baulieu E. Virilisme cliniquement tardif avec excretion de pregnanetriol et insuffisance de la production du cortisol. Ann Endocrinol (Paris) 1957; 18:416.

28. Frasier SD, Thorneycroft IH, Weill BA, Horton R. Elevated amniotic fluid concentration of 17-hydroxyprogesterone in congenital adrenal hyperplasia. J Pediatr 1975; 86:310.

29. Levine LS, Dupont B, Lorenzen F, et al. Cryptic 21-hydroxylase deficiency in families of patients with classical congenital adrenal hyperplasia. J Clin Endocrinol Metab 1980; 51: 1316.

30. Kohn B, Levine LS, Pollack MS, et al. Late-onset steroid 21-hydroxylase deficiency: a variant of classical congenital adrenal hyperplasia. J Clin Endocrinol Metab 1982; 55:817.

31. Rosenwaks Z, Lee PA, Jones GS, Migeon CJ, Wentz AC. An attenuated form of congenital virilizing adrenal hyperplasia. J Clin Endocrinol Metab 1979; 49:335.

32. Pollack MS, Levine LS, O'Neill GJ, et al. HLA linkage and B14,DR1,BfS haplotype association with the genes for late onset and cryptic 21-hydroxylase deficiency. Am J Hum Genet 1981; 33:540.

33. Laron Z, Pollack MS, Zamir R, et al. Late onset 21-hydroxylase deficiency and HLA in the Ashkenazi population; a new allele at the 21-hydroxylase locus. Hum Immunol 1980; 1:55.

34. Levine LS, Dupont B, Lorenzen F, et al. Genetic and hormonal characterization of cryptic 21-hydroxylase deficiency. J Clin Endocrinol Metab 1981; 53:1193.

35. Blankstein J, Faiman C, Reues FI, Schroeder ML, Winter JSD. Adult-onset familial adrenal 21-hydroxylase deficiency. Am J Med 1980; 68:441.

36. Migeon CJ, Rosenwaks Z, Lee PA, Urban MD, Bias WB. The attenuated form of congenital adrenal hyperplasia as an allelic form of 21-hydroxylase deficiency. J Clin Endocrinol Metab 1980; 51:647.

37. Speiser PW, Dupont B, Rubinstein P, Piazza A, Kastelan A, New MI. High frequency of nonclassical steroid 21-hydroxylase deficiency. Am J Hum Genet 1985; 37:650–667.

38. Dumic M, Brkljacic L, Speiser PW, et al. An update on the frequency of nonclassic deficiency of adrenal 21-hydroxylase in the Yugoslav population. Acta Endocrinol (Copenh) 1990; 122:703–710.

39. Temeck JW, Pang S, Nelson C, New MI. Genetic defects of steroidogenesis in premature pubarche. J Clin Endocrinol Metab 1987; 64:609.

40. Hawkins LA, Chasalow FI, Blethen SL. The role of adrenocorticotropin testing in evaluating girls with premature adrenarche and hirsutism/oligomenorrhea. J Clin Endorinol Metab 1992; 74:248–253.

41. New MI, Gertner JM, Speiser PW, del Balzo P. Growth and final height in classical and nonclassical 21-hydroxylase deficiency. J Endocrinol Invest 1990; 12:91–95.

42. Lucky AW, Rosenfield RL, McGuire J, Rudy S, Helke J. Adrenal androgen hyperresponsiveness to adrenocorticotropin in women with acne and/or hirsutism: adrenal enzyme defects

and exaggerated adrenarche. J Endocrinol Metab 1986; 62: 840.

43. Rose LI, Newmark SR, Strauss JS, Pochi PE. Adrenocortical hydroxylase deficiencies in acne vulgaris. J Invest Dermatol 1976; 66:324.

44. O'Driscoll JB, Anderson DC. Untreated congenital adrenal hyperplasia presenting with severe androgenic alopecia. J R Soc Med 1993; 86:229.

45. Pang S, Lerner AJ, Stoner E, et al. Late-onset adrenal steroid 3β-hydroxysteroid dehydrogenase deficiency. A cause of hirsutism in pubertal and postpubertal women. J Clin Endocrinol Metab 1985; 60:428.

46. Child DF, Bullock DE, Anderson DC. Adrenal steroidogenesis in hirsute women. Clin Endocrinol (Oxf) 1980; 12:595.

47. Gibson M, Lackritz R, Schiff I, Tulchinsky D. Abnormal adrenal responses to adrenocorticotropic hormone in hyperandrogenic women. Fertil Steril 1980; 33:43.

48. Lobo RA, Goebelsmann U. Adult manifestation of congenital adrenal hyperplasia due to incomplete 21-hydroxylase deficiency mimicking polycystic ovarian disease. Am J Obstet Gynecol 1980; 138:720.

49. Chrousos GP, Loriaux DL, Mann DL, Cutler GB. Late-onset 21-hydroxylase deficiency mimicking idiopathic hirsutism or polycystic ovarian disease. An allelic variant of congenital virilizing adrenal hyperplasia with a milder enzymatic defect. Ann Intern Med 1982; 96:143.

50. Chrousos GP, Loriaux DL, Mann D, Cutler GB. Late-onset 21-hydroxylase deficiency is an allelic variant of congenital adrenal hyperplasia characterized by attenuated clinical expression and different HLA haplotype association. Horm Res 1982; 16:193–200.

51. Chetkowski R, DeFazio J, Shamonki I, Judd HL, Chang RJ. The incidence of late-onset congenital adrenal hyperplasia due to 21-hydroxylase deficiency among hirsute women. J Clin Endocrinol Metab 1984; 58:595.

52. Kuttenn F, Coullin P, Girard F, et al. Late-onset adrenal hyperplasia in hirsutism. N Engl J Med 1986; 313:224.

53. Chrousos GP, Loriaux DL, Sherines RJ, Cutler GB. Unilateral testicular enlargement resulting from inapparent 21-hydroxylase deficiency. J Urol 1981; 126:127.

54. Wischusen J, Baker HWG, Hudson B. Reversible male infertility due to congenital adrenal hyperplasia. Clin Endocrinol (Oxf) 1981; 14:571.

55. Bonaccorsi AC, Adler I, Figueiredo JG. Male infertility due to congenital adrenal hyperplasia: testicular biopsy findings, hormonal evaluation, and therapeutic results in three patients. Fertil Steril 1987; 47:664–670.

56. Augartan A, Weissenberg R, Pariente C, Sack J. Reversible male infertility in late onset congenital adrenal hyperplasia. J Endocrinol Invest 1991; 14:237–240.

57. Mokshagundam S, Surks MI. Congenital adrenal hyperplasia diagnosed in a man during workup for bilateral adrenal masses. Arch Intern Med 1993; 153:1389–1391.

58. Jaresch S, Kornely E, Kley HK, Schlaghecke R. Adrenal incidentaloma in patients with homozygous or heterozygous congenital adrenal hyperplasia. J Clin Endocrinol Metab 1992; 74:685–689.

59. Jones HW, Verkauf BS. Congenital adrenal hyperplasia: age at menarche and related events at puberty. Am J Obstet Gynecol 1971; 109:292.

60. Klingensmith GJ, Garcia SC, Jones HW, Migeon CJ, Blizzard RM. Glucocorticoid treatment of girls with congenital adrenal hyperplasia: effects on height, sexual maturation, and fertility. J Pediatr 1977; 90:966.

61. Pang S, Kenny FM, Foley TP, Drash AL. Growth and sexual maturation in treated congenital adrenal hyperplasia. In: Lee PA, Plotnick LP, Kowarski AA, Migeon CJ, eds. Congenital Adrenal Hyperplasia. Baltimore: University Park Press, 1977: 233.

62. Ghali I, David M, David L. Linear growth and pubertal development in treated congenital adrenal hyperplasia due to 21-hydroxylase deficiency. Clin Endocrinol (Oxf) 1977; 6:425.

63. Reiter EO, Grumbach MM, Kaplan SL, Conte FA. The response of pituitary gonadotropes to synthetic LRF in children with glucocorticoid-treated congenital adrenal hyperplasia: lack of effect of intrauterine and neonatal androgen excess. J Clin Endocrinol Metab 1975; 40:318.

64. Kirkland J, Kirkland R, Librik L, Clayton G. Serum gonadotropin levels in female adolescents with congenital adrenal hyperplasia. J Pediatr 1974; 84:411.

65. Wentz AC, Garcia SC, Klingensmith GJ, Migeon CJ, Jones GS. Hypothalamic maturation in congenital adrenal hyperplasia. In: Lee PA, Plotnick LP, Kowarski AA, Migeon CJ, eds. Congenital Adrenal Hyperplasia. Baltimore: University Park Press, 1977:379.

66. Levin JH, Carmina E, Lobo RA. Is the inappropriate gonadotropin secretion of patients with polycystic ovary syndrome similar to that of patients with adult-onset congenital adrenal hyperplasia? Fertil Steril 1991; 56:635–640.

67. Pescovitz OH, Comite F, Cassorla F, et al. True precocious puberty complicating congenital hyperplasia: treatment with a luteinizing hormone-releasing hormone analog. J Clin Endocrinol Metab 1984; 58:857.

68. Dacou-Voutetakis C, Karidis N. Congenital adrenal hyperplasia complicated by central precocious puberty: treatment with LHRH-agonist analogue. Ann NY Acad Sci 1993; 687:250–254.

69. Wilkins L, Crigler JF, Silverman SH, Gardner LI, Migeon CJ. Further studies on the treatment of congenital adrenal hyperplasia with cortisone. II. The effects of cortisone on sexual and somatic development, with an hypothesis concerning the mechanism of feminization. J Clin Endocrinol Metab 1952; 12:277.

70. Klingensmith GJ, Wentz AC, Meyer WJ, Migeon CJ. Gonadotropin output in congenital adrenal hyperplasia. J Clin Endocrinol Metab 1976; 43:933.

71. Kiesslin GW, Schwarz G. Zur genese des hypogonadismus beim kongenitalen adrenogenitalen syndrome. Arch Klin Dermatol 1966; 228:684.

72. Kirkland RT, Keenan BS, Clayton GW. Long-term follow-up of patients with congenital adrenal hyperplasia in Houston. In: Lee PA, Plotnick LP, Kowarski AA, Migeon CJ, eds. Congenital Adrenal Hyperplasia. Baltimore: University Park Press, 1977:273.

73. Richards GE, Styne DM, Conte FA, Kaplan SL, Grumbach MM. Plasma sex steroids and gonadotropins in pubertal girls with congenital adrenal hyperplasia: relationship to menstrual disorders. In: Lee P, Plotnick LP, Kowarski AA, Migeon CJ, eds. Congenital Adrenal Hyperplasia. Baltimore: University Park Press, 1977:233.

74. Richards GE, Grumbach MM, Kaplan SL, Conte FA. The effect of long acting glucocorticoids on menstrual abnormalities in patients with virilizing congenital adrenal hyperplasia. J Clin Endocrinol Metab 1978; 47:1208.

75. Grayzel EF. Postpubertal adrenogenital syndrome: treatable cause of infertility. NY State J Med 1974; 74:1038.

76. Granoff AB. Treatment of menstrual irregularities with dexamethasone in congenital adrenal hyperplasia. J Adolesc Health Care 1981; 2:23.

77. Rosenfield RL, Bickel S, Razdan AK. Amenorrhea related to progestin excess in congenital adrenal hyperplasia. Obstet Gynecol 1980; 56:208.

78. Riddick DH, Hammond CB. Adrenal virilism due to 21-hydroxylase deficiency in the postmenarchial female. Obstet Gynecol 1975; 45:21.

79. Speroff L. The adrenogenital syndrome and its obstetrical aspects: a review of the literature and case report. Obstet Gynecol Surv 1965; 20:185.

80. Mori M, Miyakama I. Congenital adreogenital syndrome and successful pregnancy: report of a case. J Obstet Gynecol 1970; 35:394.

81. Mulaikal RM, Migeon CJ, Rock JA. Fertility rates in female patients with congenital adrenal hyperplasia due to 21-hydroxylase deficiency. N Engl J Med 1987; 316:178–182.

82. Stewart JSS. A fertile male with untreated congenital adrenal hyperplasia. Acta Endocrinol Suppl (Copenh) 1960; 51: 661.

83. Urban MD, Lee PA, Migeon CJ. Adult height and fertility in men with congenital virilizing adrenal hyperplasia. N Engl J Med 1978; 299:1392.

84. Molitor JT, Chertow BS, Fariss BL. Long-term follow-up of a patient with congenital adrenal hyperplasia and failure of testicular development. Fertil Steril 1973; 24:319.

85. Bahner F, Schwarz G. Congenitale nebennierenrinden hyperplasie beim mann mit normaler keimdrusenfunktion und fertilitat. Acta Endocrinol (Copenh) 1961; 38:236.

86. Wilkins L, Blizzard RM, Migeon CJ. The Diagnosis and Treatment of Endocrine Disorders in Childhood and Adolescence, 3rd ed. Springfield, IL: Charles C. Thomas, 1965:410.

87. Raiti S, Maclaren N, Akesode F. Gonadotropin-adrenal-testicular axis in males with congenital adrenal hyperplasia and idiopathic sexual precocity. In: Lee PA, Plotnick LP, Kowarski AA, Migeon CJ, eds. Congenital Adrenal Hyperplasia. Baltimore: University Park Press, 1977:403.

88. Blumberg-Tick J, Boudou P, Nahoul K, Schaison G. Testicular tumors in congenital adrenal hyperplasia: steroid measurements from adrenal and spermatic veins. J Clin Endocrinol Metab 1991; 73:1129–33.

89. Schoen EJ, DiRaimondo V, Dominguez OV. Bilateral testicular tumors complicating congenital adrenocortical hyperplasia. J Clin Endocrinol Metab 1961; 21:518.

90. Miller EC, Murray HL. Congenital adrenocortical hyperplasia: case previously reported as "bilateral interstitial cell tumor of the testicle." J Clin Endocrinol Metab 1962; 22:655.

91. Glenn JF, Boyce WH. Adrenogenitalism with testicular adrenal rests simulating interstitial cell tumor. J Urol 1963; 89:456.

92. Radfar N, Bartter FC. Easley R, Kolins J, Javadpour N, Sherins RJ. Evidence for endogenous LH suppression in a man with bilateral testicular tumors and congenital adrenal hyperplasia. J Clin Endocrinol Metab 1977; 45:1104.

93. Srikanth MS, West BR, Ishitani M, Isaacs H Jr, Applebaum H, Costin G. Benign testicular tumors in children with congenital adrenal hyperplasia. J Pediatr Surg 1992; 27:639–641.

94. Rutgers JL, Young RH, Scully RE. The testicular "tumor" of the adrenogenital syndrome. Am J Surg Pathol 1988; 12:503–513.

95. Chakraborty J, Franco-Saenz R, Kropp K. Electron microscopic study of testicular tumor in congenital adrenal hyperplasia. Hum Pathol 1983; 14:151–157.

96. Dupont B, Oberfield SE, Smithwick EM, Lee TD, Levine LS. Close genetic linkage between HLA and congenital adrenal hyperplasia (21-hydroxylase deficiency). Lancet 1977; 2: 1309–1311.

97. Levine LS, Zachmann M, New MI, et al. Genetic mapping of the 21-hydroxylase-deficiency gene within the HLA linkage group. N Engl J Med 1978; 299:911–915.

98. Klouda PT, Harris R, Price DA. HLA and congenital adrenal hyperplasia. Lancet 1978; 2:1046.

99. Pucholt V, Fitzsimmons JS, Gelsthorpe K, Pratt RF, Doughty TW. HLA and congenital adrenal hyperplasia. Lancet 1978; 2:1046–1047.

100. Pollack MS, Levine LS, Zachmann M, et al. Possible genetic linkage disequilibrium between HLA and the 21-hydroxylase deficiency gene (congenital adrenal hyperplasia). Transplant Proc 1979; 11:1315–1316.

101. Speiser PW, New MI. Genotype and hormonal phenotype in nonclassical 21-hydroxylase deficiency. J Clin Endocrinol Metab 1987; 64:86–91.

102. White PC, Grosberger D, Onufer BJ, New MI, Dupont B, Strominger JL. Two genes encoding steroid 21-hydroxylase are located near the genes encoding the fourth component of complement in man. Proc Natl Acad Sci USA 1985; 82:1089–1093.

103. Carroll MC, Campbell RD, Porter RR. The mapping of 21-hydroxylase genes adjacent to complement component C4 genes in HLA, the major histocompatibility complex in man. Proc Natl Acad Sci USA 1985; 82:521–525.

104. White PC, New MI, Dupont B. Structure of the human steroid 21-hydroxylase genes. Proc Natl Acad Sci USA 1986; 83: 5111–5115.

105. Higashi Y, Yoshioka H, Yamane M, Gotoh O, Fujii-Kuriyama Y. Complete nucleotide sequence of two steroid 21-hydroxylase genes tandemly arranged in human genome. Proc Natl Acad Sci USA 1986; 83:2841–2845.

106. White PC, New MI. Genetic basis of endocrine disease. 2. Congenital adrenal hyperplasia due to 21-hydroxylase deficiency. J Clin Endocrinol Metab 1992; 74:6–11.

107. Wedell A, Ritzen EM, Haglund-Stengler B, Luthman H. Steroid 21-hydroxylase deficiency: three additional mutated alleles and establishment of phenotype-genotype relationships of common mutations. Proc Natl Acad Sci USA 1992; 89:7232–7236.

108. Speiser PW, Dupont J, Zhu D, et al. Disease expression and molecular genotype in congenital adrenal hyperplasia due to 21-hydroxylase deficiency. J Clin Invest 1992; 90:584–595.

109. Bormann M, Kochhan L, Knorr D, Bidlingmaier F, Olek K. Clinical heterogeneity of 21-hydroxylase deficiency of sibs with identical 21-hydroxylase genes. Acta Endocrinol (Copenh) 1992; 126:7–9.

110. Werkmeister JM, New MI, Dupont B, White PC. Frequent deletion and duplication of the steroid 21-hydroxylase genes. Am J Hum Genet 1986; 39:461–469.

111. White PC, Vitek A, Dupont B, New MI. Characterization of frequent deletions causing steroid 21-hydroxylase deficiency. Proc Natl Acad Sci USA 1988; 85:4436.

112. Rumsby G, Carroll MC, Porter RR, Grant DB, Hjelm M. Deletion of the steroid 21-hydroxylase and complement C4 genes in congenital adrenal hyperplasia. J Med Genet 1986; 23:204–209.

113. Rodrigues NR, Dunham I, Yu CY, Carroll MC, Porter RR, Campbell RD. Molecular characterization of the HLA-linked steroid 21-hydroxylase B gene from an individual with congenital adrenal hyperplasia. EMBO J 1987; 6:1653–1661.

114. Owerbach D, Ballard AL., Draznin MB. Salt-wasting congenital adrenal hyperplasia: detection and characterization of mutations in the steroid 21-hydroxylase gene, CYP21, using the polymerase chain reaction. J Clin Endocrinol Metab 1993; 74:553–558.

115. Tajima T, Fujieda K, Fujii-Kuriyama Y. De novo mutation causes steroid 21-hydroxylase deficiency in one family of HLA-identical affected and unaffected siblings. J Clin Endocrinol Metab 1993; 77:86–89.

116. Speiser PW, New MI, White PC. Molecular genetic analysis of nonclassic steroid 21-hydroxylase deficiency associated with HLA-B14,DR1. N Engl J Med 1988; 319:19–23.

117. Tusie-Luna MT, Speiser PW, Dumic M, New MI, White PC. A mutation (Pro-30 to Leu) in CYP21 represents a potential nonclassic steroid 21-hydroxylase deficiency allele. Mol Endocrinol 1991; 5:685–692.

118. Owerbach D, Sherman L, Ballard AL, Azziz R. Pro-453 to Ser mutation in CYP21 is associated with nonclassic steroid 21-hydroxylase deficiency. Mol Endocrinol 1992; 6:1211–1215.

119. Pang S. Worldwide experience in newborn screening for classical congenital adrenal hyperplasia due to 21-hydroxylase deficiency. Pediatrics 1988; 81:866.

120. New MI, Lorenzen F, Lerner AJ, et al. Genotyping steroid 21-hydroxylase deficiency: hormonal reference data. J Clin Endocrinol Metab 1983; 57:320–326.

121. Zerah M, Ueshiba J, Wood E, et al. Prevalence of nonclassical steroid 21-hydroxylase deficiency based on a morning salivary 17-hydroxyprogesterone screening test: a small sample study. J Clin Endocrinol Metab 1990; 70:1662–1667.

122. Zerah M, Pang S, New MI. Morning salivary 17-hydroxyprogesterone is a useful screening test for nonclassical 21-hydroxylase deficiency. J Clin Endocrinol Metab 1987; 65: 227.

123. Kutten F, Late-onset adrenal hyperplasia (letter). N Engl J Med 1986; 314:450.

124. Jeffcoate TNA, Fleigner JRH, Russell SH, Davis JC, Wade AP. Diagnosis of the adrenogenital syndrome before birth. Lancet 1965; 2:553.

125. New MI, Levine LS. Congenital adrenal hyperplasia. In: Harris H, Hirschhorn K, eds. Advances in Human Genetics. New York: Plenum Press, 1973:251.

126. Levine LS. Prenatal detection of congenital adrenal hyperplasia. In: Milunsky A, ed. Genetic Disorders and the Fetus. New York: Plenum Press, 1986:369–385.

127. Nagamani M, McDonough PG, Ellegood JO, Mahesh VB. Maternal and amniotic fluid 17-hydroxyprogesterone levels during pregnancy: diagnosis of congenital adrenal hyperplasia in utero. Am J Obstet Gynecol 1978; 130:791.

128. Hughes IA, Laurence KM. Antenatal diagnosis of congenital adrenal hyperplasia. Lancet 1979; 2:7.

129. Pang S, Levine LS, Cederqvist LL, et al. Amniotic fluid concentration of Δ^5 and Δ^4 steroids in fetuses with congenital adrenal hyperplasia due to 21-hydroxylase deficiency and in anencephalic fetuses. J Clin Endocrinol Metab 1980; 51:223.

130. Hughes IA, Laurence KM. Prenatal diagnosis of congenital adrenal hyperplasia due to 21-hydroxylase deficiency: amniotic fluid steroid analysis. Prenat Diagn 1982; 2:97.

131. Blankstein J, Fujieda K, Reyes FI, Faiman C, Winter JSD. Cortisol, 11-deoxycortisol and 21-desoxycortisol concentrations in amniotic fluid during normal pregnancy. Am J Obstet Gynecol 1980; 137:781.

132. Frasier SD, Weiss BA, Horton R. Amniotic fluid testosterone: implications for the prenatal diagnosis of congenital adrenal hyperplasia. J Pediatr 1974; 84:738–741.

133. Mornet E, Boue J, Raux-Demay M, et al. First trimester prenatal diagnosis of 21-hydroxylase deficiency by linkage analysis of HLA-DNA probes and by 17-hydroxyprogesterone determination. Hum Genet 1986; 73:358–364.

134. Speiser PW, Laforgia N, Kato K, et al. First trimester prenatal treatment and molecular genetic diagnosis of congenital adrenal hyperplasia (21-hydroxylase deficiency). J Clin Endocrinol Metab 1990; 70:838–848.

135. Owerbach D, Draznin MB, Carpenter RJ, Greenberg F. Prenatal diagnosis of 21-hydroxylase deficiency congenital adrenal hyperplasia using the polymerase chain reaction. Hum Genet 1992; 89:109–110.

136. Rumsby G, Honour JW, Rodeck C. Prenatal diagnosis of congenital adrenal hyperplasia by direct detection of mutations in the steroid 21-hydroxylase gene. Clin Endocrinol (Oxf) 1993; 38:421–425.

137. Forest MG, Betuel H, David M. Traitement antenatal de l'hyperplasie congenitale des surrenales par deficit en 21-hydroxylase: etude multicentrique. Ann Endocrinol (Paris) 1987; 48:31–34.

138. Dorr HG, Sippell WG, Haack D, Bidlingmaier F, Knorr D. Pitfalls of prenatal treatment of congenital adrenal hyperplasia (CAH) due to 21-hydroxylase deficiency. Program and Abstract, 25th Annual Meeting of the European Society for Paediatric Endocrinology, Zurich, August 1986.

139. Evans MI, Chrousos GP, Mann DW, et al. Pharmacologic suppression of the fetal adrenal gland in utero. JAMA 1985; 253:1015.

140. Speiser P, Mercado AB, New MI. Prenatal treatment of congenital adrenal hyperplasia. Program and Abstracts, Fourth Joint Meeting, Lawson Wilkins Pediatric Endocrine Society and European Society for Paediatric Endocrinology, June 1993, San Francisco, California. Pediatr Res 1993; 33:S4/11.

141. Charnvises S, Fencl MD, Osathanondh R, Zhu MG, Underwood R, Tulchinsky D. Adrenal steroids in maternal and cord blood after dexamethasone administration at midterm. J Clin Endocrinol Metab 1985; 61:1220.

142. Dorr HG, Sippell WG, Bidlingmaier K, Knorr D. Experience with intrauterine therapy of CAH due to 21-hydroxylase deficiency. Program and Abstracts, Endocrine Society, 70th Annual Meeting, New Orleans, Louisiana, June 1988.

143. Goldman AS, Shapior BH, Katsumata M. Human foetal palatal corticoid receptors and teratogens for cleft palate. Nature 1978; 272:464.

144. Pang S, Clark AT, Freeman LC, et al. Maternal side effects of prenatal dexamethasone therapy for fetal congenital adrenal hyperplasia. J Clin Endocrinol Metab 1992; 75:249–253.

145. Mininberg DT, Levine LS, New MI. Current concepts in congenital adrenal hyperplasia due to 11b-hydroxylase deficiency. Clin Endocrinol (Oxf) 1980; 12:257.

146. Laragh JH. Aldosteronism in man: factors controlling secretion of the hormone. In: Christy NP, ed. The Human Adrenal Cortex. New York: Harper and Row, 1971:483.

147. Bartter FC. Adrenogenital syndromes from physiology to chemistry (1950–1975). In: Lee PA, Plotnick LP, Kowaraski AA, Migeon CJ, eds. Congenital Adrenal Hyperplasia. Baltimore: University Park Press, 1977:9.

148. Rosler A, Levine LS, Schneider B, Novogroder M, New MI. The interrelationship of sodium balance, plasma renin activity and ACTH in congenital adrenal hyperplasia. J Clin Endocrinol Metab 1977; 45:500.

149. Pang S, MacGillivray M, Wang M, et al. 3α-Androstandiol glucuronide in virilizing congenital adrenal hyperplasia: a useful serum metabolic marker of integrated adrenal androgen secretion. J Clin Endocrinol Metab 1991; 73:166–174.

150. Winter JSD. Current approaches to the treatment of congenital adrenal hyperplasia. J Pediatr 1980; 97:81.

22

Adrenal Cortex
Hypo- and Hyperfunction

Claude J. Migeon
Johns Hopkins University School of Medicine, Baltimore, Maryland

Roberto L. Lanes
Hospital de Clinicas Caracas, Caracas, Venezuela

I. INTRODUCTION

The adrenal gland is made of two parts, the cortex and the medulla, which have different embryonic origins. By 4–5 weeks of fetal life, cells from the mesoderm aggregate to form a primitive cortex between the posterior part of the dorsal mesentery and the gonadal ridge (1). Shortly thereafter, this primitive cortex becomes surrounded by a narrow band of cells termed permanent cortex. By 7–8 weeks of fetal life, the primitive cortex is invaded by chromaffin cells that develop rapidly and eventually replace most of the primitive cortical cells, forming the medulla (1). At that time, the adrenal gland is in close relation with the cranial part of the primitive kidney and not far from the genital ridge.

The adrenal medulla, which originates from ectodermal cells, has an entirely different function from the mesodermal adrenal cortex. In this chapter only the latter is discussed.

In the adult, the adrenal cortex is made of three distinctive zones. The outer zona glomerulosa secretes adlosterone; the middle zona fasciculata and the inner zona reticularis together are involved in the secretion of the cortisol and adrenal androgens (1). We first discuss the physiologic function of the adrenal cortex. Then we consider the disorders related to the hyposecretion and hypersecretion of adrenal cortical hormones.

II. PHYSIOLOGY

A. Biosynthesis of Adrenocortical Steroids

1. The Enzymes

Cholesterol is the precursor of all steroids of both gonadal and adrenocortical origin (2). The biosynthetic pathway of adrenal steroids is shown in Figure 1. The conversion of cholesterol to the various hormones requires the sequential action of a series of six enzymes, as listed in Table 1. All but 3β-hydroxysteroid dehydrogenase are members of a family of enzymes termed cytochromes P450. They are heme-containing proteins that act as mixed-function oxidases (3). Three of these enzymes have a very similar structure: cholesterol side-chain cleavage enzyme encoded by the gene CYP11A, 11β-hydroxylase encoded by CYP11B1, and aldosterone synthetase encoded by CYP11B2. The last two genes are contiguous on the long arm of chromosome 8.

The cholesterol side-chain cleavage enzyme has the ability to add a hydroxyl group on carbons 20 and 22 of the cholesterol molecule as well as remove a side chain between carbons 20 and 22 (4). The 3β-hydroxysteroid dehydrogenase (3β-HSD) converts pregnenolone to progesterone as well as 17α-hydroxypregnenolone to 17α-hydroxyprogesterone; this is accomplished by reduction of the 3β-hydroxyl group into a 3-ketone and isomerization of the 5,6 double bond to a 3,4 double bond. The 17α-hydroxylase enzyme has the ability of both 17α-hydroxylation and 17,20-lyase. The latter activity transforms steroids with a carbon 21 into steroids with a carbon 19. 21-Hydroxylase (CYP21) and 11β-hydroxylase (CPY11B1) are specific for the function of adding a hydroxyl group in carbons 21 and 11, respectively. Aldosterone synthetase (CYP11B2) adds an 11β-hydroxyl group and an 18-hydroxyl group and is also capable of 18-oxidation (5). Whereas the CYP11A, 3β-HSD, and CYP21 genes are expressed in all the zones of the adrenal cortex, the CYP17 and CYP11B1 genes are expressed only in the zona fasciculata-reticularis and the CYP11B2 gene is expressed only in the zona glomerulosa. This accounts for the specificity of steroid production by the various zones of the cortex.

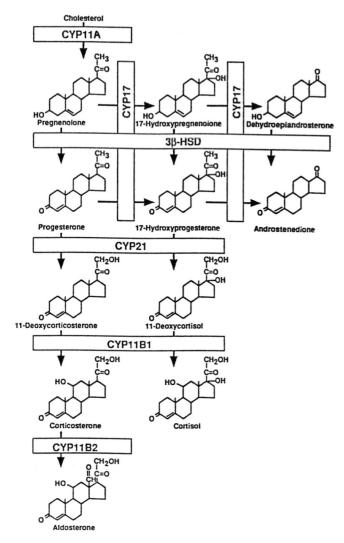

Figure 1 Biosynthesis of adrenocortical steroids. The pathway from cholesterol to cortisol, aldosterone and adrenal androgens requires the action of five cytochrome P450 (CYP11A, CYP17, CYP21, CYP11B1, and CYP11B2) and one dehydrogenase (3β-hydroxysteroid dehydrogenase). (From Ref. 2.)

Table 1 Nomenclature for the Various Steroid Biosynthetic Enzymes and the Respective Genes

Enzyme activity	Gene	Chromosomal locus
Cholesterol side-chain cleavage enzyme (20-hydroxylase, 22-hydroxylase, 20,22-lyase)	CYP11A	15q23–q24
3β-Hydroxysteroid dehydrogenase	3β-HSD	1p13.1
17α-Hydroxylase and 17,20-lyase	CYP17	10q24–q25
21-Hydroxylase	CYP21	6p21
11β-Hydroxylase (some 18-hydroxylation)	CYP11B1	8q22
Aldosterone synthetase (11β-hydroxylation, 18-hydroxylation, and 18-oxidation)	CYP11B2	8q22

2. Subcellular Location of the Various Enzymes

As shown in Figure 2, cholesterol is stored in the adrenal cell as cholesterol esters. Under the influence of an esterase, cholesterol becomes available and is transported to the mitochondria, where it is converted to pregnenolone (2). This steroid then moves into the endoplasmic reticulum, where 3β-hydroxysteroid dehydrogenase, 21-hydroxylase, and 17-hydroxylase enzymes are located. The resulting steroids include 11-deoxycorticosterone (DOC) and 11-deoxycortisol as well as two C-19 carbon steroids, androstenedione and dehydroepiandrosterone (DHA). At that point, DOC and 11-deoxycortisol return to the mitochondria, where they are converted into corticosterone and cortisol,

respectively. This is basically the end of the biosynthetic process in the cells of the zona fasciculata.

In the cells of the zona glomerulosa, there is no 17-hydroxylase activity and, therefore, no formation of cortisol or androgens. However, the mitochondria of these cells include CYP11B2 enzyme, which transforms DOC into corticosterone, 18-hydroxycorticosterone, and aldosterone.

Finally, it must be noted that the activity of all cytochrome P_{450} enzymes requires a gain of electrons. These electrons are transferred from NADPH. In the mitochondria this transfer is made via two intermediaries, adrenodoxin and adrenodoxin reductase, whereas in the microsomes the transfer requires only the presence of an adrenodoxin (2).

3. The Placental-Fetal Adrenal Unit

Early in fetal life, the adrenal cortex is capable of the secretion of steroids. It lacks 3β-hydroxysteroid dehydrogenase however, and the major hormones secreted include pregnenolone, 17α-hydroxypregnenolone, DHA, and 16α-hydroxy-DHA. All these steroids circulate as sulfate conjugates, which are then transferred to the placenta (1). This organ is rich in sulfatase, which makes the native steroids available to the greatly active placental 3β-hydroxysteroid dehydrogenase. The resulting progesterone and 17α-hydroxyprogesterone are returned in part to the fetus and are used by the fetal adrenal to make aldosterone and cortisol and by the fetal gonad to make testosterone.

The placental 3β-hydroxysteroid dehydrogenase also transforms DHA and its 16α-hydroxylated derivative into androstenedione and its 16α-hydroxylated derivative. In the next step, placental aromatase transforms androstenedione into estrone and estradiol, whereas 16α-hydroxyandrostenedione is metabolized into estriol. Most of these estrogens are excreted by the mother. It is of interest to note that the large

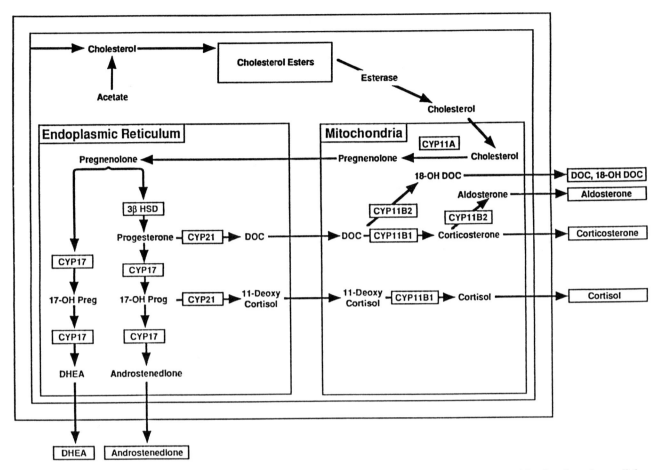

Figure 2 Subcellular location of the various steps of steroidogenesis in an adrenal cell. Cholesterol from blood or from intracellular synthesis is stored as cholesterol esters. An esterase makes cholesterol available when needed. CYP11A is located in the mitochondria. The pregnenolone formed moves to the endoplastic reticulum where it is submitted to the effects of 3β-HSD, CYP17, and CYP21. The resulting 11-deoxycorticosterone (DOC) and 11-deoxycortisol return to the mitochondria where the CYP11B1 and CYP11B2 cytochromes are located. The main steroids secreted by the adrenal cortex are shown outside of the adrenal cell. (From Ref. 2.)

amounts of estriol excreted by the mother are related to the large amounts of 16α-OH-DHA secreted by the adrenal cortex of the fetus.

B. Control of Adrenal Steroid Secretion

1. Regulation of Cortisol Secretion

The ability of the adrenal gland to synthesize cortisol is dependent upon the secretion by the hypothalamus of corticotropin-releasing hormone (CRH). By the use of the short loop of the portal vessel system from the hypothalamus to the anterior pituitary, CRH reaches the corticotrophs and triggers the secretion of adrenocorticotropic hormone (ACTH).

a. CRH and ACTH. CRH is a 41 amino acid straight-chain peptide (6). It is secreted mainly by the median eminence. However, it has also been detected in the cortical part of the brain. CRH binds with high affinity to receptors located on the membrane of the corticotrophs of the anterior

pituitary. This in turn activates the formation of cyclic AMP, which then activates a series of protein kinases, resulting in increased transcription of the proopiomelanocortin gene; appropriate processing of this mRNA results in ACTH formation.

ACTH has a half-life in blood of a few minutes. Although the native hormone has 39 amino acid residues, the first 1–24 amino acid sequence has as much activity as the ACTH itself (7). Like other peptide hormones, ACTH binds to specific membrane receptors of the adrenocortical cells to increase the formation of cyclic AMP and activation of various protein kinases.

The ACTH stimulation of cortisol secretion includes an acute and chronic phase (2). In the acute phase, which takes only a few minutes, cholesterol is made available for steroidogenesis by activating the effect of an esterase on stored cholesterol esters. The more chronic phase is related to a stimulation of transcription of the various cytochrome P450 genes. A "steroidogenetic factor 1" (SF-1) appears to be

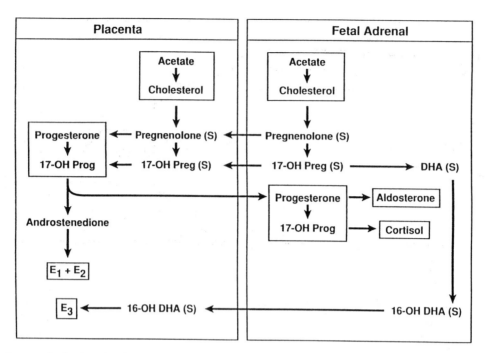

Figure 3 The placenta–fetal adrenal unit. The fetal adrenal can readily synthesize pregnenolone, 17-hydroxypregnenolone and 16-hydroxy-DHA. However, it has little or no 3β-HSD. The placenta, which is rich in this enzyme, transforms the fetal steroids into progesterone, 17-hydroxyprogesterone, and estriol. In the next step, progesterone and 17-hydroxyprogesterone are returned to the fetal adrenal which can then synthesize aldosterone and cortisol. (From Ref. 1.)

responsible for this stimulation (8). Of great interest is the recent finding that SF-1 is also necessary for the formation of steroidogenic tissues, specifically the adrenal glands and the gonads (9).

b. Mechanisms Regulating Cortisol Secretion. Three physiologic mechanisms play an important role in the secretion of cortisol: pulsatile secretion and diurnal variation, stress, and negative feedback.

i. Pulsatile secretion and diurnal variation in cortisol.
The collection of blood samples at frequent intervals has shown that cortisol is secreted in a pulsatile manner (10). Previously (11) it was observed that the plasma concentration of cortisol showed a specific diurnal variation, the highest peak taking place between 4 and 6 a.m. The concentrations then tend to decrease for the rest of the day, being at their lowest in the evening and during the night (Fig. 4).

ii. Stress. Surgical stress, such as trauma and tissue destruction, medical stress, such as acute illness, fever, and hypoglycemia, and emotional stress related to psychologic upset result in most cases in an important increase in cortisol secretion. How these various types of stress influence steroid output is not clear. However, studies of the immune system have shown that leukocytes secrete a series of peptide hormones, the interleukins (12). Their formation is markedly increased during stress, and two of them, interleukin-1 and interleukin-6, have been shown to stimulate CRH secretion and therefore to increase cortisol secretion (13).

iii. Negative feedback. Another important physiologic mechanism controlling cortisol secretion is negative feed-

back. Under normal conditions, there is equilibrium between the rate of secretion of ACTH and that of cortisol. When the plasma concentration of cortisol increases markedly, it has a negative effect on the secretion of CRH and ACTH. By this mechanism, cortisol levels in blood regulate the rate of output of CRH and ACTH.

c. Cortisol Secretion Rate. In normal children of various ages and in adult subjects, the rate of cortisol secretion increases with body size (14). When the values are corrected for body surface area, the rates are similar at various ages; the average ± standard deviation (SD) is 12.1 ± 1.5 mg/m^2/24 h (Fig. 5). However, there is a large range of variation from one individual to the other. In infants born by vaginal delivery, the secretion corrected for body surface area is slightly greater during the first 5–10 days of life.

2. Regulation of Aldosterone Secretion

Aldosterone is secreted by the cells of the zona glomerulosa of the adrenal cortex. It is mainly under the control of angiotensin II. As shown in Figure 6, the liver produces a large protein, angiotensinogen, which is cleaved by a proteolytic enzyme, renin, which is secreted by the juxtaglomerular cells of the kidney. A converting enzyme then transforms angiotensin I into angiotensin II.

Potassium concentration in plasma and ACTH also play a role in the control of aldosterone secretion. The effect of ACTH is an acute stimulation related to the rapid increase in availability of cholesterol from the cholesterol ester reserve

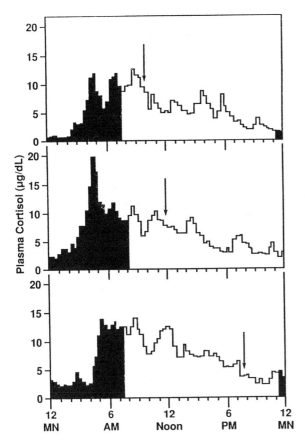

Figure 4 Diurnal variation of plasma cortisol in three normal adult subjects. Black areas represent periods of sleep. (From Ref. 105.)

(15). As shown in Figure 7, an intravenous (IV) injection of ACTH very quickly raises plasma aldosterone levels, but after 60 minutes the levels tend to decrease.

3. Regulation of Adrenal Androgen Secretion

Adrenal androgens are secreted in large amounts during fetal life. Their production decreases rapidly after birth and is not resumed until puberty. The factor that triggers the pubertal secretion of adrenal androgens is not ACTH because its levels are not different before and after puberty. However, large amounts of ACTH given chronically markedly increase the secretion of adrenal androgens. It has been postulated that a pituitary peptide other than ACTH but not yet characterized is responsible for this stimulation, and it has been named adrenal androgen stimulating hormone (16).

C. General Metabolism

As shown in Figure 8, adrenal steroids are transported by blood to reach their target tissues. The liver is one of the target tissues as well as an important site for the catabolism of the steroids.

The main glucocorticoid is cortisol. Between 80 and 90% is bound to a specific glycosylated α-globulin known as corticosteroid binding globulin (CBG), also called transcortin (17). Transcortin has a very high affinity for cortisol, but it can also bind progesterone, prednisolone, and, with less affinity, aldosterone (18). Another 7% of the total circulating cortisol is loosely bound to albumin, and about 2–3% is not bound to protein. This unbound cortisol is the fraction of the total that is available to target cells. In these cells, cortisol binds to a specific glucocorticoid receptor. The receptor-steroid complex binds to the glucocorticoid receptor elements located in the promoter area of responsive genes. By activating the transcription of such genes, glucocorticoids express their biologic activity.

The main mechanism of catabolism is a reduction of the steroid molecule and eventually conjugation with glucorinic or sulfuric acid to make products that are water soluble and readily excreted by the kidney as urinary metabolites.

Although aldosterone can bind to CBG, most of the binding sites of this protein are occupied by cortisol. For this reason, aldosterone is physiologically mainly bound to albumin. Its half-life in blood is about 20–30 minutes, compared with 60–80 minutes for cortisol. In target cells, aldosterone binds to its own specific receptor, the mineralocorticoid receptor. The mode of action of this steroid-receptor complex is similar to that described for cortisol.

D. Tests of Adrenocortical Function

Many types of tests have been proposed for the determination of adrenocortical function. In what follows, we outline only the tests considered important and practical for diagnostic purposes.

1. Tests Related to Glucocorticoid Function

a. 8 a.m. Plasma Cortisol Concentrations. It is necessary to obtain plasma levels of cortisol at a specific time of the day because of the diurnal variation discussed earlier. However, even this precaution may not be sufficient because of the episodic secretion of the steroid. In general, a single plasma value is of limited clinical significance.

There are conditions for which one must determine the plasma concentrations of cortisone and corticosterone. Normally, their concentrations are approximately one-tenth that of cortisol at 8 a.m. Changes in the ratios of these steroids to cortisol in a single blood sample may therefore be indicative of a specific abnormality of adrenal secretion.

b. Urinary 17-Hydroxycorticosteroids (17-OHCS). About 25% of secreted cortisol is excreted as 17-OHCS. For this reason, determination of their 24 h urine excretion gives a good indication of the 24 h cortisol secretion. Indeed, this test is of interest in ruling out Cushing's disease. In normal subjects, the mean ± SD urinary 17-OHCS is 2.9 ± 1.2 mg/m^2/24 h (14).

c. Urinary Free Cortisol. Approximately 0.25–0.5% of secreted cortisol is excreted as cortisol itself. Because urinary free cortisol reflects the amount of unbound cortisol

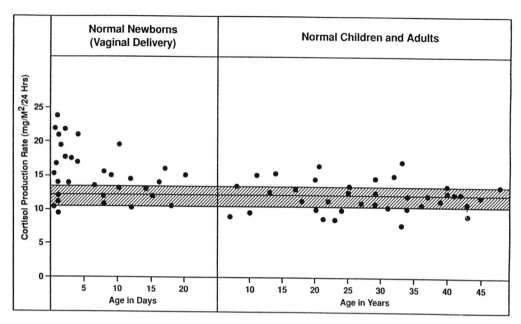

Figure 5 Cortisol secretion rate in newborn infants, children and adults. The values have been corrected for body surface area. The rates expressed in mg/M²/24 hours, were fairly constant throughout life except in the first few days when they were somewhat higher. (From Ref. 1.)

available to target cells (i.e., non–protein-bound cortisol), this test is considered of greater biologic importance than that of urinary 17-OHCS. In our opinion, however, both tests should be obtained in a single 24 h urine specimen when screening for Cushing syndrome.

d. ACTH Test. At present, the standard technique involves the IV bolus administration of 0.25 mg 1,24-ACTH (Cortrosyn). Blood samples are obtained at 0, 60, and 120 minutes after ACTH injection. As seen in Figure 7, plasma cortisol increases to about 30 μg/dl (15).

A normal baseline and a normal increment by 120 minutes rule out primary adrenal insufficiency. This test is also useful when determining the mineralocorticoid function of the adrenals.

e. Metyrapone (Metopirone) Test. Given acutely, Metopirone has the property of blocking 11β-hydroxylation. This results in decreased secretion of cortisol and corticosterone with a decrease in negative feedback on the hypothalamic-pituitary axis. As a consequence, there is an increase in ACTH secretion with an increased secretion of 11-deoxysteroid, specifically 11-deoxycortisol (compound S) and 11-deoxycorticosterone. The present standardized test consists of the administration of a single oral dose of Metopirone (300 mg/m²/per dose) at midnight and measurement the next day at 8 a.m. of plasma 11-deoxycortisol. If adrenocortical function is normal and if the pituitary is capable of increasing its ACTH secretion, the plasma concentration of 11-deoxycortisol rises to values of 7–22 μg/dl (19).

There is the possibility that Metopirone may not be available commercially in the near future. If this occurs, it is

probable that the acute ACTH test described earlier can give similar information.

f. Dexamethasone Suppression Test. Dexamethasone is a potent glucocorticoid that, given in small amounts, suppresses ACTH secretion and secondarily decreases cortisol secretion. The suppressing effects of the test are measured either by the determination of plasma ACTH and cortisol or by the determination of urinary excretion of free cortisol and total 17-OHCS.

In the low-dose or single-dexamethasone suppression test, 1.25 mg dexamethasone/m²/24 h is administered for 2 days. In the high-dose or triple-dexamethasone suppression test, 3.75 mg dexamethasone/m²/24 h is administered for an additional 2 days.

g. The CRH Test. Following the IV administration of CRH (100 μg/dose), there is a moderate but significant increase in both plasma cortisol and ACTH, the maximum response being about 60 minutes after injection. In Cushing's disease, there is a greatly exaggerated response of both plasma cortisol and ACTH, whereas in ectopic ACTH syndrome there is no change, as shown in Figure 9 (20).

2. Tests Related to Mineralocorticoid Secretion

a. Plasma Aldosterone and 11-Deoxycorticosterone. Concentrations of plasma aldosterone are quite variable, changing rapidly in relation to body posture, the standing values being greater than those while supine (15). Plasma concentrations of aldosterone are also influenced by chronic changes in sodium intake, the concentration being 15–30 ng/dl on a low-sodium diet (less than 17 mEq/24 h) and 2–12 ng/dl on a normal sodium diet (150–200 mEq/24 h in adults).

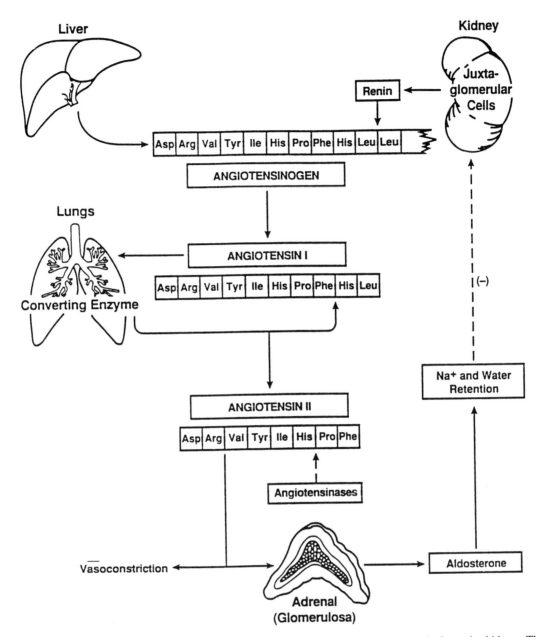

Figure 6 Control of aldosterone secretion. Angiotensinogen of hepatic origin is cleaved by renin from the kidney. The resulting angiotensin I is further cleaved into angiotensin II, an 8 amino- acid peptide which has properties of vasoconstriction on vessels and of activating secretion of aldosterone by the cells of the glomerulosa. (From Ref. 1.)

The plasma concentrations of DOC, like those of aldosterone, tend to be higher in early infancy (from 8 to 5 ng/dl) than later in childhood (5–10 ng/dl), as reported by Lashansky et al. (21).

As shown in Figure 7, ACTH acutely increases aldosterone concentration. There is also a three- to fivefold increase in DOC.

b. Urinary Excretion of Aldosterone and DOC. A small fraction of secreted aldosterone is excreted as a 21-oxoglucoronide conjugate. Following hydrolysis at pH 1.0,

aldosterone is freed and is measured by radioimmunoassay. Under normal sodium intake, the values are 3–10 μg/24 h, and on a low-sodium diet, they are 20–50 μg/24 h.

III. HYPOADRENOCORTICISM

Adrenal insufficiency can be caused by an abnormality of the adrenal glands (primary adrenocortical insufficiency) or by a decreased secretion of hypothalamic CRH and pitu-

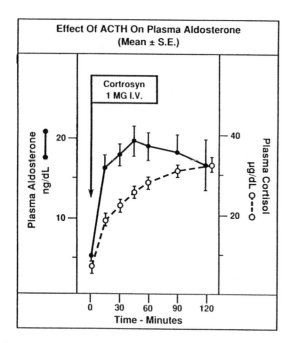

Figure 7   Effects of 1,24-ACTH on the plasma concentration of cortisol and aldosterone in 16 normal subjects. (From Ref. 15.) Copyright, the Endocrine Society.

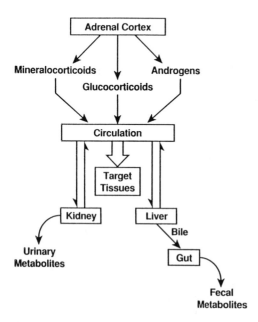

Figure 8   General metabolism of adrenal steroids. In the blood circulation, the steroids are mainly bound to specific proteins. The small unbound fraction is available to target tissues where the steroids express their biological effects. At the same time, steroids are metabolized and conjugated by the liver. The conjugates are returned to the circulation and excreted in bile by the kidney as urinary metabolites. (From Ref. 1.)

itary ACTH (hypoadrenocorticism secondary to deficient CRH and/or ACTH secretion). In rare cases the insufficiency is related to an inability of the target organs to respond to adrenal steroids (hypoadrenocorticism related to end-organ unresponsiveness). The classification of these various disorders is outlined in Table 2.

A.   Primary Adrenocortical Insufficiency

There are many causes of primary adrenal insufficiency (Table 2). In some cases, there has been a lack of differentiation of the glands (congenital adrenal aplasia) or inappropriate development (X-linked adrenal hypoplasia). In other cases, a mutation of the ACTH receptor on the membrane of the adrenocortical cells does not permit adequate stimulation of adrenal secretion (adrenocortical unresponsiveness to ACTH). Another group of abnormalities involves a mutation of one of the enzymes necessary for steroid biosynthesis (congenital adrenal hyperplasia, adrenoleukodystrophy, acid lipase deficiency, steroid sulfatase deficiency, and mineralocorticoid deficiency). Finally, there can be postnatal destruction of the adrenal cortex, either acute (adrenal hemorrhage) or chronic (addison's disease).

1. Congenital Adrenal Aplasia

This is believed to be caused by a developmental disorder of the adrenal anlage during fetal life. Symptoms occur shortly after birth and are characterized by acute shock with tachycardia, hyperpyrexia, cyanosis, and rapid respiration. Untreated, it evolves to total vascular collapse and death.

The symptoms of congenital adrenal aplasia are quite similar to those present in other conditions, such as septicemia and intracranial hemorrhage. The rapid evolution of adrenal aplasia to death is the reason it is often diagnosed at autopsy.

2. X-Linked Adrenal Hypoplasia Congenita

Among families presenting multiple cases of adrenal insufficiency, several suggested the possibility of a X-linked trait. In 1980, Guggenheim et al. (22) reported an association of glycerol kinase deficiency (GKD) with Duchenne muscular dystrophy (DMD) and adrenal hypoplasia congenita (AHC). Later, these disorders were reported to be associated with Xp21 interstitial deletion (23).

a. Pathophysiology.   The deletions of the X chromosome associated with AHC, GKD, and DMD have permitted mapping the locus of these three disorders, as well as the locus of chronic granulomatous disease, retinitis pigmentosa, and ornithine transcarbamylase deficiency, the last locus being the closest to the centromere and AHC being the closest to the end of Xp (24). However, it is not clear how the deletion of the AHC locus results in hypoplastic adrenals. The adrenal cortex in patients studied at autopsy shows a small number of large adrenocortical cells, hence the name cytomegalic adrenal hypoplasia given by pathologists.

b. Clinical Manifestations and Mapping of Xp21. AHC appears early in infancy with signs of acute adrenal insufficiency. However, the signs may occur later in

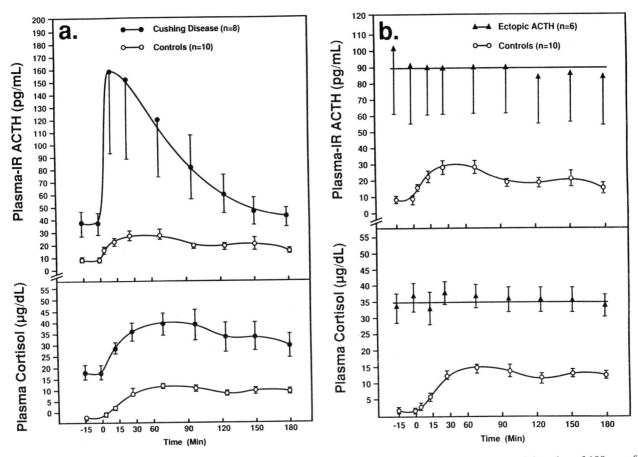

Figure 9 The CRH stimulation test. The figure shows the response of plasma cortisol and ACTH to IV administration of 100 μg of CRH in adult controls and in patients with Cushing's disease (a) and in patients with Cushing's due to ectopic ACTH (b). (From Ref. 20.)

childhood and be somewhat milder. Growth failure with short stature is often observed. In AHC caused by a deletion involving other genetic loci, such as GKD and DMD, signs of glycerol kinase deficiency and myopathy are also present.

In a series of patients presenting with the association of AHC, GKD, and DMD, mental retardation was reported in most of the cases, suggesting the existence of a contiguous locus involved in mental function (25). However, it must be considered that subjects with adrenal insufficiency may have intrinsic reasons for mental retardation in relation to hypoglycemic episodes and abnormal electrolyte balance. A number of such patients are also known. In addition, several patients with the karyotype 46, XY, Xp21 del have presented with testicular abnormalities, including anorchia, cryptorchidism, and hypogonadotropic hypogonadism (26). This has led to the suggestion of a locus for hypogonadotropic hypogonadism (HH locus) near the AHC locus (27). More recently, duplication of a DSS locus contiguous to the AHC locus was observed in subjects with male to female sex reversal (28).

c. Laboratory. Hormonal and electrolyte studies are characteristic of adrenocortical insufficiency: low basal cortisol and aldosterone levels responding poorly to an ACTH test, elevated ACTH concentrations, and hyponatremic, hyperkalemic acidosis.

GKD association is demonstrated by elevated serum and urine glycerol levels. Because glycerol is measured in the triglyceride assay, there is pseudohypertriglyceridemia. Muscle biopsy showing elevated serum creatine kinase confirms Duchenne muscular dystrophy. A luteinizing hormone-releasing hormone (LHRH) test helps in determining hypogonadotropic hypogonadism.

d. Genetics. The clinical abnormalities of AHC and associated disorders in cases with Xp21del most probably demonstrate a relation of cause to effects between the chromosomal deletion and the specific symptoms.

All cases of AHC, GKD, and DMD associated with an X deletion occurred in male subjects, suggesting X-linked recessive traits. Unaffected mothers of patients have been shown to be heterozygous for the deletion Xp21 del (23). However, one female case has been reported (25).

e. Treatment. Steroid replacement for both glucocorticoids and mineralocorticoids is necessary. If GKD

Table 2　Classification of Syndromes of Hypoadrenocorticism

Primary adrenocortical insufficiency
　Congenital adrenal aplasia
　X-linked adrenal hypoplasia
　Adrenocortical unresponsiveness to ACTH
　　(deficient ACTH receptor)
　Congenital adrenal hyperplasia (CAH)
　Adrenoleukodystrophy/adrenomyeloneuropathy
　Wolman disease (acid lipase deficiency)
　Steroid sulfatase deficiency (X-linked ichthyosis)
　Mineralocorticoid CMOI or CMOII (CYP11B2) deficiency
　Adrenal hemorrhage of the newborn
　Adrenal hemorrhage of acute infection
　Chronic hypoadrenocorticism (Addison's disease)
Secondary to deficiency CRH and/or ACTH secretion
　Hypopituitarism
　Cessation of glucocorticoid therapy
　Removal of a unilateral cortisol-producing tumor
　Infants born to steroid-treated mothers
　Respiratory distress syndrome
　Anencephaly
Related to end-organ unresponsiveness
　Cortisol resistance (deficient glucocorticoid receptor)
　Aldosterone resistance (deficient mineralocorticoid receptor)

is present, appropriate therapy must be given. Unfortunately, Duchenne muscular dystrophy is not treatable at this time.

3. Adrenocortical Unresponsiveness to ACTH (Deficient ACTH Receptor)

a. Pathogenesis. This disorder is caused by an inability of the adrenal cells of the zona fasciculata and reticularis to respond to ACTH. The lack of ACTH response is caused by a genetic abnormality of the ACTH receptor (29).

b. Clinical Manifestations. It is characterized by feeding problems in early life, failure to thrive, hypoglycemia, and hyperpigmentation of the skin (30). In some cases, the symptoms seem to occur later in infancy, perhaps because the frequent feedings of the neonatal period avoided major hypoglycemic episodes.

c. Laboratory. As already noted, glucose levels are quite low but there is no electrolyte abnormality. During a hypoglycemic episode, a blood sample demonstrates high growth hormone and low insulin concentrations with low cortisol levels. ACTH measurement shows elevated values, even when cortisol values are low.

d. Genetics. Recently the gene for the ACTH receptor was isolated and sequenced (31). The coding sequence does not contain an intron. The product of this gene is a 297 amino acid protein with seven transmembranic domains, a cytosolic COOH terminus that can react with a G protein to activate adenyl cyclase activity, and an extracellular NH_2 terminus with two possible glycosylation sites.

The disorder is an autosomal recessive trait. In one

family, both parents were heterozygous for the same mutation, the proband being hemozygous for this mutation (32), whereas in another family the parents had different mutations, the patient being an allelic compound (33). A postreceptor mutation has also been reported (34).

e. Treatment. Patients require only glucocorticoid replacement therapy, the mineralocorticoid function being normal.

f. Other Disorders. Although more than 30 cases of adrenocortical unresponsiveness to ACTH have been reported in the literature, it is probable that some of these patients presented with a different disorder. Some cases who presented with neurologic symptoms (35) were probably unrecognized cases of adrenoleukodystrophy. Other patients presented with sodium loss (36). In the past 15 years, several cases of an association of adrenal insufficiency, achelasia, and alacrima (triple A syndrome) have been reported (37,38). This may be a parasympathetic disorder of currently unknown etiology.

4. Congenital Adrenal Hyperplasia

There are five major forms of congenital adrenal hyperplasia (CAH), each of them being caused by a mutation of one of the five enzymes required for the biosynthesis of cortisol. In each of these forms of CAH the decrease in cortisol secretion results in a decrease in negative feedback at the level of the hypothalamus-pituitary (1,2). The resulting increase in ACTH output attempts to return the cortisol secretion to normal if the mutation permits some degree of enzymatic activity. At the same time, the increased ACTH secretion results in a markedly elevated production of the cortisol precursors before the mutant block. The five forms of CAH are 21-hydroxylase deficiency (salt-losing form, simple virilizing form, and attenuated form), 11β-hydroxylase deficiency related to a mutation of CYP11B1, 17-hydroxylase deficiency (hypertensive form) related to CYP17, 3β-HSD deficiency and lipoid adrenal hyperplasia related to a mutation of CYP11A. These disorders are discussed in a separate chapter of this book.

5. Adrenoleukodystrophy (ALD) and Adrenomyeloneuropathy (AMN)

This disorder has also been called diffused cerebral sclerosis associated with adrenal insufficiency.

a. Pathophysiology. It is also known as Siemerling-Creutzfeldt or Schilder's disease. The basic biochemical abnormality is an elevation in plasma and various tissues of the concentration of the very long chain fatty acids (VLCFA), C_{24}, C_{25}, and C_{26}. They probably accumulate because of a defect in their normal breakdown in cellular organelles known as peroxisomes. Pathologically, the adrenal cortex at first shows cytoplasmic striations containing cholesterol esterified with VLCFA. Later the adrenal cells appear to be filled with the abnormal cholesterol esters, and in the final stage the cells tend to atrophy and die (39).

b. Clinical Manifestations. This is a progressive disease of the brain that manifests itself in its early stage by mild symptoms, such as unusual behavior, a mild decrease in visual acuity, and a loss of muscle strength in some limbs. Over a period of a few years, the symptoms progress to dementia, blindness, and quadriparesis and end in death. At various times during this degenerative process, symptoms of adrenal insufficiency may occur, involving both cortisol and aldosterone function.

c. Genetics. The locus of adrenoleukodystrophy maps to the long arm of the X chromosome (Xq28) (40,41). Because of the location of the gene on the X chromosome, the disorder is expressed only in male subjects. Recently the ALD gene was identified (42). It encodes a 745 amino acid protein that includes six membrane-spanning segments and an ATP binding domain. The role of the ALD protein may be to transport the VLCFA-CoA synthetase. Different mutations have been reported in different families, including six detectable deletions, nine point mutations, three frameshift mutations, and one splicing mutation (43).

d. Various Clinical Forms. Most commonly, the symptoms of adrenoleukodystrophy appear at around 7 years of age. In such patients the neurologic deterioration is somewhat rapid, leading to a bedridden state in 2–3 years. There is also a group of boys in whom the illness appears between 12 and 20 years of age: in these subjects, the neurologic deterioration is usually slower. Finally, the neurologic symptoms may occur after 21 years of age (44). This form of the disorder is called adrenomyeloneuropathy (AMN) because the neurologic manifestations involve the peripheral nerves rather than the brain. However, some AMN patients may have early symptoms of mild adrenal insufficiency. These men also present with primary gonadal failure (45).

It must also be noted that some cases present with either only neurologic manifestations or only addisonian symptoms. Furthermore, a few subjects with the biochemical abnormality of ALD present no clinical features of the disorder, at least for a long period of time. All the forms mentioned earlier are considered allelic and are all X-linked recessive traits.

Except in the rare cases of de novo mutation, the mothers of ALD patients are obligate heterozygotes. These women are free of symptoms, but some of them may present with neurologic abnormalities late in life, usually between 40 and 50 years of age.

e. Autosomal Recessive Forms. Whereas ALD is an X-linked trait, there are also autosomal recessive forms that express themselves in the neonatal period. The biochemical defect appears to be similar to that seen in X-linked ALD, but the symptoms of adrenal insufficiency and central nervous system manifestation are more acute. The Neonatal ALD is caused by a marked decrease in peroxisomes, in contrast to X-linked ALD, which presents with a normal number of peroxisomes. In Zellweger syndrome (cerebrohepatorenal form), the peroxisomes are almost completely absent. Normal peroxisomes are seen in Pseudoneonatal ALD, and such a case has been reported to present with a deletion of the peroxisomal acyl-CoA oxidase gene (46).

The treatment of ALD has been very disappointing. Efforts have been made to change the diet by decreasing the amount of very long chain fatty acids. There have also been attempts at supplementation with glycerol trioleate oil as well as addition of glycerol trierucate oil. Although such drugs appear to improve the condition temporarily, the amelioration is not sustained. Attempts have also been made to treat by bone marrow transplantation but without clear success.

6. Wolman Disease (Acid Lipase Deficiency)

Wolman disease is caused by a deficiency of lysosomal acid lipase (47). This enzyme is an esterase that hydrolyzes cholesterol esters and triglycerides. In such patients the normal esterified lipids accumulate in various cells. It is also called generalized xanthomatosis with calcified adrenals.

Symptoms occur in the first month of life as failure to thrive, anemia, hepatomegaly, and splenomegaly. There is also vomiting and diarrhea as well as jaundice. Shortly thereafter, one can notice the calcified, enlarged adrenal gland and decreased cortisol secretion.

The locus for lysosomal acid lipase deficiency has been mapped to chromosome 10 (48). This is an autosomal recessive trait. There is no treatment for this extremely rare disorder, which ends in death quite rapidly.

7. Steroid Sulfatase Deficiency (X-Linked Ichthyosis)

A deficiency of steroid sulfatase results in the accumulation of sulfated products, such as 3β-hydroxysteroids (particularly DHA-S) and cholesterol sulfate. The ichthyosis is thought to be related to the accumulation in the skin of a large amount of cholesterol sulfate (49). This syndrome is not an adrenocortical insufficiency because cortisol and aldosterone secretions are normal. The normal fetus has a low steroid sulfatase activity and relies on the placenta to accomplish this function. Because the placenta is made of maternal cells and at least one of the maternal X chromosomes is normal, the steroid sulfatase activity is adequate during pregnancy.

The steroid sulfatase gene has been mapped to the X chromosome (Xp22.3) near the pseudoautosomal region of the terminal part of the short arm. Large deletions of the X chromosome in the area of the steroid sulfatase gene have been associated with hypogonadotropic hypogonadism and anosmia (Kallmann syndrome).

8. Mineralocorticoid Deficiency Caused by Mutations of CYP11B2 Gene

As previously discussed, the cytochrome P_{450} encoded by the CYP11B2 gene is capable of making the conversion of DOC to aldosterone by a series of three enzymatic steps: addition of the 11β-hydroxyl group to form corticosterone, 18-hydroxylation (also called corticosterone methyloxydase type I) to form 18-hydroxycorticosterone, and 18-dehydrogenation (also called corticosterone methyloxidase type II) to form aldosterone. Although the same enzyme appears to be involved, two types of aldosterone deficiency, 18-hydroxylase and 18-dehydrogenase, have been reported in the literature.

a. 18-Hydroxylase Deficiency. These patients present with a general failure to thrive related to mild salt wasting. Laboratory studies show decreased aldosterone and 18-hydroxycortisterone with a concomitantly elevated secretion of corticosterone and DOC (50,51). Mineralocorticoid replacement therapy results in the resumption of normal growth in infancy and early childhood. Later in life, treatment becomes unnecessary. Only a few patients have been reported with this disorder.

b. 18 Dehydrogenase Deficiency. The onset of this disorder is also in infancy or early childhood. It is characterized by a failure to thrive and symptoms of mineralocorticoid deficiency, including hyponatremia, hyperkalemia, and acidosis. However, these patients rarely present in acute adrenal crisis. This is probably because some of the precursors of aldosterone that have some sodium-retaining activity are produced in increased amount. Hormonal study shows an increase in plasma renin activity as well as an increase in DOC, corticosterone, and 18-hydroxycorticosterone, along with low aldosterone (52). It is of interest that these patients present with an increased excretion of urinary 17-OHCS; this is because the urinary metabolites of 18-hydroxycorticosterone give the Porter-Silber reaction (53). A very large Iranian Jewish pedigree has been reported with this salt-wasting disorder (54,55). Recently, mutations in the CYP11B2 gene were reported by Pascoe et al. (56).

Treatment consists of mineralocorticoid replacement therapy. It is of interest to note that later in life many of these patients have successfully withdrawn from treatment.

9. Adrenal Hemorrhage of the Newborn

Adrenal hemorrhage occurs more often after prolonged labor and a traumatic delivery, usually of a large male infant. The normal adrenal has a rich network of small vessels between the capsule and the cortex. This is the site of bleeding in adrenal hemorrhage.

Children with massive bilateral adrenal hemorrhage appear in acute shock caused by adrenal insufficiency and incipient blood loss. On the other hand, if the hemorrhage is unilateral, there are usually no adrenal symptoms. The typical laboratory finding is hypoglycemia with hyponatremic, hyperkalemic acidosis. On physical examination a mass can be felt in the flanks. Sonography reveals a mass that tends to displace the kidney downward (57). Residual calcification may be visible on x-ray of the abdomen 3–6 weeks after the bleeding occurred and as the hemorrhage resolves. With time, the calcifications themselves disappear.

The differential diagnosis includes renal vein thrombosis. An ACTH test is useful in differentiating this condition from bilateral adrenal hemorrhage.

10. Adrenal Hemorrhage of Acute Infection

An adrenal crisis may occur during an acute infection, such as fulminating meningococcemia, pneumococcal, streptococcal, haemophilus, and diphtheric infections. The acute adrenal insufficiency occurring with meningococcemia has

also been called Waterhouse-Friderichsen syndrome. The subcapsular hemorrhage is thought to be related to the effects of arterioantitoxin.

Such an acute adrenal crisis occurring at the time of a fulminating infection has an extremely poor prognosis. It is clear that rapid and energetic treatment of the infection, as well as therapy with adrenal steroids in stress doses (IV Solucortef), is necessary.

11. Addison's Disease (Chronic Hypodrenocorticism)

In the days of Thomas Addison, tuberculosis was the most common pathogenesis. Other infections have been reported, such as fungal infections (histoplasmosis and coccidiomycosis). Recently, it was also reported associated with human immunodeficiency virus infection (58). At present, the most important mechanism of destruction of the adrenals is an autoimmune disorder (59).

Addison's disease is much less frequent in children than in adult subjects. The clinical features are directly related to the decreased production of adrenal steroids. All or some of the symptoms of adrenal insufficiency outline in Table 3 may appear. Initially, there is usually general fatigue, muscle pain, weight loss, gastrointestinal symptoms, and hypotension related to salt loss. An acute adrenal crisis may occur at the time of a minor infection or febrile illness. The skin hyperpigmentation is distributed mainly in pressure areas (axillae and groin), as well as in the buccal and vaginal mucosa, the creases of the hand, and the nipples. This hyperpigmentation is related to the increased pituitary secretion of β-lipotropin, which occurs concomitantly with the increased ACTH secretion.

Depending on the etiology of Addison's disease, some other specific symptoms can be expected. In cases involving

Table 3 Signs and Symptoms of Adrenal Insufficiency

Glucocorticoid deficiency
    Fasting hypoglycemia
    Increased insulin sensitivity
    Decreased gastric acidity
    Gastrointestinal symptoms (nausea, vomiting)
    Fatigue
Mineralocorticoid deficiency
    Muscle weakness
    Weight loss
    Fatigue
    Nausea, vomiting, anorexia
    Salt craving
    Hypotension
    Hyperkalemia, hyponatremia, acidosis
Adrenal androgen deficiency
    Decreased pubic and axillary hair
    Decreased libido
Increased β-lipotropin levels
    Hyperpigmentation

---

an infectious agent, there are also signs of this infection in other sites. If the etiology is an autoimmune syndrome, then one usually finds positive adrenal antibodies. In this latter case, the pathology is a progressive lymphocytic infiltration of the adrenal cortex. In such cases, Addison's disease is often associated with other autoimmune disorders, resulting in a polyglandular syndrome (59). Two types of autoimmune disease associations have been described. Type I includes mucocutaneous candidiasis, hypoparathyroidism, and Addison's disease. In addition, one can also observe pernicious anemia, alopecia, vitiligo, and chronic progressive hepatitis. In type II, the association includes Addison's disease and chronic lymphocytic thyroiditis. This association has also been called Schmidt syndrome. If insulin-dependent diabetes also occurs, it is then called Carpenter syndrome.

The diagnosis of Addison's disease is made on the demonstration of a low cortisol concentration in plasma concomitantly with elevated ACTH levels. Early in the development of the disorder, the cortisol levels may be normal because of adrenal hyperstimulation by high levels of ACTH. The short ACTH test described earlier shows a low or normal cortisol baseline but no increase on ACTH stimulation. Because of the consequences of establishing a diagnosis of Addison's disease, we usually advise also carrying out an intramuscular (IM) ACTH test (25 mg/m^2 every 8 h for 3 days). Urine samples are collected before and on the third day of stimulation for the determination of urinary 17-OHCS and free cortisol.

The typical treatment is replacement of the missing hormone, specifically glucocorticoids and mineralocorticoids. In children, the glucocorticoids are replaced by oral cortisol or prednisone (see Table 4), whereas mineralocorticoids are replaced with Florinef (fludrocortisone). In adolescent and adult females, the lack of adrenal androgens may need to be compensated for by administration of a mild androgenic preparation to improve the libido and the growth of pubic hair.

Table 4 Maintenance and Stress Dose of Glucocorticoid and Mineralocorticoid in Treatment of Adrenal Insufficiency

Therapy	Maintenance mean (range)		Stress
Glucocorticoid replacement, mg/m^2/24 h			
Oral cortisol (one-third dose every 8 h)	24	(18–30)	75
Oral cortisone acetate (one-third dose every 8 h)	30	(24–36)	100
Oral prednisone (one-half dose every 12 h)	5	(4–6)	15
IM cortisone acetate	15	(12–18)	45
Mineralocorticoid replacement, mg/day			
Oral fludrocortisone acetate (Florinef)	0.1	(0.05–0.125)	0.1

B. Hypoadrenocorticism Secondary to Deficient CRH and/or ACTH Secretion

Unless there is an organic abnormality of the hypothalamus or the anterior pituitary, it is often difficult to determine whether a deficient ACTH secretion is related to a deficient output of CRH.

1. Hypopituitarism

Hypopituitarism is characterized by a deficient secretion of one, some, or all pituitary hormones (60). In infancy and childhood the main deficiencies are those of growth hormone, thyroid-stimulating hormone, and ACTH. A deficiency of gonadotropins and prolactin is detected only at puberty. In this chapter we consider ACTH deficiency.

a. Pathophysiology. Various congenital malformations of the brain, particularly midline defects, can result in a deficiency of secretion of hypothalamic hormones, including CRH. The most frequently recognized malformation is the septooptic dysplasia as originally described by de Morsier. This condition includes agenesis of the septum pellucidum, hypoplasia or aplasia of optic nerves and chiasma resulting in various degrees of visual impairment, and abnormality of the hypothalamus causing secondary hypopituitarism. The midline defects may be mild, with partial hypopituitarism and no eye disorder. It may also be extensive and associated with cleft palate and cleft lip. An absence of gonadotropin secretion during fetal life may result in micropenis in male infants. Congenital malformation of the pituitary gland can also occur and may be the cause of empty sella turcica.

Head trauma either at delivery or later in life may result in hemorrhage in the area of the hypothalamus or pituitary gland. This in turn may cause hypopituitarism with ACTH deficiency.

Disorders that result in the destruction of normal tissues (hemochromatosis, sarcoidosis, and histiocytosis) can cause hypothalamic and/or pituitary dysfunction. A similar situation can occur following various types of infections, such as meningitis or encephalitis. Similarly, tumors arising in the sella (craniopharyngioma) or the hypothalamus result in hypopituitarism. Radiation of a brain tumor may have the same effect.

In some patients, no specific cause for the hypopituitarism can be detected. Such cases can involve several hormones of the anterior pituitary (idiopathic panhypopituitarism) or, on rare occasions, only ACTH secretion (idiopathic isolated ACTH deficiency).

b. Clinical Manifestations. The congenital malformations described earlier can be manifested by hypoglycemia if ACTH and cortisol secretion are deficient. The hypoglycemia may be more marked if there is concomitant growth hormone secretion deficiency. Persistent hypoglycemia in a newborn requires the collection of a blood sample for the determination of true glucose, cortisol, growth hormone, and insulin concentrations. In hypopituitarism the concentration of all these hormones is very low. In contrast, in nesidioblastosis, the concentration of insulin, growth hormone, and cortisol is markedly elevated concomitantly with low glucose levels.

When the diagnosis of hypopituitarism is established, magnetic resonance imaging (MRI) of the head may show some of the characteristics of septooptic dysplasia or other brain malformation or injury. In head trauma, the MRI shows evidence of hemorrhage. Brain tumors can also be visualized by MRI studies. Various degrees of impairment of mental development can be present, particularly in hypopituitarism secondary to meningitis or encephalitis.

Because hypopituitarism can involve various combinations of tropic hormones, the clinical manifestations in childhood may include symptoms of growth hormone deficiency and hypothyroidism.

Aldosterone secretion is controlled by the renin angiotensin system, so that there are usually no electrolyte or water abnormalities in hypopituitarism. When a destructive process has taken place, however, there can be involvement of the neuronal cells that secrete antidiuretic hormone (ADH), resulting in a disturbance of electrolytes and water balance characteristic of diabetes insipidus. In addition, following neurosurgery, inappropriate ADH secretion can occur that results in electrolyte abnormalities.

By definition, patients with idiopathic isolated ACTH deficiency have normal thyroid function as well as normal growth and normal sexual maturation at puberty (61). Because females rely on adrenal androgens for the development of pubic hair at puberty, women with idiopathic isolated ACTH deficiency present with scant pubic hair.

c. Laboratory Diagnosis. It is expected that a decreased cortisol secretion would result in hypoglycemia. Indeed, hypoglycemia is quite marked in patients who have a combined deficiency of ACTH and growth hormone but is usually mild in the absence of growth hormone deficiency. A low cortisol concentration in an 8 a.m. blood sample may be observed, but values are often low normal to normal.

A single oral dose of Metopirone (metyrapone) given at midnight and an 8 a.m. plasma sample obtained the next morning show a decreased response of plasma 11-deoxycortisol (compound S) in subjects with ACTH deficiency. However, most subjects can respond to the marked stress resulting from the administration of IV Metopirone or IV pyrogen (62,63). When reviewing a large group of patients with hypopituitarism, Brasel et al. (64) found that about 50% of the patients had normal adrenocortical function; most of the others had normal basal cortisol but a poor response to the regular Metopirone test. Among the latter subjects, only those who had an organic lesion could not respond to the IV Metopirone test.

It was reported recently that Metopirone soon may not be available commercially. As a substitute, we suggest the test with 1,24-ACTH given as an IV bolus and measurements of cortisol and aldosterone before and 1 and 2 h after injection.

Finally, in hypopituitarism it is important to check the function of all pituitary hormones.

d. Treatment. Treatment consists of appropriate replacement of the deficient hormones. If basal cortisol levels are abnormally low, then maintenance as well as stress therapy is required, whereas when basal levels are normal but the oral Metopirone test is inappropriate, then stress therapy only is needed.

In addition, patients who have thyroid-stimulating hormone and/or growth hormone deficiency need appropriate replacement. Finally, in ADH deficiency, intranasal desmopressin (DDAVP) is necessary.

2. Cessation of Glucocorticoid Therapy

It is well established that the administration of glucocorticoids suppresses the secretion of CRH by the hypothalamus and of ACTH by the pituitary gland, resulting in secondary adrenal cortex atrophy. When the dose is less than the replacement level, however, for whatever period of time, or if the dose is greater than replacement but for a duration of less than 4 weeks, then no adrenocortical atrophy is expected. By contrast, if the dosage is greater than replacement and the duration of treatment is greater than 4 weeks, then suppression is expected. Experience has shown that recovery occurs within 6 weeks in about half of patients and within 6 months in all subjects (65).

a. Clinical Features. Hypoglycemia may be observed in some patients. Growth delay is mainly related to the duration of glucocorticoid therapy rather than its cessation (60). The greatest problem may occur at the time of a major medical or surgical stress.

b. Laboratory Tests. A Metopirone test is necessary to determine whether the patient has recovered normal adrenocortical function. As mentioned for hypopituitarism, an ACTH test can be simpler and as informative.

c. Treatment. Clearly there is no need for any treatment for subjects who have been treated for less than 4 weeks or for those who have received less than replacement therapy for any period of time. For other patients, treatment is required only at times of stress using a dosage equivalent to two to four times replacement and only for the period of stress. Because more than 90% of subjects recover adrenocortical function after 6 months of cessation of therapy, additional stress doses of steroid are not required after this period of time.

3. Removal of a Unilateral Adrenal Tumor

Tumors that produce excessive amounts of cortisol usually secrete steroids independently of ACTH stimulation. For this reason, such a subject usually presents with suppressed CRH/ACTH secretion and an atrophic contralateral adrenal. During the surgical removal of such tumors, the patient should receive stress dosages of glucocorticoids. After surgery, the dosage should be decreased progressively and the patient should then be considered as those discussed earlier for cessation of glucocorticoid therapy.

4. Infants Born to Mothers Treated with Glucocorticoids

Cortisol administered during pregnancy can cross the placenta, but the fetal concentration is only about 10% of maternal levels. This is in part because the placenta is rich in the enzyme that transforms cortisol into cortisone. This same enzyme transforms prednisolone into prednisone.

Experience has shown that pregnant women treated with prednisone at a dosage of two to five times replacement therapy gave birth to infants whose cortisol secretion rate was normal shortly after birth (66). Nevertheless, such infants should be followed for the possible development of hypoglycemia. Because of the physiology of the control of aldosterone secretion, no electrolyte abnormality is expected in infants born of mothers treated with glucocorticoids.

In contrast to cortisol or prednisone, dexamthasone readily crosses from the mother to the fetus and is used for fetal therapy.

5. Respiratory Distress Syndrome (RDS)

There are some differences of opinion on the optimal use of surfactant and glucocorticoids in the treatment of RDS. If steroids are used, dexamethasone is the choice because it readily crosses the placenta. Therapy may be continued for a period of time in the neonatal period and may therefore result in suppressed adrenocortical function when treatment is stopped (67). In such cases, therapy might be needed at times of stress.

6. Anencephaly

Adrenal glands are very small in patients with anencephaly, probably secondary to the absence of pituitary tissue, leading to adrenal insufficiency.

C. Hypoadrenocorticism Secondary to End-organ Unresponsiveness

Cortisol and aldosterone, like all other steroids, express their effects by binding to a protein specific for each steroid, called a receptor. Receptor abnormalities can cause steroid resistance.

1. Cortisol Resistance

This is a rare disorder that has been discovered in a small number of families (68,69). In all cases the resistance appeared partial: none of the affected subjects completely lacked glucocorticoid activity. The main laboratory characteristics of cortisol resistance are markedly increased plasma concentrations of cortisol and ACTH, as well as elevated excretion of urinary free cortisol and total 17-hydroxycorticosteroids. In addition, a standard dexamethasone suppression test is partially negative. Such laboratory findings are typical of patients with Cushing's disease, yet subjects with cortisol resistance do not present with any of the symptoms of this disorder. The elevated levels of ACTH result in increased secretion not only of cortisol but also of deoxycorticosterone and corticosterone. These two steroids are responsible for the signs of mineralocorticoid excess, including hypertension, hypokalemia, and metabolic alkalosis. As previously mentioned, the genesis of the resistance syndrome is related to an abnormal glucocorticoid receptor. The gene for this receptor has been mapped

to chromosome 5q31–q32 (70). In one family, a point mutation was found in the receptor gene. In all the families reported with this condition, the mode of inheritance has been found to be autosomal dominant.

2. Aldosterone Resistance

Aldosterone resistance is most probably a heterogeneous group of disorders that express themselves clinically as an unresponsiveness of the kidney to aldosterone. One of the first patients described in 1958 by Cheek and Perry (71) presented with a salt-losing syndrome that responded poorly to mineralocorticoid therapy but was adequately corrected by sodium chloride supplementation.

A large number of these patients have shown an improvement with age and often did not require further therapy after 1 or 2 years of age. In other affected subjects, however, therapy had to be continued.

Aldosterone resistance represents at least two different entities since autosomal dominant and autosomal recessive modes of inheritance have been reported (72,73). The gene encoding the mineralocorticoid receptor was cloned recently and mapped to chromosome 4q31 (74). This new knowledge should help us in understanding better the various forms of this disorder.

D. Treatment of Hypoadrenocorticism

1. Acute Adrenal Insufficiency

In the acute adrenal crisis, a deficiency of cortisol and aldosterone as well as dehydration must be considered. Fluid and electrolyte replacement to expand blood volume and increase blood pressure must be instituted immediately, particularly in the neonate or small child, who otherwise may decompensate rapidly. During the first hour of therapy, the patient should receive 20 ml/kg of 0.9% sodium chloride in 5% glucose solution. The intravenous solution should then be continued to deliver 60 ml/kg over the following 24 h.

In general, serum electrolytes improve, plasma concentrations of sodium and chloride returning to normal but serum potassium often remaining elevated. At some time during the period of fluid replacement therapy, steroid replacement is instituted. Cortisol sodium succinate (Solucortef) is given as a IV bolus at a dose of 25 mg/m^2 and is followed by a similar dose added to the 24 h IV maintenance fluid solution. Note that 20–35 mg Solucortef has a mineralocorticoid activity equivalent to 0.1 mg Florinef. After the acute crisis, maintenance therapy is instituted.

2. Maintenance Therapy

a. Glucocorticoid Replacement. Cortisol is the drug of choice because it is the major glucocorticoid secreted physiologically by the adrenal cortex. In infancy and childhood, synthetic preparations with high potency are not recommended for replacement treatment because their proper dosage is difficult to adjust. Furthermore, cortisol has some mineralocorticoid activity, whereas the synthetic preparations have little or none.

On the basis of a cortisol secretion of rate of 12 ± 1.5 mg/m^2/24 h, a dose similar to this secretion given over a 24 h infusion should be a maintenance dose. The oral dosage is approximately twice the physiologic secretion rate, because some oral cortisol is destroyed by the gastric acidity. Because of the short half-life of cortisol, the total 24 h dose must be given in thirds every 8 h. Cortisone acetate is slightly less potent and is given orally at 30 mg/m^2/24 h.

Experience has shown that children of school age and adolescents have problems in remembering to take the midday dose. Prednisone, which has a longer half-life than cortisol, can be used, half of the daily dose being given every 12 h (see Table 4).

Cortisone acetate administered intramuscularly is resorbed slowly, and the daily dose is 15 mg/m^2/24 h. It may also be given every third day using three times the daily replacement dose. This mode of administration is particularly helpful for infants from birth to 18 months of age because it eliminates the risk of drug regurgitation. Some families have elected to continue the IM therapy through childhood and adolescence, finding it more practical than the multiple doses of oral preparations.

b. Mineralocorticoid Replacement. As previously noted, the secretion rate of aldosterone in human subjects is similar from 2 weeks of age to adulthood. Therefore, replacement therapy remains constant regardless of the age of the patient. The only preparation availabe is 9α-fluorocortisol acetate (fludrocortisone, Florinef). It is given orally as a single dose of 0.05–0.150 mg/24 h. Mineralocorticoid therapy is effective only if salt is ingested simultaneously. Infant formulas are very low in salt (about 8–10 mEq/day), and such patients may require a modest sodium chloride supplement (10–20 mEq/day), particularly when they show serum electrolyte abnormalities and elevated plasma renin levels. When the infants start tasting regular table food, the additional salt becomes unnecessary.

3. Therapy During Stress

Subjects who receive glucocorticoid therapy for more than 1 month have an unresponsive hypothalamic-pituitary-adrenal axis. As a result, they require additional glucocorticoids during stress. For minor infection with low-grade fever, increased medication may not be required. In moderate stress the dosage is increased to twice maintenance, and in more severe stress to 3–4 times replacement (see Table 4). If a patient is unable to retain oral therapy during an acute illness, the parents must administer an IM injection of Solucortef (50 mg/m^2). Following the IM injection, the parents are advised to discuss the problem with their physician or to attend the hospital emergency room. If this cannot be done within 8 h following the first injection, then another IM Solucortef is required every 8 h.

4. Treatment at Time of Surgery

At present we advise using Solucortef. A dose of 25 mg/m^2 is given IV just before the start of anesthesia. This is followed by a second dose of 50 mg/m^2 administered as a constant infusion throughout the surgical procedure. A third 50 mg/m^2 dose of Solucortef is then given at a constant rate for the rest of the first 24 h period. During the time that the patient is unable to take oral treatment, constant infusions of Solucortef are continued at 50–75 mg/m^2/24 h.

In both medical and surgical stress it is important to limit the time of increased dose of glucocorticoid to the period of acute stress and to return to maintenance therapy as soon as improvement occurs. Otherwise, the patient may be overtreated and will then present with symptoms of Cushing's disease.

IV. HYPERADRENOCORTICISM

The syndromes of hyperadrenocorticism can be divided into four subgroups, depending on the predominance of a specific type of adrenocortical steroid. In each of these entities, however, other steroids can also be elevated.

1. Hypercortisolism, characterized by elevated cortisol secretion
2. Adrenogenital syndrome, characterized by abnormal secretion of adrenocortical androgens
3. Feminizing syndrome, related to increased estrogen secretion
4. Hyperaldosteronism, caused by excessive aldosterone secretion

A. Hypercortisolism

1. Pathophysiology

Except for the iatrogenic hypercortisolism related to glucocorticoid therapy given in pharmacologic doses, this disorder is quite rare in the newborn period and in childhood. Its frequency increases in adolescence. Harvey Cushing described patients with hypercortisolism related to a pituitary adenoma (75), and the condition has been termed Cushing's disease. When the hypercortisolism is related to an adrenal tumor, it is termed Cushing syndrome. In adults and rarely in children, malignant tumors not necessarily related to an endocrine gland can produce an excessive amount of ACTH, in which case the disorder is called ectopic ACTH syndrome. On occasion, the tumor may produce CRH, which in turn results in increased ACTH secretion and cortisol secretion. Also in adults, chronic alcoholism has been shown to result in increased CRH secretion, which in turn increases ACTH and cortisol output.

2. Clinical Manifestations

The symptoms of hypercortisolism are similar whatever the etiology. Because of the ubiquitous effects of glucocorticoid on general metabolism, the symptoms are multiple and varied (76). In muscle cells, cortisol increases the breakdown of proteins into amino acids but decreases glucose uptake, resulting in decreased glycogen storage and muscle wasting. In fat cells, cortisol increases lipolytic enzymes, resulting in hyperlipidemia, hypercholesterolemia, and redistribution of fat with truncal obesity and moon facies. In liver cells, cortisol increases gluconeogenetic enzymes and aminotransferases, resulting in hyperglycemia, glycosuria, and what is termed insulin-resistant diabetes. In bone cells, cortisol increases the resorption of the protein matrix. Simultaneously, cortisol decreases the synthesis of a specific calcium binding protein, resulting in the inhibition of vitamin D-mediated calcium absorption from the gut; in turn, this produces hypocalcemia, osteomalacia, and growth retardation. These effects of cortisol on bone are further aggravated by an increased renal calcium excretion. Because cortisol has some mineralocorticoid activity, hypercortisolism increases sodium retention and potassium loss along with water retention, resulting in often marked hypokalemia but only slight hypernatremia and mild hypertension.

In addition to increasing cortisol secretion, ACTH increases androgen secretion. Hence, when the hypercortisolism is caused by elevated ACTH secretion, the patients present with signs of virilism.

Hypercortisolism increases gastric acidity, which in turn may result in peptic ulcers. However, this is seen more frequently in adults than in children.

Also note that hypercortisolism can affect the central nervous system, resulting in emotional instability that alternates between depression and euphoria.

3. Laboratory Diagnosis

a. Demonstrate the Presence of Hypercortisolism. This is more reliably done by obtaining a 24 h urine specimen and determining both total urinary 17-hydroxycorticosteroids and free cortisol. In children and adults, the urinary excretion of 17-OHCS is similar when the values are corrected for body size. The normal value is 2.9 ± 1.2 mg/m^2/24 h (mean $\pm$ SD), as shown by the shaded area in Figure 10. Therefore, values of the urinary 17-OHCS below 5.5 mg/m^2/24 h and urinary free cortisol of less than 70 μg/m^2/24 h rule out hypercortisolism. Among obese subjects, about 30% (Fig. 10) have urinary 17-OHCS values above 5.5 mg/m^2/24 h (14). Such subjects require a low-dose dexamethasone suppression test (1.25 mg dexamethasone/m^2/24 h for 2 days). A good suppression suggests obesity and lack of it, hypercortisolism.

b. Determine the Etiology of the Disorder. This is done by carrying out a CRH stimulation test (20) and/or a high-dose dexamethasone suppression test (3.75 mg/m^2/24 h for 2 days). The response of plasma ACTH and cortisol to CRH administration is presented in Figure 9. A marked response in the CRH stimulation test and a good suppression in the high-dose dexamethasone suppression test suggest an hypercortisolism that is pituitary dependent, that is, Cushing's disease. In contrast, a lack of response to the CRH stimulation and a lack of suppression (20) to the high-dose dexamethasone suppression test strongly favor the etiology of the hypercortisolism caused by an adrenal tumor or possibly a tumor producing ectopic ACTH.

c. MRI of the Head and Abdomen. Theoretically, MRI of the head is expected to demonstrate the presence of a tumor in pituitary adenoma. Unfortunately, the adenoma can be very small and is visualized in about only one-third to one-half of cases. MRI of the abdomen visualizes adrenal tumors 1 cm or more in diameter. In hypersecretion of ACTH, bilateral adrenal hyperplasia is observed by MRI in some cases.

d. Bilateral Petrosal Sinus Sampling. This has been

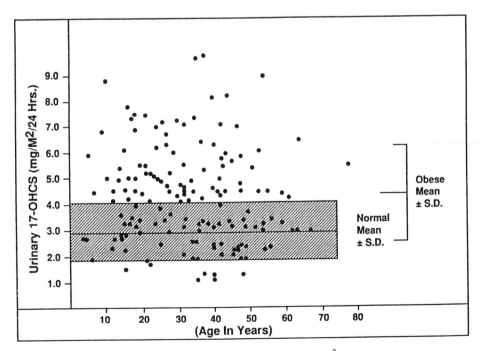

Figure 10 Urinary 17-hydroxycorticosteroids corrected for body surface area (mg/m^2/24 h) in 160 obese individuals of various age. Their values are compared to the mean $\pm$ SD of control subjects (shaded area). About 30% of obese subjects had excretions above the control mean $+2$ SD. (From Ref. 14.)

proposed as a means to localize a small pituitary adenoma that is not visible on the MRI scan. Catheters are place in the left and right inferior petrosal sinuses, and blood samples are obtained before and 10 and 30 minutes after administration of CRH (100 mg/m^2). High baseline concentrations of ACTH are expected. The differential in ACTH increase following CRH should help to determine the location of the microadenoma on the left or right side of the pituitary gland. Although this technique has been reported by some investigators to be successful (77), others have found it to be traumatic for the patient, resulting in a fair amount of body radiation, and not always accurate.

4. Treatment

Clearly, the treatment is dictated by the etiology of the hypercortisolism.

The treatment of Cushing syndrome caused by an adrenal tumor is surgical. An adenoma or well-encapsulated carcinoma without metastasis offers the best opportunity for a complete cure. By contrast, the prognosis of malignant adrenal tumors that produce glucocorticoids is generally poor.

If the tumor is localized before surgery, a transthoracic approach affords excellent exposure and ease of removal. If the tumor is not well localized, a transperitoneal approach is indicated. Patients with metastasis can be treated with the drug mitotane (o,p'-DDD), but results have been disappointing and the drug is not always well tolerated. Cis platin has also been used with limited results.

Autonomous adrenal tumors secrete cortisol in high concentrations and suppress ACTH secretion, resulting in atrophy of the contralateral adrenal gland. Therefore, we advise the following therapy at the time of surgery: an IV dose of 25 mg/m^2 of Solucortef is administered stat just before the start of anesthesia; this is followed by a constant-rate infusion of 50 mg/m^2 of Solucortef throughout surgery; after surgery an additional IV constant-rate infusion of 50 mg/m^2 is given for the rest of the first 24 h period. On postsurgical days, a constant infusion of Solucortef is continued at $50 \text{ mg/m}^2/24 \text{ h}$ until oral therapy can be given at three to four times replacement dose. After the acute period, it may be necessary to continue oral therapy at three-fourths to one-fourths replacement therapy for a few months.

In Cushing's disease with bilateral adrenal hyperplasia, several forms of therapy have been used. In the past, bilateral adrenalectomy was widely employed, resulting in immediate cure of hypercortisolism but also in adrenal insufficiency that required glucocorticoid and mineral corticoid replacement for life and the possibility of development of a pituitary tumor (78). Radiation of the sella turcica has also been used quite extensively in adults but not in children because it often results in destruction of growth hormone-secreting cells; however, newer techniques of delivery of radiation have given good results (79).

Transphenoidal microsurgery is now used to remove pituitary microadenomas and has been successful in bringing about complete cures in many patients (80,81). This form of therapy requires an experience neurosurgical team to obtain the best chances of success (82). In a few patients, surgery

has resulted in panhypopituitarism. Recurrence of the pituitary adenomas can also occur (83).

Several drugs have been used in the treatment of Cushing's disease. Cyproheptadine, a serotonin antagonist, can suppress ACTH secretion, but it is generally not recommended as long-term medical management of the disease and it often does not return the cortisol secretion rate to normal. Bromocriptine, a dopamine agonist, although useful for the treatment of prolactin and growth hormone-secreting pituitary adenomas, has not been of value in ACTH-secreting pituitary tumors. The drugs Metopirone and aminoglutethimide, which suppress adrenal secretion, have been recommended for the short-term, presurgical treatment of Cushing's disease.

Treatment of ectopic ACTH syndrome consists of the removal of the ACTH-secreting tumor. For iatrogenic Cushing syndrome, stopping the excessive glucocorticoid therapy is recommended.

B. Adrenogenital Syndrome

The adrenogenital syndrome is characterized by an abnormally elevated secretion of adrenal androgens. Hence, the virilizing forms of congenital adrenal hyperplasia, mainly 21-hydroxylase and 11-hydroxylase deficiency, are part of the syndrome. However, the excessive androgen secretion of CAH is secondary to an increased ACTH secretion, itself secondary to a deficiency of one of the enzymes required for cortisol biosynthesis. For this reason, CAH is considered a form of hypoadrenocorticism, and the only etiology of adrenogenital syndrome is a virilizing adrenal tumor, a rare condition in childhood.

1. Clinical Manifestations

These tumors result in masculinization of prepubertal children. In boys, it produces a pseudoprecocious puberty (84, 85). Sexual hair—pubic, axillary, and sometimes facial hair—develops whereas the penis is enlarged to adult size, with frequent erections. However, the testes remain prepubertal or slightly enlarged. In girls, this masculinizing syndrome is characterized by pubic and axillary hair with an enlarged and erectile clitoris (Fig. 11).

In both sexes, the excessive secretion of androgens accelerates growth, with an advancement of height age and bone age along with an increase in muscle mass.

An association of such a tumor with body hemihypertrophy and congenital malformations of the urogenital tract has been reported (86). If the clinical picture includes signs of hypercortisolism caused by increased cortisol secretion, then the patient should be considered as presenting with Cushing syndrome. This distinction is important because the prognosis of purely virilizing tumors and mixed tumors is different.

2. Pathology

Virilizing adrenal tumors are usually carcinomas containing malignant cells. Experience shows that the degree of malignancy is low, however, and it is rare to observe metastasis at the time of surgery. In cases of long standing, the tumor may invade the capsule of the adrenal and may metastasize to kidneys, liver, lungs, and bones. On occasion, an adre-

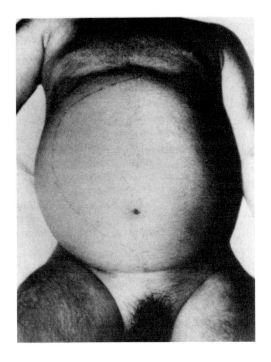

(a)

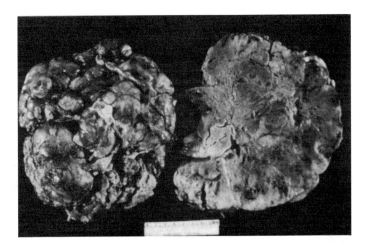

(b)

Figure 11   (a) Abdomen of a 4-year-old girl with virilizing adrenocorticol carcinoma; (b) Surgical specimen. (From Ref. 106.)

nal adenoma may also be virilizing. However, it is often difficult to determine microscopically whether the tumor is malignant or benign. Moreover, the clinical evolution does not always parallel the pathologic appearance.

3. Laboratory Studies

These tumors secrete large amounts of androgens, as demonstrated by the elevated urinary excretion of total 17-

ketosteroids and of dehydroepiandrosterone, along with abnormally high plasma concentrations of DHA and DHA sulfate (87). The latter two steroids are typical markers of virilizing adrenal tumors. There is also hypersecretion of androstenedione. The peripheral metabolism of DHA and androstenedione to testosterone is the cause of the virilism.

In contrast with congenital adrenal hyperplasia, the excessive androgen secretion of virilizing adrenal tumors is not suppressed by dexamethasone administration. In premature adrenarche, the increase in DHA, DHA sulfate, and androstenedione is at or below adult values and can also be suppressed by dexamethasone.

The differential diagnosis also includes virilizing gonadal tumors. In boys, Leydig cell tumors produce mainly testosterone with minimal amounts of DHA and DHA sulfate. In girls, virilizing ovarian tumors occur only after puberty and include the various types of tumors seen in adult women (adrenal rest tumor, hilar cell tumor, and arrhenoblastoma).

Although ultrasound study of the abdomen is usually excellent for the detection of ovarian tumors, it is not very sensitive as far as adrenal tumors are concerned. A computed tomographic (CT) scan or MRI without and with contrast is necessary to localize an adrenal mass.

4. Treatment

The tumor should be excised carefully, without damaging its capsule. Every effort should be made to remove the tumor in bloc. If present, metastases should be removed as completely as possible. In such cases, radiotherapy or chemotherapy with o,p-DDD can be attempted.

Glucocorticoid therapy should be used during and after surgery until the status of the contralateral adrenal gland is determined. Theoretically, such treatment should not be needed if the tumor does not secrete excessive cortisol. Practically, it is easy and safer to administer glucocorticoid.

As previously noted, the prognosis of purely virilizing tumors that are well encapsulated is usually excellent, whereas that of tumors that also secrete excessive amounts of cortisol is generally poor.

C. Feminizing Adrenal Tumors

These tumors are even rarer than virilizing adrenal tumors in infants and children. Extrapolating from experience in adults, approximately half of feminizing adrenal tumors are malignant (88).

1. Clinical Manifestations

In boys, the major sign is gynecomastia; the testes are prepubertal in size, but pubic hair is often present, being related to the concomitant secretion of androgens and estrogens by the tumor. In girls, there is breast development, as seen in precocious puberty; pubic hair can be present, and breakthrough vaginal bleeding may occur. In both sexes, there is rapid statural and osseous development, height age and bone age being significantly advanced.

2. Pathology

For virilizing adrenal tumors, the diagnosis of malignancy is often quite difficult.

3. Laboratory Diagnosis

Urinary and plasma estrogen levels are usually elevated. Most of the tumors also secrete an excess of androgens, resulting in increased urinary 17-ketosteroids and plasma DHA, DHA sulfate, androstenedione, and, to some extent, testosterone. This excessive secretion of steroids is not dexamethasone suppressible. Often the laboratory results are usually not characteristic.

CT scan and/or MRI is needed to make the definitive diagnosis of adrenal tumor.

4. Differential Diagnosis

Because of the lack of specificity of the clinical signs and hormone assays, the diagnosis of feminizing adrenal tumor is usually difficult.

Gynecomastia is a physiologic finding in pubertal males, and it is not easy to differentiate the breast enlargement that accompanies precocious puberty in a young boy from that of a feminizing adrenal tumor. A modest increase in testicular size in precocious puberty may not be differentiated from infantile testes in feminizing tumor. An LHRH test may be useful, showing a pubertal increase in LH in precocious puberty.

In prepubertal girls, a feminizing adrenal tumor must be differentiated from premature thelarche and idiopathic sexual precocity. Estrogens are markedly increased in an adrenal tumor but not in premature thelarche. A positive LHRH test should be helpful in determining sexual precocity.

5. Treatment

The tumor should be removed surgically promptly after the diagnosis has been established. If the tumor did not secrete excessive amounts of cortisol or 11-deoxycortisol, the prognosis is usually good.

D. Hyperaldosteronism

The various syndromes of hyperaldosteronism are outlined in Table 5.

1. Secondary Hyperaldosteronism

An increase in plasma renin activity with increased aldosterone secretion is a physiologic mechanism for the mainte-

Table 5 Syndromes of Hyperaldosteronism

1. Secondary hyperaldosteronism
     Physiologic attempts to maintain serum
     Electrolytes and fluid volumes
2. Primary hyperreninemia
     Renal ischemia
     Juxtaglomerular cell tumor
3. Primary hyperaldosteronism
     Adrenocortical adenoma
     Bilateral glomerular hyperplasia
4. Bartter syndrome
5. Dexamethasone-suppressible hyperaldosteronism
6. Apparent mineralocorticoid excess: Familial
     11β-dehydrogenase deficiency

nance of serum electrolyte concentrations and fluid volume. It occurs with sodium loss, potassium retention, or decreased intravascular volume. Sodium loss occurs during diarrhea or excessive sweating. It also happens with administration of diuretics, in patients with renal tubular acidosis or salt-losing nephritis. The edema of the nephrotic syndrome or the ascites of cirrhosis of the liver causes a decrease in blood volume that results in compensatory increased aldosterone secretion. In all these conditions, the hyperaldosteronism is an attempt to reestablish an electrolyte-water balance, and this is termed secondary hyperaldosteronism. It may also occur in hypertension related to a unilateral renal disease with increased plasma renin activity. The increased aldosterone secretion characteristic of the non–salt-losing form of 21-hydroxylase deficiency can also be considered a secondary hyperaldosteronism because it occurs in response to the salt-losing tendency created by excessive secretion of 17-hydroxyprogesterone and progesterone.

2. Primary Hyperreninemia

The most common cause is renal ischemia, whether unilateral or bilateral. Such ischemia results in excessive secretion of renin by the juxtaglomerular apparatus.

Tumors of the juxtaglomerular apparatus have also been reported as a rare cause of renin excess (89).

3. Primary Hyperaldosteronism

In 1955, Conn (90) described a disorder termed primary aldosteronism that was caused by a aldosterone-producing tumor of an adrenal gland. The symptoms included arterial hypertenson, hypokalemic alkalosis, muscle weakness, and polyuria. Subsequently it was demonstrated that the plasma renin activity was markedly decreased. This syndrome is encountered mainly in adulthood, and only a very few cases have been reported in childhood.

a. Clinical Manifestations. The full clinical picture of this disorder is directly related to the hyperaldosteronism. Aldosterone increases potassium excretion, resulting in hypokalemia. This in turn results in muscle weakness with various types of paresthesias and sometimes unusual types of periodic paralysis. It is thought that the chronic hypokalemia is also responsible for the polyuria and resulting polydipsia. Aldosterone increases the retention of sodium, but the hypernatremia is largely compensated for by increased water retention. In turn, the increase in blood volume results in hypertension, both systolic and diastolic.

b. Laboratory Diagnosis. The typical finding is a high aldosterone secretion with low plasma renin activity. Administration of a high-sodium diet or of DOCA fails to suppress aldosterone secretion. The low plasma renin activity differentiates the syndrome from the high renin levels seen in secondary hyperaldosteronism.

A CT scan or MRI is necessary for demonstrating the presence of a mass in one of the adrenals. Because the adrenocortical tumor may be quite small, it may not be seen by MRI. Catheterization of the renal veins and selective adrenal vein sampling for measurement of aldosterone may demonstrate a very large secretion on one side and a lack of aldosterone on the other.

c. Pathology. In most cases, the tumor is an adenoma, but on occasion it can be a carcinoma (91). There can also be bilateral nodular hyperplasia of the adrenal cortex or focal hyperplasia of normal glomerular cells arranged in a nodular fashion.

d. Treatment. The adrenal tumor should be removed. Because it does not secrete cortisol, there is usually no need for glucocorticoid therapy during surgery.

In bilateral nodular hyperplasia, bilateral adrenectomy may be considered. In such cases, however, medical treatment with spironolactone, an inhibitor of aldosterone biosynthesis, is preferable if it can control the hypertension.

4. Bartter Syndrome

This disorder is thought to be related to a renal tubular defect of chloride reabsorption. This results in passive loss of sodium, which in turn activates the renin-angiotensin-aldosterone system. In addition, the hyperaldosteronism results in hypokalemic alkalosis.

Patients usually present in infancy with failure to thrive, vomiting, weakness, and dehydration. The blood pressure is normal. There is hypochloremic metabolic alkalosis with hypokalemia and usually normal blood sodium. Plasma renin activity and aldosterone are elevated. One finds an increased urinary excretion of chloride and potassium with elevated excretion of prostaglandin. Renal biopsy shows hyperplasia of the juxtaglomerular apparatus (92).

There is no specific therapy, and an attempt is made to correct the electrolyte abnormalities. In some patients, the use of prostaglandin synthetase inhibitors, such as indomethacin or salicylates, can be beneficial.

5. Dexamethasone-Suppressible Hyperaldosteronism (Glucocorticoid-Remediable Aldosteronism)

In 1966, Sutherland et al. (93) reported a clinical condition characterized by hypertension, increased aldosterone secretion, and low plasma renin activity that was fully relieved by administration of dexamethasone (93,94). Most recent progress in the molecular biology of steroid biosynthesis has been able to demonstrate that this disorder was related to a chimeric gene encoding for a cytochrome P_{450} possessing aldosterone synthetase activity but capable of responding to ACTH stimulation (Fig. 12). It is inherited as an autosomal dominant trait.

a. Clinical Manifestation. Symptoms and laboratory abnormalities in this disorder are identical to those found in primary hyperaldosteronism caused by an adrenal adenoma (93,94). They include hypertension, hypokalemia, elevated plasma aldosterone concentrations, and low plasma renin activity. However, and in contrast to primary hyperaldosteronism, the hypertension, hypokalemia, increased aldosterone secretion, and low plasma renin activity can be returned to normal by the administration of dexamethasone. It has been noted that affected subjects

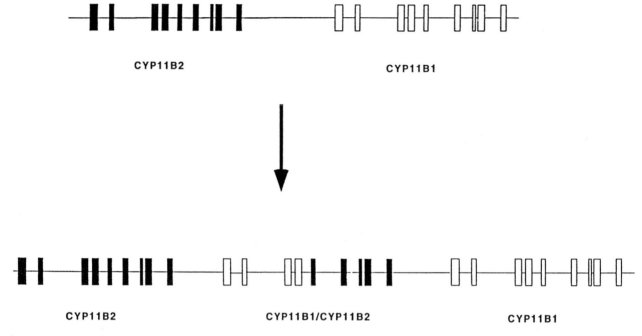

Figure 12 Gene organization of the CYP11B1 and CYP11B2 genes (upper part of the figure) and organization of the hybrid CYP11B1/CYP11B2 gene resulting from unequal crossing-over (lower part of the figure). The resulting hybrid gene can be stimulated by ACTH as it includes the promotor of the B1 gene and can form aldosterone as it includes the 3′ end of the B2 gene. (From Ref. 2.)

always present with hypertension, but the degree of hypokalemia is quite variable.

b. Pathogenesis. There are two genes, CYP11B1 and CYP11B2, that encode for a cytochrome P_{450} possessing 11β-hydroxylase activity. However, CYP11B1 is mainly expressed in the zona fasciculata, under ACTH control, and CYP11B2 is mainly expressed in the zona glomerulosa, under angiotensin II control. The product of the CYP11B2 gene is also called aldosterone synthetase, which is capable of activating 18-hydroxylation and 18-oxidation in addition to 11β-hydroxylation. Both genes are located on chromosome 8q22.

It was recently proposed that a hybrid gene, CYP11B1/CYP11B2, as shown in Figure 12, is the cause of the disorder (95–97). The promotor of the hybrid gene is derived from the CYP11B1 and is therefore responsive to ACTH, but the chimeric protein encoded by this gene has the function of the aldosterone synthetase, hence the reason for the ACTH-dependent hyperaldosteronism. Because the chimeric gene is expressed in the zone fasciculata, which also expresses the CYP17 gene, there can be secretion of cortisol, which has also been hydroxylated in the carbon 18. Indeed, the secretion of 18-hydroxy and 18-oxocortisol is characteristic of dexamethasone-suppressible hyperaldosteronism. A series of recent reports have indeed identified such a chimeric gene, which includes the 5′ sequences of the CYP11B1 gene and the 3′ sequences from the CYP11B2 gene.

c. Treatment. As expressed by the name of the syndrome, dexamethasone or other glucocorticoid

administration in replacement doses turns off ACTH secretion, which in turn blocks aldosterone secretion as well as cortisol output.

6. Familial Deficiency of 11β-Dehydrogenase

This congenital disorder is characterized by an apparent mineralocorticoid excess (98,99). A gene encoding 11β-dehydrogenase has been cloned and mapped to chromosome 1 (100). This enzyme has the property of metabolizing cortisol into cortisone. In blood, the ratio of cortisol to cortisone is 5:1 to 10:1. In contrast, the kidney is rich in 11β-dehydrogenase, and only cortisone is found in this organ (101,102). Under physiologic conditions the receptor protein for mineralocorticoids has equal affinity for cortisol and aldosterone, but cortisone does not bind.

a. Pathophysiology. In this syndrome, a deficiency of 11β-hydroxysteroid dehydrogenase in the kidneys results in binding of cortisol to the mineralocorticoid receptor. In view of the large concentration of cortisol relative to aldosterone, there is sodium retention and water retention. The increased blood volume results in hypertension, and the increased mineralocorticoid activity generates hypokalemia. Under such conditions, plasma concentrations of aldosterone and renin activity are low.

b. Treatment. The severe hypertension in this disorder is generally resistant to any medical therapy. Dexamethasone binds to the glucocorticoid receptor with high activity but does not interact with the mineralocorticoid receptor. The full suppression of cortisol secretion by dexamethasone does not improve the hypertension, however, suggesting that the increased mineralocorticoid activity of the syndrome is mediated by both the renal glucocorticoid receptor and the mineralocorticoid receptor (103).

It has been reported that subjects who ingest large amounts of licorice develop hypertension and hypokalemia, with low levels of plasma aldosterone and plasma renin activity. It has been shown (104) that licorice contains glycyrrhizic acid, which has the property of inhibiting 11β-hydroxysteroid dehydrogenase activity.

REFERENCES

1. Migeon CJ, Donohoue PA. Adrenal Disorders In: Kappy MS, Blizzard RM, Migeon CJ, eds. Wilkins Diagnosis and Treatment of Endocrine Disorders in Childhood and Adolescence. Springfield, IL: Charles C. Thomas, 1994:717–856.

2. Donohoue PA, Parker K, Migeon CJ. Congenital adrenal hyperplasia. In: Scriver CR, et al., eds. The Metabolic Basis of Inherited Disease. New York: McGraw-Hill, 1995:2929–2966.

3. Gotoh O, Tagashira Y, Iizuka T, Fujii-Kuriyaman Y. Structural characteristics of cytochrome P-450. Possible location of the heme-binding cysteine is determined amino-acid sequences. J Biochem 1983; 93:807.

4. Miller WL. Structure of genes encoding steroidogenic enzymes. J Steroid Biochem 1987; 27:759.

5. Curnow KM, Tusie-Luna MT, Pascoe L, et al. The product of the CYP11B2 gene is required for aldosterone biosynthesis in the human adrenal cortex. Mol Endocrinol 1991; 5:1513.

6. Vale W, Spiess J, Rivier C, Rivier J. Characterization of a 41-residue ovine hypothalamic peptide that stimulates secretion of corticotropin and β-endorphin. Science 1981; 213:1394.

7. Li CH, Geschwind II, Cole RD, Raacke ID, Harris JI, Dixon JS. Amino acid sequence of alpha corticotropin. Nature 1955; 176:687.

8. Lala DS, Rice DA, Parker KL. Steroidogenic factor I, a key regulator of steroidogenic enzyme expression, is the mouse homolog of Fushi-Tarazu-factor 1. Mol Endocrinol 1992; 6:1249.

9. Luo X, Ikeda Y, Parker KL. A cell-specific nuclear receptor is essential for adrenal and gonadal development and sexual differentiation. Cell 1994; 77:481.

10. Weitzman ED, Fukushima D, Nogeire C, Roffwarg H, Gallagher TF, Hellman L. Twenty-four hour pattern of the episodic secretion of cortisol in normal subjects. J Clin Endocrinol Metab 1971; 33:14–22.

11. Migeon CJ, Tyler FH, Mahoney JP, et al. The diurnal variation of plasma levels and urinary excretion of 17- hydroxycorticosteroids in normal subjects, night workers and blind subjects. J Clin Endocrinol Metab 1956; 16:622–633.

12. Dinarello CA, Mier JW. Current concepts. Lymphokines. N Engl J Med 1987; 317:940.

13. Sapolsky R, Rivier C, Yamamoto G, et al. Interleukin I stimulates the secretion of hypothalamic corticotropin releasing factor. Science 1987; 238:522.

14. Migeon CJ, Green OC, Eckert JP. Study of adrenocortical function in obesity. Metabolism 1963; 12:718.

15. Kowarski A, Lacerda L, Migeon CJ. Integrated concentration of plasma aldosterone in normal subjects: correlation with cortisol. J Clin Endocrinol Metab 1975; 40:205.

16. Sklar CA, Kaplan SL, Grumbach MD. Evidence for dissoci-

17. Dunn JF, Nisula BC, Rodbard D. Transport of steroid hormones. J Clin Endocrinol Metab 1981; 53:58–68.

18. Orth DN, Kovacs WJ, DeBold CR. The adrenal cortex. In: Wilson JD, Foster DW, eds. Williams Textbook of Endocrinology, 8th ed. Philadelphia: WB Saunders, 1992:489.

19. Meikle AW. Secretion and metabolism of the corticosteroids and adrenal function testing. In: DeGrott LJ, et al., eds. Endocrinology. Philadelphia: WB Saunders, 1989:1610.

20. Chrousos GP, Schulte HM, Oldfield EH, et al. The corticotropin-releasing factor stimulation test. N Engl J Med 1984; 310:622.

21. Lashansky G, Saenger P, Fishman K, et al. Normative data for adrenal steroidogenesis in a healthy pediatric population: age- and sex-related changes after adrenocorticotropin stimulation. J Clin Endocrinol Metab 1991; 73:674–686.

22. Guggenheim MA, McCabe ERB, Roig M, et al. Glycerol kinase deficiency with neuromuscular, skeletal, and adrenal abnormalities. Ann Neurol 1980; 7:441.

23. Bartley JA, Patil S, Davenport S, et al. Duchenne muscular dystrophy, glycerol kinase deficiency, and adrenal insufficiency associated with Xp21 interstitial deletion. J Ped 1986; 108:189.

24. Franke U, Ochs HD, DeMartinville B, et al. Minor Xp21 chromosome deletion in a male associated with expression of Duchenne muscular dystrophy, chronic granulomatous disease, retinitis pigmentosa and McLeod syndrome. Am J Human Genet 1985; 37:250.

25. Wise JE, Matalon R, Morgan AM, McCabe ERB. Phenotypic features of patients with congenital adrenal hypoplasia and glycerol kinase deficiency. Am J Dis Child 1987; 141:744.

26. Prader A, Zachmann M and Illig R. Luteinizing hormone deficiency in hereditary congenital adrenal hypoplasia. J Pediatr 1975; 86:421.

27. Goonewardena P, Dahl N, Ritzen M, et al. Deletion in Xp associated with glycerol kinase deficiency, adrenal aplasia and hypogonadotropic hypogonadism. Cytogenet Cell Genet 1987; 46:621.

28. Bardoni B, Zanaria E, Guioli S, et al. A dosage sensitive locus at chromosome Xp21 is involved in male to female sex reversal. Nature Genetics 1994; 7:497–501.

29. Migeon CJ, Kenny FM, Kowarski A, et al. The syndrome of congenital adrenocortical unresponsiveness to ACTH. Report of six cases. Pediat Res 1968; 2:501–513.

30. Shepherd TH, Landing BH, Mason DG. Familial Addison's disease. Am J Dis Child 1959; 97:154–162.

31. Mountjoy KG, Robbins LS, Mortrud MT, Cone RD. The cloning of a family of genes that encode the melanocortin receptors. Science 1992; 257:1248–1251.

32. Clark AJL, McLoughlin L, Grossman A. Familial glucocorticoid deficiency associated with point mutation in the adrenocorticotropin receptor. Lancet 1993; 341:461–462.

33. Tsigos C, Arai K, Hung W, Chrousos GP. Hereditary isolated glucocorticoid deficiency is associated with abnormalities of the adrenocorticotropin receptor gene. J Clin Invest 1993; 92:2458–61.

34. Yamaoka T, Kudo T, Takuwa Y, et al. Hereditary adrenocortical unresponsiveness to adrenocorticotropin with post- receptor defect. J Clin Endocrinol Metab 1992; 75:270–274.

35. Franks RC, Nance WE. Hereditary adrenocortical unresponsiveness to ACTH. Pediatrics 1970; 45:43.

36. Stempfel RS, Jr., Engel FL. A congenital familial syndrome

of adrenocortical insufficiency without hypoaldosteronism. J Pediatr 1960; 57:443.

37. Allgrove J, Clayden GS, Grant DB, Macaulay JC. Familial glucocorticoid deficiency with achalasia of the cardia and deficient tear production. Lancet 1978; (i):1284–1286.

38. Lanes R, Plotnick L, Bynum TE, et al. Glucocorticoid and partial mineralocorticoid deficiency associated with achalasia. J Clin Endocrinol Metab 1980; 50:268–271.

39. Powers JM, Schaumburg HH, Johnson AB, et al. A correlative study of the adrenal cortex in adrenoleukodystrophy—evidence for a fatal intoxication with very long chain saturated fatty acids. Invest Cell Pathol 1980; 3:353.

40. Fanconi A, Prader A, Isler W, et al. Morbus Addison mit Hirnsklerose in Kindersalter. Ein hereditares Syndrom mit X-chromosomaler Verebung? Helv Paediat Acta 1964; 18:480.

41. Migeon BR, Moser HW, Moser AB, et al. Addrenoleukodystrophy: evidence for x-linkage inactivation, and selection favoring the mutant allele in heterozygous cells. Proc Natl Acad Sci USA 1981; 78:5066.

42. Mosser J, Douar AM, Sarde C-O, et al. Putative X-linked adrenoleukodystrophy gene shares unexpected homology with ABC transporters. Nature (London) 1993; 361:726–730.

43. Fanen P, Guidoux S, Sarde C-O, et al. Identification of mutations in the putative ATP-binding domain of the adrenoleukodystrophy gene. J Clin Invest 1994; 94:516–520.

44. Griffen JW, Goren E, Schaumberg H, et al. Adrenomyeloneuropathy: a probable variant of adrenoleukodystrophy. Neurology 1977; 27:1107.

45. Libber SM, Migeon CJ, Brown FR, III, et al. Adrenal and testicular function in 14 patients with adrenoleukodystrophy or adrenomyeloneuropathy. Hormone Res 1986; 24:1.

46. Fournier B, Saudubray J-M, Benichou B, et al. Large deletion of the peroxisomal Acyl-CoA oxidase gene in pseudoneonatal adrenoleukodystrophy. J Clin Invest 1994; 94:526–531.

47. Patrick AD, Lake BD. Deficiency of an acid lipase in Wolman syndrome. Nature 1969; 222:1067.

48. Koch GA, Lalley PA, McAvoy M, et al. Assignment of LIPA, associated with human acid lipase deficiency to chromosome 10 and comparative assignment to mouse chromosome 19. Somat Cell Genet 1981; 7:345.

49. Ballabio A, Shapiro LJ. Steroid sulfatase deficiency and X-linked ichthyosis. In: Scriver CR, et al., eds. The Metabolic Basis of Inherited Disease. New York: Mc-Graw-Hill, 1995, p. 2999.

50. Visser HKA and Cost WS. A new hereditary defect in the biosynthesis of aldosterone: Urinary C_{21}-corticosteroid pattern in three related patients with a salt-losing syndrome, suggesting an 18-oxidation defect. Acta Endocrinol 1964; 47:589.

51. Degenhart HJ, Frankena L, Visser HKA, Cost WS, Van Setters AP. Further investigation of a new hereditary defect in the biosynthesis of aldosterone: Evidence for a defect in the 18-hydroxylation of corticosterone. Acta Physiol Pharmacol Neerl 1966; 14:88.

52. Ulick S, Gautier E, Vetter KK, et al. An aldosterone biosynthesis defect in a salt-losing disorder. J Clin Endocrinol Metab 1964; 24:669.

53. David R, Golan S, Drucker W. Familial aldosterone deficiency: Enzyme defect, diagnosis and clinical course. Pediatrics 1968; 41:403.

54. Rösler A, Rabinowitz D, Theodor R, Ramirez LC, Ulick S. The nature of the defect in a salt-wasting disorder in Jews of Iran. J Clin Endocrinol Metab 1977; 44:279–291.

55. Globerman H, Rösler A, Theodor R, New MI, White PC. An inherited defect in aldosterone biosynthesis caused by a mutation in or near the gene for steroid 11-hydroxylase. N Engl J Med 1988; 319:1193.

56. Pascoe L, Curnow KM, Slutsker L, Rösler A, White PC. Mutations in the human CYP11B2 (aldosterone synthetase) gene causing corticosterone methyloxidase II deficiency. Proc Natl Acad Sci USA 1992; 89:4996.

57. Ferran JL, Couture A, Cabissole MA, et al. Hematome de la glande surrenale chez un noveau-ne: diagnostic et surveillance par echographie. Ann Pediatr (Paris) 1980; 27:391.

58. Dobs AS, Dempsey MA, Ladenson PW, et al. Endocrine disorders in men infected with human immunodeficiency virus. Am J Med 1987; 84:611.

59. Winter WE. Autoimmune endocrinopathies. In: Kappy MS, Blizzard RM, Migeon CJ, eds. Wilkins Diagnosis and Treatment of Endocrine Disorder in Childhood and Adolescence. Springfield, IL: Charles C. Thomas, 1994:317–382.

60. Blizzard RM, Johanson A. Disorders of growth. In: Kappy MS, Blizzard RM, Migeon CJ, eds. Wilkins Diagnosis and Treatment of Endocrine Disorders in Childhood and Adolescence. Springfield, IL: Charles C. Thomas, 1994:383–455.

61. Cleveland WW, Green OC, Migeon CJ. A case of proved andrenocorticotropin deficiency. J Pediatr 1960; 57:376.

62. Aarskog D, Blizzard RM, Migeon CJ. Response to methopyrapone (Su4885) and pyrogen test in idiopathic hypopituitary dwarfism. J Clin Endocrinol 1965; 25:439–444.

63. Keenan BS, Beitins IZ, Lee PA, Kowarski AA, Blizzard RM, Migeon CJ. Estimation of ACTH reserve on normal and hypopituitary subjects. Comparison of oral and intravenous metyrapone with insulin hypoglycemia. J Clin Endocrinol Metab 1973; 37:540–549.

64. Brasel JA, Wright JC, Wilkins L, et al. An evaluation of seventy-five patients with hypopituitarism beginning in childhood. Am J Med 1965; 38:484.

65. Migeon CJ, Weldon VV, Guild HG. Adolescent Endocrinology. New York: Appleton-Century-Crofts, 1970:149.

66. Kenny FM, Preeyasombat C, Spaulding JS, Migeon CJ. Cortisol production rate. IV. Infants born of steroid-treated mothers and of diabetic infants with trisomy syndrome and with anencephaly. Pediatrics 1966; 37:34.

67. Alkalay AL, Pomerance JJ, Puri AR, et al. Hypothalamic-pituitary-adrenal axis function in very low birth weight infants treated with dexamethasone. Pediatrics 1990; 86:204.

68. Vingerhoeds ACM, Thijssen JHH, Schwarz F. Spontaneous hypercortisolism without Cushing syndrome. J Clin Endocrinol Metab 1976; 43:1129.

69. Chrousos GP, Vingerhoeds AMC, Loriaux DL, et al. Primary cortisol resistance: a family study. J Clin Endocrinol Metab 1983; 56:1243.

70. Francke U, Foellmer BE. The glucocorticoid receptor gene is in 5q31–q32. Genomics 1989; 4:610.

71. Cheek DB, Perry JW. A salt-wasting syndrome in infancy. Arch Dis Child 1958; 33:252.

72. Kuhnle U, Nielsen MD, Tietze HU, et al. Pseudohypoaldosteronism in eight families: different forms of inheritance are evidence for various genetic defects. J Clin Endocrinol Metab 1990; 70:638.

73. Hanukoglu A. Type I pseudohypoaldosteronism includes two clinically and genetically distinct entities with either renal or multiple target organ defects. J Clin Endocrinol Metab 1991; 79:936.

74. Morrison N, Harrap SB, Arriza JL, et al. Regional chromosomal assignment of the human mineralocorticoid receptor gene to 4q31.1. Hum Genet 1990; 85:130.

75. Cushing H. Basophil adenoma of the pituitary body. Bull Johns Hopkins Hosp 1932; 50:137.

76. Liddle GW, Shute AM. The evolution of Cushing syndrome as a clinical entity. Adv Intern Med 1969; 15:155.

77. Oldfield EH, Schulte HM, Chrousos GP, et al. CRH stimu-

lation in Nelson's syndrome: response of ACTH secretion to pulse injection and continuous infusion of CRH. J Clin Endocrinol Metab 1986; 62:1020–1026.

78. Grua JR, Nelson DH. ACTH-producing tumors. Endocrinol Metab Clin North Am 1991; 20:319–369.

79. Jennings AS, Liddle GW, Orth DN. Results of treating childhood Cushing's disease with pituitary irradiation. N Engl J Med 1977; 297:957–962.

80. Tyrrell JB, Brooks RM, Fitzgerald PA, et al: Cushing's disease: selective transsphenoidal resection of pituitary microadenomas. N Engl J Med 1978; 298:753–758.

81. Mampalam TJ, Tyrrell JB, Wilson CB. Transsphenoidal microsurgery for Cushing's disease: a report of 216 cases. Ann Intern Med 1988; 109:487–493.

82. Styne DM, Grumbach MM, Kaplan SL, et al. Treatment of Cushing's disease in childhood and adolescence by transsphenoidal microsurgery. N Engl J Med 1984; 310:889–893.

83. Tindall GT, Herring CJ, Clark RV, et al. Cushing's disease: results of transsphenoidal microsurgery with emphasis on surgical failures. J Neurosurg 1990; 72:363–369.

84. Kenny FM, Haskida Y, Askari A, et al. Virilizing tumors of the adrenal cortex. Am J Dis Child 1968; 115:445.

85. Ribeiro RC, Sandrini-Neto RS, Schell MJ, et al. Adrenocortical carcinoma in children: a study of 40 cases. J Clin Oncol 1990; 8:67.

86. Fraumeni JE, Miller RW. Adrenocortical neoplasms with hemihypertrophy, brain tumors and other disorders. J Pediatr 1967; 70:129.

87. Saez JM, Rivarola MA, Migeon CJ. Studies in patients with adrenocortical tumors. J Clin Endocrinol Metab 1967; 27:615.

88. Gabrilove JL, Sharma DC, Wotiz HH, et al. Feminizing adrenocortical tumors in male: a review of 52 cases including a case report. Medicine (Baltimore) 1965; 44:37.

89. Conn JW, Cohen EL, Lucas CP, et al. Primary reninism: hypertension, hyperreninemia, and secondary aldosteronism due to renin-producing juxtaglomerular cell tumors. Arch Intern Med 1972; 130:682.

90. Conn JW. Primary aldosteronism, a new clinical syndrome. J Lab Clin Med 1955; 45:3.

91. Melby JC. Diagnosis of hyperaldosteronism. Endocrinol Metab Clin North Am 1991; 20:247–255.

92. Bartter FC, Pronove P, Gill JR, Jr., et al. Hyperplasia of the juxtaglomerular apparatus with hyperaldosteronism and hypokalemic alkalosis: a new syndrome. Am J Med 1962; 33:811.

93. Sutherland DJ, Ruse JL, Laidlaw JC. Hypertension, increased aldosterone secretion and low plasma renin activity relieved by dexamethasone. Can Med Assoc J 1966; 95:1109.

94. New MI, Peterson RE. A new form of congenital adrenal hyperplasia. J Clin Endocrinol Metab 1967; 27:300.

95. Pascoe L, Curnow KM, Slutsker L, et al. Glucocorticoid-suppressible hyperaldosteronism results from hybrid genes created by unequal crossovers between CYP11B1 and CYP11B2. Proc Natl Acad Sci USA 1992; 89:8327.

96. Lifton RP, Dluhy RG, Powers M, et al. Hereditary hypertension caused by chimaeric gene duplications and ectopic expression of aldosterone synthase. Nature Genet 1992; 2:66.

97. Miyahara K, Kawamoto T, Mitsuuchi Y, et al. The chimeric gene linked to glucocorticoid suppressible hyperaldosteronism encodes a fused P-450 protein possessing aldosterone synthase activity. Biochem Biophys Res Commun 1992; 189:885.

98. Ulick S, Levine LS, Gunczler P, et al. A new syndrome of acquired mineralocorticoid excess associated with defects in the peripheral metabolism of cortisol. J Clin Endocrinol 1979; 44:757.

99. Stewart PM, Corrie JET, Shackleton CHL. Syndrome of apparent mineralocorticoid excess. A defect in the cortisol-cortisone shuttle. J Clin Invest 1988; 82:340.

100. Tannin GM. The human gene for 11B-hydroxysteroid dehydrogenase, structure, tissue distribution, and chromosomal localization. J Biol Chem 1991; 266:16653.

101. Monder C. Corticosteroids, receptors, and the organ-specific function of 11β-hydroxysteroid dehydrogenase. FASEB J 1991; 5:3047.

102. Walker BR, Campbell JC, Williams BC, Edwards CR. Tissue-specific distribution of the NAD(+)-dependent isoform of 11 beta-hydroxysteroid dehydrogenase. Endocrinology 1992; 131:970.

103. Funder JW, Pearce PT, Myles K, et al. Apparent mineralocorticoid excess, pseudohypoaldosteronism, and urinary electrolyte excretion: toward a redefinition of mineralocorticoid action. FASEB J 1990; 4:3234.

104. Farese RV Jr, Biglieri EG, Shackleton CHL, Irony I, Gomez-Fontex R. Licorice-induced hypermineralocorticoidism. N Engl J Med 1991; 325:1223.

105. DeLacera L, Kowarski A, Migeon CJ. Integrated concentration and diurnal variation of plasma contisol. J Clin Endocrinol Metab 1993; 36:227. Copyright, the Endocrine Society.

106. Lanes R, Gonzalez S, Obregon O. Adrenal cortical carcinoma in a 4 year old child. Clin Pediatr 1982; 21:164–166.

23

Sexological Considerations in Patients with a History of Ambisexual Birth Defect

John Money
Johns Hopkins University School of Medicine and Johns Hopkins Hospital, Baltimore, Maryland

Marco Danon
Maimonides Medical Center and State University of New York Health Science Center at Brooklyn, Brooklyn, New York

I. NEONATAL SEX ANNOUNCEMENT

One effect of the sexual taboo is that knowledge in the public domain includes little or nothing about the occurrence of birth defects of the sex organs. Thus, very few parents of a newborn baby have a precedent to guide them when they are told that their baby's sex cannot be decided by visual inspection alone. In the vast majority of circumstances, those present at the delivery also have no precedent. Since ambiguity of the genitalia is a surprise event at delivery, an attempt to assign the "most likely" sex is made by the involved physician and nurses. This assignment is seldom wise and should be avoided. The team at delivery should restrain from assigning sex and should inform the parents that "the sex the baby is meant to be cannot be determined yet." Thus, it is common for parents to receive arbitrary, and in many instances contradictory, opinions as to the announcement, or renouncement, of their baby's sex. From the time at delivery, the baby should be named "*Baby Smith*" or "*Baby so and so*" and should be referred to by everyone as "the baby." Efforts should be made to transfer the child to a special-care nursery or neonatal intensive-care unit for appropriate workup. Extra efforts are to be made by all involved in this baby's care to explain the importance of postponing the name and sex assignment until diagnostic steps are taken. Even after the time required to establish a diagnosis, experts do not necessarily agree as to the sex of assignment. In one school of thought, the criterion of assignment is the genetic and gonadal sex. In another, the criteria are the morphological characteristics of the external genitalia and the prognosis for the child's successful hormonal and surgical habilitation in the sex assigned, with the fewest possible surgical procedures in infancy and childhood, to minimize the extent of what is experienced by hospitalized children as nosocomial abuse (1).

Professional disagreement regarding assigned sex is generated more often when the ambiguously sexed baby proves to be chromosomally and gonadally male rather than female. Disagreement centers particularly around the syndrome of male hermaphroditism with 5-alpha-reductase deficiency, and it is based on a famous pedigree from the remote rural mountains of the Dominican Republic. One doctrine (2–4) holds that the masculinizing hormones of puberty preordain psychological masculinization, regardless of the sex assignment; and another (5–7) that community stigmatization as half-boy, half-girl, together with lack of surgical and hormonal intervention, prevents normalization as either a girl or a boy at puberty.

When experts disagree regarding the sex of a baby with ambiguous genitalia, it is rarely possible to conceal this disagreement from the parents. It is also ethically unwise to do so and could result in a costly malpractice charge, even years later. Moreover, parents are unable to commit themselves unequivocally to rearing their child as either a son or a daughter unless they have the conviction that they are doing the right thing. They are able to achieve this conviction by sharing the information used by the experts on assignment. Only then will they be prepared to be successful in explaining their baby's diagnosis, treatment, and prognosis to their relatives, friends, neighbors, and their own children, and only then will they be prepared to respond to their child's subsequent imperative need for knowledge of its own clinical history and condition.

II. TELLING OTHERS

There are too many vocal or written sources of potential disclosure, either inadvertent or contrived, for it to be feasible to maintain complete secrecy regarding a child's birth defect of the sex organs. Even if the baby's announced sex does not need to be changed, the attempt at secrecy is an intolerable burden on the parents. No matter how trusting their relationship, when desperation threatens, each needs someone else to confide in. They are, therefore, much in need of a clinical vocabulary and explanation of their baby's sex. This need is fulfilled by giving the parents an elementary course in the embryology of sexual differentiation, diagrammatically illustrated. Two diagrams in the literature (8–12) illustrate the initial neutrality of indifferentiation of the embryonic genitalia, external and internal, and the homologous nature of the various male and female parts of the genital anatomy.

The book *Sex Errors of the Body* (9), which contains both the diagrams and their explanation, is a useful reference source for parents. This book can be used again in later years when the child needs an explanation of his or her own status at birth and subsequent treatment. It can also be used to explain the new baby's congenital sexual ambiguity to older siblings. They should never be overlooked, especially in cases of sex renouncement. Otherwise, they are at risk of developing the fantasy and hypothesis that they too might become candidates for genital mutilation and an imposed change of sex.

The neglect of older siblings, young cousins, and the children of close neighbors is widespread. It is also foolhardy, for these are the young people who, if inadequately advised, may later tell the affected child that he (or she) used to be a girl (or boy).

In the past, it used to be popular to advise parents whose hermaphroditic child's sex was reannounced that they should abandon family, friends, and work and begin life anew in a far-distant place. It is virtually impossible to cut all ties with one's own past. In the case of having an ambiguously sexed child, it is also not necessary to do so. People gossip when they are mystified. They are fishing to find out what is being withheld from them. If their curiosity is satisfied at the outset, it is possible for them to conform to a request to respect a child's future integrity by not talking about the neonatal ambiguity of its sex. Some parents have found it possible to educate their friends and neighbors about their sex-reassigned child themselves (13). Others have enlisted the help of a community resource—a nurse, physician, teacher, or church leader. The policy of being open instead of secretive has a great advantage in its application to the child growing up with a history of birth-defective sex organs, for it eradicates the dread lest the child somehow be aware of his or her ambiguous beginnings. Beginning early in life, one mother told her daughter that she had been born with her female organs covered over with skin. Therefore, the doctors and nurses had thought as first that maybe she was a boy. Then they discovered that she was a girl. It was unnecessary for anyone in the family, or in the clinic, to be secretive with this girl about her clinical history. She was not vulnerable, for there was no secret knowledge to make her so.

III. PARENTAL SEX LIVES AND GENETIC COUNSELING

The subjective and emotional trauma of having produced an abnormal baby is not necessarily shared equally by each parent. Therefore, it is necessary to provide both of them with an opportunity to talk alone, as well as together. It is virtually universal for a mother to assimilate unto herself the blame for any pregnancy that produced a less than perfect child, regardless of her knowledge and intellectual sophistication. However, a father may also be afflicted with self-blame, perhaps interpreting the baby's defect as a penalty of a prior sexual indiscretion.

Although blame of the other partner rarely surfaces overtly, it may take its toll covertly. Eventually, it may be responsible for deterioration of the marital relationship into an adversarial one, with a possible culmination in separation and divorce. One warning signal is the deterioration of the couple's sexual life. Therefore, it is advantageous to provide an opportunity for each partner to talk about the effect on current sexual function of having another possibly defective baby. This concern can be countered rationally, with etiological and genetic explanations. However, rationality alone does not resolve emotional trauma, which, in some cases, is pervasive and persistent.

Probability statistics are of little value to a mother (or father) who wants to know if her (or his) next baby will have the same syndrome as the one already affected. Advice about the wisdom of attempting a new pregnancy requires consideration not only of probability statistics, but also of the morbidity risk specific to the syndrome and the therapeutic prognosis. Also to be considered is the possibility of prenatal diagnosis with the option of abortion or, in the case of the 46,XX adrenogenital syndrome, prenatal glucocorticoid therapy (14). Anything that medical technology has to offer, however, is contingent on the personal emotional, religious, and ethical concerns and obligations of the parents concerned. Rationality is not the sole consideration.

IV. THE PATIENT'S SEXUALITY

The power of the sexual taboo in our society is such that most parents of an ambiguously sexed new baby follow the standard assumption that there will be time enough in adolescence for sex to be discussed. They assume that all they need to know now is whether the baby is a boy or girl, and whether the problem can be appropriately corrected. Their first concern is personal, namely, of deciding their baby's correct sex. It is as if the decision regarding the correct sex will be a guarantee of future fertility and copulatory ability. Their secondary concern, if they have one, is whether their child's birth defect is what will cause him or her to become a homosexual or transsexual.

In response to this concern, the answer is that children born with ambiguous genitalia grow up, as a general rule, although not invariably, to develop the gender identity and role (G-I/R) of the sex to which they are assigned and reared and in which they are surgically and hormonally habilitated. This prognosis cannot be given with the certainty of a prophecy, partly because the prognosis of G-I/R is affected by the degree of emancipation that the parents themselves bring to their growing child's sexual learning and sexual rehearsal play, as well as to the child's developmental need for self-knowledge concerning his or her clinical history and prognosis. Many of the best-intentioned parents fail in this respect, victims of their own sexual upbringing and of the resurgence of antisexualism socially and politically characteristic of the present era.

There is still insufficient research information to warrant a prediction or prophecy in individual cases as to the effects of either excess or insufficiency of prenatal androgenization of the sexual brain relative to postnatal clinical and social determinants of the sex of rearing. Some individuals with the 46,XX syndrome of female pseudohermaphroditism with congenital virilizing adrenal hyperplasia (CVAH) grow up, if assigned and reared as girls, to fall in love as lesbians, or to have bisexual imagery and ideation, with or without actual bisexual experience, which those assigned and reared as boys do not have (15,16).

Studies of females with CVAH support the notion that intrauterine androgenization occurs. Females with CVAH marry with a lower frequency, have fewer children when they do marry, and have a higher incidence of lesbian behavior (17). A controlled psychological survey found that females with CVAH tend to have a more negative body image, less sexual activity, and less interest in sexual activity (18). The contributions of fetal androgenization, parental hesitations about sex assignment, and trauma of genital surgery have not been quantified and accurately assessed. An important issue that is commonly forgotten is the possible psychological trauma of vaginal examinations and procedures, including dilation, that these patients undergo during childhood years.

Some individuals with the 46,XY syndrome of insufficiently masculinized hermaphroditism, if assigned and reared as girls, fall in love with a girl and demand a sex reassignment, regardless of whether they spontaneously undergo a puberty that leaves them feminized, masculinized, or eunuchized (19), whereas relatively fewer of those assigned and reared as boys do the reverse (20). Individuals with the complete 46,XY androgen insensitivity syndrome, virtually all of whom are assigned and reared as girls, feminize at puberty. They fall in love and get married as women (21–23) and may have a family by adoption.

V. CHILDHOOD COUNSELING

Ideally, all children with a history of a birth defect of the sex organs should be followed throughout childhood and adolescence, and indeed through adulthood, since so little is known of the long-term natural history of these syndromes. The following is a schedule or checklist of topics to be alert to in age-graded counseling and caring for the affected child in individual, private, and confidential counseling sessions:

> Knowledge and explanation of the reason for clinic visits and long-term follow-up
>
> Self-knowledge of diagnosis, prognosis, and treatment rationale
>
> Overt or suspected knowledge of neonatal sexual indecision and/or sex reannouncement
>
> Experience of sibling or playmate teasing and/or gossip based on past clinical history
>
> Social problems related to being too tomboyish as a girl or not sufficiently macho as a boy
>
> Personal decisions and consequences regarding clinical experience and knowledge confided to or withheld from siblings, other relatives, and friends
>
> Reactions to exposure of nudity to spectators in physical examinations and medical photography
>
> Clinical examinations and procedures and hospital admissions experienced as nosocomial abuse
>
> Experience with parents or others as neglecting or providing for normal childhood sexual learning, explicit and by diffuse assimilation, and its consequences relative to the child's conception of his or her genital anatomy and prognosis regarding coital adequacy
>
> Experience with age mates of nudity, genital inspection, genital stigmatization, and childhood sexual rehearsal play
>
> Concepts and uncertainties of future status of parenthood by way of pregnancy, donor insemination (sperm bank), adoption, or stepchildren
>
> Concepts and fantasies regarding future sex life in marriage

Ideally, the parents will take a participatory role in the foregoing. However, they cannot be assigned the total responsibility, because parents and professionals serve different functions, and the child needs both. Moreover, many parents are entrapped in the social tradition that prescribes that they spare the child from the ostensible trauma of speaking about the unspeakable. Actually it is themselves they are sparing. What they fail to mention becomes, in fact, a monster in the child's life. It leads to a variable degree of elective mutism when the child is in the clinic, as well as to phobic aversion to the clinic and to the people in it. To help alleviate the child's distress, one plans for the child and each parent to have separate interviews, and then, in a joint interview, to share information in common—though only with prior informed consent and respect of the child's right to confidentiality. In some instances, the phobic barrier in parents and/or child is too resistant for the child's distress to be effectively alleviated.

In addition to taboo-ridden and unspeakable topics, there are others that parents are not intellectually trained to deal with. They must rely on outside help. These topics include:

Talking about chromosomal and gonadal sex (see below)

Personal problems secondary to medication or illicit drug effects

Academic status relative to IQ and cognitive abilities, impairment of which may be syndrome-specific in some varieties of 46,XY hermaphroditism, whereas by contrast, intellectual superiority is syndrome-specific in other varieties, notably in 46,XX (CVAH) pseudohermaphroditism

Personal problems and/or psychopathology relative to family psychopathology, parental feuding, or parental breakup

VI. TEENAGE COUNSELING

Two of life's great adjustments come to the foreground of the agenda of teenage counseling: autonomy and sexuality. Sexuality includes falling in love, and autonomy includes preparation for economic independence. Autonomy sometimes gets in the way of clinical compliance. Problems of compliance exist at any age. In infancy and childhood, the responsibility is with an adult. In teenage years, responsibility becomes progressively transferred to or demanded by the patient.

Teenage noncompliance may represent a so-called denial of illness—a magic sort of belief that not taking medication signifies being well. When the medication is a sex hormone, noncompliance may signify rejection of becoming sexually mature or protest against one's hormonally induced status as male instead of female, or female instead of male.

It is not too far-fetched to say that in our society, teenage sex is widely regarded not only as an evil, but also as a disease; teenagers and adults both recognize the communicational wedge that splits them. Unable to dislodge this wedge, some teenagers with a history of genital ambiguity are also unable to confide in their peers. Except in the clinic, they have no one with whom to share their romantic and erotic fears and apprehensions, such as what to reveal to a boyfriend or girlfriend, or what to expect from sexual intercourse.

VII. PARABLE TECHNIQUE

In the clinic, the parable technique is a way of circumventing the communication impasse. The counselor narrates a story derived from the case of a person of the same age and the same diagnosis as the patient. The story may also be derived from a composite of cases. The topic of the story is presumed to apply to the listener, who, even though afflicted with elective mutism, ascertains that the narrator is an informed and a safe listener with whom to reopen the topic at a later date. The parable technique is suitable for topics such as the timing of the onset of hormonal replacement therapy and the timing of reconstructive genital surgery. It applies also to such touchy subjects as: diagnostic self-knowledge, particularly about chromosomal and gonadal sex; masturbation; paraphilic erotic imagery and ideation; wet dreams; bisexual or homosexual attraction; ideas of sex change; impaired or defective

genital function in sexual intercourse; sterility, fertility, and unwed pregnancy; revealing to a lover the prognosis of sterility; hereditary transmission, telling siblings and others about the possibility of future transmission in the family pedigree; fear of rejection by intimates or officials and bureaucrats; lovesickness; suicide.

The great advantage of the parable technique is its nonjudgmentalism. It does not require the listener either to admit or to deny the relevance of a given topic, but simply indicates that the topic is safe to talk about and to be listened to, as need be.

When the parable technique is used, the agenda is fixed but the inquiry is open-ended and not stilted. Open-endedness allows the respondent free rein to define the topic in terms of what it means to him or her personally. Subsequently, the inquiry becomes less open-ended, until eventually each particular topic may be closed with an interrogatory, employing forced-choice questions. Such questions are designed to get specific responses to specific details of chronology, prevalence, location, frequency, measurements, and so on.

An open-ended inquiry may be as straightforward as an announcement of the next topic on the standardized schedule of inquiry, for example, "Play. Tell me about your child's play." This straightforward approach is based on the premise that the topic is in the public domain and poses no threat of stigmatization, self-incrimination, or breach of confidentiality.

In some instances, it is necessary to specify, not assume, that a topic is indeed in the public domain, even though it is also partly in the private domain. For example: "The bombing of abortion clinics has been in the news recently." If a patient is familiar with this news, she or he can be encouraged to verbalize her/his ideas about it. Thereafter, it becomes feasible to lead into more personal references with respect to past history and future prospects regarding decisions about abortion (24).

It is when a topic is not in the public domain, but is taboo-ridden and potentially stigmatizing and self-incriminating, that the parable technique is especially valuable.

The sportscaster technique with a detailed play-by-play account is one method to use when the informant is recounting a personal experience or encounter. Otherwise the account becomes too global and diffuse. Especially if the account involves an adversarial relationship, the raw data become lost in inferential attribution of motivations and intent, in which there is a hidden agenda, namely, to cast the interviewer in the role of juror and to win a judgment against the adversary. To establish maximum impartiality, one should interview the adversary, who also should adopt the sportscaster technique of reporting.

VIII. CHROMOSOMAL AND GONADAL SEX

The parable technique lends itself to the transmission of information that consistently plagues professionals, namely, discordance between the patient's diagnostic, chromosomal, and/or gonadal status and the status of the G-I/R. The androgen insensitivity syndrome is a prime example, because it is also known by the stigmatizing terms *testicular feminizing syndrome* and *male hermaphroditism* (or *pseudohermaphroditism*). All these terms are likely to become known to a patient with the syndrome. Proverbially, the walls in a hospital have ears. Inadvertently or otherwise, a patient has access to his or her own record, or to excerpts from it; or to a letter to another physician; or to an insurance form or clinic list on which the diagnosis appears.

The national media frequently carry medical stories from which a patient recognizes parallels with his or her own case or has information passed on by siblings or friends—not to mention high school and college texts or biology courses in which, with oneself as the subject, sex-chromatin testing is a laboratory assignment. Many older patients use libraries in the search for diagnostic self-information, and many know about the Freedom of Information Act, which entitles them legally to have access to their own hospital records. It is anachronistic for any health care provider to assume that nosological information can be perpetually hidden from a patient. The attempt at hiding simply forces a patient into simulation of ignorance in order not to confront the doctor with his or her own professional dissimulation—a less than ideal doctor-patient relationship. Moreover, withholding of information may be subject to malpractice litigation.

With respect to chromosomal status, a parable that avoids dissembling is one that tells how a patient, in this case a teenaged young lady, who gained access to her own record, learned that there are XY girls and women, XX boys and men, and many other chromosomal variants in both sexes, such as XXX, XXY, XYY, XO, as well as a multiplicity of mosaic combinations. In the case of, for example, an XY girl or woman, it makes no subjective sense to follow the standard idiom that dichotomizes XY as male and XX as female, for if the XY chromosomal pair cannot function as male, then it is not manifestly male. Rather the Y is functioning as if an X with one of its arms broken off.

The parable continues with this young lady having learned also that there are gonads which have differentiated so as to appear, under the microscope, more like testicles than ovaries (or vice versa) but which are actually neither, as they are not able to do the complete work of one or the other. Although these gonads are in fact·defective, doctors and scientists still cling anachronistically to the policy of classifying them as either male or female, and of using this classification as the basis of their diagnostic term, namely male and female hermaphroditism (or pseudohermaphroditism).

The young lady of this parable was mortified at first, but she did, in fact, make peace with the terminology in her hospital record. In her own thinking and conversation, she always changed testis into gonad or sex gland. She realized not only that it was incapable of doing male work, but also that its hormones had an ultrafeminizing effect on her body, which completely resisted androgen, more than the ordinary woman's body could do. The end of the story was that she was never again held hostage by the wording of her hospital record.

IX. COMPLIANCE

Even though the parable technique does not impose the demand of a response, it does, except when used by phone or in writing, require the presence of the listener in person. A teenager cannot, however, be forced to consent to an appointment for any kind of treatment. Some do refuse, either on their own account or in complicity with one or both parents. Others have an aversion to being stigmatized as abnormal by being in the presence of a psychologist, psychiatrist, or sexologist. Some have an aversion to talking explicitly about themselves sexually or have an aversion to burdening their parents with a bill they know they have neither the cash nor the insurance to pay. There are some who need help, but on whom compliance cannot be forced, or for whom it must be postponed until they are ready to accept the help that is available—possibly years later. The door must always be kept open.

X. UNIVERSALS OF THE AGENDA

Children with a history of birth defect of the genitalia need, in the language of childhood, "a cutting doctor, a needle doctor, and a talking doctor." The pediatric surgeon's services are usually time-limited, even though they may not be completed until the teenage years or young adulthood. The pediatric endocrinologist's services are of variable duration, according to the diagnosis: from birth onward in cases of CVAH, from the age of puberty onward in cases of gonadectomy or gonadal failure, and maybe not at all after puberty in cases of spontaneous onset of puberty concordant with the gender identity. The follow-up coverage of genetic females with CVAH is prolonged. Untreated, they are exposed from fetal life onward to high levels of androgen and they have a birth history of masculinized external genitalia. Parents must be reassured that surgical correction and long-term treatment with cortisol starting at birth will enable the female patient to grow up looking like a normal girl of her age with a gender identity that is expected to be female. Girls with CVAH often are predisposed to a high level of physical energy expenditure. Tomboyish characteristics may be related to the prenatal history of high levels of androgen exposure and may be brought up for discussion during clinic visits.

The "talking doctor" may be either a psychologist or psychiatrist, provided he or she has specialty training in sexological medicine and psychoendocrinology. His or her services, like those of a pediatrician or family physician, should be available on demand, throughout childhood and adulthood. The frequency of demand is quite variable from one individual to another, and at different periods of the life span. The fewer the clinical and/or social complications of development, the longer the interval between appointments with the doctor, and the greater the appropriateness of defining the visits as preventive, not therapeutic. The purpose of the visit, as defined, is to give a progress report. Progress reports are spaced preferably at intervals no longer than annually. To ensure complete coverage in the progress report, the agenda encompasses the five universal exigencies of being human (25,26). These exigencies constitute a template against which to analyze the progress and trace the continuity of any biography in all of its components, clinical and nonclinical. They constitute also a template that, in its five categories, allows a place for all the variables that may affect the development of an individual human life. Although the template does not guarantee that all the variables will be discovered, it does offer a guarantee against inadvertent omissions in the agenda of a schedule of inquiry.

The five universal exigencies of being human are:

1. Pairbondage, which pertains to parent-child and lover-lover bonding
2. Troopbondage, which pertains to becoming a member of a flock, herd, troop, or family
3. Abidance, which pertains to food, shelter, and clothing and to abiding and being sustained in an ecological niche
4. Ycleptance (a recycled Elizabethan term), which pertains to being named, nicknamed, classified, branded, labeled, or typecast
5. Foredoomance, which pertains to mortality and vulnerability to injury, defect, disease, and death, either one's own or someone else's

For individuals with a history of a birth defect of the sex organs, it goes without saying that, especially in adolescence and young adulthood, the pairbondage universal has special clinical significance. To establish a sexual and erotic pairbond is, in their case, to be confronted with questions and anxieties not only regarding one's fertility and parenthood, but also regarding the very adequacy of one's genitalia for copulation. For parts of the body other than the genitalia, there are explicit rehabilitation services and procedures, whereas even audiovisual demonstrations of explicit copulatory normality are subject to neglect, if not severe moral or even legal sanction, in most institutions. For the most part, even explicitly reading or talking is avoided, particularly with teenagers. The pervasiveness of the sexual taboo affects patients so thoroughly that some teenagers who do have the option of explicit love education and sex education are unable to accept it. Some of them become more sophisticated with age, but some remain sexologically permanently crippled.

The other universal exigency that has particular significance for those counseling patients with a history of birth defects of the sex organs is ycleptance. Ycleptance is the past participle of the verb "to clepe," meaning "to name, call, or style." Human beings have named and typecast one another since recorded time. The terms range from the haphazard informality of nicknames to the systematic formality of biomedical nomenclature and diagnostic terms that prognosticate our futures and shape our lives. They affect our self-image, and all too often can be brutally stigmatizing (27).

XI. PSYCHOBIOLOGICAL ASPECTS OF HUMAN SEXUAL ORIENTATION

Emphasis on the sexual dimorphism in normal mammalian brain development is currently made by accumulating available data mostly from animal experiments. This dimorphism is mediated, at least in part, by fetal testicular androgens. In the human species, androgen mediation has been implicated by studies in intersex disorders. The degree to which the human brain is sexually dimorphic, and the timing and concentrations of testosterone necessary, remain unknown.

The identification of a gene that ostensibly predisposes males to homosexuality points to the possibility that sexual orientation has a genetic component. A "gay gene" on the X chromosome may be located on Xq28, according to a study using DNA linkage analysis (28).

Neither plasma hormone values nor other endocrine tests can reliably distinguish groups with regard to sexual orientation (29). However, morphological characteristics of hypothalamic structures have been described in brains of homosexual individuals (30–32), suggesting a brain difference associated with sexual orientation. The origin and timing of the development of this difference, whether in prenatal or postnatal life, remain unknown (9).

REFERENCES

1. Money J, Lamacz M. Nosocomial stress and abuse exemplified in a case of male hermaphroditism from infancy through adulthood: coping strategies and prevention. Int J Family Psychiatry 1986; 7:71–105.
2. Imperato-McGinley J, Guerrero L, Gautier T. Peterson RE. Steroid 5-alpha-reductase deficiency in man: an inherited form of male psuedohermaphroditism. Science 1974; 186:1213–1215.
3. Imperato-McGinley J, Peterson RE. Male pseudohermaphroditism: the complexities of male phenotypic development. Am J Med 1976; 61:251–272.
4. Imperato-McGinley J, Peterson RE, Gautier T, Sturla E. Androgens and the evolution of male-gender identity among male pseudohermaphrodites with 5-alpha-reductase deficiency. N Engl J Med 1979; 300:1233–1237.
5. Rubin RT, Reinisch JM, Haskett RF. Postnatal gonadal steroid effects on human sexually dimorphic behavior: a paradigm of hormone-environment interaction. Science 1981; 211:1318–1324.
6. Money J. Gender identity and hermaphroditism. Science 1976; 191:872.
7. Money J. The development of sexuality and eroticism in humankind. Q Rev Biol 1981; 56:379–404.
8. Money J. Psychologic disorders associated with genital defects. In: Cooke RE, Levine S, eds. The Biologic Basis of Pediatric Practice, Vol 11. New York: McGraw-Hill, 1968.
9. Money J. Sex Errors of the Body and Related Syndromes: A Guide to Counseling Children, Adolescents, and Their Families, 2nd ed. Baltimore: Paul H. Brookes, 1994.
10. Money J. Psychologic aspects of endocrine and genetic disease in children. In: Gardner LI, ed. Endocrine and Genetic Diseases of Childhood, 2nd ed. Philadelphia: WB Saunders, 1975.
11. Money J, Ehrhardt AA. Man and Woman, Boy and Girl: Differentiation and Dimorphism of Gender Identity from Conception to Maturity. Baltimore: Johns Hopkins University Press, 1972.
12. Money J, Hampson JG, Hampson JL. Hermaphroditism: recommendations concerning assignment of sex, change of

sex, and psychologic management. Bull Johns Hopkins Hosp 1955; 97:284–300.

13. Money J, Potter R, Stoll CS. Sex reannouncement in hereditary sex deformity: psychology and sociology of habilitation. Soc Sci Med 1969; 3:207–216.

14. Pang S, Pollack MS, Marshall RN, Immken LD. Prenatal treatment of congenital adrenal hyperplasia due to 21-hydroxylase deficiency. N Engl J Med 1990; 322:111–115.

15. Money J, Schwartz M, Lewis VG. Adult erotosexual status and fetal hormonal masculinzation and demasculinization: 46,XX congenital virilizing adrenal hyperplasia and 46,XY androgen-insensitivity syndrome compared. Psychoneuroendocrinology 1984; 9:405–414.

16. Money J, Daléry J. Iatrogenic homosexuality: gender identity in seven 46,XX chromosomal females with hyperadrenocortical hermaphroditism born with a penis, three reared as boys, four reared as girls. J Homosexual 1976; 1:357–371.

17. Mulaikal RM, Migeon CJ, Rock JA. Fertility rates in female patients with congenital adrenal hyperplasia due to 21-hydroxylase deficiency. N Engl J Med 1987; 316:178–182.

18. Kuhnle U, Bollinger M, Schwarz HP, Knorr D. Partnership and sexuality in adult female patients with congenital adrenal hyperplasia. First results of a cross-sectional quality-of-life evaluation. J Steroid Biochem Mol Biol 1993; 45:123–126.

19. Money J, Devore H, Norman BF. Gender identity and gender transposition: longitudinal outcome study of 32 male hermaphrodites assigned as girls. J Sex Marital Ther 1986; 12:165–81.

20. Money J, Norman BF. Gender identity and gender transposition: longitudinal outcome study of 24 male hermaphrodites assigned as boys. J Sex Marital Ther 1987; 13:75–81.

21. Lewis VG, Money J. Gender-identity role [G-I/R]:XY (androgen-insensitivity) syndrome and XX (Rokitansky) syndrome of vaginal atresia compared. In: Dennerstein L, Burrows GD,

22. Lewis VG, Money J. Sexological theory, H-Y antigen, chromosomes, gonads, and cyclicity: two syndromes compared. Arch Sex Behav 1986; 15:467–474.

23. Money J, Lewis VG. Gender-identity/role [G-I/R]: a multiple sequential model of differentiation. In: Dennerstein L. Burrows GD, eds. Handbook of Psychosomatic Obstetrics and Gynecology. Amsterdam: Elsevier Biomedical Press, 1983.

24. Money J. Longitudinal studies in clinical psychoendocrinology: methodology. Dev Behav Pediatr 1986; 7:31–34.

25. Money J. Reinterpreting the Unspeakable: Human Sexuality 2000—The Complete Interviewer and Clinical Biographer, Exigency Theory, and Sexology for the Third Millennium. New York: Continuum, 1994.

26. Money J. Five universal exigencies, indicatrons and sexological theory. J Sex Marital Ther 1984; 10:229–238.

27. Money J. Psychologic considerations in patients with ambisexual development. Semin Reprod Endocr 1987; 5:307–313.

28. Hamer DH, Hu S, Magnuson VL, Hu N, Pattatucci AML. A linkage between DNA markers on the X chromosome and male sexual orientation. Science 1993; 261:321–327.

29. Friedman RC, Downey JI. Homosexuality. N Engl J Med 1994; 331:923–930.

30. LeVay S. A difference in hypothalamic structure between heterosexual and homosexual men. Science 1991; 253:1034–1037.

31. Allen LS, Gorski RA. Sexual orientation and the size of the anterior commissure in the human brain. Proc Natl Acad Sci USA 1992; 89:7199–7202.

32. Swaab DF, Hofman, MA. An enlarged suprachiasmatic nucleus in homosexual men. Brain Res 1990; 537:141–148.

eds. Handbook of Psychosomatic Obstetrics and Gynecology. Amsterdam: Elsevier Biomedical Press, 1983:51–67.

24
Disorders of the Adrenal Medulla

Mary L. Voorhess
State University of New York at Buffalo and Children's Hospital of Buffalo, Buffalo, New York

I. INTRODUCTION

The adrenal gland is composed of two distinct components, each of which functions as a separate endocrine organ. The outer portion, the adrenal cortex, secretes steroid hormones. The inner section, the adrenal medulla, secretes catecholamines and accounts for about 10% of the weight of each gland.

The adrenal medulla is derived from embryonic neural crest cells that migrate from the neural tube, differentiate into chromaffin cells, and invade the substance of the adrenal cortex at 6–7 weeks of fetal life. Other chromaffin cells, extraadrenal in location, are widely distributed within the sympathetic nervous system. Their function is not well established. A large mass called the organ of Zuckerkandl is located near the origin of the inferior mesenteric artery. The extraadrenal chromaffin tissues dominate during fetal life and early infancy, and then most involute as the adrenal medulla matures.

Functionally, the adrenal medullae are part of the sympathetic nervous system, and together they comprise the sympathoadrenal system, which is under direct control of the central nervous system. Neurochemical transducers (the catecholamines) convert neuronal activity into physiologic responses. Each medulla may be thought of as a specialized sympathetic ganglia that is innervated by preganglionic sympathetic fibers from the splanchnic nerves. The postganglionic neurons are the granule-containing cells within the medulla that secrete predominantly epinephrine and smaller amounts of norepinephrine and dopamine into the adrenal veins.

II. THE CATECHOLAMINES

A. Synthesis

Catecholamine synthesis takes place primarily within the sympathetic nerve endings, the adrenal medullae, and certain portions of the brain. The primary pathway for dopamine, norepinephrine, and epinephrine formation is shown in Figure 1. Tyrosine is transported from the bloodstream into catecholamine-secreting neurons and is converted to dopa and then dopamine within the cytoplasm of the neuron by tyrosine hydroxylase and aromatic L-amino acid decarboxylase, respectively. Dopamine then enters the granules, where it is converted to norepinephrine by dopamine β-hydroxylase. Some norepinephrine remains stored in the granules, and the rest is released into the cytoplasm of the cell. Synthesis stops here in the extraadrenal sympathetic neurons, but in the adrenal medulla the enzyme phenylethanolamine-*N*-methyltransferase (PNMT) catalyzes the conversion of norepinephrine to epinephrine. The activity of PNMT appears to depend on glucocorticoids, which are carried to the medullary cells via blood draining from the adrenal cortex. Epinephrine accounts for about 80% of the catecholamines released into the circulation from the adrenal medullae. Smaller amounts of norepinephrine and even less dopamine are released. The major source of norepinephrine in blood is the sympathetic nerve endings. In brain, the largest amount of dopamine is in the basal ganglia and median eminence; norepinephrine is concentrated in the hypothalamus. The amounts of epinephrine in brain and sympathetic neurons are small.

The rate-limiting step in catecholamine synthesis is the tyrosine to dopa step, which is catalyzed by tyrosine hydroxylase. This enzyme is subject to feedback inhibition by dopamine and norepinephrine, so there is endogenous control of amine synthesis. Such compounds as α-methyl-*p*-tyrosine also inhibit tyrosine hydroxylase and thus decrease the rate of catecholamine synthesis. Medullary norepinephrine and epinephrine are stored in granules together with ATP, lipid, and proteins, including chromogranin A. The catecholamines, ATP, and granular protein are all released together by exocytosis in response to physiologic and pharmacologic stimuli. Circulating levels of chromogranin A may reflect

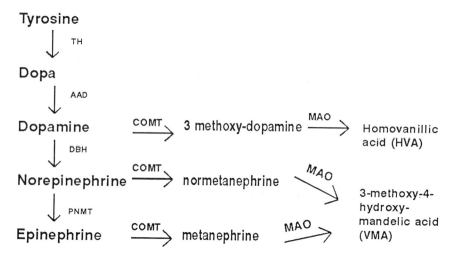

Figure 1 Principal pathways for catecholamine synthesis and metabolism. TH, tyrosine hydroxylase; AAD, aromatic amino acid decarboxylase; DBH, dopamine β-hydroxylase; PNMT, phenylethanolamine *N*-methyltransferase; COMT, catechol-*O*-methyltransferase; MAO, monoamine oxidase.

sympathoadrenal activity and also be a marker for pheochromocytoma (1,2).

B. Metabolism: Major Pathways

The major portion of norepinephrine released from sympathetic nerve endings is biologically inactivated by reuptake into the neuron granules. Monoamine oxidase located near mitochondria is the major enzyme in the intraneuronal degradation of norepinephrine. Circulating norepinephrine and adrenal medullary epinephrine are primarily O-methylated by catechol-*O*-methyltransferase (COMT) to normetanephrine and metanephrine, respectively, and excreted in urine. Most of the rest is oxidized by monoamine oxidase (MAO) to form 3-methoxy-4-hydroxymandelic acid (VMA), the catecholamine metabolite in greatest abundance in urine. Dopamine is also inactivated by MAO and COMT to form homovanillic acid, a major urinary metabolite (Fig. 1). Only small quantities of free dopamine, norepinephrine, and epinephrine appear in the urine.

C. Physiologic Effects

The physiologic effects of dopamine, norepinephrine, and epinephrine are mediated by specific receptors on the surface of the effector cell membrane. This hormone-receptor interaction triggers a series of events that lead to the biologic responses distinct to each amine by controlling the synthesis or release of second messengers.

There are two classes of adrenergic receptors, α and β, which have been further subdivided into α_1 and α_2 and β_1 and β_2 subtypes. Both β receptors stimulate the adenylate cyclase system through mediation of a G protein. α_1 Receptors are concerned with increases in intracellular calcium ion concentration; α_2 receptor activation inhibits adenylyl cyclase by interacting with an inhibitory G protein. In general, activation of α receptors is excitatory and activation of β receptors is inhibitory, except that stimulation of α receptors relaxes intestinal muscles and decreases insulin secretion but stimulation of β receptors in the myocardium is excitatory. β_1 Receptors enhance cardiac contractility, heart rate, and atrioventricular conduction. β_2 Receptors are concerned with vasodilation and bronchodilation but also increase insulin release. There are specific vascular receptors for dopamine (DA1). Activation of DA1 receptors induces vasodilation primarily in renal, mesenteric, coronary, and cerebral arterial beds; DA2 receptors are concerned with inhibition of norepinephrine (NE) release from sympathetic nerve endings and inhibition of prolactin release. Receptor responses to the catecholamines may be altered in response to drugs and in various diseases. Furthermore, autoantibodies to surface hormone receptors have been described that may simulate or inhibit hormone action.

The catecholamines help maintain a constant internal environment and are important in circulatory, visceral, and metabolic functions. Briefly, norepinephrine primarily functions as a neurotransmitter released from the axon terminals of sympathetic postganglion neurons at the effector cell, where it stimulates α receptors and causes constriction of arterioles and venules and a rise in systolic and diastolic blood pressure. In unusual stress, it may also function as a hormone (transported in the bloodstream from site of origin to site of action). Epinephrine exhibits both α- and β-adrenergic activity and has the following physiologic effects: increases heart rate and myocardial conduction rate, increases ventricular contractility, relaxes bronchial musculature, promotes glycogenolysis, and releases free fatty acids from adipose tissue. Its effect on the β cells of the pancreas depends on the balance between α and β activity, but it is usually inhibitory. The catecholamines also stimulate growth hormone, renin, glucagon, and parathyroid hormone secretion (3).

D. Biochemical Analyses

It is important to ask laboratory personnel whether drugs and other compounds will interfere with the analyses before urine or plasma samples are collected. Otherwise there may be serious errors in interpretation of results. For example, diazoxide and theophylline may stimulate endogenous catecholamine release. Exogenous catecholamines, such as nose drops, bronchodilators, and cough remedies, can be measured in the assay. Methylglucamine in radiographic contrast dye interferes with metanephrine analysis when Pisano methodology is used. Labetalol metabolites interfere in all tests. Phenothiazines and tricyclic antidepressants can cause variable changes. Clearly it is best to discontinue all medications for 7–10 days before specimens are collected, if possible (4).

1. Urine

Measurements of catecholamines and metabolites in *urine* have been used in clinical medicine for many years. Urinary free catecholamine excretion provides an integrated assessment of amine secretion over time and is usually analyzed by high-performance liquid chromatographic (HPLC) methodology. The determination of dopamine, norepinephrine, and epinephrine by HPLC has very high sensitivity. The metabolites are separated by chromatography and then measured by spectrophotometry. 24 h urine samples are preferable to random single void specimens, in which the catecholamine or metabolite output is expressed per milligram creatinine excretion. This is particularly important in infants and young children, in whom daily creatinine excretion is not constant. Normal values for various age groups should be established by the laboratory doing the analyses. The daily urinary output of catecholamines and metabolites increases with age but, if standardized by body surface area, is similar among children and adolescents (Table 1) (5,6).

2. Plasma

Plasma dopamine, norepinephrine, and epinephrine concentrations can be determined by radioenzymatic isotope assays or by HPLC. Collection of samples and preparation for analysis require meticulous attention to detail. Circulating catecholamines have a short half-life (30–60 s), and there is considerable biologic variation in plasma concentrations

Table 1 Urinary Catecholamine Excretion in Children[a]—μg per 24 hr

Age	NE (mean $\pm$ SD)	E (mean $\pm$ SD)	VMA (mean $\pm$ SD)
Birth to 1 year	10.6 $\pm$ 3.4	1.3 $\pm$ 1.2	569 $\pm$ 309
1–5 years	18.8 $\pm$ 7.0	3.2 $\pm$ 2.7	1348 $\pm$ 443
6–15 years	37.4 $\pm$ 16.6	4.8 $\pm$ 2.4	2373 $\pm$ 698
Over 15 years	50.7 $\pm$ 15.7	7.1 $\pm$ 3.3	3192 $\pm$ 669

[a]SD, standard deviation; NE, norepinephrine; E, epinephrine; VMA, vanillylmandelic acid (3-methoxy-4-hydroxymandelic acid).
Source: From Reference 5.

among healthy individuals. Physical and mental stress, decrease in plasma sodium and glucose levels, change in position from supine to erect, drugs, and a host of other factors influence plasma catecholamine concentrations. Thus, interpretation of measurements may be very difficult even under physiologic conditions, particularly if a single plasma sample is obtained. Elevated plasma catecholamine levels occur in any acute illness, in diabetic ketoacidosis, and in acute heart failure. Some patients with essential hypertension have plasma catecholamine levels that overlap those of patients with hypertension caused by a pheochromocytoma.

III. DISORDERS OF THE ADRENAL MEDULLA

The primary disorders of the adrenal medulla in childhood are neoplasms. The neuroblastoma arises from intra- or extraadrenal sympathetic nervous tissue; the pheochromocytoma develops from chromaffin cells wherever they are located. The neuroblastoma is highly malignant and found primarily in infancy and early childhood; the pheochromocytoma is rarely malignant in childhood and occurs at any age, with peak frequency at 20–30 years. Abnormally high levels of catecholamines are found in plasma and urine of most affected individuals with either neoplasm and serve as tumor markers.

Adrenal medullary hyperplasia has been described, particularly in association with multiple endocrine neoplasia type II syndromes. It may be a forerunner of pheochromocytoma.

No apparent diseases are caused by adrenal medullary insufficiency. Epinephrine deficiency has been reported in some infants with hypoglycemia, but it seems likely other factors were causative because the adrenal medulla is not necessary for euglycemia. In fact, patients who have had bilateral adrenalectomy recover similarly to healthy controls following acute insulin-induced hypoglycemia (7).

A. Pheochromocytoma

The pheochromocytoma is a rare tumor of children and adolescents whose diagnosis and localization often represent a challenge, even to the experienced physician. Signs and symptoms of catecholamine excess usually bring the patient to medical attention. Tumors have been found in the neonate, but the incidence generally peaks at age 9–12 years and boys are affected more often than girls.

Bilateral and multiple adrenal tumors are more common in children than adults, but malignant pheochromocytomas are rare in the pediatric population. The neoplasm can arise wherever chromaffin cells are located, from the base of the skull to the urinary bladder and rectum. Intrathoracic pheochromocytomas are rare in children. Tumors located outside the adrenal medulla are often called functional paragangliomas. Extraadrenal tumors, familial pheochromocytomas, and multiple endocrine neoplasia syndromes have been reported more frequently in children with pheochromocytoma than in adults. In a review of four series of pediatric patients with pheochromocytomas, familial associations were present in 31–57% of patients ($N = 45$) (8).

1. Clinical Presentation

Hypertension, headache, and excessive perspiration are the most common clinical manifestations of pheochromocytoma, the severity varying considerably among patients.

Hypertension is usually sustained in children, but episodic attacks suggestive of the intermittent release of catecholamines by tumor may occur. Sometimes the paroxysms are precipitated by excitement or a particular physical activity, such as bending over or lifting a heavy object. A dramatic history is given by the patient with a pheochromocytoma of the urinary bladder who becomes symptomatic during micturition. Sometimes children with sustained hypertension also have paroxysmal episodes. Other times they are normotensive between attacks. Pallor rather than flushing usually occurs during an episode because there is constriction of the vascular bed, not dilation. Very rarely hypotension (and flushing) occurs because the tumor produces only epinephrine or vasodilating peptides.

Nausea, vomiting, abdominal pain, constipation, polyuria, and polydipsia are less common features. Affected children often are emotionally labile and have an anxious expression. Sometimes they are labeled hyperactive, with an "attention deficit disorder." When hypertension is severe and of long standing, mottling of the skin and cold extremities with acrocyanosis result from peripheral constriction of blood vessels (Table 2). Bone lesions have been described following changes in the microcirculation in association with pheochromocytoma. Orthostatic hypotension may be found related to an inability to activate sympathetic reflexes on standing and to decreased blood volume. Excessive production of catecholamines may lead to dilated or hypertrophic cardiomyopathy and congestive heart failure mediated primarily by the α-adrenergic receptor system. Hypertensive retinopathy and hypertensive encephalopathy, although rare in children, may mimic a brain tumor. Pheochromocytoma can also masquerade as hypertension of other causes, such as thyrotoxicosis, primary renal disease, diabetes mellitus, an emotional disorder, or essential hypertension (8–27,150). Alternatively, acute mercury poisoning may mimic pheochromocytoma (28).

Pheochromocytoma sometimes occurs in association with other disorders, including neurofibromatosis (29), Cushing syndrome (30–33), cerebellar hemangioblastoma (34) and astrocytoma (35), intracerebral aneurysms (36), von Hippel-Lindau syndrome (37), polycythemia (38), sarcoidosis (39), and multiple endocrine neoplasia syndromes (see next section). Pheochromocytomas are inherited in generations of

some families in a dominant pattern (40). The tumor may be "silent" until a stressful event, such as induction of anesthesia or the labor of pregnancy, causes a rapid release of catecholamines and an unexpected hypertensive crisis (41,42). The pheochromocytoma may be an incidental finding at postmortem examination, especially in the elderly patient (43).

2. Diagnosis

a. Biochemical Tests. Although the clinical findings just described may cause the physician strongly to suspect a pheochromocytoma, definitive diagnosis depends on demonstration of excess catecholamine secretion. The most commonly used diagnostic procedure is measurement of urinary catecholamines and their metabolites, the metanephrines, and 3-methoxy-4-hydroxymandelic acid. These compounds are best determined in a 24 h urine sample, which is analyzed by sensitive and specific biochemical techniques. If all values are normal, pheochromocytoma is unlikely. Some investigators have reported valid results from random urine samples of 8–12 h collections in which the output of metabolite is expressed as concentration per milligram creatinine. A potential problem in interpretation of results occurs because creatinine excretion is not constant from day to day in young children. Furthermore, the tumor may release catecholamine intermittently. The physician should always check with the laboratory so that dietary products, medications, and other substances that can interfere with the assay are eliminated beforehand. Some techniques for measuring VMA, particularly, are nonspecific and give falsely elevated values. The daily excretion of catecholamines and metabolites is much less in healthy children than adults, so that appropriate control data are essential.

If the patient has intermittent episodes of hypertension, it is best to collect a timed urine specimen during an attack and compare the findings with excretion of catecholamines and metabolites during an asymptomatic interval. It is seldom necessary to perform provocative tests (see Sec. III.A.2.b).

In most patients with pheochromocytoma, the urinary output of total catecholamines, the metanephrines, and VMA is remarkably elevated above normal. Measurement of urinary metanephrine is the best screening test. When excretion of metabolites is equivocably abnormal, catecholamine output should be checked. Fractionation into norepinephrine and epinephrine is helpful. High epinephrine levels suggest that the tumor is intraadrenal or in the organ of Zuckerkandl, although exceptions have been reported. Likewise, epinephrine has potent β-adrenergic effects that may cause tachyarrhythmias and hypermetabolic syndromes. Interestingly, the predominant catecholamine excreted by children with pheochromocytoma is norepinephrine, in contrast to adults, in whom both norepinephrine and epinephrine output may be high. The pattern of catecholamine excretion does not differentiate benign from malignant pheochromocytomas. Although urinary excretion of dopamine and homovanillic acid (HVA) is often remarkably elevated in patients with malignant tumors, it also may be abnormally high in association with benign pheochromocytomas (44–46). Tumor size and cate-

Table 2 Signs and Symptoms of Pheochromocytoma in Children

Hypertension, usually sustained	Fatigue
Headache	Emotional lability
Diaphoresis	Polyuria, polydipsia
Nausea and vomiting	Constipation
Weight loss	Visual disturbances
Abdominal pain	Cold digits

cholamine output do not correlate well. Small tumors often release large amounts of norepinephrine and epinephrine directly into the circulation; large tumors may degrade the amines within the tumor and release large amounts of metabolites. In most patients with a pheochromocytoma, the total urinary catecholamine excretion by HPLC determination is elevated more than twofold above normal.

Most patients with pheochromocytomas have markedly elevated plasma catecholamine concentrations if samples are obtained when the individual is hypertensive. Normal values of norepinephrine and cpinephrine may be found during asymptomatic intervals. Overlap of plasma catecholamine levels has been reported between patients with and without tumor. Furthermore, sample collections and analysis require strict attention to detail. Many medications interfere with the assay, as noted previously. The patient should rest supine for 20–30 minutes after the needle is inserted in the vein, before the specimen is collected; the sample requires special handling and storage. Physicians who order plasma studies should be thoroughly familiar with the procedure and interpretation of results to avoid diagnostic errors. In some individuals, norepinephrine and epinephrine levels may reach "tumor range" in association with the stress of blood drawing. This is a particular problem in young children. Generally, total plasma catecholamine levels over 2000 pg/ml are indicative of pheochromocytoma.

Measurement of *both* urinary catecholamines and metabolites as well as plasma NE and epinephrine may lead to diagnosis when the clinical findings strongly suggest a pheochromocytoma and individual urine or plasma test results are equivocal. Studies should be repeated several times if the clinical picture and the biochemical findings are disparate (47–50). Simultaneous measurement of dihydroxyphenylglycol, the deaminated product of NE metabolism within sympathetic neurons, and norepinephrine (in urine or plasma) may be helpful when diagnosis is difficult. Because the norepinephrine from pheochromocytoma is extraneuronal in origin, norepinephrine levels are disproportionately elevated compared with DHPG when a tumor is present (51,52).

Pheochromocytoma can also produce vasoactive intestinal polypeptide (VIP) (25,53–55), adrenomedullin (56), parathyroid hormone (57), adrenorphin (58), adrenocorticotropic hormone (ACTH) (30–33), serotonin (54), renin (59,60), enolase enzymes (61) and growth hormone-releasing factor (62). Lactic acidosis has been reported in patients with pheochromocytoma, probably secondary to the effect of catecholamines on intermediary metabolism and the peripheral circulation (63). Carcinoid syndrome and pheochromocytoma may occur together (64). No wonder the clinical manifestations of a pheochromocytoma are so variable!

b. Pharmacologic Tests. Pharmacologic tests seldom have a role in the diagnosis of pheochromocytoma in children. They are potentially dangerous (especially the provocative tests, such as histamine and tyramine) and are associated with a high number of false positive and false negative results that serve only to confuse the physician. In rare cases, phentolamine administration can differentiate a hypertensive crisis as a result of catecholamine excess from "essential" hypertension; that is, the pressure drops if the hypertension is caused by catecholamines because the drug is an α-adrenergic blocker.

The clonidine suppression test may be useful in certain patients when biochemical studies are equivocable. Clonidine is a central-acting α2-adrenergic agonist. The drug suppresses plasma catecholamine levels of patients with essential hypertension (neurologically mediated catecholamines), whereas catecholamines released into the circulation from pheochromocytomas bypass normal storage and release mechanisms and are not suppressed. Hypotension is a potential risk in both patients with essential hypertension and those with a pheochromocytoma because clonidine inhibits central sympathetic outflow. It is critical that the catecholamine assay employed measure only plasma free catecholamines because the half-life of conjugated amines is long and may lead to a false positive clonidine test. False negative results have also been reported (65,66).

3. Localization of Tumor

After the biochemical studies have established the diagnosis of a catecholamine-producing tumor(s), investigative procedures are directed toward anatomic localization of the lesion. Before these studies are done, it is best to protect the patient from the potential risk of sudden catecholamine release by the tumor by use of α-adrenergic blockers if invasive procedures are contemplated.

Computed axial tomography (CT) and magnetic resonance imaging (MRI) are used for preoperative localization of tumor (Fig. 2). The third- and fourth-generation CT scanners can detect tumors in the adrenal that are >1.0 cm accurately, and the test is less expensive than MRI. However, MRI is helpful in distinguishing pheochromocytoma from other adrenal lesions because the T2-weighted images have a high signal intensity in pheochromocytoma. MRI may be more desirable for extraadrenal locations and in pregnant patients. Ultrasonography can be a helpful adjunct in children, who have less retroperitoneal fat.

If abdominal imaging results are negative, scintigraphic localization with ^{123}I or ^{131}I MIBG (metaiodobenzylguanidine) is indicated. This is the examination of choice for recurrent or metastatic disease because it permits whole-body imaging. This radiopharmaceutical accumulates in chromaffin tissue and thus can indicate the location of a pheochromocytoma. Some physicians routinely perform preoperative MIBG scanning in children in a complementary fashion with the CT to aid in localization of extraadrenal tumors. The test has a false negative rate of up to 10%, predominantly caused by limited uptake by tumor cells. False positive scans are rare.

Venography and selective arteriography very seldom are required for localization of tumor. They should be used only when imaging studies fail to identify a lesion and biochemical studies indicate the presence of a catecholamine-producing tumor. Venography is usually a safe procedure. Blood samples are obtained at different levels of the inferior or superior

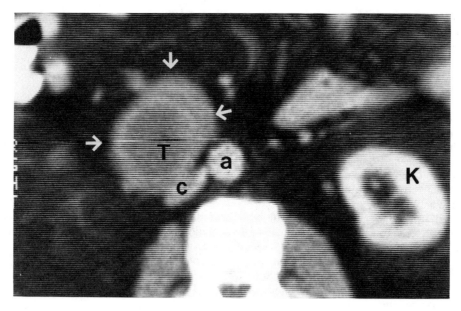

Figure 2 Abdominal CT showing an extraadrenal pheochromocytoma (arrows). The low central attenuation with peripheral enhancement suggests central necrosis; a, aorta; c, vena cava; K, kidney. (Courtesy of E. Afshani, M.D., Department of Radiology, Buffalo Children's Hospital.)

vena cava or other veins for assay of plasma catecholamine concentrations in an effort to delineate the site of a functioning tumor. The data must be interpreted carefully because blood flow patterns and intermittent release of hormones from normal adrenal glands or tumor influence the plasma levels of norepinephrine and epinephrine. At times it is difficult to differentiate abnormally high from normal values. Arteriography is a risky procedure because the contrast material required for visualization may cause the release of catecholamine by a pheochromocytoma. It is best to establish α blockade before angiography is done or to have phentolamine available for emergency intravenous administration (24,67–74).

4. Treatment

The objective of therapy is to remove the excess catecholamines that are produced by the pheochromocytoma. Surgical excision is the treatment of choice. It is essential that patients scheduled for surgery have stable blood pressure and be adequately protected from a sudden discharge of catecholamines during the induction of anesthesia and the operative procedure by adequate preoperative α blockade alone or in combination with β blockade. Such therapy has changed surgery of children with pheochromocytomas from high risk to a resection as safe as that of other tumors within the chest and abdomen (23). Preoperative normalization of blood pressure and resolution of symptoms are associated with a favorable outcome (75). When excision is not possible, that is, in patients who have a malignant pheochromocytoma, pharmacologic agents can be used to inhibit catecholamine synthesis or to establish adrenergic blockade (see Sec. III.B)

5. Preoperative Treatment

Preoperative pharmacologic therapy for 2–3 weeks is usually required to control hypertension and the other physiologic and metabolic consequences of high levels of circulating catecholamines, depending on the severity of the problem. Some patients require longer preparation. α-Adrenergic blocking agents should be administered to control hypertension. The amount of medication required to achieve adequate blockade varies from patient to patient and is achieved by gradually increasing the daily dose until the desired response is obtained. Phenoxybenzamine hydrochloride (Dibenzyline) is a long-acting oral preparation that has been prescribed for years and has proven to be an excellent drug to control the pressor effects of the catecholamines in children. Phenoxybenzamine, 5 mg every 12 h, orally (PO), is an appropriate starting dose in a young child; an older child may require 10 mg every 12 h PO. The daily dose can be increased every 3–4 days, as necessary. Some physicians calculate the dose based on body weight, that is, phenoxybenzamine at 0.25–4 mg/kg per day (23,24). Undesirable side effects of phenoxybenzamine therapy include nasal congestion, gastrointestinal irritation, and hypotension. Prazosin (Minipress) is used to prepare adults with pheochromocytoma for surgery, but information about its benefit in children is sparse. Nifedipine and labetalol have been prescribed alone or in combination with phenoxybenzamine in children, but these drugs have not been as successful as phenoxybenzamine in controlling hypertension and the clinical symptoms of catecholamine excess.

Phentolamine mesylate (Regitine) is a short-acting α-adrenergic blocking agent that is particularly effective for intravenous use to control blood pressure rapidly during hypertensive crises, diagnostic imaging, or surgery. Phentolamine, 1 mg per dose, intravenously or intramuscularly, is appropriate therapy for a child. The drug can also be titrated intravenously to provide short-term control of hypertension. Phentolamine can be administered orally, but it must be given every 4–6 h because of its short duration of action. Furthermore, this drug often causes gastrointestinal irritation, nasal stuffiness, and weakness in children, so that oral therapy is seldom prescribed.

When tachyarrhythmias are present, usually from release of epinephrine by a pheochromocytoma, treatment with β blocking drugs may be necessary. β-Adrenergic antagonists should not be given before adequate α blockade has been achieved to protect the heart from unopposed α-adrenergic stimulation. Propranolol is the primary drug that has been used. It can be given intravenously for acute control of arrhythmias or orally for long-term therapy. Propranolol, 1 mg, administered intravenously over 1 minute, with electrocardiographic monitoring, is usually sufficient for a therapeutic response. The initial oral dose of propranolol is 5–10 mg every 6–8 h. The doses should be titrated upward as necessary to achieve the desired effect. Patients with catecholamine cardiomyopathy require careful monitoring because they may be particularly sensitive to β-adrenergic antagonists (76–77).

When adrenergic blockade does not control the pressor and metabolic effects of excessive catecholamine production by a pheochromocytoma, treatment with α-methyl-p-tyrosine (AMPT; Demser, Merck) may be given to inhibit the synthesis of dopamine, norepinephrine, and epinephrine. An initial dose of AMPT, 5–10 mg/kg per day, orally in divided doses every 6 h, is usually effective. It may be titrated upward as necessary to control the symptoms. The usual side effects are sedation and gastrointestinal disturbances, although high doses of the drug have the potential to cause tremor, muscle stiffness, and depression from dopamine deficiency (78).

In addition to protecting the patient from the risks of hypertension and sudden catecholamine release by a pheochromocytoma during surgery, preoperative α blockade permits reexpansion of the intravascular space, which often is constricted by chronic adrenergic hyperactivity. Thus, the potential danger of hypovolemic shock following excision of the tumor and sudden expansion of the vascular bed is obviated (79). Some surgeons prefer that adrenergic blocking drugs be discontinued 12–24 h before operation so that increases in blood pressure during manipulation of tumor at operation can be used as a guide to its location and the presence of multiple pheochromocytomas.

6. Intraoperative Treatment

It is critical that the anesthesiologist and the surgeon understand the pathophysiology of norepinephrine and epinephrine excess and that the blood pressure and cardiac function of the patient be monitored carefully from induction of anesthesia to the end of the operative procedure. Short-acting drugs, such as phentolamine or sodium nitroprusside, are effective for management of intraoperative hypertension. Propranolol can be used to control tachydysrhythmias. Hypotension is uncommon after tumor excision if the patient has been properly prepared with α-adrenergic antagonists. Rapid administration of volume-expanding fluids should be given if hypotension occurs. Hydrocortisone is required if both adrenals are excised for removal of bilateral adrenomedullary pheochromocytomas.

7. Postoperative Care

Close monitoring of blood pressure and cardiac function is mandatory until the patient is completely stable. Hypertension often continues for 24–48 h postoperatively because of the release of stored catecholamines from adrenergic granules in the sympathetic nerve endings. Persistent hypertension may signal fluid overload, the presence of residual pheochromocytomas, or renovascular problems. If the hypertension abates following intravenous administration of phentolamine, it is likely another tumor(s) is present. Furosamide can be administered to reduce intravascular volume, if necessary.

Hypoglycemia, which can be corrected by intravenous dextrose therapy, may occur 2–3 h after surgery. It is thought to be caused by increased insulin release from β cells of the pancreas and is a transient phenomenon.

In all patients who have had excision of a pheochromocytoma urinary catecholamines and metabolites (metanephrine and VMA) should be measured 4–6 weeks after surgery, looking for residual tumor. Likewise, long-term medical follow-up is important because additional tumors may appear years later. The prognosis after removal of benign pheochromocytomas is usually excellent. Family members and the patient should also be checked for the presence of multiple endocrine neoplasia syndromes (79–82).

B. Malignant Pheochromocytomas

About 10% of pheochromocytomas of adults are malignant, but a malignant tumor is very rare in children (83). Diagnosis is difficult because benign tumors can be extraadrenal and multicentric, and pleomorphic cells, blood vessel involvement, and capsular invasion are found in benign tumors. There are no characteristic biochemical features of benign or malignant tumors. Elevated urinary dopamine and HVA levels have been found more often in association with malignant tumors, but they can be present with benign pheochromocytomas as well (84). Conclusive diagnosis of malignancy is made when functioning pheochromocytomas are located in areas where chromaffin cells normally are not found. Iodine 131 MIBG scintigraphy is a valuable aid in localization of metastatic pheochromocytoma (72,73). Sites include the skeleton, liver, lung, lymph nodes, brain, spinal cord, and pleura.

Malignant pheochromocytomas are generally resistant to chemotherapy and radiation therapy. Iodine 131 MIBG may be beneficial in certain patients when tumors are in soft tissue and concentrate the agent (85). A combination of cyclophosphamide, vincristine, and dacarbazine has been used with some success (86). Long-term treatment with α- and β-adrenergic blockade or α-methyl-p-tyrosine is effective in controlling the clinical manifestations of catecholamine excess. In addition, AMPT has been reported to cause a reduction in size of pulmonary metastases (87,88). Survival may continue for many years.

IV. MULTIPLE ENDOCRINE NEOPLASIA SYNDROMES

Adrenal medullary hyperplasia and pheochromocytoma are components of multiple endocrine neoplasia (MEN) syndromes IIa and b. MEN syndromes are familial disorders characterized by hyperplasia or tumor involving more than one endocrine gland. The clinical findings are variable and reflect the functional status of the hormone-producing tissue. At times, it takes many years for the clinical manifestations to evolve from single-gland endocrinopathy to multiple-organ involvement. The changes may be benign or malignant. The disorders are generally inherited in an autosomal dominant pattern, with high penetrance and variable expressivity. Most tumors of the MEN syndromes arise from cells of the APUD (amine precursor uptake and decarboxylation) series. Some of the cells are derived from neural crest; others appear to have endodermal or mesodermal origins. Awareness of the syndromes and preventive screening have led to diagnosis in increasingly younger children.

A. Multiple Endocrine Neoplasia IIa (Sipple Syndrome)

MEN IIa is composed of medullary carcinoma of the thyroid, pheochromocytoma, and parathyroid hyperplasia or tumor (89,90). Recently, primary cutaneous lichen amyloidosis was reported in several families (91). The frequency of the syndrome is difficult to ascertain because both pheochromocytoma and medullary thyroid carcinoma may appear as sporadic cases or familial disorders. The clinical course develops over years (92). The specific genetic defect is linked to chromosome 10 (93,94), and DNA-based diagnostic screening permits prediction of the gene carrier status with 90–99% certainty in informative families (95–97).

Medullary thyroid carcinoma (MTC) arises from the C cells of the thyroid gland and is transmitted as an autosomal dominant from generation to generation to children of either sex. Usually there is no evidence of thyroid disease on physical examination unless metastases are present. Rarely iodine 131 MIBG scintigraphy identifies MTC (71,98). The tumor is not thyroid-stimulating hormone dependent. The C cells of the thyroid and MTC produce the hormone calcitonin. High basal plasma calcitonin levels or abnormal calcitonin secretion in response to provocative testing with calcium infusion or pentagastrin stimulation helps to identify patients with MTC. Systematic screening of first-degree relatives of patients with MTC using calcitonin provocative tests has resulted in early diagnosis, early treatment, and long-term survival. It is recommended that screening begin before age 1 year for children in kindreds with MEN IIa. The combination of biochemical testing and determination of the gene carrier status permits the clinician to focus pentagastrin testing on those children at highest risk for MTC. In such individuals,

the test should be performed at least annually, depending on the calcitonin levels. Because 5–10% of a random population have abnormal calcitonin test results, DNA analysis is an important tool for diagnosis of MTC in MEN IIa kindreds (99,151). The reader should seek the latest information about MTC for appropriate management of patients. Total thyroidectomy is the treatment for MTC (100–106).

Pheochromocytomas are usually bilateral or multifocal within the adrenal glands in MEN IIa, developing gradually over the years in more than 50% of these patients. In fact, many surgeons recommend bilateral adrenalectomy when a diagnosis of pheochromocytoma is made, whether or not tumors are evident in both adrenal glands (107). The diagnosis of MTC usually precedes that of a pheochromocytoma. Yearly measurement of urinary norepinephrine and epinephrine is recommended for prospective screening, but the tumor may not secrete sufficient amine for detection until it has reached considerable size. It is likely that adrenal medullary hyperplasia precedes formation of a pheochromocytoma, per se (90). In some patients, 24 h urinary epinephrine excretion or the ratio of epinephrine to norepinephrine is more apt to be abnormal than 24 h urinary norepinephrine excretion. Computed tomography or MRI and MIBG scintigraphy are recommended to locate a tumor when catecholamine levels are abnormally increased (71,108). A careful search for a pheochromocytoma always should be performed preoperatively in patients who have other components of an MEN syndrome so that the tumor, if present, can be excised first.

Hypercalcemia, often insidious in onset, leads to the diagnosis of hyperparathyroidism. Hyperplasia rather than adenoma is the more common parathyroid disorder. The incidence and etiology are not clear. Treatment is surgical.

The cutaneous skin lesions that occur with MEN IIa appear to be a distinct but rare clinical variation. They usually evolve over a period of years, often beginning in childhood as an area of pruritus located over the upper back between the scapulae. This leads to intense scratching, hyperkeratosis, hyperpigmentation, and, finally, development of cutaneous lichen amyloidoses (89, 109).

B. Multiple Endocrine Neoplasia IIb

The major components of MEN IIb syndrome are multiple neuromas, medullary thyroid carcinoma, and pheochromocytoma. The gene is located on chromosome 10 as in MEN IIa. The syndrome can usually be diagnosed based on the physical examination.

Affected individuals often have a marfanoid body build, but in contrast to patients with Marfan syndrome, they do not have aortic or lens abnormalities. Dorsal kyphosis, pectus excavatum, pes cavus, and other skeletal disorders may be present. The presence of neuromas may cause thick "bumpy lips," nodules of the tongue and buccal mucosa, as well as of the eyelids and conjunctivae. Hypertrophied corneal nerves may be seen on slit lamp examination. When significant intestinal ganglioneuromatosis occurs, the patient often has diverse gastrointestinal manifestations of disease, including diarrhea alternating with constipation and obstruction. Diagnosis is confirmed by biopsy and histologic examination. Mucosal neuromas are not subject to carcinomatous change but may be a significant cosmetic problem. There is no specific treatment for the multiple neuromas (110–114).

Medullary thyroid carcinoma and pheochromocytoma were reviewed previously in this chapter. MTC is usually diagnosed before pheochromocytoma in MEN IIb (115–118). In fact, MTC appears at a young age, so that children born to affected families should be screened soon after birth. Usually the phenotypic appearance of affected patients identifies those at risk for MTC so that testing can be performed promptly.

C. Multiple Endocrine Neoplasia I and Mixed Type Syndromes

MEN I syndrome (tumors of the anterior pituitary, pancreas, and parathyroids) is beyond the scope of this chapter. The reader who desires information is referred to recent reviews (119,120).

Overlap between the various MEN syndromes has been described (121). In addition, ectopic secretion of ACTH, VIP, and prostaglandins has been reported, particularly in association with medullary thyroid carcinoma (102). Tumors of the adrenal cortex, carcinoids, thymomas, schwannomas, and other neoplasias have been reported in adults. There appears to be a spectrum of endocrinopathies and tumors among the MEN syndromes (122).

V. NEUROBLASTOMA

The neuroblastoma and pheochromocytoma are embryologically related tumors because both arise from neural crest ectoderm. Neuroblastomas derive from the primitive sympathoblasts within the sympathoadrenal system that normally differentiate to form sympathetic ganglion cells. The tumor has been found in the fetus and newborn infant and has a peak incidence before the age of 3 years. Most patients less than 1 year of age at diagnosis are cured of neuroblastoma, whereas children over 2 years of age at diagnosis usually succumb with widespread metastases. Recent investigations have shown a significant association between N-myc oncogene amplification and rapid progression of the tumor (123). Neuroblastomas have the highest spontaneous regression of any tumor in the human and also have the capacity to differentiate and mature to ganglioneuroblastomas and, thence, to benign ganglioneuromas. Like pheochromocytoma, they may occur in more than one member in a family. The basis for these intriguing characteristics is not understood (124–129).

It is beyond the scope of this chapter to include a detailed description of neuroblastoma and its management. The reader is referred to an in-depth current perspective on the tumor (130). The following is a general summary of the results of biochemical analyses of body fluids and tumor tissue of patients with neuroblastoma.

Abnormally high levels of catecholamines and/or their metabolites are found in the urine of approximately 95% of children with neuroblastomas and ganglioneuroblastomas. Although there is a similar histologic appearance among each tumor type, there is no consistent pattern in urinary excretion of catecholamines and metabolites by patients with these neoplasms. Most children (80–85%) excrete abnormally large amounts of dopamine, homovanillic acid, norepinephrine, and 3-methoxy-4-hydroxymandelic acid. About 15%, however, have high HVA and *normal* VMA output in urine (44,131). In rare cases, no abnormality in the urinary excretion of the catecholamines or their metabolites is found, particularly when the neuroblastoma arises from dorsal root ganglia (132). Thus, measurement of VMA alone is not an ideal screening test because a normal value does not rule out neuroblastoma (133). Determination of both HVA and VMA should detect most cases (134). Urinary epinephrine excretion is normal in patients with neuroblastoma and ganglioneuroblastoma because the tumors are unable to synthesize this amine.

Children with neuroblastoma usually excrete much smaller amounts of norepinephrine than those with ganglioneuroblastoma or pheochromocytoma. Even when the pressor amine excretion is as high or higher than that found in association with pheochromocytoma, patients with neuroblastoma and ganglioneuroblastoma usually do not have hypertension or paroxysmal attacks suggesting excess catecholamine release from the tumor. Weinblatt et al. (135), found hypertension in 19% of 59 children with neurogenic tumor. At the time of diagnosis or with progression of disease, there was no correlation of hypertension with urinary catecholamine levels. Compared with pheochromocytoma, most neuroblastomas have a paucity of storage granules and low tissue levels of catecholamine, suggesting an ineffective storage mechanism. Unbound catecholamines are easily metabolized by COMT and MAO to nonpressor compounds. The granular abnormality may also disrupt the synthesis of norepinephrine from dopamine and account for the large urinary dopamine and HVA excretion compared with norepinephrine and VMA in some patients with neuroblastoma (44).

There is no specific relation between the pattern of urinary catecholamine excretion and regression of tumor or survival with neuroblastoma, except that patients with advanced metastatic disease may have a better prognosis when the VMA/HVA ratio is high, suggesting that tumors that are unable to synthesize large amounts of norepinephrine are more malignant. Persistent tumor or recurrence of tumor is associated with abnormally high levels of catecholamines and/or metabolites, so that serial measurements are helpful in following the response to therapy. Sometimes mild elevation of HVA and/or VMA may be found when patients are in remission (136). Both primary tumors and metastases are capable of producing catecholamines.

A variety of compounds have been measured in plasma and urine of patients with neuroblastoma in an attempt to understand the biology of the tumor and to identify the ideal tumor marker. Discussion here has focused on those substances that can be measured in most hospital or reference laboratories. In addition to catecholamines, studies suggest that nervous system-specific enolase (137,138), serum ferritin (139), serum lactic dehydrogenase (140), a tumor-associated ganglioside (141), and neuropeptide Y (142) are useful in the detection of tumor and evaluation of therapy. MIBG scintigraphy and ^{31}P nuclear magnetic resonance spectroscopy also appear to have potential as useful markers of growth or regression of neuroblastoma (72,73,143).

Mass screening for neuroblastoma in the newborn period and early infancy is being performed in several countries using urine-saturated filter paper to determine HVA and VMA by a HPLC technique. Japan has the longest follow-up experience concerning the effectiveness of mass screening. The early detection of neuroblastoma has improved the prognosis for patients by increasing the number of cured patients and decreasing the number of deaths. Late-onset neuroblastoma is probably not picked up by screening in infancy (144–146).

VI. GANGLIONEUROMA

The ganglioneuroma is a benign tumor composed of mature ganglion cells that usually develops during childhood and young adulthood. It most likely represents a neuroblastoma that has progressed through the ganglioneuroblastoma stage and became a completely differentiated tumor. Serial sections of tissue are required to be certain nests of neuroblasts are not present. Patients harboring a completely mature ganglioneuroma seldom have abnormally elevated urinary catecholamines and metabolites except when accompanied by the syndrome of chronic diarrhea.

VII. NEURAL TUMORS AND CHRONIC DIARRHEA

Rarely, a patient with ganglioneuroblastoma or ganglioneuroma has a syndrome of failure to thrive, intractable watery diarrhea, and hypokalemia. Abdominal distension and metabolic acidosis may also be present. Water and electrolyte losses through the intestinal tract persist until the tumor is removed. The diarrhea then ceases abruptly, and the patient quickly improves.

The secretory diarrhea is caused by production of vasoactive intestinal peptide by the tumor. Many of these patients also excrete large amounts of catecholamines and metabolites in the urine. Prostaglandins are abnormally high in some patients (147,148).

Measurements of plasma VIP and urinary catecholamines should be performed in children with severe, intractable watery diarrhea. If levels of either or both are abnormally high, a search should be made for a neural crest tumor. Although the syndrome usually occurs with the more mature tumor, that is, ganglioneuroblastoma or ganglioneuroma, it has been reported in an infant with a neuroblastoma following chemotherapy. Interestingly, pathologic examination of the tumor revealed a maturing ganglioneuroblastoma (149).

Treatment is surgical excision of the tumor. Sometimes even partial resection results in reduction in VIP levels and cessation of diarrhea. Use of α-methyltyrosine may be beneficial when the tumor is nonresectable.

REFERENCES

1. O'Connor DT, Bernstein KN. Radioimmunoassay of chromogranin A in plasma as a measure of exocytotic sympathoadrenal activity in normal subjects and patients with pheochromocytoma. N Engl J Med 1984; 311:769–770.
2. O'Connor DT, Deftos LJ. Secretion of chromogranin A by peptide-producing endocrine neoplasms. N Engl J Med 1986; 314:1145–1151.
3. Bravo EL, Gifford RW Jr. Pheochromocytoma. Endocrinol Metab Clin North Am 1993; 22:329–341.
4. Sheps SG, Jiang N, Klee GG. Diagnostic evaluation of pheochromocytoma. Endocrinol Metab Clin North Am 1988; 17:397–414.
5. Voorhess ML. Urinary catecholamine excretion by healthy children. Daily excretion of dopamine, norepinephrine, epinephrine and 3-methoxy-4-hydroxymandelic acid. Pediatrics 1967; 39:252–257.
7. Gitlow SE, Mendlowitz M, Wilk EK, Wilk S, Wolf RL, Bertani LM. Excretion of catecholamine catabolites by normal children. J Lab Clin Med 1968; 72:612–620.
7. Ensinck JW, Walter RM, Palmer JR, Brodows RG, Campbell RG Glucagon responses to hypoglycemia in adrenalectomized man. Metabolism 1976; 25:227–232.
8. Caty MG, Coran AG, Thompson NW. Current diagnosis and treatment of pheochromocytoma in children. Arch Surg 1990; 125:978–981.
9. Tevetoglu F, Lee C-H. Adrenal pheochromocytoma simulating diabetes insipidus. Am J Dis Child 1956; 91:365–379.
10. Hume DM. Pheochromocytoma in the adult and in the child. Am J Surg 1960; 99:458–496.
11. Stackpole RH, Melicow MM, Uson AC. Pheochromocytoma in children. Report of 9 cases and review of the first 100 published cases with follow-up studies. J Pediatr 1963; 63:315–330.
12. Gifford RW Jr, Kvale WF, Maher FT, Roth GM, Priestley JT. Clinical features, diagnosis and treatment of pheochromocytoma: a review of 76 cases. Mayo Clin Proc 1964; 39:281–302.
13. Freier DT, Tank ES, Harrison TS. Pediatric and adult pheochromocytomas. Arch Surg 1973; 107:252–255.
14. Schwartz EL, Mao P, Hernried P, Born EE, Waldmann EB. Catecholamine-secreting paraganglioma. The problem of classification. Arch Intern Med 1975; 135:978–985.
15. Gibbs MK, Carney JA, Hayles A, Telander RL. Simultaneous adrenal and cervical pheochromocytomas in childhood. Ann Surg 1977; 185:273–278.
16. Hodgkinson DJ, Telander RL, Sheps SG, Gilchrist GS, Crowe JK. Extra-adrenal intrathoracic functioning paraganglioma (pheochromocytoma) in childhood. Mayo Clin Proc 1980; 55:271–276.
17. Karasov RS, Sheps SG, Carney JA, van Heerden JA, DeQuattro V. Paragangliomatosis with numerous catecholamine-producing tumors. Mayo Clin Proc 1982; 57:590–595.
18. Melicow MM. One hundred cases of pheochromocytoma (107 tumors) at the Columbia-Presbyterian Medical Center 1926–1976: a clinipathological analysis. Cancer 1977; v.40 1987–2004.
19. Schaffer MS, Zuberbuhler P, Wilson G, Rose V, Duncan WJ, Rowe RD. Catecholamine cardiomyopathy: an unusual presentation of pheochromocytoma in children. J Pediatr 1981; 99:276–279.

20. Imperato-McGinley J, Gautier T, Ehlers K, Zullo MA, Goldstein DS, Vaughan ED Jr. Reversibility of catecholamine-induced dilated cardiomyopathy in a child with pheochromocytoma. N Engl J Med 1987; 316:793–797.

21. David TE, Lenkei SC, Marquez-Julio A, Goldberg JA, Meldrum DAN. Pheochromocytoma of the heart. Ann Thorac Surg 1986; 41:98–100.

22. Marshall DG, Ein SH. Two boys with four pheochromocytomas each. J Pediatr Surg 1986; 21:815–817.

23. Kaufman BH, Telander RL, van Heerden JA, Zimmerman D, Sheps SG, Dawson B. Pheochromocytoma in the pediatric age group: current status. J Pediatr Surg 1983; 18:879–884.

24. Deal JE, Sever PS, Barratt TM, Dillon MJ. Phaeochromocytoma—investigation and management of 10 cases. Arch Dis Child 1990; 65:269–274.

25. Herrera MF, Stone E, Deitel M, Asa SL. Pheochromocytoma producing multiple vasoactive peptides. Arch Surg 1992; 127:105–108.

26. Greene JP, Guay AT. New perspectives in pheochromocytoma. Urol Clin North Am 1989; 16:487–503.

27. Hoeffel JC, Gallon MA, Worms AM, Marcon F, Masel J. Brachydactyly secondary to pheochromocytoma. Am J Dis Child 1993; 147:260–261.

28. Henningsson C, Hoffmann S, McGonigle L, Winter JSD. Acute mercury poisoning (acrodynia) mimicking pheochromocytoma in an adolescent. J Pediatr 1993; 122:252–253.

29. Bolande RP. The neurocristopathies. Hum Pathol 1974; 5:409–429.

30. Williams GA, Crockett CL, Butler WWS III, Crispell KR. The coexistence of pheochromocytoma and adrenocortical hyperplasia. J Clin Endocrinol Metab 1960; 20:622–631.

31. Spark RF, Connolly PB, Gluckin DS, White R, Sacks B, Landsberg L. ACTH secretion from a functioning pheochromocytoma. N Engl J Med 1979; 301:416–418.

32. Beaser RS, Guay AT, Lee AK, Silverman ML, Flint LD. An adrenocorticotropic hormone-producing pheochromocytoma: diagnostic and immunohistochemical studies. J Urol 1986; 135:10–13.

33. Sakurai H, Yoshike Y, Isahaya S, et al. Case report: a case of ACTH-producing pheochromocytoma. Am J Med Sci 1987; 294:258–261.

34. Chapman RC, Diaz-Perez R. Pheochromocytoma associated with cerebellar hemangioblastoma. JAMA 1962; 182:1014–1017.

35. Nibbelink DW, Peters BH, McCormick WF. On the association of pheochromocytoma and cerebellar astrocytoma. Neurology 1969; 19:455–460.

36. DeSouza TG, Berlad L, Shapiro K, Walsh C, Saenger P, Shinnar S. Pheochromocytoma and multiple intracerebral aneurysms. J Pediatr 1986; 108:947–949.

37. Neumann HPH, Berger DP, Sigmund G, et al. Pheochromocytomas, multiple endocrine neoplasia type 2, and von Hippel-Lindau disease. N Engl J Med 1993; 329:1531–1538.

38. Waldmann TA, Bradley JE. Polycythemia secondary to a pheochromocytoma with production of an erythropoiesis stimulating factor by the tumor. Proc Soc Exp Biol Med 1961; 108:425–427.

39. Murray KM, Schillaci RF. Sarcoidosis and pheochromocytoma. West J Med 1987; 146:745–747.

40. Levine C, Skimming J, Levine E. Familial pheochromocytomas with unusual associations. J Pediatr Surg 1992; 27:447–451.

41. Brenner WE, Yen SSC, Dingfelder JR, Anton AH. Pheochromocytoma: serial studies during pregnancy. Am J Obstet Gynecol 1972; 113:779–788.

42. Taubman I, Pearson OH, Anton AH. An asymptomatic catecholamine-secreting pheochromocytoma. Am J Med 1974; 57:953–956.

43. St John Sutton MG, Sheps SG, Lie JT. Prevalence of clinically unsuspected pheochromocytoma. Review of a 50-year autopsy series. Mayo Clin Proc 1981; 56:354–360.

44. Voorhess ML. Neuroblastoma-pheochromocytoma: products and pathogenesis. Ann NY Acad Sci 1974; 230:187–194.

45. Proye C, Fossati P, Fontaine P, et al. Dopamine-secreting pheochromocytoma: an unrecognized entity? Classification of pheochromocytoma according to their type of secretion. Surgery 1986; 100:1154–1161.

46. Tippett PA, McEwan AJ, Ackery DM. A re-evaluation of dopamine excretion in phaeochromocytoma. Clin Endocrinol (Oxf) 1986; 25:401–410.

47. Bravo EL, Tarazi RC, Gifford RW Jr, Stewart BH. Circulating and urinary catecholamines in pheochromocytoma. Diagnostic and pathophysiologic implications. N Engl J Med 1979; 301:682–686.

48. Ratge D, Baumgardt G, Knoll E, Wisser H. Plasma free and conjugated catecholamines in diagnosis and localization of pheochromocytoma. Clin Chim Acta 1983; 132:229–243.

49. Bravo EL, Gifford RW Jr. Pheochromocytoma: diagnosis, localization and management. N Engl J Med 1984; 311:1298–1303.

50. Cryer PE. Phaeochromocytoma. Clin Endocrinol Metab 1985; 14:203–220.

51. Duncan MW, Compton P, Lazarus L, Smythe GA. Measurement of norepinephrine and 3,4-dihydroxyphenylglycol in urine and plasma for diagnosis of pheochromocytoma. N Engl J Med 1988; 319:136–142.

52. Lenders JWM, Willemsen JJ, Beissel T, et al. Value of plasma norepinephrine/3,4-dihydroxyphenylglycol ratio for the diagnosis of pheochromocytoma. Am J Med 1992; 92:147–152.

53. Fisher BM, MacPhee GJA, Davies DL, et al. A case of watery diarrhoea syndrome due to an adrenal phaeochromocytoma secreting vasoactive intestinal peptide with coincidental autoimmune thyroid disease. Acta Endocrinol (Copenh) 1987; 114:340–344.

54. Nigawara K, Suzuki T, Tazawa H, et al. A case of recurrent malignant pheochromocytoma complicated by watery diarrhea, hypokalemia, achlorhydria syndrome. J Clin Endocrinol Metab 1987; 65:1053–1056.

55. Sparagana M, Feldman JM, Molnar Z. An unusual pheochromocytoma associated with an androgen secreting adrenocortical adenoma. Evaluation of its polypeptide hormone, catecholamine and enzyme characteristics. Cancer 1987; 60:223–231.

56. Kitamura K, Kangawa K, Kawamoto M, et al. Adrenomedullin: a novel hypotensive peptide isolated from human pheochromocytoma. Biochem Biophys Res Commun 1993; 192:553–560.

57. Kimura S, Nishimura Y, Yamaguchi K, et al. A case of pheochromocytoma producing parathyroid hormone-related protein and presenting with hypercalcemia. J Clin Endocrinol Metab 1990; 79:1559–1563.

58. Yanase T, Nawata H, Kato K, Ibayashi H, Matsuo H. Studies on adrenorphin in pheochromocytoma. J Clin Endocrinol Metab 1987; 64:692.

59. Vetter H, Vetter W, Warnholz C, et al. Renin and aldosterone secretion in pheochromocytoma. Effect of chronic alpha-adrenergic receptor blockade. Am J Med 1976; 60:866–871.

60. Hung W, August GP. Hyperreninemia and secondary hyperaldosteronism in pheochromocytomas. Pediatrics 1979; 94:215–217.

61. Yoneda M, Takatsuki K, Yamanchi K, et al. Determination of enolase isozymes in various adrenal gland tumours. Clin Endocrinol (Oxf) 1987; 26:303–310.

62. Roth KA, Wilson DM, Eberwine J, et al. Acromegaly and pheochromocytoma: a multiple endocrine syndrome caused by a plurihormonal adrenal medullary tumor. J Clin Endocrinol Metab 1986; 63:1421–1426.

63. Bornemann M, Hill SC, Kidd GS II. Lactic acidosis in pheochromocytoma. Ann Intern Med 1986; 105:880–882.

64. Warner RRP, Blaustein AS. Coexistence of pheochromocytoma and carcinoid syndrome produced by metastatic carcinoid of the ileum. Mt Sinai J Med 1970; 36:536–548.

65. Taylor HC, Mayes D, Anton AH. Clonidine suppression test for pheochromocytoma: examples of misleading results. J Clin Endocrinol Metab 1986; 63:238–242.

66. Sjoberg RJ, Simcic KJ, Kidd GS. The clonidine suppression test for pheochromocytoma. Arch Intern Med 1992; 152:1193–1197.

67. Sheps SG, Jiang N-S, Klee GG, van Heerden JA. Recent developments in the diagnosis and treatment of pheochromocytoma. Mayo Clin Proc 1990; 65:88–95.

68. Sisson JC, Frager MS, Valk TW, et al. Scintigraphic localization of pheochromocytoma. N Engl J Med 1981; 305:12–16.

69. Swensen SJ, Brown ML, Sheps SC, et al. Use of ^{131}I-MIBG scintigraphy in the evaluation of suspected pheochromocytoma. Mayo Clin Proc 1985; 60:299–304.

70. Quint LE, Glazer GM, Francis IR, Shapiro B, Chenevert TL. Pheochromocytoma and paraganglioma: comparison of MR imaging with CT and I-131 MIBG scintigraphy. Radiology 1987; 165:89–93.

71. Ansari AN, Siegel M, DeQuattro V, Gazarian LH. Imaging of medullary thyroid carcinoma and hyperfunctioning adrenal medulla using iodine-131 metaiodobenzylguanidine. J Nucl Med 1986; 27:1858–1860.

72. Shulkin BL, Shen SW, Sisson JC, Shapiro B. Iodine 131 MIBG scintigraphy of the extremities in metastatic pheochromocytoma and neuroblastoma. J Nucl Med 1987; 28:315–318.

73. Bomanji J, Levison DA, Flatman WD, et al. Uptake of iodine-123 MIBG by pheochromocytomas, paragangliomas and neuroblastomas: a histopathological comparison. J Nucl Med 1987; 28:973–978.

74. Brown MJ, Fuller RW, Lavender JP. False diagnosis of bilateral phaeochromocytoma by iodine-131-labelled meta-iodobenzyl guanidine (MIBG). Lancet 1984; 1:56–57.

75. Turner MC, Lieberman E, DeQuattro V. The perioperative management of pheochromocytoma in children. Clin Pediatr (Phila) 1992; 31:583–589.

76. Manger WM, Gifford RW Jr. Hypertension secondary to pheochromocytoma. Bull NY Acad Med 1982; 58:139–158.

77. Hull CJ. Phaeochromocytoma—diagnosis, preoperative preparation and anaesthetic management. Br J Anaesth 1986; 58:1453–1468.

78. Robinson RG, DeQuattro V, Grushkin CM, Lieberman E. Childhood pheochromocytoma. Treatment with alpha methyl tyrosine for resistant hypertension. J Pediatr 1977; 91:143–147.

79. Brunjes S, Johns VJ, Crane MG. Pheochromocytoma, postoperative shock and blood volume. N Engl J Med 1960; 262:393–396.

80. Shapiro B, Fig L. Management of pheochromocytoma. Endocrinol Metab Clin North Am 1989; 18:443–481.

81. Benowitz NL. Diagnosis and management of pheochromocytoma. Hosp Pract 1990; 251:163–177.

82. Young WF. Pheochromocytoma: 1926–1993. Trends Endocrinol Metab 1993; 4:122–127.

83. Phillips AF, McMurtry RJ, Taubman J. Malignant pheochromocytoma in childhood. Am J Dis Child 1976; 130:1252–1255.

84. Tippett PA, West RS, McEwan AJ, Middleton JE, Ackery DM. A comparison of dopamine and homovanillic acid excretion, as prognostic indicators in malignant phaeochromocytoma. Clin Chim Acta 1987; 166:123–133.

85. Sisson JC, Shapiro B, Beierwaltes WH, et al. Radiopharmaceutical treatment of malignant pheochromocytoma. J Nucl Med 1984; 24:197–206.

86. Averbuch SD, Steakley CS, Young RC, et al. Malignant pheochromocytoma: effective treatment with a combination of cylcophosphamide, vincristine and dacarbazine. Ann Intern Med 1988; 109:267–273.

87. Scott HW, Reynolds V, Green N, Page D, Oates JA, Robertson D. Clinical experience with malignant pheochromocytomas. Surg Gynecol Obstet 1982; 154:801–818.

88. Serri O, Comtois R, Bettez P, Dubuc G, Buu NT, Kuchel O. Reduction in the size of a pheochromocytoma pulmonary metastasis by metyrosine therapy. N Engl J Med 1984; 310:1264–1265.

89. Keiser HR, Beaven MA, Doppman J, Wells SA Jr, Buja LM. Sipples syndrome: medullary thyroid carcinoma, pheochromocytoma and parathyroid disease. Ann Intern Med 1973; 78:561–579.

90. Carney JA, Sizemore GW, Tyce GM Bilateral adrenal medullary hyperplasia in multiple endocrine neoplasia, type 2. The precursor of bilateral pheochromocytoma. Mayo Clin Proc 1975; 50:3–10.

91. Robinson MF, Furst EJ, Nunziata V, et al. Characterization of the clinical features of five families with hereditary primary cutaneous lichen amyloidosis and multiple endocrine neoplasia type 2. Henry Ford Hosp Med J 1992; 40:249–252.

92. Gagel RF, Tashjian AH, Cummings T, et al. The clinical outcome of prospective screening for multiple endocrine neoplasia type 2a. An 18 year experience. N Engl J Med 1988; 318:478–484.

93. Mathew CGP, Chin KS, Easton DF, et al. A linked genetic marker for multiple endocrine neoplasia type 2a on chromosome 10. Nature 1987; 328:527–528.

94. Simpson NE, Kidd KK, Goodfellow PJ, et al. Assignment of multiple endocrine neoplasia type 2A to chromosome 10 by linkage. Nature 1987; 328:528–530.

95. Sobol H, Narod SA, Nakamura Y, et al. Screening for multiple endocrine nepolasia type 2a with DNA-polymorphism analysis. N Engl J Med 1989; 321:996–1001.

96. Gagel RF. The impact of gene mapping techniques on the management of multiple endocrine neoplasia type 2. Trends Endocrinol Metab 1991; 2:19–25.

97. Gagel RF, Robinson MF, Donovan DT, Alford BR. Clinical review 44. Medullary thyroid carcinoma: recent progress. J Clin Endocrinol Metab 1993; 76:809–814.

98. Ansari AN, Siegel ME, DeQuattro V, Grazarian LH. Imaging of medullary thyroid carcinoma and hyperfunctioning adrenal medulla using iodine-131 metaiodobenzylguanidine. J Nucl Med 1986; 27:1858–1860.

99. Landsvater RM, Rombouts AGM, teMeerman GJ, et al. The clinical implication of positive calcitonin test for C-cell hyperplasia in genetically unaffected members of MEN2A kindred. Am J Hum Genet 1993; v.52 335–342.

100. Gagel RF, Jackson CE, Block MA, et al. Age-related probability of development of hereditary medullary thyroid carcinoma. J Pediatr 1982; 101:941–946.

101. Telander RL, Zimmerman D, van Heerden JA, Sizemore GW. Results of early thyroidectomy for medullary thyroid carcinoma in children with multiple endocrine neoplasia type 2. J Pediatr Surg 1986; 12:1190–1194.

102. Brunt LM, Wells SA Jr. Advances in the diagnosis and treatment of medullary thyroid carcinoma. Surg Clin North Am 1987; 67:263–279.

103. Ponder BAJ, Coffey R, Gagel RF, et al. Risk estimation and screening in families of patients with medullary thyroid carcinoma. Lancet 1988; 1:397–401.

104. Pommier RF, Brennan MF. Medullary thyroid carcinoma. Endocrinologist 1992; 2:393–405.

105. Colson YL, Carty SE. Medullary thyroid carcinoma. Am J Otolaryngol 1993; 14:73–81.

106. Libroia A, Muratori F, Verga U, et al. Evaluation of children with medullary thyroid carcinoma. Henry Ford Hosp Med J 1992; 40:281–283.

107. Lairmore TC, Ball DW, Baylin SB, Wells SA Jr. Management of pheochromocytoma in patients with multiple endocrine neoplasia type 2 syndromes. Ann Surg 1993; 217:595–603.

108. Valk TW, Frager MS, Gross MD, et al. Spectrum of pheochromocytoma in multiple endocrine neoplasia. A scintigraphic portrayal using ^{131}I-metaiodobenzylguanidine. Ann Intern Med 1981; 94:762–767.

109. Bugalho MJGM, Limbert E, Sobrinho LG, et al. A kindred with multiple endocrine neoplasia type 2a associated with pruritic skin lesions. Cancer 1992; 70:2664–2667.

110. Carney JA, Go VLW, Sizemore GW, Hayles AB. Alimentary-tract ganglioneuromatosis. A major component of the syndrome of multiple endocrine neoplasia, type 2b. N Engl J Med 1976; 295:1287–1291.

111. Carney JA, Hayles AB. Alimentary tract manifestations of multiple endocrine neoplasia, type 2b. Mayo Clin Proc 1977; 52:543–548.

112. DeSchryver-Kecskemeti K, Clouse RE, Goldstein MN, Gersell D, O'Neal L. Intestinal ganglioneuromatosis. A manifestation of overproduction of nerve growth factor? N Engl J Med 1983; 308:635–639.

113. Khan AH, Desjardius JG, Youssef S, Gregoire H, Seidman E. Gastrointestinal manifestations of Sipple syndrome in children. J Pediatr Surg 1987; 22:719–723.

114. Griffiths AM, Mack DR, Byard RW, Stringer DA, Shandling B. Multiple endocrine neoplasia 2b: an unusual cause of chronic constipation. J Pediatr 1990; 116:285–288.

115. Kaufman FR, Roe TF, Isaacs H, Weitzman JJ. Metastatic medullary thyroid carcinoma in young children with mucosal neuroma syndrome. Pediatrics 1982; 70:263–267.

116. Jones BA, Sisson JC. Early diagnosis and thyroidectomy in multiple endocrine neoplasia, type 2b. J Pediatr 1983; 102:219–223.

117. Vasen HFA, van der Feltz M, Raue F, et al. The natural course of multiple endocrine neoplasia type 2b. Arch Intern Med 1992; 152:1250–1252.

118. Sizemore GW, Carney JA, Gharib H, Capen CC. Multiple endocrine neoplasia type 2b: eighteen-year follow-up of a four-generation family. Henry Ford Hosp Med J 1992; 40:236–244.

119. Brandi ML, Marx SJ, Aurbach GD, Fitzpatrick LA. Familial multiple endocrine neoplasia type 1: a new look at pathophysiology. Endoc Rev 1987; 8:391–405.

120. Friesen SR. Tumors of the endocrine pancreas. N Engl J Med 1982; 306:580–590.

121. Hansen OP, Hansen M, Hansen HH. Multiple endocrine adenomatosis of mixed type. Acta Med Scand 1976; 200:327–331.

122. Filling A, Decker H, Roehr H-D. Unusual features of multiple endocrine neoplasia. Henry Ford Hosp Med J 1992; 40:253–255.

123. Seeger RC, Brodeur GM, Sather H, et al. Association of multiple copies of the N-myc oncogene with rapid progression of neuroblastoma. N Engl J Med 1985; 313:1111–1116.

124. Goldstein MN, Burdman JA, Journey LJ. Long term tissue culture of neuroblastomas. II. Morphologic evidence of differentiation and maturation. J Natl Cancer Inst 1964; 32:165–199.

125. Alterman K, Schueller EF. Maturation of neuroblastoma to ganglioneuroma. Am J Dis Child 1970; 120:217–222.

126. Chatten J, Voorhess ML. Familial neuroblastoma. Report of a kindred with multiple disorders including neuroblastomas in four siblings. N Engl J Med 1967; 277:1230–1236.

127. Griffin ME, Bolande RP. Familial neuroblastoma with regression and maturation to ganglioneurofibroma. Pediatrics 1969; 43:377–382.

128. Kushner BH, Gilbert F, Helson L. Familial neuroblastoma: case reports, literature review and etiologic considerations. Cancer 1986; 57:1887–1893.

129. Ho PTC, Estroff JA, Kozakewich H, et al. Prenatal detection of neuroblastoma: a ten-year experience from Dana-Farber Cancer Institute and Children's Hospital. Pediatrics 1993; 92:358–364.

130. Tracy T, Weber TR. Current concepts in neuroblastoma. Surg Ann 1992; 24:227–245.

131. Von Studnitz W, Kaser H, Sjoerdsma A, Spectrum of catecholamine biochemistry in patients with neuroblastoma. N Engl J Med 1963; 269:232–235.

132. Voorhess ML. Neuroblastoma with normal urinary catecholamine excretion. J Pediatr 1971; 78:680–683.

133. Johnsonbaugh RE, Cahill R. Screening procedures for neuroblastoma: false negative results. Pediatrics 1975; 56:267–270.

134. Tuchman M, Morris CL, Ramnaraine ML, Bowers LD, Krivit W. Value of random urinary homovanillic acid and vanillylmandelic acid levels in the diagnosis and management of patients with neuroblastoma: comparison with 24-hour urine collections. Pediatrics 1985; 75:324–328.

135. Weinblatt ME, Heisel MA, Siegel SA. Hypertension in children with neurogenic tumors. Pediatrics 1983; 71:947–951.

136. Horn M, Blatt J. Continued remission in children with neuroblastoma despite elevations of urinary catecholamine metabolites. Am J Pediatr Hematol/Oncol 1992; 14(4):312–319.

137. Ishiguro Y, Kato K, Ito T, et al. Nervous system-specific enolase in serum as a marker for neuroblastoma. Pediatrics 1983; 72:696–700.

138. Zeltzer PM, Parma AM, Dalton A, et al. Raised neuron-specific enolase in serum of children with metastatic neuroblastoma. Lancet 1983; 2:361–363.

139. Evans AE, D'Angio GJ, Propert K, Anderson J, Hann HWL. Prognostic factors in neuroblastoma. Cancer 1987; 59:1853–1859.

140. Quinn JJ, Altman AJ, Frantz CN. Serum lactic dehydrogenase, an indicator of tumor activity in neuroblastoma. J Pediatr 1980; 97:89–91.

141. Ladish S, Wu ZL. Detection of a tumour-associated ganglioside in plasma of patients with neuroblastoma. Lancet 1985; 1:136–138.

142. Rascher W, Kremens B, Wagner S, et al. Serial measurements of neuropeptide Y in plasma for monitoring neuroblastoma in children. J Pediatr 1993; 122:914–916.

143. Maris JM, Evans AE, McLaughlin AC, et al. 31-P nuclear magnetic resonance spectroscopic investigation of human neuroblastoma in situ. N Engl J Med 1985; 312:1500–1504.

144. Sawada T. Past and future of neuroblastoma screening in Japan. Am J Pediatr Hematol/Oncol 1992; 14(4):320–326.

145. Woods WG, Tuchman M, Bernstein ML, et al. Screening for neuroblastoma in North America: 2-year results from the

Quebec project. Am J Pediatr Hematol/Oncol 1992; 14(4): 312–319.

146. Craft AW, Parker L, Dale G, et al. A pilot study of screening for neuroblastoma in the north of England. Am J Pediatr Hematol/Oncol 1992; 14(4):337–341.

147. Kaplan SJ, Holbrook CT, McDaniel HG, Buntain WL, Crist WM. Vasoactive intestinal peptide secreting tumors of childhood. Am J Dis Child 1980; 24:21–24.

148. Voorhess ML. Functioning tumors. Am J Dis Child 1980; 134:14–15.

149. Cooney DR, Voorhess ML, Fisher JE, et al. Vasoactive intestinal peptide producing neuroblastoma. J Pediatr Surg 1982; 17:821–825.

150. Bravo EL. Evolving concepts in the pathophysiology, diagnosis and treatment of pheochromocytoma. Endocr Rev 1994; 15:356–368.

151. Thomas PM, Gagel RF. Advances in genetic screening for multiple endocrine neoplasia type 2 and the implications for management of children at risk. The Endocrinologist 1994; 4:140–146.

25

Thyroid Disorders in Infancy

Pavel F. Fort
North Shore University Hospital, Manhasset, New York

Rosalind S. Brown
University of Massachusetts Medical School, Worcester, Massachusetts

I. CONGENITAL HYPOTHYROIDISM

Disorders affecting the thyroid gland are among the most common endocrinopathies encountered in newborns. It has long been known that the prevalence of congenital hypothyroidism (CH) in the United States approximates 1:4000 live births, surpassing other endocrine and metabolic aberrations (1). More recently, large variations in the prevalence of CH have been found among the states, which may be related to the ethnic diversity in each state (2).

Although mandatory screening for the detection of CH has helped physicians in the early diagnosis of this disorder, by no means has the physician's role been diminished. It is the primary physician's responsibility to ensure that there are no unnecessary delays in the final diagnosis and treatment of patients with CH. Early detection of CH warrants the earliest possible treatment, which is of utmost importance to the patient. In this chapter we review current knowledge to ensure the best care of young infants with aberrations of the thyroid gland.

A. Thyroid Ontogenesis

When evaluating a child for possible CH, one should be acquainted with both the normal development of the thyroid gland and normal values for various thyroid parameters in early postnatal life.

Fetal thyroid activity usually begins during gestational week 8, when synthesis of thyroglobulin begins. About 2 weeks later, trapping of iodine occurs, followed by iodination of tyrosine. Colloid formation appears at week 12 of fetal life, and at that time, the fetal pituitary gland begins to secrete thyrotropin-stimulating hormone (TSH). In the early 1970s, it was shown that by midgestation the fetal hypothalamic-pi-

tuitary-thyroid axis was already functional and was independent of the maternal axis (3). The human placenta may allow the passage of small quantities of maternal levothyroxine (T_4) to the fetus (4); however, such transfer is usually insufficient to mitigate the effects of hypothyroidism on the fetus. Neonates with hypothyroidism are usually symptom free because of sufficient thyroxine deiodinase activity in the brain, and probably other tissues, to provide some triiodothyronine (T_3) for local hormone action (5).

Shortly after delivery, the following events take place (Fig. 1). TSH, perhaps as a result of cooling and stress, rises rapidly, reaching levels of 60–80 μU/ml within 30 minutes after delivery, and then slowly declines over the next few days to approximate levels in older children (<8 μU/ml; <8 mU/L) by 5–7 days. The elevation in TSH is followed by a rise in both T_4 and T_3 to "thyrotoxic levels" by 24 h of life. The T_4 levels are in the 15–19 μg/dl (193–245 nM) range and T_3 levels in the 300 ng/dl (4.6 nM) range. This phenomenon is frequently referred to as physiologic hyperthyroidism. These changes in thyroid hormone concentrations must be kept in mind when evaluating a newborn's thyroid function. Failure to interpret these values correctly in relation to the time after birth can lead to a false diagnosis of hyperthyroidism, or hypothyroidism may be missed. It must be kept in mind that normal values of thyroid function tests applicable to older children therefore cannot be used in newborn infants.

Children with CH can be identified in utero by measurement of fetal thyroid hormones (6). Recently, Davidson et al. reported a baby with fetal goitrous hypothyroidism in whom fetal thyroid hormones were monitored by percutaneous umbilical vessel sampling (cordocentesis) before and after intraamniotic L-thyroxine administration (7). Because cordocentesis is not without risk, however, and most infants with CH do well despite postnatal diagnosis and treatment, it seems

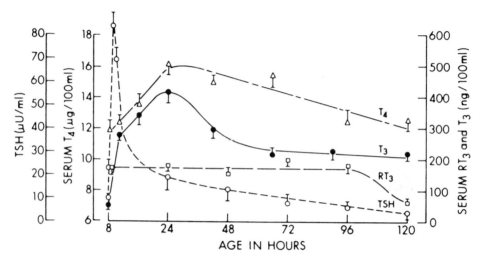

Figure 1 Changes (mean and standard error of the mean) in serum thyroid hormone and TSH concentrations in the immediate neonatal period. (From Fisher DA. In: *Perinatal Endocrinology*. Mead Johnson Symposium on Prenatal and Developmental Medicine, No. 8, 1975:42.)

prudent to reserve its use for exceptional instances, at least until further data become available.

B. Thyroid Screening in Newborns

The recommended guidelines for newborn screening for CH were recently reviewed by the American Academy of Pediatrics Committee on Genetics and the American Thyroid Association Committee on Neonatal Screening (8). There are basically two different approaches to newborn screening for CH: one is to measure the serum T_4 concentration, followed by determination of TSH if the T_4 value is low. The other method is to measure the serum TSH level only. Most North American screening programs favor the measurement of T_4 as an initial screening test, whereas the majority of European and Japanese programs prefer the determination of TSH as a primary screening test for CH (8). Both approaches have their advantages and disadvantages. For example, in infants screened by the T_4 measurement, hypothyroidism can be missed. This occurs when the T_4 level is "normal" but TSH is elevated (compensated hypothyroidism). In addition, there are infants in whom thyroid function may decompensate after the newborn period as occurs in infants with Down syndrome, for example (9). On the other hand, infants with CH may also be missed when screened by the TSH measurement only. The patients who may be missed if T_4 levels are not measured include those with hypothalamic-pituitary hypothyroidism, other rare instances of primary hypothyroidism with delayed TSH response, congenital thyroxine binding globulin (TBG) deficiency, and neonatal hyperthyroidism, although it should be possible to demonstrate a suppressed TSH in the latter if a third-generation "ultrasensitive" TSH assay were used (10). Moreover, in many United States institutions, the routine is to discharge newborns within 24–48 h of life, at which point the serum TSH levels may by physiologically elevated (Fig.

1). Thus, it would be ideal to have all newborns screened by both T_4 and TSH measurements. However, because this may be neither practical nor financially feasible, most screening programs choose a method (8) and deal with possible failures based upon their experience and by reliance on clinical supervision of all newborns after discharge from the hospital.

The current newborn screening for CH in the state of New York consists of T_4 measurements obtained from a newborn at the time of discharge. Blood samples are collected in the so-called PKU (phenylketonuria) cards and mailed to the New York State Laboratory for analysis. All samples with T_4 levels below the 10th percentile but within 2 standard deviations (SD) of the mean for the assay are redone. On retest, those with T_4 levels above 2 SD of the mean are considered normal, and no further testing is done. Those samples with T_4 levels below 2 SD of the mean are evaluated further by measuring TSH levels in the same sample. The newborns who are found to have a low T_4 value with normal or mildly elevated TSH levels (20–25 μU/ml; 20–25 mU/L) are requested to undergo a second screening test (PKU cards). When the TSH level is above 25 μU/ml, the physician is notified immediately and advised to consult with a pediatric endocrinologist for further workup (11). About 1% of the newborns are recalled for retesting because of low T_4 levels with either normal or only mildly elevated TSH levels on the initial screening specimen (11). In newborns with birth weight less than 1500 g, the recall rate is 17–35 times higher than for newborns with normal birth weight.

One must keep in mind, however, that even those children with normal T_4 and TSH levels may develop hypothyroidism in the first few weeks of life (late-onset CH) (8). For this reason, several states routinely retest at 2–6 weeks of age all infants who had normal serum thyroxine levels on the initial screening for CH. They report that another 10% of all affected infants are detected by the second screening only

(12). This approximates a prevalence of CH of 1:30,000 resulting from the second screening. The severity of CH in such infants is usually, but not always, less pronounced than in those detected by the initial screen (13). Therefore, the American Academy of Pediatrics currently recommends repeating thyroid function tests during infancy whenever there is a clinical suspicion of hypothyroidism, when there is a history of thyroid disease in pregnancy, or when there is a family history of thyroid dyshormonogenesis (8). Also, all infants with Down syndrome should be routinely retested at 2–3 months of life because of the high prevalence of late-onset CH, with or without aberrations on the initial thyroid function tests.

Although various safeguards have been developed and implemented by state thyroid screening programs, the possibility exists that a child born with CH can be missed. It has been reported that 2 cases of CH were missed for every 1 million infants screened. The most common reason was a laboratory error during the assay (14).

In 1988, the attitude of primary care physicians—their concerns as well as their suggestions for the managing of patients with CH—were reviewed (15). Primary care physicians prefer autonomy in the management of such infants. In fact, fewer than half of the physicians deemed an endocrine consultation necessary. However, the data showed that there is great variability among physicians for the therapeutic goals once hypothyroidism is confirmed. Because of this variability in standard of care, all CH patients benefit from the pediatric endocrinologist's experience. Even the busiest primary care physician does not see more than a few such children during his or her professional life, whereas the average pediatric endocrinologist has a much wider experience and, hence, a more uniform approach to management. Thus, in our opinion, the pediatric endocrinologist must be involved to provide such children with optimal care and allow continuous development of a broad expertise in the management of CH.

C. Clinical Conditions Associated with Abnormal Screening Test Results

Newborns whose T4 levels on initial screening are decreased can be categorized into two groups, depending on their TSH levels (Table 1). Serum TSH may be normal (less than 20 μU/ml; 20 mU/L) or elevated (more than 20 μU/ml; 20

mU/L). The classification of such patients is outlined in Table 2 and discussed here.

1. Low T4 with Normal TSH Levels

a. Transient Hypothyroxinemia of the Newborn of Undetermined Etiology. Full-term infants with appropriate birth weight whose initial screening reveals diminished T4 levels without elevation in TSH and whose repeat testing at 2–3 weeks of life show normal T4 and TSH levels are considered to have "transient hypothyroxinemia of undetermined etiology." These patients are clinically euthyroid, have normal levels of thyroid hormone binding proteins, and are considered, for practical purposes, to be normal. The cause of transient thyroid function alterations in these children is not clear. It may represent a laboratory error, or it may also be that the sample was not collected appropriately or that the baby had an illness. It may also suggest transiently impaired thyrotropin-releasing hormone or TSH secretion leading to transient hypothyroxinemia (16).

Between July 1978 and June 1993, we evaluated and followed 60 such infants who had low serum T4 levels (less than 2 SD below the mean for the assay) on the New York State Screening Program for CH; the mean $\pm$ SD was 7.2 $\pm$ 2.5 μg/dl (93 $\pm$ 32 nM). All these infants had normal, that is, below 20 μU/ml (20 mU/L), TSH levels on the initial screening test. None of the children showed any clinical signs or symptoms suggestive of hypothyroidism, and all were growing and developing appropriately. The possibility of congenital thyroxine binding globulin deficiency was ruled out by appropriate testing. There was no family history of CH, and none of the mothers demonstrated any thyroid dysfunction when tested. On follow-up evaluation, all these children normalized the serum T4 levels by an average of 11 weeks with no treatment. At that time, their mean $\pm$ SD serum T4 and TSH levels were 7.9 $\pm$ 2.6 μg/dl (102 $\pm$ 33 nM) and 4.5 $\pm$ 4.1 μU/ml (4.5 $\pm$ 4.1 mU/L), respectively.

In our experience, 18% of full-term newborns referred to our clinic emerged with the diagnosis of transient hypothyroxinemia of undetermined etiology (Table 2). Although the thyroid dysfunction in these children is only temporary, diminished T4 levels in early life should not be ignored. Further studies evaluating the effects of transient hypothyroxinemia during the newborn and early infancy period on a child's neuropsychologic development remain as yet uninvestigated.

Table 1 Clinical Conditions Associated with Abnormal Screening Test Results in Relation to Serum TSH Values

Normal TSH[a]	Elevated TSH
Transient hypothyroxinemia of undetermined etiology	Primary hypothyroidism
Low birth weight infants	Transient primary hypothyroidism of the newborn
Hypopituitary-hypothalamic hypothyroidism	Compensated hypothyroidism
Congenital thyroxine binding globulin deficiency	
Late-onset primary hypothyroidism	

[a]Normal: <20 μU/ml (<20 mU/L).

Table 2 Classification of Infants with Abnormal Newborn Thyroid Screening

Screening	Definite testing (at 2–3 wk of age)	Diagnosis	No. of patients at NSUH[a]
L T$_4$ N TSH	N T$_4$ N TSH	Transient hypothyroxinemia of undetermined etiology	47 full-term 17 LBW
L T$_4$ E TSH	N T$_4$ E TSH	Compensated hypothyroidism	25
L T$_4$ E TSH	L T$_4$ E TSH	Primary hypothyroidism	40
L T$_4$ E TSH	N T$_4$ N TSH	Transient hypothyroidism	67 full-term 19 LBW
L T$_4$ N TSH	L T$_4$ N TSH	Congenital TBG deficiency	41
L T$_4$ L TSH	L T$_4$ L TSH	Pituitary-hypothalamic hypothyroidism	1
			Total 257

L, low <2 SD below mean; N, normal < 20 μU/ml TSH; E, elevated >20 μU/ml; [a]experience at North Shore University Hospital from 1978 through 1987; LBW, low-birth-weight infants; TBG, thyroxine-binding globulin.

b. Low Birth Weight Infants. Transient hypothyroxinemia without elevated serum TSH levels is frequently found in infants with low birth weight, with or without prematurity. Such neonates, especially when ill, may have very low T$_4$ and T$_3$ levels, yet they remain clinically euthyroid. At times, a physician must decide whether such patients are truly hypothyroid and, thus, in need of thyroid hormone replacement, or whether low levels of thyroid hormones represent merely a protective mechanism by which the organism is able to reduce its metabolic rate during illness (17–19). Many such infants are ill, with a myriad of clinical symptoms that may be reminiscent of a hypothyroid state. Mercado et al. (20) reported eight preterm infants with low T$_4$ and normal TSH levels who developed clinical characteristics similar to those seen in CH. These babies exhibited prolonged jaundice, hypoactivity, lethargy, constipation, edema, and hoarse cry. Thyroid replacement was given for a short period, resulting in a prompt resolution of the symptoms. The authors pointed out that thyroid replacement therapy may be beneficial in premature infants demonstrating low T$_4$ levels and clinical symptoms suggestive of hypothyroidism. However, no beneficial effects of thyroid therapy on growth and development of premature infants with low T$_4$ values were found in another double-blind study (19). Wilson et al. suggested that measurement of free T$_4$ level may be of value in differentiating between true hypothyroid and euthyroid sick patients, obviating unnecessary treatment (21).

The cause of low T$_4$ levels in low birth weight infants is not clear. In some situations, it has been attributed to an iodine deficiency state particularly prevalent in certain geographic areas (22) or to increased urinary losses of iodine secondary to renal immaturity (23). Others have postulated a low rate of synthesis of thyroglobulin and a partial organification defect caused by the immaturity of the thyroid gland (24) or an accelerated peripheral utilization of thyroid hormones under stress (25). Because the negative feedback mechanism between T$_4$ and TSH is operational in healthy premature infants (26), these explanations do not account for the "normal" TSH seen. An additional abnormality, such as hypothalamic or pituitary immaturity, must also be implicated (18,27). Perhaps the most plausible explanation is that different serum levels of thyroid hormones in preterm infants may be a result of the various serum TBG concentrations in these infants (28).

Our own experience with premature infants is summarized as follows: The mean ± SD serum T$_4$ level in 46 healthy, preterm infants seen in our institution (Table 2) was 5.4 ± 2.4 μg/dl (69 ± 31 nM) at a mean age of 23 ± 14 days. In all instances, serum TSH levels were normal. None of these children exhibited any signs or symptoms of hypothyroidism, and the serum free T$_4$ levels, when measured, were above 1.5 ng/dl (19.2 pM). The thyroid binding globulins were also normal. The serum T$_4$ and TSH levels normalized spontaneously by age 9 ± 3 weeks (8.9 ± 3.2 μg/dl; 115 ± 41 nM), and TSH levels remained normal (5.0 ± 3.4 μU/ml; 5.0 ± 3.4 mU/L). As with term infants with transient hypothyroxinemia, it remains to be seen whether the low birth weight infants with transiently low serum T$_4$ levels in early life may be adversely affected later in life.

Screening for CH as well as for other metabolic diseases in premature babies is often delayed until the time of discharge. Therefore, it is recommended that thyroid function tests in infants who have prolonged hospitalizations be tested within a few days of life to avoid missing the diagnosis of CH. Our present approach to such infants is summarized in Table 3.

c. Hypopituitary-Hypothalamic Hypothyroidism. This condition, also referred to as secondary-tertiary hypothyroidism, can be confused with abnormalities observed in low birth weight infants. Hypopituitary-hypothalamic hypothyroidism is rare, with a frequency ranging from 1:50,000 to 1:150,000 live births (8). However, the 10 year experience in the Northwest Regional Screening Program estimated the frequency of this condition as 1:29,000 (29). The authors pointed out that the optimal strategy for detecting such infants is a combination of T_4 with supplemental TSH screening measurements, coupled with the recognition of clinical features of hypopituitarism. Patients with hypoglycemia, persistent jaundice, hypogonadism, micropenis, diabetes insipidus, midline defects, and various ocular abnormalities must be worked up to rule out hypopituitarism. The onset of hypothyroidism in these patients is often insidious, because the TSH deficiency is usually partial.

d. Congenital Thyroxine Binding Globulin Deficiency. Changes in TBG levels are usually inherited as X-linked dominant traits with at least two different mutations (30). In a full-term newborn with persistently low T_4 levels but normal TSH and no clinical signs or symptoms of hypothyroidism or panhypopituitarism, congenital TBG deficiency should be strongly suspected. This is a rather frequent defect, affecting 1:5,000 to 1:10,000 live births (1,8). Failure to recognize TBG deficiency may lead to an erroneous diagnosis of CH and consequent unnecessary treatment. Free T_4 levels in

patients with TBG deficiency are within the normal range; definitive diagnosis of this entity is established by determining TBG levels. A simple screening method for estimating thyroxine binding proteins is to measure the T_3 resin uptake, which is elevated in patients with TBG deficiency. Family studies can identify other affected members.

In the past several years, we have followed 58 such infants (Table 2). Their mean initial serum T_4 levels were low (4.6 ± 2.1 μg/dl; 59 ± 27 nM), whereas their T_3 resin uptake levels were elevated (mean 56%; range 38–75%). All children had normal serum TSH and free T_4 levels and decreased thyroxine binding protein levels. Such infants are, for practical purposes, considered normal and do not require further workup or follow-up.

e. Late-Onset Primary CH. Late-onset primary hypothyroidism without initial hyperthyrotropinemia has been described (31). Characteristically, the rise in TSH occurs weeks to months after the decrease in T_4 in affected infants. The prevalence of this condition has been reported as 1:50,000 to 1:100,000 (8). The exact mechanism of the normal initial TSH levels in the face of diminished serum T_4 levels and normal thyroxine binding proteins and which babies with hypothyroxinemia are at risk are not clear; however, a delay in the TSH increase has been postulated (8). Although rare,

Table 3 Screening for and Evaluation of Thyroid Aberrations in Low Birth Weight Newborns and Infants

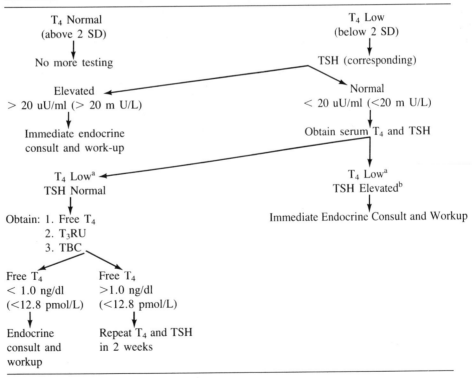

[a] T_4 in healthy premies <7.0 ug/dl (< 90 nmol/L)

T_4 in "sick" premies <5.0 ug/dl (< 5.0 ug/dl (< 64 nmol/L)

[b] **TSH > 7.0 uU/ml (> 7.0 mU/L)

this condition reemphasizes the need for a comprehensive evaluation, preferably by a pediatric endocrinologist. This may be particularly important in children with Down syndrome: such patients may present with only minimal chemical abnormalities on the initial neonatal screening. We found that the prevalence of CH in such children is about 28 times more common than in the general population (9).

2. Low T4 with Elevated TSH Levels

a. Primary Hypothyroidism. In almost all newborns with primary hypothyroidism hyperthyrotropinemia is detected by the initial screening test for CH. This may vary for moderate (20–60 μU/ml; 20–60 mU/L) to marked TSH elevation (>60 μU/ml; >60 mU/L). Most of these patients exhibit a progressive decompensation of thyroid function manifested by a further drop in T_4 and a rise in TSH levels during the first few weeks of life. Therefore, all patients with low T_4 and elevated TSH levels must be promptly treated. If a conclusive diagnosis of CH cannot be established at once, such patients should be treated for the first 3 years of life, after which the treatment can be safely discontinued and the patient reevaluated. The need for immediate action is especially important when a child presents with TSH levels above 60 μU/ml (60 mU/L). The risk of severe CH because of agenesis of thyroid gland is high. In our institution, most newborns presenting with primary CH had TSH levels well above 60 μU/ml (60 mU/L) on both the initial and repeat testing. The highest serum TSH levels were observed in patients with agenesis of thyroid gland. The various causes of primary CH are outlined in Table 4.

i. Embryogenic defects. The great majority of infants with primary CH have agenesis, dysgenesis, or ectopia of the thyroid gland; this accounts for up to 80% of all cases of CH (1,32). Thyroid agenesis is almost always nonhereditary, although studies of twins have suggested a genetic predisposition with a trigger in the environment in utero (33). There is no evidence of thyroid autoimmunity or of an increased incidence of thyroid disorders in mothers or among relatives

of such patients. In general, patients with agenesis of the thyroid gland appear to have lower T_4 and higher TSH levels than those with a dysgenetic gland (Table 4). Children born with an ectopic thyroid gland present with various degrees of thyroid dysfunction at birth.

The diagnosis of thyroid agenesis is made by thyroid scan with either ^{123}I uptake or technetium. The scan typically fails to visualize the thyroid gland, whereas visualization of salivary glands and gastric mucosa is apparent. On the other hand, the diagnosis of a dysgenetic or ectopic gland may be difficult because infants' necks are relatively small and the patients must be completely still during the procedure for an accurate visualization. Dysgenetic thyroid gland can be either in a normal position or ectopic but not fully matured. In such cases, a remnant of thyroid tissue can be visualized by the scan. The ectopic gland is the one that remains in the upper portion of the neck or elsewhere. The gland may be visualized as a mass in the back of the tongue, and the scan may show uptake of iodine in the upper neck. In our experience, infants with a normally positioned dysgenetic gland had either normal or moderately elevated TSH levels. However, patients with an ectopic thyroid gland always showed elevated TSH values (Table 4). Recently, investigators reported that infants with agenesis of the gland could be distinguished from those with dysgenesis by measurements of plasma thyroglobulin (34,35), although such findings have been disputed by others (36).

ii. Dyshormonogenesis. About 10–15% of all cases of congenital hypothyroidism are caused by an enzymatic defect in thyroid hormone synthesis, generally referred to as dyshormonogenesis (1,37). These conditions, unlike those associated with defective embryogenesis, are transmitted genetically, usually in an autosomal recessive manner. A total of 10 inborn errors of thyroid hormogenesis are recognized (38), an organification defect being the most common. An enzymatic defect is suspected whenever low T_4 and elevated TSH levels are accompanied by an increased early radioiodine thyroid uptake or evidence of a normally situated thyroid gland on ultrasound, with or without a clinically detectable

Table 4 Final Diagnosis of Infants with Congenital Primary Hypothyroidism (NSUH, 1979–1992)[a]

Diagnosis	No.	Screening T_4 (μg/dl; nM)/TSH (μU/ml; mU/L)[b]	Confirmatory T_4 (μg/dl; nM)/TSH (μU/ml; mU/L)[b]
Thyroid agenesis	23	4.2 ± 2.3/120 to >200 (54 ± 30)	2.6 ± 2.0/51 to >300 (33 ± 26)
Thyroid dysgenesis	13	6.3 ± 3.1/20 to >200 (81 ± 40)	6.7 ± 3.5/6 to >1000 (86 ± 45)
Thyroid ectopia	12	6.9 ± 3.1/35 to >200 (89 ± 40)	6.2 ± 2.4/40 to >1000 (80 ± 31)
Thyroid dyshormonogenesis	25	9.6 ± 3.2/21 to >200 (124 ± 41)	7.9 ± 3.2/29 to >600 (102 ± 41)

[a]$n = 73$.

[b]Data as mean ± SD.

goiter. Not all dyshormonogenetic defects are genetically determined. A mother who takes antithyroid drugs, such as propylthiouracil or methimazole (Tapazole) may give birth to a child with goitrous hypothyroidism, because such drugs readily cross the placenta. A specific diagnosis of the dyshormonogenetic defect may require a more demanding workup, such as a perchlorate discharge test, and should be carried out in conjunction with an experienced endocrinologist. This may be postponed to after 3 years of life when treatment is safely stopped for a short period of time.

In our clinic, over 30% of children diagnosed to have primary CH were considered to have a defect in thyroid hormonogenesis. Unlike patients with embryogenic aberrations, biochemical changes were less severe on both the initial and confirmatory tests (Table 4).

b. Transient Hypothyroidism of the Newborn. Children with transient, primary hypothyroidism have low serum T_4 and elevated TSH levels at the time of the initial screening, which subsequently normalize spontaneously. These patients differ from those classified as having transient hypothyroxinemia because they show an elevated TSH level when a low T_4 concentration is detected. They are usually placed on thyroid replacement therapy, only to be found to have normal thyroid function later in life (39). Causes to be considered are maternal iodine, antithyroid drug, or dietary goitrogen. Recently, transient CH as a result of the transplacental passage of TSH receptor blocking antibodies has been described (40). Infants with this disorder are indistinguishable at birth clinically from those with thyroid dysgenesis because they frequently have severe hypothyroidism, no goiter is palpable in either the baby or mother, and thyroid uptake on radionuclear scan is significantly reduced or absent (41,42). Unlike sporadic thyroid dysgenesis, however, babies with blocking antibody-induced CH tend to have transient disease, and the disorder has a high recurrence risk in subsequent offspring because of the tendency of these antibodies to remain elevated for a long time in maternal serum (41,42). The disease has usually been reported in babies of mothers with nongoitrous thyroiditis (also known as primary myxedema) but can also occur in mothers with a past history of Graves' disease (41,43). Like the thyroid-stimulating antibodies of Graves' disease, these IgGs are antibodies to the TSH receptor (44) but appear to bind to a different portion of the receptor (45). Rarely, mothers may have mixtures of stimulating and blocking antibodies (46,47). In these cases, the functional state of the fetus and newborn is determined by which type of antibody predominates. Because of the importance of distinguishing these babies from those with permanent thyroid dysgenesis, TSH receptor antibodies should be measured in all babies with evidence of abnormal thyroid function at birth whose mothers have autoimmune thyroid disease, particularly if a thyroid gland is demonstrable on clinical examination or ultrasound (see also later).

Congenital primary hypothyroidism caused by maternal deficiency of iodine, although still prevalent in some parts of the world, has been eliminated in the United States by increased dietary intake of iodine. On the other hand, because iodine readily crosses the placenta, an excessive maternal exposure (such as following vaginal douches with povidone iodine or use of iodine-containing radiocontrast agents) may suppress the fetal thyroid gland, resulting in CH manifested by low T_4 with increased TSH levels and diminished radioactive iodine (by radioimmunoassay, RIA) intake (48). Although CH in these patients is transient in nature, such infants may require treatment to prevent the adverse effects of diminished levels of thyroid hormones on mental development. A similar situation may arise if the newborn is exposed to excess iodine in the immediate postnatal period. Indeed, transient thyroid dysfunction may occur following repeated skin cleansing with iodine-containing substances, particular in premature (49) or very low birth weight infants or those with a large area of exposure, such as those with an omphalocele (50).

c. Compensated Hypothyroidism. The term "compensated hypothyroidism" has been reserved for patients whose T_4 and T_3 levels are normal but whose serum TSH levels are elevated. Such patients are clinically asymptomatic as long as their T_4 levels remain normal. Elevated serum TSH may persist for an indefinite period, with a possible spontaneous normalization later in life, or such patients may decompensate and develop full-blown chemical and clinical hypothyroidism. It is impossible to predict the course a patient may follow, and therefore any child whose TSH remains elevated on repeat testing should be thoroughly evaluated and treated because he or she may have a hypometabolic state despite normal serum T_4 levels (51).

Our experience with 27 children with compensated hypothyroidism is summarized in Table 5. Although the repeat T_4 levels were within the normal range for age, the serum TSH levels remained elevated, with a mean ± SD of 16 ± 13 μU/ml during the first month of life. Radionuclear studies revealed the diagnosis of dyshormonogenesis (normally positioned gland with elevated RIA uptake) in 17 infants and ectopic thyroid gland in 5 infants. In the infants who had a TSH above 7.0 μU/ml, there was a decreased basal metabolic rate despite normal serum T_4 levels. Following thyroid therapy, basal metabolic rate promptly returned to normal (51).

Another approach to such infants is to assess the TSH response to thyrotropin releasing hormone (TRH). Recently, Rapaport et al. reported the TSH response to TRH in 68 infants (22 premature) who presented in early life with "mildly abnormal thyroid function tests." They concluded that such a test, utilizing a single 30 minute post-TRH TSH value, is a valuable clinical tool in the evaluation of infants suspected of having primary hypothyroidism, because those with a TSH response over 35 mU/L were found to be at risk for hypothyroidism, whereas infants with a TSH response to TRH of less than 35 mU/L were considered normal (52). However, because TSH levels were measured by standard RIAs, it remains to be seen whether the employment of a third-generation ultrasensitive TSH assay (10) without the TRH stimulation would delineate infants at risk for hypothyroidism from normals.

Table 5 Infants with Compensated Hypothyroidism[a]

Screening[b]		Definite testing[b]				
T$_4$ (μg/dl)	TSH (μU/ml)	T$_4$ (μg/dl)	TSH (μU/ml)	Age (weeks)	Final diagnosis (no.)	Treatment age (weeks)
10.5 ± 4.0 (134 ± 51)	30 ± 9.7	10.2 ± 2.6 (131 ± 33)	16 ± 13	4.5 ± 2.5	Dyshormogenesis (17) Ectopic (5) Dysgenesis (5)	4.5 ± 2.6

[a]n = 27. Normal T$_4$ but elevated TSH on definite testing.
[b]Data as mean ± SD.

The future outcome of these children in terms of their need for continuing treatment is not clear. It is conceivable that some of these children may be taken off thyroid replacement after 2–3 years of life. However, this remains to be studied.

The foregoing approach to patients with compensated hypothyroidism may not be followed by all pediatric endocrinologists; some choose to follow these patients closely without therapy. It is our opinion that this may be risky: a hypometabolic state may be present in these infants, and the neurodevelopmental outcome is not known. Further studies must be done to provide the necessary data on which to base more rational diagnostic and therapeutic guidelines in such infants.

D. Clinical Findings in Newborns and Infants with Congenital Hypothyroidism

The symptoms of hypothyroidism characteristic of older children are often mild or absent during the first few weeks of life. Only 10–15% of hypothyroid newborns present with a clinical picture that alerts an examining physician to possible hypothyroidism (Table 6) (53). One of the most reliable signs of congenital hypothyroidism in the newborn is a patent posterior fontanelle with widely opened cranial sutures resulting from a prenatal lag in skeletal maturation. In our patient population, most hypothyroid children had delayed skeletal maturation and an open posterior fontanelle. Delayed skeletal maturation, as determined by radiologic assessment of the distal femoral surface of the knee, is not only of diagnostic importance, but it also reflects the severity and duration of the disease in utero. In some studies, but not others, it has been associated with a less favorable outcome in terms of mental development (53,54).

The next most frequent symptom of CH is umbilical hernia. Other indications of CH are less specific; therefore, they are more likely to be overlooked. Most of our patients had large for gestional age birth weight (above 3.5 kg with a gestation period more than 40 weeks). Fewer than half of our children with CH presented with significant jaundice in the early days of life. In contrast to the generally held view that CH is more common in girls than in boys, there was no sex difference in the occurrence of CH in our patient population. Additional infrequently observed signs and symptoms include constipation, hypotonia, hoarse cry, feeding or sucking difficulties, and skin mottling. The so-called CH Apgar score (Table 6) summarizes the most frequently seen signs and symptoms of congenital hypothyroidism.

It appears that infants with CH have a higher incidence of other congenital anomalies, the significance of which is unclear. Bamforth et al. reported various congenital anomalies, such as congenital heart disease, chromosomal aberrations, bone abnormalities, and split hair syndrome, in CH infants identified through the hypothyroid screen program (55).

E. Treatment

It is essential that thyroid replacement, preferably with L-thyroxine, begin as soon as possible. If an error in diagnosis has been made, the treatment may be discontinued. If a firm laboratory diagnosis cannot be made but there is a strong suspicion of CH, a prudent approach is to ensure euthyroidism by replacement therapy until after 3 years of age, when treatment can be safely stopped and the child's condition

Table 6 Apgar Scores in Hypothyroidism[a]

Symptom	Score
Hernia, umbilical	2
Y chromosome absent (female)	1
Pallor, coldness, hypothermia	1
Edematous: typical facies	2
Enlarged tongue	1
Hypotonia	1
Yellow (icterus > 3 days)	1
Rough, dry skin	1
Open, posterior fontanelle	1
Inactive defecation	2
Duration of gestation > 40 weeks	1
Birth weight > 3.5 kg	1
Total	15

[a]Score > 5 suggests hypothyroidism.

reevaluated. Treatment should be monitored closely by periodic thyroid function tests. The current guidelines recommend assessment 2 and 4 weeks after initiation of treatment, every 1–2 months in the first year of age, every 2–3 months between 1 and 3 years, and less frequently thereafter (8). A bone age should be obtained before therapy is begun and at 1 year of age. The most important single biochemical value to follow is the serum T_4 concentration, which should be maintained in the upper half of the normal range (usually between 10 and 15 $\mu g/dl$; 129 and 193 nM). The normalization of serum T_4 levels is often accompanied by a rapid decline in TSH values. In some patients, however, the TSH remains elevated despite normal T_4 levels and clinical euthyroidism. This may be the result of an abnormal feedback mechanism between circulating thyroid hormones and pituitary-hypothalamic receptors (56) or noncompliance. An attempt to normalize the elevated TSH may, in some patients, result in iatrogenic hyperthyroxinemia. In one report, early treatment with oral T_4 in a dose of 10–15 $\mu g/kg$ per day resulted in the normalization of serum T_4 within 3–4 weeks; however, in 8 of the 19 patients reported, the serum T_4 values reached levels above 15.0 $\mu g/dl$ (193 nM) without necessarily normalizing TSH values (57). A daily starting dose of 10–15 $\mu g/kg$ body weight of L-thyroxine (Synthroid Sodium) is recommended by the American Thyroid Association Committee of Neonatal Screening (8,58). The use of T_3 (liothyronine sodium) is not generally recommended because most brain T_3 is obtained by local intracellular conversion from T_4.

F. Mental Development

During fetal and early postnatal life, thyroid hormones are crucial for growth and development of the central nervous system. Both cell number and normal development of neurons are adversely affected by diminished levels of circulating thyroid hormones. In addition, the development of synaptic contacts among brain cells is impaired (59–61). Therefore, the newborn screening program for the detection of CH represents a major step in preventive medicine. The longer the diagnosis of CH is delayed, the higher is the risk of mental retardation and various neurologic sequelae, such as poor motor coordination, ataxia, spastic diplegia, muscular hypotonia, strabismus, learning disability, and diminished attention span (62).

One study has reported that if the replacement therapy is begun before 3 months of age, such patients reach a mean intelligence quotient (IQ) of 89. This number drops to 70 if the treatment is instituted between 3 and 6 months of age. After 6 months of postnatal life, the average IQ is only 54 (63).

The time at which treatment is started is not the only determinant of the prognosis, however. The cause of CH is another important factor. Infants with agenesis of thyroid gland are much more compromised in terms of mental function, if not properly treated, than those with an ectopic gland. Specifically, only 41% of patients with agenesis of the thyroid gland have an IQ above 85, whereas 44–78% of those

with dyshormonogenesis and ectopic gland have an IQ above 85 when not treated properly (64).

Although there is universal agreement that mental retardation caused by CH can be eradicated by early diagnosis and therapy, whether more subtle psychomotor dysfunction may persist, particularly in the most hypothyroid infants, is controversial at present. Glorieux et al. (65) described a prospective study of the mental development of hypothyroid infants detected by the Quebec newborn screening program. The mean age at initiation of thyroid hormone therapy in 45 infants was 27 days. The mental development of these infants was assessed at 12, 18, and 36 months and compared with that of healthy controls. There were no statistically significant differences in the various test scores between the two populations at 12 months of age. At 18 and again at 36 months of age, however, the hypothyroid infants had lower scores in hearing-speech performance scales and practical reasoning. More recently, the same author (66) reported follow-up at age 12 years. Those children with the most severe hypothyroidism at birth and the most retarded bone ages had a significantly lower IQ than those with less severe hypothyroidism. Similar results were reported by Richiccioli et al., who reported higher grade detention rates as well as lower scores in mathematics in children with CH (67). The worsening of academic performance was associated with lower serum T_4 levels at birth, smaller bone surface area, lower IQ at 4 and 7 years of age, decreased fine motor coordination, and lower socioeconomic level.

In contrast, the IQ and elementary school performance of 72 children with congenital hypothyroidism assessed by the New England Congenital Hypothyroidism Studies (68) was not significantly different from these parameters in control patients. Also, the percentage of children in need of extra help in school was the same for patients and control groups. Compared with the Quebec group, these children were detected and treated at an earlier age and received a higher replacement dosage of levothyroxine sodium (10–15 versus 6–8 $\mu g/dl$; 129–193 versus 77–103 nM), and in them serum T_4 and TSH concentrations normalized at an earlier age. The mean IQ and overall achievement score in patients were not statistically different from those in control subjects. The authors concluded that children with CH have no apparent specific impediments to learning unrelated to intelligence.

The relationship of intellectual performance of CH children to the serum T_4 levels during the first 2 years of life was evaluated in 46 Norwegian patients with CH (69). Children with mean serum thyroxine levels above 14 $\mu g/dl$ (180 nM) during the first year had a significantly higher mental developmental index at 2 years and verbal IQ at 6 years of age than children with serum thyroxine values below 10 $\mu g/dl$ (129 nM). The authors concluded that thyroxine levels above the upper reference range during the first 2 years were related to improved intellectual development at 2 and 6 years.

In summary, more studies are needed to evaluate the long-term mental development in these subjects. Current data suggest that although mental retardation has been eradicated, even early postnatal treatment may not prevent more subtle intellectual deficits, particularly in newborns with the most severe hypothyroidism in utero as reflected by clinical signs and symptoms, extremely low T_4 levels (less than 2.5 μg/dl; 32 nM), and delayed bone age. Whether earlier, more aggressive therapy will result in a more favorable outcome without producing untoward effects or whether administration of thyroxine in utero will be required remains to be determined.

G. Conclusion

Congenital hypothyroidism is a relatively frequently encountered condition. Because the physical signs and symptoms of hypothyroidism in the newborn period are few, and often nonspecific, the diagnosis in the past was often delayed beyond the time when treatment would be most effective. The screening program for congenital hypothyroidism is therefore a significant advance in the prevention of the devastating effects on mental development in such children. Although many infants with borderline abnormal screening results are found to have normal thyroid function when retested, no abnormal values can be ignored because of the possibility of delayed development of hypothyroidism and the severe consequences to the baby if treatment is delayed. All such children require an immediate workup, preferably by an experienced pediatric endocrinologist, followed by appropriate therapy.

II. NEONATAL THYROTOXICOSIS

Neonatal hyperthyroidism is a relatively rare condition, estimated to occur once in every 25,000 pregnancies (47). Most such patients are born to mothers with active Graves' disease, but the disease can also occur in mothers who are hypothyroid or euthyroid because of concomitant autoimmune thyroiditis, radioactive iodine ablation therapy, or surgery. Therefore, it is of utmost importance that physicians be aware of babies at risk and of the various manifestations of the disease. This becomes increasingly important because both clinical and biochemical symptoms of neonatal thyrotoxicosis can be suppressed for several days because of the effect of maternal antithyroid therapy. Although in most infants thyrotoxicosis is transient, some patients may suffer from severe and long-lasting disease. The mortality in the latter group may reach 20% if vigorous therapy is not instituted immediately. Moreover, severe brain damage may occur among patients who survive, primarily as a result of the hypermetabolic state and premature closure of the cranial bones, as well as the direct effect of excess thyroid hormones on brain maturation (70,71).

Because most infants presenting with neonatal thyrotoxicosis are born to mothers with Graves' disease, it is important that such mothers be followed and managed during their pregnancies, not only by an obstetrician but also by an experienced endocrinologist. The outcome of the offspring often reflects the management of their mothers' hyperthyroidism. For example, mothers who are overtreated with antithyroid drugs during the pregnancy may give birth to children with hypothyroidism. On the other hand, mothers who are undertreated may have children born prematurely and with low birth weight. It is beyond the scope of this chapter to discuss the management of hyperthyroid women during pregnancy, and the reader is referred to the appropriate literature (72).

A. Etiology

The neonatal form of Graves' disease is believed to be caused by the transplacental passage of thyrotropin (TSH) receptor antibodies (TRAbs), which mimic the action of TSH in stimulating thyroid growth and function (43,73–75). Only 2–3% of mothers with Graves' disease have affected babies. Because only babies born to mothers with the most potent stimulating activity have affected babies (76), measurement of maternal TRAbs in the third trimester in mothers requiring a high dosage of antithyroid medication and mothers whose thyroids have been ablated has been recommended to identify infants at risk. In the majority of babies, thyrotoxicosis is transient and usually resolves within a few weeks. Rarely, the disease may be more long lasting, as in the cases described by Hollingsworth and Mabry (77), who reported several patients with a strong family history of Graves' disease in whom thyrotoxicosis developed soon after birth and persisted for a prolonged period. In these cases it is likely that the babies not only had received transplacentally acquired maternal TRAbs but had developed classic Graves' disease themselves as well. Thus, there are at least two distinct groups of infants with congenital thyrotoxicosis: those with transient hyperthyroidism and, rarely, those in whom thyrotoxicosis runs a protracted course, similar to that seen in older children and adults (71). In yet other rare cases, mothers may have both stimulating and blocking TSH receptor antibodies. In these cases, babies develop either hyperthyroidism or hypothyroidism, depending on whether stimulating or inhibiting immunoglobulins predominate (43). In addition, the TRAbs can have a biphasic effect, whereby large amounts can suppress the thyroid gland and small amounts stimulate the gland (78).

B. Symptoms

Unlike newborns with CH, who are frequently postmature with increased birth weight, patients with neonatal Graves' disease are often born before term (71). If the mother was receiving antithyroid drugs, which readily cross the placenta, such infants may be asymptomatic for the first few days of life until the drug has been cleared from the baby's circulation. Thus, all babies born to mothers with Graves' disease should be closely followed for signs of thyrotoxicosis for at least the first week of postnatal life. Caution is advisable because of the poor prognosis, including developmental impairment or even death (71,73,77) if the diagnosis is missed. Unlike older children with Graves' disease, goiter and exophthalmos are infrequent features of neonatal thyrotoxicosis, although large goiters sufficient to cause respiratory impairment may occur secondary to large doses of propylthiouracil in the mother. More often, such patients have tachycardia and respiratory distress.

Hypermetabolic symptoms may eventually lead to heart failure. Other features include hyperkinesis, restlessness, diarrhea, and a poor weight gain despite increased caloric intake (71). Bone maturation is accelerated and may result in premature craniosynostosis (70). Usual features described in such patients include jaundice, pitting edema, hepatospleno-megaly, thrombocytopenia, enlargement of the reticuloendo-thelial system, the hyperviscosity syndrome, and ventricular estrasystoles (79).

C. Laboratory Diagnosis

As discussed previously, normal values of thyroid hormone levels in early life are different from those seen later. Thus, to arrive at the correct diagnosis, one must be acquainted with normal values (Fig. 1). Once a diagnosis of neonatal hyper-thyroidism is suspected, free thyroxine index (or free T_4), T_3 RIA, and TSH should be determined as early as possible. Typically, such patients have a marked elevation in both T_4 and T_3 RIA levels, although in rare instances so-called T_3 toxicosis may occur in which T_4 levels are only slightly elevated or are normal. The TSH values are low and are clearly distinguishable from normal if a third-generation ultrasensitive assay is used. Thyrotropin-releasing hormone stimulation demonstrates a flat TSH response, but this test is no longer necessary in most cases. The RIA thyroid uptake with ^{123}I at both 4 and 24 h is elevated; in rare cases in which the diagnosis is unclear, the lack of suppressibility with liothyronine (Cytomel; T_3) may be shown, but this test must be performed with caution and has been largely replaced by measurement of TSH receptor antibodies. Because, as dis-cussed earlier, mixtures of stimulating and blocking antibod-ies may exist, screening can be performed by a radioreceptor assay, which is less expensive and easier to perform. How-ever, when such antibodies are detected, further characteriza-tion of the antibody activity by bioassay should be performed to predict the likely nature of the clinical course. The

radiologic assessment of bone maturation often reveals ad-vancement of the fetal bone age. Untreated or inadequately treated neonatal hyperthyroidism may result in further ad-vancement of the bone maturation and craniosynostosis (80).

Not all infants with elevated T_4 and T_3 RIA levels have thyrotoxicosis. As shown in Table 7, several other conditions manifested by hyperthyroxinemia must be taken into consider-ation, especially when an infant is clinically euthyroid. In these cases, the TSH is not suppressed. These include alterations of binding proteins (including TBG excess rather than deficiency) and thyroid hormone resistance. The former conditions can be diagnosed by measuring various binding proteins, free T_4, and T_3 resin uptake in both the patient and family.

D. Treatment

An infant with clinical and biochemical symptoms and signs of hyperthyroidism represents a medical emergency (71). The first important aspect of the treatment is to combat the overstimulation of the cardiovascular system. This is done by administering β-adrenergic blockers, such as propranolol, 1–2 mg/kg per day in three divided doses. The next step, which should be undertaken simultaneously, is to suppress the hypersecretion of thyroid hormones using a saturated solution of potassium iodide and thioamides. Iodides may be administered as 10% potassium iodide solution, 1 drop every 8 h. If necessary, propylthiouracil in a total daily dosage of 5–10 mg/kg in three doses can be added but will not be effective for several days. This drug blocks the organification of iodine and, in addition, conversion of T_4 to T_3. If no clinical improvement takes place in 1 or 2 days, the dosage of iodine and propylthiouracil can be doubled. Severely affected infants may also benefit from glucocorticoids. Recently, a new therapeutic approach using sodium ipodate for combating the hyperthyroid state in neonates has been reported (81). Any of these treatment modalities can result in a hypothyroid state, however. There-

Table 7 Differential Diagnosis of Increased T_4 Levels in Infants

Syndrome	Total T_4	RT_3U^a	TBG^b	FT_4I^c	Free T_4	Total T_3	Free T_3
Thyrotoxicosis	↑	↑	N	↑	↑	↑	↑
TBG excess	↑	↓	↑	N	N	↑	N
Familial euthyroid hyperthyroxinemia							
Increased T_4 binding to albumin	↑	N	N	↑	N	N	N
Increased T_4 binding to prealbumin	↑	↓ (N)	N	↑	N	N	N
T_4 resistance	↑	↑	N	↑	↑	↑	↑
I_2 contamination	±	N	N	N	N	↑	N

↑ = increased
↓ = decreased
N = normal
^{a}RTB = T_3 Resin Uptake
^{b}TBG = Thyroxine Binding Globulin
^{c}FT$_4$I = Free Thyroxine Index

fore, when needed, L-thyroxine can be used to maintain clinical and chemical euthyroidism or the dosages of the other medications can be tapered. Careful follow-up is necessary for proper adjustment of the medication, because both hypo- and hyperthyroid states can interfere with the normal sequence of central nervous system maturation (70). In addition, a complete neurologic assessment is necessary in all these children periodically.

REFERENCES

1. Fisher DA, Dussault JH, Foley TP, et al. Screening for congenital hypothyroidism: results of screening one million North American infants. J Pediatr 1979; 94:700–705.
2. Toublanc J-E. Comparison of epidemiological data on congenital hypothyroidism in Europe with those of other parts in the world. Horm Res 1992; 38:230–235.
3. Fisher DA. Thyroid physiology in the fetus and newborn: current concepts and approaches to perinatal thyroid disease. In: New MI, Fisher RH, eds. Diabetes and Other Endocrine Disorders During Pregnancy and in the Newborn. New York: Alan R. Liss, 1976:221–233.
4. Dussault JH. Transplacental transport of thyroid hormone: possible clinical implications. In: Oppenheimer JH, ed. Thyroid Today. Lincolnshire, IL: Boots Pharmaceuticals, April/May/June 1992:1–7.
5. Calvo R, Obregon MJ, Ruiz de Ona C, Escobar del Rey F, Morreale de Escobar G. Congenital hypothyroidism as studied in rats: crucial role of maternal thyroxine but not 3,5,3^1-triiodothyronine in the protection of the fetal brain. J Clin Invest 1990; 86:889–899.
6. Romero R, Pilu G, Jeanty P, Ghidini A, Hobbins JC. Prenatal Diagnosis of Congenital Anomalies. Norwalk, CT: Appleton and Lange, 1988:119–120.
7. Davidson KM, Richards DS, Schatz DA, Fisher DA. Successful in utero treatment of fetal goiter and hypothyroidism. N Engl J Med 1991; 324:543–546.
8. American Academy of Pediatrics, American Thyroid Association. Newborn screening for congenital hypothyroidism: recommended guidelines. Pediatrics 1993; 91:1203–1209.
9. Fort P, Lifshitz F, Bellisario R, et al. Abnormalities of thyroid function in infants with Downs Syndrome. J Pediatr 1984; 104:545–549.
10. Nicoloff JT, Spencer CT. The use and misuse of sensitive thyrotropin assays. J Clin Endocrinol Metab 1990; 71:553–558.
11. Bellisario R, Brown SK, Beblowski D, Hedden MB, Potulka J. Newborn screening for hypothyroidism is New York State. In: Therrell BL Jr, ed. Advances in Neonatal Screening. Amsterdam: Excerpta Medica, 1987:35–39.
12. Council of Regional Networks for Genetics Services Newborn Screening Report for 1990. Meaney FJ, Chair; Riggle SM, Data Coordinator. New York: Council of Regional Networks for Genetic Services, 1992.
13. LaFranchi SH, Hanna CE, Krainz PL, Skeels MR, Miyahira RS, Sesser DE. Screening for congenital hypothyroidism with specimen collection at two time periods: results of the Northwest Regional Screening Program. Pediatrics 1985; 76:734–740.
14. Holtzman C, Slazyk WE, Cordero JF, Hannon WH. Descriptive epidemiology of missed cases of phenylketonuria and congenital hypothyroidism. Pediatrics 1986; 78:553–558.
15. Allen DB, Hendricks A, Sieger J, et al. Screening programs for congenital hypothyroidism. Am J Dis Child 1988; 142:232–236.
16. Bellisario R, Carter TP. Results of New York State Newborn Hypothyroidism Screening Program. In: Porter IH, Hatcher NH, Wieley AM, eds. Perinatal Genetics: Diagnosis and Treatment. Orlando, FL: Academic Press, 1986:219–242.
17. Oddie TH, Fisher DA, Bernard B, Lam RW. Thyroid function at birth in infants of 30 to 45 weeks gestation. J Pediatr 1977; 90:803–806.
18. Klein AH, Foley TP, Kenny FM, Fisher DA. Thyroid hormone and thyrotropin responses to parturition in premature infants with or without the respiratory distress syndrome. Pediatrics 1979; 63:380–385.
19. Chowdhry P, Scanlon JW, Auerbach R, Abassi V. Results of controlled double-blind study of thyroid replacement in very low birth weight premature infants with hypothyroxinemia. Pediatrics 1984; 73:301–305.
20. Mercado M, Szymonowicz W, Yu VYH, Gold H. Symptomatic hypothyroxinemia with normal TSH levels in preterm infants. Clin Pediatr (Phila) 1987; 26:343–346.
21. Wilson DM, Hopper AO, McDougall IR, et al. Serum free thyroxine values in term, premature, and sick infants. J Pediatr 1982; 101:113–117.
22. Sava L, Delange F, Belfiore A, Purrello F, Vigneri R. Transient impairment of thyroid function in newborn from an area of endemic goiter. J Clin Endocrinol Metab 1984; 59:90–95.
23. Delange F, Bourdoux P, Senterre J. Evidence of a high requirement of iodine in preterm infants. Pediatr Res 1984; 18:106.
24. Etling N. Concentration of thyroglobulin, iodine contents of thyroglobulin and of iodoaminoacids in human neonates thyroid gland. Acta Paediatr Scand 1977; 66:97–102.
25. Gregerman RI, Soloman N. Acceleration of thyroxine and triiodothyronine turnover during bacterial pulmonary infections and fever: implications for the functional state of the thyroid during stress and in senescence. J Clin Endocrinol Metab 1967; 27:93–105.
26. Cuestas RA. Thyroid function in healthy premature infants. J Pediatr 1982; 92:963–967.
27. Klein AH, Fisher DA. Thyroid physiology in full-term and premature infants. In: Dussalt JH, Walker P, eds. Congenital Hypothyroidism. New York: Marcel Dekker, 1983:127–143.
28. Jacobsen BB, Peitersen B, Andersen HJ, Hummer L. Serum concentration of thyroxine-binding globulin, prealbumin and albumin in healthy fulltern, small-for-gestational age and preterm infants. Acta Paediatr Scand 1979; 68:49–55.
29. Hanna CE, Drainz PL, Skeels MR, Miyahir RS, Sesser DE, LaFranci SH. Detection of congenital hypopituitary hypothyroidism: ten-year experience in the Northwest Regional Screening Program. J Pediatr 1986; 109:959–964.
30. Nusynowitz ML, Clark RF, Strader WJ III, Estrin HM, Seal US. Thyroxine-binding globulin deficiency in three families and total deficiency in a normal woman. Am J Med 1971; 50:458–464.
31. Mitchell ML, Bapat V, Larsen RP, Lind H, Lungren RB, Miliner R. Pitfalls in screening for neonatal hypothyroidism. Pediatrics 1982; 70:16–20.
32. Price DA, Ehrlich RM, Walfish PG. Congenital hypothyroidism. Clinical and laboratory characteristics in infants detected by neonatal screening. Arch Dis Child 1981; 56:845–851.
33. Greig WR, Henderson AS, Boyle JA, McGirr EM, Hutchinson JH. Thyroid dysgenesis in two pairs of monozygotic twins and in a mother and child. J Clin Endocrinol 1966; 26:1309–1316.
34. Pacini F, Lari R, LaRicca P, et al. Serum thyroglobulin determination in the differential diagnosis of congenital hypothyroidism. J Endocrinol Invest 1984; 7:29–33.

35. Leger J, Tar A, Schlumberger M, Czernichow P. Control of thyroglobulin secretion in patients with ectopic thyroid gland. Pediatr Res 1988; 23:266–269.

36. Muir A, Daneman D, Daneman A, Ehrlich R. Thyroid scanning, ultrasound, and serum thyroglobulin in determining the origin of congenital hypothyroidism. Am J Dis Child 1988; 142:214–216.

37. DeGroot LJ, Stranbury JB. The Thyroid and Its Diseases, 4th ed. New York: Wiley, 1975.

38. Lever EG, Medeiros-Neto GA, De Groot LJ. Inherited disorders of thyroid metabolism. Endocr Rev 1983; 4:213–239.

39. LaFranchi SH, Buist NRM. Transient neonatal hypothyroidism detected by newborn screening program. Pediatrics 1977; 60:538–541.

40. Matsuura N, Yamada Y, Nohara Y et al. Familial neonatal transient hypothyroidism due to maternal TSH-binding inhibitor immunoglobulins. N Engl J Med 1980; 303:738–741.

41. Connors MH, Styne DM. Transient neonatal "athyreosis" resulting from thyrotropin-binding inhibitory immunoglobulins. Pediatrics 1986; 78:287–289.

42. Francis G, Riley W. Congenital familial transient hypothyroidism secondary to transplacental thyrotropin-blocking autoantibodies. Am J Dis Child 1987; 141:1081–1083.

43. Fort P, Lifshitz F, Pugliese M, Klein I. Transient neonatal thyroid disease: differential expression in three successive offspring. J Clin Endocrinol Metab 1988; 66:645–647.

44. Brown RS, Keating P, Mitchell E. Maternal thyroid-blocking immunoglobulins in congenital hypothyroidism. J Clin Endocrinol Metab 1990; 70:1341–1346.

45. Nagayama Y, Wadsworth HL, Russo D, et al. Binding domains of stimulatory and inhibitor thyrotropin (TSH) receptor autoantibodies determined with chimeric TSH-lutropin/chorionic gonadotropin receptors. J Clin Invest 1991; 88:336–340.

46. Zakarija M, McKenzie JM, Hoffman WH. Prediction and therapy of intrauterine and late-onset neonatal hyperthyroidism. J Clin Endocrinol Metab 1986; 62:368–371.

47. Fisher DA. Neonatal thyroid disease in the offspring of women with autoimmune thyroid disease. Thyroid Today 1986; 9(4): 1.

48. Bachrach LK, Burrow GN, Gare DJ. Maternal-fetal absorption of povidone iodine. J Pediatr 1984; 104:158–159.

49. Smendely P, Lim A, Boyage SC, et al. Topical iodine-containing antiseptics and neonatal hypothyroidism in very-low-birthweight infants. Lancet 1989; 2:661–664.

50. Jackson HJ, Sutherland RM. Effects of povidone iodine on neonatal thyroid function. Lancet 1981; 2:992.

51. Alemzadeh R, Friedman C, Fort P, Recker B, Lifshitz F. Is there compensated hypothyroidism in infancy? Pediatrics 1992; 90:207–211.

52. Rapaport R, Sills I, Patel U, et al. Thyrotropin-releasing hormone stimulation tests in infants. J Clin Endocrinol Metab 1993; 77:889–894.

53. Price DA, Ehrlich RM, Walfish PG. Congenital hypothyroidism. Clinical and laboratory characteristics in infants detected by neonatal screening. Arch Dis Child 1981; 56:845–851.

54. Letarte J, Dussault JH, Guyda H, Fouron JC, Glorieux J. Clinical and laboratory investigation of early detected hypothyroid infants. In: Collu R, et al., eds. Pediatric Endocrinology. New York: Raven Press, 198,:433–464.

55. Bamforth JS, Hughes I, Lazarus J, John R. Congenital anomalies associated with hypothyroidism. Arch Dis Child 1986; 61:608–609.

56. Redmond GP, Soyka LF. Abnormal TSH secretory dynamics in congenital hypothyroidism. J Pediatr 1981; 98:83–85.

57. Fisher DA, Foley BL. Early treatment of congenital hypothyroidism. Pediatrics 1989; 83:785–789.

58. Germak JA, Foley TP Jr. Longitudinal assessment of L-thyroxine therapy for congenital hypothyroidism. J Pediatr 1990; 117:211–219.

59. Holt AB, Cheek DB, Kerr GR. Prenatal hypothyroidism and brain composition in a primate. Nature 1973; 243:413–415.

60. Nunez J. Differential expression of microtubule components during brain development. Dev Neurosci 1986; 8(3):125–141.

61. Munoz MA, Rodriguez-Pena A, Perez-Castillo A, Ferreiro B, Sutcliffe JG, Bernal J. Effects of neonatal hypothyroidism on rat brain gene expression. Mol Endocrinol 1991; 5(4):273–280.

62. MacFaul R, Dorner S, Brett EM, Grant DB. Neurological abnormalities in patients treated for hypothyroidism from early life. Arch Dis Child 1978; 53:611–619.

63. Klein AH, Meltzer S, Kenny FM. Improved prognosis in congenital hypothyroidism treated below age three months. J Pediatr 1972; 81:912–915.

64. Maenpaa J. Congenital hypothyroidism: aetiological and clinical aspects. Arch Dis Child 1972; 47:917–923.

65. Glorieux J, Dussault JH, LeTarte J, Guyda H, Morisette J. Preliminary results on the mental development of hypothyroid infants detected by the Quebec Screening Program. J Pediatr 1983; 102:19–22.

66. Glorieux J, Dussault JH, Van Vliet G. Intellectual development at age 12 years of children with congenital hypothyroidism diagnosed by neonatal screening. J Pediatr 1992; 121: 581–584.

67. Richiccioli P, Roge B, Alexandre F, Tauber MT. School achievement in children with hypothyroidism detected and birth and search for predictive factors. Horm Res 1992; 38:236–240.

68. New England Congenital Hypothyroidism Collaborative, Klein RZ, et al. Elementary school performance of children with congenital hypothyroidism. J Pediatr 1990; 116:27–32.

69. Heyerdahl S, Kase BF, Lie SO. Intellectual development in children with congenital hypothyroidism in relation to recommended thyroxine treatment. J Pediatr 1991; 118:850–857.

70. Daneman D, Howard NJ. Neonatal thyrotoxicosis: intellectual impairment and craniosynostosis in later years. J Pediatr 1980; 97:257–259.

71. Howard CP, Hayles AB. Neonatal Graves' disease. Clin Endocrinol Metab 1978; 7:131–134.

72. Hollingsworth DR. Hyperthyroidism in pregnancy. In: Ingbar SH, Braverman LE, eds. Werner's the Thyroid, 5th ed. Philadelphia: J. B. Lippincott, 1986:1043–1063.

73. Ditmikis SM, Munro DS. Placental transmission of thyroid stimulating immunoglobins. BMJ 1975; 2:665–666.

74. Fisher DA. Pathogenesis and therapy of neonatal Graves' disease. Am J Dis Child 1976; 130:133–134.

75. McKenzie JM, Zakaria M. Fetal and neonatal hyperthyroidism due to maternal TSH receptor antibodies. Thyroid 1992; 2:155–159.

76. Zakaria M, McKenzie JM. Pregnancy-associated changes in the thyroid-stimulating antibody of Graves' disease and the relationship to neonatal hyperthyroidism. J Clin Endocrinol Metab 1983; 57:1036–1040.

77. Hollingsworth DR, Mabry CC. Congenital Graves' disease. Am J Dis Child 1976; 130:148–155.

78. Yoshida S, Takamatsu J, Kuma K, Ohsawa N. Thyroid-stimulating antibodies and thyroid stimulation-blocking antibodies during the pregnancy and postpartum period: a case report. Thyroid 1992; 2(1):27–29.

79. Singer J. Neonatal thyrotoxicosis. J Pediatr 1977; 91:749–751.

80. Cove DH, Johnston P. Fetal hyperthyroidism: experience of treatment in four siblings. Lancet 1985; 1:430–432.

81. Transue D, Chan J, Kaplan M. Management of neonatal Graves' disease with iopanoic acid. J Pediatr 1992; 121:472–474.

26
Thyromegaly

John S. Dallas
University of Texas Medical Branch and Children's Hospital of Galveston, Galveston, Texas

Thomas P. Foley, Jr.
University of Pittsburgh and Children's Hospital of Pittsburgh, Pittsburgh, Pennsylvania

I. INTRODUCTION

Thyromegaly is a common clinical disorder during childhood and adolescence. Prospective studies in the United States and Japan have shown that thyromegaly may occur in up to 6% of school-age children living in iodine-sufficient areas (1–3). A child presents with either diffuse or nodular thyromegaly, although diffuse enlargement is more common. The enlargement can be either symmetric or asymmetric. According to the World Health Organization, diffuse thyromegaly is present in a child if the lateral lobes of the gland are larger than the terminal phalanx of the child's thumb (4). A nodular thyroid contains one or more solid or cystic masses that have a consistency different from that in the remainder of the gland. Thyromegaly usually occurs during adolescence with a female-male predominance (5). (For discussion of autoimmune thyrotoxicosis: Graves' disease and its pathogenesis, see Chap. 28.)

II. PATHOGENESIS OF THYROMEGALY

Enlargement of the thyroid gland may occur as a result of stimulation, infiltration, and/or inflammation of the gland (Table 1) (5). Stimulation of follicular cell growth, either hyperplasia or hypertrophy, can be mediated by thyrotropin (TSH), various TSH receptor antibodies, and other growth factors (see Table 2 for abbreviations) (6–9). Increased TSH secretion is usually the result of an impairment in the production or release of the major thyroid hormones, T_4 and T_3. Rarely, increased TSH secretion results from a TSH-producing pituitary adenoma or from pituitary resistance to thyroid hormone; in these conditions the patient presents with mild to moderate thyromegaly, normal to elevated serum levels of TSH, and elevated serum levels of total and free T_4 and T_3.

A variety of TRAb have been identified in patients with autoimmune thyroid disease. Some of these antibodies stimulate thyroid function and, possibly, thyroid follicular cell growth through interactions with membrane-bound TSH receptors (6–8). Whether there are specific thyroid growth-stimulating antibodies that mediate their mitogenic effect via the TSH receptor or other cell membrane receptors remains controversial (10–12). To date there have been no reports of direct stimulation of human follicular cell growth (increase in cell number or DNA content). Reports of increased thymidine incorporation and the S phase of the cell cycle in nonhuman thyroid cells by antibodies and other growth factors have provided indirect evidence for TGAb, although these observations could be effects upon thymidine transport, metabolism, and other nonmitogenic processes in the cell cycle (12,13).

Infiltration of the thyroid gland may occur from a neoplastic (i.e., adenoma or carcinoma) or a nonneoplastic (i.e., cyst) process. During childhood, a thyroid neoplasm, whether benign or malignant, usually presents as an isolated nodule in the thyroid gland. Recently, two mutations were reported in the intracellular domain of the TSH receptor in tumor tissue from patients with hyperfunctioning thyroid adenomas (14). These mutations cause constitutive activation of the G_s protein that is coupled to the receptor to cause an unregulated activation of the adenylyl cyclase-cAMP cascade in tumor tissue from these patients (14). Rarely, thyromegaly is found in patients with histiocytosis X or lymphoma because of cellular infiltration of the gland (15).

Although a variety of infectious agents (bacterial, viral, and fungal) can cause acute or subacute inflammation and enlargement of the thyroid gland, infectious thyroiditis rarely

Table 1 Pathogenesis of Thyromegaly

Stimulation
  Thyrotropin
    Inhibition of thyroidal hormonogenesis
    Excessive hypothalamic and pituitary secretion
  Thyrotropin receptor antibodies
    Thyroid-stimulating antibodies
    Thyroid growth-stimulating antibodies
Infiltration
  Neoplasia
    Adenoma
    Carcinoma
    Lymphoma
    Histiocytosis
  Nonneoplasia: cysts
Inflammation
  Infection
    Bacterial
    Viral
    Other pathogens
  Noninfection: lymphocytic (autoimmune)

Table 3 Causes of Thyromegaly

Diffuse thyromegaly
  Autoimmune (Hashimoto's) thyroiditis
  Thyrotoxicosis
    Graves' disease
    Toxic thyroiditis
    TSH-secreting pituitary adenoma
    Pituitary resistance to thyroid hormone
  Goitrogen ingestion
    Antithyroid drugs
    Antithyroid agents and foods
  Iodine deficiency
  Familial dyshormonogenesis
  Acute and subacute thyroiditis
  Idiopathic (simple) thyromegaly
Nodular thyromegaly
  Autoimmune (Hashimoto's) thyroiditis
  Thyroid cyst
  Thyroid tumors
    Adenoma
      Hyperfunctioning (hot): hyperthyroid or euthyroid
      Nonfunctioning (cold)
    Carcinoma
    Other tumors
  Nonthyroidal masses
    Lymphadenopathy
    Branchial cleft cyst
    Thyroglossal duct cyst

occurs during childhood (15). However, autoimmune chronic lymphocytic thyroiditis, including the goitrous variant known as Hashimoto's disease, is the most common cause of thyromegaly during childhood in nonendemic goiter regions of the world (1–3,9). In this disease, lymphocytic infiltration of the thyroid may be diffuse and cause generalized enlargement of one or both lobes or may be localized and cause nodular enlargement of the gland (5). The latter entity may be difficult to distinguish from tumors of the thyroid gland.

Disorders associated with thyromegaly during childhood can be classified depending on whether thyromegaly is diffuse or nodular (Table 3). The child initially presents for evaluation based upon the physical examination of the thyroid gland, and thus the differential diagnosis and laboratory investigation should be considered according to the physical characteristics of the gland and the surrounding structures in the neck.

Table 2 Abbreviations

TSH	thyrotropin; thyroid-stimulating hormone
TRH	thyrotropin-releasing hormone
T_4	L-thyroxine
T_3	3,3'5-L-triiodothyronine
TgAb	thyroglobulin antibodies
TRAb	thyrotropin receptor antibodies
TSAb	thyroid-stimulating antibodies
TGAb	thyroid growth antibodies
IDDM	insulin-dependent (type I) diabetes mellitus

III. CAUSES OF DIFFUSE THYROMEGALY

A. Autoimmue Thyroid Disease: Thyroiditis

1. Pathogenesis of Autoimmune Thyroid Diseases

Recent advances in immunology have led to a greater understanding of the basic abnormalities in cellular and humoral immune systems that result in autoimmune thyroid diseases. The underlying defects appear to be genetically linked defects in immunoregulation that result from an abnormal activation of an organ-specific population of suppressor T lymphocytes by HLA-related genes (7,16). In the genetically predisposed individual with the immune defect, the clinical disease may be triggered and aggravated by an environmental insult, such as a viral infection, or some form of stress, either biologic or psychologic.

In Graves' disease, the immune defect results in the production of immunoglobulin G (IgG) antibodies that bind to and stimulate the TSH receptor to cause an increase in the function and size of the thyroid gland. These effects are responsible for the clinical findings of thyrotoxicosis and goiter in Graves' disease (7,8,16). In some patients, Graves' and Hashimoto's diseases coexist, and the antibody production is polyclonal rather than monoclonal (7,8,16). As a result, more than one form of TRAb may be present, and the TRAb have been classified according to their method of analysis by in vitro assays. Antibodies that stimulate thyroid cell function are known as TSAb, or thyroid-stimulating immunoglobulins (TSI). Antibodies that displace labeled TSH from binding to TSH receptors are known as thyrotropin binding inhibitory immunoglobulins (TBII); in most instances, when tested in the TSI assays, the TBII are stimulatory (6). TSH receptor blocking antibodies may be found in patients with Hashimoto's disease or inactive Graves' disease. These immunoglobulins inhibit TSH-stimulated adenylate cyclase activity by thyroid cells or membranes.

Cytotoxic mechanisms in autoimmune thyroiditis cause the chronic inflammatory reaction so characteristic of the disease. Thyroid cell damage is probably mediated either by thyroid antibody-dependent cell mediated cytotoxicity (17) or by direct cytotoxicity from sensitized effector T lymphocytes, or both mechanisms in association with production of destructive cytokines (7,8,16).

2. Chronic Lymphyocytic Thyroiditis of Childhood and Adolescence

a. Classification. The autoimmune-mediated mechanisms cause the histologic changes in the thyroid that are the basis for the classification of the disease during childhood. These mechanisms result in the characteristic histologic abnormalities of lymphocytic infiltration and lymphoid follicles that are typical of juvenile autoimmune thyroiditis, including Hashimoto's disease. The usual histologic appearance during childhood and adolescence is follicular cell hyperplasia with minimal fibrosis (15). The fibrous variant of the disease is characterized by epithelial destruction and fibrosis (15).

b. Clinical Manifestations. Most patients with autoimmune thyroiditis present with an asymptomatic enlargement of the thyroid gland, but an occasional patient may complain of pain or a sensation of fullness in the area of the thyroid. Less often the disease becomes manifest after the onset of hypothyroidism, which may present during childhood with deceleration of linear growth and other clinical features associated with the onset of hypothyroidism during childhood (see Chap. 27). The child with thyroiditis rarely presents initially with symptoms and signs of thyrotoxicosis; in this presentation, a transient phase of hyperthyroidism occurs early in the course of autoimmune thyroiditis (toxic thyroiditis) and the patient presents with a mild disease without exophthalmos. Whereas thyrotoxicosis of Graves' disease results from excessive production and secretion of thyroid hormones caused by TRAb stimulation of TSH receptors, the thyrotoxicosis of toxic thyroiditis results from the release of excessive amounts of preformed thyroid hormones as a result of inflammatory destruction of thyroid follicular cells. These two disorders may be difficult to distinguish on clinical criteria alone, unless the exophthalmos of Graves' disease is present or TRAb are detected in serum. Autoimmune thyroiditis frequently occurs in patients with other autoimmune diseases, particularly IDDM (18,19), but also Addison's disease, alopecia, pernicious anemia, and the collagen vascular diseases (Chap. 50) (20).

On examination, the thyroid gland is either symmetrically or asymmetrically enlarged and usually nontender and firm in consistency. The surface texture may be finely granular (seedy) or discretely nodular (pebbly or crenated). Lymphoid follicles may be palpable as single or multiple nodules within one or both lobes of the gland. The gland should move freely with swallowing and should not be affixed to adjacent tissues. Nontender regional lymphadenopathy may be present (15).

c. Laboratory Evaluation. An elevated titer of thyroid antibodies is the characteristic laboratory abnormality that permits a presumptive diagnosis of autoimmune thyroiditis. Thyroid peroxidase (formerly known as microsomal antigen) and thyroglobulin antibodies are the two generally available thyroid antibody tests. More sensitive radioassay methods than previously available can detect thyroperoxidase and thyroglobulin antibodies in a grater number of children with clinical autoimmune thyroiditis (21). Antibody titers in normal children are lower than in normal adults; especially in women, these may be as high as in 30% of the general population. Occasionally, a child with autoimmune thyroiditis presents with low or absent titers of thyroid antibodies, yet on repeat determinations 3–6 months later the titers are distinctly abnormal. Transient elevations in thyroid antibodies may occur during the course of other thyroid disorders (e.g., subacute thyroiditis); therefore, a positive titer may not be indicative of chronic thyroiditis.

Although most children with autoimmune thyroiditis are clinically euthyroid, serum TSH levels should be determined to exclude primary hypothyroidism. Additional studies may be needed for patients with an atypical clinical presentation. For the child with mild symptoms of hyperthyroidism, important initial tests should include serum T_3 and TRAb determinations (6). In the child with symptoms of hyperthyroidism, serum T_3 should be elevated unless the patient either is severely ill or has experienced very poor or negligible nutritional intake for several days before testing. Further diagnostic tests are needed infrequently. The TRH test and the [^{123}I]iodide uptake test (6) may be helpful to differentiate toxic thyroiditis from early Graves' disease and other causes of hyperthyroidism. When symptoms of hyperthyroidism are present, T_4, free T_4, and T_3 values are elevated, TSH is suppressed, and thyroid antibody titers are abnormal, the patient usually does not need additional diagnostic tests. A careful follow-up evaluation for the next 1–2 months is important because the patient with toxic thyroiditis in association with autoimmune thyroiditis will improve, whereas the patient with Graves' disease usually does not.

Adults with Hashimoto's thyroiditis often have an elevated early (2–6 h) thyroidal uptake of [^{123}I]iodide with a greater than 20% release of the accumulated [^{123}I]iodide within 1 h after the oral administration of potassium perchlorate (17). This positive perchlorate discharge test indicates a defect in the intrathyroidal oxidation of iodide to iodine and may occur in anywhere from 10 to 50% of adults with autoimmune thyroiditis. This test is usually not required unless the patient has persistent clinical features of thyroiditis

Table 4 Spectrum of Thyroid Function in Autoimmune Thyroid Disease

Clinical thyroid function	T_4	T_3	TSH	TSH response to TRH
Primary hypothyroidism	Low	Low or normal	Increased	Exaggerated
Compensated hypothyroidism	Normal	Normal	Increased	Exaggerated
Euthyroidism with decreased thyroid reserve	Normal	Normal	Normal	Exaggerated
Goitrous and nongoitrous euthyroidism	Normal	Normal	Normal	Normal
Nonsuppressible euthyroidism	Normal	Normal	Normal	Blunted
Thyrotoxicosis with limited thyroid reserve	Mildly increased	Increased	Undetectable	Absent
Thyrotoxic phase of thyroiditis	Increased	Increased	Undetectable	Absent
T_3 thyrotoxicosis	Normal	Increased	Undetectable	Absent
Thyrotoxicosis	Increased	Increased	Undetectable	Absent

and negative thyroid antibodies on repeated determinations. The need for a thyroid biopsy in children with diffuse thyromegaly is very rarely necessary unless coexisting malignancy of the thyroid gland is suspected, as in a child with an asymptomatic, enlarging nonfunctional nodule within a diffusely enlarged thyroid gland in whom serum thyroid antibodies are negative.

d. Clinical Course and Management. i. Toxic Thyroiditis. The rare patient who presents with autoimmune toxic thyroiditis may gradually return to a euthyroid state within 1–2 months or may experience mild hypothyroidism before recovery. The duration of the hypothyroid phase of toxic thyroiditis is variable; it may last for a few weeks to several months, or it may be permanent. Patients who experience only mild symptoms during the thyrotoxic phase usually require no treatment, but low doses of propranolol (10 mg three or four times daily) can relieve symptoms in patients with more severe thyrotoxicosis. Antithyroid drugs are not indicated in the treatment of toxic thyroiditis. It is important to monitor serum thyroid function tests during the recovery phase of toxic thyroiditis. If hypothyroidism develops, the child should be treated with L-thyroxine. Because this phase is usually transient, the child can be given a trial off medication after 3–6 months of treatment and reevaluated 4–6 weeks later. If serum TSH is elevated, L-thyroxine replacement therapy should be resumed indefinitely. If clinically and chemically euthyroid, however, the child should be assessed annually with serum TSH to monitor for hypothyroidism, which may develop during the course of chronic lymphocytic thyroiditis.

ii. Chronic Lymphocytic Thyroiditis. Although most patients with euthyroid goiter secondary to autoimmune thyroiditis remain euthyroid, approximately 10% of patients subsequently develop hypothyroidism; for this reason, an annual clinical evaluation and assessment of serum TSH values are advised to identify the development of hypothy-

roidism during the preclinical stage (5). Once hypothyroidism develops in a previously euthyroid child, the disease is usually permanent rather than transient. Further discussion of the management of primary hypothyroidism may be found in Chapter 27.

B. Acute and Subacute Thyroiditis

Acute thyroiditis, a rare disease, is easy to recognize but difficult to manage. Classically, the child presents with an acute onset of pain in the area of the thyroid gland associated with fever, chills, dysphagia, hoarseness, and sore throat. The onset is usually preceded by an upper respiratory tract infection. On examination, the skin over the thyroid may be warm and erythematous, and regional lymphadenopathy may be present. The thyroid is asymmetrically or diffusely enlarged and extremely tender, and the child resists efforts to extend the neck. Although the child may appear "toxic" from the infectious process, he or she is not thyrotoxic. Laboratory investigation reveals leukocytosis and an elevated erythrocyte sedimentation rate. Serum thyroid function tests are usually normal at presentation and remain normal throughout the course of the disease. In fact, the disease is actually a perithyroiditis rather than an intrathyroidal infectious process. Antimicrobial therapy should be instituted promptly once appropriate cultures are obtained. A variety of aerobic and anaerobic organisms have been identified on culture of thyroid aspirates (22), and a Gram stain of the aspirate may help to determine initial antibiotic therapy pending culture results. Serial ultrasonography of the gland should be used to detect early abscess formation, at which time surgical intervention becomes indicated. Most of the recently reported cases of acute thyroiditis have been associated with an internal fistulous tract between the left pyriform sinus and the corresponding parathyroidal space (23, 24). Therefore, any child who presents with acute thyroiditis primarily involving the left lobe or who experiences recurrent acute thyroiditis should have a barium esophagram once he or she has recovered from the acute infectious process. If a fistula is identified, operative excision of the entire epithelial tract and adjacent thyroid tissue is essential to prevent recurrent thyroiditis and abscess (24).

Subacute thyroiditis also is rarely diagnosed during childhood and adolescence. The disease presumably results from a viral infection of the thyroid gland, often after a recent upper respiratory tract infection. There are two different clinical presentations (25). In the classic form, the patient presents with pain in the region of the thyroid that radiates to the jaws or ears. The patient may be clinically euthyroid or thyrotoxic. In the other form, known as painless or "silent" thyroiditis, the patient usually presents with symptoms of mild thyrotoxicosis without cervical or thyroidal pain. With either form there often are systemic symptoms of an inflammatory disease, such as fever, weakness, fatigue, and malaise. On examination, the patient with the classic form has a tender, firm, enlarged thyroid and resists efforts to extend the neck. Tenderness varies from mild to severe, and enlargement may be localized or diffuse. In the silent form, the thyroid is not tender and may or may not be enlarged.

During the early phase of the disease, one finds normal to elevated levels of total and free T_4 and T_3, normal or undetectable levels of TSH, either negative or low titers of thyroid antibodies, and a low or absent uptake of radioactive iodine. The erythrocyte sedimentation rate is usually markedly elevated in the classic form but may be normal to slightly elevated in the painless form.

Although variable, the clinical course of subacute thyroiditis often progresses through three phases (toxic thyroiditis, euthyroid goiter, and mild hypothyroidism) before the patient finally recovers, with completely normal thyroid function. The transient phase of hypothyroidism during recovery varies in length and severity, but full recovery is expected. After complete recovery, late recurrences are rare in the painful form of the disease but may occur in the painless variety after months or even years (25).

Symptomatic therapy may be necessary during the initial phase of the disease. Propranolol may alleviate symptoms of hyperthyroidism, and therapeutic doses of salicylates may provide some symptomatic relief if local pain and tenderness of the thyroid gland persist. Prednisone therapy is infrequently necessary to control symptoms. Should hypothyroidism develop, the patient can be treated with L-thyroxine (50–100 μg daily) for 3–6 months, after which time the medication dose should be tapered and discontinued. Permanent hypothyroidism rarely occurs (5).

C. Iodine Deficiency

Iodine deficiency remains the most common cause of thyromegaly worldwide (4) and is especially prevalent in the mountainous regions of South America and Central Asia (26). It has been virtually eradicated in the United States since the introduction of iodized salt in the 1920s. Iodine deficiency can occur, however, in patients with chronic renal diseases from excessive urinary loss of iodine or nutritional diseases

or in patients consuming iodine-deficient diets (less than 50 μg iodine daily). The optimal daily iodine requirement is estimated as between 150 and 300 μg, and a nutritional intake of iodine between 50 and 1000 μg/day is adequate (15). A diagnosis of iodine deficiency is confirmed if the urinary excretion of iodine is less than 50 μg/g of creatinine excretion (4,26).

D. Goitrogens

A variety of chemicals, drugs, and foods can interfere with thyroid gland function and inhibit thyroid hormone synthesis. Inhibition of hormone synthesis leads to a reduction in serum thyroid hormone levels, a compensatory increase in TSH secretion, and thyromegaly. Common goitrogens include the antithyroid drugs (propylthiouracil, methimazole, carbimazole, and iodine), sulfisoxazole, and lithium. Such foods as cassava, cabbage, cauliflower, brussels sprouts, turnips, and maize contain goitrogenic compounds. Although chronic ingestion of these substances alone may lead to goiter formation, patients with preexisting thyroid disease or iodine deficiency are more susceptible to the antithyroid effects of these agents (27). Therefore, complete dietary and medication histories should be included in the clinical evaluation of thyromegaly.

E. Idiopathic Goiter

This form of goiter, also referred to as simple, colloid, adolescent, or nonspecific goiter, usually occurs in adolescent females. The patient presents with an asymptomatic diffuse enlargement of the thyroid and is clinically and biochemically euthyroid. The history is negative for iodine deficiency or goitrogen ingestion. Serum thyroid antibodies are negative. Although some of these patients may have early atypical autoimmune thyroiditis, the cause remains uncertain in many. Recent reports suggest the presence of TGAb in approximately 40–70% of patients with idiopathic goiter (9–13). Whether these immunoglobulins directly stimulate thyroid follicular cell growth in the absence of other inhibitory factors is unclear. If TGAb are proven to be the only goitrogenic substance, then a large number of patients with idiopathic goiter may have a variant of autoimmune thyroiditis.

IV. CAUSES OF NODULAR THYROMEGALY (See Also Chaps. 29 and 30)

Localized enlargement of the thyroid gland may occur in a lobe or in the isthmus of the gland. Although a localized enlargement in the form of a single nodule may be seen in autoimmune thyroiditis or idiopathic goiter, a mass in the thyroid must be evaluated to determine whether it represents a benign or a malignant lesion.

There are a number of benign lesions, both thyroidal and nonthyroidal, which present as a thyroid nodule. These include cysts and papillary or follicular adenomas. Nonthyroidal masses include teratomas, branchial cleft and thyroglossal duct cysts, lymphadenopathy, hemangiomas, lymphangiomas, and neurofibromas. Hemiagenesis of the thyroid may also present as a nodular goiter (28). It should be remembered that the first clinical sign of metastatic thyroid carcinoma may be regional lymphadenopathy.

Certain historical features, symptoms, and signs in the child increase the suspicion that a lesion is malignant. The clinician should strongly suspect a malignant lesion whenever a patient presents with a solitary firm, painless nodule in an otherwise normal gland when there is prior irradiation to the head or neck or a family history of thyroid malignancy. Likewise, a rapidly enlarging solid mass in the region of the thyroid, especially in association with hoarseness and/or dysphagia, is indicative of thyroid carcinoma. Although most malignancies of the thyroid are carcinomas, other malignant tumors, such as lymphoma and sarcoma, occur rarely. With recent immigration to North America of children exposed to high levels of radiation from the Chernobyl nuclear power plant accident in 1986, clinicians must be aware of the dramatic rise in papillary carcinoma of the thyroid among this population of children, especially those who were very young or in utero after the first trimester of pregnancy at the time of the accident (29–31). The thyroid of these children should be carefully examined annually and ultrasound performed if a nodule is detected on palpation. The unusual susceptibility of the thyroid of very young children to the tumorigenic and carcinogenic effects of radiation is puzzling. It may be related to the residual growth potential of the thyroid follicular cell in very young children, in contrast to older children and adults

(32). Furthermore, the iodine deficiency that was prevalent in Belarus and Ukraine at the time of the accident increased the radiation dose effect of radioisotopes of iodine on the thyroid.

The most important studies for the patient with a thyroid nodule are those designed to determine the structure and consistency of the thyroid gland, namely, ultrasonography to distinguish between solid and cystic lesions and the radionuclide ($[^{123}$I]iodide or $[^{99m}$Tc]technetium) scan to determine whether the nodule is functioning (hot) or nonfunctioning (cold). Almost all malignant thyroid tumors appear as a solid, nonfunctioning mass, although cystic components may also be seen. However, small cystic lesions (less than 2 cm in diameter) without a solid component and functioning nodules are almost invariably benign.

Malignancy of the thyroid gland is usually not associated with abnormalities of thyroid function. Therefore, the solitary nodule in a patient with symptoms of hyperthyroidism and an elevated serum T_3 level is usually a functioning, benign adenoma. Hyperfunctioning thyroid carcinomas are exceedingly rare. Likewise, primary hypothyroidism and elevated titers of thyroid antibodies are strong evidence against the diagnosis of thyroid malignancy and are very suggestive of autoimmune thyroiditis as the cause of nodular goiter.

Further discussion of the evaluation, management, and prognosis of thyroid nodules and thyroid malignancies can be found in Chapters 29 and 30.

Table 5 Evaluation of the Patient with Thyromegaly[a]

Clinical presentation	Etiology	Thyroid function tests	Additional diagnostic tests
Diffuse, smooth symmetric enlargement	1. Family history 2. Goitrogen and drug history 3. Serum thyroid antibodies 4. Serum TRAb, TSAb, and TGAb	1. Serum T_3 (thyrotoxicosis) 2. Serum T_4 (hypothyroidism and hyperthyroisism) 3. Serum free T_4 4. Serum TSH (hypothyroidism)	1. $[^{123}$I]iodide uptake at 4–6 and 24 h 2. TRH test 3. Perchlorate discharge 4. Urinary iodide excretion 5. Serum thyroglobulin
Firm, irregular enlargemment	1. Family history 2. Serum thyroid antibodies	1. Serum TSH (hypothyroidism) 2. Serum T_4 (hypothyroidism and hyperthyroidism)	1. $[^{123}$I]iodide uptake at 2–4 h with image 2. Perchlorate discharge
Thyroid nodule	1. Radiation exposure 2. Ultrasonography of neck 3. Thyroid image with $[^{123}$I]iodide or technetium 99m 4. Serum thyroid antibodies 5. Thyroid excisional biopsy	1. Serum T_3 (thyrotoxicosis) 2. Serum T_4 (hypothyroidism and hyperthyroidism) 3. Serum TSH (hypothyroidism)	1. T_3 suppression test to evaluate autonomous hypersecretion 2. Serum thyroglobulin 3. Serum calcitonin response to pentagastrin and calcium infusions

[a]Serum TSH is the most sensitive diagnostic test for primary hypothyroidism.
Free thyroxine tests are necessary to exclude abnormalities of the thyroxine binding proteins and drugs.

V. SUMMARY: EVALUATION OF PATIENTS WITH THYROMEGALY (Table 5)

Evaluation of the patient with thyromegaly depends upon the initial history and results of an examination of the thyroid gland (15). The child with a symmetric, diffusely enlarged, smooth thyroid gland should be investigated for hyperthyroidism and primary hypothyroidism. The determination of serum thyroid antibodies is important to identify autoimmune thyroid disease. The most sensitive test for hyperthyroidism is the serum TT_3 determination; however, this test is not necessary if the patient has obvious exophthalmic goiter with hyperthyroidism. Only in the presence of mild, equivocal thyrotoxicosis of undetermined cause are additional tests indicated. For the patient with a firm, irregular thyroid gland, the evaluation should be directed toward the diagnosis of autoimmune thyroiditis by determining serum thyroid antibodies and thyroid function (serum TSH and free T_4).

Most children with autoimmune thyroiditis are clinically and biochemically euthyroid. Although they infrequently may present with toxic thyroiditis, the most common abnormality of thyroid function in autoimmune thyroiditis is hypothyroidism, which may develop anytime during the course of the disease and can best be detected by the annual measurement of serum TSH. When a serum TSH value is slightly elevated, a second specimen should be tested and, if elevated again, the patient started on L-thyroxine therapy. Mild primary hypothyroidism in patients with autoimmune thyroiditis may be transient or permanent, particularly if the disease presents with toxic thyroiditis.

REFERENCES

1. Rallison M, Dobyns B, Keating F, Rall J, Tyler F. Occurrence and natural history of chronic lymphocytic thyroiditis in children. J Pediatr 1975; 86:675.
2. Inoue M, Taketani N, Sato T, Nakajima H. High incidences of chronic lymphocytic thyroiditis in apparently healthy school children: epidemiological and clinical study. Endocrinol Jpn 1975; 22:483–488.
3. Trowbridge FL, Matovinovic J, McLaren GD, Nichaman MZ. Iodine and goiter in children. Pediatrics 1975; 56:82.
4. Stanbury JB, Hetzel BS, eds. Endemic Goiter and Endemic Cretinism. Iodine Nutrition in Health and Disease. New York: John Wiley and Sons, 1980:164.
5. Foley TP Jr. Goiters in adolescents. Endocrinol Metab Clin North Am 1993, 22(3):593–606.
6. Foley TP Jr, White C, New A. Juvenile Graves disease: usefulness and limitations of thyrotropin receptor antibody determinations. J Pediatr 1987; 110:378–386.
7. DeGroot LJ, Quintans J. The causes of autoimmune thyroid disease. Endocr Rev 1989; 10:537–562.
8. Smith BR, McLachlan SM, Furmaniak J. Autoantibodies to the thyrotropin receptor. Endocr Rev 1988; 9:106–121.
9. Fisher DA, Pandian MR, Carlton E. Autoimmune thyroid disease: an expanding spectrum. Pediatr Clin North Am 1987; 34(4):907.
10. Valente WA, Vitti P, Rotella CM, et al. Antibodies that promote thyroid growth: a distinct population of thyroid stimulating autoantibodies. N Engl J Med 1983; 309:1028.
11. Van der Gaag RD, Drexhage HA, Wiersinga WM, Brown RS. Further studies on thyroid growth-stimulating immunoglobulins in euthyroid nonendemic goiter. J Clin Endocrinol Metab 1985; 60:972.
12. Dumont JE, Roger PP, Ludgate M. Assays for thyroid growth immunoglobulins and their clinical implications: methods, concepts, and misconceptions. Endocr Rev 1987; 8:448–452.
13. Maurer HR. Potential pitfalls of [^{3}H]thymidine techniques to measure cell proliferation. Cell Tissue Kinet 1981; 14:111.
14. Parma J, Duprez L, Van Sande J, et al. Somatic mutations in the thyrotropin receptor gene cause hyperfunctioning thyroid adenomas. Nature 1993; 365:649–651.
15. Foley TP Jr. Acute, subacute and chronic thyroiditis. In: Kapan SA, ed. Clinical Pediatric and Adolescent Endocrinology. W. B. Saunders Company, Philadelphia: 1982:96–109.
16. Weetman AP. Thyroid autoimmune disease. In: Braverman LE, Utiger RD, eds. Werner and Ingbar's the Thyroid, 6th ed. Philadelphia: J. B. Lippincott. 1991; 1295–1310.
17. Bogner U, Wall JR, Schleusener H. Cellular and antibody mediated cytotoxicity in autoimmune thyroid disease. Acta Endcrinol (Copenh) Suppl 1987; 281:133.
18. Drash AL, Becker DJ, Villalpando S, et al. The incidence of clinical subclinical thyroid and adrenal disease and their association with antibodies to endocrine tissues in children with juvenile diabetes mellitus. J Pediatr 1975; 93:310.
19. Neufeld M, Maclaren NK, Riley WJ, et al. Islet cell and other organ-specific antibodies in U.S. caucasians and blacks with insulin-dependent diabetes mellitus. Diabetes 1980; 29:589.
20. Neufeld M, Maclaren N, Blizzard R. Autoimmune polyglandular syndromes. Pediatr Ann 1980; 9:154.
21. Hopwood NJ, Rabin BS, Foley TP Jr. Peake RL. Thyroid antibodies in children and adolescents with thyroid disorders. J Pediatr 1978; 93:57.
22. Abe K, Taguchi T, Okuno A, et al. Acute suppurative thyroiditis in children. J Pediatr 1979; 94:912.
23. Abe K, Fujita H, Matsuura N, et al. A fistula from pyriform sinus in recurrent acute suppurative thyroiditis. Am J Dis Child 1981; 135:178.
24. Miller D, Hill JL, Sun CC, et al. The diagnosis and management of pyriform sinus fistulae in infants and young children. J Pediatr Surg 1983; 18:377.
25. Nikolai TF. Silent thyroiditis and subacute thyroiditis. In: Braverman LE, Utiger RD, eds. Werner and Ingbar's the Thyroid, 6th ed. Philadelphia: J. B. Lippincott. 1991:710–727.
26. Delange F, Ermans AM. Iodine deficiency. In: Braverman LE, Utiger RD, eds. Werner and Ingbar's the Thyroid, 6th ed. Philadelphia: J. B. Lippincott. 1991:368–390.
27. Green WL. Extrinsic and intrinsic variables: antithyroid compounds. In: Braverman LE, Utiger RD, eds. Werner and Ingbar's, the Thyroid, 6th ed. Philadelphia: J. B. Lippincott. 1991:322–335.
28. Hopwood NJ, Carroll RG, Kenny FM, Foley TP. Functioning thyroid nodules in childhood and adolescence. J Pediatr 1976; 89:710–718.
29. Kazakov VS, Demidchik EP, Astakhova LN. Thyroid cancer after Chernobyl. Nature 1992; 359:21.
30. Baverstock K, Egloff B, Pinchera A, Ruchti C, Williams D. Thyroid cancer after Chernobyl. Nature 1992; 359:21–22.
31. Williams ED. Biologic effects of radiation on the thyroid. In: Braverman LE, Utiger RD, eds. Werner and Ingbar's, the Thyroid, 6th ed. Philadelphia: J. B. Lippincott, 1991:421–436.
32. Williams ED. Radiation-induced thyroid cancer (commentary). Histopathology 1993; 23:387–389.

27

Hypothyroidism

John S. Dallas
University of Texas Medical Branch and Children's Hospital of Galveston, Galveston, Texas

Thomas P. Foley, Jr.
University of Pittsburgh and Children's Hospital of Pittsburgh, Pittsburgh, Pennsylvania

I. HISTORICAL REVIEW

Endemic goiter and cretinism have been recognized for over 2000 years, as evidenced by Andean sculptures of goitrous dwarfs dating from the fourth century BCE (1) and by descriptions recorded in Europe during the first century BCE (2,3). Medical reports of nonendemic cretinism, however, did not appear until 1850, when Curling described two children who had no detectable thyroid tissue at autopsy (4). In 1871, Fagge used the term "sporadic cretinism" to describe four children with cretinism, one being a 16-year-old female with classic symptoms and signs of hypothyroidism, absence of thyromegaly, and "mental faculties unimpaired" (5). In 1878, W. M. Ord associated the term "myxedema" with his descriptions of the supraclavicular "fatty tumors" found in hypothyroid middle-aged women (6). The Committee of the Clinical Society of London was nominated in 1883 to study hypothyroidism and presented its report in 1888 describing lymphocytic infiltration and atrophy of the thyroid gland (Fig. 1) (7). This first description of chronic lymphocytic thyroiditis preceded Hashimoto's classic discussions of asymptomatic goiter (8) by 24 years.

During the last decade of the nineteenth century were several reports of successful treatment of hypothyroidism so elegantly described by Sir William Osler (9):

> That we can to-day rescue children otherwise doomed to helpless idiocy—that we can restore to life the hopeless victims of myxoedema—is a triumph of experimental medicine for which we are indebted very largely to Victor Horsley and to his pupil Murray. Transplantation of the gland was first tried; then Murray used an extract subcutaneously. Hector Mackenzie in London and Howitz in Copenhagen introduced the method

of feeding. We now know that the gland, taken either fresh, or as the watery or glycerin extract, or dried and powdered, is equally efficacious in a majority of all the cases of myxoedema in infants or adults. . . . The results, as a rule, are most astounding—Unparalleled by anything in the whole range of curative measures. Within six weeks a poor, feeble-minded, toad-like caricature of humanity may be restored to mental and bodily health.

Photographs depicting hypothyroid children before and after the initiation of thyroid extract therapy began to appear in textbooks soon thereafter (Fig. 2) (10).

During the twentieth century, our understanding of the biochemical and physiologic functions of the thyroid gland has expanded considerably. The pathogenesis of autoimmunity, the most common cause of hypothyroidism in North America, has been elucidated with the pioneering serologic studies of Roitt et al. (11) and the experimental studies of Rose and Witebsky (12). More recently, competitive binding assays, thyroid epithelial cell culture systems, and advances in molecular biology have provided improved methods to study thyroid hormone secretion and action and expanded our knowledge into the etiology and pathogenesis of autoimmunity and other causes of hypothyroidism.

II. CLASSIFICATION AND ETIOLOGY

A. Classification

Normal thyroid hormone secretion depends on an intact hypothalamic-pituitary-thyroid axis. In normals, thyrotropin-releasing hormone (TRH) modulates the release of thyrotropin

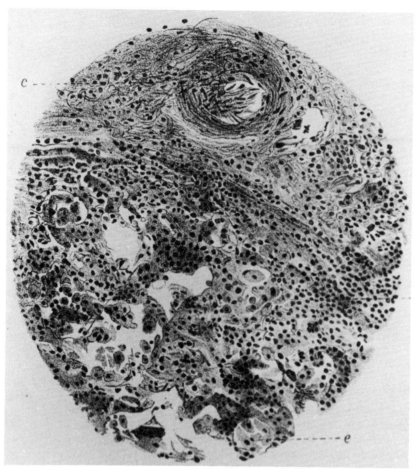

Figure 1   Lymphocytic infiltration of the thyroid gland of an adult with myxedema reported in 1888, or 4 years before the description by Hashimoto (7,8).

(TSH) from the pituitary gland. TSH then binds to TSH receptors on the thyroid gland and stimulates the production and the release of predominately L-thyroxine (T$_4$) and, in smaller molar concentrations, 3,3′,5-L-triiodothyronine (T$_3$). An abnormality at any point within this axis may result in decreased thyroid hormone secretion and cause hypothyroidism. By convention, hypothyroidism is classified according to the anatomic location within this axis where the abnormality occurs (13). For example, hypothyroidism resulting from thyroid gland failure, such as occurs with autoimmune destruction in Hashimoto's thyroiditis, is referred to as primary hypothyroidism. Likewise, secondary and tertiary hypothyroidism refer to hypothyroidism resulting from disorders at the level of the pituitary and the hypothalamus, respectively. These diseases are generally referred to as pituitary and hypothalamic hypothyroidism.

Selective peripheral resistance to thyroid hormone is a very rare cause of hypothyroidism (14). In this syndrome, the hypothalamic-pituitary-thyroid axis is normal but peripheral tissues do not adequately respond to T$_3$ and patients have symptoms and signs of hypothyroidism from an early age.

Basal serum TSH, thyroid hormone levels, and TSH responses to TRH are normal. An explanation of why only the peripheral tissue is resistant, not the pituitary, is not known.

B.   Etiology

Hypothyroidism during childhood and adolescence can result from a variety of congenital or acquired defects (Table 1). In North America, the majority of children with congenital primary hypothyroidism are detected through neonatal thyroid screening programs, but in some patients with ectopic or hypoplastic thyroid glands or with inborn errors of thyroid hormone synthesis (Fig. 3), hypothyroidism may not be recognized until later in infancy or childhood. In general, ectopic and hypoplastic glands occur sporadically, whereas the inborn errors of hormone synthesis (thyroid dyshormonogenesis) are inherited as autosomal recessive disorders (15). Recently, specific gene defects were reported to explain the abnormal or absent proteins involved in the specific steps of hormonogenesis (16).

Autoimmune chronic lymphocytic thyroiditis is the most

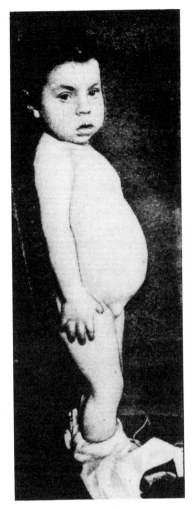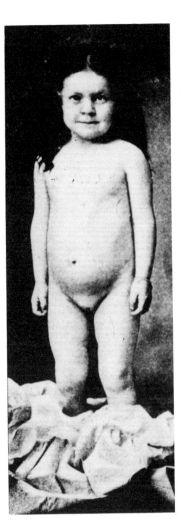

Figure 2 An early example of the effects of thyroid hormone therapy in a 7-year-old girl with the onset of hypothyroidism around age 3 years.

common cause of acquired primary hypothyroidism in North America. The disease usually occurs during childhood or adolescence and more often in girls than boys. However, it may present during infancy with symptoms and signs of hypothyroidism that are subtle, of short duration, and beginning as early as 6–9 months of age (17). The disease also occurs with increased frequency in other autoimmune-mediated diseases, especially insulin-dependent diabetes mellitus, the polyglandular autoimmune syndrome, and Down, Turner, and Klinefelter syndromes. Other causes include irradiation of thyroid tissue, surgical removal of thyroid tissue, goitrogen ingestion, and iodine deficiency (Table 2). Transient primary hypothyroidism may occur during the recovery phase of subacute and toxic thyroiditis.

Secondary and tertiary hypothyroidism result from deficiencies in TSH and TRH, respectively. Most children with secondary or tertiary (also known as central) hypothyroidism have other pituitary or hypothalamic homone deficiencies, but an isolated deficiency of either TSH or TRH can occur as an idiopathic familial or sporadic disease (18) and gene defects have been reported in a few families (19). Malformation syndromes, such as septooptic dysplasia, or midline facial anomalies, such as cleft lip or palate, can be associated with central hypothyroidism. Trauma, neoplasms, infectious or inflammatory processes, irradiation, and surgery can damage the hypothalamus or pituitary and cause TRH, TSH, and other hormone deficiencies. These diseases are discussed in further detail elsewhere.

III. PATHOPHYSIOLOGY

In primary hypothyroidism, abnormalities of the thyroid gland, or of thyroid gland function, impair thyroid hormone production and/or release. Early in the course of thyroid gland failure, a slight decrease in the serum T4 level occurs, but the

Table 1 Causes of Juvenile Primary Hypothyroidism

Congenital hypothyroidism: mild, late onset
  Ectopic thyroid dysgenesis
  Familial thyroid dyshormonogenesis
  Peripheral resistance to thyroid hormone action
Acquired primary hypothyroidism
  Chronic autoimmune thyroiditis
    Lymphocytic thyroiditis of childhood and adolescence
      with thyromegaly
    Hashimoto's thyroiditis with thyromegaly (struma
      lymphomatosa)
    Chronic fibrous variant
  Drug-induced hypothyroidism
  Endemic goiter
    Iodine deficiency
    Environmental goitrogens
  Irradiation of the thyroid
    Therapeutic radioiodine
    External irradiation of nonthyroid tumors
  Surgical excision
  Subacute thyroiditis: Transient phase

level usually remains within the normal range for age. The fall in serum T_4 leads to minor reductions in pituitary free T_4 concentrations and a subsequent decrease in the intrapituitary conversion of T_4 to T_3 (20). With the fall in pituitary T_3 concentration, there is stimulation of TSH production and release to cause increased serum TSH levels. This increased TSH secretion stimulates the thyroid gland to increase thyroid hormone synthesis and release. As thyroid gland failure progresses, however, increased TSH secretion is no longer able to stimulate hormone synthesis and serum thyroid hormones decrease to abnormal levels. Because serum TSH levels rise before serum thyroid hormone levels decrease to abnormal levels, the measurement of serum TSH is the most sensitive test for primary hypothyroidism.

Pituitary TSH synthesis and secretion are directly controlled by serum levels of free or unbound T_4 (FT_4) and T_3. This control occurs by negative feedback; that is, rising serum levels of FT_4 and T_3 inhibit, whereas decreasing FT_4 and T_3 levels enhance TSH synthesis and secretion. Through TRH and somatostatin secretion, the hypothalamus modulates this negative feedback system and determines the "set point" for TSH secretion (21). TRH secretion enhances TSH release, and somatostatin inhibits TSH release. Thus, patients with TRH deficiency have a decreased release of TSH, causing a decrease in thyroid hormone production. However, TRH deficiency is associated with increased pituitary stores of TSH with exaggerated, although usually delayed, TSH responses to TRH in experimental animals and patients (22).

IV. CLINICAL PRESENTATION

Children with hypothyroidism may have a variety of clinical presentations (Table 2) as well as a family history of thyroid or pituitary disease that may provide important diagnostic information. Some children present with an asymptomatic goiter, whereas others may present with mild tenderness or a sensation of fullness in the anterior neck. Other presenting symptoms are often nonspecific and include weakness, lethargy, decreased appetite, cold intolerance, constipation, and dry skin. Although children with hypothyroidism may have mild obesity, hypothyroidism generally does not cause morbid obesity. The course of hypothyroidism is often so insidious that neither the child nor the parents are aware of the physical changes that have occurred, and these children may experience marked growth retardation before the disease is recognized. This emphasizes the importance of serial growth measurements in all children. Whereas children with hypothyroidism before age 3 years may suffer irreversible central nervous system damage and developmental delay, onset of hypothyroidism after age 3 years does not cause mental retardation.

Infants with acquired autoimmune-mediated infantile hypothyroidism present with symptoms and signs similar to those in infants with congenital hypothyroidism (17). Deceleration of linear growth is an additional sign that may be helpful to recognize this disease.

Most adolescents with untreated primary hypothyroidism have delayed pubertal development, although an occasional patient presents with precocious puberty. Girls may also have galactorrhea, usually with an elevated serum prolactin level, and boys may have macroorchidism. This syndrome was originally postulated to occur as a result of increased luteinizing hormone (LH) and follicle-stimulating hormone (FSH) secretion through an "overlap" in the pituitary regulation of TSH secretion (23). Recent studies suggest that hyperprolactinemia, which presumably results from chronic TRH stimulation of the pituitary, plays a major role in this syndrome through an inhibition of gonadal stimulation by LH, but not FSH, thereby resulting in sustained stimulation of the gonad by FSH (24). More recently, Kohn's group reported that COS-7 cells transfected with the hCG receptor cDNA show increased cAMP and inositol phosphate levels with TSH stimulation at 10^{-11} and 10^{-9} M concentrations, respectively (25). Based on these results, they suggest that elevated TSH levels are the responsible factor in the precocious puberty of juvenile hypothyroidism (25). The adolescent female who acquires hypothyroidism after menarche often experiences excessive and irregular menstrual bleeding.

Children with severe primary hypothyroidism may present to a neurosurgeon or an endocrinologist for evaluation of sella turcica enlargement or a pituitary tumor as identified by skull x-rays, a computed tomographic scan, or magnetic resonance image (MRI) of the head. This pituitary mass may represent hypertrophy and hyperplasia of thyrotrophs in response to a lack of negative feedback by thyroid hormones (26). Therefore, these patients usually have very elevated serum TSH levels with low serum levels of thyroid hormones, in contrast to patients with hypothalamic and pituitary hypothyroidism, who usually have normal but may have mildly elevated serum TSH levels (27) with low serum levels of FT_4. Pituitary enlargement usually resolves with adequate thyroid

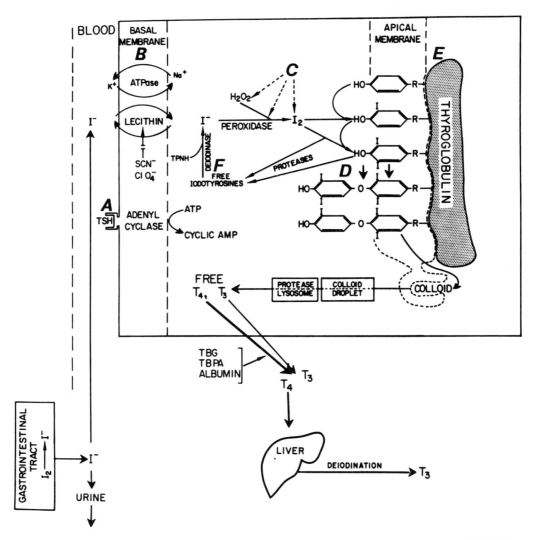

Figure 3 Thyroid hormone synthesis and the sites of the most frequent abnormalities seen in patients with familial dyshormonogenesis (15,16). (A) Impaired thyroid response to TSH; (B) iodide transport defect; (C) iodide oxidation and tyrosyl iodination defects, including Pendred syndrome; (D) iodotyrosine coupling defect; (E) thyroglobulin synthetic defects; (F) iodotyrosine deiodinase defect. Each defect is associated with thyromegaly except A. An increase in [123I]iodide uptake occurs in each defect except A and B. A rapid discharge of [123I]iodide from the thyroid after oral perchlorate occurs in the iodide oxidation and tyrosyl iodination defects.

Table 2 Clinical Features of Juvenile Hypothyroidism

Growth retardation with delayed skeletal maturation
Delayed dental development and tooth eruption
Onset of puberty usually delayed; rarely precocious
Galactorrhea: elevated prolactin
Increased skin pigmentation
Sellar enlargement
Pseudotumor cerebri
Myopathy and muscular hypertrophy

hormone replacement. Recently, primary hypothyroidism with enlargement of the sella and pituitary gland was reported in a boy in whom an empty sella and hypopituitarism developed after thyroid hormone replacement (28). Visual field defects may be detected in these patients (29).

Children with hypothalamic and pituitary hypothyroidism can present with the same nonspecific symptoms found in primary hypothyroidism, as well as with symptoms suggestive of other hormone deficiencies. Patients with organic defects may also present with symptoms of increased intracranial pressure, such as headaches, morning vomiting, and decreased visual acuity.

Features of hypothyroidism on physical examination include bradycardia, decreased pulse pressure, short stature with an increased upper-lower body ratio, delayed dentition, mild obesity, facial puffiness and dull facial expression, coarse hair, cool, dry, carotenemic skin, and delayed relaxation of deep tendon reflexes. The majority of patients with primary hypothyroidism have thyromegaly, but some patients with autoimmune thyroiditis and ectopic or hypoplastic glands do not have detectable thyroid enlargement. Thyromegaly is not associated with hypothalamic or pituitary hypothyroidism. These children may have an abnormal optic fundus examination (i.e., papilledema), and visual field defects may be found.

V. DIAGNOSTIC EVALUATION

Patients with nongoitrous, acquired primary hypothyroidism require very few diagnostic tests before therapy. Serum determinations of TSH, total T_4 (TT_4), FT_4, and thyroid antibodies should be obtained. If positive, the presence of thyroid antibodies permits a presumptive diagnosis of auto-immune thyroiditis. Some patients with autoimmune thyroiditis have negative thyroid antibodies on initial evaluation but, on repeat determinations 3–6 months later, have elevated thyroid antibody titers (30). Similar thyroid function tests should be performed in patients with goitrous hypothyroidism because the most common cause is autoimmune thyroiditis. If thyroid antibodies are negative on repeated determinations in a child with persistent thyromegaly, however, the following additional tests may be useful to determine the etiology of hypothyroidism:

1. Radioiodide uptake tests with perchlorate discharge at 2–4 h after dose, salivary-plasma ratio of radioiodide 2 h after the dose, and serum thyroglobulin (to identify inborn errors of thyroid hormone synthesis)
2. Urinary iodine excretion (to identify iodine deficiency)
3. Thyroid biopsy, if progressive asymptomatic enlargement of the thyroid occurs despite treatment with full replacement or suppressive doses of L-thyroxine (to identify rare malignant infiltrative diseases

In addition to serum thyroid function tests, a TRH test should be performed in patients with suspected hypothalamic or pituitary hypothyroidism. In children with hypothalamic hypothyroidism, the peak serum TSH response to TRH is often delayed beyond 30 minutes, and the TSH response may be prolonged with serum TSH values that remain elevated for 2–3 h. The TSH response to TRH is low or absent in patients with pituitary thyrotroph deficiency (23,31).

The euthyroid sick or nonthyroidal illness syndrome refers to the various alterations in thyroid function that often accompany such conditions as acute or chronic illnesses, surgery, trauma, malnutrition, and starvation. The magnitude of change in thyroid function tends to correlate directly with the severity of systemic illness or tissue injury. Although there are exceptions, the typical pattern of serum thyroid function

tests that allows the diagnosis of this syndrome includes low T_3, low to normal T_4, increased T_3 resin uptake, normal to high $3,3',5'$-L-triiodothyronine or reverse T_3 (rT_3), and normal TSH (32). The serum FT_4 is usually normal, but regardless of the assay method used, low serum FT_4 values have been reported, especially in the most severely ill patients (33). The direct dialysis method to measure FT_4 in serum is the most accurate determination and rarely is associated with false positive or false negative results (34).

Various factors contribute to the changes in thyroid hormone economy that occur in this syndrome. In the normal state, peripheral tissue conversion of T_4 to T_3 is the major source of circulating T_3, and conversion occurs through monodeiodination via the $5'$-deiodinase pathway. This pathway also converts rT_3 to T_2. In the euthyroid sick syndrome, $5'$-deiodinase activity is decreased in the peripheral tissues, and this leads to decreased production of T_3 and decreased clearance of rT_3. Therefore, decreased $5'$-deiodinase activity accounts for the low serum T_3 and elevated serum rT_3 levels in these patients. The increased T_3 resin uptake indicates a reduction in available serum thyroid hormone binding sites. The concentrations of thyroxine binding globulin (TBG) and transthyretin (TTR), also known as thyroxine binding pre-albumin, and the binding capacity of TBG are decreased in these patients, and these changes are largely responsible for the reduction in available binding sites. A nondialyzable substance that inhibits thyroid hormone binding to TBG and TTR may appear in the serum during severe illness (35). Decreased T_4 binding to serum proteins leads to an increased percentage of FT_4 in serum and accounts for normal FT_4 levels even when TT_4 levels are low. The factors responsible for low TT_4 levels are less well understood. Although decreased serum binding of T_4 may contribute, accelerated disposal of T_4 and decreased TSH secretion are probably the major factors leading to low TT_4 levels. Accelerated disposal of T_4 occurs through the 5-deiodinase pathway, which converts T_4 to rT_3 and through nondeiodinative pathways (32). The mechanisms responsible for the decreased TSH secretion are unknown but may reflect abnormal hypothalamic-pituitary function during severe illness (36).

Thyroid function tests are often obtained in severely ill infants and children for evaluation of such clinical findings as hypothermia, weakness, lethargy, and growth failure. Not only can the underlying illness or injury produce alterations in thyroid function, but the severely ill child is often receiving medications, such as dopamine, glucocorticoids, and phenytoin, that can also alter thyroid hormone economy (32). Whereas the ill child with low serum T_3 but normal serum TT_4 and FT_4 levels usually does not pose a diagnostic problem, the question of hypothyroidism frequently arises in the ill child with low serum levels of T_3 and TT_4. In this situation, a normal serum FT_4 is used as evidence against central hypothyroidism, especially when measured by direct dialysis methods (34). In the child with a low serum TT_4, an elevated rT_3 and normal TSH often serve to suggest the diagnosis of the euthyroid sick syndrome and distinguish it from hypothyroidism. An elevated serum TSH level in a severely ill patient usually indicates primary hypothyroidism

(32,33). Modest elevations in TSH may occur during recovery from illness (32), however, and serial TSH measurements may be required to establish the correct diagnosis (33,36).

Children with hypothalamic or pituitary hypothyroidism generally have normal TSH levels in the presence of low serum thyroid hormone levels, including rT3. These children may develop severe systemic illness, and it may be difficult to differentiate them from severely ill patients with the euthyroid sick syndrome. The history and physical examination may help to distinguish between the two disorders, but a more extensive evaluation, including a MRI study of the hypothalamic-pituitary region and pituitary function testing, may be necessary. The TSH response to TRH in the euthyroid sick syndrome can be normal, delayed, or blunted and may not be useful in differentiating the euthyroid sick syndrome from hypothalamic or pituitary hypothyroidism (32,33). Determination of rT3 is not always helpful because the level may be normal in sick hypothyroid children (32,33).

Thyroid hormone replacement is not recommended in the treatment of the euthyroid sick syndrome unless the FT4, preferably by direct dialysis, is low. Management should be directed toward supportive or specific treatment of the underlying illness. To date, studies that have evaluated the effects of T4 or T3 replacement in patients with this syndrome have not demonstrated increased survival with replacement therapy (37). However, controversy still exists about whether the euthyroid sick syndrome represents an adaptive and beneficial response to severe illness or a functional type of secondary hypothyroidism produced by severe illness (32–37).

VI. CLINICAL COURSE AND MANAGEMENT

A. Primary Hypothyroidism

L-thyroxine is the most effective thyroid preparation for the treatment of hypothyroidism in children and adolescents (38). Other thyroid preparations, such as thyroid extract, desiccated thyroid, and T4-T3 combination drugs, offer no advantage over L-thyroxine and may have some disadvantages when therapy is monitored by thyroid function tests. Generic preparations of L-thyroxine should be prescribed cautiously because some may have variable potencies and therefore may provide inconsistent replacement therapy (39). This emphasizes the importance of prescribing reliable L-thyroxine preparations for the treatment of hypothyroidism. L-thyroxine is prescribed orally as a single daily dose and should be taken at least 1/2 h before food intake to maximize absorption. The estimated dosage for children and adolescents is based on age and body weight (Table 3).

To minimize central nervous system damage, children under 3 years of age require prompt treatment with L-thyroxine in full replacement doses. Rapid achievement of euthyroidism is not as essential in the older child and adolescent; in fact, children with chronic or severe hypothyroidism often experience undesirable side effects, such as irritability, restlessness, decreased attention span, and restless sleep or insomnia, when L-thyroxine is prescribed in full replacement doses at diagnosis. For these children it is preferable to restore

euthyroidism gradually by initiating treatment with 25 μg for 2 weeks and then increasing the dose by 25 μg every 2–4 weeks until the desired dose is achieved. This regimen is not necessary for children with mild hypothyroidism or clinical symptoms of short duration. It is important to avoid excessive therapy, however, and prudent to select the lower dose per kilogram body weight for age on initiation of therapy.

In patients with compensated hypothyroidism, defined as an elevated serum TSH level but normal concentrations of TT4 and FT4, it is worthwhile to confirm that the process is persistent by repeating the serum TSH before initiating long-term therapy. This is especially important in patients with negative thyroid antibodies and no apparent etiology for the elevated TSH value. Some children have persistent hyperthyrotropinemia of unknown etiology without symptoms or signs of hypothyroidism. This observation may occur in children with Down syndrome, and the measurement of thyroid antibodies is important to differentiate it from autoimmune thyroiditis, which also occurs with greater frequency in Down syndrome than in the general population. Thyroxine therapy is indicated in compensated hypothyroidism (40) when there a known cause for hypothyroidism is identified in the evaluation or when serial TSH measurements steadily increase, especially with declining FT4 concentrations.

Serum thyroid function tests should be monitored annually to determine adequacy of therapy, anytime symptoms of hypothyroidism or hyperthyroidism occur, and 2–3 months after the dosage is changed. Serum TSH is the most useful test to monitor primary hypothyroidism, and levels should be maintained between 0.1 and 5.5 mU/L using sensitive TSH methods that can accurately distinguish normal and suppressed levels with a sensitivity of 0.05 mU/L or lower. Serum total and free T4 levels are usually adequate to determine whether the patient is receiving excessive L-thyroxine therapy; for some children, however, particularly those with congenital hypothyroidism, serum T3 and, rarely, rT3 levels may help to determine if the L-thyroxine dose is excessive.

Table 3 Guidelines for Sodium L-Thyroxine Therapy[a]

Age	Daily Dose (μg/kg)	Daily dose range (μg/day)	Weight range (kg)
<6 months	6–10	25 – 50	3– 9
6–12 months	5– 8	37.5– 75	6– 12
1–5 years	4– 6	50 –100	9– 23
5–12 years	3– 5	50 –125	15– 55
12–18 years	2– 3	75 –175	30– 90
Adult	1– 2	100 –200	50–100

[a]The dose of L-thyroxine must be determined for each patient because the rates of absorption and metabolism vary among patients of the same body weight. These doses approximate 100 μ/m²/day. In general, patients with hypothalamic hypothyroidism seem to require a lower dose per kg than patients with primary hypothyroidism. L-thyroxine is usually manufactured in 25, 50, 75, 100, 125, 150, and 200 μg tablets. Tablets should be given at least 0.5–1 h before a meal.

The child with primary nongoitrous hypothyroidism who has had serum TSH levels greater than 20 mU/L on two separate occasions generally does not recover normal thyroid function spontaneously. Therefore, this child should be treated with L-thyroxine indefinitely. On the other hand, there are reports indicating that approximately 20% of patients with autoimmune goitrous hypothyroidism may revert to the euthyroid state (41,42). These children may be given a 2–3 month trial off L-thyroxine treatment if the thyroid size and consistency become normal during treatment. The serum TSH should be determined at the end of this trial, or sooner if symptoms of hypothyroidism develop. If the serum TSH level is normal, the child should be monitored every 3 months for a year and then annually thereafter if thyroid antibody titers remain abnormal. If the TSH level becomes abnormal, L-thyroxine therapy should be resumed indefinitely. It is also important to monitor serum TSH in children receiving lithium carbonate or similar drugs that block thyroid function (43). If these children also have autoimmune thyroiditis, they very likely will develop primary hypothyroidism during lithium treatment (44).

Prepubertal children with severe hypothyroidism and short stature usually experience a period of catch-up growth after initiation of L-thyroxine replacement therapy, but despite adequate treatment, some have incomplete catch-up and never reach their full genetic growth potential (45). The mechanisms responsible for this incomplete catch-up growth have not been clearly defined, but delay in treatment of hypothyroidism may be a critical factor (45).

B. Disorders of Thyrotropin Secretion

Hypothyroidism, either hypothalamic or pituitary, may be present at the time of initial diagnosis of hypopituitarism or may develop at any time during replacement growth hormone therapy. To avoid any confusion in the differential diagnosis between hypothalamic or pituitary hypothyroidism and the euthyroid sick or nonthyroidal illness syndrome that occurs during severe illness, serum FT_4 and, if possible, rT_3 levels should be determined. The FT_4 and rT_3 levels are low in hypothyroidism, whereas the FT_4 is usually normal (33) and the rT_3 is normal or elevated (32) in the euthyroid sick syndrome. These measurements may be extremely helpful in patients with central nervous system tumors who are in a catabolic state following surgery. In general, patients with the euthyroid sick syndrome do not require L-thyroxine replacement, whereas patients with hypothyroidism do. As mentioned earlier, the TRH tests can often differentiate between hypothalamic and pituitary hypothyroidism (31).

Children with hypothalamic or pituitary hypothyroidism often require less L-thyroxine than children with congenital or acquired primary hypothyroidism. Serum levels of TT_4, FT_4, and T_3 should be monitored during L-thyroxine therapy. It is unnecessary to monitor TSH levels during treatment of patients with hypothalamic or pituitary hypothyroidism. Once the dose has been established and the patient is clinically and biochemically euthyroid, further serum thyroid function tests need only be obtained annually to assure compliance and reliability of the medication.

Although children with hypothalamic or pituitary hypothyroidism and short stature may exhibit a period of catch-up growth after initiation of L-thyroxine therapy, the course is often complicated by deficiencies of growth hormone, gonadotropins, and sex hormones, and many fail to reach their full genetic height potential. Because L-thyroxine therapy increases the metabolic clearance rate of cortisol, patients with deficient hypothalamic-pituitary-adrenal function should begin cortisol replacement with initiation of L-thyroxine replacement to avoid precipitation of an adrenal crisis.

REFERENCES

1. Gaitan E. Iodine deficiency and toxicity. In: White PL, Selvey N, eds. Proceedings of the Western Hemisphere Nutrition Congress, IV. Acton, MA: Publishing Sciences Group, 1975: 56–63.
2. Cranefield PF. The discovery of cretinism. Bull Hist Med 1962; 36:489–511.
3. Thompson J. Historical notes. In: Smithers D, ed. Tumours of the Thyroid, Vol. 6, Neoplastic Diseases at Various Sites. Edinburgh: Livingstone, 1970.
4. Curling TB. Two cases of absence of the thyroid body. Med Chir Trans 1850; 33:303–306.
5. Fagge CH. On sporadic cretinism, occurring in England. Med Chir Soc Lond 1871; 54:155–169.
6. Ord WM. On myxoedema, a term proposed to be applied to an essential condition in the "cretinoid" affection occasionally observed in middle-aged women. Med Chir Trans 1878; 61:57.
7. Report of a Committee of the Clinical Society of London, nominated December 14, 1883 to investigate the subject of myxedema. Trans Clin Soc Lond (Suppl) 18888; 21:1–202.
8. Hashimoto H. Zur Kenntniss der lymphomatösen Veränderung der Schilddrüse (struma lymphomatosa). Arch Klin Chir 1912; 97:219.
9. Osler W. The Principals and Practice of Medicine, 3rd ed. D. Appleton and Co., 1898:843.
10. Sajour CED. The Internal Secretions and the Principals of Medicine, 8th ed. London: F. A. Davis, 1919:198–201.
11. Roitt IM, Doniach D, Campbell RN, Hudson RV. Autoantibodies in Hashimoto's disease. Lancet 1956; 2:820.
12. Rose NR, Witebsky E. Studies on organ-specificity. V. Changes in the thyroid glands of rabbits following active immunization with rabbit thyroid extract. J Immunol 1956; 76:417.
13. Braverman LE, Utiger RD. Introduction to hypothyroidism. In: Braverman LE, Utiger RD, eds. Werner and Ingbar's the Thyroid, 6th ed. Philadelphia: J. B. Lippincott. 1991:919–920.
14. Kaplan MM, Swartz SL, Larsen PR. Partial peripheral resistance to thyroid hormone. Am J Med 1981; 70:1115–1121.
15. Dumont JE, Vassart G, Refetoff S. Thyroid disorders. In: Scriver CR, Beaudet AL, Sly WS, et al., eds. The Metabolic Basis of Inherited Disease, 6th ed. New York: McGraw-Hill. 1989:1843.
16. Medeiros-Neto GA, Billerbeck AEC, Wajchenberg BL, Targovnik HM. Defective organification of iodide causing hereditary goitrous hypothyroidism. Thyroid 1993; 3:143–159.
17. Foley TP Jr, Abbassi V, Copeland KC, Draznin MB. Acquired autoimmune mediated infantile hypothyroidism: a pathologic entity distinct from congenital hypothyroidism. N Engl J Med 1994; 330:466–468.

18. Foley TP Jr. Congenital hypopituitarism. In: Dussault JH, Walker P, eds. Congenital Hypothyroidism, New York: Marcel Dekker, 1983:331–348.

19. Tatsumi K-I, Miyai K, Tsugunori N, et al. Cretinism with combined hormone deficiency caused by a mutation in the PIT1 gene. Nature Genet 1992; 1:56–58.

20. Larsen PR. Thyroid-pituitary interaction. N Engl J Med 1982; 306:23–32.

21. Scanlon MF. Neuroendocrine control of thyrotropin secretion. In: Braverman LE, Utiger RD, eds. Werner and Ingbar's the Thyroid, 6th ed. Philadelphia: J. B. Lippincott, 1991:230–256.

22. Foley TP Jr, Owings J, Hayford JR, Blizzard RM. Serum thyrotropin (TSH) responses to synthetic thyrotropin releasing hormone (TRH) in normal children and hypopituitary patients: a new test to distinguish primary pituitary hormone deficiency. J Clin Invest 1972; 51:431–437.

23. Van Wyk JJ, Grumbach MM. Syndrome of precocious menstruation and galactorrhea in juvenile hypothyroidism. An example of hormonal overlap in pituitary feedback. J Pediatr 1960; 59:416.

24. Castro-Magana M, Angulo M, Canas A, Sharp A, Fuentes B. Hypothalamic-pituitary-gonadal axis in boys with primary hypothyroidism and macroorchidism. J Pediatr 1988; 112:397–402.

25. Hidaka A, Minegishi T, Kohn LD. Thyrotropin, like luteinizing hormone (LH) and chorionic gonadotropin (CG) increases cAMP and inositol phosphate levels in cells with recombinant human LH/CG receptor. Biochem Biophys Res Commun 1993; 196:187–195.

26. Yamada T, Tsukaii T, Ikejiri K, et al. Volume of sella turcica in normal subjects and in patients with primary hypothyroidism and hyperthyroidism. J Clin Endocrinol Metab 1976; 42:817.

27. Illig R, Krawczy'nska H, Torresani T, Prader, A. Elevated plasma TSH and hypothyroidism in children with hypothalamic hypopituitarism. J Clin Endocrinol Metab 1975; 41:722–728.

28. LaFranchi SH, Hanna CE, Krainz PL. Primary hypothyroidism, empty sella, and hypothyroidism. J Pediatr 1986; 108:571–573.

29. Yamamoto K, Saito K, Takai T, et al. Visual field defects and pituitary enlargement in primary hypothyroidism. J Clin Endocrinol Metab 1983; 57:283.

30. Foley TP Jr. Acute, subacute, and chronic thyroiditis. In: Kaplan SA ed. Clinical Pediatric and Adolescent Endocrinology. Philadelphia: W. B. Saunders, 1982: III, 96–109.

31. Fisher DA. Acquired juvenile hypothyroidism. In: Braverman LE, Utiger RD, eds. Werner and Ingbar's the Thyroid, 6th ed. Philadelphia: J. B. Lippincott. 1991:1228–1236.

32. Fisher DA. Euthyroid low thyroxine (T4) and triiodothyronine states in prematures and sick neonates. Pediatr Clin North Am 1990; 37:1297.

33. Foley TP Jr, Malvaux P, Blizzard RM. Thyroid disease. In: Kappy MS, Blizzard RM, Migeon CJ, eds. Wilkins the Diagnosis and Treatment of Endocrine Disorders in Childhood and Adolescence, 4th ed. Springfield, IL: Charles C. Thomas, 1994:513–515.

34. Nelson JC, Wilcox RB, Pandian MR. Dependence of free thyroxine estimates obtained with equilibrium tracer dialysis on the concentration of thyroxine-binding globulin. Clin Chem 1992; 38:1294–1300.

35. Oppenheimer JH, Schwartz HL, Mariash CN, Kaiser FE. Evidence for a factor in the sera of patients with nonthyroidal disease which inhibits iodothyronine binding by solid matrices, serum proteins, and rat hepatocytes. J Clin Endocrinol Metab 1982; 54:757–766.

36. Wehmann RE, Gregerman RI, Burns WH, et al. Suppression of thyrotropin in the low-thyroxine state of severe nonthyroidal illness. N Engl J Med 1985; 312:546–552.

37. Becker RA, Vaughan GM, Ziegler MG, et al. Hypermetabolic low triiodothyronine syndrome of burn injury. Crit Care Med 1982; 10:870–875.

38. Foley TP Jr. Thyroid disease. In: Gellis SS, Kagan BM, ed. Current Pediatric Therapy, Vol. 12. Philadelphia: W. B. Saunders, 1986:301–306.

39. Rees-Jones RW, Rolla AR, Larsen PR. Hormone content of thyroid replacement preparations. JAMA 1980; 243:549.

40. LaFranchi S. Thyroiditis and acquired hypothyroidism. Pediatr Ann 1992; 21:29–39.

41. Sklar CA, Qazi R, David R. Juvenile autoimmune thyroiditis; hormonal status at presentation and after long-term follow-up. Am J Dis Child 1986; 140:877–880.

42. Maenpaa J, Raatikka M, Rasanen J, Taskinen E, Wager O. Natural course of juvenile autoimmune thyroiditis. J Pediatr 1985; 107:898–904.

43. Levy RP, Jensen JB, Laus VG, et al. Serum thyroid hormone abnormalities in psychiatric disease. Metabolism 1981; 38:1060.

44. Bocchetta A, Bernardi F, Burrai C, et al. The course of thyroid abnormalities during lithium treatment: a two-year follow-up study. Acta Psychiat Scand 1992; 86:38–41.

45. Rivkees SA, Bode HH, Crawford JD. Long-term growth in juvenile acquired hypothyroidism: the failure to achieve normal adult stature. N Engl J Med 1988; 318:599–602.

28
Hyperthyroidism

John S. Dallas
University of Texas Medical Branch and Children's Hospital of Galveston, Galveston, Texas

Thomas P. Foley, Jr.
University of Pittsburgh and Children's Hospital of Pittsburgh, Pittsburgh, Pennsylvania

I. INTRODUCTION

Thyrotoxicosis is an uncommon disorder of childhood and is characterized by accelerated metabolism of body tissues resulting from excessive levels of unbound circulating thyroid hormones. Graves' disease accounts for at least 95% of cases in children (1). Other causes are rare and are listed in Table 1.

II. PATHOGENESIS

Thyrotoxicosis results when excessive levels of unbound thyroid hormones are present in the circulation. Mechanisms that can produce thyrotoxicosis include thyroid follicular cell hyperfunction with increased synthesis and secretion of thyroxine (T_4) and triiodothyronine (T_3), thyroid follicular cell destruction with release of preformed T_4 and T_3, and ingestion or administration of thyroid hormone or iodide preparations.

Hyperfunction of thyroid follicular cells can either be autonomous or mediated through stimulation of thyrotropin receptors by such substances as thyrotropin (thyroid-stimulating hormone, TSH) or thyrotropin receptor antibodies (TRAb). Autonomous hyperfunction of thyroid follicular cells is rarely seen during childhood and is represented by toxic adenoma, hyperfunctioning thyroid carcinoma, and the hyperthyroidism of the McCune-Albright syndrome.

Stimulation of thyrotropin receptors by TRAb produces the diffuse toxic goiter of Graves' disease and accounts for the majority of childhood thyrotoxicosis. Rarely, increased TSH secretion resulting either from a TSH-producing pituitary adenoma or from pituitary resistance to thyroid hormone can produce thyrotoxicosis. Another glycoprotein hormone, human chorionic gonadotropin (hCG), also binds to the TSH receptor and stimulates thyroid cell function (2). The thyrotropic potency of hCG is much less than that of TSH, but extremely high serum levels of hCG, such as those seen in individuals with hydatidiform moles or other trophoblastic tumors, can lead to hyperthyroidism (3). Although extremely rare, the possibility of a molar pregnancy should be considered in adolescent females with thyrotoxicosis.

Inflammation of thyroid follicular cells can be associated with viral or autoimmune processes, and extensive destruction can release large amounts of preformed T_4 and T_3 into the circulation. The resultant thyrotoxicosis tends to be mild and transient, usually lasting only a few weeks to a few months. Examples include the toxic thyroiditis of Hashimoto's disease and subacute thyroiditis.

Acute or chronic ingestion of thyroid hormone preparations, such as L-thyroxine or desiccated thyroid, can produce excessive levels of circulating thyroid hormones. Ingestion may be surreptitious, iatrogenic, or accidental. Ingestion or parenteral administration of iodides may also result in thyrotoxicosis. This phenomenon, known as Jod-Basedow, most frequently occurs in iodine-deficient areas when supplemental iodides are added to the diet. The underlying mechanisms are unknown, but iodine-induced hyperthyroidism generally occurs in thyroid glands functioning independently of TSH stimulation (4).

III. ETIOLOGY

A. Neonatal Graves' Disease

Neonatal thyrotoxicosis is uncommon and accounts for less than 1% of childhood hyperthyroidism (Chap. 25) (5). It usually occurs in association with maternal Graves' disease,

Table 1 Etiology of Thyrotoxicosis in Childhood and Adolescence

---

Graves' disease
   Neonatal Graves' disease
   Graves' disease of childhood
Autonomous functioning nodule(s)
   Toxic adenoma
   Hyperfunctioning papillary or follicular carcinoma
   McCune-Albright syndrome
TSH-induced hyperthyroidism
   TSH-producing pituitary adenoma
   Pituitary resistance to thyroid hormone
Thyroiditis
   Subacute thyroiditis
   Toxic thyroiditis of Hashimoto's disease
Exogenous thyroid hormone
Iodine-induced hyperthyroidism (Jod-Basedow)
Tumor-produced thyroid stimulators
   Hydatidiform mole
   Choriocarcinoma

---

and studies have demonstrated that thyrotoxicosis occurs in the offspring of women with the highest thyroid-stimulating immunoglobulin G (TSI) concentrations (6). Neonatal thyrotoxicosis has also been reported in infants born to euthyroid women with a history of previous Graves' disease and euthyroid or hypothyroid women with Hashimoto's thyroiditis (7). Approximately 1 in every 70 pregnant women with a history of Graves' disease delivers a clinically affected infant, and there is equal frequency of the disease in males and females (8).

There appear to be two types of neonatal thyrotoxicosis. The first and more common type is caused by placental transfer of maternal TSI to the infant. Thyrotoxicosis usually presents shortly after birth, but the onset of disease may be delayed for several days and, in rare cases, for as long as 4–6 weeks (9). Spontaneous recovery generally begins within 3 months and is usually complete by 6 months, and recurrence has not been reported. The second type may or may not be present at birth but has its onset during infancy. This type tends to be more severe and may persist for years. Treatment is often difficult, and recurrences have been reported (5). Most of these cases have occurred in families with a strong history of Graves' disease, suggesting that affected infants have an inherited, early-onset Graves' disease similar to that seen in older children. Late sequelae, such as craniosynostosis, microcephaly, mental retardation, learning disorders, advanced bone age, and short stature, have been reported in infants with the second type (5).

The clinical manifestation are similar in the two types. Affected infants are often preterm or low birth weight, appear anxious, and are restless and irritable. They may be febrile, and often the skin is flushed and warm. Tachycardia is a consistent finding and may be accompanied by cardiomegaly and heart failure. Eye signs are usually present and include stare, periorbital edema, lid retraction, and proptosis. Thyromegaly is almost always present and at times may cause tracheal compression and respiratory distress. Poor weight gain or excessive weight loss may occur despite a voracious appetite. Hepatosplenomegaly, jaundice, petechiae, thrombocytopenia, lymphadenopathy, and the hyperviscosity syndrome are less common manifestations of the disease (10).

Neonatal Graves' disease must be considered in any infant born to a woman with a history of Graves' disease. Prenatal measurements of maternal TSI and thyrotropin binding inhibitory immunoglobulin (TBII) levels may help to identify those infants at greatest risk for developing thyrotoxicosis (11,12). Further, the presence of fetal tachycardia (heart rate > 160 beats/minute) after 22 weeks gestation may be used as evidence for thyrotoxicosis in the at-risk fetus (13). Clinical evidence of disease may not become apparent until 5–10 days after birth in those infants whose mothers received antithyroid drugs (i.e., propylthiouracil) during pregnancy. Serum thyroid function tests (total T_4, free T_4, FT_4, and T_3) are useful in confirming the diagnosis and should be obtained in all infants suspected of having the disease. The normal levels of serum thyroid hormones in newborns and infants are different from those observed in older children and adolescents, and this should be considered when interpreting thyroid function tests in neonates and infants (see Chap. 25).

Treatment aimed at controlling hyperthyroidism should begin as soon as the disease becomes apparent. This usually is accomplished using an antithyroid drug with or without iodide. Either propylthiouracil (PTU) or methimazole may be used in doses of 5–10 or 0.5–1.0 mg/kg/day, respectively. The antithyroid drug should be given orally or by nasogastric tube in divided doses every 8 h. When used, iodides should be started within a few hours after the first dose of the antithyroid drug. Either Lugol's solution or a 10% solution of potassium iodide may be used, and the initial dose of either preparation is 1 drop every 8 h. Iodides have the advantage of promptly inhibiting the further release of preformed T_4 from the thyroid. If a therapeutic response is not observed within 24–48 h, the dose of one or both drugs can be increased by 50–100%. Fetal thyrotoxicosis has been treated by administering antithyroid medicine (e.g., PTU) to the mother in doses sufficient to maintain the fetal heart rate at around 140 beats/minute (14).

More recently, the radiographic contrast agents, sodium ipodate and iopanoic acid, have been used to treat neonatal Graves' disease (15–17). These agents, along with propranolol, can be used either alone or in combination with the thioureas to treat affected infants successfully. Both sodium ipodate and iopanoic acid block the peripheral conversion of T_4 to T_3 and inhibit the thyroidal secretion of T_4 and T_3. They are given enterally and can be administered either once daily or once every 3 days. The recommended starting dose for either agent approximates 0.6 g/m^2/day, with reported doses ranging from 125 mg/day to 500 mg once every 3 days (15–17). Serum T_3 levels decrease rapidly (as much as 50% in 24 h) following initiation of treatment; T_4 levels decrease more gradually. No adverse reactions have been reported with the use of these agents in the treatment of neonatal Graves' disease.

Propranolol hydrochloride in a dose of 2 mg/kg/day given in three divided doses is effective in controlling the symptoms of sympathetic hyperresponsiveness, such as tachycardia. Digitalization may be necessary if cardiac failure occurs; in this case the dose of propranolol should be reduced or discontinued. In severe cases, use of glucocorticoids (prednisone, 2 mg/kg/day in three divided doses) may be warranted, because they apparently inhibit the secretion of thyroid hormone in Graves' disease (18). Glucocorticoids also inhibit the peripheral conversion of T_4 to T_3. Supportive therapy, including temperature control and adequate fluid and caloric intake, is important in all affected infants. When the thyroid gland causes tracheal compression, elevation and extension of the infant's head may improve breathing. Rarely, surgical intervention may be necessary to relieve tracheal obstruction.

Careful assessment of thyroid function during treatment is important to assure adequate, but to avoid excessive, therapy. Once the patient has been successfully tapered off medication, it is necessary to follow the patient for several months because the disease may relapse after withdrawal of therapy.

B. Graves' Disease of Childhood

Graves' disease is an immunogenetic disorder characterized clinically by thyromegaly, hyperthyroidism, and infiltrative ophthalmopathy. A family history of autoimmune thyroid disease is present in up to 60% of patients (19). Genetic studies have shown it to be a polygenic disorder, and most of the genes that have been implicated appear to be involved in immunoregulation (20). Patients with Graves' disease have an increased incidence of HLA haplotypes A1, B8, and DR3 (21).

The concordance rate between monozygotic twins is no more than 50%, implying that environmental factors play a role in the development of the disease. The extent to which chemicals, drugs, infections, and psychologic stress can alter immunoregulatory genes is unknown. However, the existence of a two-way interaction between the immune and neuroendocrine systems may provide a mechanism by which biologic and psychologic stresses can affect lymphocyte subpopulations and immunoregulation (22).

The exact incidence of Graves' disease in childhood is unknown, but it is uncommon and has been reported to account for less than 5% of cases seen in most thyroid clinics (23). Except for neonatal Graves' disease, the incidence increases during childhood and peaks during adolescence. More than two-thirds of childhood cases occur between the ages of 10 and 15 years (1). It occurs more frequently in females in a ratio of 3:1 to 5:1 (19).

1. Pathogenesis: Thyrotropin Receptor and Thyrotropin Receptor Antibodies

The thyrotropin (TSH) receptor is a member of the large family of guanine nucleotide binding (G) protein-coupled receptors and represents the primary target antigen for au-

toantibodies that mediate the hyperthyroidism and thyromegaly of Graves' disease. The cDNA encoding the human TSH receptor was recently cloned and characterized (24,25). As deduced from the cDNA sequence, the mature receptor is a glycoprotein with a single polypeptide chain of 744 amino acids. Like all other G protein-coupled receptors, the TSH receptor has an extracellular domain, seven transmembrane domains, and an intracellular domain. The TSH and other glycoprotein hormone (i.e., luteinizing hormone (LH),CG, and follicle-stimulating hormone, [FSH]) receptors each have relatively large extracellular domains, and this characteristic differentiates them from the other G protein-coupled receptors. The TSH, LH/CG, and FSH receptors are closely related structurally and share about 70 and 45% homology in their transmembrane and extracellular domains, respectively (26).

The extracellular domain of the TSH receptor (398 amino acids) represents the amino-terminal end and the transmembrane and intracellular domains (346 amino acids) represent the carboxyl-terminal end of the protein. The extracellular domain contains six potential N-glycosylation sites and nine leucine-rich repeats of a loosely conserved 25 amino acid residue motif. Proper glycosylation appears to be important both for normal expression of the receptor on the thyroid cell membrane and for normal hormone-receptor interactions (24,25). The leucine-rich repeats, which have the potential to form amphipathic α helices, are believed to be involved in protein-protein or protein-membrane interactions. Recent studies confirmed that both TSH and autoantibodies to the TSH receptor bind to the extracellular domain (24,25). The transmembrane and intracellular domains are involved in signal transduction, acting through G protein to stimulate the production of cyclic AMP by adenylyl cyclase (24,25).

The hyperthyroidism and thyromegaly of Graves' disease are mediated through immunoglobulin G (IgG) that bind to the extracellular domain of the TSH receptor and stimulate follicular cell function and growth. In addition to the stimulating TSH receptor antibodies, sera from patients with Graves' disease may also contain other IgGs to the TSH receptor that block thyroid cell function and growth. Stimulating TRAbs are restricted to the IgG_1 subclass, suggesting that they are either oligo- or monoclonal in origin (27). On the other hand, blocking TRAbs appear to be polyclonal in origin and may be of IgG_1, IgG_2, IgG_3, or IgG_4 subclass (28). Current evidence suggests that disease caused by the immune system (i.e., autoimmune disease) results from a restricted immune response involving B and/or T lymphocytes against one or a few epitopes of the target antigen (29). These observations therefore support the importance of stimulating TRAbs in Graves' disease and imply that blocking TRAbs, much like antithyroglobulin and antithyroid peroxidase, arise as a result of thyroid tissue damage. Nevertheless, blocking TRAbs can still modulate the biologic effects of stimulating TRAbs. Therefore, a patient's clinical presentation and course may be determined by the net biologic effect of the simultaneous interaction of various stimulating and blocking TRAbs with the TSH receptor.

Several investigators have proposed that the functional effect(s) a particular TRAb exhibits is determined by the specific region to which the antibody binds on the TSH receptor (30,31). Following the successful cloning of the TSH receptor, numerous studies have attempted to identify binding sites for the various TRAbs. To date, the major experimental approaches to define TRAb epitopes have included (1) transfecting mammalian cells with mutant cDNA of the TSH receptor and (2) using synthetic peptides derived from the predicted amino acid sequence of the TSH receptor (24,25). Some of these studies have localized functional epitopes to a few relatively narrow regions of the extracellular domain (32); others have identified multiple regions throughout the entire extracellular domain that appear to be involved in TRAb binding (33). Although controversy still exists regarding the specific sites that compose TRAb epitopes, data from several laboratories support the concept that the amino acid region 25–60 contains residues important for the binding of at least some stimulating TRAbs (24,32,34,35). Moreover, amino acid region 370–400 contains residues important for the binding of some inhibitory TRAbs (24,32,36). Despite these recent advances, the exact mechanisms by which stimulating and blocking TRAbs exert their biologic effects remain unknown. The precise determination of TRAb epitopes, as well as the study of molecular mechanisms, requires the development of human, disease-associated monoclonal antibodies.

The major source of thyrotropin receptor antibody production appears to be intrathyroidal lymphocytes (31), but lymphocytes in the spleen, lymph nodes, bone marrow, and peripheral blood may also produce these antibodies (37,38). The mechanisms and control of stimulating TRAb production are uncertain, but several hypotheses have been proposed. One hypothesis suggests that a deficiency of specific suppressor T cell function accounts for TRAb production (39), whereas a second hypothesis suggests that a breakdown in the idiotype-antiidiotype network of B lymphocyte immunoregulation is responsible (40). An increased frequency of antibodies to certain serotypes of *Yersinia enterocolitica* has been reported in patients with Graves' disease (41), and infection with this bacterium has been proposed as an important initiating event in the development of the disease (42). *Y. enterocolitica* has a specific, saturable binding site for TSH, and antibodies produced against this site may cross-react with the TSH receptor on the thyroid follicular cell membrane (41). A fourth hypothesis relies on the fact that thyroid follicular cells can express HLA-DR antigens and are therefore endowed with the capacity to present other antigenic material to primed T lymphocytes. Through this mechanism, the follicular cell could present the TSH receptor as antigen and direct the synthesis of TRAb (43). Although experimental evidence exists for each of the preceding hypotheses, none can fully account for all aspects of TRAb production, and further studies are necessary to identify the responsible mechanisms.

Currently, two major types of assays are used to measure TRAbs. Receptor assays assess the ability of Graves' IgG to inhibit labeled TSH from binding to thyroid membranes, and antibodies detected by this method have been designated thyrotropin binding inhibitory immunoglobulins. Current receptor assays, which employ a combination of detergent-solubilized porcine TSH receptors and receptor-purified [^{125}-I]-labeled bovine TSH, are both sensitive and specific, and they provide a reproducible, inexpensive means of measuring TRAb in unextracted serum (30,44). Studies using these receptor assays have detected TRAb in 82–100% of adults (31) and 93% of children (45) with untreated, active Graves' disease. TRAb can also be detected by receptor assays in small numbers (10–20%) of patients with Hashimoto's thyroiditis (31,45,46). More recently, Chinese hamster ovary (CHO) cells transfected with the cDNA of the human TSH receptor have been used in the receptor assay for TRAbs (47,48). Overall, the results from assays employing the recombinant human TSH receptor show highly positive correlations with assays employing the porcine TSH receptor (48).

Bioassay methods constitute the other major type of assay currently used to measure TRAb. Most commonly, these assays employ isolated thyroid cells in culture to assess the ability of immunoglobulin concentrates from patient sera to stimulate thyroid cell production of cAMP. These assays can be performed using cells taken from human or porcine thyroid tissue, as well as from the immortal rat thyroid line, FRTL-5 cells. More recently, transfected mammalian cells (e.g., COS-7 and Chinese hamster ovary cells) expressing the recombinant human TSH receptor have been used to detect stimulating TRAbs (24,49). Antibodies detected by these assays have been designated thyroid-stimulating immunoglobulins. The bioassays show sensitivity and specificity similar to those of the receptor assays, but they are less precise and more expensive and time consuming (30,31).

Although some reports have demonstrated highly positive correlations between TRAb levels detected by the receptor and bioassay methods (50), most have demonstrated no such correlation (30). Some investigators suggest the lack of correlation between TBII and TSI levels in patient sera is a result of the presence of different populations of TRAbs that exhibit different degrees of TSH agonist activity (51). Others suggest the poor correlation results from the coexistence of both stimulating and blocking TRAb in some patients' sera (52).

2. Graves' Ophthalmopathy

Ophthalmic abnormalities are clinically evident in over half of children and adolescents with Graves' disease. In most of these patients, the signs and symptoms are relatively mild and include lid lag, lid retraction, stare, proptosis, conjunctival injection, chemosis, and periorbital and eyelid edema. Less commonly, patients may complain of eye discomfort, pain, or diplopia. Severe ophthalmopathy, associated with marked chemosis, severe proptosis, periorbital ecchymosis, corneal ulceration, eye muscle paralysis, and optic atrophy, is extremely rare during childhood and adolescence. The clinical onset of eye disease usually coincides with that of thyroid dysfunction, but it can precede or follow it by several months to years (53).

Lid lag, lid retraction, and stare most commonly result directly from thyrotoxicosis with enhanced sympathetic stimulation of Müller's muscle of the upper lid. These features can be found in patients with thyrotoxicosis of any etiology and generally improve with normalization of thyroid hormone levels. The other signs and symptoms, however, are characteristic of Graves' ophthalmopathy and can be explained by the mechanical effects of an increase in tissue volume within the bony orbit. Histologic examination reveals accumulation of glycosaminoglycans (GAGs) in the connective tissue components of the orbital fat and muscles, as well as lymphocytic infiltration of the orbital tissues. The GAGs are hydrophilic macromolecules produced by orbital fibroblasts, and their accumulation results in enlargement of the extraocular muscles and surrounding fat (54). Enlargement of these tissues within the fixed space of the bony orbit leads to forward displacement of the globe (proptosis or exophthalmos). Chemosis and periorbital edema result from decreased venous drainage from the orbit and intraorbital inflammation. Extraocular muscle dysfunction results from accumulation of GAGs, edema, inflammation, and fibrosis of the endomysial connective tissues investing the muscle fibers (54).

The cause of Graves' ophthalmopathy remains unknown, but it also appears to be an organ-specific autoimmune disorder. Current evidence supports that either orbital fibroblasts or extraocular muscle cells are the primary targets of autoimmune attack (54,55). Although the nature of the autoantigen(s) in the eye disease remains undetermined, the close association of ophthalmopathy with autoimmune thyroid disease strongly suggests that it (they) may share unique structural characteristics with antigens of the thyroid gland. Thus far, thyroid peroxidase and thyroglobulin have not been detected in orbital tissues (53). Recently, several groups have used the polymerase chain reaction to detect mRNA encoding the extracellular domain of the TSH receptor in orbital fibroblasts from patients with ophthalmopathy (53–55). If the TSH receptor is expressed on fibroblast membranes, then it could be recognized by T lymphocytes or activated by TRAbs, thus providing the pathogenic link between the eye and thyroid diseases. However, it remains to be seen whether TSH receptors are indeed expressed in the orbit, whether they are functional, and whether autoantibodies from patients with ophthalmopathy activate cellular processes through this mechanism. Although the majority of clinical studies have shown a higher prevalence of TRAb positivity in patients with ophthalmopathy than in patients without clinical evidence of eye disease, there is poor correlation between absolute levels of TRAb and the severity of eye disease (55). Other candidate autoantigens include the insulin-like growth factor type I receptor, a 64 kD eye muscle membrane protein, and a 23 kD orbital fibroblast protein (53–55).

Both humoral and cellular immune mechanisms appear to be important in the pathogenesis of Graves' ophthalmopathy. IgG from patients' sera have been shown to stimulate both the growth of extraocular myoblasts and the secretion of GAGs from orbital fibroblasts (54,55). Further, cytokines that can be released by activated T lymphocytes (e.g., interleukin-1α, tumor necrosis factor β, and interferon-γ) have been shown to stimulate GAG production by orbital fibroblasts (54,55).

Because ophthalmopathy is relatively mild and self-limited in the vast majority of affected children and adolescents, specific treatment is usually not necessary. In general, eye findings improve in association with control of the hyperthyroidism. Occasionally, local measures may be used to treat symptoms. For example, eyedrop or ointment preparations containing methylcellulose may be necessary to prevent corneal drying. Sleeping with the head elevated may help reduce chemosis and periorbital edema. Other forms of treatment, such as oral corticosteroids, orbital irradiation, and surgical decompression, are rarely indicated in children and should be reserved for those with severe ophthalmopathy.

3. Clinical Manifestations

During childhood and adolescence, most patients with Graves' disease present with the classic symptoms and signs (19). Early during the course of the disease, the symptoms and signs specific to children (Table 2) may be minimal because the disease usually develops insidiously over several months (19). Often the initial awareness of any problem is in school, where teachers notice changes in behavior and academic performance. Insomnia, restless sleep, and nocturia are common and are often associated with easy fatiguability and lethargy during the day. The symptoms of hyperthyroidism in Graves' disease, although variable, tend to be more severe than in other causes of hyperthyroidism.

Ophthalmic abnormalities are present in over one-half of patients (see earlier), and thyromegaly is almost invariably present. In fact, the absence of goiter raises serious doubt about the diagnosis of Graves' disease, and other causes of hyperthyroidism should be sought. The thyroid gland is usually symmetrically enlarged, smooth, soft, and nontender. Less often, and usually in association with coexisting Hashimoto's thyroiditis, the gland may be firm, bosselated, and asymmetrically enlarged. Other diseases have been observed in association with Graves' disease and include Hashimoto's thyroiditis, vitiligo, systemic lupus erythematosus, rheumatoid arthritis, Addison's disease, insulin-dependent diabetes mellitus, myasthenia gravis, and pernicious anemia (1).

Table 2 Common Symptoms and Signs of Graves' Disease in 290 Children and Adolescents

	(% Affected)
Goiter	98
Tachycardia	82
Nervousness	82
Increased pulse pressure	80
Proptosis	65
Increased appetite	60
Tremor	52
Weight loss	50
Heat intolerance	30

Source: Reference 19.

4. Laboratory Evaluation

Important initial laboratory tests for the child or adolescent with hyperthyroidism include serum T_4, an indirect or direct assessment of the free T_4, T_3, and TSH. The serum TSH level, as measured with the newer assays (sensitivity < 0.05 mU/L), is very useful in the patient who presents with mild symptoms of hyperthyroidism and a slight elevation in the serum T_3 values. In all causes of hyperthyroidism, except the very rare inappropriate pituitary secretion of TSH, the TSH level should be undetectable. Further, the TSH response to administered thyrotropin-releasing hormone (TRH) is very blunted or absent. Rarely, a patient presents with thyrotoxicosis and an elevated serum T_3 but normal serum T_4 (T_3 toxicosis). This may occur early in the course of the disease because the rise in the serum T_3 concentration is the first and most specific abnormality of serum thyroid function tests in hyperthyroidism. Conversely, patients with thyrotoxicosis may have mild clinical manifestations and normal serum T_3 values in the presence of chronic illness, starvation, or malnutrition.

When antithyroid drugs are selected as therapy, a baseline complete blood count with differential white blood count should be obtained, because leukopenia occurs in untreated thyrotoxicosis and granulocytopenia is an occasional toxic reaction to antithyroid drugs. Measurement of TRAb, which is now available in commercial laboratories, is not routinely necessary but is a useful additional test for patients in whom the diagnosis is uncertain. Antibodies to thyroglobulin and/or thyroid peroxidase are present in the majority of patients.

Patients with mild hyperthyroidism and no exophthalmos may require additional diagnostic tests to exclude other causes of thyrotoxicosis. Toxic thyroiditis associated with Hashimoto's disease and subacute thyroiditis with a nontender thyroid gland may be differentiated from those with Graves' disease by a normal or low radioiodine uptake and very elevated titers of thyroid antibodies in serum.

5. Clinical Course and Management

The thyrotoxicosis of untreated Graves' disease usually persists and progresses unless the thyroid gland has limited responsiveness as a result of coexisting chronic lymphocytic thyroiditis (4). The duration of thyrotoxicosis, however, is variable and unpredictable. Therapeutic intervention is recommended for the symptomatic patient. Despite recent advances in our knowledge of the TSH receptor and TRAbs, none of the currently available treatments is specifically directed against the underlying immunologic abnormality that causes Graves' disease. The three acceptable methods of therapy (antithyroid drugs, radioiodine ablation, and subtotal thyroidectomy) merely interrupt the disease process at the level of the thyroid gland, although treatment with thioureas has been reported to reduce levels of TRAb. Each method is associated with specific advantages and disadvantages.

The antithyroid drugs for long-term therapy of children in the United States include PTU and methimazole (MTZ). In addition to these two agents, a methimazole derivative, carbimazole, is available in Europe (56). These drugs block the incorporation of oxidized iodide into tyrosine residues of thyroglobulin by serving as substrates for thyroid peroxidase. The drugs are iodinated and degraded within the gland, thus diverting oxidized iodide away from thyroglobulin (57). Further, they block the coupling of iodotyrosyl residues in thyroglobulin to form T_4 and T_3. They do not interfere with the thyroid gland's ability to concentrate iodide, nor do they block the release of stored thyroid hormone into the circulation (57). Because they do not block the release of preformed, stored thyroid hormones, most patients require 4–8 weeks of antithyroid drug therapy before a euthyroid state is achieved. PTU, but not methimazole or carbimazole, also inhibits the peripheral conversion of T_4 to T_3 (57). Because of this, many clinicians tend to use PTU initially in patients with more severe hyperthyroidism.

In addition to their direct effects on thyroid hormone synthesis, the thioureas also appear to have immunosuppressive activity. Several investigators have reported significant reductions in circulating TRAbs during antithyroid drug treatment (58). Some studies suggest that thioureas have direct effects on thyroid autoantibody-producing lymphocytes, whereas others suggest that these drugs primarily act by reducing the antigenicity of thyrocytes. A recent review presents these studies in detail and clearly outlines the evidence that supports the immunosuppressive activity of these drugs (58).

Except in very young children, the initial dosage of PTU ranges between 300 and 450 mg/day in three divided doses every 8 h. The equivalent dosages for MTZ and carbimazole are one-tenth of the PTU dosage. The initial dosage of PTU for very young children is 5–10 mg/kg/day in three divided doses every 8 h. Once clinical and chemical euthyroidism is achieved, maintenance therapy may proceed by either of two methods: (1) reduce the dosage by one-third to one-half to maintain iodothyronine levels in the normal range, or (2) continue the initial therapeutic dosage to induce hypothyroidism, and initiate L-thyroxine therapy. The latter method is preferred by many clinicians for children because it reduces the need for frequent monitoring of thyroid function for the development of hypothyroidism, which is an undesirable side effect in the growing child. Further, a recent report from Japan demonstrated that the combined use of antithyroid drugs and L-thyroxine decreased both the production of TRAbs and the frequency of recurrence of hyperthyroidism in adult patients (59). Although the results of this study have yet to be substantiated in other patient groups, they currently tend to support the use of combined antithyroid drug and L-thyroxine therapy in children.

After 1–3 years of therapy, either the medication is slowly tapered or a T_3 suppression of serum T_4 using exogenous doses of oral T_3 (1.5 μg/kg/day in three divided doses) is performed (45,60). The administration of exogenous T_3 for 3 weeks to normal children or patients in remission with Graves' disease causes a decrease in the serum T_4 concentration to values below the normal range. The test is performed as follows:

1. While the patient is still receiving the antithyroid drug, T_3 is started at the dosage just listed. L-thy-

roxine therapy must be discontinued in those patients on combined therapy.

2. Serum T_4 and free T_4 levels are evaluated 3 weeks later.

   a. If the results are normal or elevated, antithyroid drug therapy is continued.

   b. If the results are below normal, discontinue the antithyroid drug and exogenous T_3 therapy.

3. Repeat the serum T_4 values 1 or 2 weeks later.

   a. If normal or elevated, resume antithyroid drug therapy.

   b. If the serum T_4 values are low, discontinue T_3 therapy and monitor serum T_4 and T_3 levels at 3 months intervals for the next year and annually thereafter. If relapse occurs, antithyroid therapy may be resumed or the patient may be offered the choice of surgical or radioiodine therapy (19).

In adults, the presence of TRAb during antithyroid drug therapy may be associated with clinical relapse of disease on termination of therapy (40). Furthermore, the predictability of relapse using an analysis of TRAb values and HLA-DR3 typing was accurate in 95% of patients in one study (61), but these results were not confirmed in another similar study (62). However, several recent reports reveal that patients (adults and children) with negative TRAb values during antithyroid drug therapy remain in remission after cessation of therapy (6,45,62). One study in children with Graves' disease compared TRAb values and the clinical course with the results of the T_3 suppression tests (45). TRAb values correctly predicted the subsequent clinical course in 72%, and the T_3 suppression tests accurately predicted the course in 64% of patients. Furthermore, the TRAb values and the T_3 suppression tests were in agreement 75% of the time. This study suggests that TRAb values are as effective as T_3 suppression tests in determining when antithyroid drug therapy can be discontinued. However, both tests are limited in their ability to predict accurately the clinical course of the disease, and patients continue to require periodic clinical evaluations and laboratory assessment after discontinuation of antithyroid drug therapy.

The major disadvantages of antithyroid drug therapy are duration of therapy and the risk of toxic side effects (Table 3) (19,57). When any serious toxic effect of the antithyroid

Table 3 Toxic Side Effects of Antithyroid Drug Therapy

Granulocytopenia	Edema
Dermatitis, urticaria	Conjunctivitis
Arthralgia, arthritis	Thrombocytopenia
Lupus-like syndrome	Hypoprothrombinemia
Lymphadenopathy	Toxic psychosis
Peripheral neuritis	Disseminated intravascular coagulation
Fever	Sensorineural hearing loss
Hepatitis	Loss of taste sensation

drugs is suspected, therapy must be stopped promptly. Except in severe systemic side effects, an alterntive antithyroid drug may be initiated once the toxic reaction has resolved..

β-Adrenergic blockade with propranolol has become an important and very effective modality for control of adrenergic symptoms during the thyrotoxic course of the disease. In addition, propranolol or one of its metabolites reduces the conversion of T_4 to T_3 by inhibiting the 5'-deiodination pathway, thus producing some decrease in serum T_3 levels (63). In reasonably low dosages (10–20 mg every 6–8 h), the distressing adrenergic symptoms and signs of restlessness, tachycardia, heat intolerance, tremor, hyperhidrosis, diarrhea, and myopathy may be decreased; however, metabolic rate and oxygen consumption are not significantly altered by propranolol therapy alone.

Therapy with [^{131}I]iodide for juvenile Graves' disease is becoming more acceptable as long-term experience in its use accumulates (64–67). Radioiodine has been the treatment of choice for patients who are poor surgical candidates or have experienced toxic reactions with the antithyroid drugs. Radioiodine is administered as an oral solution or capsule containing Na ^{131}I. After absorption by the gastrointestinal tract, it is concentrated into the thyroid gland and organified. β Emissions from the ^{131}I result in extensive tissue damage and ablation of the gland within 6–18 weeks (56). Some children experience transient, mild exacerbation of hyperthyroid symptoms as a result of increased release of preformed thyroid hormones. These symptoms can generally be controlled with β-adrenergic blockers. Rarely, the thyroid gland may become swollen and tender following radioiodine treatment. Hypothyroidism eventually develops in most children after radioiodine treatment, and T_4 treatment is indicated when this occurs. When ablative dosages of radioiodine are used, the risk of future thyroid neoplasia should not differ from its occurrence in the general population. There is currently no evidence for an increased risk of leukemia or other cancers, and there does not appear to be any teratogenic effect among the progeny of treated patients (66,67). Both hypo- and hyperparathyroidism have been reported in patients following radioiodine therapy for hyperthyroidism (68).

Graves' disease can be treated very effectively with subtotal thyroidectomy by an experienced pediatric thyroid surgeon (69). Once hyperthyroidism is controlled with antithyroid drugs and propranolol, potassium iodide or Lugol's solution (5% iodine and 10% iodide) is started for 10–14 days before surgery to decrease the vascularity of the gland. Relapse of thyrotoxicosis is an uncommon but distinct disadvantage of this procedure. The risks of thyroidectomy increase with subsequent operations and include hypoparathyroidism and damage to the recurrent laryngeal nerve. More than one-half of patients develop hypothyroidism at some time following surgery.

C. Autonomous Thyroid Nodule

The autonomously functioning thyroid nodule is a discrete thyroid nodule that functions independently of normal pituitary control. The pathogenesis has not yet been established in all cases, but recent evidence suggests that somatic mutations of the α subunit of G protein ($G_{s\alpha}$; see later) and the third intracellular loop of the TSH receptor are probably responsible for the development of some cases (70,71). In both situations, the mutations result in constitutive activation of adenylyl cyclase and unregulated production of cAMP. The unregulated cAMP production is responsible for the subsequent tissue hyperplasia and hyperthyroidism.

This disorder predominantly occurs in adults, is rare during childhood, but has been reported in a child as young as 22 months (72). Most children with a thyroid nodule come to the attention of a physician because of a mass in the region of the thyroid gland. The majority of patients with autonomous thyroid nodules are clinically euthyroid, and in contrast to adults, clinical hyperthyroidism occurs very rarely in children. Autonomously functioning nodules that cause hyperthyroidism are almost invariably benign adenomas (toxic adenoma), but very rarely hyperthyroidism caused by hyperfunctioning papillary or follicular carcinoma has been reported (73). These patients usually have extensive metastatic disease, and the diagnosis of carcinoma has been established before the onset of hyperthyroidism.

The hyperthyroidism of the McCune-Albright syndrome (MAS) is also associated with single or multiple hyperfunctioning adenomatous nodules. This syndrome is characterized by polyostotic fibrous dysplasia, multiple café au lait spots, and endocrine hyperfunction. The most common endocrinopathy is isosexual precocious puberty, but hyperthyroidism, acromegaly, Cushing syndrome, and hyperparathyroidism have been reported (74). In contrast to polyostotic fibrous dysplasia and precocious puberty, which occur more commonly in girls with the syndrome, hyperthyroidism occurs with equal frequency in boys and girls. The age of onset of hyperthyroidism tends to be between 3 and 12 years (75), and this is somewhat younger than the usual age of onset of hyperthyroidism caused by hyperfunctioning nodules in other individuals. The hyperthyroidism is clearly caused by autonomous function of the thyroid gland; basal TSH levels are suppressed and the TSH response to TRH is blunted, thyroid-stimulating antibodies are undetectable, and T_3 treatment fails to suppress radioactive iodide uptake by the thyroid.

Current evidence indicates that the receptors for each of the hormones (i.e., LH, FSH, TSH, growth hormone-releasing hormone, adrenocorticotropic hormone, and parathyroid hormone) that might otherwise be implicated in the observed endocrinopathies of MAS are all coupled to G proteins. The G proteins are heterotrimers composed of an α subunit and a tightly coupled $\beta\gamma$ dimer (76). The α subunit contains the guanine nucleotide binding site and has intrinsic GTPase activity. In the normal situation, the binding of one of these stimulatory hormones to its receptor facilitates the exchange of GTP for GDP in the guanine nucleotide binding site of the α subunit (Gsα). This results in the release of the G protein from the receptor and its dissociation into free Gsα GTP and free $\beta\gamma$ dimer. Free Gsα GTP stimulates adenylyl cyclase activity, with the subsequent production of intracellular cAMP. After a preset time, the intrinsic GTPase of Gsα hydrolyzes GTP to GDP, and the Gsα GDP reassociates with the $\beta\gamma$ dimer. The G protein is thus returned to its inactive state and can now reassociate with its receptor and participate in another cycle (76). Recent studies have identified mutations in the Gsα gene in endocrine organs, bone, and skin from patients with MAS (76,77). These mutations involve amino acid residues (Arg^{201} or Gln^{227}) that are critical for the intrinsic GTPase activity of Gsα. Therefore, a mutation involving either of these amino acids results in the constitutive activation of adenylyl cyclase and unregulated production of intracellular cAMP. In some cases, the mutation has been found in abnormal sections of tissue but not in histologically normal sections from the same tissue (76). This observation tends to explain the development of hyperfunctioning nodules within the thyroid gland.

The amount of thyroid hormone an autonomously functioning nodule produces appears to be related to its size. In adults with single autonomous nodules, hyperthyroidism usually occurs only when the nodule measures greater than 2.5–3 cm in diameter (78). Both T_4 and T_3 can be produced in excess, but an elevated serum T_3 level is frequently the only chemical abnormality. The T_3 level may be elevated enough to inhibit the TSH response to TRH but not enough to cause clinical hyperthyroidism (79).

A radionuclide image, preferably using [^{123}I]iodine, should be included in the evaluation of the hyperthyroid child with a thyroid nodule. The radioiodine image allows one to study both trapping and organification by the nodule. Technetium images demonstrate only trapping by the nodule, and the images are not always identical to those obtained with iodine. The diagnosis of a hyperfunctioning or "hot" nodule is established when the image reveals increased accumulation of the radioisotope in the nodule and decreased or absent uptake in the surrounding thyroid tissues.

Surgical removal is the preferred method of treatment for the toxic thyroid nodule and is accomplished by simple excision or lobectomy. Significant surgical complications are not expected, and postoperative hypothyroidism seldom occurs. Recurrence of hyperthyroidism postoperatively has not been reported. Because the hyperthyroidism produced by the autonomous nodule is usually mild, a long preoperative preparation with antithyroid drugs is seldom necessary. Propranolol may be used to decrease the symptoms of hyperthyroidism. The administration of iodides is not indicated in the preoperative treatment of the autonomous nodule. More recently, percutaneous intranodular ethanol injection under ultrasound guidance has been employed for the ablation of autonomous thyroid nodules (80). This approach appears to be safe and effective in adults and may prove to be a practical alternative to surgical treatment in children.

D. TSH-Induced Hyperthyroidism

Hyperthyroidism from increased TSH secretion can occur as the result of either a TSH-secreting pituitary adenoma or selective pituitary resistance to thyroid hormone. Although both are rare, each has been reported in childhood or adolescence (81). Unlike Graves' disease, the sex ratio in patients with TSH-induced hyperthyroidism is 1:1. Most cases of TSH-producing pituitary adenoma occur sporadically, but familial cases have been reported (82). Pituitary resistance to thyroid hormone appears to be familial, with an autosomal dominant pattern of inheritance (81). The etiology of pituitary resistance to thyroid hormone has not been established for all cases, but most probably represent forms of the syndrome of generalized resistance to thyroid hormone (GRTH; see later) (83). The syndrome of GRTH is caused by a mutation in one of the thyroid hormone receptor genes (c-erbAβ) (84). Although the reasons remain unclear, affected members within a family can exhibit different degrees of resistance to thyroid hormone, and various tissues (e.g., heart, liver, bone, and pituitary) can be affected to a greater or lesser degree (85). Therefore, the pituitary gland in such individuals is relatively more resistant to thyroid hormones than other tissues in the body. Pituitary thyrotroph resistance in these individuals is selective for thyroid hormones: there is normal inhibition of pituitary TSH secretion by glucocorticoids and dopaminergic agents (81).

Criteria essential for the diagnosis of this disorder include evidence of increased peripheral metabolism, diffuse thyromegaly, elevated free thyroid hormone levels, and inappropriately elevated serum levels of TSH (82). Although the TSH level may not be elevated above the normal range, it is always detectable, even in highly sensitive and specific immunoassays. In all other causes of hyperthyroidism, sensitive immunoassays reveal very suppressed or undetectable serum levels of TSH.

The clinical presentation is often very similar to that in Graves' disease, and a high degree of suspicion is needed to make the diagnosis. The patient with pituitary adenoma, however, may present with visual complaints caused by compression of optic nerve tracts by the adenoma. Increased pituitary secretion of growth hormone and prolactin has also been reported in patients with TSH-secreting tumors (82).

Once the diagnosis of TSH-induced hyperthyroidism has been established, the clinician must determine whether the increased TSH secretion results from a pituitary tumor or from pituitary resistance to thyroid hormone to determine the proper course of therapy. The TRH and T_3 suppression test may help differentiate these two disorders. In general, serum TSH levels do not increase in response to TRH when a pituitary tumor is the cause of hyperthyroidism. In contrast, the TSH response to TRH tends to be normal or exaggerated in pituitary resistance to thyroid hormone (81). Pharmacologic doses of T_3 cause significant TSH suppression in patients with pituitary resistance but fail to reduce TSH levels in patients with TSH-secreting pituitary adenomas.

Determination of serum levels of the free α subunit of the glycoproteins, including TSH, can also aid in differentiating these conditions; patients with TSH-secreting pituitary tumors generally have elevated (greater than 1) molar α subunit/TSH ratios, whereas this ratio tends to be less than 1 in patients with pituitary resistance to thyroid hormone (82). The measured α subunit is usually expressed in ng/ml, whereas TSH is usually expressed in μU/ml. To determine the α subunit/TSH molar ratio, one assumes a molecular weight for TSH of 28,000 D, a molecular weight for α subunit

of 13,600 D, and a specific activity for human TSH of 5 μU/ng (86). This results in a conversion factor of (28,000/13,600)/0.2, or approximately 10 (87). Therefore, [α subunit (ng/ml)/TSH (μU/ml)] $\times$ 10 = molar ratio. Computed tomographic scan and MRI studies of the pituitary region can also help to establish the diagnosis and to guide treatment.

Treatment for TSH-secreting adenomas consists of selective adenonectomy or radiotherapy, or a combination of the two. In the past, a brief course of antithyroid drugs was used to render the patient euthyroid before surgery. More recently, the somatostatin analog, octreotide, has proven useful in the management of TSH-producing pituitary tumors (85). This drug normalizes thyroid hormone levels in most patients and causes a decrease in tumor size in some. Because of tachyphylaxis, however, octreotide cannot be considered definitive treatment. The current approach to managing the TSH-producing pituitary tumor consists of achieving a euthyroid state with octreotide, followed by surgical resection of the tumor.

Treatment of patients with pituitary resistance to thyroid hormone is more difficult. Ideally, treatment should be aimed at reducing TSH secretion by the pituitary. A number of agents including L-T_3, D-T_4, bromocryptine, and triiodothyroacetic acid (Triac), have been advocated (82,85,88–90). To date, each agent has been used in a limited number of patients, and the overall efficacy of each has not been determined. Octreotide has not been useful in the long-term treatment of these patients (85). Propranolol may be used to decrease the symptoms of hyperthyroidism. Although antithyroid drugs reduce serum thyroid hormone levels, they also increase TSH secretion and goiter size. Because prolonged TSH hypersecretion may lead to thyrotroph hyperplasia and eventually to the development of a TSH-secreting pituitary adenoma (91), prolonged treatment with antithyroid drugs is discouraged. Likewise, subtotal thyroidectomy and radioiodine therapy should not be used in patients with pituitary resistance to thyroid hormone.

E. Subacute and Hashimoto's Thyroiditis

Subacute or granulomatous thyroiditis is a self-limited, presumably viral inflammation of the thyroid gland. This entity is rarely seen in children, occurring more frequently between the third and fifth decades of life. Mild symptoms of thyrotoxicosis may occur, but they are often overshadowed by malaise, fever, and tenderness of the thyroid gland. The erythrocyte sedimentation rate is consistently elevated. Thyroid antibodies are usually negative early in the disease, but titers may rise transiently to abnormal levels during recovery. The thyrotoxic phase of this disease probably results from destruction of thyroid follicular cells with release of large amounts of preformed thyroid hormones.

The toxic thyroiditis of Hashimoto's disease occurs early in the course of chronic lymphocytic thyroiditis and probably results from extensive autoimmune destruction of thyroid follicular cells. The child may present with mild symptoms of thyrotoxicosis and a slightly enlarged, sometimes tender, thyroid gland. Thyroid antibodies are usually positive.

Laboratory evaluation of both disorders reveals elevated

serum T_4, free T_4, and T_3 levels and undetectable TSH levels. The TSH response to TRH is either blunted or absent. The radioiodine uptake is typically low or absent during the thyrotoxic phase of these disorders and helps to differentiate toxic thyroiditis from Graves' disease.

Treatment of these disorders is symptomatic. Antithyroid drugs are not indicated in the treatment, but propranolol can be used to relieve the symptoms of thyrotoxicosis in both. The pain and tenderness of the thyroid gland may be relieved by therapeutic doses of salicylates, but on occasion glucocorticoids may be required. These disorders have been discussed in detail in Chapter 26.

F. Exogenous Thyroid Hormone

Thyrotoxicosis may result from the ingestion, usually chronic, of excessive quantities of thyroid hormone preparations (92). The term "thyrotoxicosis factitia" has been used to describe this situation. In children and adolescents, this ingestion may be surreptitious, iatrogenic, or accidental. Although therapeutic thyroid hormone preparations are the most obvious source, the clinician should keep in mind that ground meats and diet pills have reportedly been contaminated with large amounts of thyroid hormones and implicated in the thyrotoxicosis factitia in some patients (92).

Although acute accidental or intentional overdoses of thyroid hormones can produce marked elevations in serum T_4 levels, the majority of children who take as much as 5–10 mg L-T_4 in a single dose have few or no symptoms of thyrotoxicosis (93). When symptoms of thyrotoxicosis develop in these cases, they are usually mild and consist of fever, tachycardia, irritability, vomiting, diarrhea, and "hyperactive" behavior. Although more serious reactions, such as seizures, have been reported, these occur very infrequently and several hours to days after the acute overdose (94). When preparations containing significant levels of T_3 have been ingested, the onset of symptoms is within 6–12 h. The onset of symptoms following acute ingestion of L-T_4 is generally within 12–48 h but may be as late as 7–10 days after ingestion. The delayed onset of symptoms may be explained by the conversion of T_4 to its biologically active metabolite, T_3. Serum levels of T_4 and/or T_3 following acute ingestion correlate poorly with development of toxicity (95). Because the majority of these cases are relatively benign and symptoms are absent or delayed, initial therapy should be limited to gastric decontamination with syrup of ipecac followed by activated charcoal and/or a cathartic (96). Patients who have ingested thyroid hormone accidently can then be followed closely at home pending the onset of symptoms. As in other accidental poisonings, the parents should be counseled on child safety measures. Only when symptoms develop should hospitalization or further treatment be considered. Propranolol is helpful in controlling tachycardia as well as improving symptoms of nervousness, diaphoresis, or tremor. Acetaminophen may be useful for control of fever. Psychiatric evaluation may be indicated for patients with acute intentional overdoses.

Chronic ingestion of thyroid hormone preparations can produce symptoms similar to those of hyperthyroidism of thyroid origin. However, thyromegaly is not present unless the patient also has a coincident thyroid disease, such as Hashimoto's thyroiditis. Likewise, infiltrative ophthalmopathy is absent; however, as in other causes of thyrotoxicosis, lid lag and stare may be present. The diagnosis of this disorder is not difficult if the clinician is able to obtain a history of thyroid hormone ingestion. This history may be difficult to obtain, however, especially in cases of surreptitious ingestion. Nevertheless, the clinician should still be able to diagnose this disorder using a limited number of tests. Thyroid function test results depend on the type of preparation responsible for the thyrotoxicosis. If the preparation is composed mainly of T_4, the patient has elevated serum T_4 and free T_4 levels. If the preparation is T_3 or has a high T_3/T_4 ratio, the patient has a low to normal serum T_4 level. In both cases the serum T_3 level is elevated. The radioiodine uptake is low to reflect the suppression of thyroid gland activity induced by exogenous thyroid hormone. Unlike all other causes of thyrotoxicosis, the plasma thyroglobulin level in this disorder is undetectable or extremely low. Therefore, the plasma thyroglobulin level may be extremely helpful in differentiating this disorder from other causes of thyrotoxicosis.

Treatment of thyrotoxicosis resulting from chronic ingestion of thyroid hormone preparations should be guided by the circumstances surrounding ingestion. For example, in patients receiving excessive replacement for treatment of hypothyroidism the dose should be reduced. The patient who is taking thyroid hormone surreptitiously should be advised to discontinue the medication; in some cases, psychotherapy may be necessary.

IV. EUTHYROID HYPERTHYROXINEMIA

The term "euthyroid hyperthyroxinemia" is used to describe the various conditions in which the serum T_4 level, either total or free, is elevated in the absence of thyrotoxicosis. The causes are listed in Table 4 and can be divided into three major categories: increased T_4 binding by serum proteins, generalized resistance to thyroid hormones, and impaired peripheral conversion of T_4 to T_3.

Alterations in any of the serum thyroid hormone binding proteins can produce elevations in the total T_4 level, but the free T_4 level remains normal. Increased thyroxine binding globulin (TBG) concentration results from a variety of causes (Table 5) and produces concurrent elevations of the serum total T_4 and T_3 levels. Familial dysalbuminemic hyperthyroxinemia (FDH) is caused by the presence of significant amounts of serum albumin with an unusually high affinity for T_4. Because this albumin binds T_3 only weakly, the serum T_3 level remains normal. FDH is inherited in an autosomal dominant fashion and is expressed equally in males and females. Increased serum concentration or binding affinity of thyroxine binding prealbumin or transthyretin can produce elevated serum total T_4 levels, but as in FDH, the serum T_3 level remains normal. The presence of endogenous antibodies directed against T_4 can produce either true or spurious elevations in serum total T_4 levels.

Table 4 Conditions Causing Hyperthyroxinemia in the Absence of Thyrotoxicosis

Increased T_4 binding by serum proteins
   Increased concentration of TBG
   Familial dysalbuminemic hyperthyroxinemia
   Increased T_4 binding by transthyretin
   Anti-T_4 antibodies
Generalized (pituitary and peripheral tissues) resistance to thyroid hormone
Impaired conversion of T_4 to T_3
   pathophysiologic conditions (e.g., type I deiodinase deficiency and certain nonthyroidal illnesses)
   pharmacologic agents (e.g., amiodarone, propranolol, heparin, iodine contrast agents, amphetamines, L-thyroxine)

The serum free T_4 is normal in the disorders of protein binding when it is determined by equilibrium dialysis or the two-step coated tube method. Determination of the free T_4 by an analog-based "free T_4" method gives falsely high results in patients with FDH and endogenous anti-T_4 antibodies. This occurs because the variant albumin or anti-T_4 antibodies in the serum readily bind the analog tracer used in these competitive immunoassays and thereby decrease the amount of tracer available to compete for the assay antibody. The low binding of tracer by the assay antibody gives the false impression of a high free T_4 concentration.

The FT_4 index, as usually calculated from the resin T_3 uptake test, accurately reflects the FT_4 level only when increased T_4 binding is caused by TBG excess. T_4 and T_3 share the same binding site on TBG. When the concentration of TBG is increased, the available binding sites for both T_4 and T_3 are increased. The resin T_3 uptake is inversely proportional to the number of available binding sites for T_3; that is, when the available serum binding sites for T_3 are increased, the resin T_3 uptake is decreased. The FT_4 index, when calculated as the product of the T_4 and the resin T_3 uptake, is usually normal in TBG excess because the elevated T_4 is offset by the decreased resin T_3 uptake. However, when increased serum T_4 binding results because of FDH or increased T_4 binding by TBPA or anti-T_4 antibodies, the resin T_3 uptake remains normal because none of these proteins bind significant amounts of T_3. Consequently, the FT_4 index values are spuriously elevated. Therefore, one should always consider the possibility of an abnormal T_4 binding protein when

Table 5 Factors Associated with Increased TBG Concentration

Pregnancy
Neonatal state
Estrogens
Oral contraceptives
Acute intermittent porphyria
Infectious and chronic active hepatitis
Perphenazine
Genetic determination

serum T_3 and resin T_3 uptake results are normal in the face of an elevated serum T_4 level. It should be emphasized that patients with elevated serum T_4 levels resulting from abnormal serum binding proteins are euthyroid, and no antithyroid treatment is indicated.

Generalized (pituitary and peripheral tissues) resistance to thyroid hormone is a rare disorder characterized by thyromegaly, elevated serum total and free T_4 and T_3 levels, a preserved TSH response to TRH, and absence of the usual symptoms and signs of thyrotoxicosis. Although this syndrome is probably congenital, it is rarely diagnosed at birth and more often recognized during childhood and adult life (97). In the majority of affected individuals, it is inherited in an autosomal dominant fashion, but recessive transmission has also been reported (97). The male-female ratio in GRTH is close to 1. The tissue resistance to thyroid hormones is selective, and studies have shown that the pituitary thyrotrophs and peripheral tissue fibroblasts respond normally to dopaminergic drugs and/or glucocorticoids (98,99). Pituitary secretion of TSH is responsible for the thyromegaly, increased thyroid gland activity, and excessive thyroid hormone synthesis and secretion seen in this syndrome. Although the serum TSH level may not always be elevated, it is always detectable, and administration of TRH produces a further increase in TSH levels. On the other hand, administration of supraphysiologic doses of exogenous T_3 suppresses pituitary secretion of TSH in virtually all affected patients.

The syndrome of GRTH results from mutations in one of the thyroid hormone receptor genes (84). There are two thyroid hormone receptor genes, c-erbAβ and c-erbAα, which are located on chromosomes 3 and 17, respectively (100). By alternative splicing of primary transcripts, these two genes code for four main isoforms of the thyroid hormone receptor (TRα1 and c-erbAα2 and TRβ1 and TRβ2). With the exception of the c-erbAα2 isoform, each of these proteins has both T_3 binding and DNA binding domains and functions as a thyroid hormone receptor (100). All molecular genetic studies on patients with GRTH have revealed mutations in the T_3 binding domain of the c-erbAβ gene, and to date, no patients with GRTH have been described with defects in the c-erbAα gene (84). These mutations result in thyroid hormone receptors with defective T_3 binding. Patients who inherit this disorder in an autosomal recessive fashion have mutations in both alleles of the c-erbAβ gene. On the other hand, those patients who inherit GRTH in an autosomal dominant fashion have a wild-type allele, as well as a mutant allele for the receptor. Although the mechanisms are not completely defined, these mutations are dominant negative in that the mutant receptors inhibit the function of the normal β receptor (from wild-type allele) and the normal α receptor (84).

Despite the elevated levels of circulating thyroid hormones, most patients with GRTH are clinically euthyroid. Although the symptoms and signs of hypo- or hyperthyroidism are generally absent, a few patients have been reported with retarded bone age, mental retardation, stunted growth, and hearing defects (101). Similarly, persistent tachycardia, tremor, anxiety, and hyperactivity have been observed in some patients (102). These findings suggest that the degree of resistance to thyroid hormone is not the same in all tissues.

The diagnosis of GRTH requires elevated serum levels of T_4 and free T_4. Serum T_3 and reverse T_3 levels are also elevated. The TBG level is normal, and the resin T_3 uptake is elevated. As mentioned earlier, serum TSH is always detectable, and the TSH response is either normal or exaggerated (81). The radioiodine uptake is increased. Laboratory tests of metabolic status, such as basal metabolic rate, serum cholesterol and triglycerides, and carotene, are usually normal.

Most patients with GRTH require no treatment, but resistance to thyroid hormone may vary from tissue to tissue. Some patients may benefit from treatment with pharmacologic doses of T_4 or T_3; this is especially true when the peripheral tissues are more resistant than the pituitary thyrotrophs. Affected children should be monitored closely for growth deceleration, delayed bone maturation, and impaired mental development, and thyroid hormone treatment should be instituted as necessary. Any therapeutic maneuvers that may reduce the elevated circulating thyroid hormone levels are contraindicated in GRTH and should be avoided.

Peripheral conversion of T_4 to T_3 occurs through the activity of 5'-deiodinase. A variety of pathophysiologic conditions and pharmacologic agents have been associated with impaired T_4 to T_3 conversion. The clinical syndrome of type I iodothyronine-deiodinase deficiency has been reported but appears to be extremely rare (103). The reported patient was clinically euthyroid and had elevated serum levels of T_4 and reverse T_3, along with normal serum T_3 and TSH levels (104).

Alterations in serum thyroid hormone levels often accompany nonthyroidal illnesses. Although the T_4 level is typically low or normal, on occasion it may be elevated. The euthyroid sick or nonthyroidal illness syndrome is discussed in Chapter 27.

Various drugs have been found to cause an elevation in serum T_4 levels in adults, but the majority of these agents are seldom, if ever, used in children or adolescents. Examples include amiodarone, propranolol, heparin, oral cholecystographic agents, and amphetamines.

Elevated serum T_4 levels are sometimes seen in clinically euthyroid children who are receiving replacement or suppressive therapy with L-T_4. In these children, the serum T_3 level is normal. The mechanism responsible for normal T_3 levels despite increased T_4 concentrations has not been completely defined but may be explained by the fact that 5'-deiodinase activity in peripheral tissues appears to be autoregulated by the levels of circulating T_4. Thus, as the serum T_4 concentration increases from low to elevated levels, the peripheral generation of T_3 from T_4 decreases, as reflected in the steady decline in the serum T_3/T_4 ratio (92). Therefore, in patients receiving L-T_4 therapy, the serum T_3 level is a better indicator of metabolic status than the serum T_4 level.

REFERENCES

1. Hayles AB, Zimmerman D. Graves' disease in childhood. In: Ingbar SH, Braverman LE, Werner's the Thyroid, 5th ed. Philadelphia: J. B. Lippincott, 1986: 1412–1428.
2. Tomer Y, Huber GK, Davies TF. Human chorionic gonadotropin (hCG) interacts directly with recombinant human TSH receptors. J Clin Endocrinol Metab 1992; 74:1477.
3. Seely BL, Burrow GN. Thyrotoxicosis in pregnancy. Endocrinologist 1991; 1:409.
4. Ingbar SH. The thyroid gland. In: Wilson JD, Foster DW, eds. William's Textbook of Endocrinology, 7th ed. Philadelphia: W. B. Saunders, pp 1985:682–815.
5. Hollingsworth DR, Mabry CC. Congenital Graves' disease: four familial cases with long-term follow-up and perspective. Am J Dis Child 1976; 130:148.
6. Zakarija M, McKenzie JM. Pregnancy associated changes in the thyroid stimulating antibody of Graves' disease and the relationship to neonatal hyperthyroidism. J Clin Endocrinol Metab 1983; 57:1036.
7. Fisher DA. Neonatal thyroid disease in the offspring of women with autoimmune thyroid disease. Thyroid Today, 1986; 9(4):1–7.
8. Hawe P, Francis HH. Pregnancy and thyrotoxicosis. BMJ 1962; 2:817.
9. Zakarija M, McKenzie JM, Hoffman WH. Prediction and therapy of intrauterine and late onset neonatal hyperthyroidism. J Clin Endocrinol Metab 1986; 62:368.
10. Singer J. Neonatal thyrotoxicosis. J Pediatr 1977; 91:749.
11. McKenzie JM, Zakarija M. The clinical use of thyrotropin receptor antibody measurements. J Clin Endocrinol Metab 1989; 69:1093.
12. Matsura N, Konishi J, Fujieda K, et al. TSH-receptor antibodies in mothers with Graves' disease and outcome in their offspring. Lancet 1988; 1:14.
13. Pekonen F, Teramo K, Ikonen E, et al. Prenatal diagnosis and treatment of thyrotoxicosis. Acta Endocrinol (Copenh) 1983; 256(Suppl 103):111.
14. Cove DH, Johnston P. Fetal hyperthyroidism: experience of treatment in four siblings. Lancet 1985; 1:430.
15. Karpman BA, Rapoport B, Filetti S, Fisher DA. Treatment of neonatal hyperthyroidism due to Graves' disease with sodium ipodate. J Clin Endocrinol Metab 1987; 64:119.
16. Transue D, Chan J, Kaplan M. Management of neonatal Graves' disease with iopanoic acid. J Pediatr 1992; 121:472.
17. Joshi R, Kulin HE. Treatment of neonatal Graves' disease with sodium ipodate. Clin Pediatr (Phila) 1993; 32:181.
18. Williams DE, Chopra IJ, Orgiazzi J, et al. Corticosteroid-induced acute reduction in thyroid secretion in Graves' disease. Clin Res 1975; 23:244A.
19. Clayton GW. Thyrotoxicosis in children. In: Kaplan SA, ed.

Clinical Pediatric and Pediatric and Adolescent Endocrinology. Philadelphia: W. B. Saunders, 1982:110–117.

20. Farid NR. Immunogenetics of autoimmune thyroid disorders. Endocrinol Metab Clin North Am 1987; 16:229.

21. Farid NR, Stenszky V, Balazs C, et al. The major histo-compatibility complex and autoimmune thyroid disease. Mt Sinai J Med 1986; 53:6.

22. Smith EM, Morrill AC, Meyer WJ III, et al. Corticotropin releasing factor induction of leukocyte-derived immunoreactive ACTH and endorphins. Nature 1986; 32:881.

23. Hayles AB, Chaves-Carballo E. Diagnosis and treatment of exophthalmic goiter in children. Clin Pediatr (Phila) 1967; 6:681.

24. Nagayama Y, Rapoport B. The thyrotropin receptor 25 years after its discovery: new insight after its molecular cloning. Mol Endocrinol 1992; 6:145.

25. Vassart G, Dumont JE. The thyrotropin receptor and the regulation of thyrocyte function and growth. Endocr Rev 1992; 13:596.

26. Vassart G, Parmentier M, Libert F, Dumont J. Molecular genetics of the thyrotropin receptor. Trends Endocrinol Metab 1991; 2:151.

27. Weetman AP, Yateman ME, Ealey PA, et al. Thyroid-stimulating antibody activity between different immunoglobulin G subclasses. J Clin Invest 1990; 86:723.

28. Kraiem Z, Cho BY, Sadeh O, et al. The IgG subclass distribution of TSH receptor blocking antibodies in primary hypothyroidism. Clin Endocrinol (Copenh) 1992; 37:135.

29. Davies TF. New thinking on the immunology of Graves' disease. Thyroid Today 1992; 15(4):1–11.

30. Gupta MK. Thyrotropin receptor antibodies: advances and importance of detection techniques in thyroid diseases. Clin Biochem 1992; 25:193.

31. Rees Smith B, McLachlan SM, Furmaniak J. Autoantibodies to the thyrotropin receptor. Endocr Rev 1988; 9:106.

32. Kosugi S, Ban T, Akamizu T, Kohn LD. Identification of separate determinants on the thyrotropin receptor reactive with Graves' thyroid-stimulating antibodies and with thyroid-stimulating blocking antibodies in idiopathic myxedema; these determinants have no homologous sequence on gonadotropin receptors. Mol Endocrinol 1992; 6:168.

33. Nagayama Y, Wadsworth HL, Russo D, et al. Binding domains of stimulatory and inhibitory thyrotropin (TSH) receptor auto-antibodies determined with chimeric TSH-lutropin/chorionic gonadotropin receptors. J Clin Invest 1991; 88:336.

34. Nagayama Y, Rapoport B. Thyroid stimulatory antibodies in different patients with autoimmune thyroid disease do not all recognize the same components of the human thyrotropin receptor: selective role of receptor amino acids Ser_{25}-Glu_{30}. J Clin Endocrinol Metab 1992; 75:1425.

35. Kosugi S, Ban T, Kohn LD. Identification of thyroid-stimulating antibody-specific interaction sites in the N-terminal region of the thyrotropin receptor. Mol Endocrinol 1993; 7:114.

36. Dallas JS, Desai RK, Cunningham SJ, et al. TSH interacts with multiple discrete regions of the TSH receptor: polyclonal rabbit antibodies to one or more of these regions can inhibit TSH binding and function. Endocrinology 1994; 134:1437.

37. Weetman AP, McGregor AM. Autoimmune thyroid disease: developments in our understanding. Endocr Rev 1984; 5:209.

38. Valente WA, Vitti P, Yavin Z, et al. Monoclonal antibodies to the thyrotropin receptor: stimulating and blocking antibodies derived from the lymphocytes of patients with Graves' disease. Proc Natl Acad Sci USA 1982; 79:6680.

39. Volpe R. Suppressor T lymphocyte dysfunction is important in the pathogenesis of autoimmune thyroid disease: a perspective. Thyroid 1993; 3:345.

40. Zakarija M, McKenzie JM, Banovac K. Clinical significance of assay of thyroid-stimulating antibody in Graves' disease. Ann Intern Med 1980; 93:28.

41. Weiss M, Ingbar SH, Windblad S, et al. Demonstration of a saturable binding site for thyrotropin in *Yersinia enterocolitica*. Science 1983; 219:131.

42. Tomer Y, Davies TF. Infection, thyroid disease, and autoimmunity. Endocr Rev 1993; 14:107.

43. Londei M, Lamb JR, Botazzo GF, et al. Epithelial cells expressing aberrant MHC class II determinants can present antigen to cloned human T cells. Nature 1984; 312:639.

44. Southgate K, Creagh FM, Teece M, et al. A receptor assay for the measurement of TSH receptor antibodies in unextracted serum. Clin Endocrinol (Oxf) 1984; 20:539.

45. Foley TP Jr, White C, New A. Juvenile Graves' disease: usefulness and limitations of thyrotropin receptor antibody determinations. J Pediatr 1987; 110:378.

46. Takasu N, Yamada T, Katakura M, et al. Evidence for thyrotropin (TSH)-blocking activity in goitrous Hashimoto's thyroiditis with assays measuring inhibition of TSH receptor binding and TSH-stimulated thyroid adenosine 3′,5′-monophosphate responses/cell growth by immunoglobulins. J Clin Endocrinol Metab 1987; 64:239.

47. Filetti S, Foti D, Costante G, Rapoport B. Recombinant human thyrotropin (TSH) receptor in a radioreceptor assay for the measurement of TSH receptor autoantibodies. J Clin Endocrinol Metab 1991; 72:1096.

48. Costagliola S, Swillens S, Niccoli P, et al. Binding assay for thyrotropin receptor autoantibodies using the recombinant receptor protein. J Clin Endocrinol Metab 1992; 75:1540.

49. Vitti P, Elisei R, Tonacchera M, et al. Detection of thyroid-stimulating antibody using Chinese hamster ovary cells transfected with cloned human thyrotropin receptor. J Clin Endocrinol Metab 1993; 76:499.

50. Creagh F, Teece M, Williams S, et al. An analysis of thyrotropin receptor binding and thyroid stimulating activities in a series of Graves' sera. Clin Endocrinol (Oxf) 1985; 23:395.

51. Ginsberg J, Shewring G, Rees Smith B. TSH receptor binding and thyroid stimulation by sera from patients with Graves' disease. Clin Endocrinol (Oxf) 1983; 19:305.

52. Zakarija M, McKenzie JM. The spectrum and significance of autoantibodies reacting with the thyrotropin receptor. Endocrinol Metab Clin North Am 1987; 16:343.

53. Perros P, Kendall-Taylor P. Pathogenesis of thyroid-associated ophthalmopathy. Trends Endocrinol Metab 1993; 4:270.

54. Bahn RS, Heufelder AE. Pathogenesis of Graves' ophthalmopathy. N Engl J Med 1993; 329:1468.

55. Burch HB, Wartofsky L. Graves' ophthalmopathy: current concepts regarding pathogenesis and management. Endocr Rev 1993; 14:747.

56. Ross DS. Current therapeutic approaches to hyperthyroidism. Trends Endocrinol Metab 1993; 4:281.

57. Cooper DS. Antithyroid drugs. N Engl J Med 1984; 311:1353.

58. Wartofsky L. Has the use of antithyroid drugs for Graves' disease become obsolete? Thyroid 1993; 3:335.

59. Hashizume K, Ichikawa K, Sakurai A, et al. Administration of thyroxine in treated Graves' disease. N Engl J Med 1991; 324:947.

60. Lee WNP, Mpanias PD, Wimmer RJ, et al. Use of I-^{123} in early radioiodide uptake and its suppression in children and adolescents with hyperthyroidism. J Nucl Med 1978; 19:985.

61. McGregor AM, Rees Smith B, Hall R, et al. Prediction of relapse in hyperthyroid Graves' disease. Lancet 1980; 1:1101.

62. Allannic H, Fauchet R, Lorcy Y, et al. A prospective study of the relationship between relapse of hyperthyroid Graves' disease after antithyroid drugs and HLA haplotype. J Clin Endocrinol Metab 1983; 57:719.

63. Wiersinga WM. Propranolol and thyroid hormone metabolism. Thyroid 1991; 1:273.

64. Safa AM, Schumacher OP, Rodriquez-Antunez A. Long term follow-up in children and adolescents treated with radioactive iodine (^{131}I) for hyperthyroidism. N Engl J Med 1975; 292:167.

65. Freitas JE, Swanson DP, Gross MD, Sisson JG. Iodine 131: optimal therapy for hyperthyroidism in children and adolescents. J Nucl Med 1979; 20:847.

66. Shumacher OP, Safa AM. Long-term follow up results in children and adolescents treated with radioactive iodine (131-I) for hyperthyroidism. Pediatr Res 1978; 12:366A.

67. Farrar JJ, Toft AD. Iodine-131 treatment of hyperthyroidism: current issues. Clin Endocrinol, (Copenh) 1991; 35:207.

68. Zimmerman D, Gan-Gaisano M. Hyperthyroidism in children and adolescents. Pediatr Clin North Am 1990; 37:1273.

69. Howard CP, Hayles AB. Hyperthyroidism in childhood. Clin Endocrinol Metab 1978; 7:127.

70. Lyons J, Landis CA, Harsh G, et al. Two G protein oncogenes in human endocrine tumors. Science 1990; 249:655.

71. Parma J, Duprez L, Van Sande J, et al. Somatic mutations in the thyrotropin receptor gene cause hyperfunctioning thyroid adenomas. Nature 1993; 365:649.

72. Namba H, Ross JL, Goodman D, Fagin JA. Solitary polyclonal autonomous thyroid nodule: a rare cause of childhood hyperthyroidism. J Clin Endocrinol Metab 1991; 72:1108.

73. Hamilton CR, Maloof F. Unusual types of hyperthyroidism. Medicine (Baltimore) 1973; 52:195.

74. DiGeorge AM. Albright syndrome: is it coming of age? J Pediatr 1975; 87:1018.

75. Samuel S, Gilman S, Maurer HS, Rosenthal IM. Hyperthyroidism in an infant with McCune-Albright syndrome: report of a case with myeloid metaplasia. J Pediatr 1972; 80:275.

76. Schwindinger WF, Levine MA. McCune-Albright syndrome. Trends Endocrinol Metab 1993; 4:238.

77. Spada A, Vallar L, Faglia G. G protein oncogenes in pituitary tumors. Trends Endocrinol Metab 1992; 3:355.

78. Molnar GD, Wilber RD, Lee RE, et al. On the hyperfunctioning solitary thyroid nodule. Mayo Clin Proc 1965; 40:665.

79. Ridgeway EC, Weintraub BD, Cevallos JL, et al. Suppression of pituitary TSH secretion in the patient with a hyperfunctioning thyroid nodule. J Clin Invest 1973; 52:2783.

80. Paracchi A, Ferrari C, Livraghi T, et al. Percutaneous intranodular ethanol injection: a new treatment for autonomous thyroid adenoma. J Endocrinol Invest 1992; 15:353.

81. Weintraub BD, Gershengorn MC, Kourides IA, Fein H. Inappropriate secretion of thyroid-stimulating hormone. Ann Intern Med 1981; 95:339.

82. Kourides IA. TSH-induced hyperthyroidism. In: Ingbar SH, Braverman LE, eds. Werner's the Thyroid, 5th ed. Philadelphia: J. B. Lippincott, 1986:1064–1071.

83. Beck-Peccoz P, Forloni F, Cortelazzi D, et al. Pituitary resistance to thyroid hormones. Horm Res 1992; 38:66.

84. Usala SJ. Molecular diagnosis and characterization of thyroid hormone resistance syndromes. Thyroid 1991; 1:361.

85. Magner JA. TSH-mediated hyperthyroidism. Endocrinologist 1993; 3:289.

86. Kourides IA, Ridgway C, Weintraub BD, et al. Thyrotropin-induced hyperthyroidism: use of alpha and beta subunit levels to identify patients with pituitary tumors. J Clin Endocrinol Metab 1977; 45:534.

87. Oppenheim DS. TSH- and other glycoprotein-producing pituitary adenomas: alpha-subunit as a tumor marker. Thyroid Today 1991; 14(3):1–11.

88. Rosler A, Litvin Y, Hage C, et al. Familial hyperthyroidism due to inappropriate thyrotropin secretion successfully treated with triiodothyronine. J Clin Endocrinol Metab 1982; 54:76.

89. Klett M, Schonberg D. Congenital hyperthyroidism due to inappropriate secretion of thyroid stimulating hormone. In: Proceedings of the 26th Annual Meeting of the European Society for Paediatric Endocrinology, Toulouse, September 6–8, 1987, Abstract 178.

90. Beck-Peccoz P, Piscitelli G, Cattaneo MG, Faglia G. Successful treatment of hyperthyroidism due to non-neoplastic pituitary TSH hypersecretion with 3,5,3'-triiodothyroacetic acid (TRIAC). J Endocrinol Invest 1983; 6:217.

91. Furth J, Moy P, Hershman JM, Ueda G. Thyrotropic tumor syndrome. Arch Pathol 1973; 96:217.

92. Cohen JH III, Ingbar SH, Braverman LE. Thyrotoxicosis due to ingestion of excess thyroid hormone. Endocr Rev 1989; 10:113.

93. Litovitz TL, White JD. Levothyroxine ingestions in children: an analysis of 78 cases. Am J Emerg Med 1985; 3:297.

94. Kulig K, Golightly LK, Rumack BH. Levothyroxine overdose associated with seizures in a young child. JAMA 1985; 254:2109.

95. Lehrner LM, Weir MR. Acute ingestions of thyroid hormones. Pediatrics 1984; 73:313.

96. Golightly LK, Smolinske SC, Kulig KW, et al. Clinical effects of accidental levothyroxine ingestion in children. Am J Dis Child 1987; 141:1025.

97. Jaffiol C, de Boisvilliers F, Baldet L, Torresani J. Thyroid hormone generalized resistance. Horm Res 1992; 38:62.

98. Cooper DS, Ladenson PW, Nisula BC, et al. Familial thyroid hormone resistance. Metabolism 1982; 31:504.

99. Murata Y, Refetoff S, Horowitz AL, Smith TJ. Hormonal regulation of glycosaminoglycan accumulation in fibroblasts from patients with resistance to thyroid hormone. J Clin Endocrinol Metab 1983; 57:1233.

100. Chin WW. Current concepts of thyroid hormone action: progress notes for the clinician. Thyroid Today 1992; 15(3):1–9.

101. Refetoff S, Salazar A, Smith TJ, Scherberg NH. The consequences of inappropriate treatment due to failure to recognize the syndrome of pituitary and peripheral tissue resistance to thyroid hormone. Metabolism 1983; 32:822.

102. Bode HH, Danon M, Weintraub BD, et al. Partial target organ resistance to thyroid hormone. J Clin Invest 1973; 52:776.

103. St Germain DL. Iodothyronine deiodinases. Trends Endocrinol Metab 1994; 5:36.

104. Kleinhaus N, Faber J, Kahana L, et al. Euthyroid hyperthyroxinemia due to generalized 5'-deiodinase defect. J Clin Endocrinol Metab 1988; 66:684.

29

Thyroid Nodules in Children and Adolescents

Max Salas

University Of Medicine and Dentistry of New Jersey–Robert Wood Johnson Medical School,
New Brunswick, New Jersey

I. INTRODUCTION

Thyroid nodules are firm, palpable, and distinct localized masses of the thyroid gland. These are frequently asymptomatic and can occur singly or multiply. Benign, nonneoplastic nodules are far more common than malignant tumors. However, because of the possibility, malignancy thyroid nodules require a careful and complete evaluation. Because of the anatomic structure of the neck, the thyroid nodule may be clinically undetected for some time. Therefore, a careful physical examination is need. The functional status of the nodule varies. Most thyroid nodules are hypofunctional. A few produce hormones, such as thyroxine (T_4), triiodothyronine (T_3), and, in selected cases, calcitonin (medullary carcinoma of the thyroid): nodules producing high quantities of thyroid hormones could block the release of thyrotropin (thyroid-stimulating hormone, TSH) and produce hyperthyroidism. Nodules may also hypertrophy as a result of TSH stimulation in a generally hypoactive gland (1). Therefore, when examining a child, it is important to examine the neck and thyroid gland. If a nodule is felt, an assessment of the patient is needed to determine the thyroid status as well as the nature of the nodule.

II. INCIDENCE

Thyroid nodules are common in the adult population (3–5%), with a gradual increase from 1% in the second decade to 5% in the sixth decade and beyond (2–4). The incidence is higher in women (6.4%) than in men (1.5%) (5,6). These figures, however, underestimate the magnitude of the problem (7). In one study done by sonogram, the incidence in normal glands was 21% in women (8), and in autopsies nodules are present in 37–57% (9,10). The exact incidence is difficult to determine because a single type of abnormality is reported in most studies (11). However, thyroid nodules occur infrequently in children (1.5% or less) (12–14). The significance of the thyroid nodules in children became apparent in the 1950s when a sharp increase in thyroid neoplasia occurred associated with irradiation to the head, neck, pharynx, and upper thorax (15–19). Radiation for a variety of childhood disorders, such as enlarged thymus and tonsils, acne, and hemangiomas, was a commonly accepted therapy until the 1950s.

The increment in the incidence of thyroid carcinomas peaked in 1954, and by 1960 it had decreased by half (11). Because of the studies linking head and neck irradiation with thyroid malignancies, it ceased to be an accepted practice; however, irradiation to the area for therapeutic reasons (primary malignant tumors) continues to be frequently associated with secondary neoplasms (20,21). According to Schneider et al. (22), a radiation dosage of 750 rad or more is needed for a thyroid neoplasia to develop, and its incidence increases 10 years after the patient is exposed to the radiation. In a large-scale study, the same author found a 30% incidence of thyroid nodules in irradiated children, of which 36% were malignant (papillary and papillary-follicular carcinomas). In a long-term study, deVathaire et al. (23) reported 396 children followed after 11–43 years of being exposed to thyroid irradiation for skin angiomas. The frequency of nodules was 6%, and the absolute incidence rate of thyroid nodules was 1.8 per 10^3py Gy-person-years (100 rad-person-years). The risk increased significantly with the total dose of radiation to the thyroid delivered in a short period of time. Before the 1950s, the incidence of thyroid carcinoma in children was very low. From 1900 to 1930, Hayles et al. (24,25) found no cases in 57 patients seen at the Mayo Clinic for thyroid nodules but detected 57% in 121 patients from 1930 to 1955. On the other hand, Rallison et al. (14) found thyroid nodules in only 1.8% of 5179 children examined, of which 31 were thyroiditis, 31 adolescent goiter, and only 2 were carcinoma.

Rallison et al. believed that the risk of thyroid malignancy in normal children in whom nodularity is incidentally discovered by physical examination is approximately 2%.

III. CLINICAL APPROACH

The clinical approach to solitary nodules in children and adolescents varies, but it requires careful evaluation. Because thyroid nodules can be confused with other neck masses in children, the diagnostic assessment is distinct from that in adults, because the etiology and frequency differ. In chidren, infections and congenital defects (cysts and ectopia) are more common, whereas trauma and malignancy are less common (26). Because thyroid nodules are uncommon in children before puberty, a nodule discovered in such an age group should be viewed with suspicion (6,12,27). The incidence of cancer in thyroid nodules before adolescence varies from 20 to 73% (6), and therefore the approach should be more aggressive in children.

Some authors believe that all thyroid nodules are potentially malignant and therefore should be excised as soon as possible (25,28–30). Others believe that because of the low incidence and degree of malignancy and the high level of suppressibility with thyroid therapy, the risk of death and disability as a result of surgery is too high to justify it (31,32). At present, most physicians take the intermediate approach and individualize the diagnosis and the management of these patients (33). We recommend the following consideration when a patient is found to have a thyroid nodule: Analysis of the patient with a thyroid nodule must be organized and systematized (Fig. 1). Malignant causes include a variety of thyroid cancers, as reviewed in Chapter 31. Benign causes are lobulation of normal thyroid tissue, Hashimoto's thyroiditis (chronic lymphocytic thyroiditis, CLT), thyroid cysts, thyroglossal duct cysts, ectopic thyroid tissue, thyroid teratoma (11), adenoma, adenomatous nodule, hypertrophy of one lobe because of congenital agenesis of the other lobe, nonthyroid disease, abscess, and adenoma associated with CLT (4,11–14,33–36).

The history of irradiation to the neck and other surrounding areas (diagnostic or therapeutic) (37), as well as recent growth of a nodule, should make one consider the possibility of malignancy. One must also consider whether the patient comes from an area in which goiter is endemic, consumes goitrogenic foods, or has received goitrogens (38). Detailed information about the rate of growth of the nodule should be obtained, as well as the presence of local signs of compression, such as dysphagia, dysphonia (39), dyspnea, and hemoptysis (6). The association of thyroid nodules and congenital deafness should raise the diagnostic possibility of Pendred syndrome, which is frequently familial and in which goiter quite often develops during puberty. The history of thyroid carcinoma, pheochromocytoma, or multiple endocrine neoplasia (MEN) in other members of the family should make one think of medullary carcinoma. After a careful history, the physical examination is the first crucial step in the diagnosis of thyroid nodules (39,40). Examination of the neck, thyroid gland, lymph nodes, and salivary glands should be done very carefully. The size and morphologic structure can be assessed by inspection, as the patient swallows. In a thin person, a thyroid gland of normal size may be interpreted as enlarged, and the compensated hypertrophy of a hemiagenetic thyroid or the normal pyramidal lobe may be felt as a nodule. Careful palpation by the fingers and thumb of each lobe, while the trachea is mobilized sideways by the other hand, helps localize small nodules. Also, as the patient swallows, it is important to exclude low midline nodules and extension of the retrosternum by palpating the inferior and lateral aspects of the thyroid gland. Nodules larger than 1 cm in diameter should be detected during the examination; on the other hand, those smaller than 0.5 cm are difficult to detect (6).

The cervical lymph nodes should also be palpated, looking for enlargement. Any abnormal findings should be recorded in a drawing of the anatomic area on adhesive paper tape, taped to the neck of the patient and then placed in the chart for future reference. Clinical symptoms and signs suggestive of malignancy are recent, rapid, or painful enlargement of the thyroid; hoarseness or symptoms of obstruction; a single nodule in a normally sized gland; fixation of the thyroid or a nodule to the trachea or muscle; evidence of obstruction or compression; and cervical lymphadenopathy.

The key points to consider are whether the nodule is present in an otherwise unenlarged thyroid gland or whether it is part of a diffusely enlarged gland. The latter is most likely a benign process, such as thyroiditis, and in the former a differential diagnosis should include neoplasia. A well-defined nodule of normal consistency is very likely a benign process, such as thyroiditis, cyst, or cystic adenoma; a firm or stony hard nodule, especially if fixed to surrounding structures (not moving with swallowing), is highly suggestive of carcinoma (43–90% of thyroid carcinomas are hard) (33). Carcinoma is also suggested when paralysis of the vocal cords is present (33,34).

The presence of hoarseness requires direct visualization of the vocal cords by laryngoscope. Dysphagia also deserves consideration and examination by endoscopy. A tender nodule could be an inflammatory reaction or hemorrhage. The presence of regional lymphadenopathy should arouse the suspicion of malignancy. Soft nodules are usually benign (10% are malignant). The presence of multiple mucosal neuromas, whitish nodules of the tongue, palpebral conjunctiva, and commissures of the lips suggests medullary carcinoma (39). The rate of growth of the nodule is also important, because one stable in size for years is usually benign. A rapidly growing nodule that increased in size while the patient was in suppressive thyroid therapy is suggestive of autonomy and therefore of malignancy (6).

Laboratory tests are necessary to identify the nature of the thyroid nodule, because none of the historical or physical findings are sufficient to make a definitive diagnosis. It is possible to arrive at a reasonably accurate diagnosis using several diagnostic techniques and laboratory methods. The following are the most important.

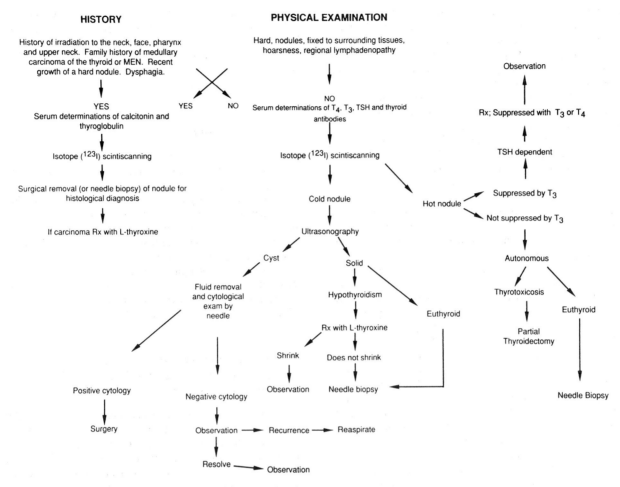

Figure 1 Analysis of the patient with a solitary thyroid nodule.

A. Ultrasonography or Echography

This noninvasive diagnostic technique is most useful for determining whether nodules are solid or cystic. However, it provides more anatomic than functional information. It may be useful to the pediatrician to determine whether there is a nodule in the thyroid. Often it may be difficult to differentiate with certainty the presence of thyroid nodules from cervical lymphadenopathy in the thyroid region. A sonogram assists the clinician in determining the presence or absence of a thyroid nodule before subjecting the patient to unnecessary referrals or more complicated testing. Ultrasonography consists of the transmission of sound (frequency 2–5 million cps) through a tissue and the analysis of the response (by the echo wave reflected by interfaces of tissue borders). Fluid (as in a cyst) produces a homogeneous echo, and solid tissue produces many interfaces. The solid nodules that become hemorrhagic and, therefore, partially cystic can be distinguished from simple cysts and solid tumors (33,35,36,40,41). Ultrasonography can also disclose nodules smaller than 1 cm in diameter, as well as changes in the trachea, lymph nodes, carotid vessels, and surface of the neck. It has the advantage that it does not use radioactive agents. Thyroid cysts are rarely malignant, but complex partially solid cysts may be malignant. In one study (30), half of the patients with thyroid carcinoma had cystic lesions. Echography can be helpful in planning needle aspiration or the surgical approach. It can also be useful in the follow-up of thyroid lesions (cystic nodules, nodule size, and recurrence).

B. Isotope Scintiscanning with Radioactive Iodine

This is probably the most useful of the laboratory procedures in the differential diagnosis of the thyroid nodule, including such anomalies as agenesis of a thyroid lobe with compensatory enlargement of the contralateral lobe presenting as a solitary nodule (42). It allows the thyroid nodules to be classified into two major groups, hot or functioning and cold or nonfunctioning, depending on the quantity of radioactivity in the nodule compared with the rest of the thyroid. A hot nodule has a very small possibility of being malignant (less than 5%).

A cold nodule in a normal child is strongly suggestive of carcinoma; a 50% chance of being malignant is expected.

The limitation of the thyroid scan is that it is a two-dimensional scanning technique (superimposition of normally functional thyroid tissue and abnormal nodular tissue) (7) that does not differentiate definitely benign from malignant lesions (42) and does not detect a nodule smaller than 1 cm in diameter (30,43–45). The functional status of the thyroid nodule can also be defined using an iodine isotope, which can measure trapping and organification, as opposed to technetium, which measures only trapping. There are many reports citing functional discrepancies between technetium and iodine scans: nodules that appear hot or warm on ^{99m}Tc scans are cold on radioiodine scans (3–8%) (7,46,47). (1) As a general principle, radioactive iodine uptake determines thyroid function and thyroid scan analyzes the anatomic integrity of the thyroid gland. Iodine 123 is better for use in children than ^{131}I because it is 100 times less radioactive (43); (2) and is the only radioisotope of iodine that should be used in children for diagnostic purposes.

The next step in the diagnosis of the hot nodules is to determine whether they are autonomous or TSH dependent. The autonomously functioning thyroid nodules in children and adolescents are unusual and have a more rapidly progressive course than those found in adults. They are independent of TSH and may appear as solitary nodules, patchy areas, or multiple nodules (48). The administration of T_3, 25 μg three times a day for 10–13 days, suppresses the TSH-dependent nodule and decreases its size as well as the ^{123}I uptake. When the nodule is not suppressed by T_3, the term "autonomous" is used. The scan and uptake measurements must be taken before and after the suppression test for comparison. It is important to compare the activity in the nodule with the activity of the rest of the parenchyma, because this ratio is stable in the TSH-dependent, but not in the autonomous, nodules (44). The clinical course of the autonomous nodules is quite variable, but basically it can be divided into five groups: (1) no change in the function of the thyroid, autonomy persists; (2) nodule changes from hot to warm, autonomy persists; (3) TSH dependence is reestablished; (4) TSH dependence is reestablished, and there is degeneration of the nodule; and (5) transformation from nontoxic to toxic (1,49–52). However, it must be remembered that carcinoma has been found in one in four cases of autonomously functioning nodules, and hence this diagnostic procedure is of limited value (43).

Cold or nonfunctioning nodules are important in children but are nonspecific. Causes include cysts, adenomas, thyroiditis, nontoxic nodular goiter, and carcinoma (1). The possibility that a discrete, cold nodule is a carcinoma in a child with a normal-appearing gland is about 50% (53). Cold nodules can be discovered by scintiscanning only if they are at least 8 mm in diameter, and they may go undetected if the uptake of the isotope by the thyroid gland is low or if the nodules are located on the periphery of the gland (44). Occasionally a hot nodule is actually a cold nodule when it is located on the posterior or anterior surface of the thyroid and has functioning thyroid tissue in front of or behind it. Here, an oblique view shows the difference (54,55). These patients are the most difficult in terms of diagnosis because

the delineation between a benign and a potentially dangerous lesion becomes less distinct. Many other radioisotopes besides ^{123}I, ^{131}I, and ^{99m}Tc have been used in the diagnosis of cold nodules. These include ^{32}P, ^{75}Semethionine, ^{67}Ga, ^{67}Ga citrate, ^{197}HgCl, and ^{131}CeCl (44), but none have proved to be more specific or more sensitive.

C. Serum Determinations of T$_4$, T$_3$, TSH, and Thyroid Antibodies

Elevation of TSH, with or without low levels of T_4 and T_3, in a patient with a thyroid nodule suggests hypothyroidism and is practically diagnostic of Hashimoto's thyroiditis. This reduces the possibility of malignancy, but it does not eliminate it (see Chap. 31) (56). Thyroiditis can be confirmed by the presence of thyroid antibodies (antimicrosomal and antithyroglobulin). On the other hand, the elevation in T_4 and T_3 is seen in nodules that are autonomous and hyperfunctioning. These are usually benign. Sometimes the patients are clinically euthyroid, and the elevated levels of T_3, which cause no response of TSH to thyrotropin-releasing hormone (TRH) (57), may be the only manifestation of thyroid dysfunction (58).

D. Serum Determinations of Calcitonin (Pentagastrin or Calcium Induced), Histamine, and Thyroglobulin

High levels of calcitonin and histamine indicate medullary carcinoma of the thyroid. Thyroglobulin may be elevated in papillary or follicular carcinoma, but it can also be elevated in benign conditions, such as thyroiditis and hyperthyroidism. Therefore, the specificity of thyroglobulin as a diagnostic tool is poor and should not be used except as a follow-up for a patient with thyroid resection for carcinoma.

E. Needle Biopsy in the Diagnosis of Thyroid Nodules

In the past, when a histologic diagnosis was necessary, surgical removal of the thyroid nodule was standard procedure. Since 1956 (Hamlin and Vickery), however, the needle biopsy has proven to be a reliable tool, with up to 94% accuracy. The procedure is safe and accurate and avoids unnecessary operations (and surgical scars) in most patients (59–64). The sensitivity is 86.3%, with 2.4% false negative results when suspicious cytologic findings are considered positive rather than negative (65.7 and 6.5%, respectively) (64).

In other studies the sensitivity varied from 71.5 to 95%, the specificity from 75 to 97.5%, predictive value for a positive and negative results 97%, and accuracy 82.2% (65–68). However, conventional analysis of sensitivity and specificity can be misleading and confusing. Ideally, the procedure should be able to determine whether a nodule is benign or malignant. Unfortunately, needle biopsy is unable to distinguish differentiated follicular thyroid cancer from a cellular or microfollicular adenoma (7,69–72). There can be four different results from a biopsy: malignant, benign, nondiagnostic, and indeterminate or suspicious. The indeterminate or suspicious category comprises about 20% of all biopsies. A major limiting factor is that invasion is rarely detected by needle biopsy and only surgical removal of the nodule can ascertain its noninvasive nature. To complicate matters, there is a great deal of confusion because of a nonuniform nomenclature for cytopathologic description (73). Cytologic false negative results range from 1 to 6% (74), mainly the results of misdiagnosis or sampling errors (75) because of small size (less than 1 cm), large size (more than 4 cm), hemorrhage, multinodular glands, or inadequate biopsy specimens (76–78); 10% of the results are positive, of which 3–6% are falsely positive.

With both fine and large needles, the complications are negligible in experienced hands, and the accuracy of the two methods is similar. Therefore, when histologic diagnosis is important, it is preferable to obtain the tissue specimen by needle biopsy instead of by surgical excision. This, of course, depends on the availability of an experienced surgeon as well as a competent cytopathologist. Aspiration of fluid is the procedure of choice in the diagnosis and treatment of a cyst.

F. Clinical Approach

In the presence of a solitary thyroid nodule, with the foregoing history and physical findings, the following guidelines are of value.

The first step is the measurement of serum T_4, T_3, TSH, and thyroid antibodies to determine the functional status of the thyroid because it is important to exclude hypothyroidism most likely caused by Hashimoto's thyroiditis or hyperthyroidism caused by a toxic nodule. The thyroid antibodies are useful when considering the diagnosis of Hashimoto's thyroiditis. This first step is followed by the isotope scintiscanning using ^{123}I or ^{131}I. If the nodule is warm (isofunctional), it is more likely benign and should be given a trial of thyroid suppressive therapy to determine change in size over time (57). If the nodule is hot, the differential diagnosis includes thyroiditis, adenoma, hyperplasia, and, rarely carcinoma (12). It can also be seen in agenesis of the contralateral lobe of the thyroid. In this case, the thyroid scan needs to be repeated following TSH stimulation and ultrasound (39). Single hot nodules may be thyrotoxic or nontoxic, and some may become toxic gradually; they also may or may not be autonomous. If the scanning reveals a cold nodule, ultrasonography is then indicated. When ultrasound shows a cyst, removal of the fluid by needle and its cytologic analysis is in order. If the cytology result is negative for malignant cells and the cyst resolves, only observation is necessary. If it recurs, reaspiration is indicated. When the result of the cytologic examination is positive or suspicious, surgical removal is mandatory (79). If the nodule is small (less than 4 cm in diameter) and the cytologic appearance is benign, it may be observed only every 4–6 months. If the nodule is solid and there is hypothyroidism, therapy with L-thyroxine is instituted and observation is the logical course. The most likely diagnosis is Hashimoto's thyroiditis, especially if

antibodies are present (although test results may be negative at some stages of the disease). If the nodule decreases with thyroid treatment, no further action is necessary. On the other hand, if it does not decrease in size, a needle biopsy is indicated. An enlarging cyst, a mixed solid-cystic nodule, and a solid nodule should be excised surgically. If the nodule is solid and the patient is euthyroid, suppressive therapy without further diagnostic studies is contraindicated because of the possibility of malignancy. According to Molitch et al. (80), the major weakness of this therapeutic trial is that there is a low initial probability of carcinoma, yet many benign nodules do not reduce in size. On the other hand, some malignancies decrease in size with thyroxine treatment. Failure to respond to medication increases the possibility of malignancy by only 10%, whereas shrinkage of the nodule reduces it by only 7–10%. In a more recent study, Gharib et al. (81) and Reverter et al. (82) observed no significant decrease in diameter of the nodule after 6 months of therapy. In these cases, aspiration biopsy or surgical removal of the nodule is indicated for diagnosis and treatment (34).

IV. TREATMENT

The patient with a TSH-dependent nodule can be treated with either L-thyroxine (75–100 μg/day) or L-triiodothyronine (50–75 μg/day), depending on age. There is some evidence that T_3 is more effective (33,83). Observation is necessary. The size of the nodule must be assessed very accurately by careful measurements and by repeat sonograms (33). Suppressive therapy is maintained for a minimum of 3 months, at which time the nodule is reassessed. During suppressive therapy, the nodule should regress over a 12 month period. Failure of suppressive therapy is indicated by (1) continued growth of the nodule, (2) reduction in size of less than 50%, and (3) reduction in ^{123}I or ^{131}I uptake to no less than 3%. If there is no suppression, the nodule is autonomous and requires surgical therapy.

The rationale behind the suppressive medical therapy is based upon clinical evidence as well as in vitro studies. These have shown that thyroid tissue, including some neoplasias, decrease in size when TSH is suppressed and grow under the effects of TSH. It is believed that a nodule that does not decrease in size when TSH is suppressed adequately is no longer under neuroendocrine control and therefore is potentially malignant. On the other hand, malignancy cannot be excluded when a nodule shrinks while under suppression; however, the malignancy is likely to remain inactive and, therefore, not destructive (33). Surgical excision of a benign tumor or cyst is usually curative and requires no additional therapy. If the nodule is histologically a lymphoid follicle and represents chronic lymphocytic thyroiditis, the patient should be evaluated for the development of primary hypothyroidism.

The management of thyroid malignancy depends upon the histologic character and location of the neoplastic tissue (see Chap. 31).

A chest x-ray should be performed preoperatively to determine whether there are pulmonary metastasis. In the presence of localized metastatic disease, some clinicians advocate ablative therapy with radioiodine after thyroidectomy and surgical excision of metastatic disease. In all instances the patient must be maintained on thyroid suppressive therapy with a dosage of L-thyroxine that maintains the serum T_4 value slightly above the upper limit of the normal range and a suppressed serum TSH level between 0.1 and 0.6 μU/ml.

Because no differentiated thyroid cancer takes up radioiodine in the presence of any significant amount of normal thyroid tissue, it is important that every patient with thyroid cancer be evaluated for metastases after total thyroidectomy. This is done by a body scan following the administration of ^{131}I while the patient is chemically hypothyroid (84). Thus, after total thyroidectomy the patient should be given no treatment until the TSH levels are high and the patient can undergo the body scan. If the patient was already started on thyroid replacement therapy, this should be stopped before the patient is restudied. The treatment of such patients is first switched to triiodothyronine (Cytomel) replacement. After 3–4 weeks, this is discontinued and TSH levels are evaluated. Usually, within 1–2 weeks a body scan can be performed (49).

Patients with medullary carcinoma of the thyroid should undergo total thyroidectomy and periodic evaluation for other associated tumors in the multiple endocrine neoplasia syndromes IIA and IIB. These tumors include pituitary adenoma, parathyroid adenoma, pheochromocytoma and adrenocortical tumors for MEN IIA, and gastrointestinal neuromas and pheochromocytoma in MEN IIB. The secretion of calcitonin after pentagastrin stimulation is useful to determine the presence of persistent medullary carcinoma following surgery. Similar tests should be performed in immediate family members because the disease is inherited as an autosomal dominant trait.

In patients who have a nodule and become hyperthyroid, a partial thyroidectomy is indicated. In these patients the diagnosis of Plummer syndrome is made. They usually do not undergo symptomatic remission while receiving antithyroid medication, although they may be suppressed and be maintained euthyroid until thyroidectomy can be done. Therapy with ^{131}I in the latter situation is not indicated because the rest of the gland would be exposed to the radioisotope (52). Carcinoma has been reported in a patient with a thyroid nodule treated with ^{131}I (59).

V. CONCLUSIONS

The previous guidelines are by no means definitive, and there is still a great deal of discussion about the management of the solitary thyroid nodule in children and adolescents. DeGroot summarized the difficulty in the diagnosis and management of patients with thyroid nodules (85).

Finding an inactive thyroid nodule does not significantly increase the likelihood of distinguishing the 5–10% malignant lesions from the 90–95% benign lesions. Functioning warm nodules can be malignant. Hot nodules are hardly every

malignant. The distinction between solid and cystic nodules is seldom clear-cut. Even when sonography is combined with fine-needle aspiration and cytologic examination, the diagnosis often remains unclear. Needle aspiration is rarely complete, and questions are raised about the remaining material. In about 10% of aspirations, the number of follicular cells is inadequate. A positive diagnosis can be made in 5–10% of the cases, but the diagnosis is uncertain in 10–20% of the samples. Using all techniques available, a reliable diagnosis in a benign thyroid nodule can be made in 60–70% of all the cases.

Many physicians believe that surgical resection of the nodule (hot or cold) is indicated only in the following situations: (1) rapid growth; (2) regional lymphadenopathy; (3) rock-like hardness; (4) dysphagia, hoarseness, or evidence of vocal cord paralysis; (5) history of irradiation to the face, neck, pharynx, and upper thorax; and (6) lack of suppression of the nodule while receiving T_3 therapy. Other investigators, however, because of the possibility of carcinoma, firmly believe that all nodules should be excised when adequate surgical facilities are available (27,43,83). We agree with such an approach, particularly for children and adolescents in whom the likelihood of malignancies is higher.

The most important studies for the patient with a solitary thyroid nodule are those designed to determine the structure and consistency of the thyroid gland: ultrasound to distinguish between solid and cystic lesions and the radionuclide scan to determine whether the nodule is functioning (hot) or nonfunctioning (cold). To ensure that the thyroid nodule is not associated with a nonsurgical lesion, such as Hashimoto's thyroiditis, serum thyroid antibody determinations are important. Because malignancy of the thyroid gland is usually not associated with abnormalities of thyroid function, laboratory tests to exclude hyperthyroidism (a serum T_3 determination) and hypothyroidism (a serum TSH) are important at the time of initial evaluation.

Additional tests are usually not necessary unless the patient has mild hyperthyroidism with an autonomously functioning nodule; the T_3 suppression test and TRH test are often useful. Rarely, the TSH stimulation test is helpful to determine suppressed thyroid tissue throughout the remainder of the gland.

Children with a solitary, solid, nonfunctioning (cold) nodule require surgical excisional biopsy. This procedure should not be performed, however, until all laboratory test results are available.

In conclusion, thyroid nodules are uncommon in children and adolescents. When a thyroid nodule is detected in a young patient, a decreased possibility of benign disease exists. It is therefore imperative to rule out malignancy.

REFERENCES

1. Hamburger JI. Evolution of toxicity in solitary autonomously functioning thyroid nodules. J Clin Endocrinol Metab 1980; 50:1089–1093.
2. Rojeski MT, Gharib H. Nodular thyroid disease. N Engl J Med 1985, 313:428–436.

3. Maxon HR, Thomas JR, Saenger EL, et al. Ionizing irradiation and the induction of clinically significant disease in the human thyroid gland. Am J Med 1977; 63:967–978.

4. Hansen GA, Komorowski RA, Cerlett JM, Wilson SD. Thyroid gland morphology in young adults: normal subjects versus those with prior low-dose neck irradiation in childhood. Surgery 1983; 94:984–988.

5. Vander JB, Gaston EA, Dawber TR. The significance on non-toxic thyroid nodules. Ann Intern Med 1968; 69:537–540.

6. Ridgway EC. Clinical evaluation of solitary thyroid nodules. In: Braverman LE, Utige R, eds. Werner and Inghar's the Thyroid, 6th ed. Philadelphia: J. B. Lippincott, 1991:1197–1203.

7. Ross DS. Evaluation of the thyroid nodule. J Nucl Med 1991; 32:2181–2192.

8. Carroll BA. Asymptomatic thyroid nodules. AJR 1982; 138:499–501.

9. Rice CO. Incidence of nodules in the thyroid. Arch Surg 1932; 42:505–515.

10. Mortensen JD, Woolner LB, Bennett WA. Gross and microscopic findings in clinically normal thyroid gland. J Clin Endocrinol Metab 1955; 15:1270–1280.

11. White AK, Smith RJH. Thyroid nodules in children. Otolaryngol Head Neck Surg 1986; 95:70.

12. Scott MD, Crawford JD. Solitary thyroid nodules in childhood: is the incidence of thyroid carcinoma declining? Pediatrics 1976; 58:521–525.

13. Kirkland RT, Kirkland JL, Rosenberg HS, et al. Solitary thyroid nodules in 30 children and report of a child with a thyroid abscess. Pediatrics 1973; 51:85–90.

14. Rallison ML, Dobyns BM, Keating R, et al. Thyroid nodularity in children. JAMA 1975; 233:1069–1072.

15. Duffy BJ, Fitzgerald PJ. Cancer of the thyroid in children. A report of 28 children. J Clin Endocrinol Metab 1950; 10:1296.

16. De Groot LJ, Paloyan E. Thyroid carcinoma and radiation, a Chicago epidemic. JAMA 1973; 225:487.

17. Favus MJ, Schneider AB, Stachura ME, et al. Thyroid cancer as a late consequence of head-neck irradiation: evaluation of 1056 patient. N Engl J Med 1976; 294:1019.

18. Hempelmann JH. Risk of thyroid neoplasms after irradiation in childhood: studies of population exposed to radiation in childhood show a dose-response over a wide dose range. Science 1968; 160:159.

19. Refetoff S, Harrosin J, Karanfilsski BT, et al. Continuing occurence of thyroid carcinoma after irradiation to the neck in infancy and childhood. N Engl J Med 1975; 269:171.

20. Vane D, King DR, Coles ET. Secondary thyroid neoplasms in pediatric cancer patients: increased risk with improved survival. J Pediatr Surg 1984; 19:855–859.

21. Tang TT, Holcenberg JS, Duck SC, et al. Thyroid carcinoma following acute lymphoblastic leukemia. Cancer 1980; 46:1572–1576.

22. Schneider AB, Farne MJ, Stachura ME, et al. Incidence prevalence and characteristics of radiation-induced thyroid tumors. Am J Med 1978; 64:243.

23. DeVathaire F, Fraga P, Francois P, et al. Long-term effects on the thyroid of irradiation for skin angiomas in childhood. Pediatr Res 1993; 133:381–386.

24. Hayles AB, Kennedy RL, Woolner LB, et al. Nodular lesions of the thyroid gland in children. J Clin Endocrinol Metab 1956; 16:1580.

25. Hayles AB, Johnson ML, Beahrs OH, et al. Carcinoma of the thyroid in children. Am J Surg 1963; 106:735.

26. Gorlin JB, Sallan SE. Thyroid cancer in children. Endocrinol Clin North Am 1990; 19:649–662.

27. Silverman SH, Nussbaum M, Rausen AR. Thyroid nodules in children: a ten year experience at one institution. Mt Sinai J Med 1979; 46:460–463.

28. Goephert H, Dichtel WJ, Saaman NA. Thyroid cancer in children and teenagers. Arch Otolaryngol 1984; 110:72–75.

29. Adams HD. Nontoxic nodular goiter and carcinoma of the thyroid in children 15 years of age and younger. Surg Clin North Am 1967; 47:601–605.

30. Desjardins JG, Khah AH, Montupet P, et al. Management of thyroid nodules in children: a 20 year experience. J Pediatr Surg 1987; 22:736–739.

31. Van Vliet G, Glinoer D, Velelst J, et al. Cold thyroid nodules in children: is surgery always necessary? Eur J Pediatr 1987; 146:378–382.

32. Studer H, Gebel F. Simple and sporadic goiter. In: Werner SC, Ingbar SH, eds. The Thyroid, 5th ed. Hagerstown, MD: Harper & Row, 1986: 696–704.

33. Blum M. Management of the solitary thyroid nodule. A selective approach. Thyroid Today 1978; 1(9):1–6.

34. Ingbar SH, Woeber KA. The thyroid gland. In: Williams RE, ed. Textbook of Endocrinology, 7th ed. Philadelphia: W. B. Saunders, 1985:801–803.

35. Hamburger JI. The autonomously functioning thyroid nodule. Endocr Rev 1987; 8:439–447.

36. Rosenbloom AL, Moore MM. Hyperfunctioning thyroid adenoma in a euthyroid adolescent. South Med J 1973; 66:1247.

37. Pillay R, Graham-Pole J, Miraldi E, et al. Diagnostic x-irradiation as a possible etiologic agent in thyroid neoplasms in childhood. J Pediatr 1982; 101:566–568.

38. Belfiore A, LaRosa GL, LaPorta GA, et al. Cancer risk in patients with thyroid nodules; relevance of iodine intake, sex, age and multinodularity. Am J Med 1992; 93:363–369.

39. Hung W. Nodular thyroid disease and thyroid carcinoma. Pediatr Ann 1992; 21:50–57.

40. Topliss DJ, Halff V, Johnson WR, et al. Thyroid mass and nodules: evolution and management. Med J Aust 1986; 145:334–338.

41. Croom RD, Thomas CG, Roddick RL. Autonomously functioning thyroid nodules in childhood and adolescence. Surgery 1987; 102:1101–1108.

42. Hung W, Anderson KD, Chandra RS, et al. Solitary thyroid nodules in 71 children and adolescents. J Pediatr Surg 1992; 27:1407–1409.

43. Hopewood NJ, Carroll RG, Kenny FM, Foley TP. Functioning thyroid masses in childhood and adolescence. Clinical surgical and pathological correlations. J Pediatr 1976; 89:710–718.

44. Johnson PM. Thyroid and whole body scanning. In: Werner SC, Ingbar SH, eds. The Thyroid, 5th ed. Hagerstown, MD: Harper & Row, 1986:458–478.

45. Sykes D. The solitary thyroid nodule. Br J Surg 1981; 68:510–512.

46. Turner JW, Spencer RP. Thyroid carcinoma presenting as a pertechnetate "hot" nodule but without ^{131}I uptake: a case report. J Nucl Med 1976; 17:22–23.

47. Erjavec M, Movrin T, Auersperg M, et al. Comparative accumulation of ^{99m}Tc and ^{131}I in the thyroid nodules: case report J Nucl Med 1977; 18:346–347.

48. Thomas CB, Croom RD. Current management of the patient with autonomously nodular goiter. Surg Clin North Am 1987; 67:315–328.

49. Silverstein GE, Burke G, Cogan R. The natural history of the autonomous hyperfunctioning thyroid nodule. Ann Intern Med 1967; 67:539.

50. Campbell WL, Santiago HE, Perzin KH, Johnson PM. The autonomous thyroid nodule: correlation of scan appearance and histopathology. Radiology 1968; 107:133.

51. Wiener JD. Autonomously functioning thyroid nodules. J Pediatr 1977; 91:682–683.

52. Hamburger JI, Meier DA. Cancer following treatment of an autonomously functioning thyroid nodule with sodium iodine I^{131}. Arch Surg 1971; 103:762.

53. Fisher DA. Thyroid nodules in childhood and their management. J Pediatr 1976; 89:866–868.

54. Godden JO, Volpe R. Assessment and Management of Thyroid Dysfunction. Amer. Educ. Inst. 1975.

55. Nelson RL, Wahner HW, Gorman CA. Rectilinear thyroid scanning as a predictor of malignancy. Ann Intern Med 1978; 88:41–44.

56. McConahey WM, Hay ID, Woolner LB, et al. Papillary cancer treated at the Mayo Clinic 1946 through 1970: initial manifestations, pathological findings, therapy and outcome. Mayo Clin Proc 1986; 61:978–996.

57. Ridgeway EC, Weintraub BD, Cevallos JL, et al. Suppression of pituitary TSH secretion in the patient with a hyperfunctioning thyroid nodule. J Clin Invest 1973; 52:2783.

58. Pompa BH, Cloutier MD, Hales AB. Thyroid nodule producing T$_3$ toxicosis in a child. Mayo Clin Proc 1973; 43:273.

59. Wang C. Management of thyroid disease based on needle biopsy pathology. Clin Endocrinol Metab 1981; 10:293–298.

60. Patnaik JK, Satpathy PC, Dan BS, Bose TK. Role of scintiscan and aspiration cytology in the diagnosis of the hypofunctioning thyroid nodules. Indian J Med Res 1987, 85:53–60.

61. Gagneten CB, Roccatagliata G, Lowenstein A, et al. The role of fine needle aspiration biopsy cytology in the evaluation of the clinically solitary thyroid nodules. Acta Cytol 1987; 31:595–598.

62. Miller JM, Hamburger JI, Kini SR. The needle biopsy diagnosis of papillary thyroid carcinoma. Cancer 1981; 48:989–993.

63. Pretorious HT, Katikineni M, Kinsella TJ, et al. Thyroid nodules after high-dose external radiotherapy. Fine-needle aspiration cytology in diagnosis and management. JAMA 1982; 247:3217–3220.

64. Hawkins F, Bellido D, Bernal C, et al. Fine needle aspiration biopsy in the diagnosis of thyroid cancer and thyroid disease. Cancer 1987; 59:1206–1209.

65. Piromalli D, Martelli G, Del Prato I, et al. The role of the fine needle aspiration in the diagnosis of thyroid nodules: an analysis of 795 consecutive cases. J Surg Oncol 1992; 50:247–250.

66. Bouvet M, Feldman JI, Gill GN, et al. Surgical management of the thyroid nodule: patient selection based on the results of fine needle aspiration cytology. Laryngoscope 1992; 102:1353–1356.

67. Ongphiphadhanakul B, Rajanatavin R, Chiemchanya S, et al. Systemic inclusion of clinical and laboratory data improves diagnostic accuracy of fine-needle aspiration biopsy in solitary thyroid nodules. Acta Endocrinol (Copenh) 1992; 126:233–237.

68. Bisi H, Asato de Camargo RY, Fiho Longatto A. Role of fine needle aspiration cytology in the management of thyroid nodules. Diagn Cytol 1992; 8:504–510.

69. Mazzaferi EL. Thyroid cancer in thyroid nodules: finding a needle in the haystack. Am J Med 1992; 93:359–362.

70. Gharib H, Geeliner JR, Zinsmeister AR, et al. Fine needle aspiration biopsy of thyroid. The problem of suspicious cytologic findings. Ann Intern Med 1984; 101:25–28.

71. Block MA, Dalley GE, Robb JA: Thyroid nodules indeterminate by needle biopsy. Ann Surg 1983; 146:72–78.

72. Ramacciotti CE, Pretorious HT, Chu EW, et al. Diagnostic accuracy and use of aspiration biopsy in the management of thyroid nodules. Arch Intern Med 1984; 144:1169.

73. Rosen IB, Wallace C, Strawbridge HG, et al. Reevaluation of needle aspiration cytology in detection of thyroid cancer. Surgery 1981; 90:747–756.

74. Caruso D, Mazzaferri EL. Fine needle aspiration biopsy in the management of thyroid nodules. Endocrinologist 1991; 1:194–202.

75. Hall TL, Layfield LJ, Phillippe A, et al. Sources of diagnostic error in fine needle aspiration of the thyroid. Cancer 1989; 63:718–725.

76. Mazzaferri EL. Management of the solitary thyroid nodule. N Engl J Med, 1992; 328:553–559.

77. Gharib H, Mazzaferri EL. A strategy in the solitary thyroid nodule. Hosp Pract 1992; 27:53–60.

78. Sheppard MC, Franklyn JA. Management of the single thyroid nodule. Clin Endocrinol (Copenh) 1992; 401. 37:398–401.

79. Mahoney CP. Differential diagnosis of goiter. Pediatr Clin North Am 1987; 34:891–905.

80. Molitch ME, Bede JR, Dreisman M, et al. The cold thyroid nodule: an analysis of diagnostic and therapeutic options. Endocr Rev 1984; 5:185–199.

81. Gharib H, James EM, Carboneau JW, et al. Suppressive therapy with levothyroxine for solitary thyroid nodules. N Engl J Med 1987; 317:70–75.

82. Reverter JL, Lucas A, Salinas I, et al. Suppressive therapy with levothyroxine for solitary nodules. Clin Endocrinol (Copenh) 1992; 36:25–28.

83. Mazzaferri EL. Solitary thyroid nodule. Postgrad Med 1981; 70:98–117.

84. Leeper RD, Shimaoka K. Treatment of metastatic thyroid cancer. Clin Endocrinol Metab 1980; 9:383–404.

85. DeGroot LJ. Management of thyroid nodules. How far have we come? Hosp Pract 1986; 21:9–10.

30

Carcinoma of the Thyroid in Children and Adolescents

Joseph N. Attie

Albert Einstein School of Medicine, Bronx, New York

I. INTRODUCTION

Carcinoma of the thyroid in a child was first reported in 1902 (1), and by 1948 only 62 cases were reported in the world literature. Between 1948 and 1970, Winship and Rosvoll (2) collected a total of 878 cases of thyroid carcinoma in patients 15 years of age or younger: 411 published cases and 467 unpublished cases from many parts of the world. The number of reported cases rose sharply in 1945, reached a peak in 1957, and declined in the next 10–12 years (Fig. 1). This rise and fall in the incidence of thyroid cancer paralleled the prevalence of the use of radiation of the head and neck in children.

II. INCIDENCE

Thyroid carcinoma is rare, constituting 0.6 and 1.6% of malignant tumors in men and women, respectively. Because of its good prognosis, thyroid cancer causes only 0.14 and 0.3% of cancer deaths in men and women, respectively. Approximately 12,700 new cases were expected to occur in the United States in 1993. It is estimated that 10% of differentiated thyroid cancers occur in patients under the age of 20. A recent study by the National Cancer Institute (3), based on surveillance of registries in five states and six metropolitan areas covering 10% of the U.S population, revealed that between 1973 and 1977 there was a 50% increase in the incidence of papillary and follicular carcinoma. It was the third most common cause of cancer in girls 15–19 years of age. There has been no satisfactory explanation for this increased incidence.

The sex distribution is different from that in adults. In large published series of thyroid cancer in adults, women outnumber men 4:1. In children below 15 the ratio of girls to boys is 1.5:1; in patients aged 15–20 the ratio is 3:1.

Carcinoma of the thyroid has been reported at all ages. In Winship's collected series 14 patients had tumors at birth that later proved to be carcinoma of the thyroid. Our patients with thyroid cancer ranged in age from 3 to 19 (Fig. 2).

Authors of series of childhood and adolescent thyroid carcinomas selected different upper age limits in their studies, varying from 15 to 20 years of age. We arbitrarily used age 19 as our upper age limit, because most of these patients were admitted to the department of pediatrics.

III. ETIOLOGY

The relationship of thyroid carcinoma to other preexisting thyroid abnormalities is inconclusive. In countries where endemic goiter is rare, the thyroid glands in patients with thyroid cancers do not show a higher incidence of benign nodules or thyroiditis than sex- and age-comparable individuals. There is evidence, however, that Graves' disease may influence the development and behavior of thyroid carcinoma (4). Thyroid carcinoma occurs with greater frequency in patients with Graves' disease, especially in those with palpable nodules. Tumors in patients with Graves' disease are often larger and behave more aggressively than those in other patients (5). It may be that thyroid-stimulating hormones or possibly thyroid-stimulating antibodies support the growth and function of thyroid cancer. Exogenous thyroid hormone routinely used in the treatment of thyroid cancer does not inhibit thyroid-stimulating hormone in patients with coexisting Graves' disease and may increase thyroid-stimulating antibody formation, thereby enhancing tumor growth.

The relationship of radiation to the head and neck to the development of thyroid cancer has been well established. It was first noted by Duffy and Fitzgerald who reported a series of 28 children with thyroid cancer, of whom 9 received radiation in infancy. Clark (7) stated that of 15 children he encountered with thyroid carcinoma, all had been subjected to prior irradiation to the head and neck. Fetterman (8) found that of 10 children and adolescents with thyroid cancer seen at University of Pittsburgh, 8 had received radiation 3–12 years before the diagnosis. In series of 878 cases of thyroid

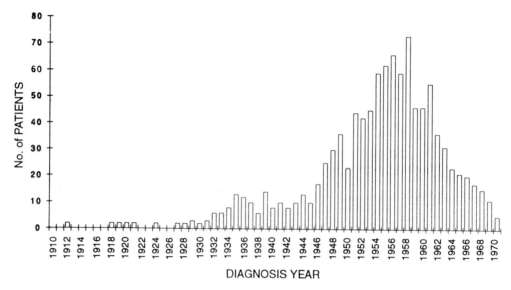

Figure 1   Number of childhood cancers seen annually between 1910 and 1970. (After Winship and Roswoll.)

cancer reviewed by Winship, an attempt to obtain a history of irradiation was made in 476 patients; of these, 76% had received x-ray treatment to the head and neck 3–14 years previously. In several other reported series of thyroid carcinoma in children, a significant percentage of the cases received prior radiation to the head and neck (Table 1). The treatment of benign conditions with radiation therapy was common until about 1970 and included radiation for enlarged thymus in infants, radiation of tonsils and adenoids, treatment of tinea capitis, acne, tuberculous lymphadenitis, and eczema. The dosage involved in patients developing thyroid carcinoma varied but was usually low, with a threshold level of about 180 rad. Ron et al. (18) showed that children who received 6 cGy to the thyroid during radiation for tinea capitis had four times the rate of thyroid cancer as the controls. The interval between irradiation and the appearance of thyroid cancer varied from 3 to 35–40 years.

An attempt was made by Schneider et al. (19) to determine the incidence of thyroid cancer developing in a group of children irradiated at ages 2–8 with 750–900 rad to the throat. Of a total of 5266 subjects who received radiation, 1712 participated in the screening program 20–35 years after treatment. Of these, 520 (30%) had nodular thyroids; of 350 operated upon, 108 (32%) had carcinoma of the thyroid. The majority of the cancers were papillary, multicentric, and bilateral. Simpson and Hemperman (20) studied 2333 children who had received irradiation to the thymus in infancy and used as controls 2622 of the irradiated children's siblings who had not received x-ray therapy. In the former group, thyroid carcinoma developed in 11 cases, whereas in the control sibling group no cases of thyroid cancer were found. An increased incidence of thyroid cancer has also been reported following external radiation for Hodgkin's disease (21).

Nonmedullary thyroid carcinoma is occasionally seen in

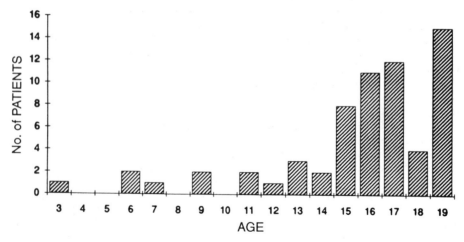

Figure 2   Age distribution of 65 childhood thyroid carcinomas.

Table 1 Radiation History in Childhood Thyroid Cancer

Author	No. cases	No. irradiated (%)
Clark (7)	15	15 (100)
Fetterman (8)	10	8 (80)
Tawes and deLormer (9)	34	14 (41)
Hayles et al. (10)	19	15 (78)
Harness et al. (11)	58	29 (50)
Crile (12)	18	11 (61)
Buckwalter et al. (13)	69	14 (20)
Nishiyama et al. (14)	36	17 (47)
Duffy and Fitzgerald (15)	28	10 (36)
Wilson et al. (16)	37	16 (43)
Hagler et al. (17)	15	14 (93)

families. Well-differentiated thyroid cancer may be associated with lipomas, osteomas, intestinal polyposis or carcinoma in Gardner syndrome, with autosomal dominant inheritance (22). Altered oncogenes have been found in a number of thyroid cancers of follicular cell origin and suggest that oncogene expression may be the cause of some or all thyroid cancers. An oncogene, *ptc*, has been isolated from human papillary thyroid cancers; it is located on the proximal long arm of chromosome 11 (23). Mutated forms of *ras* oncogenes are found in thyroid neoplasms (24). Because they occur in benign as well as malignant tumors, they are not of diagnostic use. Altered forms of ras oncogenes are nonspecific, having been found in pancreatic and colon carcinoma as well as thyroid cancer. We showed that the *c-myc* oncogene is expressed more often in malignant than in benign follicular neoplasms (25). Recently we found that there is a significant difference in the expression of several genes in follicular and Hürthle cell thyroid cancers (26), suggesting that they should be considered separate entities. A *ret* protooncogene has been found in papillary cancer (27) and a *fos* protooncogene in follicular carcinoma (28). In papillary cancer, a rearrangement of *ret* protooncogene results in expression of the tyrosine kinase portion driven by promoter sequences from another gene, H-4. This rearranged gene is probably responsible for the development of 20–30% of papillary cancers (29).

Medullary thyroid carcinoma (MTC) in children is usually seen as a component of multiple endocrine neoplasia (MEN) type II, which is genetic with autosomal dominant inheritance and incomplete penetrance. MTC is a malignancy derived from the parafollicular or C cells, which migrate into the thyroid anlage in utero from the ultimobranchial bodies and probably constitute the only lateral contributions to the thyroid gland. The C cells secrete calcitonin and calcitonin gene-related peptide. They are distributed in the upper portions of both lobes of the thyroid, with the greatest concentration in the junction region between the upper third and the middle third of the lobes, thus explaining the usual location of most hereditary medullary cancers. It is believed that C cell hyperplasia is a frequent precursor of medullary carcinoma.

The disease gene for MEN IIa has been mapped to the centrometric region of chromosome 10. There is an inclusion of the *ret* protooncogene (which is a receptor of the tyrosine kinase class) in a 500,000 base pair region containing the MEN IIa gene (29). A total of 20 different mutations within the *ret* protooncogene have been identified as those probably responsible for the development of MEN IIa (30). It has been suggested (31) that, as in other neoplasms, the development of medullary cancer occurs in two stages: inactivation of a tumor-suppressor gene on chromosome 10, causing C cell hyperplasia, followed by deletion of another gene on chromosome 1 (where a high incidence of deletions have been reported in both MTCs and pheochromocytomas), resulting in frank tumor formation (32). The mutations in the *ret* protooncogene activate the *ret* tyrosine kinase receptor and cause cell growth (23). One mutation of *ret* protooncogene has been identified as responsible for MEN IIb.

It is now possible to perform genetic screening of family members of patients with MEN II. The analysis of restriction fragment length polymorphism patterns in affected families carries a 90% accuracy at present. This technique can point to individuals likely to develop MTC (50% of family members). Some thyroidectomies have been performed on the basis of this finding without prior demonstration of elevation of calcitonin levels after pentagastrin stimulation. It is best to identify patients with MEN II before the age of 6, which is the youngest age in which metastatic medullary cancer has been reported (33).

IV. CLINICAL PICTURE

The usual presentation of thyroid carcinoma is that of a solitary asymptomatic mass in the thyroid gland. It may be soft or firm, usually mobile, but sometimes hard, irregular, or fixed to surrounding tissues. Multiple nodules may be felt. Rarely, there are preoperative criteria for malignancy, such as hardness, fixation, hoarseness, or cervical lymphadenopathy. Occasionally, the palpated nodule proves to be benign upon removal, but at surgery another nonpalpable lesion is found that is malignant.

In a series of 58 children up to age 15 with thyroid cancer reported by Harness et al. (11), the most common presenting sign was cervical lymphadenopathy (63%). In some patients the enlarged lymph nodes were observed for more than 5 years; the average duration of lymphadenopathy before biopsy was over 2 years. A palpable thyroid nodule was the presenting finding in only 37% of cases. Recurrent laryngeal paralysis was present in 4 patients when first seen, and 2 had extensive pulmonary metastasis on first examination.

The clinical presentation of the 702 patients in the collected series of Winship was varied (2). Cervical node metastasis was found at the first examination in 74% of the patients; the nodal disease was bilateral in 32% of cases. In 41 patients the thyroid primary lesion was not clinically palpable. Pulmonary metastasis was present in 103 (14.4%) of the patients on initial examination and appeared at a later time in 37 others (5.2%); in 9 patients lung involvement was the presenting symptom.

The incidence of thyroid carcinoma in nodular thyroids is much higher in children than in adults. Ward (34) found only 7% of nodular thyroids in patients of all ages to be malignant, but 47% of thyroid nodules in patients younger than 15 years were carcinomas. Because the results of treatment are best in patients whose cancer is in an early stage (intrathyroid with no evidence of metastasis), it is important to select for surgical exploration those patients with nodular thyroids most likely to yield early carcinoma.

The method of evaluation and management of the child or adolescent with a thyroid nodule is discussed in chapter 26. In general, patients with nodular thyroid glands with a history of radiation in infancy, those with suspicious or definite diagnosis of carcinoma on aspiration cytology, those with no response or increase in size while on suppression with thyroid hormone, those presenting with a palpable lymphadenopathy associated with the thyroid mass, and those who have clinical criteria of cancer (hardness, hoarseness, or fixation) are candidates for surgery.

In a personal series of 256 thyroidectomies performed in patients 19 years or younger, 64 proved to have carcinoma (Table 2). The presenting sign in the 64 thyroid cancers is shown in Table 3. Of 148 who presented with nodular thyroid glands, 41 (28%) proved to be malignant. Because this is a surgical series, it is difficult to estimate how many nodules were evaluated before those referred for surgical treatment were selected. In reported series the incidence of carcinoma in nodular thyroids varied from 17 to 50% (Table 4).

Although diffuse thyroid enlargement rarely harbors malignant tumors, we found two cancers in patients with Hashimoto's thyroiditis ages 15 and 19 and three in cases of Graves' disease 15, 16, and 17 years of age. The cancers in the patients with thyroiditis were extensive and multicentric and, in one patient, involved lateral lymph nodes. The three carcinomas associated with hyperthyroidism were occult cancers (under 6 mm) and were found incidentally on microscopy. The coexistence of carcinoma and Graves' disease raises the possibility that thyroid-stimulating antibodies play a part in the pathogenesis and progression of thyroid neoplasms (41).

Table 3 Presenting Sign in Children with Thyroid Carcinoma

Sign	Number of patients
Solitary adenoma	35
"Cold" nodule 29	
"Hot" nodule 3	
Aspiration biopsy 3	
Thyroid mass and lateral node palpable	13
Multinodular thyroid	6
Lateral node palpable, thyroid gland nonpalpable	4
Elevated calcitonin in MEN II, no thyroid mass	3
Carcinoma in Graves' disease	2
Thyroglossal cyst	1

Papillary thyroid carcinoma has been found in the walls of thyroglossal cysts; Fernandez et al. (42) reported 110 cases as of 1991. I have encountered 3 cases of papillary carcinoma in thyroglossal cysts, 2 in adults and 1 in a 16 year old. The behavior of papillary cancer arising in a thyroglossal cyst is similar to that of other papillary cancers. It generally remains localized in the neck; occasionally other foci may occur in the thyroid gland.

V. PATHOLOGY AND BEHAVIOR

The classification of malignant tumors of the thyroid gland is as follows:

1. Papillary
   a. Papillary and follicular
   b. Pure papillary
   c. Occult (or micro) cancer
   d. Follicular variant of papillary
2. Follicular
3. Hürthle cell
4. Medullary
5. Anaplastic carcinoma
6. Lymphoma

Table 2 Diagnosis in 256 Thyroidectomies in Patients Under 19 Years

Diagnosis	Number of patients
Single adenoma	86
Diffuse toxic thyroid	76
Carcinoma	64
Multinodular thyroid	17
Hashimoto's thyroiditis	8
Toxic adenoma	4
Undescended thyroid	1

Table 4 Incidence of Carcinoma in Childhood Nodular Thyroids

Author	No. nodular thyroids	No cancers (%)
Scott and Crawford (35)	36	6 (17)
Adams (36)	44	9 (21)
Hayles et al. (10)	138	69 (50)
Kirkland et al. (37)	30	12 (40)
Hung et al. (38)	35	5 (18)
Valentin et al. (39)	49	10 (20)
Desjardins et al. (40)	58	12 (21)
Attie	148	41 (28)

7. Metastatic
8. Miscellaneous (sarcoma, teratoma, and epidermoid carcinoma)

In our series of 64 patients, the distribution of the types of thyroid carcinoma can be seen in Table 5. The TNM (tumor, node, metastases) classification of thyroid carcinoma is shown in Table 6.

A. Papillary Carcinoma

This is the most common type of thyroid carcinoma, constituting more than 80% of all cancers of the thyroid gland. Most cases are mixed papillary and follicular; pure papillary carcinomas are less frequent. The tumor usually occurs in otherwise normal thyroid parenchyma and is often multicentric and bilateral. Papillary carcinoma progresses very slowly and may remain localized for as long as 20 or 30 years before metastasizing via the bloodstream. In rare cases the lesion appears histologically to be nearly purely follicular, but the so-called ground-glass (Orphan Annie) appearance of the nuclei is characteristic of papillary tumors; these have been labeled the follicular variant of papillary cancer. Capsular and/or vascular invasion may be found, and psammoma bodies occur within or adjacent to the lesion. Mixed papillary and follicular tumors behave as papillary even if they are predominantly follicular in appearance. Lymph node metastases frequently occur early, are often bilateral, and are more common in children and young adults. The pattern of lymph node metastasis is unpredictable. The earliest involved nodes may be paratracheal, precricoid, or jugular. An enlarged lymph node may be the first sign of the disease; the primary tumor is such cases may be very small and nonpalpable. There were four such cases in our series of childhood thyroid cancer. Cady et al. (43) emphasized that the prognosis in children with nodal metastases is as favorable as in those without node involvement. Distant metastases may occur in approximately 10% of adults and 20% of children. The most common sites of distant spread are lungs and bone.

Papillary carcinoma in children and adolescents is less aggressive and less frequently fatal than in adults. Only one of our patients, a 17-year-old male who presented with a massive lesion and bilateral extensive nodal metastases, died of papillary cancer four years after surgery. Goepfert et al.

Table 5 Classification of Thyroid Carcinoma in 64 Patients

Classification	Number of patients
Papillary	51
Papillary and follicular 34	
Pure papillary 13	
Microcarcinoma (<1 cm) 4	
Follicular	8
Medullary (MEN II)	5

Table 6 TNM Classification of Thyroid Carcinoma

T	primary tumor	
	T0	No palpable tumor
	T1	Single tumor confined to gland; no deformity
	T2	Multiple tumors or single tumor with deformity
	T3	Tumor extending beyond the gland
N	regional lymph nodes	
	N0	No palpable nodes
	N1	Movable homolateral nodes
		N1a nodes not considered to contain growth
		N1b nodes considered to contain growth
	N2	Movable contralateral or bilateral nodes
		N2a nodes not considered to contain growth
		N2b nodes considered to contain growth
	N3	Fixed nodes
M	distant metastaes	
	M0	No evidence of distant metastases
	M1	Distant metastases present

(44) reported no cancer-related deaths in a series of 66 patients 20 years or younger; 84% of these had nodal metastasis, and 12% also had pulmonary metastases that disappeared after radioactive treatment. Buckwalter et al. (45) assert that there is no difference in life expectancy between children treated for papillary thyroid cancer and the normal population of the same age group. Schlumberger et al. (46) pointed out, however, that when the resection was incomplete, relapses were five times as frequent: 8% of their children died of cancer, all of whom had inadequate resections. Two reports (7,47) emphasize the improved results following total thyroidectomy and adequate nodal dissection.

In patients with papillary lesions larger than 1 cm in diameter, we prefer total thyroidectomy with removal of paratracheal nodes because of the frequent occurrence of mutlicentricity and bilateral foci of cancer. Postoperative radioiodine uptake studies of the neck, as well as total-body scans, can then be done, and microfoci of distant metastases may be successfully treated with ablative doses of radioactive iodine. In the absence of normal thyroid tissue, patients may be followed by annual thyroglobulin studies to detect possible recurrence. Total thyroidectomy was performed in 43 and near-total thyroidectomy in 5 patients without recurrent nerve damage or permanent hypoparathyroidism.

Our youngest patient treated with papillary carcinoma was a 6 year old with extensive bilateral lymph node involvement. She was treated by total thyroidectomy and bilateral modified radical neck dissection followed by radioiodine treatment. She required a temporary tracheostomy (6 months) postoperatively. She is living and free of disease 10 years.

B. Follicular Carcinoma

Follicular carcinoma is rare in children. Winship and Rosvoll (2) found 17% of their collected cases to be follicular. Crile (12) reported only 1 instance of follicular carcinoma in 18 children with thyroid cancer. Thompson et al. (47) believe that the follicular variant of papillary carcinoma is often classified as follicular carcinoma and that 20% of follicular cancers are so misdiagnosed; as mentioned earlier, this type behaves similarly to papillary cancer and has an excellent prognosis.

Differentiation between follicular adenoma and follicular carcinoma is often difficult; the histologic appearance may be identical, and the diagnosis depends on the finding of capsular and/or vascular invasion. Fine-needle aspiration biopsy merely shows follicular cells, and frozen section is usually reported as "follicular neoplasm": the final diagnosis is often made days later, when capsular invasion is discovered. The prognosis varies with the degree of capsular invasion. Follicular carcinoma is relatively slow growing and is rarely multicentric. Metastasis to lymph nodes is infrequent. Vascular invasion is common, and distant metastases to lungs and bones were found in 30–40% of patients. Metastatic foci may be functional, and cases of hyperthyroidism in the absence of the normal thyroid gland have been reported. The resemblance of such metastases to normal thyroid follicles resulted in their being called benign metastasizing struma. The ability of such functional metastases to take up radioactive iodine has been useful in the treatment of these foci with large doses of radioactive iodine after total ablation of the thyroid gland. Total thyroidectomy is the treatment of choice; it allows total-body scans postoperatively to detect and treat occult metastases (before they are detectable by x-rays or computed tomographic scans).

C. Hürthle Cell Carcinoma

Hürthle cell tumors are extremely rare in childhood. Most Hürthle cell tumors are benign and were previously known as oxyphil carcinomas. The malignant Hürthle cell tumors behave like follicular carcinomas but are more aggressive and have a worse prognosis. They almost never spread to lymph nodes; metastases occur to lungs, bone, brain, and liver. In a series of 42 patients studied by Brondeson et al. (44B), only 1 was under the age of 20. There was no case of Hürthle cell cancer in our series.

D. Medullary Carcinoma

This carcinoma may occur in either a sporadic or hereditary form. The sporadic form is rare in childhood and adolescence. When hereditary, medullary thyroid cancer may occur in one of the three forms: (1) multiple endocrine neoplasia IIa, characterized by MTC, pheochromocytoma, and occasional hyperthyroidism; (2) multiple neoplasia IIb characterized by MTC, multiple mucosal neuromas, and ganglioneuromas with occasional marfanoid habitus; and (3) familial non-MEN MTC, in which hereditary MTC occurs without associated endocrinopathies. In all types, hereditary MTC is autosomal dominant, so that half the siblings and children of affected individuals contract the disease.

The cells of MTC arise from the C cells ("parafollicular cells"), which secrete calcitonin, a peptide hormone. Calcitonin is readily measured in the blood by radioimmunoassay. Using this marker, it is possible to confirm the presence of MTC before operation based on the increased concentration of calcitonin in affected subjects. By using calcium, pentagastrin, or both intravenously, one can stimulate calcitonin levels and thereby make it possible to detect patients with clinically occult MTC (49). It has been demonstrated (50) that MTC was discovered at an earlier stage and had a higher cure rate if the thyroid neoplasm was diagnosed biochemically rather than clinically (i.e., with a palpable thyroid mass). Some of the clinically negative cases prove to have C cell hyperplasia, a precursor of medullary cancer. Because C cells are predominantly found in the upper pole regions of the thyroid lobes, most medullary cancers are in these locations. Nearly all patients with MTC have bilateral tumors.

It is important to study all members of families of patients diagnosed as having medullary carcinoma. Once the disease is identified as familial, kindred are then screened annually to detect elevations in calcitonin. One of the largest such families studied was the J family; 83 of the 89 living members of the kindred in three generations were studied at the New England Medical Center (51): 12 had elevated serum calcitonin levels after calcium infusion, and all were subjected to total thyroidectomy. All had bilateral carcinoma, 7 with local lymph node metastasis, although none of the 12 had palpable thyroid nodules or abnormal radioactive iodine scans. Subsequently, all members of the fourth generation of the J family were screened annually by calcium infusion of pentagastrin-provoked plasma calcitonin elevation, starting at age 4 (52). The initial calcitonin levels in all patients were normal. Patients in whom calcitonin levels rose above 0.55 ng/ml after two separate provocative tests 6 months apart were subjected to total thyroidectomy. A total of 17 children were operated upon. The thyroid gland was not palpable in any of the patients: 8 had medullary carcinoma, 8 had C cell hyperplasia, and in 1 patient the thyroid gland was normal. The age range was 8–18 years.

Many families have been screened in a similar manner. At the Mayo Clinic (53), 219 relatives of 36 patients with "sporadic" MTC (no family history of the thyroid tumor) were studied for calcitonin elevation. A total of 57 new affected members in seven families were found.

Two of my patients, ages 6 and 7, were siblings with MEN IIa and MEN IIb, respectively, whose mother had MEN II manifested by MTC and pheochromocytoma and died of disease. In both children the thyroid nodules were not palpable. One of the children had three foci of MTC as well as paratracheal lymph node involvement; the other child proved to have a minute focus of MTC in the pyramidal lobe measuring about 2 mm. The youngest patient in our series was operated on at age 2½, when elevated serum calcitonin levels were found on pentagastrin stimulation; a 2 mm medullary carcinoma in the pyramidal lobe was the only focus of disease. She is living free of disease 6 years. I had operated upon the mother, one aunt, and the grandfather; the last two had pheochromocytoma as well as MTC. The great grandmother had died many years earlier of "thyroid malignancy."

Annual screening of family members of calcitonin elevation, preferably starting at age 2, detects MTC or C cell hyperplasia early and results in a better cure rate. Genetic screening is now available and should be instituted in these families to detect which members possess the defective gene on chromosome 10 and indicate who should have calcitonin assays.

E. Anaplastic Carcinoma

Anaplastic or undifferentiated thyroid carcinomas are generally advanced when first seen, involving most structures in the midcompartment of the neck. They are rare, comprising fewer than 3% of all thyroid cancers. Most of them are of the large cell or giant cell variety. Small cell cancers have been described; most of these on careful review prove to be lymphomas. Anaplastic cancers rarely metastasize to lymph nodes and are usually nonresectable when first diagnosed. They occur in older patients, usually with a long history of thyroid mass; they are extremely rare in children and young adults. Some of these tumors respond to radiation and chemotherapy. In the Winship and Rosvoll series of 878 childhood cancers (2), there were 14 instances of small cell cancer and only 2 patients had the giant cell variety. There were no undifferentiated carcinomas in our series.

F. Lymphoma

Lymphoma occasionally presents as a solitary thyroid nodule. It is usually part of a generalized lymphoma but may be confined to the thyroid gland. Most cases are non-Hodgkin's lymphoma. In rare instances the neoplasm arises in preexisting Hashimoto's (lymphocytic) thyroiditis. The youngest patient I could find in several large series was aged 21. We have not encountered lymphoma of the thyroid in a child.

G. Metastatic Carcinoma

Metastasis to the thyroid is rare. The most common primary tumors that spread to the thyroid are renal carcinoma and breast and lung cancer. We have not seen any cases of carcinoma metastasizing to the thyroid in a child.

H. Miscellaneous

Fibrosarcomas have been rarely reported in the thyroid gland. Teratomas (tumors derived from three germ layers) are usually benign in children and malignant in adults. Primary epidermoid carcinomas of the thyroid are extremely rare and highly malignant, with few long-term survivors.

VI. TREATMENT

The management of the solitary thyroid nodule was discussed in the preceding chapter. In view of the high incidence of carcinoma in nodular thyroids in childhood and adolescence (41 cancers in 148 patients with nodular thyroids in my experience, or 28%), surgical treatment is indicated for nearly all solitary and discrete nodules in children.

Most thyroid carcinomas should be treated by total thyroidectomy. Because of the possibility of paratracheal lymph node involvement, total thyroidectomy should include resection of the paratracheal lymph nodes. Papillary and mixed papillary and follicular carcinomas are often multicentric and bilateral. Clark et al. (54) reported foci in the opposite lobes in 30% of patients in whom the lobe was routinely studied and in 82% of those studied by subserial section. When only hemithyroidectomy was performed, clinical recurrence in the opposite lobe was seen in 24% of their patients followed for 2–18 years. Long-term survival rates following total thyroidectomy for papillary carcinoma are higher than in patients undergoing less than total thyroidectomy (55,56).

Some have advocated performance of nearly total thyroidectomy, followed by ablation of the stump with radioactive iodine instead of total resection. However, not all papillary cancers concentrate the radioiodine and are thereby destroyed. Leeper (57) has reported a high death rate from anaplastic transformation of some of these remnants.

The advantage of total thyroidectomy in the treatment of follicular carcinoma is that one can detect and possibly treat metastatic foci with radioactive iodine when the normal thyroid tissue has been completely removed. Occult metastatic foci may be detected before they are discernible by x-ray and treated successfully. Treatment of large lung metastases is not always successful; furthermore, the pulmonary fibrosis following treatment of such foci may cause significant pulmonary dysfunction and has occasionally resulted in fatality.

In medullary carcinoma, especially in patients with MEN II, total thyroidectomy is mandatory because the disease is usually bilateral and multicentric. In addition to the medullary cancer, there is often C cell hyperplasia, which may, if not removed, lead to new foci of carcinoma.

Many surgeons have been reluctant to perform total thyroidectomy because of the increased risk of permanent hypoparathyroidism. Using an improved technical approach to preserve the parathyroid glands and their blood supply, Attie and Khafif (58) reduced the incidence of hypoparathyroidism to nearly zero. We studied a large number of our patients postoperatively with radioiodine and demonstrated the feasibility of total thyroidectomy (59).

Spread to the jugular lymph nodes from thyroid carcinoma occurs often and early, especially in young patients. In our 64 cases of thyroid carcinomas in patients age 19 and under, 33 had modified radical neck dissections, and in these, 28 had positive jugular lymph nodes, 3 bilaterally. With proper surgical treatment, the spread to lateral nodes did not adversely affect long-term survival. Only 1 of our patients with papillary carcinoma metastatic to lateral neck nodes bilaterally is known to have died of distant metastases, 4 years postoperatively. Cady et al. (43) reported better survival rates in children with extensive nodal involvement than in the series of papillary cancer as a whole. Whether this resulted from more adequate surgical treatment in that group of patients is not clear. The authors do not advocate routine total thyroidectomy in all patients. However, of those patients who developed local recurrences, only 38% survived for 5 years or longer.

Until 1983, because of the high incidence of nodal involvement in papillary carcinoma, we performed elective (i.e., no palpable nodes) modified radical neck dissection in patients with large or aggressive papillary cancers (60). During the past 10 years we have changed our approach. We now perform a modified radical neck dissection only in patients with palpable or proven metastatic nodal disease. During the thyroidectomy, the carotid sheath is opened and nodes are inspected and biopsied, and if positive for carcinoma, neck dissection is performed. The operation is done through a single transverse incision. The sternomastoid, the spinal accessory nerve, and the entire cervical plexus are preserved (61). In our patients under 19 years, 14 of 18 who underwent elective neck dissections had positive nodes (78%).

After total thyroidectomy, the patient is allowed to become hypothyroid (high thyroid-stimulating hormone) and a neck and total-body scan are performed. If the uptake in the thyroid bed is over 2% or there is evidence of distant metastatic foci, the patient is treated with radioactive iodine. Some authors routinely use radioactive iodine postoperatively in the treatment of papillary and follicular thyroid cancer.

Following total or nearly total thyroidectomy, the patient is placed on lifelong exogenous thyroid medication (62). The preferred synthetic hormone is levo-thyroxine. The dose varies from 50 to 400 μg daily. Excessive doses may result in hyperthyroid manifestations and increase loss of bone density later in life. The value of thyroid hormone in the prevention of recurrence in patients with sufficient thyroid left to maintain a euthyroid condition remains to be proven.

Since 1954, I have operated on 64 patients with carcinoma of the thyroid, ages 3–19. None of the patients had evidence of distant metastasis at the time of operation. The procedures carried out are shown in Table 7. During the early years of our experience, some patients were treated by less than total thyroidectomy. After we developed an operative technique in which we preserved the parathyroids with their blood supply (58), all patients were treated by total thyroidectomy (except for 2 cases of incidental microcancers discovered during subtotal thyroidectomy for Graves' disease).

In follow-ups varying from 6 months to 39 years, two of our patients died of distant metastasis, one with papillary and follicular carcinoma (age 18) and the other of medullary carcinoma, MEN II (age 17). There has been no instance of local or nodal recurrence in our series.

Table 7 Operations performed on 64 Patients with Thyroid Carcinoma

Operation	Number of patients
Total thyroidectomy	22
Total thyroidectomy and unilateral neck dissection	18
Total thyroidectomy and bilateral neck dissection	3
Nearly total thyroidectomy and unilateral neck dissection	5
Hemithyroidectomy and unilateral neck dissection	7
Bilateral subtotal thyroidectomy	4
Hemithyroidectomy	4
Partial thyroidectomy (thyroglossal cyst plus pyramidal)	1

REFERENCES

1. Ehrhardt O. Zur anatomie und Klinik der Struma maligna. Beitr Klin Chir 1902; 35:343.
2. Winship T, Rosvoll R. Thyroid carcinoma in childhood: final report on a 20 year study. Clin Proc Child Hosp DC 1970; 26:237–238.
3. Brennan MF, Bloomer WD. Cancer of the endocrine system. In: DeVita VT Jr, Hellman S, Rosenberg SA, (eds.) Cancer: Principles and Practice of Oncology. Philadelphia: J. B. Lippincott, 1982:973.
4. Mazzaferri EL. Thyroid cancer and Graves' disease. J Clin Endocrinol Metab 1990; 70:826–829.
5. Belfiore A, Garofalo MR, Giuffrida D, et al. Increased aggressiveness of thyroid cancer in patients with Graves' disease. J Clin Endocrinol Metab 1990; 70:830–835.
6. Duffy BJ, Fitzgerald PJ. Cancer of the thyroid in children—a report of 28 cases. J Clin Endocrinol 1950; 10:1296–1308.
7. Clark DE. Association of irradiation with cancer of the thyroid in children and adolescents. JAMA 1955; 159:1007–1009.
8. Fetterman GH. Carcinoma of the thyroid in children-a report of 10 cases. J Dis Child 1956; 92:581–587.
9. Taws RL, deLorimer AA. Thyroid carcinoma during youth. J Pediatr Surg 1968; 3:210–218.
10. Hayles AB, Kennedy RL, Beahrs OH, Woolner LB. Management of the child with thyroidal carcinoma. JAMA 1960; 173:21–28.
11. Harness JK, Thompson NW, Nishiyama RH. Childhood thyroid carcinoma. Arch Surg 1971; 102:278–284.
12. Crile G Jr. Carcinoma of the thyroid in children. Ann Surg 1959; 150:959–964.
13. Buckwalter JA, Gurll NJ, Thomas CG. Cancer of the thyroid in youth. World J Surg 1981; 5:15–25.
14. Nishiyama RH, Schmidt RW, Batsakis JG. Carcinoma of the thyroid in children and adolescents. JAMA 1962; 181:1034–1038.
15. Duffy BJ, Fitzgerald PJ. Thyroid cancer in childhood and adolescence. Report on 28 cases. Cancer 1950; 3:1018–1032.
16. Wilson GM, Kilpatrick R, Eckert H, et al. Thyroid neoplasms following irradiation. BMJ 1958; 2:929–934.
17. Hagler AB, Rosenblum P, Rosenblum A. Carcinoma of the

thyroid in children and young adults: iatrogenic relation to previous radiation. Pediatrics 1966; 38:77–81; Am J Surg 1963; 106:735–743.

18. Ron E, Modan, B, Preston D, et al. Thyroid neoplasia following low-dose radiation in childhood. Radiat Res 1989; 120:516–531.

19. Schneider AB, Pinsky S, Bekerman C, Ryuo V. Characteristics of 108 thyroid cancers detected by screening in a population with a history head and neck irradiation. Cancer 1980; 46:1218–1227.

20. Simpson CL, Hempelmann LH (cited by Duffy BJ Jr). Can radiation cause thyroid cancer? Trans Am Goiter Assoc 1957; 17:1384–1388.

21. Hancock SL, Cox RS, McDougall IR. Thyroid diseases after the treatment of Hodgkin's disease. N Engl J Med 1991; 325:599–605.

22. Lote K, Andersen K., Nordal E, et al. Familial occurrence of papillary thyroid carcinoma. Cancer 1980; 46:1291–1297.

23. Grieco M, Santoro M, Berlingieri MT, et al. PTC is a novel rearranged form of the ret proto-oncogene and is frequently detected in human thayroid papillary carcinomas. Cell 1990; 60:557–563.

24. Wright P, Lemoine NR, Mayall ES, et al. Papillary and follicular carcinomas show a different pattern of ras oncogene mutation. Br J Cancer 1989; 60:576–577.

25. Auguste LJ, Masood S, Westerband A, Belluco C, Valderamma E, Attie JN. Oncogene expression in follicular neoplasms of the thyroid. Am J Surg 1992; 164:592–593.

26. Masood, S, August L, Westerband A, Belluco C, Valderama E, Attie J. Differential oncogenic expression in thyroid follicular and hürthle cell carcinomas. Am J Surg 1993; 166:366–368.

27. Ishizaka Y, Itoh F, Tahira T, et al. Presence of aberrant transcripts of ret protooncogene in a human thyroid carcinoma cell line. Jpn J Cancer Res 1989; 80:1149–1152.

28. Wyllie FS, Lemoine NR, Williams ED, Wynford-Thomas D. Structure and expression of nuclear oncogenes in multi-stage thyroid tumorigenesis. Br J Cancer 1989; 60:561–565.

29. Gardner E, Papi L, Easton DF, et al. Genetic linkage studies map the multiple endocrine neoplasia type 2 loci to a small interval on chromosome 10q11.2. Hum Mol Genet 1993; 2:241–246.

30. Mulligan LM, Kwok JBJ, Healey CS, et al. Germ-line mutations of the RET proto-oncogene in multiple endocrine neoplasia type 2A. Nature 1993; 363:458–460.

31. Matthew, CGP, Smith BA, Easton DF, et al. Deletion of genes on chromosome 1 in endocrine neoplasia. Nature 1987; 328:524–526.

32. Nelkin BD, de Bustros AC, Mabry M, Baylin SB. The molecular biology of medullary thyroid carcinoma. JAMA 1989; 261:3130–3135.

33. Gagel RF, Robinson MF, Donovan DT, Alford BR. Medullary thyroid carcinoma: recent progress. J Clin Endocrinol Metab 1993; 76:809–814.

34. Ward R. Cancer of the thyroid in children. Am J Surg 1955; 90:338–344.

35. Scott MD, Crawford JD. Solitary thyroid nodules in childhood: is the incidence of thyroid carcinoma declining? Pediatrics 1976; 58:521–525.

36. Adams HD. Nontoxic nodular goiter and carcinoma of the thyroid in children 15 years of age and younger. Surg Clin North Am 1967; 47:601–604.

37. Kirkland RT, Kirkland JL, Rosenberg HS, Harberg FJ, Librik L, Clayton GW. Solitary thyroid nodules in 30 children and a report of a child with a thyroid abscess. Pediatrics 1973; 51:85–90.

38. Hung W, August GP, Randolph JG, Schisgall, RM, Chandra R. Solitary thyroid nodules in children and adolescents. J Pediatr Surg 1981; 17:225–229.

39. Valentin L, Ramirez C, Valentin WH, Figueroa I. Thyroid nodules in children. Bol Asoc Med PR 1986; 78:92–94.

40. Desjardins JG, Khan AH, Montupet P, et al. Management of thyroid nodules in children: a 20 year experience. J Pediatr Surg 1987; 22:736–739.

41. Filetti S, Belfiore A, Daniels GH, Ippolito O, Vigneri R, Ingbar SH. The role of thyroid stimulating antibodies of Graves' disease in differentiated thyroid cancer. N Engl J Med 1988; 318:753–759.

42. Fernandez JF, Ordoñez NG, Schultz PN, Samaan NA, Hickey RC. Thyroglossal duct carcinoma. Surgery 1991; 110:928–935.

43. Cady B, Sedgwick CE, Meissner WA, Rookwalter JR, Romagosa V, Werber J. Changing clinical, pathologic, therapeutic and survival patterns in differentiated thyroid carcinoma. Ann Surg 1976; 184:541–554.

44. Goepfert H, Dichtel WJ, Samaan NA. Thyroid cancer in children and teenagers. Arch Otolaryngol 1984; 110:72–75.

45. Buchwalter JA, Thomas CG, Freeman TB. Is thyroid cancer a lethal disease? Ann Surg 1975; 181:632–639.

46. Schlumberg M, DeVathaire F, Travagli JP, et al. Differentiated thyroid carcinoma in childhood: long term follow up of 72 patients. J Clin Endocrinol Metab 1987; 65:1088–1094.

47. Thompson NW, Nishijama RH, Harness JK. Thyroid carcinoma: current controversies. Curr Prob Surg 1978; 15:1–67.

48. Bondeson L, Bondeson AG, Ljunberg O, Tibblin S. Atypical tumors of the thyroid. Ann Surg 1981; 194:677–680.

49. Tashjian AH Jr, Hawland BG, Melvin KEW, Hill CS. Immunoassay of human calcitonin. Clinical measurement, relation to serum calcium and studies in patients with medullary thyroid carcinoma. N Engl J Med 1970; 283:890–895.

50. Wells SA, Baylin SB, Gann DS, et al. Medullary thyroid carcinoma: relationship to method of diagnosis to pathologic staging. Ann Surg 1978; 188:337–388.

51. Melvin KEW, Miller HH, Tashjian AH. Early diagnosis of medullary carcinoma of thyroid gland by means of calcitonin assay. N Engl J Med 1971; 285:115–120.

52. Leape LL, Miller HH, Graye K, et al. Total thyroidectomy for occult familial medullary carcinoma of the thyroid in children. J Pediatr Surg 1976; 11:831–837.

53. Sizemore GW, Carney JA, Heath H III. Epidemiology of medullary carcinoma of the thyroid gland—a five year experience (1971–1976). Surg Clin North Am 1977; 57:633–645.

54. Clark RL, White EC, Russell ED. Total thyroidectomy for cancer of the thyroid. Significance of intraglandular dissemination. Ann Surg. 1959; 149:858–866.

55. Mazzaferri EL, Young RL. Papillary thyroid carcinoma: a ten year follow-up of the impact of therapy in 576 patients. Am J Med 1981; 70:511–518.

56. Samaan NA, Maheshwan YK, Nader S, et al. Impact of therapy for differentiated carcinoma of the thyroid. J Clin Endocrinol Metab 1983; 56:1131–1138.

57. Leeper RD. Controversies in the treatment of thyroid cancer: the NY Memorial Hospital approach. Thyroid Today, 1982; July/August.

58. Attie JN, Khafif RA. Preservation of parathyroid glands during total thyroidectomy: improved technique utilizing microsurgery. Am J Surg 1975; 130:399–402.

59. Attie JN, Moskowitz GW, Marguleff D, Levy LM. Feasibility

of total thyroidectomy in the treatment of thyroid carcinoma. Postoperative radioactive iodine evaluation in 140 cases. Am J Surg 1979; 138:555–560.

60. Attie JN, Khafif RA, Steckler RM. Elective neck dissection in papillary carcinoma of the thyroid. Am J Surg 1971; 122:464–471.

61. Attie JN. Modified neck dissection in treatment of thyroid cancer: a safe procedure. Eur J Cancer Clin Oncol 1988; 24:315–324.

62. Clark OH. TSH suppression in the management of thyroid nodules and thyroid cancer. World J Surg 1981; 5:39–47.

31
Hypoparathyroidism and Min...

Jaakko Perheentupa
Children's Hospital, University of Helsinki,
Helsinki, Finland

I. INTRODUCTION

Hypoparathyroidism (HP) refers to a spectrum of disorders with deficient parathyroid hormone (PTH) effect. It comprises deficient secretion of PTH (HP) and defects in its effector mechanism collectively called pseudo-HP (PHP). Delay in the recognition of these disorders may lead to permanent brain damage or even death. An effective therapy is available. It is not, however, a real substitution therapy but employs calciferol sterols, which lack the renal effects of PTH and are potentially toxic. Therefore, the therapy must be carefully monitored.

II. PHYSIOLOGIC BACKGROUND

The homeostasis of calcium (Ca) and phosphate concentrations in the extracellular fluid (1) is maintained by a finely integrated regulation of their absorption from the intestine, reabsorption from the glomerular filtrate, and mobilization from the skeleton. The parathyroid glands (PTG) are the regulatory center. Their action is mediated by PTH, directly and indirectly via the steroid hormone calcitriol.

A. Parathyroid Glands and Hormones

Most people have four PTG, with an average total weight of 120 mg in the adult. The lower pair arise in association with thymus from the third branchial pouch and migrate caudally to separate from the thymus at the 18 mm embryo stage and assume a variable final location, commonly at the lower pole of the thyroid gland but sometimes mediastinally even at the level of the pericardium. The upper pair derive from the more caudal fourth branchial pouch and remain stationary, with final location at the upper pole of the thyroid. Chief cells, the major cells of the glands, are arranged in cords and sheets.

PTH (1) is a single-chain 9500 molecular weight 84 amino acid polypeptide (Fig. 1) produced by two enzymatic cleavages at the amino terminus of its preprohormone (115 amino acids). The gene, located in chromosome 11p15, most likely near the border of bands 11p15.4 and 11p15.3 (3), consists of four introns and three exons. It has been sequenced (4) and cloned (5). Several polymorphisms of the gene have been reported, which allows linkage studies (6–8).

PTH(1–34) possesses the full adenylyl cyclase stimulating activity of the hormone, residues 1 and 2 being necessary for this potency and residues 10–34 for binding to a specific cell membrane receptor (9). PTH molecule lacking residues 1 and 2 is a competitive inhibitor of the hormone in vitro, lacking the biologic potency but having full receptor binding activity. The molecule appears to have two other regions with different biologic activities (Fig. 1); there may be other receptors for these regions (2).

PTH-related peptide, another hormone produced by PTG, and PTH are very similar in their regions of the first 13 amino acids and less so in their 14–34 regions as to amino acid sequence, action, and receptor affinity (Fig. 1). The rest of the two molecules differ almost completely (2,10). The PTH-related peptide (PTHrP) gene resides on chromosome 12p in a location analogous to that of PTH gene on 11p. The PTHrP gene can serve as a template for three different forms of PTHrP, formed by alternative splicing of the last three coding regions of the primary messenger RNA transcript. These forms consist of 139, 141, and 173 amino acids, being identical in their 1–139 region. The 75–85 region exerts a strong placental Ca transport stimulating activity (Fig. 1), and fetal parathyroidal PTHrP is thought to be the circulating PTH of the mammalian fetus that maintains the fetal-maternal calcemia gradient, among other functions (2). PTHrP is widely distributed in human fetal epithelia (11) and presumably has other functions besides its role in Ca homeostasis.

1. Regulation of Parathyroid Hormone Synthesis and Secretion

The secretion, synthesis, and intraparathyroid degradation of PTH are all regulated most importantly by the extracellular

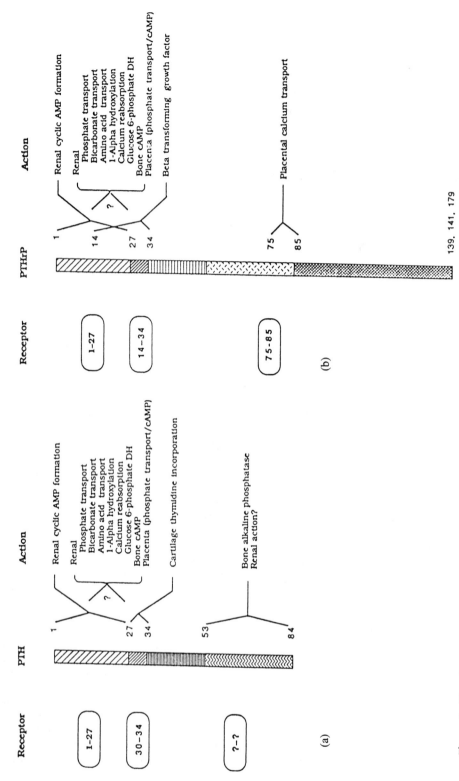

Figure 1 Functional regions of PTH (a) and PTH-related peptide (b) and their documented or postulated receptors. Different shadings indicate the approximate extent of the functional domains that can be differentiated. (From Ref. 2.)

Ca^{2+} concentration through complex mechanisms that have not been completely clarified. The chief cells of PTG are exquisitely sensitive to Ca^{2+} (12,13). Low Ca^{2+} enhances PTH release, probably via a mechanism that includes activation of protein kinase C as the principal component (14). Production of cAMP is also involved. PTG adenylyl cyclase has an absolute requirement for Mg^{2+}, is stimulated by low Ca^{2+} concentration, and has a sensitivity to inhibition by high Ca^{2+} concentrations, some 100- to 200-fold higher than this enzyme in other cell types. High Ca^{2+}, perhaps through a "Ca^{2+} receptor," enhances cellular membrane phospholipid hydrolysis, producing inositol triphosphate and diacylglycerol. These act to increase intracellular Ca^{2+} levels, thereby activating proteolysis of PTH. Both the proteolysis of PTH and simultaneous inactivation of protein kinase C are probably a result of activation by Ca^{2+} of protease calpain (14). These two responses mediate a rapid decrease in the release of intact PTH. At normal extracellular Ca^{2+} levels, PTG synthesizes PTH at a nearly maximal rate, and changing the Ca^{2+} concentration has no rapid effects on PTH mRNA expression. The primary control of availability of PTH is probably achieved via the effect of Ca^{2+} on PTH secretion and degradation. At high Ca^{2+} levels a smaller proportion of the secretion of PTG is intact PTH and a larger proportion PTH fragments. There is an inverse sigmoidal relationship between extracellular Ca^{2+} concentration and the release of intact PTH, with the normal set point (the 50% response) at approximately 1.25 mmol/L. A Ca^{2+}-independent, nonsuppressible baseline component of PTH secretion is also present.

Both positive and negative regulatory elements exist in the 5' flanking region of the PTH gene (5). Cytoplasmic levels of preproPTH mRNA may be directly regulated by Ca^{2+}, and Ca^{2+} probably modifies PTH gene transcription. Calcitriol is also a potent downregulator of the expression of the gene. A normal extracellular concentration of Mg^{2+} (9) is a prerequisite of normal PTH secretion, and both hypermagnesemia and hypomagnesemia inhibit it. Statistically, persons with low borderline plasma Mg concentration recover more slowly from induced reduction of plasma Ca^{2+} than persons with high normal plasma Mg (15).

Newborn infants under 3 days of postnatal age have poorer PTH secretory responses to hypocalcemia than older infants. Postnatal age has here a dominant effect over gestational age (16).

2. Parathyroid Hormone in the Circulation

Intact PTH, its active amino-terminal fragment, and its inactive carboxyl-terminal fragment are present in plasma. In normocalcemia, their respective proportions of the total circulating PTH immunoreactivity are 10, 10, and 80% (1). At low extracellular Ca^{2+} levels large quantities of the intact hormone are secreted, and at high levels more of the carboxyl-terminal fragment.

3. Cellular Mechanism of Parathyroid Hormone Action

The cAMP effector system of the cellular actions of PTH is the best known (Fig. 2). A heterotrimeric guanine nucleotide binding or G protein (previously called N protein) couples the receptor to adenylyl cyclase. A family of G proteins

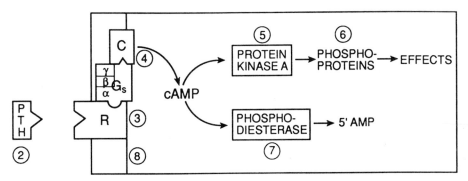

Figure 2 Effector cascade of PTH in a cell of the proximal renal tubule. Activation of adenylyl cyclase by binding of PTH to its specific receptor (R) in the basolateral cell membrane is mediated by the G$_s$ (stimulatory guanyl nucleotide) protein. The G$_s$ protein consists of three subunits, of which the α subunit binds guanyl nucleotide and interconverts between inactive GDP binding and active GTP binding forms. In the presence of PTH, a PTH-receptor complex is formed, binds to the G$_s$ protein, and induces such a change in the conformation of the α subunit that this rejects GDP and allows GTP to enter. The G$_s\alpha$-GTP complex then dissociates from the rest of the G$_s$ protein and activates adenylyl cyclase. Cyclic AMP (cAMP) is produced and binds to the regulatory subunit of protein kinase A, liberating the catalytic subunit of the kinase (C). The kinase thus activated then phosphorylates specific effector proteins, resulting in inhibition of the cotransport of phosphate and Na$^+$ among other effects. The PTH effect is reflected by an increase in cAMP in blood plasma and urine. The PTH signal is automatically switched off because the G$_s$ protein has an intrinsic GTPase activity (built-in device of deactivation) and cytosolic phosphodiesterase hydrolyzes cAMP. Many other polypeptide hormones use the same effector cascade, only the hormone receptor and the effector proteins being specific to the cell type. The circled numbers indicate different potential locations of defect in the signal cascade that may lead to failure of the PTH effect: 1 is deficiency of PTH; 8 refers to the possibility that inhibitory G protein G$_i$, also present in these cells, could carry a defect leading to constant inhibition of adenylyl cyclase.

mediates numerous transmembrane hormone and sensory transduction processes in eukaryotic cells (17). The α subunit, which is distinctive to each G protein, contains a GTP binding site, confers specificity for binding of the G protein to specific membrane-associated receptors, and has GTPase activity. The β and γ subunits are essential for efficient coupling of the α subunit to the receptor and are important for modulation of effectors (18). A receptor-inhibitory G protein (G_i) complex mediating inhibitory signals to the adenylyl cyclase is present in many cells, including the epithelial cells of proximal renal tubules (19). The phospholipase C/protein kinase C signaling cascade is also involved in the regulation of proximal tubular cells by PTH (20). It is not clear whether this cascade is linked to the same or a different PTH receptor as the adenylyl cyclase/protein kinase A pathway (21). The phospholipase C/protein kinase C cascade may be predominant (22) in the actions of PTH on bone remodeling and Ca reabsorption in the distal renal tubule (23–25).

The cDNA encoding a 585 amino acid receptor for PTH and PTHrP(1–27) has been cloned (26,27). The molecule has seven putative membrane-spanning regions, as is common to receptors associated with adenylyl cyclase. It has a striking homology with the calcitonin receptor and secretin receptor and a lack of homology with other G protein-linked receptors. Other PTH and PTHrP receptors are likely to exist. A PTH-sensitive adenylyl cyclase has been identified in skin fibroblasts, cardiac cells, and vascular smooth muscle. PTH may regulate cytosolic Ca^{2+} in these cells (25).

There is a single 13 exon $G_s\alpha$ gene spanning 20 kilobases in chromosome 20q13.11. It produces four isoforms of the protein with slightly different amino acid sequences as a result of alternative splicing of the gene transcript. Two of them are long (52 kD) and two short (45 kD). These isoforms may have different functions in the cell (28).

B. Calcitriol (1,25-Dihydroxycalciferol)

The inactive prohormone vitamin D or calciferol is obtained from synthesis in sun-exposed skin and from food. It is hydroxylated in the liver to 25-hydroxyvitamin D [25(OH)*D*], a partially active compound, and in the kidney (and placenta, bone cells, keratinocytes, and breast and granulomatous tissue) further to the hormone calcitriol [1,25-dihydroxyvitamin D, 1,25(OH)$_2$D] or, alternatively, to 24,25(OH)$_2$D (24, 25-dihydroxyvitamin D), a less active compound of unclear significance. These hydroxylations in the kidney are the key points in the regulation of the hormone synthesis.

Vitamins D$_2$ and D$_3$ and their corresponding metabolites are equally potent in humans.

Calcitriol acts on the kidneys, skeleton, intestine, and PTG, and has other important functions. It regulates the activity of T lymphocytes and is a growth factor for many types of cells, both normal and tumoral (29).

1. Calcitriol Production and Its Regulation (30–32)

Vitamins D$_2$ and D$_3$ are absorbed from the duodenum and jejunum into the lymphatic channels. In states of fat malabsorption this absorption may fail. Both prohormones are stored in adipose tissue and muscle. The amount stored is simply a function of the intake. Their hydroxylated metabolites are less fat soluble and less likely to be stored in amounts that may be harmful. Conversion to 25(OH)D depends directly on the quantity of circulating vitamin D.

The synthesis of the 1- and 24-hydroxylases is regulated reciprocally so that conditions that favor the synthesis of one inhibit the synthesis of the other (33,34). The regulators are PTH, calcitriol, and extracellular concentrations of phosphate and Ca. Manipulation of Ca intake within the normal range has a pronounced effect on circulating calcitriol levels through modifying the secretion of PTH (35). Low extracellular concentrations of phosphate promote the synthesis of calcitriol, and high phosphate concentrations inhibit it. These effects are independent of PTH. In turn, calcitriol stimulates mobilization of phosphate from bone and its absorption from the intestine. Thus a plasma phosphate-calcitriol feedback loop exists regulating plasma phosphate concentration independently of the Ca^{2+}-PTH-calcitriol loop.

Glucocorticoids appear to interfere with the effects of calcitriol without altering its synthesis.

2. Calciferol Sterols in Plasma

Normally, the total concentration of D$_2$ and D$_3$ in plasma is 2.6–26 nmol/L (1–10 ng/ml), and their half-lives in the circulation are about 24 h. The major circulating form is the 25(OH)D, with an average plasma concentration of 75 nmol/L and a circulating half-life of about 15 days. Calcitriol circulates at almost 1000-fold lower concentrations (Table 1), with a half-life of approximately 15 h (36). These sterols are bound to a specific α-globulin, vitamin D binding protein, of which only 1–3% is saturated at physiologic levels of the sterols. The protein also appears to have a storage function. When bound to this carrier, calcitriol is the most freely dissociable of the group.

3. Cellular Mechanism of Calcitriol Action

Like other steroid hormones, calcitriol binds in its target cells to a specific cytoplasmic 427 amino acid receptor, the vitamin D receptor (VDR). The complex is then translocated to the nucleus, where it binds to response elements on specific DNA and activates gene transcription. The VDR gene is a member of the steroid receptor supergene family.

4. Synthetic Analogs

Two synthetic vitamin D analogs are therapeutically important, 1α(OH)D$_3$ and dihydrotachysterol (DHT). These do not need the 1-hydroxylation for activation and are therefore potent in states of reduced 1-hydroxylation activity, such as HP. 1α(OH)D$_3$ is similar in potency to the hormone, presumably after 25-hydroxylation in the liver. DHT is rapidly hydroxylated to 25(OH)DHT. DHT was the active component of AT-10, a drug notorious historically for its unreliable composition and potency.

C. The Kidneys

Regulation of urinary excretion plays an important role in the homeostasis of minerals, especially phosphate (1). This

Table 1 Reference Values for Parameters of Mineral Metabolism

Parameter	SI			Conventional			Conversion factor
Calcium, serum							
Ionized	1.18–	1.30	mmol/L	4.7 –	5.2	mg/dl	0.25
Total	2.20–	2.65	mmol/L	8.8 –	10.6	mg/dl	
Calcitriol, plasma	35 –	160	pmol/L	15 –	67	pg/ml	2.40
25(OH)D, plasma	20 –	120	nmol/L	8 –	48	ng/ml	2.50
Magnesium, serum							
Newborn	0.75–	1.15	mmol/L	1.82–	2.80	mg/dl	0.41
Child and adult	0.70–	1.00	mmol/L	1.70–	2.40	mg/dl	
Parathyroid hormone, intact, serum (immunoradiometric assay)	15 –	60	ng/L	15 –	60	pg/ml	
Phosphate (as P), serum							
Newborn	1.40–	3.05	mmol/L	4.3 –	9.4	mg/dl	0.32
1–5 months	1.55–	2.60		4.8 –	8.1		
6–24 months	1.30–	2.20		4.0 –	6.8		
2–3 years	1.16–	2.10		3.6 –	6.5		
Prepubertal child	1.16–	1.80		3.6 –	5.6		
Puberty	1.07–	1.95		3.3 –	6.0		
After puberty	0.80–	1.40		2.5 –	4.3		
T_mP/GFR[a]							
Newborn	1.30–	3.46	mmol/L	4.0 –	10.7	mg/dl	0.32
3 months	1.30–	3.07		4.0 –	9.5		
6 months	1.30–	2.62		4.0 –	8.2		
Child	1.30–	2.58		4.0 –	8.0		
Puberty: gradual decrease to adult values							
Adult	0.71–	1.45		2.2 –	4.5		

[a]From: References 38a and 39.

regulation is mediated by PTH. The PTG-kidney axis also indirectly regulates the intestinal absorption of Ca^{2+} and phosphate by determining the rate of synthesis of calcitriol.

1. Effects of Parathyroid Hormone

PTH has three main actions on the kidneys (Fig. 3). The total rate of phosphate excretion is always less than its filtered load, normally 5–20%. Phosphate is reabsorbed in the proximal tubules by a pH- and Na^+-dependent, active, saturable mechanism involving a Na^+/phosphate cotransporter (20,37). Hence this reabsorption has a maximum rate (T_mP). If other factors remain unaltered, increased PTH secretion reduces T_mP and decreased secretion enhances it. T_mP in turn determines the fasting plasma phosphate concentration, which is maintained close to the value of the quotient of T_mP and the glomerular filtration rate (T_mP/GFR, Fig. 4 and Table 1). This quotient is also called the phosphate threshold. T_mP/GFR is the best laboratory indicator of renal PTH action (38,38a,39). In response to an injection of PTH, an abrupt increase in phosphate excretion occurs within minutes. HP results in an increased T_mP/GFR and thus an elevated plasma phosphate level. Similarly, PTH reduces the reabsorption of bicarbonate, and in HP plasma bicarbonate levels are often elevated.

In normal circumstances tubular Ca^{2+} reabsorption is extremely efficient: only 1–3% of the filtered load is excreted. Reabsorption takes place at multiple sites: approximately 67% is absorbed in the proximal tubule, 25% in the loop of Henle, and the rest in the distal tubule. The reabsorption mechanisms are different (Fig. 3) (39a). The proximal process is unsaturable and strongly linked to Na^+ reabsorption. Hence, factors that enhance the delivery of Na^+ to the distal tubule (high Na^+ intake and furosemide) lead to a decrease in the fractional absorption of Ca^{2+} in the proximal tubule. The distal Ca^{2+} absorption mechanism is saturable, independent of Na^+ transport, and sensitive to PTH. It is the distal reabsorption that is adjusted by PTH, and the Ca^{2+} messenger system may be involved in mediation of this PTH action (22,24). Normocalcemic patients with HP excrete about threefold more Ca^{2+} than normal subjects (24,40). Saline diuresis (except when induced by thiazide diuretics) is accompanied by an increase in Ca^{2+} excretion, because the distal reabsorptive capacity is overwhelmed by the increased distal delivery of Ca^{2+}.

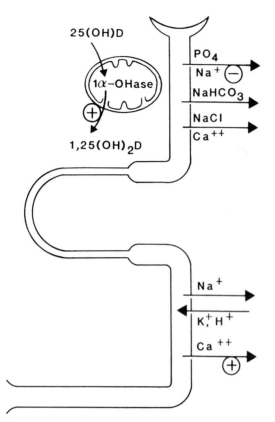

Figure 3 Effects of PTH in the kidney. The three effects are marked + (stimulation) and − (inhibition): (1) inhibition of the reabsorption of phosphate and Na$^+$ in the proximal tubule, (2) stimulation of the synthesis of 1-hydroxylase in the proximal tubule and, thereby, production of calcitriol [1,25(OH)₂D], and (3) stimulation of reabsorption of Ca^{2+} in the distal tubule. The proximal tubule has a different mechanism for reabsorption of Ca^{2+}; this is associated with the absorption of the NaCl and is not affected by PTH.

2. Effects of Calcitriol

Calcitriol suppresses the synthesis of the 1-hydroxylase and induces the synthesis of 24-hydroxylase in the cells of the proximal tubules.

Both PTH and calcitriol are needed for normal control of fractional Ca^{2+} excretion (41). A calcitriol-inducible Ca^{2+} binding protein, calbindin-D$_{28k}$, may be involved in the PTH-mediated Ca^{2+} reabsorption (32,42). Calcitriol does not appear to exert a direct influence on T_mP, but it has a permissive role in the phosphaturic effect of PTH. When used in the treatment of HP, vitamin D sterols reduce phosphate reabsorption from elevated to normal levels. This results largely from an increase in plasma Ca^{2+}, which directly reduces proximal tubular phosphate reabsorption. Calcitriol may be involved in the inherent ability of the nephrons to adapt to altered plasma phosphate levels. This adaptability is independent of PTH but appears to be more efficient in the presence of calcitriol than in its absence (37).

D. The Skeleton

The skeleton serves as a store of Ca^{2+} and phosphate through two metabolic systems, the homeostatic and the remodeling system. In the homeostatic system, surface osteocytes alter on a minute-by-minute basis the flux of mineral between the skeletal surface compartment and the extracellular fluid. The remodeling system consists of osteoclasts resorbing old bone and osteoblasts laying down new bone. PTH regulates both these systems with calcitriol in a permissive role, especially in the homeostatic system (43). During sustained hypocalcemia these hormones inhibit osteoblastic bone formation while activating osteoclasts and increasing their number. Calcitriol appears to influence the entire gene apparatus that regulates the maturation of osteoclasts from their precursor cells. The osteoclasts lack the PTH receptor, and the action of PTH on the osteoclast appears to be secondary to an effect on the osteoblast.

Modest elevations of plasma concentration of calcitriol, for example to 70 pg/ml, are not associated with hypercalcemia, which develops with elevations in the range of 125 pg/ml (1).

Calcitriol also induces the synthesis of alkaline phosphatase and osteocalcin in the osteoblasts and inhibits the synthesis of type I collagen. In normal mineralization calcitriol appears to act only by maintaining an adequate ion product of Ca and phosphate, not by a direct action on bone cells.

E. The Intestine

The intestinal absorption of Ca^{2+} is precisely regulated. The active absorption of Ca^{2+} is regulated by calcitriol, and PTH is involved only as the regulator of the synthesis of calcitriol. Calcitriol induces in the intestinal mucosa the synthesis of a Ca binding protein, calbindin$_{9k}$, possibly a transporter (42). The Ca^{2+} absorption system is independent of phosphate transport, although phosphate is the anion that normally accompanies Ca^{2+}. Net Ca^{2+} absorption normally averages about 20% of Ca^{2+} intake but can vary over the range of 15–75%, depending on the calcitriol status. The absorption of phosphate and magnesium is a linear function of their dietary intake (44). Both are absorbed predominantly by (separate) active carrier-mediated transport mechanisms, but also by passive diffusion. The proportion of phosphate absorbed is about threefold larger than that of Ca^{2+}.

F. Calcium, Phosphate, and Magnesium in Plasma

1. Calcium

The total content of Ca in plasma (Table 1) consists of three fractions: Ca^{2+} (normally about 43%), protein-bound Ca (47%, 70% being bound to albumin), and Ca complexed to phosphate, citrate, and so on (10%). Ca^{2+} is the regulated, physiologically important fraction.

The regulation of plasma Ca concentration is so precise that it normally fluctuates by <0.025 mmol/L (<0.1 mg/dl) in either direction from its "set" value. The skeletal and renal

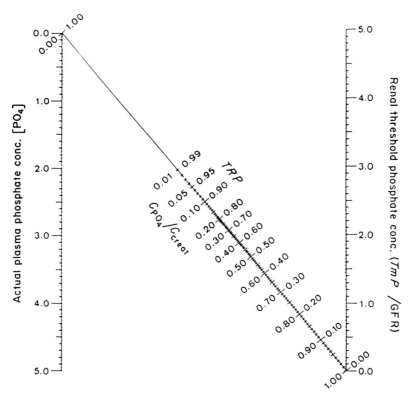

Figure 4 Nomogram for determination of T_mP/GFR. Traditional units (mg/dl) are used. T_mP/GFR is obtained by drawing a straight line from the serum phosphate concentration on the left vertical scale through the value on the lower diagonal scale of the quotient of phosphate and creatinine clearances (C_{PO_4}/C_{creat}), calculated as (U-P × S-Cr)/(S-P × U-Cr), where U is urine, S is serum and Cr is creatinine. The point of intersection of this line and the right vertical scale indicates the value of T_mP/GFR. For reference values, see Table 1. (From Ref. 38.)

effects of PTH make up a fast-acting short-loop feedback system. The renal-intestinal effect provides a slower (12–24 h) long-loop feedback system (1).

The binding of albumin is pH dependent: the concentration of Ca^{2+} decreases in acute alkalosis and increases in acute acidosis. If plasma albumin concentration decreases by 50%, the total Ca concentration is reduced by about 20%. Also, for every 10 g/L (g/dl) reduction in plasma albumin, the total Ca is decreased by approximately 0.25 mmol/L (1.0 mg/dl). These changes as such do not alter the Ca^{2+} concentration. Total Ca varies only slightly with age, the actual extent depending on the protein concentration.

A decrease in the concentration of Ca^{2+} increases Na^+ permeability and enhances the excitability of all excitable cells. An increased concentration has the reverse effect.

Hypocalcemic challenges are of varying severity. A 12–15 h fast is a mild challenge. Because of continued Ca^{2+} loss via the urine, the plasma Ca^{2+} concentration decreases slightly and is rapidly corrected by increased entry from the kidneys and skeleton, induced by a minor increase in PTH secretion (Fig. 5). A stronger challenge, such as an extra urinary loss of Ca^{2+} after administration of a large dose of furosemide, calls for a moderate increase in PTH secretion and part of the response is an increase in the synthesis of

calcitriol. The increased PTH activity also decreases renal reabsorption of phosphate, and this rids the extracellular fluid of the extra phosphate. Plasma levels of Ca and phosphate are thus normalized, but a mild secondary hyperparathyroidism persists, the improved intestinal absorption of minerals replacing the initial need for skeletal mobilization.

Hypercalcemia, even a slight rise in plasma Ca^{2+}, is combated by suppression of PTH secretion. This leads to increased urinary loss of Ca^{2+} and reduced entry of minerals from the skeleton and, through suppression of the synthesis of calcitriol, from the intestine. Hypercalcemia raises the concentration of calcitonin in plasma, but calcitonin does not appear to contribute importantly to the protection against hypercalcemia. A limit to the protection against hypercalcemia is set by the excretory capacity of the kidneys. This may be impaired by a vicious cycle based on the fact that hypercalcemia leads to excessive urinary loss of water and hence tends to cause dehydration.

2. Phosphate

The plasma phosphate concentration is more variable than the Ca concentration. It is influenced by age (Table 1), diet, and some hormones. No known endocrine factor protects it as a primary function. An adequate ion product of Ca^{2+} and

Normal protection
against hypocalcemia

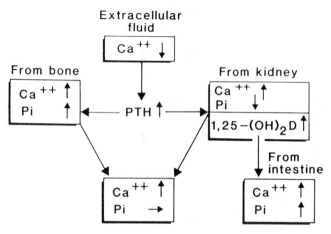

Figure 5 Sequence of adjustments (long arrows) in response to hypocalcemia. Pi, inorganic phosphate. Short arrows indicate directions of change in concentrations in the extracellular fluid (middle), in release from the skeleton (left), in retrieval in the kidneys, and in absorption from the intestine (right).

phosphate is required for normal mineralization of the skeleton. Of the total plasma phosphate, about 52% is ionized, about 35% is complexed to Na^+, Ca^{2+}, and Mg^{2+}, and about 13% is protein bound. The role of the kidneys is paramount in the maintenance of a normal plasma phosphate level, which tends to be close to T_mP/GFR (Sec. II.C.1).

A decrease in plasma phosphate leads to activation of the renal synthesis of calcitriol and thereby to increased intestinal absorption of Ca and a slight rise in its plasma level. Suppression of PTH secretion follows, leading to reduction of renal phosphate clearance and enhancement of Ca clearance. Within 3–4 days of phosphate withdrawal, phosphate excretion may be virtually abolished, and even the phosphaturic response to exogenous PTH becomes blunted. An excess of plasma phosphate is cleared rapidly by normal kidneys because the filtered phosphate load exceeds the renal threshold.

3. Magnesium

Plasma Mg is also less narrowly regulated than Ca. It is determined principally by the renal threshold for Mg excretion. The proportional distribution of plasma Mg to three fractions is similar to that of Ca. The mechanisms of Mg homeostasis are poorly understood. PTG responds similarly to changes in plasma Mg^{2+} as to changes in plasma Ca^{2+}, but less sensitively.

III. MANIFESTATIONS OF DEFICIENT PARATHYROID HORMONE ACTION

A. Chemical Effects

Deficiency of PTH action leads to decreased production of calcitriol, resulting in a bihormonal deficiency. Hypocalcemia

and hyperphosphatemia are pathognomonic to frankly deficient PTH action. Hypocalcemia results from reduced osteocytic Ca transfer as a result of both deficiencies, reduction of PTH-dependent osteoclastic bone resorption and distal tubular Ca reabsorption, and impaired intestinal Ca absorption caused by calcitriol deficiency. Hyperphosphatemia results from increased renal tubular phosphate reabsorption caused by the absence of its adequate inhibition by PTH. Hyperphosphatemia further lowers calcemia by physicochemical means, and further reducing calcitriol synthesis.

1. Hypocalcemia

Severity of deficiency of PTH action varies. Consequently, the plasma Ca concentration in different patients ranges from 1.25 mmol/L (5 mg/dl) to normal (45). In all cases the stability of the plasma Ca level is impaired. It fluctuates with changes in Ca intake and reciprocally with changes in plasma phosphate concentration (46). In the mildest cases the reserve capacity of the calcemia homeostatic system is limited, but normocalcemia is maintained by its maximal activity. In the next degree of severity normocalcemia is maintained in normal situations, but periodic hypocalcemia ensues with fasting or an otherwise unusually low Ca intake, and with excessive phosphate influx from the intestine or breakdown of intracellular organic phosphate compounds during febrile illness. With more severe failure, hypocalcemia is continuous and minor hypocalcemic factors evoke symptoms.

Hypocalcemic patients are hypocalciuric, although their Ca excretion is high relative to the plasma Ca level.

2. Hyperphosphatemia

This is a much less constant feature than hypocalcemia, because (1) less PTH effect is needed to maintain a normal renal phosphate threshold (Sec. II.C) than to maintain normocalcemia (45), and (2) phosphate flow from the skeleton and intestine is subnormal owing to the deficiency of the PTH effect.

3. Other

Because a deficiency of the PTH effect also causes increased renal reabsorption of bicarbonate, plasma bicarbonate levels and blood pH may be elevated (47). Bone remodeling is reduced, and this is reflected by decreased urinary excretion of hydroxyproline in a majority of patients (48). Plasma alkaline phosphatase activity is subnormal only in a few patients, but plasma osteocalcin levels are usually subnormal (48–50).

B. Clinical Manifestations

The main cause of clinical manifestations (51) of deficient PTH effect is hypocalcemia, largely as a result of increased irritability of the central and peripheral nervous systems. Manifestations are more likely to appear when plasma Ca level is falling rapidly than during steady hypocalcemia. Low concentrations of Mg^{2+} and H^+ (alkalosis) and high concentrations of K^+ predispose to tetany. Moderate hypocalcemia may be symptomless.

1. Tetany

Tetany refers to the entire complex of manifestations of increased neural excitability. It ranges from signs evocable by testing (latent tetany) and minor tingling sensations and numbness of the hands to abdominal pain and major convulsive seizures with loss of consciousness. A typical attack of tetany (4) begins with increasing tingling, which starts in the fingertips, around the mouth and sometimes in the feet, and spreads proximally and over the face. Numbness may follow. The muscles then feel tense and go into spasm in the same pattern as the sensory symptoms. The hands and forearms are the parts of the body most commonly involved. First, the thumbs become adducted, followed in order by flexion of the metacarpophalangeal joints, extension of the interphalangeal joints, and flexion of the wrist and elbow, the classic "obstetrician's hand" posture. The muscle spasm causes pain, which may be severe. A similar spasm in the feet is less common, with plantar flexion of the toes, arching of the feet, and contraction of the calf muscles. With a severe attack the face may become involved, with wrinkling of the forehead, a staring gaze, and pursed lips. Hypocapnia and increased epinephrine secretion (caused by panic) worsen the tetany. Hyperventilation is a common feature of hypocalcemic tetany, and hysteria is often incorrectly diagnosed.

a. Atypical Tetany. Patients may experience cramps, stiffness, or clumsiness. With long-standing hypocalcemia they may have frequent mild paresthesias and cramps instead of clearly defined attacks of tetany or may have carpal spasm only during prolonged use of the hand and forearm. Symptoms may be provoked by hyperventilation as a result of emotional stress or exercise. The symptoms may be exclusively sensory. Limping and falling may occur as a result of leg spasms. The symptoms may be unilateral. Laryngeal spasm may occur, causing stridor, crowing respiration, and cyanosis. Minor difficulties in vocalization are not uncommon. Smooth muscle spasms may cause dysphagia, abdominal pain, biliary colic, and wheezing with shortness of breath. Persistent diarrhea may occur (52). Infants are unlikely to develop carpopedal spasms but are prone to tremors and twitches.

b. Signs of Latent Tetany. Signs of latent tetany remain useful in diagnosis and in adjusting therapy. Chvostek's sign is elicited by tapping the facial nerve with a fingertip as a hammer, 1–2 cm anterior to the earlobe just below the zygomatic process. It consists of twitching of the muscles innervated by the facial nerve and is graded (1) twitching of the upper lip at the corner of mouth only, (2) twitching of the alae nasi also, (3) contraction of the orbicularis oculi also, and (4) contraction of all the muscles of that side. The relative sensitivity with which these signs are elicited varies individually. A grade 1 sign is said to be found in >25% of normal children (51). Trousseau's sign is evoked by a sphygmomanometer cuff on the upper arm when inflated to above the systolic pressure for up to 3 minutes.

The sensory and motor manifestations of tetany develop to a typical carpal spasm within 2 minutes. In the mildest cases the patient can overcome the spasm. In the severest not even the examiner can overcome it. Only the severe grade of the sign is abnormal with certainty because the milder grade occurs in a small percentage of normal subjects. The sign depends on induction of ischemia of the ulnar nerve.

c. Seizures. Seizures resembling epilepsy occur. These are of two distinct types. First, because hypocalcemia lowers the threshold for preexisting subclinical epilepsy, epileptic seizures of any type may occur (53). The other type consists of generalized tetany followed by prolonged tonic spasms. It may be preceded by the sensory symptoms of tetany. During the seizure there may be tongue biting, loss of consciousness, and incontinence, and postictal confusion may occur. Hypocalcemia is frequently associated with characteristic changes in the electroencephalogram (54); in severe hypocalcemia, these may be irregular sharp spike-and-wave patterns. These changes may not disappear for some days after restoration of normocalcemia, and abnormal background activity may continue for several weeks.

2. Other

a. Basal Ganglion Calcification and Extrapyramidal Signs. In patients with HP or especially PHP untreated for many years, small irregular calcifications may be seen in the basal ganglia in skull radiographs, particularly on computed tomographic scans (55). These lesions may cause various extrapyramidal signs, including chorioathetosis, dystonic spasms, and classic parkinsonism.

b. Papilledema and Raised Intracranial Pressure. In long-standing untreated HP there may be swelling of the optic disks. This may develop within as little as 2 weeks after the onset of HP as seen following thyroid surgery. It is moderate in degree (≤3 diopters) and unaccompanied by hemorrhage or impaired vision. It may cause unfounded suspicion of an intracranial tumor. The papilledema usually begins to subside within a few days of normocalcemia but may take several weeks to disappear.

c. Psychiatric Disorders. Impaired mental functioning occurs in patients with long-standing HP or PHP. Psychiatric disorders of many kinds have also been described.

d. Dermal and Dental Changes. The skin may be dry and scaling, the nails brittle and fissured, and the hair coarse, dry, fractured, and easily shed. Eruption of teeth may be delayed, and their roots may be blunted. These nail and tooth changes are distinct from the ectodermal dystrophy of autoimmune polyendocrinopathy-candidiasis-ectodermal dystrophy (APECED; Sec. IV.B.1).

e. Cataracts. Lenticular cataracts are a common complication of chronic hypocalcemia. They first appear as discrete punctate or lamellar opacities in the cortex, separated by a clear zone from the capsule (56). They may develop in distinct layers, more in the posterior pole than the anterior, and within 5–10 years they become confluent, with total opacification of the lens. Control of hypocalcemia arrests their progression.

   f. Cardiovascular and Muscle Disorders. Hypocalcemia delays ventricular depolarization and prolongs the $Q-T_c$ and ST intervals on the electrocardiogram. A 2:1 heart block may develop. Ca^{2+} exerts a positive ionotropic effect on the myocardium, but hypocalcemia rarely causes clinical cardiac problems. However, congestive heart failure occurs in children with HP (57) and sudden death caused by cardiac tetany is possible.

   Myopathy, in mildest cases reflected by markedly supranormal plasma creatine kinase levels, has been reported in several hypocalcemic patients (58,59).

IV.   CAUSES OF HYPOPARATHYROIDISM

Congenital HP may be caused by a specific defect in the synthesis or cellular processing of PTH or by aplasia or hypoplasia of PTG. PTG aplasia and hypoplasia occur as isolated defects and as part of sets of anomalies. Depending on its severity, congenital HP may manifest neonatally or only (even several years) later. Late manifestation may be caused by failure of growth of hypoplastic PTG: hence it may be difficult to distinguish between inborn and acquired forms of HP, and the inborn defects should be considered in HP manifesting at any age (Table 2) (52).

A.   Familial Isolated Hypoparathyroidism

Familial isolated HP is a heterogeneous group of conditions fulfilling these criteria: no demonstrable wider anatomic cause, no evidence for APECED (Sec. IV.B), and no (other) developmental defects (60). The group probably includes entities with PTG aplasia and hypoplasia, but anatomic information is meager. Pedigrees with autosomal dominant, autosomal recessive, and X-linked inheritance have been reported. Age at manifestation varies even within pedigrees, often from neonatal to adult (60–62), or there may be no manifestation at all (63).

   Two general molecular mechanisms cause inborn HP. Mutations in or near the preproPTH gene may account for autosomal HP, but such mutations are uncommon (6). Mutations of distant loci that affect embryologic development, cellular composition, or homeostatic regulation of PTG could cause X-linked or autosomal HP (6). Such mutations are the predominant cause of familial isolated HP.

1.   Autosomal Dominant Isolated Hypoparathyroidism

Autosomal dominant familial isolated HP is a heterogeneous group of conditions. A single base mutation was present in the PTH gene in one kindred, resulting in substitution of Arg for Cys in the midst of the hydrophobic signal sequence, which presumably impairs translocation of the molecule across the endoplasmic reticulum (62). Mutation of the PTH gene has been excluded in several families (6,60,64).

2.   Autosomal Recessive Isolated Hypoparathyroidism

In one kindred with autosomal recessive isolated HP, a donor splice mutation was detected at the exon 2/intron 2 boundary, resulting in a loss of exon 2 in the PTH mRNA. Because exon 2 encodes the initiation codon and the signal peptide, a loss of this exon presumably prevents translation of the PTH mRNA and translocation of the peptide. Affected members of the kindred were homozygous for this mutation (65). Mutation of the PTH gene has been excluded in some kindreds (60).

3.   X-Linked Isolated Hypoparathyroidism

Two large kindreds with X-linked recessive isolated HP have been reported from eastern Missouri (66,67). Affected boys had seizures during infancy. In a careful search at autopsy of one of the patients who died accidentally while a teenager, no PTH tissue could be identified (68). The mutant gene, which thus appears to cause defective development of PTG, was localized to Xq26–27 (69).

4.   Other Isolated Hypoparathyroidism

The largest subgroup of patients seems to have circulating PTG antibodies and includes a majority of females. The HP usually manifests at 2–10 years of age. In about one-quarter of cases there is evidence of autosomal recessive inheritance (70). The possibility of APECED cannot be excluded, and one should look for features of ectodermal dystrophy and candidiasis (Sec. IV.B.1).

B.   Autoimmune Polyendocrinopathy-Candidiasis-Ectodermal Dystrophy

This condition is known by many names, including polyglandular autoimmune disease type I; multiple endocrine deficiency, autoimmunity, and candidiasis; and hypoparathyroidism, Addison's disease, and moniliasis (71,72). I prefer APECED (73) because it includes ectodermal dystrophy (a distinguishing feature) and does not include specific endocrinopathies (none of these is constant) (74). This autosomal recessive disease (75,76) manifests as a widely variable combination of three groups of components (74): autoimmune destruction of tissues, predominantly endocrine glands; consequences of a defect of cell-mediated immunity, most commonly chronic superficial candidiasis; and ectodermal dystrophy.

1.   Clinical Picture

This description is based mainly on my experience with 68 patients (Table 3) (74).

   a. Ectodermal Changes. All three groups of disease components include ectodermal changes. These herald the danger of life-threatening manifestations. Chronic oral candidiasis precedes endocrine failure in most cases. It commonly appears during the first year of life, the incidence then slowly decreasing but continuing into the third decade. The oral candidiasis is of variable severity, ranging from intermittent or continuous angular cheilosis (perlèche;

Table 2   Causes of Postneonatal Hypoparathyroidism

I.	Familial isolated PTH deficiency
	A. Autosomal dominant
	B. Autosomal recessive
	C. X-linked
	D. Other
II.	Autoimmune polyendocrinopathy-candidiasis-ectodermal dystrophy (APECED)
III.	PTH deficiency of dysmorphic syndromes
	A. DiGeorge malformation complex
	B. Partial monosomy 10p
	C. Kenny syndrome
	D. Congenital HP, mental retardation, severe growth failure, and dysmorphic features (Sanjad syndrome)
	E. Autosomal dominant HP, deafness, and renal dysplasia
	F. Familial nephrosis, nerve deafness, and HP
	G. Autosomal recessive HP-renal insufficiency-developmental delay
	H. Congenital lymphedema, HP, nephropathy, facial dysmorphism, prolapsing mitral valve, and brachytelephalangy
	I. Other syndromes
IV.	Other congenital isolated PTH deficiency
V.	Transient PTH deficiency
	A. Critical illness
	B. Transient congenital hypoparathyroidism
	C. Maternal hyperparathyroidism
	D. Magnesium depletion
	E. Toxic influence
VI.	Other acquired PTH deficiency
	A. Surgical removal or lesion of PTG
	B. Radiation damage
	C. Infiltration of PTG
	D. Other
VII.	Pseudohypoparathyroidism
	A. Type I (defects proximal to cAMP production)
	1. Type IA (multiple hormone resistance with AHO[a])
	a. Type IAα (G$_s\alpha$ protein defect)
	b. Type IAc (adenylyl cyclase defect)
	2. Type IB (isolated PTH resistance, without AHO): type IBr (PTH receptor defect)
	B. Type II (defects distal to cAMP production)

[a]Albright hereditary osteodystrophy (see text).

fissuring and whitish coating of the labial commissures, Fig. 6) to acute inflammation of the oral mucosa and hyperplastic chronic candidiasis, with thick white coating of the tongue. There may also be atrophic disease with scant coatings and a scarred and thin mucosa (77). Even mild oral candidiasis may cause a burning sensation in the mouth, especially when the patient eats sour foods. Chronic mucosal candidiasis is carcinogenic and should be carefully suppressed by good dental care and oral hygiene, with local antimycotics and, when necessary, systemic antifungal therapy (78). Vulvovaginal candidiasis is common in pubertal and postpubertal patients. Nail and skin candidiasis may also develop. The affected nails are darkly discolored, thickened, or eroded (Fig. 6). Candidal eczema of the hands tends to develop if the hands are frequently wetted and may even spread to the face. Dystrophy of the enamel of the permanent teeth also occurs in almost all patients, but the teeth may be faultless (77). In most patients all the permanent teeth have hypoplastic enamel: either transverse hypoplastic bands alternating with zones of well-formed enamel (Fig. 6), or hypoplasia of all the enamel. In contrast with what has been generally accepted, enamel hypoplasia is not associated with HP. Four closely monitored patients with extensive enamel hypoplasia dating from birth to 10 years had no HP at ages 14–24 years (77). Pitted nail dystrophy is another characteristic in most patients. Although a minor abnormality, it helps to identify patients with otherwise insufficient diagnostic features.

Atrophy of the tympanic membranes is a common,

Table 3　Prevalence of Components of APECED in 68 Patients During Follow-up According to Age[a]

Characteristic	Age (years)									Total
	1	2	5	10	15	20	30	40	50	
No. in age group	67	67	67	61	53	44	19	9	4	68
No. females	31	31	31	28	25	22	9	1	1	31
No. deaths	0	0	0	1	3	5	5	6	6	9
No. endocrine components per patients, %										
≥1	0	6	31	64	79	86	89	89	100	96
≥2	0	0	6	18	43	55	47	25	75	60
≥3	0	0	0	18	43	55	47	25	75	60
None	100	94	39	36	21	14	11	11	0	4
Endocrine components, %										
Hypoparathyroidism	0	6	31	57	70	80	74	56	100	79
Adrenal failure	0	0	3	23	51	66	58	33	25	72
Insulin-dependent diabetes mellitus	0	0	3	2	2	9	11	22	50	12
Parietal cell atrophy	0	0	0	2	6	9	16	33	75	13
Hypothyroidism	0	0	0	0	0	5	5	0	0	4
Ovarian failure[b]	—	—	—	—	36	55	56	0	0	60
Testicular failure[c]	—	—	—	—	4	14	20	25	67	14
Nonendocrine components, %										
Candidiasis[d]	18	31	55	89	94	95	100	100	100	100
Alopecia	0	0	0	13	25	32	44	44	33	29
Vitiligo	1	1	4	5	8	16	26	11	0	13
Keratopathy	1	4	10	23	32	30	26	33	25	35
Hepatitis	—	—	—	—	—	—	—	—	—	12
Intestinal malabsorption	—	—	—	—	—	—	—	—	—	18
Enamel hypoplasia[e]	—	—	—	—	—	—	—	—	—	77
Tympanic membrane calcification[f]	—	—	—	—	—	—	—	—	—	33
Nail dystrophy[g]	—	—	—	—	—	—	—	—	—	52

[a]Because the present ages of the patients range from 10 months to 53 years and some patients have died, the number of observations shown decreases with increasing age. Dashes indicate that data according to age were unavailable. Ovarian and testicular failure were not diagnosed before puberty, and the development of the components shown at the bottom was not monitored systematically.

[b]Calculated for females ≥ 13 years of age.

[c]Calculated for males ≥ 15 years of age.

[d]For 10 patients, the age at onset of candidiasis was taken as 10 years because it developed earlier but exact dating was impossible. Includes oral, dermal, and ungual candidiasis.

[e]Based on 44 patients who could be evaluated.

[f]Based on 42 patients who could be evaluated.

[g]Based on 50 patients who could be evaluated.

Source: From Reference. 74.

although less clearly defined, anomaly. Many patients have conspicuous Ca deposits in the tympanic membranes (79).

Alopecia showed its highest incidence at ages 5–15 years. It appears as hairless patches (Fig. 6) and may proceed to complete baldness and lack of eye and body hair. It results from autoimmune injury to the hair follicles, as evidenced by their lymphocytic infiltration. Vitiligo appears as unpigmented patches that tend to grow slowly.

b. Endocrinopathies. Hypoparathyroidism appeared at ages 1.6–44 years. Its incidence in patients at risk was highest, 0.09 cases per patient year, at ages 2–4 years. It then decreased slowly to 0.05 per patient-year at ages 15–19 years. In some patients, there was progression of HP from a latent to a severe form during a period of some months.

Addison's disease appeared at ages 4.3–41 years. Its incidence in the patients at risk increased from 0.01 cases per patient year at ages 2–4 years to a maximum of 0.08 cases/year at ages 10–14 years, thereafter slowly decreasing. Deficiencies of cortisol and aldosterone often appeared independently of each other (separated by as much as 6 years), and in random order. In some patients the transition from normal cortisol secretion to severe failure occurred within a few months, but the destruction may be much slower (80).

Hypogonadism developed in 60% of our female patients at risk and only 14% of the male patients at risk. It was caused by a primary gonadal lesion in all but one patient, a male with secondary hypogonadism. Half the females with ovarian atrophy had failure of pubertal development and primary amenorrhea. Slow destruction of the ovaries has been described (81).

Insulin deficiency has now occurred in 15% of our patients, with an even incidence throughout the age range 1–40 years.

Thyroid disease appeared only in the form of primary atrophic hypothyroidism and was relatively uncommon. Several other patients had significant titers of circulating thyroid antibodies. We are not aware of any certain cases of Graves' or Hashimoto's disease.

Antidiuretic hormone deficiency has been described in two patients (82,83); circulating antibodies reacting with the cytoplasmic components of vasopressin-secreting cells were observed in one of them (82). A male patient of ours and another (84) had gonadotropin deficiency. Adrenocorticotropic hormone (ACTH) deficiency has been reported in three patients (84,85), but differentiation from primary Addison's disease was not convincing.

c. Ocular Disease. Keratopathy developed between the ages of 0.8 and 18 years. It appears as a sensation of having sand in the eyes and increased sensitivity to light. If not carefully treated (with local application of cortisol and, with secondary infections, antibiotics), it causes a permanent decrease in visual acuity (≤ 0.25 in 42% of the affected eyes) (86) and even total blindness. Keratopathy occurs independently of HP.

Additional problems were iritis in two of our patients, cyclitis in one, and optic atrophy in two (86). Papilledema, cataract, retinitis pigmentosa, pseudoptosis, and exotropia have been described (87).

d. Others. Periodic intestinal fat malabsorption occurs through an unknown mechanism. It has been associated with HP and hypocalcemia in all our patients. Steatorrhea was part of the initial manifestation of APECED in most of our patients who have it. It tends to recur whenever the patients become hypocalcemic and renders the control of hypocalcemia difficult. However, other patients with a comparable degree of hypocalcemia maintain normal fat absorption. Hypocalcemia caused by vitamin D deficiency secondary to steatorrhea may be erroneously diagnosed in these patients. This condition includes secondary hyperparathyroidism and thus should be easily differentiated from HP by measurements of serum phosphate (high in HP and low in vitamin D deficiency) and serum PTH (low in HP and high in vitamin D deficiency) (52).

Gastric parietal cell failure with vitamin B_{12} malabsorption necessitates vitamin B_{12} injections as permanent replacement therapy. It is essential that the macrocytic anemia these patients may develop not be mistakenly diagnosed as resulting from folate deficiency (often associated with fat malabsorption). Folate therapy may temporarily correct the anemia and thus allow the neurologic manifestations of vitamin B_{12} deficiency to develop (52). Pure red cell aplasia has been observed in a few cases; in one patient gammaglobulin therapy led to complete recovery (88).

Hepatitis was chronic in all but two patients, who died of fulminant hepatic failure at ages 7 and 17 years. Chronic hepatitis was the presenting manifestation in a boy of 0.7 years.

Dermal vasculitis was part of the presenting picture of our patient with early hepatitis. Rheumatoid arthritis developed in a severe form in one of our patients in her late twenties.

e. Course and Prognosis (74). Most of the patients (75% in our series) develop a clear nonendocrine manifestation (oral candidiasis in 62%, alopecia in 10%, and keratopathy in 3%) before the first endocrinopathy. In our series this interval was 0.1–33.3 (median 4.1) years. At least one endocrinopathy was present in 96% of the patients (this figure is certainly an overestimate, because of obvious nonascertainment of patients lacking endocrinopathy). Whether some patients remain free of endocrinopathy is unknown. In patients with endocrinopathy, the initial failure was HP in 75% and Addison's disease in 18%. Both appeared simultaneously in 7%. In the others who had both failures, the interval between the manifestations was 0.3–28 (median 5.5) years. Apparently, the risk of developing new components continues throughout life, although it decreases continuously. Patients in whom the disease has not been diagnosed are at risk of death from HP, Addison's disease, diabetes mellitus, hepatitis, and, perhaps, tuberculosis. Patients in whom the diagnosis has been made must be monitored for the appearance of additional disease components. Teenage patients with multiple disease components suffer from a great psychic burden, and their management may be especially difficult. Kidney damage during periods of hypercalcemia caused by oversubstitution for HP is also a risk. The therapy for hepatitis is unsatisfactory, as may be that for rheumatoid arthritis. Oral carcinoma is another risk; 4 of our patients have developed it.

2. Immune System Abnormalities

a. Autoantibodies. The autoimmune destruction of endocrine glands (evidenced by lymphocytic infiltration) is reflected by circulating autoantibodies against the affected tissues. Only a few laboratories have succeeded in demonstrating anti-PTG antibodies (89). Adrenal and steroidal cell antibodies are predictive of Addison's disease, steroidal cell antibodies also of ovarian failure (81). The antigens recognized by the adrenal and steroidal cell antibodies are varyingly cytochrome P_{450} enzymes $P_{450}scc$, $P_{450}c17$, and $P_{450}c21$ (90,91). Antiparietal cell antibodies precede parietal cell atrophy. High

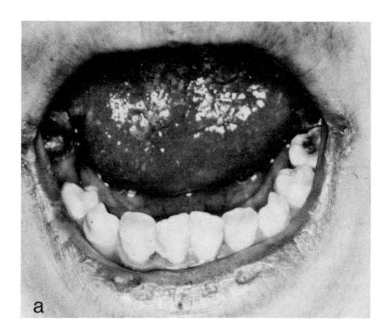

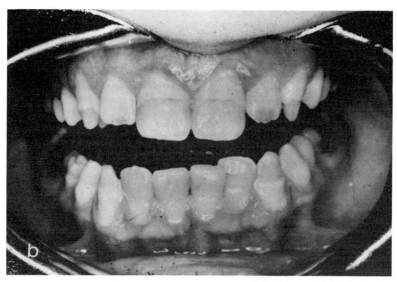

Figure 6 Ectodermal manifestations of APECED: (a) angular cheilosis with candidal coating of the tongue; (b) transverse ridges of enamel hypoplasia in permanent teeth; (c) pitted nail dystrophy; (d) eroding nail candidiasis; and (e) patches of vitiligo and alopecia.

titers of antibodies reacting with glutamic acid decarboxylase (GAD65) and the pancreatic islet cells are common, but their value in predicting diabetes is poor (92,92a); the same is true for antithyroidal antibodies in predicting hypothyroidism. Antibodies against vasopressin-secreting cells have been reported in 1 case (83). Antimelanocyte antibodies have been reported in vitiligo (93) and antibodies against hair follicles in alopecia (94).

b. Lymphocyte Abnormalities. The basic defect underlying the autoimmunity and defective immunoprotection

against *Candida* remains unknown; it is probably a disorder of immunoregulation. Part of the ignorance is because heterogeneous groups of patients with different polyendocrinopathies have been studied (95). No abnormal feature seems to be universally present in all patients with APECED. The most common feature is a selective defect in the T cell-mediated immunity against *Candida*, evidenced by an absent or deficient delayed cutaneous hypersensitivity response to *Candida* antigen. A wider failure of delayed hypersensitivity has been observed in some patients

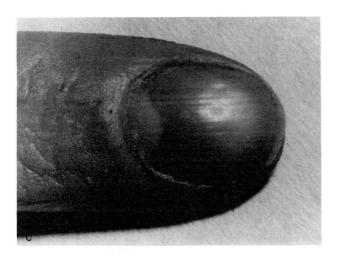

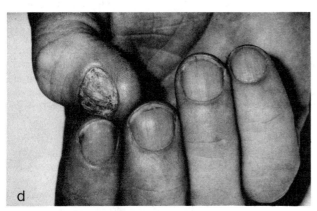

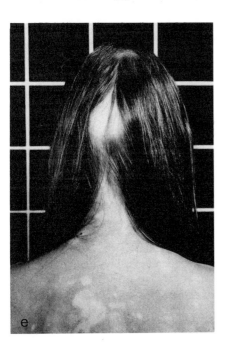

(84,85,95). Lymphocytes responded normally in vitro to stimulation by *Candida albicans* (85). Subnormal suppressor cell activity has been reported (96). An increased frequency of a number of mild lymphocyte abnormalities has been observed (97). Circulating levels of immunoglobulins show variable abnormalities; some patients have IgG and IgA hyperimmunoglobulinemia, and others have IgA deficiency.

c. Genetics. APECED is transmitted by an autosomal recessive mutant gene located in chromosome 21q22.3 (97a). HLA-A28 antigen shows an association with the components HP, keratopathy, and alopecia (98). Insulin deficiency is not associated with HLA-DQ or DR (92a).

C. Hypoparathyroidism of Dysmorphic Syndromes

1. DiGeorge Malformation Complex (DMC, Dysbranchiogenesis)

Congenital aplasia and hypoplasia of PTG occur in association with cardiac abnormalities predominantly of the outflow tract, aplasia or hypoplasia of thymus, and characteristic facial dysmorphism. DMC is a causally heterogeneous developmental field defect of the third and fourth pharyngeal pouches (99). In most cases it is part of a wider, poorly delineated "Catch 22" spectrum of phenotypes caused by a microscopic or submicroscopic deletion within chromosome 22q11. This spectrum includes the velocardiofacial syndrome (100,101), "conotruncal anomaly face," and cases of isolated conotruncal heart defects (102–104). The possibility of HP and immune defect should be kept in mind in apparently isolated cases of such defects, particularly truncus arteriosus communis, D transposition of the great vessels, Fallot's tetralogy (105), and supracristal ventricular septal defect. DMC may also originate from other causes, such as fetal exposure to alcohol or retinoic acid, maternal diabetes mellitus, and chromosome 10p monosomy (Sec. IV.C.2). There is evidence that the common denominator of these conditions, the dysmorphogenetically reactive unit, is a population of cephalic neural crest cells (99).

a. Incidence and Types. More than 300 cases of DMC have been reported (104,106). Minimum diagnostic criteria are at least three of cardiac defect, HP, evidence of thymus hypoplasia, and characteristic facial dysmorphism (107). Evidently, the prevalence of these components may have become overestimated because DMC has been delineated by studying series of patients selected according to these criteria. Patients are often labeled as cases of complete (with thymus aplasia) or partial DMC (thymus hypoplasia). This division does not correlate with the presence or absence of other anomalies, except that PTG aplasia is commonly associated with thymus aplasia (106). Patients with complete DMC die early (108). Reliable diagnosis of thymic aplasia can only be made at autopsy.

b. Manifestation. In 83% of cases the disease became manifest in the neonatal period, mostly because of cardiac problems, and in one-third of cases as convulsions. Sometimes the first symptoms appeared only at school age. In several cases DMC was diagnosed in an asymptomatic adult patient because of symptomatic disease in an offspring

(109). In the 1960s and 1970s some 80% of recognized patients died within a year of birth, a majority from cardiac causes and one-fifth from infection (106).

c. Endocrine Defects. Hypocalcemic convulsions occurred in 61% and hypocalcemia in 85% of reported cases (104,106). Hypocalcemia was reported to have resolved in 26 of 40 cases (104). However, the capacity to tolerate hypocalcemic stress was not tested, and latent HP is presumably prevalent in these patients (110,111). In 85 patients PTG were searched for at autopsy. In 41 no PTG tissue was found by careful serial sectioning of the area. In 30 patients hypoplastic PTG were observed (106).

A malformation of the thyroid gland is also common (106), and at least 2 of 44 patients were hypothyroid (104). Thyroid C cells, also derivatives of the third and fourth branchial pouches (cephalic neural crest cells), are deficient in numbers in patients with DMC (112,113).

d. Cardiac Defects. Approximately 90% of recorded patients have had a cardiac defect, half of them an anomaly of the aortic arch, most commonly a type B interrupted arch or right aortic arch. One-fifth have truncus arteriosus communis (104,106,108). Hypoplastic left heart and coarctation of the aorta also occur. The right outflow tract is affected in some 12% of the patients, predominantly by obstructive anomalies, and a similar proportion have Fallot's tetralogy. An associated ventricular septal defect is present in a majority of the patients, and associated valve anomalies are common. In contrast, isolated septal defects and valve anomalies are infrequent. One-quarter of the patients have an aberrant right subclavian artery, which may cause dysphagia. The spectrum of circulatory anomalies ranges from left heart hypoplasia to a harmless abnormality of subclavian artery.

e. Immune Defect. Infections are relatively rare causes of early death in DMC patients, but susceptibility to infections becomes more prominent with increasing age. Half of the 20 patients, who died at age 5–12 months, succumbed to pneumonia or sepsis (106). Bacteria and *C. albicans* were the common agents. Only 2 cases of malignant neoplasm seem to be on record (106). Failure of the descent of thymus is extremely common, but immunodeficiency that requires correction occurs in only approximately 25% of the cases. Such patients can be identified by CD4$^+$ T cell enumeration and an in vitro proliferation response to phytohemagglutinin (114, 115). Approximately three-quarters of the patients have low T cell counts or evidence of thymus hypoplasia. Of 85 patients tested, only 5 had completely normal immune function. In the others the findings varied greatly. In 71% total blood lymphocyte count was normal. B lymphocyte counts were supranormal in half of the patients, but antibody production capacity was subnormal in one-third. IgG responses to immunization with bacterial polysaccharides may be particularly impaired (116). Diversification of the immunoglobulin V$_H$ gene repertoire is restricted (117). Many patients have hypergammaglobulinemia (117). Transplantation with fetal thymus tissue or bone marrow has given promising results (106).

f. Dysmorphic Features. All patients have some facial dysmorphism, but the features that are most helpful for the diagnosis are ear shape, prominence of nasal root, and, in the younger child, small mouth (104). The ears are set low and posteriorly rotated with deficient upper helices, along with an increase in anteroposterior diameter, giving a relatively circular ear (Fig. 7). At least one-quarter of the patients have a hearing deficit. The root and bridge of the nose are wide and prominent (Fig. 7), and there is a marked indentation on either side of the nasal tip above the midpoint of each nostril. Most patients have micrognathia, and about one-quarter have palatal clefts. The lips are often prominent and U shaped, and the philtrum is short and poorly modeled. Lateral displacement of the inner canthi is frequent. The palpebral fissures are often short, but the angle is variable (Fig. 7).

A great number of other variable malformations have been reported. Among these, different renal and urinary tract anomalies are most common. Other frequent sites are the pharynx, gastrointestinal tract, lungs, spleen, skeleton, brain, and genitals (104,106).

g. Development and Growth. Of surviving patients, at least one-half have had moderate to severe developmental delay, in some series all (108). Hypoxic episodes may have contributed to this (104), and management of hypocalcemia and avoidance of hypoxia are important in the prevention of developmental problems. Growth is said to be retarded, with stature below the third percentile (106).

h. Genetics. In 88% of the patients deletions were observed within chromosome 22q11 (segmental monosomy). Only a majority have a microscopic deletion (118). The others can be identified with fluorescent in situ hybridization by probes and cosmids from the "DiGeorge critical region" (119–123). Some patients have monosomy of the entire chromosome 22 (124).

Familial cases are on record (124,125). In approximately 25% of the couples one of the parents has the deletion (104), and for such couples the risk of any child being affected is 50%.

2. Hypoparathyroidism as Part of Partial Monosomy 10p
Monosomy of the tip of the short arm of chromosome 10 (p13-ter) is a rare condition (1 case among 27,500 consecutive births in Tokyo) (126) that appears to be one of the causes of the DiGeorge malformation complex (127). More than 20 cases have been reported; congenital HP was observed in 5 (128–132), but it may be a more frequent component. Approximately 80% of cases have been a result of de novo mutation. In the others a parent is the carrier of a balanced translocation (128). Severe mental and motor retardation have been nearly constant features. Typically, the patients have an abnormally shaped, usually microcephalic skull, prominent forehead, downslanting palpebral fissures, bilateral epicanthus, everted nostrils, prominent upper lip, low-set dysplastic ears, high-arched or cleft palate, and short neck. Prenatal- or postnatal-onset growth deficiency is common. Such eye abnormalities as fundus anomalies, arteria hyaloidea persistens, microphthalmus, strabismus, exudative maculopathy, astigmatism, cataract, and amblyopia occur frequently. Half

the patients had genital or urinary tract abnormalities: kidney aplasia, hypoplasia, or dysplasia, hydronephrosis, ureter duplex, ureteral stenosis, hypoplastic penis and scrotum with cryptorchidism, and hypospadias. Limb anomalies include syndactyly, clinodactyly, clubhands and clubfeet, short terminal phalanges, short upper limbs, proximally implanted or broad thumbs, and preaxial polydactyly. Half the patients have had heart defects, septal defects, patent ductus arteriosus, pulmonary stenosis, coarctation of aorta, or truncus arteriosus. Approximately one-third of the patients died neonatally of cardiac failure. Postmortem observations included hypoplasia or aplasia of the olfactory bulbs and tracts and hypoplasia of the cerebellum and brain stem (129). A partial functional T lymphocyte defect was observed in a few patients (130,131). Two patients had hypothyroidism.

3. Kenny Syndrome

Congenital HP occurs as a frequent (>70%) component of the rare Kenny (Kenny-Caffey) syndrome, which includes severe growth failure, slender long bones with medullary stenosis and cortical thickening, macrocephaly, absent diploid space in calvaria, delayed closure of the anterior fontanelle, and eye abnormalities (often microphthalmia and papillary pseudoedema) (132a–135). In 1 of 24 patients serum PTH levels were high measured by N-terminal assay but undetectable by carboxyl-terminal assay. The other patients examined had inappropriately low or undetectable levels. No PTG was found at the one autopsy that has been reported (132a).

The syndrome is heterogeneous. Of the 24 patients 22 had short stature; this was short limbed in three families and proportional in the others. Six of the reported families included more than one case. Three of these families were consistent with autosomal dominant inheritance. Three others were suggestive of autosomal recessive transmission.

4. Congenital Hypoparathyroidism, Mental Retardation, Severe Growth Failure, and Dysmorphic Features (Sanjad Syndrome)

A total of 21 children have been described with congenital HP, severe retardation of growth and mental development, and characteristic facial dysmorphism. All were of Middle Eastern origin, and 19 were offspring of cousins; the disease is clearly autosomal recessive (136–138). All patients were microcephalic (head circumference standard deviation, SD, score –4.0 to –9.1 at 1–12 years), and 13 were severely, 6 moderately, and 2 mildly mentally retarded. Height SD scores were –5 to –12 at 1–12 years of age. The characteristic face included deep-set eyes, depressed nasal bridge with beaked nose, prominent forehead, long philtrum, thin upper lip, and micrognathia. Several patients had floppy earlobes, low-set and/or posteriorly rotated ears, microphthalmos, esotropia, small hands and feet, and micropenis. None had congenital heart defect. There were some differences between the two main reports. In Sanjad's series (137), all patients had tetany or convulsions, 9 of 12 neonatally, none had medullary stenosis, and immune system abnormalities were not observed. In the Richardson and Kirk series (136,136a) convul-

sions were not mentioned, although all patients presented with hypocalcemia neonatally, 7 of 8 patients had medullary stenosis, 3 patients had neonatal septicemia, and there were 3 probable additional cases in the families who had died in neonatal sepsis; all 4 patients tested had subnormal T lymphocyte counts.

5. Autosomal Dominant Hypoparathyroidism, Deafness, and Renal Dysplasia (139)

Two sisters aged 9 and 10 years and their father and paternal uncle had asymptomatic HP incidentally discovered, with sensorineural hearing loss noted at ages varying from infancy to adulthood. The girls had renal dysplasia with subnormal filtration rate; the adults had a renal cyst without insufficiency. The two brothers of the girls had renal dysplasia, and one of them had died neonatally. Of the two half-brothers (same father), one had died suddenly in infancy and the other had had hypocalcemia. A father and son have been reported with symptomatic hypocalcemia and sensorineural hearing loss (139).

6. Familial Nephrosis, Nerve Deafness, and Hypoparathyroidism

Four male siblings died at age 3–8 years of a disease consisting of nephrotic syndrome, HP, and nerve deafness (140). At autopsy the PTG were absent or small and fibrotic. The paternal grandmother, one of her sisters, and two of her brothers became deaf at an early age, but none of them had any known evidence of renal disease or HP.

7. Autosomal Recessive Hypoparathyroidism, Renal Insufficiency, and Developmental Delay

Two boys and two girls in a large Asian kindred died by age 15 months of a disease that included HP and renal insufficiency with tubular acidosis and developmental delay. Autopsy was obtained in one case; no PTG were found. Two of the patients had hyperoxaluria, which was thought to be secondary to malabsorption. Two of them had evidence of nerve deafness. The same patients had excess fecal fat excretion. Transmission was clearly autosomal recessive (141).

8. Congenital Lymphedema, Hypoparathyroidism, Nephropathy, Facial Dysmorphism, Prolapsing Mitral Valve, and Brachytelephalangy (142)

In two brothers persistent swelling of all limbs was noted shortly after birth; it increased after they began walking. They were seen at age 26 and 17 years because of bilateral cataracts and dry itchy skin, respectively, and were found to have HP with inappropriately low plasma PTH levels. Both had lymphedema of all limbs and, probably, pulmonary lymphangiectasia. Intravenous urography revealed small, inadequately functioning kidneys. In the elder brother, renal failure progressed and led to successful renal transplantation. Both brothers had identical facial dysmorphism: medial flare of eyebrows, broad nasal bridge with lateral displacement of the inner canthi, and hypertrichosis of the face and forehead. Both also had short nail beds, brachydactyly, and an increased carrying angle. Echocardiography showed prolapsing mitral

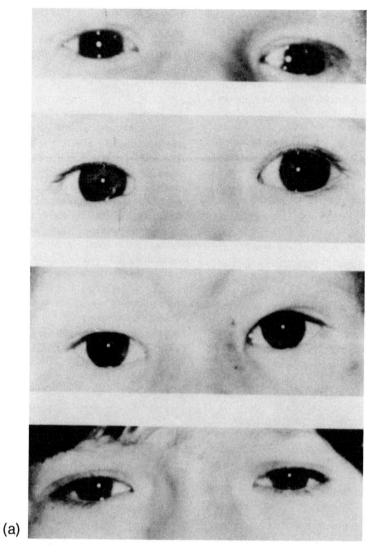

(a)

Figure 7 Characteristic facial features in patients with the DiGeorge malformation complex. (a) Nasal root and eyes (from the top) of a baby, an infant, a young child, and a teenager. (b) The tip of the nose, philtrum, and mouth. Age increases from neonate to young child in the top row and on into teenage years on the bottom row. Length of philtrum, size of mouth, and thickness of lips are variable. (c) Abnormalities of the ear, from neonate (top left) to adult (bottom right). (From Ref. 104.)

valve. The disease was thought to be transmitted by an X-linked recessive gene; the parents and the other siblings, a brother and a sister, had no feature of the disease (142).

9. Other Syndromes
A single case with hypoparathyroidism has been observed in association with the Dubowitz syndrome (143,144), the Hallermann-Streiff syndrome (145,146), mulibrey nanism (147), and the Russell-Silver syndrome (148).

D. Other Congenital Isolated PTH Deficiency
Isolated PTG hypoplasia (transient congenital hypoparathyroidism or transient congenital parathyroid gland dysplasia) (149,150) may become manifest as late neonatal tetany or may

not appear until the age of several weeks. Calcemia is then usually normalized within weeks or months. However, the PTH reserves may be permanently subnormal (latent HP), tetany may recur any time during hypocalcemic stress, and permanent HP may develop after several years (111,143,151, 152).

E. Transient Hypoparathyroidism
Hypoparathyroidism limited to the neonatal period is discussed in Chapter 31.

1. Critical Illness
Hypocalcemia is frequently associated with critical illness in children (153–155), and some of these children have PTH deficiency (153,156). Of 145 patients admitted to the pediat-

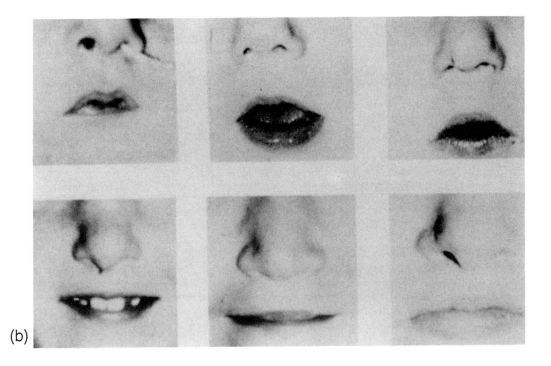

(b)

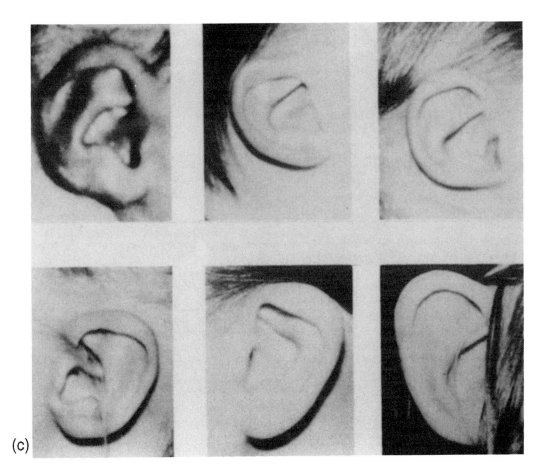

(c)

ric intensive care unit at the Massachusetts General Hospital (53 after major surgery and 92 for acute medical problems), 71 had subnormal total serum Ca. Subnormal serum Ca^{2+} was observed in 26, but many others presumably had it because Ca^{2+} could not be predicted from total Ca. As a group these 26 patients were more critically ill than the rest; 17 had an inappropriately low plasma PTH level (153). No information was given on magnesemia, although hypomagnesemia is very common in the critically ill (157). According to others hypocalcemia in critically ill children was often associated with hypercalcitoninemia (155) or hypermagnesemia (154). These dysmineralemias predict high mortality (153,154), and their correction may improve the outcome. The mechanisms and therapeutic implications of these observations should be clarified.

2. Maternal Hyperparathyroidism

Hypoparathyroidism is common in infants born to hyperparathyroid mothers; the maternal disease is often undiagnosed. Symptoms usually appear within the first 2 weeks but may be delayed (158). Complete recovery is the rule, but the condition may be prolonged or even permanent (159). Presumably this HP develops because of suppression of the fetal PTG by fetal hypercalcemia maintained by excessive placental transfer of Ca from the hypercalcemic mother.

3. Magnesium Depletion

Hypoparathyroidism is a frequent manifestation of Mg depletion. The mechanism involves impaired secretion of PTH (160,161), target cell resistance to PTH, and independent disturbance of the blood-bone equilibrium. Magnesium depletion may be caused by an inborn error of metabolism, a specific defect in the intestinal absorption of Mg, called primary congenital hypomagnesemia (162). It usually manifests as tetany at 1–4 months of age. Serum Mg levels are <0.4 mmol/L (1.0 mg/dl), distinct from the less severe hypomagnesemia frequently encountered in late neonatal hypocalcemia (163). The hypocalcemia can only be controlled by continuous Mg substitution. Magnesium deficiency may also occur as an acquired problem in nonspecific intestinal malabsorption (chronic diarrhea, Crohn's disease, or large resection of small bowel) (164), or it may result from a renal reabsorption defect of Mg^{2+} (gentamicin toxicity) (52). This type of HP can only be corrected by Mg repletion (Fig. 8).

4. Toxic Influence

Transient HP developed during cytotoxic therapy that included asparaginase in a child with acute lymphoblastic leukemia (165). The condition was complicated by acute renal failure and hypomagnesemia, and the role of the drugs and various metabolic derangements in the causation of the HP was unclear. Several other cases of HP during cytotoxic therapy of malignancy have been reported. Again, the relative roles of hypomagnesemia and the various drugs could not be established. Asparaginase was not used, and the authors suspected doxorubicin and cytarabine (166).

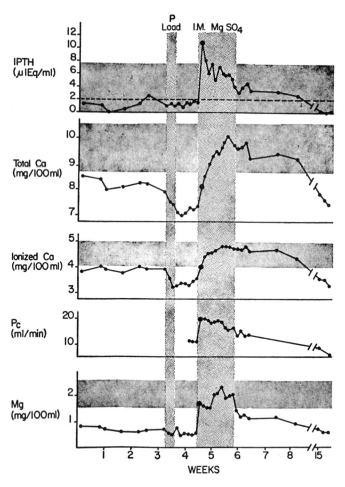

Figure 8 Plasma concentrations of immunoreactive PTH (IPTH), total Ca, Ca^{2+}, and Mg and renal phosphate clearance (P_c) in a patient with HP caused by severe hypomagnesemia. First, hypocalcemia was made more severe by an oral phosphate challenge; this did not result in increased secretion of PTH. Mg was then replenished by intramuscular injections of Mg sulfate. The shaded areas indicate the normal ranges. (From Ref. 160.)

L-asparaginase leads to necrosis of chief cells in rabbit PTG, with ensuing HP (167).

F. Other Acquired Hypoparathyroidism

1. Surgical Removal or Lesion of PTG

This condition, the most common variety of HP in adults (51,167), is rare in children. After thyroid surgery hypocalcemia is relatively frequent and must not be equated with HP. A sudden transition from the hyperthyroid to the euthyroid state, with reversal of negative bone Ca balance, is often associated with the "hungry bone" phenomenon. Such hypocalcemia disappears spontaneously within 24–48 h and is unlikely to cause tetany.

If caused by parathyroidectomy, tetany rarely occurs within 3 days of the operation and is often delayed for a week.

It has been reported to manifest months and even years later (168). The prevalence of HP is highest after thyroidectomy for cancer, in which all the PTGs may have to be removed. Otherwise, it seems to depend on PTG injury caused by ischemia, and it probably reflects the extent of dissection and hemostasis (51).

Patients who recover from postoperative HP usually recover within a few weeks to 6 months but occasionally only after years. Latent HP may persist, with intermittent relapses during hypocalcemic stress. This is inevitable after delayed recovery (51).

2. Irradiation Damage
Permanent combined HP and hypothyroidism has occurred in the infant after ^{131}I treatment of the hyperthyroid pregnant mother (169). Otherwise, irradiation HP is rare because the PTG are relatively resistant to radiation.

3. Infiltration
Iron storage in the PTG is a rare cause of HP; it is usually associated with similar destruction induced by hemosiderosis of the thyroid gland, gonads, pancreatic islets, liver, myocardium, and, occasionally, pituitary gland. This condition may complicate any disease in which blood transfusions are frequently required, such as thalassemia major and hypoplastic anemia. In β-thalassemia major HP commonly manifests in the second decade of life, but latent HP may develop much earlier (170,171).

HP may also develop in Wilson's disease, presumably because of deposition of copper in PTG (172).

Destructive infiltration by a metastasizing neoplasm or by amyloid is rare at pediatric ages.

4. Other
Sporadic cases of acquired HP of unknown or autoimmune cause are rare (Sec. IV.A.4).

Among 212 cases collected from the literature of the Kearns-Sayre syndrome associated with a distinct defect of mitochondrial genome, 14 had HP. Of these patients 4 were hypomagnesemic, 5 had hypogonadism, 4 diabetes mellitus, and 2 hypothyroidism. These associated endocrinopathies were no more prevalent than in the non-HP patients (173).

G. Pseudohypoparathyroidism

PHP is a heterogeneous group of diseases with deficient PTH action but supranormal plasma levels of PTH, indicating end-organ resistance. The resistance can be further proven by giving a test intravenous injection of PTH: phosphaturic, calcemic, and calcitriolemic responses are absent or markedly blunted.

1. Types of Pseudohypoparathyroidism
Because of the complexity of the signal transduction cascade of PTH in the proximal kidney tubule, there are many possible sites of defect causing failure of the cascade (Fig. 2). Several kinds of basic defects have indeed been identified in PHP,

and others will certainly follow. There is some confusion in the literature about the classification of PHP, the same name (for example IB) being used for different types. The primary basis for classification of these defects is their location proximal or distal to the generation of cAMP. Defects that are proximal are identified by the absence or marked blunting of the response of plasma and urinary cAMP to exogenous PTH stimulation, and this is the criterion for type I PHP. In this type the renal mechanism of response to cAMP is intact as evidenced by responsiveness to injected (dibutyryl) cAMP (174). In patients with distal defects, plasma and urinary cAMP responses to exogenous PTH are normal and basal urinary cAMP excretion may be supranormal; such patients have type II PHP. The second basis for classification is the extent of the consequences of the defect. Although PTH shares some components of the cellular signal transduction cascade with other hormones (the G_s protein complex and adenylyl cyclase), a part of the cascade is specific to PTH (and PTHrP) by structure (PTH receptor) or cell type (effector phosphoproteins of the cascade). Defects of the shared components cause resistance to several hormones. It appears practical to call them collectively type IA. Most of the known cases are caused by a deficiency of the α component of the G_s protein; these could be named type IAα. In other cases a normal quantity of $G_s\alpha$ has been observed; in one such patient a mutation of the adenylyl cyclase was identified (175). Cyclase defects could be called IAc (instead of IC) (176) and the rest IA$_?$ until the specific defect has been defined. PHP caused by defects of the specific cascade components should be called type IB. In study of patients with type IB, the skin fibroblasts of most were selectively resistant to PTH with respect to cAMP response, and a defective PTH receptor was deemed likely (177). Because type IB is also clearly heterogeneous, the subtype caused by receptor defects could be called type IBr.

There is evidence for the occurrence in some patients with type I PHP of a circulating PTG-derived antagonist of PTH action (23,178,179). The plasma of such patients was observed to have a higher PTH bioactivity when assayed in a metatarsal chondrocyte bioassay than when assayed in a renal bioassay (179,180). Such an antagonist could be an aberrant PTH molecule capable of binding to the receptor but incapable of activating it. This could be a cause of type IB PHP.

Theoretically, HP could be caused by a defect in the synthesis of PTH, which would lead to an aberrant form of PTH with immunoactivity in assays but without bioactivity. Patients with such a defect would be identified by normal responses to exogenous PTH and thus do not have PHP. No undisputed cases have been reported.

2. Type IA Pseudohypoparathyroidism
In a great majority of PHP patients the basic defect is in the protein G_s-adenylyl cyclase complex; thus these patients belong to type IA. Approximately 60% have been reported to have a G_s protein defect (181,182); the largest of all PHP subgroups is thus type IAα. Because types other than IA are rare and less well characterized, it is unclear how much of the information given here may also be true of the other types.

a. Renal Resistance. Renal resistance to PTH is the hallmark of PHP. In the proximal tubules, all responses to PTH are impaired in type 1A PHP: production of cAMP and calcitriol and excretion of phosphate and bicarbonate. The lack of a phosphaturic response to PTH leads to hyperphosphatemia, which probably further inhibits the production of calcitriol, aggravating its deficiency. The calcitriol response to an acute lowering of plasma phosphate level is also subnormal, in clear contrast to patients with PTH deficiency. There is no such difference in calcitriol response to dibutyryl cAMP injection. This suggests that there is abnormality in the 1α-hydroxylase system. Apparently, many features of the disease are secondary to the calcitriol deficiency. One such secondary defect is in the distal tubular Ca reabsorption response to PTH; it is normalized by correction of hypocalcemia and the calcitriol deficiency (Fig. 9) (24). The primary renal resistance thus seems to be confined to the proximal tubular actions of PTH.

Significantly stronger calciuria and lower plasma PTH levels have been observed in type I PHP patients without Albright hereditary osteodystrophy (AHO) than in those with AHO, despite similar calcemia levels (183). This observation is consistent with the normal PTH responsiveness of the distal tubules.

b. Skeletal Resistance. Whether skeletal resistance to PTH is an innate part of PHP has been a matter of dispute. The remodeling system appears active, and there is even evidence for its acceleration as a result of the supranormal levels of PTH. In contrast to patients with PTH deficiency and similar degrees of hypocalcemia and hypocalcitriolemia, PHP patients as a group have subnormal bone density (184) and more than doubly larger urinary excretion of hydroxyproline (an index of osteoclastic bone degradation) (48,184). Half of the PHP patients excrete supranormal amounts of hydroxyproline (48). Patients with PHP respond to exogenous PTH by an increase in hydroxyproline excretion similarly to patients with HP (184). During substitution therapy, an inverse correlation was observed between the plasma Ca level and hydroxyproline excretion, and this excretion normalized in most patients during normocalcemia (48). However, plasma alkaline phosphatase activity and osteocalcin concentration (markers of osteoblastic bone formation) are normal in PHP, in contrast to supranormal levels in primary hyperparathyroidism, although plasma PTH levels are more elevated in PHP (48). In HP, osteocalcin levels are subnormal. Despite the higher plasma PTH levels in patients with PHP than in patients with hyperparathyroidism, none of the three markers of bone turnover was different between these patient groups, suggesting that the remodeling system has some degree of resistance to PTH in PHP (48).

Radiologic evidence of hyperparathyroidism, subperiosteal resorption, and/or cysts has been reported in PHP but is rare (167,184–187). Of 18 patients with such changes, 7 had a slipped femoral head epiphysis (187). Histologic hyperparathyroid changes (osteitis fibrosa) are much more common; they disappear during adequate therapy (187).

The increased bone turnover in response to high PTH levels may contribute to the maintenance of calcemia. Estrogen, which blocks PTH-mediated bone resorption, has induced hypocalcemia in women with normocalcemic PHP (176).

The other skeletal metabolic system, mineral homeostasis, is unresponsive to PTH, but this may be secondary to the calcitriol deficiency (188,189). Prolonged treatment with pharmacologic doses of vitamin D has restored the calcemic responsiveness to PTH in some patients to normal (188,189), and physiologic amounts of calcitriol normalize calcemia (190,191). In fact, the PTH resistance of this system is part of the pathophysiology in D deficiency rickets (192). Presumably, this osteocytic system is more calcitriol dependent than the osteoclastic-osteoblastic remodeling system (184).

In conclusion, if there is skeletal resistance to PTH in PHP, it is only partial in contrast to the complete resistance of the proximal renal tubules.

c. Clinical Picture and Its Variability. For unknown reasons most patients maintain normocalcemia for several years: hypocalcemia and hyperphosphatemia develop at

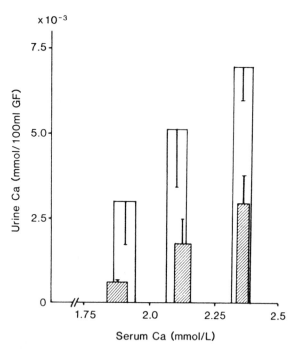

Figure 9 Comparison of urinary Ca excretion (vertical scale) at three different concentration ranges of calcemia (horizontal scale; the width of each column represents the mean ± SD of the individual concentrations) between patients with PHP (shaded columns) and HP (nonshaded columns) during therapy with different doses of 1α(OH)D₃. Mean and SD values are indicated. Normal controls had the same mean values as the normocalcemic patients with PHP. The patients with HP (in contrast to patients with PHP) have marked hypercalciuria at all levels of plasma Ca. (From Ref. 24. Copyright © 1988 by the Endocrine Society.)

variable ages, rarely before the age of 3 years. The average age at onset of symptoms is 8 years (185). Clinical manifestations may occur only at adult ages. Often, hypocalcemia or hyperphosphatemia has been noted incidentally.

Besides symptoms of hypocalcemia, often grand mal seizures, the disease may present with primary nongoitrous hypothyroidism that may be congenital (193–195), menstrual irregularities, female delayed menarche, incomplete development of female secondary sexual characteristics, primary amenorrhea or infertility, subcutaneous ossifications and bone pain (196), and slipped femoral head epiphysis (187) caused by cystic disease of skeleton. Convulsions seem to be more prevalent in PHP than HP, occurring in as many as 60% of the patients and mostly resembling grand mal seizures.

Albright's hereditary osteodystrophy (AHO) is the collective name of the abnormal features of habitus that most patients have (Fig. 10) (185): short stature, round or moon-shaped face, depressed nasal bridge, thickset, stocky or obese body, and bone anomalies—selective shortness and stubbyness of metacarpals (brachymetacarpia of, in decreasing order of prevalence, metacarpals IV, V, I, III, and, rarely and never alone, II), metatarsals (brachymetatarsia IV, V, III, I), and phalanges (brachyphalangia, most often of distal phalanx I leading to a thumbnail width-length ratio > 2.0), radius curvus, cubitus valgus, coxa vara, and genu valgum (197). Short digits arise from early closure of the epiphyses, preceded by a decrease in longitudinal growth. Cone-shaped epiphyses may be formed, and phalangeal rudimentary or pseudoepiphyses occur (167). Hand and foot abnormalities generally are not apparent before 4 years of age, and AHO habitus may only appear slowly, to be clear by school age. It may become more pronounced in successive generations (198).

Ossified plaques and nodules, also called osteomas, occur frequently in subcutaneous tissues, brain, and heart; they may be present at birth and years before hypocalcemia develops (198,199). Calcifications of the basal ganglia have been observed in up to 100% of adult patients (55). This finding has often given the first clue to the diagnosis of PHP (55).

Selective brachymetacarpia or brachymetatarsia and/or heterotopic soft tissue ossifications and absence of tall stature have often been used as the minimum criteria for AHO (200).

Dental abnormalities are common: enamel hypoplasia, small crowns, enlarged pulp chambers, root canals with open apices, pulp stones, blunted roots, delayed eruption of deciduous and permanent teeth, hypodentia, thickening of the lamina dura, and early tooth loss caused by caries (201).

In patients with type IAα, height SD score correlates with the activity of the G_s protein (202). Bone age is often advanced rather than retarded, unless hypothyroidism is present.

A mild to moderate mental retardation occurs in 50–75% of patients; it is also associated with deficiency of G_s activity (203). Subnormal senses of smell (elevated detection and recognition thresholds for all vapors) and taste (detection and recognition thresholds supranormal for sour and bitter and

normal for salt and sweet) are part of the picture (167,204). Olfaction is known to be mediated by $G_{olf}\alpha$ protein, which shows 88% amino acid identity to $G_s\alpha$ (205,205a).

The dermatoglyphic pattern may include frequent hypothenar patterns and distally located triradii (206). Degenerative changes occur in the hip joints, even necrosis of the femoral head (207). Spinal cord compression has developed as a result of a combination of abnormal vertebral fusion, shortened vertebral lamina, and soft tissue calcifications within the spinal canal (208). Hypertension is common in adult patients (209).

Some patients have completely normal habitus and mental functions.

d. Metabolic Background and Clinical Variation. The defective cAMP response to PTH has been demonstrated in early infancy (207); it is present to a milder degree before the development of hypocalcemia and during spontaneous remissions (210). That hypocalcemia develops only after the first few years of life and may alternate with normocalcemia suggests that the resistance may be acquired and depend on factors other than the primary defect (185), particularly deficiency of calcitriol, as described earlier for the skeletal homeostatic system and the distal tubular Ca reabsorption. Spontaneous normocalcemia recovery periods seem not to be associated with an increase in calcitriolemia (210).

Pregnancy, despite the high estrogen levels associated with it, has temporarily improved the Ca homeostasis of the PHP patients. This may be because of production of calcitriol by the fetally derived trophoblastic portion of placenta.

The regulation of PTH secretion is qualitatively normal, and persistent hypocalcemia maintains a supranormal secretion of PTH. Plasma PTH levels show an inverse correlation with plasma Ca levels (48). Spontaneously normocalcemic patients may also have supranormal plasma PTH (48,207). During substitution with active vitamin D analogs, plasma PTH is normalized only when plasma Ca^{2+} levels are brought to the upper normal range; this indicates an elevated set point of suppression of PTH secretion (49), presumably caused by involvement of the G_s protein-cAMP system in PTG.

In some patients the secretion of PTH may be suppressed secondary to calcitriol deficiency (207). The G_s protein defect cannot alone explain the endocrine problems, because patients with pseudo-pseudohypoparathyroidism (PPHP) have a similar G_s protein defect.

e. Other Endocrine Abnormalities. Resistance to other hormones is frequent but variable, even between siblings affected with type IA PHP (185,201,207,211–213).

Clinical hypothyroidism as a result of thyroidal resistance to thyroid-stimulating hormone (TSH) is quite common. It was observed in 15 of 26 patients (181), and the TSH response to thyrotropin-releasing hormone (TRH) was exaggerated in nearly all patients. Hypothyroidism may even be the first and congenital manifestation (193,194).

Clinical hypogonadism is common in female patients, caused by ovarian gonadotropin resistance. A spectrum of menstrual dysfunction occur, ranging from amenorrhea to a normal menstrual cycle (213). Fertility may be subnormal in

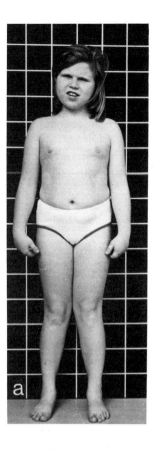

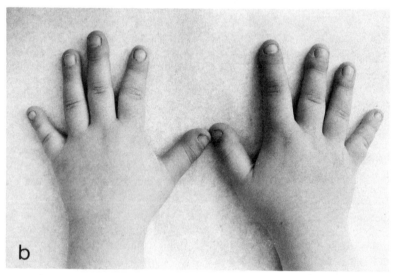

Figure 10   Abnormal features of habitus in Albright hereditary osteodystrophy (AHO) in an 11-year-old girl: (a) short stocky habitus with round face; (b and c) plump hands; and (d) feet with short metatarsals. A bone was excised from this girl's upper eyelid.

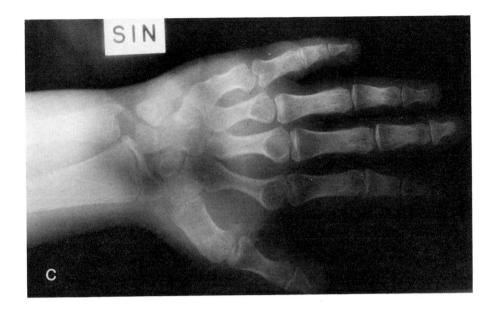

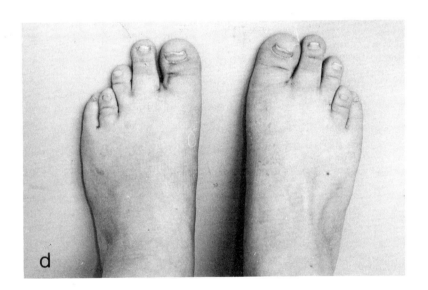

male patients, because few of them seem to have reproduced (185).

As a group, the patients have a significantly subnormal plasma cAMP response to a glucagon test, indicating subnormal hepatic cAMP (although normal glucose) responsiveness to glucagon (213). Prolactin deficiency is less common (214). Growth hormone secretion has usually been reported as normal, but there may be exceptions to this (195,215). Single cases have been reported of resistance to antidiuretic hormone (216) and ACTH (217).

In one pedigree five members of three generations had AHO, and two of them, belonging to the third generation, had primary hypothyroidism. They all had normal $G_s\alpha$ protein bioactivity, which is difficult to explain (198).

Why PHP is the dominant clinical consequence of deficiency of the protein G_s-adenylyl cyclase complex and why there is great interindividual variation in the clinical manifestation are unclear. Some possible explanations are that the amount of cAMP required to activate a given protein kinase varies from tissue to tissue and other genes may influence the picture.

3. Pseudo-pseudohypoparathyroidism

Patients with PPHP have the AHO habitus but no endocrine abnormality and an approximately normal cAMP response to PTH. The last feature distinguishes PPHP from patients in normocalcemic phase of or with incompletely expressed PHP type IA. Pedigrees with G_s protein deficiency commonly include both members with PPHP and those with PHP, and the level of G_s is similarly deficient in the cell membranes of both kinds of patients (218,219).

4. Type IB Pseudohypoparathyroidism

Type IB appears to be the second most common type of PHP and is probably heterogeneous. Patients have normal appearance and intelligence (203), and hormone resistance is limited to PTH. Short stature is common (213). Regulation of cytosolic Ca^{2+} concentration in fibroblasts is abnormal, and the defect may be in the PTH receptor that activates the Ca^{2+} messenger system (25). Prolactin deficiency may occur (214, 220).

A patient had severe osteitis fibrosa cystica with bone pain, which resolved only after parathyroidectomy. Osteoblast-like cells cultured from her trabecular bone showed normal responses to PTH and calcitriol (196).

Hypertension may be common in adult patients (209).

5. Type II Pseudohypoparathyroidism

At least 20 patients of PHP type II have been reported (185). It appears heterogeneous and is acquired in at least some cases. Hence, all reported features may not be universally true. In contrast to patients with type I, patients with type II have normal Na^+ and bicarbonate excretory responses to PTH. After prolonged normocalcemia has been maintained by Ca infusion or vitamin D administration, some of these patients have developed a normal phosphaturic response to PTH (200,221). This suggests that the primary defect is absence of a response to PTH in the renal cell membrane permeability to Ca^{2+}. Age at onset of this disease varied from 1.8 to 70 years (185). In 1 patient clinical manifestation occurred only during the hypocalcemic stress of the second half of her pregnancies (222). This is in contrast to the improvement in Ca homeostasis experienced during pregnancy by patients with type I PHP.

Type II PHP may develop with vitamin D deficiency (223,224). Sjögren syndrome may include type II PHP, presumably by an autoimmune mechanism (225).

Hyperparathyroid bone disease has been reported in some patients (185a).

6. Genetics of Pseudohypoparathyroidism

Inheritance of type IA PHP commonly follows the autosomal dominant pattern, but autosomal recessive traits may also exist (182).

In type IAα PHP, steady-state levels of the mRNA encoding the $G_s\alpha$ protein are subnormal by approximately 50% in fibroblasts of the affected members of some pedigrees, suggesting that one allele of the $G_s\alpha$ gene is defective (226,227). However, in other similar pedigrees the levels were normal (227). There was no difference between members affected with type IAα PHP or pseudo-PHP (227–230).

This was in contrast to previous findings of a more commonly, although not universally, reduced bioactivity of $G_s\alpha$ in the patients (181). Patients with normal mRNA levels have been found to have reduced levels of the protein by both

bioassay and immunoassay, just as those with subnormal mRNA levels (229). This suggests that in some pedigrees the mRNA may be defective.

At least seven different mutations have been identified in the $G_s\alpha$ gene of AHO patients (228,231,232), each in one pedigree. One of the pedigrees included a patient with type IAα PHP and another with PPHP; both had the same gene defect. One of the mutations caused production of a variant $G_s\alpha$ protein lacking the normal amino-terminal end of the protein; an antiserum specific to the carboxyl terminus of the $G_s\alpha$ protein detected normal $G_s\alpha$ activity in patients of the pedigree with that mutation (228). None of the three first mutations was found in any of 33 unrelated patients examined by the same groups of workers or a third group (233). Great molecular heterogeneity of the defect has thus been established.

G_s deficiency cosegregates with AHO in pedigrees affected by type IAα PHP; these pedigrees include patients with both PHP and pseudo-PHP (182,219).

Davies and Hughes were able to ascertain 31 published families in which AHO occurred in two or more generations and the affected parent could be confirmed (234). A total of 33 mothers had transmitted the gene, but only 3 fathers. Irrespective of the expression of the AHO gene in the parent, of 66 affected offspring full expression (AHO with PHP) occurred only in maternally transmitted cases; all paternally transmitted cases were of AHO alone. This suggests genomic inprinting in the expression of the dominant gene. The well-known excess of AHO females could be explained by increased ascertainment of transmitting mothers through their fully affected children.

Both familial (214,235) and apparently sporadic (177) cases of type IB PHP have been reported.

In type II PHP only a single familial instance has been reported; two brothers were affected (224). This type is presumably mostly acquired.

IV. DIAGNOSIS (Fig. 11)

A. Diagnosis of Hypocalcemia

The Chvostek test (Sec. III.B.1) is very useful for obtaining immediate evidence for or against hypocalcemia. A sign $\geq$ grade 2 argues in favor of hypocalcemia; the more so, the stronger it is. Absence of the sign argues against hypocalcemia but does not exclude it. In a convulsing patient with some evidence of hypocalcemia, it may be advisable to give a Ca gluconate infusion (Sec. VI.A) after inserting a venous catheter and taking a sample for determination of glucose and Ca. For definitive diagnosis, determinations must be obtained of Ca (preferably Ca^{2+}), Mg, phosphate, total protein, and urea or creatinine in serum.

B. Diagnosis of Deficient Parathyroid Hormone Effect

A manifestly deficient PTH effect is recognizable from the coexistence of hypocalcemia and hyperphosphatemia (Fig.

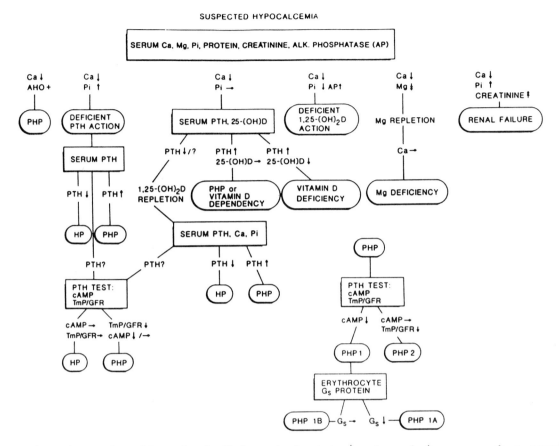

Figure 11 Diagnostic procedure of hypocalcemia. Pi, inorganic phosphate; ↓, subnormal; ↑, supranormal; →, normal; AHO, Albright hereditary osteodystrophy; TmP/GFR, quotient of maximum rate of tubular phosphate reabsorption and glomerular filtration rate (relative decrement of this quotient is the best index of PTH effect on tubular reabsorption of phosphate [Sec. II.C.1; Fig. 4]. Plasma cAMP measurement may be preferable to urine cAMP in the PTH test (Fig. 12). In a normocalcemic patient with suspicion of latent HP, perform EDTA test (Table 4).

11). Primary renal failure must be excluded by determination of serum creatinine or urea, because it may produce similar plasma mineral changes. Serum Mg should be measured to exclude severe hypomagnesemia as a cause of PTH deficiency.

In milder cases the serum phosphate concentration may be normal. In the mildest cases, even hypocalcemia may be transient, occurring during periods of hypocalcemic stress caused by fasting, exceptionally low Ca intake or high phosphate intake, or furosemide therapy. Children with "transient" neonatal HP should be followed with an EDTA infusion test (Table 4) to identify those at risk of recurrence in hypocalcemic stress (111,144,151,152). Also, cases of latent HP may be found by similar testing of persons with other features of syndromes associated with HP, such as DiGeorge syndrome (236).

C. Differentiation of Hypoparathyroidism and Pseudohypoparathyroidism

Features of AHO in the habitus and radiographic evidence of hyperparathyroidism strongly suggest PHP. Characteristics of

a specific form of HP (DiGeorge syndrome, Kenny syndrome, hypomagnesemia, APECED, or surgical HP) may suggest or even give a definite diagnosis. Differentiation of HP and PHP can be made by simultaneous measurement of serum Ca and PTH concentrations; a reliable assay of human intact PTH (237) or PTH(1–32) is necessary. Several measurements should be obtained during hypocalcemia (induced by cessation of therapy or by an EDTA infusion; Table 4), because this increases plasma PTH in PHP and accentuates the contrast between subnormal levels in HP and supranormal levels in PHP. Importantly, subnormal levels include levels within the "normal range" during hypocalcemia. Serum 25-hydroxyvitamin D should also be measured to exclude vitamin D deficiency because it may cause PTH resistance (224). Hypomagnesemia may have to be corrected to reveal the supranormal PTH levels of PHP (237a). Some patients with PHP may show the characteristic supranormal plasma PTH levels only after repletion of calcitriol (207).

The PTH test (Fig. 12) may help to confirm or exclude PHP, besides being the key to the type diagnosis of PHP. This test may not differentiate between HP and PHP type II,

Table 4   EDTA Infusion Test of PTG Reserve

Procedure

  After an overnight fast, infuse over 2 h disodium EDTA intravenously, 75 mg/kg (not exceeding 3 g) in 200–500 ml (depending on the size of the patient) 5% glucose solution containing 0.1 mg/kg of lidocaine.

  Obtain blood samples for determinations of serum Ca^{2+} and PTH just before the infusion and at 30, 60, 120, 180, and 240 minutes

Assessment

  Normal PTG reserve indicated by a clear rise in serum PTH even at 30 minutes and full recovery of serum Ca^{2+} by 240 minutes

  Defective reserve reflected by absent or subnormal rise in serum PTH and delayed recovery of serum Ca^{2+} levels

Source: From References 110 and 167.

however, because the cAMP response is normal in both and the phosphaturic response, which should distinguish between these two conditions, is not quite reliable but may give both false positive and false negative results even when the ideal response index, relative decrement in T_mP/GFR, is used (238,239).

An alternative approach is testing whether the kidneys respond to the PTH test dose by an increase in plasma calcitriol. In a small series of mostly adult patients, all 14 patients with HP showed a 24 h increment in plasma calcitriol of at least 24 pmol/L (10 pg/ml), whereas the responses of all 4 patients with PHP was below this limit (240). Another method is observing whether the skeleton responds to a trial treatment with PTH over some days by an increase in calcemia.

D.   Diagnosis of Specific Forms of Hypoparathyroidism

To diagnose transient neonatal and surgical HP, substitution therapy should be interrupted in the young infant with HP (the first time at 6 weeks after its introduction) and in surgical HP (the first time 3 weeks after its introduction), with close observation of the patient for recurrence of hypocalcemia. Absence of recurrence proves the transient nature of the disorder. However, a permanent decrease in PTH reserves should be tested for.

HP secondary to maternal hyperparathyroidism is confirmed by definite diagnosis of the mother's disease and the transient nature of the infant's HP.

HP secondary to Mg depletion is confirmed if hypomagnesemia is severe and Mg repletion corrects the HP.

APECED is confirmed or likely if the patient has, in addition to HP, at least one of the following: a sibling with APECED, chronic mucocutaneous candidiasis (angular cheilitis), definite enamel hypoplasia, alopecia, vitiligo, Addison's disease (or adrenocortical antibodies), hypogonadism [or steroid cell antibodies (81)], gastric parietal cell atrophy

(or parietal cell antibodies, or B_{12} hypovitaminemia), and chronic or recurrent fat malabsorption.

Isolated idiopathic HP can be positively differentiated from APECED only if the patient belongs to a kindred with clear case(s) of isolated idiopathic HP. Otherwise the patient should be examined for the presence of ectodermal signs of APECED and followed for the appearance of antibodies against other endocrines and the development of other components of APECED.

E.   Type Diagnosis of Pseudohypoparathyroidism and Diagnosis of Pseudo-pseudohypoparathyroidism

The type of PHP should be determined for assessing the risk of hypothyroidism and hypogonadism and for purposes of genetic counseling. It requires the PTH test be performed with biosynthetic fragments of human PTH, such as PTH(1–34) or PTH(1–38), with determination of plasma and/or urinary cAMP response (Fig. 12) (238,239). The patient should have a steady water diuresis during the test (241). A deficient cAMP response identifies type I and normal response type II. Type IA is recognized from evidence of other hormone resistance, most readily by a supranormal TSH response to a TRH test. The diagnosis of type IAα requires demonstration of subnormal activity of the G_s protein in cell membranes (241a).

The definition of PPHP is the presence of AHO with a normal cAMP response to the PTH test (Fig. 12).

VI.   THERAPY

A.   Tetany

A patient who is convulsing or has laryngeal stridor or severe tetany should be given a prompt intravenous injection of 10% Ca gluconate solution. This solution contains 0.23 mmol/ml (9.4 mg/ml) of Ca. The most rapid effect can be attained by injection of 0.25 ml/kg (0.06 mmol; 2.3 mg/kg) over ≥2 minutes. This may ameliorate the tetany for 15 minutes to several hours; if not, the injection may be repeated. A continuous infusion should then follow, 1.7 ml/kg (0.4 mmol; 16 mg Ca per kg) of the 10% solution over 6–12 h (242). Extravasation of the solution should be strictly avoided, because of the risk of tissue necrosis. It should preferably be given diluted, for example 1:10 in 5% glucose solution. Oral administration of Ca salts is quite efficient for the control of hypocalcemia and is perferable to prolonged infusion. Liberal amounts should be given orally, for example 50 mg Ca per kg per 24 h in four to five divided doses. To sequestrate phosphate in the intestine, doses may be fourfold higher. The Ca content of oral preparations varies: carbonate, 40%, chloride, 36%, lactate, 13%, gluconate, 8.8%, and glucobionate, 6.5%. Thus, 2.5, 2.8, 7.7, and 11.0 g is required, respectively, to provide 1.0 g Ca. Chloride can only be given in dilute (2%) solution (preferably in fruit juice) because it irritates the gastric mucosa. During steatorrhea the effect of oral administration may be poor.

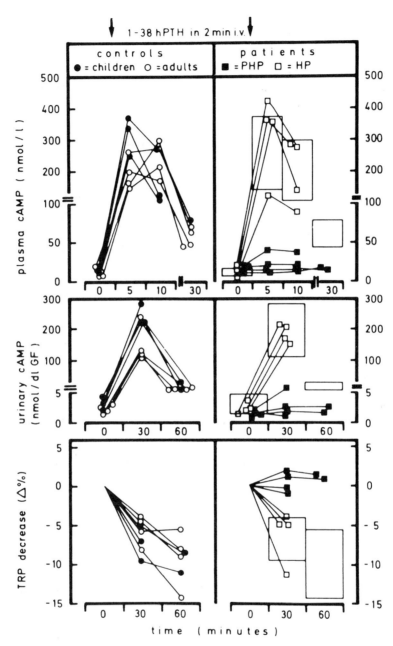

Figure 12 PTH test: effect of an intravenous injection of human PTH [0.5 μg/kg of PTH(1–38) over 2 minutes] on cAMP concentration in plasma (upper panels, nmol/L) and urine (middle panels, nmol/dl glomerular filtrate), and on tubular reabsorption of phosphate (TRP, lower panels, decrease in %) in controls (left) and in patients with PHP and HP (right). The rectangles on the right indicate the ranges of controls. (From Ref. 238.)

B. Long-Term Therapy

1. General Aspects

The aim of therapy of patients with HP is to maintain the plasma Ca at around the lower limit of the normal concentration range, at 2.1–2.25 mmol/L (8.5–9.0 mg/dl), so that, on the one hand, hypocalcemic manifestations are limited to the mildest symptoms and, on the other hand, harmful hypercalcemia and hypercalciuria are avoided. Preferably, plasma phosphate levels should also be normal. If therapy is successful HP does not disturb the patient's life, and long-term complications are avoided. The most serious risk to avoid most carefully is hypercalcemia. It easily remains unnoticed yet in a few weeks may cause irreparable kidney damage. In addition to drugs, therapy includes the regular intake of relatively large amounts of fluid (to avoid low urine flow) and normal food, with particular avoidance of fasting and high phosphate intake.

In patients with PHP, in contrast to those with HP, therapy should aim at maintaining plasma Ca at a high normal level (48). The basic differences between these two conditions dictating this difference in therapy are (1) normocalcemia causes hypercalciuria in HP but not in PHP, and (2) in PHP even low normal calcemia is associated with secondary hyperparathyroidism, which may harm the skeleton.

Two principles of long-term drug therapy are possible in HP: (1) PTH replacement with a calciferol sterol is a necessity, (2) oral Ca supplementation is a recommended adjunct therapy. The dose of the sterol must be carefully adjusted and frequently readjusted, because the need may fluctuate even after long periods of steady normocalcemia. Serum Ca and phosphate levels and urinary Ca excretion must be regularly monitored. Responsibility for control of calcemia lies with the family. The patients should carry a physician-alert sign identifying the disease.

2. Sterol Therapy

Calciferol sterols (Table 5) are the only drugs available for long-term replacement therapy. Hypocalcemia can be effectively controlled with them and the desired level of calcemia can be maintained, because they increase the flow of Ca^{2+} from the intestine and skeleton (Fig. 13). Normocalcemia, in itself, restores the inherent ability of the kidneys to adjust the excretion of phosphate to phosphatemia. Reaching a sustained decrease in plasma phosphate levels requires, on average, 2 months (243). However, the sterols lack one important renal action of PTH: stimulation of the distal tubular reabsorption of Ca^{2+}. Hence, normocalcemic patients with HP excrete on average threefold more Ca in urine than normal persons (Fig.

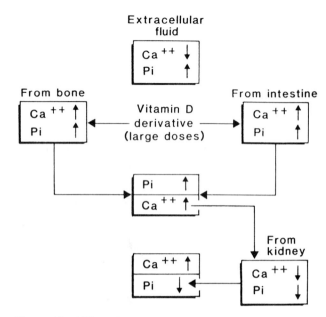

Figure 13 Effect of therapy with calciferol sterols in HP. For explanations and comparison, see Figure 5; this therapy is not complete replacement of PTH because the calciferols lack the renal effects of PTH.

9). This poses a risk of Ca sedimentation in the kidneys. It is to avoid this danger that plasma Ca levels should be maintained no higher than the lower border of the normal range, and measurements of urinary Ca excretion are a part of the routine monitoring of therapy. In contrast, patients with PHP normalize calciuria with therapy (Fig. 9). Presumably, their endogenous PTH stimulates the distal tubular absorption of Ca^{2+} as soon as their calcitriol levels are normalized.

Even an optimized sterol therapy does not substitute for normal PTH secretion, which varies greatly according to mineral balance.

Vitamin D (D_2 and D_3 are identical in effect) has a slow, prolonged, and cumulative action. These sterols involve a risk of severe prolonged hypercalcemia, even after years of stable maintenance of normocalcemia, because they are stored in the adipose tissue. Stores may become large enough to maintain replacement therapy for as much as half a year (52). Therefore, vitamin D is not recommended for routine replacement therapy, especially not for labile patients and when regular laboratory monitoring cannot be guaranteed. Probably, the effect of vitamin D is based on the generation of large amounts of 25(OH)D, which has a low affinity for the receptors of calcitriol.

25(OH)D_3 is available in the United States and some other countries. It has little to recommend it, if its cost remains very high.

Calcitriol and 1α(OH)D are the fastest and shortest acting derivatives and probably are good alternatives for treatment. Two very favorable reports have appeared on the long-term use of calcitriol in children with HP. None of them had APECED (in which HP may be very labile and the longer

Table 5 Calciferol Sterols Used in the Therapy of HP and PHP

Sterol	Average dosage[a] (μg/kg-day)	Average $T_{1/2}$ (days)	Comments
1,25(OH)$_2$D	0.03	1	Limited experience
1α(OH)D	0.06	2	Limited experience
DHT	20	7	Highly recommended
25(OH)D	4	15	Questionable value
D$_2$ and D$_3$	50	30	Risk of cumulative action

[a]Individual variation in requirement is great. Therapy should be initiated with about half this dosage, and the dosage carefully adjusted according to response. Frequent monitoring of serum Ca and phosphate levels and 24 h urinary Ca is mandatory, even in patients with stable response (see text). Clear onset of action is usually evident in approximately $T_{1/2}$, a plateau in $2-4T_{1/2}$, and after discontinuation of the drug, its action continues for $2-3T_{1/2}$, but this may be much longer for the D vitamins.

acting DHT may therefore be the drug of choice). In a report on 10 children (243), the dose, initially 0.25 μg/day, was raised in increments of 0.25–0.5 μg until normocalcemia was achieved, over a minimum of 3 days. The final dose was 0.50–1.25 μg/day, given in two or three divided doses. It was neither weight nor age related. Hypercalcemia was observed eight times during a total of 35 patient-years; it was controlled by an interruption of therapy for 3 days. Hypocalcemia was registered 10 times, half of them transient and related to intercurrent febrile illness. In a report of four children (244), the dose required to maintain plasma Ca at levels > 2.0 mmol/L (>8.0 mg/dl) was 0.75–1.00 μg/day. Only two hypercalcemic and two hypocalcemic periods were observed during a total of 21 patient-years.

In a comparative study of therapy in adults with HP or PHP (245), the mean daily dosages required were similar for calcitriol (1.5 μg) and DHT (450 μg). In contrast, consistently in several studies (24,245,246), more 1α(OH)D was required in HP (4μg) than in PHP (2 μg). This may reflect a pathophysiologic difference between these two diseases. The long-term safety of 1α(OH)D has been established (247).

Dihydrotachysterol (crystalline) is an intermediate-acting derivative and an excellent drug for long-term therapy. This vitamin D derivative has multiple advantages for use in patients requiring pharmacologic doses, as in HP (248). The crystalline form of this drug is active and has an ideal duration of action.

It is important to become well acquainted with the use of one drug, and to establish clear rules for it, which must also be given to the patient and parents. The author's rules for DHT therapy are given here as an example. The full effect of a dose of DHT is reached in 10–20 days. In regular therapy, one daily dose is given or, in the case of a very small dose (<0.05 mg), one dose every second day. Therapy is started with a dose that is likely to be too small rather than too large. The dose is increased at intervals of 10–14 days as necessary to maintain the ideal serum Ca level. For fine adjustment the increments or decrements in the dose should be around 10%. At the start of therapy and whenever the dose is increased, an extra dose is given that is sevenfold the increment. Whenever the dose must be adjusted slightly downward, a similar omission (sevenfold the decrement) is made at once. In moderate hypercalcemia (≥11.0 mg/dl or ≥2.75 mmol/L) the DHT intake is discontinued for a few days and restarted only when a repeat serum Ca determination shows normalization of the level.

3. Refractoriness to Sterol Therapy

Some patients become refractory to oral sterol therapy. This is not uncommon in patients with APECED, and another kind of case is on record (248,249). In APECED one contributing factor is fat malabsorption. Patients with this problem must be monitored very carefully. Usually, however, maintenance of normocalcemia keeps the malabsorption under control. Fat malabsorption leads to a vicious cycle of effects: like other lipids, the sterol is poorly absorbed, and this causes impairment of hypocalcemia with more severe fat malabsorption.

The cycle can be broken by increasing the oral dose of the sterol and Ca^{2+} and by decreasing fat intake or replacing ordinary fat by medium-chain triglycerides, which are more completely absorbed in this situation than ordinary fats (52).

It is important to use the shorter acting derivatives in the oral therapy of these patients, because very high doses (even 20-fold the regular dose) may be needed. In these situations serum Ca must be checked several times weekly so that the dose may be immediately reduced when the calcemia starts to improve. In very severe problem cases I have added intramuscular injections of vitamin D_3 in oil (250,000–500,000 IU at 3–4 week intervals) to oral DHT to provide a basal therapy level. Calcitriol has not proved better than DHT as therapy in these situations (52). An attempt to decrease the malabsorption by intravenous Ca infusion failed, because the large amount of Ca passed rapidly into the urine.

Mg deficiency may sometimes be a factor in the resistance (52). We have never observed hypomagnesemia in our patients with APECED. However, according to others (52, 248), $MgCl_2$ in doses up to 2 mmol/kg-day orally has reduced the sterol requirements of some refractory patients.

Other factors may be involved. One patient of ours, who has had no clear steatorrhea, has been resistant to oral therapy with both DHT and 9α-fluorocortisol.

4. Calcium Supplementation

Ca supplementation should be used at least as long as the patient is expected to be hypocalcemic (for example, for a week after an increase in the DHT dose). The ideal long-term therapy of HP probably also includes a Ca supplement of approximately 20 mg/kg-day (up to the total dose of 1.0 g/day), given as one of the oral preparations (Sec. VI.A), the most palatable of which may be effervescent tablets. This supplementation is desirable because in HP (in contrast to PHP, Fig. 9), an excess of Ca continues to be lost in the urine. Hence, this therapy may also help to maintain normophosphatemia. In situations of hypocalcemic stress (Sec. II.F.1) or hypocalcemia, the dose may be increased twofold or more. If continuous regular Ca supplementation cannot be reliably maintained or is thought to be too stressful to the patient, it should not be prescribed at all; an irregular Ca intake causes fluctuation in the mineral balance. Furthermore, a good balance can usually be achieved without long-term Ca supplementation.

5. Therapy of Hyperphosphatemia

The foregoing therapy commonly leads (within approximately 2 months) to normalization of phosphatemia, because normocalcemia directly reduces the supranormal tubular phosphate reabsorption. Furthermore, normalization of calcitriol activity may partially restore the inherent tubular ability to adapt to phosphatemia (Sec. II.C.2), but in some patients this normalization fails. It is advisable at the beginning of therapy to restrict the ingestion of milk and cheese for 2 months to reduce phosphate intake. The corresponding amount of Ca should be replaced with one of the oral Ca preparations. In patients who remain hyperphosphatemic on a regular diet, these restrictions should be continued. Aluminum hydroxide and carbonate, a dose with each meal, have been used for intestinal binding of phosphate in patients with chronic uremia. These chemicals carry a risk of aluminum toxicity. Furthermore, my personal experiences with this therapy in HP have not been successful.

6. Therapy of Magnesium Deficiency

In HP secondary to Mg depletion, initial therapy consists of $MgSO_4$, 0.2 ml/kg of 25% solution (50% $MgSO_4 \cdot 12H_2O$), given intramuscularly at 6 h intervals for four to five doses. The therapy is then continued with oral Mg chloride, citrate, or lactate, 2 mmol/kg daily (up to a total daily dose of 1.0 g of Mg or 40 mmol) in four divided doses (52).

7. Laboratory Follow-up

Serum Ca and phosphate determinations should routinely be done together. The accuracy and precision of Ca determinations are often less than excellent, and an unexpected value should be confirmed before being taken as a basis for adjustment of therapy. Measurements of plasma Ca^{2+} are preferable to measurements of total Ca (243). It is our rule to have these determinations done at maximum intervals of 6 weeks even in patients with stable levels. During labile periods repeats may be needed even twice weekly. Frequent determinations of 24 h urinary Ca are recommended for checking that the kidneys are not at risk for hypercalciuria, which is not reliably reflected by calcemia (52). Shorter collection periods are not recommended, because of inconsistent diurnal variation in calciuria. The excretion should remain ≤ 0.1 mmol/kg (4 mg/kg). If this rate is exceeded, calcemia should be maintained at a lower level. We do most of the laboratory checking by having the laboratory closest to the patient's home take the blood samples and mail the serum to our laboratory. Similarly, 24 h urines are collected at home and, with a few ml of glacial acetic acid added, a sample from the measured total mixed volume mailed to the laboratory. This is clearly more reliable than the use of unknown laboratories.

Serum creatinine levels should be checked periodically even in patients with no known hypercalcemic periods.

Plasma total Ca may change postprandially, depending on the nature of the meal. Therefore, measurements after an overnight fast are preferable to random measurements. Also, prolonged application of a tourniquet leads to spurious elevation of plasma Ca. Normal plasma phosphate levels depend on age (Table 1). Increments and decrements ≥ 1.0 mg/dl may occur after phosphate- or carbohydrate-rich meals, respectively. Therefore, samples for routine determinations should be taken after an appropriate fast (overnight for all but infants).

8. Control by the Patient or Parents

Parents and cooperative patients must be familiar with the symptoms of hypocalcemia and, especially, hypercalcemia (headache, increased nocturnal urine flow, thirst, anorexia, nausea, vomiting, constipation, lethargy, weakness, and alterations of mental status) to be able to react to these without delay. They need detailed written information about the

disease and these symptoms, including the immediate steps to be taken if they should appear. These steps include having a blood sample taken without delay for checking the serum Ca and phosphate levels, contacting the physician, and, if this fails, first-aid adjustment of the drug therapy according to rules that are included with the instructions. They should be taught to perform the Chvostek test (Sec. III.B.1.b). The value of this test needs to be established individually: in some cases, even the grade 1 sign may be useful. Some patients have devised personal methods for recognizing hypocalcemia.

9. Patients with Associated Addison's Disease

In patients who also have Addison's disease, it is important to anticipate a decrease in Ca absorption, and consequently hypocalcemia, whenever the cortisol substitution dose is increased even slightly, and the opposite may occur after a decrease in dose. (Also, unexpected hypercalcemia may be the first signal of the development of Addison's disease.)

10. Special Aspects in Pseudohypoparathyroidism

In patients with PHP, maintenance of normocalcemia is likely to improve endogenous Ca mobilization and bring about a decrease in the sterol requirement. In contrast to patients with HP, patients with PHP during adequate sterol therapy have normal calciuria (Fig. 9). Hence, they should not need continuous Ca supplementation.

It is essential that hypothyroidism, which is frequently associated with PHP type 1A, be diagnosed and treated.

11. Therapy of Complicating Hypercalcemia

Intervening hypercalcemia should be prevented through adequate monitoring, even during prolonged periods of stable normocalcemia, and through an anticipatory decrease in replacement therapy in hypercalcemic risk situations. In hypercalcemia it is particularly important to maintain a relatively large fluid intake. Ca supplementation must be interrupted, and foods with a high Ca content should be eliminated: milk, cheese, fish with bones (canned salmon or sardines, e.g.), leafy greens, and almonds. Mild hypercalcemia in a patient receiving a short- or intermediate-acting sterol may be controlled by a 3–7 day break in sterol therapy, followed by continuation with a decreased dose. In moderate hypercalcemia (≥ 2.75 mmol/L or ≥ 11.0 mg/dl), it is advisable to delay reintroduction of the sterol until serum Ca has returned to normal. This is mandatory during therapy with vitamin D. During this therapy, and even during therapy with DHT, the patient may be unusually sensitive to reintroduction of the drug after the hypercalcemic period.

Some patients enter a vicious cycle in which hypercalcemia causes increased urine flow and hyponatremic dehydration, which in turn aggravates the hypercalcemia. In these situations rapid rehydration is mandatory, with a physiologic Na^+ solution. Rehydration and natriuresis usually rapidly alleviate the hypercalcemia.

In severe hypercalcemia (> 3.0 mmol/L or > 12.0 mg/dl), stronger measures are needed. Available alternatives are therapies with calcitonin and glucocorticoids (20–40 mg/m^2

per 24 h of prednisolone in four daily doses to inhibit intestinal absorption of Ca), maintaining natriuresis with an intravenous infusion of physiologic Na$^+$ solution, and furosemide (which increases calciuria, in contrast to thiazide diuretics).

12. Risk Situations

Febrile illness and fasting predispose to hypocalcemia. The stress of a febrile illness may cause breakdown of intracellular organic phosphate compounds, with an increase in extracellular inorganic phosphate leading to a decrease in the Ca^{2+} level (52). Fasting reduces the inflow of Ca. Immobility, because of bed rest for illness, predisposes patients to the development of hypercalcemia. If motility is markedly reduced, as in transition from a normally moving to a motionless state, a preventive reduction in the sterol dosage should be considered and plasma Ca and phosphate levels should be followed closely.

Introduction of therapy with thiazide diuretics or anticonvulsants is another hypercalcemogenic intervention; these drugs reduce calciuria. The opposite is true of furosemide. A decrease in the glucocorticoid dose also elevates calcemia, and an increase does the reverse.

REFERENCES

1. Kronenberg HM, Bringhurst FR, Nussbaum S, et al. Parathyroid hormone: biosynthesis, secretion, chemistry, and action. In: Mundy GR, Martin TJ, eds. Handbook of Experimental Pharmacology, Heidelberg: Springer, 1993:185–201.
2. Mallette LE. The parathyroid polyhormones: new concepts in the spectrum of peptide hormone action. Endocr Rev 1991; 12:110–117.
3. Tonoki H, Narahara K, Matsumoto T, Niikawa N. Regional mapping of the parathyroid hormone gene by cytogenetic and molecular studies. Cytogenet Cell Genet 1991; 56:103–104.
4. Vasicek TJ, McDevitt BE, Freeman MW, et al. Nucleotide sequence of the human parathyroid hormone gene. Proc Natl Acad Sci USA 1983; 80:2127–2131.
5. Reis A, Hecht W, Gröger R, et al. Cloning and sequence analysis of the human parathyroid hormone gene region. Human Genet 1990; 84:119–124.
6. Miric A, Levine MA. Analysis of the preproPTH gene by denaturing gradient gel electrophoresis in familial isolated hypoparathyroidism. J Clin Endocrinol Metab 1992; 74:509–516.
7. Mullersman JE, Shields JJ, Saha BK. Characterization of two novel polymorphisms at the human parathyroid hormone gene locus. Hum Genet 1992; 88:589–592.
8. Parkinson DB, Shaw NJ, Himsworth RL, Thakker RV. Parathyroid hormone gene analysis in autosomal hypoparathyroidism using an intragenic tetranucleotide (AAAT)$_n$ polymorphism. Hum Genet 1993; 91:281–284.
9. Habener JF, Rosenblatt M, Potts JT. Parathyroid hormone: biochemical aspects of biosynthesis, secretion, action, and metabolism. Physiol Rev 1984; 64:985–1053.
10. Goltzman D, Hendy GN, Banville D. Parathyroid hormone-like peptide: molecular characterization and biological properties. Trends Endocrinol Metab 1989; 1:39–50.
11. Moseley JM, Hayman JA, Danks JA, et al. Immunohistochemical detection of parathyroid hormone-related protein in human fetal epithelia. J Clin Endocrinol Metab 1991; 73:478–484.
12. Copp DH. Parathyroids, calcitonin and control of plasma calcium. Recent Prog Horm Res 1964; 20:59–88.
13. Brown EM. Four-parameter model of the sigmoidal relationship between parathyroid hormone release and extracellular calcium concentration in normal and abnormal parathyroid tissue. J Clin Endocrinol Metab 1983; 56:572–581.
14. Watson PH, Hanley DA. Parathyroid hormone: regulation of synthesis and secretion. Clin Invest Med 1993; 16:58–77.
15. Ratzmann GW, Zöllner H. Relative Nebenschilddruesen-insuffizienz bei Hypomagnesiämie. Kinderartzl Prax 1991; 59: 380–383.
16. Dincsoy MY, Tsang RC, Laskarzewski P, et al. The role of postnatal age and magnesium on parathyroid hormone response during "exchange" blood transfusion in the newborn period. J Pediatr 1992; 100:277–283.
17. Spiegel AM. Albright's hereditary osteodystrophy and defective G-proteins. N Engl J Med 1990; 322:1461–1462.
18. Schmidt CJ, Thomas TC, Levine MA, Neer EJ. Specificity of G protein beta and gamma subunit interactions. J Biol Chem 1992; 267:13807–13810.
19. Reed RR. G protein diversity and the regulation of signaling pathways. New Biol 1990; 2:957–960.
20. Murer H. Cellular mechanisms in proximal tubular P$_i$ reabsorption: some answers and more questions. J Am Soc Nephrol 1992; 2:1649–1695.
21. Muff R, Fischer JA, Biber J, Murer H. Parathyroid hormone receptors in control of proximal tubule function. Annu Rev Physiol 1992; 54:67–79.
22. Rasmussen H. Ca and cAMP as Synarchic Messengers. New York: John Wiley & Sons, 1981.
23. Radeke HH, Auf'Mkolk B, Jüppner H, Krohn H-P, Keck E, Hesch R-D. Multiple pre- and postreceptor defects in pseudohypoparathyroidism (a multicenter study with twenty four patients). J Clin Endocrinol Metab 1986; 62:393–401.
24. Yamamoto M, Takuwa Y, Masuko S, Ogata E. Effects of endogenous and exogenous parathyroid hormone on tubular reabsorption of calcium in pseudohypoparathyroidism. J Clin Endocrinol Metab 1988; 66:618–624.
25. Gupta A, Martin KJ, Miyauchi A, Hruska KA. Regulation of cytosolic calcium by parathyroid hormone and oscillations of cytosolic calcium in fibroblasts from normal and pseudohypoparathyroid patients. Endocrinology 1991; 128:2825–2836.
26. Jüppner H, Abou-Samra AB, Freeman M, et al. A G-protein-linked receptor for parathyroid hormone and parathyroid hormone-related peptide. Science 1991; 254:1024–1026.
27. Jüppner H, Schipani E, Bringhurst FR, et al. The extracelluler amino-terminal region of the parathyroid hormone (PTH)/PTH-related peptide receptor determines the binding affinity for carboxy-terminal fragments of PTH-(1–34). Endocrinology 1994; 134:879–884.
28. Kozasa T, Itoh H, Tsukamoto T, Kaziro Y. Isolation and characterization of the human G$_s\alpha$ gene. Proc Natl Acad Sci USA 1988; 85:2081–2085.
29. Reichel H, Koeffler HP, Norman AW. The role of the vitamin D endocrine system in health and disease. N Engl J Med 1989; 320:980–981.
30. DeLuca HF, Schnoes HK. Vitamin D: Recent advances. Annu Rev Biochem 1983; 52:411–439.
31. Bell NH. Vitamin D-endocrine system. J Clin Invest 1985; 76:1–6.
32. Norman AW, Roth J, Orci L. The vitamin D endocrine system: steroid metabolism, hormone receptors, and biological response. Endocr Rev 1982; 3:331–366.

33. Bresnau NA. Normal and abnormal regulation of 1,25-(OH)$_2$D synthesis. Am J Med Sci 1988; 296:417–425.

34. Henry HL, Dutta C, Cunningham N, et al. The cellular and molecular regulation of 1,25(OH)$_2$D$_3$ production. J Steroid Biochem Mol Biol 1992; 41:401–407.

35. Adams ND, Gray RW, Lemann J. The effects of oral CaCO$_3$ loading and dietary calcium deprivation on plasma 1,25-dihydroxyvitamin D concentrations in healthy adults. J Clin Endocrinol Metab 1979; 48:1008–1016.

36. Kumar R. Metabolism of 1,25-dihydroxyvitamin D$_3$. Physiol Rev 1984; 64:478–504.

37. Mizgala CL, Quamme GA. Renal handling of phosphate. Physiol Rev 1985; 65:431–466.

38. Walton RJ, Bijvoet OLM. Nomogram for derivation of renal threshold phosphate concentration. Lancet 1975; 2:309–310.

38a. Kruse K, Kracht U, Göpfert G. Renal threshold phosphate concentration (TmPO$_4$/GFR). Arch Dis Child 1982; 57:217–223.

39. Bistarakis L, Voskaki I, Lambadaridis J, Sereti H, Sbyrakis S. Renal handling of phosphate in the first six months of life. Arch Dis Child 1986; 61:677–681.

39a. Ng RCK, Rouse D, Suki WN. Calcium transport in the rabbit superficial proximal convoluted tubule. J Clin Invest 1984; 74:834–842.

40. Nordin BEC, Peacock M. Role of kidney in regulation of plasma calcium. Lancet 1969; 2:1280–1282.

41. Yamamoto M, Kawanobe Y, Takahashi H, Shimazawa E, Kimura S, Ogata E. Vitamin D deficiency and renal calcium transport in the rat. J Clin Invest 1984; 74:507–513.

42. Christakos S, Gabrielides C, Rhoten WB. Vitamin D-dependent calcium binding proteins: chemistry distribution, functional considerations, and molecular biology. Endocr Rev 1989; 10:3–26.

43. Rasmussen H, Bordier P. Vitamin D and bone. Metab Bone Dis 1978; 1:7–17.

44. Wasserman RH. Intestinal absorption of calcium and phosphorus. Fed Proc 1981; 40:68–72.

45. Parfitt AM. The spectrum of hypoparathyroidism. J Clin Endocrinol Metab 1972; 34:152–158.

46. Parfitt AM. The actions of parathyroid hormone on bone: relation to bone remodelling and turnover, calcium homeostasis and metabolic bone disease. Part 2, PTH and bone cells: bone turnover and plasma calcium regulation. Metabolism 1976; 25:909–955.

47. Barzel US. Systemic alkalosis in hypoparathyroidism. J Clin Endocrinol Metab 1969; 29:917–918.

48. Kruse K, Kracht U, Wohlfart K, Kruse U. Biochemical markers of bone turnover, intact serum parathyroid hormone and renal calcium excretion in patients with pseudohypoparathyroidism and hypoparathyroidism before and during vitamin D treatment. Eur J Pediatr 1989; 148:535–539.

49. Kruse K, Kracht U. Evaluation of serum osteocalcin as an index of altered bone metabolism. Eur J Pediatr 1986; 145:27–33.

50. Price PA, Parthemore JG, Deftos LJ. New biochemical marker of bone metabolism. Measurement of radioimmunoassay of bone Gla protein in the plasma of normal subjects and patients with bone disease. J Clin Invest 1980; 66:878–883.

51. Parfitt AM. Surgical, idiopathic, and other varieties of parathyroid hormone-deficient hypoparathyroidism. In: DeGroot LJ, Besser GM, Marshall JC, et al., eds. Endocrinology, 2nd ed. Philadelphia: W.B. Saunders, 1989:1049–1064.

52. Harrison HE, Harrison HC. Disorders of Calcium and Phosphate Metabolism in Childhood and Adolescence. Philadelphia: W.B. Saunders, 1979.

53. Frame B. Neuromuscular manifestations of parathyroid dis-ease. In: Vinken PB, Bruyn GW, eds. Handbook of Clinical Neurology, Vol. 27. Amsterdam: North Holland, 1976.

54. Swash M, Rowan AJ. Electroencephalographic criteria for hypocalcemia and hypercalcemia. Arch Neurol 1972; 26:218–228.

55. Illum F, Dupont E. Prevalences of CT-detected calcification in the basal ganglia in idiopathic hypoparathyroidism and pseudohypoparathyroidism. Neuroradiology 1985; 27:32–37.

56. Ireland AW, Hornbrook JN, Neale FC, et al. The crystalline lens in chronic surgical hypoparathyroidism. Arch Intern Med 1968; 122:408–411.

57. Aryanpur I, Farhoudi A, Zangeneh F. Congestive heart failure secondary to idiopathic hypoparathyroidism. Am J Dis Child 1974; 127:738–739.

58. Kruse K, Scheunemann W, Baier W, Schaub J. Hypocalcemic myopathy in idiopathic hypoparathyroidism. Eur J Pediatr 1982; 138:280–282.

59. Battistella PA, Pozzan GB, Rigon F, Zancan L, Zacchello F. Autoimmune hypoparathyroidism and hyper-CK-emia (letter). Brain Dev 1991; 13:61.

60. Ahn TG, Antonarakis SE, Kronenberg HM, Igarashi T, Levine MA. Familial isolated hypoparathyroidism: a molecular genetic analysis of 8 families with 23 affected persons. Medicine (Baltimore) 1986; 65:73–81.

61. Barr DGD, Prader A, Esper U, et al. Chronic hypoparathyroidism in two generations. Helv Paediatr Acta 1971; 26:507–521.

62. Arnold A, Horst SA, Gardella TJ, Baba H, Levine MA, Kronenberg HM. Mutation of the signal peptide-encoding region of the preproparathyroid hormone gene in familial isolated hypoparathyroidism. J Clin Invest 1990; 86:1084–1087.

63. De Campo C, Piscopello L, Noacco C, Da Col P, Englaro GC, Benedetti A. Primary familial hypoparathyroidism with an autosomal dominant mode of inheritance. J Endocrinol 1988; 11:91–96.

64. Schmidtke J, Kruse K, Pape G, Sippel G. Exclusion of close linkage between parathyroid hormone gene and a mutant gene locus causing idiopathic hypoparathyroidism. J Med Genet 1986; 23:217–219.

65. Parkinson DB, Thakker RV. A donor splice site mutation in the parathyroid hormone gene is associated with autosomal recessive hypoparathyroidism. Nature Genet 1992; 1:149–152.

66. Peden VH. True idiopathic hypoparathyroidism as a sex-linked recessive trait. Am J Hum Genet 1960; 12:323–337.

67. Whyte MP, Weldon VV. Idiopathic hypoparathyroidism presenting with seizures during infancy: X-linked recessive inheritance in a large Missouri kindred. J Pediatr 1981; 99: 608–611.

68. Whyte MP, Kim GS, Kosanovich M. Absence of parathyroid tissue in sex-linked recessive hypoparathyroidism. J Pediatr 1986; 109:915.

69. Thakker RV, Davies KE, Whyte MP, Wooding C, O'Riordan JLH. Mapping the gene causing X-linked recessive idiopathic hypoparathyroidism to Xq26–Xq27 by linkage studies. J Clin Invest 1990; 86:40–45.

70. Spinner MW, Blizzard RM, Gibbs J, et al. Familial distribution of organ-specific antibodies in the blood of patients with Addison's disease and hypoparathyroidism and their relatives. Clin Exp Immunol 1969; 5:461–468.

71. Whitaker JA, Landing BH, Esselborn VM, Williams RR. Syndrome of familial juvenile hypoadrenocorticism, hypoparathyroidism and superficial moniliasis. J Clin Endocrinol Metab 1956; 16:1374–1387.

72. Neufeld M, Maclaren NK, Blizzard RM. Two types of autoimmune Addison's disease associated with different polyglandular autoimmune syndromes. Medicine (Baltimore) 1981; 60:355–362.

73. Perheentupa J. Autoimmune polyendocrinopathy candidosis-ectodermal dystrophy (APECED). In: Eriksson AW, Forsius HR, Nevanlinna HR, Workman PL, Norio RK, eds. Population Sructure and Genetic Disorders. New York: Academic Press, 1980; 583–587.

74. Ahonen P, Myllärniemi S, Sipilä I, Perheentupa J. Clinical variation of autoimmune polyendocrinopathy-candididiasis-ectodermal dystrophy (APECED) in a series of 68 patients. N Engl J Med 1990; 322:1829–1836.

75. Spinner MW, Blizzard RM, Childs B. Clinical and genetical heterogeneity in idiopathic Addison's disease and hypoparathyroidism. J Clin Endocrinol Metab 1968; 28:795–804.

76. Ahonen P. Autoimmune polyendocrinopathy-candidosis-ectodermal dystropy (APECED): autosomal recessive inheritance. Clin Genet 1985; 27:535–542.

77. Myllärniemi S, Perheentupa J. Oral findings in the autoimmune polyendocrinopathy-candidosis syndrome (APECED) and other forms of hypoparathyroidism. Oral Surg 1978; 45:721–729.

78. Ahonen P, Myllärniemi S, Kahanpää A, Perheentupa J. Ketokonazole is effective against the mucocutaneous candidosis of autoimmune polyendocrinopathy-candidosis-ectodermal dystrophy (APECED). Acta Med Scand 1987; 220:333–339.

79. Perheentupa J, Ahonen P, Grahne B. Tympanic membrane atrophy and calcification in autoimmune polyendocrinopathy-candidiasis-ectodermal dystrophy (unpublished).

80. Leisti S, Ahonen P, Perheentupa J. The diagnosis and staging of adrenocortical failure in progressing autoimmune adrenalitis. Pediatr Res 1983; 17:861–867.

81. Ahonen P, Miettinen A, Perheentupa J. Adrenal and steroidal cell antibodies in patients with autoimmune polyglandular disease type I and risk of adrenocortical and ovarian failure. J Clin Endocrin Metab 1987; 64:494–500.

82. Clifton-Bligh P, Lee C, Smith H, Posen S. The association of diabetes insipidus with hypoparathyroidism, Addison's disease and mucocutaneous candidiasis. Aust NZ J Med 1980; 10:548–551.

83. Scherbaum WA, Bottazzo GF. Autoantibodies to vasopressin cells in idiopathic diabetes insipidus. Lancet 1983; 1:897–901.

84. Arvanitakis C, Knouss RF. Selective hypopituitarism, impaired cell-mediated immunity and chronic mucocutaneous candidiasis. JAMA 1973; 225:1492–1495.

85. Castells S, Fikrig S, Inamdar S, Orti E. Familial moniliasis, degective delayed hypersensitivity, and adrenocorticotropic hormone deficiency. J Pediatr 1971; 79:72–79.

86. Tarkkanen A, Merenmies L, Perheentupa J. Ocular changes in autoimmune polyendocrinopathy-candidosis-ectodermal dystrophy syndrome. R Soc Med Int Cong Symp Ser 1981; 50:677–681.

87. Wagman RD, Kazdan JJ, Kooh AW, Fraser D. Keratitis associated with the multiple endocrine deficiency, autoimmune disease, and candidiasis syndrome. Am J Ophthalmol 1987; 193:569–575.

88. Mandel M, Etzioni A, Theodor R, Passwell JH. Pure red cell hypoplasia associated with polyglandular autoimmune syndrome type I. Isr J Med Sci 1989; 25:138–141.

89. Blizzard RM, Chee D, Davis W. The incidence of parathyroid and other antibodies in the sera of patients with idiopathic hypoparathyroidism. Clin Exp Immunol 1966; 1:119–128.

90. Uibo R, Aavik E, Peterson P, et al. Autoantibodies to cytochrome P_{450} enzymes $P_{450}scc$, $P_{450}c17$, and $P_{450}c21$ in autoimmune polyglandular disease types I and II and in isolated Addison's disease. J Clin Endocrinol Metab 1994; 78:323–328.

91. Uibo R, Perheentupa J, Ovod V, Krohn KJE. Characterization of adrenal autoantigens recognized by sera from patients with autoimmune polyglandular syndrome type I. J Autoimmun 1994; 7:399–411.

92. Ahonen P, Miettinen A, Perheentupa J. Cytoplasmic islet cell antibodies in patients with autoimmune polyendocrinopathy-candidosis-ectodermal dystrophy (APECED). Acta Endocrinol Suppl (Copenh) 1985; 270:78.

92a. Tuomi T, Björses P, Falorni A, et al. Antibodies to glutamic acid decarboxylase in diabetic and nondiabetic patients with APECED. 1995; submitted.

93. Hertz KG, Gazze LA, Kirkpatrick CH, et al. Autoimmune vitiligo: detection of antibodies to melanin-producing cells. N Engl J Med 1977; 297:634–637.

94. Nunzi E, Hamerlinck F, Cormane RH. Immunopathological studies on alopecia areata. Arch Dermatol Res 1980; 269:1–11.

95. Wilson PW, Buckley CE III, Eisenbarth GS. Disordered immune function in patients with polyglandular failure. J Clin Endocrinol Metab 1981; 52:284–288.

96. Arulanantham K, Dwyer JM, Genel M. Evidence for defective immunoregulation in the syndrome of familial candidiasis endocrinopathy. N Engl J Med 1979; 300:164–168.

97. Ahonen P, von Willebrand E, Miettinen A, Perheentupa J. Lymphocyte abnormalities in patients with autoimmune polyglandular disease, type I. (unpublished)

97a. Aaltonen J, Björses P, Sandkuijl L, Perheentupa J, Peltonen L. An autosomal locus causing autoimmune disease: autoimmune polyglandular disease type I assigned to chromosome 21. Nature Genetics 1994; 8:83–87.

98. Ahonen P, Koskimies S, Lokki M-L, Tiilikainen A, Perheentupa J. The expression of autoimmune polyglandular disease type I (APG I) appears associated with several HLA-A antigens but not with HLA-DR. J Clin Endocrinol Metab 1988; 66:1152–1157.

99. Lammer EJ, Opitz JM. The DiGeorge anomaly as a developmental field defect. Am J Med Genet Suppl 1986; 2:113–127.

100. Stevens CA, Carey JC, Shigeoka AO. DiGeorge anomaly and velocardiofacial syndrome. Pediatrics 1990; 85:526–530.

101. Motzkin B, Marion R, Goldber R, Shprintzen R, Saenger P. Variable phenotypes in velocardiofacial syndrome with chromosomal deletion. J Pediatr 1993; 123:406–410.

102. Hall JG. Catch 22 (editorial). Med Genet 1993; 30:801–802.

103. Scambler PJ. Deletions of human chromosome 22 and associated birth defects. Curr Opin Genet Dev 1993; 3:432–437.

104. Wilson DI, Burn J, Scambler P, Goodship J. DiGeorge syndrome: part of CATCH 22. J Med Genet 1993; 30:852–856.

105. Radford DJ, Thong YH. Facial and immunological anomalies associated with teralogy of Fallot. Int J Cardiol 1989; 22:229–239.

106. Belohradsky BH. Thymusaplasie und -hypoplasie mit Hypoparathyreoidismus, Herz—und Gefässmissbildungen—DiGeorge (Syndrom). Ergeb Inn Med Kinderheilkd 1985; 54:36–105.

107. Carey JC. Spectrum of the DiGeorge "syndrome" (letter). J Pediatr 1980; 96:955.

108. Müller W, Peter HH, Wilken M, et al. The DiGeorge syndrome. I. Clinical evaluation and course of partial and complete forms of the syndrome. Eur J Pediatr 1988; 147:496–502.

109. Maaswinkel-Mooij PD, Papapoulos Se, Gerritse EJ, Mudde AH, Van de Kamp JJ. Facial dysmorphia, parathyroid and thymic dysfunction in the father of a newborn with the DiGeorge complex. Eur J Pediatr 1989; 149:179–183.

110. Hasegawa T, Hasegawa Y, Yokoyama T, Koto S, Asamura S, Tsuchiya Y. Unmasking of latent hypoparathyroidism in a child with partial DiGeorge syndrome by ethylenediaminetetraacetic acid infusion. Eur J Pediatr 1993; 152:316–318.

111. Bainbridge R, Mughal Z, Mimouni F, Tsang RC. Transient congenital hypoparathyroidism: how transient is it? J Pediatr 1987; 111:866–868.

112. Palacios J, Gamallo C, Garcia M, Rodriguez JI. Decrease in thyrocalcitonin-containing cells and analysis of other congenital anomalies in 11 patients with DiGeorge anomaly. Am J Med Genet 1993; 46:641–646.

113. Pueblitz S, Weinberg AG, Albores-Saavedra J. Thyroid C cells in the DiGeorge anomaly: a quantitative study. Pediatr Pathol 1993; 13:463–473.

114. Bastian J, Law S, Vogler L, et al. Prediction of persistent immunodeficiency in the DiGeorge anomaly. J Pediatr 1989; 115:391–396.

115. Hong R. The DiGeorge anomaly. Immunodefic Rev 1991; 3:1–14.

116. Schubert MS. Moss RB. Selective polysaccharide antibody deficiency in familial DiGeorge syndrome. Ann Allergy 1992; 69:231–238.

117. Haire RN, Buell RD, Litman RT, et al. Diversification, not use, of the immunoglobulin VH gene repertoire is restricted in DiGeorge syndrome. J Exp Med 1993; 178:825–834.

118. De la Chapelle A, Herva R, Koivisto M, Aula P. A deletion in chromosome 22 can cause DiGeorge syndrome. Hum Genet 1981; 57:253–256.

119. Scambler PJ, Carey AH, Wyse RKH, et al. Microdeletions within 22q11 associated with sporadic and familial DiGeorge syndrome. Genomics 1991; 7:201–206.

120. Carey AH, Clausen U, Ludecke HJ, et al. Investigation of deletion in DiGeorge syndrome detected from microclones from 22q11. Mammal Genome 1992; 3:101–105.

121. Desmaze C, Scambler P, Prieur M, et al. Routine diagnosis of DiGeorge syndrome by fluorescent in situ hybridization. Hum Genet 1993; 90:663–665.

122. Driscoll DA, Salvin J, Sellinegr B, et al. Prevalence of 22q11 microdeletions in DiGeorge and velocardiofacial syndromes: implications for genetic counselling and prenatal diagnosis. J Med Genet 1993; 30:813–817.

123. Lindsay EA, Halford S, Wadey R, Scambler PJ, Baldini A. Molecular cytogenetic characterization of the DiGeorge syndrome region using fluorescence in situ hybridization. Genomics 1993; 17:403–407.

124. McKusick VA. Mendelian Inheritance in Man, 10th ed. Baltimore: Johns Hopkins University Press, 1992.

125. Keppen LD, Fasules JW, Burks AW, Gollin SM, Sawyer JR, Miller CH. Confirmation of autosomal dominant transmission of the DiGeorge malformation complex. J Pediatr 1988; 113:506–507.

126. Higurashi M, Oda M, Iijima K, et al. Livebirth prevalence and follow-up of malformation syndromes in 27,472 newborns. Brain Dev 1990; 12:770–773.

127. Obregon MG, Mingarelli R, Giannotti A, di Comite A, Spedicato FS, Dallapiccola B. Partial deletion 10p syndrome. Report of two patients. Ann Genet 1992; 35:101–104.

128. Gencík A, Brönniman V, Tober R, Auf Der Maur P. Partial monosomy of chromosome 10 short arms. J Med Genet 1983; 20:107–111.

129. Koenig R, Kessel E, Schoenberger W, Partial monosomy 10p syndrome. Ann Genet 1985; 28:173–176.

130. Greenberg F, Valdes C, Rosenblatt HM, Kirkland JL, Ledbetter DH. Hypoparathyroidism and T cell immune defect in a patient with 10p deletion syndrome. J Pediatr 1986; 109:489–492.

131. Monaco G, Ciccimarra F, Pignata C, Garofalo S. T cell immunodeficiency in a patient with 10p deletion syndrome (letter). J Pediatr 1989; 115:330.

132. Lai MM, Scriven PN, Ball C, Berry AC. Simultaneous partial

monosomy 10p and trisomy 5q in a case of hypoparathyroidism. J Med Genet 1992; 29:586–588.

132a. Fanconi S, Fischer JA, Weiland P, et al. Kenny syndrome: evidence for idiopathic hypoparathyroidism in two patients and for abnormal parathyroid hormone in one. J Pediatr 1986; 109:489–492.

133. Bergada I, Schiffrin A, Abu Srair H, et al. Kenny syndrome: description of additional abnormalities and molecular studies. Hum Genet 1988; 80:39–42.

134. Abdel-Al YK, Auger LT, El Gharbawy F. Kenny-Caffey syndrome, case report and literature review. Clin Pediatr (Phila) 1989; 28:175–179.

135. Franceschini P, Testa A, Bogetti G, et al. Kenny-Caffey syndrome in two sibs born to consanguineous parents: evidence for an autosomal recessive variant. Am J Med Genet 1992; 42:112–116.

136. Richardson RJ, Kirk J. Short stature, mental retardation, and hypoparathyroidism: a new syndrome. Arch Dis Child 1991; 65:1113–1117.

136a. Richardson RJ, Kirk J. A new syndrome of congenital hypoparathyroidism, severe growth failure, and dysmorphic features (letter). Arch Dis Child 1991; 66:1365.

137. Sanjad SA, Sakati NA, Abu-Osba YK, Kaddoura R, Milner RD. A new syndrome of congenital hypoparathyroidism, severe growth failure, and dysmorphic features. Arch Dis Child 1991; 66:193–196.

138. Kalam MA, Hafeez W. Congenital hypoparathyroidism, seizure, extreme growth failure with developmental delay and dysmorphic features—another case of this new syndrome. Clin Genet 1992; 42:110–113.

139. Bilous RW, Murty G, Parkinson DB, et al. Autosomal dominant familial hypoparathyroidism, sensineural deafness and renal dysplasia. N Engl J Med 1992; 327:1069–1974.

140. Barakat AY, D'Albora JB, Martin MM, Jose PA. Familial nephrosis, nerve deafness and hypoparathyroidism. J Pediatr 1977; 91:61–64.

141. Shaw NJ, Haigh D, Lealmann GT, Karbani G, Brocklebank JT, Dillon MJ. Autosomal recessive hypoparathyroidism with renal insufficiency and development delay. Arch Dis Child 1991; 66:1191–1194.

142. Dahlberg PJ, Borer WZ, Newcomer KL, Yutuc WR. Autosomal or X-linked recessive syndrome of congenital lymphedema, hypoparathyroidism, nephropathy, prolapsing mitral valve and brachytelephalangy. Am J Med Genet 1983; 16:99–104.

143. Kuster W, Mahewski F. The Dubowitz syndrome. Eur J Pediatr 1986; 144:574–578.

144. Lerman-Sagie T, Merlob P, Shuper A, et al. New findings in a patient with Dubowitz syndrome: velopharyngeal insufficiency and hypoparathyroidism. Am J Med Genet 1990; 37:241–243.

145. Chandra RK, Jogleker S, Antonio Z. Deficiency of humoral immunity and hypoparathyroidism associated with the Hallerman-Streiff syndrome, clinical note. J Pediatr 1978; 93:892–893.

146. Cohen MM Jr. Hallermann-Streiff syndrome: a review. Am J Med Genet 1991; 41:488–499.

147. Perheentupa J, Lipsanen-Nyman M. Hypoparathyroidism in an infant with Mulibrey nanism. 1994; unpublished.

148. Tanner JM, Lejarraga H, Cameron N. The natural history of the Silver-Russel syndrome: a longitudinal study of thirty-nine cases. Pediatr Res 1975; 9:611–623.

149. Fanconi A, Prader A. Transient congenital idiopathic hypoparathyroidism. Helv Paediatr Acta 1967; 22:342–359.

150. Rosenbloom AL. Transient congenital idiopathic hypoparathyroidism. South Med J 1973; 66:666–668.

151. Kooh SW, Binet A. Partial hypoparathyroidism: a variant of transient congenital hypoparathyroidism. Am J Dis Child 1991; 145:877–880.

152. Cruz ML, Mimouni F, Tsang RC. "Transient" congenital hypoparathyroidism. J Pediatr 1992; 120:332.

153. Cardenas-Rivero N, Chernow B, Stoiko MA, Nussbaum SR, Todres ID. Hypocalcemia in critically ill children. J Pediatr 1989; 114:946–951.

154. Broner CW, Stidham GL, Westenkirchner DF, Tolley EA. Hypermagnesemia and hypocalcemia as predictors of high mortality in critically ill pediatric patients. Crit Care Med 1990; 18:921–928.

155. Gauthier B, Trachtman H, Di Carmine F, et al. Hypocalcemia and hypercalcitonemia in critically ill children. Crit Care Med 1990; 18:1215–1219.

156. Zaloga GB. Hypocalcemia in critically ill patients. Crit Care Med 1992; 20:251–262.

157. Ryzen E. Magnesium homeostasis in critically ill patients. Magnesium 1989; 8:201–212.

158. Hanukoglu A, Chalew S, Kowarski A. Late-onset hypocalcemia, rickets, and hypoparathyroidism in an infant of a mother with hyperparathyroidism. J Pediatr 1988; 112:751–754.

159. Bruce J, Strong JA. Maternal hyperparathyroidism and parathyroid deficiency in the child. Q J Med 1955; 24:307–319.

160. Anast CS, Mohns JM, Kaplan SL, et al. Evidence for parathyroid failure in magnesium deficiency. Science 1972; 177:606–608.

161. Anast S, Winnacker JL, Forte LR, Burns TW. Impaired release of parathyroid hormone in magnesium deficiency. J Clin Endocrinol Metab 1976; 42:707–717.

162. Suh SM, Tashjian AH, Matsuo N, et al. Pathogenesis of hypocalcemia in primary hypomagnesemia: normal end-organ responsiveness to parathyroid hormone, impaired parathyroid gland function. J Clin Invest 1973; 52:153–160.

163. Woodard CJ, Webster PD, Carr AA. Primary hypomagnesemia with secondary hypocalcemia, diarrhea and insensitivity to parathyroid hormone. Am J Dig Dis 1972; 17:612–618.

164. Allgrove J, Adami S, Fraher L, Reuben A, O'Riordan JLH. Hypomagnesaemia: studies of parathyroid hormone secretion and function. Clin Endocrinol (Oxf) 1984; 21:435–449.

165. Wandrup J, Kancir C. Complex biochemical syndrome of hypocalcemia and hypoparathyroidism during cytotoxic treatment of an infant with leukemia. Clin Chem 1986; 32:706–708.

166. Freedman DB, Shannon M, Dandona P, Prentice HG, Hoffbrand AV. Hypoparathyroidism and hypocalcemia during treatment of acute leukemia. BMJ 1982; 284:700–702.

167. Nagant De Deuxchaisnes C, Krane SM. Hypoparathyroidism. In: Alvioli CV, Krane SM, eds. Metabolic Bone Disease, Vol. II. New York: Academic Press, 1978:218–445.

168. Thompson NW, Harness JK. Complications of total thyroidectomy for carcinoma. Surg Gynecol Obstet 1970; 131:861–868.

169. Richards GE, Brewer ED, Conley SB, Saldana LR. Combined hypothyroidism and hypoparathyroidism in an infant after maternal ^{131}I administration. J Pediatr 1981; 99:141–143.

170. Gertner JM, Broadus AE, Anast CS, Grey M, Pearson H, Genel M. Impaired parathyroid response to induced hypocalcemia in thalassemia major. J Pediatr 1979; 95:210–213.

171. De Sanctis V, Vullo C, Bagni B, Chiccoli L. Hypoparathyroidism in beta-thalassemia major. Clinical and laboratory observations in 24 patients. Acta Haematol (Basel) 1992; 88:105–108.

172. Carpenter TO, Carnes DL, Anast CS. Hypoparathyroidism in Wilson's disease. N Engl J Med 1983; 309:873–877.

173. Harvey JN, Barnett D. Endocrine dysfunction in Kearns-Sayre syndrome. Clin Endocrinol (Oxf) 1992; 37:97–103.

174. Bell NH, Avery S, Sinha T, Clark LC Jr, Alle DO, Johnston C Jr. Effects of dibutyryl cyclic adenosine 3',5'-monophosphate and parathyroid extract on calcium and phosphorus metabolism in hypoparathyroidism and pseudohypoparathyroidism. J Clin Invest 1972; 51:816–823.

175. Barrett D, Breslau NA, Wax MB, Molinoff PB, Downs RW Jr. A new form of pseudohypoparathyroidism with abnormal catalytic adenylate cyclase. Am J Physiol 1989; 257:E277–283.

176. Breslau NA. Pseudohypoparathyroidism: current concepts. Am J Med Sci 1989; 298:130–140.

177. Silve C, Santore A, Breslau N, Moses A, Spiegel A. Selective resistance to parathyroid hormone in cultured skin fibroblasts from patients with pseudohypoparathyroidism type Ib. J Clin Endocrinol Metab 1986; 62:640–644.

178. Loveridge N, Fischer JA, Nagant de Deuxchaisnes C, et al. Inhibition of cytochemical bioactivity of parathyroid hormone by plasma in pseudohypoparathyroidism type I. J Clin Endocrinol Metab 1982; 54:1274–1275.

179. Bradbeer JN, Dunham J, Fischer JA, Nagant de Deuxchaisnes C, Loveridge N. The metatarsal cytochemical bioassay of parathyroid hormone: validation, specificity, and application to the study of pseudohypoparathyroidism type I. J Clin Endocrinol Metab 1988; 67:1237–1243.

180. Nagant de Deuxchaisnes C, Fischer JA, Dambacher MA, et al. Dissociation of parathyroid hormone bioactivity and immunoreactivity in pseudohypoparathyroidism type I. J Clin Endocrinol Metab 1981; 53:1105–1109.

181. Farfel Z, Brickman AS, Kaslow HR, Brothers VM, Bourne HR. Defect of receptor-cyclase coupling protein in pseudohypoparathyroidism. N Engl J Med 1980; 303:237–242.

182. Farfel Z, Brothers VM, Brickman AS, Neer R, Bourne HR. Pseudohypoparathyroidism: inheritance of deficient receptor cyclase coupling activity. Proc Natl Acad Sci USA 1981; 78:3098–3102.

183. Mizunashi K, Furukawa Y, Sohn HE, Miura R, Yumita S, Yoshinaga K, Heterogeneity of pseudohypoparathyroidism type I from the aspect of urinary excretion of calcium and serum levels of parathyroid hormone. Calcif Tissue Int 1990; 46:227–232.

184. Breslau NA, Moses AM, Pak CYC. Evidence for bone remodeling but lack of calcium mobilization response to parathyroid hormone in pseudohypoparathyroidism. J Clin Endocrinol Metab 1983; 57:638–644.

185. Drezner MK, Neelon FA. Pseudohypoparathyroidism. In: Stanbury JB, Wyngaarden JB, Frederickson DS, et al. eds. The Metabolic Basis of Inherited Disease. New York: McGraw-Hill, 1983:1508–1527.

185a. Kolb FO, Steinbach HL. Pseudohypoparathyroidism with secondary hyperparathyroidism and osteitis fibrosa. J Clin Endocrinol Metab 1962; 22:59–70.

186. Allen EH, Millard FJC, Nassim JR. Hypo-hyperparathyroidism. Arch Dis Child 1968; 43:295–301.

187. Kidd GS, Schaaf M, Adler RA, Lassman MN, Wray HL. Skeletal responsiveness in pseudohypoparathyroidism. A spectrum of clinical disease. Am J Med 1980; 68:772–781.

188. Stögmann W, Fischer JA. Pseudohypoparathyroidism: disappearance of the resistance to parathyroid extract during treatment with vitamin D. Am J Med 1975; 59:140–144.

189. Drezner MK, Neelon FA, Haussler M, McPherson HT, Lebowitz HE. 1,25-Dihydroxycholecalciferol deficiency: the probable cause of hypocalcemia and metabolic bone disease in pseudohypoparathyroidism. J Clin Endocrinol Metab 1976; 42:621–628.

190. Werder EA, Kind HP, Egert F, Fischer JA, Prader A. Effective long term treatment of pseudohypoparathyroidism

with oral 1α-hydroxy- and 1,25-dihydroxyvitamin D. J Pediatr 1976; 89:266–268.

191. Davies M, Hill LF, Taylor CM, Stanbury SW. 1,25-Dihydroxycholecalciferol in hypoparathyroidism. Lancet 1977; 1:55–58.

192. Metz SA, Baylink DJ, Hughes MR, Haussler MR, Robertson RP. Selective deficiency of 1,25-hydroxycholecalciferol: a cause of isolated skeletal resistance to parathyroid hormone. N Engl J Med 1977; 297:1084–1089.

193. Levine MA, Jap TS, Hung W. Infantile hypothyroidism in two sibs: an unusual presentation of pseudohypoparathyroidism type Ia. J Pediatr 1985; 107:919–922.

194. Weisman Y, Golander A, Spirer Z, Farfel Z. Pseudohypoparathyroidism type 1a presenting as congenital hypothyroidism. J Pediatr 1985; 107:413–415.

195. Shima M, Nose O, Shimizu K, Seino Y, Yabuuchi H, Saito T. Multiple associated endocrine abnormalities in a patient with pseudohypoparathyroidism type 1a. Eur J Pediatr 1988; 147:536–538.

196. Murray TM, Rao LG, Wong MM, et al. Pseudohypoparathyroidism with osteitis fibrosa cystica: direct demonstration of skeletal responsiveness to parathyroid hormone in cells cultured from bone. J Bone Miner Res 1993; 8:83–91.

197. Poznanski AK, Werder EA, Giedion A. The pattern of shortening of the bones of the hand in PHP and PPHP—a comparison with brachydactyly E, Turner syndrome, and acrodysostosis. Radiology 1977; 123:707–718.

198. Izraeli S, Metzker A, Horev G, Karmi D, Merlob P, Farfel Z. Albright hereditary osteodystrophy with hypothyroidism, normocalcemia, and normal G_s protein activity: a family presenting with congenital osteoma cutis. Am J Med Genet 1992; 43:764–767.

199. Prendiville JS, Lucky AW, Malory SB, Mughal Z, Mimouni F, Langman CG. Osteoma cutis as a presenting sign of pseudohypoparathyroidism. Pediatr Dermatol 1992; 9:11–18.

200. Van Dop C. Pseudohypoparathyroidism: clinical and molecular aspects. Semin Nephrol 1989; 9:168–178.

201. Faull CM, Welbury RR, Paul B, Kendall-Taylor P. Pseudohypoparathyroidism: its phenotypic variability and associated disorders in a large family. Q J Med 1991; 78:251–264.

202. Saito T, Akita Y, Fujita H, et al. Stimulatory guanine nucleotide binding protein activity in the erythrocyte membrane of patients with pseudohypoparathyroidism type I and related disorders. Acta Endocrinol (Copenh) 1986; 111:507–515.

203. Farfel Z, Friedman E. Mental deficiency in pseudohypoparathyroidism type I is associated with N_s-protein deficiency. Ann Interna Med 1986; 105:197–199.

204. Weinstock RS, Wright HN, Spiegel AM, Levine MA, Moses AM. Olfactory dysfunction in humans with deficiency guanine nucleotide-binding protein. Nature 1986; 322:635–636.

205. Pace V, Hanski E, Salomen Y, Lanset D. Odorant-sensitive adenylate cyclase may mediate olfactory reception. Nature 1985; 316:255–258.

205a. Jones DT, Reed RR. G_{olf}: an olfactory neuron-specific G protein involved in odorant signal transduction. Science 1989; 244:790–795.

206. Forbes AP. Fingerprints and palmprints (dermatoglyphics) and palmar flection creases in gonadal dysgenesis, pseudohypoparathyroidism, and Kleinfelter's syndrome. N Engl J Med 1964; 270:1268–1277.

207. Werder EA. Pseudohypoparathyreodism. Adv Intern Med Pediatr 1979; 42:191–221.

208. Van Dop C, Wang H, Mulakai WJ III, Tolo VT, Rosenbaum AE. Pseudohypoparathyroidism with spinal cord compression. Pediatr Radiol 1988; 18:429–431.

209. Brickman AS, Stern N, Sowers JR. Hypertension in pseudohypoparathyroidism type I. Am J Med 1988; 85:785–792.

210. Breslau NA, Notman D, Canterbury JM, Moses AM. Studies on attainment of normocalcemia in patients with pseudohypoparathyroidism. Am J Med 1980; 68:856–860.

211. Carlson HE, Brickman AS, Burns TW, Langley PE. Normal free fatty acid response to isoproterenol in pseudohypoparathyroidism. J Clin Endocrinol Metab 1985; 61:382–384.

212. Farfel Z, Bourne HR. Pseudohypoparathyroidism: mutation affecting adenylate cyclase. Miner Electrolyte Metab 1982; 8:227–231.

213. Levine MA, Downs RW Jr, Moses AM, et al. Resistance to multiple hormones in patients with pseudohypoparathyroidism and deficient guanine nucleotide regulatory protein. Am J Med 1983; 74:545–556.

214. Carlson HE, Brickmann AS, Bottazzo GF. Prolactin deficiency in pseudohypoparathyroidism. N Engl J Med 1977; 296:140–144.

215. Wägar G, Lehtovuori J, Salven I, Backman R, Sivula A. Pseudohypoparathyroidism associated with hypercalcitoninemia. Acta Endocrinol (Copenh) 1980; 93:43–48.

216. Brickman AS, Weitzman RE. Renal resistance to arginine vasopressin in pseudohypoparathyroidism. Clin Res 1977; 26:164.

217. Ridderskamp P, Schlaghecke R. Pseudohypoparathyreoidismus und Nebennierenrindeninsuffizienz. Klin Wochenschr 1990; 68:927–931.

218. Fischer JA, Bourne HR, Dambacher MA, et al. Pseudohypoparathyroidism: inheritance and expression of deficient receptor-cyclase coupling protein activity. Clin Endocrinol (Oxf) 1983; 19:747–754.

219. Levine MA, Tjin-Shing J, Mauseth RS, Downs RW, Spiegel AM. Activity of the stimulatory guanine nucleotide-binding protein is reduced in erythrocytes from patients with pseudohypoparathyroidism and pseudopseudohypoparathyroidism: biochemical, endocrine, and genetic analysis of Albright's hereditary osteodystrophy in six kindreds. J Clin Endocrinol Metab 1986; 62:497–502.

220. Kruse K, Gutekunst B, Kracht U, Schwerda K. Deficient prolactin response to parathyroid hormone in hypocalcemic and normocalcemic pseudohypoparathyroidism. J Clin Endocrinol Metab 1981; 52:1099–1105.

221. Rodriquez HJ, Villareal H, Klahr S, Slatopolski E. Pseudohypoparathyroidism type II. Restoration of normal renal responsiveness to parathyroid hormone by calcium administration. J Clin Endocrinol Metab 1974; 39:693–701.

222. Saito H, Saito M, Saito K, et al. Case report. Subclinical pseudohypoparathyroidism type II: evidence for failure of physiologic adjustment in calcium metabolism during pregnancy. Am J Med Sci 1989; 297:247–250.

223. Matsuda I, Takekoshi Y, Tanaka M, Matsuura M, Nagai B, Seino Y. Pseudohypoparathyroidism type II and anticonvulsant rickets. Eur J Pediatr 1979; 132:303–308.

224. Rao DS, Parfitt AM, Kleerekoper M, Pumo PS, Frame B. Dissociation between effects of endogenous parathyroid hormone on adenosine 3′,5′-monophosphate generation and phosphate reabsorption in hypocalcemia due to vitamin D depletion: an acquired disorder resembling pseudohypoparathyroidism type II. J Clin Endocrinol Metab 1985; 61:285–290.

225. Yamada K, Tamura Y, Tomioko H, Kumagai A, Yoshida S. Possible existence of anti-renal tubular plasma membrane autoantibody which blocked parathyroid hormone-induced phosphaturia in a patient with pseudohypoparathyroidism type II and Sjögren's syndrome. J Clin Endocrinol Metab 1984; 58:339–343.

226. Carter A, Bardin C, Collins R, Simon C, Bray P, Spiegel A. Reduced expression of multiple forms of the α subunit of the stimulatory GTP-binding protein in pseudohypoparathyroidism type Ia. Proc Natl Acad Sci USA 1978; 84:7266–7269.

227. Levine MA, Ahn TG, Klupt SF, et al. Genetic deficiency of the α subunit of the guanine nucleotide-binding protein G_s as the molecular basis for Albright hereditory osteodystrophy. Proc Natl Acad Sci USA 1988; 85:617–621.

228. Patten JL, Johns DR, Valle D, et al. Mutation in the gene encoding the stimulatory G protein of adenylate cyclase in Albright's hereditary osteodystrophy. N Engl J Med 1990; 322:1412–1419.

229. Patten JL, Levine MA. Immunochemical analysis of the α-subunit of the stimulatory G-protein of adenylyl cyclase in patients with Albright's hereditary osteodystrophy. J Clin Endocrinol Metab 1990; 71:1208–1214.

230. Schuster V, Eschenhagen T, Kruse K, Gierschik P, Kreth HW. Endocrine and molecular biological studies in a German family with Albright hereditary osteodystrophy. Eur J Pediatr 1993; 152:185–189.

231. Weinstein LS, Gejman PV, Friedman E, et al. Mutations of the G_s α-subunit gene in Albright hereditary osteodystrophy detected by denaturing gradient gel electrophoresis. Proc Natl Acad Sci USA 1990; 87:8287–8290.

232. Miric A, Vechio JD, Levine MA. Heterogeneous mutations in the gene encoding the α-subunit of the stimulatory G protein of adenylyl cyclase in Albright hereditary osteodystrophy. J Clin Endocrinol Metab 1993; 76:1560–1568.

233. Lin CK, Hakakha MJ, Nakamoto JM, et al. Prevalence of three mutations in the G_s alpha gene among 24 families with pseudohypoparathyroidism type Ia. Biochem Biophys Res Commun 1992; 189:943–949.

234. Davies SJ, Hughes HE. Imprinting in Albright's hereditary osteodystrophy. J Med Genet 1993; 36:101–103.

235. Winter JSD, Hughes JA. Familial pseudohypoparathyroidism without somatic anomalies. Can Med Assoc J 1980; 123:26.

236. Gidding SS, Minciotti AL, Langman CB. Unmasking of hypoparathyroidism in familial partial DiGeorge syndrome by challenge with disodium edetate. N Engl J Med 1988; 319:1589–1591.

237. Kruse K, Kracht U, Wohlfart K, Kruse U. Evaluation of intact serum parathyroid hormone (PTH 1–84) in the diagnosis of disorders of calcium metabolism. Acta Endocrinol Suppl (Copenh) 1988; 287:64–65.

237a. Allen DB, Friedman AL, Greer FR, Chesney RW. Hypomagnesemia masking the appearance of elevated parathyroid hormone concentrations in familial pseudohypoparathyroidism. Am J Med Genet 1988; 31:153–158.

238. Kruse K, Kracht U. A simplified diagnostic test in hypoparathyroidism and pseudohypoparathyroidism type I with synthetic 1–38 fragment of human parathyroid hormone. Eur J Pediatr 1987; 146:373–377.

239. Mallette LE. Synthetic human parathyroid hormone 1–34 fragment for diagnostic testing. Ann Intern Med 1988; 109:800–804.

240. Miura R, Ymita S, Yoshinaga K, Furukawa Y. Response of plasma 1,25-dihydroxyvitamin D in the human PTH(1–34) infusion test: an improved index for the diagnosis of idiopathic hypoparathyroidism and pseudohypoparathyroidism. Calcif Tissue Int 1990; 46:309–313.

241. Yamamoto M, Furukawa Y, Konagaya Y, et al. Human PTH(1–34) infusion test in differential diagnosis of various types of hypoparathyroidism: an attempt to establish a standard clinical test. Bone Miner 1989; 6:199–212.

241a. Levine MA, Downs RW Jr, Singer M, Marx SJ, Aurbach GD, Spiegel AM. Deficient activity of guanine nucleotide regulatory proteins in erythrocytes from patients with pseudohypoparathyroidism. Biochem Biophys Res Commun 1980; 94:1319–1324.

242. Marx SJ. Hypoparathyroidism. In: Krieger DT, Bardin CW, eds. Current Therapy in Endocrinology and Metabolism. Toronto: B.C. Decker, 1985:329–333.

243. Markowitz ME, Rosen JF, Smith C, DeLuca HF. 1,25-Dihydroxyvitamin D_3-treated hypoparathyroidism: 35 patient years in 10 children. J Clin Endocrinol Metab 1982; 55:727–733.

244. Chan JCM, Young RB, Hartenberg MA, Chinchilli VM. Calcium and phosphate metabolism in children with idiopathic hypoparathyroidism or pseudohypoparathyroidism: effect of 1,25-dihydroxyvitamin D_3. J Pediatr 1985; 106:421–426.

245. Okano K, Furukawa Y, Morii H, Fujita T. Comparative efficacy of various vitamin D metabolites in the treatment of various types of hypoparathyroidism. J Clin Endocrinol Metab 1982; 55:238–243.

246. Mizunashi K, Furukawa Y, Miura R, Yumita S, Sohn HE, Yoshinaga K. Effects of active vitamin D_3 and parathyroid hormone on the serum osteocalcin in idiopathic hypoparathyroidism and pseudohypoparathyroidism. J Clin Invest 1988; 82:861–865.

247. Halabe A, Arie R, Mimran D, Samuel R, Liberman UA. Hypoparathyroidism—a long-term follow-up experience with 1α-vitamin D_3 therapy. Clin Endocrinol (Oxf) 1984; 40:303–307.

248. Harrison HE, Lifshitz F, Blizzard RM. Comparison between crystalline dihydrotachysterol and calciferol in patients requiring pharmacologic vitamin D therapy. N Engl J Med 1967; 276:894–900.

249. Dent CE, Morgans ME, Harper CM, et al. Insensitivity to vitamin D developing during treatment of postoperative tetany. Its specificity as regards the form of vitamin D taken. Lancet 1955; 2:687–690.

32

Neonatal Calcium and Phosphorus Disorders

Ronald R. Bainbridge
Maimonides Medical Center and State University of New York Health Science Center at Brooklyn, Brooklyn, New York

Winston W. K. Koo
University of Tennessee at Memphis, Memphis, Tennessee

Reginald C. Tsang
University of Cincinnati and Children's Hospital Medical Center, Cincinnati, Ohio

I. PHYSIOLOGY

A. Calcium and Phosphorus

Calcium (Ca) and phosphorus (P) form the major inorganic constituents of bone and serve a vital role in cell function and cell metabolism. Calcium is the most abundant mineral in the body. At all ages, 98% of total body Ca is in the bone. About 89% of the total body P is in the bone, 9% in skeletal muscle, and the remainder is in viscera and extracellular fluid. Bone mineral exists in two physical forms, amorphous and crystalline. The initial amorphous form consists mainly of brushite ($CaHPO_4 \cdot 2H_2O$) and tricalcium phosphate [$(Ca_3(PO_4)_2$]; there is a gradual transition to the crystalline form. In the crystalline form, the lattice structure is similar to that of naturally occurring geological minerals called apatites: mainly hydroxyapatite [$Ca_{10}(PO_4)_6(OH)_2$] with traces of fluorapatite ($Ca_{10}(PO)_6F_2$] (1,2).

In the fetus, most of the Ca and P accretion occurs from 24 weeks to term gestation. Calcium and P accretion occurs in a relatively constant proportion during the third trimester, being approximately 2:1 (by weight) for bone and approximately 1.7:1 for total body accretion, including soft tissues. This accretion reaches a peak of approximately 117 mg Ca and 74 mg P/kg/day at 34 to 36 weeks of gestation. In newborn infants, the total body Ca and P content is approximately 28 g and 16 g, respectively. This is approximately 2.2% of the total body content of these minerals in an adult. After birth, infancy has the next most (after late fetal age) rapid rate of Ca and P accretion (3,4).

In the circulation, the fraction of Ca and P is less than 1% of the total body content; however, disturbances in serum concentrations of Ca and P may be associated with disturbances of physiological function. Chronic and severely lowered serum concentrations of these minerals may reflect the presence of a deficiency state.

Serum Ca is found in three forms: approximately 40% is bound predominantly to albumin, approximately 10% is chelated and complexed to small molecules, and approximately 50% is ionized; complexed and ionized Ca are "ultrafiltrable." Early neonatal serum Ca concentrations increase with increasing gestational age. Serum total Ca concentrations may be as high as 3 mmol/L (conversion 1 mmol/L = 4 mg/dl) in cord blood from infants born at term, and they are significantly higher than paired maternal values at delivery (5,7). Serum total Ca reaches a nadir during the first 2 days after birth (8,9); thereafter, it increases and stabilizes generally above 2.0 mmol/L. In infants exclusively fed human milk, the mean serum total Ca increases from 2.3 to 2.7 mmol/L over the first 6 months postnatally (10). Serum total Ca concentrations in infants and children generally remain slightly higher than adult values (10,11). Normally, serum total Ca concentrations in children and adults remain stable, with a diurnal range of <0.13 mmol/L (12). During the third trimester of pregnancy a modest reduction in serum total Ca concentration (average 0.1 mmol/L) occurs concomitant with a decrease in serum albumin concentration (13).

Serum ionized calcium (Ca^{2+}) is the physiologically active form of calcium. Early neonatal serum Ca^{2+} increases with gestational age, and similar to total serum Ca, cord serum

Ca^{2+} levels are higher than paired maternal values (6). There is a decline in Ca^{2+} in the first 48 hr of life with a nadir at 24 hr in term neonates (14). Serum Ca^{2+} also decreases in the presence of high serum albumin, phosphorus, magnesium, and alkalosis (15–17). Excessive amounts of heparin in venipuncture syringes may artefactually lower Ca^{2+} (18). With the use of ion-selective electrodes normal serum concentrations of Ca^{2+} range from 1.05 to 1.36 mmol/L (4.2 to 5.44 mg/dl) in the first 48 hr of life and from 1.2 to 1.3 mmol/L (conversion, 1 mmol/L = 4 mg/dl) in adults (19,20). In term infants serum Ca^{2+} concentrations average 1.25 mmol/L with 95% confidence limits of 1.1–1.4 mmol/L (4.4–5.6 mg/dl) (14). Therefore, defining neonatal hypocalcemia as a serum Ca^{2+} concentration of less than 1.1 mmol/L (4.4 mg/dl) seems rational. Whether this definition applies for preterm infants is unknown.

Serum Ca^{2+} concentrations remain generally slightly higher in infants and children than in adults (11). In adults, a circadian rhythm for serum Ca^{2+} has been reported, with a peak occurring at 10:00 A.M.; the maximal change between peak and trough values is small, averaging 0.08 mmol/L (0.32 mg/dl) (12). Serum Ca^{2+} is stable and normal during pregnancy (13,21).

The Ca messenger system is a nearly universal means by which extracellular messengers regulate cell function. Cellular enzyme cascades are activated with a transient increase in intracellular Ca^2 concentration (22). The concentration of Ca^{2+} is critical to many important biological functions, and there is a finely tuned regulation of extracellular Ca^{2+} concentration and maintenance of an extremely large Ca^{2+} concentration gradient across the plasma membrane. In the cell, distribution of Ca is not uniform. The cytosolic compartment contains 50–150 nmol of Ca per liter of water; a larger intramitochondrial Ca pool contains 500–10,000 nmol of Ca per liter of cell water. In contrast, extracellular fluid Ca^{2+} is 1 million nM. At least two adenosine triphosphate (ATP)–dependent mechanisms are involved in the maintenance of the Ca concentration gradient across the plasma membrane.

The total P in serum can be divided into an acid-insoluble fraction, comprising mainly phospholipids, and an acid-soluble fraction, comprising a small amount of organic ester phosphate and all of inorganic phosphate. Normally, more than 90% of the inorganic phosphate is diffusible.

Cord serum P concentrations at term ranges from 1.8 to 2.3 mmol/L (conversion, 1 mmol/L = 3.1 mg/dl). There are large variations in postnatal serum P concentrations. In most newborn infants there is a rise in serum P over the first 48 hr after birth (7–9), probably unrelated to intestinal absorption of P because dietary P intake is limited at this age. Renal excretion of P is low and contributes to the maintenance of high serum P concentrations. Serum P concentrations are high during infancy [(2.3 ± 0.2 mmol/L mean ± standard deviation (M ± SD)] compared with those in adults of 0.9–1.5 mmol/L, and there is a rough correlation between the rate of skeletal growth and serum P concentration during development (23). In adults, serum P has a biphasic diurnal rhythm, with peaks in the afternoon and at 3:00 A.M.; maximal change

between peak and trough values is <0.4 mmol/L (12). Serum P concentrations also fall by about 0.1 mmol/L after a meal (24). During pregnancy, maternal serum P concentration remains stable (13).

In the cell, phosphate is the principal intracellular anion and is mostly in the form of organic phosphate. The intracellular inorganic phosphate is normally in equilibrium with both extracellular phosphate and intracellular glyceraldehyde-3-phosphate, an intermediate compound in the regeneration of ATP. The cellular phosphorus/nitrogen ratio is relatively constant. For example, it is 0.07 (by weight) in muscle, and gains or losses of nitrogen by the body are usually accompanied by corresponding gains or losses of extraosseus P (25). The relationship between potassium, the major intracellular cation, and P is more variable.

B. Parathyroid Hormone

Parathyroid hormone (PTH) is synthesized in the parathyroid gland. It is an 84-amino-acid polypeptide with a relative molecular mass (Mr) of 9500. It is derived from its precursor, prepro- and pro-PTH, through cleavage by specific proteases. Recent advances in the molecular biology of native PTH and the isolation of parathyroid hormone–related peptide (PTHrP) have increased our understanding of the physiology of PTH (26–28). The PTH genes and cDNAs have been isolated and characterized in the human, bovine, rat, and mouse species. In humans, the PTH gene, like the genes for insulin, β globin, and calcitonin, is located on the short arm of chromosome 11, and restriction site polymorphisms near the PTH gene have been detected (29,30). The initial translational product of the mRNA is a 115-amino-acid prepro-PTH (31). Prepro-PTH then undergoes two proteolytic cleavages to form PTH. About 50% of the newly generated PTH is also proteolytically degraded intracellularly (32). The 1–34 fragment (Mr 3500–4000) from the amino (NH_2)-terminal of PTH appears to be the potent fraction for bioactivity; the carboxyl (COOH)-terminal fragment (Mr 6000–7000) is bioinactive.

Current radioimmunoassay (RIA) techniques show that the intact molecule and NH_2-terminal fragment constitute a small percentage of PTH immunoreactivity in the peripheral circulation; NH_2-terminal measurements generally are useful in assessing acute fluctuations in PTH secretion. The COOH-terminal fragment predominates in the peripheral circulation and, although bioinactive, generally reflects chronic steady-state secretion of the parathyroid gland. The clearance of the latter is inversely related to renal function (33). The interpretation of circulating PTH concentrations often is made difficult because antisera produced by different investigators may detect different parts of the hormones, and each antiserum may contain several antibodies against PTH (34). Thus, the normal range of serum PTH concentrations is variable among laboratories. There is a nocturnal peak (about twice the basal concentration) in serum PTH, but no major fluctuation of peripheral blood immunoreactivity of PTH during daylight hours (35). The half-life ($t_{1/2}$) of circulating intact PTH is short (<20 min) because of its degradation by proteolytic enzymes in the blood and because of its peripheral metabolism in the kidney, liver, gastrointestinal tract, and possibly other organs (36,37). Serum PTH concentrations in cord blood are frequently low, but they increase postnatally coincident with the fall in serum Ca (21,38,39). Serum intact PTH concentrations peak at 24 hr in both healthy term and hypocalcemic preterm infants and then decline slowly over several days (21,39).

Umbilical venous blood assay for both PTH-like bioactivity (bio PTH) and intact PTH (iPTH) revealed elevated bio PTH in nondiabetic term and preterm newborns and suppression in five term infants compared to normal adults (39), while iPTH was low in all three groups. The precise reason for this observed difference in unclear. However, it is possible that the immunoradiometric assay may detect bioinactive PTH fragments. Further, human cord blood PTHrP is higher than maternal serum PTHrP and two- to threefold higher than in the human adult, which may explain this discrepancy (40). Serum PTH concentrations are similar for children and adults, but increase in elderly persons; whether this is related to alternations in the intracellular messenger system or to end-organ responsiveness to PTH is not certain (41). Small amounts (about 5%) of perfused fragments (35–84,44–68, and 65–84 amino acids), but probably not the intact PTH, have been reported to cross the human placenta (42). There is no correlation between PTH concentrations in cord blood and maternal blood (13). Physiological maternal hyperparathyroidism has been reported by some, but not all, authors in the third trimester of pregnancy (13,21).

In physiological terms, PTH is the most important regulator of extracellular Ca concentration. It increases serum Ca concentration through mobilization of Ca from bone, probably synergistic with 1,25-dihydroxyvitamin D [1,25(OH)$_2$D]; increases renal distal tubular reabsorption of Ca but decreases proximal tubular reabsorption of sodium, calcium, phosphate, and bicarbonate; and increases intestinal Ca absorption probably secondary to stimulating 1,25(OH)$_2$D production (Fig. 1; 43); however, in vitro studies have shown a direct PTH effect on the intestinal Ca absorption (44). Although PTH action on bone results in an increase in serum P concentrations, its potent phosphaturic effect overwhelms the bone effect and results in lowered serum P concentrations.

The functional effects of PTH are dependent on the amount of PTH (33) and whether PTH is administered on a continuous or an intermittent basis (45). Parathyroid hormone is bound to specific membrane-bound protein receptors such as those present in renal tubular (46) and bone cells (47). A cDNA encoding a 585-amino-acid PTH/PTHr P receptor has been reported (48). The hormone receptor interacts with a coupling nucleotide regulatory protein (N); when bound to guanosine triphosphate (GTP), N protein (also called G) is able to stimulate adenylate cyclase activity, which catalyzes the conversion of ATP to cyclic adenosine monophosphate (cAMP). The Ca-dependent second-messenger system, and possibly other intracellular factors, may be involved in the expression of the PTH hormonal effects (49). The jejunal adenylate cyclase system appears to be insensitive to PTH, and the intestinal P absorptive mechanism is resistant to

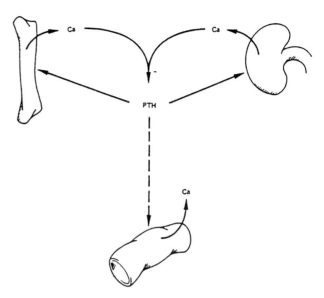

Figure 1 Parathyroid hormone (PTH) increases bone mobilization of Ca, increases renal Ca reabsorption, and possibly increases Ca absorption in the intestine (probably through effects on vitamin D metabolism, see Fig. 3). Increased serum Ca suppresses PTH production. (From Ref. 162.)

cAMP (50). Urinary cAMP excretion is an indicator of PTH activity. The absolute amount of cAMP excreted depends on both the amount of PTH acting on the tubules and the number of tubules. It is usually expressed as the quantity of cAMP excreted per minute per deciliter glomerular filtration rate (GFR). A very small amount of excreted cAMP is not produced by the tubules but, rather, is filtered from the blood by the glomeruli. Thus, the most accurate measure of renal "tubular" cAMP production is the "nephrogenous cAMP," or total cAMP excreted per unit time minus (GFR × plasma cAMP), all divided by GFR (51).

Extracellular Ca in turn is the most potent regulator of PTH secretion. Recently a 5.3-kb cDNA encoding a 120-kDa extracellular Ca^{2+} sensing receptor has been cloned from bovine parathyroid (52). This bovine parathyroid Ca^{2+} sensing receptor (BoPCaR1) has a large extracellular domain coupled to a seven-membrane-spanning domain similar to those in the G-protein-coupled receptor superfamily. The extracellular domain of this receptor contains a high density of acidic residues, which potentially could be involved in Ca^{2+} binding. The BoPCaR1, however, has an apparent low affinity for extracellular Ca. On Northern analysis transcripts of similar size to BoPCaR1 cDNA have been found in bovine kidney cortex and medulla; thyroid and brain. The human homolog of the BoPCaR1 has been mapped to chromosome 3 (53). The PTH secretion in response to decreased serum Ca is rapid and is most pronounced when serum Ca is in the mildly hypocalcemic range. Thus, there is a sigmoidal type of PTH secretion response to serum Ca concentration. An acute decrease in serum magnesium (Mg) concentration also can stimulate PTH secretion, although chronic hypomagnesemia inhibits PTH secretion. Hypercalcemia and hypermagnesemia both are able to block PTH release.

In magnesium-deficient patients intravenous administration of magnesium results in an immediate rise in serum intact PTH, with a twofold increase in 5 min (54). Impaired PTH secretion appears to be a major factor contributing to hypocalcemia in magnesium deficiency (54). Vitamin D metabolites, in particular $1,25(OH)_2D$, can regulate PTH gene transcription (55) and suppress PTH production (56). Hyperphosphatemia stimulates PTH secretion, probably by lowering the serum Ca concentration. Other systemic factors (catecholamines, prostaglandins, growth hormone, calcitonin, estrogen, progesterone, cortisol, and somatostatin) and local factors (interleukin-1) modulate PTH secretion and function (57,58). However, their role in the regulation of calcium metabolism under physiological conditions is not clear. Recently, the amino acid sequence of PTH-related protein (PTHrP) has been completed. The precise function of PTHrP in healthy human newborns is unknown. However, PTHrP concentrations, which are normally low or undetectable, are elevated in individuals with humoral hypercalcemia of malignancy (HHM) (28). Several PTHrP assays with varying sensitivities and specificities have been developed (28). The stability of PTHrP in plasma samples may be enhanced if sample collection is done in the presence of protease inhibitors. However, the variability reported between assays suggests that we are still early in their development, and at present PTHrP measurement is of clinical utility only as a tumor marker in HHM. PTHrP mRNA is expressed in high quantities in the mammary glands and PTHrP is present in the milk of a number of species, including humans (40). Immunoreactivity for PTHrP mRNA has been identified in kidney, bone, placenta, uterus, and fetal smooth and skeletal muscle. The isolation of PTHrP in several tissues suggests that it functions at a local level to regulate Ca concentration.

PTHrP cDNA encodes a 177-amino-acid protein. The N-terminal 1–13 region has eight of 13 residues similar to PTH. The amino acids 34–111 segment is highly conserved among species while amino acid 118 to the C-terminus is poorly conserved.

C. Calcitonin

Calcitonin (CT) monomer is a 32-amino-acid peptide with a Mr of 3400. Its precursors are prepro- and pro-CT. The larger prohormones include peptides linked to the NH_2- and COOH-terminals of the CT sequence. Calcitonin and equimolar amounts of non-CT secretory peptides, corresponding to these flanking peptides, are generated during precursor processing. In addition, similar processing of a CT gene–related precursor results in a CT gene–related peptide (CGRP), which is a 37-amino-acid peptide sequence with a Mr of 4000, and additional flanking peptides (59–62).

The gene (CALC-1) encoding for CT is located adjacent to the gene encoding PTH, on the short arm of chromosome 11 in the human (30); on chromosome 1 in the rat (63); and on chromosome 7 in the mouse (64). The CT gene has also been isolated and characterized in the chicken. Alternative

processing of the initial gene transcript results in the production of two distinct RNA-encoding precursors of CT and CGRP. There is probably at least one other gene (CALC-II) encoding a second human CGRP (hCGRP-2). In contrast to CALC-1, CALC-II does not seem to be alternatively expressed, and human CT-like mRNA cannot be demonstrated (62). The 75 NH_2-terminal residues of each preprohormone for CT and CGRP are predicted to be identical. Procalcitonin is a 116-amino-acid peptide, whereas the pro-CGRP is a 103-amino-acid peptide (65). Bioactivity of human calcitonin (hCT) is present in the full 32-amino-acid structure or its smaller fragments, such as hCT (8–32) and hCT (9–32); the ring structure of CT enhances, but is not essential for, hormonal action.

Calcitonin is secreted from thyroid C cells (these cells are also found in the brain and pituitary) and, probably, from the mammary gland (60,62,66). The CGRP is found predominantly in nerve fibers in the central and peripheral nervous system, blood vessels, thyroid and parathyroid glands, liver, spleen, heart, and lung, and possibly bone marrow (60,67–69). Both CT and CGRP are present in the fetus (70,71). In healthy adult men CGRP demonstrates diurnal variability (72).

There are distinct but overlapping effects of CT and CGRP. For example, CT has a potent hypocalcemic effect and inhibits bone resorption, whereas CGRP is about three orders of magnitude less potent than CT (73); CGRP affects catecholamine release, vascular tone (and blood pressure), and cardiac contractility (60–62,67). Both CT and CGRP inhibit gastric acid secretion and food intake (60,74). Thus, the influence of CGRP on Ca and P homeostasis is probably minor compared with CT. The clinical significance of CGRP based on its vasoactive or neurotropic effects, or possibly its use as a tumor marker, and other potential functions remain to be defined (60–62,75,76). The physiological function of flanking peptides such as the COOH-terminal adjacent peptide (CCAP also named PDN-21 in humans) is not known (73).

Current measurements of immunoreactive calcitonin (iCT) are not specific for monomeric CT. Immunoreactive calcitonin concentrations are expressed in gravimetric or molar equivalents of synthetic CT monomer, unless the samples are first prepared using multiple procedures including gel chromatography, immunoextraction, and high-performance liquid chromatography (HPLC). Thus, the resultant measurement of iCT concentrations usually represents the aggregate immunoreactivity of multiple forms of calcitonin that may vary in number and proportion (66,77).

In the rat, the number of thyroid C cells and secretion of CT increase from fetal life to suckling (78), which are periods of rapid growth. There is probably no placental crossover of CT; the human placental tissue is able to produce CT in response to the presence of Ca in the culture medium (79). In human neonates, the CT content in crude tissue preparations of thyroid is larger than that of the adult thyroid (70). Serum CT concentrations are high at birth compared with paired maternal CT concentrations. Serum CT concentrations further increase during the first few days after birth and may reach five- to 10-fold higher than adult CT concentrations. Serum CT concentrations increase after birth in both healthy normal term infants and infants of diabetic mothers (IDM) regardless of serum calcium levels (80).

The precise role of CT in calcium homeostasis in the neonate is still unclear as there is neither an identifiable hypocalcemic response to the postnatal surge in serum CT nor a blunting of CT secretion in the presence of hypocalcemia.

Serum CT concentrations decrease progressively during infancy; in several-month-old preterm infants, the mean serum CT concentration still may be twice the adult values (81). There is also a small peak of serum CT concentration during late childhood. In human adults, the basal serum CT concentration may be lower in women than in men, but it is not affected by old age (82). The CT secretory response to Ca infusion is lower in women and with old age (82).

The sex difference in serum CT concentrations probably results from lower rates of CT secretion in females (82). Unlike the rat (83), there is no diurnal variation in serum CT concentrations in the human (35). Serum CT concentrations are variable during pregnancy (13). The kidney appears to be the dominant organ in the metabolism of human CT. A small percentage of the metabolic clearance rate of CT in humans may be accounted for by enzymatic degradation owing to the presence of a heat-labile factor in blood. Injected hCT monomer disappears from the blood in vivo with a $t_{1/2}$ of approximately 10 min; in contrast, the $t_{1/2}$ of hCT in plasma incubated in vitro at 37°C may be longer than 20 hr (84). Depending on the animal species, other sites, such as liver, intestine, and bone, may be involved in the metabolism of CT (2,74).

Calcitonin and P are two physiological inhibitors of bone resorption. Calcitonin also decreases renal tubular reabsorption of Ca, Mg, P, and Na and increases free water clearance in humans. In physiological concentration, CT probably does not influence intestinal absorption of Ca and P. The net effect of CT is a lowering of serum Ca and P concentrations (Fig. 2). Thus, the bioactivity of CT is frequently opposite that of PTH: CT probably modulates the effect of PTH on organs. Developmentally, calcitonin-containing cells and parathyroid gland cells are suggested to have a similar tissue origin from the neural crest (85). Calcitonin may activate the 1-hydroxylase system independently of PTH (86). The physiological significance of this action is unknown.

The actions of CT are frequently, but not always, mediated by the adenylate cyclase system (74,87) after attachment of CT to membrane receptors in various target organs (88). A cDNA has been cloned for the 482-amino-acid CT receptor. This receptor apparently is homologous to the PTH/PTHrP receptor, indicating that the receptors for the hormones regulating Ca homeostasis represent a new family of G-protein-coupled receptors (88). In the rat, calcitonin gene expression in vivo is regulated by the administration of $1,25(OH)_2D_3$ but not by chronic changes in serum Ca although acute changes in serum Ca result in a transient increases in calcitonin mRNA levels (89).

In vitro, cAMP can induce transcription of the CT gene

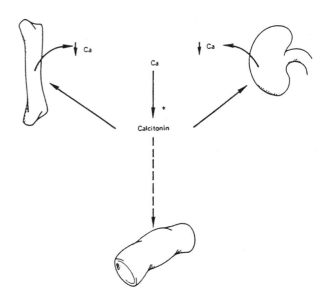

Figure 2 Calcitonin decreases Ca mobilization from bone and increases Ca excretion in the kidney; intestinal effects are uncertain. Ca stimulates the production of calcitonin. (From Ref. 162.)

(90); whether or not this forms a part of the amplification system for CT production is unknown. Secretion of CT is stimulated by an increase in serum Ca and Mg concentrations and by gastrin, glucagon, and cholecystokinin, along with several other structural analogs of these hormones, for example, pentagastrin and prostaglandin E_2 (2,74,91). Propanol, an adrenergic antagonist, and somatostatin may inhibit the secretion of CT.

D. Vitamin D

Vitamin D undergoes several major metabolic conversion steps and under in vivo conditions produces at least 20 vitamin D metabolites, with or without putative functions (92). Vitamin D_2 is a plant steroid, and vitamin D_3 is endogenously synthesized in animals. In the mammal, vitamins D_2 and D_3 appear to metabolize along the same pathway, and there is no functional difference between their metabolites. The term "vitamin D" is frequently used generically to describe vitamins D_2 and D_3 and, correspondingly, their metabolites. Vitamin D_3 (Mr 384) is synthesized in the skin from its precursors provitamin D_3 (7-dehydrocholesterol), after chemical photolysis under ultraviolet B (UVB) irradiation at 280–300 nm wavelength, produces provitamin D_3; provitamin D_3 undergoes thermal isomerization to vitamin D_3 (93). Dietary vitamin D_3 (or D_2) (1 mg = 40 I.U.) is absorbed by the intestinal lymphatics (94), and about 50% of the vitamin D in chylomicron is transferred to vitamin D–binding globulin in blood before uptake by the liver (95).

Vitamin D is catalyzed to 25-hydroxyvitamin D [25(OH)D] by a cytochrome P_{450}-like enzyme (96) almost entirely in hepatic microsomes and mitochondria. Regulation of vitamin D25-hydroxylase activity by vitamin D and 25(OH)D is limited. At high concentrations of vitamin D, the mitochondrial enzyme will form significant quantities of 25(OH)D. Thus, the circulating 25(OH)D (1nmol/L = 0.4 ng/ml) concentration is a useful index of vitamin D reserves. The physiological significance of decreased plasma concentration of 25(OH)D after administration of 1,25(OH)$_2$D in vivo is unclear (97). Serum P changes do not alter serum 25(OH)D concentrations. Phosphate depletion increases 25(OH)D-1α-hydroxylase activity and serum 1,25(OH)$_2$D concentration (98); conversely, P ingestion decreases serum 1,25(OH)$_2$D (99,100). 25-Hydroxyvitamin D is metabolized to 1,25(OH)$_2$D, the hormonal form of vitamin D. This process, catalyzed by a cytochrome P$_{450}$-like mixed-function oxidase [25(OH)D-α-hydroxylase], occurs predominantly in the mitochondria of the proximal tubules of the nephron (100,101). The production of 1,25(OH)$_2$D is tightly regulated in children (102) and in adults (103). The physiological significance of extrarenal synthesis of 1,25(OH)$_2$D in normal individuals is not clear (104).

Parathyroid hormone and deficiencies in Ca and P increase, whereas Ca, P, and 1,25(OH)$_2$D decrease, the activity of the 25(OH)D-1α-hydroxylase enzyme or circulating 1,25(OH)$_2$D concentration (see Figs. 3 and 4). Other factors, such as sex steroids, prolactin, growth hormone, pregnancy, CT, and possibly thyroid hormone, also may increase the enzyme activity of circulating 1,25(OH)$_2$D. In contrast with the rapid increase in PTH secretion and serum PTH concentrations, measurable alteration in serum

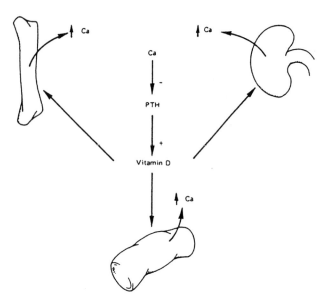

Figure 4 Vitamin D [through its most active metabolite 1,25(OH)$_2$D] acts on the intestine to increase Ca absorption, mobilizes Ca from bone, and reabsorbs Ca in the kidney. The feedback loop might be completed by inhibition of PTH production by Ca, which in turn results in decreased production of 1,25(OH)$_2$D (see Fig. 3). (From Ref. 162.)

1,25(OH)$_2$D concentrations usually occurs some hours after exposure to an appropriate stimulus (2,43,86).

The circulating $t_{1/2}$ of 25(OH)D is 2–3 weeks, depending on the vitamin D status of the individual; it is decreased in vitamin D–deficient individuals (105). 1,25-Dihydroxyvitamin D has a much shorter $t_{1/2}$ of several hours (106). Additional metabolic alterations of 25(OH)D and 1,25(OH)$_2$D occur in the kidney, liver, intestine, and other organs. For example, 25(OH)D undergoes 24-R-hydroxylation to 24R,25(OH)$_2$D or oxidation at C-23 and C-26, which ultimately leads to 25R-OH-26,23S-lactone or possible side-chain cleavage of 25(OH)D to form 23-carboxyltetranorvitamin D [C-23 acid of 25(OH)D] (107). 1,25-Dihydroxyvitamin D is metabolized by side-chain cleavage to 1,23(OH)$_2$-24,25,26,27-tetranorvitamin D (C-23 alcohol) (108) and to 1-hydroxy-23 carboxytetranorvitamin D (calcitroic acid, C-23 carboxylic acid), a major metabolite of 1,25(OH)$_2$D in the kidney. 24-Hydoxylation of 1,25(OH)$_2$D results in 1,24,25(OH)$_3$D; a number of other metabolites are also produced including polar metabolites such as 1,25(OH)$_2$D monoglucuronide in bile (108,109). Biliary excretion is another route of excretion for vitamin D metabolites (106). Metabolites of 25(OH)D and 1,25(OH)$_2$D may undergo enterohepatic circulation after exposure to intestinal β-glucuronidase.

The physiological role of enterohepatic circulation of vitamin D metabolites has not been precisely quantitated (109,110).

Vitamin D and its metabolites are protein bound, mainly to vitamin D–binding protein (DBP; about 85%) and to

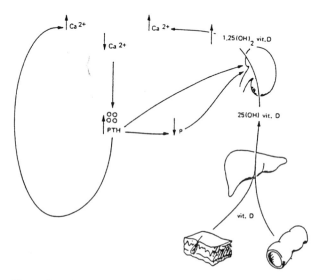

Figure 3 Vitamin D metabolic pathway and its interrelationship with PTH and Ca. The PTH increases in response to hypocalcemia. PTH directly (or through hypophosphatemia) stimulates 1,25(OH)$_2$D (the active metabolite of vitamin D) production from 25(OH)D. Both increased 1,25(OH)$_2$D and increased PTH act to restore serum Ca to normal levels. Vitamin D (D$_3$) is synthesized in the skin or ingested (D$_2$ or D$_3$). (From Ref. 208.)

albumin (about 15%) (111,112). The DBP gene is located on the long arm (q11–13) of human chromosome 4. It is a member of a gene family that includes serum albumin and α-fetoprotein (113).

Vitamin D–binding protein is a globulin with a Mr of approximately 52,000 Da in the rat and approximately 58,000 Da in the human; it is normally <5% saturated with vitamin D metabolite (111,112). Its affinity to vitamin D metabolites depends inversely on the distance between the 3B-hydroxy group and other hydroxyl groups on each vitamin D metabolite. Thus, its affinities for $25(OH)D_3, 24,25(OH)_2D_3$ and $25,26(OH)_2D_3$ are greater than for vitamin D_3 and $1,25(OH)_2D_3$ (114).

It has been suggested that DPB functions in the transport of vitamin D_3 from skin to circulation (93). In addition, the amount of DBP may influence the concentration of "free" $1,25(OH)_2D$ in plasma. The concentration of free hormone appears important in determining the bioactivity of the hormone (112). However, it is possible that some vitamin D and its metabolites may be taken up into target organs when bound to DBP, since liver and kidney readily take up radiolabeled DBP and DBP-actin complexes (115). Thus DBP may aid in the internalization of vitamin D sterols. It binds strongly to actin (111,112) and plasma clearance of the DBP-actin complex appears to be faster than that of DBP alone (115).

Measurements of circulating vitamin D and its metabolites may be complicated by differences in the pharmacokinetics between vitamins D_2 and D_3 (and between their respective metabolites) in their affinity to DBP and receptors; D_2 and D_3 have different chromatographic behavior on various preparative chromatographic systems (116).

Thus, great care must be taken in assay techniques when dealing with patients who have significant vitamin D_2 intake, and appropriate vitamin D standards need to be utilized for standard curve generation when performing competitive protein-binding assays of these compounds to ensure reliable results. Values from different laboratories cannot be compared without making direct comparison of the assay procedures. Interlaboratory coefficients of variation for the measurement of $25(OH)D$, $24,25(OH)_2D$, and $1,25(OH)_2D$ may range between 35% and 52% (117).

Maternofetal transfer of vitamin D and its metabolites varies depending on the species. In humans, cord serum vitamin D is very low and may be undetectable, thought to be related to poor maternofetal crossover; $25(OH)D$ is directly correlated with, but is lower than, maternal values, consistent with placental crossover of this metabolite; $1,25(OH)_2D$ concentrations are also lower than maternal values, but there is no agreement on the maternofetal relationship of this and other dihydroxylated vitamin D metabolites (2,5,13,118). In vivo some placental crossover may occur after maternal exposure to massive pharmacological doses of vitamin D (119). In vitro experiments demonstrate that $25(OH)D$ and $1,25(OH)_2D$ may cross the perfused human placenta (120). In one report of human pregnancy, with consistently elevated (10 times normal) maternal plasma $1,25(OH)_2D$ concentrations from pharmacological doses of $1,25(OH)_2D$ resulted in

similarly elevated cord serum $1,25(OH)_2D$ concentrations at delivery (121). However, the placenta, like the kidney, produces $1,25(OH)_2D$, making it difficult to ascertain just how much fetal $1,25(OH)_2D$ results from placental crossover versus placental synthesis. Seasonal and racial variations in (presumably) endogenously produced serum $25(OH)D_3$ concentrations (lower in winter and in black persons) and $1,25(OH)_3D$ concentrations (higher in blacks) in the mother may be reflected in cord serum values (118,122). The vitamin D metabolite $24,25(OH)_2D$ also crosses the placenta and varies with the seasons, being highest in autumn (123). The significance of this finding is unclear as $24,25(OH)_2D$ may be a metabolic product of $25(OH)D$ to prevent vitamin D toxicity. It appears, therefore, that normally in the human fetus, vitamin D metabolism probably "begins" with $25(OH)D$ and not with vitamin D. Neonates receiving standard supplementary vitamin D intake can achieve adult serum $25(OH)D$ values (2,124).

Serum $1,25(OH)_2D$ concentrations in the newborn become elevated within 24 hr after delivery; thereafter, it appears to vary according to Ca and P intake (2,124–126). Blacks have higher $1,25(OH)_2D$ concentrations than whites in infancy and early childhood (124,127), but not in the older pediatric or adult population (128).

Human milk vitamin D, but not $25(OH)D$ concentration, correlates with maternal vitamin D intake (129,130). Infant serum $25(OH)D$ concentration does not correlate with either human milk vitamin D or $25(OH)D$ concentrations. Sunshine exposure or vitamin D supplementation is the major source of vitamin D in human milk-fed infants (129,130).

In normal adults, serum $1,25(OH)_2D$ concentrations are relatively constant and are maintained within approximately 20% of their overall 24-hr mean (131).

Serum $1,25(OH)_2D$ concentrations decrease with old age in adults, possibly in part related to a decrease in the responsiveness of $25(OH)D-1\alpha$-hydroxylase enzyme activity (132) and, speculatively, low vitamin D production in Northern latitudes (133).

Although a number of vitamin D metabolites may have activity, it is generally agreed that $1,25(OH)_2D$ is the most active vitamin D metabolite. The molecular effects of $1,25(OH)_2D$ are mediated by vitamin D receptors (VDRs). The VDRs are ligand-inducible intracellular transcription factors. Specific $1,25(OH)_2D$ receptors are present in intestinal tissue. Free receptors occur in the cytoplasm, whereas occupied receptors are localized in the nuclei (134). Avian (58–60 kDa) and mammalian (52–55 kDa) $1,25(OH)_2D$ receptor proteins are approximately 75% homologous, based on amino acid sequences produced from cDNAs, and they belong to an enlarging superfamily of gene regulatory proteins that include the steroid, thyroid, and retinoic acid receptors, all of which exhibit a common structural architecture.

The vitamin D receptor gene is located on chromosome 12 in humans [12q (12–14)] and chromosome 7 in rats (135,136). The VDRs are up-regulated by $1,25(OH)_2D$ at both the mRNA and protein levels (137,138). They are increased during growth, gestation, and lactation, but show an age-dependent decrease in mature animals (139); presumably, this implies that VDRs may be up- or down-regulated depending on Ca needs.

Vitamin D receptors are present in an increasingly extensive list of tissues and organs (140). Thus, the list of potential target organs and functional effects of 1,25(OH)$_2$D also increases beyond the target organs of intestine, bone, and kidney. The availability of monoclonal antibodies against VDRs should further enhance the understanding of the mechanism and regulation of 1,25(OH)$_2$D function.

Two basic clinical functions define the major classic action of vitamin D. The first is that vitamin D is required to prevent rickets in children and osteomalacia in adults. The second is the prevention of hypocalcemic tetany (92).

Bone mineralization of skeleton is thought to be predominantly secondary to the action of 1,25(OH)$_2$D in increasing the intestinal absorption of Ca and independently of P; these two actions, thereby, elevate plasma Ca and P concentrations.

Intestinal absorption of Ca and P consists of a passive (concentration-dependent) and active component (2,43,141). Classic vitamin D–dependent active Ca absorption in the intestine is effected largely by a nuclei-mediated process involving transcription and translation of the specific genes that code for Ca and P transport proteins (92). Messenger RNA levels for Ca-binding protein increase after the administration of 1,25(OH)$_2$D. Thus, the synthesis of Ca-binding protein and other membrane and intracellular proteins is important in the movement of Ca across the intestinal cell layer. In addition, 1,25(OH)$_2$D induction of brush border enzyme activities, such as alkaline phosphatase (142) and calcium-dependent ATPase activity at the basolateral membrane, is probably important in the movement of Ca across cell membranes. There are conflicting reports on 1,25(OH)$_2$D-induced changes in membrane fluidity from altered lipid composition of intestinal cell membranes.

Partly on kinetic grounds of extremely rapid onset of action (within minutes after exposure to 1,25(OH)$_2$D), as well as on lack of inhibition by actinomycin D, it is suggested that there is nongenomic, receptor-mediated action of 1,25(OH)$_2$D on intestinal Ca transport (transcaltachia) (44,143). Finally, other factors such as the availability of sodium are important for the active transport of Ca.

There are at least two vitamin D–dependent Ca-binding proteins (CaBP, or calbindin D) and their expression depends on the animal species and the organ studied. In mammals, the 7.5 to 10-kDa CaBP (calbindin D 9K) is found mainly in the duodenum, whereas the 28-kDa CaBP (calbindin D 28K) is found mainly in the kidney and cerebellum (144–147). In avian species, such as the chicken, calbindin D 28K is found in the intestine (148). The calbindin genes among various species have significant homology, but they are not identical (149,150). There is an age-dependent decrease in calbindin D 9K in the rat and human intestine (151). This occurs despite a corresponding increase in intestinal mRNA for calbindin D 9K. Both calbindin D 28K and its mRNA show an age-dependent decrease in the rat kidney (146,152).

In the human, calbindin D 28K gene is located on chromosome 8 (149). The gene for calbindin D 28K is markedly different from the gene for other calcium-binding proteins such as the calmodulin family (149). Calbindin proteins bind Ca with high affinity and undergo conformational changes with the addition of Ca. Analogous to rat and chicken, the human calbindin D 28K also contains six EF-hand-like domains, and there are at least four functional binding sites for Ca (146,148,149). In the rat, a low-P diet may increase calbindin D 28K mRNA along with a corresponding increase in serum 1,25(OH)$_2$D concentrations and 1,25(OH)$_2$D receptor mRNA; a low-Ca diet results in increased serum 1,25(OH)$_2$D concentrations only (153).

Active transport processes of P across the intestine include: (1) a saturable, sodium-dependent Na$^+$,K$^+$-ATPase that involves the endoplasmic reticulum, (2) an unsaturable and sodium-independent component for brush border uptake and basolateral membrane exit processes, and (3) a Ca^{2+}- and vitamin D–dependent component (2,43,154). The vitamin D–dependent mechanism may not be important, except in vitamin D–deficiency states (2). Intestinal P absorption is well established in infants of human and animal species and may be as high as 90% of P intake. In preterm infants (155) as in neonatal rats (156), P absorption appears not to be significantly affected by vitamin D intake.

The effect of vitamin D and its various metabolites on ion transport is much less marked on the kidney than on the intestine. In humans, conflicting data have been reported on the effect of vitamin D and its metabolites on renal excretion of Ca and P, probably because of the difficulty in controlling the many variables that may influence renal handling of these minerals (2,43,100).

In animal experiments, when the vitamin D and PTH status and the serum Ca concentrations are controlled independently, it appears that vitamin D deficiency decreases the effect of PTH to stimulate renal tubular Ca reabsorption, and that vitamin D deficiency per se decreases tubular reabsorption of Ca (157). Receptors for 1,25(OH)$_2$D and vitamin D–dependent CaBP are found in the distal tubule, and the latter may be an important site of vitamin D action on tubular Ca reabsorption. There is a change in cell membrane potential in proximal renal tubular cells within minutes after exposure to 1,25(OH)$_2$D$_3$ (158); however, the role of this nongenomic effect of 1,25(OH)$_2$D in the renal tubule is unclear.

In the normocalcemic, normophosphatemic rat model, vitamin D depletion is associated with decreased renal P reabsorption that is corrected rapidly by physiological amounts of 1,25(OH)$_2$D, probably from stimulation of sodium-dependent P transport in the brush border membrane of proximal tubules (159) and possibly from changes in the lipid composition of tubular membrane (160).

Larger doses of 1,25(OH)$_2$D produce hypercalcemia, hyperphosphatemia, and phosphaturia (100). It appears that PTH and 1,25(OH)$_2$D function closely to maintain stable serum Ca concentration and to be able to react quickly to abrupt changes in serum Ca concentrations. Parathyroid hormone serves as a component of rapid response to hypocalcemia, whereas 1,25(OHD$_2$D, with its major effect on elevating intestinal absorption of Ca, is responsible for a slower, but more sustained effort in maintaining normocalcemia.

II. DISTURBANCES IN SERUM CALCIUM AND PHOSPHORUS CONCENTRATIONS

A. Hypocalcemia

Neonatal hypocalcemia may be defined as a serum total Ca concentration below 2 mmol/L (conversion, 1 mmol/L = 4 mg/dl) in term infants and 1.75 mmol/L in preterm infants, with Ca^{2+} concentrations below 0.75 to 1.1 mmol/L, depending on the particular ion-selective electrode used. These definitions are taken from a clinical viewpoint; physiological dysfunctions, for example through echocardiographic studies, may or may not be demonstrated at these serum values (93,161). However, serum Ca concentrations are maintained within narrow ranges under normal circumstances, and the potential risk for disturbances of physiological function is likely to increase as the serum Ca concentration further decreases.

1. Causes

There are two peaks in the occurrence of neonatal hypocalcemia (Table 1; 162,163). An early form typically occurs during the first few days of life, with the lowest concentrations of serum Ca being reached at 24–48 hr of age; late neonatal hypocalcemia occurs toward the end of the first week of life and generally presents as neonatal tetany. Nevertheless, the lowest serum Ca concentration in the human infant may occur at fewer than 12 hr after birth (38,164) or not until after the first few weeks of life (165).

Early neonatal hypocalcemia occurs primarily in preterm infants. Approximately 30–90% of preterm neonates may have hypocalcemia; the frequency of hypocalcemia varies

Table 1 Neonatal Hypocalcemia

Early neonatal hypocalcemia
    Preterm infants
    Infants with birth asphyxia
    Infants of insulin-dependent, diabetic mothers
    Infants of mothers with hyperparathyroidism (?)
    In utero exposure to anticonvulsants (?)
    Phototherapy (?)
Late neonatal hypocalcemia
    High dietary phosphate load
    Phosphate enemas
    Intestinal calcium malabsorption
    Hypomagnesemia
    Hypoparathyroidism (sporadic, associated with other
       defects, e.g., DiGeorge syndrome, inherited forms)
    Infants of mothers with hyperparathyroidism (?)
Decreased ionized calcium
    Exchange blood transfusion (citrated donor blood)
    Increased free fatty acid (intravenous lipid infusions)
    Alkalosis
    In utero exposure to narcotics (?)

Source: Modified from Ref. 162.

inversely with birth weight and gestational age (38,138,164). Hypocalcemia also occurs in infants who have suffered birth asphyxia (one-third; 8,166) and in infants of mothers with insulin-dependent diabetes (one-half; 167). Neonatal hypocalcemia has been reported to occur during the use of phototherapy and after intrauterine exposure to anticonvulsant drugs. Infants with intrauterine growth retardation may have hypocalcemia if they are also preterm or have experienced birth asphyxia; otherwise, there is apparently no increased incidence of hypocalcemia related to growth retardation per se (168).

Late neonatal hypocalcemia occurs toward the end of the first week of life and, in the United States, occurs less frequently than early neonatal hypocalcemia. Apart from phosphate imbalance from cows' milk–derived formulas, other potentially more common clinical circumstances associated with hypocalcemia include intestinal malabsorption of Ca, hypomagnesemia, and hypoparathyroidism of the transient or permanent form (169–173).

Although neonatal hypocalcemia may occur at different postnatal ages, the mechanisms of hypocalcemia are varied and frequently interrelated (Table 2). The physiological bases for the development of hypocalcemia were discussed in Section I. A predisposing factor to early neonatal hypocalcemia can be inadequate Ca intake when the placental supply of Ca to the neonate is abruptly discontinued at delivery. We found no seasonal differences in Cincinnati in the rate of early hypocalcemia (174), but an increased incidence of hypocalcemia in Caucasian versus African-American neonates. Postnatally, even if there is maximal intestinal absorption of about 60% (175, 176), Ca retention with milk feeding is probably only 15 mg/kg body weight on the first day of life, rising to 45 mg/kg on the third day of life; these amounts are significantly lower than in utero Ca accretion rates. In sick infants, there is further limitation in milk and Ca intake.

Any chronic diarrheal condition, especially if associated with steatorrhea, is generally associated with intestinal malabsorption of Ca. In addition, there is possibly impaired enterohepatic circulation of vitamin D and vitamin D metabolites.

High serum P concentration in the neonatal period also may decrease serum Ca through physicochemical effects, blunting of the action of PTH, or augmentation of the action of CT.

Excessive dietary P load from ingestion of cows' milk-type formulas (9), or the early neonatal introduction of cereals (177), is typically associated with the late onset of hypocalcemia. This form of hypocalcemia occurs during or after the second week of life, when oral intake is well established. Feeding infants with "humanized" cows' milk formula, with a lower P content and a relative increase in Ca/P ratio, apparently has not completely eliminated the occurrence of this form of hypocalcemia (178).

The high P content of formula proteins and the low solubility of Ca salts in solution result in relatively higher serum P and lower serum Ca in formula-fed infants versus human milk-fed infants (178). Decreased serum Ca and increased P may, however, stimulate PTH secretion, which

Table 2 Possible Mechanisms Involved in Neonatal Hypocalcemia

Agent	Problem	Specific condition
Ca supply	Decreased	Inadequate intake or malabsorption
Mg	Decreased	Maternal hypomagnesemia or specific Mg malabsorption (rare)
P	Increased	Dietary and endogenous phosphate loading
pH	Increased	Respiratory/metabolic alkalosis
Parathyroid hormone	Decreased	Decreased responsivity to hypocalcemia
Calcitonin	Increased (?)	Clinical significance (?)
Vitamin D metabolites	Decreased (?)	Late neonatal hypocalcemia

Source: From Ref. 162.

in turn minimizes the hypocalcemic effect of hyperphosphatemia. The presence of maternal vitamin D deficiency may theoretically enhance the effect of hyperphosphatemia (179), either because of secondary maternal hyperparathyroidism (with resultant fetal and neonatal hypoparathyroidism) or because of disturbances in neonatal vitamin D metabolism. The neonatal hypocalcemia in this situation appears to be compounded by seasonal variations in maternal sunlight exposure, increased maternal age and parity, and poor socioeconomic class (179).

Transient decreases in serum Mg concentrations have been reported in infants of diabetic mothers (167). In these infants, the hypomagnesemia is often associated with hypocalcemia. However, it is unclear whether the decrease in both serum Mg and Ca is the result of a common insult or whether the decrease in serum Mg leads to, or aggravates, hypocalcemia. The decrease in serum Mg in these infants apparently returns to normal ranges spontaneously.

Specific intestinal malabsorption of Mg (54) may lead to Mg depletion and, secondarily, to hypocalcemia, which can be corrected only when the Mg disturbance is corrected. The most common cause of intestinal malabsorption of Mg is surgical resection of large segments of small bowel, with or without fistula losses of various minerals.

Higher fecal loss of Mg with lower net absorption and retention may not occur in low-birth-weight infants fed a higher P (106–120 mg/100 kcal) and a fixed Ca (180 mg/100 kcal) content formula (180). On the contrary, P depletion may be associated with hypermagnesuria; hypomagnesemia occurs in rats with P depletion (54). Hypomagnesemia may contribute to neonatal hypocalcemia by inhibiting formation of $1,25(OH)_2D$ (54) or inhibiting PTH secretion.

In clinical practice, administration of sodium bicarbonate in the therapy of neonatal acidosis has been frequently associated with early neonatal hypocalcemia (8,166). During acidosis in these infants, Ca is possibly mobilized from bone to extracellular fluid and then lost through renal excretion. During alkali therapy, it is suggested that decreased bone release of Ca may trigger hypocalcemia and tetany. Each of the Ca-regulating hormones [PTH, CT, and $1,25(OH)_2D$] has been implicated in the development of hypocalcemia. New

born infants increase their serum PTH concentrations after birth (38). The increase is coincidental, with a fall in serum total and ionized Ca concentrations, presumably reflecting abrupt withdrawal of the pregnancy-related maternofetal Ca transfer. In situations of induced hypocalcemia, such as during an exchange transfusion, the response of the parathyroid gland in the neonate may be transient (181) or delayed. However, the ability of the neonatal parathyroids to respond to a hypocalcemic stress increases with postnatal age (181) and, presumably, reflects increasing adaptation to extrauterine existence.

Temporary neonatal hypoparathyroidism may be a problem, accentuating and perpetuating the tendency toward decreased serum Ca concentrations in preterm infants (164, 181) and in infants of diabetic mothers (IDM). However, infants in both groups may be able to increase serum PTH concentrations, to some degree, in response to hypocalcemic stresses.

In contrast, more severe and prolonged hypocalcemia may occur with parathyroid suppression from maternal hyperparathyroidism (165), neonatal parathyroid hypoplasia, or neonatal parathyroid agenesis (169–173). In the first instance, the diagnosis of maternal hyperparathyroidism is often made because of the infant's condition. In the latter two conditions, hypocalcemia may be permanent and may require continuous therapy. Hypoparathyroidism may occur sporadically or as sex-linked inheritance, or it may be associated with congenital dysplasia of the structures of the third and fourth pharyngeal pouches (DiGeorge syndrome). Recently a deletion within chromosome 22q11 has been identified in patients with DiGeorge and velocardiofacial/shprintzen syndromes (172, 182). Both syndromes may be associated with transient congenital hypoparathyroidism (TCHP) or neonatal hypocalcemia and may represent different degrees of the same disorder. There is now also growing evidence that neonates previously diagnosed with TCHP may have recurrence of their hypoparathyroidism in later childhood (171–173). Autosomal-dominant familial hypoparathyroidism with and without associated hypomagnesemia has also been reported (170, 171).

The exact role of elevated CT concentration in the

pathogenesis of neonatal hypocalcemia is not known. In both healthy term and IDM neonates serum CT appears not to correlate with serum Ca (80). Postnatal increases in serum CT concentrations occur in full-term infants, low-birth-weight infants (38), IDM (167,183), and infants with birth asphyxia (7). The stimulus for the postnatal rise in serum CT, despite falling serum Ca concentration, is unknown. There are conflicting reports on the effect of Ca supplementation to suppress the nostanatal surge in CT secretion (38,183). However, serum CT concentration is increased after an intravenous bolus injection of Ca during exchange blood transfusion (184).

Increased postnatal serum concentrations of $1,25(OH)_2D$ can be associated temporally with an increase in serum PTH concentrations, presumably secondary to decreased serum Ca levels. It is possible that there is an end-organ resistance to $1,25(OH)_2D$ action to elevate serum Ca in vivo and in vitro (185), particularly in the small preterm infant, and this phenomenon may be a factor in the high prevalence of neonatal hypocalcemia in such infants.

Decreases in serum Ca^{2+} can occur without decreases in serum total Ca concentration. Agents that complex Ca in the blood would be expected to decrease Ca^{2+}. Such agents include citrate, which is used as an anticoagulant for blood storage. During "exchange" blood transfusion, serum Ca^{2+} concentrations can be decreased to 0.5 mmol/L, in spite of administration of conventional amounts of Ca (i.e., 0.5–1 ml of 10% calcium gluconate for each 100 ml of blood exchanged) during the transfusion (181,184); increases in long-chain free fatty acids also can complex Ca in vitro and lower Ca^{2+} (186).

Alkalosis from overtreatment with alkali, or hyperventilation from overuse of respirators, can result in shifts or Ca from the ionized state to the protein-bound fraction. Because alkalosis per se (187) increases neuromuscular hyperirritability, the combination of decreased serum Ca^{2+} and alkalosis may precipitate clinical tetany in an infant with borderline serum Ca status. For reasons unclear, infants born to narcotic-using mothers have been described to have a lower serum Ca^{2+} if they develop withdrawal symptoms (188).

Hypocalcemia in neonates receiving phototherapy is thought to result from the stimulation of a complex system of extraretinal photoreception, which results in neuroendocrine sequelae and hypocalcemia (189). The anticonvulsant drugs phenytoin and phenobarbital are known to induce hepatic microsomal enzyme activity, which results in an increased hydroxylation of vitamin D or D metabolites to biologically inactive metabolites (190). Transplacental anticonvulsant drugs may persist in high concentrations in the neonate because maturation of the hepatic parahydroxylating capacity for metabolism of anticonvulsant is thought to be low in the first days of life. The risk of neonatal hypocalcemia theoretically may be greater if there is preexisting maternal vitamin D deficiency.

2. Diagnosis

Suspicion of hypocalcemia should be confirmed with the measurement of serum total Ca and Ca^{2+} and by the clinical response to administration of Ca. A history of Ca-related disorders may be present (Table 3). A maternal history suggestive of hyperparathyroidism (nausea, vomiting, polyuria, hypertension, and renal stones) may be confused with pregnancy-related complications. The clinical manifestation of neonatal hypocalcemia in infants also may be easily confused with other neonatal disorders, such as hypoglycemia, sepsis, meningitis, anoxia, intracranial bleeding, and narcotic withdrawal. The neonate with hypocalcemia also may be asymptomatic; the less mature the infant, the more subtle and varied are the clinical manifestations.

Significant clinical signs are tremulousness, apnea, cyanosis, and seizures; infants also may be lethargic, feed poorly, vomit, and develop abdominal distension. Frank convulsions are more commonly seen with late neonatal hypocalcemia. The degree of "irritability" of the infants does not appear to correlate with serum Ca values. The classic signs of peripheral hyperexcitability of motor nerves, carpopedal spasm (spasm of the wrists and ankles), and laryngospasm (spasm of the vocal cord) are uncommon in newborn infants.

Measurement of serum total Ca should be performed in all infants suspected of having hypocalcemia; measurements of Ca^{2+} are preferable. At physiological concentrations of H^+ and K^+, tetany may develop in older infants at Ca^{2+} concentrations of <0.8 mmol/L and will almost always be manifested (possibly with the exception of preterm infants) at Ca^{2+} concentrations <0.6 mmol/L. If serum albumin concentrations are normal, the corresponding serum total Ca concentrations are <1.8 mmol/L (187). Serum Ca^{2+} concentrations may not decrease to the same extent as total Ca in the preterm infant (164,191), presumably related in part to

Table 3 Diagnostic Workup for Hypocalcemia

History	Familial
	Pregnancy (maternal illness, e.g., diabetes mellitus, hyperparathyroidism, intrapartum events, and infant's gestational age)
	Dietary intake of infant
Physical examination	Jitteriness
	Seizures
	Associated features (infant of diabetic mother, prematurity, birth asphyxia, congenital heart defect)
Investigations	Serum, Ca, Mg, P, Ca^{2+}, glucose
	Vitamin D metabolites
	Parathyroid hormone
	Calcitonin
	Acid-base balance
	ECG (Q-Tc > 0.4 sec or Q-oTc > 0.2 set)
	Chest X-ray film (thymic shadow aortic arch position)
	Chromosomal analysis for 22q 11 deletion.
	Others: Urine drug screen, malabsorption workup, maternal/family screening

the low serum albumin concentrations and frequent acidosis found in premature infants. The sparing effect of the lowered albumin concentrations on Ca^{2+} concentrations may partially explain the frequent lack of signs of hypocalcemia in premature infants. Serum total Ca and Ca^{2+} concentrations are correlated (14,164,191), but one cannot accurately predict Ca^{2+} from total Ca concentrations in the infant. The standard nomogram relating serum total Ca and total protein to Ca^{2+} has not been predictive of neonatal serum Ca^{2+}. The value of electrocardiographic QT intervals, corrected for heart rate (191,192), is also of little value for prediction of neonatal hypocalcemia.

Assays of calciotropic hormones and 25(OH)D may be useful in the diagnosis of uncommon causes of neonatal hypocalcemia, such as primary hypoparathyroidism, malabsorption, and disorders of vitamin D metabolism. Chromsomal analysis for 22q11 deletion should be considered especially if there is a family history suggestive of velocardiofacial/shprintzen or DiGeorge syndromes. Other investigations listed in Table 3 also may be important in the diagnosis and understanding of the mechanisms for hypocalcemia.

Confirmation of hypocalcemia as the cause of clinical symptomatology is the reversibility of clinical signs when serum total Ca or Ca^{2+} has been increased to the normal range.

3. Therapy

Any neonate with seizures should have blood drawn for diagnostic tests before therapy. Intravenous administration of Ca salts is the most effective and most rapid means of elevating serum Ca concentration. Seizures suspected to be caused by hypocalcemia should be treated with intravenous 10% calcium gluconate (1 ml/kg) administered over 10 min with constant monitoring of the heart rate. A gradual or abrupt decrease in heart rate during the infusion would necessitate slowing or stopping the infusion. Intravenous Ca therapy may be complicated by acute hypercalcemia; extravasation of Ca solution leads to skin sloughs, tissue necrosis, and calcification.

Intravenous Ca boluses over 10 min result in a transient decrease in blood pH, increased serum osmolality, and decreased serum P while having no effect on serum free bilirubin (193). The clinical significance of these biochemical changes in unclear. The effect on serum osmolality is not observed when 5% calcium gluconate is infused. If umbilical vein catheters are used, the tips should not be too close to the heart because of possible accidental administration of Ca directly into the heart. Direct admixture with bicarbonate or phosphate solution is not permitted because of precipitation.

There is little information on comparative efficacy of Ca preparations, but 10% $CaCl_2$ (0.3 ml/kg) also may be used with the same precautions as above. Prolonged use of $CaCl_2$ in high doses may be associated with acidosis and probably should be avoided. Further Ca therapy would depend on symptomatic response, and repeated measurement of serum total Ca and Ca^{2+} concentrations may be necessary.

After the resolution of the seizures, intravenous Ca solutions may be continued at 75 mg elemental Ca per kilogram per day until the serum Ca concentrations have remained consistently in the normal range.

Thereafter, the intravenous Ca solution can be reduced in stepwise fashion (50% of maintenance dose for a day, 25% dose for another day, before discontinuation). With intravenous therapy, continuous infusion is probably more efficacious than intermittent therapy (194), presumably because renal loss of Ca may be greater with the latter method. Anecdotal cases of massive sloughing of soft tissue in the areas perfused by arteries receiving Ca infusion have been reported, and inadvertent administration into a mesenteric artery can theoretically lead to necrosis of intestinal tissue. However, the infusion of Ca-containing parenteral nutrition solutions through the umbilical artery catheter is a common practice in neonatal intensive care units, and the Ca content has not been specifically implicated as a cause of significant complications.

Oral Ca therapy in the same dosage (75 mg/kg/day in four to six divided doses) may be used for maintenance therapy. Oral Ca preparations with syrup base contain a high sucrose content, which may be a significant carbohydrate and osmolality load for very small infants. It has the advantage of being concentrated (for example, calcium glubionate and calcium gluceptate have 115 and 90 mg elemental Ca per 5 ml, respectively) if the infant is under fluid restriction. In general, a solution such as 10% calcium gluconate (intravenous preparation) is well tolerated orally and would be the agent of choice. However, all Ca preparations are hypertonic, and there is a theoretical potential for precipitating necrotizing enterocolitis in infants at risk for this condition. Also, increase in frequency of bowel movements can be expected, especially with syrup bases (195).

The duration of supplemental Ca therapy varies with the cause of hypocalcemia; in most situations it might require only 2–3 days, such as for early neonatal hypocalcemia, or therapy might be prolonged for hypocalcemia caused by malabsorption or hypoparathyroidism. The serum Ca concentrations need to be measured on two or more occasions each day during the first few days of treatment and for a day after discontinuation to detect any "rebound" phenomenon.

Vitamin D Metabolites. $1,25(OH)_2D$ at 0.05–0.2 $\mu g/kg/day$, intravenously or orally (196); $1\alpha(OH)D_3$, an analog of $1,25(OH)_2D$ at 0.33 μg b.i.d. orally (197); and exogenous PTH (166) have been used in the treatment of neonatal hypocalcemia. However, there is no practical advantage to the use of these agents in the treatment of acute hypocalcemia, and their use should be considered experimental. 1,25-Dihydroxyvitamin D is commonly used in maintenance therapy for chronic conditions that cause hypocalcemia (e.g., hypoparathyroidism).

The successful management of neonatal hypocalcemia also depends on the resolution, if possible, of the primary cause of hypocalcemia. For example, in P-induced hypocalcemia, high-phosphate formulas and solids should be discontinued, and breast milk or a low-phosphate formula should be substituted. Use of aluminum hydroxide gel to bind intestinal P should be avoided because of potential risk for aluminum toxicity (198). Removal of complexing agents will resolve conditions caused by complexing of Ca. Because of the effect of increased pH on serum Ca^{2+}, it would be advisable to prevent alkalosis in high-risk infants with borderline serum Ca concentrations. Magnesium depletion and hypoparathyroidism should be considered in patients refractory to standard Ca therapy, and specific therapy should be instituted after appropriate diagnosis (43,163).

Neonatal hypocalcemia may resolve spontaneously (9, 194). Thus, it is possible that asymptomatic neonatal hypocalcemia may not require treatment. However, because of the major physiological importance of Ca in all cellular systems, especially its role as a second messenger for the initiation of intracellular enzymatic cascades (22), hypocalcemia potentially can alter important cellular functions and probably should be corrected. Infusion of a single bolus of 18 mg of elemental Ca per kilogram has been shown to increase heart rate and blood pressure in preterm infants with hypocalcemia (199). Treatment of asymptomatic hypocalcemia can be instituted with oral or intravenous Ca salts, using the same regimen as just described.

Pharmacological prevention of neonatal hypocalcemia has primarily focused on the prophylactic use of Ca salts or the vitamin D metabolites. Prophylactic oral Ca supplementation (75 or 80 mg/kg/day of elemental Ca, given in four divided doses each day) has been used in preterm infants and in infants with birth asphyxia, with good results and no deleterious effects on serum P, Mg, PTH, or 25(OH)D (195). In low-birth-weight infants, continuous intravenous infusion of 1–1.5 mg/kg/hr of elemental Ca sustains low-normal serum Ca concentrations (200,201); doses approximating the oral doses appear to be well tolerated in clinical practice.

Vitamin D_3 30 μg (conversion, 1 μg = 40 IU)/day orally, 25(OH)D at 10 μg/kg per day orally (201,202), 1α-hydroxyvitamin D_3 at 0.05–0.1 μg/kg/day intravenously (203), and 1,25(OH)$_2$D at 0.5–1 μg/day orally or 0.1–4 μg/kg/day intramuscularly or intravenously (164,204) have been used in attempts to prevent neonatal hypocalcemia with variable degrees of success. In small preterm infants, serum Ca was normalized only at pharmacological doses of 1,25(OH)$_2$D. Early feeding, and delivery of Ca to the gut, has been suggested to be important in enhancing the ability of vitamin D metabolites in the prevention of neonatal hypocalcemia.

Thus, the most effective prevention of neonatal hypocalcemia is preventing the primary causes, such as prematurity and birth asphyxia, judicious use of bicarbonate therapy, and minimizing the occurrence of respiratory alkalosis from excessive mechanical ventilation. The practice of early feeding and, if necessary, the use of oral or parenteral supplement of Ca salts also are useful measures. Maintenance of normal maternal vitamin D status with exogenous vitamin D supplement, if needed, may theoretically be helpful in maintaining normal vitamin D status and, secondarily, in prevention of late hypocalcemia in some neonates.

B. Hypercalcemia

An infant can be considered to be hypercalcemic when serum total Ca concentrations are >2.7 mmol/L or when Ca^{2+} concentrations are >1.4 mmol/L (11,14). In pathological situations of hypercalcemia, elevation of serum Ca^{2+} concentrations usually occurs simultaneously with elevation of total Ca. However, elevated serum total Ca may occur without elevation of Ca^{2+}. Elevation of protein available to bind Ca—for example, in situations of prolonged application of tourniquet before venipuncture, with transudation of plasma water into tissues, in patients with multiple myeloma, and possibly in situations of adrenal insufficiency—may result in elevation of serum total Ca. A change in serum albumin of 1 g/dl generally results in a parallel change in total Ca of about 0.2 mmol/L. Conversely, reduced albumin binding of Ca may result in normal serum total Ca in the presence of elevated Ca^{2+} (43).

Hypercalcemia is the result of imbalance between fluxes of Ca into and out of extracellular fluid. An increase in net Ca mobilization from the skeleton is generally the primary cause of hypercalcemia. Although the kidney and gastrointestinal tract are involved in total body Ca homeostasis, and sometimes in maintaining hypercalcemia, there are few hypercalcemic disorders that are thought to be primarily due to Ca hyperabsorption by the intestine or reabsorption by the kidney.

Hypercalcemia in infants is rare. It is frequently iatrogenic and may be discovered by serendipity on a routine "chemistry panel." Its onset may be at birth or delayed for weeks or months. The most common clinical cause of hypercalcemia in infants (Table 4) is a relative deficiency in the P supply with hypophosphatemia, during inappropriate parenteral nutrition (205), or enteral human milk feeding in preterm infants (206). Hypophosphatemia can result in elevated circulating 1,25(OH)$_2$D with theoretical attendant increased intestinal absorption of Ca. Phosphorus deficiency results in increased bone resorption and decreased bone formation; Ca cannot be deposited in bone in the absence of P and contributes to hypercalcemia. A number of other pathological situations with increased PTH or vitamin D may increase bone turnover, intestinal Ca absorption, and renal Ca reabsorption and may result in hypercalcemia.

Neonatal hyperparathyroidism frequently results in marked hypercalcemia, but there is a range of manifestations. Hyperparathyroidism may be congenital and inherited as an autosomal-dominant or autosomal-recessive trait, or it may be secondary to maternal hypoparathyroidism (207). In affected infants, serum Ca concentrations may be markedly elevated (>3.7 mmol/L), whereas serum P concentration is frequently <1.2 mmol/L. The serum alkaline phosphatase activity may be normal or increased. Unexplained anemia, splenomegaly, and hepatomegaly may be present. Radiographic skeletal demineralization, subperiosteal resorption, and pathological fractures are frequently present. Renal calcinosis is also common. The characteristic pathological finding in the parathyroid glands is clear cell hyperplasia (208).

Table 4 Neonatal Hypercalcemia

Phosphate deficiency
   Parenteral nutrition
   Very-low-birth-weight infants fed human milk or
   (less commonly) standard formula
Hypervitaminosis D
   Excessive maternal vitamin D intake
Hyperparathyroidism
   Congenital parathyroid hyperplasia
   Maternal hypoparathyroidism
   Maternal and neonatal renal tubular acidosis
Mutations in Ca^{2+}-sensing receptor gene
   Neonatal, severe (primary) hyperparathyroidism
   Familial, hypocalciuric hypercalcemia
Uncertain pathophysiological mechanism
   Idiopathic infantile hypercalcemia
   Severe infantile hypophosphatasia
   Subcutaneous fat necrosis
   Blue diaper syndrome
Chronic maternal hypercalcemia (?)
   Thyrotoxicosis
   Chronic thiazide diuretic, lithium therapy
   Vitamin A intoxication

Source: Modified from Ref. 163.

Neonatal hyperparathyroidism has also been reported to occur in the presence of maternal and neonatal renal tubular acidosis and with familial hypocalciuric hypercalcemia (209–211). Familial hypocalciuric hypercalcemia (FHH) has been reported in patients from 2 hr to 82 years of age (212). It is usually diagnosed in infants as part of a "screening" procedure after the diagnosis of a family member with hypercalcemia of familial multiple endocrine neoplasia. It is inherited as an autosomal-dominant trait with high degree of penetrance. There is usually significant hypophosphatemia and a modest increase in serum Mg concentrations. There is now, in fact, compelling evidence that both neonatal severe hyperparathyroidism (NSHPT) and FHH are caused by mutations in the human Ca^{2+}-sensing receptor gene (53,213). Both the human Ca^{2+}-sensing receptor gene and the NSHPT/FHH locus map to chromosome 3. It has been proposed that the mutated Ca^{2+}-sensing receptor in NSHPT/FHH patients decreases the sensitivity of parathyroid cells to extracellular Ca^{2+}. Patients with FHH are probably heterozygous and those with NSHPT homozygous for the mutant human Ca^{2+}-sensing receptor gene (213). Mutated receptors might interfere with the function of the normal receptors or be nonfunctional. Alternativity, gene mutations might cause a decrease of cell surface Ca^{2+} receptors. DNA markers linked to both chromosomes 3q and 19p have been identified in families with FHH (213). However, only one in 16 families map to 19p and may have more mild hypercalcemia than those mapped to 3q.

Neonatal hyperparathyroidism that resolves spontane-

ously over several months has been reported in three affected infants (211).

Chronic excessive exposure to vitamin D or its metabolites in a mother during pernancy, such as that which occurs during treatment of maternal hypocalcemic disorders or by self-medication, may result in neonatal hypercalcemia (43). Other causes of neonatal hypercalcemia in which no specific defect of vitamin D or PTH physiology has been demonstrated include idiopathic infantile hypercalcemia, often considered part of a syndrome of hypercalcemia, mental retardation, "elfin facies," and supravalvular aortic stenosis (Williams syndrome). Various combinations of the major manifestations of the syndrome may occur and there may be pre- and postnatal growth failure. Several chromosomal abnormalities have been described in patients with Williams syndrome (214). More recently mutations in the elastin gene on the long arm of chromosome 7 has been reported in these patients (215). Hemizygosity at the elastin locus has been identified in four familial and five sporadic cases of Williams syndrome. This suggests that deletions involving an elastin allele cause Williams syndrome. The presence of hypercalcemia in infants with Williams syndrome is variable and serum calcium may be normal, but the presence of nephrocalcinosis and soft-tissue calcifications in some of these infants suggests that hypercalcemia may have occurred previously. Exaggerated response to pharmacological doses of vitamin D_2 (18,000–100,000 IU) and a blunted calcitonin response to calcium loading may contribute to the pathogenesis of hypercalcemia of idiopathic infantile hypercalcemia (43).

Severe infantile hypophosphatasia is associated with hypercalcemia and is a rare autosomal-recessive disorder associated with low serum alkaline phosphatase levels because of an absence of alkaline phosphatase from bone, endochondral defect in ossification with severe radiographic bone demineralization, and elevated urinary phosphoethanolamine. The condition may be lethal in utero or shortly after birth because of inadequate bony support of the thorax and skull (216).

Neonates with extensive subcutaneous fat necrosis may develop hypercalcemia, usually occurring after a period of low or normal serum Ca concentrations. Hypercalcemia usually occurs at the end of the first week of life, with the neonate experiencing complications in the majority of reported cases (217). The most often reported clinical sign in these infants is failure to thrive with 15 percent mortality (217). Increased prostaglandin E activity, increased release of Ca from fat tissues, and unregulated production of $1,25(OH)_2D$ from marcrophages infiltrating the fatty lesions have been postulated to be responsible for the hypercalcemia in this condition (43,218). Blue diaper syndrome is a rare familial disorder, with malabsorption of tryptophan (219). There is increased urinary excretion of indican, an end-product of intestinal degradation of unabsorbed tryptophan and hepatic metabolism of its intermediate metabolites. The blue discoloration of the urine is due to the hydrolysis and oxidation of urinary indican. Hypercalcemia and nephrocalcinosis usually are not manifested until some months after birth. Theoretically, causes of chronic maternal hypercalcemia, including thyrotoxicosis, chronic thiazide diuretics, lithium therapy, and vitamin A intoxication, may predispose newborn infants to hypercalcemia (43).

Neonates with hypercalcemia may be asymptomatic, and the diagnosis is made on routine screening because of the known predisposing factors, or the babies may have serious symptomatology requiring urgent treatment. Symptoms and signs of neonatal hypercalcemia are frequently nonspecific and include lethargy, irritability, polyuria, vomiting, constipation, dehydration, and failure to thrive. Hypertension, nephrocalcinosis, and band keratopathy of the limbus of the eye may be present in severely affected instances. Anatomical anomalies (e.g., elfin facies and evidence of congenital heart disease) may be present on physical examination. A maternal dietary and drug history during pregnancy should be obtained, as should a family history for evidence of disturbed Ca metabolism.

Laboratory investigations include serum total Ca and Ca^{2+}, P, and alkaline phosphatase; PTH, 25(OH)D, and 1,25(OH)$_2$D; urinary Ca, P, and cAMP levels; and radiograph of hands and wrists for evidence of hyperparathyroidism; these measurements are useful in the differential diagnosis of hypercalcemia. Measurement of nephrogenous cAMP may also be useful. Other tests, such as renal function, abdominal ultrasound for nephrocalcinosis, and ophthalmological examination, may refect the extent of the effect of hypercalcemia.

Therapy of neonatal hypercalcemia includes removal of specific underlying causes (e.g., large vitamin D intake). Often nonspecific therapy is the only one available. Treatment for chronic conditions includes restriction of dietary intake of vitamin D and Ca, as well as minimizing exposure to sunlight to lower endogenous vitamin D production. For short-term treatment of acute hypercalcemic episodes, expansion of the extracellular compartment with 10–20 ml/kg of 0.9% sodium chloride, intravenously, followed by an intravenous injection of a potent loop diuretic, such as 1–2 mg/kg of furosemide, may be effective. One should take care to avoid fluid and electrolyte imbalance. Further intravenous fluid should replace urine losses of water, Na, and K, which are measured at 4–6-hr intervals. Furosemide may be repeated at 2–4-hr intervals. Prolonged diuresis also requires replacement of Mg losses. Phosphate supplements of 0.5–1 mmol/kg of elemental P per day, in divided doses, in patients with low serum P levels may normalize the serum P concentration and lower serum Ca concentrations; excessive amounts of P may result in diarrhea and hypocalcemia and a theoretical possibility of metastatic calcification (43,175,208).

Minimal information is available on the use of hormonal and other drug therapy for neonatal hypercalcemia. Short-term treatment with CT at 4–8 IU/kg subcutaneously or intramuscularly, every 12 hr, or prednisone 0.5–1 mg/kg/day, or a combination, may be useful on a short-term basis. Onset of action of these therapies is slow and ranges from hours for CT to days for glucocorticoid; their hypocalcemic effect may be variable, and "escape" from the hypocalcemic effect of CT may occur. Other hormones, such as estrogen and progesterone, and drugs, such as plicamycin (mithramycin), an antineoplastic agent that inhibits RNA synthesis, biphos-

phonates (e.g., etidronate disodium, a synthetic inhibitor of osteoclast function), can have unacceptable side effects and are not used for infants.

Because some instances of neonatal hypercalcemia may resolve spontaneously, the need for treatment should be reassessed at regular intervals. Family screening for hypercalcemia should be done, unless a specific, nonfamilial cause for hypercalcemia in the index case is established. Parathyroidectomy may be indicated in severely affected neonates with primary hyperparathyroidism.

C. Hypophosphatemia

An infant can be considered to be hypophosphatemic when serum P concentration is <1.3 mmol/L (conversion, 1 mmol/L = 3.1 mg/dl). Hypophosphatemia may occur within days of birth and may persist for many months. Usually, it has a "nutritional" basis (Table 5) and occurs most frequently in infants receiving low P intake from parenteral nutrition (125,126) and in preterm infants fed human milk (206).

In infants receiving parenteral nutrition, hypophosphatemia is exaggerated if there is an associated rapid increase in delivery of carbohydrates (glucose). This is probably the result of transcellular shift of P in addition to a relative or absolute deficiency in P intake. Hypophosphatemia occurs with administration of glucose, and it may be accentuated during starvation (221). The "refeeding syndrome," from overzealous increase in the delivery of calories, can be associated with multiple electrolyte abnormalities, including hypophosphatemia, hypokalemia, and hypomagnesemia, and life-threatening complications (221,222). In malnourished states, glucose and P are utilized initially to meet muscle needs, and this is partly responsible for the compartmental shift of P from extracellular fluid (221,223). Insulin lowers serum P by facilitating the intracellular movement of glucose and P, with secondary decrease in renal phosphate filter load and decrease in urinary phosphate excretion (224). Respira-

Table 5 Causes of Neonatal Hypophosphatemia

Nutritional
  Low phosphorus intake
    Parenteral nutrition; human milk or standard formula
      feeding (preterm infants)
  Trancellular shift
    Refeeding syndrome in malnutrition
  Low phosphorus absorption
    Vitamin D deficiency; malabsorption (e.g., short gut)
      syndromes
  Excessive nutrient intake
    Sodium, calcium, glucose, amino acids
Nonnutritional
  Hyperparathyroidism
  X-linked hypophosphatemic rickets
  Fanconi's syndrome
  Chronic diuretic therapy

tory alkalosis, liver disease, and hypokalemia also may contribute to "shift hypophosphatemia."

Hypophosphatemia from decreased intestinal P absorption can be an early manifestation of vitamin D deficiency (225,226). Theoretically, any severe and prolonged malabsorption syndrome may be associated with hypophosphatemia. Excessive nutrient intake, including Na, glucose, amino acids, and Ca, particularly if they are delivered intravenously, can result in hypophosphatemia (175,205,227). The mechanism for the development of hypophosphatemia is not fully understood, but, in part it may be related to extracellular fluid volume expansion or to interference with renal tubular P reabsorption. The excretion of these nutrients (including P) is interdependent, and they are effected by sodium-dependent cotransport systems. Thus, interference with renal tubular transport of any of these nutrients potentially can affect the renal tubular P reabsorption (43,228).

Nonnutritional causes of neonatal hypophosphatemia are much less frequent than nutritional causes. The primary mechanism of hypophosphatemia in non-nutritional-related hypophosphatemia is probably decreased renal tubular P reabsorption and may or may not be secondary to elevated PTH. The causes include primary hyperparathyroidism, X-linked hypophosphatemic rickets, Fanconi's syndrome (idiopathic or secondary to inborn errors of metabolism such as cystinosis and tyrosinosis), and chronic diuretic treatment (43).

Hypophosphatemia may be an early manifestation of P deficiency. Phosphorus deficiency may have multiple clinical consequences affecting hematological, immunological, cardiorespiratory, neuromuscular, skeletal, peripheral, and central nervous systems (229). In most cases of neonatal hypophosphatemia, the diagnosis can be made with a careful review of the history and a few laboratory investigations. Hypophosphatemia in neonates is usually asymptomatic and may be diagnose from routine screening because of a family history of disturbances in mineral metabolism.

Clinical signs attributed to hypophosphatemia are usually noted when the serum P concentration is <0.7 mmol/L. However, many of the clinical signs of P deficiency are masked by the underlying illness or by the therapy administered to the infant; for example, bronchopulmonary dysplasia and hypophosphatemia may occur simulateneously, and it may be difficult to distinguish the relative contribution of each to the respiratory failure in an affected infant; multiple blood transfusion may mask the effect of decreased oxygen delivery associated with hypophosphatemia. More dramatic skeletal manifestations of prolonged and severe hypophosphatemia, such as rickets and osteomalacia, usually are not present until after the neonatal period (230). In other situations, such as neonatal primary hyperparathyroidism, the presenting symptoms and signs are usually unrelated to hypophosphatemia (see Sec. II.B). Laboratory investigations should include determination of serum concentrations of P, total Ca and Ca^{+2}, Na, K, and creatinine, urine Ca, P, Na, and creatinine, serum PTH, 25(OH)D, and 1,25(OH)$_2$D, and measurement of renal tubular reabsorption of P (phosphate clearance × 100% divided by creatinine clearance), and urine glucose and amino acid screening. Radiographs of hands and wrists for evidence of rickets and osteopenia may be helpful in determining the cause and effect of hypophosphatemia. Hypophosphatemia from nutritional causes may be severe (serum P < 0.7 mmol/L) and is typically associated with hypercalcemia, almost total absence of P in the urine, and renal tubules that are resistant to the phosphaturic effects of PTH.

Nutritional hypophosphatemia may be treated with P supplementation at 0.5–1.5 mmol/kg of elemental phosphorus per day (175). Calcium supplementation (see Sec. II.A) is useful because it may minimize the fall in serum Ca concentration during P treatment, and it would alleviate Ca deficiency, which also occurs frequently in these infants (2,175). Standard vitamin D supplementation of 400 IU/day is adequate therapy for vitamin D–deficient rickets in infancy (124,226). Therapy of nonnutritional hypophosphatemia is similar, in addition to treatment of the underlying disorder.

D. Hyperphosphatemia

An infant can be considered to be hyperphosphatemic when the serum P concentration is >2.6 mmol/L (conversion, 1 mmol/L = 3.1 mg/dl). This condition can have nutritional or nonnutritional causes (Table 6). Nutritional causes usually occur with the infusion of excessive P content (125) or an unusual combination of Ca and P delivered from parenteral nutrition solution (205). Ingestion of cows' milk–type formulas (9) and early introduction of high-P-containing cereals (177) may lead to neonatal hyperphosphatemia. Vitamin D toxicity may result in hyperphosphatemia, in addition to hypercalcemia (43), primarily because of increased intestinal absorption of Ca and P. Nonnutritional causes include perinatal asphyxia with release of intracellular P to the extracellular compartment, together with a low renal glomerular filtration. Hyerphosphatemia can occur during the first few days after delivery (8,166). Renal failure (33,43), usually from intrinsic renal failure, such as congenitally dysplastic kidneys, and hypoparathyroidism (208) may be associated with hyperphosphatemia. The use of P-containing enemas in early infancy has been reported to result in hyperphosphatemia and hypocalcemia (231).

Hyperphosphatemia may be asymptomatic, or it may be manifested because of its associated hypocalcemic effects (see

Table 6 Neonatal Hyperphosphatemia

Nutritional
  High P load from parenteral nutrition, cows' milk-type
    formula, cereals
  Hypervitaminosis D
Nonnutritional
  Perinatal asphyxia
  Renal failure
  Hypoparathyroidism
  Phosphate enema

Sec. II.A), except in the situation of hypervitaminosis D when hypercalcemia accompanies hyperphospatemia. Therapy consists of treatment of the underlying cause, for example eliminating or minimizing the P load with the use of "humanized" formulas with low P content and a "high" Ca/P ratio of about 2:1, and temporarily discontinuing the use of cereals. A brief period of Ca supplementation may be necessary if there is associated hypocalcemia.

III. REQUIREMENTS FOR CALCIUM AND PHOSPHORUS IN INFANTS

A. Enteral Requirements

The requirements for Ca and P in an infant vary with growth rate. They primarily concern the need to meet demands for bone mineralization and to maintain normal ranges of serum concentrations of these minerals. Calcium and P needs during the first 6 months after birth for an infant born at term may be met by the amount delivered from human milk. Human milk Ca content remains fairly stable during the first few months after delivery (232,233); the P content decreases by about 20% during the first 6 months of lactation (10). During the first 6 months after delivery, the estimated intake of a breast-fed infant is approximately 50–60 mg Ca and 28–32 mg P per kilogram each day, which is the recommended daily intake (234).

For preterm infants, the recommended daily intakes of Ca and P per unit body weight are higher (235,236) than those for term infants, and they are usually based on intrauterine accretion rates. The exact amount and duration of Ca and P required for preterm infants probably varies with gestational age and infant weight. The two reports that indicated success in matching postnatal changes in bone mineral content to "fetal" rates delivered total Ca intake of 210–250 mg/kg and total P intake of 112–125 mg/kg/day (237,238). The duration of Ca and P supplementation also may be important because a "conventional" 6-week period of Ca and P supplementation may fail to prevent the development of radiographic rickets in small preterm infants with birth weights of less than 1 kg (230). It now seems reasonable to recommend an intake of Ca and P that may match the intrauterine accretion of these minerals. Allowing for variability in Ca and P retention, an intake of up to 230 mg calcium and 140 mg phosphorus per kg per day may be needed to achieve Ca and P retention rates comparable to in utero accretion (235,236). This intake may be continued for 8–10 weeks or until the infant's body weight reaches 2–2.5 kg (i.e., near the time of discharge from hospital) and should meet the Ca and P needs of the small preterm infant. Phosphorus intake may need to be slightly more than half the amount of Ca intake to allow for P demand from soft tissue growth (see Sec. I.A).

For infants receiving human milk feeding, Ca and P supplementation may be attained by using Ca-and-P-fortified "preterm infant formulas" as a complement, powdered cows' milk–based fortifier for human milk (so-called human milk fortifier), or lyophilized human milk powdered as fortifier

(175). The latter is not freely available in North America. It should be pointed out that the major problem of bone demineralization and rickets, associated with Ca and P deficiency in preterm infants, occurs primarily in infants who are severely ill with multiple clinical complications (2,230). In such infants, there are practical difficulties in ingestion of intake to match intrauterine mineral accretion.

B. Parenteral Requirements

The goal of nutrient delivery to infants who cannot be fed enterally is to achieve growth rates of all tissues similar to those in infants fed normally. The technical difficulties in maintaining relatively large quantities of Ca and P in solution have led to a wide range of reported Ca (10–200 mg/kg/day) and P (9–109 mg/kg/day) intake from parenteral nutrition, with Ca/P ratios that have ranged from 4:1 to 1:8 (175).

Parenteral nutrition solutions with "high" content of 50–60 mg of Ca and 39–47 mg of P per dl (Ca/P ratio of 1:1 to 1.3:1 by molar ratio and 1.3:1 to 1.7:1 by weight) can result in a stable metabolic milieu, as indicated by normal and stable serum concentrations of $1,25(OH)_2D$ and normal and stable renal tubular reabsorption of P in preterm and term infants (125,126,236). These Ca and P contents were calculated to approximate the range of intake from human milk–fed term infants. In these studies, the calciuria generally associated with the use of parenteral nutrition solutions was not increased with the relatively high Ca and P contents in the intravenous solutions. However, higher contents of P may result in hyperphosphatemia and possibly hypocalcemia (175).

C. Calcium/Phosphorus Ratio

The Ca/P ratio varies widely in foods from a high of 2.8:1 (by weight) in green vegetables to a low of 0.06:1 in meat. The approximate ratio by weight for human milk is 2:1, for cows' milk it is 1.2:1, for commercial infant formula it is 1.3–1.5:1, and for commercial preterm infant formula it is 2:1 (175). In general, infants are remarkably tolerant of a wide range of Ca/P ratios in their diet.

Theoretically, a number of factors may influence the development of symptoms and signs in infants receiving varying dietary intakes of Ca and P: (1) the absolute quantity of Ca and P delivered in their diet: for example, a grossly "imbalanced" Ca/P ratio in a single food item (e.g., green leafy vegetable or meat), ingested in limited quantities, will have little impact on Ca and P homeostasis; (2) the maturity of intestinal absorption; and (3) the renal excretory system since the more mature infant theoretically will have greater capacity to excrete excess minerals and, thereby, minimize the disturbance to the body homeostasis. Human milk with its low P content and a Ca/P ratio of approximately 2:1 by weight appears most appropriate for Ca and P homeostasis, at least for term infants.

For the preterm infant, the ideal Ca/P ratio in the diet is unknown. There is a wide range of "optimal" Ca/P ratios to promote Ca and P retention. For example, in preterm infants receiving enteral feeding, Ca/P ratios of 2.0:1 to 3.8:1 (by weight) with an intake of 250 mg/kg Ca and 66–128 mg/kg P per day are reported to result in better Ca and P retention, compared with the Ca/P ratios of 1.4:1 or 2.6:1 (by weight) at a lower absolute Ca and P intake (239); in preterm infants receiving parenteral nutrition, a Ca/P ratio of 1.7:1 (by weight) with an intake of 76 mg/kg of Ca and 45 mg/kg of P per day is reported to result in better Ca and P retention than the use of Ca/P ratios of 1.3:1 or 2:1 (240). It is difficult to draw conclusions from these studies on the optimal Ca/P ratios, because the absolute amounts of either or both Ca and P content must be altered, sometimes to extreme levels to manipulate the Ca/P ratio. Furthermore, the difference in the amounts of Ca and P retained may reflect only the difference in the absolute quantities of intake, and the percentage of Ca and P retention compared with intake were similar within a range of Ca/P ratios tested (239,240). Nevertheless, a reverse Ca/P ratio of less than 1 or alternating Ca and P infusion to achieve greater intravenous delivery may result in marked disturbances of Ca and P homeostasis and should not be used (241). A parenteral nutrition infusate containing 60–80 mg of Ca and 47–62 mg of P per deciliter (Ca/P ratio 1.3:1 by weight or 1:1 by molar ratio) appears satisfactory for use in infants when used with caution. The lower content of Ca and P probably can be used for larger preterm and term infants and higher amounts for small preterm infants. Careful evaluation of serum Ca and P concentrations should be performed when these relatively high Ca and P content solutions are used. "Stepwise" increase in Ca and P content over the first few days of parenteral nutrition would minimize the potential risk of hypercalcemia and hyperphosphatemia and their sequelae (241,242).

ACKNOWLEDGMENT

The authors thank Ms. Nilda Barbieri for her assistance in preparing this manuscript.

REFERENCES

1. Parfitt AM, Kleerekoper M. The divalent ion homeostatic system-physiology and metabolism of calcium, phosphorus, magnesium and bone. In: Maxwell MH, Kleeman CR, eds. Clinical Disorders of Fluid and Electrolyte Metabolism, 3rd ed. New York: McGraw-Hill, 1980:269–398.
2. Koo WWK, Tsang R. Bone mineralization in infants. Prog Food Nutr Sci 1984; 8:229–302.
3. Sparks JW. Human intrauterine growth and nutrient accretion. Semin Perinatol 1984; 8:74–93.
4. Trotter M, Hixon BB. Sequential changes in weight, density, and percentage ash weight of human skeletons from an early fetal period through old age. Anat Rec 1974; 179:1–18.
5. Steichen JJ, Tsang RC, Gratton TL, Hamstra A, DeLuca HF. Vitamin D homestasis in the perinatal period 1,25-dihydrox-yvitamin D in maternal, cord and neonatal blood. N Engl J Med 1980; 302:315–319.
6. Pitkin RM, Cruikshank DP, Schauberger CW, Reynolds WA, Williams GA, Hargis GK. Fetal calcitropic hormones and neonatal calcium homeostasis. Pediatrics 1980; 66:77–82.
7. Venkataraman PS, Tsang RC, Chen IW, Sperling MA. Pathogenesis of early neonatal hypocalcemia: studies of serum calcitonin, gastrin, and plasma glucagon. J Pediatr 1987; 110:559–603.
8. Tsang RC, Oh W. Neonatal hypocalcemia in low birth weight infants. Pediatrics 1970; 45:773–781.
9. Snodgrass GJAI, Stemmler L, Went J, Abrams ME, Will EJ. Interrelations of plasma calcium, inorganic phosphate, magnesium and protein over the first week of life. Arch Dis Child 1973; 48:279–285.
10. Greer FR, Tsang RC, Levin RS, Searcy JE, Wu R, Steichen JJ. Increasing serum calcium and magnesium concentrations in breast fed infants: longitudinal studies of minerals of human milk and in sera of nursing mothers and their infants. J Pediatr 1982; 100:59–64.
11. Specker BL, Lichtenstein P, Mimouni F, Gormley C, Tsang RC. Calcium regulating hormones and minerals from birth to 18 months: a cross sectional study. II. Effects of sex, race, age, season and diet on serum minerals, parathyroid hormone, and calcitonin. Pediatrics 1986; 77:891–896.
12. Markowitz M, Rotkin L, Rosen JR. Circadian rhythm of blood minerals in humans. Science 1981; 213:672–674.
13. Pitkin RM. Calcium metabolism in pregnancy and perinatal period: a review. Am J Obstet Gynecol 1985; 151:99–109.
14. Loughead JL, Mimouni F, Tsang RC. Serum ionized calcium concentrations in normal neonates. Am J Dis Child 1988; 142:516–518.
15. Mimouni A, Mimouni F, Mimouni C, Mou S, Ho M. Effects of albumin on ionized calcium in vitro. Pediatr Emerg Care 1991; 7:149–151.
16. Lehmann M, Mimouni F, Tsang R. Effect of phosphate concentration on ionized calcium concentration in vitro. Am J Dis Child 1989; 143:1340–1341.
17. Liu C, Mimouni F, Ho M, Tsang R. In vitro effect of magnesium on ionized calcium concentration in serum. Am J Dis Child 1988; 142:837–838.
18. Forman D, Lorenzo L. Ionized calcium: its significance and clinical usefulness. Ann Clin Lab Sci 1991; 21:297–304.
19. Wandrup J, Kancir C, Norgaard-Pederson B. The concentration of free calcium ions in capillary blood from neonates on a routine basis using the ICA1. Scand J Clin Lab Invest 1984; 44:19–24.
20. Bowers GN, Jr., Brassard C, Sena SF. Measurement of ionized calcium in serum with ion selective electrodes: a mature technology that can meet the daily service needs. Clin Chem 1986; 32:1437–1447.
21. Saggese S, Baroncelli G, Bertelloni S, Cipolloni C. Intact parathyroid hormone levels during pregnancy, in healthy term neonates and in hypocalcemic preterm infants. Acta Pediatr Scand 1991; 80:36–41.
22. Rasmussen H. The calcium messenger system. N Engl J Med 1986; 314:1094–1101, 1164–1170.
23. Meites S. Pediatric Clinical Chemistry. A Survey of Normals, Methods, and Instrumentation, with Commentary, 1st ed. Washington, DC: American Association for Clinical Chemistry, 1977:176–177.
24. Annino JS, Relman AS. The effect of eating on some of the clinically important chemical constituents of blood. Am J Clin Pathol 1959; 31:155–159.
25. Baldwin D, Robinson PK, Zierler KL, Lilenthal JL. Jr. Interrelations of magnesium, potassium, phosphorus, and creatine in skeletal muscle of man. J Clin Invest 1952; 31:850–858.
26. Kemper B. Molecular biology of parathyroid hormone. CRC Crit Rev Biochem 1986; 19:353–379.
27. Burtis WJ: Parathyroid hormone-related protein: structure, function, and measurement. Clin Chem 1992; 38:2171–2183.

28. Bilezikian JP: Clinical utility of assays for parathyroid hormone-related protein. Clin Chem 1992; 38:179–181.

29. Kronenberg HM, Igarashi T, Freeman MW, Okazaki T, Brand SJ, Wiren KM, Potts JT. Jr. Structure and expression of the human parathyroid hormone gene. Recent Prog Horm Res 1986; 42:641–663.

30. Meyers DA, Beaty TH, Maestri NE, Kittur SD, Antonarakis SE, Kazazian HH. Jr. Multipoint mapping studies of six loci on chromosome 11. Hum Hered 1987; 37:94–101.

31. Wiren KM, Freeman MW, Potts JT, Kronenberg HM. Preproparathyroid hormone. A model for analyzing the secretory pathway. Ann NY Acad Sci 1987; 493:43–49.

32. Cohn DV, Kumarasamy R, Kemp WK. Intracellular processing and secretion of parathyroid gland proteins. Vitam Horm 1986; 43:283–316.

33. Klahr S, Slatopolsky E. Toxicity of parathyroid hormone in uremia. Annu Rev Med 1986; 37:71–78.

34. Armitage EK. Parathyrin (parathyroid hormone): metabolism and methods of assay. Clin Chem 1986; 32:418–424.

35. Robinson MF, Body JJ, Offord KP, Heath H III. Variation of plasma immunocreactive parathyroid hormone and calcitonin in normal and hyperparathyroid man during daylight hours. J Clin Endocrinol Metab 1982; 55:538–544.

36. MacGregor RR, Jilka RL, Hamilton JW. Formation and secretion of fragments of parathormone. Identification of cleavage sites. J Biol Chem 1986; 261:1929–1934.

37. Balabanova S, Modinger C, Wolf AS, Teller WM. Degradation of parathyroid hormone by placental homogenate. Acta Obstet Gynecol Scand 1986; 65:775–777.

38. David L, Salle BL, Putet G, Grafmeyer DC. Serum immunoreactive calcitonin in low birth weight infants. Description of early changes; effect of intravenous calcium infusion; relationship's with early changes in serum calcium, phosphorus, magnesium, parathyroid hormone and gastrin levels. Pediatr Res 1981; 15:803–808.

39. Rubin L, Posillico J, Anast C, Brown E: Circulating levels of biologically active and immunoreactive intact parathyroid hormone in human neonates. Pediatr Res 1991; 29:201–207.

40. Hillman LS, Forte LR, Veum T, et al: Effect of parathyoid hormone-related peptide supplementation of soy protein formulas in the neonatal pig model. J Bone Miner Res 1994; 9:1047–1052.

41. Scarpace PJ, Armbrecht HJ. Adenylate cyclase in senescence: catecholamine and parathyroid hormone pathways. Rev Clin Basic Pharm 1987; 6:105–118.

42. Balabanova S, Lang T, Wolfe AS, et al. Placental transfer of parathyroid hormone. J Perinat Med 1986; 14:243–250.

43. Koo WWK, Tsang RC. Calcium and magnesium metabolism. In: Werner M, ed. CRC Handbook of Clinical Chemistry, Vol. 4. Orlando FL: CRC Press, 1989:51–91.

44. Nemere I, Norman AW. Parathyroid hormone stimulates calcium transport in perfused duodena of normal chicks: comparison with the rapid effect of 1,25-dihydroxyvitamin D_3. Endocrinology 1986; 199:1406–1408.

45. Tam CS, Heersche JNM, Murray TM, Parsons JA. Parathyroid hormone stimulates the bone apposition rate independently of its resorptive action: differential effects of intermittent and continuous administration. Endocrinology 1982; 110:506–512.

46. Brennan DP, Levine MA. Characterization of soluble and particulate parathyroid hormone receptors using a biotinylated bioactive hormone analog. J Biol Chem 1987; 262:14795–14800.

47. Teitelbaum AP, Silve CM, Nyiredy KO, Arnaud CD. Down regulation of parathyroid hormone (PTH) receptors in cultured bone cells is associated with agoinist specific intracellular

processing of PTH receptor complexes. Endocrinology 1986; 118:595–602.

48. Juppner H, Abou-Samra A-B, Freeman M, et al. A G protein-linked receptor for parathyroid hormone and parathyroid hormone-related peptide. Science 1991; 254:1024–1026.

49. Rasmussen H, Kojima I, Apfeldorf W, Barrett P. Cellular mechanism of hormone action in the kidney: messenger function of calcium and cyclic AMP. Kidney Int 1986; 29:90–97.

50. Lee DB, Welling MW, Palant CE, Tallos E. Jejunal phosphate transport is not regulated by PTH adenylate cyslase system. Further studies on the contrasting features between intestinal and renal phosphate transport mechanisms. Miner Electrolyte Metab 1986; 12:293–297.

51. Broadus AE. Nephrogenous cyclic AMP. Recent Prog Horm Res 1981; 37:667–701.

52. Brown E, Gamba G, Riccardi D, et al. Cloning and characterization of an extracellular Ca^{2+} sensing receptor from bovine parathyroid, Nature 1993; 366:575–580.

53. Pollak M, Brown E, Chou Y, et al. Mutations in the human Ca^{2+}, sensing receptor gene cause familial hypercalciuric hypercalcemia and neonatal severe hyperparathyroidism. Call 1993; 75:1297–1303.

54. Paunier L. Effect of magnesium on phosphorus and calcium metabolism. Monatsschr. Kinderheilkd 1992; 140 (Suppl): S17–S20.

55. Silver J, Naveh-Many T, Mayer H, Schmelzer HJ, Popovtzer MM. Regulation by vitamin D metabolites of parathyroid hormone gene transcription in vivo in the rat. J Clin Invest 1986; 78:1296–1301.

56. Cantley LK, Russell JB, Lettieri DS, Sherwood LM. Effects of vitamin D_3, 25-hydroxyvitamin D_3 and 24, 25-dihydroxyvitamin D_3 on parathyroid hormone secretion. Calcif Tissue Int 1987; 41:48–51.

57. Dewhirst FE, Ago JM, Peros WJ, Stashenko P. Synergism between parathyroid hormone and interleukin I in stimulating bone resorption in organ culture. J Bone Miner Res 1987; 2:127–134.

58. Greenberg C, Kukreja SC, Bowser EN, Hargis GK, Henderson WJ, Williams GA. Parathyroid hormone secretion. Effect of estradiol and progesterone. Metabolism 1987; 36:151–154.

59. Birnbaum RS, Mahoney W, Roos BA. Purification and amino acid sequence of a noncalcitonin secretory peptide derived from preprocalcitonin. J Biol Chem 1983; 258:5463–5466.

60. Fischer JA, Born W. Novel peptides from the calcitonin gene: expression, receptors and biological function. Peptides 1985; 6(Suppl 3):265–271.

61. Goodman EC, Iversen LL. Calcitonin gene-related peptide: novel neuropeptide. Life Sci 1987; 38:2169–2178.

62. Steenbergh PH, Hoppener JW, Zandberg J, Visser A, Lips CJ, Jansz HS. Structure and expression of the human calcitonin/CGRP genes. FEBS Lett 1986; 209:97–103.

63. Todds S, Yoshida MC, Fang XE, et al. Genes for insulin I and II, parathyroid hormone, and calcitonin are on rat chromosome I. Biochem Biophys Res Commun 1985; 131:1175–1180.

64. Lalley PA, Sokaguchi AY, Eddy RL. Mapping polypeptide hormone genes in the mouse: somatostatin, glucagon, calcitonin, parathyroid hormone. Cytogenet Cell Genet 1987; 44:92–97.

65. Gkonos PJ, Born W, Jones BN, et al. Biosynthesis of calcitonin gene related peptide and calcitonin by a human medullary thyroid carcinoma cell line. J Biol Chem 1986; 261:14386–14391.

66. Bucht E, Telenius-Berg M, Lundell G, Sjoberg HE. Immunoextracted calcitonin in milk and plasma from totally thyroid-

ectomized women. Evidence of monomeric calcitonin in plasma during pregnancy and lactation. Acta Endocrinol 1986; 113:529–535.

67. Jansen I, Uddman R, Hocherman M, et al. Localization and effects of neuropeptide Y, vasoactive intestinal polypeptide, substance P, and calcitonin gene-related peptide in human temporal arteries. Ann Neurol 1986; 20:496–501.

68. Zabel M, Biela-Jacek I. Surdyk J, Dietel M. Studies on localization of calcitonin gene-related peptide (CGRP) in the thyroid-parathyroid complex. Virchows Arch 1987; 411:569–573.

69. Nakamuta H, Fukuda Y, Koida M, et al. Binding sites of calcitonin gene related peptide (CGRP): abundant occurence in visceral organs. Jpn J Pharmacol 1986; 42:175–180.

70. Wolfe HJ, DeLellis RA, Volkel EF, Tashjan AH. Distribution of calcitonin-containing cells in the normal neonatal human thyroid gland: a correlation of morphology with peptide content. J Clin Endocrinol Metab 1975; 41:1076–1081.

71. Nitta K, Kito S, Kubota Y, et al. Ontogeny of calcitonin gene-related peptide and calcitonin in the rat thyroid. Histochemistry 1986; 84:139–143.

72. Trasforini G, Margutti A, Portaluppi F, Menegatti M, et al. Circadian profile of plasma calcitonin gene-related peptide in healthy man. J Clin Endocrinol Metab 1991; 73:945–951.

73. Roos BA, Fischer JA, Pignat W, Alander CB, Raisz LG. Evaluation of the in vivo and in vitro calcium regulating actions of non calcitonin peptides produced via calcitonin gene expression. Endocrinology 1986; 118:46–51.

74. Austin LA. Health H III. Calcitonin, physiology and pathophysiology N Engl J Med 1981; 304:269–278.

75. New HV, Mudge AW. Calcitonin gene-related peptide regulates muscle acetycholine receptor synthesis. Nature 1986; 323:809–811.

76. Zhou ZC, Villanueva ML, Noguchi M, Jones SW, Gardner JD, Jensen RT. Mechanism of action calcitonin gene-related peptide in stimulating pancreatic enzyme secretion. Am J Physiol 1986; 233:G391–397.

77. Gharib H, Kao PC, Health H III. Determination of silica purified plasma calcitonin for the detection and management of medullary thyroid carcinoma: comparison of two provocative tests. Mayo Clin Proc 1987; 62:373–378.

78. Garel JM,, Besnard P, Rebut-Bonneton C. C cell activity during the prenatal and postnatal periods in the rat. Endocrinology 1981; 109:1573–1577.

79. Balabanova S, Kruse B, Wolfe AS. Calcitonin secretion by human placental tissue. Acta Obstet Gynecol Scand 1987; 66:323–326.

80. Mimouni F, Loughead J, Tsang R, Khoury J. Postnatal surge in serum calcitonin concentrations: no contribution to neonatal hypocalcemia in infants of diabetic mothers. Pediatr Res 1990; 28:493–495.

81. Hillman LA, Hoff N, Walgate J, Haddad JG. Serum calcitonin concentrations in premature infants during the first 12 weeks of life. Calcif Tissue Int 1982; 34:470–473.

82. Tiegs RD, Body JJ, Barta JM, Health H III. Secretion and metabolism of monomeric human calcitonin: effects of age, sex and thyroid damage. J Bone Miner Res 1986; 1:339–349.

83. Hirsch PF, Hagaman JR. Feeding regimen, dietary calcium, and the diurnal rhythms of serum calcium and calcitonin in the rat. Endocrinology 1982; 110:961–968.

84. Huwyler R, Born W, Ohnhaus EE, Fischer JA. Plasma kinetics and urinary excretion of exogenous human and salmon calcitonin in man. Am J Physiol 1979; 236:E15–19.

85. Burke BA, Johnson D, Gilbert EF, Drut RM, Ludwig J, Wick MR. Thyrocalcitonin containing cells in the DiGeorge anomaly. Hum Pathol 1987; 19:355–360.

86. Kawashima H, Torikai S, Kurokawa K. Calcitonin selectively stimulates 25-hydroxyvitamin D_3-1α-hydroxylase in the proximal straight tubule of rat kidney. Nature 1981; 291:327–329.

87. Nicosia S, Guidobono F, Musanti M, Pecile A. Inhibitory effects of calcitonin on adenylate cyclase activity in different rat brain areas. Life Sci 1986; 39:2253–2262.

88. Lin HY, Harris TL, Flannery MS, et al. Expression cloning of an adenylate cyclase-coupled calcitonin receptor. Science 1991; 254:1022–1024.

89. Naveh-Many T, Raue F, Grauer A, Silver J. Regulation of calcitonin gene expression by hypocalcemia, hypercalcemia, and vitamin D in the rat. J Bone Miner Res 1992; 7:1233–1237.

90. deBustros A, Baylin SB, Levine MA, Nelkin BD. Cyclic AMP and phorbol esters separately induce growth inhibition, calcitonin secretion, and calcitonin gene transcription in cultured human medullary thyroid carcinoma. J Biol Chem 1986; 261:8036–8041.

91. Gottfried H, Mamikunian G, Falkmer S, Emdin SO, Landaw E, Dadourian B. Structural analysis of the molecular evolution of some gastro-entero-pancreatic hormones. Acta Paediatr Scand 1977; 270(Suppl)26–36.

92. DeLuca HF. The metabolism and functions of vitamin D. Adv Exp Med Biol 1986; 196:361–375.

93. Holick MF. The cutaneous photosynthesis of previtamin D_3: a unique photo-endocrine system. J Invest Dermatol 1981; 77:51–58.

94. Blomhoff R, Helgerud P, Dveland S, Berg T, Pedersen JI. Lymphatic absorption and transport of retinol and vitamin D_3 from rat intestine: evidence of different pathways. Biochim Biophys Acta 1984; 772:109–116.

95. Dueland S, Peterson JJ, Helgerud P, Drevon CA. Transport of vitamin D_3 from rat intestine: evidence for transfer of vitamin D_3 from chylomicrons to α-globulins. J Biol Chem 1982; 257:146–150.

96. Yoon PS, DeLuca HF. Resolution and reconstitution of soluble component of rat liver microsomal vitamin D_3-25-hydroxylase. Arch Biochem Biophys 1980; 203:529–541.

97. Bell NH, Shaw S, Turner RT. Evidence that 1,25-dihydroxyvitamin D_3 inhibits the hepatic production of 25-hydroxyvitamin D in man. J Clin Invest 1984; 74:1540–1544.

98. Lufkin EG, Kumar R, Heath H III. Hyperphosphatemic tumoral calcinosis: effects of phosphate depletion on vitamin D metabolism and of acute hypocalcemia on parathyroid secretion and action. J Clin Endocrinol Metab 1983; 56:1319–1322.

99. Van Der Berg CJ, Kumar R, Wilson DM, Heath H III, Smith LH. Orthophosphate therapy decreases urinary calcium excretion and serum 1,25-dihydroxyvitamin D concentrations in idiopathic hypercalciuria. J Clin Endocrinol Metab 1980; 51:998–1001.

100. Kawashima H, Kurokawa K. Metabolism and sites of action of vitamin D in the kidney. Kidney Int 1986; 29:98–107.

101. Henry HL, Lunato EM, Dutta CD, Cunningham NS, Kain SR. Current models for studying the regulation of 250HD3 metabolism. In: Norman AW, Schaefer K, Grigolait HG, Herrath DV, eds. Vitamin D: Molecular, Cellular and Clinical Endocrinology. Berlin: Walter de Gruyter, 1988:157–165.

102. Markestad T, Hesse V, Siebenhuner M, et al. Intermittent high dose vitamin D prophylaxis during infancy: effect on vitamin D metabolites, calcium and phosphorus. Am J Clin Nutr 1987; 46:652–658.

103. Stern PH, De Olazabal J, Bell NH. Evidence for abnormal regulation of circulating 1α 25-dihydroxyvitamin D in patients with sarcoidosis and normal calcium metabolism. J Clin Invest 1980; 66:852–855.

104. Merke J, Ritz E, Boland R. Are recent findings on 1,25-dihydroxycholecalciferol metabolism relevant for the pathogenesis of uremia? Nephron 1986; 42:277–284.

105. Stanbury SW, Mawer EB, Taylor CM, DeSilva P. The skin, vitamin D and the control of its 25-hydroxylation: an attempted intergration. Miner Electrolyte Metab 1980; 3:51–60.

106. Seeman E, Kumar R, Hunder GG, Scott M, Health H III, Riggs BL. Production, degradation and circulating levels of 1,25-dihydroxyvitamin D in health and in chronic glucocorticoid excess J Clin Invest 1980; 66:664–666.

107. Reddy GS, Tserng KY. Isloation of 23-carboxyltetranorvitamin D₃. A renal metabolite of 250HD₃. Proceedings 7th Workshop on Vitamin D. 1988:28.

108. Reddy GS, Tserng KY, Thomas BR, Dayal R, Norman AW. Isolation and identification of 1,23-dihydroxy-24,25,26,27-tetranorvitamin D₃, a new metabolite of 1,25-dihydroxyvitamin D₃ produced in rat kidney. Biochemistry 1987; 26:324–331.

109. Kumar R. Hepatic and intestinal osteodystrophy and the hepatobiliary metabolism of vitamin D. Ann Intern Med 1983; 98:662–663.

110. Clements MR, Chalmers TM, Fraser DR, Enterohepatic circulation of vitamin D: a reappraisal of the hypothesis. Lancet 1984; 1:1376–1379.

111. Haddad JG. Nature and functions of the plasma binding proteins for vitamin D and its metabolites. In: Kumar R, ed. Vitamin D: Basic and Clinical Aspects. Boston: Martinus Nijhoff, 1984:383–396.

112. Bikle DD, Siiteri PK, Ryzen E. Haddad JG, Gee E. Serum protein binding of 1,25-dihydroxyvitamin D: a reevaluation by direct measurement of free metabolite levels. J Clin Endocrinol Metab 1985; 61:969–975.

113. Cooke NE, David EV. Serum vitamin D binding protein in a third member of the albumin and alpha-fetoprotein gene family. J Clin Invest 1985; 76:2420–2426.

114. Revelle L, Solan V, Londowski J, Bollman S, Kumar R. The synthesis and biologic activity of a C-ring analog of vitamin D₃: biologic and protein binding propertites of 1α hydroxyvitamin D₃. Biochemistry 1984; 23:1981–1987.

115. Dueland S, Blomhoff R, Pedersen JI. Uptake and degradation of vitamin D binding protein-actin complex in vivo in the rat. Proceedings 7th Workshop on Vitamin D. 1988:163.

116. Hollis BW. Comparison of equilibrium and disequilibrium assay conditions for ergocalciferol, cholecalciferol and their major metabolities. J Steroid Biochem 1984; 21:81–86.

117. Jongen MJM, Van Ginkel FC, van der Vijgh WJF, Kuiper S, Netelenbos JC, Lips P. An international comparison of vitamin D metabolite measurements. Clin Chem 1984; 30: 399–403.

118. Hollis BW, Pittard WB III. Evaluation of the total fetomaternal vitamin D relationship at term: evidence for racial differences. J Clin Endocrinol Metab 1984; 59:652–657.

119. Greer FR, Hollis BW, Napoli JL. High concentrations of vitamin D₂ in human milk associated with pharmacologic doses of vitamin D₂. J Pediatr 1984; 105:61–64.

120. Ron M, Levitz M, Chuba J, Davies J. Transfer of 25-hydroxyvitamin D₃ and 1,25-dihydroxyvitamin D₃ across the perfused human placenta. Am J Obstet Gynecol 1984; 148: 370–374.

121. Marx SJ, Swart EG Jr, Hamstra AJ, DeLuca HF. Normal intrauterine development of the fetus of a woman receiving extraordinarily high doses of 1,25-dihydroxyvitamin D₃. J Clin Endocrinol Metab 1980; 51:1138–1142.

122. Verity CM, Burman D, Beadle PC, Holton JB, Morris A. Seasonal changes in perinatal vitamin D metabolism: maternal and cord blood biochemistry in normal pregnancies. Arch Dis Child 1981; 56:943–948.

123. Nehama H, Weintroub S, Eisenberg Z, Birger A, Milbauer B, Weisman Y. Seasonal variation in paired maternal newborn serum 25 hydroxyvitamin D and 24, 25 dihydroxyvitamin D concentrations in Israel. Isr J Med Sci 1987; 23:274–277.

124. Specker BL, Greer F, Tsang RC. Vitamin D. In: Tsang RC, Nichols BL, eds. Nutrition During Infancy. Philadelphia: Hanley and Belfus, 1988:264–276.

125. Koo WWK, Tsang RC, Steichen JJ, et al. Parenteral nutrition for infants: effect of high versus low calcium and phosphorus content. J Pediatr Gastroenterol Nutr 1987; 6:96–104.

126. Koo WWK, Tsang RC, Succop P, Krug-Wispe SK, Babcock D, Oestreich AE, Minimal vitamin D and high calcium and phosphorus needs of preterm infants receiving parenteral nutrition. J Pediatr Gastroenterol Nutr 1989; 8:225–233.

127. Lichtenstein P, Specker BL, Tsang RC. Mimouni F, Gormley C. Calcium regulating hormones and minerals from birth to 18 months of age: A cross-sectional study. I. Effects of sex, race, age, season and diet on vitamin D status. Pediatrics 1986; 77:883–890.

128. Chesney RW, Rosen JF, Hamstra AJ, Smith C, Mahaffey L, DeLuca HG. Absence of seasonal variation in serum concentrations of 1,25-dihydroxyvitamin D despite a rise in 25-hydroxyvitamin D in summer. J Clin Endocrinol Metab 1981; 53:139–142.

129. Specker B, Tsang R, Hollis B. Effect of race and diet on human milk vitamin D and 25 hydroxyvitamin D. Am J Dis Child 1985; 139:1134–1137.

130. Specker B, Valanis B, Hertzberg V, Edwards N, Tsang R. Sunshine exposure and serum 25. Hydroxyvitamin D concentrations in exclusively breast fed infants. J Pediatr 1985; 107:372–376.

131. Halloran BP, Portale AA, Castro M, Morris RC Jr., Goldsmith RS. Serum concentrations of 1,25-dihydroxyvitamin D in the human: diurnal variation. J Clin Endocrinol Metab 1985; 60:1104–1110.

132. Tsai KS, Heath H III. Kumar R, Riggs BL. Impaired vitamin D metabolism with aging in women: possible role in pathogenesis of senile osteoporosis. J Clin Invest 1984; 73:1668–1672.

133. Bouillon RA, Auwerx JH, Lissens WD, Pelemans WK. Vitamin D status in the elderly: seasonal substrate deficiency causes 1,25-dihydroxycholecalciferol deficiency. Am J Clin Nutr 1987; 45:755–763.

134. Pike JW, Haussler MS. Association of 1,25-dihydroxvitamin D₃ with cultured 3T6 mouse fibroblasts: cellular uptake and receptor-mediated migration to the nucleus. J Biol Chem 1983; 259:8554–8560.

135. Szpirer J, Szpirer RC, Riviere M, et al. The SP 1 transcription factor gene (SP1) and the 1,25 dihydroxyvitamin D₃ receptor gene (VDR) are colocalized on human chromosome arm 12q and rat chromosome 7. Genomics 1991; 11:168–173.

136. Labuda M, Ross M, Fujiwara T, et al. Two hereditary defects related to vitamin D metabolism map to the same region of human chromosome 12q (abstract). Cytogenet Cell Genet 1991; 58:1978.

137. Haussler MR. Vitamin D hormone receptors: structure, regulation and molecular function. Proceedings 7th Workshop on Vitamin D. 1988:45.

138. Pike JW. Structure and function of vitamin D receptors. Proceeding 7th Workshop on Vitamin D. 1988:45.

139. Horst RL, Reinhardt TA. Changes in intestinal, 1,25-dihydroxyvitamin D receptor during aging, gestation and pregnancy in rats. Proceedings 7th Workshop on Vitamin D. 1988:47.

140. Haussler MR. Vitamin D receptor: nature and function. Annu Rev Nutr 1986; 6:527–562.

141. Bronner F. Current concepts of calcium absorption: an overview. J Nutr 1992; 122:641–643.

142. Lucas PA, Ben Nasr L, Monet JD, Drueke T. Stimulation of rat duodenum activity within 10 minutes of in vivo calcitriol administration. Proceedings 7th Workshop on Vitamin D. 1988:90.

143. Nemere I, Norman AW. The rapid, hormonally stimulated transport of calcium (transcaltachia). J Bone Miner Res. 1987; 2:167–169.

144. Davie M. Calcium-ion-binding activity in human small-intestinal mucosal cytosol: purification of two proteins and interrelationship of calcium fractions. Biochem J 1981; 197:55–61.

145. Staun M, Noren O, Sjostrom H. Ca^{2+} binding from human kidney: purification and properties. Biochem J 1984; 217:229–237.

146. Thomasset M, Parkes CO, Cuisinier-Gleizes P. Rat calcium-binding proteins: distribution, development and vitamin D dependence. Am J Physiol 1982; 243:E483–E488.

147. Dechesne CJ, Brehier A, Thomasett M, Sans A. Calbindin-D 28K (CaBP 28K) localization in the peripheral vestibular system of various vertebrates and comparison with its distribution during development of the mouse and man. Proceedings 7th Workshop on Vitamin D. 1988:120.

148. Gross MD, Nelsestuen G, Sykes B, Kumar R. Nuclear magnetic resonance and terbium fluorescence studies on the vitamin D dependent 28 kilodalton chick intestinal calcium binding protein: evidence for calcium dependent conformational charges. Proceedings 7th Workshop on Vitamin D. 1988:118.

149. Bendik I, Hunziker W. The human calbindin D28 gene. Proceedings 7th Workshop on vitamin D. 1988:118.

150. Mifflin TE, Pearson WR, Reinhart J, Bruns DE, Bruns ME. Molecular cloning and sequencing of calbindin-D_{9K} cDNA from mouse placenta. Proceedings 7th Workshop on Vitamin D. 1988:109.

151. Ebeling PR. Evidence of an age related decrease in intestinal responsiveness to vitamin D: relationship between serum 1,25 dihydroxy vitamin D_3 and intestinal vitamin D receptor concentrations in normal women. J Clin Endocrinol Metab 1992; 75:176–182.

152. Armbrecht HJ, Bolz M, Strong R, Bruns MEH, Christakos S. Expression of calbindin D decreases with age in intestine and kidney. Proceedings 7th Workshop on Vitamin D. 1988:116.

153. Christakos S, Pike JW, Huang YC. Modulation of rat calbin-din-D_{28K} and 1,25(OH)$_2$$D_3$ receptor gene expression by 1,25(OH)$_2$$D_3$ and dietary alteration. Proceedings 7th Workshop on Vitamin D. 1988:109.

154. Ghishan FK, Arab N. Phosphate transport by intestinal endoplasmic reticulum during maturation. Pediatr Res 1988; 23:612–615.

155. Senterre J, Salle B. Calcium and phosphorus ecomony of the preterm infant and its interaction with vitamin D and its metabolites. Acta Paediatr Scand 1982; 296(Suppl):85–92.

156. Aloia JF, Yeh JK. Phosphate transport in the intestine of rats during early development: role of viamin D. Proceedings 7th Workshop on Vitamin D. 1988:129.

157. Yamamoto M, Kawanobe Y, Takahashi H, Shimazawa E, Kimura S, Ogata E. Vitamin D deficiency and renal calcium transport in the rat. J Clin Invest 1984; 74:507–513.

158. Edelman A, Thil CL, Garabedian M, Anagnostopoulos T, Balsam S. Genome independent effects of 1,25-dihydroxyvit-amin D_3 on membrane potential. Biochim Biophys Acta 1983; 732:300–303.

159. Kurnik BR, Hruska KA. Effects of 1,25-dihydroxycholecal-ciferol on phosphate transport in vitamin D-deprived rats. Am J Physiol 1984; 247:F177–182.

160. Kurnik BRC, Hruska KA. Mechanism of stimulation of renal phosphate transport by 1,25-dihydroxycholecalciferol. Biochim Biophys Acta 1985; 817:42–50.

161. Venkataraman PS, Wilson DA. Sheldon RE, Rao R, Parker MK. Effect of hypocalcemia on cardiac function in very low birth weight preterm neonates: studies of blood ionized calcium, echocardiography, and cardiac effect of intravenous calcium therapy. Pediatrics 1985; 76:543–550.

162. Tsang RC, Steichen JJ, Chan GM. Neonatal hypocalcemia Mechanism of occurrence and management. Crit Care Med 1977; 5:56–61.

163. Koo WWK, Tsang RC. Calcium and magnesium homeotasis in the newborn. In: Avery GB ed. Neonatology—Pathophysiology and Management of the Newborn, 3rd ed. Philadelphia: JB Lippincot, 1987:710–723.

164. Venkataraman PS, Tsang RC, Steichen JJ. Early Neonatal hypocalcemia in extremely preterm infants: high incidence, early onset, and refractoriness to supraphysiologic dose of calcitrol. Am J Dis Child 1986; 140:1004–1008.

165. Hanukoglu A, Chalew S, Kowardski AA. Late onset hypocalcemia, rickets and hypoparathyroidism in an infant of a mother with hyperparathyroidism. J Pediatr 1988; 112:751–754.

166. Tsang RC, Chen I, Hayes W, Atkinson W, Atherton H, Edwards N. Neonatal hypocalcemia in infants with birth asphyxia. J Pediatr 1974; 84:428–433.

167. Mimouni F, Tsang RC, Hertzberg VS, Miodovnik M. Polycythemia, hypomagnesemia and hypocalcemia in infants of diabetic mothers. Am J Dis Child 1986; 140:798–800.

168. Namgung R, Tsang R, Specker B, Sierra R, Ho M. Reduced serum osteocalcin and 1,25 dihydroxyvitamin D concentrations and low bone mineral content in small for gestational age infants: evidence of decreased bone formation rates. J Pediatr 1993; 122:269–275.

169. Barr DGD, Prader A, Esper U, Rampini S, Marrian VJ, Forfar JO. Chronic hypoparathyroidism in two generations. Helv Paediatr Acta 1971; 26:507–521.

170. Conley ME, Beckwith JB, Mancer JFK, Tenckoff L. The spectrum of the DiGeorge syndrome. J Pediatr 1979; 94:883–890.

171. Bainbridge R, Mughal Z, Mimouni F, Tsang RC. Transient congential hypoparathyroidism: how transient is it? J Pediatr 1988; 111:866–868.

172. Paul E, Fleischman A, Greig F, Saenger P. Transient congenital hypoparathyroidism: resolution and recurrence. Pediatr Res 1994; 35:206A.

173. Kooh S, Binet A. Partial hypoparathyroidism. A variant of transient congenital hypoparathyroidism. Am J Dis Child 1991; 145:877–880.

174. Mimouni F, Mimouni C, Loughead J, Tsang R. A case control study of hypocalcemia in high risk neonates: racial, but no seasonal differences. J Am Coll Nutr 1991; 10:196–199.

175. Koo WWK, Tsang RC. Calcium, magnesium and phosphorus. In: Tsang RC, Nichols BL, eds. Nutrition in Infancy. Philadelphia: Hanley and Belfus, 1988:175–189.

176. Hillman LS, Tack E, Covell DG, Vieira NE, Yergey AL. Measurement of true calcium absorption in premature infants using intravenous [46]Ca and oral [44]Ca. Pediatr Res 1988; 23:589–594.

177. Pierson JD, Crawford JD. Dietary dependent neonatal hypocalcemia. Am J Dis Child 1972; 123:472–474.

178. Specker B, Tsang R, Ho M, Landi T, Gratton T. Low serum calcium and high parathyroid hormone levels in neonates fed humanized cow's milk-based formula. Am J Dis Child 1991; 145:941–945.

179. Watney PJM, Chance GW, Scott P, Thompson JM. Maternal

factors in neonatal hypocalcemia: a study in three ethnic groups. Br Med J 1971; 2:432–436.

180. Rodder S, Mize C, Forman L, Uauy R. Effects of increased dietary phosphorus on magnesium balance in very low birthweight babies. Magnes Res 1992; 5:273–275.

181. Dincsoy MY, Tsang RC, Laskarzewski P, et al. The role of postnatal age and magnesium on parathyroid hormone responses during "exchange" blood transfusion in the newborn period. J Pediatr 1982; 100:277–283.

182. Driscoll D, Salvin J, Sellinger B, et al. Prevalence of 22q 11 microdeletions in DiGeorge and velocardiofacial syndromes: implications for genetic counselling and prenatal diagnosis. J Med Genet 1993; 30:813–817.

183. Salle BL, David L, Chopard JP, Grafmeyer DC, Renand H. Prevention of early neonatal hypocalcemia in low birth weight infants with continuous calcium infusion. Effect on serum calcium, phosphorus, magnesium and circulating immunoreactive parathyroid hormone and calcitonin. Pediatr Res 1977; 11:1180–1185.

184. Dincsoy MY, Tsang RC, Laskarzewski P, Ho M, et al. Serum calcitonin response to administration of calcium in newborn infants during exchange blood transfusion. J. Pediatr 1982; 100:782–786.

185. Ravid A, et al. Mononuclear cells from human neonates are partially resistant to the action of 1,25 dihydroxyvitamin D. J Clin Endocrinol Metab 1988; 67:755–759.

186. Whitsett J, Tsang RC. In vitro effects of fatty acids on serum ionized calcium. J Pediatr 1977; 91:233–236.

187. Harrison HE. Tetany. In: Behrman R, Vaughan VC, eds. Nelson Textbook of Pediatrics, 12th ed. Philadelphia: WB Saunders, 1983:249–250.

188. Oleske JM. Experience with 118 infants born to narcotic-using mothers. Does a lower serum ionized calcium level contribute to the symptoms of withdrawal? Clin Pediatr 1977; 16:418–423.

189. Gutcher GR, Odell GB. Hypocalcemia associated with phototherapy in newborn rats: light source dependence. Photochem Photobiol 1983; 37:177–180.

190. Hahn TJ, Hendin BA, Scharp CR, Boisseau VC, Haddad JG. Serum 25-hydroxycholecalciferol levels and bone mass in children on chronic anticonvulsant therapy. N Engl J Med 1975; 292:550–554.

191. Scott SM, Ladenson JH, Aguanna JJ, Walgate J, Hillman LS. Effect of calcium therapy in the sick premature infant with early neonatal hypocalcemia J Pediatr 1984; 104:747–751.

192. Colleti RB, Pan MW, Smith EWP, Genel M. Detection of hypocalcemia in susceptible neonates, the QoTc interval. N Engl J Med 1974; 290:931–935.

193. Venkataraman P, Sanchez G, Parker M, Altmiller D. Effect of intravenous calcium infusions on serum chemistries in neonates J Pediatr Gastroenter Nutr 1991; 13:134–138.

194. Brown R, Steranko BH, Taylor FH. Treatment of early onset neonatal hypocalcemia: effects on serum calcium and ionized calcium. Am J Dis Child 1981; 135:24–28.

195. Brown DR, Tsang RC, Chen IW. Oral calcium supplementation in premature and asphyxiated neonates. J Pediatr 1976; 89:973–977.

196. Kooh SW, Fraser D, Toon R, DeLuca HF. Response of protracted neonatal hypocalcemia to 1α, 25-dihydroxyvitamin D3. Lancet 1976; 2:1105–1107.

197. Barak Y, Milbauer B, Weisman Y, Edelstein S, Spirer Z. Response of neonatal hypocalcemia to 1α, 25-dihydroxyvitamin D3. Arch Dis Child 1979; 54:642–643.

198. Koo WWK, Kaplan LA. Aluminum and bone disorders: with specific reference to aluminum contamination of infant nutrients. J Am Coll Nutr 1988; 7:199–214.

199. Salsburey DJ, Brown DR. Effect of parenteral calcium treatment on blood pressure and heart rate in neonatal hypocalcemia. Pediatrics 1982; 69:605–609.

200. Nervez CT, Shott RJ, Bergstrom WH, Williams ML. Prophylaxis against hypocalcemia in low birth weight infants requiring bicarbonate infusion. J Pediatr 1975; 87:439–442.

201. Salle BL, David L, Glorieux FA, Delvin E, Senterre J, Renaud H. Early oral administration of vitamin D and its metabolites in premature neonates. Effect on mineral hemeostasis. Pediatr Res 1982; 16:75–78.

202. Fleischman AR, Rosen JF, Nathenson G. 25-Hydroxycholecalciferol for early neonatal hypocalcemia. Occurrence in premature newborns. Am J Dis Child 1978; 132:973–977.

203. Petersen S, Christensen NC, Fogh-Andersen N. Effect on serum calcium of 1α hydroxyvitamin D3 supplementation in infants of low birth weight with perinatal asphyxia and infants of diabetic mothers. Acta Paediatr Scand 1981; 70:897–901.

204. Chan GM, Tsang RC, Chen IW, DeLuca HF, Steichen JJ. The effect of 1,25(OH)2 vitamin D3 supplementation in premature infants. J Pediatr 1978; 93:91–96.

205. Kimura S. Nose O, Seino Y, et al. Effects of alternate and simultaneous administrations of calcium and phosphorus on calcium metabolism in children receiving total parenteral nutrition. J Parenter Enteral Nutr 1986; 10:513–516.

206. Lyon AJ, McIntosh N, Wheeler K, Brooke OG. Hypercalcemia in extremely low birthweight infants Arch Dis Child 1984; 59:1141–1144.

207. Loughead J, Mughal F, Mimouni F, Tsang R, Oestreich A. Spectrum and natural history of congenital hyperpapathyroidism secondary to maternal hypocalcemia. Am J. Perinatol 1990; 7:350–355.

208. Tsang RC, Noguchi A, Steichen JJ. Pediatric parathyroid disorders. Pediatr Clin North Am 1979; 26:223–249.

209. Savani R, Mimouni F, Tsang R. Maternal and neonatal hyperparathyroidism as a consequence of maternal renal tubular acidosis. Pediatrics 1993; 91:661–663.

210. Igarashi T, Sekine Y, Kawato H, Kamoshita S, Saigusa Y. Transient neonatal distal renal tubular acidosis with secondary hyperparathyroidism. Pediatr Nephrol 1992; 6:267–269.

211. Wilkinson H, James J. Self limiting neonatal primary hyperparathyroidism associated with familial hypocalciuric hypercalcemia. Arch Dis Child 1993; 69:319–321.

212. Marx SJ, Spiegel AM, Levine MA, et al. Familial Hypocalciuric Hypercalcemia. The relation to primary parathyroid hyperplasia. N. Engl. J. Med. 1982; 307:416–426.

213. Pollack MR, Chou Y-H, Marx SJ, et al. Familial hypocalciuric hypercalcemia and neonatal severe hyperparathyroidism: effects of mutant gene dosage on phenotype, J Clin Invest 1994; 93:1108–1112.

214. Telvi L, Pinard J, Ion R, et al. De novo t(X;21)(q28;q11) in a girl with phenotypic features of Williams-Beuren syndrome. J Med Genet 1992; 29:747–749.

215. Ewart AK, Morris CA, Atkinson D, et al. Hemizygosity at the elastin locus in a developmental disorder, Williams syndrome. Nature Genet 1993; 5:11–16.

216. Fraser D. Hypophosphatasia. Am J Med 1957; 22:730–746.

217. Hicks M, Levy M, Alexander J, Flaitz C. Subcutaneous fat necrosis of the newborn and hypercalcemia: case report and review of the literature. Pediatr Dermatol 1993; 10:271–276.

218. Finne PH, Sanderud J, Aksnes L, Bratlid D, Aarskog D. Hypercalcemia with increased and unregulated 1,25-dihydroxyvitamin D production in a neonate with subcutaneous fat necrosis. J Pediatr 1988; 112:792–794.

219. Drummond KN, Michael AF, Ulstrom RA, Good RA. The blue diaper syndrome: familial hypercalcemia with nephrocalcinosis and indicanuria. Am J Med 1964; 37:928–948.

220. Koo WWK, Sherman R, Succop P, Ho M, Buckley D, Tsang RC. Sequential serum vitamin D metabolites in very low birth weight infants with and without fractures, and rickets. J Pediatr 1989; 114:1017–1022.

221. Corredor DG, Sabeb G, Mendelsohn LV, Wasserman RE. Sunderman JH, Danowski TS. Enhanced postglucose hypophosphatemia during starvation therapy of obesity. Metabolism 1969; 18:754–763.

222. Weinsier RL, Krumdieck CL. Death resulting from overzeolous total parenteral nutrition: the refeeding syndrome. Am J Clin Nutr 1980; 34:393–399.

223. Hill GL, Guinn EJ, Dudrick SJ. Phosphorus distribution in hyperalimentation induced hypophosphatemia. J Surg Res 1976; 20:527–531.

224. DeFronzo RA, Cooke CR, Andres R. The effect of insulin on renal handling of sodium, potassium, calcium and phosphate in man. J Clin Invest 1975; 55:845–855.

225. Arnaud SB, Stickler GB, Haworth JC. Serum 25-hydroxyvitamin D in infantile rickets. Pediatrics 1976; 57:221–225.

226. Venkataraman PS, Tsang RC, Buckely DD, Ho M, Steichen JJ. Elevation of serum 1,25-dihydroxyvitamin D in response to physiologic doses of vitamin D in vitamin D deficient infants. J Pediatr 1983; 103:416–419.

227. Al-Jurf AS, Chapmann-Furr F. Phosphate balance and distribution during total parenteral nutrition: effect of calcium and phosphate additives. J Parenter Enteral Nutr 1986; 10:508–512.

228. Rabito CA. Sodium cotransport process in renal epithelial cell lines. Miner Electrolyte Metab 1986; 12:32–41.

229. Knochel JP. Deranged phosphorus metabolism. In: Seldin DW, Giebisch G, eds. The Kidney: Physiology and Pathophysiology. New York: Raven Press, 1985:1397–1416.

230. Koo WWK, Sherman R, Succop P, et al. Fractures and rickets in very low birth weight infants: conservative management and outcome. J Pediatr Orthop 1989; 9:326–330.

231. Davis RF, Eichner JM, Bleyuer WA, Okamoto G. Hypercalcemia, hyperphosphatemia and dehydration following a single hypertonic phosphate enema. J Pediatr 1977; 90:484–485.

232. Lemons JA, Moye L, Hall D, Simmons MA. Differences in the composition of preterm and term human milk during early lactation. Pediatr Res 1982; 16:113–117.

233. Steichen JJ, Krug Wispe SK, Tsang RC. Breastfeeding the low birthweight infant. Clin Perinatol 1987; 14:131–171.

234. National Academy of Sciences Food and Nutrition Board: National Research Council recommended dietary allowances. In: Pediatric Nutrition Handbook. Elk Grove Village, IL: American Academy of Pediatrics, 1993:345–347.

235. American Academy of Pediatrics Committee on Nutrition: Calcium, phosphorus, and magnesium. In: Pediatric Nutrition Handbook. Elk Grove Village, IL: American Academy of Pediatrics, 1993:111–124.

236. Koo WWK, Tsang RC. Calcium, magnesium, phosphorus, and vitamin D. In: Tsang RC, Lucas A, Uauy R, Zlotkin S, eds. Nutitional Needs of the Preterm Infant. Baltimore: Williams & Wilkins, 1993:135–155.

237. Steichen JJ, Gratton TL, Tsang RC. Osteopenia of prematurity: the cause and possible treatment. J Pediatr 1980; 96:528–534.

238. Greer FR, Steichen JJ, Tsang RC. Effects of increased calcium, phosphorus, and vitamin D intake on bone mineralization in very low birth weight infants fed formula with polycose and medium chain triglycerides. J Pediatr 1982; 100:951–955.

239. Giles MM, Fenton MH, Shaw B, Elton RA, Clarke M, Lang M, Hume R. Sequential calcium and phosphorous balance studies in preterm infants. J Pediatr 1986; 110:591–598.

240. Pelegano JF, Carey DE, Rowe JC, et al. Calcium, phosphorus ratio of 1.7:1 in parenteral nutrition promotes efficient calcium and phosphorus retention in preterm infants. J Bone Miner Res 1988; 3 (Suppl 1):S165.

241. Koo WWK. Calcium, phosphorus, and vitamin D requirements of infants receiving parenteral nutrition. J Perinatol 1988; 8:263–268.

242. Greene HL, Hambidge KM, Schanler R, Tsang RC. Guidelines for the use of vitamins, trace elements, calcium, magnesium, and phosphorus in infants and children receiving total parenteral nutrition. Report of subcommittee from the Commitee in Clinical Practice Issue of American Society for Clinical Nutrition. Am J Clin Nutr 1988; 48:1324–1342.

33
Hyperparathyroidism in Children

Scott A. Rivkees
Riley Hospital for Children, Indianapolis, Indiana

I. INTRODUCTION

Although accounting less than 1% of total-body calcium stores, extracellular calcium plays a critical role in mammalian physiology. Proper levels of the circulating divalent cation are necessary for normal cell membrane electrical potential, neurotransmitter release, renal function, and cardiovascular tone. Thus, maintenance of calcium levels in the normal range is a fundamental homeostatic mechanism (Chap. 31). The task of maintaining circulating calcium levels in the normal range is the domain of the parathyroid glands. Elevation in calcium levels, as in hyperparathyroidism, impairs renal function and can affect other organ systems. Thus, proper recognition and treatment of hyperparathyroidism are essential.

II. THE PARATHYROID GLANDS

The parathyroid glands are paired structures located behind the superior and inferior aspects of the thyroid (1). In 84% of individuals, four parathyroid glands are present (1). The superior pair of glands is 1 cm above the recurrent laryngeal nerve and inferior thyroidal arteries, behind the upper thyroid. The inferior glands are located behind the inferior poles of the thyroid. In 13% of individuals, a fifth gland is present in the region of the thymus (1,2). Each gland is small, measuring less than 6 × 5 × 2 mm in adulthood (3).

The parathyroids are encapsulated by fibrous connective tissue (1). Within the glands, fibrovascular bundles divide the stroma into cord-like structures. Chief cells, of epithelial origin, are typically the only cell type recognized within the glands before puberty (4). After puberty, fat deposition occurs within the glands, and fat content may reach 10–50% of parathyroid cell mass in adults (5). Oxyphilic cells are rare in children and make up less than 5% of parathyroid tissue in adults (6).

Parathyroid embryogenesis occurs during early gestation (4). During gestation week (GW) 6, the dorsum of the third pharyngeal pouch differentiates into the inferior parathyroid glands. The ventral region of this pouch differentiates into the thymus. The thymic and parathyroid primordia are contiguous until GW 10, when the parathyroids separate from the thymus. The fourth pharyngeal pouch gives rise to the superior parathyroid glands. At GW 10, both pairs of glands come to lie on the dorsal surface of the thyroid gland, which completes its migration from the foramen cecum to the pretracheal region by GW 8 (4).

There may be excessive migration of both the superior and inferior parathyroid glands (1). Thus, the final resting location of each gland pair may be inferior to the normal position. The superior glands may migrate to the region of the lower thyroid, and the inferior glands may migrate below the suprasternal notch to within the thymus (1). Parathyroid tissue may also migrate to within thyroid tissue (7).

The factors involved in parathyroid formation and migration are unknown. Transgenic animal study suggests that the homeobox gene Hox-1.5 may be involved in parathyroid development. The selective deletion of Hox-1.5 in mice results in abnormal differentiation of the third and fourth branchial arches and a phenotype similar to DiGeorge syndrome (parathyroid hypoplasia, cardiac abnormalities, and thymic hypoplasia) (8).

Chief cells differentiate during the embryonic period and are functional during fetal life (4). Oxyphil cells do not differentiate until 6 years after birth (6). After birth, parathyroid hormone (PTH)-related peptide levels fall and PTH levels increase (9).

III. PARATHYROID HORMONE AND THE PARATHYROID HORMONE RECEPTOR

A gene on the short arm of chromosome 11 in humans encodes PTH (10,11). A preprohormone of 115 amino acids is encoded, which is cleaved to an 84 amino acid peptide in its final form (12). PTH secretion is regulated largely by external calcium levels (13). At low calcium levels PTH secretion is stimulated, whereas PTH release is suppressed at high levels. In vivo and in vitro studies suggest that the ionized calcium concentration required to achieve half-maximal suppression of PTH secretion is 0.99 mmol/L (14,15). In normal physiology, circulating levels of intact PTH range between 10 and 65 pg/ml (16). During hypocalcemia, levels may rise fivefold (17,18). During hypercalcemia, levels are undetectable, or less than 10 pg/ml (17,18).

Hypomagnesemia may also stimulate PTH secretion (19). However, when magnesium levels drop below 1.5 mg per 100 mg/dl, PTH secretion may be impaired (Chap. 37) (19). Hyperphosphatemia may increase PTH secretion; however, this effect is secondary to phosphate-induced suppression of calcium levels (18). The vitamin D metabolites, 1,25-dihydroxy vitamin D and 24,25-dihydroxyvitamin D, can directly inhibit PTH secretion (20,21).

Evidence suggests that PTH is stored and then degraded within the parathyroid glands after synthesis. Circulating PTH levels reflect an alteration in the intrinsic rate of PTH degradation within the parathyroids rather than changes in PTH gene expression (21–23). PTH degradation falls with the lowering of the serum calcium, making additional hormone available for release into the circulation (22). Parathyroid tissue reserves are sufficient to produce sustained elevated levels of circulating PTH for about 2 h after a hypocalcemic stimulus (21).

Parathyroid hormone exerts its potent biologic effects via specific cell surface receptors. The recent cloning of a parathyroid hormone receptor has enhanced the understanding of PTH action (24,25). As suggested by earlier biochemical studies, the PTH receptor is a monomeric protein of 585 amino acids, with seven transmembrane spanning domains. The receptor couples with guanine nucleotide binding proteins (G proteins). Receptor occupation activates adenylate cyclase, leading to intracellular cAMP accumulation. Receptor activation also stimulates phospholipase C, resulting in intracellular accumulation of inositol phosphates and diacylglycerol and the release of intracellular calcium. Ligand binding studies reveal the high affinity of the receptor for PTH. The equilibrium dissociation constant of PTH for its receptor is about 4 nM.

IV. MECHANISM OF PARATHYROID HORMONE ACTION

PTH is the principal regulator of calcium metabolism and acts on kidney, bone, and gut to increase the net flow of calcium into the extracellular fluid space. PTH effects on the kidneys are the most important factor in the moment-to-moment regulation of serum calcium levels (26,27). About 8000 mg

calcium/m^2 is filtered by the kidneys each day (13,28). The vast amount of filtered calcium is reabsorbed, with only about 5% eliminated in the urine (150–250 mg/m^2/day (29,30). During hypercalcemia, urinary calcium excretion may increase more than fourfold, whereas excretion falls during hypocalcemia (29). About 60% of filtered calcium is reabsorbed in the proximal tubule (31). The remaining calcium is reabsorbed by the loop of Henle or distal tubules, where PTH-stimulated calcium reabsorption acts to maintain serum calcium levels in the normal range (31).

While promoting calcium reabsorption, PTH induces renal phosphate wasting (32). Thus, following bone dissolution calcium returns to the circulation and phosphate is excreted in the urine. The effects of PTH on renal phosphate handling occur at the proximal tubule (33,34).

PTH also influences the tubular reabsorption of bicarbonate, glucose, and amino acids (13,33). Bicarbonate, glucose, and amino acid wasting attend hyperparathyroidism, resulting in a clinical picture similar to renal tubular acidosis or Fanconi syndrome (35,36). During hypoparathyroidism, there is excessive bicarbonate reabsorption resulting in metabolic alkalosis (13).

In the kidneys, PTH directly stimulates the enzyme 25-hydroxyvitamin D-1α-hydroxylase, promoting the formation of 1,25-dihydroxyvitamin D (calcitriol) (20). Calcitriol is the most potent vitamin D metabolite, acting on gut to promote calcium absorption (20).

Each day approximately 15 mg/kg of calcium is ingested and 12 mg/kg is excreted in the feces, yielding a net calcium absorption of 3 mg/kg/day (28,37). The absorbed calcium is either deposited in the skeleton or excreted in the urine. At calcium intakes above 10 mg/kg/day, the net calcium absorption increases only slightly (28).

Several target sites of PTH action on bone have been identified (38). Following peripheral injection of PTH, osteoclast proliferation and activity are induced, leading to bone dissolution and calcium and phosphate release (39). These effects occur more than 12 h after PTH administration and do not acutely influence calcium levels. Another pool of endosteal cells are believed to mediate the acute effects of PTH on bone. Activation of these cells induces calcium release from bone within a few hours (38,40). However, it is important to emphasize that the effects of PTH on kidney, rather than on bone, are responsible for the acute regulation of serum calcium levels.

V. PATHOGENESIS OF HYPERPARATHYROIDISM

Hyperparathyroidism results when PTH is released independently of calcium levels or the "set point" for calcium-induced suppression of PTH secretion is elevated (41,42). Hyperparathyroidism is typically a disease of adulthood, presenting between 40 and 60 years of age (43,44). It is more common in women than in men, and the incidence in the population is between 0.05 and 0.5%. Of individuals with hyperparathyroidism 85% have parathyroid adenomas (43,44). The remaining individuals have diffuse parathyroid hyperplasia.

Over the past several years, there have been important advances in our understanding of hyperparathyroidism. Recent data suggests that parathyroid adenomas result from the clonal expansion of individual parathyroid cell lines (45). In some individuals a candidate oncogene (PRDA1) has been found to be abnormally rearranged within the PTH chromosome locus (11q13) (46). This gene encodes a 295 amino acid "cyclin" protein, which may be important in cell cycle regulation (46,47). It has been postulated that the overexpression of PRAD1 plays a role in the development of parathyroid adenomas (48). Recently, abnormalities of the retinoblastoma gene were also found in parathyroid adenomas (49).

The pathogenesis of parathyroid hyperplasia involves different mechanisms. Diffuse hyperplasia of the parathyroid gland may occur for unknown reasons or following long-standing stimulation of parathyroid activity in response to hypocalcemia. Individuals with chronic hyperphosphatemia from renal failure or exogenous phosphate administration may develop secondary hyperparathyroidism, which is reversible with normalization of the serum calcium in the early stages (50).

Over time, the calcium concentration needed to suppress PTH secretion gradually increases, leading to a new steady state in which the serum calcium is maintained at a higher level (51). Ionized calcium concentrations of 1.1–1.4 mmol/L may be needed to achieve half-maximal suppression of PTH secretion (normal = 0.99 mmol/L) (51). Eventually, PTH secretion may not be suppressible even by high circulating levels of calcium. Supporting this hypothesis, individuals with tertiary hyperparathyroidism may show a spectrum of evolving parathyroid dysfunction. In one of our patients with multiglandular hyperplasia, for example, the set points for PTH suppression of three distinct glands were 1.1, 1.4, and 1.6 mmol/L, respectively. In the fourth gland, PTH secretion was not suppressible even by high calcium levels (52).

VI. DIFFERENTIAL DIAGNOSIS OF HYPERPARATHYROIDISM

Hyperparathyroidism is rare in pediatric patients. Thus, other causes should be sought in the hypercalcemic child. In the newborn period, idiopathic hypercalcemia of infancy, or Williams syndrome, must be considered (53). These individuals typically have hypercalcemia but do not have hypophosphatemia. Affected children may be small for gestational age and have a characteristic facial appearance and supravalvular aortic stenosis. Parathyroid hormone levels are suppressed in this disorder.

Familial hypocalciuric hypercalcemia (FHH) presents with hypercalcemia and hypocalciuria (54,55). This disorder may be difficult to distinguish from hyperparathyroidism. However, there are several distinguishing features. In FHH, serum phosphate levels are normal. Parathyroid hormone levels are usually normal but also may be slightly elevated. Patients with FHH have exceedingly high renal calcium reabsorption. More than 99% of filtered calcium is reabsorbed in FHH, whereas 95% of filtered calcium may be reabsorbed

in hyperparathyroidism. A familial history also aids in the diagnosis of FHH, because the disorder is transmitted by autosomal dominant inheritance. It is important to note that primary hyperparathyroidism has been described in FHH kindreds (56). However, in such individuals PTH levels are significantly elevated (56).

Vitamin D intoxication may induce hypercalcemia at doses more than 100 times the physiologic requirement (20). Excessive vitamin D fortification of dairy milk (up to 10,000 u/L; normal 400 u/L) has led to epidemic hypercalcemia in local communities (57). Excessive vitamin D supplementation of infant formulas has also been described (58). During vitamin D intoxication, PTH levels are suppressed and serum phosphate values are normal.

Other causes of hypercalcemia have also been described, including immobilization, granulomatous disease, and thiazide diuretic therapy. These topics have been reviewed elsewhere (44).

VII. HYPERPARATHYROIDISM: RECOGNITION AND DIAGNOSIS

Because hyperparathyroidism may result in serious adverse effects on several organ systems, recognition of hyperparathyroidism in the early stages is important. When hypercalcemia is present, hyperparathyroidism can be suspected from serum and urinary calcium and phosphate values (59). The combination of hypercalcemia, hypophosphatemia, and phosphaturia suggests hyperparathyroidism (44,60). In some individuals, however, calcium elevations may be episodic (61). In individuals with hyperphosphatemia or those receiving phosphate therapy, hypercalcemia may also be masked (52).

The tubular reabsorption of phosphate [TRP = $(1 - U_P \times S_{Cr}/U_{Cr} \times S_P)$ 100%] is normally greater than 85%, and levels of phosphate in the urine are <50 mg/dl (13,28). During hyperparathyroid states, the TRP may fall to as low as 50% and the urinary phosphate concentration is high (13,44). However, in up to 40% of individuals with hyperparathyroidism, hypophosphatemia may not be present, and the TRP may be normal (44).

The urinary excretion of calcium typically falls during hyperparathyroidism. In normal individuals, urinary calcium excretion increases about fivefold when the serum calcium rises from 10 to 11mg/dl (62). This corresponds with increased urinary calcium-creatinine ratios (mg/mg) from 0.2 to 1.0. In states of hyperparathyroidism, urinary calcium excretion may not increase despite high calcium levels, and the tubular reabsorption of calcium may be $>95\%$ [$(1 - U_{Ca} \times S_{Cr}/U_{Cr} \times S_{Ca})$ 100%] (30).

Both calcium and phosphate excretion can be assessed from "spot" urine samples if the creatinine concentration is also determined in the sample. This avoids the need for 24 h urine collections, which are often difficult to obtain in children. Urinary calcium excretion is normally 2 mg/kg/day, and hypercalciuria is defined as >4 mg/kg/day (21). Over the 24 h day, 10–15 mg/kg of creatinine is excreted in the urine (63). Thus, in children, the urinary calcium-creatinine ratio is normally less than 0.1, with a ratio > 0.2 defined as hypercalciuria.

A suspected diagnosis should be confirmed by assessment of circulating PTH levels. Measurement of the intact PTH molecule by radioimmunoassay is now recommended (normal values 10–65 pg/ml) (16,64). The presence of intact parathyroid hormone in the hypercalcemic patient is inappropriate and indicative of hyperparathyroidism. In 90% of individuals with hyperparathyroidism, PTH levels are clearly elevated (65). In 10%, PTH levels may be close to the normal range yet are inappropriate for the calcium levels (65).

Preoperative localization of hyperactive parathyroid tissue is difficult. Using high-resolution ultrasonography (66), computed axial tomography, magnetic resonance imaging (67), and radionuclide scanning (68), it has been possible to localize parathyroid tissue. However, these methods may not localize small glands with great fidelity. Thus, because 85% of individuals have four normally positioned parathyroid glands, preoperative localization of the parathyroids is not routinely performed (1). In comparison with these noninvasive methods, arteriography and selective venous sampling have the greatest likelihood of localizing abnormal tissue (69,70) and are recommended in cases requiring repeated surgery.

VIII. PRIMARY HYPERPARATHYROIDISM IN PEDIATRICS

Fewer than 100 cases of isolated primary hyperparathyroidism have been reported in children (71–76). Both parathyroid adenomas and multiglandular hyperplasia have been described. It is postulated that primary hyperparathyroidism in children represents early presentation of the sporadic form of hyperparathyroidism that typically affects adults. No clear-cut pattern of inheritance is generally found, although several kindreds have been reported in whom primary hyperparathyroidism affects several generations (77).

Hyperparathyroidism also may present as a pernicious disorder in newborns. This disorder may be transmitted in an autosomal dominant manner (78,79). There have also been reports of neonatal hyperparathyroidism in families with FHH (56). The resultant hypercalcemia is severe and may result in fatality. Serum calcium levels may be more than 15 mg/dl and have been reported to be as high as 30 mg/dl. This is a life-threatening condition requiring emergency parathyroidectomy (79).

Hyperparathyroidism may also be a feature of multiple hereditary endocrinopathy syndromes (Chap. 50) (80–83). Hyperparathyroidism is the most common presenting feature of multiple endocrine neoplasia type I (MEN I, 97% of cases), which is also associated with tumors of the pancreas (40%) and pituitary (20%). Hyperparathyroidism may occur in 20% of cases of MEN II (84,85). This disorder is also associated with medullary carcinoma of the thyroid and adrenal tumors (pheochromocytomas). These disorders are transmitted in an autosomal dominant manner. Hyperparathyroidism typically presents during adulthood, although cases have been reported

in children. MEN IIb (III) is not associated with primary hyperthyroidism (44).

Radiation exposure may be associated with the development of hyperparathyroidism. An increased incidence of hyperparathyroidism has been reported in adult survivors of the Hiroshima atomic blast (86). It has been suggested that the incidence of hyperparathyroidism is greater three decades after head and neck radiotherapy (87,88). Hyperparathyroidism has also been reported in a few patients treated with radioiodine for Graves' disease (89–91).

Primary hyperparathyroidism has been described in neonates following gestational hypoparathyroidism in the mother (87,88). Primary hyperparathyroidism has also been described in one infant with congenital hypothyroidism (92).

Carcinoma of the parathyroid glands can present with biochemical features similar to those of primary hyperparathyroidism. Although there are very few reports of parathyroid carcinoma in children (93), parathyroid carcinoma has been reported in adolescents with familial hyperparathyroidism (94,95).

IX. SECONDARY AND TERTIARY HYPERPARATHYROIDISM IN CHILDREN

Secondary and tertiary hyperparathyroidism are most commonly seen in hypocalcemic and/or hyperphosphatemic states. An appropriate response to hypocalcemia (secondary hyperparathyroidism) may evolve into autonomous parathyroid hyperactivity (tertiary hyperparathyroidism) following prolonged stimulation of parathyroid activity.

In the newborn period, secondary hyperparathyroidism may be seen in children born to a hypocalcemic mother. This typically resolves within several months of birth (96,97). We also recently cared for a newborn infant with transient hyperparathyroidism (Ca^{2+}, 12 mg/dl) whose mother did not have hypocalcemia. In this child, the hypercalcemia resolved at 3 months of age.

Vitamin D-deficient and vitamin D-dependent rickets, which can result in hypocalcemia, may be associated with biochemical hyperparathyroidism (98,99). Whereas PTH levels are not elevated in the first stage of vitamin D-deficient rickets, PTH levels increase in the second and third stages (100). Diffuse parathyroid hyperplasia has also been described in these patients (101).

Chronic elevation of serum phosphate levels may be the most common cause of secondary hyperparathyroidism in children. Phosphate-induced depression of the serum calcium may appear to be clinically insignificant ($<10\%$) but may be sufficient to stimulate PTH secretion (102). The inability of the kidneys to excrete phosphate places individuals with renal failure at risk for hyperparathyroidism (50,103,104). This is especially troublesome for a skeletal system already at risk for metabolic bone disease (105). Thus, parathyroid function must be routinely monitored during chronic renal failure, and parathyroidectomy is needed when hyperparathyroidism develops (104,106).

The treatment of familial hypophosphatemic rickets

(vitamin D-resistant rickets or X-linked hypophosphatemic rickets) with phosphate may also result in hyperparathyroidism (Chap. 34) (52,102). Hypophosphatemic rickets is characterized by renal phosphate wasting and hypophosphatemia. In the untreated state serum calcium levels are normal and PTH is usually not elevated (102). Oral phosphate therapy, however, may result in significant elevations of circulating phosphate levels and falls in the serum calcium, leading a secondary hyperparathyroidism (102). With long-term phosphate therapy, secondary hyperparathyroidism may evolve into tertiary hyperparathyroidism (52). Furthermore, even in the setting of abnormal parathyroid regulation, phosphate therapy may continue to stimulate parathyroid hormone secretion, contributing to progression of parathyroid disease (52). Because oral phosphate lowers the serum calcium even in the presence of high PTH levels, hypercalcemia may not be detected in the hyperparathyroid patient, delaying recognition of hyperparathyroidism.

Careful assessment of phosphate and PTH levels in individuals with hypophosphatemic rickets is needed, and care should be taken to use less than 2 g/day of inorganic phosphate. In addition, adjunctive therapy with calcitriol may prevent or reverse secondary hyperparathyroidism in the early stages (107,108). However, after the development of significant parathyroid hyperplasia, hyperparathyroidism is not reversible and surgical treatment is needed (52).

X.   COMPLICATIONS OF HYPERPARATHYROIDIMS AND HYPERCALCEMIA

The adverse effects of hyperparathyroidism are related to bone dissolution and hypercalcemia. Excessive PTH activity leads to skeletal demineralization and osteopenia. In adults with hyperparathyroidism, demineralization is readily recognized on standard radiographs in up to 30% of patients (44). Bone densitometry studies show reduced mineralization in more than 75% of affected individuals (109,110).

Hyperparathyroidism affects the kidneys in several ways. Hypercalcemia can directly reduce the glomerular filtration rate (111). Long-standing hypercalcemia may lead to deposition of calcium in the tubules, especially during hyperphosphatemia, resulting in nephrocalcinosis (111). Nephrocalcinosis can be detected by ultrasound, which should be performed in individuals with hyperparathyroidism (112). Whereas nephrolithiasis has been well described in adults with hyperparathyroidism (44), there are few reports of renal stones in children with hyperparathyroidism. Calcium levels in excess of 15 mg/dl also may result in polyuria secondary to nephrogenic diabetes insipidus (111).

Hypercalcemia also affects other systems. Hypercalcemia may induce increased cardiovascular tone and hypertension (113). High calcium levels may lead to heart block and shortening of the ST segment (113). The central nervous system is also sensitive to the effects of calcium at high levels (114). Impaired mentation and convulsions may occur at levels above 13 mg/dl (114). Muscle weakness and

hyporeflexia may occur (115). Gastric ulcers and constipation may reflect hypercalcemia (116). Anorexia may attend hypercalcemia. Patients are also at increased risk for pancreatitis (117, 118).

XI.   TREATMENT OF HYPERPARATHYROIDISM AND HYPERCALCEMIA

Acute therapy of hypercalcemia is indicated for symptomatic individuals or when the total calcium exceeds 13 mg/dl (44). Treatment with intravenous saline (3000 m/m^2/day; 200–400 ml/kg/day) and furosemide (1 mg/kg every 4–6 h) lowers calcium levels within hours (40,119). After correction of acute hypercalcemia, a high sodium diet promotes continued renal calcium excretion. Oral furosemide therapy (1–2 mg/kg/day divided in three doses) may also be of benefit.

Adjunctive therapy with prednisone is not effective in hyperparathyroidism (44). Calcitonin may initially lower serum calcium levels, but patients with hyperparathyroidism often "escape" from the effects of calcitonin. The use of diphosphonates, which inhibit hydroxyapatite dissolution, is not effective in hyperparathyroidism (44).

Oral or intravenous phosphate therapy can lower circulating calcium levels (44). However, raising serum phosphate levels leads to precipitation of calcium and phosphate salts in the vascular system and kidneys, and thus phosphate therapy is not recommended. Continued oral phosphate therapy, however, may maintain the calcium in an acceptable range in phosphate-treated patients awaiting parathyroidectomy (52).

Although experimentally effective, PTH antagonists are not clinically available (120). Selective ablation of parathyroid glands by embolization has been shown to be effective only for some ectopic parathyroid glands (121). Thus, surgery is the current definitive cure for hyperparathyroidism.

In adults, treatment of the asymptomatic patient with hyperparathyroidism has been the subject of debate (44,122, 123). Surgery is recommended for asymptomatic individuals with evidence of demineralization, nephrolithiasis, or nephrocalcinosis. However, surgery may be postponed in individuals without evidence of complications. In such patients renal function, bone density, and gastrointestinal status should be assessed regularly (44,123).

Children and adolescents with hyperparathyroidism face the prospect of progressive skeletal mineral loss and the adverse effects of long-term hypercalcemia on the kidneys. Thus, surgical treatment should be strongly considered for pediatric patients with this disorder (124).

Postsurgical hypoparathyroidism is readily managed using calcitriol. Thus, total parathyroidectomy should be considered unless a solitary adenoma can be identified (125). Transplantation of excised tissue to the forearm should be considered in patients undergoing total parathyroidectomy (126). If autotransplantation is successful, functional activity can be detected within 6 weeks of surgery. PTH levels are greater in venous blood obtained from the brachial vein from the recipient arm than in blood from the other arm. In addition, excised parathyroid tissue should be cryopreserved (127) for future autotransplantation, if necessary.

When a subtotal parathyroidectomy is performed, the remaining parathyroid tissue that was previously suppressed by hypercalcemia will become functional 30 h after surgery (128).

XII.   MANAGEMENT AFTER PARATHYROIDECTOMY

After successful resection of hyperactive parathyroid tissue, serum calcium levels may fall rapidly. Intraoperatively, in hypocalcemic patients Chevostek's sign may be elicited by tapping over the facial nerve at the temporal-mandibular region. Patients may also develop laryngospasm.

Intravenous infusions of calcium should be started to maintain the calcium level in the lower range of normal (50 mg/kg/day) of elemental calcium. If hypocalcemia persists beyond the first postoperative day, oral calcitriol therapy should be started (0.025–0.5 μg twice per day). This potent vitamin D metabolite has a rapid onset of action (20). The dose may be advanced 0.5 μg each day until serum calcium levels stabilize (up to 3 μg/day). When serum calcium levels are stable and intravenous therapy is no longer needed, the calcitriol dose can be gradually reduced. Care should be taken to avoid hypercalcemia during vitamin D therapy. Single episodes of hypercalcemia can induce permanent renal damage in children.

Serum magnesium levels also should be determined because hyperparathyroidism may deplete total-body magnesium stores. When the serum magnesium concentration is <1.5 mg/dl, there may be impaired PTH secretion from residual parathyroid tissue (19,129). Of the available oral magnesium supplements, Magonate (Flemming, Fenton, MO) is the most palatable.

If the patient receives a diet including liberal amounts of dairy products, calcium supplementation is not necessary. Despite widespread belief to the contrary, oral calcium supplements do not greatly increase net intestinal calcium absorption in children or adults (130). Furthermore, hyperphosphatemia spontaneously corrects with normalization of the serum calcium. Thus, phosphate binding agents are not needed.

In patients without gross skeletal demineralization, intravenous calcium infusions often can be discontinued 5–7 days after surgery (131). However, individuals with significant skeletal demineralization are at risk for "hungry bone syndrome" and may require prolonged intravenous infusion of calcium (131).

The growing child with hyperparathyroidism is at special risk for hungry bone syndrome. We have cared for two adolescent females who required intravenous calcium infusion for 3 months after total parathyroidectomy to prevent symptomatic hypocalcemia (52). Preoperatively, gross demineralization was noted in radiographs of the hands. To facilitate discharge from the hospital, indwelling central venous catheters were placed, allowing infusions at home. After 45 days,

it was possible to administer calcium during the night, allowing schooling during the day. Following the appearance of urinary calcium (calcium/creatinine ratio > 0.02), it was possible to stop intravenous therapy within a few weeks (52).

XIII.   SUMMARY

Childhood primary hyperparathyroidism is a rare disorder that may present as a severe disorder in neonates, sporadically in children, or as part of MEN syndromes. Secondary and tertiary hyperparathyroidism may develop in children with chronic hyperphosphatemia from renal disease or phosphate therapy. The constellation of hypercalcemia, hypophosphatemia, and renal phosphate wasting suggests PTH excess. By measuring intact PTH levels, hyperparathyroidism can be readily diagnosed. Hyperparathyroidism leads to skeletal demineralization and renal damage. Thus, surgery is indicated for pediatric patients. Postoperatively, children with demineralization may be at risk for hungry bone syndrome and require prolonged intravenous calcium infusions. The child rendered hypoparathyroid by surgery can be readily managed with oral calcitriol therapy.

REFERENCES

1. Wolfe HJ. The anatomy of the parathyroids. In: DeGroot LM, ed. Endocrinology. Philadelphia: W.B. Saunders, 1989: 844–847.
2. Nathaniels EK, Nathaniels AM, Wang CA. Mediastinal parathyroid tumors: a clinical and pathological study of 84 cases. Ann Surg 1970; 171:165–170.
3. Dufour DR, Wilkerson SV. The normal parathyroid revisited: Percentage of stomal fat. Hum Pathol 1982; 92:814–821.
4. Moore KL. The Developing Human. Philadelphia: W.B. Saunders, 1973.
5. Dekker A, Dunsford HA, Geyer SJ. The normal parathyroid gland at autopsy: the significance of stromal fat in adult patients. J Pathol 1979; 128:127–132.
6. Christie AC. The parathyroid oxyphil cells. J Clin Pathol 1967; 20:591–602.
7. Spiegel AM, Marx SJ, Doppman JL, et al. Intrathyroidal parathyroid adenoma or hyperplasia. An occasionally overlooked cause of surgical failure in primary hyperparathyroidism. JAMA 1975; 234:1029–1033.
8. Chisaka O, Capecchi MR. Regionally restricted developmental defects resulting from targeted disruption of the mouse homeobox gene hox-1.5. Nature 1991; 350:473–479.
9. Burton PB, Moniz C, Quirke P, et al. Parathyroid hormone-related peptide: expression in fetal and neonatal development. J Pathol 1992; 167:291–296.
10. Naylor SL, Sakaguchi AY, Szoka P, et al. Human parathyroid hormone gene (PTH) is on short arm of chromosome 11. Somat Cell Genet 1983; 9:609–616.
11. Vasicek TJ, McDevitt BE, Freeman MW, et al. Nucleotide sequence of the human parathyroid hormone gene. Proc Nat Acad Sci USA 1983; 80:2127–2131.
12. Kemper B, Habener JF, Potts JT Jr, et al. Proparathyroid hormone: identification of a biosynthetic precursor to parathyroid hormone. Proc Nat Acad Sci USA 1972; 69:643–647.
13. Bringhurst FR. Calcium and phosphate distribution, turnover,

and metabolic actions. In: DeGroot LJ, ed. Endocrinology. Philadelphia: W.B. Saunders, 1989:805–843.

14. Brown EM. PTH secretion in vivo and in vitro. Regulation by calcium and other secretagogues. Miner Electrolyte Metab 1982; 8:130–150.

15. Brown EM, Wilson RE, Thatcher JG, Marynick SP. Abnormal calcium-regulated PTH release in normal parathyroid tissue for patients with adenomas. Am J Med 1981; 71:565–570.

16. Nussbaum SR, Potts JT Jr. Immunoassays for parathyroid hormone 1–84 in the diagnosis of hyperparathyroidism. J Bone Miner Res 1991; 6(Suppl 2):S43–50.

17. Blum JW, Mayer GP, Potts JT Jr. Parathyroid hormone responses during spontaneous hypocalcemia and induced hypercalcemia in cows. Endocrinology 1976; 95:84–91.

18. Sherwood LM, Mayer GP, Ramberg CF Jr, et al. Regulation of parathyroid hormone secretion: proportional control by calcium, lack of effect of phosphate. Endocrinology 1968; 83:1043–1051.

19. Anast CS, Mohs JM, Kaplan SL, et al. Evidence for parathyroid failure in magnesium deficiency. Science 1972; 177:606–608.

20. Holick MF. Vitamin D. Biosynthesis, metaoblism, and mode of action. In: DeGroot LM, ed. Endocrinology. Philadelphia: W.B. Saunders, 1989:902–926.

21. Rosenblatt M, Kronenberg HM, Potts JT Jr. Parathyroid hormone. Physiology, chemistry, biosynthesis, secretion, metabolism, and mode of action. In: DeGroot LM, ed. Endcrinology. Philadelphia: W.B. Saunders, 1989:848–891.

22. Habener JF, Kemper B, Potts JT Jr. Calcium-dependent intracellular degradation of parathyroid hormone: a possible mechanism for the regulation of hormone stores. Endocrinology 1975; 97:431–441.

23. Russell J, Lettieri D, Sherwood LM. Direct regulation by calcium of cytoplasmic messenger ribonucleic acid coding for pre-proparathyroid hormone in isolated bovine parathyroid cells. J Clin Invest 1983; 72:1851–1855.

24. Juppner H, Abou-Samra AB, Freeman M, et al. A G protein-linked receptor for parathyroid hormone and parathyroid hormone-related peptide. Science 1991; 254:1024–1026.

25. Schipani E, Karga H, Karaplis AC, et al. Identical complementary deoxyribonucleic acids encode a human renal and bone parathyroid hormone (PTH)/PTH-related peptide receptor. Endocrinology 1993; 132:2157–2165.

26. Aurbach GD, Heath DA. Parathyroid hormone and calcitonin regulation of renal function. Kidney Int 1974; 6:331–345.

27. Nordin BE, Peacock M. Role of kidney in regulation of plasma-calcium. Lancet 1969; 2:1280–1283.

28. Neer R. Calcium and inorganic phosphate homeostasis. In: DeGroot LM, ed. Endocrinology. Philadelphia: W.B. Saunders, 1989:927–953.

29. Peacock M, Nordin BE. Tubular reabsorption of calcium in normal and hypercalciuric subjects. J Clin Pathol 1968; 21:353–358.

30. Nordin BE, Hodgkinson A, Peacock M. The measurement and the meaning of urinary calcium. Clin Orthop 1967; 52:293–322.

31. Lassiter WE, Gottschalk CW, Mylle M. Micropuncture study of renal tubular reabsorption on calcium in normal rodents. Am J Physiol 1963; 204:771–775.

32. Kenny AD, Pang Pk. Phosphaturic response to parathyroid hormone (letter). N Engl J Med 1983; 308:1362.

33. Wang CA, Guyton SW. Hyperparathyroid crisis: clinical and pathologic studies of 14 patients. Ann Surg 1979; 190:782–790.

34. Nordin BE, Bulusu L. Plasma-phosphate and tubular reabsorption of phosphate. Lancet 1970; 1:998.

35. Coe FL, Firpo JJ, Jr. Evidence for mild reversible hyperparathyroidism in distal renal tubular acidosis. Arch Intern Med 1975; 135:1485–1489.

36. Coe FL. Magnitude of metabolic acidosis in primary hyperparathyroidism. Arch Intern Med 1974; 134:262–265.

37. Phang JM, Berman M, Finerman GA, et al. Dietary perturbation of calcium metabolism in normal man: compartmental analysis. J Clin Invest 1969; 48:67–77.

38. Norimatsu H, Yamamoto T, Ozawa H, et al. Changes in calcium phosphate on bone surfaces and in lining cells after the administration of parathyroid hormone or calcitonin. Clin Orthop 1982; 164:271–278.

39. Robertson WG, Peacock M, Atkins D, et al. The effect of parathyroid hormone on the uptake and release of calcium by bone in tissue culture. Clin Sci 1972; 43:714–718.

40. Norimatsu H, Wiel CJ, Talmage RV. Morphological support of a role for cells lining bone surfaces in maintenance of plasma clacium concentration. Clin Orthop 1979; 139:254–262.

41. Murray TM, Peacock M, Powell D, et al. Non-autonomy of hormone secretion in primary hyperparathyroidism. Clin Endocrinol 1972; 1:235–246.

42. Mayer GP, Habener JF, Potts JT Jr. Parathyroid hormone secretion in vivo. Demonstration of a calcium-independent nonsuppressible component of secretion. J Clin Invest 1976; 57:678–683.

43. Barbier J, Kraimps JL, Denizot A, et al. Primary hyperparathyroidism. Results of a French multicenter study. Bull Acad Natl Med 1992; 176:1033–1047.

44. Habener JF Potts JT Jr. Primary hyperparathyroidism. Clinical features. In: DeGroot LM, ed. Endocriniology. Philadelphia: W.B. Saunders, 1989:954–966.

45. Arnold A, Staunton CE, Kim HG, et al. Monoclonality and abnormal parathyroid hormone genes in parathyroid adenomas. N Engl J Med 1988; 318:658–662.

46. Arnold A, Motokura T, Bloom T, et al. PRAD1 (cyclin D1): a parathyroid neoplasia gene on 11q13. Henry Fod Hosp Med J 1992; 40:177–180.

47. Motokura T, Bloom T, Kim HG, et al. A novel cyclin encoded by a bcl1-linked candidate oncogene. Nature 1991; 350:512–515.

48. Motokura T, Arnold A. Cyclin D and Oncogenesis. Curr Opin Genet Dev 1993; 3:5–10.

49. Cryns VL, Thor A, Xu HJ, et al. Loss of the retinoblastoma tumor-suppressor gene in parathyroid carcinoma. N Eng J 1994; med 330:257–761.

50. Ramirez JA, Goodman WG, Gornbein J, et al. Direct in vivo comparison of calcium-regulated parathyroid hormone secretion in normal volunteers and patients with secondary hyperparathyroidism. J Clin Endocrinol Metab 1993; 76:1489–1494.

51. El-Hajj Fuleihan G, Chen CJ, Rivkees SA, et al. Calcium-dependent release of N-terminal fragments and intact immunoreactive parathyroid hormone by human pathological parathyroid tissue in vitro. J Clin Endocrinol Metab 1989; 69:860–867.

52. Rivkees SA, el-Hajj-Fuleihan G, Brown EM, et al. Tertiary hyperparathyroidism during high phosphate therapy of familial hypophosphatemic rickets. J Clin Endocrinol Metab 1992; 75:1514–1518.

53. Lowe KG, Henderson JL, Park, WW, McGreal DA. The idiopathic hypercalcaemic syndromes of infancy. Lancet 1954; 1:101–110.

54. Marx SJ, Stock JL, Attie MF, et al. Familial hypocalciuric hypercalcemia: recognition among patients referred after unsuccessful parathyroid exploration. Ann Intern Med 1980; 92:351–356.

55. Marx SJ, Spiegel AM, Brown EM, et al. Circulating parathyroid hormone activity: familial hypocalciuric hypercalcemia

versus typical primary hyperparathyroidism. J Clin Endocrinol Metab 1978; 47:1190–1197.

56. Page LA, Haddow JE. Self-limited neonatal hyperparathyroidism in familial hypocalciuric hypercalcemia. J Pediatr 1987; 111:261–264.

57. Jacobus CH, Holick MF, Shao Q, et al. Hypervitaminosis D associated with drinking milk. N Engl J Med 1992; 326:1173–1177.

58. Holick MF, Shao Q, Liu WW, et al. The vitamin D content of fortified milk and infant formula. N Engl J Med 1992; 326:1178–1181.

59. Mallette LE, Bilezikian JP, Heath DA, et al. Primary hyperparathyroidism: clinical and biochemical features. Medicine (Baltimore) 1974; 53:127–146.

60. Girard RM, Belanger A, Hazel B. Primary hyperparathyroidism in children. Can J Surg 1981; 282:1023.

61. Siperstein AE, Shen W, Chan AK, et al. Normocalcemic hyperparathyroidiam. Biocemical and symptom profiles before and after surgery. Arch Surg 1992; 127:1157–1156.

62. Peacock M, Robertson WG, Nordin BE. Relation between serum and urinary calcium with particular reference to parathyroid activity. Lancet 1969; 1:384–386.

63. Graystone JE. Creatinine excretion during growth. In: Cheek DB, ed. Human Growth. Philadelphia: Lea and Febiger, 1968: 182–197.

64. Hackeng WH, Lips P, Netelenbos JC, et al. Clinical implications of estimation of intact parathyroid hormone (PTH) versus total immunoreactive PTH in normal subjects and hyperparathyroid patients. J Clin Endocrinol Metab 1986; 63:447–453.

65. Hollenberg An, Arnold A. Hypercalcemia with low-normal serum intact PTH: a novel presentation of primary hyperparathyroidism. Am J Med 1991; 91:547–548.

66. Simeone JF, Mueller PR, Ferrucci JT Jr, et al. High-resolution real-time sonography of the parathyroid. Radiology 1981; 141:745–751.

67. Kier R, Blinder RA, Herfkens RJ, et al. MR imaging with surface coils in primary hyperparathyroidism. J Comput Assist Tomog 1987; 11:863–868.

68. Zwas ST, Czerniak A, Boruchowsky S, et al. Preoperative parathyroid localization by superimposed iodine-131 toluidine blue and technetium-99m pertechnetate imaging. J Nucl Med 1987; 28:298–307.

69. Reitz RE, Pollard JJ, Wang CA, et al. Localization of parathyroid adenomas by selective venous catheterization and radioimmunoassay. N Engl J Med 1969; 281:348–351.

70. Powell D, Murray TM, Pollard JJ, et al. Parathyroid localization using venous catheterization and radioimmunoassay. Arch Intern Med 1973; 131:645–648.

71. Steendijk R. Metabolic bone disease in children. Clin Orthop 1971; 77:247–275.

72. Latham SC. Mild hyperparathyroidism in a girl aged 10 years 6 months. Proc R Soc Med 1969; 62:909.

73. Latham SC, Bordier P, Doyle FH, et al. A case of mild hyperparathyroidism in childhood. Arch Dis Child 1969; 44:521–526.

74. Girard RM, Belanger A, Hazel B. Primary hyperparathyroidism in children. Can J Surg 1982; 25:11–13.

75. Allen DB, Friedman AL, Hendricks SA. Asymptomatic primary hyperparathyroidism in children. Newer methods of preoperative diagnosis. Am J Dis Child 1986; 140:819–821.

76. Nolan RB, Hayles AB, Woolner NB. Adenoma of the parathyroid glands in children: report of case and brief review of the literature. Am J Dis Child 1960; 99:622–627.

77. Marx SJ, Powell D, Shimkin PM, et al. Familial hyperpara-

thyroidism. Mild hypercalcemia in at least nine members of a kindre. Ann Intern Med 1973; 78:371–377.

78. Ross AJ, Cooper A, Attie MF, et al. Primary hyperparathyroidism in infancy. J Pediatr Surg 1986; 21:493–499.

79. Blair JW, Carachi R. Neonatal primary hyperparathyroidism—a case report and review of the literature. Eur J Pediatr Surg 1991; 1:110–114.

80. Kraimps JL, Duh QY, Demeure M, et al. Hyperparathyroidism in multiple endocrine neoplasia syndrome. Surgery 1992; 112:1080–1086.

81. Miller SS, Sizemore GW, Sheps SG, et al. Parathyroid function in patients with pheochromocytoma. Ann Intern Med 1975; 82:372–375.

82. Jackson CE, Boonstra CE. The relationship of hereditary hyperparathyroidism to endocrine adenomatosis. Am J Med 1967; 43:727–734.

83. Van Heerden JA, Kent RB, Sizemore GW, et al. Primary hyperparathyroidism in patients with multiple endocrine neoplasia syndromes. Surgical experience. Arch Surg 1983; 118:533–536.

84. Benson L, Ljunghall S, Akerstrom G, et al. Hyperparathyroidism presenting as the first lesion in multiple endocrine neoplasia type 1. Am J Med 1987; 82:731–737.

85. Benson L, Rastad J, Ljunghall S, et al. Parathyroid hormone release in vitro in hyperparathyroidism associated with multiple endocrine neoplasia type 1. Acta Endocrinol (Copenh) 1987; 114:12–17.

86. Fujiwara S, Sposto R, Ezaki H, et al. Hyperparathyroidism among atomic bomb survivors in Hiroshima. Radiat Res 1992; 130:372–378.

87. Landing BH, Kamoshita S. Congenital hyperparathyroidism secondary to maternal hypoparathyroidism. J Pediatr 1970; 77:842–847.

88. Bronsky D, Kiamko RT, Moncada R, et al. Intra-uterine hyperparathyroidism secondary to maternal hypoparathyroidism. Pediatrics 1968; 42:606–613.

89. Bondeson AG, Bondeson L, Thomspon NW. Hyperparathyroidism after treatment with radioactive iodine: not only a coincidence? Surgery 1989; 106:1025–1027.

90. Esselstyn CB Jr, Schumacher OP, Eversman J, et al. Hyperparathyroidism after radioactive iodine therapy for Graves' disease. Surgery 1982; 92:811–813.

91. Kawamura J, Tobisu K, Sanada S, et al. Hyperparathyroidism after radioactive iodine therapy for Graves' disease; a case report. Acta Urol Jpn 1983; 29:1513–1519.

92. Holcomb GW, Perloff LJ. Primary hyperparathyroidism in a hypothyroid child. Surgery 1990; 108:588–592.

93. Wang CA, Gaz RD. Natural history of parathyroid carcinoma. Diagnosis, treatment, and results. Am J Surg 1985; 149:522–527.

94. McHenry CR, Rosen IB, Walfish PG, et al. Parathyroid crisis of unusual features in a child. Cancer 1993; 71:1923–1927.

95. Mallette LE, Bilezikian JP, Ketcham AS, et al. Parathyroid carcinoma in familial hyperparathyroidism. Am J Med 1974; 57:642–648.

96. Lnading BH, Kamoshita S. Congenital hyperparathyroidism secondary to maternal hypoparathyroidism. J Pediatr 1970; 77:842–847.

97. Goldberg E, Winter ST, Better OS, Berger A. Transient neonatal hyperparathyroidism associated with maternal hypothyroidism. Isr J Med Sci 1976; 12:199–201.

98. Falls WF Jr, Carter NW, Rector FC Jr, et al. Familial vitamin D-resistant rickets. Study of six cases with evaluation of the pathogenetic role of secondary hyperparathyroidism. Ann Intern Med 1968; 68:553–560.

99. Arnaud C, Glorieux F, Scriver CR. Serum parathyroid hor-

mone levels in acquired vitamin D deficiency of infancy. Pediatrics 1972; 49:837–840.

100. Lloyd HM, Aitken RE, Ferrier TM. Primary hyperparathyroidism resembling rickets of late onset. BMJ 1965; 5466:853–856.

101. Steendijk R. Vitamin D and the pathogenesis of rickets and osteomalacia. Folia Med Neer 1968; 11:178–186.

102. Arnaud C, Glorieux F, Scriver C. Serum parathyroid hormone in X-linked hypophosphatemia. Science 1971; 173:845–847.

103. Pletka PG, Strom TB, Hampers CL, et al. Secondary hyperparathyroidism in human kidney transplant recipients Nephron 1976; 17:371–381.

104. Hanley DA, Sherwood LM. Secondary hyperparathyroidism in chronic renal failure. Pathophysiology and treatment. Med Clin North Am 1978; 62:1319–1339.

105. Cochran M, Bulusu L, Horsman A, et al. Hypocalcaemia and bone disease in renal failure. Nephron 1973; 10:113–140.

106. Bessell JR, Proudman WD, Parkyn RF, et al. Parathyroidectomy in the treatment of patients with chronic renal failure: a 10-year review. Br J Surg 1986; 80:40–42.

107. Costa T, Marie PJ, Scriver CR, et al. X-linked hypophosphatemia: effect of calcitriol on renal handling of phosphate, serum phosphate, and bone mineralization. J Clin Endocrinol Metab 1981; 52:463–472.

108. Glorieux FH, Marie PJ, Pettifor JM, et al. Bone response to phosphate salts, ergocalciferol, and calcitriol in hypophosphatemic vitamin D-resistant rickets. N Engl J Med 1980; 303:1023–1031.

109. Pak CYC, Stewart A, Kaplan R, et al. Photon absorptiometric analysis of bone density in primary hyperparathyroidism. Lancet 1975; 2:7–8.

110. Mautalen C, Reyes HR, Ghiringhelli G, et al. Cortical bone mineral content in primary hyperparathyroidism. Changes after parathyroidectomy. Acta Endocrinol (Copenh) 1986; 111:494–497.

111. Gamble JL. Chemical Anatomy, Physiology and Pathology of Extracellular Fluid. Cambridge, UA: Harvard University Press, 1947.

112. Verge CF, Lam A, Simpson JM, et al. Effects of therapy in X-linked hypophosphatemic rickets. N Engl J Med 1991; 325:1843–1848.

113. Klein I, Ojamaa K. Clinical review 36: Cardiovascular manifestations of endocrine disease. J Clin Endocrinol Metab 1992; 75:339–342.

114. Petersen P. Psychiatric disorders in primary hyperparathyroidism. J Clin Endocrionl Metab 1968; 28:1491–1495.

115. Patten BM, Bilezikian JP, Mallette LE, et al. Neuromuscular disease in primary hyperparathyroidism. Ann Intern Med 1974; 80:182–193.

116. Barreras RF. Calcium and gastric secretion. Gastroenterology 1973; 64:1168–1184.

117. Bess MA, Edis AJ, van Heerden JA. Hyperparathyroidism and pancreatitis. Chance or a causal association? JAMA 1980; 243:246–247.

118. Sitges-Serra A, Alonso M, de Lecea C, et al. Pancreatitis and hyperparathyroidism. Br J Surg 1988; 75:158–160.

119. Watson L. Diagnosis and treatment of hypercalcaemia. BMJ 1972; 2:150–152.

120. Caporale LH, Rosenblatt M. Parathyroid hormone antagonists effective in vivo. Adv Exp Med Biol 1986; 208:315–327.

121. Doppman JL, Marx SJ, Spiegel AM, et al. Treatment of hyperparathyroidism by percutaneous embolization of a mediastinal adenoma. Radiology 1975; 115:37–42.

122. Mitlak BH, Daly M, Potts JT Jr, et al. Asymptomatic primary hyperparathyroidism. J Bone Miner Res 1991; 6(Suppl. 2): S103–110.

123. Potts JT Jr. Clinical review 9: Management of asymptomatic hyperparathyroidism. J Clin Endocrinol Metab 1990; 70:1489–1493.

124. Ross AJ. Parathyroid surgery in children. Prog Pediatr Surg 1991; 26:48–59.

125. Wang CA. Surgery of the parathyroid glands (review) Adv Surg 1971; 5:109–127.

126. Wells SA, Gunnells JC, Shelburne JD, et al. Transplantation of the parathyroid glands in man: clinical indications and results. Surgery 1975; 78:34–44.

127. Brennan MF, Brown EM, Sears HF, et al. Human parathyroid cryopreservation: in vitro testing of function by parathyroid hormone release. Ann Surg 1978; 187:87–90.

128. Brasier AR, Wang CA, Nussbaum SR. Recovery of parathyroid hormone secretion after parathyroid adenomectomy. J Clin Endocrinol Metab 1988; 66:495–500.

129. David L, Anast CS. Calcium metabolism in newborn infants. The interrelationship of parathyroid function and calcium, magnesium, and phosphorus metabolism in normal, "sick," and hypocalcemic newborns. J Clin Invest 1974; 54:287–296.

130. Peacock M. Calcium absorption efficiency and calcium requirements in children and adolescents. Am J Clin Nutr 1991; 54:261S–265S.

131. Brasier AR, Nussbaum SR. Hungry bone syndrome: clinical and biochemical predictors of its occurrence after parathyroid surgery. Am J Med 1988; 84:654–660.

34

Rickets and Other Disorders of Vitamin D and Phosphate Metabolism

Joseph M. Gertner

New York Hospital–Cornell University Medical Center, New York, New York

I. INTRODUCTION

The recognition of rickets as a deforming bone disease of childhood is centuries old. Early in the twentieth century, Huldschinsky (1), in Vienna, made the critical observation that artificial sunlight could cure and prevent rickets, and Mellanby, working in England, showed that a lipid-soluble substance made in the skin or ingested in the diet was necessary to prevent rickets (2). This substance was classified among the essential food factors and called vitamin D, although it differs from true vitamins in that mammals, including humans, can synthesize it in vivo. The most recent 30 years have seen the recognition that vitamin D needs to be activated, via hepatic and renal hydroxylations, to 1,25-dihydroxyvitamin D (calcitriol) and that the latter is a hormone the production of which is sensitive to hormonal, metabolic, and nutritional regulation. Calcitriol is a sterol derived from cholesterol with considerable structural homology to the adrenal and gonadal steroids. Its principal actions are mediated by the binding of calcitriol to a specific intracellular receptor of the steroid, thyroid, retinoic acid class, followed by interaction of the hormone-receptor complex with the nucleus, where it acts to regulate the transcription of certain specific genes.

In the midtwentieth century, Winters in North Carolina and Prader in Zurich described forms of rickets that did not respond to standard replacement therapy with vitamin D. Winter's discovery eventually led to an appreciation of the role of non–vitamin D-dependent mineral (particularly phosphate) metabolism in skeletal development, and the observation by Prader opened a field of inquiry that would eventually link the pathophysiology of vitamin D metabolism and calcitriol-receptor interactions to skeletal disorders in childhood. The present chapter covers the morphologic manifestations of rickets and the associated skeletal histopathology. The specific clinical and biochemical features of rickets as a result of disorders of nutrition, vitamin D metabolism, and calcitriol-receptor interaction are then reviewed. Next, I cover the skeletal effects of phosphate depletion, particularly renal phosphate wasting. Finally, rickets and rickets-like conditions caused by renal failure and less common nutritional, metabolic, and genetic disorders are reviewed.

A. Nomenclature

Rickets can be caused by a number of distinct abnormalities of vitamin D intake and metabolism and of mineral homeostasis. As the underlying causes of the varieties of rickets are discovered, more rational names can be applied to individual rachitic syndromes. The names "vitamin D-resistant rickets" and "renal rickets" are no longer used because they may be applied to a number of conditions that do not resolve with nutritionally adequate doses of vitamin D or that are attributable to a variety of defects in renal function, respectively. International consultations designed to develop a logical and uniformly acceptable nomenclature are currently being held. The names of the various kinds of rickets given in this chapter have been selected as the most unambiguous and informative with regard to etiology.

B. Definition

Rickets is a bone disease of childhood resulting from the undermineralization of the cartilaginous epiphyseal growth plate. Rickets is confined to childhood because the growth plate exists only when the skeleton is growing. Widening and flaring of the epiphysis is seen with all forms. Softening of the skull (craniotabes) leading to permanent frontal bossing occurs when the onset is in infancy. The ribs (costochondral junctions), ankles, wrists, and knees are other sites commonly affected in growing children. The severity of involvement of particular epiphyses depends on the relative growth rate, which varies with age. The equivalent in adults is a generalized softening of the skeleton caused by a reduction in mineralization, known as osteomalacia. Children with rickets often also suffer from osteomalacia, so that the shafts of the long bone as well as the growth plates are affected (Fig. 1).

C. Structural and Clinical Pathology

Although some characteristics of rickets vary with the cause, the widening and flaring of the epiphysis is seen with all forms. Frontal bossing occurs when the onset is in infancy. The ribs (costochondral junctions), ankles, wrists, and knees are other sites commonly affected in growing children. The severity of involvement of particular epiphyses depends on the relative growth rate, which varies with age.

Deformity as a result of uneven epiphyseal growth and softening of the long bones is common in severe cases. The nature of the deformity is age dependent. The arms may be affected when used for weight bearing in babies. The typical lower limb deformity is genu varum when the age of onset is under 3 or 4 years and genu valgum when rickets starts in school-age children. These differences may be caused by the changing relative rates of growth at various epiphyses.

D. Extraskeletal Clinical Features

The structural and orthopedic features of the various types of rickets are similar, but this is not true of the extraskeletal manifestations of the conditions that lead to rickets. Hypocalcemia leading to tetany and seizures occurs in vitamin D deficiency and related disorders but not in rickets because of phosphate depletion. Many types of rickets are associated with weakness and myopathy; others are not. Other nonskeletal tissues are also involved in selected forms of rickets, including the hair in calcitriol resistance and the teeth in familial hypophosphatemia. Because of this heterogeneity, nonskeletal manifestations are described under the heading of each individual type of rickets.

II. NUTRITIONAL RICKETS

Although nutritional deficiencies of calcium and phosphate can give rise to rickets, the term "nutritional rickets" is generally reserved for the disease that results from a deficiency of vitamin D. Nutritional rickets, once the scourge of poorer children in industrial northern countries, is now largely a disease of developing nations. However, cases occur in the United States and other advanced industrial countries, posing a significant challenge to preventative health services in these countries.

A. Symptomatology

Vitamin D deficiency rickets can present at any age during childhood. In severely endemic areas, the deformities and hypocalcemia of rickets may exist at birth (neonatal rickets). When it presents at birth, the softening of the skull (craniotabes) and the neuromuscular consequences of hypocalcemia dominate the clinical picture. More typically, it appears in toddlers aged between 1 and 2 years with a triad of deformity, weakness, and bone pain (Fig. 2). Most frequently, there is enlargement of the epiphyseal growth plates at the ankles and wrists and expansion of the growth plates at the costochondral junctions (rachitic rosary). The lower limbs may be bowed (genu varum), especially if the child is walking. Because of the proximal muscle weakness of vitamin D deficiency and possibly because of bone pain, a child who had been walking may become reluctant to walk and revert to crawling or

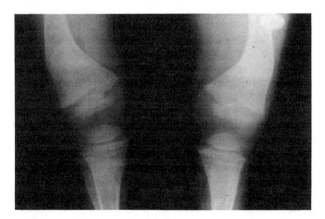

Figure 1 Widening of the epiphyses indicates rickets, and the bending of the lower femoral shafts demonstrates the accompanying osteomalacia in a 5-year-old boy with Fanconi syndrome as a result of cystinosis.

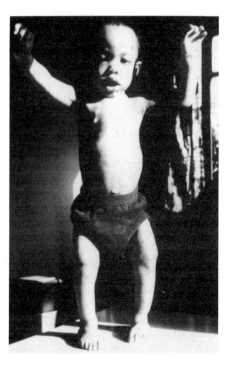

Figure 2 Long-standing nutritional rickets. Note the frontal bossing, rachitic rosary of the costochondral junctions, and deformities of the lower limbs.

shuffling. There may be tenderness on pressure over the long bones. Growth and weight gain may be impaired either because of a specific deficit in long bone growth because of vitamin D deficiency or generalized undernutrition of which the vitamin D deficiency is only a part. Associated hypocalcemia may lead to tetany or seizures.

In older children the presentation of nutritional rickets tends to be more subtle, with the gradual appearance of genu varum up to the middle of the first decade and with a knock-kneed or genu valgum deformity occurring in preadolescents. In this age group, as in infants, vitamin D deficiency may also present with hypocalcemia with little or no physical or radiologic evidence of skeletal disease. Such children may have a hypocalcemic seizure, or they may complain of distressing paresthesias or tetany.

B. Radiology

The characteristic radiologic changes of rickets are widening, cupping, and fraying of the epiphyses (Fig. 3), together with metaphseal distortion from osteomalacia with malalignment of the long bones resulting from both the epiphyseal and metaphyseal changes. The sites at which these changes are seen vary with the age of the patient and with the etiology of the rickets. In infants the wrists and ankles are most likely to show abnormalities, along with the costochondral junctions. In metabolic bone disease of prematurity rickets is often detected at chest x-ray, not only from the costochondral junctions but also because of abnormalities of the proximal humeral and medial clavicular epiphyses. In older children the major epiphyseal changes are more often seen at the knees and hips. The last epiphysis to fuse at adolescence is the iliac

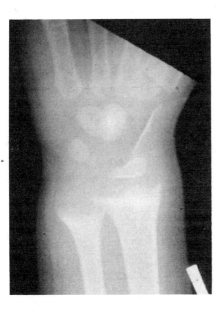

Figure 3 Cupping, fraying, and widening of the epiphyses at the wrist in a young child with nutritional rickets.

crest, which may therefore show rachitic changes in mature teenagers when all other epiphyses are closed. When rickets is treated the widened epiphyses calcify, often to a density higher than seen in the x-rays of healthy children.

In familial hypophosphatemic rickets (FHR), the upper limbs and costochondral junctions tend to be spared and the major impact falls on the lower limbs. The fraying of the upper tibial epiphysis is often much more marked medially than laterally.

The osteomalacic bending of long bones (Fig. 1) is not often seen today except in long-standing disease or in those varieties of rickets (such as calcitriol resistance) that have no effective treatment. Malaligment of the lower limbs, on the other hand, is common. Young children tend to show a bowlegged deformity (genu varum), but rickets of onset in an older age group often gives rise to the opposite, knock-kneed (genu valgum) deformity. In contrast to the epiphyseal changes, the changes in alignment do not resolve rapidly with treatment. They may resolve slowly, however, as remodeling and growth proceed over the years following successful treatment of the rickets.

C. Biochemical Changes (Table 1)

The biochemical abnormalities in nutritional rickets are a subset of the biochemical disturbances seen in rickets generally. In almost all cases of rickets, bone turnover rates are increased and the attempt to synthesize new osteoid is accompanied by an elevation in serum alkaline phosphatase levels. Serum calcium is usually low, although cases of significant vitamin D deficiency rickets may have normal serum calcium, presumably as a result of parathyroid compensation. The hyperparathyroidism leads to phosphaturia and hypophosphatemia. Eventually parathyroid compensation becomes inadequate and serum calcium falls. Finally, the renal tubule may lose its sensitivity to parathyroid hormone (3), with the result that the renal tubular threshold for phosphate rises with a corresponding increase in serum phosphorus (4). Vitamin D metabolite levels reflect the nutritional deprivation. The most abundant metabolite in the plasma, the level of which most closely reflects vitamin D nutritional status, is calcidiol.

D. Epidemiology

A dietary history may reveal prolonged breast-feeding, a failure to take prescribed vitamin supplements, or, in countries where milk is fortified with vitamin D, an aversion to or intolerance for milk. Disorders of the alimentary tract may also contribute to nutritional rickets, most notably gluten-sensitive enteropathy (5), biliary atresia (6), and surgical short-gut syndromes (7).

Anticonvulsant rickets is a special case of vitamin D deficiency rickets. Patients taking phenobarbital and phenytoin were noted over 20 years ago to have an increased incidence of raised alkaline phosphatase and an increased risk of rickets. (8). Subsequent work has shown that phenytoin may be responsible for a variety of relatively mild distur-

Table 1 Biochemical Abnormalities in Various Types of Rickets[a]

Type of rickets	Ca^{2+}	Phosphate	Alkaline phosphatase	HCO$_3^-$	PTH	Cacifediol	Calcitriol
Nutritional	↓	↓ N or ↑	↑	N	↑	↓	↓ N or ↑
1α-Hydroxylase deficiency	↓	↓	↑	N	↑	N	↓
Calcitriol resistance	↓	↓	↑	N	↑	N	↑
Familial hypophosphatemic	N	↓	↑	N	N or ↑	N	N
HHRH	N	↓	↑	N	↓	N	↑
Tumor rickets	N	↓	↑	N	N	N	↓ or N
McCune-Albright syndrome	N	↓	↑	N	N	N	N
Uremia	↓ N or ↑	↑	↑	↓	↑↑	N	↓
Fanconi syndrome	N	↓	↑	↓	↑	N	↓ or N
Hypophosphatasia	N	↑	↓	N	N	N	N
Epiphyseal dysplasia	N	N	N	N	N	N	N

bances of calcium and bone mineral metabolism. These are not necessarily related to vitamin D. Phenobarbital, however, by inducing enzymes that catalyze the hepatic conjugation of vitamin D metabolites, can increase the rate of loss of vitamin D from the body, giving rise to vitamin D deficiency in subjects with marginal states of vitamin D nutrition.

E. Treatment

The treatment of vitamin D deficiency rickets is to provide adequate but not excessive replacement doses of vitamin D. With the recommended daily allowance of vitamin D in childhood at 400 IU (10 μg) we have found that four to five times this dose (i.e., 1600–2000 IU/day) almost always reverses the biochemical and structural changes of vitamin D deficiency. Alkaline phosphatase may rise initially (the so-called flare effect) but after 2–4 weeks begins to fall toward normal. This approach to treatment constitutes a "diagnosis by therapy" because unusual and unexpected forms of resistance to standard doses of vitamin D do not respond to replacement doses and then become the focus of more extensive investigations. Treatment may be discontinued when all physical, radiologic, and biochemical fractures of rickets have been reversed and the family counseled on dietary and lifestyle changes that can provide the child with the recommended daily allowance (RDA) of vitamin D.

One group of patients who do not respond to vitamin D in doses of four to five times the RDA is that with severe malabsorption syndrome. In such patients vitamin D should be given intramuscularly, using 100,000–200,000 units. If the malabsorption cannot be reversed by specific therapy, the dose can be repeated after some weeks or months as biochemical indices of osteomalacia begin to worsen again. There is no place for using the hydroxylated metabolites of vitamin D

(calcidiol and calcitriol) in the treatment of rickets caused vitamin D deficiency.

F. Prevention

Vitamin D deficiency rickets can be prevented in healthy children by permitting adequate exposure to sunlight and/or by ensuring an adequate dietary intake of the vitamin. Although the majority of the U.S. population is believed to receive most of its vitamin D from solar irradiation (9), this may not apply to impoverished persons living in crowded surroundings or to those immobilized by disability. To target these children and others who may be at risk, the U.S. government has ordered the fortification of milk with vitamin D since the 1930s. In many other advanced countries this policy is not followed, and this difference in public policy may well account for the higher incidence of vitamin D deficiency in the United Kingdom and other European counties compared with the United States. Children who do not receive dairy milk may be at increased risk for vitamin D deficiency unless they receive adequate sunshine exposure. This includes infants and lactose-intolerant, vegan, or other milk-averse individuals. Formula-fed infants can be assumed to be receiving adequate nutritional vitamin D. Breast-fed babies, however, can receive dietary vitamin D only insofar as the mother is herself adequately nourished. Most of the infantile rickets seen in the United States comes from this breast-fed group. Breast-fed babies and milk-avoiding growing children should receive vitamin D supplementation according to the RDA, which is 400 IU.

Although U.S. Food and Drug Administration guidelines specify that milk should be fortified with 400 IU per quart (~900 ml), recent reports from Holick and colleagues have shown that many milk samples are inadequately or far too heavily fortified (10). In some cases this has led to vitamin

D intoxication and consequent hypercalcemia in heavy drinkers of milk (11).

III. DISORDERS OF VITAMIN D METABOLISM (TABLE 2)

As noted, Vitamin D is activated by two hydroxylation steps catalyzed by the hepatic microsomal cytochrome P_{450} enzyme, vitamin D 25-hydroxylase, and the renal mitochondrial cytochrome P_{450}, 25-hydroxyvitamin D 1α-hydroxylase, respectively. Defective activation can occur if sufficient enzyme-bearing tissue is not available, if enzyme activity is inhibited by the hormonal and ionic milieu, and when genetic disease has reduced or destroyed enzyme activity. In practice, much redundancy exists in the availablity of enzyme for the 25-hydroxylation of vitamin D, so that hepatic cirrhosis is not accompanied by a deficiency of calcidiol unless associated biliary obstruction leads to fat malabsorption causing substrate (vitamin D) deficiency. No genetic syndrome caused by a deficiency of vitamin D 25-hydroxylase has been recognized to date.

The formation of calcitriol in the kidney is tightly regulated and can be pathologically inhibited by a lack of renal tissue or by an excessive extracellular fluid concentration of inorganic phosphate. These conditions prevail in renal failure, which is discussed later. Rarely, however, the 1α-hydroxylation of calcidiol may be defective in the absence of any other renal dysfunction. The types of rickets attributable to disorders of vitamin D nutrition and metabolism are summarized in Table 1.

A. Calciferol Deficiency Rickets (Vitamin D Dependency Type I, or Pseudodeficiency Rickets)

In 1961, Prader and colleagues (12) described an autosomal recessively inherited form of persistent infantile rickets they named pseudodeficiency rickets. The name arises from the close resemblance of the disease to vitamin D deficiency, the major clinical differences lying in the early onset and severity of the rickets and the failure to respond to replacement doses of vitamin D. A few years later, Fraser, Scriver, and colleagues noted that pseudodeficiency rickets, also called vitamin D dependency rickets, could be treated with small doses of calcitriol. The condition thus became the first inborn error of vitamin D deficiency to be recognized as such (13). The concept of an abnormality of 1α-hydroxylation was supported when radioreceptor assays for vitamin D metabolites showed patients with pseudodeficiency rickets to have normal levels of calcidiol and very low levels of calcitriol. The presumption is that the disease is caused by a mutation of the gene for the 1α-hydroxylase. Although the trait for

Table 2 Classification of Hypophosphatemic Rickets

Class of rickets	MIM no.[a]	Inheritance	Comment
Isolated phosphaturia			
Low urine calcium			
Familial hypophosphatemic rickets	307800	X-linked dominant	Relatively common
Autosomal hypophosphatemic rickets	241520	Autosomal recessive	Very rare, phenotypically identical to 307800
Tumor rickets	—	Not familial	
McCune-Albright syndrome	174800	Not familial	Activation of receptor G proteins
High urine calcium: hereditary hypophosphatemic rickets with hypercalciuria	241530	Autosomal recessive	Mile cases may have nephrolithiasis only
Fanconi syndrome (proximal tubular failure			
Cystinosis	219800	Autosomal recessive	Lysosomal cystine storage; progressive uremia
Dent's disease	310468	X linked	May be a variant of "X-linked nephropathy"

[a]McKusick, V. A., Mendelian Inheritance in Man, Catalogs of Autosomal Dominant, Recessive, and X-Linked Phenotypes, (Tenth Edition) Vol. 1., The Johns Hopkins University Press, Baltimore and London, 1992.

pseudodeficiency rickets has been mapped to 12q13–14 (14), the hydroxylase had, in mid-1994, not yet been cloned.

Undiagnosed or untreated Vitamin D dependency; type I can lead to severe deformity, accompanied by hypocalcemia and weakness. However, the disease is readily amenable to treatment with physiologic replacement doses of calcitriol (0.5–2.0 μg/day).

B. Vitamin D Dependency Type II: Calcitriol Resistance (Vitamin D-Dependent Rickets Type II)

In 1978, two groups independently described patients who appeared to have vitamin D dependency type I but in whom circulating levels of calcitriol were very high. The patients of Marx et al. (15) were siblings with severe hypocalcemic rickets who responded to treatment with high doses of vitamin D_2 or of calcitriol. Three families were described independently 2 years later (from Israel, the United States, and Japan) in which this type of rickets was associated with severe alopecia. The inheritance pattern of the disease and the high frequency of consanguinity in affected kindreds strongly suggest recessive inheritance. The biochemical features resemble those of calcitriol deficiency except that calcitriol levels are high. The patient's condition resists the administration of calcitriol, although some patients respond to doses as high as 12.5–20 μg/day. Carefully conducted therapeutic trials have shown that the osteopathy of vitamin D dependency type II can be sharply improved by the intravenous infusion of calcium (16). This is of practical importance because resistance to vitamin D metabolites may be nearly complete in affected patients, offering no other chance for normal bone development. The finding is also of theoretical importance because it implies that the major contribution of calcitriol to skeletal mineralization is the provision of ionized calcium to the extracellular milieu rather than a direct action of calcitriol on bone cells.

The pathogenetic mechanism underlying vitamin D dependency type II is resistance to calcitriol, which has been demonstrated at the subcellular level. The calcitriol receptor may fail to bind hormone because of a mutation at the hormone binding site (17). Alternatively, receptor binding may be normal but hormone action is prevented by impaired interaction of the hormone-receptor complex with the nucleus because of mutations of the DNA binding "zinc fingers" (18). In other cases of clear-cut calcitriol resistance, mutations are apparently absent from both the hormone and the DNA binding regions (19). It is of interest that alopecia accompanies cases of calcitriol resistance of various genetic causes, indicating that normal hair growth may have a direct requirement for functional calcitriol receptors.

IV. PHOSPHATE HOMEOSTASIS AND ITS DISORDERS

A. Physiology of Phosphate Homeostasis

Phosphorus exists in the body largely as phosphate ion bound to organic molecules to form organophosphates. In the serum,

about two-thirds of circulating phosphate forms part of such organic molecules bound to protein, but one-third is unbound and is measured after separation from the bound form as "inorganic phosphate (P_i)." Concentrations of phosphate in the serum are given in molar units or in mass units, which refer to the quantity of elemental phosphorus within molecules of inorganic phosphate.

The systems that control phosphate homeostasis tend to regulate total-body phosphate content rather than, as in the case of calcium, absolute ionic concentration in the extracellular fluid. This difference accords with the different extracellular roles of calcium and phosphate. Tight control of extracellular Ca^{2+} is essential for the correct function of calcium-dependent cellular activation processes. In contrast, the function of extraskeletal phosphate is mostly as intracellular organophosphates providing intermediaries in energy metabolism, signaling systems, and the genetic code. In accord with these observations is that no well-characterized hormonal system operates primarily to regulate serum phosphate concentration. Instead it is total-body phosphate that is sensed and regulated.

The intestinal absorption of dietary phosphate is largely unregulated, about two-thirds of the phosphate content of digested foodstuffs being absorbed. The regulation of phosphate balance lies almost entirely at the level of the proximal renal tubule, which can vary the rate at which filtered P_i is reabsorbed from the tubular fluid. This reabsorption, which normally accounts for 85–95% of filtered P_i, is facilitated by one or more saturable, sodium-dependent transporters located on the brush-border membrane. Two genes coding for such transporters in the human were recently cloned. Theoretically, the causes of disorders of phosphate homeostasis could be attributable to intrinsic disorders of one or more of these transporter systems or to dysregulation of their function.

1. Dietary Regulation

The renal tubular reabsorption of P_i is extraordinarily sensitive to the dietary intake of phosphorus, specifically to the relationship of the intake of phosphate to that of total calories. In classic studies defining the phosphate-deprived state, Lotz et al. found a sharp reduction in urinary phosphate excretion, increased calciuria, and such symptoms as muscle weakness (20). The reduction in urinary phosphate excretion is rapid, occurring before there is time for serum phosphate to fall significantly, thus leading to the view that there exists a diet-sensitive hormonal system regulating urinary phosphate excretion. The mechanism whereby such a system might influence renal tubular phosphate transport is not known.

2. Parathyroid Hormone (PTH) and PTH-Related Protein (PTHrP)

Although primarily functioning as a regulator of Ca^{2+}, PTH also affects renal phosphate control by inducing phosphaturia. Patients with hyperparathyroidism are hypophosphatemic, and conversely, hypoparathyroidism is associated with hyperphosphatemia. PTHrP, circulating in excess in patients with humoral hypercalcemia of malignancy, leads to hypophosphatemia, presumably because of the interaction of PTHrP with renal PTH receptors.

3. Vitamin D Endocrine System

The adequacy of phosphate nutrition and the level of P_i in the serum are major regulators of the renal 1α-hydroxylation of calcidiol to calcitriol. Calcitriol levels are generally high during phosphate deprivation and in the face of hypophosphatemia and are depressed by phosphate excess. Although phosphate regulates the activation of vitamin D, the converse, a vitamin D effect on phosphate homeostasis, appears to play only a minor part in normal physiology.

4. Insulin, Growth Hormone, and Insulin-like Growth Factor Type I (IGF-I)

Generally, the injection of insulin is accompanied by a profound fall in serum phosphate as phosphate moves into the intracellular compartment. The direct effect of insulin on renal phosphate control was shown to be antiphosphaturic in clamp studies in which glucose was held constant during insulin infusion (21). In diabetic ketoacidosis, renal phosphate losses tend to be high because of the osmotic diuresis and a degree of competition between the proximal tubular transport systems for phosphate and glucose. The shift of phosphate into the intracellular compartment upon treatment with insulin can lead to profound hypophosphatemia in these phosphate-depleted patients.

Growth hormone has an antiphosphaturic effect, seen during growth hormone treatment of deficient children and in the disease acromegaly, which is caused by a growth hormone-secreting pituitary tumor. It is now known whether the effect of growth hormone upon the renal tubule is direct or whether it is mediated by the growth hormone-dependent protein insulin-like growth factor I. Exogenously administered IGF-I has an antiphosphaturic action in the human (22), but this does not exclude a parallel direct action of growth hormone.

Physical growth is itself associated with increased serum phosphate levels as a result of an increase in the threshold for tubular phosphate reabsorption during phases of rapid growth. For this reason, normal values for serum phosphate are substantially higher in growing children than in adults. It is now known whether the changes in phosphate threshold at puberty are mediated by IGF-I or growth hormone (GH). Serum phosphate is also high during the rapid growth period of early infancy, but GH, especially IGF-I levels, are quite low in this age group compared with older children.

B. Disordered Control of Serum Phosphate

Because the control of serum phosphate resides primarily in the proximal renal tubules, it follows that disorders of phosphate control are a result of primary tubular dysfunction or that they are secondary to processes that impact upon tubular function. They can be divided broadly into phosphate-retaining and phosphate-wasting states.

1. Hyperphosphatemia

The pathologic states relating to hypoparathyroidism and parathyroid hormone resistance are covered in Chapter N. From the clinical point of view, the most important phosphate-retaining disorder is uremia, which leads to a complex bone disease known as uremic osteodystrophy.

a. Uremic Osteodystrophy. Uremic osteodystrophy (UOD) is a cause of growth failure and limb deformity in children with renal glomerular failure. The symptoms and associated radiologic signs may be present from a very young age and are particularly prominent in congenital obstructive uropathy, which is more common in male infants. Affected children may manifest muscular weakness in addition to growth failure and rickets-like limb deformities. Radiologically the changes may closely resemble rickets, but there is a prominent element of hyperparathyroid bone disease, manifest as subcortical erosions, often at the epipyseal corners. In extreme cases the entire femoral head may become necrotic and disintegrate (the so-called rotting stump appearance). Skeletal sclerosis of the long bones or vertebrae may also be seen. Although there are many causes of growth failure in childhood uremia, UOD is undoubtedly one of the contributing factors (23).

Most of the biochemical abnormalities leading to UOD can be attributed to phosphate retention. This tends to depress serum calcium directly and also indirectly by its inhibitory effect on calcitriol formation (24). In addition, because calcitriol synthesis occurs almost entirely within the kidney, a reduction in renal tissue mass further reduces the capacity to synthesize calcitriol. The bone disease is thus a consequence of chronic parathyroid hypersecretion and the lack of calcitriol. Other etiologic factors in the development of osteodystrophy include the chronic acidosis of uremia.

The observed biochemical abnormalities thus comprise hyperphosphatemia, hyperphosphatasia (as in all states with high skeletal turnover), hyperparathyroidism, and calcitriol deficiency. The development of UOD can be detected noninvasively at an early stage by measuring serum intact PTH(1–84) and can be confirmed by histomorphometric examination of bone biopsy samples (25). Calcitriol levels are suppressed, but calcifdiol levels, reflecting vitamin D nutrition, are generally normal.

The treatment of uremic osteodystrophy consists largely in limiting the accumulation of serum inorganic phosphate and providing supplements of calcitriol. In addition, care must be taken to ensure adequate nutrition, particularly of calcium. Short of renal transplantation, hyperphosphatemia is minimized by dialysis and/or by giving a low-phosphate diet with an oral agent designed to bind phosphate insolubly in the intestine to prevent its absorption. In the past aluminum hydroxide gel was used as a phosphate binder, but because of abundant, if controversial, evidence that aluminum itself contributes to osteodystrophy, its use has largely been abandoned. Recently calcium carbonate, combined with small doses of calcitrol, has replaced aluminum as the phosphate binder of choice (26).

b. Tumoral Calcinosis (Fig. 4). The name of this inherited disorder refers to the lumps or "tumors" of ectopic, amorphously calcified material found in the soft tissues of affected persons, especially around the joints (Fig. 2) and in subcutaneous tissues (27). Affected patients also have dental abnormalities, with hypoplasia of the dental roots. Most but not all cases described in the United States have been in blacks, and the disease may be relatively frequent in parts of Africa (28).

Pathophysiologically, the disease appears to be caused by an inappropriately high "set point" for renal tubular phosphate reabsorption. Serum phosphate is very high, but calcium, calcitriol, and PTH levels are normal and respond in the expected way to phosphate deprivation and phosphate loading. The ectopic calcification is presumably a result of the precipitation of calcium phosphates in a milieu that has a much higher calcium phosphate ion product than healthy extracellular fluid.

Tumoral calcinosis is very rare but is of considerable theoretical importance, not least because its pathophysiology is a mirror image of that the more common phosphate-wasting condition, familial hypophosphatemic rickets. Although the inheritance pattern is recessive in most families, it appears to be an autosomal dominant in at least one large and well-described kindred (29).

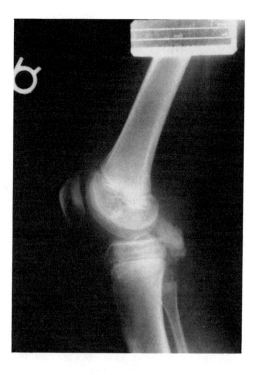

Figure 4 Tumoral calcinosis in a 13-year-old boy. Amorphous calcium phosphate has accumulated in the popliteal space. Serum phosphate was persistently elevated because of excess renal tubular phosphate reabsorption. Renal function and calcitropic hormone levels were normal.

2. Phosphate-Wasting States

These are listed in Table 3. Because they lead to hypophosphatemia, their chief manifestations, when chronic, are rickets and osteomalacia, the general features of which have been discussed. Primary and secondary hyperparathyroidism are discussed under hypercalcemia (Chap. ?) and vitamin D deficiency, respectively.

3. Primary Renal Causes of Hypophosphatemia

a. Familial Hypophosphatemic Rickets. Familial hypophosphatemic rickets, a condition dominated by proximal renal tubular phosphate wasting, is by far the most common cause of this type of phosphaturic rickets.

Rickets appears in the first year of life. The skeletal changes resemble those of vitamin D deficiency, but the lower limbs are much more severely impacted than the upper and the rachitic rosary is not seen. Frontal cranial bossing is common, and rarely there may be a degree of craniosynostosis. There is a striking absence of muscular weakness. Dental deterioration and dental abscess formation are common and may constitute presenting symptoms of the disease. Physical growth is impaired. Untreated, the disease results in severe growth retardation and deformity in males, who are hemizygotes. The course is more variable in heterozygous females, some being seriously affected; in others, short stature or the biochemical finding of a reduced renal tubular resorptive capacity for phosphorus may be the only manifestation.

The biochemical findings (Table 1) are dominated by hypophosphatemia with normocalcemia. The renal tubular phosphate threshold is always subnormal in hypophosphatemic rickets. The normal calcitriol concentration is the face of hypophosphatemia (which generally stimulates calcitriol formation) suggests that the fundamental defect involves vitamin D metabolism as well as renal tubular phosphate transport. This concept is supported by observation that calcitriol formation stimulated by PTH infusion (30) or by phosphate deprivation (31) is impaired in subjects with FHR relative to normal individuals.

FHR is usually inherited as an X-linked dominant (Fig. 5), but there are quite credible reports of similar phenotypes inherited as autosomal dominant and recessive (32) traits. A good animal model for FHR (the *hyp* mouse) exists, but the etiology is still unknown in both the mouse and human disorders. Although the mutation responsible for FHR has been mapped to the Xp.21 region of the X chromosome, the actual gene and its product remain to be identified. Recent evidence derived from work on the *hyp* mouse suggests that the renal tubular phosphate leak is secondary to the action of humeral factors on the kidney rather than to an intrinsic defect of the kidney itself (33).

The aims of treatment in FHR are to reduce deformity and optimize statural growth while minimizing the side effects of therapy. The recognition that FHR is primarily a disease of phosphate wasting led Glorieux et al. (34) to propose a regimen of high-dose phosphate replacement. Such regimens form the mainstay of modern treatment and are always supplemented with a vitamin D preparation, usually calcitriol.

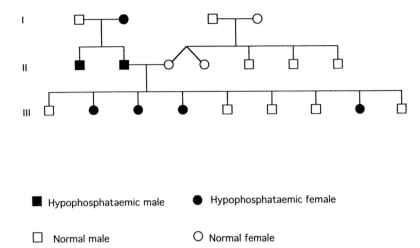

■ Hypophosphataemic male   ● Hypophosphataemic female

□ Normal male   ○ Normal female

Figure 5   Pedigree of a large kindred bearing the trait for familial hypophosphatemic rickets. Note dominant inheritance with absence of male-to-male transmission, typical of an X-linked trait. All affected persons are short and hypophosphatemic, but some of the heterozygote females do not have rachitic deformities.

Phosphate is given as a soluble buffered sodium and/or potassium salt. The dose is calculated in terms of elemental phosphorus and ranges from 0.5 to 1.5 g/day depending on the size of the patient. Emphasis has been placed on the need to space doses as widely as possible over the 24 h to maximize the period over which phosphate concentrations are enhanced. This usually involves waking a young child at night to give five doses every 4 h each day. Calcitriol is given for two reasons: first, even though calcitriol levels are generally normal in untreated FHR, additional supplementation may promote skeletal mineralization. Second, hyperparathyroidism, an unwanted consequence of phosphate supplementation, is minimized by the additional intestinal calcium absorption that follows calcitriol supplementation. The latter is assessed by measuring serum alkaline phosphatase, the most readily accessible marker of bone turnover, urinary calcium excretion, and PTH levels. In affected children, alkaline phosphatase should be below the pediatric upper limit, high levels generally indicating active osteomalacia and requiring higher doses of phosphate. Urinary calcium and PTH measure opposite ends of the spectrum of desirable calcitriol supplementation. This should be increased (and/or the phosphate dose decreased) if PTH is elevated and decreased if urinary calcium excretion is excessive (above 4 mg/kg/day). Occasionally it is impossible to find a therapeutic combination that achieves all these goals. Hyperparathyroidism is unusual in untreated FHR, although the author has observed asymptomatic cases. During phosphate treatment, however, prolonged secondary hyperparathyroidism is common and may lead to autonomous gland hyperfunction. Rarely this has necessitated parathyroidectomy (35). Nephrocalcinosis and occasionally nephrolithiasis occur frequently in affected children. These renal changes are probably consequences of excessive urinary calcium excretion during therapy (36); they rarely lead to significant renal glomerular impairment. Thiazide diuretics, which reduce urinary calcium

excretion, have been used to reduce the chance of renal damage from hypercalciuria, but they are not widely used in treatment. The results of treatment of FHR have been surprisingly controversial. Most modern authors are convinced that deformity is reduced and, perhaps less confidently, that treatment leads to improved adult stature. A trial of human growth hormone showed improvement in growth velocity but a worsening in alkaline phosphatase, reflecting activity of the rickets. Further studies with growth hormone are in progress. Future directiosn in the treatment of FHR include the possible use of 24,25-dihydroxycholecalciferol or syntetic analogs of calcitriol that may aid bone mineralization and reduce secondary hyperparathyroidism during treatment. IGF-I is a potent antiphosphaturic substance (37) and could be tried for a potential effect in FHR. Finally, the characterization of the gene and product responsible for FHR may lead to the design of more rational therapy directly targeted at the celluar cause of the phosphaturia.

b. Hereditary Hypophosphatemic Rickets with Hypercalciuria and Dent's Disease. A low urinary calcium excretion is a biochemical feature common to most types of rickets, including vitamin D deficiency, vitamin D dependency and resistance, and X-linked hypophosphatemia. However, two apparently separate syndromes are known in which hypophosphatemic rickets is accompanied by hypercalciuria.

In 1985, Tieder et al. (38) described an inbred Bedouin family, many members of which had short stature with rickets of infantile onset. Affected subjects had profound hypophosphatemia, parathyroid suppression, elevated calcitriol levels, and marked hypercalciuria, in contrast to FHR patients suffer from severe muscular weakness. In other described cases, the rickets may be relatively mild, without significant growth impairment.

This form of hypercalciuric rickets, hereditary hypophosphatemic rickets with hypercalciuria (HHRH), is a rare, autosomal recessive inherited condition in which renal phosphate wasting leads to the "expected" elevation in calcitriol concentrations. Thus, the condition stands in contrast to FHR, in which calcitriol levels are low despite phosphate wasting and hypophosphatemia. As a consequence of elevated calcitriol levels affected subjects may hyperabsorb calcium, which leads to the excessive urinary calcium excretion with resulting nephrolithiasis. Most cases have been described in Middle Eastern and North African populations, but the apparently sporadic cases have been seen in North Americans of English and Irish backgrounds.

Unlike X-linked familial hypophosphatemic rickets, HHRH has proved relatively easy to control with oral phosphate. Because calcitriol levels are high in the disease and PTH is suppressed, there is no need to supplement with a vitamin D metabolite and no danger of secondary or autonomous hyperparathyroidism. In the author's limited experience and in published reports, the response to therapy has been excellent in terms of increased strength, prevention of deformity, and statural growth.

Another type of hypercalciuric rickets, now named Dent's disease, was first described by Dent and Friedman (39). Here hypophosphatemic hypercalciuric rickets is associated with generalized tubulopathy and eventual renal failure. The disease is inherited as an X-linked recessive trait.

c. Tumor (or Oncogenous) Rickets. Hypophosphatemic rickets is occasionally found in children and adults bearing a small mesenchymal tumor, usually benign (40). The tumor is often classified as a hemangiopericytoma, but benign fibromas, some malignant tumors, and nontumorous conditions, such as the linear nevus sebaceus syndrome, have been linked to this type of hypophosphatemia. Resection of the tumor from affected individuals has resulted in complete and rapid resolution of the hypophosphatemia, leading to the inescapable conclusion that the tumor, often very small, must be secreting an intensely phosphaturic substance. Such a substance was recently partially characterized (41). The hypophosphatemia is accompanied by inappropriately low levels of calcitriol, and the degree of osteomalacia or rickets may be severe. Clarification of the mechanism of phosphaturia and the nature of any phosphaturic substance in these cases continues because the condition is clearly of great theoretical importance.

d. McCune-Albright Syndrome. Also called polyostotic fibrous dysplasia, this is a pervasive multisystemic disease of childhood onset that appears to be nonfamilial. Patients show a progressive fibrosis and deformity of bone affecting noncontiguous parts of the skeleton, although completely normal bony architecture is preserved elsewhere. The fibrous dysplasia may lead to pain, weakness, and fractures, with associated disturbances of gait. Children with fibrous dysplasia often manifest hyperactivity of one or more endocrine systems, particularly precocious puberty, thyrotoxicosis, and acromegaly. They also show large, irregularly shaped pigmented skin nevi that are characteristic of the disease. Many of these children have a phosphaturic

state that can lead to rickets and osteomalacia, with worsening of the bone pain and deformity.

Recent work, recognizing that most of the manifestations of the disease can be explained by hyperresponsiveness of cyclic AMP-dependent hormone receptors, demonstrated that McCune-Albright syndrome is caused by somatic mutations in the gene coding for the α_s subunit of the G proein gene that controls the regulation of such receptors (42). The receptors are thus constitutively activated even though the target organs are not exposed to high levels of the hormonal or other stimulus that would normally be required for activation. In this model the hypophosphatemia would presumably be a result of activation of renal tubular PTH receptors in the absence of excessive PTH concentrations.

e. Generalized Tubulopathies. This group of disorders is characterized by excessive urinary losses of all the factors primarily reabsorbed from the proximal tubular fluid. These include glucose, phosphate, bicarbonate, and amino acids. Genetic causes are generally responsible for proximal tubular failure in children.

i. Cystinosis. Severe Fanconi syndrome is seen in cystinosis, an autosomal recessive lysosomal storage disease in which cystine accumulates intracellularly. The onset is in infancy, with failure to thrive and rickets. Affected children are hypophosphatemic and acidotic and go on to develop proressive renal glomerular failure. Treatment with phosphate supplements, calcitriol, and alkalinizing agents, such as the citrates of sodium, potassium, or magnesium, can ameliorate the bone disease. However, until recently only renal transplantation could prevent early death from uremia. The introduction of cysteamine and related sulfur-containing compounds to reverse lysosomal cystine overload and preserve renal cell function has greatly improved the prognosis in this formerly fatal disease (43).

ii. Other Causes of Fanconi syndrome. Genetic conditions in which the impact of the associated Fanconi syndrome is relatively minor include Lowe syndrome (cause of tubular failure unknown) and Wilson's disease and type I glycogen storage disease, recessive conditions of copper and carbohydrate metabolism, respectively. Another form of Fanconi syndrome that has attracted interest recently is Dent's disease.

C. Nonrenal Disorders: Dietary Phosphate Insufficiency Including Metabolic Bone Disease of Prematurity (MBDP)

Dietary phosphate deficiency is very uncommon in adults and older children and is usually seen in association with the abuse of aluminum-containing antacid gels, which bind phosphorus in the gastrointestinal tract. In the premature infant, however, a bone disease that encompasses a spectrum of disturbances resulting in rickets, osteomalacia, and osteoporosis may occur as a result of an oral or parenteral intake insufficient in phosphorus. The spectrum of severity of milder MBDP is reflected in the classification shown in Table IV. Milder cases may show only biochemical changes. The frequency of MBDP varies depending on the diagnostic criteria. In one prospective radiologic survey, fractures were detected in 20% of newborns with a birth weight of less than 1500 g and gestational age less than 34 weeks. Subclinical disease may be more common, as suggested by the prevalence of elevated serum alkaline phosphatase and decreased bone mineral content. Biochemical abnormalities may be detectable as early as 2 weeks after birth, with radiologic changes noted as early as 4 weeks and or late as 20 weeks of life. The long-term prognosis of MBDP is quite good, with little evidence of persistent skeletal morbidity as these infants grow on into childhood.

The primary cause of MBDP is a deficiency of phosphate and calcium as a result of decreased intake (Fig. 6). Initial reports of MBDP involved infants fed human milk and parenterally fed sick neonates often with respiratory disease. Human milk is relatively low in calcium and phosphate. Infants on parenteral alimentation are at risk because of the low mineral concentration in the infusion fluid.

Of calcium and phosphate accretion for the fetal skeleton, 80% occurs during the third trimester by active transport across the placenta (Fig. 4). After premature delivery an infant taking 150–200 ml/kg/day of human milk receives each day only 25–50% of the phosphorus and 35–70% of the calcium accumulated daily in utero during the third trimester. A standard formula provides only 55–90% of the phosphorus and 45–100% of the calcium. Adequate mineral delivery via total parenteral nutrition (TPN) is confounded by the difficulty of maintaining the solubility of concentrated mixtures of calcium and phosphorus.

Biochemical tests may detect early MBDP. An alkaline phosphatase level that is more than five times the maximum adult level may suggest MBDP even in an infant who is not on TPN and has no radiologic bone disease. Most preterm

infants, including those with bone disease, appear to have normal levels of calcidiol and calcitriol and are able to absorb calcium and phosphorus efficiently from the intestine. In some cases with MBDP, calcitriol levels are elevated, probably because of the stimulation by hypophosphatemia.

The prevention and treatment of MBDP have been the subject of extensive investigation. The Committee on Nutrition of the American Academy of Pediatrics (44) recommended calcium and phosphorus supplementation of the formula used to feed premature infants to match the expected fetal accretion rate of these minerals. Special formulas for this purpose are available despite the difficulty of maintaining high concentrations of calcium and phosphates in solution together. The recommendation for infants weighing 800–1200 g is for a calcium intake of 210 mg/kg/day; in parenterally fed babies, 30–40 mg/kg/day of both calcium and phosphorus should be given.

V. RICKETS-LIKE CONDITIONS

A. Hypophosphatasia

This term is used for a group of inherited diseases characterized by variable defects in bone mineralization, absent or subnormal serum alkaline phosphatase (ALP) activity, and an excess of natural ALP substrates in the blood or urine. The severity is inversely related to the age of onset, which ranges from perinatal to adult. In addition to rickets-like bone deformity, affected children frequently show early loss of teeth. Serum ALP levels are low, but levels may fluctuate and may not correlate closely with clinical severity. Urinary excretion of phosphoethanolamine and inorganic pyrophos-

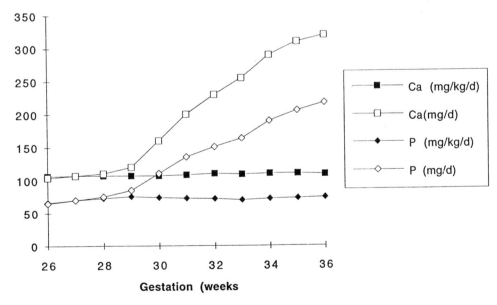

Figure 6 Accumulation of calcium and phosphorus in the normal fetus approaching term. Note that mineral needs on a weight-adjusted basis are stable but that in absolute terms demands rise steeply after 30–32 weeks. Reproduced with permission from Oski, FA, DeAngelis, CD, Feigin, RD, McMillan, JA, and Warshaw, JB (ed.), Principles and Practice of Pediatrics, F. A. Oski (ed.), J. B. Lippincott Co., Philadelphia, 1989 (2nd Edition), pp. 448–458.

phate is increased, and in severe forms, serum pyridoxal 5′-phosphate levels are also high. All these appear to be naturally occurring substrates for tissue-nonspecific alkaline phosphatase (TNSALP). The disease is caused by homozygosity or compound heterozygosity for deletions or mutations in the TNSALP gene (45).

The alkaline phosphatases are a family of enzymes that hydrolyze organic phosphates at alkaline pH. Recent advances permit a clearer understanding of the relationship between the ALPs and some insight into the reasons that ALP levels are elevated or depressed in cerain disease states. Five members of the ALP family are recognized: tissue nonspecific, placental, placental-like, and intestinal. The tissue nonspecific form is further subdivided into bone, liver, and renal forms. The TNSALPs appear to be coded by a gene localized to 1p36.1-p34, and the others have been mapped to 2q34–q37. The differences between forms arising from the same gene (e.g., bone and liver) are a result of tissue-dependent posttranslational modifications. Although assays for the ALPs are among tissue-dependent posttranslational modifications. Although assays for the ALPs are among the oldest established and most performed of clinical chemistry measurements, the lack of enzymic specificity limits the value of such assays in evaluating skeletal disorders. Specificity for bone alkaline phosphatase can be enhanced by heat inactivation of the enzyme before assay because bone ALP is much less stable than the liver enzyme at 65°C. The development of radioimmunoassays specific for bone ALP has further improved the specificity of assay for bone ALP. Serum levels of alkaline phosphatase are expressed in units based on the rate of hydrolysis of an artificial substrate. Levels are higher in growing children than in adults, with a generally accepted upper limit of three times the upper margin for adults.

B. Epiphyseal Dysplasias

These types of deforming bone disease are generally inherited as autosomal dominant trails. Until recently they were not classified as metabolic bone diseases and their etiology was completely mysterious. In the last few years, work combining gene-mapping techniques with an examination of appropriately located candidate genes has shown that mutations in genes coding for collagen and possibly other bone matrix proteins can explain these skeletal dysplasias (46). The nosology and classification of these diseases is beyond the scope of this chapter. However, it should be mentioned that at least one of the skeletal dysplasias, epiphyseal dysplasia, Schmidt type, may be confused radiologically with some types of chronic metabolic rickets. The distinction can be made on simple biochemical grounds because these patients never show abnormalities of calcium, phosphate, or alkaline phosphatase. Appropriate diagnosis is important for the prevention of unneccessary procedures aimed at identifying the more classic "metabolic bone diseases" and for the provision of accurate genetic counseling.

REFERENCES

1. Huldschinsky K. Heilung von Rachitis durch künstliche Hohensonne. Dtsch. Med. Wochenschr. 1919; 45:712–713.
2. Mellanby E. An experimental investigation on rickets. Lancet 1919; 1:407–412.
3. Kruse K, Bartels H, Kracht U. Parathyroid function in different stages of vitamin D deficiency rickets. Eur J Pediatr 1984; 141:158–162.
4. Robinson D, Flynn D, Dandona P. Hyperphosphataemic rickets in an Asian infant. BMJ 1985; 290:1318–1319.
5. Stenhammar L. Coeliac disease presenting as vitamin D deficiency rickets in a vegetarian child (letter). Acta Paediatr Scand 1985; 74:972–973.
6. Vanderpas JB, Koopman BJ, Cadranel S, et al. Malabsorption of liposoluble vitamins in a child with bile acid deficiency. J Pediatr Gastroenterol Nutr 1987; 6:33–41.
7. Touloukian RJ, Gertner JM. Vitamin D. deficiency rickets as a late complication of the short gut syndrome during infancy. J Pediatr Surg 1981; 16:230–235.
8. Kruse K, Bartels H, Gunther H. Serum alkaline phosphatase isoenzymes in epileptic children receiving anticonvulsant drugs. Eur J Pediatr 1977; 126:237–242.
9. McKenna MJ. Differences in vitamin D status between countries in young adults and the elderly. Am J Med 1992; 93:69–77.
10. Holick MF, Shao Q, Liu WW, Chen TC. The vitamin D content of fortified milk and infant formula. N Engl J Med 1992; 326:1178–1181.
11. Jacobus CH, Holick MF, Shao Q, et al. Hypervitaminosis D associated with drinking milk. N Engl J Med 1992; 326:1193–1197.
12. Prader A, Illig R, Heierli E. Eine besondere Form der primaeren Vitamin-D-resistenten Rachitis mit Hypocalcaemie und autosomal-dominantem Erbgang: die hereditaere Pseudo-Mangelrachitis. Helv Paediatr Acta 1961; 16:452–468.
13. Fraser D, Kooh SW, Kind HP, Holick MF, Tanaka Y, DeLuca HF. Pathogenesis of hereditary vitamin-D-dependent rickets. An inborn error of vitamin D metabolism involving defective conversion of 25-hydroxyvitamin D to 1 alpha, 25-dihydroxyvitamin D. N Engl J Med 1973; 289:817–822.
14. Labuda M, Fujiwara TM, Ross MV, et al. Two hereditary defects related to vitamin D metabolism map to the same region of human chromosome 12q13–14. J Bone Miner Res 1992; 7:1447–1453.
15. Marx SJ, Spiegel AM, Brown EM, et al. A familial syndrome of decrease in sensitivity to 1,25-dihydroxyvitamin D. J Clin Endocrinol Metab 1978; 47:1303–1310.
16. Hochberg Z, Tiosano D, Even L. Calcium therapy for calcitriol-resistant rickets. J Pediatr 1992; 121:803–808.
17. Kristjansson K, Rut AR, Hewison M, O'Riordan JL, Hughes MR. Two mutations in the hormone binding domain of the vitamin D receptor cause tissue resistance to 1,25 dihydroxyvitamin D3. J Clin Invest 1994; 92:12–16.
18. Hughes MR, Malloy PJ, Kieback DG, et al. Point mutations in the human vitamin D receptor gene associted with hypocalcemic rickets. Science 1988; 242:1702–1705.
19. Hewison M, Rut AR, Kristjansson K, et al. Tissue resistance to 1,25-dihydroxyvitamin D without a mutation of the vitamin D receptor gene. Clin Endocrinol (Oxf.) 1993; 39:663–670.
20. Lotz M, Zisman E, Bartter FC. Evidence for a phosphorus-depletion syndrome in man. N Engl J Med 1968; 278:409–415.
21. DeFronzo RA, Cooke CR, Andres R, Faloona GR, Davis PJ. The effect of insulin on renal handling of sodium, potassium, calcium, and phosphate in man. J Clin Invest 1975; 55:845–855.

22. Walker JL, Ginalska-Malinowska M, Romer TE, Pucilowska JB, Underwood LE. Effects of the infusion of insulin-like growth factor I in a child with growth hormone insensitivity syndrome (Laron dwarfism). N Engl J Med 1991; 324:1483–1488.

23. Chantler C. Growth and metabolism in renal failure. The Teale Lecture 1987. J R Coll Phys Lond 1988; 22:69–73.

24. Bikle DD, Rasmussen H. The ionic control of 1,25-dihydroxyvitamin D$_3$ production in isolated chick renal tubules. J Clin Invest 1975; 55:292–298.

25. Fanconi A, Prader A. Die Hereditäre Pseudomangel Rachitis. Helv Paediatr Acta 1969; 24:423–447.

26. Juppner H, Hoyer PF, Latta K, Winkler L, Offner G, Brodehl J. Efficacy of calcium carbonate and low-dose vitamin D/1,25(OH)$_2$D$_3$ in reducing the risk of developing renal osteodystrophy in children on continuous ambulatory peritoneal dialysis. Pediatr Nephrol 1990; 4:614–617.

27. Slavin RE, Wen J, Kumar D, Evans EB. Familial tumoral calcinosis: a clinical, histopathological, and ultrastructural study with an analysis of its calcifying process and pathogenesis. Am J Surg Pathol 1993; 17:788–802.

28. McClatchie S, Bremner AD. Tumoural calcinosis—an unrecognized disease. BMJ 1969; 1:153–155.

29. Lyles KW, Burkes EJ, Ellis GJ, Lucas KJ, Dolan EA, Drezner MC. Genetic transmission of tumoral calcinosis: autosomal dominant with variable clinical expressivity. J Clin Endocrinol Metab 1985; 60:1093–1096.

30. Lyles KW, Drezner MK. Parathyroid hormone effects on serum 1,25-dihydroxyvitamin D levels in patients with X-linked hypophosphatemic rickets: evidence for abnormal 25-hydroxyvitamin D-1-hydroxylase activity. J Clin Endocrinol Metab 1982; 54:638–644.

31. Insogna KL, Broadus AE, Gertner JM. Impaired phosphorus conservation and 1,25 dihydroxyvitamin D generation during phosphorus deprivation in familial hypophosphatemic rickets. J Clin Invest 1983; 71:1562–1569.

32. Perry W, Stamp TCB. Hereditary hypophosphataemic rickets with autosomal recessive inheritance. J Bone Joint Surg [Br] 1978; 60:430–434.

33. Nesbitt T, Coffman TM, Griffiths R, Drezner MK. Cross-transplantation of kidneys in normal and Hyp mice. Evidence that the Hyp mouse phenotype is unrelated to an intrinsic renal defect. J Clin Invest 1994; 89:1543–1459.

34. Glorieux FH, Scriver CR, Reade TM, Goldman H, Roseborough A. Use of phosphate and vitamin D to prevent dwarfism and rickets in X-linked hypophosphatemia. N Engl J Med 1972; 287:481–487.

35. Rivkees SA, El-Hajj-Fuleihan G, Brown EM, Crawford JD. Tertiary hyperparathyroidism during high phosphate therapy of familial hypophosphatemic rickets. J Clin Endocrinol Metab 1992; 75:1514–1518.

36. Verge CF, Lam A, Simpson JM, Cowell CT, Howard NJ, Silink M. Effects of therapy in X-linked hypophosphatemic rickets. N Engl J Med 1991; 325:1843–1848.

37. Hirschberg R, Brunori G, Kopple JD, Guler HP. Effects of insulin-like growth factor I on renal function in normal men. Kidney Int 1993; 43:387–397.

38. Tieder M, Modai D, Samuel R, et al. Hereditary hypophosphatemic rickets with hypercalciuria. N Engl J Med 1985; 312:611–617.

39. Dent CE, Friedman M. Hypercalciuric rickets associated with + renal tubular damage. Arch Dis Child 1964; 39:240–249.

40. Harrison HE, Oncogenous rickets: possible elaboration by a tumor of a humoral substance inhibiting tubular reabsorption of phosphate. Pediatrics 1975; 52:432–434.

41. Cai C, Hodgson SF, Kao PC, et al. Inhibition of renal phosphate transport by a tumor product in a patient with oncogenic osteomalacia. N Engl J Med 1994; 330:1654–1649.

42. Weinstein LS, Shenker A, Gejman PV, Merino MJ, Friedman E, Spiegel AM. Activating mutations of the stimulatory G protein in the McCune-Albright syndrome. N Engl J Med 1991; 325:1688–1695.

43. Markello TC, Bernardini IM, Gahl WA. Improved renal functon in children with cystinosis treated with cysteamine. N Engl J Med 1993; 328:1157–1162.

44. American Academy of Pediatrics Committee on Nutrition. Nutritional needs of low-birth-weight infants. Pediatrics 1985; 75:976.

45. Weiss MJ, Cole DE, Ray, K, et al. Missense mutation in the human liver/bone/kidney alkaline phosphatase gene causing a lethal form of hypophosphatasia. Proc Natl Acad Sci USA 1988; 85:7666–7669.

46. Lee B, Vissing H, Ramirez F, Rogers D, Rimoin D. Identification of the molecular defect in a family with spondyloepiphyseal dysplasia. Science 1989; 244:978–980.

35
Metabolic Bone Disease

Salvador Castells

State University of New York Health Science Center at Brooklyn, Brooklyn, New York

I. INTRODUCTION

Metabolic bone disease is mostly the consequence of a genetic change causing the metabolism of bone to be deranged. This group of diseases has an origin in the bone itself, or they may occur because of abnormalities in vitamin, hormonal, or mineral metabolism. Other groups of metabolic bone disease can be acquired, such as a nutritional deficiency of vitamin D, causing rickets.

II. CLINICAL MANIFESTATIONS

Bone pain, fracture, deformity, and growth retardation are common manifestations of metabolic bone diseases in children. The cause of bone pain in some metabolic bone diseases is not well understood. Pain may result from stretching of the periosteum, which is rich with nerve fibers, or from micro- or macrofractures. The differential diagnosis of persistent localized skeletal pain in the absence of fractures is from sarcoma.

The symptoms of fracture depend on the bone involved. They occur after minor trauma and manifest with mild pain in osteogenesis imperfecta. Fractures also occur in osteopetrosis, and bone pain follows. The differential diagnosis between child abuse and metabolic bone disease is important (1).

Deformities may result from multiple fractures or from bone softening. The deformities of rickets in childhood include knock-knees and bowlegs, bossing of the skull, and enlarged epiphyses. Anomalies of the body proportions are found in several metabolic bone diseases. A low upper segment-lower segment ratio is found in homocystinuria, mucopolysaccharidosis type IV, and Marfan syndrome. A high upper segment-lower segment ratio is found in familial hyphosphatemia, achondroplasia, and dysplasia epiphysialis multiplex.

Deformities of the spine are important features. Changes in the spine in osteogenesis imperfecta are very similar to changes occurring in juvenile osteoporosis. The vertebrae are biconcave and osteoporotic and show evidence of multiple compression fractures. A common change is the thoracic kyphosis of juvenile osteoporosis, the sternum becoming prominent and a transverse crease developing across the abdomen.

The most devastating clinical manifestation of metabolic bone disease is growth retardation. In osteogenesis imperfecta congenita, growth retardation produces marked dwarfism that is permanent. Growth retardation is also present in rickets and improves with vitamin D treatment in the vitamin D-responsive types. Osteoporosis is another cause of severe growth retardation.

Muscular weakness, especially weaknesses of the proximal muscles, may be the presenting complaint in hyperparathyroidism. Muscular weakness is also a feature of vitamin D deficiency and is also found in osteogenesis imperfecta. Tetany consists of muscular spasms affecting the hands and the feet. Any disorder that causes hypocalcemia (rickets, hypoparathyroidism, or alkalosis) can cause tetany. Several standard tests have been designed to produce muscle spasm in patients with latent tetany. Trousseau's sign is produced by ischemia of the forearm when a sphygmomanometer cuff applied to the arm is inflated above the systolic blood pressure for 4 minutes. Chvostek's sign is elicited by tapping the branches of the facial nerve in the parotic area.

Finally, specific clinical features provide clues to particular metabolic bone disorders. The astute clinician should meticulously examine a child suspected of metabolic bone disease. The appearance of the face may be diagnostic, such as the elfin face of idiopathic hypercalcemia. The eyes may be the clue to the diagnosis, such as the "snowstorm" appearance in rickets, the cystine crystal corneal deposits in cystinosis, and blue sclerae of osteogenesis imperfecta, the lateral dislocation of the lens in Marfan syndrome, or the downward displacement in homocystinuria.

III. DIAGNOSIS

A. Biochemical Investigations

Several biochemical investigations are used in the study of patients with suspected metabolic bone disease. Fasting blood and urine samples for analysis should be taken in the morning between 8:00 and 9:00 a.m. because of the changes secondary to circadian rhythm in the concentration of substances in blood. Serum calcium, inorganic phosphorus, and alkaline phosphatase are the most routine investigations. The normal fasting serum calcium concentration does not vary with age. The amount of protein in the blood is important because almost half of the serum calcium is bound to protein, mostly to albumin, and the binding is influenced by pH. The use of a calcium ion-selective electrode has become a valuable technique for measurement of ionized calcium. In contrast with calcium, the intestinal absorption of phosphate plays a minor role in phosphate homeostasis. Phosphate metabolism is regulated mostly by renal excretion of phosphate (2). Serum inorganic phosphorus concentration varies with age, and it is higher in infancy (3). Urinary mineral excretion rates given by glomerular filtration and mass concentration calculated from serum and urinary creatinine concentrations require only a random urine collection obtained during fasting and a simultaneously obtained blood sample (4). A low serum phosphate concentration is found in hyperparathyroidism, vitamin D deficiency, hypophosphatemic rickets, cystinosis, and acquired renal tubular defects, such as tyrosinemia. Hyperphosphatemia occurs in renal insufficiency. The level of serum alkaline phosphatase is increased in childhood compared with adulthood, and it reaches the highest serum concentration during the accelerated growth of adolescence. The total serum alkaline phosphatase is formed by enzymes derived from the liver, bone, kidney, and gut. High serum alkaline phosphatase levels might be a result of liver disease, hereditary hyperphosphatemia, Paget's disease, metastatic tumor in bone, osteogenic sarcoma, rickets, hyperparathyroidism, and fracture healing. Other serum measurements are parathyroid hormone and two vitamin D metabolites, 25-hydroxyvitamin D_3 [25(OH)D], synthesized by the liver, and $1\alpha,25$-dihydroxyvitamin D_3 [1,25(OH)$_2$D], synthesized by the kidney. Serum calcitonin concentration in children is increased in medullary thyroid carcinoma.

Bone proteins found to be present in blood are becoming important for the diagnosis of metabolic bone disease. Osteocalcin, a calcium binding protein of the bone matrix, plays an important role in the regulation of mineral deposition and the remodeling process of bone. Osteocalcin is found in all osseous tissues, comprising approximately 1–2% of the total bone protein; its appearance coincides with histologically detectable bone mineralization, and it is synthesized by bone (5–7). The osteocalcin content of bone increases linearly with increasing bone density (8). It can be measured in plasma and is elevated in the plasma of patients with bone diseases in which there is an increased bone turnover (9).

Endopeptidases cleave procollagen to amino (NH$_2$)-terminal extension peptide (pColl-N) and a carboxyl (COOH)-terminal extension peptide (pColl-I-C). Serum levels of pColl-I-C in patients with different forms of metabolic bone disease may become an important index of bone formation (10,11).

Balance studies require prolonged hospitalization of several weeks, and they must be carefully performed by specialized nurses, dietitians, and technicians. Balance studies in children have no place in the routine investigation of metabolic bone diseases and should be confined to research projects in specialized metabolic units.

B. Bone Biopsies

The problem of evaluating bone biopsies in children is that the architecture and structure of bone are undergoing change by growth, ossification, and remodeling. These changes, occurring at different ages, require normal controls and an experienced pathologist, available in only a few medical centers. Bone is a microfibrillar network of collagen, mucopolysaccharides, and noncollagen protein impregnated by apatite minerals. Bone is rich in cells, including fibroblasts, chondroblasts, osteoblasts, osteoclasts, and osteocytes.

C. Bone Density

Visual radiography is a poor technique for the early diagnosis of osteoporosis; quantitative methods offer a greater advantage. There are different methods for quantitating bone density (12). We have been using the radiographic method of photodensitometry (absorptiometry) of Colbert et al. (13,14), which by using the left hand and wrist permits simultaneous measurements of bone age and bone density. This method automatically compares the minimal value of the patient's middle phalanges with that of age- and sex-matched peer norms. A computer-controlled microdensitometer scans 1 mm "slices" of the image of each phalanx on a conventional nonscreen radiograph of the hand and wrist. For the baseline study and each subsequent determination, a pair of radiographs (exposed at 50–60 KVp) is obtained with an aluminum allow reference wedge included in the field to permit correction for day-to-day variation in radiographic exposure and energy spectrum. The ratio of bone mineral mass to bone image area is the mineral concentration, expressed in computer units. The diagnosis of osteoporosis requires radiologic evidence of bone loss greater than the normal skeletal mass for the age, race, and sex of the person.

The mineral content of long bones may also be estimated by single-photon absorptiometry (15), dual-photon absorptiometry (16), and quantitative computed tomography (17,18). Recent studies showed that bone density in the radius, oscalcis, and forearm predicts future fracture rate. Rectilinear single-photon absorptiometry is fast, inexpensive, and accurate and can assess the radius (15).

D. Regulation of Bone Remodeling

Bone remodeling comprises resorption and formation of new bone. Bone remodeling is an endocrine process regulated by hormones and a local process regulated by growth factors.

The hormones regulating bone remodeling are (1) the polypeptide hormones parathyroid hormone, calcitonin, insulin, and growth hormone, (2) the steroid hormones 25-hydroxyvitamin D, 1,25-dihydroxyvitamin D, glucocorticoids, and sex steroids, and (3) thyroid hormones. The local factors are growth factors and prostaglandins synthesized by bone cells under the direction of the circulating hormones (19,20).

The measurement of circulating hormones and growth factor may be important in the diagnosis and management of metabolic bone diseases. The skeletal system is a major target of insulin-like growth factor (IGF) action by increasing cartilage and bone formation and decreasing matrix absorption (21). Information about the diagnosis and therapeutic value of IGFs in bone diseases is still in the research area.

Rickets is described in Chapter 34.

IV. OSTEOPOROSIS

Osteoporosis in children is a heterogeneous group of metabolic bone diseases that have in common a loss of bone mass manifested by skeletal brittleness and rarefaction of bone with normal mineral metabolism. It is the loss of bone tissue that secondarily affects bone mineral by increasing the liberation of calcium and phosphorous into blood and urine. In some cases of osteoporosis, secondary hypercalcemia, hyperphosphatemia, and hypercalciuria may be found. Age influences the turnover of bone, with two periods of very rapid bone gain—from birth to 2 years and during adolescence. Puberty is a period of increased bone mineral content. The significant difference in bone mass at different ages reflects a greater net formation relative to net resorption, resulting in a larger skeletal mass than that at a previous age. This may explain why in some types of childhood osteoporosis, such as osteogenesis imperfecta and Down syndrome, there is significant clinical and radiologic improvement during adolescence. In osteoporosis, accelerated bone resorption overtakes bone formation, and the result is a loss of bone mass. Osteoporosis in children is characterized by a reduction in bone mass below the norm for the age, sex, and race of a child.

A. Classification

Table 1 is a classification of osteoporosis, representing a heterogeneous group of disorders, in children. Some are caused by primary metabolic bone disease; others are secondary to other metabolic disorders.

B. Laboratory Examination

1. Serum Concentration of Calcium, Phosphate, and Alkaline Phosphatase

Serum concentrations of calcium, phosphate, and alkaline phosphatase are normal in most children with osteoporosis. An exception is the hypercalcemia found in the acute osteoporosis of disuse in children (22–24). Some diseases with osteoporosis may have characteristic changes in serum phosphate levels. In Cushing's disease, for example, the serum phosphate level is low because of the effect of glucocorticoids

Table 1 Classification of Osteoporosis

Idiopathic juvenile osteoporosis
Immobilization
Osteoporosis associated with accelerated bone formation
　(juvenile Paget's disease of bone)
Congenital
　Osteogenesis imperfecta
　Osteolysis
Endocrine disorders
　Hypopituitarism with growth hormone deficiency
　Hypogonadism
　Hyperthyroidism
　Juvenile diabetes
　Acromegaly
　Hyperadrenocorticism
　Progeria
Arthritic disorders
　Juvenile arthritis
　Rheumatoid arthritis
Genetic disorders
　Turner syndrome (ovarian agenesis)
　Down syndrome
Metabolic disorders
　Hemocystinuria
　Marfan syndrome
　Ehlers-Danlos syndrome
　Menke syndrome
　Riley-Day syndrome
　Cystic fibrosis
Blood disorders
　Waldenström's macroglobulinemia
　Lymphoma
　Leukemia
　Multiple myeloma
　Heparin therapy
Malnutrition
　Anorexia nervosa
　Scurvy
　Protein deficiency

in the renal tubule, lowering the tubular reabsorption of phosphate.

Urine calcium measurements are also of little value in the diagnosis of osteoporosis. Hypercalciuria is found in the osteoporosis of immobilized children (22–25). Normal urine calcium excretion in children has been reported to be less than 4 mg/kg boy weight per 24 h (26). The urinary calcium-creatinine concentration ratio in random samples is a good index for screening for hypercalciuria. The normal values are variable between ambulatory children and hospitalized and partially immobilized children (27–29).

There is increased fecal calcium excretion in osteoporosis. This has been observed in idiopathic juvenile osteoporosis and in the osteoporosis of immobilization (27–29). The increase in fecal calcium in osteoporosis appears to be caused by diminution of dietary calcium absorption, not by an increase in calcium secretion into the intestine. The difficulty of measuring fecal calcium and doing calcium balance studies makes this measurement useless to the clinician.

The serum alkaline phosphatase concentration is normal or slightly above the norm for age, with a temporary elevation during fractures.

2. Serum Concentrations of Osteocalcin

Human osteocalcin is a calcium ion (Ca^{2+}) binding protein of the bone matrix (30,31) that contains three carboxyglutamic acid (Gla) residues among its 40 amino acids at positions 17, 21, and 24 (31). The amino acid Gla side chain is directly involved in Ca^{2+} binding and the absorption of osteocalcin to hydroxyapatite surfaces in vivo and in vitro (31). Osteocalcin is present in developing bone at the onset of mineralization and may participate in bone formation (30). It may come from the proteolytic processing of a higher molecular weight "prohormone" (32). Osteocalcin can be detected in serum by radioimmunoassay (33), and its concentration may correlate with metabolic bone diseases; high plasma levels are observed in growing children (34). The synthesis of osteocalcin appears to be modulated by vitamin D. The bones of vitamin D-deficient chicks contain 50% less osteocalcin than normal bones (35). The renal metabolite of vitamin D, $1,25(OH)_2D$, stimulates osteocalcin synthesis and secretion in osteosarcoma cells in culture (36), and the administration of $1,25(OH)_2D_3$ to experimental animals results in the elevation of serum osteocalcin (37).

Osteocalcin plays an important role in the regulation of mineral deposition and remodeling of bone. Studies of plasma levels of this peptide are helpful for understanding some of the underlying changes observed in metabolic bone diseases and to provide a biochemical marker to monitor the effects of therapy with such agents as calcitonin, vitamin D_3, and calcitriol. We have found that plasma osteocalcin levels are elevated in osteogenesis imperfecta (38); they return toward normal levels during treatment with calcitonin (39). The elevation of plasma osteocalcin in osteogenesis imperfecta is age dependent. It is high in the first decade but becomes normal during puberty (40). In all types of rickets, we have found decreased plasma osteocalcin levels (41), and during treatment with vitamin D_3 or calcitriol, a rapid increase in plasma osteocalcin concentrations occurs (41,42). Thus, plasma osteocalcin concentrations can differentiate between the osteoporosis of osteogenesis imperfecta and osteomalacia secondary to rickets, and these concentrations also allow the clinician to follow the response to treatment with calcitonin or vitamin D_3. In some other types of osteoporosis, for example those caused by growth hormone deficiency, serum plasma levels of osteocalcin have been reported to be lower compared with those in normal children and to increase toward normal with treatment with human growth hormone (43). In juvenile idiopathic osteoporosis, plasma osteocalcin concentrations have been reported as normal or elevated (44).

C. Idiopathic Juvenile Osteoporosis

Idiopathic juvenile osteoporosis is a rare disorder of prepubertal children that manifests clinically between the ages of 8 and 14 years. The frequency of juvenile osteoporosis, compared with postmenopausal or senile osteoporosis, is certainly uncommon. The disorder may be more common if kyphosis is taken as a manifestation of the disease (45). More boys than girls (3:1) seem affected (46). From the evidence now available, there is no suggestion of a hereditary factor.

1. Clinical Manifestations of the Disease

Bone pain seems to be the main symptom. The bone pain, which can be localized in the lower extremities, increases further with walking. It is described by the patients as a constant, dull ache that makes walking difficult. Another frequent location of the pain is the spine. The backache is generalized.

In other cases, the clinical onset of the disease is manifested by a fracture of one or more bones, usually from minimal trauma. Scheuermann's kyphosis is considered a form of juvenile osteoporosis (47). Like idiopathic juvenile osteoporosis, it tends to be self-limiting and appears between the ages of 8 and 14 years. The arcuate deformity of Scheuermann's juvenile kyphosis is caused by wedge-shaped deformities of the vertebrae (46).

2. Mechanism of the Osteoporotic Process

Roentgenorgraphic and clinical studies seem to indicate that bone formation is normal; they suggest a predominance of bone resorption over formation. Microradiographic studies indicate that there is an increase in resorption surface compared with that in age-matched controls (48). The clinical improvement coincides with a decrease in the abnormally increased bone resorption (49). Further histologic evidence for increased bone resorption has been presented (50,51). However, other investigators have reported a reduction in bone formation rather than an increase in bone resorption (52,53).

Plasma calcium, phosphate, and alkaline phosphatase have been reported as normal in some patients, but some authors have found that plasma alkaline phosphatase and urinary total hydroxyproline levels were slightly increased in some patients compared with their age-matched controls (54,55).

A deficiency of 1,25-dihydrocholecalciferol has been suggested in the pathogenesis of juvenile osteoporosis (56, 67). Dihydrotachysterol and vitamin D_2, or its active metabolites have been used to correct the calcium malabsorption in this disease (58,59). Because hypercalciuria has been reported in some cases, some clinicians have been reluctant to use vitamin D_2 or calcitriol in the treatment of idiopathic juvenile osteoporosis, but supplemental calcitriol therapy has been used in selected patients (56,57). Calcium supplements to maintain a 1 g calcium intake have been advocated. The use of sex hormones has been recommended based on the theoretical assumption that a temporary hormonal disturbance is associated with the hormonal changes of puberty. No laboratory evidence for such an abnormality has been found. Calcitonin has been used in a few patients (60), as has bisphosphonate (51).

Because of the self-limited course of this disease, with spontaneous recovery, we advise a conservative approach consisting of physical therapy, appropriate amounts of calcium intake, and vitamin D_2 supplementation in the diet.

D. Osteoporosis of Immobilization

Long-standing immobilization may produce bone demineralization, hypercalcemia, and, occasionally, diminished renal function (61–63). The symptoms of immobilization hypercalcemia may occur early or late during immobilization or may appear suddenly or insidiously. The symptoms include headaches, sometimes described as migraine attacks, anorexia, malaise, nausea and vomiting, abdominal pain, constipation, and weight loss. Polydipsia and polyuria may be found in some patients. If the patient is not treated, renal insufficiency, hypertension, seizures, and hearing loss may develop. Blood chemistry evaluations show elevated serum calcium with normal phosphate concentrations, metabolic alkalosis, hypercalciuria, hyperphosphaturia, normal to elevated alkaline phosphatase levels, and a decreased glomerular filtration rate and creatinine clearance. The serum parathyroid hormone concentration has been normal in all cases. The rise in serum calcium concentration during immobilization is more clear when determinations of serum ionized calcium are made (64).

The osteoporosis and hypercalcemia of immobilization have been explained by an increase in bone resorption, the rise in serum calcium coming from bone (65,66). There is also an increase in calcium excretion, which causes a negative calcium balance, with more calcium excreted than taken in by diet (65). The increase in bone resorption may be accompanied by decreased osteoblastic bone formation (66). Four mechanisms—lack of mechanical stress, poor vascularity, metabolic bone changes, and denervation—have been suggested as pathophysiologic mechanisms for these changes (67–69).

Bronner et al. (70) have reported similar results, with a decreased rate of bone deposition in patients with scoliosis who are immobilized in a cast, whereas the rate of bone resorption increased. It appears that, in immobilized children and adolescents, the first response to the immobilized bone is increased bone resorption and decreased bone formation secondary to the loss of mechanical factors stimulating bone during ambulation. Hypercalcemia is a consequence of the increased rate of calcium resorption from bone. After the loss of bone mineral, osteoporosis appears.

The diagnosis of this condition requires serial measurements of serum calcium, phosphate, and alkaline phosphatase during immobilization. Urinary calcium excretion should also be followed. Normal urinary calcium excretion in children is less than 4 mg/kg of body weight per 24 h. The calcium-creatinine ratio (Ca/Cr) concentration ratio (mg/mg), determined from a randomly collected urine sample, can be also used to screen for hypercalciuria.

Moore et al. (27) and Stapelton et al. (28) have shown

that the normal Ca/Cr ratio in random urine samples of children from 3 months to 18 years of age ranged from 0.01 to 0.73 mg/kg with a mean ± standard deviation of 0.06 ± 0.06. Ratios greater than 0.18 require a 24 h urine collection to demonstrate urinary calcium excretion of more than 4 mg/kg body weight. Calcium is filtered by the glomerulus and reabsorbed in the tubules. There is an increase in the filtered load of calcium in immobilized children, which is responsible for hypercalciuria (71).

The treatment of hypercalcemia and hypercalciuria is crucial to prevent the severe complications of renal damage, with hypertension and seizures. Osteoporosis and hypercalcemia of immobilization can be prevented by mobilization at the earliest possible time. The most effective treatment for osteoporosis and hypercalcemia of immobilization is remobilization. Hypercalcemia responds quickly to weight-bearing mobilization. Recovery proceeds at a rapid rate after reambulation is initiated, contrary to studies that question the reversibility of mineral loss caused by immobilization. Oral phosphates to decrease serum calcium levels has been recommended in the treatment of hypercalcemia (72). Supplemental oral phosphate reduces urinary calcium excretion but does not prevent osteoporosis during immobilization (72), making oral phosphatase therapy of little value for the treatment of hypercalcemia of immobilization. Rapid diuresis induced by furosemide be useful for short-term treatment of hypercalcemia (73). Furosemide, a potent natriuretic agent, also increases calcium excretion in direct proportion to the sodium excretion (73). The careful replacement of water and electrolyte losses is essential. Steroid therapy, 25–40 mg/m^2 per 24 h of prednisone for 1–2 weeks, is regarded as an effective treatment. Mithramycin also produces a decrease in serum calcium concentrations (74) by reducing bone resorption. We have had good results with salmon calcitonin (Calcimar) when administered at a dose of 2–4 MRC (Medical Research Council) units subcutaneously per kilogram body weight. The plasma calcium concentrations should be followed carefully, and the administration of salmon calcitonin should be repeated if increases above the normal values occur in plasma calcium concentrations.

E. Juvenile Paget's Disease of Bone

Paget's disease usually is not detected before the age of 40 years. Although uncommon in the pediatric- and adolescent-aged groups, several cases have been reported in children (75,76).

Initially there is excessive bone resorption followed by excessive and disorganized new bone formation. Paget's disease goes through various phases of activity and may become dormant. Serum alkaline phosphatase concentrations are elevated, and high rates of urinary hydroxyproline excretion occur. Radiologic evidence for abundant bone formation, with thickening of the cortex, osteosclerosis, and osteoporosis, is characteristic. Bone biopsies in children reveal resorption and formation of bone as described in adult patients with Paget's disease.

Calcitonin is effective in the treatment of adult patients

with Paget's diseases (77,78); similar results have been reported in the juvenile form (79).

The differential diagnosis of juvenile Paget's disease is from congenital hyperphosphatasia (hyperostosis corticalis deformans juvenilis). The disease is a rare disorder in children characterized by a high serum alkaline phosphatase concentration and bowing of the long bones. In juvenile Paget's disease the classic mosaic pattern is characteristic, and it is not seen in cases of congenital hyperphosphatasia.

F. Osteogenesis Imperfecta

Osteogenesis imperfecta is an inherited disorder of connective tissue that primarily affects the skeletomuscular system. The genetic disorder causes generalized osteoporosis. The generalized osteoporosis determines bone fragility, multiple fractures, and deformities of the skeleton.

Patients with osteogenesis imperfecta tarda associated with bowing have tarda type I (OIT I); patients without bowing have tarda type II (OIT II).

Silence et al. (81) classify osteogenesis imperfecta in four groups, considering tarda or congenita, mode of inheritance, and the presence of blue sclerae (see Table 2). More recently, as clinical studies have progressed, both type I and IV have been expanded to include varieties in which dentinogenesis imperfecta is either present or absent; autosomal dominant and autosomal recessive varieties have been included in type III; type II is now thought to be heterogeneous (82).

Initially, many of the genetic diseases appeared to be simple homogeneous entities, but as more biochemical and genetic knowledge about the disorders developed, several fundamentally distinct disorders were differentiated. The clinical classification helps the clinician predict the natural history of an infant with osteogenesis imperfecta. However, it is still difficult to distinguish those infants with the congenital form, who may survive for a few days, weeks, or years. The clinical classification does not yet provide a basis to determine the type of inheritance. We hope that the biochemical studies of collagen metabolism in osteogenesis imperfecta will finally provide a way to coordinate the clinical, genetic, and biochemical groups.

The prevalence of osteogenesis imperfecta has been determined accurately for Edinburgh to be 5.77×10^{-5} (83); for Sweden, 4.0×10^{-5} (84); and for Australia, 3.5×10^{-5}; the overall prevalence of osteogenesis imperfecta identifiable at birth is therefore about 1:20,000 total births.

Osteogenesis imperfecta is a disease of the connective tissue with abnormalities in the structure or biosynthesis of the fibrillar collagens. The discovery in the last few years of the heterogeneity of the collagens and the biosynthetic steps leading to fibrillogenesis (85–87) explains the variable degrees of increased urinary hydroxyproline excretion, with lack of normal cortical remodeling and bone deformities.

1. Classification

Clinically, two varieties have been distinguished: the congenita and the tarda forms (Table 2). In osteogenesis imperfecta congenita, the osteoporosis is already present in fetal life and is so severe that minor trauma to the fetus produces numerous intrauterine fractures. The victim is born with multiple fractures at different stages of callus formation. The

Table 2 Classification of Osteogenesis Imperfecta

Type	Inheritance	Clinical findings
Clinical[a]		
Congenital		
Tarda type I		
Tarda type II		
Genetic[b]		
I	Autosomal dominant	Bone fragility and blue sclerae
		Scoliosis and growth retardation
		Hearing loss
		Walking independently
II	Autosomal dominant or recessive	Marked bone fragility in utero
		Blue sclerae
		Perinatal death
III	Autosomal dominant or recessive	Bone fragility and growth retardation
		Mild blue sclerae
IV	Autosomal dominant	Osteoporosis, bone fragility, and fractures with variable deformity of long bone
		Normal sclerae

[a]From Reference 80.
[b]From Reference 81.

cranium is soft and membranaceous. There are multiple wormian bones in the membranous skull. The extremities are short and clumsy. The affected infant has a characteristic appearance, with striking micromelia and a disproportionately large head.

In osteogenesis imperfecta tarda, the disease is not manifested at birth but the fractures and deformities appear during or after the first year of life. Falvo et al. (80) proposes that the tarda group be subdivided according to the existence of expressivity and clinical complexity of the inherited connective tissue disorders. Osteogenesis imperfecta is not considered, along with Ehlers-Danlos syndrome, Marfan syndrome, and possibly the chondrodystrophies, as a genetic disorder of collagen structure and biosynthesis. A number of osteogenesis imperfecta types have been extensively studied at the biochemical molecular levels of collagen structure and biosynthesis (88–108). Cultures of skin fibroblasts from patients with osteogenesis imperfecta have indicated mutations of one or two genes encoding type I procollagen (109,110). The genetic defects are within two groups: one is consistent with reduced collagen production and the other leads to structural defects in the collagen helix. The defect in collagen production reduces the production of type I collagen to one-half the normal amounts. The clinical manifestations are mildly comparable to the structural defects in collagen.

The osteoporotic process in osteogenesis imperfecta is caused by increased bone resorption. Several studies (111–113) have used tetracycline-based measurements of bone dynamics in patients with osteogenesis imperfecta to demonstrate an increased bone turnover at endosteal surfaces. We have undertaken a study of calcium kinetics in patients with osteogenesis imperfecta by using ^{47}Ca. Our results also indicate that bone resorption in osteogenesis imperfecta is more generalized throughout the skeleton than had until now been demonstrated (114).

The fractures in patient with osteoporosis imperfecta heal as fast as in normal individuals.

Failure to grow is an important manifestation of the disease. It appears to correlate with the severity of the osteoporotic process. The marked shortness of the lower extremities is partly a result of skeletal deformities, bowing, and multiple fractures of long bones. Also, multiple microfractures at the growth plate may interfere with bone growth. Another important factor may be a decreased responsiveness of the growth plate to growth factors. Growth hormone and IGF-I serum levels have been reported as normal in osteogenesis imperfecta. We have seen several patients with marked short stature who have neither skeletal deformities nor a history of fractures. The growth retardation in these patients can be explained only by an unresponsiveness of the growth plate to growth factors secondary to the osteoporotic process. Scoliosis and kyphoscoliosis may develop as a result of laxity of ligaments, as well as of vertebral osteoporosis. The vertebrae develop a characteristic "codfish" or "hourglass" deformity because of the pressure of the normally elastic nucleus pulposus on the abnormally osteoporotic vertebrae. The scoliosis is often extreme and appears to progress during adolescence, when the number of fractures markedly decreases.

Prenatal osteogenesis imperfecta can be detected very early in the second trimester by sonographic studies (115–117).

The management of patients with osteogenesis imperfecta includes medical and surgical treatment.

2. Medical Treatment

Because the osseous manifestations greatly outweigh the other manifestations in clinical importance, all attempts to treat the disease have been directed toward correcting the generalized osteoporosis. It is expected that if mineralization of the bone can be increased, its resistance to trauma would improve. The primary difficulty in osteogenesis imperfecta is that the evaluation of therapeutic programs for children with this disorder has been complicated by extreme differences in the clinical manifestations of bone fragility and variations in the natural course of the disease.

The role of sex hormones in the treatment of osteogenesis imperfecta has been based on the clinical observation that in this disorder there is a decrease in the prevalence of fractures observed at puberty and an increase in this prevalence after menopause, but considering the severity of the side effects of anabolic steroids and their failure to produce increased deposition of calcium in the bone, they should not be administered to either children or adults with osteogenesis imperfecta.

The use of fluoride in the treatment of osteogenesis imperfecta is based on observations suggesting that sodium fluoride, when given over a prolonged period, has beneficial effects in osteoporosis (118–126), multiple myeloma (127), and Paget's disease (128).

Albright and Grunt (129) treated 13 patients who had osteogenesis imperfecta of different severities with sodium fluoride. The dose ranged from 0.25 to 0.90 mg/kg body weight per day. Calcium and phosphate balance studies did not vary significantly during the period of sodium fluoride therapy. Although the incidence of fractures decreased in some patients during the period of fluoride therapy, the authors believed that the overall results did not warrant the general use of fluoride for the treatment of patients with osteogenesis imperfecta.

The use of magnesium oxide for the treatment of osteogenesis imperfecta is based on the work of Solomons and Styner (130), who found that the bone collagen of patients with osteogenesis imperfecta is a potent inhibitor of calcification in vitro. This inhibition was removed by treatment of the collagen from these patients with pyrophosphate in the presence of magnesium ions. It was also found that serum and urinary levels of inorganic pyrophosphate were elevated in 281 patients with osteogenesis imperfecta, but the precise role of pyrophosphate metabolism in this disorder is still unclear.

Calcitonin is a polypeptide hormone secreted in mammals by the parafollicular cells of the thyroid gland and, in other animals, by the ultimobranchial body (131). The major action of calcitonin is to inhibit bone resorption (132). In adults, calcitonin seems to be more effective in treating diseases with an abnormally high rate of bone resorption.

The possibility that calcitonin may also be beneficial in

the treatment of osteogenesis imperfecta is based on the presence of increased bone resorption in this disease and on the decrease in abnormally high bone absorption rates by calcitonin administration. Logic suggests that treatment directed at decreasing bone resorption may improve the osteopenia of osteogenesis imperfecta. Salmon calcitonin may provide a more convenient and more effective form of long-term therapy of osteogenesis imperfecta than porcine calcitonin.

For several years, we have used synthetic salmon calcitonin to treat 50 patients who have osteogenesis imperfecta. The patients were classified as having osteogenesis imperfecta congenita or tarda (types I and II) according to the clinical classifications of Falvo et al. There was a significant improvement in fracture rate and in bone density during treatment with the salmon calcitonin (133). The major disadvantage in the use of salmon calcitonin in children has been the need to be given by multiple subcutaneous or intramuscular injections. Recent advances in the administration of calcitonin by intranasal spray and in the proof of its effectiveness in osteogenesis imperfecta may make the drug an acceptable form of therapy (134).

V. OSTEOLYTIC DISEASES

Osteolytic diseases are manifest by accelerated destruction of bone, localized mainly in the extremities. In the advanced forms of the diseases, there are characteristic deformities of the hands and feet, which appear foreshortened and clawlike. There is a progressive shortening of the limbs that makes the term "vanishing limbs" appropriate. The joints are swollen, tender, and stiff. Fractures are frequently present, and kyphoscoliosis is found in many patients. Growth retardation is marked. Roentgenographic studies reveal osteoporosis with destruction of the distal portion of long bones. There are at least six different forms of osteolytic disease (Table 3).

There is an increased bone resorption in patients with osteolysis. One patient had an increased exchangeable calcium of 17.20 g (normal in control children, 9.70 ± 2.4)

Table 3 Types of Osteolytic Disease

Carpal and tarsal osteolysis
   Cranioskeletal dysplasia with acroosteolysis (135)
   Acroosteolysis alone (136)
Multicentric osteolysis
   Hereditary (137)
   Nonfamilial with nephropathy (138–141)
Massive osteolysis (142)
Angiomatosis of bone (lymphangiomatosis, hemangiomatosis with osteolysis) (143)
Skin lesions and corneal opacities with osteolysis Winchester syndrome (144–147)
Selective muscle fiber hypoplasia and epiphyseal osteolysis (148)

(135). The cause of the accelerated osteolytic process is unknown. The etiology may be multiple, such as a genetic disorder, a biochemical abnormality of fibroblasts and muscle fibers, and renal and hemangiomatosis disorders.

Physical therapy and orthopedic treatment of fractures and deformities until now have been the only available modalities of treatment.

Calcitonin seems to be an effective medical treatment. We treated one patient with synthetic salmon calcitonin at 2 MRC units/kg, 3 days per week, with oral supplementation of calcium. The patient had a marked improvement during calcitonin therapy with less bone pain (148).

VI. OSTEOPETROSIS

Osteopetrosis is a disease characterized by bone sclerosis, with involvement of other organ systems. Hematologic, neurologic, and immunologic complications are part of the spectrum of clinical presentations. Juvenile and adult forms with dominant-recessive-autosomal inheritance have been described. Variable degrees of severity are found in each variant.

The prevalence of all the variants of osteopetrosis has been estimated as between 1:100,00 and 1:500,000 inhabitants (149). A recent epidemiologic study reveals that the prevalence of the benign autosomal dominant form of osteoporosis is 5.5:100,000 inhabitants (150).

The histologic studies on the osteopetrotic bone suggest that different conditions can produce the characteristic bone sclerosis by a common mechanism of decreased rate of bone and cartilage formation and resorption (151–155).

A heterogeneous group of disorders has been grouped under the term "osteopetrosis." With the advent of new therapeutic modalities, such as high-dose calcitriol and bone marrow transplantation, a complete characterization of each individual patient is necessary to develop a rational therapeutic approach (156,157).

A. Etiology

The animal studies and the clinical reports on osteopetrosis, together with recent studies on the biology of the osteoclasts, seem to corroborate the notion that the osteopetrotic phenotype is the end result of multiple genetic defects. The osteoclast originates by differentiation from a stem cell, described as a lymphoid-like mononuclear precursor. Local and systemic factors are necessary to activate the resorptive apparatus of the osteoclasts. In this sequence of events, there are many potential sites of dysfunction, for which clinical examples have already been reported (158–163). Transplantation studies in osteopetrosis have been particularly helpful in clarifying the origin of the osteoclasts and have established the stem cell dysfunction as one of the causal factors in osteopetrosis.

B. Histologic Findings

Bone histologic studies in patients with osteopetrosis have shown abnormalities in the cortex, marrow, matrix, and osteoclasts. The separation between the cortex and the marrow becomes indistinct because of an excess of wide bony trabeculae with a core of cartilage. Osteoid seams may be present. Decreased hematopoiesis is frequent, and myelofibrosis is occasionally observed. The collagen fibers in the matrix are usually normal, but a patient with anomalous collagen fibers and a decreased number of the round vesicles associated with mineralization has been reported. Studies of the cellular components of the bone revealed normal osteoblasts. The osteoclasts showed different types of abnormalities (164–167). Their number can be decreased, normal, or increased. Most of the time, the osteoclasts are properly juxtaposed to bone but do not seem active in resorption. Howship's lacunae, ruffled borders, clear zones, and enzymatic secretion are frequently absent. In some of the osteoclasts, an increased number of nuclei, large vacuoles (which may be abnormal lysosomes), and abnormal mitochondria may be seen.

Studies of bone metabolism in osteopetrosis have yielded inconsistent results. Serum concentrations of calcium and phosphorus have been reported as normal or low. Serum concentrations of alkaline and acid phosphatase have been found to be normal or elevated. The serum concentration of calcitonin is usually normal, but the levels of parathyroid hormone (PTH) and $1,25(OH)_2D_3$ may be normal or elevated. Calcium balance studies done in some patients with osteopetrosis have been reported to be positive.

C. Malignant Osteopetrosis

Malignant osteopetrosis, inherited as an autosomal recessive trait, represents the most severe form of osteopetrosis (158–160). Skeletal sclerosis and bone fractures have been detected in utero (168). Affected infants have progressive leukoerythroblastic anemia and marked hepatosplenomegaly secondary to extramedullary erythropoiesis (169). Deficiencies in immune function and neurologic abnormalities are also present.

The skeletal abnormalities that may be found in the osteopetrotic skeleton include macrocephaly (caused by thickening of the cranial foramina and associated hydrocephalus) (169); trapezoidal head (caused by thickening of the frontal and parietal bones) (170); frontal bossing, hypertelorism, proptosis, flattened nasal bridge, and choanal atresia (171–172); hypoplastic or hyperplastic mandible and maxilla; delayed linear growth; delayed dentition; and rickets (173).

Pathologic fractures are common because despite its dense composition, the osteopetrotic bone is brittle (167–170).

Roentgenographic findings generally include increased density of all bones, decreased remodeling with evidence of increased cortical thickness, widened shafts, and decreased marrow space in long bones.

Hematologic derangements are very common in malignant osteopetrosis because the skeletal sclerosis is associated with obliteration of the marrow cavities and increasing marrow fibrosis. The fibrosis promotes extramedullary erythropoiesis, with hepatosplenomegaly and subsequent hypersplenism.

Neurologic impairment is frequent in the patients with malignant osteopetrosis (174, 175). Progressive bony encroachment on cranial nerve foramina causes direct compression of the nerve, vascular occlusion, and gradual deterioration of neural function. The optic nerve, vestibulocochlear nerve, facial nerve (unilateral or bilateral), and trigeminal nerve (mandibular division) are the most frequently affected.

D. Benign Osteopetrosis

The benign form of osteopetrosis is transmitted as an autosomal dominant trait. Incomplete penetrance and heterogeneity in clinical expression are seen, even among siblings within the same family (176,177). In almost half of the cases, the patients are asymptomatic and the disorder is discovered incidentally by finding increased density in bone. A normal life span can be expected. Hematologic complications are rare. Symptoms, when present, include fractures (40%), bone pain (20–25%), cranial enlargement of the cranial vault and mandible, tall stature, genu valgum, clubbing of the long bones, and proptosis. Osteomyelitis of the mandible (178, 179) and, to a lesser extent, of the maxilla (180) can also occur.

E. Intermediate Osteopetrosis

Both autosomal dominant and autosomal recessive inheritance have been found in cases associated with intermediate symptomatology (181). There is an autosomal recessive form of osteopetrosis that differs from the malignant autosomal recessive form by the relative mildness of clinical symptoms during infancy and childhood. Children with the disorder present with recurrent fractures, cranial nerve compression, and osteomyelitis (182,183).

Mild to moderate anemia may be present; however, marked hepatomegaly and severe anemia are absent. Survival into adult life is the rule. Radiographic evidence of disease is present. In many cases, parental consanguinity is ascertained, and in all cases only one generation is affected. It may be clinically indistinguishable from the "benign" autosomal dominant form. Family evaluation and pedigree analysis are the only reliable methods of determining the pattern of gene transmission (181).

F. Osteopetrosis Associated with Renal Tubular Acidosis and Calcification

This variant of osteopetrosis has been described in 21 patients from 12 unrelated families (184,185). It is inherited in an autosomal recessive manner. The biochemical hallmark is an almost complete deficiency of the enzyme carbonic anhydrase type II (CAII) in the erythrocytes of homozygotic patients and decreased levels of the enzyme in obligate heterozygotes. The course is milder than that found in malignant osteopetrosis. Failure to thrive, hypotonia, and short stature may appear in infancy and midchildhood as the result of chronic systemic acidosis.

G. Osteopetrosis in Association with Other Disorders

There have been reports of osteopetrosis associated with non-Hodgkin's lymphoma (186). Crohn's disease (187), bronchogenic carcinoma (188), ichthyosis, and neuronal storage disease. The importance of these associations in the pathogenesis of the disease is unknown.

H. Treatment

Allogenic bone marrow transplantation from HLA-matched sibling donors offers the greatest hope for long-term survival in infants with malignant disease (189–192). In a series of 14 marrow transplantations for infantile osteopetrosis, 6 proved successful. In those successfully treated, significant reversal of osseous abnormalities was achieved, with improvement in hematologic status and immune function. The failure of successful bone marrow transplantation in some infants may reflect the heterogeneity in the etiology of the disorder. Hormonal therapy is an alternative for those patients who are unwilling or unable, for lack of an appropriate donor, to undergo bone marrow transplantation. Potent stimulators of bone resorption, for example high-dose calcitriol $[1,25(OH)_2D_3]$ (193) and bovine parathyroid hormone, have been utilized to induce osteoclast function.

Studies suggest a dual role for calcitriol in inducing bone resorption in patients with osteopetrosis. In vitro exposure to $1,25(OH)_2D_3$ stimulates cellular differentiation of the monocyte (and human myeloid leukemic cell) to cells capable of bone resorption (193,194).

Further, administration of 1α-hydroxlated vitamin D_3 stimulates functional osteoclasts to resorb bone at a higher rate than normal (194). Thus, the action of calcitriol is mediated both by its ability to increase the differentiation of precursors into competent bone-resorbing cells as well as by directly stimulating cells to resorb bone more effectively. Cellular resistance to calcitriol is suggested by the need for very high dose therapy in these patients (16–32 αg/day) despite high basal levels of circulating $1,25(OH)_2D$ (195, 196).

Brief clinical trials with intravenous infusion of parathyroid extract or bovine PTH for patients with severe disease have been unable to provide conclusive evidence of the therapeutic efficacy. Short-term (1–6 months) therapy with high-dose intravenous methylprednisone (197) has induced regression of hepatosplenomegaly, increased the peripheral leukocyte and platelet count, normalized the hemoglobin concentration, and improved bone marrow cellularity. Potential side effects of high-dose steroid therapy include severe growth retardation, increased susceptibility to infection, and lowering of serum calcium.

REFERENCES

1. Hurwitz A, Castells S. Misdiagnosed child abuse and metabolic diseases. Pediatr Nurs 1987; 13:33–36.
2. Broadus AE. Physiological functions of calcium, magnesium and phosphorous and mineral ion balance. In: Favus MJ, ed. Primer on the Metabolic Bone Diseases and Disorders Mineral Metabolism, 2nd ed. New York: Raven Press, 1993:41–46.
3. De Wijn TF. Changing levels of blood constituents during growth. In: Van der Werft Ten Bosch JJ, Haak A, eds. Somatic Growth of the Child. Leiden: Stenfert Kroese, 1966:99–118.
4. Lemann J Jr. Urinary excretion of calcium, magnesium, and phosphorus. In: Favus MJ, ed. Primer of the Metabolic Bone Diseases and Disorders of Mineral Metabolism, 2nd ed. New York: Raven Press, 1993:50–54.
5. Hauschka PV, Gallop PM. Purification and calcium-binding properties of osteocalcin, the γ-carboxyglutamate-containing protein of bone. In: Wasserman RH, Carradino RA, Carafoli E, et al., eds. Calcium Binding Proteins and Calcium Functions. New York: North Holland, 1977:338.
6. Hauschka PV, Frenkel J, DeMuth R, Gundberg CM. Presence of osteocalcin and related higher molecular weight carboxyglutamic acid-containing proteins in developing bone. J Biol Chem 1983; 250:176.
7. Nishimoto SK, Price PA. Proof that the γ-carboxyglutamic acid-containg bone protein is synthesized in calf bone. J Biol Chem 1979; 254–447.
8. Lian JB, Roufosse AH, Reit B, Glimcher MJ. Concentrations of osteocalcin and phosphoprotein as a function of mineral content and age in cortical bone. Calif Tissue Int 1982; 34:S82.
9. Price PA, Parthemore JG, Deftos LJ. New biochemical marker for bone metabolism: measurement by radioimmunoassay of bone Gla protein in the plasma of normal subjects and patients with bone disease. J Clin Invest 1980; 66:878.
10. Karfitt AM, Simon LS, Villanueva AR, Krane SM. Procollagen type I carboxyterminal extension peptide in serum as a marker of collagen biosynthesis in bone. Correlation with iliac bone formation rates and comparison with total alkaline phosphatase. J Bone Miner Res 1987; 2:427–436.
11. Simon LS, Slovik DM, Neer RM, Krane SM. Changes in serum levels of type I and III procollagen extension peptides during infusion of human parathyroid hormone fragment (1–34). J Bone Miner Res 1988; 3:241–246.
12. Genant HK, Block JE, Steiger P, Glueer CC, Ettinger B, Harris ST. Appropriate use of bone densitometry. Radiology 1989; 170:817–822.
13. Colbert C, Spruit JJ, Davila LR. Biophysical properties of bone: determining mineral concentration from the x-ray image. Trans NY Acad Sci 1967–1968; 30:271.
14. Colbert C, Bachtell RS. Radiographic absorptimetry (photodensitometry). In: Cohn SH, ed. Non-invasive Measurements of Bone Mass and Their Clinical Application. Boca Raton, FL: CRC Press, 1981:51–84.
15. Nilas L, Norgaard H, Podenphant J, Gotfredsen A, Christiansen C. Bone composition in the distal forearm. Scand J Clin Lab Invest 1987; 47:41–47.
16. Wahner HW, Brown ML, Dunn WL, Hauser MF, Morin RL. Comparison of quantitative digital radiography and dual photon absorptiometry for bone mineral measurement of the lumbar spine, In: Dequeker J, Geusens P, Wahner HW, eds. Bone Mineral Measurement by Photon Absorptiometry: Methodological Problems. Leuven: Leuven University Press, 1988: 419–426.
17. Revak CS. Mineral content of cortical bone measured by computed tomography. J Comput Assist Tomogr 1980; 4:342–350.
18. Genant HK, Block JE, Steiger P, Glueer CC, Smith R. Quantitative computed tomography in assessment of osteoporosis. Semin Nucl Med 1987; 17:316–333.
19. Canalis E. The hormonal and local regulation of bone formation. Endocr Rev 1983; 4:62–77.

20. Canalis E, McCarthy TL, Centrella M. Growth factors and cytokines in bone cell metabolism. Annu Rev Med 1991; 42:17–24.

21. Canalis E. Growth factors and their potential clinical value. J Clin Endocrinol Metab 1992; 75:1–4.

22. Dodd K, Grawbarth H, Rapoport S. Hypercalcemia nephropathy and encephalopathy following immobilization. Pediatrics 1952; 6:124–130.

23. Evans RA, Bridgeman M, Hilis E, Dunstan CR. Immobilization hypercalcemia. Miner Electrolyte Metab 1984; 10:244–248.

24. Winters JL, Kleinschmidt AG Jr, Frensilli JJ, Sutton M. Hypercalcemia complicating immobilization in the treatment of fractures. J Bone Joint Surg [Am] 1966;48:1182–1184.

25. Hulley SB, Vogel JM, Donaldson CL, Bayers JH, Friedman RJ, Rosen SN. The effect of supplemental oral phosphate on the bone mineral changes during prolonged bed rest. J Clin Invest 1971; 50:2506–2518.

26. Langman CB, Moore ES. Hypercalcemia in clinical pediatrics. Clin Pediatr (Phila) 1984; 23:135–137.

27. Moore ES, Coe FL, McMann BJ, Favus MJ. Idiopathic hypercalcemia in children: prevalence and metabolic characteristics. J Pediatr 1978; 92:906–910.

28. Stapelton FB, Noe HN, Jerkins G. Urinary excretion of calcium following an oral calcium loading test in healthy children. Pediatrics 1982; 69:594–597.

29. Rose A. Immobilization osteoporosis. A study of the extent, severity and treatment with bendrofluazide. Br J Surg 1966; 53:769–777.

30. Price PA, Otsuka AA, Poser JW, Kristaponis J, Raman N. Characterization of a γ-carboxyglutamic acid-containing protein from bone. Proc Natl Acad Sci USA 1976; 73:1447–1451.

31. Price PA, Otsuka A, Poser JW. Comparing γ-carboxy-glutamic acid-containing proteins from bovine and swordfish bone: primary structure and Ca^{2+} binding. In: Wasserman RH, Carradino RA, Carafoli E, Kretsinger RH, McLennan DH, Siegel FL, eds. Calcium-Binding Proteins and Calcium Functions. New York: North Holland, 1977:333–337.

32. Nishimoto SK, Price PA. Secretion of the vitamin K-dependent protein of bone by rat osteosarcoma cells. J Biol Chem 1980; 255:6579–6583.

33. Price PA, Parthemore JG, Deftos LJ. New biochemical marker for bone metabolism: measurement by radioimmunoassay of bone Gla protein in the plasma of normal subjects and patient with bone disease. J Clin Invest 1980; 66:879–883.

34. Gundberg CM, Lian JB, Gallop PM. Measurements of γ-carboxyglutamate and circulating osteocalcin in normal children and adults. Clin Chim Acta 1983; 128:1–8.

35. Lian JB, Glimcher MJ, Roufosse AH, et al. Alteration of the carboxyglutamic acid and osteocalcin concentrations in vitamin D-deficient chick bone. J Biol Chem 1982; 257:4999–5003.

36. Price PA, Baukol SA. 1,25-Dihydroxy-vitamin D_3, increases synthesis of the vitamin K-dependent bone protein by osteosarcoma cells. J Biol Chem Commun 1980; 255:1660–1663.

37. Price PA, Buakol SA. 1,25-Dihydroxy-vitamin D_3 increases serum levels of the vitamin K-dependent bone protein.

38. Castells S, Yasumura S, Fusi MA, Colbert C, Bachtell RS, Smith S. Plasma osteocalcin levels in patients with osteogenesis imperfecta. J Pediatr 1986; 109:88–91.

39. Castells S, Yasumura S, Smith S, Casas J. Calcitonin suppresses elevated plasma levels of osteocalcin in children with osteogenesis imperfecta. Pediatr Res 1986; 20:327A.

40. Brenner RE, Schiller B, Vetter U, Ittner J, Teller WM. Serum concentration of procollagen IC-terminal propeptide, osteocalcin and insulin-like growth factor-I in patients with non-lethal osteogenesis imperfecta. Acta Paediatr 1993; 82:764–767.

41. Greig F, Casas J, Castells S. Changes in plasma osteocalin concentrations during treatment of rickets. J Pediatr 1989; 114:820–823.

42. Castells S, Greig F, Fusi MA, et al. Severely deficient binding of 1,25-dihydroxyvitamin D to its receptors in a patient responsive to high doses of this hormone. Clin Endocrinol Metab 1986; 63:252–256.

43. Delmas DD, Chatelain P, Malaval L, Bonne G. Serum bone Gla-protein in growth hormone deficient children. J Bone Miner Res 1986; 1:333–338.

44. Cole DEC, Carpenter TO, Gundberg CM. Serum osteocalcin concentrations in children with metabolic bone disease. J Pediatr 1985; 106:770–776.

45. Bradford DS, Brown DM, Moe JH, Winter RB, Towsey J. Scheuermann's kyphosis: a form of juvenile osteoporosis. Clin Orthop 1976; 118:10–15.

46. Jones ET, Hesinger RN. Spinal deformity in idiopathic juvenile osteoporosis. Spine 1981; 6:1–4.

47. Bradford DS, Moe JH. Scheuermann's juvenile kyphosis. Clin Orthop 1975; 110:45.

48. Jowsey J, Johnson KA. Juvenile osteoporosis: bone findings in seven patients. J Pediatr 1972; 81:511–517.

49. Cloutier MD, Hayles AB, Riggs BL, Jowsey J, Bickel WH. Juvenile osteoporsis: report of a case including a description of some metabolic and microradiographic studies. Pediatrics 1967; 40:649–655.

50. Jowsey J, Johnson KA. Juvenile osteoporosis: bone findings in seven patients. J Pediatr 1972; 81:511–517.

51. Hoekman K, Pappapoulos SE, Peters ACB, Bijvoet OL. Characteristics and bisphosphonate treatment of a patient with juvenile osteoporosis. J Clin Endocrinol Metab 1985; 61:952–956.

52. Evans RA, Dunstan CR, Hill E. Bone metabolism in idiopathic juvenile osteoporosis: a case report. Calif Tissue Int 1983; 35:5–8.

53. Smith R. Idiopathic osteoporosis in the young. J Bone Joint Surg [Br] 1980; 620:417–427.

54. Teotia M, Teotia SPS, Singh RK. Idiopathic juvenile osteoporosis. Am J Dis Child 1979; 133:894–900.

55. Lapatsanis P, Kavadias A, Uretos K. Juvenile osteoporosis. Arch Dis Child 1971; 46:66–71.

56. Marder HK, Tsang RC, Hug G, Crawford AC. Calcitriol deficiency in idiopathic juvenile osteoporosis. Am J Dis Child 1982; 136:914–917.

57. Saggese G, Bertelloni S, Baroncelli G, Perri G, Calderazzi A. Mineral metabolism and calcitriol therapy in idiopathic juvenile osteoporosis. Am J Dis Child 1991; 145:457–461.

58. Dent CE, Friedman M. Idiopathic juvenile osteoporosis. QJ Med 1965; 34:177–210.

59. Evans RA, Bridgeman M, Hills E, Dunstan CR. Immobilization hypercalcemia. Miner Electrolyte Metab 1984; 10:244–248.

60. Jackson EC, Strife CF, Tsang RC, Marder HK. Effect of calcitonin replacement therapy in idiopathic juvenile osteoporosis. Am J Dis Child 1988; 142:1237–1239.

61. Halvorsen L. Osteoporosis, hypercalcemia and nephropathy following immobilization in children. Acta Med Scand 1954; 149:401–408.

62. Root AW, Bongiovanni AM, Eberlein WR. Measurement of the kinetics of calcium metabolism in children and adolescents utilizing nonradioactive strontium. J Clin Endocrinol Metab 1966; 26:537–544.

63. Maynard FM. Immobilization hypercalcemia following spinal cord injury. Arch Phys Med Rehabil 1986; 67:41–44.

64. Health H, Earll JM, Schaaf M, Piechocki JT, Li TK. Serum ionized calcium during bed rest in fracture patients and normal men. Metabolism 1972; 21:633–640.

65. Hyman LR, Boner G, Thomas JC, Segar WE. Immobilization hypercalcemia. Am J Dis Child 1972; 124:723–727.

66. Minairie P, Meunier P, Edouard C, Bernard J, Courpron P, Bourret J. Quantitative histologic data on disuse osteoporosis; comparison with biological data. Calcif Tissue Res 1974; 17:57–73.

67. Becker RO. Electrical osteogenesis-pro and con. Calcif Tissue Res 26:93–97.

68. Hardt AB. Early metabolic responses of bone to immobilization. J Bone Joint Surg [Am] 1972; 54:119–124.

69. Geiser M, Trueta J. Muscle action, bone rarefraction and bone formation; an experimental study. J Bone Joint Surg [Br] 1958; 40:282–311.

70. Bronner F, Richelle WJ, Saville PD, Nicholas JS, Cobb JR. Quantitation of calcium-metabolism in postmenopausal osteoporosis and in scoliosis. J Clin Invest 1963; 42:898–905.

71. Van Zuiden L, Anguist KA, Schachar N, Kastelen N. Immobilization hypercalcemia. Can J Surg 1982; 25:646–649.

72. Goldsmith RS, Ingbar SH. Inorganic phosphate treatment of diverse etiologies. N Engl J Med 1966; 24:1–7.

73. Enkoyan G, Suki WN Martinez-Maldonaddo M. Effect of diuretics on urinary excretion of phosphate, calcium, and magnesium in thyroparathyroidectomized dogs. J Lab Clin Med 1970; 76:257–268.

74. Singer FR, Neer RM, Murray TM, Keutmann HT, Deftos LJ, Potts JT Jr. Mithramycin treatment of intractable hypercalcemia due to parathyroid carcinoma. N Engl J Med 1970; 282:634–636.

75. Choremis C, Yannakos D, Papadotos C, Baroutsou E. Osteitis deformans (Paget's disease) in an 11 year old boy. Helv Paediatr Acta 1958; 13:185–188.

76. Irving RE. Familial Paget's disease with early onset. J Bone Joint Surg [Br] 1953; 35:106–111.

77. DeRose J, Singer FR, Avvramides A, et al. Response of Paget's disease to porcine and salmon calcitonins: effects of long term treatment. Am J Med 1974; 56:858–866.

78. Goldfield EB, Braiker BM, Prendergat JJ, Kolb FO. Synthetic salmon calcitonin: treatment of Paget's disease and osteogenesis imperfecta. JAMA 1972; 22:1127–1129.

79. Doyle FH, Woodhouse NJY, Glen ACA, Jopin FG, McIntryre I. Healing of the bone in juvenile Paget's disease treated with human calcitonin. Br J Radiol 1974; 47:9–15.

80. Falvo KA, Root L, Bullough PG. Osteogenesis imperfecta: clinical evaluation and management. J Bone Joint Surg [Am] 1974; 56:783–793.

81. Silence DO, Senn A, Danks DM. Genetic heterogeneity in osteogenesis imperfecta. J Med Genet 1979; 16:101–116.

82. Byers PH, Bonadio JF, Steinman B. Invited editorial comment. Osteogenesis imperfecta: updata and prospective. Am J Med Genet 1984; 17:429–435.

83. Wynne-Davis R, Gormley J. Clinical and genetic patterns in osteogenesis imperfecta. Clin Orthop 1981; 159:26–35.

84. Gunnar S, Osteogenesis Imperfecta in Sweden. Stockholm: Scandinavia University Books, 1961.

85. Miller EJ. A review of biochemical studies on the genetically distinct collagens of the skeletal system. Clin Orthop 1973; 92:260.

86. Rowe DW, Poirier M, Shapiro J. Osteogenesis imperfecta: a genetic probe to study type I collagen biosynthesis. In: Veiw A, ed. The Chemistry and Biology of Mineralized Connective Tissues. New York: Elsevier–North Holland, 1981:155–162.

87. Bornstein P. Structurally distinct collagen types. Annu Rev Biochem 1980; 49:957–1003.

88. Sykes B, Francis MJ, Smith R. Altered relation of two collagen types in osteogenesis imperfecta. N Engl J Med 1977; 296:1200–1203.

89. Barsh GS, David KE, Pyers PH. Type I osteogenesis imperfecta: a nonfunctional allele for pro α_1(I) chains of type I procollagen. Proc Natl Acad Sci USA 1982; 79:3838–3842.

90. Trelstad RL, Rubin D, Gross J. Osteogenesis imperfecta congenita: evidence for a generalized molecular disorder of collagen. Lab Invest 1971;36:501–508.

91. Barsh GS, Byers PH. Reduced secretion of structurally abnormal type I procollagen in a form of osteogenesis imperfecta. Proc Natl Acad Sci USA 1981; 78:5142–5146.

92. Williams C, Prockop DJ. Synthesis and processing of a type I procollagen containing shortened pro α_1(I) chains by fibroblasts from a patient with osteogenesis imperfecta. J Biol Chem 1983; 258:5915–5921.

93. Kirsch E, Glanville RW, Krieg T, Muller P. Analysis of cyanogen bromide peptides of type I collagen from a patient with lethal osteogenesis imperfecta. Biochem J 1983; 211:599–603.

94. Dewet WG, Pihlajaniemi T, Myers J, Kelly TE, Prockop DJ. Synthesis of a shortened pro-α_2(I) chain and decreased synthesis of pro-α_1(I) chains in a proband with osteogenesis imperfecta. J Biol Chem 1983; 258:7721–7728.

95. Batman JF, Mascara T, Chan D, Cole WG. Abnormal type I collagen metabolism by cultured fibroblasts in fetal preinatal osteogenesis imperfecta. Biochem J 1984; 217:103–115.

96. Steinmann B, Rao VH, Vogel A, Bruchner P, Gitzelmann R, Byers PH. Cysteine in triple-helical domain of one allelic product of the α_1(I) gene of type I collagen produces of lethal form of osteogenesis imperfecta. J Biol Chem 1984; 259:1129–1138.

97. Bonadio J, Holbrook KA, Gelinas RE, Jacob J, Byers PH. Altered triple-helical structure of type I procollagen in lethal perinatal osteogenesis imperfecta. J Biol Chem 1985; 260:1734–1742.

98. Pope FM, Cheah KSE, Nicholls AC, Price AB, Grosveld FG. Lethal osteogenesis imperfecta congenita and a 300 base pair gene deletion for an α_1(I)-like collagen. BMJ 1984; 288:431–434.

99. Sykes BC, Ogilvie DJ, Wordsworth BP. Lethal osteogenesis imperfecta and a collagen gene deletion. Length polymorphism provides and alternative explanation. Hum Genet 1985; 70:35–37.

100. Chu ML, Williams CJ, Pepe G, Hirsch JL, Prockop DJ, Ramirez F. Internal deletion of agene in a perinatal lethal form of osteogenesis imperfecta. Nature 1983; 304:78–80.

101. Ramirez F, Sangiorgi FO, Tsipouras P. Human collagens. Biochemical molecular and genetic features in normal and diseased states. In: Blasi F, ed. Human Genes and Diseases. Chichester: John Wiley & Sons, 1986:341–375.

102. Peltonen L, Palotie A, Prockop DJ. A defect in the structure of type I procollagen in a patient who had osteogenesis imperfecta: excess mannose in the COOH-terminal propeptide. Proc Natl Acad Sci USA 1980; 77:6179–6183.

103. Pope FM, Nicholls AC. Heterogeneity of osteogenesis imperfecta congenita. Lancet 1980; 1:820–821.

104. Deak S, Chu ML, Meyers TC, et al. A term of osteogenesis imperfecta in which the mRNA for pro-α_2(I) is inefficiently translated in fibroblasts. Fed Proc 1982; 41:825A.

105. Chu ML, Rowe D, Nicholls AC, Pope FM, Prockop DJ. Presence of translatable mRNA for pro-α_2(I) chains in fibroblasts from a patient with osteogenesis imperfecta where type I collagen does not contain α_2 (I) chains. Collagen 1984; 4:389–394.

106. Byers PH, Shapiro JR, Rowe DW, David KE, Holbroo KA. Abnormal α_2 chain in type I collagen from a patient with a form of osteogenesis imperfecta. J Clin Invest 1983; 71:689–694.

107. Byers PH, Bonadio JF, Steinmann B. Osteogenesis imperfecta: update and prospective. Am J Med Genet 1984; 17:429–435.

108. Tsipouras P, Myers JC, Ramirez F, Prockop DJ. Restriction fragment length polymorphism associated with the pro-α_2(I) gene of human type I procollagen. Application to a family with an autosomal dominant form of osteogenesis imperfecta. J Clin Invest 1983; 72:1262–1267.

109. Kuivaniemi H, Tromp G, Prockop DJ. Mutations in collagen genes because of rare and some common diseases in humans. FASEB J 1991; 5:2052–2060.

110. Byers PH, Steiner RD. Osteogenesis imperfecta. Annu Rev Med 1992; 43:269–282.

111. Jett S, Ramser JR, Forst HM, Villaneuva AR. Bone turnover and osteogenesis imperfecta. Arch Pathol 1966; 81:112–116.

112. Lee WR. A quantitative microscopic study of bone formation in a normal child and 2 children suffering from osteogenesis imperfecta. In: Proceedings of the Second Symposium of Calcified Tissues. Leige, 1965:451.

113. Ramser JR, Villanueva AR, Pirok D, Frost HM. Tetracyclin-based measurement of bone dynamics in 3 women with osteogenesis imperfecta. Clin Orthop 1966;49:151–162.

114. Castells S, Lu C, Baker RK, Wallach S. Effects of synthetic salmon calcitonin in osteogenesis imperfecta. Curr Ther Res 1974; 16:1–13.

115. Shapiro JE, Phillips JA III, Byers PH et al. Prenatal diagnosis of lethal preinatal osteogenesis imperfecta (01 type II). J Pediatr 1982; 100:127–133.

116. Elejalde BR, de Eljalde MD. Prenatal diagnosis of perinatally lethal osteogenesis imperfecta. Am J Med Genet 1983; 14: 353–359.

117. Hobbins JC, Bracken MB, Mahoney MJ. Diagnosis of fetal skeletal dysplasia with ultrasound. Am J Obstet Gynecol 1982; 142:306–312.

118. Bernstein DS, Cohen P. Use of sodium fluoride in the treatment of osteoporosis. J Clin Endocrinol Metab 1967; 27:197–210.

119. Cass RM, Croft JD Jr, Perkins P, Nye W, Waterhouse C, Terry R. New bone formation in osteoporosis following treatment with sodium fluoride. Arch Intern Med 1966; 118:111–116.

120. Cohen MB, Rubini ME. The treatment of osteoporosis with sodium fluoride. Clin Orthop 1965; 40:147–152.

121. Geal MG, Beilin LJ. Sodium fluoride and optic neuritis. BMJ 1964; 2:355–356.

122. Rich C, Ensinck J. Effect of sodium fluoride on calcium metabolism of human beings. Nature 1961; 191:184–195.

123. Slayton R, Ensinck J, Ivanovich P. The effects of sodium fluoride on calcium metabolism of subjects with metabolic bone disease. J Clin Invest 1964; 43:545–556.

124. Rich C, Ivanovich P. Response to sodium fluoride in severe primary osteoporosis. Ann Intern Med 1965; 63:1069–1074.

125. Rose GA. Study of the treatment of osteoporosis with fluoride therapy and high calcium intake. Proc R Soc Med 1965; 58:436–440.

126. Cohen P, Gardner FH. Induction of skeletal fluorisis in two common demineralizing disorders. JAMA 1964; 195:962–963.

127. Neer RM, Zipkin I, Carbone PP, Rosenberg LE. Effect of sodium fluoride therapy on calcium metabolism in multiple myeloma. J Clin Endocrinol Metab 1966; 26:1059–1068.

128. Higgens BA, Nassim JR, Alexander R, Hilb A. Effect of sodium fluoride on calcitonin, phosphorus, nitrogen balance in patients with Paget's disease. BMJ 1965; 1:1159–1161.

129. Albright JA, Grunt JA. Studies of patients with osteogenesis imperfects. J Bone Joint Surg [Am] 1971; 53:1415.

130. Solomons CC, Styner J. Osteogenesis imperfecta. Effect on magnesium administration of pyrophosphate metabolism. Calcif Tissue Res 1969; 3:318–326.

131. Hirsch PF, Munson PL. Thyrocalcitonin. Physiol Res 1969; 49:547.

132. Rasmussen H, Tenenhous A. Thyroacalcitonin, osteoporosis, and osteolysis. Am J Med 1967; 43:711–726.

133. Castells S, Colbert C, Chakrabarti C, Bachtell RS, Kassner EG, Yasumura S. Therapy for osteogenesis imperfecta with synthetic salmon calcitonin. J Pediatr

134. Nishi Y, Hamamoto K, Kajiyama M, Onoh, Kihara M, Jinno K. The effect of long-term calcitonin therapy by injection and nasal spray on the incidence of fractures in osteogenesis imperfecta. J Pediatr 1992; 121:477–480.

135. Chawla S. Cranio-skeletal dysplasia with acro-osteolysis. Br J Radiol 1964; 37:702–705.

136. Cheney WD. Acro-osteolysis. AJR 1985; 94:595–607.

137. Kohler E, Babbitt D, Huizenga B, Good TA. Hereditary osteolysis. Pediatr Radiol 1973; 108:99–105.

138. Mahoudeau D, Dubrisay J, Elissalde B, Sraer C. Osteolyse essentielle nephrite. Bull Mem Soc Med Hop 1961; 77:229–234.

139. Marie J, Leveque B, Lyon G, Bebe M, Watchi TM. Acro-osteolyse esentielle compliquee de'insuffisanse renale d'evauation fetale. Presse Med 1963; 71:249–252.

140. Torg JS, Steel HH. Essential osteolysis with nephropathy. A review of the literature and case report of an unusual syndrome. J Bone Joint Surg 1958; 50:1629–1638.

141. Shurtleff DB, Sparkes RS, Clawson K, Gutheroth WG, Mottet NK. Hereditary osteolysis with hypertension and nephropathy. JAMA 1964; 188:133–118.

142. Gorham L, Wright AW, Shultz HH, Maxon FC Jr. Disappearing bone: a rare form of massive osteolysis. Am J Med 1954; 17:674–682.

143. Halliday DR, Dahlin DC, Pugh DG, Young HH. Massive osteolysis and angiomatosis. Radiology 1964; 82:637–644.

144. Winchester P, Grossman H, Lim WN, Danes BS. A new acid mucopolysaccharidosis with skeletal deformities stimulating rheumatoid arthritis. AJR 1968; 106:121–128.

145. Brown SI, Kuwabara T. Peripheral corneal opacification and skeletal deformities. Arch Ophthalmol 1970; 83:667–577.

146. Hollister DW, Rimoin DL, Lachman RS, Cohen AH, Reed WB, Westin GW. The Winchester syndrome: a nonlysosomal connective tissue disease. J Pediatr 1974; 84:701–709.

147. Cohen AH, Hollister DW, Reed WB. The skin in the Winchester syndrome: histological and ultrastructural studies. Arch Dermatol 1975; 111:230–136.

148. Castells S, Sher J, Rose J, Anderson HC, Shafig S, Hashemia SE. Selective muscle fiber hypoplasia and epiphyseal osteolysis. Pediatr Res 1977; 2:920–928.

149. Johnson CC Jr, Lavy N, Lord T, Vellios F, Merritt AD, Deiss WP. Osteopetrosis: clinical, genetic, metabolic, and morphologic study of the dominantly inherited, benign form. Medicine (Baltimore) 1968; 47:149–167.

150. Bollerslev J. Osteopetrosis: a genetic and epidemiological study. Clin Genet 1987; 31:86–90.

151. Frost HM, Villanueva AR, Jett S, Eyring E. Tetracycline based analysis of bone remodeling in osteopetrosis. Clin Orthop 1969; 65:203–217.

152. Walker DG. Osteoporosis cured by temporary parabiosis. Science 1973; 180:875.

153. Walker DG. Bone resorption restored in osteopetrotic mice by transplants of normal bone marrow and spleen cells. Science 1975; 190:784–787.

154. Bonucci E. New knowledge on the origin, function and fate of osteoclasts. Clin Orthop 1981; 158:252–269.

155. Marks SC. Osteopetrosis—multiple pathways for the interception of osteoclast function. Bone Pathol Appl Pathol 1987; 5:172–183.

156. Coccia PF, Krivit W, Cervenka J, et al. Successful bone-marrow transplantation for infantile malignant osteopetrosis. N Engl J Med 1980; 302:701–708.

157. Key L, Carnes D, Cole S, et al. Treatment of congenital osteopetrosis with high dose calcitriol. N Engl J Med 1984; 310:409–415.

158. Ambler MW, Trice J, Grauerholz J, O'Shea PA. Infantile osteopetrosis and neuronal storage disease. Neurology 1983; 33:437–441.

159. Sly WS, Hewett-Emmett D, Whyte MP, Yu YL, Tashian RE. Carbonic anhydrase II deficiency identified as the primary defect in autosomal recessive syndrome of osteopetrosis with renal tubular acidosis and cerebral calcification. Proc Natl Acad Sci USA 1983; 80:2752–2756.

160. Sly WS, Whyte MP, Sundaram V et al. Carbonic anhydrase II deficiency in 12 families with the autosomal recessive syndrome of osteopetrosis with renal tubualr acidosis and cerebral calcification. N Engl J Med 1985; 313:139–145.

161. Glorieux FH, Pettifor JM, Marie PJ, Delvin EE, Travers R, Shepard N. Induction of bone resorption by parathyroid hormone in congenital malignant osteopetrosis. Metab Bone Dis 1981; 3:143–150.

162. Shapiro F, Glimcher MJ, Haltrop ME, Tashjian AH, Brickley-Parsons D, Kenzora JE. Human osteopetrosis. J Bone Joint Surg [Am] 1980; 62:384–399.

163. Reeves J, Arnaud S, Gordon S, et al. The pathogenesis of infantile malignant osteopetrosis: bone mineral metabolism and complications in five infants. Metab Bone Dis 1981; 3:135–142.

164. Teitelbaum SL, Coccia PF, Brown DM, Kahn AJ. Malignant osteopetrosis: a disease of abnormal osteoclast proliferation. Metab Bone Dis 1981; 3:99–105.

165. Horton WA, Schimke RN, Iyama T. Osteopetrosis: further heterogeneity. J Pediatr 1980; 97:580–585.

166. Bonucci E, Sartori E, Spina M. Osteopetrosis fetalis: report of a case with special reference to ultrastructure. Virchows Arch [A] 1975; 368:109–121.

167. El Khanzen N, Tanerly D, Vamos E, et al. Lethal osteopetrosis with multiple fractures in utero. Am J Med Genet 1986; 23:811–819.

168. Mathur BP, Karan S. Non-immune hydrops fetalis due to osteopetrosis congenita. Indian Pediatr 1984; 21:651–653.

169. Friede H, Mananligod JR, Rosenthal IM. Craniofacial abnormalities in osteopetrosis with precocious manifestations: report of a case with serial cephalometric roentgenograms. J Craniofac Genet Dev Biol 1985; 5:247–257.

170. Chudhuri JN, Banerjee S, Koshnia BR, Chatterji P, Soni NK. Marble bone disease in a child. J Laryngol Otol 1986; 100:935–938.

171. Marula AA, Ambegaikar AG. Choanal atresia: early management and an association with marble bone disease. J Laryngol Otol 1986; 100:959–963.

172. Oliveira G, Boechat MI, Amaral SM, Young LW. Osteopetrosis and rickets: an intriguing association. Am J Dis Child 1986; 140:337–338.

173. McClearly L, Rovit RJ, Murali R. Case report: Myelopathy secondary to congenital osteopetrosis of the cervical spine. Neurosurgery 1987; 20:487–489.

174. Miyamoto RT, House WF, Brackmann DE. Neurotologic manifestations of the osteopetroses. Arch Otolaryngol 1980; 106:210–214.

175. Bajaj S, Gupta SC, Nigam DK. Osteopetrosis with bilateral facial nerve palsy. J Assoc Physicians India 1986; 34:529–530.

176. Andersen PE Jr, Bollerslev J. Heterogeneity of autosomal dominant osteopetrosis. Radiology 1987; 164:223–225.

177. Silvestrini G, Ferracciolli GF, Quaini F, Palummeri E, Bonnucci E. Adult osteopetrosis: study of two brothers. Appl Pathol 1987; 5:184–189.

178. Gupta DS, Gupta MK, Borle RM. Osteomyelitis of the mandible in marble bone disease. Int J Oral Maxillofac Surg 1986; 15:201–205.

179. Steiner M, Gould AR, Means WR. Osteomyelitis of the mandible associated with osteopetrosis. J Oral Maxillofac Surg 1983; 41:395–405.

180. Crokett DM, Stanley RB, Lubka R. Osteomyelitis of the maxilla in a patient with osteopetrosis (Albers-Schonberg's disease). Otolaryngol Head Neck Surg 1986; 95:117–121.

181. Adeloye A. The syndrome of osteopetrosis in siblings: its occurrence in two sisters in Nigeria. Childs Nerv Syst 1987; 3:128–131.

182. Ohlsson A, Cumming WA, Paul A, Sly WS. Carbonic anhydrase II deficiency syndrome: recessive osteopetrosis with renal tubular acidosis and cerebral calcification. Pediatrics 1986; 77:371–381.

183. Cumming WA, Ohlsson A. Intracranial calcification in children with osteopetrosis caused by carbonic anhydrase Ii deficiency. Radiology 1985; 157:325–327.

184. Ohlsson A, Stark G, Sakati N. Marble bone disease: recessive osteopetrosis, renal tubular acidosis and cerebral calcification in three Saudi Arabian families. Dev Med Child Neurol 1980; 22:72–84.

185. Whyte MP, Murphy WA, Fallon MD, et al. Osteopetrosis, renal tubular acidosis and basal ganglia calcification in three sisters. Am J Med 1980; 69:64–74.

186. Shibuya H, Suzuki T, Matsusaka S, Suzuki S. Non-Hodgkin's lymphoma in a patient with osteopetrosis. Lymphology 1986; 19:90–92.

187. Henderson RG, Long PJ, Al-Nafussi AI, Coombs RR, Gibson RN. Paget's disease with benign osteopetorosis and Crohn's disease. JR Soc Med 1985; 78:766–768.

188. Sand JJ, Biller J, Aschenbrener CA. Nonbacterial thrombotic endocarditis and nondisseminated malignancy associated with osteopetrosis. Eur Neurol 1987; 27:167–172.

189. Sieff CA, Chessells JM, Levinsky RJ, et al. Allogeneic bone-marrow transplantation in infantile malignant osteopetrosis. Lancet 1983; 1:437–441.

190. Nisbet NW. Bone marrow transplantation in precocious osteopetrosis (editorial). BMJ 1987; 294:463–464.

191. Eischer A, Griscelli C, Friedrich W, et al. Bone-marrow transplantation for immuno deficiencies and osteopetrosis: European survey 1968–1985. Lancet 1986; 2:1080–1084.

192. Sorell M, Kapoor N, Kirkpatrick D, et al. Marrow transplantation for juvenile ostepetrosis. Am J Med 1987; 70:1280–1287.

193. Miyaura C, Abe E, Kuribayshi T, et al. 1α,25-Dihydroxyvitamin D$_3$ induces differentiation of human myeloid leukemia cells. Biochem Biophys Res Commun 1981; 102:937–943.

194. Bar-Shavit Z, Teitelbaum SL, Reitsma P, et al. Induction of monocyte differentiation and bone resorption of 1,25-dihydroxyvitamin D$_3$. Proc Natl Acad Sci USA 1983; 80: 5907–5911.

195. Tinkler SMB, Williams DM, Johnson NW. Osteoclast formation in response to intraperitoneal injection of 1α-hydroxycholecalciferol in mice. J Anat 1981; 133:91–97.

196. Blazar BR, Fallon MD, Teitlebaum SL, Ramsay NK, Brown DM. Calcitriol for congenital osteopetrosis (letter). N Engl J Med 1984; 311:55.

197. Ozsoylu S. High dose intravenous methylprednisolone in treatment of recessive osteopetrosis (letter). Arch Dis Child 1987; 62:214–215.

36

Metabolic Bone Disease in Total Parenteral Nutrition

Adib Moukarzel

Maimonides Medical Center and State University of New York Health Science Center at Brooklyn, Brooklyn, New York

I. INTRODUCTION

Parenteral nutrition (PN) is a technique for providing the body's nutritional needs through the intravenous route. The nutrients that are typically administered consist of water, dextrose, amino acids, lipid emulsion, minerals, vitamins, and trace metals. Intravenous nutrition has been available for the past 25 years and has become a well-accepted medical practice. For the newborn and infant, intravenous nutrition is usually given continuously. Children and adolescents usually receive nightly cyclic therapy over 10–14 h, which allows a more normal life in a home setting when the PN is thought to be necessary for a prolonged period. However, metabolic, mechanical, and infectious complications can occur with its use. Bone disease is a well-known complication of prolonged PN therapy and has been reported in patients of all ages (1–5).

In the past, a clinical syndrome seen in patients on long-term PN consisting of potentially severe bone pain and fractures, hypercalcemia with normal serum phosphate, 1,25-dihydroxyvitamin D, and 25-dihydroxyvitamin D was associated with aluminum toxicity (3–7). This symptomatic bone disease has not been seen in patients who receive crystalline amino acid solutions contaminated with small amounts of aluminum (8). Today, the prevalence of this bone disease is unknown. Reports suggest that 40–100% of subjects receiving long-term PN have histological features of bone disease or decreased bone density (5), but many of these are asymptomatic. The incidence of PN-related bone disease would be significantly higher using more sensitive measurements of bone mineralization such as bone densitometry or neutron activation or with the use of biochemical criteria of elevated serum alkaline phosphatase activity and abnormal serum calcium (Ca) and phosphorus (P) concentrations (9).

Premature infants may develop a condition called osteopenia of prematurity, which is characterized by decreased bone mineralization. In most instances, it is subclinical and is often diagnosed only after the development of bone fractures or overt rickets (10). It is currently believed that deficiencies of calcium and phosphorus are responsible for the osteopenia, rather than a defect in vitamin D metabolism (11). Fluoride deficiency has also been implicated in its pathogenesis (12).

Osteopenia in the premature infant can be assessed by measuring the serum alkaline phosphatase level. Elevations exceeding six times the adult normal value warrant further evaluation. In infants, bone disease may result in considerable morbidity (1,10,13). Newborns with the lowest gestational ages and birth weights tend to develop osteopenia after a much shorter period of PN support compared to older children. The bone disease may be diagnosed as early as 2–4 months after birth (10). The effects of underlying illnesses and associated nutritional deficiencies, including disturbed mineral homeostasis (14) and low bone mineral content (15,16), paradoxically may become more prominent as the general nutritional status of the patient improves. For example, in adults, symptomatic bone disease often occurs after significant weight gain, and the pain improves when PN is stopped (3). In infants, nutritional rickets tends to develop during the period of postnatal "catchup" growth during recovery from serious illnesses (10). Severe intestinal malabsorption increases the risk of bone abnormalities. Hylander and colleagues (17,18) reported that 53% of 118 patients with Crohn's disease had decreased calcium absorption and reduced bone density before starting PN. In a report of eight infants who received at least 6 months of home PN, three of them had radiographic evidence of rickets or had one or more abnormal biochemical abnormalities consistent with the presence of bone disease (1).

II. BONE MINERALIZATION

Numerous factors may affect bone mineralization. However, few published reports control for the multiple confounding variables that affect the dynamic process of bone mineralization in patients receiving PN. These include parenteral intake of multiple nutrients, nonnutritional factors including the underlying disease processes that dictate the need for PN, and therapeutic interventions such as chronic diuretic therapy. The single most important contributor to the bone disease is the negative calcium balance, with increased urinary calcium losses and decreased mineral intake (9,10,19). The former seem to be related to the PN itself; the latter may be induced by low calcium supplementation in part due to the incompatibility of the high level of calcium and phosphorus in the PN solution.

Whether current total PN formulations contribute to the syndrome of bone pain and fractures remains controversial. A longitudinal assessment (20) involving 14 patients evaluated bone mass for 7–61 months by single and dual photon absorptiometry and by bone biopsy. The mean bone density of these patients was significantly below expected values when they entered the study, but during observation, PN produced no consistent positive or negative effects on bone health. Deterioration was noted in some patients, improvements or no change in others. The authors concluded that current PN formulations that are low in aluminum and vitamin D are not necessarily detrimental to the bones.

It is important to remember that PN is an unphysiological route of nutrient supply that bypasses the phylogenetic means of food processing and distribution, i.e., the gastrointestinal tract and the portal system. The effects of continuously administering nutrients directly into venous blood are largely unknown and appear to be associated with many alterations of bone and mineral metabolism. Thus, the different biochemical anomalies probably do not arise from a single cause, nor are the bone pain and fractures experienced by many patients necessarily manifestations of a single abnormality. The role in PN-related bone disease of a number of nutrients and toxins present in PN solutions in current use is shown in Table 1.

A. Increased Urinary Losses

Administration of a PN solution has been shown to induce increased urinary mineral losses (19). Protocols using different PN solutions evaluated the effects of varying the quantity of glucose, the amount of amino acids, or the quantity of calcium present in the PN solution. Urinary excretion was studied during PN infusion and when subjects were not infused (Table 2).

In comparison of measurements during the PN infusion with those during the daytime hours with no infusion, there was a 33% increase in endogenous creatinine clearance during the infusion period. More calcium, sodium, phosphate, and magnesium was excreted at night during the infusion than during the daytime hours when no infusions were given. After calcium was removed from the PN solution, there was a rapid reduction in the fractional excretion of calcium, and the urinary values returned quickly to the previous levels upon readdition of calcium to the infusion with no change in endogenous creatinine clearance rate. As calcium was either added to or removed from the PN solution, there were no significant changes in the fractional excretion of sodium, magnesium, or phosphate.

The effects of reducing the amino acid concentrations in the PN solution from 3% to 0.6% are also shown in Table 2. There was a small but significant decrease in the fractional excretion of calcium with the reduction of protein intake, during the PN infusion. The fractional calcium excretion tended to increase on return to the higher amount of protein. The fractional excretion rates for sodium, phosphate, and magnesium were unchanged. The effect of varying the quantity of glucose in the PN infusion on the fractional excretion of calcium was studied. Changing the quantity of glucose over a wide range had no effect on the fractional excretion of calcium. However, the presence of glucose in the PN solution affected the pattern of phosphate excretion. When glucose was removed from the PN solution, there was a greater fractional phosphate excretion during the infusion hours with glucose-free PN solution compared to the hours without the infusion, but there was no significant difference in fractional excretion of phosphate during the infusion hours with a glucose-containing PN solution compared to the noninfusion hours.

Additionally, there was a direct relationship between the total daily urinary calcium excretion and the amount of calcium given in the PN solution. In adults receiving 90 g amino acids/day, urinary calcium excretion often, but not invariably, exceeded the quantity administered; clearly, calcium excretion exceeded the amount administered when calcium was totally withdrawn from the solution. In the children receiving 30 g amino acids/day, total urinary calcium excretion was substantially lower than the quantity given in PN.

In summary, many factors related to the PN contribute to measured urine mineral loss (21–23), including excessive infusion of intravenous fluid or vitamin D and increased filtered load of sodium, magnesium, Ca, amino acids, or P. Patients receiving cyclic PN have significantly greater urinary calcium exertion during the hours of infusion (19,24–26). Suppression of the secretion of parathyroid hormone by the calcium present in the PN solution or the resistance of the parathyroid hormone associated with P deficiency might cause

Table 1 Pathogenesis of Parenteral Nutrition–Related Bone Disease

Nutrients
   Deficiency: copper, calcium, phosphorus
   Excess: vitamin D
Toxins: aluminum
Potential agents[a]
   Nutrients: vitamin A ↑, vitamin C ↓, zinc ↓ ↑,
       manganese ↓, silicone ↓ ↑, fluoride ↑ ↓,
       boron ↓
   Toxins: cadmium, strontium
   Drugs: furosemide, heparin, acetate

[a]Down or up arrows indicate deficiency or excess, respectively.

Table 2 Renal Function and Urinary Mineral Content in Response to Alterations of PN Solutions

	Urine volume (ml/min)	[c]Creat[a] (ml/min) (1.73 m^2)	Fractional Excretion[b]			
			Na (%)	Ca (%)	Mg (%)	P (%)
Normal Protein, Normal Calcium[c]						
Adults[d]						
Infusion	2.29 ± 0.20	78 ± 8	0.99 ± 0.12	8.89 ± 0.91	41.2 ± 3.1	38.5 ± 5.1
Off inf.	0.61 ± 0.05	62 ± 7	0.29 ± 0.05	2.38 ± 0.36	15.2 ± 1.8	28.7 ± 4.2
Children						
Infusion	0.54 ± 0.22	95 ± 5	0.68 ± 0.08	2.87 ± 1.43	20.4 ± 4.1	5.8 ± 1.9
Off inf.	0.07 ± 0.02	66 ± 8	0.17 ± 0.07	0.10 ± 0.03	2.3 ± 0.7	6.6 ± 1.3
Normal Protein, No Calcium[c]						
Infusion	2.59 ± 0.46	73 ± 9	0.86 ± 0.22	3.94 ± 1.02	39.5 ± 5.0	51.5 ± 5.9
Off inf.	0.78 ± 0.10	60 ± 12	0.64 ± 0.03	1.83 ± 1.02	24.2 ± 4.3	40.3 ± 7.7
Low Protein, Normal Calcium[c]						
Infusion	2.78 ± 0.50	70 ± 14	1.11 ± 0.21	6.65 ± 1.52	40.9 ± 9.0	57.2 ± 15.3
Off inf.	0.76 ± 0.14	61 ± 15	0.28 ± 0.09	187 ± 1.18	17.8 ± 6.5	26.8 ± 11.3
Low Protein, No Calcium[c]						
Infusion	2.67 ± 0.55	67 ± 13	0.72 ± 0.25	2.88 ± 0.89	38.1 ± 7.4	55.8 ± 9.5
Off inf.	0.70 ± 0.10	59 ± 16	0.26 ± 0.11	0.93 ± 0.41	16.2 ± 6.5	27.3 ± 14.2

[ac]Creat-creatinine clearance.

[b]Fractional excretion-percentage of the filtered load appearing in the urine (in % for Na, Ca, Mg, P).

[c]Type of PN infusion. The PN infusion was given during a 12-h period, from 7 P.M. to 7 A.M. The "off-infusion" period represents urine collection between 9 A.M. and 7 P.M. Serum values are those that follow the infusion or the off-infusion period.

[d]All patients who had calcium or protein reduced in the PN solution were adults.

physiological hypoparathyroidism. This would lead to decreased renal tubular reabsorption of calcium and contribute to the higher fractional excretion of calcium. Several observations suggest the presence of a "physiological" hypoparathyroidism with long-term PN. Serum iPTH levels have generally been subnormal or in the low range of normal in most patients treated with PN. Moreover, blood levels of ionized calcium are sometimes low (3,27) and are associated with intermittent mild hyperphosphatemia during long-term PN.

Large amounts of protein enhance urinary calcium excretion and may lead to a negative calcium balance (28). The high protein load in parenteral formulas may contribute to this hypercalciuria by using calcium carbonate stored in bone as a buffer for the acid load generated in the metabolism of sulfur-containing and neutral amino acids (5,29). Also the D-lactic acidosis that occurs in a small number of patients on PN with bacterial overgrowth syndromes may contribute to Ca losses (30). Acetate is added to current PN solutions to minimize this effect (31). Acidosis can affect bone mineralization and bone cell metabolism and is a potential risk factor in the development of PN-related bone disease. Thus, the maintenance of acid-base balance is also important to minimize the risk of developing PN-related bone disease.

Hypertonic dextrose infusions and high sodium loads can also contribute to calciuresis (19). Calciuria at greater than 50% of Ca intake can occur in infants receiving PN despite low Ca and P intake (22,32). The calciuria with P deficiency may be reduced by as much as 75% when P delivery is increased to correct hypophosphatemia and produce phosphaturia; more than 1 mmol of P/kg/day may be necessary to achieve this effect (21,22).

In addition, nonnutritional factors, including furosemide, spironolactone, and occasionally thiazide and theophylline, also increase urine Ca loss and theoretically may be associated with disturbed bone mineralization. Animal studies (33) suggest that small bowel resection, but not PN alone, is associated with increased urinary calcium loss. Thus the lack of participation of the gut in regulating calcium metabolism in PN may be a significant factor in PN-induced metabolic bone disease. Other explanations for the hypercalciuria include aluminum and vitamin D toxicity (5,34). The role of these two elements in metabolic bone disease is discussed below.

Urinary loss of Mg and P also may be increased in PN due to similar factors that affect urinary loss of Ca, thereby playing a role in metabolic bone disease. However, renal handling of Mg appears to be unaffected by the quantity or type of amino acids infused, as well as independent of the Ca and P content of the currently used PN solution or the urinary excretion of Ca, P, and sodium. In infants receiving low P intake, the renal tubular reabsorption of phosphate may approach 100%. Urinary phosphate excretion tends to parallel urinary Ca excretion in patients receiving PN, although the rate of negative P balance appears to be less than the negative Ca balance (9,19). In adults receiving PN, maintenance of Ca and P balance may not be possible in all patients at the Ca intake of 180–540 mg/day and at the P intake of 500–700 mg/day (3,6,34).

B. Decreased Calcium, Phosphorus, and Magnesium Intake

The failure to provide adequate Ca and P is critical in the development of nutrition-related bone disorders (5,10,18). Studies of infants with bone disease frequently report the presence of hypophosphatemia, elevated serum alkaline phosphatase activity, decreased urinary P, and increased urinary Ca loss. These findings are consistent with the presence of mineral deficiency, particularly P deficiency (18). In children receiving long-term PN, there is a correlation between the daily parenteral calcium intake and the degree of osteopenia assessed by computerized tomography of the trabecular bone of the lumbar vertebra (35). The higher the calcium intake, the lower the osteopenia. The severity of the osteopenia increases with the duration of the PN (Figs. 1 and 2). The PN-related bone disease indicated by standard biochemical and radiographic findings is less severe when the Ca and P delivered in PN solutions is doubled to 1.36 mmol (54.4 mg) Ca and 1.22 mmol (37.8 mg) P/kg/day (36).

The range of recommended daily intakes of electrolytes and minerals for PN solutions in infants and children is shown on Tables 3 and 4. Higher parenteral Ca and P intake, similar to the recommended intake of 12.5–15 mmol (500–600 mg)/L Ca and 13–14.5 mmol (400–450 mg)/L P(19) delivered at 120–150 ml/kg per day, is reported to result in stable normal serum concentrations of Ca, P, parathyroid hormone, calcitonin, vitamin D metabolites (25-hydroxyvitamin D and 1,25-dihydroxyvitamin D), and normal renal tubular reab-

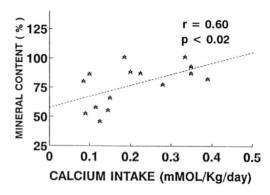

Figure 2   Significant correlation between the trabecular mineral content (in % of controls) and average parenteral calcium intake (in mmol/kg/day) for the total duration of the parenteral nutrition (2–14 years).

sorption of phosphate (10,37). Additional data supporting the use of these levels of Ca and P content of PN solutions include several balance studies (Table 5) demonstrating a mean fractional retention of 88–94% for Ca and 83–97% for P in clinically stable infants receiving 1.45–1.9 mmol (58–76 mg)/kg/day Ca and 1.23–1.74 mmol (38–54 mg)/kg/day P from PN (38–40). With these solutions a 60–70% of the interoaccretion of Ca and P can be achieved.

Ca and P ratios may be important to achieve optimal mineral retention in infants requiring PN therapy. PN solutions with extremes of Ca:P ratios by weight from 4:1 to 1:8 have been used without apparent side effects (41). A Ca:P ratio of <0.78:1 by molar ratio or <1:1 by weight has a potential risk for disturbance of Ca and P homeostasis, specifically hyperphosphatemia and hypocalcemia (22). Although the most appropriate Ca:P ratio in PN solution is not well defined, the optimal ratio in terms of maintaining Ca and P homeostasis and maximizing Ca and P retention appear to be solutions with Ca:P ratios of 1:1 to 1.3:1 by molar ratio or 1.3:1 to 1.7:1 by weight (10,38,40).

The use of alternate PN infusions of Ca and P to increase the delivery of these minerals while avoiding Ca-P precipitation in the solutions resulted in lower Ca and P retention (42–63%) (22,42,43) as compared to the rates attained when these minerals are infused simultaneously (83–97%) (38–40,42). In addition, hypercalcemia and hypophosphatemia may occur during high Ca infusion, whereas hyperphosphatemia and hypocalcemia may occur during high P infusion (42). Therefore, infusion of both calcium and phosphorus should occur simultaneously as long as they are given in stable calcium and phosphorus concentrations (42). There are no documented major complications associated with the currently recommended higher Ca and P intake for premature infant receiving PN. Serial abdominal ultrasound examinations showed that biliary sludge did not occur with greater frequency in infants receiving the higher Ca-P solution compared with those with lower mineral intake. Biliary sludge appeared to resolve upon enteral feeding. In the absence of chronic diuretic therapy, abnormal renal ultrasound findings

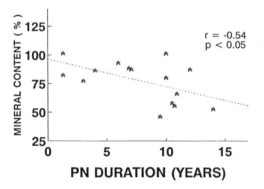

Figure 1   Significant correlation between the trabecular mineral content (in percentage value of age-and-gender-matched controls) and the duration in years of the parenteral nutrition in 15 children receiving long-term parenteral nutrition.

Table 3 Daily Intravenous Electrolyte Requirements in Patients with Adequate Renal Function

	Usual adult dose per 24 h	Pediatric dose per kg/24 h	Infant dose per kg/24 h
Sodium	100–150 mmol	3–4 mmol	2–8 mmol
Potassium	60–120 mmol	2–3 mmol	2–6 mmol
Chloride	100–150 mmol	2–4 mmol	0–6 mmol
Calcium[a]	4.5–11 mmol	0.25–0.5 mmol	0.45–1.15 mmol
			200–500 mg[a]
Phosphate[a]	15–30 mmol	2 mmol	1–1.5 mmol
Magnesium[c]	4–12 mmol	0.125–0.25 mmol	0.125–0.25 mmol[b]

[a]The product obtained by multiplying the total number of mEq of calcium per liter by the total number of mEq of phosphate per liter must not exceed 200 to prevent precipitation of the calcium phosphate complex. Must include calcium and phosphate content of base solutions. Increased concentration of administration on the basis of fluid restriction may result in precipitation.

[b]Given as calcium gluconate salt, 430.5 mg/mmol = 2 mEq = 40 mg calcium: maximum for infants 2 g/24 h.

[c]Given as magnesium sulfate salt; 120.3 mg/mmol = 2 mEq = 24 mg.

such as nephrocalcinosis have not been reported with the higher Ca and P intake (10,37).

Fluctuations in serum concentration of Mg can occur secondarily to changes in the amount of Mg delivered in PN solution, losses from gastrointestinal fluid, and the presence of underlying renal dysfunction. PN solutions containing 1 mmol (24 mg) Mg/L resulted in hypomagnesemia (44). In contrast, PN solutions with 4 mmol (96 mg) Mg/L delivering an average of 0.5 mmol (12 mg) Mg/kg/day resulted in transient hypermagnesemia (37). None of these reports used Mg replacement for gastrointestinal fluid losses, which can have Mg contents as high as 7 mmol/L (21,44). Parenteral nutrition solutions with Mg content of 3 mmol/L that deliver approximately 0.3–0.4 mmol (7.2–9.6 mg) Mg/kg/day appear to maintain stable serum Mg concentrations. Transient hyper-

magnesemia may occur in premature infants at this level of intake (10), presumably in part due to a delay in adaptive renal excretory response to the intravenous Mg load. A balance study of Mg (45) reported an average Mg retention of 61% in preterm infants receiving a total daily Mg intake of 0.51 mmol from solutions containing 3.4 mmol (80 mg)/L. This amount is approximately twice the in utero accretion rate for Mg.

C. Calcium and Phosphorus Solubility

Precipitation of calcium and phosphate in PN solutions has been a continual problem. It is particularly prevalent in solutions for neonates because their calcium and phosphate needs are high, yet fluid requirements are restricted and amino

Table 4 Advisable Parenteral Intake for Calcium (Ca), Magnesium (Mg), Phosphorus (P), and Vitamin D in Preterm Infants

	Ca	Mg	P	Vitamin D[b]
mmol/L	12.5–15.0	1.5–2.0	12.5–15.0	
(mg/L)	(500–600)	(36–48)	(390–470)	250–1,000 IU
mmol/kg/day[a]	1.5–2.25	0.18–0.30	1.5–2.25	
(mg/kg/day)	(60–90)	(4.3–7.2)	(47–70)	40–160 IU/kg

[a]Based on an intake of 120–150 ml/kg/day. For Ca, Mg, and P, concentration-based (mmol/L or mg/L), as per kg per day, recommendations should be used since alterations of fluid volumes by clinical circumstances (such as restriction) could inadvertently result in high mineral concentrations and precipitation of minerals. Ca and P could be adjusted accordingly to biochemical measurements within the range of 1:1 to 1,3:1 molar ratio or 1.3:1 by weight.

[b]Maximum daily total 400 IU.

Conversion: Ca 1 mmol = 40 mg = 430.5 mg calcium gluconate. Mg 1 mmol = 24 mg = 120.3 mg magnesium sulfate. P 1 mmol = 31 mg.

Table 5 Calcium and Phosphorus Balance in Preterm Infants Receiving Parenteral Nutrition

	Pelegano et al. (38) (n = 5)	Chessex et al. (39) (n = 16)	Pelegano et al. (40) (n = 16)	Pelegano et al. (40) (n = 12)	Pelegano et al. (40) (n = 13)
Vitamin D (IU/day)	100–200	200	100–200	100–200	100–200
Ca content (mmol/L)	14.5(580)	12.8(510)	15.0(600)	15.0(600)	10.1(400)
Ca intake (mmol/kg/day)	1.79(72)	1.80(72)	1.90(76)	1.90(76)	1.45(58)
Urinary Ca excretion (mmol/kg/day)	0.10(4)	0.23(9)	0.13(5)	0.10 4)	0.10(4)
Ca retention (mmol/kg/day)	1.39(56)	1.58(63)	1.79(72)	1.80(72)	1.35(54)
Ca retention (%)	91%	88%	93%	94%	93%
P content (mmol/L)	11.0(341)	12.7(394)	9.7(282)	11.3(350)	11.0(341)
P intake (mmol/kg/day)	1.32(41)	1.74(54)	1.23(38)	1.45(45)	1.45(45)
Urinary P excretion (mmol/kg/day)	0.13(4)	0.06(2)	0.10(3)	0.13(4)	0.23(7)
P retention (mmol/kg/day)	1.17(36)	1.67(52)	1.13(35)	1.32(41)	1.23(38)
P retention (%)	89%	97%	92%	90%	83%

Number in parentheses is in mg. Conversion: Ca 1 mmol = 40 mg; P 1 mmol = 31 mg.

acid concentrations are low (46). To minimize the risk of precipitation, recommendations for Ca and P intake are based on concentration per liter of solution rather than in amount per kilogram. Of note, calcium and phosphorus requirements in some preterm infants may exceed the solubility of these two elements in the PN solutions. This typically occurs during fluid restriction when the ideal amount of calcium and phosphorus cannot be provided. Factors that enhance precipitate formation include high calcium and phosphate concentrations, decreased amino acid concentration, increased environmental temperature, higher pH of the amino acid mixture and of the PN solution, and prolonged hanging time (47,48).

Calcium gluconate is traditionally used instead of calcium chloride in parenteral fluids because it is far less likely than calcium chloride to react with phosphate. Calcium glycerophosphate has been shown to be more soluble than calcium gluconate plus phosphate (49). Limited information exists on the use of alternate sources of inorganic (39,46) and organic salts (49,50) of Ca and P in PN solutions.

The titratable acidity of the PN solution offers a protective effect on calcium phosphate compatibility. The higher the concentration of amino acids, the lower the PH and the greater amount of calcium and phosphorus that can be admixed to the solution without precipitation (47). Of note, the titratable acidity and pH of the commercially available amino acid solutions varies. In this regard, the pediatric amino

acid mixtures (TrophAmine and Aminosyn), which have an acidic pH to allow for adequate amounts of calcium and phosphorus to be added to the solutions, are of particular benefit (38,41,48). Also, other additives normally used in clinical practice, such as magnesium, can influence the calcium phosphate reaction (47). As the pH rises, the more soluble monobasic phosphate salt is converted to dibasic phosphate salt, which is available to bind calcium and precipitate. Acidification of the solution by adding cysteine hydrochloride can improve solubility. However, cysteine and other sulfate-containing amino acids have detrimental effects on calcium balance during parenteral nutrition (23,51). Admixture of alkaline drugs such as aminophylline in a PN solution may result in calcium phosphate precipitation in solutions containing low amounts of amino acids (52). The pH of the solution may also be increased by the addition of lipid emulsion (47). However, pH changes in the solution due to aminophylline or lipid emulsion are less appreciable as the amino acid concentration increases from 1 to 2% (52). Of concern, the addition of sodium bicarbonate to acidic PN solutions has the potential for causing carbon dioxide formation, with loss of the bicarbonate ion and formation of insoluble calcium and magnesium carbonates (53). As a result, most clinicians use acetate salts, which serve as precursors to bicarbonate.

At room temperature, conventional dextrose–amino acid mixtures (e.g., 25% dextrose and 4–5% amino acids) rarely

Table 6 Highest Compatible Concentration for Calcium and Phosphate[a] (storage 37°C for 24 h)

1% TrophAmine 10% Dextrose		2% TropAmine 20% Dextrose		2% TrophAmine 20% Dextrose cysteine[b]	
Phosphate (mmol/L)	Calcium (mEq/L)	Phosphate (mmol/L)	Calcium (mEq/L)	Phosphate (mmol/L)	Calcium (mEq/L)
25	5	50	5	70	14
20	5	40	6	55	15
15	9	30	6	45	18
12	10	25	7	31	25
10	15	20	9	21	30
9	40	15	10	18	40
7	50	13	15		
		11	20		
		9	35		
		9	60		

[a]Due to the individual nature of formulations and mixing techniques, these should be used as guidelines.
[b]50 mg cysteine HCl per gram protein.

pose an incompatibility problem if calcium gluconate concentrations are 5 mmol/L or less and phosphate concentrations are 30 mmol/L or less. However, insoluble complexes may precipitate when the PN solution is warmed, as in infusing the solution into the patient (54).

After millions of patient-days of PN delivery, reported adverse events appear to be rare (55) when appropriate procedures in the preparation and delivery of PN are followed. If symptoms of acute respiratory distress, pulmonary embolus, or interstitial pneumonitis develop, the infusion should be stopped immediately and thoroughly checked for precipitates. Appropriate medical intervention should be instituted.

D. Role of Vitamin D

The role of vitamin D in the development of PN-related bone disease remains controversial. In adults receiving PN solutions, vitamin D intake of 500 IU on alternate days was implicated in the development of symptomatic bone disease (27,34). The discontinuation of vitamin D in PN solutions for 6 months or more was associated with significant decline in urinary Ca and P excretion, decreased bone pain, healing of fractures, and significantly increased mineralization surface, as indicated by increased tetracycline uptake on bone biopsies (34). However, in another study, removal of vitamin D from the PN solutions resulted in low serum levels of 25-(OH)D but no clinical or histological manifestions of bone disease (56). Larchet et al. (57) completely withdrew the vitamin D in children given PN. This resulted in a marked decrease in serum 25-(OH)D concentrations into the vitamin D–deficient range, but serum concentrations of 1,25(OH)$_2$D, Ca, and P remained normal. There were no consistent changes in urine Ca and P excretion and no apparent clinical effects were detected up to 2 years. Another study failed to demonstrate

osteomalacia even though patients were receiving very small amounts of vitamin D (24).

PN solutions with a vitamin D content of 250 IU/L can maintain normal vitamin D status in preterm infants for longer than 3 months as indicated by normal serum 25-(OH)D concentrations (58). Based on systematic studies of preterm infants receiving PN solution with high Ca and P content of 12.5–15 mmol/L each (37–40), these amounts of Ca and P appear suitable for use in preterm infants for at least the first 6 months of life. In contrast, recent studies have demonstrated that an intravenous vitamin D intake as low as 30 IU/kg is adequate to maintain normal vitamin D status while the infant is receiving Ca and P–containing PN solutions (58). A higher dose of 160 IU of vitamin D/kg/day with a maximum of 400 IU/day has not been associated with complications while maintaining the serum 25-(OH)D concentrations within the reference range for term infants fed orally. This is the currently recommended dose of vitamin D intake for infants requiring PN (59).

In summary, the vitamin D requirement is minimal for patients requiring total PN and does not appear to be greater that the recommended dose for patients receiving a normal diet, i.e., 200 IU/day for adults and 400 IU/day for pediatric patients. Since it is well known that chronic vitamin D deficiency can result in bone disease, it would seem prudent to maintain normal vitamin D status in patients receiving PN. This practice complements the general goal of maximizing the absorption and retention of any enteral nutrients tolerated by these patients because vitamin D metabolite promotes the intestinal absorption of Ca and P. Thus, until further evidence becomes available, the complete discontinuation of vitamin D supplementation for patients requiring PN is not recommended.

E. Role of Aluminum

Although insufficient provision of calcium or phosphate may be primarily responsible for the osteopenia, aluminum loading may be a complicating factor (7,9,60–65). In humans, the trace metal aluminum (Al) has no known physiological function and it is regarded as a potential toxin (60–65), particularly in patients with impaired renal function. However, the role of Al in the pathogenesis of bone disease requires further study.

Klein et al. first reported Al to be a contaminant of casein hydrolysate, which is no longer used as a nitrogen source in PN solutions (6). However, extensive Al contamination (Table 7) persisted in PN solutions for infants because of Al contamination of other nutrients, mainly in calcium and phosphate salts, heparin, and albumin (60,65). These sources can result in PN solutions containing 30–306 μg/L of Al (61). Adults receiving 2–3 mg of Al/day from casein hydrolysate-based PN solutions developed symptoms of bone pain within 2–36 months after initiation of PN (3,4). Trabecular bone area and bone formation rates were decreased with an increased amount of stainable Al on bone biopsy and high plasma and urinary Al concentrations (47,60,61). Discontinuation of PN resulted in reduction of bone pain and hyper-

Table 7 Sources of Aluminum in Common Intravenously Administered Products

Solution	Number of lots tested	Aluminum content[a] (μg/L)
Potassium phosphate	3	16,598 ± 1801
Sodium phosphate	1	5977
10% calcium gluconate	5	5056 ± 335
Heparin (100 μ/ml)	3	684 ± 761
25% albumin	4	1822 ± 2503
Trace metal solution	7	972 ± 108

[a]Values are given as mean ± SD.

calciuria, improvement in bone formation rate, and return of serum concentrations of $1,25(OH)_2D$ to normal (3,4,7,62). Low turnover bone disease and decreased bone formation also are reported in adults (61,63) and children (64) with no Al staining on bone biopsy and normal or elevated (9,19) plasma Al concentration. Autopsy specimens of vertebrae from two infants who died while receiving PN revealed a positive stain for aluminum at the level of the mineralization front. On the basis of the above findings, some investigators have speculated that Al in the circulation reduces bone formation even before it accumulates in bone (4).

The amount of Al received by the infants is about 20–40 μg/kg/day, depending (49,61) on the mineral content of the PN solutions. This is somewhat less than the amount of Al (about 60 μg/kg/day) received by adult patients with normal renal function who had elevated bone Al and abnormal bone histomorphometric parameters (4,6,7). The risk of Al retention may be increased because the renal function in infants is developmentally reduced and may attain 50–75% of the intravenous Al load (60,61). Of note, adult patients receiving long-term PN with crystalline amino acids instead of casein hydrolysate received only 1 μg/kg/day. The latter groups had no evidence of elevated serum, urine, or bone content of aluminum.

In conclusion, bone pathology may result from high Al loading with PN solutions. The current use of crystalline amino acid solutions as a nitrogen source has resulted in a significant overall reduction of Al content. However, Al contamination of other components of PN solutions, especially the minerals, continues to exist and results in tissue accumulation and/or elevated plasma and urine Al concentrations. Whether the lower Al loading from currently used PN solutions has a precipitating or additive effect on the development of PN-related bone disease remains to be determined. It is to be noted that recently, we evaluated the aluminum content of PN solution manufactured at UCLA Medical Center and found no significant contamination, although the patients had asymptomatic ostepenia (8).

F. Role of Other Nutrients and Toxins

A recent report in children after 9 years of PN therapy demonstrated a significant osteopenia (35). All children were

receiving crystalline amino acid PN solution, i.e., how Al intake and an adequate amount of vitamin D. A similar study in adults (16) confirmed that factors other than vitamin D and Al intake were important in the pathogenesis of PN-related bone disease.

However, there exist limited data on the role of trace metal (25,26) known to affect bone cell function and/or mineral metabolism in the pathogenesis of PN-related bone disease. These include nutrients known to be essential for PN (59) such as vitamin A (66), vitamin C (67), zinc (68), copper (69,70), and manganese (71), nutrients without adequate data to have specific recommendation for use in PN such as fluoride (12,72) silicon (73–75) vanadium (75,76), and boron (76–79), and toxins such as cadmium (80) and strontium (81). Thus, it is also possible that unrecognized deficiency or excess of any of those nutrients or substances or unrecognized toxic contaminants may contribute to the development of PN-related bone disease. Fluoride has a special role. In a prospective study of children receiving long-term PN for an average of 9 years, the serum fluoride level was within normal limits (3.2 ± 0.8 μmol/L), however there was a significant correlation between the plasma fluoride level and the bone density (12).

Deficiencies of copper, magnesium, and boron can impair bone formation. Enteric copper and magnesium losses are increased in patients with short bowel syndrome, steatorrhea, and steroid administration. Copper deficiency impairs collagen synthesis and hence formation of bone. Magnesium deficiency results in decreased PTH levels, decreased 1,25-dihydroxyvitamin D formation, and increased bone resistance to PTH activity. Boron impairs PTH function and thereby interferes with the metabolism of calcium, phosphorus, magnesium, and vitamin D. Decreased levels of boron are associated with secondary hyperparathyroidism, hypercalciuria, and osteoporosis (79). Animal studies have shown an increased need for boron in coexistent magnesium deficiency. Recently, the influence of boron supplementation on the prevention of calcium loss and bone demineralization was shown in postmenopausal women (77).

Contrary to the hypothesis of boron deficiency, the mean serum boron (14.5 μg/ml) in PN patients was significantly higher than that of controls (11.5 μg/ml) and correlated with the duration of PN. A significant contamination of boron in glucose–amino acid solutions and in fat emulsion was observed. The subjects were receiving daily 9.4–30 mg parenteral boron. The mineral content correlated with the duration of the PN but not with serum boron. Thus there is enough boron contamination in PN solutions to maintain serum boron at or above normal levels (78).

Silicon's primary effect in bone and cartilage appears to be on the formation of the organic matrix. Bone and cartilage abnormalities are associated with a reduction in matrix components, resulting in the establishment of a requirement for silicon in collagen and glyconsaminoglycan formation (74,75). Additional support for silicon's metabolic role in connective tissue is provided by the finding that silicon is a major ion of osteogenic cells, especially high in the metabolically active state of the cell. Recently (73), the serum silicon levels in children receiving long-term PN were found to be lower than those of controls but the mineral content correlated significantly with the duration of the PN and poorly with the silicon level. However, further investigation is warranted to determine whether patients on PN may be deficient in this essential mineral.

The use of copper-free PN solution is reported to result in bone disease in infants (70), but there is limited information on the status of various trace metals in pediatric patients with nutrition-related bone disease. In one study, children who received PN therapy from early infancy had normal serum concentrations of iron, copper, and manganese; elevated serum zinc; and lower serum selenium, chromium, nickel, rubidium, and bromine compared with healthy children of similar age range (82). The PN solutions contained added zinc and copper and intermittently added iron. However, both the lipid-free PN solutions and the 20% lipid emulsion used for the PN therapy were shown to have a varying extents of contamination of all trace metals measured. There were no obvious clinical signs or symptoms attributable to trace metal deficiency. In small, preterm infants with nutrition-related bone disease, serum zinc, copper, and ceruloplasmin concentrations were similar to those in matched infants without bone disease (68,69).

Heparin has been shown to promote bone resorption (83) when used in large doses (15,000–30,000 units) for 8–60 months, is associated with the development of spontaneous fractures of vertebrae and ribs, and is reported to result in osteomalacia, but this dose is many times the usual content of 1 unit heparin per milliliter of PN solution.

III. TREATMENT AND PREVENTION

Every attempt should be made to provide, especially to premature infants, as much calcium and phosphate as permitted through the PN solution.

Until manufacturers reduce the aluminum content of the products used for PN, periodic monitoring of infants receiving this treatment for evidence of bone disease is recommended. Determinations of serum levels of calcium, phosphorus, PTH, 25-OHD, and 1,25(OH)$_2$D can identify associated hyperparathyroidism and vitamin D deficiency. If bone disease persists despite maximal calcium and phosphate supplementation, and if 24-h urine excretion of calcium and phosphorus does not exceed intake, then aluminum in plasma, in urine, and in the PN solution should be assessed. Specimens must be collected in plastic containers and sent to a specialized laboratory for analysis.

Plasma aluminum concentration exceeding 100 μg/L and/or urine aluminum/creatinine (μg/mg) greater than 0.3 requires analysis of the components of the PN solution for aluminum content. Although deferoxamine therapy has been useful in chelating aluminum from the bones of adults with dialysis osteomalacia, its use in infants is inappropriate because of its nonspecific chelating action. It can chelate and therefore lead to the loss of important nutrients, including iron, copper, zinc, cobalt, magnesium, and calcium (84). Its use in one infant resulted in hypocalcemia, and prolonged

therapy were deferoxamine is reported to result in other major complications (85).

Interrelation of various nutrients, for example, calcium, phosphorus, and vitamin D, in their effects on bone mineralization, demands simultaneous assessment of the role of multiple nutrients and increases the difficulty in defining the role of a single nutrient in the development of bone disease.

Nonnutritional factors, including chronic use of potent loop diuretic and altered acid-base status, can affect bone mineralization, particularly in infants, Current evidence indicates that the cause of PN-related bone disease is multifactorial, and the prevention of PN-related bone disease awaits better delineation of the exact sequence of pathogenic events. However, some factors such as Ca and P requirement may be more important. A team approach including a PN pharmacist would be best to deal with the management of this particular osteopenia.

ACKNOWLEDGMENT

This work was partially funded by the Maimonides Research Foundation.

REFERENCES

1. Cannon RA, Byrne WJ, Ament ME, et al. Home parenteral nutrition in infants. J Pediatr 1980; 96:1098–1104.
2. Gefter WB, Epstein DM, Anday EK, et al. Rickets presenting as multiple fractures in premature infants on hyperalimentation. Radiology 1982; 142:371–374.
3. Klein GL, Ament ME, Bluestone R, et al. Bone disease associated with total parenteral nutrition. Lancet 1980; 2: 1041–1044.
4. Foldes J, Rimon B, Muggia-Sullam M, et al. Progressive bone loss during long-term home total parenteral nutrition. J Parenter Enter Nutr 1990; 14:139–142.
5. Hurley DL, McMahon M. Long-term parenteral nutrition and metabolic bone disease. Endocrinol Metab Clin North Am 1990; 19:113–131.
6. Klein GL, Alfrey AC, Miller NL, et al. Aluminum loading during total parenteral nutrition. Am J Clin Nutr 1982; 35:1425–1429.
7. Ott SM, Maloney NA, Klein GL, et al. Aluminum is associated with low bone formation in patients receiving chronic parenteral nutrition. Ann Intern Med 1983; 98:910–914.
8. Moukarzel A, Ament ME, Vargas J, et al. Parenteral nutrition bone disease in children. Clin Res 1990; 3:190A.
9. Winston WKK. Parenteral nutrition–related bone disease. J Parenter Enter Nutr 1992; 16:386–394.
10. Koo WWK, Tsang RC, Succop P, et al. Minimal vitamin D and high calcium and phosphorus needs of preterm infants receiving parenteral nutrition. J Pediatr Gastroenterol Nutr 1989; 8:225–233.
11. Tsang RC. The quandary of vitamin D in the newborn infant. Lancet 1983; 1:1370–1372.
12. Moukarzel AA, Ament ME, Vargas J; et al. Is fluoride deficiency related to the bone disease of parenteral nutrition? Clin Nutr 1990; 9:65.
13. Klein GL, Cannon RA, Diament M, et al. Infantile vitamin

D–resistant rickets associated with total parenteral nutrition. Am J Dis Child 1982; 136:74–76.

14. Epstein S, Traberg H, Levine G, et al. Bone and mineral status of patients beginning total parenteral nutrition. J Parenter Enter Nutr 1986; 10:263–264.

15. Koo WWK, Sherman R, Succop P, et al. Sequential bone mineral content in very low birth weight infants with and without fractures and rickets. J Bone Miner Res 1988; 3:193–197.

16. Saitta JC, Lipkin EW, Ott SM, et al. Longitudinal measurements of bone histomorphology and bone density in parenteral nutrition with solutions low in aluminum and vitamin D₂. J Parenter Enter Nutr 1991; 15:20S.

17. Hylander E, Ladefoged K, Jarnum S. The importance of the colon in calcium absorption following small intestine resection. Scand J Gastroenterol 1980; 15:55–59.

18. Hylander E, Ladefoged K, Madsen S. Calcium balance and bone mineral content following small intestine resection. Scand J Gastroenterol 1981; 16:167–170.

19. Klein L, Ament ME, Slatopolsky E, Coburn JW. Urinary Mineral Excretion During Long-Term Total Parenteral Nutrition in Metabolic Bone Disease in Total Parenteral Nutrition. Baltimore: Urban & Schwarzenberg. 1985:101–128.

20. Saitta JC, Ott SM, Sherrard DJ, et al. Metabolic bone disease in adults receiving long-term parenteral nutrition: Longitudinal study with regional densitometry and bone biopsy. J Parenter Enter Nutr 1993; 17:214–219.

21. Koo WWK, Tsang RC. Mineral requirements of low-birth-weight infants. J Am Coll Nutr 1991; 10:474–486.

22. Chessex P, Pineault M, Zebiche H, Ayotte RA. Calciuria in parenterally fed preterm infants: Role of phosphorus intake. J Pediatr 1985; 107:794–796.

23. Cole DEC, Zlotkin SH. Increased sulfate as an etiological factor in the hypercalciuria associated with total parenteral nutrition. Am J Clin Nutr 1983; 37:108–113.

24. Shike M, Shils ME, Heller A, et al. Bone disease in prolonged parenteral nutrition: Osteopenia without mineralization defect. Am J Clin Nutr 1986; 44:89–98.

25. Lipkin EW, Ott SM, Chestnut CH, et al. Mineral loss in the parenteral nutrition patient. Am J Clin Nutr 1988; 47:515–518.

26. Wood RJ, Bengoa JM, Sitrin MD, et al. Calciuretic effect of cyclic versus continuous total parenteral nutrition. Am J Clin Nutr 1985; 41:614–617.

27. Shike M, Strutridge WC, Tam CS, et al. A possible role of vitamin D in the genesis of parenteral nutrition induced metabolic bone disease. Ann Intern Med 1981; 95:560–568.

28. Kim Y, Linkswiler HM. Effect of level of protein intake on calcium metabolism and on parathyroid and renal function in the adult human male. J Nutr 1979; 109:1399–1404.

29. Goodman WG, Lemann J, Lennon EJ, et al. Production, excretion and net balance of fixed acid in patients with renal acidosis. J Clin Invest 1966; 44:495–497.

30. Karton MA. Rettmer R, Lipkin EW, et al. D-Lactate and metabolic bone disease in patients receiving long-term parenteral nutrition. J Parenter Enter Nutr 1989; 13:132–135.

31. Berkelhammer CH, Wood RJ, Rosenberg IH, et al. Alkalization with acetate reduces hypercalciuria during total parenteral nutrition. Clin Res 1986; 34:792A.

32. Ricour C, Millot M, Balsan S. Phosphorus depletion in children on long-term total parenteral nutrition. Acta Paediatr Scand 1975; 64:385–392.

33. Chu RC, Barkowski SM, Buhac J. Small bowel resection-associated urinary calcium loss in rats on long-term parenteral nutrition. J Parenter Enter Nutr 1990; 14:64–67.

34. Shike M, Sturtridge WC, Tam CS, et al. A possible role of vitamin D in the genesis of parenteral nutrition induced metabolic bone disease. Ann Intern Med 1981; 95:560–568.

35. Moukarzel A, Ament ME, Vargas J, et al. Non aluminum dependent osteopathy in children on long term parenteral nutrition. Am J Clin Nutr 1990; 51:520.

36. MacMahon P, Blair ME, Treweeke P, Kovar IZ. Association of mineral composition of neonatal intravenous feeding solutions and metabolic bone disease of prematurity. Arch Dis Child 1989; 64:489–493.

37. Koo WWK, Tsang RC, Steichen JJ, et al. Parenteral nutrition for infants: Effect of high versus low calcium and phosphorus content. J Pediatr Gastroenterol Nutr 1987; 6:96–104.

38. Pelegano JF, Rowe JC, Carey DE, et al. Simultaneous infusion of calcium and phosphorus in parenteral nutrition for premature infants: Use of physiologic calcium/phosphorus ratio. J Pediatr 1989; 114:115–119.

39. Chessex P, Pineault M, Brisson G, et al. Role of the source of phosphate salt in improving the mineral balance of parenterally fed low birth weight infants. J Pediatr 1990; 116:765–772.

40. Pelegano JF, Rowe JC, Carey DE, et al. Effect of calcium/phosphorus ratio on mineral retention in parenterally fed premature infants. J Pediatr Gastroenterol Nutr 1991; 12:351–355.

41. Lenz GT, Mikrut BA. Calcium and phosphate solubility in neonatal parenteral nutrient solutions containing Aminosyn-PF or Trophamine. Am J Hosp Pharm 1988; 45:2367–2371.

42. Kimura S, Nose O, Seino Y, et al. Effects of alternate and simultaneous administration of calcium and phosphorus on calcium metabolism in children receiving total parenteral nutrition. J Parenter Enter Nutr 1986; 10:513–516.

43. Hoehn GJ, Carey DE, Rowe JC, et al. Alternate day infusion of calcium and phosphate in low birth weight infants: Wasting of the infused mineral. J Pediatr Gastroenterol Nutr 1987; 6:752–757.

44. Koo WWK, Tsang RC. Calcium, magnesium, phosphorus, and vitamin D. In: Tsang RC, ed. Nutritional Needs of the Preterm Infant. New York: Caduceus Medical Publishers, 1992:135–156.

45. Koo WWK, Tsang RC. Calcium, magnesium and phosphorus. In: Tsang RC, Nichols BL, eds. Nutrition in Infancy. Philadelphia: Hanley and Belfus, 1988:175–189.

46. MacMahon P, Mayne PD, Blair M, et al. Calcium and phosphorus solubility in neonatal intravenous feeding solutions. Arch Dis Child 1990; 65:352–353.

47. Niemiec PW, Vanderveen TW: Compatibility considerations in parenteral nutrient solutions. Am J Hosp Pharm 1984; 41:893–911.

48. Dunham B, Marcuard S, Khazanie PG, Meade GT, Nichols K. The solubility of calcium and phosphorus neonatal in total parenteral nutrition solutions. J Parenter Enter Nutr 1991; 5:608–611.

49. Hanning RM, Atkinson SA, Whyte RK. Efficacy of calcium glycerophosphate vs conventional mineral salts for total parenteral nutrition in low-birth weight infants: A randomized clinical trial. Am J Clin Nutr 1991; 54:903–908.

50. Draper HH, Yuen DE, Whyte RK. Calcium glycerophosphate as a source of calcium and phosphorus in parenteral nutrition solutions. J Parenter Enter Nutr 1991; 15:176–180.

51. Schmidt GL, Baumgartner TG, Fischlishweiger W, et al. Cost containment using cysteine HCl acidification to increase calcium/phosphate solubility in hyperalimentation. J Parenter Enter Nutr 1986; 10:203–207.

52. Kirkpatrick AE, Holcombe BJ, Sawyer WT. Effect of retrograde aminophylline administration on calcium and phosphate solubility in neonatal total parenteral nutrient solutions. Am J Hosp Pharm 1989; 46:2496–2500.

53. Henann NE, Jacks TT. Compatibility and availability of

sodium bicarbonate in total parenteral nutrient solutions. Am J Hosp Pharm 1985; 42:2718–2720.

54. Robinson LA, Wright BT. Central venous catheter occlusion caused by body-heat-mediated calcium phosphate precipitation. Am J Hosp Pharm 1982; 39:120–121.

55. Knowles JB, et al. Pulmonary deposition of calcium phosphate crystals as a complication of home total parenteral nutrition. J Parenter Enter Nutr 1989; 13:209–213.

56. Jeejeebhoy KN, Shike M, Sturtridge WC, et al. TPN bone disease at Toronto. In: Coburn JW, Klein GL, eds. Metabolic Bone Disease in Total Parenteral Nutrition. Baltimore: Urban & Schwarzenberg, 1985:17–29.

57. Larchet M, Garabedien M, Bourdeau A, et al. Calcium metabolism in children during long-term total parenteral nutrition: The influence of calcium, phosphorus, and vitamin D intakes. J Pediatr Gastroenterol Nutr 1991; 13:367–375.

58. Koo WWK, Tsang RC, Steichen JJ, et al. Vitamin requirement in infants receiving parenteral nutrition. J Parenter Enter Nutr 1987; 11:172–176.

59. Greene HL, Hambidge KM, Schanler R, et al. Guidelines for the use of vitamins, trace elements, calcium, magnesium, and phosphorus in infants and children receiving total parenteral nutrition: Report of the Subcommittee on Pediatric Parenteral Nutrient Requirements from the Committee on Clinical Practice Issues of the American Society for Clinical Nutrition. Am J Clin Nutr 1988; 48:1324–1342.

60. Sedman AB, Klein GL, Merritt RJ, et al. Evidence of aluminum loading in infants receiving intravenous therapy. N Engl J Med 1985; 312:1337–1343.

61. Koo WWK, Kaplan LA, Krug-Wispe SK, et al. Response of preterm infants to aluminum in parenteral nutrition. J Parenter Enter Nutr 1989; 13:516–519.

62. Klein GL, Horst RL, Alfrey AC, et al. Serum levels of 1,25 dihydroxyvitamin D in children receiving parenteral nutrition with reduced aluminum content. J Pediatr Gastroenterol Nutr 1985; 4:93–96.

63. DeVernejoul MC, Messing B, Modrowski D, et al. Multifactorial low remodeling bone disease during cyclic total parenteral nutrition. J Clin Endocrinol Metab 1985; 60:109–113.

64. Heyman MB, Klein GL, Wong A, et al. Aluminum does not accumulate in teenagers and adults on prolonged parenteral nutrition containing free amino acids. J Parenter Enter Nutr 1986; 10:86–87.

65. ASCN/ASPEN Working Group on Standards for Aluminum Content of Parenteral Nutrition Solutions: Parenteral drug products containing aluminum as an ingredient or a contaminant: Response to FDA notice of intent. Am J Clin Nutr 1991; 53:399–402.

66. Frame B, Jackson CE, Reynolds WA, et al. Hypercalcemia and skeletal effects in chronic hypervitaminosis A. Ann Intern Med 1974; 80:44–48.

67. Clemetson CAB. Clinical and Pathological Findings in Ascorbic Acid Deficiency, Vol II. Boca Raton FL: CRC Press, 1989:1–248.

68. Koo WWK, Succop P, Hambidge KM. Serum alkaline phosphatase and serum zinc concentrations in preterm infants with rickets and fractures. Am J Dis Child 1989; 143:1342–1345.

69. Koo WWK, Succop P, Hambidge KM. Sequential serum copper and ceruloplasmin concentrations in preterm infants with rickets and fractures. Clin Chem 1991; 37:556–559.

70. Heller RM, Kirchner SG, O'Neill JA, Jr, et al. Skeletal changes of copper deficiency in infants receiving total parenteral nutrition. J Pediatr 1978; 92:947–949.

71. Mena I. Manganese. In: Bronner F, Coburn JW, eds. Disorders of Mineral Metabolism, Vol 1. New York: Academic Press, 1981:236–264.

72. Riggs BL, Hodgson SF, O'Fallon WM, et al. Effect of fluoride treatment on the fracture rate in postmenopausal women with osteoporosis. N Engl J Med 1990; 322:802–809.

73. Moukarzel A, Song MK, Haddad I, et al. Is silicon deficiency involved in the pathogenesis of metabolic bone disease of children receiving parenteral nutrition? J Parenter Enter Nutr 1992; 16(1):31S.

74. Carlisle EM, Silicon as a trace nutrient. Sci Total Environ 1988; 73:95–106.

75. Nielson FH. Newer trace elements in human nutrition. Food Technol 1974; 28:38–52.

76. Nielsen FH. Nutritional requirements for boron, silicon, vanadium, nickel, and arsenic: Current knowledge and speculation. FASEB J 1991; 5:2661–2667.

77. Nielsen FH, Hunt CD, Mullen LM, Hunt JR. Effect of dietary boron on mineral, estrogen, and testosterone metabolism in post-menopausal women. FASEB J 1987; 1:394–397.

78. Moukarzel AA, Buchman AL, Song M, et al. Osteopenia of parenteral nutrition bone disease in children: Boron deficiency is not an etiological factor. Clin Res 1992; 40:60A.

79. Nielsen FH. Studies on the relationship between boron and magnesium which possibly affects the formation and maintenance of bones. Magnes Trace Elem 1990; 9:61–69.

80. Nomiyama J. Recent progress and perspectives in cadmium health studies. Sci Total Environ 1980; 14:199–232.

81. Omdahl JL, DeLuca HF. Strontium induced rickets: Metabolic basis. Science 1971; 174:949–951.

82. Dahlstrom KA, Ament ME, Medhin MG, et al. Serum trace elements in children receiving long-term parenteral nutrition. J Pediatr 1986; 109:625–630.

83. Griffith GC, Nichols G, Jr, Asher JD, et al. Heparin osteomalacia. JAMA 1965; 193:91–94.

84. Klein GL, Snodgrass WR, Griffin MP, et al. Hypocalcemia complicating deferoxamine therapy in an infant with parenteral nutrition associated aluminum overload: Evidence for a role of aluminum in the bone disease of infants. J Pediatr Gastroenterol Nutr 1989; 9:400–403.

85. Nebeker HG, Andress DL, Ott SM, et al. Treatment of aluminum related bone disease with deferoxamine: Results in 51 cases. Xth International Congress of Nephrology, London, July 1987 (abstract).

37

Pediatric Magnesium Disorders

Francis B. Mimouni

Maimonides Medical Center and State University of New York Health Science Center at Brooklyn, Brooklyn, New York

I. INTRODUCTION

The field of magnesium (Mg) metabolism is expanding as a considerable amount of research is accomplished daily. Two major international newspapers are exclusively dedicated to Mg research, with many other articles on Mg published in various subspecialty journals covering the fields of metabolism, nutrition, endocrinology, bone diseases, and others. Because of the relative rarity of Mg disorders in humans, however, very few physicians acquire expertise in the recognition and/or management of clinical entities related to magnesium alterations. Pediatricians and pediatric endocrinologists often seek help with a patient with an abnormality in serum Mg and cannot readily find answers in standard textbooks. The purpose of this chapter is to familiarize the reader with Mg disorders encountered in pediatric practice and to suggest practical approaches that will facilitate their recognition and management. We focus mostly on the impact of Mg (deficiency or excess) on bone and mineral metabolism, with a brief reminder of the role of Mg in carbohydrate metabolism and diabetes mellitus.

II. MAGNESIUM METABOLISM

A. Role of Mg in Health

Mg is mostly known for its interactions with the calcium (Ca)-parathyroid hormone (PTH) system (1). It seems, however, that the intracellular *functions* of Mg are considerably more diverse and still incompletely understood. Because of its contribution to the tridimensional structure of many enzymes, Mg is an important cofactor to their function, which means a key role in the metabolism of carbohydrates, lipids, and proteins (2). Similarly, Mg is an important cofactor in protein and DNA synthesis (2); its deficiency is teratogenic in several animal models (3) and possibly also in humans (4). Considerable interest in Mg has been developed in topics as

diverse as hypertension (5), pregnancy-induced hypertension (6), myocardial infarction (7), or sudden infant death syndrome (8,9); however, the best documented disorders of Mg metabolism relate to the field of bone and mineral metabolism and, to a lesser extent, carbohydrate metabolism.

B. Mg Distribution

Mg is the fourth most abundant metal in humans, and has three major compartments (10): the mineral phase of the skeleton contains 65% of total body stores, 34% are in the intracellular space, and approximately 0.3–1% is in the extracellular fluid (1). It is generally estimated that nearly 75–85% of plasma Mg exists in the ionic or complexed (as salts) form (filterable) and the remainder is bound to protein (nonfilterable) (1). The ionic form alone may constitute up to 70% of total plasma Mg (11).

C. Magnesium Absorption

Most of the intestinal absorption of Mg occurs in the duodenum and jejunum; the colon may also have Mg-absorbing capability (10). Magnesium is absorbed in part by simple diffusion in a linear fashion and according to a concentration gradient (10). A facilitated diffusion mechanism is also in place, however, which is saturable and consumes energy (10). Digestive secretions also contain Mg, and it is estimated that the intestinal Mg secretion amounts to 25% of the intestinal absorption flow (10). Ca and Mg compete for intestinal absorption, which has the potential of reducing Mg absorption when Ca intake is high (12). The percentage of ingested Mg that is absorbed (fractional absorption) is variable and is frequently quoted as approximate 40–60% based upon the results of balance studies (13). Using a stable isotope of Mg (^{25}Mg), Schuette et al. showed that in full-term infants, the fractional absorption of Mg varies between 44 and 64% and is proportional to the amount of Mg ingested (14). Phytates, fiber, or the presence of nonabsorbed fat may reduce intestinal Mg absorption (10,15).

D. Mg Excretion

The kidney is considered the main organ controlling Mg balance, because urinary Mg excretion adjusts dramatically to Mg intake changes (16). The renal tubular reabsorption of Mg in humans occurs in the ascending limb of Henle's loop and is influenced by PTH, calcitonin, glucagon, insulin, and antidiuretic hormone but also by glycemia, magnesemia, and calcemia (10). Such drugs as furosemide, digoxin, gentamicin, and cyclosporines inhibit tubular Mg reabsorption and may induce Mg deficiency (10).

E. Mg Requirements

There are no data on the exact Mg requirements in infants and young children. Because the approximate breast milk intake of a 6-month-old infant is 750 ml and human milk contains 28–48 mg Mg per liter (17), the average daily Mg intake of a breast-fed infant is 30 mg. To allow for variations in growth, the recommended dietary allowance (RDA) was established at 40 mg/day, to be increased to 60 mg/day for the second 6 months of life (15). Based upon studies by Schwartz, the RDA in childrem 1–15 years was established at 6.0 mg/kg/day (15).

F. Assessment of Mg Status

1. Measurements of Serum Mg

The gold standard is atomic absorption spectrometry (18). This method has the greatest accuracy and reproducibility and has a coefficient of variation of less than 1% (18). In clinical use and because of automation needs, calorimetric methods are often used, which are usually considered less accurate and reproducible (19). An enzymatic assay (glucokinase activation) was recently developed, appears to be quite accurate and reproducible, and may easily be automated (20). Regardless of the method used, serum Mg is often criticized as a means to assess Mg status (18). Its limitations are of two kinds: (1) the measurement of total Mg does not indicate the ionized fraction (presumably the active fraction); and (2) there is a significant zone of overlap between the normal and the deficient range. This may be related to the fact that the plasma compartment represents only 0.3–1% of total body stores, which makes it an imperfect estimate of intracellular stores (15). During the neonatal period, the normal "range" is reported to be 1.6–2.8 mg/day (21,22); we believe that numbers comprised between 1.4 and 1.8 mg/day can be seen in infants in a state of Mg sufficiency as well as deficiency (23). In later childhood the normal range is reported to be 1.75–2.40 mg/dl (24).

2. Ionized Mg Measurements

Recently, a novel ion-selective electrode was developed for ionized Mg measurements (iMg) in whole blood, plasma, or serum (11). Using this electrode, Altura et al. found that 71%

of total magnesium in blood circulates in the ionized form. Studies are being conducted to determine the clinical usefulness of this methodology. Although iMg measurement directly evaluates the active fraction of serum Mg, there are no data showing that serum iMg is an accurate reflection of intracellular Mg.

3. Measurements of Intracellular Mg

Because of the relative inadequacy of serum Mg measurements to assess intracellular Mg stores accurately, many investigators have attempted to measure intracellular Mg directly in erythrocytes (25) or in mononuclear blood cells (26) using atomic absorption spectrometry after cell lysis (25,26) or nuclear magnetic resonance (27,28). These methods are time consuming and expensive and remain restricted to research laboratories. It appears that erythrocyte Mg concentration is genetically regulated (23) and little influenced by dietary intake (25). In one study, in which Mg depletion in humans was created by dietary restriction, red blood cell-free Mg determined by nuclear magnetic resonance fell significantly, but so did serum Mg concentration. Whether these methods will be useful clinically remains to be demonstrated.

4. Magnesium Loading Tests

It has been suggested by some investigators that a Mg loading test may be used to demonstrate a deficiency state (29). The test is based on the principle that the fractional tubular reabsorption of Mg is maximized in Mg deficiency, leading to maximal retention of an intramuscular load of Mg (16). Caddell et al. (29) utilized a 6 mg elemental Mg/kg body weight intramuscular dose, followed by a 24–32 h urine collection. The percentage retention is calculated from the dose given and the amount excreted in urine. This test has been used as described or with some modifications by several investigators. It may be particularly helpful in Mg-wasting disorders originating in the gut (30). In contrast, when the source of Mg wasting is the kidney, as in diabetes mellitus or in various tubular disorders, urinary Mg excretion can be high, even in the presence of severe Mg deficit. Moreover, in the neonatal period, the interpretation of this test may be difficult, because newly born infants tend to retain a large proportion of the Mg given (regardless of their Mg status), maybe because of a low glomerular filtration rate (9).

III. MG DEFICIENCY AND HYPOMAGNESEMIA IN PEDIATRICS

A. Endocrine Consequences of Mg Deficiency

The endocrine consequences of Mg deficiency relate primarily to calcium and carbohydrate metabolism.

1. Effect on Mineral Metabolism

Mg has been labeled the mimic antagonist of Ca (1). This is particularly true when it relates to PTH secretion. In Mg sufficiency, Mg mimics Ca: acute hypermagnesemia (pharmacologically induced) or hypomagnesemia stimulates or inhibits PTH secretion, respectively (1,31). In contrast, in chronic Mg deficiency (usually associated with hypomagnesemia), PTH secretion *and* action are deficient, probably because both require a Mg-dependent adenylate cyclase (1,32). As soon as Mg stores are restored by a Mg infusion, serum Mg rises rapidly, followed by a use in serum PTH (23). Thus, Mg deficiency leads to functional hypo- and-pseudohypoparathyroidism, with subsequent hypocalcemia. Because the consequences of hypocalcemia and hypomagnesemia on nerve conduction and neuromuscular function are very similar, the two conditions potentiate each other; this aggravates the risk for tetany or seizures, as described in greater detail in Chapters 31 and 32.

2. Magnesium, Glucose Homeostasis, and Diabetes Mellitus

Magnesium deficiency may occur in children with poorly controlled diabetes mellitus (33,34), and results from increased Mg losses secondary to glycosuria, as shown in humans and in experimental diabetes in rats (35). In vitro and in vivo studies have pointed out the role of Mg in insulin action (36). Mg deficiency may cause insulin resistance (37); this may be particularly important during diabetic ketoacidosis, during which severe hypomagnesemia may develop, in particular after fluid and insulin therapy has been started (38). Also, because insulin plays an important role in Mg entry into the cells (38), insulin deficiency or resistance may theoretically lead to intracellular Mg deficiency, which in turn may increase insulin resistance.

Recently, a panel of experts from many countries, which was convened by the American Diabetes Association, summarized and published a consensus statement (39). It was generally agreed that there is a great need for "well designed prospective studies demonstrating the safety and beneficial results of magnesium replacement therapy" (39). The panel recommended attempting to identify Mg deficiency in patients with diabetes at risk for deficiency, among them patients with poorly controlled diabetes and during the treatment of diabetic ketoacidosis. Although it is theoretically conceivable that Mg replacement should improve insulin sensitivity and shorten the treatment of ketoacidosis, this remains to be demonstrated in a rigorous, scientific manner (39).

B. Renal Causes of Mg Deficiency

1. Acquired Causes

These causes are mostly related to diuretic treatment (loop diuretics and chlorothiazides) and as a consequence of alcoholism (10). Although chronic alcoholism as a cause of Mg deficiency is probably very rare in childhood, infants born to alcoholic mothers may present with symptomatic hypomagnesemia. Other agents can cause urinary Mg losses, among them such antibiotics as aminoglycosides, such antifungal agents as amphotericin B, immunosuppressants, such as cyclosporin A, or antineoplastic agents, such as mithramycin (10). The chronic use of these drugs mandates the routine evaluation of serum Mg, together with Mg supplementation whenever required.

Any tubular disorder has the potential for causing Mg deficiency. Acute tubular necrosis, in its polyuric phase, can induce profound salt losses, in particular Mg losses (22). Theoretically, acute tubular necrosis may contribute, through urinary Mg loses, to the hypocalcemia frequently found in the asphyxiated infant.

Neonatal hypocalcemia in infants of diabetic mothers is believed to be caused by Mg deficiency (40). Indeed, in diabetes mellitus, osmotic diuresis as a result of hyperglycemia and glycosuria causes urinary Mg losses in the mother (41). This leads to maternal Mg deficiency, which is followed by fetal deficiency. Amniotic fluid Mg concentrations are decreased in diabetic pregnancy, which is interpreted as a decreased urinary Mg excretion by the fetus, an index of Mg deficiency (42). In normal pregnancies, following birth and clamping of the umbilical cord, the Ca transport from mother to fetus is abruptly interrupted, and neonatal Ca concentrations start to decrease (43). The parathyroid glands are stimulated by decreasing serum Ca, and serum PTH rises to stop the decrease in serum Ca (44). In infants of diabetic mothers, Mg deficiency prevents an adequate rise in serum PTH, and neonatal hypocalcemia may follow (40,45).

2. Congenital or Inherited Causes

Both Bartter and Gitelman syndromes may be causes of renal tubular Mg wastage (46). These two conditions are characterized by hypokalemic metabolic alkalosis. There is a generalized wastage of water, chloride, sodium, and potassium, much more pronounced in Bartter than in Gitelman syndrome (46). Increased plasma renin activity is found in both (43). The two conditions are probably genetically inherited, because parental consanguinity and other affected siblings have been reported (46). In general, Bartter syndrome appears to be a more severe condition presenting in infancy; it is sometimes preceded by polyhydramnios and preterm delivery and is followed by significant postnatal failure to thrive. In contrast, Gitelman patients are usually diagnosed after 6 years of age because of a febrile seizure or a tetanic episode, or even by chance (random serum electrolyte measurements) (46). The two conditions have a component of renal Mg wastage, although this is much more pronounced in Gitelman than in Bartter syndrome. In one study, 7 of 18 patients with Bartter syndrome and 16 of 16 patient with Gitelman syndrome had significant hypomagnesemia (46). A significant biochemical difference between the two syndromes is an increased calciuria in Bartter patients, with urinary molar Ca/creatinine ratios > 0.20; patients with Gitelman syndrome have hypocalciuria (molar calcium/creatinine ratio < 0.20) (46). The pathophysiology of the two syndromes is not very well understood; loop diuretics, which bind to and inhibit the luminal sodium-potassium-chloride cotransporter in the thick ascending loop of Henle (47), may cause biochemical changes mimicking Bartter syndrome; it was therefore suggested by some authors that some inherited structural or functional disturbance of this cotransporter is the cause of Bartter syndrome (46). In contrast, thiazide diuretics, which bind and inhibit the luminal sodium chloride carrier protein in the distal convoluted tubule (47), cause biochemical disturbances mimicking Gitelman syndrome. It has been suggested that a structural or functional disturbance of this cotransporter may be the cause of Gitelman syndrome (46).

The congenital Mg-losing kidney is a separate, genetically inherited entity, characterized by chronic, often severe urinary Mg wastage with hypocalcemic tetany (48,49); some patients also have a hearing loss, and some males also have oligospermia (48,49). Renal biopsy, when performed, shows patchy interstitial fibrosis and glomerular sclerosis, with medullary nephrocalcinosis (48). Hypocalcemia and chronic urinary potassium wasting may also be present (48,49). It is not clear whether the renal biopsy findings are cause or consequence of the Mg wastage. One patient, described by Zelikovic et al., also had severe rickets and hyperphosphatemia, probably on the basis of renal failure and defective 1,25-dihydroxyvitamin D production (49).

Renal tubular acidosis may lead to significant Mg losses (50). During its correction with alkali therapy, a syndrome similar to the "hungry bone syndrome" may occur, with significant hypomagnesemia and tetany (51).

C. Intestinal Causes of Mg Deficiency

Mg deficiency may occur in childhood or infancy as a consequence of decreased intestinal magnesium absorption arising from malabsorption syndromes, steatorrhea, prolonged diarrhea, laxative abuse, short gut, or intestinal fistula (21).

In chloride-losing diarrhea, characterized by a specific defect of ileal chloride transport, patients present with a neonatal watery diarrhea, often preceded by maternal polyhydramnios (52). Subsequently, hypochloridemia, hypokalemia, and metabolic alkalosis develop. In this condition, a significant Mg deficiency may occur, presumably as a result of chronic, secondary hyperaldosteronism and increased magnesuria. The treatment of chloride-losing diarrhea consists of sodium and potassium chloride supplements.

Mg deficiency can also occur as a primary and isolated defect of intestinal Mg absorption, as initially described by Paunier et al. (53) and recently reviewed by Dudin and Tecbi (54). Among the approximate 30 cases reported in the literature, most have been males, with a male-female ratio of 4:1 (54). Parental consanguinity was found in 3 of 28 families reported, and the condition was diagnosed among siblings in 2 families; thus the exact transmission is unclear. It has been hypothesized by Mettey and Hoppler (55) that an autosomal recessive gene coding for the defect is modulated by another gene on the short arm of chromosome X. Indeed, one female patient affected and reported by Meyer et al. (56) had a balanced translocation 46, XX, t(9; X) (q12:p22); in general, the normal X is preferentially inactivated in most balanced X-autosome translocations (54).

The clinical features of primary Mg malabsorption were summarized by Dudin and Tecbi (54). Briefly, the syndrome manifests itself in early infancy, from 2 weeks to 4 months, or even in early adolescence in some mild cases. Revealing symptoms are those of hypocalcemia and hypomagnesemia, documented by seizures and/or tetany and often preceded by irritability and poor sleeping patterns. Calcium salt therapy relieves the symptoms only partially and/or momentarily, but Mg therapy alone leads to a complete correction of both hypocalcemia and hypomagnesemia (54). The doses of Mg required are well in excess of 4–20 times the normal daily requirements, however, and Mg supplementation is required for life (50).

D. Hypomagnesemia with Hypocalcemia: Differential Diagnosis

The presence of late-onset hypocalcemia (>3 days of age) associated with hypomagnesemia creates a clinical dilemma. Indeed, such a combination may exist as a result of Mg deficiency (as discussed), but it may also be seen in congenital hypoparathyroidism or in phosphorus intoxication.

In congenital hypoparathyroidism, serum Mg is generally low, without necessarily indicating Mg deficiency, similar to low serum Ca not necessarily indicating a Ca deficiency; this may be confusing, because Mg deficiency leads to a functional defect of PTH secretion and to PTH resistance. Thus, in both hypoparathyroidism and Mg deficiency, serum PTH is low in the presence of hypocalcemia and hypomagnesemia. Furthermore, treatment with Ca salts, appropriate in hypoparathyroidism, is not in Mg deficiency. Indeed, if given orally, Ca salts inhibit intestinal Mg absorption and, if given intravenously, inhibit tubular Mg reabsorption and may aggravate the Mg deficit (12). We propose to treat such patients with Mg salts first, which leads to a correction of serum Ca and an increase in serum PTH in Mg deficiency, although it corrects neither in hypoparathyroidism. In symptomatic hypocalcemia with hypomagnesemia, the thought of administering Mg alone may be of concern; however, Turner et al. showed that late-onset hypocalcemic seizures can be stopped with Mg sulfate faster than when Ca salts or phenobarbital are given (57). An additional concern to the endocrinologist is that of hypoparathyroidism treated with Ca salts and vitamin D metabolites with persisting hypomagnesemia. Such patients may have a concomitant Mg deficit. Treatment of these patients with Mg salts often decreases their vitamin D and calcium requirements, suggestive of resistance to treatment induced by the Mg deficit.

Phosphorus intoxication can be differentiated from hypoparathyroidism and from Mg deficiency because in phosphorus intoxication serum PTH is appropriately elevated, rather than decreased (58). Phosphate-induced hypocalcemia is very rare nowadays and has been reported only in some infants fed a high-phosphorus–containing formula (58); once serum Ca is corrected using intravenous or oral Ca salts, its treatment consists of switching the infant to a low-phosphorus–containing formula, such as SMA (Wyeth Laboratories, Philadelphia).

E. Treatment of Mg Deficiency

The treatment of Mg deficiency is rendered complicated by the number of Mg salt preparations available. To avoid confusion we recommend that all calculations be made in terms of elemental Mg, and that mg and mEq not be confused. Table 1 shows the Mg content of various preparations.

In most situations of renal or intestinal Mg wasting, oral Mg salts suffice to maintain serum Mg concentrations within normal limits. However, several points are important. First small but frequently administered doses are more likely not to cause gastrointestinal upset than larger doses administered less frequently. Second, it is preferable to use a schedule of increasing doses over several days to improve gastrointestinal tolerance. Finally, although some controversy exists in regard to which form of Mg salts is preferred, in our experience enterically coated forms of magnesium chloride allow a greater degree of gastrointestinal tolerance while providing an excellent degree of bioavailability. Coated tablets are impractical in infants, however, in whom a liquid preparation of Mg sulfate is most often utilized.

In symptomatic hypomagnesemia, in particular when there are seizures, the intramuscular or the intravenous route may be required. Doses of 6 mg elemental Mg per kg body weight (in the form of 50% Mg sulfate) raise the serum concentrations by an average of 1 mg/dl (23). We recommend that parenteral correction of Mg deficiency be done under electronic cardiac and blood pressure monitoring, in view of the potential cardiac effects of hypermagnesemia (see later).

IV. HYPERMAGNESEMIA

A. General Consequences

One of the first consequences of hypermagnesemia is neuromuscular hypoexcitability with progressive loss of tendon reflex and muscle hypotonia but also somnolence. At higher degrees of hypomagnesemia, successive paralysis of the voluntary and respiratory muscles may occur; ultimately, during severe intoxication, death may occur after cardiac arrest in diastole as a result of atrioventricular dissociation (10).

B. Neonatal Hypermagnesemia

Parenteral Mg is used frequently in pregnancy. The two main indications are preeclampsia, in which Mg salts are used to prevent seizures (59,60), and preterm labor, because Mg acts as an excellent tocolytic agent (61,62). In both situations Mg

Table 1 Elemental Magnesium Content of Various Mg Preparations

Mg salt	Elemental Mg content	
	mg/g	mEq/g
$MgSO_4 \cdot 7H_2O$	97.56	8.13
$MgCl \cdot 6H_2O$	116.00	9.75
MgO	550.00	46.00
$Mg(C_2H_3O_2) \cdot 4H_2O$	112.10	9.35

sulfate is utilized to reach serum concentrations very close to the toxic range (4–8 mg/dl).

1. Consequences to the Mother

It is important to understand the fluctuations in serum ionized Ca and Mg during Mg administration in obstetrics. In a landmark study by Cholst et al. (62), women were treated for preterm labor with a loading dose followed by a continuous infusion of Mg sulfate. While the serum Mg concentration rose, serum total and ionized Ca declined. Serum PTH abruptly declined after the Mg load and then returned within hours to the baseline values. This return to the baseline may be considered insufficient because serum ionized Ca concentrations measured at the same time were relatively low (62). This observation is consistent with an inhibitory effect of acute hypermagnesemia on PTH production and with the observation that isolated parathyroid glands perfused in vitro with a medium enriched with Mg have a decreased PTH output (1).

2. Consequences to the Fetus and the Newborn

Compared with control infants, infants born to hypermagnesemic mother are also hypermagnesemic (59,63); however, their serum Ca and serum ionized Ca concentrations between birth and 72 h are increased compared with controls, despite that serum PTH concentrations are more often detectable in hypermagnesemic infants than in control infants (63). Thus, the rise in serum ionized Ca is not driven by PTH but rather inhibits PTH production (64). It has been speculated that, as previously shown in cultured bone in vitro, excessive Mg transported to the fetus competes with Ca at the bone surface, which leads to a rise in serum ionized Ca concentration and subsequently to blunted PTH secretion (63).

Additionally, we showed recently that Mg added in vitro to serum or serum ultrafiltrate leads to an increase in serum or ultrafiltrate ionized Ca concentration, consistent with competition of Mg with Ca bound to albumin or complexed to salt (65). Recently, Lamm et al. reported five infants whose mothers had received several weeks of Mg sulfate therapy (66). Of the five infants, two presented with congenital rickets, which is consistent with the theory of heteroionic exchange of Mg with Ca at the bone. Alternatively, the authors of this report speculated that chronic maternal hypermagnesemia results in inhibition of PTH production in both mother and the fetus, chronic hypocalcemia, and inadequate Ca supply to the bone (66). The most likely explanation, however, has been presented by Wians et al., who showed that hypermagnesemia increases in vivo serum osteocalcin concentrations (67), confirming previous in vitro results that demonstrated that Mg is a potent inhibitor of osteocalcin binding to hydroxyapatite (68). Osteocalcin is a protein synthesized by osteoblasts that plays a significant role in bone formation (69); thus, the inhibition of its action by Mg ions is likely to cause profound disturbances in bone metabolism.

C. Other Causes of Hypermagnesemia

The other causes of hypermagnesemia are mostly decreased glomerular filtration rate caused by either acute or chronic renal failure (10). Another related situation is that of preterm infants on total parenteral nutrition. Indeed, preterm infants have very low glomerular filtration rates and a much lesser capability to excrete excess Mg (70). In our experience, Mg intakes below 6 mg/kg/dl have not led to any significant hypermagnesemia in preterm infants on total parenteral nutrition, as long as their kidney function was adequate.

Finally, hypermagnesemia has been reported as a side effect of overdosage of a Mg-containing laxative or antacid (71,72). The chronic use of these medications requires routine monitoring of serum Mg concentrations, in particular in patients with renal disease.

D. Treatment

In most cases, when the renal function is normal, adequate hydration and discontinuation of Mg intake suffice and serum Mg gradually falls. Diuretic therapy may help hasten normalization of serum Mg but should be reserved to cases with neuromuscular depression. In severe cases, exchange transfusion with citrated blood may be of help.

When the renal function is impaired, hemodialysis with a Mg-free medium may be required. This is usually efficient in returning the serum Mg concentrations within safe limits in 4–6 h (73).

In a life-threatening event, such as cardiorespiratory depression or cardiac arrhythmia, 10% calcium gluconate as a slow push (1–2 ml/kg body weight) is the drug of choice (74).

ACKNOWLEDGMENTS

Supported in part by a grant from the Maimonides Medical Center Research Foundation.

REFERENCES

1. Levine BS, Coburn, JW. Magnesium, the mimic/antagonist of calcium. N Engl J Med 1984; 310:1253–1255.
2. Ebel H, Gunther T. Magnesium metabolism: a review. J Clin Chem Clin Biochem 1980; 18:257–270.
3. Gunther T., Hirsch W. Embryotoxic effects produced by magnesium deficiency in rats. Adv Exp Med Biol 1972; 27:295–300.
4. Mimouni F, Miodovnik M, Tsang RC, Holroyde J, Dignan PS, Siddiqi TA. Decreased maternal serum magnesium concentration and adverse fetal outcome in insulin-dependent diabetic women. Obstet Gynicol 1987; 70:85–88.
5. Westea PO, Dyckner T. Magnesium and hypertension. J Am Coll Nutr 1987; 6:321–328.
6. Conradt A, Weindinger H, Algayer H. Magnesium therapy decreased the rates of intrauterine growth retardation, premature rupture of membranes and premature delivery in high risk pregnancies treated with beta-mimetics. Magnesium 1985; 4:20–28.
7. Teo KK, Yusuf S, Gollins R, Held PH, Peto R. Effects of intravenous magnesium in suspected acute myocardial infarction: overview of randomized trials. BMJ 1991; 303:1499–1503.
8. Caddell JL. Magnesium therapy in premature neonates with apnea Neonatorum. J Am Coll Nutr 1988; 7:5–16.
9. Tsang RC, Mimouni F. Editorial. J Am Coll Nutr 1988; 7:1–3.
10. Speich M, Bousquet B. Magnesium: recent data on metabolism, exploration, pathology and therapeutics. Magnes Bull 1991; 13:116–121.
11. Altura BT, Shirey TL, Young CC, et al. A new method for the rapid determination of ionized Mg^{2+} in whole blood, serum and plasma. Methods Find Exp Clin Pharmacol 1992; 14:297–304.
12. Alcock N, MacIntyre I. Interrelation of calcium and magnesium absorption. Clin Sci 1962; 22:185–193.
13. Schwartz R, Spencer H, Wentworth RA. Measurement of magnesium absorption in man using stable ^{22}Mg as a tracer. Clin Chim Acta 1978; 87:265–273.
14. Schuette SA, Ziegler EE, Welson SE, Janghorhani M. Feasibility of using the stable isotope ^{25}Mg to study Mg metabolism in infants. Pediatr Res 1990; 27:36–40.
15. Subcommittee on the Tenth Edition of the RDAs. Minerals. In: Recommended Dietary Allowances, 10th ed. Washington DC: National Academy Press, 1989: pp. 174–194.
16. Shils ME. Experimental production of magnesium deficiency in man. Ann NY Acad Sci 1969; 162:847–855.
17. Lemons JA, Moye L, Hall D, Simmons M. Differences in the composition of preterm and term human milk during early lactation. Pediatr Res 1982; 16:113–117.
18. Wills MR, Sunderman FW, Savory J. Methods for the estimation of serum magnesium in clinical laboratories. Magnesium 1986; 5:317–27.
19. Cohen SA, Daza IE. Calmagite method for determination of serum magnesium modified. Clin Chem 1980; 26:783.
20. Fossati P, Sirtoli M, Tarenghi G, Giacheti M, Bert G. Enzymatic assay of magnesium through glucokinase activation. Clin Chem 1989; 35:2212–2216.
21. Tsang RC. Neonatal magnesium disturbances. Am J Dis Child 1972; 124:282–293.
22. Mimouni F, Tsang RC. Perinatal magnesium metabolism: personal data and challenges for the 1990s. Magnes Res 1991; 4:109–117.
23. Shaul PW, Mimouni F, Tsang RC, Specker BL. The role of magnesium in neonatal calcium homeostasis: effects of magnesium infusion on calciotropic hormones and calcium. Pediatr Res 1987; 22:319–323.
24. Specker BL, Lichtenstein P, Mimouni F, Gormley C, Tsang RC. Calcium-regulating hormones and minerals from birth to 18 months of age: a cross-sectional study. II. Effects of sex, race, age, season, and diet on serum minerals, parathyroid hormone, and calcitonin. Pediatrics 1986; 77:891–896.
25. Moser PB, Issa CF, Reynolds RD. Dietary magnesium intake and the concentration of magnesium in plasma and erythocytes of postpartum women. J Am Coll Nutr 1983; 4:387–396.
26. Elin R, Hosseini JM. Magnesium content of mononuclear blood cells. Clin Chem 1985; 31:377–320.
27. Ryzen E, Servis KL, DeRusso P, Kershaw A, Stephen T, Rude RK. Determination of intracellular free magnesium by nuclear magnetic resonance in human magnesium deficiency. J Am Coll Nutr 1989; 8:580–587.
28. Santarromana M, Delepicare M, Feray JC, Franck G, Garay R, Henrotte JG. Correlation between total and free magnesium levels in human red blood cells: influence of HLA antigens. Magnes Res 1989; 2:281–283.
29. Caddell JL, Byrne PA, Triska RA, McElfresh AE. The magnesium load test. III. Correlation of clinical and laboratory data in infants from one to six months of age. Clin Pediatr (Phila) 1975; 14:478–848.
30. LaSala MA, Lifshitz F, Silverberg M, Wapnir RA, Carrera E. Magnesium metabolism studies in children with chronic inflammatory disease of the bowel. J Pediatr Gastoenterol Nutr 1985; 4:75–81.
31. Habener JF, Potts JT Jr. Relative effectiveness of magnesium

and calcium on the secretion and biosynthesis of parathyroid hormone in vitro. Endocrinology 1976; 98:197–202.

32. Matsuzaki S, Dumont JE. Effect of calcium ions on horse parathyroid gland adenyl cyclase. Biochim Biophys Acta 1972; 284:227–234.

33. Ponder SW, Bronkard BH, Travis LB. Hyperphosphaturia and hypermagnesuria in children with IDDM. Diabetes Care 1990; 13:437–441.

34. Fort P, Lifshitz F. Magnesium status in children with insulin-dependent diabetes mellitus. J Am Coll Nutr 1986; 5:69–78.

35. Fort P, Lifshitz F, Wapnir IL, Wapnir RA. Magnesium metabolism in experimental diabetes mellitus. Diabetes 1977; 26:882–886.

36. Lostroh AJ, Krahl ME. Magnesium a second messenger for insulin: ion translocation coupled to transport activity. Adv Enzyme Regul 1974; 12:73–81.

37. Durlach J, Rayssiguer Y. Magnesium et glucides I. Donnees cliniques et therapeutiques, Magnesium 1983; 2:192–224.

38. Moles KW, McMullen JK. Insulin resistance and hypomagnesemia: case report. BMJ 1982; 285:262.

39. Americam Diabetes Association. Magnesium supplementation in the treatment of diabetes: a consensus statement. Diabetes Care 1992; 15:1065–1067.

40. Mimouni F, Loughead J, Miodovnik M, Khoury J, Tsang RC. Early neonatal predictors of neonatal hypercalcemia in infants of diabetic mothers: an epidemiologic study. Am J Perinatol 1990; 7:203–206.

41. Mimouni F, Tsang RC, Hertzberg VS, Neuman V, Ellis K. Parathyroid hormone and calcitiol changes in normal and insulin dependent diabetic pregnancies. Obstet Gynecol 1989; 74:49–54.

42. Mimouni F, Miodovnik M, Tsang RC, Callahan J, Shaul P. Decreased amniotic fluid magnesium concentration in diabetic pregnancy. Obstet Gynecol 1987; 69:12–14.

43. Loughead JL, Mimouni F, Tsang RC. Serum ionized calcium concentrations in normal neonates. Am J Dis Child 1988; 142:516–518.

44. Loughead JL, Mimouni F, Ross R, Tsang RC. Postnatal changes in serum osteocalcin and parathyroid hormone concentration. J Am Coll Nutr 1990; 9:358–362.

45. Loughead JL, Mimouni F, Tsang RC, Khaury JC. A role for magnesium in neonatal parathyroid gland function? J Am Coll Nutr 1991; 10:123–126.

46. Bettinell A, Bianchetti MG, Girardin E, et al. Use of calcium excretion values to distinguish two forms of primary renal tubular hypokalemic alkalosis: Bartter and Gitelman syndromes. J Pediatr 1992; 120:38–43.

47. Breyer J, Jacobson HR. Molecular mechanisms of diuretic agents. Annu Rev Med 1990; 41:265–275.

48. Evans RA, Carter JN, George CRP, et al. The congenital "magnesium losing kidney." Q J Med 1981; 197:39–52.

49. Zelikovic I, Dabbagh S, Friedman AL, Goelzer ML, Chesney RW. Severe renal osteodystrophy without elevated serum immunoreactive parathyroid hormone concentrations in hypermagnesemia due to renal magnesium wasting. Pediatrics 1987; 79:403–407.

50. Bianchetti MG, Oetlier OH, Lutschg J. Magnesium deficiency in primary distal tubular acidosis. J Pediatr 1993; 122:833.

51. Fisch L, Mimouni F. Hypermagnesemia following correction of metabolic acidosis: a case of hungry bones. J Am Coll Nutr 1993; 12:710–713.

52. Holmberg C. Congenital chloride diarrhea. Clin Gastroenterol 1986; 92:583–587.

53. Paunier L, Raddle IC, Kooh SW, Conen PE, Frazer D. Primary hypomagnesemia with secondary hypocalcaemia in an infant. Pediatrics 1968; 4:385–392.

54. Dudin KI, Tecbi AS. Primary hypomagnesemia. Eur J Pediatr 1987; 146:303–305.

55. Mettey R, Hoppler A. Les deficits magnesiens de l'enfant. Arch Fr Pediatr 1982; 39:837–844.

56. Meyer M, Mattei JF, Vialard JL, Goumy P, Dastugue B, Malpuech G. Hypocalcemie magnesodependante par trouble specifique de l'absorption du magnesium, associee a une anomalie chromosomique. Rev Fr Endocrinol Clin 1978; 19:101–108.

57. Turner TL, Cockburn F, Forfar JO. Magnesium therapy in neonatal tetany. Lancet 1977; 1:283–284.

58. Venkataraman PS, Tsang RC, Greer FR, Noguchi A, Laskarzewoki P, Steichen JJ. Late infantile tetany and secondary hyperparathyroidism in infants fed immunized cow's milk formula. Am J Dis Child 1985; 139:664–668.

59. Cruikshank DP, Pitkin RM, Reynolds WA, Williams GA, Hargis GK. Effects of magnesium sulfate treatment on perinatal calcium metabolism I. Maternal and fetal responses. Am J Obstet Gynecol 1979; 134:243–249.

60. McGuinness GA, Weinstein MM, Cruikshank DP, Pitkin RM. Effects of magnesium sulfate treatment on perinatal calcium metabolism. II. Neonatal responses. Obstet Gynecol 1980; 56:595–600.

61. Elliot JP. Magnesium sulfate as a tocolytic agent. Am J Obstet Gynecol 1983; 147:277–284.

62. Cholst IN, Steinberg SF, Tropper PJ, Fox HE, Sergre GV, Bilezkian JP. The influence of hypermagnesemia on serum calcium and parathyroid hormone levels in human subjects. N Engl J Med 1984; 310:1221–1225.

63. Donovan EF, Tsang RC, Steichen JJ, Strub RJ, Chen JW, Chen M. Neonatal hypermagnesemia: effect on parathyroid hormone and calcium homeostasis. J Pediatr 1980; 96:305–310.

64. MacManus J, Heaton FW. The influence of magnesium on calcium release from bone in vitro. Biochim Biophys Acta 1970; 215:360–367.

65. Liu CL, Mimouni F, Ho M, Tsang RC. In vitro effects of magnesium on ionized calcium concentration in serum. Am J Dis Child 1988; 142:837–838.

66. Lamm CI, Norton KI, Murphy RJC, Wilkins IA, Rabinowitz JG. Congenital rickets associated with magnesium sulfate for tocolysis. J Pediatr 1988; 113:1078–1082.

67. Wians FH, Strickland DM, Hawkins GDV, Snyder RR. The effect of hypermagnesemia on serum levels of osteocalcin in an animal model. Magnes Trace Elem 1990; 9:28–35.

68. Wians FH, Kzech KE, Haushka PV. Effects of magnesium and calcium on osteocalcin absorption to hydroxyapatite. Magnesium 1983; 2:83–92.

69. Boskey AL, Wians FH, Hauschka PV. The effect of osteocalcin on in vitro lipid-induced hydroxyapatite formation and seeded hydroxyapatite growth. Calcif Tissue Int 1985; 37:57–62.

70. Oh W. Renal function and clinical disorders in the neonate. Clin Perinatol 1981; 8:215–223.

71. Weber CA, Santiago RM. Hypermagnesemia, a potential complication during treatment of theophyllin intoxication with oral activated charcoal and magnesium-containing cathartics. Chest 1989; 95:56–59.

72. Brand JM, Greer FR. Hypermagnesemia and intestinal perforation following antacid administration in a premature infant. Pediatrics 1990; 85:121–123.

73. Alfrey AC, Terman DS, Brettschneider L, Simpson KM, Ogden DA. Hypermagnesemia after renal hemotransplantation. Ann Intern Med 1970; 73:367–372.

74. Alfrey AC. Normal and abnormal magnesium metabolism. In: Schrier RW, ed. Renal and Electrolyte Disorders, 4th ed. Boston: Little, Brown, 1992:371–404.

38

Diabetes Mellitus in the Child
Classification, Diagnosis, Epidemiology, and Etiology

Allan L. Drash

University of Pittsburgh and Children's Hospital of Pittsburgh, Pittsburgh, Pennsylvania

I. INTRODUCTION

Diabetes mellitus is a common, chronic, systemic disease with hyperglycemia as a cardinal biochemical feature. The major forms of diabetes generally can be divided into those that result from primary damage to the β cells of the pancreas, leading to partial or complete insulin deficiency, and those that are a consequence of insulin resistance occurring at the tissue level, with little or no impairment of insulin synthesis or release. These two major forms of diabetes are in fact quite different diseases in their genetic, pathologic and clinical aspects, with differing clinical courses and outcomes.

II. CLASSIFICATION

In 1979, the National Diabetes Data Group, working under the direction of the National Institutes of Health, provided a revision of the previously accepted classification of diabetes mellitus (1). This work followed shortly after the report of a working group of the World Health Organization recommending some modification in the classification and criteria of diagnosis. The widely used term "juvenile diabetes" or "juvenile-onset diabetes" has been discarded. Replacing it is the more appropriate terminology, "insulin-dependent diabetes mellitus" (IDDM), or type I diabetes, according to the European classification system. This classification clearly indicates that patients so categorized are insulin dependent secondary to β cell damage. The European terminology of type I also carries with it the understanding of an underlying autoimmune destructive process. The disorder, previously described as adult-onset diabetes or maturity-onset diabetes, is now designated "non–insulin-dependent diabetes," or type II diabetes, by the European terminology. The old diagnostic category of asymptomatic diabetes, also called chemical diabetes, subclinical or preclinical diabetes, borderline diabe-

tes, or latent diabetes, has been replaced by the category of impaired glucose tolerance. Maturity-onset diabetes of youth (MODY) is a very specific genetic form of carbohydrate intolerance that is diagnosed in childhood, usually with mild hyperglycemia and similarly affected individuals in three generations.

In our experience in Pittsburgh, with over 2000 diabetic children, we find that well over 97% of them have classic insulin-dependent diabetes mellitus secondary to β cell destruction. The remaining 3% or fewer are a combination of children and adolescents with the true maturity-onset type of diabetes associated with marked obesity, examples of the MODY type of diabetes, and rare examples of specific causes of β cell destruction, such as pancreatitis (2).

III. DIAGNOSIS OF DIABETES IN CHILDHOOD

In almost all children with newly diagnosed diabetes, this diagnosis is immediately apparent. These children have the classic triad of polyuria, polydipsia, and polyphagia, and in addition, they have weight loss and fatigue, and many have further metabolic deterioration with diabetic ketoacidosis. The blood glucose concentration is elevated far above 200 mg/dl, and glucose and ketones are present in large amounts in the urine. Such patients present no diagnostic dilemmas. The oral glucose tolerance test, a commonly used diagnostic tool in adult medicine, is primarily a research tool in pediatrics. However, it is rarely needed to confirm the diagnosis of diabetes in the child. The currently accepted tolerance criteria for the diagnosis of diabetes in the child or adolescent uses a glucose load of 1.75 g/kg ideal body weight, up to a maximum dose of 75 g. The fasting venous plasma must exceed 140 mg/dl (120 mg/dl for venous whole blood or capillary whole blood), and the 2 h value, as well as an intervening value (either 0.5 or 1 h) must exceed 200 mg/dl in venous plasma or capillary whole blood and 180 mg/dl in venous whole blood. The diagnosis of diabetes should not be made on the basis of a single observation only. Repeated values—fasting, postprandial, or oral glucose tolerance testing—should be assessed to ensure a proper diagnosis.

Persistent hyperglycemia (blood glucose values in excess of 200 mg/dl) should lead to a diagnosis of diabetes mellitus and initiation of appropriate therapy. However, one must remain aware that, even in the child, hyperglycemia may be a result of biologic processes not directly involving the β cell. The single most common cause in the pediatric age group is administration of high doses of steroids. This may be seen in patients with renal disease, rheumatoid arthritis, asthma, or leukemia. Endogenous, excessive cortisol production, as seen in adrenal hyperplasia, is a rare cause of hyperglycemia in the child. A number of pharmacologic agents, such as those used in the treatment of leukemia, may result in hyperglycemia. Pheochromocytoma may be associated with elevations of blood glucose levels, as may primary tumors of the central nervous system. Although these very rare conditions should be excluded, the initiation of therapy with insulin, if needed, should not be delayed (3).

IV. EPIDEMIOLOGY OF DIABETES IN CHILDHOOD

Although the past decade has witnessed a dramatic advance in our understanding of many basic aspects of diabetes, there has also been an explosion in the epidemiologic studies, with many investigators in various parts of the world participating in the collection and analysis of this important new information. The following section summarizes the highlights of these recent studies. The frequency of IDDM among children and adolescents is compared with that of other common, serious pediatric disorders in Table 1. It is seen that diabetes mellitus

Table 1 Risk of Type I Diabetes Compared with Chronic Disease of Children

Disease	Rate/100,000
Type I diabetes	14.8
Cancer < 15 year (overall risk)	12.2
Leukemia	3.9
Brain	2.6
Lymphoma	1.3
Other cancers	4.8
Peptic ulcer	3.5
Cystic fibrosis	3.1
Multiple sclerosis	3.0
Juvenile rheumatoid arthritis	3.0
Nephrotoc syndrome	1.3
Muscular dystrophy	1.1
Lupus erythematosus	0.2

Source: From Reference 4.

in childhood outranks cancer as one of the leading serious chronic diseases of childhood (4).

Prevalence, the determination of the total number of patients in the population with a particular disorder, expressed per thousand age- and sex-matched population, is a statistic that is fraught with potential inaccuracies because of the difficulties in complete ascertainment. Prevalence studies of IDDM in children in the United States are presented in Table 2 (4). One sees a variation from 0.6 to 2.5 cases per 1000 population. Our own prevalent figure of 1.73:1000 is very similar to the Minnesota School survey result of 1.88. Whether the great variation in prevalence of IDDM in different parts of the United States is an accurate reflection or whether it represents variations in incomplete ascertainment is not now clear.

Incidence, the determination of the number of new cases identified per year, per 100,000 population, age matched, is a far more accurate statistic. Collaborative efforts by many investigators around the world have led to the development of highly accurate incidence data on childhood diabetes, documenting a remarkable variation based on geography, race, culture, and other currently unidentified factors. Figure 1 documents most recently compiled worldwide distribution incidence figures (5).

Figure 1 displays the remarkable variation in childhood diabetes in different countries. The highest incidence is found in Finland, with a current rate of approximately 35 new cases per 100,000 per year, and the lowest in Korea and Mexico City, at under 1 per 100,000 per year.

Figure 2 presents a plot of the incidence in various countries against their geographic location in terms of latitude north or south of the equator (6). There is a high statistically positive correlation with those countries located at greater distance from the equator and a higher attack rate for diabetes in childhood. This observation was further refined by making a similar analysis with mean annual temperature. These data are presented in Figure 3 (7). This analysis further confirms that there is a very high correlation between environmental temperature and the expression of diabetes in children, those countries having the lowest mean annual temperature having the highest frequency of diabetes.

Figure 4 presents the data from Allegheny County, Pennsylvania, plotting the frequency of diagnosis based on age at time of diagnosis (8). It is clear that diabetes in childhood is uncommon in the infant and toddler, increases in frequency until adolescence, and then drops sharply at the end of the growth phase. Furthermore, the peak incidence rate is earlier in girls than in boys by approximately 18 months, entirely consistent with the earlier onset of adolescence in girls and their more rapid movement into and through adolescence. This distribution curve is duplicated in essentially all countries in which it has been studied, despite marked variations in the incidence. For example, the frequency distribution at age of onset in children in Japan, Korea, the Philippines, Israel, and many European countries essentially duplicates the shape of the curve from the Pittsburgh experience, whereas absolute numbers are remarkably different.

Table 2 Prevalence Studies of IDDM

Study	Prevalence estimate (years)	Type of study	Age range	Overall prevalence rate/1:000
National health interview study	1976	Interview	0–16	1.60
National health interview study	1976	Interview	0–16	1.50
Allegheny County, PA	1976	Estimate from incidence data	5–17	1.73
Minnesota	1978	School survey	5–17	1.88
Rochester, MN	1976	Hospital/physician records	5–18	1.02
Michigan	1972	School survey	5–17	1.61
Pennsylvania	1975	School survey	5–17	1.71
Erie County, NY	1961	Hospital/physician records	0–16	0.6
Colorado	1981	School survey	<15	1.7
Kentucky	1979	School survey	5–17	2.10
Rhode Island	1980	Random sample	<15	2.50
Utah	1981	Random sample	<15	1.20
North Dakota	1983	Outpatient records	<18	1.30

Source: From Reference 4.

A similar observation is made for the seasonal variation in the diagnosis of diabetes. It has been known for many years that diabetes in children tends to be diagnosed more frequently in winter than in the summer months (9,10). The Pittsburgh experience has been documented in many other countries, again with great variation in the overall incidence (11). An associated observation, which currently lacks careful documentation, is that of the variation in frequency of diabetic ketoacidosis at diagnosis. Diabetic ketoacidosis, at diagnosis, appears to be quite uncommon in countries near the equator and in more moderate climates, whereas the frequency increases as one moves farther away from the equator. Diabetic ketoacidosis at presentation is reported to be rare in Israel, Italy, and France, but in the Scandinavian countries, it is quite comparable to that seen in Western Pennsylvania, where approximately 40% of newly diagnosed patients are first seen with diabetic ketoacidosis.

V. MIGRANT STUDIES

Although classic, prospective, migrant studies have not been carried out in IDDM, there are a number of important and valuable observations that strongly suggest that susceptibility to IDDM may be significantly altered by changes in geography and lifestyle. These conclusions result from the study of individuals of a particular geographic or nationality group living at a distance from their natural home within a population that has an IDDM incidence significantly different from that in the study population. Such observations have documented that ethnic Japanese living in Hawaii have an IDDM incidence approximately five times greater than Japanese

children living in Japan. Similarly, there is an approximate doubling of the incidence among ethnic French, Italian, and Israeli children in Montreal, compared with the incidence in France, Italy, and Israel (12–15). The incidence of IDDM in Indian children following migration from South Africa to England showed a dramatic increase from very low levels to that comparable to English children in the same community (16).

These studies and others strongly support the thesis that environmental factors may either increase or decrease the expression of diabetes in susceptible individuals. The migrant study observations have been appropriately criticized by the absence of experiences documenting reduced risk in certain populations. However, the natural migrant drift in the past several decades is from East to West, from Third World developed countries, from poverty to affluence, and from the tropics to the temperate zones. All these moves in general involve movement of individuals from countries at lesser risk for the development of diabetes to countries where the incidence rate is higher.

VI. SECULAR TRENDS IN IDDM INCIDENCE

If the incidence of IDDM were exclusively dependent upon the frequency of the diabetes susceptibility genes within the population, one would expect that annual incidence would be remarkably similar year after year, reflecting the absence or very slow change in the distribution of diabetes-related genes in the population over time. This, in fact, is not the case. There is now substantial evidence based on carefully constructed registry data extending in many countries over the

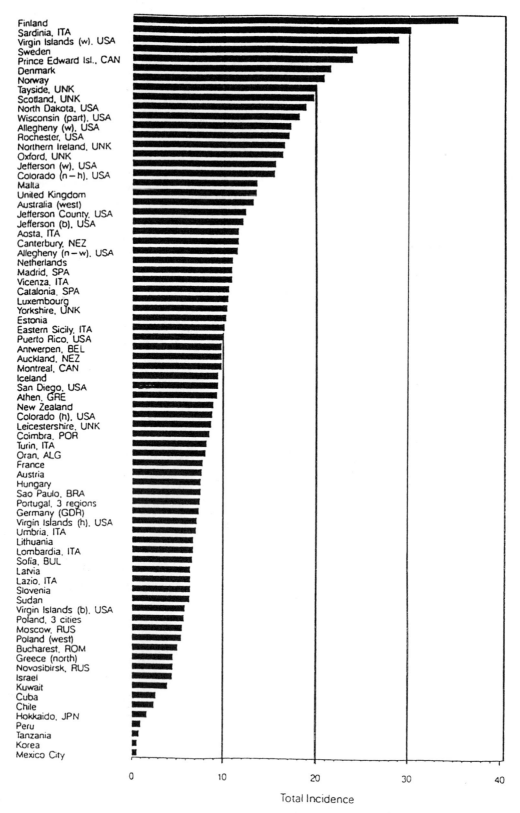

Figure 1 Age-specific incidence (per 100,000 population) of type I diabetes in age group under 15 years. Data for boys and girls have been pooled. The populations are arranged in ascending order according to the incidence. AUS, Australia; BEL, Belgium; BRA, Brazil; BUL, Bulgaria; GRE, Greece; ITA, Italy; JPN, Japan; NEZ, New Zealand; POL, Poland; POR, Portugal; SPA, Spain; UNK, United Kingdom; USA, United States of America; w, White; n-w, non-White; b, Black; h, Hispanic; n-h, non-Hispanic. (From Ref. 5.)

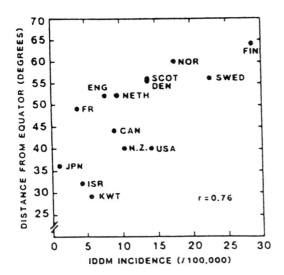

Figure 2 Relationship between IDDM incidence rates and distance from the equator. Countries are the same as in Figure 1. (From Ref. 6.)

last 20–40 years that there have been substantial increases in IDDM incidence in many locations, particularly in the Scandinavian countries. The incidence of diabetes among Finnish children has almost doubled during the past 20 years. Similar

observations have been made in Norway, Denmark, and Sweden. In our own experience in Allegheny County, Pennsylvania, we have observed an increase of approximately 1% per year in the incidence of IDDM until a more recent acute acceleration (see Table 3 and Ref. 5) (17–22).

Probably the most dramatic evidence of a secular increase is the experience on the Italian island of Sardinia. The incidence of IDDM currently in Sardinia approaches 30:100,000 per year, just below that in Finland and approximately 5 times greater than the incidence of diabetes in Italian children living on the mainland of Italy. This high incidence is "explained" by the finding of a very high frequency of homozygous nonaspartic acid genetic status in the population of Sardinia (23–25). However, a recent review of the earlier incidence of diabetes in Sardinia, not yet published or verified, suggests that the attack rate for this disease among Sardinian schoolchildren 20–30 years ago was in the neighborhood of 4–5:100,000 per year, the incidence rate now seen on the mainland of Italy. Obviously there has been no significant increase in the genetic susceptibility to diabetes in Sardinia over the past quarter-century. The increase in attack rate, if it is accurate, must reflect significant environmental changes that have occurred during this time period, almost certainly associated with industrialization, changes in lifestyle patterns, and changes in dietary habits.

VII. DIABETES EPIDEMICS

Secular changes in IDDM incidence over a period of several ayears strongly challenge the validity of a totally genetic-immunologic explanation for IDDM, but acute increases in incidence, referred to by some as diabetes epidemics, truly defy genetic explanation and must be viewed as a consequence of acute environmental changes. There are now several well-documented, abrupt increases in IDDM incidence followed by decreases back to baseline in several countries, including Poland, Latvia, and England (26–30).

Our own recent experience in Pittsburgh is particularly important in this regard. In both our Children's Hospital and Allegheny Country registry, we have continued surveillance both retrospectively and prospectively, covering approximately 40 years. We have documented a slight, just statistically significant incidence increase of about 1% per year from 1965 through 1985, and we recently observed a major increase in incidence during the interval 1985–1989. This increase in incidence is seen predominantly in males, in younger children, and in blacks (of mainly African ancestry). It is statistically correlated with chicken pox epidemics, with a lag phase between 2 and 3 years. We do not suggest that chicken pox is a primary etiologic factor in IDDM, but we believe strongly that our recent observations of a highly statistically significant increase in incidence among children in Western Pennsylvania is indicative of changing environmental stresses. Our documentation of increasing frequency of IDDM in younger children is consistent with the clinical experience of many pediatric diabetologists in various parts of the world

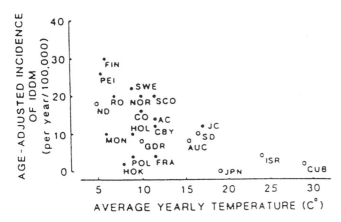

Figure 3 Correlation between age-adjusted IDDM incidence under age 15 years in various areas and average yearly temperature. FIN, Finland; PEI, Prince Edward Island, Canada; SWE, Sweden; RO, Rochester, MN; SCO, Tayside, Scotland; NOR, Norway; ND, North Dakota; CO, Colorado; AC, Allegheny County, PA; CBY, Canterbury, New Zealand; JC, Jefferson County, AL; HOL, the Netherlands; SD, San Diego, CA; Mon, Montreal; AUC, Auckland, New Zealand; GDR, German Democratic Republic; POL, Wielkopolska, Poland; FRA, Rhone, France; ISR, Israel; CUB, Cuba; HOK, Hokkaido, Japan; JPN. Japan, $r_s = -0.55$, $P < 0.005$ for untransformed data. (Open circles) Registries for which no ascertainment estimate was available. Ascertainment for Japan was 60%. (From Ref. 7.)

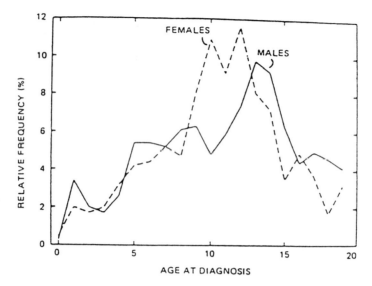

Figure 4 Overall incidence rates for IDDM in Allegheny County, Pennsylvania (white males and females). (From Ref. 4.)

and, again, suggests environmental stresses appearing at earlier ages (31).

The issue of a possible socioeconomic status (SES) relationship to IDDM remains unsettled. Our studies in Pittsburgh show no SES relationship, whereas studies in other parts of the world have shown an increased correlation with families at the affluent end of the socioeconomic scale; other studies have shown diabetes as more common in children from families of lower socioeconomic status, however (11,19, 32–34). It seems likely that these variations are not primarily socioeconomic; rather, they include other environmental or lifestyle factors (35).

In summary, epidemiologic studies carried out over the past two decades have provided important insights into the worldwide magnitude of the problem of childhood diabetes, with particular importance in terms of etiologic concepts. The findings that there are major differences in the expression of diabetes in different countries and that there are clear associations between the risk of diabetes and geographic location and national mean environmental temperature, as well as findings that migrants appear to take on the incidence experience of their adopted country and that there is evidence for "epidemics of diabetes," all point toward specific environmental factors as highly important in the expression of childhood diabetes. Our calculations suggest that approximately 75% of childhood diabetes is potentially preventable, assuming that the environmental factors can be identified and eliminated from the susceptible child's environment.

VIII. EVIDENCE FOR ENVIRONMENTAL FACTORS IN THE ETIOLOGY OF INSULIN-DEPENDENT DIABETES MELLITUS

Environmental factors may play one of several possible roles in β cell destructive processes. At one extreme, there are

undoubtedly cases of diabetes resulting directly from ingestion of β-cytotropic agents with no intervening genetic susceptibility or autoimmune mechanisms necessary, to the other extreme, in which β cell destruction results exclusively from genetically mediated autoimmune processes that are internally triggered without interphase with specific environmental stimulants. It seems likely, however, that most cases of IDDM fall in a middle ground in which environmental factors, rather than being directly causative, act to stimulate or provoke the immune system. Further, it is my belief that in the great majority of cases, IDDM does not result from a single environmental insult leading to a relentless autoimmune destructive process, but rather there are "multiple hits" from the environment, resulting in waxing and waning of the inflammatory process. What is the evidence (35–38)?

There are four general environmental categories that have been proposed as potential causative or provocative agents in IDDM expression. These include infectious agents, environmental toxins, nutrient factors, and physical and emotional stress. An additional interesting observation indicates that children who experience maternal-child blood group incompatibility are at a fourfold increased risk for IDDM (37). It is likely that genetically susceptible individuals actually develop diabetes after multiple environmental insults, possibly involving adverse experiences from each of the four general areas, and a discussion of the evidence available at present for causation is presented separately.

IX. ANIMAL STUDIES

In medicine, we have traditionally looked to animal models for insights and understanding of disease processes that cannot be fully elucidated in the human subject. Animal research has played a principal role in the study of diabetes for well over 100 years. Strangely, those stringent advocates of an exclu-

Table 3 Reported Increase in Type 1 Diabetes Incidence During 1960–1989

No temporal increase reported	Study period	Temporal increase reported	Study period
North America		North America	
United States		United States	
Allegheny County	1966–1986	Virgin Islands	1979–1988
California	1978–1981		
Colorado	1966–1986		
Jefferson	1966–1986		
North Dakota	1966–1986		
Rochester	1966–1986		
Canada			
Montreal	1966–1986		
Prince Edward Island	1975–1986		
Toronto	1976–1978		
Europe		Europe	
Estonia	1980–1988	Austria	1966–1986
Island	1970–1989	Finland	1965–1984
Latvia	1983–1988	France	1970–1989
Lithuania	1983–1988	Denmark	1949–1984
Luxembourg	1977–1986	Germany (GDR)	1960–1989
Malta	1980–1987	Hungary	1976–1985
Portugal, Coimbra	1987–1990	Norway	1973–1982
		Netherlands	1960–1970
Russia, Moscow	1970–1989	Poland	1970–1985
		Slovakia	1985–1991
Spain, Madrid	1985–1988	Sweden	1978–1987
		United Kingdom	
		Leicestershire	1966–1981
		Scotland	1966–1986
Asia		Asia	
Russia, Novosibirsk	1983–1989	Japan, Hokkaido	1966–1986
Oceania		Oceania	
Australia	1985–1989	New Zealand, white	1966–1986
New Zealand, nonwhite	1966–1986		

Source: From Reference 5.

sively internally mediated, autommune disease process accept the evidence of disease mechanisms from genetically susceptible models as important to the human condition yet reject the clear evidence of environmental manipulation in the expression of diabetes in animal models when it is moved to the human experience. The animal experience can be summarized as follows. (1) Toxic agents, for example alloxan and streptozotocin, can regularly induce β cell destruction and diabetes in both genetically susceptible and normal animals. Overt diabetes can be rapidly induced by a large dose of streptozotocin by direct toxic action of the drug or probably by autoimmune mechanisms utilizing small doses of the toxin repeatedly (this is reminiscent of the human situation with the drug Vacor, in which acute large-dose ingestion results in rapid β cell destruction but small-dose chronic ingestion appears to induce autoimmune β cell destruction) (39). (2) A variety of infectious agents can induce β cell destruction in diabetes-susceptible and nonsusceptible animal models. The identified agents include encephalomyocarditis virus, Mengo virus, and coxsackie virus B variants. The β cell destructive process may either be directly cytolytic or the induction of β cell damage leads to eventual autoimmune destruction (40). (3) Environmental manipulation alters the expression of diabetes in genetically susceptible animal strains. The BB rat and the NOD mouse strains are immunologically defective animals that are at markedly increased risk for the development of β cell destruction and overt diabetes, mimicking human IDDM in many respects. Environmental manipulation, particularly dietary alteration, can result in marked variation in the expression of disease in both animal models (41–43). This is particularly true in relationship to cow's milk protein and/or beef in the animal chow. Adding bovine serum albumin or whole milk or beef protein to the chow increases the incidence of diabetes; replacing the animal chow with synthetic proteins and amino acids reduces the expression of diabetes to near zero. This evidence strongly suggests that cow's milk protein or beef has a specific provocative effect on the immune system of these animals, resulting in progressive β cell destruction (Chap. 41). (4) A variety of immunosuppressive or modulatory strategies introduced well before β cell damage reduce the expression of diabetes in genetically susceptible animal models. These observations provide some optimism that immunologic intervention before diabetes may prevent diabetes in the human condition (44–47).

X. INFECTIOUS DISEASES

A number of viral infections have been associated with the development of IDDM, based on either epidemiologic surveys or individual case reports. The association between mumps infection and IDDM has a history of approximately 100 years duration, with episodic case reports appearing in the literature associating diabetes in individual cases to mumps occuring a few weeks previously. Coxsackie virus infections, particularly B3 and B4, have been associated with IDDM both in disease surveillance statistics and in a few isolated but highly important individual cases. Cytomegalovirus (CMV) has also been associated with carbohydrate intolerance and diabetes, and insulitis has been identified in the pancreas of infants dying with disseminated CMV infection. The best documented association between a specific viral infection and IDDM is that associated with the congenital rubella syndrome. Rubella infection, acquired by the fetus as a result of transplacental passage, results in a generalized rubella infection, which may have devastating effects on the fetus. In the great majority of cases, the infection "burns out" soon after delivery. However, it leaves behind an autoimmune destructive process that over a period of 5–20 years results in β cell destruction and overt diabetes. HLA studies indicate that diabetes eventually develops in those rubella syndrome children who have the genetic predisposition to disease. In fact, the eventual development of diabetes may approach 100% in those individuals who are HLA-DR3 and/or DR44. No DQ α or β studies have been reported on this group of patients, but this should be accomplished. The congenital rubella syndrome-diabetes association is strong evidence of a virus-induced autoimmune phenomenon leading to β cell destruction. The recent studies by Yoon et al. documenting an increased frequency of CMV viral fragments in the genome of children with IDDM suggests either that such patients acquired CMV infections very early in life, and that this initiated a β cell destructive process or that IDDM is associated with persistence of the infection (48–55).

XI. ENVIRONMENTAL TOXINS

It is well documented that a number of chemical agents have β cell destructive properties. Streptozotocin, the agent used to induce diabetes in laboratory animals, has been used to destroy the pancreas in humans with severe hypoglycemia

resulting from inoperable islet cell malignancy. The rodenticide Vacor is highly β cell toxic, resulting in an acute induction of diabetic ketoacidosis following large-dose oral ingestion (56,57). Inadvertent chronic small-dose ingestion, as apparently occurred in Korea when the rat poison was mixed with feed, is strongly reminiscent of the low-dose streptozotocin-induced autoimmune destruction in laboratory animal models. Nitrosamines, produced as a consequence of curing food by smoking techniques, has been implicated in cases of IDDM in Iceland (58–59). The possibility that the widely used grilling or barbecuing of beef may be a factor needs investigation. Further, almost nothing is known about the health hazards of a large number of industrial environmental contaminants as they enter our food and water supply. The recent finding that the apparently benign, inert silicone breast implants may be associated with autoimmune disease should raise increasing concern about the health hazards of "biologic advances" in our society.

XII. NUTRIENTS

There is increasing evidence that nutrients play either a protective or provocative role in the development of IDDM (Chap. 41). Of special interest is the accumulating evidence that early introduction of cow's milk protein may be an important factor in the later expression of diabetes in genetically susceptible infants (60–62).

The recent studies of Karjalainen et al. (63) focused attention on the possible relationship between the early ingestion of bovine serum albumin and the later development of diabetes in genetically susceptible individuals. They document that antibody to a specific fragment of bovine serum albumin, referred to as Abbos, is present in 100% of newly diagnosed diabetic Finnish children but essentially is never present in nondiabetic children or normal adults. The Abbos epitope is immunologically cross-reactive with a β cell autoantigen, P69, which may explain by virtue of molecular biologic mimicry why ingestion of this compound may induce β cell inflammatory responses (63). Recent attempts in another laboratory to confirm the Abbos finding have been unsuccessful (64).

It is well documented that the antioxidant potential of the islet tissue of the pancreas is inherently deficient compared with most of the other tissues and organs of the body. This means that the islet tissue is at increased risk of free radical damage. The balance between oxidant and antioxidant concentrations within the body fluids and tissues is delicate. Free radical excess or antioxidant deficiency results in disease. Nutritional intake is an important factor in this balance, with antioxidant ingestion becoming increasingly important as a preventive approach to human disease. It is possible that the lower content of naturally occurring antioxidants that characterizes the Western diet may be inadequate to neutralize free radical accumulation, thus increasing the likelihood of β cell damage and clinical diabetes mellitus. Conversely, the considerably lower incidence of diabetes in Asia may be at least partially related to the high dietary intake of antioxidant compounds (65–74).

XIII. STRESS

The relationship between acute emotional stress and the induction of thyrotoxicosis has been widely accepted among endocrinologists for many years. The anecdotal association between the two is convincing. Only recently has research begun to explore the complexities of the interrelationship between the endocrine and the immunologic systems. It is now quite clear that alterations in the hypothalamic-pituitary-adrenal axis, through the release of both adrenocorticotropic hormone and adrenal steroids, can result in major alterations in the effectiveness of the immunologic surveillance system. The anecdotal association between emotional trauma and the onset of IDDM is not as strong in diabetes as it is in thyrotoxicosis, but there are a number of studies suggesting such a cause-and-effect relationship (75–78).

XIV. ETIOLOGY OF INSULIN-DEPENDENT DIABETES MELLITUS

The advances in knowledge of the multifactorial nature of the etiology of insulin-dependent diabetes mellitus over the past two decades is one of the highlights of modern medicine. We now know that IDDM is not genetic in the usual mendelian sense. Rather, a number of genetic alterations, most but probably not all of which are located on chromosome 6 within the major histocompatibility complex, result in an increased likelihood of β cell damage (38,79–87).

The mechanism of β cell damage and destruction is autoimmune in nature. Substantial evidence suggests that antigens released from the β cell are seen as foreign protein by the macrophage or antigen presenting cell, which presents the altered antigen to a highly specialized HLA-linked receptor in a helper T cell. This process then initiates an active cellular and humoral response involving antibody production and lymphokine release. The final biochemical mediator of this toxic process is probably nitric oxide (88–93). (For a complete discussion of the autoimmune nature of IDDM, see Chap. 50.)

XV. THE FUTURE

The possibility of curing or preventing insulin-dependent diabetes mellitus rests solely on the continued accumulation of knowledge into causation. This includes a more complete understanding of the several genetic alterations that may be associated with either increasing risk for diabetes or protection against β cell inflammation. Much more must be learned about the normal immunologic system and the alterations that occur in individuals who later develop IDDM. There is increasing focus on the development of new immunosuppressive or immunomodulatory mechanisms that may alter the immune reaction and thus prevent β cell destruction. In addition, efforts must continually be directed toward further defining environmental risk factors and the development of epidemiologic methods for reducing these risks with a major collaborative effort involving basic and clinical scientists. One can

look forward to the future with optimism (94–96). (See Chap. 44 for a detailed discussion of preventive strategies.)

This chapter is partially derived and adapted from References 97 and 98.

REFERENCES

1. National Diabetes Data Group. Classification and diagnosis of diabetes mellitus and other categories of glucose intolerance. Diabetes 1979; 28:1039–1057.
2. Drash AL. The classification of diabetes mellitus in children and adolescents. Acta Paediatr Jpn 1987; 29:325–334.
3. Drash AL. Clinical Care of the Diabetic Child. Chicago: Yearbook Medical, 1987.
4. Cruickshanks KJ, LaPorte RE, Dorman JS, et al. The epidemiology of insulin-dependent diabetes mellitus: etiology and prognosis. In: Ahmad PI, Ahmad N, eds. Coping with Juvenile Diabetes. Springfield, IL: Charles C. Thomas, 1985:332–357.
5. Karvonen M, Tuomilehto J, Liebman I, LaPorte R. A review of the recent epidemiologic data on the world-wide incidence of type I (insulin-dependent) diabetes mellitus. Diabetologia 1993; 36:883–892.
6. LaPorte RE, Tajima N, Akerbloom HR, et al. Geographic differences in the risk of insulin dependent diabetes mellitus: the importance of registries. Diabetes Care 8(Suppl) 1985; 101–108.
7. Diabetes Epidemiology Research International Group. Geographic patterns of childhood insulin-dependent diabetes mellitus. Diabetes 1988; 37:1113–1119.
8. LaPorte RE, Fishbein HA, Kuller LH, et al. The Pittsburgh insulin-dependent (IDDM) registry: the incidence of insulin-dependent diabetes mellitus in Allegheny County, Pennsylvania (1965–1976) Diabetes 1981; 30:279–284.
9. Adams SF. Seasonal variation in the onset of acute diabetes: age and sex factors in 1000 diabetic patients. Arch Intern Med 1926; 37:361–864.
10. Fleegler FM, Rogers KD, Drash AL, et al. Age, sex and seasonal onset of juvenile diabetes in different geographic areas. Pediatrics 1979; 63:374–379.
11. Siemiatycki J, Colle E, Aubert D, Campbell S, Belmonti MM. The distribution of type I (insulin-dependent) diabetes mellitus by age, sex, secular trend, seasonality, time clusters and space time clusters: evidence from Montreal, 1971–1983. 1986; Am J Epidemiol 124:546–560.
12. Mimura G. Present status and future view of the genetics of diabetes in Japan. In: Mimura G, Baba S, Goto W, Kobberline J, eds. Clinical Genetics of Diabetes Mellitus, International Congress Series 597. Amsterdam: Excerpta Medica, 1982:13–18.
13. Kitagawa T, Fujita H, Hibi I, et al. A comparative study of the epidemiology of IDDM between Japan, Norway, Israel and the United States. Acta Paediatr Jpn 1984; 26:275–281.
14. Siemaitycki J, Colle E, Campbell S, Dewar R, Aubert D, Bellmonti MM. Incidence of IDDM in Montreal of ethnic group and by social class and comparisons with ethnic groups living elsewhere. Diabetes 1988; 37:1096–1112.
15. Laron Z, Karp M, Modan M. The incidence of insulin-dependent mellitus in Israeli children and adolescents 0–20 years of age: a retrospective study, 1971–1980. Diabetes Care 1985; 8(Suppl. 1):24–28.
16. Burden AC, Burden ML, Willimas ER, et al. Evidence of frequent epidemics of childhood diabetes. Diabetes 1991; 40:373A.
17. Diabetes Epidemiology Research International Group. Secular

trends in incidence of childhood IDDM in 20 countries. Diabetes 1990; 39:858.

18. Metcalfe M, Baum J. Incidence of insulin-dependent diabetes in children aged under 15 years in the British Isles during 1988. BMJ 1991; 302:443.

19. Joner G, Sovik O. Increasing incidence of diabetes mellitus in Norwegian children 0–14 years of age (1973–1982). Diabetologia 1989; 32:79.

20. Nystrom L, Dahlquist G, Rewers M, et al. The Swedish childhood diabetes study. An analysis of the temporal variation in diabetes incidence 1978–1987. Int J Epidemiol 1990; 19:141.

21. Tuomilehto J, Rewers M, Reunanen A, et al. Increasing trend in type I (insulin-dependent) diabetes mellitus in childhood in Finland. Analysis of age, calendar time and birth cohort effects during 1965–1984. Diabetologia 1991; 34:282.

22. Gren A, Gale EA, Patteson CC. Incidence of childhood-onset insulin-dependent diabetes mellitus, the EURODIAB ACE study. Lancet 1992; 339:905.

23. Dorman J, LaPorte R, Stone R, et al. Worldwide differences in the incidence of type I diabetes are associated with amino acid variation at position 57 of the HLA-DQ betachain. Proc Natl Acad Sci USA 1990; 87:7370.

24. Contu L, Carcassi C, Trucco M. Diabetes susceptibility in Sardinia. Lancet 1991; 338:65.

25. Muntoni S, Songini LM. High incidence rate of IDDM in Sardinia. Diabetes Care 1992; 15:1317.

26. Rewers M, LaPorte R, Walczakj M, et al. Apparent epidemic of insulin-dependent diabetes mellitus in mid-western Poland. Diabetes 1987; 36:1206.

27. Rewers M, Stone R, LaPorte R, et al. Poisson regression modeling in temporal variation in incidence of childhood insulin-dependent diabetes mellitus in Allegheny County Pennsylvania and Wielkopolska, Pland. Am J Epidmeiol 1989; 129:569.

28. Wagenknecht L, Rosemann J, Herman W. Increased incidence of insulin-dependent diabetes mellitus following an epidemic of coxsackievirus B5. Am J Epidemiol 1989; 129:569.

29. Pociot F, Norgaard K, Hobolth N, Andersen O, Nerup J. A nationwide population-based study of the familial aggregation of type I (insulin-dependent) diabetes mellitus in Denmark. Diabetologia, 1993; 36:9.

30. LaPorte RE, Tan M, Podar T, et al. Childhood diabetes, epidemics, and epidemiology—an approach for controlling diabetes. Am J Epidemiol 1992; 135:803–816.

31. Dokheel T, Pittsburgh Diabetes Epidemiology Research Group. An epidemic of childhood diabetes in the United States? Evidence from Allegheny County, Pennsylvania. Diabetes Care 1993; 16:1606–1611.

32. LaPorte RE, Orchard TJ, Kuller LH, et al. The Pittsburgh insulin-dependent diabetes mellitus registry. The relationship of insulin-dependent diabetes mellitus incidence to social class. Am J Epidemiol 1981; 114:379–384.

33. DeBono J, Johnson C, Betts P. Juvenile diabetes and social class. Lancet 1983; 1:1113–1114.

34. Tarn AC, Gorsuch AN, Spencer KM, Bottazzo GF, Lister J. Diabetes and social class. Lancet 1983; 2:631–632.

35. Orchard TJ, Dorman JS, LaPorte RE, Ferrell RE, Drash AL. Host and environmental interactions in diabetes mellitus. J Chron Dis 1986; 39:979–999.

36. Drash A. Reflection on the beta cell and its demise, diabetes in the young. Bull ISGD 1988; 19:233.

37. Dahlquist G. Etiological aspects of insulin dependent diabetes mellitus: an epidemiological prospective. Autoimmunity 1993; 15:61–65.

38. Trucco M. Immunogenetics of insulin-dependent diabetes

mellitus: the second-event hypothesis. Curr Top Diabetes Res 1993; 12:124–146.

39. Kolb H. Mouse models of insulin dependent diabetes: low doses, treptozotocin-induce diabetes in non-obese diabetic (NOB) mice. Diabetes Metab Rev 1987; 8:751.

40. Yoon J. Role of viruses in the pathogenesis of IDDM. Ann Med 1991; 23:437.

41. Elliott R, Martin J. Dietary protein: a trigger of insulin dependent diabetes in the BB rat? Diabetologia 1984; 26:297.

42. Daneman D, Fishman L, Clarson C, et al. Dietary triggers of insulin-dependent diabetes in the BB rat. Diabetes 1987; 5:93.

43. Coleman D, Kuzava J, Leiter E. Effect of diet on incidence of diabetes in non-obese diabetic mice. Diabetes 1990; 39:432.

44. Sumoski W, Baquerizo H, Rabinovitch A. Oxygen free radical scavengers protect rat islet cell from damage bycytokines. Diabetologia 1989; 32:792.

45. Drash AL, Rudert WA, Borquaye S, et al. Effect of probucol on development of diabetes mellitus in BB rats. Am J Cardiol 1988; 62(3):27.

46. Like AA, Anthony M, Buberski DL, et al. Spontaneous diabetes mellitus in the BB/W rat: effect of glcocorticoids, cyclosporin A and antiserum to rat lymphocytes. Diabetes 1983; 32:326.

47. Murase N, Lieberman I, Nalesnk M, et al. Prevention of spontaneous diabetes in the BB rat with FK-506. Lancet 1990; 336:373.

48. Harris HF. A case of diabetes mellitus following mumps. Boston Med Surg J 1987; 140:645–649.

49. Gamble DR, Taylor KW, Cumming H. Coxsackie viruses in diabetes mellitus. BMJ 1984; 4:260–262.

50. Yoon JW, Austin M, Ondera T, et al. Virus induced diabetes mellitus: isolation of a virus from the pancreas of a child with diabetic ketoacidosis. N Engl J Med 1979; 300:1173–1179.

51. Forrest JM, Menser MA, Burgess JA. High frequency of diabetes mellitus of young adults with congenital rubella. Lancet 1971; 2:332–334.

52. Drash AL. Evidence for viral infections in the etiology of insulin-dependent diabetes mellitus. In: Czernichow P, Dorchy H, eds. Diabetologie Pediatrique. Paris, 1990.

53. Roberts SS. New clues to IDDM origins: IDDM may arise from a case of mistaken identity in which the immune system mistakes a normal beta cell antigen for a virus. Diabetes Care 1992; 15:137–139.

54. Fohlman J, Friman G. Is juvenile diabetes a viral disease? Ann Med 1993; 25:569–574.

55. Hyoty H, Hiltunen M, Reunanen A, et al. Decline of mumps antibodies in type I (insulin-dependent) diabetic children and a plateau in the rising incidence of type I diabetes after introduction of the mumps-measles-rubella vaccine in Finland. Diabetologia 1993; 36:1303–1308.

56. Karam J, Prosser P, Lewitt P. Islet cell surface antibodies in a patient with diabetes mellitus after rodenticide ingestion. N Engl J Med 1979; 299:11.

57. Karam J, Lewitt P, Young C, et al. Insulinopenic diabetes after rodenticide (Vacor) ingestion: a unique model of acquired diabetes in man. Diabetes 1980; 29:971–978.

58. Helgason T, Jonnasson MR. Evidence for a food additive as a cause of ketosis-prone diabetes. Lancet 1981; 2:716.

59. Helgason T, Ewen SWB, Ross IS, Stowers JM. Diabetes produced in mice by smoked/cured mutton. Lancet 1982; 2:1017–1022.

60. Gerstein HC. Does cow's milk cause type I diabetes mellitus? A critical overview of the clinical literature. Diabetes Care 1994; 17:13–19.

61. Kostraba JN. What can epidemiology tell us about the role of

infant diet in the etiology of diabetes? Diabetes Care 1994; 17:87–91.

62. Drash AL, Kramer MS, Swanson J, Udall J. Infant feeding practices and their possible relationship to the etiology of diabetes mellitus. Pediatrics (in press).

63. Karjalainen J, Marin J, Knip M, et al. Evidence for a bovine albumin peptide as candidate trigger of type I diabetes. N Engl J Med 1992; 327:302.

64. Atkinson MA, Bowman MA, Kao KJ, et al. Lack of immune responsiveness to bovine serum albumin in insulin dependent diabetes. N Engl J Med 1993; 329:1853–1858.

65. Gey FK, Puska P, Paul J, et al. Inverse correlation between plasma vitamin E and mortality from ischemic heart disease in cross-cultural epidemiology. Am J Clin Nutr 1991; 53: 326S.

66. Gey F, Ulrich M, Jordan P, et al. Increased risk of cardiovascular disease at suboptimal plasma levels of essential antioxidas: an epidemiological up-date with special attention to carotene and vitamin C. Am J Clin Nutr in press.

67. Steinberg D, Parthasarathy S, Carew T, et al. Beyond cholesterol: modification so flow-density lipoprotein that increases its atherogenicity. N Engl J Med 1989; 320:915.

68. Riemersma R, Wood D, Macintyre CCA, et al. Risk of angina pectoris and plasma concentrations of vitamins A, C and E and carotene. Lancet 1991; 337:1.

69. Grei B. Ascorbic acid protects lipids in human plasma and low-density lipoprotein against oxidative damage. Am J Clin Med 1992; 54:113S.

70. Keizo S, Nikim E, Shimasaki H. Free radical-mediated chain oxidation of low-density lipoprotein and synergistic inhibition by vitamin E and vitamin C. Arch Biochem Biophys 1990; 279:402.

71. Halliwell B, Gutteridge J, Cross CE. Free radicals, antioxidants, and human disease: where are we now? J Lab Clin Med 1992; 119:598.

72. Olson JA, Kobayashe S. Antioxidants in health and disease: overview. Proc Soc Exp Biol Med 1992; 200:245.

73. Asayama K, Uchida N, Makane T, et al. Antioxidants in the serum of children with insulin dependent diabetes mellitus. Free Radic Biol Med 1993; 15:597–602.

74. Wolff SP. Diabetes-mellitus and free radicals. Br Med Bull 1993; 49:642–652.

75. Bateman A, Singh A, Kral T, Solomon S. The immune-hypothalamic-pituitary-adrenal axis. Endocr Rev 1989; 10:92–112.

76. Gupta D. Pathophysiology of immune-neuroendocrine network. Network Lett 1992; 14:1–19.

77. Lager J, Attvall S, Eriksson BM, von Schenk H, Smith K. Studies on the insulin antagonistic effect of catecholamines in normal man. Diabetologia 1986; 29:409–416.

78. Surwit RS, Schneider MS. Role of stress in the etiology and treatment of diabetes-mellitus. Psychosom Med 1993; 55:380–393.

79. Todd JA, Bell JI, McDevitt HO. HLA-DQ beta gene contributes to susceptibility and resistance to insulin-dependent diabetes mellitus. Nature 1987; 329:599.

80. Morel PA, Dorman JS, Todd JA, et al. Aspartic acid at position 57 of the DQ beta chain protects against type I diabetes: a family study. Proc Natl Acad Sci USA 1988; 85:9111.

81. Trucco M. To be or not to be ASP 57, that is the question. Diabetes Care 1992; 15:712.

82. Segurado OG, Arnaizvillena A, Wank R, Schendel DJ. The multi-factorial nature of MHC-linked susceptibility to insulin-dependent diabetes. Autoimmunity 1993; 15:85–89.

83. Kumar D, Gemayel NS, Deapen D, et al. North American twins with IDDM–genetic, etiological and clinical significance of disease concordance according to age, zygosity and the interval before diagnosis in first twin. Diabetes 1993; 42:1351–1363.

84. Serjentson JW, Court J, MacKay IR, et al. HLA-DQ genotypes are associated with autoimmunity to glutamic acid decarboxylase in insulin-dependent diabetes mellitus patients. Hum Immunol 1993; 38:97–104.

85. Penny MA, Micovic CH, Cavan DA, et al. An investigation of the association between HLA-DQ heterodimers and type I (insulin-dependent) diabetes mellitus in five racial groups. Hum Immunol 1993; 38:179–183.

86. Cruickshanks KJ, Jobim LF, Lawlerhevner J, et al. Ethnic differences in human leukocytes antigen markers of susceptibility to IDDM. Diabetes Care 1994; 17:132–137.

87. Vanendert PM, Liblau RS, Patel SD, et al. Major histocompatability complex-encoded antigen processing gene polymorphism in IDDM. Diabetes 1994; 43:110–117.

88. Gepts W. Pathologic anatomy of the pancreas in juvenile diabetes mellitus. Diabetes 1965; 14:619.

89. Drell DW, Notkins AL. Multiple immunologic abnormalities in patients with type I (insulin dependant) diabetes mellitus. Diabetologia 1987; 30:132.

90. Bottazzo GF. Death of a beta cell: homicide or suicide? Diabetic Med 1986; 3:119–130.

91. Eisenbarth GS. Type I diabetes mellitus. A autoimmune disease. N Engl J Med 1986; 314:1360–1368.

92. Kolb H, Kolb-Bachofen V. Nitric oxide: a pathogenic factor in autoimmunity. Immunol Today 1992; 13:157–160.

93. Laron Z, Karp M, eds. Genetic and Environmental Risk Factors for Type I Diabetes (IDDM) Including a Discussion on the Autoimmune Basis. London: Freund Publishing House, 1992.

94. Skyler JS, Marks JB. Immune intervention in type I diabetes mellitus. Diabetes Rev 1993; 1:15–42.

95. LaPorte RE, Baba S. Magic bullets, reportable disease, and the prevention of childhood diabetes. Diabetes Care 1992; 15:128–131.

96. Alberti KG. Preventing insulin dependent diabetes mellitus. BMJ 1993; 307:1435–1436.

97. Drash AL. Does beta cell death result exclusively from genetically-mediated autoimmune mechanisms? A polemic—the case for environmental factors in the etiology of insulin dependent diabetes mellitus. In: Dorman J, ed. Standardization of Epidemiologic Studies of Host Susceptibility, NATO ASI Series. New York: Plenum, (in press).

98. Drash AL. The contributions of epidemiology to the understanding of the etiology of insulin dependent diabetes. In: Cowett R, ed. Diabetes—Biochemical, Physiological, Clinical, and Epidemiological Aspects, 35th Nestle Nutrition Workshop (in press).

39

The Infant of a Diabetic Mother and Diabetes in the First Year of Life

Alicia A. Romano
New York Medical College, Valhalla, New York

I. INTRODUCTION

Developmental abnormalities of the fetal pancreas may result in anatomic or functional anomalies. Many of the anatomic malformations, for example the annular pancreas, are incidental findings and are not clinically relevant. The functional anomalies can affect the endocrine and/or exocrine pancreas and usually manifest themselves clinically. Under the influence of maternal hyperglycemia and abnormal metabolic fuels, there is an accelerated maturation of the pancreatic β cells, which in turn is responsible for many of the clinical sequelae encountered in these infants as newborns, later in childhood, and through adult life. In contrast to the infant of a diabetic mother, the infant with transient diabetes of the newborn has a delay in the maturation of the pancreatic β cells and the clinical manifestations are quite different. Like infants with transient diabetes of the newborn, infants with pancreatic dysgenesis have hyperglycemia but the exocrine pancreas is affected as well.

This chapter reviews the altered metabolism in the diabetic pregnancy, the consequences of this altered metabolism in the antenatal, perinatal, and neonatal periods, and the long-term effects on the infant of the diabetic mother. Hyperglycemia in the first year of life is presented, focusing on transient diabetes of the newborn (TDNB) and pancreatic dysgenesis. The clinical presentation, pathophysiology, diagnostic evaluation, and treatment of these entities are discussed.

II. THE INFANT OF A DIABETIC MOTHER

Although the outcome of pregnancy for women with diabetes mellitus has improved in recent years, the infant of a diabetic mother has an increased risk of major clinical problems. Consideration of diabetes in pregnancy and the consequent metabolic changes help to explain the pathogenesis of the abnormalities encountered in these infants. Appropriate medical and obstetric intervention utilizing a team approach to achieve maternal metabolic normalization can minimize many of the problems, as descriptively depicted by Farquhar in 1959 (1):

> . . . they (infants of diabetic mothers) emerge at least alive from within the fiery metabolic furnace of diabetes mellitus, but because they resemble one another so closely that they might well be related. They are plump, sleek, liberally coated with vernix caseosa, full-faced and plethoric. During their first 24 or more extra-uterine hours they lie on their backs, bloated and flushed, their legs flexed and abducted, their lightly closed hands on each side of the head, the abdomen prominent and their respiration sighing. They convey a distinct impression of having had such a surfeit of both food and fluid pressed upon them by an insistent hostess that they desire only peace so that they may recover from their excesses. And on the second day their resentment of the slightest noise improves the analogy while their trembling anxiety seems to speak of intrauterine indiscretions of which we know nothing.

A. Diabetes in Pregnancy

The actual prevalence of gestational diabetes is difficult to assess because of a variety of factors that influence the disease prevalence. These factors include racial or ethnic differences, maternal age and obesity, and different diagnostic criteria for gestational diabetes (2). It has been estimated that diabetes before pregnancy complicates 0.2–0.3% of all gestations (3) and that gestational diabetes accounts for an additional 2–3% of pregnant women (4–8). Optimal metabolic control throughout and even preceding pregnancy can reduce the fetal morbidity and mortality by severalfold (9–14).

Older retrospective studies have demonstrated that abortions, stillbirths, neonatal deaths, and abnormal survivors were significantly higher in the pregnancies of overt diabetics compared with control subjects (15). For diabetic women receiving optimal care, excluding deaths as a result of congenital malformations, the perinatal mortality rate is now as low as that observed in normal gestations. Furthermore, cost-benefit analysis of preconception care for women with established diabetes has revealed that intensive medical care before conception results in cost savings (16).

The White et al. classification (17), subsequently modified by Cornblath and Schwartz (18), is a system that categorizes the severity of maternal vascular compromise. Class A includes women with gestational diabetes and prediabetes. *Gestational diabetes* is defined as abnormal glucose tolerance during pregnancy that reverts to a normal tolerance postpartum; the *prediabetes class* includes pregnant women with normal glucose tolerance but a predisposition to the disease, including a strong family history of diabetes, a previous history of large infants (>4000 g), or unexplained stillbirth beyond 28 weeks gestation. Classes B–F include women with overt diabetes with increasing vascular compromise in the latter classes. Other more complex classification systems have been developed and may be more useful in particular circumstances: Freinkel et al.'s classification of carbohydrate intolerance during pregnancy (19) allows comparisons between the current pregnancy outcome with prior pregnancies; the Pedersen and Molsted-Pedersen "prognostically bad signs" (20), along with the degree of metabolic control and vascular compromise, are more predictive of perinatal outcome. In general, infants of mothers with gestational diabetes experience fewer perinatal problems than those of overtly diabetic mothers, and infants of mothers with vascular compromise have fetal complications different from those in infants without vascular compromise.

B. Metabolism During Pregnancy

Pregnancy, even in the normal woman, is associated with significant alterations in carbohydrate homeostasis. In the first trimester, estrogens and progesterone enhance the action of insulin (21) and result in a depression in blood glucose levels. During the second and third trimesters, glucose tolerance is reduced despite increased insulin levels. This insulin resistance is in part mediated by human placental lactogen, a hormone similar to growth hormone, that is produced by the syncytiotrophoblast of the placenta. Its concentration increases in proportion to the placental mass and is not regulated by serum glucose. The resultant increase in maternal glucose and other nutrients is presumably an adaptive mechanism to increase the availability of glucose and amino acids to the fetus during this time of rapid growth.

During normal pregnancy, these metabolic changes result in maternal β cell hypertrophy with increased insulin secretion; gestational diabetes occurs in those women with borderline β cell function. Accordingly, women with overt diabetes

require substantial increases in insulin dosage during the latter part of pregnancy.

Because insulin does not cross the placenta, the fetal metabolism of maternal substrates is entirely dependent on fetal insulin production. This classic maternal hyperglycemia-fetal hyperinsulinism theory of Pedersen (22) has been widely accepted, although we now know that the metabolic-endocrine disturbances in the diabetic pregnancy are more complex. Freinkel and Metzger modified the Pedersen hypothesis and describe pregnancy as "a tissue culture experience" (10,23) in viewing the disordered fuel metabolism in the diabetic pregnancy. In the normal pregnancy, the "physiologic" increase in maternal postprandial nutrients, especially amino acids, serves as a stimulus for the secretion of fetal insulin. In this way, fetal glucose and nutrient levels remain in the normal range. In the poorly controlled diabetic pregnancy, the maternal hyperglycemia and hyperaminoacidemia stimulate the fetal pancreas, resulting in β cell hyperplasia and fetal hyperinsulinemia. This β cell overactivity is present even when only minimal hyperglycemia has been documented (24–26) and is evidenced by a "maturation" of the fetal β cell in the infant of a diabetic mother.

In vitro studies support this precocious maturation of the fetal β cell induced by hyperaminoacidemia islet "priming" in early gestation followed by glucose enhancement in later gestation. The human fetal islet cell secretes insulin in response to selective amino acids from week 14 of gestation onward; the glucose-mediated insulin release occurs after about week 28 of gestation (27). Increased stimulated insulin secretion and maturation of the response have been demonstrated in fetal pancreases from insulin-dependent diabetic women in poor control compared with those from nondiabetic women (28). Furthermore, in the normal neonate, there is an attenuated glucose-mediated insulin release; however, in the infant of a diabetic mother, the glucose-mediated insulin release as well as nutrient-stimulated release (24,26,29) is enhanced.

C. Consequences of Altered Metabolism

Table 1 lists the abnormalities encountered in infants of diabetic mothers and divides them into problems during the antenatal, perinatal, and neonatal periods, as well as those during childhood and adolescence. Many, but certainly not all, of these abnormalities are consequences of fetal hyperglycemia and hyperinsulinemia. Other factors, such as hypoglycemia (30), hyperosmolality (31,32), hyperketonemia (33–36), disturbed myoinositol and arachidonic acid metabolism (37–39), free oxygen radicals (40,41), disturbed extracellular matrix formation (42), and somatomedin inhibitors (43–45), either singly or synergistically (34,35,46) have been shown to affect organogenesis. The abnormal metabolic intrauterine environment has also been implicated in long-term effects on the offspring of diabetic mothers. The phrase "fuel-mediated teratogenesis" (35) was coined by Freinkel et al. to convey the importance and permanence of the effects of the altered maternal metabolic milieu.

Table 1 Problems Encountered in Infants of Diabetic Mothers

Antenatal abnormalities	Perinatal abnormalities	Neonatal abnormalities	Childhood and adolescent abnormalities
Fetal death	Traumatic delivery	Metabolic disturbances	Obesity
In utero thrombosis		Hypoglycemia	Diabetes
Congenital malformations		Hypocalcemia	**Impaired intellect**
Macrosomia		Hypomagnesemia	Detectable autoantibodies
		Respiratory distress syndrome	
		Hematologic disturbances	
		Polycythemia	
		Hyperviscosity	
		Thrombosis	
		Hyperbilirubinemia	
		Cardiovascular disturbances	
		Hypertrophic cardiomyopathy	
		Persistent fetal circulation	
		Congenital heart disease	

1. Antenatal Abnormalities

a. Fetal Wastage. There is an increased incidence of fetal wastage in diabetic women (15,47). This may be attributable to maternal vascular disease, poor metabolic control, and/or fetal hyperinsulinemia, which can decrease fetal arterial O_2 content (48).

b. Congenital Malformations. Despite the decline in perinatal mortality in pregnancies complicated by diabetes mellitus, congenital malformations remain a significant problem. Earlier studies reveal a two- to fourfold increase in the rate of congenital malformations in diabetic pregnancy (49), accounting for 30–50% of the neonatal mortality in infants of diabetic mothers (50). The pathogenesis of this increase in congenital anomolies is not fully understood. Genetic factors are not operative because there is no increase in the incidence of birth defects in the offspring of diabetic fathers (51). Studies in primates also support a lack of paternal influence (52). It is generally accepted that the malformations are indeed related to the diabetic intrauterine environment during the period of organogenesis. Thus, they represent an early manifestation of fuel-mediated teratogenesis (35). Because the common anomalies in offspring of diabetic women occur before week 7 of gestation, most malformations take place before the pregnancy is recognized and the intensified diabetic treatment regimen is initiated. This explains the apparent paradox between the improved perinatal mortality and the increased incidence of anomalies despite improved antenatal care of diabetic pregnant women. Meticulous metabolic control maintained periconceptually and throughout the pregnancy, especially during the critical period of organogenesis, can reduce the rate of malformations toward rates found in the nondiabetic pregnancy (10–14). Thus, for women with pregestational diabetes, it seems prudent to offer contraceptive advice so that every pregnancy can be planned with optimum metabolic control before conception. Unfortunately, poor metabolic control in the pregestational diabetic woman before the pregnancy is recognized, or in the gestational diabetic woman before the diabetes is recognized, may have significant ramifications. For these women, even early sonographic evaluation for fetal growth delay has not been useful in predicting which infants are affected by congenital malformations (53).

A wide variety of malformations is commonly encountered in offspring of diabetic mothers. These anomolies include major malformations of the heart and brain, the caudal regression syndrome, and other multisystem associations.

Congenital heart disease, including transposition of the great vessels, coarctation of the aorta, and atrial and ventricular septal defects, is five times (54) more common in infants of diabetic mothers. Generalized myocardial hypertrophy, however, is the most common cardiac abnormality encountered in these infants. The interventricular septum seems to be most affected by the increased growth in tissue, and the morbidity is increased with increasing septal thickness (54). Diminished cardiac output, left ventricular outflow obstruction, and sudden death may occur. DiGeorge anomaly with either unilateral or bilateral renal agenesis has been described in four infants of diabetic mothers (55–57). Because of the association with renal agenesis, renal ultrasonography should be considered in offspring of diabetic pregnancies with third and fourth pharyngeal pouch cardiac defects. Evaluation of immune and parathyroid function should be considered as well. It is not clear whether all infants of diabetic mothers might benefit from routine echocardiography in the neonatal period. Certainly, many of the cardiac problems in these infants present themselves symptomatically. However, studies that describe altered diastolic function (58) indicative of poor ventricular compliance or relaxation in asymptomatic infants without ventricular or septal hypertrophy reveal subtle myocardial dysfunction that could lead to higher morbidity if these infants are exposed to stress.

Brain anomolies overrepresented in offspring of diabetic mothers include anencephaly, meningomyelocele, and holoprosencephaly (59). Septooptic dysplasia (60) and unusual brain dysplasia have also been reported (61). The caudal regression syndrome is a rare malformation strongly associated with diabetes in pregnancy. It includes a spectrum of defects involving the lower extremities and spine that range from minor abnormalities to agenesis of the sacrum and legs (62). Other reported malformations encountered in the infant of the diabetic mother include hypoglossia and hypodactylia syndrome with jejunal atresia (63); polysplenia complex with mesocardia and renal agenesis (64); biliary atresia and splenic malformation syndrome (65); and short left colon (66). Anomolies associated with in utero thrombosis and gangrene have also been reported (67).

c. Macrosomia. Macrosomia is one of the most common abnormalities in the diabetic pregnancy. Earlier studies revealed that infants of poorly controlled diabetic mothers are on average 550 g heavier and 1.5 cm longer at birth than infants born to nondiabetic mothers at 36–38 weeks gestation (68). The excess weight in the majority of infants of diabetic mothers is a result of increased subcutaneous fat and visceral enlargement, especially of the liver and heart (69–71). Despite improved metabolic control, the incidence of macrosomia remains high. Even in studies in which "tight" metabolic control was acheived in women with gestational diabetes, the incidence of macrosomia was 17.9% (72). There is increasing evidence that macrosomia is related to 1 h postprandial glucose levels in the third trimester (72,73). The current recommended target for 1 h postprandial glucose seems to be 7.3 mM (130 mg/dl) (72). Because there is an association between low maternal glucose levels and small for gestational age infants (72,74,75), long-term follow-up data are needed to optimize the target glucose level that minimizes both the risk of macrosomia and intrauterine growth retardation.

Another factor that may influence the development of macrosomia is the formation of maternal insulin antibodies. Maternal immunoglobulin G antibodies can transport insulin across the placenta into the fetal blood (76). Results of studies trying to define this relationship between maternal insulin antibodies and macrosomia have been conflicting (77,78). In a prospective controlled trial of human versus animal insulin during pregnancy, maternal or infant insulin antibody levels were not related to type of insulin used (79). However, women with type I diabetes who were randomized to human insulin before 20 weeks gestation had fewer large for gestational age infants, fewer blood glucose excursions beyond the therapeutic range, and lower infant C peptide responses to glucose and amino acid challenge at 3 months of age (79). The route of insulin administration has also been considered in the production of insulin antibodies. In another prospective controlled trial, the production of insulin antibodies was compared in women with gestational diabetes who used a jet injector versus a needle in the aministration of human insulin. The jet-injected insulin was associated with decreased antibody formation and postprandial glucose variability compared with needle-injected insulin (80).

2. Perinatal Abnormalities: Macrosomia

Fetal macrosomia is a complication that affects both the mother and the fetus. The mother of the macrosomic infant is at increased risk for labor abnormalities, cesarean section, and severe perineal lacerations (81). Macrosomia can lead to traumatic delivery because of shoulder dystocia, with resultant birth injury and/or asphyxia (82,83). Potential birth injuries include cephalohematoma, subdural hemorrhage, clavicular fracture, brachial plexus injuries, and liver and spleen lacerations. In an effort to predict risk of birth trauma in infants of diabetic pregnancies, sonographic measurement of fetal humeral soft tissue thickness was recently described (84). Because the larger shoulder circumference in these infants may produce difficulty in delivery, this measurement may be useful in distinguishing these large infants with trunchal obesity from those that are symmetrically large. Childbirth classes should place equal emphasis on both vaginal delivery and caesarean section, because caesarean delivery may be required. Close intrapartum monitoring may further minimize potential complications.

3. Neonatal Abnormalities

After birth, the infant of the diabetic pregnancy is at risk for the development of numerous clinical problems. These include the metabolic disturbances of hypoglycemia, hypocalcemia, and hypomagnesemia, respiratory distress syndrome, hematologic abnormalities of polycythemia with subsequent hyperbilirubinemia, hyperviscosity and renal vein thrombosis, and cardiovascular problems of persistent fetal circulation (PFC) or resulting from hypertrophic cardiomyopathy.

a. Hypoglycemia. The hypoglycemia that develops in the infant of a diabetic mother is multifactorial in etiology. Shortly after birth, there is rapid utilization of serum glucose by hyperinsulinemia. Because of the hyperinsulinemia, there is an inability to mobilize glucose and alternative fuels despite ample supplies of glycogen and increased amounts of adipose tissue triglycerides. Suppression of glucagon secretion (85–87) and an inability to down-regulate the number of insulin receptors on target tissues in response to the prevailing hyperinsulinism (88) may also contribute to the hypoglycemia. These factors all contribute to the significance of hyperinsulinemic hypoglycemia: there are no available alternative substrates for cerebral energy. Thus, because the hypoglycemia may be asymptomatic, blood glucose determinations should be serially followed for the first 72 h of life in all infants of diabetic mothers as well as in large for gestational age infants whose mothers lack a history of diabetes. The diagnosis of hypoglycemia should not be based on blood glucose values obtained with reagent strips in the nursery. Confounding factors, such as polycythemia and insufficient quantities of blood, can result in false negatives and positives with use of this methodology.

Symptoms and treatment of hypoglycemia in the newborn are discussed in detail in Chapter 48. In general, symptoms of hypoglycemia in the newborn include jitteriness, poor feeding, pallor, apnea, bradycardia, cyanosis, and seizures. Asymptomatic infants with documented low blood glucose values should have early feedings only. Symptomatic infants require glucagon (30 μg per kg intravenously or intramuscularly) or an intravenous bolus of dextrose (2ml per kg of 10% dextrose), followed by continuous dextrose infusion (4–8 mg per kg per minute). The infusion rate may need to be increased (8–15 mg per kg per minute of dextrose) to maintain euglycemia. Infants should be gradually weaned from intravenous dextrose to avoid rebound hypoglycemia. Other causes of hypoglycemia should be considered if higher infusion rates are required or if hypoglycemia persists for more than 72 h despite *gradual* weaning of intravenous dextrose.

b. Hypocalcemia and Hypomagnesemia. "Early" neonatal hypocalcemia (serum total calcium <1.75 mM, 7 mg/dl) occurs in approximately 50% of infants of diabetic mothers (89,90). It occurs in the first 3 days of life and is also associated with a variety of other conditions encountered in infants of diabetic pregnancies. These conditions include prematurity, birth asphyxia, birth trauma, respiratory distress, and administration of maternal magnesium sulfate. The hypocalcemia seems to be an exaggeration of the fall in serum calcium levels observed in normal infants between 24 and 48 h of life. The frequency and severity of the hypocalcemia are related to the degree of maternal diabetes control, and they are potentiated by fetal asphyxia (89). Hypocalcemia is usually associated with hyperphosphatemia and hypomagnesemia. "Functional hypoparathyroidism" (91,82) has been suggested as the etiology. Parathyroid hormone levels are usually lower and slower to rise in hypocalcemic than normocalcemic infants (93). Interestingly, bone mineral content as measured by direct photon absorptiometry is significantly decreased in infants of diabetic mothers (94). Symptoms and treatment of neonatal hypocalcemia are discussed in Chapter 48. Because hypocalcemic infants may be asymptomatic or manifest only subtle symptoms, serial serum calcium measurements should be performed in the first 72 h of life in all infants born to diabetic mothers.

c. Respiratory Distress Syndrome. Based on the retrospective analysis by Robert et al. in 1975, there is a five- to sixfold increase in the incidence of respiratory distress syndrome (RDS) in infants born of diabetic pregnancies compared with infants of nondiabetic mothers (95). This has been at least partially attributed to a higher incidence of premature delivery, cesarean section, and asphyxia at delivery. Whether hyperglycemia and/or hyperinsulinemia may also play a role in this increased incidence by delaying lung maturation is somewhat controversial. In fetal lambs, the amount of surface-active material in tracheal fluid is reduced by glucose infusion. (96). Several earlier studies also supported a delayed biochemical maturation of the fetal lung in diabetic gestation (97,98). Other studies have suggested an abnormal structure and composition of surfactant phospholipids based on normal lecithin-sphingomyelin ratios in the amniotic fluid of infants with typical RDS (99). Additionally, decreased amounts of amniotic fluid surfactant-associated protein (SAP-35), have been found in pregnant women with diabetes (99,100). Earlier studies, however, failed to demonstrate differences in fetal lung maturation (101,102), delays in maturation of the L/S ratio, or the appearance of phosphatidylglycerol (102–104), marking the final step in lung maturation. Furthermore, in a recent clinical study of 526 infants of diabetic mothers, only 5 cases of 18 with respiratory distress were caused by surfactant-deficient RDS, and these infants were all <34 weeks gestation (105). The remaining 13 cases were a result of transient tachypnea of the newborn ($n = 5$), hypertrophic cardiomyopathy ($n = 4$), polycythemia ($n = 2$), and meconium aspiration ($n = 1$). All infants of diabetic mothers must therefore be monitored carefully for signs of respiratory distress, and etiologies other than surfactant deficiency should be considered.

d. Hematologic Abnormalities. The hematologic abnormalities encountered in offspring of diabetic women include polycythemia, hyperviscosity, and hyperbilirubinemia. The polycythemia observed in the normal newborn is more pronounced in infants of diabetic pregnancies. The increased erythropoeisis in these infants is attributable to elevated erythropoietin levels (106). Plasma erythropoietin concentrations correlate directly with plasma insulin levels in both infants of diabetic mothers and controls (106). Insulin may have a direct effect on erythropoeisis as evidenced by insulin stimulation of growth in culture of late erythroid progenitors in cord blood (107), or it may indirectly increase erythropoietin through tissue hypoxia. Polycythemia may result in significant hyperviscosity, which can affect the central nervous system, lung, and renal circulations. Persistence of the fetal circulation and renal vein thrombosis (108) are sequelae of hyperviscosity prevalent in offspring of diabetic pregnancies.

The prolonged indirect hyperbilirubinemia that occurs in infants of diabetic mothers is multifactorial in etiology. There is a functional immaturity of hepatic enzymes as well as an increased catabolism of hemoglobin (109) in these infants. Polycythemia and resorption of blood from cephalohematoma or ecchymoses may augment the hyperbilirubinemia by increasing the bilirubin load.

e. Cardiovascular Abnormalities. The cardiovascular problems encountered in the infant of a diabetic mother in the neonatal period are related to any congenital heart defects or hypertrophic cardiomyopathy and an increased incidence of PFC. The susceptibility to PFC in these infants is multifactorial; they may suffer from asphyxia in utero, polycythemia, hyperviscosity, and hypoglycemia. With subsequent hypoxemia, there may be a delay in the decrease in pulmonary vascular resistance (110).

D. Prognosis

There is increasing evidence that the altered intrauterine environment created by maternal diabetes may have long-term effects on offspring. Freinkel suggested that tissues that are incapable of significant postpartum differentiation, such as fat, neural tissue, and pancreatic islets, may be permanently affected by the abnormal metabolism in the diabetic pregnancy (10). The abnormal maternal fuels could affect cells in the fetus undergoing differentiation, proliferation, or functional maturation. This expanded concept of fuel-mediated teratogenesis (35) is supported by reports of increased risk for obesity, impaired intellect, and diabetes in offspring of diabetic pregnancies.

The potential for obesity in later life has been supported by a variety of studies (111–113). The Pima are a population with a very high prevalence of non–insulin-dependent diabetes mellitus (NIDDM), and there is a strong association with maternal diabetes. Among the Pima, 60% of offspring of diabetic mothers had weights that were >140% of desired weight compared with 25% of offspring of women who developed diabetes after pregnancy and 17% of nondiabetic women (114). Other studies have correlated obesity in 6-year-old offspring of diabetic pregnancies with obesity at birth and amniotic fluid insulin levels (115). Ongoing prospective studies continue to demonstrate a marked increase in weight after 6 years of age (116).

Although some studies show favorable developmental outcome in offspring of diabetic pregnancies (117), alterations in neuropsychologic development were demonstrated in earlier studies (118,119) as well as more recent reports. Subnormal performance on developmental tests at 4–5 years of age has been associated with early fetal growth delay on ultrasound measurements at 8–14 weeks gestation, a problem linked to poor diabetes control in early pregnancy (120,121). Lower psychologic test scores at 4 years of age were detected in children of mothers with ketonuria in late pregnancy (122). A prospective study of offspring of diabetic pregnancies revealed an increased incidence of intellectual delay at 3 and 5 years and an adverse effect of acetonuria on the intellectual status of offspring at 5 years of age (123). Fasting blood glucose and glycohemoglobin in the second and third trimesters were inversely related to three (interactive, motor, and physiologic control) of four newborn behavioral dimensions of the Brazelton neonatal behavioral assessment scale (124). In the child follow-up study, the children's mental development index scores at the age of 2 years correlated inversely with the mother's third trimester plasma β-hydroxybutyrate levels and the average Stanford-Binet scores correlated inversely with third-trimester plasma β-hydroxybutyrate and free fatty acid levels (125). These associations between maternal gestational ketonemia and lower intelligence quotient in offspring certainly justify avoidance of ketoacidosis and accelerated starvation in pregnant women. The results of all these studies also emphasize the importance of continued attention and research to define more clearly the ramifications of the abnormal intrauterine environment on the neurodevelopment of offspring of diabetic pregnancies. Until then, neurodevelopmental assessments should be considered in infants of diabetic mothers with a history of early growth delay in pregnancy and in those whose developmental progress is less than anticipated.

There is an increased risk of diabetes in offspring of diabetic pregnancies compared with offspring of nondiabetic pregnancies. Impaired glucose tolerence and subsequent gestational diabetes have been reported in offspring of diabetic rats (126,127). Data from the Pima also reveal an increased risk of diabetes in offspring of diabetics. The prevalence of NIDDM by age 20–24 years in the Pima is 1.4% among children of nondiabetic mothers, 8.6% among children of mothers who were not diabetic during pregnancy but subsequently developed NIDDM, and 45% among children exposed to diabetes in utero (128). In a Swedish study of 2757 children who developed insulin-dependent diabetes mellitus (IDDM) before the age of 15, maternal diabetes had the highest odds ratio (3.90) and was identified as the most significant risk factor for the development of diabetes (129). In a recent prospective study of insulin autoantibodies (IAA) and islet cell antibodies (ICA) in offspring of diabetic mothers, most infants who were antibody positive at birth lost their antibody positivity by 9 months of age (130). At 2 years of age, however, the prevalence of IAA and ICA positivity was 7.7% (130).

More recent epidemiologic studies have provided further data on other factors that may influence the development of diabetes in offspring. Warram et al. found a decreased risk of diabetes in offspring of diabetic mothers who gave birth after age 25 compared with those who gave birth before age 25 (131). A child born to a diabetic mother greater than 25 years of age has a risk of developig IDDM (by age 20 years) almost as low as a child of nondiabetic parents. Bleich et al. found that maternal diabetes acquired during adrenarche is associated with a decreased risk of type I diabetes in offspring (132). They found that mothers who developed diabetes before age 8 transmitted diabetes at the same rate as diabetic fathers and that the sex difference in diabetes transmission is caused by a decreased transmission rate by mothers who acquired diabetes after age 8. Before this study, offspring of woman with type I diabetes were thought to have a lower risk of developing type I diabetes than offspring of diabetic fathers (by age 20 years, 1.3 versus 6.1%) (133). Thus, exposure to maternal diabetes in utero seems to have a modifying influence that may affect genetic and/or environmental determinants in the transmission of diabetes. Like the other long-term sequelae in the offspring of the diabetic pregnancy, the risk of subsequent diabetes requires more study.

III. DIABETES IN THE FIRST YEAR OF LIFE

Hyperglycemia in the first year of life is a relatively uncommon entity. In infants less than 6 months of age, the differential diagnosis primarily includes transient diabetes of the newborn and pancreatic dysgenesis. True type I insulin-dependent diabetes mellitus can be seen in this age group, but it occurs more commonly in older infants. Glucose intolerance may be seen in infants with severe prematurity, and this is most likely attributable to the functional immaturity of the pancreatic β cell to release insulin. Central nervous system (CNS) injury and overwhelming stress may also be associated with glucose intolerance, but the magnitude of the hyperglycemia is usually small relative to the seriousness of the primary illness.

This section focuses on TDNB and pancreatic dysgenesis; IDDM is covered in Chapter 40. The hyperglycemia that results from severe prematurity, CNS injury, and severe stress improves with resolution of the primary illness and may be managed as the hyperglycemia as a result of TDNB.

A. Transient Diabetes of the Newborn

TDNB is a rare disorder characterized by hyperglycemia, glycosuria, and dehydration in the first 6 weeks of life. This syndrome is also known as congenital neonatal diabetes, pseudodiabetes, congenital temporary diabetes, and infantile glycosuria. One of the first reported cases occurred in the son of a physician in 1852 (134). He presented with "honeyed napkins," polyuria, polydipsia, dehydration, and emaciation within a few days of birth. Glycosuria was detected at 14 days of life, and the infant died of a urinary tract infection at 6 months of age.

1. Clinical Presentation

Infants are typically small for gestational age, have a characteristic "open-eyed alert facies," and have marked subcutaneous fat wasting (135). Males and females are equally affected. The average age of detection is 15 days, but the range of onset may be within hours of birth to about 6 weeks of age. The onset is usually sudden, with severe dehydration, and there is no history of vomiting or diarrhea. As in all sick newborns, a complicating infection should be considered but is most likely absent.

2. Etiology

The etiology of TDNB is obscure. In a few patients studied, no characteristic pancreatic abnormalities have been detected at autopsy. The pancreatic appearance has been described as normal (136), showing reduced numbers of islet cells (137, 138), or even an excess of islets (139). There is a family history of IDDM in approximately one-third of the cases (135). Familial cases have been reported in siblings and half-siblings (140–144).

Insulin, C peptide, and insulin-like growth factor (IGF) type I levels are low in these infants during the diabetic phase but normalize with clinical remission (135,145–148). IGF-II levels seem to be normal (145). Considering the role of insulin as a growth factor in utero (149,150), this hypoinsulinemic state may explain why these infants are small for gestational age (SGA). Some mothers of these infants were found to have flat oral glucose tolerance curves. This led to speculation that this disorder is caused by hypoplastic β cells as a result of a lack of normal glucose stimulation in utero (151). This does not seem a likely explanation because the normal fetal pancreas secretes very small amounts of insulin and because insulin does not appear to play a significant role in carbohydrate homeostasis in utero. Additionally, TDNB has occurred in infants of mothers with impaired carbohydrate tolerance (152).

Data from studies on fetal pancreases and in neonates suggest that the most likely etiology of this disorder is a maturational delay in the development of cAMP-mediated insulin release. The normal fetal pancreas undergoes a maturation process, during which time the mechanisms develop enabling insulin release to specific secretogogues. The secretagogues capable of releasing insulin earliest in gestation are leucine and those agents that generate cAMP either by stimulation of adenyl cyclase (e.g., glucagon) or by increasing its concentration through inhibition of phosphodiesterase (e.g., theophylline and caffeine) (27,153). Subsequently, arginine and then glucose become effective secretogogues (27,153,154). Consistent with these data are the findings from in vivo studies. Normal newborn infants demonstrate varying degrees of decreased sensitivity of insulin release to glucose and tolbutamide (29,155). Premature infants have impaired glucagon-mediated insulin release that can be enhanced by the addition of theophylline (156). On the other hand, infants of diabetic mothers who have an accelerated maturation of the β cells have an exaggerated insulin response to glucose and release insulin in response to tolbutamide immediately after birth (28,157). Just as infants of diabetic mothers seem to have a precocious maturation of the β cell, infants with TDNB have a delayed maturation. This was demonstrated in vivo by Pagliara et al., who studied the insulin responses to tolbutamide and hyperglycemia in an infant with TDNB in the diabetic phase and after remission (158). The glucose- and tolbutamide-mediated insulin release were absent during the diabetic phase, enhanced with caffeine, and normal after clinical recovery. Because caffeine, a phosphodiesterase inhibitor, enhanced insulin release during the transient diabetic phase, the defect may indeed be related to a delayed maturation of the adenyl cyclase-cyclic adenosine monophosphate system. This is also consistent with the transient course of this illness.

3. Diagnosis

The diagnosis is based on the clinical presentation and laboratory findings of glycosuria and hyperglycemia. The hyperglycemia may be severe (blood glucose > 111 mM, 2000 mg/dl), and the rate of rise in the blood glucose may be very rapid. It is not uncommon for the blood glucose value to increase dramatically on the repeat confirmatory blood glucose specimen. Although ketonuria is usually absent, the presence of mild ketonuria should not rule out the diagnosis.

Sequential glucagon stimulation testing may help predict the clinical course and establish β cell function. Baseline insulin and C peptide levels are obtained after which glucagon, 30 μg per kg, is administered intravenously. Insulin and C peptide levels at 5 and 15 minutes are subsequently drawn. During the diabetic phase, the glucagon-mediated insulin and C peptide response is minimal. With clinical recovery, there is an increased β cell response to glucagon.

Parents of infants with an appreciable insulin response could be reassured of improving β cell function with an anticipated spontaneous recovery. On the other hand, a diminished insulin response in an infant with a prolonged insulin requirement should prompt the clinician to suspect the diagnosis of pancreatic dysgenesis and to consider further diagnostic studies (see Sec. III.B).

4. Treatment

The treatment of this disorder consists of hydration, insulin therapy, and close monitoring. Isotonic intravenous fluids are usually required to keep up with the excessive osmotic losses associated with severe hyperglycemia. Because many of these infants can be quite insulin sensitive, small frequent doses of short-acting insulin are helpful in avoiding hypoglycemia and rapid drops in blood glucose values. Daily insulin requirements vary widely, and initial doses of short-acting insulin should be conservative, that is 0.25–0.50 units per kg per dose administered subcutaneously. These doses can be repeated approximately every 4 h (every 2 h if there is no decline in hyperglycemia). Alternatively, insulin may be administered by continuous intravenous infusion. This route of administration may be especially useful in those infants with severe hyperglycemia. Infusion dosages can be quite small (i.e., 0.025 units per kg per h) but may exceed 0.2 units per kg per h in the more insulin-resistant infants. Insulin should be aggressively titrated to reduce the hyperglycemia gradually by 80–100 mg per dl per h. Blood glucose should be monitored hourly if intravenous insulin is administered and every 2 h if subcutaneous insulin is administered until hyperglycemia is stabilized.

Some infants with TDNB may require insulin for more than only a few days, so that insulin therapy should be changed to include a longer acting insulin preparation (NPH Insulin or Lente Insulin) either alone or with regular insulin. Insulin adjustments should be made based on the blood glucose values in a fashion similar to that in children with type I IDDM. Hypoglycemia should be avoided, and as the infant recovers insulin doses must be reduced.

Although many infants with TDNB undergo a spontaneous recovery before hospital discharge, some infants continue to require insulin after hospitalization. Parents should be prepared for this prospect, as well as for the possibility of a persistent need for insulin. Parents and caregivers of these infants must therefore receive diabetes education in addition to normal newborn care education. Many of these parents are initially quite reluctant to participate in their infant's diabetes care because most of these infants are quite small and are regarded as too "fragile." The education sessions should take this into consideration and emphasize the importance of insulin for the infant's growth. Close follow-up is usually required to avoid hypoglycemia as insulin requirements diminish.

B. Pancreatic Dysgenesis

Pancreatic dysgenesis encompasses a spectrum of developmental functional anomalies ranging from mild hypoplasia to agenesis. These functional anomalies of the pancreas with endocrine and exocrine insufficiences are not reported as such and exclude the following: (1) anatomic pancreatic variants (i.e., annular pancreas), (2) pancreatic aplasia associated with severe fetal gastrointestinal malformations, and (3) combined renal and pancreatic dysplasia syndromes. Pancreatic dysgenesis is more common than previously recognized and can be classified as mild, moderate, or severe. This classification system has been devised to explain atypical hyperglycemia in infants and children, and hyperglycemia attributable to "permanent neonatal diabetes mellitus" and "insulin-dependent diabetes mellitus recurring after transient diabetes of the newborn."

1. Classification

The milder cases may represent what has been termed incidental hyperglycemia and glycosuria of childhood (159), whereby mild hyperglycemia is detected in children during intercurrent illnesses. These children are typically found to have a random elevated blood sugar during the evaluation for an acute infectious process, such as pneumonia, otitis media, or gastroenteritis. They lack the usual symptoms of polyuria, polydipsia, and polyphagia, and the hyperglycemia resolves with resolution of the acute process. Some of the children may in fact be at risk for developing type I IDDM, and several studies (i.e., islet cell antibodies, HLA-DR3/DR4 heterozygosity, sequential glucose tolerance testing, and others) may help identify this subset of children. The remaining children may simply have mild pancreatic dysgenesis.

The mildest cases may not even be clinically apparent. This author has followed an infant who presented at 4 weeks of age with asymptomatic hyperglycemia (postprandial blood glucose values between 11 mM, 200 mg/dl, and 14.5 mM, 260 mg/dl; preprandial blood glucose values normal). She was not SGA at birth, and the only reason she was identified was because her mother, fearful that her baby would have diabetes like her husband, detected glycosuria. Her islet cell antibodies were negative. She could not be treated with insulin because her preprandial blood glucose values were normal, and her blood glucose values normalized over a period of 2 months. She continues to thrive (no evidence of pancreatic exocrine insufficiency) at the age of 15 months. The atypical features of TDNB (atypical in that she was not SGA and there was no acute onset or need for insulin) make mild pancreatic dysgenesis a more likely cause of hyperglycemia than TDNB.

The moderate cases of pancreatic dygenesis may be those cases of permanent diabetes developing later in childhood after TDNB during infancy. There are now nine reports of children with TDNB who subsequently developed diabetes mellitus later in childhood (144,160–167). Table 2 summarizes their clinical courses. All these patients were small for gestational age at birth and developed hyperglycemia (range 17.8–45 mM, 321–810 mg/dl) between birth and 7 weeks of age. All these children are female. Their initial hyperglycemia resolved by 12 months of age, and the hyperglycemia recurred as permanent diabetes between the ages of 8 and 20 years. One of these nine cases is well controlled on small doses of an oral hypoglycemic agent (163), and two of the remaining seven on insulin therapy are on very small doses of insulin (165). Four of the nine children have been tested for islet cell antibodies and are negative. In one of these nine children extensive studies searched for serologic evidence of autoimmunity (162). Islet cell, insulin, glutamic acid 65 and 67, thyoperoxidase, gastric parietal cell, adrenal, steroidal, and antinuclear antibodies were negative. Thus, the development of permanent diabetes following TDNB in this setting seems to be unrelated to autoimmunity and may in fact be a form of pancreatic dysgenesis.

The more severe cases of pancreatic dysgenesis are extremely rare and have been reported as pancreatic agenesis or as permanent neonatal diabetes. Most infants with pancreatic agenesis do not survive the neonatal period and have

Table 2 Cases of Diabetes Recurring after Transient Diabetes of the Newborn[a]

Sex	Birth weight (kg)	Initial blood glucose (mg/dl)	Insulin therapy	Presentation of recurrent hyperglycemia	Therapy	Islet cell antibodies	Haplotype	Other clinical data	Reference
F	2.13	800	34–51 days	Age 18 years: 4 month history of polyuria and polydipsia	Insulin	N	A2A9B12	Necrobiosis lipoidica diabeticorum	160
F	1.65	497	20 h–14 weeks	Age 9 years: asymptomatic, nonketotic hyperglycemia, good growth (50%)	Insulin (1.1 U/kg)	N	24Bw48Cw8DR	Antiinsulin, glutamic acid 65 and 67, thyroperoxidase, gastric parietal cel, adrenal, steroidal antibodies negative; ANA negative; maternal Hb A1C normal	162
F	1.5	780	14 days to 8 months	Age 12 years: 2 week history of polyuria and polydipsia	Oral agent	NA	A2B7B20	Intercurrent illness glycosuria as toddler, impaired glucose tolerance at age 5 years, on insulin first and second pregnancy, first outcome stillborn; second outcome 4.77 kg; now age 22 good control on a small dose sulfonylurea	163
F	1.7	321	12 h to 6 months	Age 13 years: DKA	Insulin	NA	NA	On minimal insulin as infant	164
F	1.9	600	5 days to 6 months	Age 10 years: enuresis, growth deceleration, elevated Hb A1C	Insulin (5–6 U/day)	N	DR3, 6	Onset seizure disorder age 5.5 years treated with valproic acid	165
F	2.4	810	7 weeks to 12 months	Age 8 years: abnormal oral glucose tolerance test	Insulin (0.6 U/kg/day)	N	DR2, 6	On haloperidol for Tourette syndrome; on insulin, height 85%, weight 35%	165
NA	IUGR	NA	NA	Age 13 years: DKA	Insulin	NA	NA	NA	166
F	1.6	445	12–34 days	Age 20 years: 1 month history of polyuria, polydipsia, weight loss, and abdominal pain; blood glucose 396 mg/dl, ketonuria	Insulin	NA	NA	NA	167
F	?	654	12–113 days	Age 15 years: DKA, coma, blood glucose 1300 mg/dl	Insulin	NA	NA	NA	144

multiple other associated anomalies (168–170), including absence of the gallbladder. However, five children [four reported (171–173) and one from this author's experience] with evidence of both pancreatic exocrine and endocrine function have survived into childhood. The clinical findings of the four reported cases are summarized in Table 3. All five children were SGA, developed hyperglycemia during infancy, and were subsequently found to have fat malabsorption. The age of diagnosis of pancreatic exocrine deficiency in these children was variable, ranging from 12 weeks to 12 years of age. Additionally, there is one report of two male siblings who were both SGA and died by 48 h: the second infant was known to have hyperglycemia, and an autopsy revealed absence of the islets of Langerhans (174). Because both infants were very young, their pancreatic exocrine function is not known.

Some children described as having permanent neonatal diabetes may in fact have pancreatic dysgenesis. Because resolution of the hyperglycemia in TDNB has occurred up to 18 months of age (175), some of the cases of permanent neonatal diabetes described in children less than 18 months of age may have been reported before a spontaneous remission. In those children whose diabetes has not resolved, their growth and/or pancreatic exocrine function is not known. Because the onset of manifestations of pancreatic exocrine deficiency is variable, their growth or lack of symptoms at initial report is not helpful in assessing whether they in fact have pancreatic dysgenesis.

2. Diagnosis

The diagnosis of pancreatic dysgenesis is a clinical diagnosis based on demonstration of both pancreatic endocrine and exocrine dysfunction. Typically, these infants initially present as infants with TDNB. They are SGA and develop hypergly-

Table 3 Cases of Pancreatic Dysgenesis[a]

Sex	Birth weight (kg)	Initial blood glucose (mM)	Age hyperglycemia detected	HLA haplotype	Other clinical data	Reference
M	1.95	>33.3	2 days	NA	Edema, hypoproteinemia, anemia and failure to thrive from age 5 months; gross fat droplets in stool and steatorrhea detected at age 18 months, no pancreatic enzyme activity after cholecystokinin infusion	171
M	1.6	NA	7 weeks	A3B7DR2 A2B7DR4	Onset seizures age 7 weeks; abnormal stools noted at age 12 weeks; steatorrhea; tolerated no insulin for 1 week intervals as a toddler; low bicarbonate in response to secretin stimulation	172
M	2	NA	5 months	A3B7DR2 A9B40Cw3DR8	Low bicarbonate in response to secretin stimulation age 13 years; increased fecal fat, depressed pancreatic amylase, and trypsin-like immunoreactivity age 20 years	172
F	1.7	26.4	9 hours	NA	Abnormal stools noted at age 10 days; steatorrhea; no visible pancreas on ultrasound; no increase in PABA after bentiramide; pancreatic enzyme replacement begun at 18 days of age; at age 4 months weight 25%, height 10%	173

[a]M, male; NA, not applicable; F, female.

cemia, glycosuria, and dehydration within the first few weeks of life. Unlike infants with TDNB, the diabetes is not transient. A persistent need for insulin beyond several months of age, an unremarkable insulin response to glucagon, abnormal stools, and/or failure to gain weight despite a high caloric intake and reasonable control of hyperglycemia with insulin should alert the clinician to the possibility of exocrine dysfunction as well. The onset of this is variable and may be quite subtle.

The diagnosis of pancreatic exocrine insufficiency in the newborn or young infant may be difficult to establish. The exocrine pancreas is quite complex and is involved in both the digestion and absorption of ingested nutrients. Assessment of pancreatic function is accomplished by methods that evaluate the ability of the pancreas to secrete digestive enzymes or the efficacy of nutrient digestion and absorption. The exocrine pancreas has a tremendous functional reserve capacity. Clinical malabsorption, detected by steatorrhea, occurs with the loss of 98–99% of pancreatic lipase and colipase activity (176). Thus, assessment of pancreatic function by recognizing the presence of maldigestion and malabsorption detects only severe impairment. Furthermore, not all diseases involving the exocrine pancreas have equal effects upon both the enzyme component and the electrolyte component of the gland's secretion. This may be of particular

importance regarding pancreatic dysgenesis because of the small number of described cases. These facts, as well as the degree of invasiveness of the tests chosen, should guide the clinician in choosing among a wide array of tools to assess pancreatic function. These tests may be classified as direct tests, indirect tests, and blood tests (177).

Direct tests evaluate the secretory capacity of the exocrine pancreas. These involve the collection (via small intestinal intubation) of pancreatic secretions, usually under stimulated conditions. Examples include the use of either exogenous hormonal stimulants, such as secretin or cholecystokinin, or nutrient stimulants, such as fatty acids or amino acids. Although these tests may be considered the gold standard for appraisal of exocrine pancreatic function, their invasive, complex nature precludes their routine use and limits their value for serial monitoring purposes.

Indirect tests detect abnormalities caused by the loss of pancreatic function by quantifying the malassimilation of specific nutrients in the feces or by measuring metabolic products in the blood, urine, or breath. Examples include 72 h stool fat balance studies, stool smears for fat, the bentiramide test, and radiolabeled breath tests. The bentiramide test is a relatively simple, useful test that was recently modified to detect pancreatic insufficiency reliably in young children (178). Bentiramide is a nonabsorbable synthetic peptide specifically cleaved by pancreatic chymotrypsin. This cleavage releases the marker *p*-aminobenzoic acid (PABA). Levels of PABA do not increase after bentiramide ingestion in those with pancreatic insufficiency.

Blood tests of pancreatic enzymes include the measurement of total amlyase or lipase, isoamylase, trypsinogen, and pancreatic polypeptide. They are somewhat limited by a lack of test specificity and because there is a variable maturation of pancreatic enzymes, especially in early infancy. However, serum immunoreactive trypsinogen levels have been evaluated in pediatric patients and seem to detect pancreatic insufficiency reliably (179).

In this author's opinion, a reasonable approach to the diagnostic evaluation of suspected pancreatic insufficiency in infants includes stool smears for fat droplets, 72 h stool fat balance studies, serum immunoreactive trypsinogen, and perhaps the bentiramide test. A clinical trial of pancreatic enzyme replacement may also be of value using weight gain and/or fecal fat balance studies as objective measures of efficacy.

3. Treatment

The treatment of this disorder consists of managing the hyperglycemia and the pancreatic insufficiency. The initial management of the diabetes is the same as that for infants with TDNB, and the same principles employed in managing the child with type I IDDM may be subsequently used. In the young infant with diabetes, however, glycosylated hemoglobin values must be interpreted with caution because hemoglobin F can interfere with some assays.

The treatment of pancreatic insufficiency consists of maintaining a diet with adequate fat intake in conjunction with optimal pancreatic enzyme replacement. Stool consistency and frequency, weight gain, and linear growth should be used to titrate the appropriate amount of pancreatic enzyme replacement. Diets should be supplemented with fat-soluble vitamins, especially vitamins A and E. They are absorbed best when ingested with fat-containing meals and pancreatic enzymes. Prothrombin time, partial thromboplastin time, and fat-soluble vitamin levels should be monitored periodically to evaluate compliance and adequacy of supplementation.

C. Summary

Glucagon stimulation testing, especially if performed sequentially, may be useful in infants with hyperglycemia to help predict their clinical course and establish β cell function. Most infants with newborn hyperglycemia have transient diabetes of the newborn, and a spontaneous remission can be anticipated. The insulin response to glucagon should improve with clinical recovery. Recurrence of hyperglycemia later in childhood should alert the clinician to the possible diagnosis of pancreatic dysgenesis rather than TDNB. Pancreatic dysgenesis may be more common than previously recognized and should be seriously considered in infants with apparent TDNB, especially if there is a prolonged insulin requirement or failure to thrive. Thus, children with newborn hyperglycemia should have careful and long-term follow-up to assess their growth, possible pancreatic exocrine insufficiency, and glucose intolerance. Only with long-term follow-up of these infants and further research in this area will we be able to understand the etiology of these disorders and predict their clinical courses.

REFERENCES

1. Farquhar JW. The child of the diabetic woman. Arch Dis Child 1959; 34:76–96.
2. Dooley AL, Metzger BE, Cho NH. Gestational diabetes mellitus. Influence of race on disease prevalence and perinatal outcome in a U.S. population. Diabetes 1991; 40(Suppl. 2):25–29.
3. Connell FA, Vadheim C, Emmanuel I. Diabetes in pregnancy: a population based study of incidence, referral for care and perinatal mortality. Am J Obstet Gynecol 1985; 151:598–603.
4. National Diabetes Data Group. Classification and diagnosis of diabetes mellitus and other categories of glucose intolerance. Diabetes 1979; 28:1039–1057.
5. Freinkel N, Josimovich J, Conference Planning Committee. American Diabetes Association Workshop—Conference on Gestational Diabetes. Summary and recommendations. Diabetes Care 1980; 3:499–501.
6. Freinkel N. Summary and recommendations of the second International Workshop—Conference on Gestational Diabetes Mellitus. Diabetes 1985; 34(Suppl. 2):123–126.
7. American Diabetes Association. Position statement: gestational diabetes mellitus. Diabetes Care 1986; 9:430–431.
8. Hod M, Merlob P, Friedman S, Schoenfeld A, Ovadia J. Gestational diabetes mellitus. A survey of perinatal complications in the 1980s. Diabetes 1991; 40(Suppl. 2):74–78.
9. Landon MB, Gabbe SG. Diabetes and pregnancy. Med Clin North Am 1988; 72:1493–1511.
10. Freinkel N. The Banting Lecture 1980: of pregnancy and progeny. Diabetes 1980; 29:1023–1035.
11. Freinkel N, Dooley SL, Metzger BE. Care of the pregnant woman with insulin dependent diabetes mellitus. N Engl J Med 1985; 313:96–101.
12. Damm P, Molsted-Pedersen L. Significant decrease in congenital malformations in newborn infants of an unselected population of diabetic women. Am J Obstet Gynecol 1989; 161:1163–1167.
13. Steel JM, Johnstone FD, Hepburn DA, Smith A. Can prepregnancy care of diabetic women reduce the risk of abnormal babies? BMJ 1990; 301:1070–1074.
14. Kitzmiller JL, Gavin LA, Gin GD, Jovanovic L, Main EK, Zigrang WD. Preconception care of diabetes: glycemic control prevents congenital anomalies. JAMA 1991; 731–736.
15. Dekaban A, Baird R. The outcome of pregnancy in diabetic women. 1. Fetal wastage, mortality, and morbidity in the offspring of diabetic and normal control mothers. J Pediatr 1959; 55:563–576.
16. Elixhauser A, Weschler JM, Kitzmiller JL, et al. Cost-benefit analysis of preconception care for women with established diabetes mellitus. Diabetes Care 1993; 16(8):1146–1157.
17. White P, Koshy P, Duckers J. The management of pregnancy complicating diabetes and of children of diabetic mothers. Med Clin North Am 1953; 37:1481–1496.
18. Cornblath M, Schwartz R. Infant of the diabetic mother. In: Cornblath M, Schwartz R, eds. Disorders of Carbohydrate Metabolism in Infancy, Major Problems in Clinical Pediatrics, Vol. 3, 2d ed. Philadelphia: W.B. Saunders, 1976:115–153.
19. Freinkel N, Metzger BE, Potter JM. Pregnancy in diabetes.

In: Ellenberg M, Rifkin H, eds. Diabetes Mellitus: Theory and Practice, 3rd ed. New York: Medical Examination, 1983:689–714.

20. Pedersen J, Molsted-Pedersen L. Prognosis of the outcome of pregnancies in diabetics. A new classification. Acta Endocrinol (Copenh) 1965; 50:70–78.

21. Kalkhoff RK, Kissebah AH, Kim HJ. Carbohydrate and lipid metabolism during normal pregnancy: relationship to gestational hormone action. Semin Perinatol 1978; 2:291–307.

22. Pedersen J. Weight and length at birth of infants of diabetic mothers. Acta Endocrinol (Copenh) 1954; 16:330–343.

23. Freinkel N, Metzger BE. Pregnancy as a tissue culture experience: the critical implications of maternal metabolism for fetal development. In: Pregnancy Metabolism, Diabetes and the Fetus. CIBA Foundation Symposium, No. 63. Amsterdam: Excerpta Medica, 1979:3–23.

24. Luyckx AS, Massi-Benedetti F, Falorni A, Lefebvre PJ. Presence of pancreatic glucagon in the portal plasma of human neonates. Differences in the insulin and glucose responses between normal infants and infants of diabetic mothers. Diabetologia 1972; 8:296–300.

25. Ogata ES, Freinkel N, Metzger BE, et al. Perinatal islet function in gestational diabetes: assessment by cord plasma C-peptide and amniotic fluid insulin. Diabetes Care 1980; 3:425–429.

26. Phelps RL, Freinkel N, Rubenstein AH, et al. Carbohydrate metabolism in pregnancy. XV. Plasma C-peptide during intravenous glucose tolerance in neonates from normal and diabetic mothers. J Clin Endocrinol Metab 1978; 46:61–68.

27. Milner RDG, Ashworth MA, Barson AJ. Insulin release from human fetal pancreas in response to glucose, leucine and arginine. J Endocrinol 1972; 52:497–505.

28. Reiher H, Fuhrmann K, Noack S, Woltanski KP, Jutzi E, Dorsche HH, Hahn HJ. Age-dependent insulin-secretion of the endocrine pancreas in vitro from fetuses of diabetic and nondiabetic patients. Diabetes Care 1983; 6:446–451.

29. Pildes RS, Hart RJ, Warner R, Cornblath M. Plasma insulin response during oral glucose tolerance tests in newborn infants of normal and gestational diabetic mothers. Pediatrics 1969; 44:76–83.

30. Buchanan T, Schemmer JK, Freinkel N. Embryotoxic effects of brief maternal insulin-hypoglycemia during organogenesis in the rat. J Clin Invest 1986; 78:643–649.

31. Cockroft DL, Coppola PT. Teratogenic effects of excess glucose on head-fold rat embryos in culture. Teratology 1977; 16:141–146.

32. Takao Y, Akazawa S, Matsumoto K, et al. Glucose transporter gene expression in rat conceptus during high glucose culture. Diabetologia 1993; 36:696–706.

33. Horton WE, Sadler TW. Effects of maternal diabetes on early embryogenesis: alterations in morphogenesis produced by the ketone body, beta-hydroxybutyrate. Diabetes 1983; 32:610–616.

34. Lewis NJ, Akazawa S, Freinkel N. Teratogenesis from beta-hydroxybutyrate during organogenesis in rat embryo organ culture and enhancement by subteratogenic glucose. Diabetes 1983; 32:11A.

35. Freinkel N, Cockroft DL, Lewis NJ, et al. The 1986 McCollum Award Lecture. Fuel-mediated teratogenesis during early organogenesis: the effects of increased concentrations of glucose, ketones or somatomedin inhibitor during rat embryo culture. Am J Clin Nutr 1986; 44:986–995.

36. Eriksson UJ. Diabetes in pregnancy: effects of post-implantation embryos. Isr J Med Sci 1991; 27:478–86.

37. Weigensberg M, Garcia-Palmer F, Freinkel N. Competition between glucose and myo-inositol for transport in the embryopathy of hyperglycemia? Clin Res 1987; 35:863A.

38. Goldman AS, Baker L, Piddington R, et al. Hyperglycemia-induced teratogenesis is mediated by a functional deficiency of arachidonic acid. Proc Natl Acad Sci USA 1985; 82:8227–8231.

39. Goto MP, Goldman AS, Uhing MR. PGE-2 prevents anomalies induced by hyperglycemia or diabetic serum in mouse embryos. Diabetes 1992; 41:1644–1650.

40. Eriksson UJ, Borg LAH. Protection by free oxygen radical scavenging enzymes against glucose-induced embryonic malformations in vitro. Diabetologia 1991; 34:325–331.

41. Eriksson UJ, Borg LAH. Diabetes and embryonic malformations. Role of substrate-induced free-oxygen radical production for dysmorphogenesis in cultured rat embryos. Diabetes 1993; 42:411–419.

42. Cagliero E, Forsberg H, Sala R, Lorenzi M, Eriksson UJ. Maternal diabetes induces increased expression of extracellular matrix components in rat embryos. Diabetes 1993; 42:975–980.

43. Sadler TW, Horton WE Jr, Hunter ES. Maternal diabetes: mechanisms of teratogenicity. Diabetes 1984; 33(Suppl. 1):43A.

44. Cockroft DL, Freinkel N, Phillips LS, Shambaugh GE III. Metabolic factors affecting organogenesis in diabetic pregnancy. Clin Res 1981; 29:577A.

45. Sadler TW, Phillips LS, Balkan W, et al. Somatomedin inhibitors from diabetic rat serum alter growth and development of mouse embryos in culture. Diabetes 1986; 35:861–865.

46. Akashi M, Akazawa S, Akazawa M, et al. Effects of insulin and myo-inositol on embryo growth and development during early organogenesis in streptozocin-induced diabetic rats. Diabetes 1991; 40:1574–1579.

47. Combs CA, Kitzmiller JL. Spontaneous abortion and congenital anomalies in diabetes. Clin Obstet Gynecol 1991; 5:315–332.

48. Carson BS, Philipps AF, Simmons MA, et al. Effects of a sustained insulin infusion upon glucose uptake and oxygenation of the ovine fetus. Pediatr Res 1980; 14:147–152.

49. Molsted-Pedersen L, Tygstrup I, Pedersen J. Congenital malformations in newborn infants of diabetic women. Lancet 1964; 1:1124–1126.

50. Gabbe SG. Diabetes mellitus in pregnancy. Have all the problems been solved? Am J Med 1981; 70:613–618.

51. Comess LJ, Bennett PH, Man MB, et al. Congenital anomalies and diabetes in the Pima Indians of Arizona. Diabetes 1969; 18:471–477.

52. Mintz DH, Chez RA, Hutchinson DL. Subhuman primate pregnancy complicated by streptozotocin induced diabetes mellitus. J Clin Invest 1972; 51:837–847.

53. Brown ZA, Mills JL, Metzger BE, et al. National Institute of Child Health and Human Development Diabetes in Early Pregnancy Study. Early sonographic evaluation for fetal growth delay and congenital malformations in pregnancies complicated by insulin-requiring diabetes. Diabetes Care 1992; 15(5):613–619.

54. Rowland TW, Hubbell JP Jr, Nadas AS. Congenital heart disease in infants of diabetic mothers. J Pediatr 1973; 83:815–820.

55. Wilson TA, Blethen SL, Vallone A, et al. DiGeorge anomaly with renal agenesis in infants of mothers with diabetes. Am J Med Genet 1993; 47:1078–1082.

56. Black F, Spanier S, Kohut R. Aural abnormalities in partial DiGeorge syndrome. Arch Otolarynol 1975; 101:129–134.

57. Gosseye S, Collaire M, Verellin G, van Lierde M, Claus D. Association of bilateral renal agenesis and DiGeorge syndrome in an infant of a diabetic mother. Helv Paediatr Acta 1982; 37:471–474.

58. Mehta S, Nuamah I, Kalhan S. Altered diastolic function in asymptomatic infants of mothers with gestational diabetes. Diabetes 1991; 40:56–60.

59. Barr M, Hanson JW, Currey K, et al. Holoprosencephaly in infants of diabetic mothers. J Pediatr 1983; 102:565–568.

60. Shammas NW, Brown JD, Foreman BW, Marutani DR, Tonner D. Septo-optic dysplasia associated with polyendocrine dysfunction. J Med 1993; 24(1):67–74.

61. Kousseff BG, Villaveces C, Martinez CR. Unique brain anomolies in an infant of a diabetic mother. Acta Paediatr Scand 1991; 80(1):110–115.

62. Rusnak SL, Driscoll SG. Congenital spinal anomolies in infants of diabetic mothers. Pediatrics 1965; 35:989–995.

63. David A, Roze JC, Remond S, Branger B, Heloury Y. Hypoglossia-hypodactylia syndrome with jejunal atresia in an infant of a diabetic mother. Am J Med Genet 1992; 43(15):882–884.

64. Gonzalez A, Krassikoff N, Gilbert-Barness EF. Polyasplenia complex with mesocardia and renal agenesis in an infant of a diabetic mother. Am J Med Genet 1989; 32(4):457–460.

65. Davenport M, Savage M, Mowat AP, Howard ER. Biliary atresia splenic malformation syndrome: an etiologic and prognostic subgroup. Surgery 1993; 113(6):662–668.

66. Philippart AJ, Reed OJ, Georgeson KE. Neonatal small left colon syndrome: intramural not intraluminal obstruction. J Pediatr Surg 1975; 10:733–739.

67. Van Allen MI, Jackson JC, Knopp RH, Cone R. In utero thrombosis and neonatal gangrene in an infant of a diabetic mother. Am J Med Genet 1989; 33(3):323–327.

68. Osler M, Pedersen J. The body composition of newborn infants of diabetic mothers. Pediatrics 1960; 26:985–992.

69. Pildes RS. Infants of diabetic mothers. N Engl J Med 1973; 289:902–905.

70. Pedersen J. The Pregnant Diabetic and Her Newborn: Problems and Management. Baltimore: Williams & Wilkins, 1967.

71. Ogata ES, Sabbagha R, Metzger BE, et al. Serial ultrasonography to assess evolving fetal macrosomia. Studies in 23 pregnant diabetic women. JAMA 1980; 243:2405–2408.

72. Combs CA, Gunderson E, Kitzmiller JL, Gavin LA, Main EK. Relationship of fetal macrosomia to maternal postprandial glucose control during pregnancy. Diabetes Care 1992; 15(10):1251–1257.

73. Jovanovic-Peterson L, Peterson CM, Reed GF, et al. Maternal postprandial glucose levels and infant birthweight: the diabetes in early pregnancy study. Am J Obstet Gynecol 1991; 164:103–111.

74. Adell DA. The significance of abnormal glucose tolerance (hyperglycemia and hypoglycemia) in pregnancy. Br J Obstet Gynaecol 1979; 86:214–221.

75. Lager O, Levy J, Brustman L, et al. Glycemic control in gestational diabetes mellitus—how tight is tight enough: small for gestational age versus large for gestational age? Am J Obstet Gynecol 1989; 161:646–653.

76. Bauman WA, Yalow RS. Transplacental passage of insulin complexed to antibody. Proc Natl Acad Sci USA 1981; 78:4588–4590.

77. Menon RK, Cohen RM, Sperling MA, et al. Transplacental passage of insulin in pregnant women with insulin dependent diabetes mellitus: its role in fetal macrosomia. N Engl J Med 1990; 323:309–315.

78. Rosenn B, Miodovnik M, Combs CA, et al. Human versus animal insulin in the management of insulin dependent diabetes: lack of effect on fetal growth. Obstet Gynecol 1991; 78:590–593.

79. Jovanovic-Peterson L, Kitzmiller JL, Peterson CM. Randomized trial of human versus animal species insulin in diabetic pregnant women: improved glycemic control, not fewer antibodies to insulin, influences birth weight. Am J Obstet Gynecol 1992; 167:1325–1330.

80. Jovanovic-Peterson L, Sparks S, Palmer JP, Peterson CM. Jet-injected insulin is associated with decreased antibody production and postprandial glucose variability when compared with needle-injected insulin in gestational diabetic women. Diabetes Care 1993; 16(11):1479–1484.

81. Susa JB. Effects of diabetes on fetal growth. In: Reece EA, Coustan DR, eds. Diabetes Mellitus in Pregnancy, Principles and Practice. New York: Churchill Livingstone, 1988:105–122.

82. Acker DB, Sachs BP, Friedman EA. Risk factors for shoulder dystocia. Obstet Gynecol 1985; 66:762–678.

83. Mimouni F, Miodovnik M, Siddiqi TA, Khoury J, Tsang RC. Perinatal asphyxia in infants of insulin-dependent diabetic mothers. J Pediatr 1988; 113:345–353.

84. Landon MB, Sonek J, Foy P, Hamilton L, Gabbe SG. Sonographic measurement of fetal humeral soft tissue thickness in pregnancy complicated by GDM. Diabetes 1991; 40(Suppl. 2):66–70.

85. Bloom SR, Johnston DI. Failure of glucagon release in infants of diabetic mothers. BMJ 1972; 4:453–454.

86. Williams PR, Sperling MA, Racasa Z. Blunting of spontaneous and alanine-stimulated glucagon secretion in newborn infants of diabetic mothers. Am J Obstet Gynecol 1979; 133:51–56.

87. Knip M, Kaapa P, Koivisto M. Hormonal enteroinsular axis in newborn infants of insulin treated diabetic mothers. J Clin Endocrinol Metab 1993; 77(5):1340–1344.

88. Neufeld ND, Kaplan SA, Lippe BM, Scott M. Increased monocyte receptor binding of [^{125}I]insulin in infants of gestational diabetic mothers. J Clin Endocrinol Metab 1978; 47:590–595.

89. Tsang RC, Kleinman LI, Sutherland JM, Light J. Hypocalcemia in infants of diabetic mothers: studies in calcium, phosphorus and magnesium metabolism and parathormone responsiveness. J Pediatr 1972; 80:384–395.

90. Mimouni F, Tsang RC, Hertzberg VS, Miodovnik M. Polycythemia, hypomagnesemia and hypocalcemia in infants of diabetic mothers. Am J Dis Child 1986; 140:798–800.

91. Tsang RC, Chen IW, Friedman MA, et al. Parathyroid function in infants of diabetic mothers. J Pediatr 1975; 86:399–404.

92. Noguchi A, Eren M, Tsang RC. Parathyroid hormone in hypocalcemic and normocalcemic infants of diabetic mothers. J Pediatr 1980; 97:112–114.

93. Parfitt AM, Kleerekoper M. Clinical disorders of calcium, phosphorus and magnesium metabolism. In: Maxwell M, Kleeman CR, eds. Clinical Disorders of Fluid and Electrolyte Metabolism, 3rd ed. New York: McGraw-Hill, 1980:947–1152.

94. Mimouni F, Steichen JJ, Tsang RC, Hertzberg V, Miodovnik M. Decreased bone mineral content in infants of diabetic mothers. Am J Perinatol 1988; 5:339–343.

95. Robert MF, Neff RK, Hubbell JP, et al. Association between maternal diabetes and the respiratory-distress syndrome in the newborn. N Engl J Med 1976; 294:357–360.

96. Warbuton D. Chronic hyperglycemia reduces surface active material flux in tracheal fluid of fetal lambs. J Clin Invest 1983; 71:550–555.

97. Tsai MY, Shultz EK, Nelson JA. Amniotic fluid phosphatidylglycerol in diabetic and control pregnant patients at different gestational lengths. Am J Obstet Gynecol 1984; 149:388–392.

98. Gluck L, Kulovich MV. Lecithin/sphingomyelin ratios in

amniotic fluid in normal and abnormal pregnancy. Am J Obstet Gynecol 1973; 115:539–546.

99. Nogee L, McMahan M, Whitsett JA. Hyaline membrane disease and surfactant protein, SAP-35, in diabetes in pregnancy. Am J Perinatol 1988; 5:374–377.

100. McMahon MJ, Mimouni F, Miodovnik M, et al. Surfactant associated protein (SAP-35) in amniotic fluid from diabetic and nondiabetic pregnancies. Obstet Gynecol 1987; 70:94–98.

101. Ferroni KM, Gross TL, Sokol RJ, et al. What affects fetal pulmonary maturation during diabetic pregnancy? Am J Obstet Gynecol 1984; 150:270–274.

102. Fadel HE, Saad SA, Nelson GH, et al. Effect of maternal-fetal disorders on lung maturation. I. Diabetes mellitus. Am J Obstet Gynecol 1986; 155:544–553.

103. Dudley DK, Black DM. Reliability of lecithin/sphingomyelin ratios in diabetic pregnancy. Obstet Gynecol 1985; 66:521–524.

104. Farrell PM, Engle JM, Curet LB, et al. Saturated phospholipids in amniotic fluid of normal and diabetic pregnancies. Obstet Gynecol 1985; 64:77–85.

105. Kjos SL, Walther FJ, Montoro M, et al. Prevalence and etiology of respiratory distress in infants of diabetic mothers: predictive value of fetal lung maturation tests. Am J Obstet Gynecol 1990; 163:893–903.

106. Widness JA, Susa JB, Garcia JF, et al. Increased erythropoiesis and elevated erythropoietin in infants born to diabetic mothers and in hyperinsulinemic rhesus fetuses. J Clin Invest 1981; 67:637–642.

107. Perrine SP, Greene MF, Lee PDK, Cohem RA, Faller DV. Insulin stimulates cord blood erythroid progenitor growth: Evidence for an aetiological role in neonatal polycythema. Br J Haematol 1986; 64:503–511.

108. Avery ME, Oppenheimer EH, Gordon NH. Renal vein thrombosis in newborn infants of diabetic mothers. N Engl J Med 1957; 256:1134–1138.

109. Stevenson DK, Ostrander CR, Hopper AO, Cohen RS, Johnson JD. Pulmonary excretion of carbon monoxide as an index of bilirubin production. IIa. Evidence for possible delayed clearance of bilirubin in infants of diabetic mothers. J Pediatr 1981; 98:822–824.

110. Gersony WM. Persistence of the fetal circulation: a commentary. J Pediatr 1973; 82:1103–1106.

111. Cummins M, Norrish M. Follow-up of children of diabetic mothers. Arch Dis Child 1980; 55:259–264.

112. Vohr BR, Lipsitt LP, Oh W. Somatic growth of children of diabetic mothers with reference to birth size. J Pediatr 1980; 97:196–199.

113. Green OC, Winter RJ, Depp R, et al. Fuel-mediated teratogenesis: prospective correlations between anthropometric development in childhood and antepartum maternal metabolism. Clin Res 1987; 35:657A.

114. Pettitt DJ, Baird HR, Aleck KA, Bennett PH, Knowler WC. Excessive obesity in offspring of Pima Indian women with diabetes during pregnancy. N Engl J Med 1983; 308:242–245.

115. Metzger BE, Silverman BL, Freinkel N, et al. Amniotic fluid insulin as a predictor of obesity. Arch Dis Child 1990; 65:1050–1052.

116. Silverman BL, Rizzo T, Green OC, et al. Long term prospective evaluation of offspring of diabetic mothers. Diabetes 1991; 40:121–125.

117. Persson B, Gentz J. Follow up of children of insulin dependent and gestational diabetic mothers. Neuropsychological outcome. Acta Pediatr Scand 1984; 73:343–358.

118. Farquhar JW. Prognosis for babies born to diabetic mothers in Edinburgh. Arch Dis Child 1969; 44:36–47.

119. Yssing M. Oestriol excretion in pregnant diabetes related to long term prognosis of surviving children. Acta Endocrinol (Copenh) 1974; 182:95–104.

120. Peterson JB, Pedersen SA, Greisen G, Pedersen JF, Molsted-Pedersen L. Early growth delay in diabetic pregnancy relation to psychomoter development at age 4. BMJ 1988; 196:598–600.

121. Pedersen JF, Molsted-Pedersen L, Mortensen JB. Fetal growth delay and maternal hemoglobin A1C in early pregnancy. Obstet Gynecol 1984; 64:351–352.

122. Churchill JA, Berendes HW, Nemore J. Neuropsychological deficits in children of diabetic mothers. Am J Obstet Gynecol 1969; 105:257–268.

123. Stehbens JA, Baker GL, Kitchell M. Outcome at ages 1, 3, and 5 years of children born to diabetic women. Am J Obstet Gynecol 1977; 127:408–413.

124. Rizzo T, Freinkel N, Metzger BE, et al. Correlations between antepartum maternal metabolism and newborn behavior. Am J Obstet Gynecol 1990; 163:1458–1464.

125. Rizzo T, Metzger BE, Burns WJ, Burns K. Correlations between antepartum maternal metabolism and intelligence of offspring. N Engl J Med 1991; 325:911–916.

126. Gauguier D, Bihoreau M, Picon L, Ktorza A. Insulin secretion in adult rats after intrauterine exposure to mild hyperglycemia during late gestation. Diabetes 1991; 40(Suppl. 2):109–114.

127. Van Assche FA, Aerts L, Holemans K. Metabolic alterations in adulthood after intraterine development in mothers with mild diabetes. Diabetes 1991; 40(Suppl. 2):106–108.

128. Pettitt DJ, Bennett PH, Saad MF, et al. Abnormal glucose tolerance during pregnancy in Pima Indian women. Long-term effects on offspring. Diabetes 1991; 40(Suppl. 2):126–130.

129. Dahlquist G, Kallen B. Maternal-child blood group incompatibility and other perinatal events increase the risk for early-onset type I (insulin-dependent) diabetes mellitus. Diabetologia 1992; 35:6671–6675.

130. Ziegler AG, Hillebrand B, Rabl W, et al. On the appearance of islet associated autoimmunity in offspring of diabetic mothers: a prospective study from birth. Diabetologia 1993; 36:402–408.

131. Warram JH, Martin BC, Krolewski AS. Risk of IDDM in children of diabetic mothers decreases with increasing maternal age at pregnancy. Diabetes 1991; 40:1679–1684.

132. Bleich D, Polak M, Eisenbarth GS, Jackson RA. Decreased risk of type I diabetes in offspring of mothers who acquire diabetes during adrenarchy. Diabetes 1993; 42:1433–1439.

133. Warram JH, Krolewski AS, Gottlieb MS, Kahn CR. Differences in risk of insulin-dependent diabetes in offspring of diabetic mothers and diabetic fathers. N Engl J Med 1984; 311:149–152.

134. Lawrence RD, McCance RA. Gangrene in an infant associated with temporary diabetes. Arch Dis Child 1931; 6:343–356.

135. Gentz JCH, Cornblath M. Transient diabetes of the newborn. Adv Pediatr 1969; 16:345.

136. Hickish G. Neonatal diabetes. BMJ 1956; 1:95–96.

137. Lewis E, Eisenberg H. Diabetes mellitus neonatorum. Am J Dis Child 1935; 49:408–410.

138. Tidd JT, Stanage WF. Congenital diabetes mellitus. S D J Med 1965; 18:15–19.

139. Osbourne GR. Congenital diabetes. Arch Dis Child 1965; 40:332.

140. Ferguson AW, Milner RDG, Naidu SH. Transient neonatal diabetes mellitus in three successive male siblings. Arch Dis Child 1971; 46:724–729.

141. Ferguson AW, Milner RDG. Transient neonatal diabetes mellitus in sibs. Arch Dis Child 1970; 45:80–83.

142. McGill JJ, Roberton DM. A new type of transient diabetes mellitus of infancy? Arch Dis Child 1986; 61:334–336.

143. Coffey JD, Womack NC. Transient neonatal diabetes mellitus in half sisters. Am J Dis Child 1967; 113:480–482.

144. Coffey JD, Killelea DE. Transient neonatal diabetes mellitus in half sisters: a sequel. Am J Dis Child 1982; 136:626–727.

145. Blethen SL, White NH, Santiago JV, Daughaday WH. Plasma somatomedins, endogenous insulin secretion, and growth in transient neonatal diabetes mellitus. J Clin Endocrinol Metab 1981; 52:144–147.

146. Halliday HL, McC Reid M, Hadden DR. C-peptide levels in transient neonatal diabetes. Diabetic Med 1986; 3:80–81.

147. Milner RDG, Ferguson AW, Naidu SH. Aetiology of transient neonatal diabetes. Arch Dis Child 1971; 46:724–726.

148. Schiff D, Colle E, Stern L. Metabolic and growth patterns in transient neonatal diabetes. N Engl J Med 1972; 287:119–122.

149. Hill DJ, Milner RDG. Insulin as a growth factor. Pediatr Res 1985; 19:879–886.

150. Philipps A, Rosenkrantz TS, Clark RM, et al. Effects of fetal insulin deficiency on growth in fetal lambs. Diabetes 1991; 40:20–27.

151. Gerrard DM, Chin WP. The syndrome of transient diabetes. J Pediatr 1962; 61:89–93.

152. Lambert AE, Junod A, Stauffacher W, Jeanrenaud B, Renold AE. Organ culture of fetal rat pancreas. I. Insulin release induced by caffeine and by sugars and some derivatives. Biochim Biophys Acta 1969; 184:529–539.

153. Espinosa-de-los Monteros MM, Driscoll SG, Steinke J. Insulin release from isolated human fetal pancreas. Science 1970; 168:1111–1112.

154. Chez RA, Mintz DH, Hutchinson DL. Effect of theophylline on glucagon and glucose mediated plasma insulin responses in subhuman primate fetus and neonate. Metabolism 1971; 20:805–815.

155. Isles TE, Dickson M, Farquhar JW. Glucose tolerance and plasma insulin in newborn infants of normal and diabetic mothers. Pediatr Res 1968; 2:198–208.

156. Grasso S, Messina A, Saporito N, Reitano G. Effect of theophylline, glucagon and theophylline plus glucagon on insulin secretion in the premature infant. Diabetes 1970; 19:837–841.

157. Velasco MSA, Paulsen EP. The response of infants of diabetic women to tolbutamide and leucine at birth, and glucose and tolbutamide at 2 years of age. Pediatrics 1969; 43:546–557.

158. Pagliara AS, Karl IE, Kipnis DB. Transient neonatal diabetes: delayed maturation of the pancreatic beta cell. J Pediatr 1973; 82:97–101.

159. Schatz DA, Kowa H, Winter WE, Riley WJ. Natural history of incidental hyperglycemia and glycosuria of childhood. J Pediatr 1989; 115:676–680.

160. Campbell IW, Fraser DM, Duncan LJP, Keay AJ. Permanent insulin-dependent diabetes mellitus after congenital temporary diabetes mellitus. BMJ 1978; 2:174.

161. Geffner ME, Clare-Salzler M. Kaufman DL, et al. Permanent diabetes developing after transient neonatal diabetes. Lancet 1993; 341:1095.

162. Gottschalk ME, Schatz DA, Clare-Salzler M, et al. Permanent diabetes without serological evidence of autoimmunity after transient neonatal diabetes. Diabetes Care 1992; 15:1273–1276.

163. Briggs JR. Permanent non-insulin dependent diabetes mellitus after congenital transient diabetes mellitus. Scott Med J 1986; 31:41–42.

164. Schield JPH, Baum JD. Is transient neonatal diabetes a risk factor for diabetes later in life? Lancet 1993; 341:693.

165. Weimerskirch D, Klein DJ. Recurrence of insulin-dependent diabetes mellitus after transient neonatal diabetes: A report of two cases. J Pediatr 1993; 122:598–600.

166. Edidin DV. Permanent diabetes developing after transient neonatal diabetes. Lancet 1993; 341:1095.

167. Croxson SCM, Burden AC. Insulin dependent diabetes following neonatal diabetes. Aust Paediatr J 1988; 24:157.

168. Dourov N, Buyl-Strovrens ML. Agenesie du pancreas. Arch Fr Pediatr 1969; 26:641.

169. Mehes K, Vamos K, Goda M. Agenesis of pancreas and gall-bladder in an infant of incest. Acta Paediatr Acad Sci Hung 1976; 17:175–176.

170. Lemons JA, Ridenhour R, Orsini EN. Congenital absence of the pancreas and intrauterine growth retardation. Pediatrics 1979; 64:255–257.

171. Howard CP, Go VLW, Infante AJ, et al. Long-term survival in a case of functional pancreatic agenesis. J Pediatr 1980; 97:786–789.

172. Winter WE. Congenital pancreatic hypoplasia: a syndrome of exocrine and endocrine insufficiency. J Pediatr 1986; 109:465–468.

173. Wright NM, Metzger DL, Clarke WL. Permanent neonatal diabetes mellitus and pancreatic exocrine insufficiency resulting from pancreatic agenesis. Am J Dis Child 1993; 147:607–608.

174. Dodge JA, Laurence KM. Congenital absence of islets of Langerhans. Arch Dis Child 1977; 52:411–419.

175. Wylie MES. A case of congenital diabetes. Arch Dis Child 1953; 28:297–299.

176. Gaskin KJ, Durie PR, Lee L, et al. Colipase and lipase secretion in childhood-onset pancreatic insufficiency. Gastroenterology 1984; 86:1–7.

177. Couper R, Durie PR. Pancreatic function tests. In: Walker WA, Durie PR, Hamilton JR, Walker-Smith JA, Watkins JB, eds. Pediatric Gastrointestinal Disease: Pathophysiology, Diagnosis, Management. Philadelphia: B. C. Decker, 1991: 1341–1353.

178. Lauffer D, Cleghorn G, Forstner G, Ellis L, Koren G, Durie P. The bentiramide test using plasma p-aminobenzoic acid for diagnosing pancreatic insufficiency in young children. The effect of two different doses and a liquid meal. Gastroenterology 1991; 101:207–213.

179. Moore DJ, Forstner GG, Largman C, Cleghorn GJ, Wong SS, Durie PR. Serum immunoreactive cationic trypsinogen: a useful indicator of severe exocrine dysfunction in the pediatric patient without cystic fibrosis. Gut 1986; 27:1362–1368.

40

Complications of Insulin-Dependent Diabetes Mellitus in Childhood and Adolescence

Dorothy J. Becker
*Children's Hospital of Pittsburgh and University of Pittsburgh,
Pittsburgh, Pennsylvania*

I. INTRODUCTION

The complications of insulin-dependent diabetes (IDDM) can be classified as (1) acute complications (usually reversible); (2) intermediate complications (probably reversible); and (3) chronic complications (questionably reversible). Chronic complications are divided into those that are considered of microvascular pathogenesis and those of macrovascular pathogenesis (Table 1). The classic triad of retinopathy, nephropathy, and neuropathy (commonly considered microvascular) are the most common chronic complications of IDDM and usually manifest clinically in early adulthood. Macrovascular disease manifesting as cerebrovascular accidents and cardiovascular and peripheral vascular disease usually occur later in adulthood. Although the pediatrician of today is usually spared the difficulties of caring for patients with these overt problems, subclinical manifestations of both micro- and macrovascular disease can already be found during adolescence.

Although there is little doubt that poor glycemic control, frequently associated with either over- or underinsulinization, is the cause of acute and some of the intermediate complications of diabetes, the pathogenesis of the chronic complications of IDDM have not been as clear. Recent intervention trials have put to rest the previous controversies regarding a direct glucotoxic pathogenesis of subclinical and clinical microvascular complications. However, there are probable additional pathogenic effects of other metabolic processes, as well as possible genetic and environmental influences.

II. ACUTE COMPLICATIONS

The most common acute complications of IDDM are hypoglycemia and ketoacidosis. These are caused by absolute or relative excess or insufficiency of circulating insulin. Both these complications are theoretically preventable through education of physicians, patients, and families, as well as meticulous monitoring of metabolic control. Unfortunately, this is not easy in practice: titration of insulin dose, food, and activity is particularly difficult in childhood. Recognition of ketosis in both the newly diagnosed and previously diagnosed child and adolescent with diabetes should enable the rapid institution of insulin therapy to prevent the development of ketoacidosis. The prevention of ketoacidosis would eliminate the most feared acute complication of IDDM, which is cerebral edema, whose pathogenesis is not yet clear. In our experience, cerebral edema and, less often, cerebral vascular thromboses are the most common causes of death in children and adolescents with IDDM (1). In contrast, hypoglycemia is a relatively rare cause of death but a major cause of morbidity. Severe hypoglycemia can cause coma and seizures and, if frequent, may probably result in some chronic central nervous system (CNS) changes, as discussed later. Increased susceptibility to infection in very poorly controlled patients is probably caused by interference with the function of the immunologic system by various mechanisms. Allergic reactions to insulin preparations appear to be less common today than previously described, probably because of the improved purity of insulin preparations. Although acute complications are not preventable in all patients, they are usually reversible with appropriate medical management. A detailed description of the acute complications of IDDM is beyond the scope of this chapter.

III. INTERMEDIATE COMPLICATIONS

Intermediate complications manifest gradually over a relatively short period of time compared with chronic complications. Most are clearly associated with poor glycemic control

Table 1 Complications of Diabetes in Childhood and Adolescence

Acute complications
   Ketoacidosis
     Dehydration
     Shock
     Cerebral edema
   Hypoglycemia
   Weight loss and weight gain
   Insulin allergy
   Susceptibility to infection
Intermediate complications
   Lipohypertrophy
   Lipoatrophy
   Limited joint mobility
   Osteopenia
   Growth failure
   Pubertal delay and menstrual disturbances
   Impaired cognitive function
   Cataracts
   Necrobiosis lipoidica diabeticorum
   Failure of glucose counterregulation
   Emotional disturbance
   Hyperlipidemia
Chronic complications
   Retinopathy ⎫
   Nephropathy ⎬ Microvascular
   Neuropathy ⎪
     Peripheral
     Autonomic
     CNS ⎫
   Cardiopathy ⎬ Micro- and macrovascular
   Macrovascular disease

because of under- or overinsulinization or inappropriate food consumption. Thus, some of these complications, such as growth failure and delayed puberty, which are specific for the pediatric age group, are easily preventable by adequate insulinization. Similarly, most of the other intermediate complications seen in this age group are preventable by appropriate insulin therapy and are also usually reversible, unless they have continued for an excessive length of time. Over the past few years, the pathogenesis and frequency of hypoglycemia unawareness, the potential reversibility of impaired counterregulation, and the decreased mental efficiency associated with hypoglycemia have been elucidated. These intermediate complications are discussed in more detail in the following subsections.

A. Lipoatrophy and Lipohypertrophy

Lipoatrophy and lipohypertrophy are subcutaneous side effects of insulin injections, and the latter remains the most common subacute complication of IDDM. Lipoatrophy,

which is an indentation or atrophy of the subcutaneous fat, should no longer occur. It most certainly is a response to the injection of a foreign material into the subcutaneous fat. The impurities of insulin preparations of two decades ago, as well as amino acid differences of beef compared with human insulin, presumably resulted in local immunologic responses. The introduction of pure pork and human insulins has resulted in a dramatic decrease in the incidence of lipoatrophy. Occasionally, one still sees very slight atrophy in children treated with either human or pork insulin, particularly in the younger age group. However, this is almost never severe and is easily corrected by giving the insulin injections around the edges of the area.

By contrast, lipohypertrophy unfortunately remains extremely common. This is highly unlikely to be a result of impurities in insulin preparation. Rather, it is caused by trauma of the insulin injection being placed in the same area of the subcutaneous tissue repeatedly, with resultant scarring and decreased sensitivity to pain. The hypertrophy results in cosmetic unsightliness that can be embarrassing to the patient. Of greater concern is the apparent interference with absorption of insulin from hypertrophied areas, causing erratic metabolic control. Hypertrophy cannot be remedied by altering insulin type. It disappears only if the site of insulin injection is changed.

B. Skeletal and Joint Abnormalities

The syndrome of limited joint mobility (LJM) was described in 1976 (2,3) and has subsequently been termed Rosenbloom syndrome. The earliest manifestations are an inability to approximate the palmar surfaces of the hands when in a prayer position, as a result of flexion contractures of the metacarpophalangeal and proximal interphalangeal joints starting with the fifth finger. These changes then spread medially and later may involve the wrist and even the elbow and other large joints, including the cervical and thoracolumbar spine. This condition may be associated with thickening of the skin reminiscent of scleroderma (4). It rarely occurs before 10 years of age, irrespective of age of onset of IDDM, and was described in 3–25% of pediatric diabetes populations. It appears to be far less common today, apparently associated with overall improved glycemic control, because the most severely affected patients usually have very poor diabetes control. However, lesser forms of the syndrome have been described, with no correlation with glycemic control in some studies. Support for a role of glycemic control in the pathogenesis of LJM was found in a study showing decreased skin thickness, measured by ultrasound, with improved metabolic control. It is thought that the biochemical basis for this manifestation of IDDM is glycosylation of protein with the formation of advanced glycosylation end products (5), particularly collagen, of the skin and joints. Most patients are unaware of any side effects from this diabetes complication. Some notice joint stiffening, however. The major interest in quantifying LJM is the association described by Rosenbloom with a risk for subsequent development of microvascular complications. It has been suggested that the presence or absence of LJM may delineate high- or low-risk groups of patients for early microvascular disease (3). In a recent study of 357 young subjects with IDDM, 26% demonstrated limited joint mobility. This study confirmed the relationship between LJM and microvascular complications of IDDM, and its relationship with retinopathy (but not nephropathy) appeared to be independent of glycosylated hemoglobin concentrations (6). LJM has also been associated with myocardiopathy and decreased pulmonary compliance (7,8).

Osteopenia is a far less frequently recognized manifestation of IDDM (3). Decreased bone mineral content is measured by photon absorption densitometry or other radiologic means. Prevalence varies between 7 and 54% of patients studied, with both a positive relationship or no correlation with duration and a direct correlation or no effect of diabetes control being reported. The exact mechanism of this osteopenia remains unclear. Excess calcium loss in poorly controlled diabetes is well known, presumably related to the presence of hyperglycemia and insulin deficiency. This is reversible by subcutaneous insulin infusion on a short-term basis. There is no agreement in the reported studies on whether parathyroid hormone levels are normal or abnormal in IDDM and whether there are alterations in vitamin D metabolites (3). The clinical significance of this osteopenia is not clear; the incidence of fractures is not increased in patients with IDDM (9). At this stage, it is also unknown whether the osteopenia is preventable or reversible by long-term improved glycemic control.

C. Growth Failure and Short Stature

Growth failure resulting from insulin deficiency represents a treatment failure of IDDM. In contrast with the experience of a few decades ago, it is now obvious that children with IDDM who receive adequate insulin doses grow perfectly normally and do not have short stature (10). Although reports of decreased growth velocity persist in the current literature, these appear to be related to underinsulinization and poor metabolic control (11,12). In contrast, normal growth velocities are the general experience in patients who are well insulinized in fairly good metabolic control (13). The extreme example of growth failure from insulin deficiency is the development of the Mauriac syndrome, or diabetic dwarfism. Children with this syndrome are short, with a decreased growth velocity. They are usually pale, with thickened skin and protuberant abdomen with hepatomegaly, and they may have a cushingoid appearance. This syndrome, which is now rarely seen in developed countries, is rapidly correctable, with improvement in growth with adequate insulin delivery. However, we suggest that in chronic underinsulinization, as in Mauriac syndrome, insulin be increased slowly, with gradual rather than rapid improvement of metabolic control. We have documented the rapid development of retinopathy during rapid increases in insulin therapy in such patients (14). Insulin, together with growth hormone and thyroxine, are all required for maintenance of normal growth. Growth failure can be prevented if subtle decreases in growth rates are detected by regular measurements of heights and weights plotted on growth charts during physician visits. As soon as a decrease in growth rate is observed, the treatment strategy should be reevaluated to reverse the situation. Obviously, other causes for growth failure, such as hypothyroidism, eating disorders and other chronic illnesses, and growth hormone deficiency, should be excluded. The growth failure of hypothyroidism, which is frequently associated with IDDM (15,16), is usually not preceded by poor weight gain. Although short-term growth failure is quickly reversible, if poor growth remains undetected into the late adolescent years complete reversal of growth failure is rarely achieved.

The mechanism of growth failure in the face of the well-documented elevations of basal and stimulated growth hormone concentrations in poorly controlled IDDM (17–19) is apparently related to decreased growth hormone binding protein levels, which reflect the extracellular moiety of the growth hormone receptor (20). The institution of effective insulin therapy decreases the growth hormone and increases the growth hormone binding protein levels (19,21,22). It seems possible that a growth hormone receptor defect can explain reports of low circulating insulin-like growth factor type I (IGF-I) levels in some (but not all) IDDM patients, with impaired "somatomedin generation" in response to exogenous growth hormone (23,24) but, again, there is normalization with adequate insulinization (25). IGF binding protein I levels are high in diabetic adolescents and correlated with metabolic control, possibly decreasing the availability of free IGF-I at the receptor level (26).

D. Delay in Sexual Maturation

Delay in sexual maturation usually occurs in association with growth failure (27). Children with IDDM who have poor growth invariably have a delayed bone age. This is almost always associated with a deficiency of insuln delivery. However, some girls with very poor glycemic control may have reasonable growth but a delay in sexual progression with late menarche (28). Once menarche occurs, poor control may be associated with irregular menstruation or secondary amenorrhea accompanied by decreased sex hormone binding globulin and IGF-I levels and an increased ratio of luteinizing hormone to follicle-stimulating hormone (28,29). There is evidence that ovarian cells have insulin and IGF-I receptors and are stimulated by insulin and IGF-I, making it likely that insulin is important for normal ovarian cycling (30–32). Although this is presumably also true for the testicle, there is less documentation in the literature. In addition, abnormalities of hormone secretion have been shown to occur throughout the hypothalamic-pituitary-gonadal axis, with abnormalities of the gonadotropin-releasing hormone (GnRH) pulse generator and a low gonadotropin response to GnRH stimulation (33,34). It appears that insulin deficiency or hyperglycemia per se may result in ovarian or testicular dysfunction by mechanisms that are not totally clear (32). In males, both decreased testosterone and sex hormone binding globulin levels have been reported (33).

E. Impaired Intellectual Development

The recent development of sensitive neuropsychologic techniques have allowed the documentation of definite impairment of neuropsychologic function in cohorts of children with IDDM, especially prevalent in those whose onset of illness was before 5 years of age (35–37). Many of these children have clear impairment of cognitive function compared with their siblings. It is postulated that either hyper- or hypoglycemic insults to the developing brain may result in permanent damage. Because most studies are retrospective, it is difficult to document the exact associations of this decreased intellectual function, but avoidance of hpoglycemia, particularly in the preschool period, appears warranted. Our data suggest that transient decreases in mental efficiency occur during even mild hypoglycemia under experimental conditions and are likely to occur at higher glycemic levels in younger children than adults (38). Recent data suggest that children with IDDM have relatively poorer school performance than their siblings (39). It is postulated that the reasons for this are multiple, such as chronic impairment of neuropsychologic function, transient cognitive difficulties as a result of asymptomatic hypoglycemia, or relatively frequent school absences. To avoid this situation, it is suggested that in very young children or those who cannot discern or express hypoglycemic symptoms, goals for glycemic control should probably be appropriately raised.

F. Cataracts

Although cataracts are not frequent, they are occasionally seen in large populations of diabetic children. The more common type of cataract, known as the sugar cataract, usually appears during recovery from an episode of ketoacidosis (40). These cataracts disappear rapidly with correction of the metabolic disorder, with subsequent normalization of the lens stucture. Occasionally, these cataracts do not disappear and persist over weeks or months, with the development of dense white opacities that may need surgical removal. The so-called sugar cataracts are thought to be a result of an abnormality of some osmotic mechanism in the lens. The "juvenile cataract" is caused by the accumulation of sorbitol in the presence of aldose reductase and ambient hyperglycemia (40). These cataracts are usually subcapsular because of the presence of aldose reductase in the lens epithelium and superficial cortical fibers. They always require surgical removal. It is not clear what characterizes those rare patients who develop cataracts under the same metabolic circumstances found in those who do not.

G. Necrobiosis Lipoidica Diabeticorum

This skin condition is thought to occur in about 0.3% of patients with IDDM, usually female, and it may actually occur before the onset of diabetes (41). It consists of round or oval indurated plaques, usually on the shins, with central atrophic areas and eventual ulceration. These lesions are painless unless they become secondarily infected. Although their pathogenesis is not understood and is thought to be unrelated to the adequacy of metabolic control, a recent study suggests a relationship with glycosylated hemoglobin. In addition, smoking, proteinuria, and retinopathy were found to be more common in patients with necrobiosis. This suggests an etiologic factor affecting the microvascular circulation. Treatment is controversial and difficult, with a number of medications being tried with varied success. The lesions are usually self-limiting (42).

H. Failure of Glucose Counterregulation and Hypoglycemic Unawareness

Hypoglycemic unawareness, usually associated with failure of the secretion of counterregulatory hormones (glucagon, catecholamines, and pancreatic polypeptide), was first described in adults with IDDM and was originally thought to be associated with prolonged duration of diabetes and possibly autonomic neuropathy (43,44). Over the past few years, the mechanism and frequency of hypoglycemia unawareness, impaired counterregulation, and decreased mental efficiency associated with hypoglycemia have been elucidated. Chronic autonomic neuropathy is unlikely to be involved but, rather, a vicious cycle of recurrent hypoglycemia inducing autonomic failure (45). Frequent mild episodes of hypoglycemia, which are often associated with very tight glycemic control as occurred in the intervention group of the Diabetes Control and Complications Trial (DCCT) (46), can, under experimental conditions, both induce failure of recognition of autonomic symptoms of hypoglycemia and impair the normal counterregulatory hormone responses to an hypoglycemic event (47). The loss of awareness of hypoglycemic symptoms, together with the inability to induce glucose counterregulation, is characteristic of subjects who have frequent and severe hypoglycemic events (48,49). Recent evidence in adults has shown that meticulous prevention of hypoglycemia for 2 weeks can reverse the abnormalities of symptom recognition and, in one study, the impaired counterregulatory hormone secretion in adults (50,51).

Most pediatricians have recognized hypoglycemic unawareness in their patients for many years. This is more frequent in very young children, presumably because of difficulty in expression of symptoms. Anecdotal experience has suggested that this syndrome is related to the presence of frequent hypoglycemia or the slow onset of hypoglycemia. Recent data suggest that hypoglycemic unawareness is more frequent than previously thought and that many children and adolescents may be totally unaware of hypoglycemic symptoms until changes in mental function occur. Although we have found little correlation between hypoglycemic symptoms and the increment of catecholamine secretion during hypoglycemia, most patients with total unawareness have poor counterregulatory hormone responses (52,53). As in adults, children with IDDM have very poor glucagon responses to hypoglycemia (54), which is stimulus specific (55). Decreased glucagon secretion is already present at diagnosis in children with IDDM (56), and its severity does not appear to be related to the duration of diabetes (54). Acute improvements in glycemic control do not affect glucagon responses to hypoglycemia, but they diminish catecholamine responses (52), similar to the situation described in adults (57). The syndromes of hypoglycemic unawareness and defective glucose counterregulation place patients with IDDM at great risk for the development of severe hypoglycemia. The exact pathogenesis of how prior hypoglycemia induces these syndromes is unknown, but these appear to be reversible in young patients by prevention of antecedent hypoglycemia.

IV. CHRONIC COMPLICATIONS

The chronic complications of IDDM relate mostly to the micro- and macrovascular systems. The most common and most devastating complications are those associated with microvascular disease of the retina and kidney. Although it is possible that microvascular disease can explain some of the pathogenesis of neuropathy, it has become increasingly clear that abnormalities of sorbitol and myoinositol metabolism play important roles. Microvascular disease, which can also be detected in the subungual capillaries of the fingers and toes (58), may explain a large proportion of heart disease seen in patients with IDDM in adulthood (59). Macrovascular disease, probably related to hyperlipoproteinemia, and abnormalities in the clotting mechanism result in peripheral vascular disease, coronary artery disease, and cerebrovascular accidents, all of which are excessively common in adults with IDDM (60).

Improved techniques for the evaluation of chronic diabetes complications have resulted in the documentation of subclinical manifestations of the chronic complications of diabetes in the childhood years. Although there is no proof that these subclinical abnormalities always predict overt clinical manifestations, it is clear that overt disease is preceded by a period of subclinical disease and that these abnormalities start in the pediatric diabetes population. Al-

though there is now clear evidence that improved glycemic control with intensive diabetes therapy can prevent or delay the progression of subclinical complications (46), a major question remains as to why some patients progress to renal failure and blindness, whereas others, with apparently similar metabolic control, escape all chronic complications of IDDM (61). The lack of uniformity in the course of diabetes complications has given rise to various hypotheses on the pathogenesis of these complications.

A. Pathogenesis

It is probable that more than one mechanism is involved in the development of the microvascular complications of IDDM. The thickened capillary basement membrane is the microscopic hallmark of the lesions of the microvasculature in IDDM. This is associated with alterations in membrane permeability and also occlusion of the microvasculature. The major clinical consequences of these lesions are seen in the retina and kidney, and possibly the nerves, although alterations in the capillaries throughout the body can be seen. A number of biochemical mechanisms that could produce these abnormalities have been postulated, which may be interactive or affect various tissues differently. As a result of insulin deficiency, there are abnormal concentrations of intermediary metabolities of glucose, fat, and amino acids (62). Hypercholesterolemia and hypertriglyceridemia, with abnormalities of high-density lipoproteins (HDL_2 and HDL_3), as well as low-density lipoproteins (LDL) and alterations of apolipoproteins, are well-known associates of insulin deficiency. These may relate to the pathogenesis of macrovascular disease in IDDM, although direct evidence of this association is not yet available (63). In addition, roles for hemodynamic, hormonal, genetic, and environmental factors are also possible (Fig. 1).

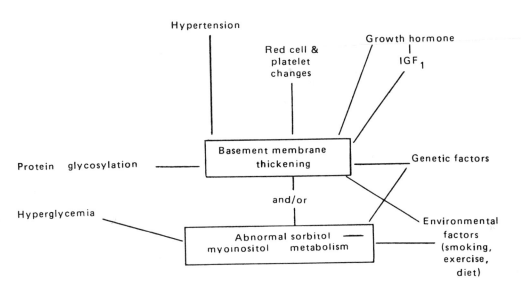

Figure 1 Postulated mechanisms of the pathogenesis of microvascular disease.

1. Glucotoxic Theory and Glycosylation

There is a large body of epidemiologic research supporting previous animal experiments that suggested that diabetes complications are a direct result of the metabolic abnormalities associated with IDDM as represented by hyperglycemia. The "glucotoxic" theory suggests that tissues are damaged by glucose excess and that glycemic control should prevent microvascular abnormalities. The recent conclusion of two large intervention studies has now provided the evidence that we needed in humans to confirm that the complications of diabetes are preventable by meticulous attention to metabolic control (46,64). Because blood and urine glucose concentrations are the easiest measures of metabolic control, glycemic control has been used synonymously with metabolic control. However, it should be remembered that IDDM is a disorder of insulin deficiency with a number of other metabolic derangements. There is considerable evidence that hyperglycemia, per se, can alter circulating and tissue proteins and affect tissue metabolism. Glycosylation of hemoglobin has been known since 1968 (65), but this phenomenon has only been used for evaluation of glycemic control since the late 1970s. Since then, it has been shown that this posttranslational nonenzymatic glycosylation involves protein of collagen, lens crystalline, nerve myelin proteins, lipoproteins, and even DNA (62,66). The Amadori glycosylation products are now known to be chemically reversible, with equilibrium reached in weeks. After prolonged hyperglycemia, probably 4–8 weeks, some of these glycosylation products undergo slow chemical rearrangements to form irreversible advanced glycosylation end products (AGP) (67,68). These AGPs accumulate slowly on extracellular matrix and vascular intracellular proteins with a low physiologic turnover rate and a nonlinear dependence on glucose concentrations. They cause structural tissue alterations, including progressive occlusion of diabetic vessels and interference with site-specific interactions among basement membrane structural components (69). Irreversible glycosylation of lipoproteins resulting in covalent cross-linking to matrix proteins may explain macrovascular disease in diabetes. This glycosylation may also account for alterations in the charge of the proteoglycan component of the basement membrane, with a persistent increase in leakage of negatively charged proteins from the plasma. Also, alterations of size-selective pores in the glomeruli could result in protein leakage. Glycosylation may account for increases in basement membrane thickness, which is a hallmark of microvascular disease in IDDM. The measurement of basement membrane thickness in the capillaries of skeletal muscle has resulted in much controversy (70,71), but it is probable that this thickening can already be identified in children with IDDM (72). There has been no clear correlation between the degree of thickness of skeletal muscle capillary basement membrane and the presence or absence of microvascular complications of IDDM, and reversibility has not been studied in childhood.

Another possibly important effect of AGPs is interference with gene transcription. Amadori products have been identified in endothelial cells from diabetic patients and may be involved in the induction of strand breakage in DNA (66,69). This may explain the "hyperglycemic memory" resulting in microvascular changes in experimental dogs 2 years after a period of hyperglycemia (73).

2. Intracellular Metabolic Abnormalities

Before the development of long-term irreversible metabolic and structural changes, hyperglycemia induces acute intracellular abnormalities. These cause abnormal vascular leakage and vasoreactivity. Microvascular hypertension occurs before the development of systemic hypertension in such organs as the kidney. The best known of the acute intracellular abnormalities involve the polyol or sorbitol pathway. Sorbitol accumulates in a number of tissues, especially lens and nerve, in the presence of hyperglycemia. Sorbitol is enzymatically formed from glucose during its metabolism to fructose under the influence of aldose reductase. The hyperglycemia-related increased flux through the polyol pathway is associated with decreased myoinositol uptake and decreased Na, K-ATPase activity. This metabolic abnormality has been described most clearly in the nerve, but it may also pertain to other tissues (62,74). Hyperglycemia is also associated with abnormalities of the diacylglycerol pathway and protein kinase C overactivity. These changes have been related to increased permeability and resultant increased pressure and leakage in blood vessels. Increased release of vasoconstrictive prostanoids is also described, and decreased Na, K-ATPase activity appears to decrease the release of the endothelium-derived relaxation factor, nitric oxide (Fig. 2) (69).

3. Rheology

Abnormalities of blood rheology associated with defective metabolism of red cells and platelets are well described and may be a mechanism by which both macro- and microvascular disease occur. There is increased red blood cell aggregation and decreased deformability, both of which could result in blockage of small capillaries. The mechanism may be glycosylation of the cell membranes or alterations of intracellular constituents. In addition, abnormalities of hemoglobin oxygen affinity, possibly caused by glycosylation or by decreased 2,3-dyphosphoglycerate, have been suggested to play a role in the development of retinopathy. Increased platelet stickiness has been described to be associated with abnormalities of the coagulation and fibrinolytic systems, with elevation of fibrinogen levels and other antithrombotic factors as well as prostaglandin metabolism (62,75,76).

4. Blood Pressure

Cross-sectional epidemiologic studies have suggested a strong relationship between the presence of hypertension and that of microvascular disease (60,77). These epidemiologic data have been strengthened by small intervention studies in which reversal of hypertension with drug therapy was shown to slow the progression of nephropathy (78). It has been shown that the mean blood pressure is higher in IDDM subjects with microvascular complications than in those who do not have complications, even at levels not conventionally defined as hypertension. Slightly increased blood pressure levels associated with both retinopathy and microalbuminuria have been

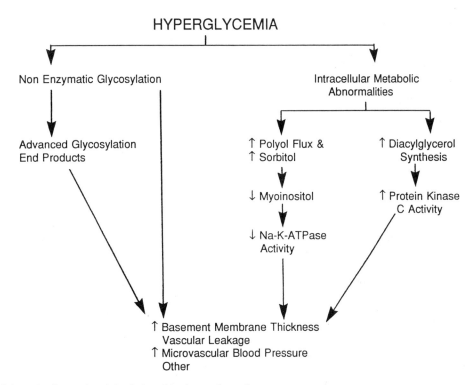

Figure 2   Potential mechanisms of toxicity induced by hyperglycemia.

described even during childhood and adolescence (79,80). It has been postulated that hemodynamics rather than metabolic factors are the major pathogenic factor resulting in diabetic glomerulopathy (81). Increased blood flow with elevated afferent arteriolar pressure, even without systemic hypertension, is suggested to play a major role in the development of nephropathy (81). These altered renal hemodynamics, which may be associated with glomerular hyperfiltration, are possibly related to protein intake (77,81). Renal hemodynamic changes may also be explained by altered prostaglandin production (82).

5. Growth Factors

Paracrine growth factors and the hormonal milieu may modulate the development of the complications of IDDM. In addition to basement membrane thickening, excessive growth of endothelial cells to form microvessels occurs in diabetes, the prime example being proliferative retinopathy. This angiogenesis is thought to be under the control of tissue growth factors, such as insulin and IGF-I. Other growth factors may also be involved including fibroblast growth factor, platelet-derived growth factor, and transforming growth factor β. Because these growth factors act in a paracrine or autocrine manner, local concentrations are not detectable in the circulation (83). The elevated growth hormone levels that are pathognomonic of poorly insulinized subjects with IDDM have long been thought to be a factor in the development of proliferative retinopathy, which has led to hypophysectomy as a treatment modality in the past (84). Although the elevated growth hormone levels described in IDDM are thought to be

related to decreased production of IGF-I, IGF-I levels have been reported as normal or low (23,24). A further apparent paradox is a report of elevated IGF-I concentrations in the serum in patients with retinopathy (85). Growth hormone, which is inceased by large amounts of protein intake and is elevated during puberty, may also play a pathogenic role in renal hyperfiltration as well as enhanced platelet aggregation (86,87). The increase in growth hormone and sex hormones associated with the onset of puberty may explain the apparent effect of puberty on the prevalence of subclinical microvascular complications. Rogers and coworkers have summarized data that show increased retinopathy in older children compared with younger children with IDDM of similar duration, and they have related this to pubertal staging (88). We and others have shown similar data for albuminuria, and an effect of puberty has been suggested in subclinical neuropathy (89–91). Our data show that postpubertal duration of diabetes has a greater relationship to the prevalence of complications than total duration (90). In addition, puberty has been associated with increased skeletal muscle capillary basement membrane width (92). The hypothesis that sex hormones play a role in the development of complications has been pursued by Williamson and associates in animal studies, showing that increased vascular permeability and abnormal polyol metabolism are sex steroid dependent in diabetic rats (93).

6. Genetic Susceptibility

Although there is increasing evidence that lower glycosylated hemoglobin levels are associated with less chronic complications of IDDM (46,80), not all patients with poor glycemic control develop severe complications of IDDM, and vice versa. It seems possible that there is variable genetic susceptibility to the metabolic effects of IDDM. The work of Marks et al. (94), showing increased basement membrane thickness in parents of children with IDDM has been interpreted to show that basement membrane thickening may be a familial characteristic unrelated to hyperglycemia. By contrast, other investigators (95) have shown increased basement membrane thickening in patients who developed IDDM as a result of the ingestion of a rodenticide, Vacor. In these subjects whose β cell destruction was caused by an exogenous agent rather than an autoimmune process, hyperglycemia appears to have been the mechanism rather than a genetic predisposition to develop IDDM.

A number of workers have attempted to find a relationship between the histocompatibility antigen (HLA) system and microvascular complications of diabetes. Although one report suggested that HLA-DR4, together with poor diabetes control, was found more often in patients with retinopathy than those with no retinopathy, other authors have not been able to confirm this relationship. There is as yet no good evidence linking the susceptibility to the development of diabetes complications to the HLA system (96,97). Another possible genetic mechanism for the predisposition to develop retinopathy and nephropathy has been explored recently. It has been suggested that markers for a genetic predisposition to the development of hypertension may be increased in patients with overt nephropathy (98,99). In these studies, sodium-lithium transport in red cells was increased in patients with nephropathy compared with those without nephropathy (99). Patients with IDDM who had a parent with hypertension had a tripled risk for the development of diabetic nephropathy (98). However, this concept is not supported by other researchers (100, 101). In a pediatric study, sodium-lithium countertransport was most strongly related to metabolic control (102). This supports our own data showing a strong relationship between circulating insulin levels and sodium-lithium countertransport (103). None of these studies were able to show a strong relationship between sodium-lithium transport and actual blood pressure.

7. Environmental Factors

There is increasing evidence suggesting familial clustering of the development of complications in IDDM (104). It is not always possible to separate the effects of genes and environment in family studies. In twin studies, lack of concordance of complications is common, suggesting environmental influences in addition to genetic inheritance (105,106). Some of our own epidemiologic data suggest that participation in team sports, physical activity, and smoking play roles in the development of complications (107–109). Although a role for smoking has been confirmed by other investigators (110), it did not appear to be a major factor in differentiating those subjects who had overt complications after 25 years of diabetes compared with those who had none (111).

It seems unlikely that anyone of the foregoing mechanisms is the sole producer of diabetic complications. More likely, there is interaction between many of the metabolic and other influences that are already known and more likely to be discovered in the future.

B. Retinopathy

Retinopathy is the most common microvascular change seen in patients with IDDM. In cross-sectional studies, more than 90% of patients eventually have some degree of retinopathy detected by sensitive techniques, such as stereo fundus photography or fluorescein angiography (80,112,113). The progression to blindness is not uniform, however, and varies between 20 and 55% in different series (60). Diabetes accounts for 10–20% of all cases of blindness and is its most frequent single cause in adults, estimated as responsible for 12,000–24,000 of new cases of blindness in the United States each year (114). Retinal photocoagulation, which began in the mid-1970s, has been a major advance in the prevention and treatment of advanced retinopathy. In the Early Treatment Diabetic Retinopathy Study, laser therapy of macular edema produced significant reductions in subsequent loss of vision (115). Although laser therapy of preproliferative retinal changes was of little benefit, this group showed major beneficial effects of laser therapy on proliferative retinopathy in the prevention of new vision loss. Therefore, it is important to detect retinopathy early and observe its progression carefully. In addition to ophthalmologic examination by the diabetes physician at each clinical examination, a well-trained diabetologist or ophthalmologist should examine the patient through dilated pupils at least annually after 5 years of diabetes duration in the postpubertal child and every 6 months once moderate background retinopathy is detected. Without dilatation, the severity of retinopathy is correctly identified in only 50% of eyes (116). It has been suggested that retinopathy is detectable approximately 2 years earlier by fundus photography or fluorescein angiography than by an expert ophthalmologist (112,117). Fluorescein angiography has the advantage over stereo fundus photography in that it is able to detect vascular leakage and is slightly more sensitive in the detection of rare microaneurysms, which are the earliest signs of retinopathy (118). Vitreous fluorophotometry has been used on a research basis to quantitate this leakage in some studies in childhood, abnormalities being found in 40% of patients fairly early in the disease (119). Nonmydriatic seven-field stereoscopic fundus photography has been reported to be as accurate and sensitive as an ophthalmologist's examination (120), although less sensitive in a community setting (121). From a clinical point of view, it is not clear whether very early detection of one or two microaneurysms is important or whether or how frequently dilated fundus photography should be performed in childhood and adolescence.

A number of systems have been developed to classify or grade diabetic retinopathy. These classifications are dependent on accurate photography using stereoscopic retinal color photographs or fluorescein angiograms. *Background retinopathy* or *nonproliferative retinopathy* is defined as the presence of microaneurysms only or as microaneurysms plus rare blot hemorrhages or hard exudates. As this progresses, there may be questionable soft exudates, venous beading, or venous dilatation. *Nonproliferative retinopathy with macular edema* includes these changes plus retinal thickening and increasing hard exudates with macular edema. The next level, which is also still considered background retinopathy, includes more hard exudates and definite soft exudates with intraretinal microvascular abnormalities (IRMA). The next stage is the more severe *preproliferative diabetic retinopathy*, with extensive hemorrhages and microanuerysms seen in a large number of photographic fields, with more soft exudates, definite venous beading, and IRMA. *Proliferative vascular disease* is the development of new vessels and fibrous proliferation on the macula and elsewhere. Although there appears to be a natural progression through these stages of retinopathy, there are as yet no longitudinal studies to determine the predictive value of any one of these stages for vision-threatening disease in childhood (Table 2).

A number of cross-sectional studies have been undertaken to document the prevalence of retinopathy in childhood IDDM. These studies have examined associations between retinopathy and demographic factors, glycemic control, and hypertension to attempt to understand factors that might affect the pathogenesis and progression of retinopathy. Despite differences in cohort selection, results of prevalence have been surprisingly similar. Most studies have found very few patients who have at least one microaneurysm within the first 2 years of the diagnosis of IDDM. Thereafter, there is a progressive increase in the prevalence of microanuerysms associated with both age and duration of IDDM, with the prevalence affected by pubertal status. Less retinopathy is seen in prepubertal children than in pubertal children with disease of long duration. Children with onset of diabetes in the older age group are more likely to develop background retinopathy earlier in the disease (88,112). Microanuerysms are seen in less than 20% of children with IDDM for fewer than 5 years. In our population of consecutive patients studied 5 years after diagnosis, in 12.7% at least one microaneurysm was detected by fluorescein angiography (122). In most studies, approximately 60% of patients with IDDM for duration of 5–10 years have background retinopathy. After 10 years, background retinopathy is seen in about 80–90% of patients (80,112,113,117).

Microanuerysms may appear and disappear because of variable perfusion and capillary remodeling, even without any change in glycemic control. Numerous epidemiologic studies in the past decade have confirmed the importance of glycemic control and blood pressure as risk factors for the frequency, severity, and progression of retinopathy (123). In our early studies of a cohort of patients between the ages of 14 and 18 years with diabetes that was diagnosed 8 years or more previously, 64% had retinopathy, with a clear relationship between the degree of retinopathy and glycemic control as measured by glycosylated hemoglobin over the prior 2 years (124). When followed over time, those patients with the highest glycosylated hemoglobin values had the most rapid advance in the retinopathy over the subsequent 2 years (125). The close correlation between the incidence and progression of diabetic retinopathy over 2–4 years has been reported in a number of studies of both adults and adolescents (126–128). The pathogenic importance of the significant associations between glycemic control and retinopathy were ultimately proven by the final outcome of the DCCT (46). In this study, intensive diabetes therapy reduced the mean glycosylated hemoglobin over a 9 year period, with a resultant significant decrease in the onset and progression of retinopathy in IDDM patients. In the 125 adolescent participants in this study, the onset of clinically important retinopathy was delayed by 50% compared with the conventionally treated group, and in those who already had some retinopathy, its progression was decreased by 59%. The results in the adolescents were very similar to those in the overall cohort (129). In this study there was initial deterioration in retinopathy after the rapid improvement in glycemic control during intensive therapy in subjects with initial high glycosylated hemoglobin levels. This has been noted in other intervention studies, and the mechanism is unclear (14,130,131).

Hypertension is a well-known risk factor for retinopathy in diabetes (132). Even slightly increased blood pressure levels, not defined as hypertension, have been associated with the incidence of retinopathy and its progression in adolescents and adults (79,80,127,133). Although it has been suggested that hypertension is a risk factor for retinopathy only in the face of nephropathy (134), antihypertensive treatment with captopril was reported to reverse abnormalities of the blood-retina barrier permeability to fluorescein (135). Thus, antihy-

Table 2 Madison Modification of Airlie House Classification of Diabetic Retinopathy

	Definitions of retinopathy levels
Level 1	No retinopathy
Level 2	Microaneurysms only
Level 3	Microaneurysms plus one more of retinal hemorrhages but < Standard Photo 2A[b], or hard exudates < Standard Photo 3, or questionable soft exudates, questionable venous beading, or other definite venous changes
Level 4	Microaneurysms plus one or more of hemorrhages/microaneurysms but ≥ Standard Photo 2A, hard exudates ≥ Standard Photo 3, definite soft exudates, definite intraretinal microvascular abnormalities, definite venous beading (but not meeting level 5 requirement)
Level 5	In retinal fields not including disk and macular regions any three of hemorrhages/microaneurysms ≥ Standard Photo 2A, definite soft exudates in ≥two fields, definite venous beading in ≥two fields, or definite intraretinal microvascular abnormalities ≥ Standard Photo 8A in ≥two fields and present four fields
Level 6	New vessels and/or fibrous proliferations on disk or elsewhere or photocoagulation scars or vitreous hemorrhage obscuring fundus

pertensive therapy may benefit retinopathy as well as nephropathy.

Proliferative retinopathy is extremely rare in prepubertal children and was reported in only 10% of adolescents with retinopathy (112). It is our experience that with improved glycemic control over the past decade, proliferative retinopathy in adolescents is now extremely rare.

Variations in the severity and prevalence of retinopathy with apparently similar long-term metabolic control have aroused interest in possible genetic or environmental risk factors. Several studies have suggested an association between retinopathy and the HLA antigens DR3 and DR4 (136,137); others have not been able to confirm these associations (138,139). If there is a role for circulating immune complexes in the development of retinopathy, this could explain the recent confirmation of an association between Gm types and retinopathy (140). The importance of genetic markers is suggested by the concordance of retinopathy in identical twins. However, those that are discordant for complications suggest nongenetic factors (105,106). Smoking is described as a risk factor for proliferative retinopathy (109).

C. Nephropathy

Renal failure remains the most common cause of death in patients with IDDM, contributing to more than 50% of deaths from diabetes at age 25–40 years in our population of childhood-onset IDDM (141). Overt nephropathy occurs in 30–40% of patients with IDDM, with the average onset of macroproteinuria at 10–15 years and renal failure by 20 years after the onset of the disorder (142). The cumulative incidence of diabetic nephropathy, as manifested by persistent albuminuria, in patients with diabetes duration of 25 years has been reported to have decreased markedly within the past decade (143). This coincides with our clinical impression of a decreasing frequency of overt proteinuria in our adolescent population. End-stage renal disease is rarely, if ever, seen in childhood IDDM. However, overt proteinuria occurs in patients with disease of long duration and usually in very poor glycemic control. The prevalence of overt proteinuria in recent studies varies between 0 and 2% (144–148). Patients with nephropathy have much poorer survival rates than those without proteinuria, with increased mortality from causes in addition to renal failure (149), and proteinuria appears to be the most important prognostic feature for morbidity and mortality in IDDM (150).

Clinically, nephropathy is defined by the leakage of large amounts of albumin in the urine. *Overt nephropathy* is defined as urinary protein excretion of 500 mg/day or more, which is equivalent to a urinary albumin excretion rate (AER) of about 300 mg/day, or 200 μg/minute. Overt nephropathy is associated with glomerulosclerosis on histopathologic examination (77). Clinical proteinuria usually identifies patients who will progress to severe renal failure within a period of 7–20 years without intervention. In patients with established nephropathy, the variable rate of progression of decreasing glomerular filtration to frank renal failure is probably influ-

enced by blood pressure and diet rather than metabolic control (77). Overt nephropathy is preceded by the excretion of smaller amounts of albumin detected by microtechniques, that is, *microalbuminuria* (77,151). This microalbuminuria is defined as a period of incipient nephropathy with urinary AER of 20–200 μg/minute or 30–300 mg/24 h. Although small prospective studies in adults suggested that microalbuminuria of varying degrees predicts subsequent development of overt nephropathy (77,152), this is not universal (153,154). In our experience of a childhood onset cohort of IDDM patients, which is similar to that of others, microalbuminuria and even overt nephropathy may regress without intervention (155, 156). However, incipient nephropathy usually progresses through a number of subclinical and clinical stages, as described in Table 3.

Because elevations of AER into the "microalbuminuria" range may be transient (147), clinically significant microalbuminuria possibly representing incipient nephropathy is defined as a urine AER in the microalbuminuric range in two of three consecutive samples. Exercise and posture affect renal albumin excretion, resulting in large day-to-day variations (151). For this reason, particularly during adolescence, a number of investigators prefer an overnight rather than a 24 h period urine collection, because this is easier to obtain and provides the least intraindividual variation (157). Single urine samples with measurement of albumin-creatinine ratio are convenient for the patient, but values predicting microalbuminuria are very variable (158). This variability is expected when one considers the variations in creatinine clearance associated with muscle mass and gender (159). We await long-term studies to determine which of these urine collection methods yields the best specificity and sensitivity for the prediction of clinical nephropathy.

Other markers of subclinical diabetic nephropathy include an increase in renal size, which may or may not correlate with increased glomerular filtration rate (GFR). An early increase of GFR of more than 150 ml/minute has been suggested as predictive of subsequent renal failure (77). This concept was confirmed in a study of children and adolescents followed for up to 20 years, in whom glomerular hyperfiltration was a risk factor for overt nephropathy as well as microalbuminuria,

Table 3 Classification of Nephropathy

Subclinical	
Stage I	Renal hypertrophy with raised GFR
Stage II	Histologic changes of basement membrane thickening and mesangial expansion
Stage III	Incipient nephropathy; albumin excretion rate 20–200 μg/minute
Overt	
Stage IV	Dipstix proteinuria with albumin excretion rate > 200 μg/minute with or without hypertension
Renal failure	
Stage V	Uremia and hypertension

irrespective of glycemic control. About 50% of the patients with increased GFR did not develop microalbuminuria or overt nephropathy, however, suggesting that glomerular hyperfiltration is one of a number of factors that are important in the pathogenesis of clinical nephropathy (160). A low or declining GFR is the hallmark of incipient renal failure. Although this is usually preceded by overt albuminuria, there is a recent report of low GFR and documented severe glomerular pathology in IDDM patients with normal urine AER (161). Creatinine clearance is the most common method for the measurement of GFR, but it consistently results in overestimations (77). Therefore, radionuclide techniques are probably far more accurate and are easier to perform than the standard insulin clearances of the last decade. Currently, radionuclide measurements of GFR remain a research tool in childhood IDDM without clinical nephropathy.

The pathogenesis of proteinuria in diabetes is related to hemodynamic factors and size- and charge-selective abnormalities of the glomerular capillary filtration barrier. Neutral dextran clearance studies have shown that in the early stages of nephropathy proteinuria is mainly a result of the loss of barrier charge selectivity (162), and this is corrected by improvement of glycemic control (163). The abnormal barrier size and charge selectivity result in increased excretion of proteins other than albumin, which are demonstrable in the adolescent age group, such as IgG and β_2-microglobulin (164), lysozyme, and N-acetyl-β-D-glucosaminidase (NAG) (165,166). In a study of young adults with intermittent or mild microalbuminuria, there was a close relationship between change in basement membrane thickening during improvement of glycemic control and the protein selectivity index (163,167).

Histopathologic glomerulosclerosis is recognized in approximately 90% of patients with IDDM for more than 15 years, irrespective of the presence of proteinuria (142). This consists of increased basement membrane thickness and expansion of the mesangium, often with the appearance of solid structures in the glomeruli. One group has reported that some histopathologic changes may be seen soon after the diagnosis of IDDM (168). There is already an accumulation of basement membrane material in the glomeruli with increased glomerular size. Progression of basement membrane thickening can occur after only a few years of IDDM, even before the presence of increased urine albumin excretion. Cross-sectional studies suggest a gradual progression of pathologic abnormalities with duration of IDDM, although this relationship is not universally found. In one small study there was no relationship between albumin excretion and structural changes (169), although in another study young adults with microalbuminuria were reported to have clear histopathologic abnormalities compared with nondiabetic subjects, which correlated with glycosylated hemoglobin (170). There is also a very close correlation in early diabetes between enlargement of the filtration surface and GFR. Glomerular occlusion is present in a variable proportion of patients with increased albumin excretion. Increased albuminuria is associated with more advanced glomerular lesions. Abnormalities of the renal arterioles progress together with the degree of

glomerular occlusion. An unusual dissociation between the degree of structural abnormalities and proteinuria has also been described, no structural parameters precisely predicting albumin excretion rate. Some patients with severe glomerulopathy have been shown to have normal AERs (161).

Like retinopathy, microalbuminuria is related to the duration of diabetes and is more common in postpubertal adolescents. Although it is rare before 5 years of IDDM duration (89,147) in clinic populations, its presence before 5 years duration has been reported from the Eurodiab Study (171,172). In a cohort study of 62 children with IDDM followed for 5 years in Pittsburgh, 21% had an albumin excretion rate of more than 20 μg/minute (122). The 5 year mean glycosylated hemoglobin measurements were slightly higher in these patients than those with a normal AER. In a later study, another group found microalbuminuria in 6 of 72 children with IDDM duration less than 5 years, with no relationship to glycemic control or blood pressure (148). The group reported microalbuminuria to be present in 10% of diabetic children under the age of 12 years, compared with 20% over this age. At 5 years duration, the albumin excretion rate was significantly higher in diabetic children older than 12 years than the younger ones (89,173). A similar relationship between microalbuminuria and puberty has been confirmed by others (144,174). Overall prevalence rates of microalbuminuria of 10–33% have been reported in a variety of studies of children and adolescents with IDDM, with the higher rates in earlier studies (89,145–147,164,175–177). The prevalence of microalbuminuria in our childhood-onset cohort followed in the Epidemiology of Diabetes Complications Study (EDC) was 14% for those less than 18 years of age and greater than 5 years diabetes duration (144). In this study with prolonged duration of diabetes up to 30 years, 80% of males and over 50% of females had either micro- or macroalbuminuria (80). Thus, with prolonged duration of IDDM, most patients have evidence of microvascular renal damage, but not all develop renal failure. This prevalence is higher than that reported from a multiclinic survey of single urine collections in Europe (171).

In the first incidence study of microalbuminuria from onset to 15 years duration in children, the cumulative incidence was 24% (148). Although there was no relationship between the relative risk of developing microalbuminuria within the first 5 years and the mean glycosylated hemoglobin in those who developed microalbuminuria after 5 years, the mean glycosylated hemoglobin was higher in the initial 5 years than in the normoalbuminuric group (148). A number of other studies have shown that there is a strong association between glycosylated hemoglobin and microalbuminuria. In the Wisconsin study, the risk of developing microalbuminuria was twice as high in patients in the highest quartile of glycosylated hemoglobin distribution compared with those in the lowest quartile (175). This type of association has been demonstrated in children attending diabetes clinics (134,178) and in a population-based study in Norway (146). In another childhood study, it has been suggested that the maintenance of glycosylated hemoglobin levels less than 1.5 times the normal range, or standard deviations above the normal mean resulted in a significantly lower risk for developing nephropathy (179). Surprisingly, the association between the level of glycemic control and microalbuminuria has not been found in a number of other investigations in the pediatric population (89,145,147). The DCCT study has finally proven that microalbuminuria and overt nephropathy can be delayed or prevented by intensive diabetes therapy (46). In the adolescent cohort of the DCCT, the occurrence of microalbuminuria was decreased by 55% over the 9 years of the study in the intensive therapy group (129). In this study there was no acceleration of albumin leakage with the onset of improved control associated, unlike the situation with retinopathy. However, we have reported the appearance of overt proteinuria in patients after rapid increases of insulin therapy who had been in very poor control (180).

Although glycemic control is important in the development and progression of microalbuminuria, a number of other factors are probably also major factors in the development of nephropathy. A significant role of hypertension in the rapid deterioration of renal function and the effectiveness of antihypertensive therapy have been shown in adult studies with decreases in the rate of decline of GFR (77). Antihypertensive treatment in both hypertensive and nonhypertensive patients has been reported to decrease AER (77,181). Similar to findings in retinopathy, increased blood pressures have been associated with microalbuminuria and its progression to overt nephropathy (80,153). As in adult studies, children and adolescents with microalbuminuria have higher blood pressures than those with normoalbuminuria (89,146,176,182, 183). In their incident study, Rudberg et al. found no difference in frequently obtained blood pressure readings in children and adolescents who developed microalbuminuria compared with those who did not (148). This supports two other studies that suggest that persistent microalbuminuria precedes elevations in blood pressure by 2–3 years (147,160, 184). Thus, incipient nephropathy may precipitate hypertension that may be exacerbated in families with a genetic predisposition to hypertension with elevated sodium-lithium countertransport. As previously mentioned, however, this concept is controversial (98–101). In an adolescent population, sodium-lithium countertransport was related to glycemic control rather than microalbuminuria, although there was a correlation between levels in IDDM subjects and their siblings (102).

Another metabolic abnormality that is associated with nephropathy is the frequent hyperlipidemia that is characteristic of IDDM. Increases in total and LDL cholesterol and triglyceride levels are well known in individuals with overt nephropathy (185). Only two of numerous cross-sectional studies have found a significantly higher LDL cholesterol level in microalbuminuric individuals (186,187). We have found that elevated LDL cholesterol and triglyceride levels are predictive of subsequent microalbuminuria in our EDC study (153). We have also found a number of patients whose overt nephropathy or microalbuminuria has regressed, the major predictive factor for this regression being decreased LDL cholesterol (156). Lipid abnormalities documented during the stage of incipient nephropathy suggest a possible role

of dyslipidemia in the pathogenesis of nephropathy. In animal models, cholesterol feeding resulted in albuminuria in spontaneously hypertensive rats and in the obese Zucker rat. Hypertriglyceridemia preceded the development of proteinuria and glomerular injury (188,189). This raises the possibility that drugs that lower cholesterol may improve albuminuria. However, a recent small placebo-controlled intervention study over 12 weeks in adults with IDDM proved negative (190).

A controversial issue is the possible relationship between protein in the diet and microalbuminuria. Although there is little disagreement on the role of low-protein diets in the treatment of chronic renal failure, a reduction in protein intake in the incipient nephropathic stage may or may not be useful. Protein restriction has been shown to decrease hyperfiltration in rats (191). In IDDM adults with overt proteinuria, protein restriction has been shown to slow the rate of decline of GFR significantly over 3–5 years (192). In microalbuminuric patients, dietary protein restriction has decreased AER in short studies (193) and in an adult study of longer duration (194). It is possible that substitution of animal protein with vegetable protein would have a similar effect as very low protein diets (195,196). There are no long-term studies of low-protein diets in children. Because of the importance of sufficient nutritional protein content in growing children, severe protein restriction below 15% of daily calories is probably not currently justified in the treatment of children and adolescents with IDDM. However, excessive protein intake should be avoided.

Although there is some controversy regarding the role of glycemic control as a risk factor for microalbuminuria in cross-sectional studies, the accumulating incidence data and the efficacy of glycemic intervention suggest an important role for glycemic control for the development of incipient and overt nephropathy. This supports findings in animal experiments in which transplantation of normal kidneys into diabetic rats resulted in the development of glomerulopathy. In addition, islet cell transplantation into diabetic rats markedly reduced the structural lesions of diabetes in the kidney. In humans, normal kidneys transplanted into diabetic recipients developed hyaline arteriolar lesions within the first few years (97). Two kidneys transplanted from diabetic subjects into nondiabetic recipients showed reversal of basement membrane thickening and mesangial expansion in renal biopsies taken 7 months later (197). Despite these data, success in reversing overt proteinuria in adults with intensive insulin therapy has been poor (198); it may be too late to reverse the structural abnormalities at this stage. Thus, prevention of progression to microalbuminuria and from microalbuminuria to overt proteinuria is important. One could conclude that glycemic control is important in the structural changes of diabetic nephropathy early in the disease. The modulating effect of hypertension, hyperlipidemia, and environmental factors, such as smoking, may occur later. Cross-sectional relationships between smoking and albuminuria have been reported in adults and in children with IDDM (109,110,153, 196,199). Cigarette smoking has been reported to be an important factor associated with progression of nephropathy in treated hypertensive type I diabetic patients (200).

D. Neuropathy

1. Peripheral Neuropathy

Clinical manifestations of peripheral neuropathy are unusual in children and adolescents with IDDM. In our large clinic population, we have seen clinical peripheral neuropathy in only two or three patients over the past 20 years, which was associated with very poor contol; symptoms markedly improved with appropriate insulin therapy. In our EDC study, careful history and physical examination elicited a clinical neuropathy prevalence of 34% in the total cohort including only 3% of 65 children less than 18 years of age, 18% between 18 and 29 years of age, and 58% over 30 years of age (201). This prevalence is similar to that found at baseline in the DCCT, a cohort that comprised a similar age range (202), and to the 20% prevalence rate reported by Allen for subjects age 16–29 years (203). The prevalence of clinical neuropathy in all studies was associated with both duration of diabetes and age.

Although clinical neuropathy is rare, subclinical neuropathy as assessed by decreased motor nerve conduction velocities and sensory changes is well described in diabetic children (91,204–206). These studies record subclinical functional changes in 50–72% of children and adolescents with close correlations with age and duration of IDDM. In addition, vibration perception threshold abnormalities were more frequent in postpubertal children (91). It is recognized that nerve conduction studies suffer from a number of sources of error, including patient variation. It is suggested that in patients with minimal symptomatology, the most susceptible nerves (i.e., the lower extremity sensory nerves) are more likely to reveal abnormalities than motor nerves. However, the absence of lower extremity abnormalities does not preclude the presence of structural abnormalities or subsequent neuropathy. Thus the prediction of the development of clinical neuropathy based on conduction impairment has not been established (207), and it appears advisable to continue to use multiple measures of neuropathy as recommended by the San Antonio Conference (208).

An independent relationship between neuropathy and glycosylated hemoglobin has been reported in some but not all studies (201,202,204,206,209) and may be limited to the postpubertal age group (91). A prospective study of 32 patients aged 12–36 years for 5 years after diagnosis showed that nerve conduction was slower, and temperature (but not vibration) thresholds were higher in the group with poorer glycemic control (210). The importance of the role of glycemic control in clinical neuropathy was underscored by the results of the DCCT in whom intensive diabetes therapy decreased clinical neuropathy by 60% (46). In the adolescent cohort, there were too few subjects with clinical neuropathy to assess an effect. However, peripheral motor and sensory nerve conduction velocities were significantly faster after 5 years of intensive therapy compared with conventional treatment (129). Some correlation between neuropathy and hyperlipidemia and smoking has also been suggested (201). No relationship has been demonstrated between the presence of motor or sensory nerve conduction abnormalities and microalbuminuria or retinopathy (204,211).

2. Autonomic Neuropathy

Clinically manifest autonomic neuropathy in childhood is even more rare than peripheral neuropathy. There are some isolated reports of gastroparesis, however, which are reversible by improved metabolic control (212,213).

Reliable measures of autonomic neuropathy are difficult. Sensitive measures of cardiovascular reflexes have been suggested as the most sensitive measures of subclinical autonomic neuropathy (214). However, these tests are difficult to carry out and expensive. Pupillometry has also been used in pediatric studies (215). The increased heart rate seen, especially in girls with IDDM, may be based on very early autonomic nervous system abnormalities (79). Autonomic neuropathy has been estimated as present in 30% of teenage subjects (215,216). It has been suggested that autonomic neuropathy may be a cause of hypoglycemic unawareness in older subjects with IDDM of long duration. However, it does not appear to be associated with this syndrome in younger and more recently diagnosed patients (45). We have failed to detect a relationship between glucose counterregulation and R-R interval measurements (211). In addition, pancreatic polypeptide responses in insulin-induced hypoglycemia, which has been described as a measure of autonomic neuropathy in adults (217), is markedly decreased in diabetic children compared with controls and shows no relationship with R-R variation (52,218).

3. CNS Changes

Central nervous system abnormalities have been detected by the increased prevalence of electroencephalographic (EEG) changes in children with IDDM (204,219–223). These changes are more likely to occur in children with diabetes onset under 5 years of age (222). Although a relationship between the amount of severe hypoglycemia experienced by the patients and the EEG abnormalities has been suspected, this has not been proved (221–223). A relationship between these EEG abnormalities and the frequency of seizures has not been shown. In studies including both children and adults, both impaired auditory and visual brain stem evoked potentials have been described (224,225). Significant abnormalities of visual evoked potentials were reported in 30% of 30 children with IDDM. Again, there was no relationship with duration of diabetes or metabolic control (226).

Cognitive impairment has been described in children with IDDM who were diagnosed under the age of 5 years (35–37). An increased frequency of neurobehavioral complications also described in adults with IDDM (227). This cognitive impairment has been confirmed by a number of groups, and although an association with prior repeated severe episodes of hypoglycemia has been reported, this is controversial (228). In a cross-sectional study of adults with IDDM who were part of our EDC cohort, IDDM subjects with one or more complications performed significantly more poorly on a cognitive battery than nondiabetic control subjects or IDDM subjects with no complications. This study confirmed an association between cognitive impairment and peripheral neuropathy but could find no independent association with recurrent hypoglycemia (228).

E. Cardiopathy

Cardiac abnormalities, eventually resulting in congestive failure, are well known in adults with IDDM (60) but are almost unknown in the pediatric age group. Ischemic heart disease and myocardial infarction are caused by changes in both the coronary and small vessels supplying the myocardium. Microvascular disease with microaneurysms, as well as thickened capillary basement membrane, have been shown in the hearts of patients with IDDM (60). These lesions probably account for the cardiomyopathy of IDDM patients. Noninvasive techniques have shown subclinical abnormalities in young children, despite the lack of symptomatology. These patients show a high prevalence of echocardiographic abnormalities, reflecting reduced myocardial performance that correlated with age but not with glycosylated hemoglobin values (7,229,230).

F. Macrovascular Disease

Macrovascular disease associated with atherosclerosis is clearly increased in diabetic patients (63). In the nondiabetic population, epidemiologic studies suggest a role for both genetic and environmental factors in the pathogenesis of antherosclerosis. A major influence of hyperlipoproteinemia associated with an increased quantity of dietary fat in the Western diet, as well as smoking and the lack of exercise, have been invoked as important risk factors. Our own studies have shown that the cardiovascular risk profile was already mildly disturbed in diabetic adolescents compared with their normal siblings (79). Slightly higher blood pressures, as well as higher total cholesterol levels, were seen. We were unable to explain these changes by the evaluation of diet, glycosylated homoglobin levels, or physical activity. Abnormalities were more common in girls than in boys. By contrast, only abnormalities of diastolic blood pressure in male diabetics compared with their siblings were reported by a British group (231). Hypercholesterolemia is frequently found in diabetic children, and most studies find a correlation with glycosylated hemoglobin values (232,233). The importance of the role of glycemic control is underscored by the findings in the adolescent participants in the DCCT, in whom total cholesterol levels were lower in the intensively than the conventionally treated groups (129). In these and other studies, HDL cholesterols were normal. Raised LDL cholesterol and reduced HDL cholesterol are also well established in adult IDDM populations (234). Cross-sectional studies have shown an association between increased lipid levels and microalbuminuria (187,235).

The risk factors for the 11-fold greater cardiovascular mortality in childhood-onset IDDM than age-matched controls (141) are thought to be related to altered lipoprotein concentrations. However, in our EDC population no lipid parameters predict coronary artery disease. Despite this, lipoprotein concentration disturbances are common and altered lipoprotein metabolism may be related to atherogenesis. Examples of potential mechanisms are glycosylation and oxidation of lipoproteins (63). Although lipoprotein (a) is increased in IDDM, our studies showing a lack of association between lipoprotein (a) levels and cardiovascular disease in IDDM

(236) have been confirmed in a number of other reports. Hypertension is another major risk factor for cardiovascular disease in IDDM. This is particularly true in the presence of renal disease with overt proteinuria, which is a major risk factor for cardiovascular mortality (149). Clinically apparent coronary artery disease is extremely rare in adolescents with IDDM. However, there is a report of fatal myocardial infarction in diabetic patients less than 20 years of age in association with hypertension and hyperlipidemia (237).

Peripheral vascular disease is also extremely rare in the pediatric age group. Subclinical abnormalities have been described, including a significantly decrease in postischemic hyperemia in 28 children with IDDM (238). Transcutaneous oximetry has also shown peripheral vascular abnormalities that do not correlate with levels of glycosylated hemoglobin in diabetic children (239).

Peripheral vascular abnormalities, as measured by the ankle-arm blood pressure ratio, is rare until 25 years of diabetes duration in our EDC population and was shown to be related to LDL cholesterol and fibrinogen levels, but not nephropathy (234). An ultrasound study of the carotid arteries in children, adolescents, and young adults with IDDM showed intimal thickening compared with controls already in the pediatric age groups. The degree of thickening in children was related to age and duration of IDDM. There was no relationship with lipids or glycosylated hemoglobin (240). This study provides clear evidence of structural changes in large vessels that are already occurring in childhood.

G. Mortality

Studies in the 1970s and 1980s showed a 15-fold excess mortality in patients with IDDM (141,241). In a long-term study, 50% of patients with IDDM onset in childhood had died by 50 years of age. With improved therapy, however, these mortality rates have decreased. A large number of patients with IDDM live 40–50 years after the diagnosis, possibly related to genetic factors and improved metabolic control. A large Danish study has shown a trend toward decreased mortality rates (242). In three different populations, mortality rates were low before 10–15 years duration. Thereafter, there was a steep rise in mortality, renal failure being the major cause of death (141,150,243,244). In patients with diabetes duration less than 15 years, death is almost uniformly a result of acute causes, most unrelated to diabetes (141,245, 246). At our institution, diabetes-related acute mortality in childhood is almost totally related to ketoacidosis, but in the Norwegian experience hypoglycemia was equally common (1,246). Recently, differences in age-specific mortality rates, up to the age of 30 years, have been described, the United States and Japan experiencing higher death rates than Finland and Israel (243).

V. CAN THE CHRONIC COMPLICATIONS OF INSULIN-DEPENDENT DIABETES MELLITUS BE PREVENTED?

The numerous observational studies showing a relationship between glycemic control and microvascular complications of IDDM suggested that improved glycemic control might prevent these complications. These epidemiologic studies led to a number of relatively short-term, small intervention studies to assess the effect of improved glycemic control on the progression of microvascular complications. Many of these studies were too small or too short to provide conclusive results (123). The 1993 reports of the DCCT and Stockholm study provided data from large and long-term studies showing the indisputable value of intensive diabetes therapy in decreasing the risk of the development of microvascular complications in subjects with disease of short duration and decreasing the progression of these complications in patients in whom these were present at baseline (46,64). Intensive therapy significantly improved overall glycemic control over the 9 years of the study in both the adult and adolescent groups in the DCCT. Although normal HbA$_1$C levels were achieved in only 2% of the adolescent population, intensive therapy significantly reduced the onset and progression of retinopathy and microalbuminuria (129). Thus, it appears that the onset of microvascular complications and their progression to overt clinical manifestations should be preventable by excellent glycemic control. Unfortunately, an analysis of the relationship between mean glycosylated hemoglobin and the rate of progression of retinopathy in the intensive group did not show a specific breakpoint below which retinopathy did not progress. However, the relatively linear relationship suggests that, even in patients with poor glycemic control, improvement in glycosylated hemoglobin is associated with decreased risk of deterioration in retinopathy. The persistent increased incidence of severe hypoglycemia in the intensively treated group remains a major barrier to the widespread institution of tight glycemic control. Despite that there were no demonstrable long-term detrimental effects of severe hypoglycemia on cognitive function and measures of psychosocial well-being, hypoglycemia remains a major concern in terms of uncomfortable symptoms and accidents. Additional barriers to the universal implementation of intensive therapy are the well-known compliance and psychosocial issues that are characteristic of many patients with IDDM. Thus, although we can theoretically prevent or decrease the complications of IDDM with tight glycemic control, this may not always be possible in practice. Therefore, other treatment modalities of subclinical complications will continue to be important in our therapeutic regimens. Research into intervention measures other than tight metabolic control has expanded in the last decade, although studies in the pediatric age group are sparse. Thus, although it is clear that glycemic control should be as tight as possible, a role for other interventions, such as the use of antihypertensive agents and protein restriction, are not yet proven.

From our current knowledge, it is clear that hypertension should be treated early and aggressively to delay the progression of both nephropathy an retinopathy. In patients with overt diabetic nephropathy, antihypertensive treatment for 32–91 months decreased the rate of decline of GFR compared with pretreatment levels (247). Angiotensin converting enzyme (ACE) inhibitors have recently received increasing support for blood pressure control in patients with micro- or macro-albuminuria. ACE inhibitors reduce blood pressure and also

have been shown to decrease intraglomerular pressures in diabetic rats. There are now a large number of studies showing decreased albuminuria during treatment with ACE inhibitors compared with other antihypertensives and placebo controls. It appears that ACE inhibitors in humans also have an effect in addition to lowering of blood pressure (248). In adults with overt nephropathy and with hypertension, in about 75% at entry, ACE inhibitors decreased the risk of doubling serum creatinine levels and decreased the risk of progression to end-stage renal disease or death by 50%. The effect was independent of blood pressure control (249). There are also several reports of smaller studies showing decreased microalbuminuria in patients with IDDM with our without hypertension and diminished rates of progression to clinical albuminuria compared with placebo-treated control subjects (181,248,250,251). However, before placing all normotensive patients on ACE inhibitors, it should be remembered that a significant number of subjects with microalbuminuria do not progress to overt nephropathy (153,154). Although side effects of ACE inhibitors in these studies, such as the induction of hyperkalemia, were rare, the widespread use of these drugs in the pediatric age group with relatively mild microalbuminuria and normotension cannot be supported at this stage. However, treatment with ACE inhibitors seems advisable in those adolescents with slightly elevated blood pressures, particularly in the face of microalbuminuria. Another indication in the pediatric age group may be moderate microalbuminuria that does not revert to normal with improved glycemic control or in a patient in whom glycemic improvement cannot be achieved.

A number of studies have shown decreased urinary albumin excretion in IDDM patients during short-term protein restriction diets. In both overt nephropathy and incipient nephropathy, AER decreased (192,193). These findings have been supported by a long-term study in adults with microalbuminuria (194). As discussed in Chapter 41, because of the risk of protein deficiency inducing growth retardation and other metabolic abnormalities, very low protein diets are not advised in the pediatric age group (252). Rather, avoidance of protein intakes above the current recommendations of 15% of the calories should be advised. It is possible that vegetable proteins have less of a detrimental effect on renal function, and the consumption of a vegetarian diet allows high protein intakes in IDDM subjects with early nephropathy (195,196).

Because the sorbitol pathway, controlled by aldose reductase, is possibly related to a number of complications of diabetes, prevention of the progression of these complications using aldose reductase inhibitors has elicited a large amount of interest. Aldose reductase inhibitors have effects on nerve conduction, myoinositol uptake, and regeneration in nerves of diabetic rats. In addition in these rats, they also prevented cataracts, reduced basement membrane thickening, and decreased albuminuria. Clinical trials in humans have concentrated on the effects of neuropathy. Although early studies were inconclusive, recent reports suggest delay in progression or even reversal of mild autonomic and peripheral neuropathy with tolrestat. Although there is some toxicity with this drug, modifications of aldose reductase inhibitors may result in improved risk benefit ratios. Trials are underway to assess the effects of new aldose reductase inhibitors on neuropathy, retinopathy, and nephropathy (253–255). Another agent currently being tested in a multicentered, randomized double-blind study is aminoguanidine. This substance, which inhibits advanced glycosylation end products, has been very effective in decreasing complications of the eye, kidney, and nerve in the rat model (68).

A cure of IDDM, with total prevention of complications, is the goal of most of our patients. Pancreas or islet cell transplantation, when successful, could improve the quality of life with possible independence from exogenous insulin injections. However, this goal is not easy to achieve. In addition, the need for chronic immunosuppression, with its own side effects, may offset any potential benefits. For example, a significant decrease in glomerular filtration in patients with pancreas transplants compared with a control group has been ascribed to cyclosporine therapy (256), results that confirm previous experience (257). Measurements of glomerular structure 5 years after pancreas transplantation did not show significant benefit compared with a group of patients treated with insulin (256). This is in contrast to shorter term studies that suggested less mesangial expansion in patients who received pancreas transplants (258). Retinopathy was also no different in successfully pancreas-transplanted subjects compared to those in whom the transplant failed (259). Neuropathy was only slightly improved by pancreas transplantation after a 42 month period (260). Thus, it appears that if transplantation is to prevent the complications of IDDM, this must be performed before the development of clinical complications that appear to be difficult to reverse. A total cure with prevention of complications can only be envisaged with successful transplantation of encapsulated or otherwise protected islets.

The DCCT has demonstrated the importance and feasibility of long-term improved glycemic control in adolescents with IDDM. Although prepubertal children appear to be somewhat protected and severe hypoglycemia is likely to be more detrimental, one cannot apply the DCCT findings to this age group. At all ages, however, therapy should be aimed at achieving the best glycemic control possible for each individual. The modulating effects of hypertension, environmental influences, and genetic background should not be forgotten in our therapeutic strategies. Excessive dietary saturated fat and protein intake should be avoided and smoking should be strongly discouraged. The initial effects of IDDM on the microvasculature and nerve fibers seem to be functional and are reversible by tight metabolic control. These abnormalities later become structural and will be reversible only by new therapeutic modalities. Therefore, it seems that if chronic complications of diabetes are to be prevented, the time of intervention should be in the early years during childhood and adolescence before structural damage has occurred. The DCCT has shown us that although glycosylated hemoglobin levels in adolescents were higher than those of the adults, the intensive efforts on the part of the patients and the health care team were worthwhile (46,129). The therapeutic strategy in childhood diabetes is still to do the best that is possible for each individual patient in terms of glycemic control, prevention of hypoglycemia, and adaptation to life with a chronic illness.

REFERENCES

1. Scibillia J, Finegold D, Dorman J, Becker D, Drash AL. Why do children with diabetes die? Acta Endocrinol (Copenh) 1986; Suppl. 279:326–333.
2. Grgic A, Rosenbloom AL, Weber FT, Giordano B, Malone J, Schuster JJ. Joint-contracture—common manifestation of childhood diabetes mellitus. J Pediatr 1976; 88:584–588.
3. Rosenbloom AL. Skeletal and joint manifestation of childhood diabetes. Pediatr Clin North Am 1984; 31:569–589.
4. Brik R, Berant M, Vardi P. The scleroderma-like syndrome of insulin-dependent diabetes mellitus. Diabetes Metab Rev 1991; 7:120–128.
5. Monnier VM, Vishwanath V, Frank KE, et al. Relation between complications of type I diabetes mellitus and collagen-linked fluorescence. N Engl J Med 1986; 314:403–408.
6. Garg SK, Chase HP, Marshall G, et al. Limited joint mobility in subjects with insulin dependent diabetes mellitus: relationship with eye and kidney complications. Arch Dis Child 1992; 67:96–99.
7. Baum VC, Levitsky LL, Englander RM. Abnormal cardiac function following exercise in young insulin dependent diabetics. Diabetes Care 1987; 10:319–323.
8. Schnapf BM, Banks RA, Silverstein JH, et al. Pulmonary function in insulin-dependent diabetes with limited joint mobility. Am Rev Respir Dis 1984; 130:930–932.
9. Bouillon R. Diabetic bone disease. Calcif Tissue Int 1991; 49:155–160.
10. Jackson RL. Growth and maturation of children with insulin-dependent diabetes mellitus. Pediatr Clin North Am 1984; 31:545–567.
11. Brown M, Ahmed ML, Clayton KL, Dunger DB. Growth during childhood and final height in type I diabetes. Diabetic Med 1994; 11(2):182–187.
12. Clarke WL, Vance ML, Rogol AD. Growth and the child with diabetes mellitus. Diabetes Care 1993; 16:101–106.
13. Wise J, Kolb E, Sauder S. Effect of glycemic control on growth velocity in children with IDDM. Diabetes Care 1992; 15:826–830.
14. Daneman D, Drash AL, Lobes LA, Becker DJ, Baker LM, Travis LB. Progressive retinopathy with improved control in diabetic dwarfism (Mauriac syndrome). Diabetes Care 1981; 4:360–365.
15. McKenna MI, Herskowitz R, Wolfsdorf JI. Screening for thyroid disease in children with IDDM. Diabetes Care 1990; 13:801–803.
16. Riley WJ, Maclaren NK, Lezotte DC, et al. Thyroid autoimmunity in insulin-dependent diabetes mellitus: the case for routine screening. J Pediatr 1981; 99:350–354.
17. Drash AL, Field JB, Garces LY, et al. Endogenous insulin and growth hormone response in children with newly diagnosed diabetes mellitus. Pediatr Res 1968; 2:94–102.
18. Edge JA, Dunger DB, Matthews DR, et al. Increased overnight growth hormone concentrations in diabetics compared with normal adolescents. J Clin Endocrinol Metab 1990; 33:1356–1362.
19. Hansen AP. Normalization of growth hormone hyper-response to exercise in juvenile diabetics after "normalization" of blood sugar. J Clin Invest 1971; 50:1086–1091.
20. Menon RK, Arslanian S, May B, et al. Diminished growth

hormone-binding protein in children with insulin-dependent diabetes mellitus. J Clin Endocrinol Metab 1992; 74:934–938.

21. Arslanian S, Menon RK, Gierl AP, et al. Insulin therapy increases low plasma growth hormone binding protein in children with new onset type I diabetes. Diabetic Med 1993; 10:833–838.

22. Tamborlane WV, Sherwin RS, Koivisto V, et al. Normalization of the growth hormone and catecholamine response to exercise in juvenile-onset diabetic subjects treated with a portable infusion pump. Diabetes 1974; 28:785–788.

23. Blethen SL, Sargaent DT, Whitelow MG, Santiago JV. Effect of pubertal stage and recent blood glucose control on plasma somatomedin C in children with insulin dependent diabetes. Diabetes 1981; 30:868–872.

24. Lanes R, Becker B, Thorpe P, Lifshitz F. Impaired somatomedin generation test in children with insulin dependent diabetes mellitus. Diabetes 1985; 34:156–160.

25. Tamborlane WV, Hintz RL, Bergman M, et al. Insulin-infusion pump treatment of diabetes. Influence of improved metabolic control on plasma somatomedin levels. N Engl J Med 1981; 305:303–307.

26. Holly JMP, Dunger DB, Edge JA, et al. Insulin-like growth factor binding protein-1 levels in diabetic adolescents and their relationship to metabolic control. Diabetic Med 1990; 7:618–623.

27. Jivani SKM, Rayner PHGH. Does control influence the growth of diabetic children. Arch Dis Child 1973; 48:109–115.

28. Kjaer K, Hagen C, Sando SH, et al. Epidemiology of menarche and menstrual disturbances in an unselected group of women with insulin-dependent diabetes mellitus compared to controls. J Clin Endocrinol Metab 1992; 75:524–529.

29. Adcock CJ, Perry LA, Lindsell AM, et al. Menstrual irregularities are more common in adolescents with type I diabetes: association with poor glycemic control and weight gain. Diabetic Med 1994; 11:465–470.

30. Dunaif A, Graf M. Insulin administration alters gonadal steroid metabolism independent of changes in gonadotropin secretion in insulin-resistant women with the polycystic ovarian syndrome. J Clin Invest 1989; 83:23–29.

31. Poretsky L, Grigorescy F, Seibel M, Mosers AC, Flier JS. Distribution and characterization of insulin and insulin-like growth factor I receptor in normal human ovary. J Clin Endocrinol Metab 1985; 61:728–734.

32. Poretsky L, Kalin MF. The gonadotropic function of insulin. Endocr Rev 1987; 8:132–141.

33. Sharp SC, Diamond MP. Sex steroids and diabetes. Diabetes Rev 1993; 1:318–42.

34. Sherman LD, Rogers DG, Gabbay KH, et al. Pulsatility of luteinizing hormone during puberty is dependent on recent glycemic control. Adol Pediatr Gynecol 1991; 4:87–93.

35. Ryan C, Vega A, Drash A. Cognitive deficits in adolescents who develop diabetes early in life. Pediatrics 1985; 75:921–927.

36. Rovet JF, Ehrlich RM, Hoppe M. Specific intellectual deficits associated with early onset insulin dependent diabetes mellitus in children. Diabetes Care 1987; 10:510–515.

37. Golden MP, Ingersall GM, Brack CJ, et al. Longitudinal relationship of asymptomatic hypoglycemia to cognitive function in IDDM. Diabetes Care 1989; 12:89–93.

38. Ryan CM, Atchison J, Puczynski S, Puczynski M, Arslanian S, Becker D. Mild hypoglycemia associated with deterioration of mental efficiency in children with insulin dependent diabetes mellitus. J Pediatr 1990; 117:32–38.

39. Kovacs M, Goldston D, Lyengar S. Intellectual development in academic performance of children with insulin dependent diabetes mellitus: a longitudinal study. Dev Psychology 1992; 28:676–684.

40. Bron AJ, Cheng H. Cataract and retinopathy: screening for treatable retinopathy. Clin Endocrinol Metab 1986; 15:971–999.

41. Alexander S. Skin disorders associated with diabetes. In: Keen H, Jarrett J, eds. Complications of Diabetes. London: Edward Arnold, 1982:205–213.

42. Kelly WF, Nicholas J, Adams J, Mahmood R. Necrobiosis lipoidica diabeticorum: association with background retinopathy, smoking, and proteinuria. A case control study. Diabetic Med 1993; 10:725–728.

43. Amiel SA, Tamborlane WV, Sacca L, Sherwin RS. Hypoglycemia and glucose counterregulation in normal and insulin-dependent diabetic subjects. Diabetes Metab Rev 1988; 4:71–89.

44. Cryer PE, White NH, Santiago JV. The relevance of glucose counterregulatory systems to patients with insulin dependent diabetes mellitus. Endocr Rev 1986; 7:131–139.

45. Cryer PE. Iatrogenic hypoglycemia as a cause of hypoglycemia-associated autonomic failure in IDDM: a vicious cycle. Diabetes 1992; 41:255–260.

46. Diabetes Control and Complications Trial Research Group. The effect of intensive treatment of diabetes on the development and progression of long-term complications in insulin dependent diabetes mellitus. N Engl J Med 1993; 329:977–986.

47. Cryer PE, Fisher JN, Shamoon H. Hypoglycemia. Diabetes Care 1994; 17:734–755.

48. Gold AE, MacLeod KM, Frier B. Frequency of severe hypoglycemia in patients with impaired awareness of hypoglycemia. Diabetes Care 1994; 17:697–703.

49. White MH, Skor DA, Cryer PE, Bier DM, Levandoski L, Santiago JV. Identification of type I diabetic patients at increased risk for hypoglycemia during intensive therapy. N Engl J Med 1983; 308:485–491.

50. Dagogo-Jack SE, Rattarasarn C, Cryer PE. Dissociation of symptomatic and neuroendocrine responses to hypoglycemia in IDDM with hypoglycemia unawareness and during reversal of unawareness by avoidance of iatrogenic hypoglycemia. Diabetes 1994; 43:141A.

51. Finelli CG, Epifano L, Rambotti AM, et al. Meticulous prevention of hypoglycemia normalizes the glycemic thresholds and magnitude of most neuroendocrine responses to symptoms and cognitive function during hypoglycemia in intensively treated patients with short-term IDDM. Diabetes 1993; 42:1683–1689.

52. Hoffman RP, Singer-Granick C, Drash AL, Becker DJ. Plasma catecholamine responses to hypoglycemia in children and adolescents with insulin dependent diabetes. Diabetes Care 1991; 14:81–88.

53. Hoffman RP, Singer-Granick C, Becker DJ. Lack of relationship between hypoglycemic awareness and catecholamine response in insulin dependent diabetes. Pediatr Res 1987; 21:342A.

54. Singer-Granick C, Hoffman RP, Kerensky K, Drash AL, Becker DJ. Glucagon responses to hypoglycemia in children and adolescents with IDDM. Diabetes Care 1988; 11:643–649.

55. Hoffman RP, Singer-Granick C, Drash AL, Becker DJ. Abnormal alpha cell hypoglycemia recognition in children with insulin dependent diabetes. J Pediatr Endocrinol 1994; 7:225–234.

56. Hoffman RP, Arslanian S, Drash AL, Becker DJ. Glucagon and epinephrine deficiency in children and adolescents with new onset IDDM. J Pediatr Endocrinol 1994; 7:235–244.

57. Amiel SA, Sherwin RS, Simonson DC, Tamborlane WV. Effect of intensive insulin therapy on glycemic thresholds for

counterregulatory hormone release. Diabetes 1988; 37:901–907.

58. Tubianna-Ruf NN, Priollet P, Levy-Marchal CC, Czernichow P. Nailfold capillary microscopy. Pediatr Adol Endocrinol 1988; 17:98–104.

59. Factor SM, Okun EM, Minase T. Capillary micro-aneurysms in the human diabetic heart. N Engl J Med 1980; 302:384–388.

60. Keen H. Chronic complications of diabetes mellitus. In: Galloway JP, Patvin JH, Shuman CR, eds. Diabetes Mellitus. Indianapolis: Eli Lilly, 1988:178–305.

61. Raskin P, Rosenstock J. Blood glucose control and diabetic complications. Ann Intern Med 1986; 105:254–263.

62. Alberti KGM, Press CM. The biochemistry of the complications of diabetes mellitus. In: Keen H, Jarrett J, eds. Complications of Diabetes. London: Edward Arnold, 1982:231–270.

63. Donahue RP, Orchard TJ. Diabetes mellitus and macrovascular complications: an epidemiological prospective. Diabetes Care 1992; 15:1141–1153.

64. Reichard P, Nilsson BY, Rosenquist U. The effect of long-term intensified insulin treatment on the development of microvascular complications of diabetes mellitus. N Engl J Med 1993; 329:304–309.

65. Rahbar S. An abnormal hemoglobin in red cells of diabetics. Clin Chim Acta 1968; 22:296–298.

66. Mullokandov EA, Franklin WA, Brownlee M. DNA damage by the glycation products of glyceraldehyde-3-phosphate and lysine. Diabetologia 1994; 37:145–149.

67. Brownlee M, Cerami A, Vlassara H. Advanced glycosylation and products in tissue and the biochemical basis of diabetic complications. N Engl J Med 1988; 318:1315–1321.

68. Brownlee M. Glycation and diabetic complications. Diabetes 1994; 43:836–841.

69. Ruderman NB, Williamson JR, Brownlee M. Glucose and diabetic vascular disease. FASEB J 1992; 6:2905–2914.

70. Kilo C, Vogler N, Williamson JR. Muscle capillary basement membrane changes related to aging and to diabetes mellitus. Diabetes 1972; 21:881–905.

71. Siperstein MD, Unger RH, Madison LL. Studies of muscle capillary basement membrane in normal subjects, diabetic and prediabetic patients. J Clin Invest 1987; 47:1973–1999.

72. Raskin P, Marks JF, Burns H Jr, Plumer MD, Siperstein MD. Capillary basement membrane width in diabetic children. Am J Med 1975; 58:365–372.

73. Engerman RL, Kern TS. Progression of incipient diabetic retinopathy during good glycemic control. Diabetes 1987; 36:808–812.

74. Greene DA, Lattimer SA, Simon AAF. Sorbitol, phosphoinositides and sodium potassium-ATPase in the pathogenesis of diabetic complications. N Engl J Med 1987; 316: 599–606.

75. Lee P, Jenkins P, Bourke C, et al. Prothrombotic and antithrombotic factors are elevated in patients with type I diabetes complicated by microalbuminuria. Diabetic Med 1993; 10:122–128.

76. Watala C. Altered structural and dynamic properties of blood cell membranes in diabetes mellitus. Diabetic Med 1993; 10:13–20.

77. Mogensen CE, Schmitz A, Christensen CK. Comparative renal pathophysiology relevant to IDDM and NIDDM patients. Diabetes Metab Rev 1988; 4:453–483.

78. Mogensen CE. Long-term anti-hypertensive treatment inhibiting progression of diabetic nephropathy. BMJ 1982; 285: 685–688.

79. Cruickshanks KJ, Orchard TJ, Becker DJ. The cardiovascular risk profile of adolescents with insulin dependent diabetes mellitus. Diabetes Care 1985; 8:118–124.

80. Orchard TJ, Dorman JS, Maser R, et al. Prevalence of complications in IDDM by sex and duration. Pittsburgh Epidemiology of Diabetes Complications Study II. Diabetes 1990; 39:1116–1124.

81. Hostetter TH, Rennke HG, Brenner BM. The case for intrarenal hypertension in the initiation and progression of diabetic and other glomerulopathies. Am J Med 1982; 72:375–380.

82. Viberti GC, Benigni A, Bognetti E. et al. Glomerular hyperfiltration and urinary prostaglandins in type I diabetes mellitus. Diabetic Med 1989; 6:219–223.

83. Yue DK, McLenna N, Turtle JR. Pathogenesis of diabetic microangiopathy: the roles of endothelial cell and basement membrane abnormalities. A review. Diabetic Med 1992; 9:218–223.

84. Kohner EM. McLeod D, Marshall J. Diabetic eye disease. In: Keen H, Jarrett J, eds. Complications of Diabetes. London: Edward Arnold, 1982:99–108.

85. Merimee TJ, Zapf J, Froesch ER. Insulin-like growth factors: studies in diabetics with and without retinopathy. N Engl J Med 1983; 309:527–530.

86. Christiansen JS. On the pathogenesis of increased glomerular filtration rate in short term insulin dependent diabetes. Dan Med Bull 1984; 31:349–361.

87. Colwell JA, Halushka PV, Sarji K, et al. Altered platelet function in diabetes mellitus. Diabetes 1976; 25(2):826–831.

88. Rogers DG, White NH, Shalwitz RA, Palmberg P, Smith ME, Santiago JV. The effect of puberty on the development of early diabetic microvascular disease in insulin-dependent diabetes. Diabetes Res Clin Pract 1987; 3:39–44.

89. Dahlquist G, Rudberg S. The prevalence of microalbuminuria in diabetic children and adolescents and its relation to puberty. Acta Pediatr Scand 1987; 76:795–800.

90. Norris-Kostraba J, Dorman JS, Orchard TJ, et al. Contribution of diabetes duration before puberty to development of microvascular complications in IDDM subjects. Diabetes Care 1989; 12:686–693.

91. Sosenko JM, Boulton AJM, Dibrusly DB, et al. The vibratory perception threshold in young diabetic patients: associations with glycemia and puberty. Diabetes Care 1985; 8:605–607.

92. Sosenko JM, Miettinen OS, Williamson JR, Gabbay KH. Muscle capillary basement membrane thickness and long-term glycemia in type I diabetes mellitus. N Engl J Med 1984; 31:694–698.

93. Williamson JR, Chang K, Tilton RG, Kilo C. Sex steroid modulation of vascular leakage and collagen metabolism in diabetic rats. Pediatr Adol Endocrinol 1988; 17:12–17.

94. Marks JR, Raskin P, Stastny P. Increase in capillary basement membrane width in parents of children with type I diabetes mellitus, association with HLA-DR. Diabetes 1981; 30:475–480.

95. Feingold KR, Lee TH, Chung MY, Siperstein MD. Muscle capillary basement membrane width in patients with Vacor-induced diabetes mellitus. J Clin Invest 1986; 78:102–107.

96. Barnett AH, Pyke DA. The genetics of diabetes complications. Clin Endocrinol Metab 1986; 15:715–726.

97. Rosenstock J, Raskin P. Diabetes and its complications: blood glucose control vs genetic susceptibility. Diabetes Metab Rev 1988; 4:417–435.

98. Krolewski AS, Canessa M, Warram JH, et al. Predisposition to hypertension and susceptibility to renal disease in insulin-dependent diabetes mellitus. N Engl J Med 1988; 318:140–145.

99. Mangili R, Bending JJ, Scott G, Li KK, Gupta A, Viberti GC. Increased sodium-lithium countertransport activity in red cells of patients with insulin dependent diabetes and nephropathy. N Engl J Med 1988; 18:146–150.

100. Elving LD, Wetzels JFM, DeNobel E, Berden JHM. Eryth-

rocyte sodium-lithium countertransport is not different in type I (insulin dependent) diabetic patients with and without diabetic nephropathy. Diabetologia 1991; 34:126–128.

101. Jensen JS, Mathiesen ER, Norgaard K, et al. Increased blood pressure and erythrocyte sodium/lithium countertransport activity are not inherited in diabetic nephropathy. Diabetologia 1990; 33:619–624.

102. Crompton CH, Balfe JW, Balfe JA, Chatzilias A, Daneman D. Sodium-lithium transport in adolescents with IDDM. Relationship to incipient nephropathy and glycemic control. Diabetes Care 1994; 17:704–710.

103. Bunker CH, Wing RR, Mellinger AG, Becker DJ, Mathews KA, Kuller LH. Cross-sectional and longitudinal relationships of sodium-lithium countertransport to obesity, insulin and blood pressure in healthy premenopausal women. J Hum Hypertens 1991; 5:381–392.

104. Seaquist ER, Goetz FC, Rich S, Barbosa J. Familial clustering of diabetic kidney disease. Evidence for genetic susceptibility to diabetic nephropathy. N Engl J Med 1989; 320:1161–1165.

105. Ganda OP, Soeldner JS, Gleason RE, et al. Monozygotic triplets with discordance for diabetes mellitus and diabetic microangiopathy. Diabetes 1977; 26:469–479.

106. Leslie RDG, Pyke DA. Diabetic retinopathy in identical twins. Diabetes 1982; 31:19–21.

107. LaPorte RE, Dorman JS, Tajima N, et al. The Pittsburgh insulin dependent diabetes mellitus morbidity and mortality study: physical activity and diabetes complications. Pediatrics 1986; 78:1027–1033.

108. Moy CS, Krisk A, LaPorte RE, et al. Insulin dependent diabetes mellitus, physical activity and death. Am J Epidemiol 1993; 137:74–81.

109. Muhlhauser I, Sawicki P, Berger M. Cigatette smoking as a risk factor for macroproteinuria and proliferative retinopathy in type I (insulin-dependent diabetes). Diabetologia 1986; 29:500–502.

110. Couper JJ, Staples AJ, Cocciolone R, et al. Relationship of smoking and albuminuria in children with insulin dependent diabetes. Diabetic Med 1994; 11:666–669.

111. Orchard TJ, Dorman JS, Maser RE, et al. Factors associated with avoidance of severe complications after 25 years of IDDM: Pittsburgh Epidemiology of Diabetes Complications Study I. Diabetes Care 1990; 13:741–747.

112. Burger W, Hovener G, Dusterhus R, Hartman R, Weber B. Prevalence and development of retinopathy in children and adolescents with type I (insulin-dependent) diabetes mellitus. A longitudinal study. Diabetologia 1986; 19:7–22.

113. Klein R, Klein BEK, Moss SE, Davis ME, DeMets DL. The Wisconsin epidemiologic study of diabetic retinopathy. II. Prevalence and risk of diabetic retinopathy when age at diagnosis is less than 30 years. Arch Ophthalmol 1984; 102:520–526.

114. Will JC, Geiss LS, Wetterhall SF. Diabetic retinopathy. N Engl J Med 1990; 323:613.

115. Early Treatment Diabetic Retinopathy Study Research Group. Photocoagulation for diabetic macular edema: Early Treatment Diabetic Retinopathy Study Report 1. Arch Ophthalmol 1985; 103:1796–1806.

116. Moss SE, Klein R, Kessler SD. Comparison between ophthalmoscopy and fundus photography in determining severity of diabetic retinopathy. Ophthalmology 1985; 92:62–67.

117. Palmberg P, Smith M, Waltman S, et al. The natural history of retinopathy in insulin dependent juvenile-onset diabetes. Ophthalmology 1981; 88:613–618.

118. Diabetes Control and Complications Trial Research Group. Color photography vs fluorescein angiography in the detection of diabetic retinopathy in the Diabetes Control and Complications Trial. Arch Ophthalmol 1987; 105:1344–1351.

119. White NH, Waltman SE, Krupin T, Santiago JV. Reversal of abnormalities in ocular fluorophotometry in insulin-dependent diabetes after five to nine months of improved diabetic control. Diabetes 1982; 31:80–85.

120. Pugh JA, Wiley R, Tuley MR, et al. Diabetic retinopathy screening: the nonmydriatic camera performs better mydriatically. Diabetes 1990; 39(Suppl 1):17A.

121. Higgs ER, Harney BA, Kelleher A, Reckless JPD. Detection of diabetic retinopathy in the community using a nonmydriatic camera. Diabetic Med 1991; 8:551–555.

122. D'Antonio JA, Ellis D, Doft BH, et al. Diabetes complications and glycemic control. The Pittsburgh Prospective Insulin-Dependent Diabetes Cohort Study. Status report after 5 years of IDDM. Diabetes Care 1989; 12:694–700.

123. Becker DJ, Orchard TJ, Lloyd CE. Control and outcome: clinical and epidemiologic aspects. In: Kellner CJH, ed. Childhood Diabetes. London: Chapman and Hall, 1995:519–538.

124. Doft BH, Kingsley LA, Orchard TJ, Kuller L, Drash AL, Becker DJ. The association between long-term diabetic control and early retinopathy. Ophthalmology 1986; 91:763–769.

125. Drash AL, Kingsley LA, Doft B, et al. Observations on the effects of changing therapeutic strategies on metabolic status and microvascular complications. Pediatr Adol Endocrinol 1988; 17:206–214.

126. Klein R, Kleins BEK, Scott M, Moss MA, Davis MD, DeMets DL. Glycosylated hemoglobin predicts the incidence and progression of diabetic retinopathy. JAMA 1988; 260:2864–2871.

127. Lloyd CE, Klein R, Maser RE, Kuller ALH, Becker DJ, Orchard TJ. The progression of retinopathy over two years: the Pittsburgh Epidemiology of Diabetes Complications Study. J Diab Compl. In Press.

128. Weber B, Burger W, Hartmann R, Hovener G, Malchus R, Oberdisse U. Risk factors for the development of retinopathy in children and adolescents with type IA (insulin-dependent) diabetes mellitus. Diabetologia 1986; 29:23–29.

129. Diabetes Control and Complications Trial Research Group. Effect of intensive diabetes treatment on the development and progression of long-term complications in adolescence with insulin dependent diabetes mellitus: Diabetes Control and Complications Trial. J Pediatr 1994; 125:177–188.

130. Ballegooie E, van Hooymans JMM, Timmerman Z, et al. Rapid deterioration of diabetic retinopathy during treatment with continuous subcutaneous insulin infusion. Diabetes Care 1984; 7:236–242.

131. Dahl-Jorgensen K, Brinchmann-Hansen O, Hansen KF, Sandvik L, Aagenaes O. Rapid tightening of blood glucose control leads to transient deterioration in retinopathy in insulin dependent diabetes mellitus—the Oslo Study. BMJ 1985; 290:811–815.

132. West KM, Erdrich LJ, Stober JA. A detailed study of risk factors for retinopathy and nephropathy in diabetes. Diabetes 1980; 29:501–508.

133. Chase HP, Garg SK, Jackson WE, et al. Blood pressure and retinopathy in type I diabetes. Ophthalmology 1990; 97:155–159.

134. Norgaard K, Storm B, Graa E, Feldt-Rasmussen B. Elevated albumin excretion and retinal changes in children with type I diabetes are related to long-term poor blood glucose control. Diabetic Med 1989; 6:325–328.

135. Parving HH, Larsen M, Hommel E, et al. Effect of antihypertensive treatment on blood-retinal barrier permeability to fluorescein in hypertensive type I (insulin-dependent) diabetic patients with background retinopathy. Diabetologia 1989; 32:440–444.

136. Cruickshanks KJ, Vadheim CM, Moss SE, et al. Genetic

marker associations with proliferative retinopathy in persons diagnosed with diabetes more than 30 years of age. Diabetes 1992; 41:879–885.

137. Dornan TL, Ting A, McPherson CK, et al. Genetic suscepti- bility to the development of retinopathy in insulin dependent diabetics. Diabetes 1982; 31:226–231.

138. Barbosa J, Saner B. Do genetic factors play a role in the pathogenesis of diabetic microangiopathy? Diabetologia 1984; 27:487–492.

139. Bodinsky HJ, Wolf E, Cudworth AG, et al. Genetic and immunologic factors in microvascular disease in type I insulin dependent diabetes. Diabetes 1982; 31:70–74.

140. Stewart LL, Field LL, Ross S, McArthur RG. Genetic risk factors in diabetic retinopathy. Diabetologia 1993; 36:1293–1298.

141. Dorman JS, LaPorte RE, Kuller LH, et al. The Pittsburgh insulin-dependent diabetes mellitus morbidity and mortality study. Mortality results. Diabetes 1984; 33:271–276.

142. Deckert T, Paulsen JE. Diabetic nephropathy: fault or destiny? Diabetologia 1981; 21:178–183.

143. Bojestig M, Arnqvist HJ, Hermansson G, Karlberg BE, Ludvigsson J. Declining incidence of nephropathy in insulin dependent diabetes mellitus. N Engl J Med 1994; 330:15–18.

144. Becker DJ, Coonrod BA, Ellis D, et al. Influence of age, sex, blood pressure and glycemic control on microalbuminuria in children and adolescents with IDDM. In: Weber B, Berger W, Danner T, eds. Structural and Functional Abnormalities in Subclinical Diabetic Angiopathy. Basel: Karger, 1992:95–107.

145. Cook JJ, Daneman D. Microalbuminuria in adolescents with insulin-dependent diabetes mellitus. Am J Dis Child 1990; 144:234–237.

146. Joner G, Brinchmann-Hansen O, Torres CG, Hanssen KF. A nationwide cross-sectional study of retinopathy and microal- buminuria in young Norwegian type I (insulin-dependent) diabetic patients. Diabetologia 1992; 35:1049–1054.

147. Mathiesen ER, Saurbrey N, Hommel E, Parving HH. Preva- lence of microalbuminuria in children with type I (insulin-de- pendent) diabetes mellitus. Diabetologia 1986; 29:640–643.

148. Rudberg S, Ullman E, Dahlquist G. Relationship between early metabolic control and the development of microalbumin- uria—a longitudinal study in children with type I (insulin-de- pendent) diabetes mellitus. Diabetologia 1993; 36:1309–1314.

149. Borch-Johnsen K, Anderson PK, Deckert T. The effect of proteinuria on relative mortality in type I (insulin-dependent) diabetes mellitus. Diabetologia 1985; 28:590–596.

150. Borch-Johnsen K, Kreiner S, Deckert T. Mortality of type I (insulin-dependent) diabetes mellitus in Denmark: a study of relative mortality in 2930 Danish type I diabetic patients diagnosed from 1933 to 1972. Diabetologia 1986; 29:767–772.

151. Rosenstock J, Raskin P. Early diabetic nephropathy. Assess- ment and potential therapeutic interventions. Diabetes Care 1986; 9:529–545.

152. Mogensen CE, Christensen CK. Predicting diabetic nephrop- athy in insulin dependent patients. N Engl J Med 1984; 311:89–93.

153. Coonrod BA, Ellis D, Becker DJ, et al. Predictors of microalbuminuria in individuals with insulin dependent diabe- tes mellitus. The Pittsburgh Epidemiology of Diabetes Com- plication Study. Diabetes Care 1993; 16:1376–1383.

154. Forsblom CM, Groop PH, Ekstrand A, Groop LC. Predictive value of microalbuminuria in patients with insulin dependent diabetes of long duration. BMJ 1992; 305:1051–1053.

155. Almdal T, Norgaard K, Feldt-Rasmussen B, Deckert T. The predictive value of microalbuminuria in IDDM: a five-year follow up study. Diabetes Care 1994; 17:120–125.

156. Ellis D, Orchard T, Lloyd C, Becker DJ. Regression or improvement of diabetic nephropathy is associated with de- creased LDL cholesterol. Submitted.

157. Gatling W, Knight C, Hill RD. Screening for early diabetic nephropathy: which sample to detect microalbuminuria? Dia- betic Med 1985; 2:451–455.

158. Marshall SM. Screening for microalbuminuria: Which mea- surement? Diabetic Med 1991; 8:706–711.

159. Connell SJ, Hollis S, Tieszen KL, McMurray JR, Dornan TL. Gender and the clinical usefulness of the albumin:creatinine ratio. Diabetic Med 1994; 11:32–36.

160. Rudberg S, Persson B, Dahlquist G. Increased glomerular filtration rate as a predictor of diabetic nephropathy—an eight year prospective study. Kidney Int 1992; 41:822–828.

161. Lane PH, Steffes MW, Mauer SM. Glomerular structure in IDDM women with low glomerular filtration rate and normal urinary albumin excretion. Diabetes 1992; 41:581–586.

162. Deckert T, Kofoed-Enevoldsen A, Vidal P, Norgaard K, Andreasen HB, Feldt-Rasmussen B. Size and charge selectiv- ity of glomerular filtration in type I (insulin-dependent) diabetic patients with and without albuminuria. Diabetologia 1993; 36:244–251.

163. Bangstad HJ, Kofoed-Enevoldsen A, Dahl-Jorgensen K, Han- sen KF. Glomerular charge selectivity and the influence of improved blood glucose control in type I (insulin-dependent) diabetic patients with microalbuminuria. Diabetologia 1992; 35:1165–1169.

164. Ellis D, Becker DJ, Daneman D, Lobes L, Drash AL. Proteinuria in children with insulin-dependent diabetes: rela- tionship to duration of disease, metabolic control and retinal changes. J Pediatr 1983; 102:673–680.

165. Miltény IM, Körner A, Tulassay T, Szabó A. Tubular dysfunction in type I diabetes mellitus. Arch Dis Child 1985; 60:929–931.

166. Walton C, Bodansky HJ, Wales JK, Forbes MA, Cooper EH. Tubular dysfunction and microalbuminuria in insulin depen- dent diabetes. Arch Dis Child 1988; 63:244–249.

167. Bangstad HJ, Osterby R, Dahl-Jorgensen K, Berg KJ, Hart- mann A, Hanssen KF. Improvement of blood glucose control in IDDM patients retards the progression of morphological changes in early diabetic nephropathy. Diabetologia 1994; 37:483–490.

168. Osterby R. Structural changes in the diabetic kidney. Clin Endocrinol Metab 1986; 15:733–751.

169. Chavers MB, Bilous RW, Ellis EN, Steffes MW, Mauer SM. Glomerular lesions and urinary albumin excretion in type I diabetes without overt proteinuria. N Engl J Med 1989; 320:966–970.

170. Bangstad HJ, Osterby R, Dahl-Jorgensen K, et al. Early glomerulopathy is present in young type I (insulin-dependent) diabetic patients with microalbuminuria. Diabetologia 1993; 36:523–529.

171. Eurodiab IDDM Complications Study Group. Microvascular and acute complications in IDDM patients: the Eurodiab IDDM Complications Study. Diabetologia 1994; 37:278–285.

172. Stephenson J, Fuller J, Eurodiab IDDM Complications Study Group and the WHO Multinational Study Group. Microalbu- minuria is not rare before five years of IDDM. Diabetes 1994; 43(Suppl 1):28A.

173. Dahlquist G, Rudberg S. Microalbuminuria in diabetic chil- dren and adolescents and its relation to puberty. Pediat Adol Endocrinol 1988; 17:153–161.

174. Salardi S, Cacciari E, Pascucci MG, et al. Microalbuminuria in diabetic children and adolescents: relationship with puberty and growth hormone. Acta Pediatr Scand 1990; 79:437–443.

175. Klein R, Klein BEK, Linton KLP, Moss SE. Microalbumin-

uria in a population based study of diabetes. Arch Intern Med 1992; 152:153–158.

176. Mortensen HB, Marinelli K, Norgaard K, et al. A nationwide cross-sectional study of urinary albumin excretion rate, arterial blood pressure and blood glucose control in Danish children with type I diabetes mellitus. Diabetic Med 1990; 7:887–897.

177. Rowe DJF, Boggs H, Betts PB. Normal variations in rate of albumin excretion and albumin-to-creatinine ratios in overnight and daytime urine collections in non-diabetic children. BMJ 1985; 291:693–694.

178. Chase HP, Jackson WE, Hoops L, Cockertran RS, et al. Glucose control and the renal and retinal complications of insulin dependent diabetes. JAMA 1989; 261:1155–1160.

179. Roe TF, Costin G, Kaufman FR, Carlson ME. Blood glucose control and albuminuria in type I diabetes mellitus. J Pediatr 1991; 119:178–182.

180. Ellis D, Avner ED, Transue D, Yunis EJ, Drash AL, Becker DJ. Diabetic nephropathy in adolescence: appearance during improved glycemic control. Pediatrics 1983; 71:824–829.

181. Mathiesen ER, Hommel E, Giese J, Parving HH. Efficacy of captopril in postponing nephropathy in normotensive insulin dependent diabetic patients with microalbuminuria. BMJ 1991; 303:81–87.

182. Davies AG, Price DA, Poslethwaite RJ, Addison GM, Burn JL, Fielding BA. Renal function in diabetes mellitus. Arch Dis Child 1985; 60:299–304.

183. Mathiesen ER, Ronn B, Jensen T, Storm B, Deckert T. Relationship between blood pressure and urinary albumin excretion in development of microalbuminuria. Diabetes 1990; 39:245–249.

184. Microalbuminuria Collaborative Study Group, United Kingdom. Risk factors for development of microalbuminuria in insulin-dependent diabetic patients: a cohort study. BMJ 1993; 306:1235–1239.

185. Jensen T, Borch-Johnsen K, Kofoed-Enevoldsen A, Deckert T. Coronary heart disease in type I (insulin-dependent) diabetic patients with and without diabetic nephropathy: incidence and risk factors. Diabetologia 1987; 30:144–148.

186. Jensen T, Stender S, Deckert T. Abnormalities in plasma concentrations of lipoproteins and fibrinogen in type I (insulin-dependent) diabetic patients with increased urinary albumin excretion. Diabetologia 1988; 31:142–145.

187. Jones SL, Close CF, Mattock MB, et al. Plasma lipid and coagulation factor concentrations in insulin dependent diabetics with microalbuminuria. BMJ 1989; 298:487–490.

188. Cooper ME, Vranes DA, Panagiotopoulos S, et al. Hyperlipidemia increases albuminuria in hypertensive and normotensive rats. Clin Exp Pharmacol Physiol 1990; 17:225–228.

189. Kasiske BL, O'Donnell MP, Keane WF. The Zucker rat model of obesity. Insulin resistance, hyperlipidemia, and renal injury. Hypertension 1992; 19:110–115.

190. Hommel E, Anderson P, Gall MA, Nielsen N, et al. Plasma lipoproteins and renal function during simvastatin treatment in diabetic nephropathy. Diabetologia 1992; 35:447–451.

191. Zatz R, Meyer TW, Rennke HG, Brenner BM. Predominance of hemodynamic rather than metabolic factors in the pathogenesis of diabetic glomerulopathy. Proc Natl Acad Sci USA 1985; 82:5963–5967.

192. Walker C, Dodds, RA, Murrells TJ, et al. Restriction of dietary protein in progression of renal failure in diabetic nephropathy. Lancet 1989; 2:1411–1444.

193. Cohen D, Dodds R, Viberti GC. Effect of protein restriction in insulin dependent diabetics at risk of nephropathy. BMJ 1987; 294:795–798.

194. Dullart RP, Beusekump BJ, Meijer S, et al. Long-term effects of protein restricted diet on albuminuria and renal function in IDDM patients without clinical nephropathy and hypertension. Diabetes Care 1993; 16:483–492.

195. Jibani MM, Bloodworth LL, Foden E, et al. Predominantly vegetarian diet in patients with incipient and early clinical diabetic nephropathy: effects on albumin excretion rate and nutritional status. Diabetic Med 1991; 8:949–953.

196. Viberti GC, Yip-Messent J, Morocutti A. Diabetic nephropathy: future avenue. Diabetes Care 1992; 15:1216–1225.

197. Abouna GM, Al-Adnani MS, Kremer GD, Kumar SA, Daddah SK, Kusma G. Reversal of diabetic nephropathy in human cadaveric kidneys after transplantation into non-diabetic recipients. Lancet 1983; 2:1274–1276.

198. Bending JJ, Viberti GC, Watkins PJ, Keen H. Intermittent clinical proteinuria and renal function in diabetes: evaluation of the effect of glycemic control. BMJ 1986; 292:83–86.

199. Chase HP, Satish KG, Marshall G, et al. Cigarette smoking increases the risk of albuminuria among subjects with type I diabetes. JAMA 1991; 265:614–617.

200. Sawicki PT, Didjurgeit U, Muhlhäuser I, et al. Smoking is associated with progression of diabetic nephropathy. Diabetes Care 1994; 17:126–131.

201. Maser RE, Steenkiste R, Dorman JS, et al. Epidemiological correlates of diabetic neuropathy: report from Pittsburgh Epidemiology of Diabetes Complications Study. Diabetes 1989; 38:1456–1461.

202. DCCT Research Group. Factors in development of diabetic neuropathy: baseline analysis of neuropathy in feasibility phase of diabetes control and complications trial (DCCT) Diabetes 1988; 37:476–481.

203. Allen C, Duck SC, Sufitrl E, et al. Glycemic control and peripheral nerve conduction in children and young adults after 5 to 6 months of IDDM. Diabetes Care 1992; 15:502–507.

204. Dorchy H, Noel P, Kruger M, et al. Peroneal motor nerve conduction velocity in diabetic children and adolescents. Relationship to metabolic control, HLA-DR antigens, retinopathy and EEG. Eur J Pediatr 1985; 144:310–315.

205. Hoffman WH, Hart ZH, Frank RN. Correlates of delayed motor nerve conduction and retinopathy in juvenile onset diabetes mellitus. J Pediatr 1983; 102:351–356.

206. Käär, M-L, Saukkonen A-L, Pitkänen, Akerblom, HK. Peripheral neuropathy in diabetic children and adolescents. A cross-sectional study. Acta Paediatr Scand 1983; 73:373–378.

207. Greene DA, Brown MJ, Brounstein SN, Schwartz SN, Asbury AK, Winegrad AL. Comparison of clinical course and sequential electrophysiological tests in diabetes with symptomatic polyneuropathy and its implications for clinical trials. Diabetes 1981; 30:139–140.

208. Consensus Statement. Report and recommendation of the San Antonio Conference on Diabetic Neuropathy. Diabetes 1988; 37:1000–1004.

209. Young RJ, Ewing DJ, Clarke BS. Nerve function and metabolic control in teenage diabetics. Diabetes 1983; 32:142–147.

210. Ziegler D, Moyer P, Mühlen H, Gries FA. The natural history of somatosensory and autonomic nerve dysfunction in relation to glycaemic control during the first five years of diagnosis of type I (insulin dependent) diabetes mellitus. Diabetologia 1991; 34:822–829.

211. Becker DJ, Greene DA, Aono SA, et al. Assessment of subclinical autonomic and peripheral neuropathy in childhood insulin-dependent diabetes mellitus. Pediatr Adol Endocrinol 1988; 17:173–178.

212. Reid B, DiLorenzo C, Trains L, et al. Diabetic gastroparesis due to postprandial antral hypomobility in childhood. Pediatrics 1992; 90:43–46.

213. White N, Waltman S, Krupi T, et al. Reversal of neuropathic and gastrointestinal complications related to diabetes mellitus

in adolescents with improved metabolic control. J Pediatr 1981; 99:41–45.

214. Pfeiffer MA, Weinberg CR, Cook DL, et al. Autonomic neural dysfunction in recently diagnosed diabetic subjects. Diabetes Care 1986; 7:447–453.

215. Barkai L, Madacsy L, Kassay L. Investigation of subclinical signs of autonomic neuropathy in the early stages of childhood diabetes. Horm Res 1990; 34:54–59.

216. Ewing DJ, Clarke BS. Diabetic autonomic neuropathy: present insight and future prospects. Diabetes Care 1986; 9:648–665.

217. Hilsted J, Masbad S, Karup T, et al. No response of pancreatic hormones to hypoglycemia in diabetic autonomic neuropathy. J Clin Endocrinol Metab 1982; 56:815–819.

218. Singer-Granick C, Hoffman R, Waters T, Becker DJ. Pancreatic polypeptide counterregulation of children with IDDM. Diabetes (Suppl) 1986; 35:4A.

219. Eeg-Olofsson O. Hypoglycemia and neurological disturbances in children with diabetes mellitus. Acta Paediatr Scand (Suppl) 1977; 270:91.

220. Halonen N, Hiekkala H, Huupponen T, Hakkinen VK. A follow up EEG study in diabetic children. Ann Clin Res 1983; 15:167–172.

221. Haumont D, Dorchy H, Pelc S. EEG abnormalities in diabetic children. influence of hypoglycemia and vascular complications. Clin Pediatr 1979; 18:750–753.

222. Singer-Granick C, Crumrine P, Drash AL, Becker DJ. Electroencephalographic abnormalities in children with insulin-dependent diabetes. Pediatr Res 1985; 19:321A.

223. Soltesz G, Acsadi G. The association between diabetes, severe hypoglycemia, and electroencephalographic abnormalities. Arch Dis Child 1989; 64:992–996.

224. Fedele D, Martini A, Cardone C, et al. Impaired auditory brainstem-evoked responses in insulin-dependent diabetic subject. Diabetes 1984; 33:1085–1089.

225. Khodori R, Soler NG, Good DC, et al. Brainstem auditory and visual evoked potentials in type I (insulin-dependent) diabetic patients. Diabetologia 1986; 29:362–366.

226. Cirillo D, Gonfiantini E, Grandis DD, Bongiovanni L, Robert JJ, Pinelli L. Visual evoked potentials in diabetic children and adolescents. Diabetes Care 1984; 7:273–275.

227. Ryan C. Neurobehavioral complications of type I diabetes: examination of possible risk factors. Diabetes Care 1988; 11:86–93.

228. Ryan CM, Williams TM, Finegold DN, Orchard TJ. Cognitive dysfunction in adults with type I (insulin dependent) diabetes mellitus of long duration: effects of recurrent hypoglycemia and other chronic complications. Diabetologia 1993; 36:329–334.

229. Lababidi ZA, Goldstein DE. High prevalence of echocardiographic abnormalities in diabetic youths. Diabetes Care 1983; 6:18–22.

230. Friedman NE, Levitsky LL, Edidin DV, et al. Echocardiographic evidence for impaired myocardial performance in children with type I diabetes mellitus. Am J Med 1982; 73:846–850.

231. Tarn AC, Drury PL. Blood pressure in children, adolescents and young adults with type I (insulin dependent) diabetes. Diabetologia 1986; 29:275–281.

232. Becker DJ, Tsalikian E, Daneman D, Hengstenberg F, Drash AL. Plasma lipids and glycosylated hemoglobin in children with insulin dependent diabetes mellitus. Pediatr Adol Endocrinol 1981; 9:205–210.

233. Sosenko J, Spack N, Breslow JL, Mientinen O, Gabbay KH. Relationship of glycosylated HGB with cholesterol and LDL-cholesterol in insulin dependent diabetes. Diabetes 1978; 27:505.

234. Maser RE, Wolfson SK, Ellis D, et al. Cardiovascular disease and arterial calcification in insulin dependent diabetes mellitus: interrelations and risk profiles. Arteriosclerosis Thromb 1991; 11:958–965.

235. Jay RH, Jones SL, Hill CE, et al. Blood rheology and cardiovascular risk factors in type I diabetes: relationship with microalbuminuria. Diabetic Med 1991; 8:662–667.

236. Maser RE, Usher D, Becker DJ, et al. Lipoprotein (a) shows little relationship to IDDM complications in the Pittsburgh Epidemiology of Diabetes Complications Study cohort. Diabetes Care 1993; 16:755–758.

237. Declue TJ, Malone JI, Root AW. Coronary artery disease in diabetic adolescents. Clin Pediatr (Phila) 1988; 27:587.

238. Ewald J, Tuvemo T. Reduced vascular reactivity in diabetic children and its relation to diabetic control. Acta Paediatr Scand 1985; 74:77–84.

239. Arslanian S, Makaroon M, Moosa H, Johnson R, Drash A. Detection of subclinical vasculopathy in children with insulin dependent diabetes. Diabetes (Suppl) 1987; 36:767.

240. Yamasaki IY, Kawamori R, Matsushima H, et al. Atherosclerosis in carotid arteries of young IDDM patients monitored by ultrasound high-resolution B-mode imaging. Diabetes 1994; 43:643–649.

241. Deckert T, Paulsen JE, Larson M. Prognosis of diabetics with diabetes onset before age thirty one. Diabetologia 1978; 14:363–370.

242. Green A, Borch-Johnsen K, Krag H, Andersen P, et al. Relative mortality of type I (insulin-dependent) diabetes in Denmark: 1933–1981. Diabetologia 1985; 28:339–342.

243. Diabetes Epidemiology Research International Mortality Study Group. Major cross-country differences in risk of dying for people with IDDM. Diabetes Care 1991; 14:49–54.

244. Modan M, Karp M, Bauman B, Gordon O, Danon YL, Laron Z. Mortality in Israeli Jewish patients with type I (insulin-dependent) diabetes mellitus diagnosed prior to 18 years of age: a population based study. Diabetologia 1991; 34:515–520.

245. Diabetes Epidemiology Research International Mortality Study Group. International evaluation of cause-specific mortality and IDDM. Diabetes Care 1991; 14:55–60.

246. Joner G, Patrick S. The mortality of children with type I (insulin-dependent) diabetes mellitus in Norway, 1973–1988. Diabetologia 1991; 34:29–32.

247. Parving HH, Andersen AR, Smidt UM, et al. Effect of antihypertensive treatment on kidney function in diabetic nephropathy. BMJ 294:1143–1147.

248. Kasiske BL, Kalil RSN, Maj A, et al. Effect of antihypertensive therapy on the kidney in patients with diabetes: a metaregression analysis. Ann Intern Med 1993; 118:129–138.

249. Lewis EJ, Unsicker LG, Bain RP, Rohde RD. Collaborative Study Group. The effect of angiotension-converting enzyme inhibition on diabetic nephropathy. N Engl J Med 1993; 329:1456–1462.

250. Cook JJ, Daneman D, Spino M, et al. Angiotensen converting enzyme inhibitor therapy to decrease microalbuminuria in normotensive children with insulin dependent diabetes mellitus. J Pediatr 1990; 117:39–45.

251. Rudberg S, Aperia A, Freyschuss U, Persson B. Enalapril reduces microalbuminuria in young, normotensive type I (insulin-dependent) diabetic patients irrespective of a hypotensive effect. Diabetologia 1990; 33:470–476.

252. Brodsky IG, Robins DC, Hiser E, et al. Effects of low protein diet on protein metabolism in insulin dependent diabetes mellitus patients with early nephropathy. J Clin Endocrinol Metab 1992; 75:351–357.

253. Giugliano D, Marfella R, Quatraro A, et al. Tolrestat for mild

diabetic neuropathy: a 52-week, randomized, placebo control trial. Ann Intern Med 1993; 118:7–11.

254. Passariello N, Sepe J, Marrazzo G, et al. Effect of aldose reductase inhibitor (Tolrestat) on urinary albumin excretion rate and glomerular filtration rate in IDDM subjects with nephropathy. Diabetes Care 1993; 16:789–795.

255. Tomlinson DR. Aldose-reductase inhibitors and the complications of diabetes mellitus: a review. Diabetic Med 1993; 10:214–230.

256. Fioretto B, Mauer SM, Bilous RW, et al. Effects of pancreas transplantation on glomerular structures in insulin dependent diabetic patients with their own kidneys. Lancet 1993; 342: 1193–1196.

257. Morel P, Sutherland DER, Armand PS, et al. Assessment of renal function in type I diabetic patients after kidney, pancreas, or combined kidney-pancreas transplantation. Transplantation 1991; 51:1184–1189.

258. Bilous RW, Mauer SM, Sutherland DER, et al. The effect of pancreas transplantation on the glomerular structure of renal allografts in patients with insulin dependent diabetes. N Engl J Med 1989; 321:80–85.

259. Ramsey RC, Goetz FC, Sutherland DER, et al. Progression of diabetic retinopathy after pancreas transplantation for insulin dependent diabetes mellitus. N Engl J Med 1988; 318:208–214.

260. Kennedy WR, Navarro X, Goetz FC, et al. Effects of pancreatic transplantation on diabetic neuropathy. N Engl J Med 1990; 322:1031–1037.

41

Nutrition and Diabetes

Fima Lifshitz and Melanie M. Smith
*Maimonides Medical Center and State University of New York Health Science Center at Brooklyn,
Brooklyn, New York*

I. INTRODUCTION

The relationship between nutrition and diabetes mellitus (DM) has been apparent since the disease was first recognized. Prior to the discovery of insulin in 1922, dietary therapy was the only means to mitigate the symptoms of the disease. Periods of starvation and high-fat diets were used to circumvent the carbohydrate alterations by maximizing fat metabolism. Today, nutrition is recognized as an important factor in three different aspects of diabetes mellitus. Nutrition may: (1) contribute to the risk of diabetes; (2) influence the manifestations or complications of diabetes; and (3) affect the daily management of diabetes. In this chapter, we will review the role of nutrition in the etiology, complications, and daily management of diabetes mellitus.

II. NUTRITION AND RISK OF DIABETES MELLITUS

It was long suspected that nutrition played a major role in the development of diabetes mellitus. As the Japanese began to "westernize" their diet and life-style, the incidence of DM was coincidentally "westernized" (1). The establishment of Israel in 1948 was also followed by an increased incidence of diabetes mellitus among the new Eastern immigrants settling in a westernized Israeli culture (2). Similar observations have been noted in native American groups (3,4), in several other countries (5,6), and among aboriginal populations (7). After these groups adopted a dietary intake akin to ours, high in calories, fat, and refined sugars, coupled with a sedentary life-style, the incidence of diabetes mellitus increased more than 10-fold.

It has long been recognized that nutrition is linked to the increased risk of developing DM largely through the problem of obesity; the greater the degree and the longer the duration of the increased adiposity, the higher the risk of developing the disease in susceptible individuals (8). The search to elucidate whether excess caloric intake, type of carbohydrate, or dietary fat is the primary culprit dates back many years (2,6,9) but has not been resolved satisfactorily. The incidence of diabetes parallels increased sugar consumption (2,8,9), but this dietary change is usually associated with other factors such as high fat and high caloric intake as well as decreased exercise. Human studies suggest that sugar and fat may not be important contributing factors to the incidence of diabetes apart from their effects on levels of caloric consumption and adiposity (10). However, experimental animal models have demonstrated that refined sugars independently increase the risk of developing DM (11). A low fiber intake also appears to enhance the risk of DM (12).

The increased risk of developing DM associated with these dietary and life-style patterns primarily relates to type II diabetes or non-insulin-dependent DM (NIDDM). However, an increased incidence of type I diabetes or insulin-dependent DM (IDDM) was noted in association with the incorporation of "Western" dietary patterns in Japan (13). The etiology of IDDM is complex and appears to involve interactions of genetic, immunological, and environmental factors. Several nutritional factors have been implicated as risk factors for IDDM including high protein feedings (14), consumption of nitrosamines (15), and childhood coffee and tea consumption (16). Nitrosamines are toxic and are related to streptozotocin, which can induce pancreatic beta-cell damage. An analytical case-control study showed a dose-response relationship between the frequency of foods containing nitrosamine and the risk of IDDM before the age of 15 (17).

Feeding patterns in infancy, specifically early exposure to nonhuman milk proteins, may also be associated with IDDM. It has been reported that a large number of diabetic children were never breast-fed and were exposed to cow's milk or soy protein early in life (18,19). An intriguing hypothesis linking early exposure to cow's milk proteins to IDDM has been proposed. Bovine serum albumin (BSA), a protein found in the whey fraction of cow's milk, shows a short region of similarity to a specific pancreatic beta-cell surface protein, ICA69 (20). Based on a hypothesis of molecular mimicry, these two antigenic determinants, ICA69 and BSA, may play a role in the induction of cow's milk–induced B-cell autoimmunity (21). A Finnish study reported elevated serum levels of BSA antibodies in 100% of newly diagnosed diabetic children compared with <4% of control children (21) whereas another study described a similiar humoral response to ovalbumin in diabetic and nondiabetic children (22). Although the relevance of anti-BSA antibodies in the pathogenesis of IDDM has been questioned (23), other studies have shown a gene-environment interaction with a markedly higher risk of IDDM in children with the HLA-DQB1 marker who received cow's milk before age 3 months (24). A recent meta-analysis of 19 studies concluded that early exposure to cow's milk proteins results in a mildly (OR = 1.5) increased risk of subsequent type I diabetes (25). Current recommendations by the American Academy of Pediatrics encourage breast feeding for all infants, and in families with a history of IDDM, the avoidance of products containing intact cow's milk protein during the first year is also recommended (26).

Specific nutritional alterations may also play a role in the development of DM. Numerous studies have found alterations in the micronutrient status of IDDM patients, and deficiencies of micronutrients in these patients have been correlated with complications of the disease (27). However, the micronutrient status in diabetes is inconsistent (Table 1). There appears to be a link between diabetes and Mg deficiency, although the exact nature of that link, especially in terms of Mg status, glucose disposition, and the possible role of Mg deficiency in diabetic complications, needs further exploration (28–30). Vitamin E– and selenium-deficient diets increase the susceptibility to diabetogenic agents that act as oxidants or free radical producers (31,32). Marasmus or kwashiorkor in infancy is sometimes associated with pancreatic calcification, which may result in diabetes in later life. Although specific dietary deficiencies may result in impaired glucose tolerance, the amount of food and the total caloric intake remain the most important factors for an increased risk of DM. A quantitative reduction in food intake without qualitative changes has been shown to improve glucose control (33).

III. NUTRITION AND THE COMPLICATIONS OF DIABETES MELLITUS

A. Short-Term Complications

Nutrition plays an important role in the acute complications of diabetes. Food intake, along with physical activity or

Table 1 Micronutrient Status of Diabetic Patients

Micronutrient	Usual Levels in Blood	
	IDDM	NIDDM
Trace Elements		
Zinc (Zn)	–	–
Calcium (Ca)	–	NL
Magnesium (Mg)	–	–
Manganese (Mn)	– or NL	+[a]
Copper (Cu)	NL	NL or +
Iron (Fe)	NL	NL
Chromium (Cr)	+	NL
Selenium (Se)	+	?[c]
Vitamins		
1,25-dihydroxycholecalciferol	–	NL
B6	NL or –	NL or –
B12	NL or –	NL
C	NL or –	NL or –
Thiamin	?[c]	NL[b]
A	?[c]	NL
E	+	+

[a]Type of diabetes not specified.
[b]Increased in Japanese diabetics.
[c]Unknown
NL = neither increased or decreased; – = decreased; + = increased.
Source: Modified from Ref. 27.

illness, determines the presence or absence of hypoglycemia or hyperglycemia. Blood glucose levels are affected by the timing of meals and snacks, the period of time between insulin injection and food intake, and the frequency and content of foods consumed. Dietary factors have also been implicated in short-term metabolic consequences such as ketonuria.

Table 2 illustrates a frequent problem in IDDM patients who eat excessively. The patient shown was being treated with insulin twice daily, but this was considered insufficient since he exhibited marked hyperglycemia and glycosuria and had high glycosylated hemoglobin level. Increased insulin dosages did not resolve the problem. Glycosuria and high fasting blood glucose levels continued, yet he gained 6 kg in 12 months. Patients who are underinsulinized are in negative nitrogen balance and do not gain weight. This patient, who is gaining excessive weight, therefore is not lacking insulin; hence he must be overeating. Without changes in dietary intake and caloric expenditures, there will be no improvement in the control of the disease. Individualized nutritional therapy was helpful; excess weight gain ceased and improved glycemic control allowed reduced insulin dosages.

B. Long-Term Complications

The results of the Diabetes Control and Complications Trial (DCCT) have confirmed the importance of appropriate control

Table 2 Overeating in IDDM (Male patient diagnosed at age 3 10/12 yr.)

Date	Age	Weight (kg)	Insulin Dose kg/units/day	Time AM NPH	Reg	PM NPH	Reg	Glucose Blood	Urine	HgbA1C
April	5 10/12	31.0	0.97	7	6	5	2	>240	>4+	9.5 (n < 6.6)
September	6 3/12	32.5	1.05	18	7	6	3	' '	' '	9.4
February	6 8/12	35.1	1.09	20	7	7	3	' '	' '	
April	6 10/12	37.0	1.03	17	7	8	6	' '	' '	
				Nutritionist						
June	7 0/12	37.0	0.92	17	7	7	3	<240	3–4+	8.4 (n < 8)

of the disease (34; this volume, Chapter 40). The DCCT showed that intensive diabetes treatment resulting in lower blood glucose and glycosylated hemoglobin levels may delay the development and slow the progression of microvascular complications of diabetes compared with the standard diabetes treatment program. There was also a trend of fewer microvascular events in the intensive-treatment group. However, these benefits came at a price. The intensive diabetes treatment was associated with increased weight gain and 300% increase in the risk of severe hypoglycemia. Furthermore, despite the efforts of the highly skilled diabetes teams, less than 5% of those in the intensive group were able to achieve the goal of maintaining the serum glycosylated hemoglobin levels in the nondiabetic range. Still, the decrease in glycosylated hemoglobin attained was associated with less retinopathy progression. As the DCCT did not include children under 13 years or those with severe complications, intensive treatment for these patients should be considered on an individual basis (34).

Independently of the diabetic control of the patients, it has long been known that some of the long-term complications of diabetes were related to nutritional intake and genetic makeup (35,36). For example, diabetics in Japan have gangrene and coronary artery disease less frequently than Western diabetics. The diabetic Navajo Indians in America, the diabetic Nigerians in Africa, and diabetic Pacific populations also have a lower incidence of microvascular disease than do other populations with this disease. This may be related to the nutritional habits of these groups, i.e., lower intake of saturated fats, and possibly to genetic factors. However, in NIDDM a higher carbohydrate content of the diet produced deterioration of glycemic control, accentuation of hyperinsulinemia, and increased triglyceride and VLDL cholesterol levels (37).

1. Hypertension

The association of hypertension with diabetes exists in both IDDM and NIDDM. The presence of hypertension in diabetes doubles the risk for atherosclerotic events and increases the progression of nephropathy (38). Nutrition plays a multifactorial role in the development of this complication. In addition to obesity and sodium intake, there are other cations that affect the blood pressure of patients with or without diabetes (39,40). Studies using sophisticated 3P-NMR techniques have

suggested that alterations in intracellular Mg levels may partially explain the well-known association of NIDDM with obesity and hypertension (41). Other studies have found lower free intracellular Mg and ionized extracellular Mg in diabetic patients (42). Thus dietary interventions should consider weight control and/or sodium restriction and ensure adequate intake of other nutrients such as magnesium, potassium, and calcium. Increased physical activity is also a critical component of hypertension management.

2. Coronary Artery Disease

Coronary artery disease is the second leading cause of death for individuals with IDDM of greater than 30 years' duration (43). Data from the Multiple Risk Factor Intervention Trial indicated that men with diabetes compared to nondiabetic men had an increased relative risk of death ranging from 2.83 to 4.46 depending on their level of serum cholesterol (44). Many of the risk factors for atherosclerosis and coronary artery disease identified in population studies are overrepresented in diabetes. Plasma VLDL, LDL, triglycerides, and cholesterol may be elevated while HDL is decreased, especially in type II diabetes. Adolescents with IDDM show disturbed cardiovascular risk profiles compared with nondiabetic siblings (45). Appropriate treatment of DM is associated with improvement in plasma VLDL and LDL concentrations and often increased HDL levels.

Nutrition and physical activity remain the basis of treatment of lipid disorders in persons with diabetes (46). Recommended treatment focuses on weight reduction when indicated, increased physical activity, and a low-saturated-fat diet. Such dietary manipulation and improvements in glycemic control have been successful in returning elevated blood fats to normal levels (47).

3. Nephropathy

Renal disease poses an even more imminent threat to IDDM individuals than coronary artery disease (Chapter 40). It accounts for one-half of all deaths in IDDM, and end-stage renal disease is the primary cause of death in children with diabetes aged between 15 and 30 years (48). There is growing evidence that protein intake may be important in increasing the risk for renal disease and for contributing to the worsening of nephropathy in DM. The increase in renal blood flow, glomerular filtration, and structural changes associated with excessive protein ingestion may all play a role in the loss of kidney function (49). It appears that high protein intake may increase the workload of the kidney, and protein restriction could restore glomerular hemodynamics before structural changes have advanced to overt nephropathy. Protein restriction at later stages of diabetic nephropathy may also be efficacious (50,51). The type of protein ingested may also play a role in the etiopathogenesis of diabetes nephropathy (52,53).

IV. NUTRITION IN THE MANAGEMENT OF DIABETES MELLITUS

Medical nutritional therapy is an integral part of diabetes management. The American Diabetes Association has recently revised its position on medical nutrition therapy for people with DM, which dramatically has altered the philosophy of the nutritional care of people with diabetes (55). Individualized dietary recommendations based on metabolism, nutrition, and life-style replace the calculated prescription. Additionally, the approach to the nutritional management of NIDDM now includes goals for optimizing glucose, blood pressure, and lipid levels, as well as weight loss. For children with IDDM a meal plan based on the individual's tastes, likes, and usual food consumption should be integrated with insulin therapy, glucose monitoring, and physical activity.

Most of the specific components of diabetes management are superimposed on the basic tenants of human nutrition, and thus it is important to be familiar with current nutrition guidelines for the general population (56–58). The 1994 recommendations make obsolete the concept of "ADA diet" (55). Patients requiring insulin therapy need to follow the general nutritional guidelines for the population at large, including protein, sucrose, and fiber intake. However, day-to-day consistency in the timing and amount of food consumed is more important for them as dietary intake must be synchronized with the time actions of insulin therapy. An exception from previous recommendations for persons with diabetes and from current advice for the general population is that a diet providing less than 30% of calories as total fat may not be recommended for every person with diabetes. Different guidelines for total fat and carbohydrate intake are suggested for individuals with different metabolic abnormalities. Diets high in monounsaturated fat may be preferable to high-carbohydrate diets for certain persons with diabetes, especially those with elevated triglyceride levels and elevated very-low-density lipoprotein (VLDL) cholesterol levels (59).

A. Energy

Energy requirements are those needed to achieve and maintain ideal body weight and normal growth and development. It is difficult to determine individual energy requirements as they may vary tremendously, especially during growth spurts or with different levels of physical activity. Individual appetite is usually the best indication of caloric needs and can be the sole determinant of total dietary intake unless excessive or inadequate weight gain is occurring. Often during periods of catchup growth, i.e., following onset of IDDM, serious illness, or ketoacidosis, considerable additional energy is required.

B. Carbohydrates

Carbohydrate restriction is no longer recommended in DM (55). This is due to the fact that the insulin requirement is more related to total fuel supply than to the amount of carbohydrate ingested. The liver readily converts glucose from a variety of substrates, i.e., protein, fat, or carbohydrate. Moreover, when the amount of carbohydrate is restricted, it is difficult to construct diets that are not high in fat, cholesterol, and protein. The amount of carbohydrate in the diet should be liberalized and individualized, potentially up to 55–60% of total calories, with the amount dependent on the impact of blood glucose, lipid levels, and individual eating patterns (55,60).

Previous recommendations stressed the use of complex carbohydrate for meeting the liberalized total carbohydrate intake. A study of NIDDM (61) has shown that simple carbohydrates from milk, fruit, and vegetables need not be restricted for adequate glycemic control. However, refined sugars should be limited in the diet of diabetics and nondiabetics alike in accordance with the general nutrition recommendations for healthy persons. Moderation is also advisable since high sugar intake may increase LDL cholesterol. Although foods rich in sucrose tend to be high in fat and low in other nutrients, it is not necessary to completely eliminate sucrose. With moderation and appropriate timing, favorite sucrose-containing foods can be included in the diet of persons with diabetes without affecting glycemic control.

Dietary fructose produces a smaller rise in plasma glucose than isocaloric amounts of sucrose and most starch carbohydrates (62) and reduces postprandial glucose levels when it replaces other carbohydrates in the diets of subjects with diabetes (63). However, this potential benefit may be overshadowed by the concern that fructose may adversely affect serum lipids, particularly LDL cholesterol (63). Based on the available data, there is no reason to recommend that people with diabetes avoid naturally occurring sources of fructose such as fruits, vegetables, or honey. However, as added sweetener, fructose may not have an advantage over other nutritive sweeteners.

C. Glycemic Index

The current dietary recommendations of the American Diabetes Association do not recommend the glycemic index classification for use in selecting starchy foods (55). The clinical utility of the glycemic index was criticized on the basis that glycemic index classification of single foods was not able to predict the ranking of glycemic response to mixed meals due to the other noncarbohydrate components (64,65).

Insulin appears to be the main factor in the alterations in glycemic response to mixed meals with various types of carbohydrate in children with IDDM (66). When a proper adjustment of insulin dose is made, the type of food in a mixed meal does not appear to have significant effects on the postprandial glycemia in children with longstanding IDDM (67). However, some of the longer-term studies have found that the reduction in the glycemic index of the diet has been associated with reductions of glycosylated proteins, LDL cholesterol, serum triglycerides, and phospholipids (68,69).

D. Fiber

An increase in dietary fiber has been associated with lower plasma postprandial glucose levels in patients with diabetes. Unrefined soluble fiber is most effective in decreasing the plasma glucose response to meals (70). However, the long-term benefits of increasing dietary fiber 2–5 times did not lead to improvement in the control of diabetic patients (71). Two studies of children with diabetes showed conflicting results: one showed improved glycemic control using beans (72), whereas another failed to find any improvement using grains, fruits, and vegetables (73). Moreover, high-fiber diets may result in abdominal cramping, discomfort, loose stools, and flatulence or interfere with mineral absorption. Careful attention must also be paid to insulin dose, because hypoglycemia can result if there is a radical change in fiber intake that reduces the carbohydrate intake. Additionally, there is concern that high-fiber diets may yield inadequate caloric intake due to unpalatability or early satiety.

Intake recommendations regarding dietary fiber are the same for diabetics and nondiabetics alike. They should be advised to gradually incorporate foods naturally rich in total fiber into their diet. The accepted nutritional guidance of increasing current intake to 20–35 g/day from a varied diet of food sources is prudent for the general public and for diabetic persons.

E. Protein

As with the other macronutrients, the amount of protein from animal and vegetable sources in the diabetic diet is being reexamined. Protein intake should be evaluated in terms of its effect on renal hemodynamics as well as growth and development and glycemic control (74). Studies indicate that high protein intake and hyperglycemia may be independently involved in the decline in renal function (75). Some studies have suggested that in the early stages, microalbuminuria may be reversed by protein restriction (76,77). With American children typically consuming more than twice the Recommended Dietary Allowances (RDA) for protein (56), there is ample room to cut back protein intakes of children with IDDM. Current recommendations, 10–20% of energy, are likely to be lower than current protein intake levels. Adolescents with microalbuminuria are candidates for protein restrictions to the RDA (0.8–1.0 g/kg), and protein intake should also be lowered in children with diabetic nephropathy to the

lowest proportion possible, which may fall below 8% of energy (78).

F. Fat

Given the increased incidence of coronary artery disease among adult diabetics, the type and amount of dietary fat should also be considered in pediatric IDDM patients. In most cases fat should range from 30% to 35% of total calories (54). No more than 10% of total calories should be ingested from saturated fat or polyunsaturated fat, with the remainder being monounsaturated fat. In cases when the carbohydrate content of the diet is moderate, monounsaturated intakes up to 20% of calories may be indicated (55). The American Heart Association does not recommend the use of fish oil supplements but does encourage one to two fish meals per week (79). It appears that fish oil supplements in IDDM, unlike NIDDM, may decrease serum triglycerides, increase HDL-2, and do not adversely affect glycemic control (80). Effects on LDL cholesterol and apolipoprotein B, however, are inconsistent (81) and further studies are necessary.

Recent studies have shown that cholesterol-lowering intervention by diet is not very effective (82–86). Meta-analysis of long-term studies showed that a total fat intake of less than 30% of calories given as individual intervention for long periods results in a net reduction of serum cholesterol of only about 2% (86). More restrictive dietary treatment (step 2) led to a lowering of LDL cholesterol levels on average of 5%, but the level of HDL cholesterol was also similarly reduced, thus offsetting the possible beneficial effects (85). Thus it is not necessary to severely restrict dietary fat in childhood (54). Children are not "little adults" and their dietary guidelines should be based on moderation, not arbitrary numerical targets (54).

G. Micronutrients

The role of vitamins and minerals in the diet of children with diabetes must be considered in the context of total dietary intake. Alterations in the micronutrient status of IDDM patients and micronutrient deficiencies have been correlated with complications (27). However, the results are inconsistent (Table 1) and vary in accordance with multiple clinical factors.

Hyperglycemia and glycosuria may be the main mechanisms for increased urinary losses of vitamins and trace minerals. Furthermore, diabetic patients maintained on restricted diets may consume inadequate amounts and high-fiber diets may also compromise vitamin and mineral status, especially magnesium and zinc. Special circumstances related to chromium, zinc, magnesium, vitamin E, vitamin B_{12}, and iron that occur in diabetics warrant review. Chromium deficiency in animal models is associated with elevated blood glucose, cholesterol, and triglyceride levels (87). Persons with impaired glucose tolerance who consumed a diet deficient in chromium for 4 weeks improved glucose tolerance with chromium supplementation (88). However, in individuals with diabetes, double-blind crossover studies on chromium supplementation did not result in improved blood glucose control (89,90).

While serum zinc levels are generally lower in diabetics compared to nondiabetic persons, zinc replacement has been shown to be beneficial in healing leg ulcers but not under other circumstances (91). Magnesium depletion has been associated with insulin insensitivity, which may improve with oral supplementation (92). There may be a need for magnesium replacement in patients with poor glycemic control or who require diuretics. The American Diabetes Association consensus statement did not advocate routine screening for Mg deficiency but recommended evaluation of Mg levels in patients at the greatest risk (92). There is no evidence of benefit from routine supplementation of vitamin B_{12} except with documented deficiency such as the polyglandular endocrinopathies associated with type I diabetes or elderly type II diabetes (93). Similarly, iron replacement should be advised after assessment of iron nutriture. Thus there is no need for people with diabetes to take vitamin/mineral supplements unless micronutrient deficiency has been documented (94).

H. Nonnutritive Sweeteners and Dietetic Foods

Special foods for individuals with diabetes are not necessary to achieve the dietary objectives recommended (95). They can be accomplished conveniently and inexpensively through prudent choices of commonly available food items. As sucrose-containing foods can be included in moderation, there are no specific therapeutic properties in dietetic or diabetic food products that can be defined on rational grounds (96). Yet there is great appeal to persons with diabetes to ingest these products. Diabetic or dietetic food products may mislead

consumers since they appear to permit consumption without regard to energy content or micronutrient composition.

Many individuals tend to use dietetic or diabetic products, and physicians and other health professionals often recommend them in the hope of achieving better control of the disease. Decisions regarding the use of these products are influenced by many factors, such as advertising, fear of sugar and other carbohydrates, and the desire for sweets. There is also a misunderstanding of the nutritional value of these products, and there is lack of available information on the comparison between dietetic and regular products (Table 3). In most instances, the consumer receives little or no nutritional benefit from costly dietetic products. Since these constitute only a fraction of total food intake, the differences in their composition have little or no effect on the relationship of nutrients consumed within a 24-h period. It has been shown that the nutritional value of a majority of these products was not different from that of regular items (97); often, the amount of calories provided by dietetic products is not significantly different from that of their regular counterparts, and the cost is usually higher. In addition, the use of dietary products may replace more nutrient-dense foods, particularly in a low-calorie food plan. Thus, the most beneficial diet is one derived from a wide variety of ordinary foods (54).

Currently, three nonnutritive sweeteners are approved for use in the United States, saccharin, aspartame, and acesulfame K. Other sweeteners used include sorbitol, mannitol, and xylitol. As with all food additives, the FDA determines an acceptable daily intake (ADI), which is defined as the amount of a food additive that can be safely consumed on a daily basis over a person's lifetime without any adverse effects and includes a 100-fold safety factor. Although nutritive and nonnutritive sweeteners are safe in portions typically con-

Table 3 Comparison of Dietetic and Regular Foods

Food item	Amount (oz)	Calories (kcal)	Carbohydrates (gm)	Fat (gm)	Cost per amount ($)
Flavor drops, dietetic	1	38	2.9	0.0	.35
Hard candy, regular	1	108	27.2	0.8	.08
Chocolate, dietetic	2	168	14.0	14.0	1.19
Chocolate, regular	2	150	16.0	9.0	.22
Ice cream, dietetic	4	87	15.6	0.9	1.00
Ice cream, regular	4	130	16.0	7.0	0.57
Pancake syrup, lite	1	60	15.0	0	0.13
Pancake syrup, regular	1	100	26.0	0	0.13
Fudge cookie, dietetic	1	120	16.0	4	.21
Fudge cookie, regular	1	124	20.0	4	.03
Applesauce, dietetic	4	50	12.0	0	.40
Apple sauce, unsweetened regular	4	46	11.0	0.1	.19

Note that the calorie content of some dietetic foods differs very slightly from the non-dietetic products. At times it may even be higher as shown for chocolate, where the dietetic product yields higher calories due to the high fat content. The cost of dietetic products is usually higher.
Source: Children's Nutrition, Lifshitz F, Moses N, Lifshitz JZ, eds., Boston: Jones and Bartlett, 1991.

sumed (98), it should be kept in mind that there is no scientific evidence that they have greatly improved the care and ease of management of diabetic individuals nor do they help to limit caloric intake and/or weight loss. However, when used in excess, they may cause osmotic diarrhea or other side effects, i.e., increased uric acid, bilirubin, and lactate levels. Oxalosis may result from sorbitol and cataracts may follow xylitol and sorbitol ingestion. In addition, the use of artificial sweeteners and special products gives the individual or family a false perception of treating the diabetes, when, in fact, the most beneficial diet is one derived from a variety of ordinary food (97). Awareness of the relationship between food composition and diabetes control is the key. Avoidance of sugar per se is not a panacea.

V. IMPLEMENTATION OF NUTRITIONAL GOALS

Achieving nutrition-related goals requires a coordinated team effort, which includes the IDDM patient and family. The exchange system has been the most widely used method of meal planning. However, no studies have addressed the long-term effectiveness of this system in children. The important feeding regimen considerations should be to guide the child to a meal plan that fits individual life-style, promotes optimal compliance, and advances the goals of euglycemia and normal lipid levels. For children with IDDM a meal plan based on the individual's usual food intake should be determined and insulin therapy should be integrated into the usual exercise and eating patterns. It is not desirable or necessary to divide meals and snacks into an artificial or unnatural pattern. Individuals also need to monitor blood glucose levels and adjust insulin doses to accommodate any deviations noted.

Intensified insulin therapy, such as multiple daily injections or the use of an insulin delivery pump, allows for considerable flexibility regarding when and what foods people eat. The decision to consider such therapies should be made on an individual basis depending on the age of the child, level of motivation, and diabetic control.

There is considerable evidence that the majority of individuals with diabetes do not follow, on a long-term basis, appropriate dietary recommendations (99,100). Issues contributing to dietary indiscretion include feeling different from other children, unrealistic diabetes treatment goals, inadequate support from parents, and underinvolved or overprotective parents. It is helpful to (1) adjust the diabetes nutrition education to the child's life-style; (2) adopt a realistic plan that includes sweets and other desired foods and provide instruction to include these items; (3) encourage parents to be positive role models; and (4) guide parents in the appropriate level of responsibility according to their child's developmental stage (101). Several different strategies have been proposed to improve dietary adherence in children and adolescents (102,103) and variations or combinations of them may prove useful in individual cases.

As eating may be a sensitive indicator of emotional state and parent/child interaction (104), it is understandable why diabetes, with its demanding meal pattern requirements, is considered a risk factor for obesity and eating disorders (Chapters 52 and 59). The prevalence of eating disorders in individuals with IDDM ranges from 7 to 35%, far exceeding the range (1–4%) reported in the general population (105). Most disturbing is induced glycosuria, a unique form of purging used by individuals with diabetes, which entails the purposeful attempt to control weight through the omission or reduction of insulin intake. Elevated glycoslyated hemoglobin levels and poor glycemic control have been reported in diabetic patients with eating disorders (106,107). The prevention of eating disorders should begin early by detecting persons at risk and providing education to reshape attitudes and behaviors. Unexplained poor control, severe hypoglycemia, or preoccupation with body weight may signal early indications of an eating problem that should be investigated further.

The ultimate goal and approach to nutrition education and counseling is to promote positive behavioral changes. For this to occur, a phased plan for nutrition counseling is recommended for the patient with IDDM and his/her family. The key components of such a plan include the initial or "survival" phase followed by an in-depth or counseling phase (Chapter 46). In the initial phase, a simplified, individualized meal plan and an introduction to the basics of meal planning are needed. This usually occurs in the hospital after diagnosis and immediately posthospitalization. In our clinic, this is achieved through two or three 45-min sessions in the hospital and one to three 45-min follow-up sessions with the patient and family in the first 2–3 months following hospitalization. Factors such as family dynamics and previous dietary patterns determine the precise number of nutrition educational sessions.

During the second in-depth and continuing phase, the person with diabetes and his family learn how to make decisions about food selection and diabetes control. The approach needs to be realistic and provide as much flexibility as possible in accordance with the general nutrition goals. Educational tools should also be appropriate for the individual, taking into account age and educational level. Because the in-depth phase requires continuing education and counseling and the nutritional needs of children are constantly evolving, the American Diabetes Association has recommended a nutrition appointment at least every 6 months, preferably every 3 months (59).

VI. FINAL CONSIDERATIONS

It is evident that nutrition and diabetes are intimately interrelated. A better understanding of this association may reduce the risk of diabetes, improve its daily management, and ameliorate some of the complications of the disease. However, further studies are needed to clarify specific nutritional issues. Reports of dietary intake of patients with diabetes are largely unreliable (108); thus it is difficult to facilitate dietary modifications for the improved overall health of diabetic individuals. We are able to obtain facts and outline goals but we are far less successful in their implementation and follow-through, largely because of the relative crudity of our motivational techniques. We must continue to support research in the behavioral aspects of dietary and life-style modification and work to achieve results within our centers.

REFERENCES

1. Fujimoto WY, Bergstrom RW, Newell-Morris LL, Leonmatti DL. Nature and nuture in the etiology of type 2 diabetes in Japanese Americans. Diabetes Metab Rev 1989; 5:607–625.
2. Cohen AM, Teitelbaum A, Saliternik R. Genetics and diet as factors in development of diabetes mellitus. Metabolism 1972; 21:235–240.
3. Knowler WC, Pettit DJ, Saad MF, Bennet PH. Diabetes mellitus in the Pima Indians: Incidence, risk factors and pathogenesis. Diabetes Metab Rev 1990; 6:1–27.
4. Ritenbaugh C, Goody CS. Beyond the thrifty gene: Metabolic implications of prehistoric migration into the New World. Med Anthrop 1989; 11:227–236.
5. West KM, Kalbfleich JM. Diabetes in Central America. Diabetes 1970; 19:656–663.
6. West KM. Diabetes in American Indians and other native populations of the world. Diabetes 1974; 23:841–844.
7. O'Dea K. Westernization, insulin resistance and diabetes in Australian aborigines. Med J Aust 1991; 155:258–264.
8. West KM, Kalbfleich JM. Influence of nutritional factors on prevalence of diabetes. Diabetes 1971; 20:99–108.
9. Cleave TL. The Saccharine Disease. Bristol, England: 1974.
10. West KM, Kalbfleich JM. Influence of nutritional factors on prevalence of diabetes. Diabetes 1971; 10:99–108.
11. Goda T, Yamada K, Sugiyama M, Moriuchi S, Howoya N: Effect of sucrose and acarbose feeding on the development of streptozotocin-induced diabetes in the rat. J Nutri Sci 1982; 28:41–56.
12. Thornburn AW, Brand JC, Trusell AS. Slowly digested and absorbed carbohydrate in traditional bushfood: A protective factor against diabetes? Am J Clin Nutr 19897; 45:98–106.
13. Miki E, Maruvama H. Childhood diabetes mellitus in Japan. In: Tsjui S, Wada M, eds. Diabetes Mellitus in Asia. Amsterdam: Excerpta Medica, 1971.
14. Elliot RB, Martin, JM. Dietary protein: A trigger of insulin dependent diabetes in the BB rat? Diabetologia 1984; 26:297–299.
15. Helgason T, Ewen SW, Ross JS, Stowers JM. Diabetes produced in mice by smoked/cured mutton. Lancet 1982; 2:1012–1022.
16. Virtanen SM, Rasanen SL, Aro A, et al. Is children's or parents' coffee or tea consumption associated with the risk of type I diabetes mellitus in children? Eur J Clin Nutr 1994; 48:279–285.
17. Dhalquist G, Blom L, Persson LA, Sandstrom A, Wall S. Dietary factors and the risk of developing insulin dependent diabetes in childhood. Br Med J 1990; 300:1302–1306.
18. Borch-Johnsen K. Relationship between breast feeding and incidence rates of insulin dependent diabetes mellitus. Lancet 1984; 2:1083–1086.
19. Fort P, Lanes R, Dahlem S, et al. Breast feeding and insulin dependent diabetes mellitus in children. J Am Coll Nutr 1986; 5:435–441.
20. Pietropaolo M, Castano L, Babu S, et al. Islet cell autoantigen 69 kDa (ICA69): Molecular cloning and characterization of a novel diabetes associated autoantigen. J Clin Invest 1993; 92:359–371.
21. Karjalainen J, Martin JM, Knip M, et al. A bovine albumin peptide as a possible trigger of insulin-dependent diabetes mellitus. N Engl J Med 1992; 327:302–307.
22. Saukkonen T, Savilahti E, Vaarala O, Virtala ET, Tuomilehto J, Akerblom HK. Children with newly diagnosed IDDM have increased levels of antibodies to bovine serum albumin but not to ovalbumin. Diabetes Care 1994; 17:970–976.
23. Atkinson MA, Bowman MA, Kao K, et al. Lack of immune responsiveness to bovine serum albumin in insulin-dependent diabetes. N Engl J Med 1993; 329:1853–1858.
24. Kostraba JN, Cruickshanks KJ, Lawler-Heavner J, et al. Early exposure to cow's milk and solid foods in infancy, genetic predisposition, and risk of IDDM. Diabetes 1993; 42:288–295.
25. Gerstein HC. Cow's milk exposure and type 1 diabetes mellitus. Diabetes Care 1994; 17:13–19.
26. Work Group on Cow's Milk Protein and Diabetes Mellitus: Infant feeding practices and their possible relationship to the etiology of diabetes mellitus. Pediatrics 1994; 94:752–754.
27. Mooradian AD, Morley JE. Miconutrient status in diabetes mellitus. Am J Clin Nutri 1987; 45:877–895.
28. Paolisso G, Scheen A, D'Onofrio F, et al: Magnesium and glucose homeostasis. Diabetologia 1990; 33:511–514.
29. Campbell RK, Nadler J. Magnesium deficiency and diabetes. Diabetes Educ 1992; 18:17–19.
30. Hatwal A, Gujral AS, Bhatia RPS, et al. Association of hypomagnesemia with diabetic retinopathy. Acta Opthalmol 1989; 67:714–716.
31. Slonim AE, Surber ML, Page DL, Sharp RA, Burr IM. Modification of chemically induced diabetes in rats by vitamin E: Supplementation minimizes and depletion enhances development of diabetes. J Clin Invest 1983; 71:1282–1288.
32. Behrens WA, Scott WS, Madere R, Trick K, Hanna K. Effect of dietary vitamin E on the vitamin E status in the BB rat during development and after the onset of diabetes. Ann Nutr Metabol 1986; 30:157–165.
33. Wing RR, Blair EH, Bononi P, Marcu M, Watanabe R, Bergman R: Caloric restriction per se is a significant factor in improvements in glycemic control and insulin sensitivity during weight loss in obese NIDDM patients. Diabetes Care 1994; 17:30–36.
34. Diabetes Control and Complications Trial Research Group. The effect of intensive treatment of diabetes on the development and progression of long-term complications in insulin-dependent diabetes mellitus. N Engl J Med 1993; 329:977–986.
35. West KM. Diabetes in American Indians and other native populations of the world. Diabetes 1974; 23:841–844.
36. Zimmet P. Epidemiology of diabetes and its microvascular manifestations in Pacific populations: The medical effects of social progress. Diabetes Care 1979; 2:144–153.
37. Garg A, Bantle JP, Henry RR, et al. Effect of varying carbohydrate content of diet in patients with non-insulin dependent diabetes mellitus. JAMA 1994; 271:1421–1428.
38. American Diabetes Association. Treatment of hypertension in diabetes (consensus statement). Diabetes Care 1993; 16:1394–1401.
39. Joffres MR, Reed DM, Yano K: Relationship of magnesium intake and other dietary factors to blood pressure: The Honolulu Heart Study. Am J Clin Nutr 1987; 45:469–475.
40. Widman L, Wester PO, Stegmar BK, et al. The dose-dependent reduction in blood pressure through administration of magnesium: A double blind placebo controlled cross-over study. Am J Hypertens 1993; 6:41–45.
41. Resnick LM, Gupta RK, Bhargava KK, et al. Cellular ions in hypertension, diabetes, and obesity: A nuclearmagnetic

resonance spectroscopic study. Hypertension 1991; 17:951–957.

42. Resnick LM, Altura BT, Gupta RK, et al. Intracellular and extracellular magnesium depletion in type 2 (non-insulin dependendent) diabetes mellitus. Diabetologia 1993; 36:767–790.

43. Klienman JC, Donahue PR, Harris MI, Finucane FF, Madans JH, Dwight BB. Mortality among diabetics in a national sample. Am J Epidemiol 1988; 89:389–401.

44. Stamler J, Vaccaro O, Neaton JD, Wenworth D, for the Multiple Risk Factor Intervention Trial Research Group. Diabetes, other risk factors, and 12-yr cardiovascular mortality for men screened in the Multiple Risk Factor Intervention Trial. Diabetes Care 1993; 16:434–444.

45. Cruickshanks KJ, Orchard TJ, Becker DJ. The cardiovascular risk profile of adolescents with insulin-dependent diabetes mellitus. Diabetes Care 1985; 8:118–124.

46. American Diabetes Association. Detection and management of lipid disorders in diabetes (consensus statement). Diabetes Care 1993; 16(Suppl 2):106–112.

47. Blanc MH, Ganda OP, Gleason RE, Soeldner JS. Improvement in lipid status in diabetic boys: The 1971 and 1979 Joslin Camp lipid levels. Diabetes Care 1983; 6:64–66.

48. Dorman JJ, Laporte RE, Kuller LH, et al. The Pittsburgh Insulin Dependent Diabetes Mellitus (IDDM) Morbidity and Mortality Study: Mortality results. Diabetes 1984; 32:274.

49. Laouri D, Kleinkneckt C, Gubler MC, Ravet U, Broyer M. Importance of proteins in the deterioration of remnant kidneys, independent of other nutrients. Int J Pediatr Nephrol 1982; 3:263–269.

50. Maschio G, Oldrizzi L, Tessitore N, et al.. Early protein and phosphorus restriction is effective in delaying progression of chronic renal failure. Kidney Int 1983; 24(Suppl 16):5273–5277.

51. Maschio G, Oldrizzi L, Tessitore N, et al. Effect of dietary protein and phosphorus restriction on the progression of early renal failure. Kidney Int 1982; 22:371–376.

52. Jibani MM, Bloodworth LL, Foden E, et al. Predominantly vegetarian diet in patients with incipient and early clinical diabetic nephropathy: Effects on albumin excretion rate and nutritional status. Diabetic Med 1991; 8:949–953.

53. Viberti GC, Yip-Messent J, Morocutti A. Diabetic nephropathy: Future avenue. Diabetes Care 1992; 15:1216–1225.

54. Lifshitz F. Children on adult diets: Is it harmful? Is it healthful? J Am Col Nutr 1992; 11S:84–90S.

55. American Diabetes Association. Nutrition recommendations and principles for people with diabetes mellitus. Diabetes Care 1994; 17:519–522.

56. Committee on Dietary Allowances. National Research Council, Recommended Dietary Allowances, 10th ed. Washington, DC: 1989. National Academy of Sciences. 1989.

57. U.S. Department of Agriculture, U.S. Department of Health and Human Services. Nutrition and Your Health: Dietary Guidelines for Americans, 3rd ed. Hyattsville, MD: USDA's Human Nutrition Information Serivce, 1990.

58. U.S. Department of Agriculture. The Food Guide Pyramid. Hyattsville, MD: USDA's Human Nutrition Information Service, 1992.

59. Franz MJ, Horton ES, Bantle JP, et al. Nutritional principles for the management of diabetes and related complications. Diabetes Care 1994; 17:490–518.

60. Committee on Nutrition. Nutritional Management of Children and Adolescents with Insulin Dependent Diabetes Mellitus. Elk Grove Village, IL: Academy of Pediatrics, 1985.

61. Coulston AM, Hollenbeck CB, Donner CC, Williams R. Choiu Y-AM, Reaven GM. Metabolic effects of added dietary sucrose in individuals with noninsulin dependent diabetes (NIDDM). Metabolism 1985; 34:962–966.

62. Bantle JP, Laine DC, Castle GW, Thomas JW, Hoogwerf BJ, Goetz FC. Postprantdial glucose and insulin responses to meals containing different carbohydrates in normal and diabetic subjects. N Engl J Med 1983; 309:7–12.

63. Bantle JP, Swanson JE, Thomas W, Laine DC. Metabolic effects of dietary fructose in diabetic subjects. Diabetes Care 1992; 15:1468–1476.

64. Hollenbeck CB, Coulston AM, Reaven GM. Comparison of plasma glucose and insulin response to mixed meals in high-, intermediate- and low-glycemic potential. Diabetes Care 1988; 111:323–332.

65. Laine DC, Thomas W, Levitt MD, Bantle JP. Comparision of predictive capabilities of diabetics exchange lists and glycemic index of foods. Diabetes Care 1987; 19:387–394.

66. Weyman-Daum M, Fort P, Recker B, Lifshitz F. Glycemic response in children with insulin dependent diabetes mellitus after high or low glycemic index breakfast. Am J Clin Nutr 1987; 46:798–803.

67. Vlachokosta FV, Piper CM, Gleason R, Kinzel L, Kahn CR. Dietary carbohydrate, a Big Mac, and insulin requirements in type I diabetes. Diabetes Care 1988; 11:330–336.

68. Fontvielle AM, Rizkalla SW, Penfornis A, Acosta M, Bornet FR, Slama G. The use of low glyscemic index foods improves metabolic control of diabetic patients over five weeks. Diabetes Med 1992; 9:440–445.

69. Brand JC, Calagiuri S, Crossman S, et al. Low-glycemic index foods improve long-term glycaemic control in NIDDM. Diabetes Care 1991; 14:95–101.

70. Vinik AL, Jenkins DJA. Dietary fiber in management of diabetes. Diabetes Care 1986; 11:160–173.

71. Hollenbeck CB, Coulston AM, Reaven GM. To what extent does increased dietary fiber improve glucose and lipid metabolism in patients with noninsulin-dependent diabetes mellitus (NIDDM)? Am J Clin Nutr 1986; 43:16–24.

72. Kinmouth AL, Angus RM, Jenkins PA, Smith MA, Blum JD. Whole foods and increased fiber improves blood glucose control in diabetic children. Arch Dis Child 1982; 10:126–132.

73. Lindsay AN, Hardy S, Jarrett L, Rallison ML. High-carbohydrate, high fiber diet in children with type I diabetes mellitus. Diabetes Care 1984; 7:63–67.

74. Wylie-Rosett J. Evaluation of protein in dietary management of diabetes mellitus. Diabetes Care 1988; 11:143–148.

75. Reynolds JW. Nutritional management of children and adolescents with insulin-dependent diabetes mellitus. Pediatr Rev 1987; 9(5):155–162.

76. Wiseman MJ, Bognetti E, Dodds R, Keen H, Viberti GC. Changes in renal function in response to protein restricted diet in type I diabetic patients. Diabetologia 1987; 30:154–159.

77. Zeller K, Whittaker E, Sullivan L, Raskin P, Jacobson HR. Effect of restricting dietary protein on the progression of renal failure in patients with insulin-dependent diabetes mellitus. N Engl J Med 1991; 324:78–84.

78. Levine SE. Renal failure: Diabetic nephropathy. In: Powers MA, ed. Handbook of Diabetes Nutritional Management. Rockville, MD: Aspen Pub., 1987:378–397.

79. Dietary Guidelines for Health Adult Americans. Dallas, TX: American Heart Association, 1988.

80. Mori TA, Vandongen R, Masarei JR, Rouse IL, Dunbar D. Comparison of diets supplemented with fish oil or olive oil on plasma lipoproteins in insulin-dependent diabetics. Metabolism 1991; 40:241–246.

81. Mori TA, Vandongen R, Masarei JR. Fish oil-induced changes

in apolipoproteins in IDDM subjects. Diabetes Care 1990; 13:725–732.

82. Wynder EL, Perenson GS, Strong WB, Williams C, eds. Coronary artery disease prevention, cholesterol, a pediatric perspective. Prev Med 1989; 18:323–409.

83. Puska P, Vartiainen E, Pallonen U, et al. The North Karelia Youth Project: Evaluation of two years of intervention on health behavior and CVD risk factors among 13–15 year-old children. Prev Med 1982; 11:550–570.

84. Walter HJ, Hofman A, Vaughan RD, Wynder EL. Modification of risk factors for coronary heart disease, five year results of a school-based intervention trial. N Engl J Med 1988; 318:1093–110.

85. Hunninghake DB, Stein EA, Dujovne CA, et al. The efficacy of intensive dietary therapy alone or combined with lovastatin in our patients with hypercholesterolemia. N Engl J Med 1993; 328; 17, 1213–1219.

86. Ramsay L, Yeo WW, Jackson PR. Dietary reduction of serum cholesterol concentrations: Time to think again. Br Med J 1991; 303:953–957.

87. Wolliscroft J, Barbosa J. Analysis of chromium induced carbohydrate intolerance in the rat. J Nutr 1977; 88:439–445.

88. Anderson RA, Polansky MM, Canary JJ. Supplemental chromium effects on glucose, insulin, glucagon, and urinary chromium losses in subjects consuming controlled low chromium diets. Am J Clin Nutr 1991; 54:909–916.

89. Rabinowitz MB, Gonick HC, Levin SR, Davidson MB. Effect of chromium and yeast supplements on carbohydrate and lipid metabolism in diabetic men. Diabetes Care 1983; 6:319–327.

90. Abraham AS, Brooks BA, Eylate U. The effects of chromium supplementation on serum glucose and lipids in patients with and without non-insulin dependent diabetes. Metab Clin Exp 1992; 41:768–771.

91. Niewoehner CB, Allan JI, Boosalis M, Levin AS, Morley JE. The role of zinc supplementation in type II diabetes mellitus. Am J Clin Nutr 1986; 81:63–68.

92. American Diabetes Association Consensus Conference. Magnesium supplementation in the treatment of diabetes mellitus. Diabetes Care 1993; 6(Suppl 2):1065–1067.

93. Trence DL, Morley JE, Handwerger BS. Polyglandular autoimmune syndromes. Am J Med 1984; 77:107–116.

94. Mooradian AD, Failla M, Hoogwerf B, Isaac R, Maryniuk M, Wylie-Rosett J. Selected vitamins and minerals in diabetes mellitus. Diabetes Care 1994; 17:464–479.

95. Talbot JM, Fisher KD. The need for special foods and sugar substitutes by individuals with diabetes mellitus. Diabetes Care 1981; 1:231–240.

96. Strefa D, Boyko E, Rabkin SW. Nutrition therapy in non-insulin dependent diabetes mellitus. Diabetes Care 1981; 4:84.

97. Wunschel IM, Sheikholislam BM. Is there a role for dietetic foods in the management of diabetes and/or obesity? Diabetes Care 1978; 1:247–249.

98. American Diabetic Association. Use of noncaloric sweeteners. Position statement. Diabetes Care 1987; 10:526.

99. Eckerling L, Kohrs MB. Research on compliance with diabetic regimens: Applications to practice. J Am Diet Assoc 1984; 84:805–809.

100. Lorenz RA, Christiansen NK, Pichert JW. Diet-related knowledge, skill, and adherence among children with insulin-dependent diabetes mellitus. Pediatrics 1985; 75:872–876.

101. Follansbee DS. Assuming responsibility for diabetes management: What age? What price? Diabetes Educ 1989; 15:347–352.

102. Pichert JW, Meek JM, Schlundt DG, et al. Impact of anchored instructions on problem-solving strategies of adolescents with diabetes. J Am Diet Assoc 1994; 94:1036–1037.

103. Loghmani E, Rickard KA. Alternative snack system for children and teenagers with diabetes mellitus. J Am Diet Assoc 1994; 94:1145–1148.

104. Satter EM. Childhood eating disorders. J Am Diet Assoc 1986; 86:357–361.

105. Stacin T, Link DL, Reuter JM. Binge eating and purging in young women with IDDM. Diabetes Care 1989; 12:601–603.

106. Wing RR, Norwalk MP, Marcus MD, et al. Subclinical eating disorders and glycemic control in adolescents with type I diabetes. Diabetes Care 1986; 9:162–167.

107. Rodin GM, Johnson LE, Garfinkel PE, Daneman D, Kenshole GM. Eating disorders in female adolescents with insulin dependent diabetes mellitus. Int J Psych Med 1986; 16:49–57.

108. Alemzadeh R, Goldberg T, Fort P, Recker B, Lifshitz F. Reported dietary intakes of patients with insulin-dependent diabetes mellitus: Limitations of dietary recall. Nutrition 1992; 8:87–93.

42

Management of the Child with Diabetes Mellitus
Clinical Course, Therapeutic Strategies, and Monitoring Techniques

Allan L. Drash

University of Pittsburgh and Children's Hospital of Pittsburgh, Pittsburgh, Pennsylvania

I. INTRODUCTION

Diabetes mellitus is a disease of insulin deficiency. Insulin deficiency may be partial or complete, and clinical symptomatology correlates well with the degree of insulin deficiency. To a smaller extent, the clinical course and outcome, in terms of diabetic complications, also probably relate to the degree of insulin deficiency. Almost all children (>95%) with diabetes mellitus have the insulin-deficient form (IDDM), whereas most persons who develop diabetes during the adult years have obesity-related non–insulin-dependent disease.

II. METABOLIC DISTURBANCES AS A CONSEQUENCE OF INSULIN DEFICIENCY

The hormone insulin has pervasive effects on overall energy homeostatis. Although diabetes mellitus is usually considered a disease of carbohydrate metabolism, in fact, equally serious alterations are present in the area of lipid and protein metabolism. The actions of insulin that are referrable to carbohydrate metabolism are multifold. Insulin promotes the translocation of glucose from the intravascular space to the intracellular space by activation of insulin receptors that promote glucose transport. Intracellularly, glucose may be utilized as a direct energy source, converted to glycogen for storage purposes (primarily in the liver, muscle, and kidney), or converted into the lipid synthesis pathway for the promotion of lipid accumulation within the cell. Furthermore, insulin inhibits the release of glucose from the liver, promoting hepatic glucose storage. The actions of insulin on lipid metabolism include the transfer of "excess dietary carbohydrate calories" into the lipid synthesis and storage pool and the inhibition of lipid mobilization from adipose tissue stores. Insulin has both direct and indirect effects on

protein metabolism. The insulin molecule, apparently through specialized cell membrane receptors, works in a coordinated fashion with pituitary growth hormone to stimulate amino acid uptake into cells and promote cell growth and multiplication. Indirectly, insulin promotes glycolysis and inhibits gluconeogenesis.

Insulin release is stimulated by dietary intake (glucose and amino acids and, to a much smaller extent, fats and ketones). The body energy economy is alternatively under the direct control of insulin during the prandial and immediate posprandial periods, whereas it is probably under the direction of glucagon and epinephrine in the distal postprandial periods, growth hormone and cortisol being added during intervals of fasting. The overall effect in the normal healthy individual is very narrow variations in the concentration of all nutrients throughout the course of each day, despite feasting and fasting cycles. These well-regulated nutrient concentrations include glucose, amino acids, triglycerides, cholesterol, ketone bodies, and a number of energy intermediates, such as lactate, pyruvate, and glycerol. The extremes of both hyper- and hypoglycemia are avoided, as are significant variations in lipid and protein concentration.

The deficiency of insulin results in a reversal of all these normal patterns. Hyperglycemia results as a consequence of impaired peripheral glucose uptake and increased hepatic glucose production, both from an increased rate of glycogenolysis and from gluconeogenesis. Hyperlipidemia results from a marked increase in the mobilization of preformed fat in adipose tissues, and ketonuria results if this process continues unabated, without intervention of insulin therapy. The concentration of several counterregulatory hormones is increased, including growth hormone, adrenocorticotropic hormone (corticotropin), cortisone, glucagon, and, in extreme stress, the catecholamines. The combination of insulin deficiency and counterregulatory hormone excess combine to complicate the metabolic picture further, exacerbating hyperglycemia and hyperlipidemia and leading to an increased rate of proteolysis and gluconeogenesis, placing the individual in negative nitrogen balance (1,2).

III. CLINICAL CORRELATES OF THE BIOCHEMICAL CONSEQUENCES OF INSULIN DEFICIENCY (3)

The child with newly diagnosed IDDM usually presents with the classic diabetic triad: polyuria, polydipsia, and polyphagia. These clinical symptoms are a direct consequence of insulin deficiency as it relates to carbohydrate homeostatis. In the absence of adequate insulin synthesis and release during the prandial period, the postprandial rise in blood glucose is excessive, exceeding the renal threshold and resulting in glucosuria. As the insulin secretory capacity continues to deteriorate, hyperglycemia in the fasting state also results, leading to continuous glucosuria.

The magnitude of the energy losses associated with untreated or uncontrolled diabetes mellitus must be appreciated. Let us consider a 10-year-old boy with newly diagnosed diabetes. The caloric requirements for a healthy 10-year-old boy are approximately 2000 cal/day, of which about 1000 is derived from carbohydrate. The patient is initially seen with a urine glucose concentration of 5% (the highest that can be read with the Clinitest) and his 24 h urine volume is 5 L. This calculates to a 24 h urine glucose loss of 250 g, or 1000 cal, derived from dietary carbohydrate that is being lost in the urine. With the high fluid and calorie losses, it is no wonder that the body attempts to compensate for them by increasing both fluid and food intake. These prodigious nutrient losses may be adequately met for various periods, but if a diagnosis of diabetes mellitus is not made at this stage, invariably the additional metabolic consequences of excess fatty acid mobilization and increased ketone body production intervene, resulting in the development of diabetic ketoacidosis, a complication seen in 20–40% of our newly diagnosed diabetic patients.

Eventually, insulin deficiency, or its metabolic consequences, adversely affect essentially all body organ systems. Although the primary focus is on the genitourinary tract, with the initial complaints frequently thought to be secondary to genitourinary infection, the gastrointestinal symptoms become involved as the metabolic status deteriorates, with the development of abdominal pain, nausea, vomiting, and constipation. Similarly, the respiratory system is involved as acidosis develops, with characteristic labored respiration—Kussmaul breathing. Cardiovascular alterations include tachycardia as a regular accompaniment of hyperglycemia; vascular collapse may result from the extreme degrees of dehydration seen in diabetic ketoacidosis (DKA), and cardiac arhythmias may be a consequence of either hypo- or hyperkalemia. Central nervous system (CNS) depression results from continuing severe acidosis, with somnolence and coma developing if proper intervention is not instituted. Cerebral edema and CNS infarction are little understood, but highly feared, complications of DKA (see Chap. 38). Visual disturbances are common at the time of the diagnosis of diabetes and usually are a result of increased glucose in the lens of the eyes. Overt cataracts are seen occasionally and are usually reversible with initiation of insulin therapy. The musculoskeletal system shows symptoms directly related to chronic insulin deficiency. Muscular weakness is a consequence of muscle glycogen depletion and potassium loss. A decline in the level of physical fitness and physical performance can usually be readily documented in the patient with a recent diagnosis of diabetes.

Growth may be adversely affected by insulin deficiency. Almost invariably, patients have lost weight during the symptomatic prediagnosis interval of several weeks. However, height status is more variable. Our own studies indicate that, on average, children who are younger than 10 years of age when the diagnosis is made are of average or above average height, whereas those older than 10 when the diagnosis is made are usually shorter than the national averages and than their own siblings, when corrected for age. These apparently divergent findings may indicate that the duration of insulin deficiency before diagnosis is considerably shorter in children younger than 10 years of age at diagnosis; consequently, no significant adverse effect of insulin deficiency is seen on linear growth. However, it is possible that in those children who develop diabetes at a later age, there has been a prolonged interval of relative insulin deficiency, possibly for several months, or even years, that results in significant slowing of linear growth during the months before diagnosis (4).

IV. THE EARLY CLINICAL COURSE

The early clinical course of diabetes in the child and the adolescent can be viewed from the perspective of endogenous insulin secretory capacity. There is substantial evidence that more than 90% of the pancreatic β cell insulin synthesis and release capacity has been destroyed or effectively inactivated before the clinical features of diabetes mellitus become evident.

The initial phase of diabetes coincides with the development of clinical symptomatology, resulting in presentation and diagnosis. Table 1 lists the presenting symptoms, important clinical signs, and laboratory alterations present at diagnosis in a group of 183 white children (of mainly European ancestry) seen by us over a 2 year period (5). The primary clinical features in both boys and girls include polydipsia, polyuria, nocturia, weight loss, fatigue, and, in many, a recent flu-like illness. The maximum duration of symptoms identified by the patient or parents before diagnosis was slightly in excess of 1 month. Glycosylated hemoglobin (HbA_1) was markedly elevated at diagnosis, indicating a relatively long-term interval of carbohydrate intolerance, probably well in excess of the 30 days identified by the families. Diabetic ketoacidosis occurred in 20% of our patients, with a strict criterion and a pH of 7.2 or less, whereas a more generally accepted criterion of a bicarbonate concentration of 15 mEq/L or less resulted in 42% of our patients

Table 1 Clinical Features at Presentation of Insulin-Dependent Diabetes Mellitus, Whites ($N = 183$)

Clinical features	Male	Female	Total	(No.)
Frequency of symptoms and recent illness, %				
Polydipsia	89	92	90	(178)
Polyuria	90	88	89	(179)
Nocturia	95	93	94	(130)
Recent weight loss	80	84	82	(158)
Fatigue	72	73	73	(135)
Recent "flu-like" infection	56	57	57	(143)
Maximum duration of symptoms, days	30	41	36	(180)
Clinical signs and laboratory mean values				
Impaired level of consciousness, %	15	19	18	(171)
Serum ketones, %	80	87	84	(153)
Blood glucose, mg/dl	415	495	457	(182)
Blood pH	7.31	7.29	7.30	(157)
Blood urea nitrogen, mg/dl	18	18	18	(139)
Serum bicarbonate, mEq/L	15	15	15	(153)
Sodium, mEq/L	133	133	133	(157)
Serum osmoles, mOsmol/L	302	307	305	(145)
C peptide, pmol/ml	0.13	0.11	0.12	(146)
Hemoglobin A_1, %	13.4	14.9	14.2	(158)
Insulin dose at hospital discharge, units/kg/day	0.81	1.14	0.98	(181)

Source: From Reference 5.

being classified as having the complication of diabetic keto-acidosis at diagnosis. We, and others, have identified some special histocompatibility antigen (HLA) relationships with the metabolic status at diagnosis. Patients with the HLA-DR4 are sicker at the time of diagnosis, with higher initial blood glucose concentrations, more frequent diabetic ketoacidosis, a higher degree of dehydration, and a threefold increase in the frequency of impaired consciousness. A preexisting history of viral infections is found in 62% of the HLA-DR4 patients and 37% of those without this antigen. The significance of these observations is unclear, but they suggest that the mechanism of β cell destruction is somewhat different in HLA-DR3 and HLA-DR4 persons or that superimposition of a viral infection in the HLA-DR4 patients results in a rapid β cell destruction and a more rapidly progressing metabolic deterioration (5).

The second phase in the early natural history of diabetes in the child is the period of clinical remission. This has also been referred to as the honeymoon phase. According to our studies, as well as those of many other investigators worldwide, significant numbers of diabetic children, whose diagnosis is recent, undergo a spontaneous decline in insulin requirement. *Partial remission* is arbitrarily defined as an insulin requirement of less than 0.5 units/kg/day, with metabolic normality (normal blood glucose variations and normal glycosylated concentration), whereas *total remission* is defined as complete metabolic normality, without the need for exogenous insulin administration. According to our studies, partial remission occurs in approximately two-thirds of all

patients, with the nadir in insulin requirements seen at about 13 weeks after diagnosis. Partial remission is much less common in the younger child, but it increases in frequency with increasing age through adolescence. Complete remission occurs much less regularly and has been seen in approximately 3% of our patients. The duration of the insulin-free interval has varied from as short as 1 month to as long as 2 years. Invariably, all our patients who have experienced complete remission have eventually returned to full insulin requirement at a relatively standard dose of insulin (6).

The mechanism that results in clinical remission is almost certainly secondary to improved β cell insulin synthesis and release after clinical stabilization of the patient. At the time of diagnosis of IDDM, most, but certainly not all, of the β cells have been destroyed by what in most cases is an autoimmune process. The few remaining cells are damaged as a consequence of the inflammatory process and produce little or no insulin. With initiation of exogenous insulin therapy, the inflammatory process appears to be abated somewhat, allowing the "sick" β cells to return toward metabolic normality, with some synthesis and release of insulin in response to dietary intake. Depending upon the magnitude of recovery, insulin secretion may be minimal or near normal, resulting in no detectable decrease in exogenous insulin requirements, to full withdrawal of external insulin.

The remission phenomenon has been exceedingly important in stimulating investigators to pursue pharmacologic mechanisms for preservation of β cell function. This work began initially with Elliot et al., who treated newly diagnosed diabetic children with high doses of prednisone (7). Soon thereafter, the important clinical trials of Stiller et al. (8) demonstrated that the potent immunosuppressive agent cyclosporin A could greatly increase the frequency of total remission, approaching 50% in an uncontrolled trial. Various other immunosuppressive and antioxidant agents have been tried, with varying success (9,10). The use of pharmacologic agents at the time of diagnosis of diabetes mellitus, which might protect the β cell against progressive inflammatory damage, must be viewed with great caution. Considerably more clinical research must be carried out before any of these agents can be recommended in the routine treatment of the newly diagnosed diabetic patient.

The third phase of the early natural history of diabetes in the child and adolescent is relapse, an interval of progressive increase in insulin requirement, resulting from a declining endogenous insulin secretory capacity, as well as from other factors, such as the development of insulin resistance. Figure 1 illustrates the changing insulin requirement over a 5 year interval after diagnosis in a group of approximately 500 adolescent children (6). One notes that insulin requirements are consistently higher for girls than for boys and that there is a linear increase in insulin dosage administered to the girls, up to a peak of 1.20 units/kg after 4 years of diabetes, with a modest decline thereafter. The adolescent boys appear to reach a plateau in their insulin requirement about 3 years after diagnosis at a dose of near 1.0 units/kg. The interval of relapse in most patients is identifiable only in retrospective analysis of insulin requirements over time. There is usually a slowly progressive increase in insulin requirement, as expressed per kilogram body weight, over a period of months or even several years. On the other hand, some children demonstrate an acute loss of the remission phase, usually associated with intercurrent illnesses or significant environmental stress.

The final stage in the early natural history of diabetes in the child and adolescent is the interval of *total diabetes*, which by strict definition refers to the period associated with complete β cell destruction, with no capacity for endogenous insulin synthesis or release. Once reached, this is an irreversible stage, only pancreas transplantation offering a hope of cure. Total diabetes may in fact be a misnomer in the sense that a significant number of patients, particularly those whose diagnosis is made in adolescence and young adult life, may have a small but definite capacity for synthesis and release of insulin for many years. From a practical point of view, however, total diabetes can be considered to be reached when the insulin requirements for the preadolescent has plateaued at approximately 0.8 units/kg per day and in the adolescent at about 1.0 units/kg per day. Interestingly, the insulin requirement of the adult with IDDM is between 35 and 40 units/day, or an insulin dosage of about 0.5 units/kg per day. This observation strongly suggests a major component of "insulin resistance" associated with adolescence, possibly explained by the insulin-resistant effects of sex hormones, the increase in growth hormone secretion, and the increased levels of stress that are characteristic of adolescence.

V. MANAGEMENT COMPONENTS FOR THE CHILD WITH DIABETES MELLITUS

Diabetes mellitus is a complex systemic, metabolic, and endocrine disorder with acute alterations reflected throughout the energy homeostatic system and chronic complications potentially involving all organ systems, with particular damage directed to the microvasculature of the eyes, kidney, and nervous system and with macrovascular damage involving the heart, kidneys, brain, and peripheral vascular systems. Proper therapy of the child and adolescent with diabetes involves the integration of insulin administration, dietary management, physical exercise and fitness, and emotional support (3,11–13).

We are currently in the midst of major, if not revolutionary, changes in the strategies, techniques, and objectives of diabetes management. A number of factors have contributed to these changes. They include the development of practical techniques for short- and intermediate-term assessment of metabolic control using capillary blood glucose monitoring and assessment of glycosylated proteins, particularly glycosylated hemoglobin determination, on a routine basis. The widespread utilization of these monitoring techniques has provided to the patient, as well as the therapeutic team, quantitative means of assessing metabolic status over time. These advances, occurring over the past 15 years, have been coupled with improvement in the purification of animal sources of insulin, the introduction of human insulin produced by DNA technology, and, more recently, the development of insulin analogs that may allow much more precise "tailoring" of an individual patient's insulin therapeutic needs based on the individual's personal lifestyle (14,15). The development of insulin infusion devices, both external and implanted, also provides the potential for more physiologic insulin delivery (16).

With these methodologic advances has come an increasing interest in attempting to normalize energy metabolism with the anticipation that this will eliminate or reduce the

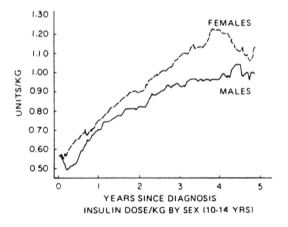

Figure 1 Comparison of mean insulin dosages in boys and girls from the diagnosis of diabetes through 5 years of disease in those diagnosed between 10 and 14 years of age. (From Ref. 6.)

serious vascular complications of diabetes. This increasingly popular therapeutic movement has been improperly referred to as "intensive insulin therapy" (17). Unfortunately, many, both physicians and patients, have concluded that the way to improve diabetes management is simply to give insulin more often. This is a serious misconception that may result in more harm than good by induction of frequent hypoglycemia.

VI. THE DIABETES CONTROL AND COMPLICATIONS TRIAL (DCCT): IMPLICATIONS FOR PATIENT MANAGEMENT

The DCCT began in 1982 as a multicenter intervention trial in which adolescents and young adults with IDDM were randomized into either traditional therapy or an experimental therapy involving overall intensification of management. Approximately 1500 patients were randomized into this study, which was completed in June 1993. The comparative results unequivocally documented that management techniques that moved the patients toward physiologic energy homeostasis were associated with significant decrease in retinopathy, nephropathy, neuropathy, and probably also large-vessel disease (18). This study finally closed the door on the long-standing argument about whether there was an identifiable relationship between metabolic control over time and the serious vascular complications of the disease.

It is essential to emphasize the absolute importance of the therapeutic team as a key factor in the success of the DCCT. The team members included (1) diabetes nurse educators, (2) dietitians, (3) behavioral scientists, and (4) diabetologists. The patient was the central figure in the therapeutic team and was involved in all aspects of therapeutic decision making. The definition of experimental or intensive therapy within the DCCT included a minimum of three insulin injections per day or use of an insulin infusion pump, but this was clearly not the primary focus of this intervention. The patients were continuously involved in ongoing education in all aspects of diabetes and its management. For most patients, intensification of dietary management was an essential feature in improvement of metabolic control. Recommendations for exercise and providing emotional support were also of major importance. The frequency of patient contact and the establishment of an open, friendly, flexible therapeutic relationship between the team and the patient proved invaluable (19,20).

The obvious benefits of intensive diabetes management as practiced within the DCCT are tempered somewhat by the threefold increase in frequency of serious hypoglycemia in those patients compared with patients in the standard treatment arm of the study. Approximately 14% of the total DCCT patient population were adolescents at entry (between 13 and 18 years of age). In a subanalysis focused on the adolescent participants in the study, the benefits in terms of reduction and delay of vascular complications were comparable to those seen in the adults, but the frequency of severe hypoglycemia in the intensively managed adolescents was approximately twice as great as in the adults (21). The other major complication of intensive management as seen within the DCCT was excessive weight gain, occurring two to three times as frequently in the intensively managed cohort. One must be concerned about this problem because it may lead to noncompliance in the short term and may adversely impact on large-vessel disease in the long term.

The DCCT results place a strong mandate on all of us who care for individuals with insulin-dependent diabetes mellitus. There is a clear obligation to work increasingly closely with our patients and their families to achieve a level of physiologic homeostasis approaching that of normality. With few exceptions, this can only be accomplished by utilizing the resources of the diabetes therapeutic team. This concept, originally introduced by Etzweiler in the late 1950s, has come to characterize university-based diabetes teaching and management programs, as well as diabetes specialty clinics (22). The diabetes therapeutic team received its maximum challenge within the DCCT and its major endorsement through the outcome of this 10 year intervention trial.

The American Diabetes Association has estimated that fewer than 5% of Americans with diabetes mellitus receive their care from a trained endocrinologist or diabetologist. My personal estimates suggest that possibly as many as 20% of children and adolescent with IDDM in the United States receive the benefits of university-based specialty care utilizing the therapeutic team concept. We are faced with both a major dilemma and an extraordinary challenge and opportunity. In a research setting with small numbers of highly selected IDDM patients and almost unlimited resources, we have learned how to improve metabolic control, which has resulted in reduction in complication rates. We must find a means of achieving the same therapeutic goals in a safe, cost-effective fashion for the general population of diabetic patients (23).

VII. THE THERAPEUTIC TEAM

Medical care of the child with diabetes is quite different from that of most other diseases handled by the pediatrician. The primary focus is on education. A major responsibility for the physician is to ensure that the patient and family members are well educated about the diversity of problems associated with diabetes. This cannot be a one-time educational experience: it must be a constantly renewed and ongoing activity. However, the attainment of knowledge is only half the battle. The knowledge gained about insulin administration, the utilization of monitoring information, dietary principles, and the incorporation of exercise into daily life must be accepted by the patient in a very personal sense, with adherence to the therapeutic regimen as a personal commitment for improved health. Each patient and family have their own unique barriers to full acceptance and incorporation of the recommended therapeutic regimen. Although most of these barriers are in the psychologic sphere, other factors, such as peer group pressures, financial problems, or unavailability of parents at appropriate times, may make the recommended therapeutic regimen difficult, if not impossible, to follow.

The physician-diabetologist must serve as captain of the therapeutic team. It is his or her responsibility to assess the unique characteristics of each patient and family and to determine the general therapeutic strategies to be used in an attempt to help the child achieve and maintain good health. Several other team members are essential for the development of an effective diabetes therapeutic program. The diabetes nurse educator plays a pivotal role. Although the physician must always be involved in reinforcing the educational components of therapy, it is a grossly inefficient utilization of his or her time to carry the primary educational activities. The nurse educator must become involved with the family as early as possible, usually during the hospitalization at the time of initial diagnosis. It is clear from a number of studies that this is not an optimal time for teaching because of the family shock at the diagnosis of diabetes. However, we believe it important to begin this process and ensure that the family have at least "survival skills" when the child is discharged from the hospital 5–7 days later. The educational process continues at each clinic visit, and if necessary, special educational sessions are set up with the diabetes educator outside the normal clinic schedule. The dietitian assesses the family's knowledge of food and nutrition at the initial hospital visit and begins constructing a diet appropriate to the particular child. At least, an annual review by the dietitian of the patient's nutritional status is desirable. Specific questions about the appropriateness of particular food substances can usually be handled by telephone consultation. The psychiatric social worker plays a special role within the diabetes therapeutic team. It is the social worker's responsibility to assess the strengths and weaknesses of the family as they relate to emotional issues, economic and community support, educational activities, and so on. It is usually the social worker's assessment and recommendations that determine whether other professionals, such as clinical psychologists and psychiatrists, become promptly involved with the family. The development of psychiatric problems over time as a consequence of the stresses of the disorder also call for the social worker's reinvolvement. The social worker can be particularly useful in families with limited financial resources, helping them to obtain support for diabetes medication and supplies, transportation to clinic appointments, and the like.

The core diabetes therapeutic team includes the physician diabetologist, diabetes nurse educator, dietitian, and psychiatric social worker. However, the central member of the therapeutic team is the patient. The patient, when old enough to be involved in a meaningful way in decisions, or the parents of the younger child, must be incorporated from the beginning in the planning of therapeutic strategies and in all other major decisions. It is not therapeutically meaningful to insist on an insulin therapy of two injections daily and a monitoring program of four blood glucose determinations daily when the patient adamantly refuses more than one injection of insulin and no monitoring. Although one continues to try to educate the patient and family about the importance of a more comprehensive approach at the same time, it is essential to deal with reality. Most patients understand and appreciate the responsibility being placed upon them as part of the therapeutic team and respond maturely and appropriately to it.

The need for the diabetes therapeutic team cannot be

minimized. Creative new ways must be found to make these resources available to all children and adolescents with IDDM. University diabetes centers must provide the leadership and direction for the development of networks of diabetes therapeutic programs across geographic areas, involving small communities with apparently limited diabetes-related resources. The local family physician or pediatrician must be reincorporated into the therapeutic team and given encouragement for periodic reeducation to function locally as the diabetes leader. In every community, it should be possible to identify nurses and dietitians who are willing to accept increased responsibility with appropriate training to become the local "diabetes educator or special diabetes dietitian." The university-based diabetes center or specialty clinic must provide outreach to the local community diabetes program by providing periodic visiting specialists, local patient and professional teaching conferences, and referral services for especially difficult management problems. Opportunities for educational renewal by the local team members must be available on a periodic basis. Such a networking program, once in place, should provide the benefits of diabetes team management to the great majority of children and adolescents with IDDM in the United States. Although initial costs of such a program will clearly be in excess of current management activities, the long-term reduction in vascular complications will greatly reduce the health care costs associated with visual loss, end-stage renal disease, peripheral vascular disease, heart attacks, and strokes.

VIII. THERAPEUTIC OBJECTIVES AND MONITORING REQUIREMENTS

It is the therapeutic goal of all of us to "put our patients right." We would like to be able to provide such comprehensive management to our patients with diabetes mellitus that they are metabolically normal, physically and emotionally healthy, and free of diabetes-related complications, both acute and chronic, as they go through life. Unfortunately, even with the advances of the DCCT, this is not now possible. We regularly find ourselves making therapeutic compromises between what we and the patients would like to achieve and what is reasonable within their personal life situations. In Table 2 are listed the principles of diabetes therapy as they have evolved over the last several years within the diabetes clinic within the Children's Hospital of Pittsburgh. Certainly, a primary therapeutic objective is to eliminate the obvious symptoms of poorly controlled diabetes, including polyuria, polydipsia, and polyphagia. Conversely, serious hypoglycemia should be avoided while understanding that mild, readily managed hypoglycemia is likely to be a concomitant of otherwise reasonable management. Careful attention to physical growth and sexual maturation is important. Inadequate insulin therapy results in slow growth and delayed maturation. Unfortunately, the achievement of these important therapeutic goals is not enough. Many patients deny symptoms of either hyper- or hypoglycemia with maintenance of normal growth and maturation while maintaining blood glucose and glycosylated

Table 2 Principles of Diabetic Therapy

Elimination of the clinical features of inadequately controlled diabetes, including polyuria, polydipsia, and polyphagia

Prevention of diabetic ketoacidosis

Avoidance of hypoglycemia

Maintenance of normal growth and sexual maturation

Prevention of obesity

Early detection of associated diseases: a number of autoimmune diseases (such as Hashimoto's thyroiditis) occur with increased frequency in patients with IDDM; routine surveillance is important to detect these conditions in the early stages

Prevention of emotional disorders: the chronic and unrelenting demands of the disease and the therapeutic regimentation necessary to achieve reasonable control result in behavioral disability in a large number of families; the therapeutic program should be designed to prevent such problems or provide prompt and effective therapy as required

Prevention of chronic vascular complications of diabetes

Table 3 Specific Therapeutic Objectives

1. Glycosylated hemoglobin (total HbA_1 or HbA_{1c}) should be obtained every 3–4 months; the goal in patients participating in an optimized management program should be an HbA_{1c} of 8% or lower; a goal of 9% for other patients is reasonable (see text)
2. Self-monitoring for blood glucose should be carried out daily before each meal and at bedtime; the blood glucose goals in optimized patients should be in the range 80–120 mg/dl in the fasting state and 80–140 mg/dl at other times (see text for goals for younger patients)
3. Urine testing: daily dipstick testing for glucose and ketones of the first voided urine in the morning; presence of ketonuria should lead to prompt consultation with the therapeutic team; quantitative 24 h urine glucose determinations should be done annually or as necessary to help improve overall diabetes management; urine glucose loss should not exceed 7% of the daily dietary carbohydrate, equivalent to approximately 20–25 glucose in the 24 h urine of the average teenager
4. Urine testing for protein: dipstick testing for gross albuminuria should be performed on a single voided specimen at each clinic visit; presence of proteinuria should promptly lead to assessment of a 24 h urine collection; in the absence of postural proteinuria, overt proteinuria should result in a detailed renal evaluation and appropriate therapeutic intervention; microalbumin methods are now becoming available and are recommended for routine assessment; a timed overnight specimen is preferred
5. Blood lipids: fasting blood should be obtained annually for determination of total cholesterol, HDL, LDL, VLDL, and triglyceride; the lipid fractions should be within the normal range for nondiabetic children and adolescents; hyperlipidemia may reflect inadequate diabetes management or genetic lipid alterations
6. Thyroid function should be assessed annually by determination of TSH, T_4, and free T_4; The presence of a goiter should indicate assessment of thyroid antibody levels as well

hemoglobin levels that are, it is clear, persistently and excessively high.

Specific therapeutic objectives are presented in Table 3. Based on the DCCT results, primary therapeutic emphasis should be placed on achieving a metabolic status that is near normal while avoiding the known complications of this approach, including hypoglycemia and excessive weight gain. The primary biochemical guides to management include glycosylated hemoglobin obtained every 3–4 months and self-monitoring for blood glucose carried out three to four times daily. A number of commercial techniques are available for determination of glycosylated hemoglobin. It is imperative that the physician be well acquainted with his or her own laboratory, its normal range, and any special peculiarities of the assay. The major assays are total HbA_1 and HbA_{1c}. The DCCT used a highly precise method for measuring HbA_{1c} that had an upper limit of normal of 6.05%. This was the therapeutic goal of the intensively managed patients, a goal achieved in only about 5%. At the close of the study, the mean HbA_{1c} in the intensively managed adults was 7.1%, compared with 9% in the conventionally treated cohort. In those individuals who entered the study as adolescents, mean values were approximately 1% higher with the intensively treated adolescents, with a mean of 8.1% and the conventional at 9.8%. Because the effectiveness of the management appears to be comparable in both adults and adolescents in terms of minimizing rates of progression of vascular change, it seems reasonable to use the HbA_{1c} value of 8.0% as a therapeutic goal for adolescents participating in an optimized management program. In those laboratories utilizing total HbA_1, the appropriate values would be 1.5–2.0% higher.

There were no patients younger than 13 years of age at entry into the DCCT, and at conclusion of the study, there were no individuals under 20 years of age. Consequently, one translates the conclusions of the DCCT to younger children with extreme caution. It is our view at this time that although

the general principle of moving all patients toward physiologic homeostasis should be embraced, specific goals should be higher in the preadolescent, particularly the preschooler. It is probably wiser to focus on blood glucose variation in these two younger groups, the glycosylated hemoglobin playing a secondary role in terms of assessing effectiveness of management.

Routine self-monitoring for blood glucose is an essential component of good diabetes management. We recommend that the patient carry out blood glucose determinations before each meal and at bedtime. In addition, periodically, blood glucose determination at 2–3 a.m. should be obtained to document whether hypoglycemia is occurring during sleep. Further, it is obvious that other blood glucose determinations should be obtained under special circumstances. For example, it is important to document symptomatic hypoglycemia by promptly doing a blood glucose determination. During illness, blood glucose monitoring probably should be more frequently obtained. Although there is a general correlation between the frequency of blood glucose determinations and control, this is true only if the individual uses this information to make informed decisions regarding alteration in insulin dosage or other aspects of management.

Practically speaking, in the past, we have not insisted that our patients obtain blood glucose values at school before lunch, but we insist that prelunch values be obtained routinely on the weekend to assess properly the need for regular insulin in the morning injection. With the move toward intensification we are now recommending that prelunch blood sugar determinations be obtained on an increasingly routine basis. Self-determinations of blood glucose should be recorded by the patient in some format that can be easily reviewed by the physician and therapeutic team on a regular basis at office or clinic visits. There are major advantages to the use of meters with extensive memory capacity, primarily to cross-check the patient's accuracy in the recording of blood glucose results. However, the use of a memory meter should not be used as an excuse for not recording the daily results in a format that is available for review by the parent as well as the team.

We are in the process of adapting the DCCT blood glucose goals for our adolescent patients who have made a commitment with us to optimize management. These blood glucose goals are directed toward achieving a normal fasting blood glucose in the range of 80–120 mg/dl. Any other daytime determination should fall in the range of 80–140 mg/dl, with 3 a.m. values in excess of 70 mg/dl. The DCCT results, based on seven-point glucose profiles done once monthly, gave a mean daily blood glucose of 153 mg/dl in the intensively management cohort compared with 230 mg/dl in the conventionally treated group. These results, although documenting the improved status of the intensively managed patients, further illustrates the difficulty in achieving blood glucose goals close to the normal range. We are pleased if our patients meet the agreed goals about 80% of the time.

We are in transition within our own clinic in attempting to come to grips with the issues surrounding the general implementation of DCCT guidelines in the younger child. At this time, in the pre-adolescent (6–13 years of age), I am recommending that fasting blood glucose goals be the same as for the adolescent, that is, 80–120 mg/dl; the other determinations, all of which are postprandial, fall in the 80–180 mg/dl range. There are obviously preadolescents patients who are stable and predictable enough in blood glucose excursion that careful management adjustments can be made to bring them into line with the adolescent recommendations. For the preschool-aged child, we strongly recommend that higher blood glucose goals be implemented to minimize the danger of hypoglycemia. Our specific recommendations are for fasting blood glucose to fall in the 100–140 mg/dl range and postprandial values in the 100–200 mg/dl range. Allowable glycosylated hemoglobin results might be 1–1.5% higher than those of the adolescent who is participating in intensified management.

With the widespread acceptance of routine self-monitoring for blood glucose, urine glucose testing has largely been relegated to an assay of historical interest only. We think that this is a mistake and that serious therapeutic errors could have been avoided by routine daily testing for urine glucose and ketones. We continue to urge our patients to perform at least one urine test daily, preferably the first void. A dipstick method is used to measure both glucose and ketones. The presence of ketonuria is always of importance. Ketonuria associated with negative or minimal glucose spill is suggestive of nighttime hypoglycemia, and the combination of high urinary glucose and ketones must be considered a strong indication of impending serious metabolic deterioration that requires careful follow-up. Under these circumstances, each successive voiding should be checked until ketonuria is clear. Communication with the therapeutic team is necessary to alter management as necessary to prevent progression to DKA.

I continue to use 24 h urine collections for quantitative urine glucose determination about once annually or as necessary to assist in changing therapeutic strategies. A maximum excretion of (7% of the daily dietary carbohydrate is a reliable index of reasonable control. This translates to 20–25 g glucose for 24 h in the average teenager. Urine protein determination is an essential component of routine management. A freshly voided specimen should be checked by one of the "dipstick" protein methods at each visit. These techniques become positive with a urinary albumin concentration of about 300 mg/L or total protein of 500 mg/L. Proteinuria at this level or higher, if related to diabetes renal damage, is indicative of significant and serious pathology. The development of more sensitive methods for albumin determination, referred to as microalbuminuria, has led to the observation that protein excretion in the range of 30–300 mg/24 h may be indicative of impending, progressive renal disease. Consequently, many centers, ourselves included, are now also routinely assaying for microalbuminuria. A carefully obtained 24 h urine specimen is probably the best choice. For practical reasons, however, a timed overnight urine specimen obtained the evening before the clinic or office visit is a reasonable compromise.

Patients with poorly controlled diabetes mellitus frequently have elevations in several of the blood lipid fractions. As a component of assessment of control, we recommend that fasting blood be obtained annually for the determination of total cholesterol, low-density lipoproteins (LDL), high-density lipoproteins (HDL), very low density lipoproteins (VLDL), and triglyceride. Total cholesterol values should be below 200 mg/dl, LDL should be below 130 mg/dl, and triglyceride below 140 mg/dl. Elevated lipid values may be a result of either inadequate diabetes management or one of the forms of genetic hyperlipidemia. If the patient's diabetes control is unsatisfactory, the first objective should be to improve overall diabetes management and determine whether the elevated lipid fractions return toward the normal range. On the other hand, if persistent hyperlipidemia is identified in individuals with satisfactory diabetes control, then an evaluation for genetic hyperlipidemia should follow. Pharmacologic therapy with lipid-lowering agents may be necessary.

Thyroid disease is commonly seen in association with IDDM. Hashimoto's thyroiditis, an autoimmune destructive process, appears to share many similarities with the mechanism of β cell destruction leading to IDDM. In our experience, approximately 40% of our patients, particularly during the adolescent years, have evidence of Hashimoto's thyroiditis, including the presence of a goiter and elevations in thyroid antibodies. Approximately 10% of these patients develop hypothyroidism, and a significantly smaller number develop hyperthyroidism. Timely diagnosis and appropriate management of these conditions are obviously important to the patient's well-being. Careful examination of the patient's neck should be a part of each clinic visit, and assessment of thyroid function should occur as specifically indicated or on an annual basis. We recommend that serum be assessed for thyrotropin-stimulating hormone (TSH), thyroxine (T_4), free T_4, and thyroid antibodies.

IX. CLINICAL ASSESSMENT AND THERAPEUTIC DECISION MAKING

Children and adolescents with insulin-dependent diabetes mellitus require regular ongoing physical, biochemical, and emotional assessment and modification in all aspects of management to meet changing needs and individual lifestyle requirements. Because of the complexity of this problem, we are convinced that this process should be carried out in a setting in which the talents of several diabetes therapeutic team members can be brought to bear on the problems of the patient and family.

In the past, we have seen our patients routinely at 4 month intervals. We are convinced that this is an inadequate frequency for the great majority of our patients if we are to be successful in achieving acceptable therapeutic goals. We are currently recommending that routine care involve a full clinic visit at 3 month intervals, with interim visits with the nurse educator or dietitian as required. The physician's routine evaluation should include a careful review of general health and diabetes management issues in the interval since the last examination. Particular inquiry in regard to frequency, severity, and management of hypoglycemia should be elicited. Symptoms of hyperglycemia, such as nocturia or urinary frequency, should be documented. Dietary management should be reviewed by the physician, and specific dietary problems should be referred to the dietitian. An evaluation of physical activity should be obtained and the patient encouraged to participate in daily exercise to achieve superior physical fitness. Psychologic issues should be reviewed, including how the patient is handling the personal problems of diabetes and its management, school performance, and interpersonal relationships at school and at home. Issues of sexuality and drug and alcohol abuse should be approached directly in a nonjudgmental fashion. Sexually active girls should be referred to a gynecologist for additional counseling.

Physical examination should be complete. Height and weight measurements should be transferred to a standard percentile growth grid in which assessment of growth parameters over time can be accurately followed. A declining growth rate or inadequate weight gain should result in a careful review to determine whether this is a reflection of inadequate diabetes management. In the adolescent patient, the physical examination should include determination of Tanner staging and information on menses in girls. Blood pressure should be carefully obtained with the patient in a relaxed state. Even modest elevations above the appropriate blood pressure range for age should lead to additional determinations during the visit and, if necessary, periodically by the school nurse. The development of persistent hypertension is a serious problem in the diabetic patient and must be aggressively evaluated and treated. The diabetologist should be comfortable and confident in carrying out a routine ophthalmologic examination, looking for the early changes indicative of background retinopathy. Insulin injection sites should be carefully examined. The presence of lipohypertrophy may result in impairment of insulin absorption and contribute to inadequate management.

A major portion of the routine visit is the review of the patient-generated blood glucose records by the diabetologist. This should be an opportunity for teaching about diabetes therapeutics and encouraging the patient's and parents' participation in therapeutic decision making. The individual's blood glucose goals in the fasting and postprandial state are reviewed, and an assessment of the interim performance is provided. The focus is on insulin adjustments, but the integration of diet and physical activity must also be emphasized in these discussions. Any therapeutic changes must be followed by a telephone conversation between the patient and the therapeutic team, which may include faxing the most recent blood glucose results. The results of the biochemical assessment (see earlier) are shared with the family and referring physician by letter within a very few days of the clinic visit. Elevations in glycosylated hemoglobin, for example, may dictate more vigorous therapeutic changes than the initial review of the patient's blood glucose record. Achievement of biochemical therapeutic goals should result in congratulations to the patient and family and encouragement to keep up the good work. Lack of achievement of goals should not be presented in a negative or punitive fashion but rather as encouragement to the patient and family to try even harder with the assistance of the therapeutic team in the future.

X. CONSULTATIONS AND REFERRALS

For the child and adolescent with diabetes mellitus, there may be several occasions on which the advice of physicians outside the therapeutic team may be especially valuable. We recommend that all children with diabetes of at least 5 years duration, as well as all patients during their adolescent years, be seen by an ophthalmologist on an annual basis. Ideally, the ophthalmologist should have experience in early diabetic retinal changes. Fundus photography, either stereo color photography or fluorescein angiography, may be appropriate as a baseline observation sometime during the adolescent years. The detection of vascular changes in the eye by either the family physician or diabetologist should promptly result in ophthalmologic referral. Although, in most cases, the ophthalmologist provides no therapeutic intervention at that time, the visit may provide an opportunity for the therapeutic team to reemphasize the importance of good diabetes management. Adolescent girls should be referred to a gynecologist, and this process should be accelerated in sexually active adolescents. The stress of diabetes and its management requirements exact a heavy toll in terms of behavioral problems and disabilities. In prospective studies carried out in our institution, nearly 50% of our patients during their movement through adolescence developed significant psychopathology (24). In most cases, this was pathologic depression, requiring professional intervention. Other problems include antisocial acting-out behaviors, eating disorders, and adjustment problems. It is essential for all therapeutic team members to be sensitive to behavioral issues and be prepared for referral to colleagues in psychiatry or psychology if necessary. There is a natural reticence on the part of most patients and families toward psychiatric referrals. By including the behavioral scientist as an integral member of the therapeutic team from the beginning and emphasizing the importance of psychologic well-being as part of the management of the patient with diabetes, the likelihood of family cooperation, if active intervention therapy is needed, is increased.

Eventually, the patient followed by the pediatric diabetes specialist must be referred for total care based on age. It is our preference to continue to work with these patients through adolescence, high school graduation being a natural time to terminate this therapeutic relationship and hand the patient over to an adult diabetologist. All too often, the young adult diabetic, following high school graduation and either entry into the workforce or departure from home for university education, is frequently lost from the health care system and may not return to it for several years. Unfortunately the return is frequently precipitated by an acute event, such as retinal hemorrhage or other diabetic complications. It is not enough simply to refer the patient back to the family doctor and assume that proper future management will be arranged locally. These patients deserve the opportunity to continue in a therapeutic environment characterized by the diabetes therapeutic team and led by a skilled internist or diabetologist. Assuring that this connection is made will go a long way toward minimizing serious complications during the young adult years.

XI. THERAPEUTIC STRATEGIES FOR THE CHILD AND ADOLESCENT WITH DIABETES MELLITUS

Successful therapeutic management of the child and adolescent with diabetes mellitus requires a highly integrated four-pronged approach: insulin administration, dietary management, physical activity and physical fitness, and emotional support. The nutritional aspects of diabetes management, as well as psychologic aspects, are covered in later chapters.

This section focuses on insulin therapeutics and exercise as components of overall management.

A. Insulin Therapy

The past 15 years have witnessed major changes in all aspects of insulin therapeutics. Improvement in manufacturing techniques have resulted in remarkably increased purity of commercially available insulins. Mixed beef and pork insulin, formerly the standard of therapy, has been basically removed from the marketplace. Highly purified pork insulin and human insulin produced by DNA technology are the choices available. The general wisdom has been that human insulin has both theoretical and practical advantages and should be the insulin of choice. Two issues have raised concern about this apparently reasonable conclusion. Several investigators, particularly European, have reported that severe hypoglycemia, usually without typical hypoglycemic symptoms, is far more common among patients treated with human insulin preparations. The suggestion is that there is something uniquely different about the body's response to human insulin that increases the likelihood of hypoglycemia. The controversy remains unresolved, with most studies not supportive of a uniquely dangerous hypoglycemic potential to human insulin (25,26). The second issue has to do with the time course of human insulin and relates to our own experience and decision to choose pork insulin as our primary insulin preparation. All the human insulin preparations appear to have a quicker onset time and a shorter duration of effect than the comparable pork insulin preparations (27). Because most of our patients are on a standard split-dose regimen of NPH Insulin plus Regular Iletin given before breakfast and the evening meal, the shorter time course of human NPH Insulin, particularly overnight, does not provide adequate glucose control for most of our patients. Increasing the dose increases the likelihood of nocturnal hypoglycemia. For this very practical reason, the great majority of our patients are managed with highly purified pork NPH Insulin and Regular Iletin. Current research of the insulin manufacturers focuses on the development of synthetic analogs that will have variable action profiles. It should be possible in the near future to tailor the individual patient's insulin management carefully to his or her lifestyle and changing requirements. The eventual availability of a family of synthetic insulins will make the demise of animal species of insulin less painful for all of us.

There has been a gradual movement toward intensification of diabetes management, climaxed by the results of the DCCT. The term "intensive insulin therapy" has unfortunately become embedded in our terminology and to the uninitiated may be interpreted to mean that overall diabetes management can be improved simply by increasing the frequency of insulin administration. The proper message, of course, is that improved results are accomplished in the great majority of patients only with intensification of all aspects of management. The "therapeutic set" of the diabetes team, with full cooperation of the patient and family, is directed toward achieving either optimal management utilizing whatever resources are available or something less. The concept of conventional versus intensive management must be set aside. We must undertake to do the very best we can with each patient, understanding that there are major differences in resources and abilities, as well as many barriers to the achievement of near metabolic normality.

At this time, essentially all our newly diagnosed IDDM patients are placed on a combination of NPH Insulin plus Regular Iletin before breakfast and the evening meal, using pork insulin as the species source. Initial insulin requirements are approximately 1.0 units/kg/day. A partial remission, identified as a decline in insulin requirement below 0.5 units/kg/day associated with very good metabolic control, occurs in more than 65% of all newly diagnosed patients during the first several weeks after diagnosis, with the nadir in insulin requirement reached on average between 12 and 16 weeks after diagnosis. During this period, insulin doses must be carefully adjusted downward to prevent hypoglycemia. In some cases, the evening dose can be entirely eliminated. This is particularly true in those children in the 6–10 year age group. In 2–3% of patients "total remission" occurs, identified by essentially normal metabolic status without the need for insulin injections. This period is usually short, a few weeks or months, but in some cases may last for as long as 2 years before insulin needs are again expressed. The future clinical course of those patients who have experienced a complete remission is in no way different from that in those patients who have a more characteristic course. Eventually, in all patients, insulin requirements begin to climb after the nadir of early remission and generally plateau at about 0.8 units/kg/day in the preadolescent and somewhat above 1.0 units/kg/day in the adolescent child.

B. Insulin Therapeutic Strategies

At this time, approximately 75% of our patients are on therapy utilizing pork insulin, with NPH Insulin and Regular Iletin given two or more times daily. Most of the remaining patients are on similar combinations but utilizing human insulin. By applying blood glucose goals derived from self-monitoring of blood glucose as defined earlier, insulin adjustments are made as necessary to attempt continually to bring the patient's glucose variation into the target range. Of course, diet and exercise alterations are also considered and applied as necessary. I use a "10% rule" in terms of insulin changes. By summing the total daily insulin dose and dividing by 10, one obtains a number of units of insulin that are generally safe to increase or decrease in a patient who requires change. However, a maximum increase is 6 units (total insulin dose of 60 units). If the patient's blood glucose levels are generally high throughout, then the distribution of the increase follows the current distribution, usually two-thirds added to the morning and one-third to the evening dosage. On the other hand, if the patient has a particular time point, for example before dinner, that is persistently out of range, then the insulin dose increment applies only to the morning insulin and the amount is determined by 10% of the morning dose. Again, the distribution between NPH Insulin and Regular Iletin depends upon the blood glucose levels. In the asymptomatic patient, we prefer to make insulin adjustments relatively slowly, after 3–5 days on a particular dose. On the other hand, if the patient is symptomatic and/or ketonuric, one must be more aggressive in moving toward acceptable blood glucose excursion.

A very common management problem is illustrated by the child whose fasting blood glucoses are consistently elevated. The usual strategy is to increase the predinner NPH Insulin until fasting glucoses are satisfactory. The common complication of this technique is that nocturnal hypoglycemia may be induced, leading to the Somogyi reaction and rebound hypoglycemia the next morning. This is particularly true with human insulin because of its shorter duration time. An alternative approach is to move the predinner NPH Insulin to bedtime. This timing alteration, without an increase in insulin dosage, may resolve the dilemma. If fasting glucose levels are still high, then careful progressive increase in the bedtime NPH Insulin is in order. In essentially all patients, excluding some toddlers, this maneuver necessitates a three injection/day program because of the need to continue covering the postprandial glucose rise after dinner with Regular Iletin insulin given 30 minutes before this meal. This change has been frequently successful and surprisingly well accepted by most patients and parents (28,29).

Within the DCCT experience, in those intensively managed patients on multiple-dose insulin (MDI) therapy, approximately two-thirds were on a combination of Ultralente Iletin and Regular Iletin insulin, with a minimum of three injections daily. Our experience with this technique has led us to begin its application in our general clinic population of adolescents who have agreed to pursue a plan for optimizing management. We are using human Ultralente Iletin and human Regular Iletin in these patients. Human Ultralente Iletin lasts approximately 30 h, with no definable peak time but rather a slow-wave action curve. By giving Ultralente Iletin twice daily, it should be possible to develop a relatively constant concentration of insulin in the circulation, similar to that in the nondiabetic individual. Regular Iletin insulin is then given before each meal to control the postprandial glucose surge. We routinely gave Regular Iletin insulin before each meal and frequently before the bedtime snack within the DCCT intensively managed patients, but we have started our clinic adolescent patients with Regular Iletin insulin given only before breakfast and dinner. In a number of these patients, however, we are finding that late hypoglycemia is a frequent accompaniment of a morning Ultralente Iletin dose that is sufficient to bring the predinner blood sugar into range. The solution in such patients is to reduce the morning Ultralente Iletin and provide a small amount of Regular Iletin insulin before lunch. This has been reasonably well accepted by the few clinic patients in whom it has been recommended. In our successful Ultralente Iletin patients, those both within the DCCT and within our general diabetes clinic, approximately 60% of the total dose is provided as Ultralente Iletin, with the remainder as Regular Iletin. We initiate the Ultralente Iletin regimen by reducing the patient's total daily NPH Insulin dose by 10% and then giving half of this with human Regular Iletin before breakfast and half with human Regular

Iletin before the evening meal. It may be necessary to move the predinner Ultralente Iletin to bedtime, again converting the patient to a three-injection insulin regimen.

C. Insulin Infusion Therapy

In the early days of insulin pumps, we developed an extensive pump experience with our adolescent patients. Their initial metabolic response was gratifying in terms of decreasing glycosylated hemoglobin and blood glucoses. As we followed these patients over time, however, their enthusiasm for living with a pump declined and their compliance with the therapeutic regimen diminished. Thus, the early successes were lost. We concluded that the rigors of insulin infusion therapy were such that few children or adolescents would adapt successfully to it and have essentially discontinued pump use in our general clinic population (30). About one-third of the DCCT intensively managed patients were on an insulin infusion device. The general experience did not clearly document a benefit of either pump or MDI therapy. However, we now have an open mind about the potential application of pump therapy in very carefully selected adolescents who are unusually mature and have made a clear commitment to improved health.

D.   Exercise as a Therapeutic Modality

There is an increasing body of scientific data that suggests, but does not definitively prove, that physical fitness is a beneficial and highly desirable state for the patient with diabetes mellitus (31–34). We have taken on faith that this is, in fact, true and, consequently, recommend to our patients that they incorporate a regular exercise program into their daily lives. Exercise increases glucose utilization, and highly fit muscles have an increased sensitivity to insulin and, consequently, glucose movement. Our clinical observations include the following. (1) Highly fit children and adolescents with diabetes usually require less insulin per level of metabolic control. (2) These individuals are generally in better metabolic control than their relatively unfit diabetic peers. (3) The physically fit individual, particularly the competitive athlete, usually has a better self-image and a better appreciation of the importance of good diabetes management. (4) Episodic exercise, as opposed to regular exercise leading to an improved level of physical fitness, may be dangerous in terms of both hypoglycemia or the induction of diabetic ketoacidosis in the very poorly controlled patient. (5) Our long-term diabetes complications studies indicate that those individuals who participated in competitive athletics during high school and college had a significant reduction in both diabetes-related morbidity and mortality when evaluated 10–30 years later.

Our recommendation to our patients is that they develop a daily exercise regimen (7 days per week) that involves a fairly vigorous level of exercise for approximately 1 h each day. This is usually most easily achieved by participating in competitive athletic programs at the child's school. If this is neither possible nor desirable, then other entirely satisfactory exercise activities can be substituted, such as vigorous walking, jogging, swimming, aerobic dancing, tennis, and golf. The patients must understand the effects of exercise on blood glucose and be ready to make necessary adjustments in either insulin dose or diet. In general, we prefer to increase caloric intake before exercise rather than reduce insulin, although either or both may be satisfactory solutions to problems of hypoglycemia associated with exercise. The very poorly controlled patient who desires to embark on an exercise program should be encouraged to improve overall metabolic control by increasing insulin dosage before embarking on an exercise regimen.

XII.   FUTURE THERAPIES

Efforts to improve the management and outcome of patients with diabetes mellitus continue to be the focus of investigators around the world. The diversity of the research is great, varying from efforts to develop safe techniques for immunologic suppression to protect the β cell from progressive damage to technologic approaches to the development of a totally implantable mechanical pancreas. The insulin manufacturers are working to manipulate the insulin molecule to tailor the timing of onset and duration of action to meet individual needs in a far more comprehensive fashion than the few varieties of insulin now available. Nutritional research is attempting to develop nutrients with a "Lente" type of action, that is, a slowly absorbed carbohydrate that could sustain modest blood glucose elevations for a period of several hours. Pharmacologic approaches to the prevention of diabetic vascular complications also show promise, and refinement of surgical techniques for pancreatic transplantation is leading to improved results.

Although the future shows great promise, it is important that those of us who care for children with diabetes continue to provide them with optimal management with the tools currently available to ensure that they can take full advantage of new advances as they become available.

REFERENCES

1.   Feldman JM. Pathophysiology of diabetes mellitus. In: Galloway JA, Potvin JH, Shuman CR, eds. Diabetes Mellitus, 9th ed. Indianapolis: Eli Lilly, 1988:28–44.
2.   Gerich JA. Hormonal control of homeostatis. In: Galloway JA, Potvin JH, Shuman CR, eds. Diabetes Mellitus, 9th ed. Indianapolis: Eli Lilly, 1988:45–64.
3.   Drash AL. Clinical Care of the Diabetic Child. Chicago: Year Book Medical, 1987.
4.   Songer TJ, LaPorte RE, Tajima N, et al. Height at the diagnosis of insulin-dependent diabetes in patients and their nondiabetic family members. BMJ 1986; 292:1419–1422.
5.   Eberhardt MS, Wagener DK, Orchard TJ, et al. HLA heterogeneity of insulin-dependent diabetes mellitus at diagnosis: the Pittsburgh IDDM study. Diabetes 1985; 34:1247–1252.
6.   Drash AL, LaPorte RE, Becker DJ, et al. The natural history of diabetes mellitus in children. Insulin requirements during the initial two years. Acta Paediatr Belg 1980; 33:66–69.

7. Elliott RB, Crossle JR, Berryman CC, et al. Partial preservation of pancreatic B cell function in children with diabetes. Lancet, 1981; 2:1–3.

8. Stiller CR, Dupre J, Gent, et al. Effects of cyclosporine immunosuppression in insulin dependent diabetes mellitus of recent onset. Science 1984; 223:1362–1367.

9. Drash AL, Arslanian SA. Can insulin-dependent diabetes mellitus be cured or prevented? A status report on immunomodulatory strategies and pancreas transplantation. Pediatr Clin North Am 1990; 1467–1487.

10. Skyler JS, Marko JB. Immune intervention in type I diabetes mellitus. Diabetes Rev 1993; 1:15–42.

11. Santiago JV. Insulin therapy in the last decade: a pediatric perspective. Diabetes Care 1993; 16(3):143–154.

12. Becker DJ. Management of insulin-dependent diabetes mellitus in children and adolescents. Curr Opin Pediatr 1991; 3:710–723.

13. Rother KT, Levitsky LL. Diabetes mellitus during adolescence. Adolescent endocrinology. Endocrinol Metab Clin North Am 1993; 22:553–572.

14. Galloway JA. New directions in drug development: mixtures, analogues, modeling. Diabetes Care 1993; 16(3):16–23.

15. Chance RE, Frank BH. Research, development, production, and safety of biosynthetic human insulin. Diabetes Care, 1993; 16(3):133–142.

16. Saudek CD. Future developments in insulin delivery systems. Diabetes Care 1993; 16(3):122–132.

17. Schade DS, Santiago JV, Skyler JS, Rizza RA. Intensive Insulin Therapy. Amsterdam: Excerpta Medica, 1983.

18. Diabetes Control and Complications Trial Research Group. The effect of intensive treatment of diabetes on the development and progression of long-term complications in insulin-dependent diabetes mellitus. N Engl J Med 1993; 329:977–986.

19. Santiago JV. Lessons of the Diabetes Control and Complications Trial. Diabetes 1993; 42:1549–1554.

20. Drash AL. The child, the adolescent and the Diabetes Control and Complications Trial. Diabetes Care 1993; 16:1515–1516.

21. Diabetes Control and Complications Trial Research Group. The effect of intensive diabetes treatment on the development and progression of long-term complications in adolescents with insulin-dependent diabetes mellitus: The Diabetes Control and Complications Trial. In press.

22. Etzwiler DD, Sines LK. Juvenile diabetes and its management: family, social, and academic implications. JAMA 1962; 191:304–308.

23. Drash AL. Clinical care of the patient with diabetes mellitus: what is the role of the diabetes professional. Diabetes Care. In press, July 1994.

24. Drash AL, Becker DJ. Behavioral issues in patients with diabetes mellitus, with special emphasis on the child and adolescent. In: Rifkin H, Porte D, eds. Ellenberg and Rifkins's Diabetes Mellitus Theory and Practice, 4th ed. New York: Elsevier, 1990:922–934.

25. Cryer P. Human insulin and hypoglycemia unawareness. Diabetes Care 1990; 13:536–538.

26. Orchard TJ, Maser RE, Becker DJ, Doman JS, Drash AL. Human insulin use and hypoglycemia: insights from the Pittsburgh Epidemiology of Diabetes Study. Diabetic Med 1991; 8:469–474.

27. Heinemann L, Richter B. Clinical pharmacology of human insulin. Diabetes Care 1993; 16(3):90–100.

28. Zinman B. Insulin regimens and strategies for IDDM. Diabetes Care 1993; 16(3):24–28.

29. Bolli GB, Peniello G, Carmine G, Famelli P, DeFeo P. Nocturnal blood glucose control in type I diabetes mellitus. Diabetes Care 1993; 16(3):71–89.

30. Becker DJ, Kerensky KM, Transue D, et al. Current status of pump therapy in childhood. Acta Paediatr. Jpn. 1984; 6:347–358.

31. LaPorte R, Dorman JS, Tajima N, et al. Pittsburgh insulin-dependent diabetes mellitus mobidity and mortality study: physical activity and diabetic complications. Pediatrics 1986; 78:1027–1033.

32. Moy CS, LaPorte RE, Dorman J, et al. Physical activity, insulin dependent diabetes mellitus and death. Am J Epidemiol 1993; 137(1):74–81.

33. Zinman B. Exercise in the patient with diabetes mellitus. In: Galloway JA, Potvin JH, Schuman CR, eds. Diabetes Mellitus, 9th ed. Indianapolis: Eli Lilly, 1988:215–224.

34. Arslanian S, Nixon PA, Becker D, Drash AL. Impact of physical fitness and glycemic control on in vivo insulin action in adolescents with IDDM. Diabetes Care 1990; 13:9–15.

43
Diabetes Ketoacidosis

David Zangen and Lynne L. Levitsky

Massachusetts General Hospital and Harvard Medical School, Boston, Massachusetts

I. INTRODUCTION

Diabetic ketoacidosis is the most severe manifestation of the metabolic decompensation induced by insulin deficiency. In the child with newly diagnosed diabetes, diabetic ketoacidosis is the result of a failure of recognition of premonitory symptoms. In the child with preexistent diabetes, it is the result of a failure of patient monitoring or response. Therapy of diabetic ketoacidosis is essential. Investigation of the cause of each episode of diabetic ketoacidosis is equally important, however, because with this information, episodes of a potentially fatal complication of diabetes mellitus may be prevented.

II. PATHOPHYSIOLOGY

Diabetic ketoacidosis is the result of insulin deficiency with concomitant increased production of the stress hormones, glucagon, epinephrine, cortisol, and growth hormone. The metabolism of glucose requires insulin in most tissues. In the absence of sufficient insulin and in the presence of excess glucagon (1), gluconeogenesis is increased, glucose from both dietary and endogenous sources is not stored, and alternative fuels (fatty acids and ketone bodies) are released to the tissues in increased amount (Fig. 1) (2).

Insulin stimulates glucose entry into muscle and fat by upregulating glucose transport into these tissues. The upregulation of the specific muscle and fat glucose transporter, glucose transporter 4 (GLUT-4) (3,4), permits lipogenesis from glucose in the adipocyte and the use of glucose for immediate energy needs and glycogen storage by muscle. In the liver and kidney cortex, insulin upregulates glucokinase and glycogen synthase, thereby enhancing glycogen synthesis, and also diminishes the activity of key enzymes of gluconeogenesis. In muscle, insulin increases amino acid uptake and stimulates muscle protein synthesis, diminishing proteolysis. Insulin inhibits endothelial lipolysis, diminishing circulating free fatty acids. Lack of insulin causes relatively increased sodium loss in the kidney and a shift of potassium from the intracellular to the extracellular compartments. Hyperglycemia produced as a result of insulin deficiency provokes an osmotic diuresis with resultant dehydration.

Hyperglucagonemia also contributes to the pathogenesis of diabetic ketoacidosis (5). Elevated glucagon levels increase gluconeogenesis and stimulate glycogenolysis. As a result more glucose is produced and sent into the circulation, causing further hyperglycemia. Glucagon enhances muscle proteolysis, providing more substrate for gluconeogenesis. It affects lipid metabolism by inhibiting acetyl-CoA carboxylase, reducing adipocyte lipogenesis and decreasing hepatic malonyl-CoA. This directs the flux of fatty acid to ketogenesis.

Epinephrine, cortisol, and growth hormone enhance gluconeogenesis in a similar manner. Cortisol stimulates proteolysis. Epinephrine increases glucagon levels and enhances lipolysis. Growth hormone increases lipolysis and inhibits glucose transport into fat, diminishing peripheral lipogenesis (6,7).

The outcome is hyperglycemia as a result of overproduction of glucose by liver and kidney and underutilization of glucose by muscle and fat. The shift to lipolysis in peripheral tissues and increased capacity for ketone body production by liver and kidney lead to ketonemia. Decreased utilization of ketones by muscle increases ketonemia. Hypertriglyceridemia results from substrate excess (free fatty acids) and decreased peripheral utilization. The renal osmotic diuresis leads to loss of electrolyte as well as water (8,9). Physiologic hyperaldosteronism because of decreased intravascular volume specifically depletes potassium. Ketone bodies are excreted, coupled with electrolytes. The kidney loses the ability to buffer the metabolic acidosis (exchange hydrogen ion) because of electrolyte loss and dehydration.

Without appropriate fluid, electrolyte, and insulin therapy, the resultant hyperglycemia, dehydration, and ketoacidosis inevitably lead to coma and death.

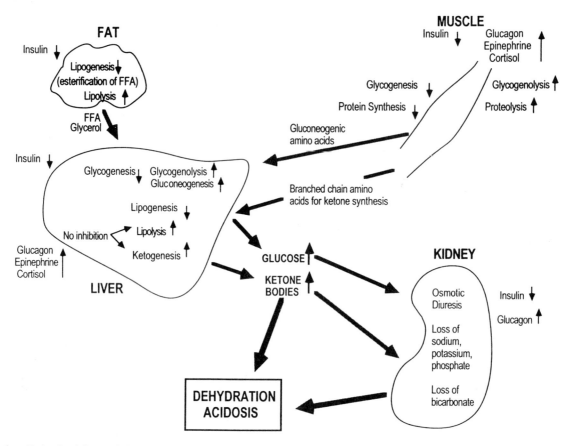

Figure 1 Pathophysiology of diabetic ketoacidosis.

III. CLINICAL PRESENTATION

The literature suggests that only 10% of episodes of diabetic ketoacidosis occur in new-onset insulin-dependent diabetes mellitus (IDDM) (10,11), whereas most episodes occur in patients with known IDDM (12). In known diabetes mellitus, diabetic ketoacidosis occurs because of failure to receive adequate insulin or insulin resistance induced by acute illness or stress (11,13). In our experience, however, diabetic ketoacidosis is infrequent in the well-controlled and well-educated patient with diabetes who has telephone access to medical advice in the event of intercurrent illness. We rarely see recurrent acidosis unless there is significant familial psychosocial disruption and failure of adult supervision.

A. History

The history in a patient with diabetic ketoacidosis should include an evaluation of the symptoms of hyperglycemia and ketoacidosis. Determination of the duration and extent of polyuria, polydipsia, new-onset nocturia or nocturnal enuresis, frequent diaper change in babies, and weight loss should be made. The duration of weakness and lethargy, nausea and vomiting, history of change in level of conciousness, and development of an increased respiratory rate with the deep

(Kussmaul) respirations typical of metabolic acidosis help to assess the severity of the ketoacidosis. A history of back pain or diffuse abdominal pain may be elicited. This pain seems related to degree of acidosis rather than to hyperglycemia and dehydration.

Precipitating factors in the development of diabetic ketoacidosis should be determined. A patient with known diabetes should be evaluated for intercurrent illness, trauma, or obscure infection. Adherence to a diabetes regimen should be examined. If the child uses a glucose meter with a memory, the memory can be downloaded and blood sugar values examined directly rather than examined as a written record. With the tools available to children with diabetes today (blood testing for glucose and urine testing for ketones), it is essentially impossible to develop severe ketoacidosis without failure of adherence to regimen, ignorance of symptoms and signs of ketoacidosis, or inability to reach medical attention. Information about general health, growth pattern, and family history, including family history of diabetes, should be obtained in every child with newly diagnosed diabetic ketoacidosis.

The duration of symptoms may predict the severity of the diabetic ketoacidosis and is, in addition, a known risk factor for the development of central nervous system complications of diabetic ketoacidosis (14–16). In the newly diagnosed child, severe diabetic ketoacidosis of long duration implies greater damage to functional β cells and less chance of a prolonged remission phase.

B. Physical Examination

Physical examination should assess the state of consciousness and the severity of dehydration and acidosis. The state of consciousness may vary from alertness to severe coma and does not always correlate with laboratory indicators of hyperglycemia or acidosis. Blood pressure, pulse rate, skin turgor, orthostatic changes, and body weight changes help in the determination of dehydration. Flushed cheeks, an acetone odor to the breath, Kussmaul respirations, and back pain or diffuse abdominal pain severe enough to suggest an acute surgical abdomen may be concomitants of severe acidosis. However, the respiratory center may not function appropriately at an arterial pH less than 7.1, so that severe acidosis may not be attended by Kussmaul respirations until therapy has elevated the arterial pH. The results of the initial thorough neurologic examination, including examination of the fundi, provide a comparison for both improvement and deterioration in neurologic status. Adherence to a diabetes regimen in a child with known diabetes may sometimes be assessed by examining blood glucose monitoring sites for puncture wounds. A careful search for infection or evidence of trauma may be helpful in planning therapy.

C. Initial Laboratory Findings

Although the history and physical examination often strongly suggest the diagnosis of diabetic ketoacidosis, laboratory confirmation is essential. Criteria for confirmation of the diagnosis of diabetic ketoacidosis include ketonuria or ketonemia, a blood glucose greater than 250 mg/dl, and a blood pH less than 7.3 or serum bicarbonate less than 20. Elevated glucose on initial bedside glucose testing with a glucose meter and a positive urine ketone strip are sufficient to begin initial rehydration therapy while awaiting the return of other laboratory tests. Bedside testing is only as good as the instrumentation and the individual performing the test, so it should be carefully observed and validated by the physician planning therapy. Essential laboratory tests are described in Table 1. We believe that venous blood gases are sufficient in most children with mild to moderate diabetic ketoacidosis and that

Table 1 Recommended Initial Laboratory Studies in Diabetic Ketoacidosis

---

1. Blood glucose, electrolytes, bicarbonate, and pH (venous pH sufficient unless patient is in coma or hemodynamically unstable, in which case arterial pH is preferable), calcium, phosphorus, BUN, and creatinine, complete blood count, and differential white blood cell count
2. Urinalysis for glucose, ketones, protein
3. Electrocardiogram for hypo- or hyperkalemia

---

only in severe diabetic ketoacidosis is it necessary to follow arterial blood gases for appropriate management. Results of initial studies are important in determining the type and rate of rehydration fluid, the insulin dose to be administered, and the need for bicarbonate therapy. The level of pH, serum bicarbonate, and P_{CO_2} may offer some special clues to management. In the event of pneumonia, respiratory compensation for metabolic acidosis may be diminished. Prolonged vomiting may produce a mixed picture with some metabolic alkalosis. Children can also present with a hyperglycemic hyperosmolar state and minimal ketosis. Acidosis may be secondary to lactic acidosis. Nonketotic hyperosmolar coma in children with diabetes, as in adults, is usually associated with some endogenous insulin release and self-rehydration with sugar-containing fluids.

Electrolyte values help in deciding appropriate fluid management and are necessary for the calculation of blood osmolality and anion gap, values that can be followed to determine response to therapy. The anion gap $[(Na + K) - (Cl + HCO_3), mEq]$ is initially greater than 12–16 mEq but should fall during therapy. The sodium is usually mildly low because of relatively increased water in the extracellular compartment as a result of hyperglycemia and hyperosmolality. Mathematic correction for the sodium value may be approximately expressed as Na (mEq) = measured Na (mEq) + 1.6[(glucose, mg/dl, – 100)/100] (2). In addition, hypertriglyceridemia (serum lipemia) causes an artifactually low sodium when expressed as concentration in total volume of serum rather than concentration in serum water. Uncorrected serum sodium should rise as ketoacidosis and hyperglycemia are corrected. Initial potassium levels neither reflect total-body potassium loss nor predict the serum potassium response to insulin and rehydration. Even if potassium levels are initially high, they may decrease to clinically dangerous levels unless potassium supplementation is given. The electrocardiogram is an important tool in the assessment of physiologic potassium status.

Blood urea nitrogen (BUN) and creatinine give an indication of the severity of dehydration. However, some chemical techniques to measure creatinine give falsely elevated values in the presence of acetoacetate (17). Newer enzymatic methods of creatinine measurement are not so affected. This should be confirmed with the laboratory.

Urinalysis reveals the presence of glucose and acetoacetate/acetone. In states of severe dehydration and acidosis, urinary ketones may be less than expected for the degree of acidosis because the acetoacetate-β-hydroxybutyrate relationship (reflecting the redox state) is altered in the direction of β-hydroxybutyrate (not identified on ketone strips) (18). The urinalysis should never be used to determine glycemia. Levels of urine glucose predict blood glucose in only the most nonspecific manner. Moreover, urine specific gravity cannot be used to assess dehydration in diabetic ketoacidosis, because urine glucose contributes to the elevated urine specific gravity and does not correlate directly with hydration state.

Complete blood count gives an indication of degree of dehydration (hemoconcentration as reflected in the hemoglobin and hematocrit) and the possibility of an acute infectious etiology of the decompensation of diabetes. Unfortunately, a polymorphonuclear leukocytosis and an increase in immature band forms must be reassessed after therapy because these findings may represent a stress response to diabetic ketoacidosis rather than infection.

Severe abdominal pain, nausea, and vomiting may provoke the physician to obtain a serum amylase. This enzyme may be elevated in diabetic ketoacidosis but seems a reflection of salivary rather than pancreatic amylase (19). This laboratory test also should be repeated as the patient's clinical status improves.

IV. THERAPY

The main strategies of therapy include appropriate replacement of water and electrolytes and treatment with insulin.

Recognition of the following additional concepts should assist in protecting the patient from adverse therapeutic outcomes:

1. Significantly compromised hemodynamic status (shock) calls for immediate rehydration with isotonic saline or other isotonic solute solution until the child is hemodynamically stable. This therapy not only restores necessary intravascular volume but also helps prevent further lactic acidosis from poor tissue perfusion.
2. Treatment should cause a *gradual* decrease in blood sugar not exceeding 75–100 mg/dl (4.2–5.6 mM) per h. This may protect the brain from large osmolar shifts that could lead to adverse central nervous system outcomes.
3. The aim of acute treatment in diabetic ketoacidosis is to restore normal hemodynamic status and normal acid-base balance, as well as slowly to correct the blood glucose to a range that is not acutely danger-

ous (200–300 mg/dl, 11.1–16.7 mM). Euglycemia should never be the goal in the first 24 h. A rapid decrease to normoglycemia in an individual who has been hyperglycemic for a prolonged period may increase central nervous system osmotic dysequilibrium.

4. Close monitoring is mandatory to fulfill these principles. A detailed record of hourly clinical status, laboratory results, fluid balance, and insulin dosage helps to avoid management errors (suggested format in Table 2).

Treatment of diabetic ketoacidosis includes the administration of fluid and salt, potassium, phosphate, and, on occasion, bicarbonate, in addition to insulin. In the following, each is discussed in detail. Abbreviated guidelines for treatment may be found in Table 3.

V. FLUID THERAPY

An initial loading dose of 20 ml/kg of 0.9% saline intravenously should be given within the first hour after diagnosis of diabetic ketoacidosis. Ringer's lactate is equally effective in initial rehydration, but lactate content eliminates the ability to use blood lactate as a measure of lactic acidosis. Blood sugar may drop 100–200 mg/dl (5.6–11.1 mM) without insulin therapy following this initial rehydration, because hyperglycemia is in part related to dehydration and failure of the kidney to continue to excrete the glucose osmotic load. If a component of markedly elevated blood sugar (greater than 500 mg/dl, or 27.8 mM) is a result of spontaneous oral self-rehydration with sugar-containing fluids (juice or soft drinks), vigorous rehydration may contribute to an even more rapid drop in the serum glucose. The rapid decrease in glycemia may be slowed or moderated by avoiding the use of unnecessary repeated intravenous boluses of fluid. This is

Table 2 Management of Diabetic Ketoacidosis

	Physical examination			Laboratory				Therapy			
Date/ time	Vital signs	Level of consciousness	Fundi, headache	Glucose	Na/K	pH/ ketonuria	HCO₃/ anion gap	Intravenous fluid	Output	Insulin	Other therapy

Table 3 Abbreviated Management Plan for Diabetic Ketoacidosis

1. Administer loading dose of 10–20 ml/kg of 0.9% NaCl. Repeat loading dose twice if necessary for shock.
2. Infuse fluid as maintenance + deficit over 24–36 h at a constant rate. Fluids should consist of 0.45% saline, potassium chloride, and potassium phosphate as described in step 4. Add 5% glucose to intravenous infusion when blood glucose is less than 300 mg/dl (16.7 mM). Switch to 10% glucose if patient is still acidotic but blood glucose is 200 mg/dl (11.1 mM) or less. Increase saline concentration to 0.9%, and decrease infusion rate if serum sodium is decreasing or remains 132 mEq or less during therapy.
3. Regular insulin should be piggybacked to intravenous infusion at a rate of 0.1 U/kg per h (made up as 1 U/kg in 100 ml of 0.9% saline). When acidosis clears (pH 7.3 or greater) and blood glucose is 300 mg/dl (16.7 mM) or less, insulin infusion rate can be decreased to 0.05 U/kg per h. It is rare to need to decrease rate further before discontinuation of intravenous therapy. If blood glucose does not decrease 75–100 mg/dl (4.2–5.6 mM) per h in first 2 h and insulin dilution is correct, insulin infusion rate can be increased to 0.2 U/kg per h. This is very unusual and indicates insulin resistance or a problem with insulin dilution.
4. Potassium should be administered as 40 mEq/L of intravenous fluids and should be given as half potassium chloride and half potassium phosphate to assure phosphate replacement.
5. Bicarbonate: 0.2 × base excess × body weight = ml NaHCO₃ over 20–30 minutes, *only* if arterial pH is less than 7.1 and clinical situation justifies it.
6. Close monitoring, with hourly vital signs, monitoring of state of consciousness, and hourly glucose and urine ketones until intravenous phase of therapy is terminated, is essential. There should be an initial electrocardiogram and a follow-up electrocardiogram at 6–8 h. Electrolytes and pH should be obtained every 2–4 h depending on severity of acidosis, for first 12 h. During recovery phase of intravenous therapy, frequency can decrease to every 6–8 h. Phosphate and calcium should be rechecked at 6–8 h and at about the time of discontinuation of intravenous therapy. Urine output should be monitored every 4–6 h.
7. Treat the underlying condition if possible.
8. Begin subcutaneous insulin therapy when the patient is ready to eat, pH is greater than 7.3, and glucose less than 300 mg/dl (16.7 mM).

particularly important in infants and toddlers because their total required rehydration volumes are smaller. In mild ketoacidosis or when dehydration is minimal, 10 ml/kg may suffice as a loading dose. On the other hand one to two repeat boluses of 20 ml/kg of 0.9% saline are indicated as necessary if dehydration compromises hemodynamic status (low blood pressure and significant tachycardia). Saline should be given until the classic hemodynamic signs of more than 10% dehydration disappear.

While the initial loading dose of saline is being infused, the fluid requirement for rehydration should be calculated. Estimated fluid deficit (as replacement of dehydration losses) and maintenance should be administered evenly over 24 h. There is no need to subtract the initial fluid bolus as long as it was administered according to the preceding guidelines. Continued urine losses are considerable in the very early phases of replacement, but no allowance should be made for the ongoing replacement of urinary losses. Replacement of urinary loss increases the risk of acute fluid overload and attendant adverse effects. The usual replacement solution should contain 0.45% saline. If there is significant hyponatremia (sodium 132 mEq or less), it is advisable to continue the correction for at least the first 6–8 h with 0.9% saline and to calculate replacement over a 36 h period. Hyponatremia, if not artifactual, may be a sign of inappropriate secretion of vasopressin and a warning of potential risk of central nervous system complications (14). If serum sodium level does not rise slowly in parallel with the decrease in glucose and lipemia during treatment, this should be taken as a warning of the potential for undesired central nervous system osmotic fluid shifts. A decrease in the rate of fluid administration and a return to 0.9% saline may be indicated. Rehydration should not exceed 2500, 3200, and 4000 ml/m² body surface area per day for 5, 7.5, and 10% dehydration, respectively. It has been suggested that administration of more than 4 L fluid/m² in 24 h is associated with increased risk for developing cerebral edema (16).

A. Introduction of Intravenous Glucose

Blood glucose levels should be monitored hourly at the bedside so that the composition of the infusion fluid can be changed as glycemia diminishes. When the blood glucose level falls to 300 mg/dl or less, 5% dextrose should be added to the infusate. If blood sugars continue to fall but acidosis is still a problem (pH less than 7.30), the intravenous fluid glucose content should be increased to 10% to avoid hypoglycemia, but the rate of insulin infusion should not be changed.

B. Potassium

Potassium loss in urine during diabetic ketoacidosis is further complicated by a shift of potassium from the extracellular to intracellular compartments during treatment (8). The mechanisms that contribute to this shift and resulting hypokalemia are (1) insulin stimulates potassium entry into cells; (2) rehydration leads to movement of potassium with water into cells; (3) correction of acidosis during treatment causes an exchange between increased intracellular hydrogen ion and relatively "increased" extracellular potassium ion; and finally (4) potassium is required for glycogen synthesis after insulin treatment.

Potassium replacement is important from the earliest stages of rehydration. However, on rare occasions the patient may present with severe dehydration, oliguria, or anuria. In these cases potassium supplementation may exacerbate mild hyperkalemia. Therefore, potassium should be added to the rehydration fluids only after the patient has urinated, serum potassium is found to be less than 6 mEq/L, and an electrocardiogram has confirmed that there are no signs of hyperkalemia. Because all patients with diabetic ketoacidosis have phosphate loss, we recommend replacement with 40 mEq/L of potassium, administered half as the chloride and half as the phosphate salt. This helps to alleviate the hyperchloremia typically seen in recovering diabetic ketoacidosis and also provides phosphate in an amount unlikely to induce hypocalcemia (20).

C. Bicarbonate

Although correction of acidosis is one of the two main therapeutic goals, administration of bicarbonate is seldom necessary. Rehydration and improvement in organ perfusion diminish the production of lactic acid and permit the continued excretion of hydrogen ion. Insulin therapy inhibits ketogenesis and stimulates the further metabolism of ketone bodies. Metabolism of ketone bodies produces endogenous buffer. There are a number of theoretical objections to administration of bicarbonate, none of which has ever been shown in clinical studies to affect therapeutic outcome. The oxyhemoglobin dissociation curve is shifted to the right because of acidosis. This leads to increased oxygen availability to peripheral tissues, despite decreased levels of 2,3-diphosphoglycerate as a result of hypophosphatemia. Rapid correction of pH shifts the oxyhemoglobin dissociation curve to the left, diminishing peripheral oxygen availability (21). Paradoxic cerebrospinal fluid and, by inference, central nervous system acidosis develops during recovery from ketoacidosis because of the difference in transport of carbon dioxide and bicarbonate ion across the blood-brain barrier. The carbon dioxide easily equilibrates between serum and the cerebrospinal fluid and dissociates in water to form a weak acid. Bicarbonate does not cross as readily into the central nervous system, leading to worsening of the central nervous system acidosis during the period of disequilibration because of insufficient bicarbonate to function as buffer. Bicarbonate therapy would potentially worsen this problem (22). Bicarbonate is also hypertonic, could contribute to hypokalemia, as well as late alkalemia as a result of overtreatment, and therefore could contribute further to central nervous system dysfunction. We argue that bicarbonate is necessary only if there is clinical reason to suspect impending ventilatory and circulatory compromise (arterial pH less than 7.1 and clinical indicators). We recommend treatment with bicarbonate sufficient to replace only one-third the calculated deficit initially. Because correction of acidosis inevitably occurs if fluid, electrolyte, and insulin replacement are administered to a patient with normal cardiovascular and respiratory status, there seems no argument for administering bicarbonate over a prolonged period of time. It should be administered over a period of less than 1 h as a resuscitation measure purely to treat or prevent impending circulatory collapse. Close laboratory follow-up of acid-base status is mandatory.

D. Phosphate

There is phosphate loss in urine during glucose-induced osmolar diuresis (23,24). Severe hypophosphatemia causes muscle weakness. Replacement of phosphate diminishes weakness and has been shown to alleviate respiratory failure in some cases. Replacement of phosphate also increases 2,3-diphosphoglycerate levels and shifts the oxyhemoglobin dissociation curve to the right, enhancing oxygen delivery to the periphery (25). Because most patients rapidly replenish circulating phosphate from endogenous stores, replacement of phosphate has not been shown significantly to affect clinical outcome in diabetic ketoacidosis. We have seen patients with profound muscle weakness as a result of phosphate depletion, however, and believe that phosphate replacement as potassium phosphate is a wise adjunct to therapy. We suggest supplementing potassium half with potassium chloride and half with phosphate because full replacement with potassium phosphate has led to hypocalcemia (20).

VI. INSULIN

A. Choice of Therapeutic Approach

Diabetic ketoacidosis can be managed using subcutaneous insulin administration at 2–4 h intervals, intramuscular insulin administration hourly, or continuous intravenous insulin administration.

1. Subcutaneous Insulin Administration

For many years, intermittent subcutaneous insulin administration was the standard of treatment for diabetic ketoacidosis. Subcutaneous insulin absorption is erratic, however, particularly if there is dehydration and poor perfusion, and this approach is no longer the treatment of choice in a controlled hospital setting.

2. Intramuscular Insulin Administration

Intramuscular insulin administration (26) in a dose of 0.1 units/kg per h, adjusted as described for continuous intravenous administration, induces a steady, controllable fall in blood sugar and improvement in acidosis. If the setting is such that continuous intravenous insulin cannot be reliably administered, this alternative may be considered. Intramuscular injections are painful, however, and can be administered using standard insulin syringes with swaged short needles only in the smallest and thinnest of children. Administration of small doses of insulin using another type of syringe introduces many opportunities for medication error.

3. Continuous Intravenous Insulin Administration

We recommend continuous intravenous infusion of regular insulin for the treatment of diabetic ketoacidosis in the hospital. The recommended initial intravenous insulin dose is 0.1 U/kg per h. There is no advantage to administering an initial intravenous bolus of insulin (27). Intravenous insulin, if the patient is reasonably hydrated (after initial intravenous therapy with bolus 0.9% saline), acts within minutes and has a circulating half-life of just over 4 minutes, so that rapid adjustments can be made in insulin dose. As in other aspects of treatment, infants should be treated more cautiously, and if the pH is greater than 7.2, therapy should be initiated with 0.05 U/kg per h. In rare patients with insulin resistance, higher doses of insulin may be necessary. If blood sugar does not diminish by 75–100 mg/dl (4.2–5.6 mM) per h, the rate of insulin infusion can be increased to 0.2 U/kg per h or even higher if necessary (28).

B. Practical Aspects of Intravenous Insulin Administration

A practical insulin administration technique is to make up 1 U/kg of insulin in 100 ml of 0.9% saline and then administer 10 ml/h (0.1 U/kg per h). This can be piggybacked into the intravenous infusion solution so that there is no risk of hypoglycemia should the intravenous rehydration fail but insulin infusion continue. The insulin infusion rate may be decreased to 0.05 U/kg per h when acidosis clears (pH greater than 7.3 and glucose of 200 mg/dl, 11.1 mM or less). However, if the blood glucose decreases to 200 mg/dl (11.1 mM) or less without clearing of acidosis, an increase in the glucose infusion rate but no decrease in insulin infusion is indicated until acidosis is resolved. Urine ketones should not be used as a criterion for altering insulin infusion rate because ketosis and ketonuria will resolve after hyperglycemia and acidosis. As acidosis improves, the equilibrium between β-hydroxybutyrate and acetoacetate shifts toward acetoacetate. Because only acetoacetate is measured by urine ketone tests, semiquantitative measures of "ketones" may actually increase during the initial phase of rehydration and insulin therapy. Table 3 offers suggested guidelines for insulin therapy and the glucose concentration of intravenous fluids during rehydration.

C. Discontinuation of Intravenous Insulin Therapy

Because of the short half-life of intravenous regular insulin, it should not be discontinued abruptly when blood sugars fall into the normal range and acidosis is alleviated. Discontinuation of insulin before initiation of subcutaneous insulin therapy may result in the return of hyperglycemia and ketoacidosis. Intravenous insulin should be continued for 30 minutes after the administration of the first dose of subcutaneous insulin.

D. Continuation of Intravenous Insulin Therapy

Fixed-rate combinations of insulin- and glucose-containing intravenous fluids offer little flexibility and are best avoided during therapy of diabetic ketoacidosis. If a patient, after recovery from ketoacidosis, must be retained on intravenous insulin and glucose therapy for a prolonged period of time, fixed combinations of 2 units regular insulin/5 g glucose (10 units regular insulin/500 ml of 5% dextrose solution with appropriate electrolyte) are sometimes useful, although individual patients vary widely in insulin need, children under 5 often requiring half this amount of insulin and adolescents or children with infection or surgical stress often requiring more insulin to maintain euglycemia.

VII. MONITORING

Meticulous therapy of diabetic ketoacidosis requires careful monitoring. Although rehydration and insulin are the effective therapies for diabetic ketoacidosis, inattention to either fluid replacement or insulin therapy may lead to hypoglycemia, severe electrolyte disturbances, unnecessary prolongation of the acidotic state, or central nervous system complications, including cerebral edema.

Using Table 2 or a similar flow sheet to summarize clinical and laboratory data and therapy is efficient and may prevent management errors. Vital signs and fundus examinations are important for later comparison and assessment of complications. Worsening state of consciousness, headache, bradycardia, or pulse pressure increase are alarm signs for increased intracranial pressure and should lead to an immediate investigative and/or treatment response. Blood glucose and amount and type of intravenous fluids, as well as insulin dosage, should be monitored hourly. Electrolytes and pH should be reassessed every 4 h or more often depending on the initial presentation. Urine output should be monitored every 4–6 h. An initial electrocardiogram should be repeated in 6–8 h. As the clinical condition improves, blood glucose monitoring and clinical assessment should continue hourly until the patient is ready to be transferred to subcutaneous insulin. Electrolytes and pH can be reassessed less frequently than during the initial 12 h of management. If possible, the underlying etiology of a recurrent episode of diabetic ketoacidosis should be identified and treated.

VIII. RECOVERY

The aim of *acute* therapy is to restore fluid volume and return acid-base status to normal, but not to achieve stable euglycemia immediately. When the patient is ready to eat and drink, the blood pH is greater than 7.3, and glucose is generally less than 300 mg/dl (16.7 mM), it is appropriate to switch from continuous intravenous insulin therapy to subcutaneous insulin.

A. Child with Previously Treated Diabetes

A patient with known diabetes can be placed back on the previous insulin regimen unless an increase in the insulin dose based upon historical blood sugar data is thought appropriate. Subcutaneous regular insulin may be administered as 20% of the total daily dose to tide the individual over for the 4–6 h until it is time for intermediate-acting insulin. Supplemental regular insulin (10–20% of daily dose) may then be administered before meals as necessary for hyperglycemia.

B. Newly Diagnosed Child with Diabetes

The first dose of subcutaneous insulin can consist of either a fraction of the total projected daily dose as regular insulin or a split-mixed dose of insulin. To begin therapy with subcutaneous regular insulin, we define the estimated total daily dose (0.5 units/kg per day in the child under 5 years and 1 unit/kg per day in the older child). This dose is then administered before each meal and at bedtime as 40% before breakfast, 20% before lunch, 30% before dinner, and 10% at bedtime. The bedtime dose may be given as an intermediate-acting insulin (NPH or Lente) to permit long duration until morning, or a small amount of supplemental regular insulin (10% of dose) may be administered at 2 A.M. for blood sugars greater than 300 mg/dl. Regular insulin could be initiated and administered at 6 h intervals, but this does not permit adequate coverage for postprandial hyperglycemia.

In a patient with newly diagnosed diabetes, the only advantage of initiating subcutaneous regular insulin is that the patient and family have more frequent opportunity to practice insulin administration. We customarily begin with a split-mixed twice daily insulin regimen of human regular insulin with NPH or Lente insulin. If the child has been severely ketoacidotic at diagnosis, we begin with a total dose of 1 U/kg per day of insulin. If acidosis has been mild and of short duration, we may assume that there is some endogenous insulin release and begin with 0.5 U/kg per day. The insulin dose is divided as two-thirds of the total dose in the morning before breakfast, with one-third of that dose as regular and the other two-thirds as intermediate (NPH or Lente) insulin. The other one-third of the total insulin dose is administered before dinner in a 1:1 mixture of regular and intermediate-acting insulin. The first meal should be served approximately 30 minutes after administration of subcutaneous insulin, and intravenous insulin may then be discontinued. Intravenous fluids may be discontinued within the next hour. There is no therapeutic advantage to graded introduction of a clear liquid diet or other limitations on oral nutritional support if the patient is awake, alert, and free from nausea. Meals should be calculated to provide appropriate calories for each child according to American Diabetes Association guidelines. Blood sugar monitoring should be performed before each meal, at bedtime, and, during initial calibration of insulin needs, at 2 A.M. These values can then be used to make anticipatory changes in insulin dose. It is our practice to give supplemental regular insulin in hospital to the newly diagnosed child only if the blood sugar is greater than 300 mg/dl (16.7 mM) and to plan most insulin adjustments for the period immediately after hospital discharge. Starting split-mixed insulin regimen immediately after acute therapy of ketoacidosis reduces the length of stay in the hospital necessary for insulin adjustment in these children.

IX. SPECIAL CONSIDERATIONS IN DIABETIC KETOACIDOSIS

A. Preoperative Patient

The patient who requires surgery because of acute illness (appendicitis, for example) or trauma should be stabilized as much as possible before anesthesia. Severe diabetic ketoacidosis is a difficult anesthetic management problem because of the danger of arrhythmia under anesthesia. Repair of diabetic ketoacidosis can usually be part of the normal stabilization process before surgical intervention. Moreover, the unexplained "surgical" acute abdomen may on occasion be alleviated with treatment of ketoacidosis.

B. Euglycemic Diabetic Ketoacidosis (29,30)

Small, malnourished children may sometimes present with relatively low (less than 300 mg/dl, or 16.7 mM) blood sugars and ketoacidosis. These young children must be distinguished from children with certain inborn errors of metabolism, who may also initially present with "ketoacidosis" and modest hyperglycemia. However, therapy with insulin, electrolyte replacement, and adequate glucose is as effective in reversing the catabolic state leading to decompensation of a genetic metabolic defect as it is in treating diabetic ketoacidosis. Therefore, treatment can proceed with early introduction of sufficient glucose into the intravenous fluids, and diagnostic studies can then be performed on blood and urine samples obtained during decompensation or after recovery.

C. Nonketotic Hyperosmolar Coma and Morbid Hyperosmolality

Diabetic coma with high blood sugar (750 mg/dl, 41.7 mM or greater) and no or minimal ketosis is seen in individuals with some residual insulin capacity and inability to achieve appropriate fluid intake when osmotically challenged by hyperglycemia. This disorder is associated with a very high mortality rate in adults because of associated preexisting conditions. The mortality rate in children is much lower but nonetheless of concern. Typically, the very young infant or the child with mental retardation presents with such severe hyperglycemia. It may also be seen as a result of drug therapy in susceptible individuals (high-dose glucocorticoids for other illness or diazoxide therapy for hypoglycemia) (31,32). Remarkable hyperglycemia without coma (blood sugars of 750 mg/dl, 41.7 mM to over 1000 mg/dl, 55.6 mM) is also seen if attempts at oral rehydration have been made entirely with sugar-containing soft drinks and juices (33). This hyperglycemia diminishes rapidly after initial hydration. Therapy for the nonketotic hyperosmolar state remains the same as that for diabetic ketoacidosis, although there may be a rapid drop in blood glucose with initial hydration and insulin infusion rate needs may be lower than for ketoacidosis.

Remarkable hyperglycemia (blood glucose greater than 1200 mg/dl, 66.7 mM) with or without ketoacidosis may be associated with a higher probability of central nervous system and other complications, such as acute renal failure and disseminated intravascular coagulation. Tertiary care is vital for these patients. They must be handled by a skilled intensive care team. Occasionally these patients may present with hyponatremia that fails to rise as blood glucose levels decline. Relatively slower correction of hyperosmolality (three-quarters normal saline in intravenous solutions, correction over 36 h) and a lower dose of intravenous insulin (0.05 units/kg or less) may prevent complications.

D. Infant and Toddler

Small infants often have a delayed diagnosis of diabetes and more severe diabetic ketoacidosis. In addition, because of the delay in diagnosis and the need for fluid and electrolyte management tailored to their low body weights, they may be at greater risk for the development of central nervous system complications. Therefore, careful monitoring and meticulous follow-up are most important in this age group.

E. Adolescent with Recurrent Diabetic Ketoacidosis

Recurrent diabetic ketoacidosis is almost always seen in young adolescents from families in whom management of diabetes has been prematurely delegated to the child. It is a result of failure of insulin administration and can be prevented if a responsible adult is given control of insulin management. Children with recurrent ketoacidosis often remain in poor glycemic control because episodes of recurrent ketoacidosis are a reflection of their emotional chaos and need for close supervision and family counseling (34).

F. Complications of Diabetic Ketoacidosis

Relatively minor problems of electrolyte imbalance, hypoglycemia, and hypophosphatemic muscle weakness during recovery are the most common complications of diabetic ketoacidosis and its treatment. Acute tubular necrosis from severe dehydration has been reported (35,36), however, as have hemolysis and myoglobinuria from acidosis (37,38). Pulmonary edema and adult respiratory distress syndrome have been seen as a result of relative therapeutic fluid overload (39). The serious cardiovascular complications of diabetic ketoacidosis in adults are rarely a problem in children. The most worrisome complications are those of the central nervous system.

The central nervous system complications of diabetic ketoacidosis are responsible for most of the deaths from diabetes in childhood. The mortality rate has been variably estimated as 2.5–10:1000 episodes (40,41). Central nervous system complications seem to be of two types: those with an unremitting course from diagnosis of diabetic ketoacidosis and associated with thrombovascular phenomena, and those occurring late in the course of repair of the metabolic abnormalities of diabetic ketoacidosis and associated with isolated cerebral edema. Cerebral edema has been reported to occur to some extent in all children being treated for diabetic ketoacidosis (40) and may even be identified before the onset of therapy (42). In a small number of children,

however, it becomes significant enough to lead to brain herniation and consequent severe brain damage or death.

Children who develop symptomatic cerebral edema seem to be recovering from diabetic ketoacidosis and are usually not very acidotic when they develop signs of acute intracranial pressure elevation (headache preceding altered consciousness, slowed pulse, and widened pulse pressure) (43). If they are treated rapidly with hyperventilation, mannitol (0.5–2 g/kg body weight at 4–6 h intervals), immediate reduction in intravenous fluid rate, and neurosurgical intervention as necessary, they may recover without sequelae. However, the time between development of signs and cerebral herniation may be so short that intervention is not successful. As many as half the children recognized clinically to have symptomatic cerebral edema may survive the episode, many with significant cerebral deficits, and the other half die. Cerebral intravascular coagulation may also lead to brain damage and death in children with diabetic ketoacidosis (44). Children with cerebral vascular thromboses tend never to have a period of recovery of consciousness but follow an unrelenting course leading to severe central nervous system damage and often death.

The etiology of cerebral edema is unknown and is probably multifactorial (16,45). It is of interest that symptomatic cerebral edema has been only rarely reported in adults with diabetic ketoacidosis. A number of etiologies have been hypothesized (43). First, many children at risk of cerebral edema demonstrate laboratory evidence of hyponatremia, and there is some support for inappropriate regulation of vasopressin secretion as a contributing factor. Second, the osmotic dysequilibrium between brain and periphery during diabetic ketoacidosis is corrected intracerebrally by the generation of hypothetical osmotically active particles termed idiogenic osmoles that serve to maintain brain tissue isosmolar with the blood (15). When recovery from diabetic ketoacidosis is rapid, dissipation of idiogenic osmoles may be inappropriately slow and influx of water into cerebral cells causes brain swelling. Experimentally, rapid influx of hypotonic fluid coupled with insulin administration leads to cerebral edema (46). Intravascular coagulation in small vessels of the brain may be found as a result of dehydration and the hypercoagulability of diabetic ketoacidosis (increased platelet "stickiness" can be measured). This may also contribute to the appearance of cerebral edema. Moreover, as the sodium-hydrogen pump functions to restore normal pH to cerebral cortical cells, water is also drawn into these cells, leading to brain swelling (47).

G. Outpatient Management of Impending Diabetic Ketoacidosis

Many episodes of impending diabetic ketoacidosis in patients with known insulin-dependent diabetes mellitus may be aborted before decompensation is severe enough to warrant a trip to the hospital emergency room. If there is appropriate parental support and the home laboratory and clinical information is deemed reliable, children with early diabetes decompensation may be treated with appropriate telephone

Table 4 Telephone Management of Impending Diabetic Ketoacidosis in Patients with Known Insulin-Dependent Diabetes Mellitus

I. Obtain history from responsible family member or older adolescent with diabetes.
   A. Present illness.
      1. Presence of fever, symptoms of intercurrent illness, history of trauma.
      2. Duration of symptoms (polyuria, polydypsia, headache, nausea, vomiting).
      3. Present state of consciousness, weakness, lethargy.
      4. Frequency of vomiting.
      5. Estimation of dehydration from moisture of oral mucosa, sunken eyes.
      5. Presence of breath acetone odor and/or rapid respirations.
      6. Exact dose of insulin, time of last injection, history of any missed insulin injections.
   B. Laboratory data.
      1. Blood sugar records for past 2–3 days.
      2. Current urine ketones and history of ketonuria.
   C. Social history.
      1. Is there a responsible adult to help with management?
      2. Are there adequate supplies of oral rehydration fluid, insulin, blood sugar, and urine ketone testing strips?
      3. Will transporation be available if the child or adolescent must come to a hospital emergency room?
II. Make an immediate decision as to whether telephone management is appropriate.
   A. Refer to emergency room immediately if the following conditions are present.
      1. Unreliable social situation, insufficient testing or rehydration supplies, or transportation will take some time to arrange.
      2. History of unexplained high fever, significant trauma, prolonged (more than 4 h) vomiting, significant dehydration, alteration of consciousness, or Kussmaul respirations.
      3. Blood sugar greater than 600 mg/dl (33.3 mM) and large urine ketones for more than 6 h.
   B. Attempt telephone management if the following conditions apply.
      1. Adequate social situation and capacity for rehydration and blood glucose and urine ketone testing; no time constraint on availability of transportation.
      2. Short duration of symptoms (one to two vomiting episodes), reasonable explanation for decompensation (error of insulin administration, self-limited illness, such as viral gastroenteritis), no alteration of consciousness or evidence for severe dehydration, normal respiratory pattern.
III. Begin telephone management:
   A. Telephone management should consist of suggesting and monitoring by telephone the following steps.
      1. Administration of extra regular insulin in addition to normal insulin regimen. Regular insulin should be given as approximately 10–20% of total daily dose subcutaneously every 4–6 h until blood sugar decreases to the normal range and symptoms of ketoacidosis clear.
      2. Oral rehydration with sips of fluid containing both electrolyte and some glucose. Initial rehydration with Nutrasweet-containing diet soft drinks only is not appropriate because the sodium content of these drinks is minimal. It is reasonable to alternate diet soft drinks with canned broth or bouillion. Table 5 lists the electrolyte content for some commonly available diet soft drinks. Children who are nauseated and vomiting do best with iced drinks in small quantities, given slowly. Replacement should be calculated as maintenance fluids and replacement for 5% loss over 24 h (see fluid management of diabetic ketoacidosis). In actuality, this means that the average *preschooler* should be taking in 2–3 ounces, the average *school-age child*, 3–5 ounces, and the *adolescent*, 5–7 ounces of fluid an hour. When blood sugars dip to 300 mg/dl (16.7 mM) or less, fluid replacement can be continued with cold iced soft drinks containing sugar (ginger ale or other non–caffeine-containing beverages). Until nausea has subsided, fruit juices and milk are inappropriate. Solid foods (crackers or toast) may be introduced in small quantities as tolerated.
      3. Blood sugar testing every 2 h, with ketone testing of each urine.
      4. Telephone contact every 2–4 h depending upon severity of symptoms, until symptoms have resolved.
   B. Telephone management should be discontinued and considered successful when the following occur.
      1. The child is eating a normal diet and no longer requiring frequent supplementation with regular insulin.
      2. Urine ketones and symptoms have cleared.

C. Telephone management should be discontinued and the child immediately sent to the emergency room if the following appear.
1. There is worsening of the state of consciousness or development of Kussmaul respirations.
2. Blood sugar continues to rise and urine ketones persist despite therapy over 4–6 h.
3. Vomiting persists longer than 6 h and prevents oral rehydration.
4. The child refuses oral rehydration.
5. The social situation changes so that continued home management is no longer feasible.

Table 5 Sodium and Potassium Content of Selected Diet Soft Drinks and Mineral Waters

Soft drink	Na$^+$ (mg/12 ounces)	K$^+$ (mg/12 ounces)	Soft drink	Na$^+$ (mg/12 ounces)	K$^+$ (mg/12 ounces)
Brewed coffee	5	240	Hoffman cola	80	NA
Perrier	7	0	Waldbaum cola	80	0[b]
Hoffman seltzer	7	NA[a]	Seven-Up	82	NA
White Rock mineral	4	NA	Cott grapefruit	83	NA
No Cal club	<15	NA	Mission grapefruit	83	NA
Canada Dry seltzer	15	NA	Cott chocolate	83	NA
Ferrarelle mineral water	14	NA	Mission chocolate	90	140
Hoffman ginger ale	16	NA	Cott cream	90	NA
Canada Dry ginger ale	22	NA	Shasta grape	90	3
No Cal ginger ale	22	0[b]	Cott orange	90	NA
No Cal orange	23	0[b]	Cott black raspberry	90	NA
No Cal cola	24	NA	Cott root beer	90	NA
No Cal grape	24	NA	Cott black cherry	92	NA
No Cal quinine	24	NA	Hoffman orange	92	NA
Tab	26	0[b]	Shasta strawberry	94	0[a]
Brewed tea	27	90	Hoffman strawberry	112	NA
Diet Coke	33	0[b]	Dr. Brown's black cherry	114	NA
Dr. Pepper	36	0[b]	Hoffman black cherry	114	NA
Canada Dry tonic water	36	0[b]	Yukon Club cola	114	NA
Canada Dry orange	39	0[b]	Hoffman grapefruit	128	NA
Canada Dry root beer	39	NA	Yukon Club root beer	128	NA[a]
Sprite	48	0	Yukon Club cream	138	NA
Hires root beer	53	NA[a]	Yukon Club orange	138	NA
Diet Rite Cola	58	0.6	Yukon Club black cherry	142	NA
RC Cola	58	NA	Hoffman grape	142	NA
Dr. Brown Celray	60	NA	Waldbaum grape	142	NA
Pepsi Cola	62	12	Dr. Brown's grape	142	NA
Fresca	62	0[b]	Key Food grape	142	NA
Hoffman coffee	64	NA	Shasta club	196	NA
Cott ginger ale	64	NA	Vichy Celestine water	434	18
Cott lemon	68	NA	⅓ normal saline	468	0
Shasta black cherry	74	0[b]	Vichy Saint-Yorre	595	NA
Shasta cola	74	0[b]	½ normal saline	655	0
Shasta cherry cola	74	0[b]	Quik Prep	1200	140
Shasta ginger ale	74	0[b]			
Shasta black raspberry	74	NA			
Shasta root beer	74	1			
Canada Dry club	75	3.3			
Cott cola	76	0[b]			
Shasta Cream	78	NA			
A & W Root Beer	79	4			

[a]NA, data not available.

[b]No added potassium except for local water content.

Source: Reprinted from Pugliese, Fort and Lifshitz, Diabetic ketoacidosis. In: Lifshitz F, ed. Pediatric Endocrinology, 2nd ed. Data from References 34, 61, 62, 63 and manufacturers. New York: Marcel Dekker, Inc., 1990:745–766.

advice and support. Telephone management should be attempted only if parental reliability is assured and there is ready access to a medical facility if such management fails. In infants and toddlers, telephone management should be carried out with great caution. Guidelines for initial telephone evaluation, treatment, and follow-up are listed in Table 4 (see also Table 5).

H. Prevention of Diabetic Ketoacidosis

The only sure way to avoid serious complications of diabetic ketoacidosis is to prevent and abort all such episodes of decompensation. In the undiagnosed child with diabetes, sensitivity to complaints of increased thirst, urination, new-onset enuresis, and malaise lead to early diagnosis before decompensation. A urine test for glucose should accompany the usual reassurance offered the family of the child with this constellation of symptoms. Children with known diabetes should remain under close adult supervision until they are late in adolescence. They and their families must be frequently reeducated about the symptoms and signs of metabolic decompensation and the value of careful record keeping. Social service support should be readily available to those families with diminished ability to cope with the large changes in behavior required when a child develops diabetes.

REFERENCES

1. Unger RH. Glucagon and the insulin:glucagon ratio in diabetes and other catabolic illnesses. Diabetes 1971; 20:834–838.
2. Fleckman AM. Diabetic ketoacidosis. Endocrinol Metab Clin North Am 1993; 22:181–207.
3. Sivitz WI, DeSautel SL, Kayano T, Bell GI, Pessin JE. Regulation of glucose transporter messenger RNA in insulin-deficient states. Nature 1989; 340:72–74.
4. James DE, Strube M, Mueckler M. Molecular cloning and characterization of an insulin-regulatable glucose transporter. Nature 1989; 338:83–87.
5. Gerich JE, Tsalikian E, Lorenzi M, Karam JH, Bier DM. Plasma glucagon and alanine responses to acute insulin deficiency in man. J Clin Endocrinol Metab 1975; 40:526–529.
6. Shamoon H, Hendler R, Sherwin RS. Altered responsiveness to cortisol, epinephrine, and glucagon in insulin-infused juvenile-onset diabetics. Diabetes 1980; 29:284–291.
7. Gerich JE, Lorenzi M, Bier DM, et al. Effects of physiologic levels of glucagon and growth hormone on human carbohydrate and lipid metabolism. J Clin Invest 1976; 57:875–884.
8. Foster DW, McGarry JD. The metabolic derangements and treatment of diabetic ketoacidosis. N Engl J Med 1983; 309:159–169.
9. Ellis EN. Concepts of fluid therapy in diabetic ketoacidosis and hyperosmolar hyperglycemic nonketotic coma. Pediatr Clin North Am 1990; 37:313–321.
10. Krentz AJ, Nattrass M. Diabetic ketoacidosis, nonketotic hyperosmolar coma and lactic acidosis. In: Williams G, ed. Textbook of Diabetes, Vol. 1. London: Blackwell Scientific, 1991:480–481.
11. Faich GA, Fishbein HA, Ellis SE. The epidemiology of diabetic acidosis: a population-based study. Am J Epidemiol 1983; 117:551–558.
12. Glasgow AM, Weissberg-Benchell J, Tynan WD, et al.
13. Readmissions of children with diabetes mellitus to a children's hospital. Pediatrics 1991; 88:98–104.
14. Snorgaard O, Eskildsen PC, Vadstrup S, Nerup J. Diabetic ketoacidosis in Denmark: epidemiology, incidence rates, precipitating factors and mortality rates. J Internal Med 1989; 226:223–228.
15. Harris GD, Fiordalisi I, Harris WL, Mosovich LL, Finberg L. Minimizing the risk of brain herniation during treatment of diabetic ketoacidemia: a retrospective and prospective study. J Pediatr 1990; 117:22–31.
16. Harris GD, Fiordalisi I, Finberg L. Safe management of diabetic ketoacidemia. J Pediatr 1988; 113:65–67.
17. Duck SC, Wyatt DT. Factors associated with brain herniation in the treatment of diabetic ketoacidosis. J Pediatr 1988; 113:10–14.
18. Todd JC, Sanford AH. Clinical chemistry. In: Davidsohn I, Henry JB, eds. Clinical Diagnosis by Laboratory Methods, 15th ed. Philadelphia: W.B. Saunders, 1974:596.
19. Marliss EB, Ohman JL Jr, Aoki TT, Kozak GP. Altered redox state obscuring ketoacidosis in diabetic patients with lactic acidosis. N Engl J Med 1970; 283:978–980.
20. Warshaw AL, Feller ER, Lee K-H. On the cause of raised serum-amylase in diabetic ketoacidosis. Lancet 1977; 1:929–931.
21. Winter RJ, Harris CJ, Phillips LS, Green OC. Diabetic ketoacidosis. Am J Med 1979; 67:897–900.
22. Bureau MA, Begin R, Berthiaume Y, Shapcott D, Khoury K, Gagnon N. Cerebral hypoxia from bicarbonate infusion in diabetic acidosis. J Pediatr 1980; 96:968–973.
23. Kaye R. Diabetic ketoacidosis—the bicarbonate controversy. J Pediatr 1979; 87:156–159.
24. Keller U, Berger W. Prevention of hypophosphatemia by phosphate infusion during treatment of diabetic ketoacidosis and hyperosmolar coma. Diabetes 1980; 29:87–95.
25. Becker DJ, Brown DR, Steranka BH, Drash AL. Phosphate replacement during treatment of diabetic ketosis. Am J Dis Child 1983; 137:241–246.
26. Fisher JN, Kitabchi AE. A randomized study of phosphate therapy in the treatment of diabetic ketoacidosis. J Clin Endocrinol Metab 1983; 57:177–180.
27. Kutsi O, Lala VR, Juan CS, AvRuskin TW. Glucagon suppression with low-dose intramuscular insulin therapy in diabetic ketoacidosis. J Pediatr 1979; 94:307–311.
28. Fort P, Waters SM, Lifshitz F. Low-dose insulin infusion in the treatment of diabetic ketoacidosis: bolus versus no bolus. J Pediatr 1980; 96:36–40.
29. Usala A-L, Madigan T, Burguera B, et al. Brief report: treatment of insulin-resistant diabetic ketoacidosis with insulin-like growth factor I in an adolescent with insulin-dependent diabetes. N Engl J Med 1992; 327:853–857.
30. Bell PM, Hadden DR. Ketoacidosis without hyperglycemia during self-monitoring of diabetes. Diabetes Care 1983; 6:622–623.
31. Munro JF, Campbell IW, McCuish AC, Duncan LJP. Euglycaemic diabetic ketoacidosis. BMJ 1973; 2:578–580.
32. Balsam MJ, Baker L, Kaye R. Hyperosmolar nonketotic coma associated with diazoxide therapy for hypoglycemia. J Pediatr 1971; 78:523–525.
33. Spenney JG, Eure CA, Kreisberg RA. Hyperglycemic, hyperosmolar, nonketoacidotic diabetes. Diabetes 1969; 18:107–110.
34. Rubin HM, Kramer R, Drash A. Hyperosmolality complicating diabetes mellitus in childhood. J Pediatr 1969; 74:177–186.
35. Golden MP, Herrold AJ, Orr DP. An approach to prevention of recurrent diabetic ketoacidosis in the pediatric population. J Pediatr 1985; 107:195–200.

35. Murdoch IA, Pryor D, Haycock GB, Cameron SJ. Acute renal failure complicating diabetic ketoacidosis. Acta Paediatr Scand 1993; 82:498–500.

36. Grenfell A. Acute renal failure in diabetics. Intensive Care Med 1986; 12:6–12.

37. Buckingham BA, Roe TF, Yoon J-W. Rhabdomyolysis in diabetic ketoacidosis. Am J Dis Child 1981; 135:352–354.

38. Chamberlain MC. Rhabdomyolysis in children: a 3-year retrospective study. Pediatr Neurol 1991; 7:226–8.

39. Hansen LA, Prakash UBS, Colby TV. Pulmonary complications in diabetes mellitus. Mayo Clin Proc 1989; 64:791–799.

40. Krane EJ, Rockoff MA, Wallman JK, Wolfsdorf JI. Subclinical brain swelling in children during treatment of diabetic ketoacidosis. N Engl J Med 1985; 312:1147–1151.

41. Bello FA, Sotos JF. Cerebral oedema in diabetic ketoacidosis in children. Lancet 1990; 2:64.

42. Hoffman WH, Steinhart CM, Gammal TE, Steele S, Cuadrodo AR, Morse PK. Cranial CT in children and adolescents with diabetic ketoacidosis. Am J Neuroradiol 1988; 9:733–739.

43. Rosenbloom AL. Intracerebral crises during treatment of diabetic ketoacidosis. Diabetes Care 1990; 13:22–33.

44. Barnett AH, Harrison JH. Disseminated intravascular coagulation in diabetic ketoacidosis. Lancet 1979; 2:103.

45. Rosenbloom AL, Riley WJ, Weber FT, Malone JI, Donnelly WH. Cerebral edema complicating diabetic ketoacidosis in childhood. J Pediatr 1980; 96:357–361.

46. Arieff AI, Kleeman CR. Studies on mechanisms of cerebral edema in diabetic comas. J Clin Invest 1973; 52:571–583.

47. Van der Meulen JA, Klip A, Grinstein S. Possible mechanism for cerebral oedema in diabetic ketoacidosis. Lancet 1987; 2:306–308.

44

Future Trends in Therapy of Diabetes Mellitus

Susan E. Stred
State University of New York Health Science Center at Syracuse, Syracuse, New York

Alberto Hayek
University of California at San Diego, La Jolla, California

I. CURRENT CONCEPTS IN PATHOGENESIS

In the individual genetically predisposed to insulin-dependent diabetes mellitus (IDDM), it is postulated that an environmental event triggers an immunologic reaction that slowly but inexorably and with exquisite specificity leads to the destruction of all insulin-producing cells within the islets of Langerhans. Elucidation of the pathophysiologic elements involved in this autoimmune insulitis may prove invaluable in designing strategies for intervention.

Since the first report of islet cell autoantibodies (ICA) (1), there has been a dramatic increase in the number of autoantibodies identified to constituents of the β cell. These include not only insulin, its main secretory product, but also cell membrane proteins, such as the glucose transporters (2), the smaller isoform of the enzyme glutamic acid decarboxylase (GAD), and two newly identified, less well characterized antigens: the bovine albumin-related 69 kD antigen and a protein of molecular weight 38,000 whose structure is thought to be consistent with a membrane protein found in the insulin secretory granule (see summary of the 12th International Immunology and Diabetes Workshop, Ref. 3).

Useful information has derived from extensive investigation of the mechanisms by which diabetes develops in two naturally occurring rodent models of autoimmune diabetes, the nonobese spontaneously diabetic NOD mouse and the BioBreeding Wistar rat. Further insights into this pathophysiology now stem from the creation of transgenic mice. Mice genetically altered to hyperexpress membrane-bound proteins or cytokines intimately involved in immune inflammatory processes have been found to develop a diabetes-like illness. The best two examples of induction of IDDM have been provided by the introduction into the islet cell of the interferon-α (4) or -γ (5) genes, leading to an insulin-deficient

state with clear evidence of islet inflammatory changes similar to those of human type I diabetes. Of great interest for potential clinical trials is the demonstration that, at least for interferon-α, treatment of the animal with a neutralizing antibody against the cytokine prevents insulitis and, more importantly, the diabetes itself. Those observations may allow integration of the known autoimmune diathesis with the observation that viral infections may be involved in some cases of IDDM. Viruses able to induce the expression of cytokines in islets may trigger the immune reaction against the β cell in a fashion similar to those observed in these mice.

An important step in understanding the antigenicity of the enzymes involved in the production of intercellular messages, such as GAD, was recently reported (6). Spontaneous development of a proliferative T cell response to GAD was noted in mice genetically predisposed to diabetes. If, on the other hand, the mice were injected with this antigen at age 3 weeks, tolerance developed and diabetes was prevented in 75% of the mice. In another interesting approach, GAD injected into the thymus in the same murine strain significantly diminished the percentage of mice developing diabetes at a later date (7). This basic research presages proposed human clinical trials in which GAD would be administered in an effort to prevent IDDM in susceptible individuals.

II. PREVENTION

A. Prediction and Early Diagnosis

The prediabetic state can now be diagnosed with some degree of certainty when the presence of specific markers of β cell antigenicity are detected in the peripheral circulation of individuals with susceptible HLA haplotypes. Because overt glucose intolerance is not likely to develop until 90% of the pancreatic islets have been destroyed, coupling antibody markers to evidence of diminished β cell function gives even stronger support to a presumptive diagnosis of latent diabetes. These screening tests may allow trials aimed at the prevention of IDDM in a population at high risk of developing the disease. Our present incomplete understanding and the possible inadvertent ill effects on children, however, dictate great caution in considering prevention programs. Despite this important precaution, most researchers believe that some preventive programs appear to offer favorable benefit-risk ratios that warrant continuing screening for liability to IDDM. A further justification for screening selected groups for autoantibodies is the reasonable hope that positive identification would sound an alarm, eliminating much of the risk to life in ketoacidosis occurring in the near future.

At very great risk of developing diabetes is the very young child possessing the IDDM-associated HLA alleles and with more than one antibody marker of high titer. For these and other at-risk groups of children, such as siblings of IDDM patients, an additional important consideration is that any protocol for prevention of diabetes must entail sufficient subjects to identify a large population to give all reasonable opportunities of yielding conclusive results.

B. Prevention Trials

Because population-based screening is not yet feasible in the United States, most studies are recruiting first-degree relatives of IDDM patients for prevention trials. The most commonly accepted criterion for entry into protocols at this time is the demonstration of islet cell autoantibodies at titers greater than a standard reference serum (>20 JDF units) (8), alone or in conjunction with evidence of diminished β cell function. The latter is determined by measuring insulin release immediately following an intravenous glucose challenge. This so-called first-phase insulin release is calculated by summing the insulin concentrations at 1 and 3 minutes after the infusion of glucose (9). Values lower than the fifth percentile of normal controls are considered evidence of β cell insufficiency, but some protocols specify the more stringent cutoff of less than the first percentile for enrollment.

Studies are already in progress to test whether continuous generalized immunosuppression prevents the high-risk individuals discussed earlier from progressing to clinical diabetes. At this time, the largest trials enrolling young people meeting these criteria for active intervention before development of overt diabetes involve the administration of either oral nicotinamide or parenteral insulin. Both nicotinamide and insulin administration appears to delay the onset of diabetes in rodent models of IDDM. Pilot human trials have indicated that these agents may be of help in preventing or delaying the onset of overt diabetes (10). Preliminary human studies have already suggested that in individuals who have both ICA and diminished first-phase insulin response, nicotinamide treatment is not effective in preventing overt diabetes (11). Whether this derivative of nicotinic acid (vitamin B₃) will be useful if administered orally before detectable diminution of β cell

function may be answered by the European nicotinamide diabetes intervention trial, a multicenter study involving 18 European countries, Israel, and Canada (12).

The exact mechanism responsible for the observed protective effect of nicotinamide in animals is not well understood. It is believed that nicotinamide may prevent cell death by interfering with DNA repair or, as shown very recently in our laboratory (13), by allowing a compensatory increase in the number of new β cells by its powerful action in inducing the differentiation and maturation of human fetal pancreatic cells in vitro. Theories proposed for the beneficial effect of insulin include induction of immune tolerance, direct stimulation of lymphocyte replication or activation of the T cell receptor, or placing the β cell at rest. The last concept holds that suppressing the release of endogenous insulin induces downregulation of presenting antigens that would otherwise be expressed on the cell surface, available to trigger antibody- or lymphocyte-mediated cytotoxicity (14).

III. PROLONGATION OF REMISSION

Once IDDM is clinically apparent, immunosuppressive therapy could be beneficial in preserving the function of any remaining islets and prolonging the "honeymoon phase" of IDDM. Past trials with generalized immunosuppressive agents, such as cyclosporin A, FK506, and azathioprine with and without glucocorticoids, were recently reviewed extensively by Skyler and Marks (10). If the end point of intervention is to eliminate dependence on injection of exogenous insulin altogether, the results, except for the cyclosporine studies, have been rather disappointing. If, however, the results of intervention are judged by such criteria as sustained C peptide production or a reduction in total insulin dose compared with control groups, the results are a bit more promising. Preserving some measure of endogenous insulin secretion may prove especially beneficial to young children, in whom the hospitalization rate for ketoacidosis is very low during the honeymoon phase but rises significantly once endogenous insulin production is entirely obliterated. Immunosuppressive agents are not without risk, however, and the value of any of these interventions in preventing the long-term complications of IDDM is entirely speculative at this time. Most effort is currently being directed to prevention trials and transplantation strategies.

IV. TRANSPLANTATION

A. Intact Pancreas

If normoglycemia independent of insulin injections is considered the goal of pancreatic transplantation for the treatment of IDDM, then the procedure itself is no longer experimental (15). Since last reviewed in this chapter, the total number of pancreas transplants for IDDM has increased by almost fivefold, from about 1000 to close to 5000. The number of transplants worldwide appears to be stabilizing at about 1000 annually according to the information available at the International Pancreas Transplantation Registry based at the University of Minnesota, where the first such transplant took place in 1966. Of all pancreas transplants, 85% occur simultaneously with a kidney transplant, 10% follow successful renal transplant, and isolated pancreas transplants currently account for only 5% of the total. The 1 year graft survival is around 80%, which equals the success of other organ transplants (16).

The most common procedure in use at this time is anastomosis of the pancreas allograft in the iliac fossa, with drainage of exocrine secretions into the urinary bladder. This allows a rapid and unique method of monitoring graft function; rejection rapidly diminishes the output of pancreatic amylase into urine. Because there may be an appreciable loss of bicarbonate into the bladder, metabolic acidosis can develop, which in turn requires reanastomosis of the pancreatic duct to an enteric site in as many as 30% of cases. Most of the complications of pancreas transplantation are related to the surgical procedure and tend to resolve spontaneously. Besides metabolic acidosis, other complications include pancreatic fistula, wound infections, hemorrhagic cystitis, and pancreatitis. Standard immunosuppression for pancreas transplants includes antilymphocytic globulin, cyclosporine, azathioprine, and prednisone. Largely because of the high potential for development of growth failure and depressed immune function with these agents, isolated pancreatic allografts are still rare in the pediatric population. However, teens already candidates for renal transplantation for diabetic nephropathy are reasonably considered candidates for simultaneous pancreas transplant.

There is evidence that pancreas transplantation does not reverse or halt the progression of severe retinopathy (17) or established nephropathy (18), but some studies have shown improvement in renal function and nerve conduction (19,20). If one extrapolates the results of the Diabetes Control and Complications Trial (21) to the transplant population, one could logically expect the improvement in glycemic control that follows pancreas transplantation to retard progression of complications in those individuals who have not yet developed overt organ failure.

Concern has been expressed regarding the availability of pancreases for transplantation. There are approximately 4500 cadaveric donors per year in the United States. Because the number of diabetic individuals receiving kidney transplants in the United States currently averages 2500 each year, the supply of cadaveric pancreases should be adequate to provide pancreases for this cohort as well. If, however, more patients with IDDM were to become eligible for a pancreatic transplant, the demand would quickly exceed the supply.

More relevant to pediatric endocrinologists is the frequent inquiry about whether a parent or an immediate relative could donate part of a pancreas for a segmental graft. At the University of Minnesota, about 80 segmental grafts have been performed with living donors (related and unrelated) (16). Graft function in the recipient has been acceptable. Of great concern, however, are the data demonstrating that hemipancreatectomy may, within a relatively short time, lead to evidence of altered pancreatic islet function in the donor (22).

Whether this may proceed to overt diabetes in the future is not known at this time, but recognition of this risk should limit consideration of this procedure until the preservation of pancreatic endocrine function in the donor can be better ensured.

In summary, pancreatic transplantation is not a therapeutic alternative for the majority of diabetic children at the present time. On the other hand, most individuals with IDDM who are candidates for renal transplants are potential pancreatic transplant recipients. An important additional consideration is that the costs of the operation, postoperative care, and subsequent immunosuppressive therapy are considerable and are not yet universally covered by insurance plans.

B. Isolated Pancreatic Islets

1. Adult Islets

Of all the strategies for cure of IDDM, islet transplantation alone remains the most appealing: only the defunct endocrine cells are replaced, without the added load of extraneous exocrine tissue. Furthermore, the majority of the techniques used to introduce isolated islets are considerably more benign than the major surgical procedure required for pancreatic transplantation. Most islet transplants have used islets isolated from adult organ donors and infused into the liver by embolization through the umbilical vein into the portal vein.

When last reviewed (in the second edition of this book), no cures were attributable to islet transplantation. There are now several reports indicating short-term successes (23) and at least one IDDM patient who has not required insulin injections for at least 3 years after the implantation of islets (24). Patterned after the International Pancreas Transplant Registry, an Islet Transplant Registry was created in 1989 at Justus-Liebig University in Giessen, Germany. Based on the information contained in the registry, Hering et al. (25) recently published a comprehensive review of the worldwide experience with clinical islet transplantation. Of the 167 adult islet transplants tallied to June 1992, about 60% had been performed at nine institutions in North America.

In the sole long-term success reported in the literature, normoglycemia occurred with the transplantation of about 10,000 islets/kg of a mixture of fresh and cryopreserved human adult islets (26), equivalent to a full adult complement of islets. A cell mass of this magnitude mandates the need for multiple donors because the yield from a single pancreas using current methods of islet isolation rarely exceeds one-half million islets (27). By contrast, islet autografts in such cases as pancreatitis require only about a quarter of a million islets (28), an amount close to the 10% pancreatic mass needed to maintain normoglycemia in partially pancreatectomized animals or humans. A clear explanation to account for this discrepancy in the number of islets needed to induce and maintain normoglycemia in the allo- and autograft situation is not available. It may well be that alloantigens interfere with engraftment and revascularization of the transplanted cells, leading to significant losses of the transplanted cells immediately after injection, or that the liver is not the optimal allograft site.

When evaluating the results of islet transplantation, it is important to take into account the differences in outcome when the transplantation is done because of autoimmune diabetes as opposed to other causes of insufficiency, such as pancreatectomy for pancreatitis or extensive abdominal tumors. In IDDM, the islet allograft faces not only simple organ rejection but the very real problem of cytotoxic immune destruction identical to that responsible for loss of the original islet mass. For some researchers the purity of the islet preparation is essential to a good outcome (25), although a recent report (29) indicates that transplantation of unpurified islets from a single pancreas leads to normoglycemia if accompanied by use of the novel immunosuppressive agent, 15-deoxyspergualin. The authors postulate that this agent enhances successful engraftment by inhibiting macrophage function in the immediate posttransplant period. Islet allografts continue to face a difficult prognosis, essentially rendering the recipient dependent on lifelong immunosuppressive therapy. As with transplant of the whole organ, islet transplant does not appear to be safe and effective for use in children until the benefits of successful transplantation outweigh the risks of immunosuppression or until functional islet grafts can be maintained without immunosuppression.

Two interesting approaches to islet transplantation that obviate the need for immunosuppressive medications merit consideration. The first is the immunoisolation of islets to create a physical barrier between the islets and the elements of the immune system. Researchers have microencapsulated individual islets, clustered them in hollow polymeric fibers, or placed them in implantable mechanical devices with vascular connections in which permselective membranes isolate the islets from the circulation. These techniques have been used successfully in reversing diabetes in rodents and dogs (reviewed in Ref. 30; see also Ref. 31). Viability of islets, normal glucose sensitivity, and promptness of insulin release have all been maintained in the isolated islets with these devices. Such techniques may allow use of plentiful xenogeneic (i.e., porcine) islets in treating human diabetes, without the need for immunosuppression.

The second approach to permit allograft survival without the need for continuous pharmacologic immunosuppression is the induction of donor-specific tissue unresponsiveness. Intrathymic inoculation of islets was originally reported (32) to induce immune tolerance in adult rats rendered diabetic chemically. A similar approach to induction of tolerance of extrathymic allogeneic transplants was recently reported (33), in which solubilized spleen cell membrane antigens injected into the rat thymus in conjunction with a single dose of antilymphocyte serum allowed rejection-free acceptance of allogeneic islets. Such strategies may hold great promise in allowing avoidance of immunosuppressive drugs. However, hurdles remain in demonstrating the reproducibility of this maneuver in humans, or nonhuman primates, whose thymuses have undergone partial or total atrophy.

2. Fetal Islets

A recent change in federal guidelines permits the use of funds in transplantation research with human fetal cells. Studies may now proceed to determine whether fetal islet cells can function as replacement pancreatic tissue for transplantation in IDDM. Although the obstacles are still formidable, newer techniques in molecular biology suggest the feasibility of development of β cell lines exhibiting decreased immunogenicity while preserving normal insulin secretion in response to glucose.

There has been more basic research using porcine fetal islets than with their human counterparts. In both species, methods of islet isolation developed to date are inadequate to provide functioning islet cells for clinical transplantation. In pigs, the islet as such forms postnatally; in humans, the yield from second-trimester fetuses is too low to allow meaningful clinical studies. Furthermore, there is a lag of approximately 12 weeks between harvest of human islets and the production of adequate glucose-stimulated insulin secretion (13), suggesting that a period in tissue culture is advisable before transplantation. Most current research is focused on developing methods for the isolation of islet precursor cells and the identification of factors that induce specific β cell differentiation. Strategies for harvest, growth and maturation, and preservation must be refined. Preliminary studies in animals suggest that islet-like fetal cell clusters allowed to mature following cryopreservation are viable for transplantation (34).

The international islet transplant registry also keeps track of fetal pancreas transplantation. A recent review (35) lists more than 1500 such transplants, most of then performed in Eastern European countries and China and unfortunately without adequate documentation to allow scientific judgment for the validity of the claims. In the United States (36) and Sweden, reports have not demonstrated beneficial effects after the transplantation of limited amounts of fetal pancreatic tissue. Xenografts of fetal pig pancreas to humans in amounts sufficient to deliver a volume of tissue similar to an adult islet human transplant embolized to the liver via the portal vein have also failed to produce evidence of adequate function to improve insulin production (35). Thus, extended basic research is required before attempts at treating IDDM using fetal tissue are entertained.

V. TECHNOLOGIC ADVANCES

In the days of epidemic paralytic poliomyelitis before the breakthrough offered by the Salk vaccine, dedicated workers in the field labored diligently to optimize the iron lung in an attempt to offer the best quality of life for their patients, for whom they could offer neither protection nor cure at that time. We face similar challenges today in IDDM, when the opportunities for prevention of the disease by immunization or cure by transplantation are tantalizingly beyond our reach. In the wake of the Diabetes Control and Complications Trial, there is increased dedication toward attempts to normalize glycemic control. Home blood glucose monitoring has been a crucial tool in striving for good metabolic control using exogenous insulin.

A. Refinement of Current Technologies

In infants and toddlers, attempts to minimize fluctuations in blood glucose values may be especially frustrating. Food consumption may be difficult to predict preceding the meal, when insulin is usually injected. If some of the meal is subsequently refused, the insulin administered may not match the food as intended. A new short-acting insulin analog, Lys(B28)Pro(B29) human insulin (Eli Lilly, Indianapolis, IN), may allow better regulation. This analog is rapidly absorbed from subcutaneous injection depots and cleared from the circulation more rapidly than regular human insulin (37,38). Thus, it may offer the opportunity to administer at least the rapidly acting component of the insulin regimen after the meal is completed, without significantly compromising postprandial glycemic excursion. This product may also minimize problems of overlap in older patients on intensive therapy using basal insulin plus premeal bolus regular insulin, who for some reason may be eating within 2–4 h of a previous dose of regular insulin.

The twice-daily use of Ultralente insulin originally proposed by Holman and Turner (39) nearly a decade ago never developed a very large following in the clinical community when animal insulins had a duration of action greater than 24 h. The development of human Ultralente insulin, with a modestly shorter duration and a more detectable peak of action than the animal source preparation (40), has led to reconsideration of this tactic (41). The experience at one of our centers, similar to that reported by Johnson et al. (42), is that Ultralente insulin administered in equal doses at intervals of approximately 12 h facilitates improvement in fasting blood glucose values without increasing symptomatic hypoglycemia. To provide more intensive therapy than those investigators, we recommend a small injection of Regular insulin at each meal (see also Ref. 41). Acceptance has been very good in children who are newly diagnosed, in individuals for whom strict daily schedules are impractical, and in our teenaged patients in whom attempts to normalize fasting values by increasing the dose of intermediate-acting insulin administered before dinner resulted in an unacceptable rate of hypoglycemic reactions during the night.

Subcutaneous pump therapy has not yet found its place in the routine treatment of the majority of children with IDDM. In the motivated adolescent, however, the pump represents an excellent vehicle to achieve improved glycohemoglobin concentrations through intensive insulin therapy. Transdermal "jet" injectors, touted to provide painless, needle-free administration of insulin, have not fulfilled their promise in clinical use in our population. At the same time, the use of finer gauge needles for intermittent subcutaneous insulin injection has diminished the discomfort of injections and improved acceptance.

B. Novel Technologies

1. Insulin Administration

Endogenous insulin is secreted into the portal vein, providing the highest concentrations on the first pass to the target organ, the liver. Because subcutaneous insulin is administered at a nonphysiologic site, insulin levels achieved in the peripheral circulation may not be optimal for hepatic function. The peritoneal mucosa offers a very large surface area over which insulin is readily absorbed directly into the portal circulation. Thus, it is not surprising that introduction of intraperitoneal catheters attached to small insulin pumps implanted in subcutaneous abdominal locations has been successful in normalizing blood glucose in pilot studies (43,44). This strategy is likely to be used for the efferent arm of a future artificial pancreas.

A novel approach to the peripheral administration of insulin is the transdermal insulin patch, analogous to those in use for sex steroids, nicotine, and vasodilators. An obvious difficulty is facilitating absorption of a large, polar molecule like insulin through skin of different thicknesses in a uniform, predictable fashion. One commercial group claimed (noted in Ref. 45) to have developed a delivery strategy to overcome this impediment. The problems of titrating doses and providing additional bolus insulin at meals remain. Costs are estimated to approximate total costs for current intermittent subcutaneous injection. Unfortunately, the proprietary nature of the development of this product has limited scientific data for review.

2. Glucose Monitoring

The necessity of pricking one's finger to obtain blood samples is uncomfortable and eventually becomes a limiting factor in obtaining frequent data points with a home blood glucose monitor. It would be a boon to intensive therapy if one could instantaneously determine the glycemic consequences of different foods, activities, and insulin doses. Monitors utilizing noninvasive, near-infrared spectroscopy to measure blood glucose across the dermal barrier of a fingertip have been under development for some time (46,47). This so-called "dream beam" may even offer the opportunity for parents to generate blood glucose data while young children are asleep without having to awaken them. The physics of the technology is well understood, but in practice, developing and calibrating a small spectroscopic device for home use has proven to be slow going. A major impediment is that the faint spectroscopic signature of glucose, although very specific, is easily obscured by the significantly brighter optical signature of the more plentiful water. Additional problems have been identified with skin temperature and positioning of the finger within the device (46). Once again, these spectrometers represent devices in which there is a substantial proprietary stake, and therefore information on the progress of clinical trials is scarce.

An alternative technique for estimating blood glucose is an implantable sensor that measures interstitial tissue glucose concentration (48). There have been preliminary reports that implantable subcutaneous electrochemical detection devices are of utility in the determination of ambient tissue glucose concentration in dogs (49). The sensitivity and speed of detection have been very reliable. Rather than being useful in the average physically active child using intermittent subcutaneous insulin injections, however, this instrument is likely to find its greatest promise in the development of an intraperitoneal closed-loop artificial pancreas, because it would obviate the need for continuous vascular access for blood glucose detection (reviewed in Ref. 50).

In conclusion, the advances in basic research, particularly new developments in immunology and molecular biology, are likely to make a significant impact on the prognosis of IDDM. Developments in somatic cell therapy and gene therapy may eventually allow intervention in the pathogenesis of the disease or enable more physiologic insulin replacement therapy. In the interim, the new models of intensified diabetes care provide a more hopeful future for the many children with this chronic disorder.

REFERENCES

1. Bottazzo GF, Florin-Christensen A, Doniach D. Islet cell antibodies in diabetes mellitus with autoimmune polyendocrine deficiencies. Lancet 1974; 7892:1279–1283.

2. Inman LR, McAllister CT, Chen L, et al. Autoantibodies to the GLUT-2 transporter of β cells in insulin-dependent diabetes of recent onset. Proc Natl Acad Sci USA 1993; 90:1281–1284.

3. Maclaren N, Lafferty K. The 12th International Immunology and Diabetes Workshop. Diabetes 1993; 42:1099–1104.

4. Stewart TA, Hultgren B, Huang X, Pitts-Meek S, Hully J, MacLachlan NJ. Induction of type I diabetes by interferon-alpha in transgenic mice. Science 1993; 260:1942–1946.

5. Sarvetnick N, Liggitt D, Pitts SL, Hansen SE, Stewart TA. Insulin-dependent diabetes mellitus induced in transgenic mice by ectopic expression of class II MHC and interferon-gamma. Cell 1988; 52:773–782.

6. Kaufman DL, Clare-Salzler M, Tian J, et al. Spontaneous loss of T-cell tolerance to glutamic acid decarboxylase in murine insulin-dependent diabetes. Nature 1993; 366:69–72.

7. Tisch R, Yang X-D, Singer SM, Liblau RS, Fugger L, McDevitt HO. Immune response to glutamic acid decarboxylase correlates with insulitis in non-obese diabetic mice. Nature 1993; 366:72–75.

8. Gleichmann H, Botazzo GF. Progress toward standardization of cytoplasmic islet cell antibody assay. Diabetes 1987; 36:578–584.

9. Bingley PJ, Colman P, Eisenbarth GS, et al. Standardization of IVGTT to predict IDDM. Diabetes Care 1992; 15:1313–1316.

10. Skyler JS, Marks JB. Immune intervention in type I diabetes. Diabetes Rev 1993; 1:15–42.

11. Eisenbarth GS, Verge CF, Allen H, Rewers MJ. The design of trials for the prevention of IDDM. Diabetes 1993; 42:941–947.

12. Pociot F, Reimers JI, Andersen HU. Nicotinamide—biological actions and therapeutic potential in diabetes prevention. Diabetologia 1993; 36:574–576.

13. Otonkoski T, Beattie GM, Mally MI, Ricordi C, Hayek A. Nicotinamide is a potent inducer of endocrine differentiation in cultured human fetal pancreatic cells. J Clin Invest 1993; 92:1459–1466.

14. Bjork E, Kampe O, Andersson A, Karlsson FA. Expression of the 64kDa/glutamic acid decarboxylase rat islet cell autoantigen is influenced by the rate of insulin secretion. Diabetologia 1992; 35:490–493.

15. Robertson RP. Pancreatic and islet transplantation for diabetes-cures or curiosities? N Engl J Med 1992; 327:1861–1868.

16. Sutherland DER. Pancreatic transplantation: an update. Diabetes Rev 1993; 1:1–14.

17. Ramsay RC, Goetz FC, Sutherland DER, et al. Progression of diabetic retinopathy after pancreas transplantation for insulin-dependent diabetes mellitus. N Engl J Med 1988; 318:208–214.

18. Fioretto P, Mauer SM, Bilous RW, Goetz FC, Sutherland DER, Steffes MW. Effects of pancreas transplantation on glomerular structure in insulin-dependent diabetic patients with their own kidneys. Lancet 1993; 342:1193–1196.

19. Bilous RW, Mauer SM, Sutherland DER, Najarian JS, Steffes MW. The effect of pancreas transplantation on the glomerular structure of renal allografts in patients with insulin-dependent diabetes. N Engl J Med 1989; 231:80–85.

20. Kennedy WR, Navarro X, Goetz FC, Sutherland DER, Najarian JS. The effect of pancreas transplantation on diabetic neuropathy. N Engl J Med 1990; 322:1021–1037.

21. DCCT Research Group. The effect of intensive treatment of diabetes on the development and progression of long-term complications in insulin-dependent diabetes mellitus. N Engl J Med 1993; 329:977–986.

22. Kendall DM, Sutherland DER, Najarian JS, Goetz FC, Robertson RP. Effects of hemipancreatectomy on insulin secretion and glucose tolerance in healthy humans. N Engl J Med 1990; 322:898–903.

23. Scharp DW, Lacy PE, Santiago JV, et al. Insulin-independence after islet transplantation into type I diabetic patient. Diabetes 1990; 39:515–518.

24. Warnock GL, Kneteman NM, Ryan EA, Rabinovitch A, Rajotte RV. Long-term follow-up after transplantation of insulin-producing pancreatic islets into patients with type I diabetes (insulin-dependent) diabetes mellitus. Diabetologia 1992; 35:89–95.

25. Hering BJ, Browatzki CC, Schultz A, Bretzel RG, Federlin KF. Clinical islet transplantation—registry report, accomplishments in the past and future research needs. Cell Transplant 1993; 2:269–282.

26. Warnock GL, Kneteman NM, Ryan E, Seelis REA, Rabinovitch A, Rajotte RV. Normoglycemia after transplantation of freshly isolated and cryopreserved pancreatic islets in type I diabetes (insulin-dependent) diabetes mellitus. Diabetologia 1991; 34:55–58.

27. Ricordi C, Lacy PE, Finke EH, Olack BJ, Scharp DW. Automated method for isolation of human pancreatic islets. Diabetes 1988; 37:413–420.

28. Pyzdrowski KL, Kendall DM, Halter JB, Nakhleh RE, Sutherland DER, Robertson RP. Preserved insulin secretion and insulin independence in recipients of islet autografts. N Engl J Med 1992; 327:220–226.

29. Gores PF, Najarian JS, Stephanian E, Lloveras JJ, Kelley SL, Sutherland DER. Insulin independence in type I diabetes after transplantation of unpurified islets from single donor with 15-deoxyspergualin. Lancet 1993; 341:19–21.

30. Lacy PE. Status of islet cell transplantation. Diabetes Rev 1993; 1:76–92.

31. Soon-Shiong P, Feldman E, Nelson R, et al. Long-term reversal of diabetes by the injection of immunoprotected islets. Proc Natl Acad Sci USA 1993; 90:5843–5847.

32. Posselt AM, Barker CF, Tomaszewski JE, Markmann JF, Choti MA, Naji A. Induction of donor-specific unresponsiveness by intrathymic islet transplantation. Science 1990; 249:1293–1295.

33. Qian T, Schachner R, Brendel M, Kong SS, Alejandro R. Induction of donor-specific tolerance to rat islet allografts by intrathymic inoculation of solubilized spleen cell membrane antigens. Diabetes 1993; 42:1544–1546.

34. Beattie GM, Otonkoski T, Lopez AD, Hayek A. Maturation and function of human fetal pancreatic cells after cryopreservation. Transplantation 1993; 56:1340–1344.

35. Andersson A, Sandler S. Fetal pancreatic transplantation. Transplant Rev 1993; 6:20–38.

36. Lafferty K, Hao L. Fetal pancreas transplantation for treatment of IDDM patients. Diabetes Care 1993; 16:383–386.

37. Woodworth J, Howey D, Bowsher R, Lutz S, Santa P, Brady P. [Lys(B28), Pro(B29)] human insulin (K): dose-ranging vs. human insulin (H). Diabetes 1993; 42(Suppl. 1):54A.

38. TerBraak EW, Bianchi R, Erkelens DW. Faster, shorter and more profound action of Lys(B28), Pro(B29) human insulin analogue compared to regular insulin irrespective of the injection site. Diabetes 1993; 42(Suppl. 1):207A.

39. Holman RR, Turner RC. A practical guide to basal and prandial insulin therapy. Diabetic Med 1985; 2:45–53.

40. Heinenmann L, Richter B. Clinical pharmacology of human insulin. Diabetes Care 1993; 16(Suppl. 3):90–100.

41. Zinman B. Insulin regimens and strategies for IDDM. Diabetes Care 1993; 16(Suppl. 3):24–8.

42. Johnson NB, Kronz KK, Fineberg NS, Golden MP. Twice-daily Humulin Ultralente insulin decreases morning fasting hypoglycemia. Diabetes Care 1992; 15:1031–1033.

43. Selam JL, Raccah D, Jean-Didier N, Lozano JL, Waxman K, Charles MA. Randomized comparison of metabolic control achieved by intraperitoneal insulin infusion with implantable pumps versus intensive subcutaneous insulin ther-apy in type I diabetic patients. Diabetes Care 1992; 15:53–58.

44. Giacca A, Caumo A, Galimberti G, et al. Peritoneal and subcutaneous absorption of insulin in type 1 diabetic subjects. J Clin Endocrinol Metab 1993; 77:738–742.

45. Experimental insulin patch stirs interest. Clin Diabetes 1993; 11:44.

46. Robinson MR, Eaton RP, Haaland DM, et al. Noninvasive glucose monitoring in diabetic patients: a preliminary evaluation. Clin Chem 1992; 38:1618–1622.

47. Steuer R. The light at the end of the meter. Diab Self-Management 1993; 10:42–44.

48. Wilson GS, Zhang Y, Reach G, et al. Progress toward the development of an implantable sensor for glucose. Clin Chem 1992; 38:1613–1617.

49. Fischer U, Rebrin K, Able P, Von Woedtke T. Usefulness of subcutaneous glucose concentration in metabolic care. Diabetes 1993; 42(Suppl. 1):248A.

50. Pickup JC. In vivo glucose monitoring: sense and sensorbility. Diabetes Care 1993; 16:535–539.

45

Psychosocial Aspects of Diabetes Mellitus

Arlan L. Rosenbloom
University of Florida College of Medicine, Gainesville, Florida

I. FUNDAMENTAL IMPORTANCE OF PSYCHOSOCIAL CONSIDERATIONS

The diagnosis and long-term management of childhood diabetes present a formidable challenge to the child and family, requiring the acquisition of knowledge and skills for insulin administration, blood testing, urine testing for ketones, interpretation of symptoms and signs, and routinization of meals, as well as providing the child and family with a tool for manipulation and control. The perception of diabetes management as the triangle of diet, insulin, and exercise tunneled the vision of therapists for the first 40 years of the insulin era. Recognition and investigation of the complex relationship between patient characteristics, family and environmental influences, physician behavior, and demands of disease management have emerged over the past 30 years (1–4).

The profound and pervasive importance of psychosocial factors in childhood diabetes was poignantly outlined at a workshop in 1981 dealing with this problem, in which diabetes was presented as a means to disrupt the family and establish psychologic problems for a child [modified from Travis (5)]:

1. Introduce a disorder of unknown cause.
2. Give it to a child who is incapable of mature understanding and, therefore, can assume that he or she is being punished.
3. Expect the child to exert inordinate self-discipline in the management of this disorder.
4. Further convince the child he or she is bad and being punished by making the treatment painful, time consuming, and frustrating.
5. Implicate heredity as a causative factor to enhance guilt in one or both parents and anger in the child.
6. Have the treatment program alter family life through regimentation, and have it disrupt the most important family ritual—eating.
7. Ask people to take care of the disease with imprecise instructions and tools.
8. Have the family deal daily with decisions that affect health and life.
9. Make certain the child, family, or both, are held responsible for any failures.
10. Assure, despite best efforts, an uncertain future involving the possibilities of impotence, difficult pregnancy, blindness, kidney failure, and early death.

Insulin-dependent diabetes mellitus (IDDM) in childhood epitomizes the shift in pediatrics from management of acute problems to the far more demanding and multifaceted involvement of the physician as a team member directing a case-management program (6). The physician has had to learn that his or her own attitude and approach can either coopt the family or isolate him or her from it. The term "therapeutic alliance" recognizes that the patient and family are the principal therapists on a day-to-day basis, with the physician and various team members as consultants. The physician's role then becomes one of understanding the effect of diabetes on the child and family, appreciating the developmental issues for each stage of childhood and their relationship to the diabetes and recognizing their influence on management decisions (Table 1) (7).

Physicians or other members of the health team should not blandly propose that one can lead a normal life with diabetes, even though in intent this is laudable—to emphasize that diabetes need not preclude achievement of life goals. However, it is certainly not normal to take injections daily to survive, to monitor blood glucose regularly, for a youngster to have to attend clinic frequently (and, often, be told how naughty he or she has been), or to be unable to serve in the military or obtain standard-rate health and life insurance.

The recently completed Diabetes Control and Complications Trial (DCCT) and the appropriate attendant publicity of the findings that intensive therapy delays the onset and slows

Table 1 Effect of Diabetes Mellitus on Child and Family and Management Implications Relative to Development Stage

	Diagnosis[a]	Major developmental issues	Management implications	
			Parent/patient	Treatment team
Infant	Sensitive to added tension with irritability	Trust; parents provide cuddling and food	Difficulty distinguishing hypo-glycemic reactions from ordi-nary upset; feeling over-whelmed and isolated	Anticipatory guidance and con-stant availability; parent-peer support system
Toddler	Regression in speech, toilet training	Beginning autonomy; exploration of environment	Temper tantrums difficult to dis-tinguish from reactions and complicate injections and glu-cose testing; emotional trauma of inflicting pain on child able to verbalize anger	As for infant; identification of least painful means of re-ducing pain of injections (ice, distractions, reward) and blood tests.
Preschool	Regression in social behavior	Body strength and wholeness; diabetes treatment as punish-ment; fear of injections and blood testing	Normal moodiness confused with reactions or with hypergly-cemia	As for infant and toddler
School-age	Regression, depression, social withdrawal; school problems, awareness of genetic factors	Curiosity; motor, intellectual, social skills; peer recognition; sense of adequacy	Self-monitoring, recognition of hypoglycemic reactions, par-ticipation in nutrition de-cisions, assistance in blood testing, drawing up and inject-ing insulin, all requiring supervision!	Begin seeing child alone during part of visit, addressing the child and reinforcing positive behaviors without scolding for negative ones
Adolescence	Adult-style grief; awareness of complications, genetics	Identity formation, intense body awareness and sexual identity; dependence struggle with de-fiance; comparison of self with peers; diabetes decreases sense of adequacy	Experimentation and risk taking: stopping insulin, blood testing, nutrition, potential for recur-rent DKA; sensitive regarding physical contact and concerned about sexuality and diabetes; capable of self-management but still requiring adult supervi-sion and involvement	Serve as patient's, not parent's doctor, assuring confidentiality and privacy; understand with-out condoning (inappropriate affect, school or work de-terioration, recurrent keto-acidosis)
Young adult	As for adolescence	Emotional ties outside family; career development; concerns about complications and effects on work and family goals	Responsible for diabetes manage-ment and sharing information with team and others in en-vironment who need to know; often marked improvement in control with independence from family	Continuing relationship and prep-aration for adult issues of po-tential complications; appropri-ate followup for monitoring for complications; often do better through college years maintain-ing relationship to pediatric di-abetes group; recognize in-dicators of need for counseling

[a]Effects on child shown. At all developmental stages parents show shock, disbelief, denial, anger, guilt, despair, and variable impairment in their ability to learn about the diabetes.
Source: Modified from Reference 7.

the progression of diabetic retinopathy, nephropathy, and neuropathy in patients with IDDM can add additional stress to the family of the child with diabetes (8,9). It must be emphasized, however, that the profound commitment and understanding required to achieve the levels of control that resulted in such effects was not considered feasible for preadolescents (under 13 years of age) and that the 20% of the cohort in the 13–19 year age group was highly selected and still unable to achieve the levels of control of older individuals (9). The results of the DCCT must be used as a motivation and inspiration rather than a bludgeon.

In the context of the therapeutic alliance between the patient-family and management team, the word *compliance* has assumed a pejorative connotation, implying an authori-tarian relationship. The substitution of *adherence* is slightly more palatable. Both terms connote a passive role for the patient, who must either comply with or adhere to the recommendations of authority (4). I have proposed the term "earnestness" to focus properly on the central role of patient and family attitude and behavior in adherence. This term, or its less archaic equivalent, "enthusiasm," provides an alliter-ative reminder of the "five Es" of diabetes control: education, eating, exercise, emotional state, and earnestness-enthusiasm (10).

II. PSYCHOLOGICAL FACTORS

Recognition of the importance of psychosocial factors in diabetes (child and adult) has led to the increasing involvement of clinical specialists and investigators in behavior. Early studies, largely anecdotal, concentrated on the personality of the patient or comparisons of persons with diabetes with healthy controls (2). Contemporary investigations are directed toward the variables that relate to coping and health status within the population of patients with diabetes, under the assumption that there is great heterogeneity in the response to the disorder and how it is managed (4). The object, in keeping with the therapeutic alliance principle, is to provide therapists with greater understanding of what is really essential in the management program and how patients and their families can be helped to participate fully. Before one dismisses this kind of research as validation of the obvious, it is useful to look at how some of our impressions have responded to inquiry.

People with diabetes have a characteristic personality. The myth of the diabetic personality (passive-resistant, hysterical, depressed, and manipulative) was the first to fall to the onslaught of behavioral investigation (2,11). There is as wide a range in personalities and coping styles among patients with diabetes as one would expect in any cross section of the child population. This does not diminish the potential for deleteriously influencing personality by inducing guilt or thwarting self-esteem either in the clinic or at home.

Self-efficacious patients (internal locus of control) do better with their diabetes. Recent studies have failed to support this notion. The complexities of diabetes management and inability of the patient (or therapist!) to explain or understand episodic or long-term instability could increase stress and instability, despite improved efforts in some individuals, negating the positive effect in others (12,13).

Anxious and unhappy youngsters have poorer control of the diabetes than less anxious and happier youngsters. Several studies have now shown that more neurotic and unhappy youngsters can have better blood glucose and glycosylated hemoglobin (HbA_{1C}) levels than their more equanimous peers and that associated distractibility may modify the anticipated negative effects of stress on diabetes metabolism (14–18).

The earlier children take responsibility for the management of their own diabetes, the more likely it is that will one see good control. Premature assignment of responsibility to the young patient is increasingly recognized as a potential cause of decreasing stability of the diabetes (17,19–21).

A quality diabetes education program will greatly enhance diabetes control. Although the provision of good information is essential at the time of diagnosis,

at follow-up visits, and during acute situations by telephone, the discrepancy between patient-parent knowledge and health status may be wide, even when subjects have acquired the knowledge that has been proffered (22). Education is critical, but it must be part of a comprehensive program (23).

The signs and symptoms of hypo- and hyperglycemia are sufficiently consistent that a checklist can be used for training health workers, teachers, and particularly patients and parents. In both adults and children, wide individuality has been described in the symptoms associated with hypo- and hyperglycemia, with very little cross-subject consistency for any single symptom. Headache and fatigue, for example, can occur with either hypo- or hyperglycemia. These studies have emphasized the importance of self-monitoring of blood glucose for determination of individual responses and for distinguishing the symptoms of simple anxiety from those of true hypoglycemia (24,25).

Adherence to the major components of the diabetes treatment regimen is essential to control, and it can be used as a surrogate for measuring control, or vice versa. Although it may be logical to equate health status with adherence to the regimen, aside from the essential behavior of taking insulin, one must be cautious. Noncompliance with blood glucose monitoring, for example, may have no deleterious effect in an individual who has good health behaviors or during the first year or so of diabetes when insulinogenic reserve can make control easier. On the other hand, demands for rigid adherence to the regimen may result in poorer control as a result of increased family stress. Sophisticated studies have now shown that there are only weak relationships, at best, between adherence and glycemic control (4,26–28). Furthermore, intelligent patients may be appropriately nonadherent to bad or unrealistic advice! Patients may also be noncompliant inadvertently because of the common problem of not understanding or recalling advice. Johnson (4) has emphasized that adherence or nonadherence should not be considered a global description of patients but that specific aspects of the regimen, and even elements of those aspects, must be separately considered. Caution is needed in reading papers that use glycemic control or health status measures to ascertain compliance, based on the assumption that regimen adherence is found only in association with good health status and that good health status can be achieved only through (global) regimen adherence (29,30).

Severe instability, with recurrent ketoacidosis, inability to work or attend school, and failing health, is often caused by management errors or unusual insulin resistance. Pediatric investigators have long recognized that once obvious management errors are excluded, severe instability results from psychosocial factors, including emotional stress, overinsulinization, and deliberate omission of insulin (31–33). This realization has been emphasized by the recent concentration of such patients in the fruitless quest for the rare subcutaneous insulin resistance syndrome (34).

The difficulties in managing diabetes in adolescents compared with younger children or adults can be entirely attributed to poor compliance in this age group. Although it is certainly true that diabetes has its greatest negative impact at the time of greatest concern with self-image, independence, and awareness of the future, there is good evidence that physiologic factors come to bear on even the most stable of adolescents, those who have gone through the stiff qualifying process for the DCCT (8,9). The more exuberant epinephrine response to a falling blood glucose concentration in children and adolescents compared with that of adults may be a contributing factor (35).

III. PSYCHOSOCIAL ASSESSMENT

In addition to reviewing a child's adjustment, peer relations, intellectual functioning, school achievement, participation in physical education, and extracurricular activities or work, there are specific issues regarding patient and family management of the diabetes that must be periodically reviewed.

A. Knowledge About Diabetes

It is generally assumed that the more knowledge a patient or parent has about the physiology and clinical management of diabetes, the more effective he or she will be. However, one is continually struck by shortcomings in patient knowledge, despite repeated exposure to the information or, as can be seen in medical personnel as well, by the hiatus between knowledge and application. There are also those patients who learn what they must to take care of their diabetes, without ever understanding the nature of the disorder, and yet achieve high degrees of control.

One of the few consistencies in the psychosocial literature of diabetes is the inadequacy of patient knowledge, in both children and adults (22,36,37). Furthermore, knowledge about different components of the diabetes regimen is often uneven (22,38). These studies emphasize the importance of periodically reviewing all aspects of diabetes management, including direct observation of the skills required, particularly the injection of insulin and blood glucose testing.

It is also important to consider the maturational level of the youngster (see Table 1). Most children are able to self-inject insulin by 9 years of age (22,39–41), but children at this age would probably not be reliable in their blood glucose monitoring, a skill more readily mastered by a 12 year old (22,38). Although children may be limited in what they can acquire in educational sessions, they should participate with the parents and learn to do whatever portion of the procedure they are capable of doing. They should not feel excluded from discussions of their management.

There are few studies of parents' knowledge about diabetes. However, there is agreement that the mother is typically the most knowledgeable individual, adolescent patients often being as knowledgeable as she is (22,42–44). The exclusion of fathers from the day-to-day management of diabetes can set the stage for family conflict. Fathers must be encouraged to participate in their child's diabetes care, to attend clinic, if possible, and to become involved in family support groups.

The recognition that the knowledge about diabetes or skills with insulin injection and blood testing cannot be assumed on the basis of assent by the patient has led to the development of more extensive methods of assessment (4,22), including information about task responsibilities within the family (45). As such assessment becomes the standard of care, the involvement of psychologists or education specialists on diabetes treatment teams will be imperative (6).

B. Earnestness-Enthusiasm (Adherence)

As has been emphasized, knowledge does not equate with effective management of the diabetes. Nonadherence may be based on a conscious decision to forego portions of the regimen thought to be unnecessary (e.g., rigid dietary constraints or monitoring at certain times of day), particularly in adolescent patients (7,10,27), or it may be inadvertent, the result of deficient knowledge or skill. The latter may be particularly common in younger children who are prematurely responsible for their own care. Withdrawal of the parent from the treatment process, even in adolescence, may trigger deterioration of control (17,19,45).

As with knowledge and skills, what patients or parents say about their adherence to daily care procedures may resemble more what the physician has prescribed or what the parent thinks the child is doing than what is actually done. Early studies found physician estimates of patient adherence to be inaccurate (46–48). More recent study, perhaps reflecting a greater sensitivity of physicians to the factors affecting adherence, has found the correlation to be high between physician ratings of patient adherence and an interviewer's ratings based on lengthy discussions with the adolescents and their mothers ($r = 0.7$) (49). Physicians have a tendency to equate compliance with control, and it is clear that control is a function of more than adherence.

The most obvious other factors are the appropriateness of the medical management program and other stressors in the children's environment and how they interpret them (4).

When asked to evaluate a youngster in poor diabetes control because it is thought that behaviors are an important contributing factor, the psychologist faces a particular challenge. Parents and children are often incapable of keeping reliable records of their diabetes management behaviors, and this is expected to be especially problematic in the situations for which consultation is sought. Furthermore, it is uncertain which of the adherence behaviors should be monitored. For these reasons, Johnson et al. (27) developed 24 h recall interviews, based on the nutritional model, to assess multiple adherence behaviors in a sample of 168 patients and their parents. Three independent interviews were conducted with each youngster and his or her parent and information obtained on 15 adherence behaviors. Parent-patient agreement was good to excellent for most of the behaviors, although agreement was influenced by the age of the child. As expected, those 10–15 years old had the most consistent agreement between parent and patient, whereas younger children were reliable about all behaviors except those involving time. This method required approximately 20 minutes per interview and could be conducted in person or by telephone. Cooperation was high in this unselected group of patients, who cut across all socioeconomic and educational categories.

In this study, an interrelationship between adherence behaviors was not found. Rather, a five-factor grouping accounted for over 70% of the variance. Regimen adherence was determined to be a complex construct in which insulin injection behaviors, exercise, type of food eaten, amount of food taken, and eating and glucose testing frequency were independent of and unrelated to each other. Thus, all components of the diabetes regimen must be assessed if one addresses compliance issues.

The relationship of coping styles to regimen adherence and metabolic control has been studied in 100 adolescents, revealing that ventilation and avoidance were associated with high stress and low family cohesion and were also negatively related to adherence. The style of using personal and interpersonal resources was not associated with adherence, however, either negatively or positively. Neither of these coping styles was in any way related to diabetes control (28). These findings seem to contrast with an earlier study showing that self-esteem, perceived competence, social functioning and the nature of behavioral symptoms, and adjustment to diabetes are predictive of adherence behaviors. This study, however, dealt only with recent-onset diabetes over a broad age range. Furthermore, adherence deteriorated over the 18 months of the study, and adolescents were less adherent than preadolescents (50).

Adherence measures and the outcome of diabetes control have varied greatly over the years as a result of improved diabetes management technology, making comparison of earlier and more recent studies problematic. For example, noncompliance with unreliable and difficult to interpret urine testing (51) has a much different significance from nonadherence to blood glucose testing. Until the advent of HbA$_{1C}$ measurement, there was no "gold standard" for diabetes control. Even this measure may obscure relationships between adherence and control, however, failing to reflect variability in blood glucose levels. A recent study suggested that measures of lipid metabolism may be more strongly associated with adherence behaviors than glucose metabolism (52).

C. Stress

The importance of physical stress, such as illness or trauma, on diabetes metabolism has been well accepted as an obvious clinical observation, despite the absence of systematic study.

The comparable observations of the destabilizing effects of psychologic stress, more difficult to quantify or identify than, for example, a fever or a urinary tract infection, have been met with greater skepticism. Among the earliest demonstrations of emotional stress effects on metabolic control was the report of a 15-year-old girl with repeated ketoacidotic episodes who kept a diary of daily stressful events that showed a striking relationship between these and the appearance of urinary ketones (53). We have made similar observations in our camp program and in our inpatient diabetes rehabilitation unit (54–56). Recent studies of adults and adolescents failed to demonstrate metabolic derangement in response to laboratory stressors, suggesting that for most patients, acute metabolic derangement does not commonly follow the stresses of daily life (57,58). These types of studies, however, can obscure subgroups of patients for whom there may be such an association. For example, Stabler et al. (59) showed that type A individuals (competitive, striving, impatient, aggressive, and hostile) have stress-hyperglycemia relationships, whereas type B youngsters do not. It is noteworthy, however, that this personality type and the glycemic responsiveness to the laboratory stressor did not predict glucose regulation as measured by HbA$_{1C}$ (60).

An early study of campers found that 9–12 year olds had higher urine glucose levels when they were exposed to a competitive as opposed to a noncompetitive camp atmosphere (61). Another study in the camp setting found that the frequency of major life events during the 12 months before camp was related to the number of illness episodes during the 3 week residential session (62). With the same social readjustment rating scale, stress was found to be associated with poor diabetes control in a sample of 32 children aged 15–18 years (63); however, these associations did not hold for older adolescents or for younger children. This finding is similar to that of a more recent study that was unable to document stress-hyperglycemia relationships in younger adolescents (mean 13 years) but did document that ketonuria during camp was related to major life events before camp, particularly in those youngsters with internal locus of control (64).

A study of 53 young adults found that those in poor control had more positive and neutral life events during the previous year, suggesting that even life changes that would be viewed as benign may result in metabolic control difficulties. Interestingly, there was no relationship of negative life events to control. Those in poor control also reported more recent symptoms of depression, anxiety, and hostility than those in moderate or very good control; these symptoms may further impair the ability to adhere to a complex care regimen. As with the younger patients, daily hassles were not disruptive of control (65).

A hypothesis for the effects of stress on diabetes control must include not only the counterregulatory hormonal stimulation induced by the stress, which tends to be more exuberant in diabetes and quite individual (33,35), but also the disruptive effect of stress on critical aspects of adherence to the regimen and on life habits (eating, sleeping). Furthermore, consideration must be given to the possibility that the physiologic effects of poor control (fatigue, decreased performance, headaches) might be stress inducing.

D. Family Stress

No physician experienced with childhood diabetes would deny that the most important factor in success in the management of diabetes is the stability and communication within the family. In the extreme, family conflict, particularly that which remains unresolved, appears to play a critical role in repeated ketoacidosis (31). Children with recurrent ketoacidosis and chronic school absence invariably stop having these problems on admission to residential rehabilitation units (54–56,66,67). Numerous studies have associated poor family circumstances with poor health in children with diabetes (1,2,68–70).

Although the literature does not provide clear evidence about what specific family elements are linked to poor health or adjustment, it is clinically apparent that chaos and lack of emotional support have a devastating effect. Four types of problem family patterns have been identified: (1) overprotective and overanxious; (2) overindulgent and overpermissive; (3) perfectionistic and controlling; and (4) indifferent and rejecting. All these patterns are associated with poor diabetic control and poor psychologic adjustment. The perfectionistic, controlling pattern may result in adequate health for a time, but psychologic problems often surface. In contrast, families with children in good diabetic control are characterized by high-stability, low-stress environments, little interpersonal conflict between the child and the parents, cooperation between the parents, and mothers who are not overwhelmed by anxiety despite strong feelings about the child's diabetes and its management (68,71). Anderson et al. (45) recently emphasized the importance of communication within the family about responsibilities, finding correlation between the levels of such communication and HbA$_{1C}$ levels.

The study of Minuchin and coworkers (31) has highlighted the importance of pathologic family patterns in describing the psychosomatic diabetic patient. The characteristics they have noted are (1) enmeshment to such an extent that individual identities and roles are unclear; (2) overprotectiveness toward all family members; (3) rigidity in maintaining the status quo; and (4) lack of conflict resolution. In these families, the child with diabetes has an important role in helping the family avoid conflict, which inevitably surfaces, leading to emotional and physiologic arousal. Such arousal frequently leads to ketoacidosis.

The classic enmeshed family is only one of the patterns seen in disturbed families of children with diabetes. Nonetheless, the work in Minuchin et al. (31) underscores the problem of inappropriate role differentiation in the problem family patterns. In the overprotective or overindulgent home, the child's role is minimized and is not permitted to develop. In the overcontrolling home, the child's role may be defined, but in a very rigid manner, with no room for independent decision making by the child. The indifferent or rejecting pattern is at the other end of the continuum, with the parents (or often single parent) so uninvolved that the youngster must fend for himself or herself or engage in attention-getting behavior that may be self-destructive. It should be apparent that many families function without overt difficulty despite

these patterns until diabetes develops in the child. The diabetes exerts constant, long-term, time-consuming, and complex demands that only unusually well organized and integrated families can handle in an entirely appropriate fashion (45,71).

IV. TREATMENT

Some of the treatment implications for the diabetes team as a whole are outlined in Table 1, relative to the developmental level and developmental tasks of the various stages of childhood and adolescence. No aspects of management can be excluded from consideration of psychosocial implications; this section reviews education, behavior therapy, family therapy, camping, residential treatment, and psychiatric referral.

A. Education

Learning is a psychologic process, and the educational effort cannot be undertaken without consideration of the context. The few studies that have been carried out on the effectiveness of diabetes education consistently demonstrate the ability to enhance knowledge of children and adolescents, as well as their parents, with a variety of techniques, including a teaching machine (72), using corrective feedback to improve urine glucose testing (73), with an instructional book and game designed for 7–12 year olds (74), and using group family-based problem solving to improve communication and metabolic status in adolescents (75). Age as a proxy for cognitive development level has been demonstrated to be an important factor in knowledge and learning (38,39).

The goal of education is to enhance adherence and improve health status. It is surprising that of 320 articles reviewed in 1981 on the education of chronically ill patients, only 30 were controlled studies that included outcome measures of both adherence and health status. These articles provided little evidence that improved health resulted from the acquisition of knowledge (76). This is consistent with the early observations of Etzwiler and Robb (72) in young patients with diabetes.

There is a growing recognition that educational programs must be individualized, recognizing a variety of contextual factors. At the time of initial diagnosis, training the child and parents to deal with the rudiments of survival (insulin administration, blood testing, and contacting the treatment team) may be all that is appropriate to convey, given the state of mind of the family (see Table 1). On the other hand, to cope with the problems, some families want to know about the physiology, etiology, epidemiology, and natural history of diabetes from the outset. In the absence of a specialized parent-care facility, this may be best accomplished in the least stressful environment, without hospitalization, provided the child does not require intravenous fluid therapy (77).

Another factor in individualization is the variation in signs and symptoms from individual to individual. A goal of education is to teach patients to detect signs of hyper- or hypoglycemia so that they can take appropriate action. As previously noted, studies have failed to demonstrate consistent symptom association with high or low blood glucose levels between patients (24,25). Some patients develop neuroglycopenia without experiencing adrenergic symptoms.

Kirscht (78) has emphasized the importance of the stages of change that determine a person's response to the acquisition of information (contemplation, decision, trial, and maintenance), as well as the personal factors (motive, information-processing capability, and resources) that influence this process. Among the resources are the behavioral repertoire of the person, his or her coping ability, family support, and access to the health care system. Individuals respond depending on how well they understand the regimen, how they interpret its value, their own sense of ability to deal with it, the environmental forces that enhance or reduce the ability to comply, and the barriers to compliance, such as complexity, cost, and convenience.

Associations between knowledge acquired and metabolic control may be difficult to demonstrate, but the critical importance of diabetes education, as previously noted, in the context of a comprehensive program, has been repeatedly demonstrated (54,75,77). Giordano et al. (77) early showed that a comprehensive program involving intensive education, frequent follow-up by telephone for support and during crises, and admission to the hospital of newly diagnosed patients only if intravenous fluids were required or the family was seriously decompensated resulted in a dramatic reduction in initial and recurrent hospitalization. Satin et al. (75) recently described a group family intervention program with problem-solving exercises designed to increase family communication and management skills for their adolescents' diabetes. Metabolic improvement was demonstrable for 6 months following the program.

B. Behavior Therapy

Large studies are not available to determine the effectiveness of behavior therapy in children with diabetes, but there are studies of small populations that indicate that behavioral techniques can modify adherence behavior. Epstein et al. (79) taught parents to use praise and reward points to improve the frequency of urine glucose testing, as well as for good urine glucose test results. Other investigators have demonstrated improvement in behavioral self-management skills in young patients with such systems (80–82). Five shy youngsters were taught to be more effective using modeling and role playing; an in vivo assessment had them respond to a waiter pressuring them to eat ice cream in a restaurant, and all refused the ice cream and explained why (83). Kaplan et al. (84) used social skills training to help adolescents resist negative peer pressure, with a control group simply learning medical facts about diabetes. The experiment group had better diabetes control, determined by HbA$_{1C}$, than the comparison group 4 months after this intervention.

Some of these studies have focused on behavior changes only (79,82), whereas others have looked at behavior and health without finding improvement in health status despite improved behavior (79,81,82). The study by Kaplan et al.

(84) looked at the outcome without assessing differences in behavior between the control and experimental group! Thus, both behavior and health status (control) must be monitored to determine whether specific adherence behaviors are important to glycemic control.

There is little information about relaxation training and biofeedback with stress-related problems in children and adolescents with diabetes. In a study of adolescents using a single-subject multiple-baseline design, relaxation training was associated with improved urinary glucose results for all five female, poorly controlled youngsters. Other measures of diabetic control were not consistently affected, and there was no reduction in stress or anxiety noted by the patients (85). Similar results have been reported in adults (86,87).

C. Family Therapy

The need for intervention by a behavior specialist reflects recognition of the failure of family processes to cope with the diabetes. Under these circumstances, the diabetes is playing a central role in the family's interaction patterns, which must be altered before diabetes management can be successful. The importance of pathologic family patterns as a cause of poorly controlled diabetes has been most effectively demonstrated in the psychosomatic family constellation (31). These original studies evolved from the observation that youngsters, usually girls, with recurrent ketoacidosis cease having problems when admitted to a residential facility, similar to observations that have been made in European residential centers since World War II (67). As noted earlier, in these psychosomatic families the child's illness plays an important role in the family's attempts to avoid conflict and maintain the status quo. Conflict necessarily occurs, however, leading to emotional and physiologic arousal, described as the "turn-on" phase, during which blood glucose and free fatty acid levels rise. In these patients, the return to normal levels of physiologic response, the "turn-off" phase, is limited by the failure of conflict resolution. Thus, the children with diabetes in such a family maintain a level of heightened physiologic response.

In such a family, there is overinvolvement by one parent, usually the mother. This leads to her providing less attention to the siblings and father, resulting in strained marital relationships and sibling hostilities. These resentments cannot be expressed because they might upset the patient and result in ketoacidosis. The parents are able to avoid intimacy and marital conflict by focusing attention on the child's problems. The goal of family therapy in this situation is to identify and change these maladaptive problems, decreasing the family's use of the child's illness as a means of avoiding family conflict.

It is often not recognized that Minuchin and associates (31) studied only seven patients and documented that these youngsters had a more spectacular free fatty acid response to stress, which returned more slowly to normal levels, than their well-adjusted peers with diabetes subjected to the same stressors. Our own experience with many youngsters with severe instability suggests that this type of family constellation, although important, accounts for only a portion of the family pathology that results in scholastic deficits and recurrent ketoacidosis. Other types of family problems, as noted earlier, predominate.

D. Camping

A camping experience can substantially aid the development of independence and self-confidence while teaching important self-care behaviors. The motto of our camp program is, "I can handle it!" Meeting other youngsters with diabetes, identifying with counselors and medical personnel with diabetes, being treated as a healthy active person, and being unable to use diabetes in a manipulative fashion are important parts of the special experience of camp. For the health professional, it is an exceptional opportunity to develop an understanding of the day-to-day problem of living with diabetes and learning to appreciate the amount of courage required of these children. Diabetes camping programs for children and adolescents are now expected to meet American Camping Association standards for the facility and the recreation program, as well as the diabetes supervision. The presence of a psychologist in camp permits the identification and early intervention in problems that may not be recognized by a nonspecialist referring physician.

The camp setting offers an exceptional opportunity for behavioral research, particularly of the effect of the camping experience. McGraw and Travis (88) found a substantial improvement in self-esteem associated with the camping experience but found a similar improvement during the same period among those who did not go to camp. Obviously, children's self-esteem improves during the summer, whether or not they go to camp. Spevack et al. (89) studied adherence in a camp population and found that the improved behaviors recorded during camp were not maintained 3 months after returning home.

Despite the inability to demonstrate long-term effects on diabetes control or psychosocial variables as a result of the camping experience, the role of camp as part of the continuum of care for children with diabetes and support for their families remains unquestioned by all participants. No other setting provides the opportunity for the development of coping mechanisms for youngsters and the unique experience for health professionals and students of day-to-day involvement with a group of youngsters with special health care needs.

E. Residential Rehabilitation

Recurrent hospitalization for ketoacidosis or hypoglycemia, homebound schooling, and frequent school absence with scholastic deficiencies affect a small, but substantial number of youngsters with diabetes. These problems are not caused by an exceptional kind of diabetes but result from pathologic and nonsupportive environments. A survey of physicians caring for children with diabetes indicated a strong need for residential facilities for 5–12% of their patients, an estimate that on a population basis would be comparable to the number of places available per capita for Danish, Dutch, and German children (66).

The European residential centers have long demonstrated the reversal of chronic hospitalization, school absenteeism, and antisocial behavior through these residential programs. When rehabilitation of the family is possible, children can be discharged after several months, but in many instances, rehabilitation of the environment is not possible, and these children remain in the residential center until adulthood (67).

The experience of the European centers emphasizes the factors that are important in successful intervention and its maintenance. Although most residential centers were established and supported by medical personnel, one of the most successful, the Danish home, had been run for 16 years by an educated couple without medical training. During this time there had never been a nurse on the staff, and a physician visited only once a month for a few hours. Nonetheless, episodes of ketoacidosis had been rare among the 115 youngsters who had gone through the home, and only 2 had required psychiatric consultation. Thus, of far greater importance than medical and psychiatric-psychologic supervision was the commitment of dedicated individuals who could provide a stable, structured environment (67).

Our own experience since 1980 with an experimental residential unit is consistent with these observations. Episodes of ketoacidosis virtually cease with admission to the unit, and children who have not attended school for extended periods resume attendance immediately and have fewer absences than those without diabetes. Conversion symptoms, often disabling, are thwarted. These benefits can only be sustained if the family participates in counseling regularly during the residential treatment period and following discharge (56). If not, alternative placement is essential. When these recommendations are not followed by local social service agencies, frequent hospitalization recurs and fatal complications may develop (23). The morbidity and mortality in the population requiring residential rehabilitation is exceptional; most of the premature death and severe complications before age 30 are seen in this group.

V. ASSOCIATED PROBLEMS

A. Psychiatric Problems

In a study of 74 newly diagnosed patients, one-third had reactions that were consistent with a psychiatric disorder, most commonly reactive-depression syndrome. The rest had milder symptoms of sadness, anxiety, a sense of friendlessness, and social withdrawal. Recovery from both the mild and more severe reactions occurred over the first 7–9 months. The more severe reactions occurred in the lower socioeconomic groups and in those families in which there was marital distress (90). Other studies are more or less equally divided between those that found an increased rate of psychiatric disorders and those that did not, as recently reviewed by Blanz et al. (91). They attributed the variability in these studies to wide age ranges and case definition. To correct for this, they examined a narrow age range of 93 IDDM adolescents 17–19 years of age and compared them to a healthy control group without diabetes matched for age-, sex-, and socioeconomic status. They found a threefold increase (33 versus 10%) in psychiatric disorders in the youngsters with diabetes, emphasizing the importance of recognizing that diabetes is a risk factor for psychiatric illness.

Although it is unclear whether psychiatric problems are more common in children with diabetes or in their families, the presence of psychiatric illness has devastating effects on diabetes management. Attempts to identify insulin resistance or cryptic explanations for associated symptoms may serve to forestall the recognition of conversion reactions, obsessive-compulsive behavior resulting in frequent and severe hypoglycemia, eating disorders, severe depression, and suicidal behavior. Of the 80 youngsters who were admitted to the residential rehabilitation unit at the University of Florida during the first decade, 10% required admission to a psychiatric facility and an equivalent number with severe psychiatric problems were seen who needed psychiatric care.

A manifestation of underlying psychiatric illness in adolescents has been the surreptitious administration of insulin, reported in six adolescents aged 12–15 years of age (92). This is the obverse of the destructive and far more common behavior of failing to take insulin (32).

B. Eating Disorders

Eating disorders have been found to be common, affecting 7% of 208 young women with diabetes and associated with a high frequency of early microvascular disease: 4 with anorexia nervosa had acute neuropathy beginning at the same time as the eating disorder (93). The problem of anorexia can also be seen in young men with diabetes, and neuropathy is a frequent concomitant. Although several other studies have confirmed the increased risk of eating disorders (94–96), some studies have not (97,98). Subclinical eating disorders may contribute to disordered diabetes control (99).

In addition to disordered eating behavior adversely affecting diabetes control and long-term prognosis, manipulation of insulin dosage to promote weight loss or avoid weight gain is not uncommon, particularly in young women (96,97,99,100).

C. Child Abuse and Neglect

One of the expressions of increased family stress in children with chronic disease is an increased prevalence of child abuse and neglect in this group, reported to be 15–20%. Although overt physical or sexual abuse is not clearly greater among youngsters with diabetes, neglect certainly has more apparent effects in the child with diabetes, and it appears to be a frequent cause of metabolic instability. In response to the provocative question of whether there is a relationship between insulin-dependent diabetes mellitus and child abuse, Horan et al. (101), although not providing an answer, tabulated family psychosocial variables that have been cited in both the child abuse and diabetes literature. These were family organization, cohesion among family members, marital discord, number of positive child contacts, degree of stress, parental ability to cope with stress, parental feelings

of inadequacy, flexibility and appropriateness of parental expectations for child behavior, tolerance for child deviations from parental control, and inadequacy of disciplinary procedures.

D. Learning Problems

The intellectual function of persons with diabetes has been of concern since the beginning of the insulin era (102). Early studies suggested impaired intellectual capability (102–104). In comparing children with diabetes with their siblings, Ack et al. (105) found no differences when the diabetes began after 5 years of age but found significantly lower intelligence quotients in those with earlier onset. Similar findings have been reported more recently, along with a disproportionate frequency of convulsions, in the younger onset group (106). These findings emphasize the importance of not applying stringent control criteria to the management of the young patient with diabetes.

Psychometric testing of children with diabetes (107) has shown poor performance at normal or somewhat less than normal blood glucose levels. Cognitive functioning in 12 patients was studied during low (60 mg/dl), normal (110 mg/dl), and high (300 mg/dl) blood glucose maintenance with a glucose-controlled insulin infusion system. Performance was impaired and the time required to solve problems increased during hypoglycemia, although reading comprehension was not affected (108). Other aspects of nervous system functioning, such as release of catecholamines and the appearance of autonomic symptoms, have been noted to occur at elevated blood glucose levels. Patients with poorly controlled diabetes or chronic hyperglycemia may have difficulty functioning even before hypoglycemic levels are reached. Cox et al. (109) recently demonstrated that adults with IDDM had impairment in cognitive tasks when blood glucose levels were lowered from 5.4 mmol (97 mg/dl) to 2.6 mmol (47 mg/dl). A motor task was not impaired. There was considerable individual variability in sensitivity to the drop in blood glucose level.

With the contemporary enthusiasm for tighter control of diabetes, heightened by the DCCT (8), the potential for inducing temporary or permanent cerebral dysfunction should not be forgotten. Patients in the DCCT experienced a threefold increase in episodes of severe hypoglycemia.

VI. CONCLUSIONS

Access to a specialized program of care and education for children and adolescents with diabetes, and their families, can no longer be considered a luxury. Just as the sophisticated means of monitoring control and the rapid pace of technical development in diabetes management require access to a specialized program, managing the critical psychosocial aspects requires this access as well. The presence of a professional with specialized training in the emotional and social issues of family interactions and reactions to chronic disease is needed, not only to deal with individual patients but to heighten the sensitivity of other members of the treatment team to the behavioral factors within the family unit that are more influential in day-to-day control than any other aspect of management. Instruments are now available for routine evaluation of family interaction and details of adherence and knowledge, and these must become a routine part of clinical evaluation of the young patient with diabetes (4,45).

The awareness of the pivotal role of psychosocial issues underlies the setting of realistic goals for diabetes management and achieving therapeutic alliance with the child and family. The treatment team must bring psychosocial issues to the forefront early, as part of the educational process, and offer anticipatory guidance as well as crisis intervention. The family routine, organization, and style must be assessed. The family experience with diabetes and attitudes toward it are critical. The parent and child roles within the family must be assessed. The way in which diabetes can affect the family structure must be explored. The treatment team should be sufficiently experienced to recognize problems and intervene early and should be diligent in monitoring relationships and attitudes as they are with blood glucose records and HbA$_{1C}$ measurements!

ACKNOWLEDGMENTS

The author is indebted to the following individuals, who have contributed greatly to the knowledge and perspective in this review and provided editorial commentary and suggestions: Suzanne B. Johnson, Ph.D., Janet H. Silverstein, M.D., Gary Geffken, Ph.D., and Marika Spevack, Ph.D.

REFERENCES

1. Koski ML. The coping process in childhood diabetes. Acta Paediatr Scand Suppl 1969; 198:1–56.
2. Johnson, SB. Psychosocial factors in juvenile diabetes: a review. J Behav Med 1980; 3:95–116.
3. Rubin RR, Peyrot M. Psychosocial problems and interventions in diabetes: a review of the literature. Diabetes Care 1992; 15:1640–1650.
4. Johnson SB. Methodological issues in diabetes research: measuring adherence. Diabetes Care 1992; 15:1658–1665.
5. Travis LB. Workshop on the psychosocial management of diabetes in children and adolescents. Lawson Wilkins Pediatric Endocrine Society 1981 (unpublished).
6. Rosenbloom AL. Primary and subspecialty care of diabetes mellitus in children and youth. Pediatr Clin North Am 1984; 31:107–117.
7. American Diabetes Association. Psychosocial problems: helping patients cope. In: Sperling MA, ed. Physician's Guide to Insulin Dependent (Type I) Diabetes: Diagnosis and Treatment. Alexandria, VA: American Diabetes Association, 1988: 89–102.
8. Diabetes Control and Complications Trial Research Group. The effect of intensive treatment of diabetes on the development and progression of long-term complications in insulin-dependent diabetes mellitus. N Engl J Med 1993; 329: 977–986.
9. Drash AL. The child, the adolescent, and the diabetes control and complications trial. Diabetes Care 1993; 16:1515–1516.
10. Rosenbloom AL. General approach to treatment of adolescents with diabetes. Q Rev Diabetes Assoc Que 1984; 26:31–36.
11. Dunn SM, Turtle JR. The myth of the diabetic personality. Diabetes Care 1981; 4:640–646.
12. Brand AH, Johnson JH, Johnson SB. Life stress and diabetic control in children and adolescents with insulin dependent diabetes. J Pediatr Psychol 1986; 11:481–495.
13. Grossman HY, Brink S, Hauser ST. Self efficacy in adolescent girls and boys and insulin dependent diabetes mellitus. Diabetes Care 1987; 10:324–329.
14. Surwit RS, Scovern AW, Feinglos MN. The role of behavior in diabetes care. Diabetes Care 1982; 5:337–342.
15. Rovet JF, Ehrlich RM, Hoppe M. Behavior problems in children with diabetes as a function of sex and age of onset of disease. J Child Psychol Psychiatry 1987; 28:477–491.
16. Rovet JF, Ehrlich RM. Effect of temperament on metabolic control in children with diabetes mellitus. Diabetes Care 1988; 11:77–82.
17. Fonagy P, Moran GS, Lindsey MKM, Kurtz AB, Brown R. Psychological adjustment and diabetic control. Arch Dis Child 1987; 62:1009–1013.
18. Lane JD, Stabler B, Ross SL, Morris MA, Litton JC, Surwit RS. Psychological predictors of glucose control in patients with IDDM. Diabetes Care 1988; 11:798–800.
19. Ingersoll GM, Orr DP, Herrold AJ, Golden MP. Cognitive maturity and self management among adolescents with insulin dependent diabetes mellitus. J Pediatr 1986; 108:620–623.
20. Follansbee DS. Assuming responsibility for diabetes management: what age? What price? Diabetes Ed 1989; 15:347–352.
21. La Greca AM, Follansbee DS, Skyler JS. Behavioral aspects of diabetes management. Child Health Care 1990; 19:132–139.
22. Johnson SB, Pollak T, Silverstein JH, et al. Cognitive and behavioral knowledge about insulin dependent diabetes among children and parents. Pediatrics 1982; 69:708–713.
23. Rosenbloom AL. Primary and subspecialty care of diabetes mellitus in children and youth. Pediatr Clin North Am 1984; 31:107–117.
24. Cox DJ, Gonder-Frederick L, Pohl S, et al. Symptoms and blood glucose levels in diabetics. JAMA 1985; 253:1558.
25. Freund A, Johnson SB, Rosenbloom AL, Alexander B, Hansen CA. Subjective symptoms, blood glucose estimation, and blood glucose concentrations in adolescents with diabetes. Diabetes Care 1986; 9:236–243.
26. Glasgow RE, McCaul KD, Schafer LC. Self care behaviors and glycemic control in type-I diabetes. J Chron Dis 1987; 40:399–412.
27. Johnson SB, Silverstein JH, Rosenbloom AL, Carter R, Cunningham W. Assessing daily management in childhood diabetes. Health Psychol 1986; 5:545–546.
28. Hanson CL, Cigrang JA, Carle DL, Haddock CK, Henggeler SW. Coping styles in youth with IDDM. Diabetes 1988; 27(Suppl. 1):19A.
29. Alonga M. Perception of severity of disease and health locus of control in compliant and non-compliant diabetic patients. Diabetes Care 1980; 3:533–534.
30. Clarke WL, Snyder AL, Nowacek G. Outpatient pediatric diabetes. 1. Current practices. J Chron Dis 1985; 38:85–90.
31. Minuchin S, Baker L, Rosman BL, Liebman R, Milman L, Todd TC. A conceptual model of psychosomatic illness in children. Arch Gen Psychiatry 1975; 32:1031–1038.
32. Malone JI, Root AW. Plasma free insulin concentrations: keystone to effective management of diabetes mellitus in children. J Pediatr 1981; 99:862–867.
33. Rosenbloom AL, Clarke DW. Excessive insulin treatment and the Somogyi effect. In: Pickup JC, ed. Brittle Diabetes, Oxford: Blackwell 1985:103–131.

34. Schade DS, Duckworth WC. In search of the subcutaneous insulin resistance syndrome. N Engl J Med 1986; 315:147–153.

35. Amiel SA, Simonson DC, Sherwin RS, Lauritano AA, Tamborlane WV. Exaggerated epinephrine responses to hypoglycemia in normal and insulin dependent diabetic children. J Pediatr 1987; 110:832–837.

36. Epstein LH, Coburn PC, Becker B, Drash A, Siminerio L. Measurement and modification of the accuracy of the determinants of urine glucose concentration. Diabetes Care 1980; 3:535–536.

37. Watkins JD, Roberts DE, Williams TF, Martin DA, Coyle V. Observations of medication errors made by diabetic patients in the home. Diabetes 1967; 16:882–885.

38. Harkavy J, Johnson SB, Silverstein JH, Spillar R, McCallum M, Rosenbloom AL. Who learns what at diabetes summer camp? J Pediatr Psychol 1983; 8:143–153.

39. Gilbert BO, Johnson SB, Spillar R, McCallum M, Silverstein JH, Rosenbloom AL. The effects of peer modeling film on children learning to self inject insulin. Behav Ther 1982; 13:186–193.

40. Kohler E, Jurwitz LS, Milan D. A developmentally staged curriculum for teaching self-care to the child with insulin dependent diabetes mellitus. Diabetes Care 1982; 5:300–304.

41. Naughten E, Smith A, Baum JD. At what age do diabetic children give their own injections? Am J Dis Child 1982; 136:690–692.

42. Etzwiler DD, Sines LK. Juvenile diabetes and its management: family, social, and academic implications. JAMA 1962; 181:94–98.

43. Garner A, Thompson C, Partridge J. Who knows best? Diabetes Bull 1969; 45:3–4.

44. Partridge JW, Garner AM, Thompson CW, Cherry T. Attitudes of adolescents toward their diabetes. Am J Dis Child 1972; 124:226–229.

45. Anderson BJ, Auslander WF, Jung KC, Miller JP, Santiago JV. Assessing family sharing of diabetes responsibilities. Diabetes Spectrum 1991; 4:263–268.

46. Caron HS, Roth HP. Patients' cooperation with a medical regimen. JAMA 1968; 203:120–124.

47. Charney E, Bynum R, Eldridge D, Frank D, et al. How well do patients take oral penicillin? A collaborated study in private practice. Pediatrics 1967; 40:188–195.

48. Davis MS. Physiologic, psychological and demographic factors in patient compliance with doctor's orders. Med Care 1968; 6:115–122.

49. Bobrow ES, AvRuskin TW, Siller J. Mother-daughter interaction and adherence to diabetes regimens. Diabetes Care 1985; 8:146–151.

50. Jacobson AM, Jauser ST, Wolfsdorf JI, et al. Psychologic predictors of compliance in children with recent onset of diabetes mellitus. J Pediatr 1987; 110:805–811.

51. Malone JI, Rosenbloom AL, Grgic A, Weber FT. The role of urine sugar in diabetic management. Am J Dis Child 1976; 130:1324–1327.

52. Johnson SM, Freund A, Silverstein J, Hansen CA, Malone J. Adherence-health status relationships in childhood diabetes. Health Psychol 1990; 9:606–631.

53. Hinkle LE, Wolf S. Experimental study of life situations, emotions, and the occurrence of acidosis in a juvenile diabetic. Am J Med Sci 1949; 217:130–135.

54. Johnson SB, Davidson N, Spillar R, Silverstein J. What determines success in a residential treatment center? Diabetes 1982; 31:17A.

55. Buithieu M, Geffken G, Silverstein JH, Johnson SB, Rosenbloom AL. Evaluation of a residential program for youngsters with insulin dependent diabetes mellitus (IDDM). Diabetes 1987; 36:19A.

56. Geffken GR, Lewis C, Johnson SB, Silverstein JH, Rosenbloom AL. Residential treatment for youngsters with difficult to manage insulin dependent diabetes mellitus: an evaluation of 52 patients. J Pediatr Endocrinol (in press).

57. Kemmer F, Bisping R, Steingruber H, et al. Psychological stress and metabolic control in patients with type I diabetes mellitus. N Engl J Med 1986; 314:1078–1084.

58. Gilbert BO, Johnson SB, Silverstein J, Malone J. Psychological and physiological responses to acute laboratory stressors in insulin-dependent diabetes mellitus adolescents and nondiabetic controls. J Pediatr Psychol 1989; 14:577–591.

59. Stabler B, Surwit S, Lane JD, Morris MA, Litton J, Feinglos MN. Type A behavior pattern in blood glucose control in diabetic children. Psychosom Med 1987; 49:313–316.

60. Stabler B, Lane JD, Ross S, Morris MA, Litton J, Surwit RS. Type A behavior pattern and chronic glycemic control in individuals with IDDM. Diabetes Care 1988; 11:361–362.

61. Weil WB, Sussman MB, Cain AJ. Social patterns and diabetic glucosuria. Am J Dis Child 1967; 113:454–460.

62. Bedell JR, Giordani B, Amour JL, Tavormina J, Boll T. Life stress and the psychological and medical adjustment of chronically ill children. J Psychosom Res 1977; 21:237–242.

63. Chase HP, Jackson GG. Stress and sugar control in children with insulin dependent diabetes mellitus. J Pediatr 1981; 98:1011–1013.

64. Hanson SL, Pichert JW. Perceived stress and diabetes control in adolescents. Health Psychol 1986; 5:439–452.

65. Karlsson JA, Holmes CS, Lang R. Psychosocial aspects of disease duration and control in young adults with type I diabetes. J Clin Epidemiol 1988; 41:535–540.

66. Rosenbloom AL. Need for residential treatment for children with diabetes mellitus. Diabetes Care 1982; 5:545–546.

67. Rosenbloom AL. Residential treatment centers in Europe for children and youth with diabetes mellitus. Clin Pediatr (Phila) 1983; 22:760–763.

68. Anderson B, Auslander W. Research on diabetes management in the family: a critique. Diabetes Care 1980; 3:671–696.

69. Anderson B, Miller J, Auslander W, Santiago J. Family characteristics of diabetic adolescents: relationship to metabolic control. Diabetes Care 1981; 4:586–594.

70. Gaff A, Smith M, Baum J. Emotional behavior and educational disorders in diabetic children. Arch Dis Child 1980; 55:371–375.

71. Johnson SB, Rosenbloom AL. Behavioral aspects of diabetes mellitus in childhood and adolescence. Psychiatric Clin North Am 1982; 5:357–369.

72. Etzwiler DD, Robb JR. Evaluation of programmed education among juvenile diabetics and their families. Diabetes 1972; 21:967–971.

73. Epstein LH, Figueroa J, Farkas GM, Beck S. The short-term effects of feedback on accuracy of urine glucose determinations in insulin dependent diabetic children. Behav Ther 1981; 12:560–564.

74. Heston JV, Lazar SJ. Evaluating a learning device for juvenile diabetic children. Diabetic Care 1980; 3:668–671.

75. Satin WS, La Greca AM, Zigo M, Skyler JS. Diabetes in adolescence: effects of multifamily group intervention and parent simulation of diabetes. J Pediatr Psychol 1989; 14:259–275.

76. Mazzura SA. Does patient education in chronic disease have therapeutic value? J Chron Dis 1982; 35:521–529.

77. Giordano B, Rosenbloom AL, Heller DR, Weber FT, Gonzales R, Grgic A. Regional services for children and youth with diabetes. Pediatrics 1977; 60:492–498.

78. Kirscht J. Promoting adherence to clinical management strategies. Symposium: New horizons for clinical management. Am Diabetes Assoc Annu Meeting, New Orleans, June 13, 1988.

79. Epstein LH, Beck S, Figueroa J, et al. The effects of targeting improvements in urine glucose on metabolic control in children with insulin dependent diabetes. J Appl Behav Anal 1981; 14:365–375.

80. Gross AM. Self-management training and medication compliance in children with diabetes. Child Fam Behav Ther 1982; 4:47–55.

81. Carney RM, Schechter K, Davis T. Improving adherence to blood glucose testing in insulin dependent diabetic children. Behav Ther 1983; 14:247–254.

82. Schafer LC, Glasgow RE, McCaul KD. Increasing adherence of diabetic adolescents. J Behav Med 1982; 5:353–363.

83. Gross AM, Johnson WG, Wildman HE, Mullet J. Coping skills training with insulin dependent pre-adolescent diabetics. Child Behav Ther 1981; 3:141–153.

84. Kaplan RM, Chadwick MW, Schimmel LE. Social learning intervention to promote metabolic control in type I diabetes mellitus: pilot experiment results. Diabetes Care 1985; 8:152–155.

85. Rose MI, Firestone P, Heick HMC, Faught AK. The effects of anxiety management training on the control of juvenile diabetes mellitus. J Behav Med 1983; 6:381–395.

86. Lammers CA, Naliboff BD, Straatmeyer AJ. The effects of progressive relaxation on stress and diabetic control. Behav Res Ther 1984; 22:641–650.

87. Feinglos MN, Hastedt P, Surwit RS. Effects of relaxation therapy on patients with type I diabetes mellitus. Diabetes Care 1987; 10:72–75.

88. McGraw RK, Travis LB. Psychological effects of a special summer camp on juvenile diabetics. Diabetes 1973. 22:275–278.

89. Spevack M, Johnson SB, Silverstein J. The effect of diabetes summer camp on patient adherence, glycemic control, and physician behavior. Diabetes 1988; 37:125A.

90. Kovacs M, Fineberg TL, Paulauskas S, Finkelstein R, Pollock N, Crouse-Novack M. Initial coping responses and psychosocial characteristics of children with insulin dependent diabetes mellitus. J Pediatr 1985; 106:827–834.

91. Blanz BJ, Rensch-Riemann BS, Fritz-Sigmund DI, Schmidt MH. IDDM is a risk factor for adolescent psychiatric disorders. Diabetes Care 1993; 16:1579–1587.

92. Orr DP, Eccles T, Lawlor R, Golden M. Surreptitious insulin administration in adolescents with insulin dependent diabetes mellitus. JAMA 1986; 256:3227–3230.

93. Steel JM, Young RJ, Lloyd GG, Clarke BF. Clinically apparent eating disorders in young diabetic women: associations with painful neuropathy and other complications. BMJ 1987; 294:859–862.

94. Rodin GM, Johnson LE, Garfinkel PE, Daneman D, Kenshole AB. Eating disorders in female adolescents with insulin dependent diabetes mellitus. Int J Psychiatry Med 1986; 16:49–57.

95. Rosmark B, Berne C, Holmgren S, Lago C, Renholm G, Sohlberg S. Eating disorders in patients with insulin-dependent diabetes mellitus. J Clin Psychiatry 1986; 47:547–550.

96. Stancin T, Link DL, Reuter JM. Binge eating and purging in young women with IDDM. Diabetes Care 1989; 12:601–603.

97. Birk R, Spencer ML. The prevalence of anorexia nervosa, bulimia, and induced glycosuria in IDDM females. Diabetes Ed 1989; 15:336–341.

98. Fairburn CG, Peveler RC, Davies B, Mann JI, Mayou RA. Eating disorders in young adults with insulin dependent diabetes mellitus: a controlled study. BMJ 1991; 303:17–20.

99. Wing RR, Norwalk MP, Marcus MD, Koeske R, Finegold D. Subclinical eating disorders and glycemic control in adolescents with type I diabetes. Diabetes Care 1986; 9:162–167.

100. La Greca A, Schwarz L, Satin W, Rafkin-Mervis L, Enfield G, Goldberg R. Binge eating among women with IDDM: associations with weight dissatisfaction, adherence and metabolic control. Diabetes 1990; 39:164A.

101. Horan PF, Gwynn C, Renzi D. Insulin dependent diabetes mellitus and child abuse. Is there a relationship? Diabetes Care 1986; 9:302–307.

102. Miles P, Root HF. Psychologic tests applied to diabetic patients. Arch Intern Med 1922; 30:767–777.

103. Tegarden FM. The intelligence of diabetic children with some case reports. J Appl Psychol 1939; 23:337–346.

104. Dashiell JF. Variations in psychomotor efficiency in a diabetic with changes in blood sugar level. J Comp Psychol 1930; 10:189–197.

105. Ack M, Miller I, Weil WB. Intelligence of children with diabetes mellitus. Pediatrics 1961; 28:764–770.

106. Rovet JF, Ehrlich RM, Hopp M. Intellectual deficits associated with early onset of insulin dependent diabetes mellitus in children. Diabetes Care 1987; 10:510–515.

107. Flender J, Lifshitz F. The effects of fluctuations on blood glucose levels on the psychological performance of juvenile diabetics. Diabetes 1975; 25:334.

108. Holmes C, Hayford J, Gonzalez J, Weydert J. A survey of cognitive functioning at different glucose levels in diabetic persons. Diabetes Care 1983; 6:180–185.

109. Cox DJ, Gonder-Frederick LA, Schroeder DB, Cryer PE, Clarke WL. Disruptive effects of acute hypoglycemia on speed of cognitive and motor performance. Diabetes Care 1993; 16:1391–1393.

46
Diabetes Education

Bridget F. Recker

Maimonides Medical Center, Brooklyn, New York

I. INTRODUCTION

Insulin-dependent diabetes mellitus (IDDM) is a serious and complex chronic disease. Children with diabetes as well as their parent(s) need ongoing educational and emotional support from those with the knowlege to provide it. In the past year, those involved in delivering health care services to children with diabetes and their families have had their beliefs validated regarding the beneficial effects of normalizing blood glucose levels and the therapeutic relationship necessary to reach this goal.

The validation of the benefits of improved blood glucose control came from the data of the Diabetes Control and Complications Trial (DCCT) published in 1993. The DCCT was a multicenter, randomized clinical trial designed to study the relationship between blood glucose control and the known complications of IDDM (Chapter 40). The data of the DCCT demonstrated that careful control of blood glucose levels approaching euglycemia effectively delayed the onset and slowed the progression of diabetic retinopathy, nephropathy, and neuropathy in IDDM (1).

The data from the DCCT group showed a 76% reduction in the adjusted mean risk for the development of retinopathy in the intensive-therapy group compared to those receiving conventional therapy. Individuals beginning the study with mild retinopathy experienced delayed advancement of this complication by 54%, with a 47% reduction in the development of proliferative or severe nonproliferative retinopathy (1). A consequence of intensive blood glucose control was a reduction in the amount of microalbuminuria and albuminuria. Decreased occurrence of clinical neuropathy was also found. These beneficial findings were not influenced by age, sex, or duration of IDDM.

Diabetes educators have long known that maintenance of blood glucose levels within the normal range is a reasonable goal in the management of IDDM. Yet, the categorical benefit to the individual with IDDM remained elusive until now. The

treatment group that received intensive management of diabetes approached IDDM's major goals, including normalization of blood glucose concentrations and normalization of glycated hemoglobin levels.

The American Diabetes Association's (ADA) position statement on the implications of the DCCT (2) stated the primary treatment goal in IDDM should be the achievement of blood glucose levels equaling those of the intensively treated group in the DCCT. These recommendations may also apply to individuals with non-insulin-dependent diabetes mellitus, although this group was not studied. No single method of controlling blood glucose or insulin management regimen was recommended by the ADA.

What, then, is the down side of the DCCT findings? Mainly, the increased incidence of severe hypoglycemia and weight gain experienced by the intensively managed group were the significant fallbacks. There were three times as many episodes of severe hypoglycemia in the intensely treated group. Severe hypoglycemic episodes occurred mainly during sleep (55% of total number of episodes). Forty-three percent of these episodes occurred between midnight and 8:00 A.M. The events that occurred during the day, amounting to 36% of all events, were infrequently accompanied by any warning signs (3). The risk of severe hypoglycemic events occurring in young children is greater because their life-style and nutritional intakes are less predictable (2). Long-term consequences of multiple episodes of severe hypoglycemia are not well described in the literature, but the development of seizures and neuropsychological sequelae have been reported. An alarming concern noted by the DCCT group was the consequence of hypoglycemia while driving an automobile (1). Three fatalities were reported with hypoglycemia possibly having a causative role. This finding was not linked specifically to the intensively managed group.

The development of weight gain in this group was also a concern. Those individuals receiving intensive management averaged a mean weight gain of 4.7 kg at 5 years. This weight

665

gain was not experienced by those in the conventional treatment group (1). The balancing of insulin needs, weight gain, and caloric intake must be continuously addressed for individuals choosing intensive management.

Another drawback was the personal effort of the patients as well as the size and commitment of the health care team needed to reach the goals for control of the disease attained by the intensively treated group of the DCCT. The study highlighted the significant increase in effort required to achieve a degree of euglycemia. Maintaining a continual state of intensively managed IDDM requires a phenomenal amount of commitment, time, and effort. "Effort" in this case is a global term that fails to define the cumulative efforts on the part of the individual, the family, and all members of the health care team. The health care team of the DCCT included diabetologists, nurses, nutritionists, behavioral specialists, and various medical subspecialists and their staff. If this is the amount of effort and resources necessary for adults involved in intensive insulin management, how much more time and effort are necessary to achieve these goals in children?

II. RISK VERSUS BENEFIT VERSUS COST

The cost of delivering the necessary health care support to achieve the degree of control of the patients included in the DCCT is immense. Before we can deliver the necessary services, educated professional personnel must be trained and available to meet the needs of individuals attempting to achieve intensive control of IDDM. Intensively treated individuals require a greater number of health care services and health care professionals. It is hoped that the promise of a healthier population of individuals with IDDM leading more productive lives due to the absence of debilitating complications will offset this cost.

However, the availability of these services for IDDM patients seems remote with our current state of managed care. In the managed-care environment, limited referrals to endocrinologists who are not the individual's primary care physicians will be covered by most health care insurance packages. Rarely will these referrals include or reimburse for other consultative services or involvement by the members of the diabetes care team needed to achieve the goals of diabetes management. The cost of intensive therapy therefore becomes an out-of-pocket expense. Thus, most patients with IDDM may actually be managed under a conventional treatment protocol with its now well-documented consequences and increased long-term health care costs.

Dr. A. Drash (4) proposed interesting recommendations for the implementation of intensive management of IDDM. Included are the development of regional centers of excellence for diabetes, expanded training programs for professional diabetes specialists, and implementation of programs for education and training of local community physicians currently caring for individuals with diabetes. Furthermore, all individuals with IDDM should have access to a multidisciplinary, highly skilled therapeutic team regardless of the health care system implemented in this country!

What was the cost of the DCCT? The overall cost of the trial was $165 million (5). The study lasted 9 years and included 1441 volunteers. There were 35,280 clinic visits in total by the study participants. Therefore, the study cost an average of $467 per clinic visit. Included in the costs are necessary laboratory studies, kidney function studies, nerve conduction studies, psychological tests, and retinal evaluations. Hypothetically, based on the DCCT findings, if one million people with IDDM managed to achieve the level of control accomplished by the intensively treated group in the DCCT, one-third fewer people would have sustained progression in retinopathy, only 12% would need laser therapy to prevent vision loss, and approximately 4% of these individuals would have specific signs of kidney disease (5).

Where do primary care and managed health care fit in this picture of intensive diabetes management? The publication of the findings of the DCCT placed physicians, nurses, nutritionists, and mental health professionals under a moral obligation to convince their patients of the importance of intensive management of IDDM. These professionals are also under an obligation to convince health-care payors that intensive treatment is necessary and, in fact, mandatory (6). Does the primary care physician have the skills and educational and experiential background as well as the supportive staff required to meet the needs of intensive-management regimes for individuals with IDDM?

Intensive management in IDDM does not mean providing more insulin or giving more shots. It means managing the interplay among insulin and diet, exercise, and self-monitoring requirements, as well as life's joys and stressors. If primary-care physicians must assume the responsibility for patients with IDDM, they must also attempt to meet the goals of glucose control as cited in the ADA's position statement. However, is it reasonable to assume or even expect a primary-care physician to address intensive management of IDDM alone? Realistically, the answer must be no. The physician responsible for the primary-care needs of many families will need to become part of a network that has the resources at its disposal to meet the needs of individuals with IDDM. The most likely network would include an endocrinologist and a diabetes treatment/education center. In our current managed-care environment, physicians should refrain from participating in turf wars and remember we are working for the benefit of the patients and not of the insurance companies. Let the patient and the family work alongside the physician/health care team to advocate for the necessary health care and educational services delineated by the DCCT. Patients can be referred to several lay articles that may clarify the findings and commitment essential to intensify management of IDDM. The local ADA office can help patients find such articles, which include a special report published by the ADA in 1993 (7) as well as many others.

III. DIABETES EDUCATION

Mastering the skills necessary to manage IDDM in the 21st century will, it is hoped, influence the overall health of children with IDDM and lead to the development of healthy life-style patterns that will be carried into adulthood. Educating children with IDDM and their parents is a necessary and multifaceted task. Often, in the enthusiasm to provide information, too much is given too soon. The diabetes care team may not always recognize the limits of some families or their ability to assimilate knowledge during the initial stages. This is particularly important when managed-care restrictions allow only for an initial encounter with a child with IDDM. The diabetes care team may feel they have only one chance, a brief time interval, in which to impart all the vital information families and individuals with IDDM need. A young patient related that she learned the real meaning of IDDM during her hospital stay when she was first diagnosed. A well-meaning staff member simplified the meaning of diabetes complications by summarizing that diabetes is like dying from the inside out. Years later repeated attempts to achieve improved blood glucose control were unsuccessful. Eventually, the patient informed us that no matter how healthy we make her outside, we are not making her any healthier inside. The initial encounter is key!

Certain facts and techniques must be learned by children with IDDM and their families. Today, education for children with IDDM and their parents must address all facets of available diabetes information. The major role in education is to interact with the children/families with IDDM so that learning is optimized.

The phases of diabetes education include survival education, self-management, and continuing education. Each phase addresses the changing needs of the child with IDDM over time. There is no specific time frame enabling the diabetes care team to determine the beginning of one phase and the end of another. Since age and duration of IDDM are not equated with knowledge, children may remain in the survival education phase until they reach adulthood. Assessments of each individual child with IDDM and the parent(s) must be made to direct the child/family into the proper care and educational setting. Intelligence and common sense should not be taken for granted during educational goal setting and delivery. Not all people learn at the same rate and not all people will think what the diabetes team members are saying is important to them. Therefore, all available resources, including assessment tools, must be utilized to meet the educational and emotional needs of each family.

A. Survival Education

Initially, survival education is provided once the diagnosis of IDDM has been established in a child (1). The education furnished during this period is critical! It can have a major impact on the future course of the patient's life, including how he/she will handle or accept the diagnosis.

At the time of diagnosis, the child and the family are under great emotional stress. They are overwhelmed by the diagnosis of IDDM. They often feel guilty, helpless, and inadequate. All of the stressors experienced by the family will influence their ability to integrate information and learn. These factors must be taken into account when providing

survival education. Survival education is the foundation for future learning.

Survival education should be clear, concise, and adapted to the patient's and family's needs. It includes the basic knowledge needed primarily by children with new-onset IDDM and their parent(s) to manage safely at home. Topics such as honeymoon phase, Somogyi effect, and sick-day rules, along with many other issues, should not be addressed during this period, unless specifically indicated.

The goals of survival education are simple and mainly technical. The diabetes care team must ensure that the child with IDDM and/or the parent(s):

1. Can demonstrate appropriate skill in the preparation and administration of both single-insulin and mixed-insulin doses.
2. Are able to demonstrate the appropriate technique for obtaining fingerstick blood glucose samples for testing.
3. Can successfully monitor urine for the presence of glucose and ketone.
4. Understand the action and duration of the insulins being given.
5. Understand the signs and symptoms of hypoglycemia, the ways to prevent its occurrence, and the actions to take when it does occur, including (8):
   a. Mild hypoglycemia (treated by self): beverage and snack.
   b. Moderate hypoglycemia (may need assistance): beverage, glucose tablet or gel, followed by a drink and snack.
   c. Severe hypoglycemia (needs assistance): glucagon given by intramuscular injection—for children under 3 years of age 0.5 mg, and for older children 1.0 mg.
7. Understand the signs and symptoms of hyperglycemia, the ways to prevent its occurrence, and actions to take when it does occur.
8. Understand that ketones are not normally found in urine, and that they are, at first, an indicator to contact the diabetes care team for further guidance.
9. Recognize the need to maintain contact with the diabetes care team for insulin adjustments.
10. Are prepared to seek further education from appropriately trained personnel in order to maintain good health.

If the foregoing skills and information can be taught and opportunities presented in a way that will enable the care team to assess the parents' and the child's ability to demonstrate these skills, survival education will have been successful.

B. Self-Management

Self-management education for children with IDDM and their parents should be geared to those who have mastered survival education. This single phase of education takes years. For many, this phase never ends. The goals are to increasse knowledge about diabetes, improve or introduce new skills, and master the adaptation of diabetes into individual healthy life-styles. It is obvious why this phase of education can last for extended periods. As children grow physiologically and mature emotionally, their needs change. For a child with IDDM these natural changes lead to changes in the management regimen. From a child's viewpoint, self-management education provides opportunities for continued learning about diabetes. Inherent in this knowledge is the opportunity to establish independence from their parents and develop self-care patterns that will be carried into adult life. This is the phase of education most affected by the results of the DCCT.

Self-management education is also the most labor-intensive phase. As children with IDDM and their parent(s) attempt to achieve normalization of blood glucose levels, the need for supportive services grows. These individuals need ongoing group and individual educational sessions in order to learn more about living with diabetes, incorporate new knowledge, and maintain a healthy life-style. Additionally, urgent situational episodes will also require the time and effort of the diabetes health care team members.

The goal of self-management education is to allow the children with IDDM and their families to become self-sufficient in the daily management of diabetes as they work along with the health care team to approach normalization of blood glucose levels and glycated hemoglobin. The educator/health care team needs to address such topics as:

1. Review and discussion of survival education basics.
2. Interplay of exercise, diet, meal timing, and insulin dose on blood glucose control.
3. Achieving euglycemia by presenting information to assist in the avoidance of hypoglycemia and hyperglycemia.
4. Discussion of treatment options including conventional, multiple injections of insulin, and continuous-infusion insulin modalities.
5. Home treatment of intercurrent illness to prevent ketoacidosis and subsequent hospital admissions.
6. Pathophysiology of diabetes, its management, and its treatment.
7. Possible influence of the Somogyi effect, honeymoon phase, or dawn phenomenon and the role of emotions on blood glucose.
8. Preventive health care behaviors, including primary care, foot care, personal hygiene, insulin injection site rotation, and diabetes care team follow-up.
9. Updates on attempts to achieve euglycemia and its impact on preventing or delaying complications.
10. The transfer of control from the parents to the child with IDDM without sacrificing glycemic control (may use developmental guidelines to approximate the timing of certain diabetes age-related tasks).
11. Psychosocial issues, such as living and coping with a chronic illness, adapting diabetes to the child's life-style, school and time schedule problems, traveling, parties, camps, sports, dining out, alcohol, and substance abuse.

Self-management education provides children with IDDM and their parent(s) advanced knowledge that, it is hoped, will enable them to establish a life-style that is free from the day-to-day stressors and problems that are a consequence of having a chronic disease such as diabetes.

C. Continuing Education

Continuing education is a form in which the interaction between people with diabetes and society is explored. These sessions are usually presented in the form of seminars, health education days, and programs sponsored by the ADA or other interest groups. They provide children with IDDM and their families an opportunity to learn about advances being made in the field of diabetes. This ongoing process consists of the presentation of current information, trends, and research by experts in the field of diabetes and related fields. Continuing education serves as a tool designed to maintain interest, provide for the exchange of information, and renew commitment to the care of diabetes after children with IDDM or their families feel they have learned all they need to learn.

This phase of education addresses group rather than individual needs. Such education can help people involved with diabetes focus on the disease and related issues, including treatment options, life issues, and research findings, that may influence how diabetes is managed. As the child with IDDM reaches adulthood, his/her needs and concerns change; therefore, the knowledge sought changes. Continuing education does not supersede self-management education, rather it enhances it and exposes those concerned to new and varied avenues of learning.

IV. INSULIN ADMINISTRATION

Once the diagnosis of IDDM has been made, the children and their families must accept the task of daily insulin administration. This responsibility should not rest solely on one family member. Both parents, if possible, should become skilled in insulin administration, as should the child once he/she is felt to be psychologically mature.

Educators must listen carefully to the family's feelings and fears about needles and injections. The task of maintaining sterile techniques is relatively simple compared with that of injecting a needle into oneself or one's child. Because needles and syringes are often seen as being in the domain of physicians and nurses, children and parents may have phobias or fears about their use.

The behaviors and concerns surrounding insulin administration need to be assessed by educators, and possible solutions to some common problems should be offered. Problems such as hesitation before skin puncture with an insulin syringe needle or lengthy periods between insulin dose preparation and administration could signal trouble.

If a child with IDDM and the parent(s) demonstrate ease and skill during insulin administration, they should be encouraged to continue this regimen. Nevertheless, insulin administration can become an overwhelming task for some children, and there are devices available that can be of use to them to make the daily regime of insulin administration less stressful. Injection aid devices may help children and parents who are afraid of needles and syringes. They can also be used to promote independence of children who are developmentally ready to inject their own insulin. If the issues surrounding insulin injections are more problematic than the solutions afforded by these devices, further investigation is warranted.

V. GLUCOSE MONITORING

A. Finger Sampling for Blood Glucose

Parents and children with IDDM should be encouraged to try different lancet devices during the initial onset of IDDM. For many reasons, a certain lancet or lancet device will be seen as less painful, easier to handle, or more acceptable to the child with IDDM or the parents. The different devices permit control over speed and depth of lancet penetration for blood glucose sampling. The child with IDDM and the parents may be less resistant to obtaining blood glucose samples if they are comfortable with the device and see it as making their lives or their child's life easier. If the procedure is seen as painful or uncomfortable, frequent fingerstick sampling and normalization of blood glucose levels will eventually suffer.

This is extremely important in young children with IDDM for whom the parent(s) is solely responsible for obtaining blood glucose samples. These children frequently resist the procedure, increasing the parent's anxiety and guilt, often leading to unhealthy patterns of behavior between the pair. Using a lancet device usually leads to obtaining an adequate sample of blood. Gadgets do not improve compliance or metabolic control of IDDM, but they can alleviate some stressors that these families face.

B. Blood Glucose Meters

Many meters are available on the market today. Many offer memory systems, printouts of results, averaging the results in the meter, the ability to mark unusual circumstances, dating of results, and timing of results. All offer acceptable reliability and accuracy of readings. Their different features may influence the educator's "favorite" or choice of meter recommended to the child with IDDM or the family. The development of managed-care plans has also influenced the choice of blood glucose meters. If the primary-care physician orders a meter, the glucose meter purchased by the family may be different than the one most suitable. Managed-care companies have contracted with certain suppliers, and this may supersede the physician's recommendation for a specific meter. The choice of meter given to a patient therefore becomes one of expediency rather than the result of a clinical, informed decision-making process. Education of families and primary-care physicians is necessary in these situations.

VI. CONCLUSION

IDDM is one of the most common chronic diseases that can affect a child. Today, there is no cure for diabetes; therefore, managing diabetes as meticulously as possible is the only way to assure that a child will grow and develop into a physically and psychologically healthy and happy person. Unlike other chronic diseases in childhood, the management of diabetes requires daily therapeutic decisions on the part of children with IDDM and/or their parents. Thus, the educational process becomes fundamental, not only for immediate survival but for incorporating diabetes management into a healthy life-style as well.

REFERENCES

1. Diabetes Control and Complications Trial Research Group. The effect of intensive treatment of diabetes on the development and progression of long-term complications in insulin-dependent diabetes mellitus. N Engl J Med 1993; 329: 977–86.
2. American Diabetes Association. Position statement on the implications of the Diabetes Control and Complications Trial. Diabetes 1993; 42:1555–1558.
3. Diabetes Control and Complications Trial Research Group. Epidemiology of severe hypoglycemia in the diabetes control and complications trial. Am J Med 1991; 90(4):450.
4. Drash AL. The child, the adolescent, and the Diabetes Control and Complications Trial. Diabetes Care 1993; 16(11):1515–1516.
5. McCarren M. And . . . it works: intensive therapy reduces the risk of diabetic eye, kidney, and nerve disease. Diabetes Forecast 1993; 46(9):49–51.
6. Dawson LY. DCCT and primary care: prescription for change. Clin Diabetes 1993; 11(4):88.
7. American Diabetes Association. DCCT: what it means to you. Diabetes Forecast Special Report, 1993.
8. Havlin C, Cryer P. Hypoglycemia: the limiting factor in the management of insulin-dependent diabetes mellitus. Diabetes Educ 1988; 14:408.

47

Diabetes Camping and Youth Support Programs

Stuart J. Brink
Newton Wellesley Hospital, Newton, and New England Diabetes and Endocrinology Center (NEDEC), Chestnut Hill, Massachusetts

As progressive urbanization of American society began, many became convinced of the value of the outdoor experience in the overall maturation process of the child. Not only did camping provide continued exposure to the out-of-doors, but also to the dynamics of group living. The camping experience is, by design, enjoyable as well as educational. The mere progress of daily life within a cabin group provides valuable lessons in interpersonal relationships. The activities of the camping program require group cooperation while fostering self-reliance and independence. It is the object of organized camping to set forth those values of living held as important to society: independence, self-reliance, sharing, democratic living within a group, and leadership training (1).

I. INTRODUCTION

Pediatric and adolescent insulin-dependent diabetes mellitus (IDDM) is unique among chronic medical conditions in that it requires ongoing behavior changes involving food, snacks, and activity, coupled with glucose monitoring, insulin injections, and the always present risk of hypoglycemia. There is no other illness so dependent upon what the child or adolescent does day in and day out, hour by hour, than diabetes. In many chronic illnesses, taking one's medications, visiting one's health care team, and hoping that the medications and treatment regimens work are what is required; not so for diabetes mellitus. Lifestyle changes in the family and for the patient are paramount for successful management (2). The complexities of chronic illness and psychosocial functioning were studied by Orr et al., who suggested that overall good psychosocial functioning occurs in such illnesses as IDDM (3). Nevertheless, what is now called self-management places enormous demands upon the child, teen, and family (4,5).

Camping and youth support programs were designed to help improve living with diabetes.

II. HISTORY OF DIABETES CAMPING

The recognition of how camping might offer opportunities to enhance self-image and serve as a respite from the rigors of such care began soon after insulin became available for the treatment of IDDM. Diabetes camping in the United States started when Dr. Leonard Wendt established the first such program in Detroit in 1925 (6). In that same summer, Elizabeth Devine, a nurse working with Drs. Eliot Joslin and Priscilla White in Boston, took one child to her summer home in Ogonquit, Maine. In 1929, Camp Ho-Mita-Koda was established by Dr. Henry John near Cleveland. In 1932, the Clara Barton Camp for Girls with Diabetes was founded in cooperation with the Universalist Church and the Joslin Clinic in Massachusetts. In 1938, Dr. Mary Olney in California set up the first "wilderness" diabetes camping program.

These four camping programs have been the forerunners of the diabetes camping experience in the United States for more than 65 years, a camping experience that now includes not only summer residential camping in cabins, tents, and "the wilderness" but also day camps, winter camps, and weekend retreats. Such endeavors involve not only the child or adolescent with diabetes but also parents, siblings, grandparents, and friends without diabetes. Bicycle touring, skiing, whitewater rafting, and wilderness backpacking diabetes programs have all taken place in recent years. In many countries around the world, diabetes associations and diabetes clinics work together to run such camping programs. Several have become international in scope, utilizing the terrific resources and support of the International Lions Clubs to gather youngsters with diabetes from different countries to live in the host country, travel with others who have diabetes, and then spend some time in a camp environment as well. Dr. Johnny Ludvigsson in Sweden has helped originate such programs in Sweden in cooperation with many others (including those cosponsored by members of ISPAD, the International Society for Pediatric and Adolescent Diabetes, formerly ISGD, the International Study Group).

The reasons for youngsters with diabetes to participate in a camping experience involve all of what Dr. Sam Wentworth wrote (as quoted in the opening extract in this chapter) but also include the need to provide respite for parents. Youngsters are provided respite from being so different from their friends and relatives. The daily demands of diabetes home management are fraught with guilt over not being able to meet such demands or with anger for even having to try. Camps for children and teenagers with diabetes allow the entire family to take a break from these demands and, at the same time, allow parents and other family members to know that the child is in a safe environment supervised by staff knowledgeble in managing the illness itself. Children and teenagers at camp frequently develop friendships that transcend the few days or weeks when they live together at camp and share the common bond of having diabetes (7).

Even though diabetes is the most common of all endocrine disorders and the third most common chronic medical condition in pediatric and adolescent medicine, the youngster with diabetes is likely to be the only one in his or her community with diabetes. Most "nondiabetic" camps have not been able to respond adequately to the health needs of the youngster with diabetes, and so children with diabetes were often excluded from the camping experience. Because there were no adequately trained health personnel at such "regular" camps and the fears of the nurses and occasionally doctors in residence—as well as the program staff—at "regular" camps often made the experience of caring for a camper with diabetes [and other chronic medical conditions (8,9), such as asthma, epilepsy, cancer (10), orthopedic problems, and cerebral palsy] frightening, youth with diabetes were often excluded from going to camp. Because not only dealing with the (likely) possibility of exercise-related hypoglycemia and intermittent hyperglycemia but also adjusting insulin and making sure food and snacks were appropriate and not delayed meant added responsibilities, camp owners as well as their staff rejected campers with diabetes.

Camps for children and teenagers with diabetes are not merely places to have fun but also places to deal with the overwhelming loneliness of an illness like diabetes (11). Many youngsters remain acutely embarrassed at having to take insulin injections, eat in a different fashion, or test urine or blood. Having diabetes makes one feel more isolated and more different from one's peers during a period in life when being similar is an important developmental task; most youngsters do not know others their own age with diabetes— unti they go to camp! Camping experiences offer these same children an opportunity to be included with peers. Diabetes becomes inclusionary rather than exclusionary in its day-to-day triumphs, when "something goes right" and even when "mistakes" occur and are shared with others. Listening to others describe their own frustrations with our still inadequate

treatment regimens makes it possible for youngsters with diabetes to return home and have a better attitude about their own treatment plan and its own ups and downs (12). Group support remains one of the most valuable aspects of diabetes camping (13).

III. EDUCATIONAL EXPERIENCES

Education at camp occurs in formal teaching sessions but more importantly takes place when a "teaching moment" occurs spontaneously. Watching how another camper or counselor deals with his or her diabetes, insulin injection technique, or a particularly difficult exercise period or seeing how food and insulin might be adjusted provides direct comparison to what the youngster might do in similar circumstances. Medical, nursing, and program staff trained to capture such teaching moments obtain great satisfaction in watching information that is often difficult to teach because of its abstract nature become incorporated into the repertoire of even the youngest campers. Peer pressure and sharing of common problems becomes part of the learning experience. Teaching occurs at the optimum moment when the information being taught is actually needed, as opposed to the lessons learned in a doctor, nurse, or dietitian's office far removed from the actual event. Such informal education never ends when groups of people living with diabetes are placed together. There is enormous value in watching a young adult or older teenager (what we call our diabetes camp "veterans") who has diabetes live with his or her diabetes and serve as a role model even if the same young adult or teen does not always take the best care of himself or herself at other times of the year. Knowing that somebody with diabetes can live long enough and productively enough to become a camp counselor, prepare for college or a job, fall in love, get married, and have children is a concrete demonstration that improves self-esteem for youngsters living with diabetes around the world (14).

Formal teaching is also enhanced because discussions among several youngsters who have diabetes are fostered. Successful diabetes camping programs invite guest speakers and also use selected staff members who are naturally adept as teachers in such roles. Specific topics (advanced meal planning, exercise rules and promotion, sick day guidelines, treatment and prevention of hypoglycemia, or avoiding peer pressure to start smoking, use drugs, or become sexually active, for example) can be covered in ways that are less tedious and more entertaining utilizing puppet shows, games with diabetes questions, songs, and skits written as parodies of major plays, movies, or television programs but with a diabetes motif. Role playing especially when parents assume the role of the child or adolescent and the child or teenagers assume the role of the parents, uses comedy as a mechanism to share the angst of the situations being presented.

The best camping programs "emphasize the resources of the natural surroundings to contribute to the camper's mental, physical, social and spiritual growth," according to American Camping Association guidelines (15), and this applies to diabetes camping as well. The best camping programs not only recruit staff to serve as role models for the younger campers but also train staff to identify problems in management technique (how to inject insulin properly, what to do to treat hypoglycemia, and what choices might be considered to counterbalance changes in activity when there is more exertion and also when plans change because of circumstances, such as the weather, which are unplanned), as well as how to identify psychosocial concerns that ought to be addressed (how to talk with friends who do not have diabetes, why wearing medical alert identifcation is not necessarily embarrassing, and how to deal with frustration, anger, guilt, depression, parental nagging, and being less than perfect all the time). The primary purpose of diabetes camp programs should always be to provide a safe environment in which fun-filled activities can take place and to ensure peer interaction that promotes a sense of well-being, a sense of what can be accomplished despite having diabetes, and to help foster such attitudes that will be useful when the camper returns home. Camps associated with academic centers use these programs to help train medical, nursing, and dietary students, as well as to train house officers and endocrine fellows.

IV. RESIDENTIAL SUMMER CAMPS

The genesis of diabetes camping experiences began as a simple respite from city life and the hassles of living with diabetes about 70 years ago, shortly after insulin injections allowed children to live for more than a few months after diagnosis. Some thought these ideas preposterous, and some local townsfolk worried about the contagious aspects of so many with diabetes living nearby, but the camps flourished. Sponsored by local diabetes clubs or societies, hospital, and clinics, and frequently with the assistance of Lions Clubs, they increased. Each locale produces its own version, a few owning their own camping properties but most renting or leasing camp sites in tandem with the nondiabetes camp or before or after the formal nondiabetes camp sessions. The children and teenagers gather at the camp, usually supervised by young adults or older teenagers in addition to other supervisory staff (camp medical directors, nurses, and program directors, as well as specialty staff if the camp is sufficiently large and diverse). Camp sessions vary from 1 to 4 weeks, depending upon the financial resources of the camp and the campers. Residential camps generally group campers by age group and sex, most are coeducational, and all involve having youngsters with diabetes live away from their families for some period of time. In general, most professionals involved with diabetes camps believe that youngsters separate from their families best around age 9–10 years, but there are some residential camps that recruit younger children as well; our own team does not encourage overnight camping experiences in which children are not with their families until after age 10 because of separation anxieties and excess homesickness in less mature children (16,17). The success of diabetes camps can often be measured by direct observation of the children and adolescents participating fully in the programs

and returning year after year, wanting to keep in touch with campers and staff between camp sessions and aspiring to help others with diabetes to know about their programs. No good scientific, objective, and unbiased study of camping programs has ever been completed, but anecdotal evidence (18,19) is enormously supportive of what camps can accomplish in promoting healthy attitudes about diabetes management and fostering self-esteem (20) in the process. Formal diabetes assessment of skills and knowledge takes place at more than 85% of camps, and youngsters participate in their own self-management directly or with assistance and guidance of staff. More than 50% of diabetes residential camp programs participated in formal scientific research programs. Whether metabolic control actually improves has been more difficult to document, and two specific studies looking at the effect of such programs did not show camp-related changes as consistent or maintained (21,22). Another study (23) failed to show any difference between adolescents with IDDM when assessed by adjustment to diabetes, self-worth, behavioral competencies, and personality functioning compared to a control group with IDDM who had not attended diabetes camp. Problem-solving behavior and locus of control were improved in studies by Moffatt and Pless (24) and Smith et al. (25).

V. DAY CAMPS

More recently, especially for the youngest children with diabetes, day camps (26) have been started to offer similar experiences but without the necessity to sleep away from family and home each night. Mostly organized by local diabetes associations and occurring during school vacations, these are run in a similar fashion but only during the daytime hours. Lunch is either included or brought from home each day. As with residential camp programs, fun-filled days and education are mixed together, often in inseparable fashion.

VI. ADVENTURE, OUTWARD BOUND, BICYCLING, SKIING, AND WILDERNESS CAMPING

Following the example established by Dr. Olney, more rustic camping experiences have increased over the past 20 years as well (27). Acknowledging that youngsters with diabetes also enjoy adventure, programs that are more challenging have been developed to offer experiences with diabetes management and control in addition to mountaineering, bicycling, skiing, and living in the wilderness. Whitewater rafting trips, Outward Bound programs, and other challenges that would have seemed impossible to propose several years ago have been initiated to deal with the specific needs of a group of people who have diabetes so that safety issues are addressed. Such programs help challenge those living with diabetes to become more self-reliant, introspective, self-assured, and confident. Most such programs are offered to teenagers who are carefully selected in association with more highly trained staff in supervisory roles. Overcoming the challenges faced by such rigorous programs, despite, not because of, diabetes, produces enormous pride and a sense of accomplishment.

VII. YOUTH GROUPS AND NONSUMMER CAMPS: FAMILY SUPPORT WEEKENDS, WACKY WEEKENDS WITH FRIENDS, GRANDPARENT WEEKENDS, TEEN RETREATS, AND YOUTH LEADERSHIP CONGRESSES

Because of the success of summer camp programs, other programs throughout the rest of the year and with an expanded focus have been developed around the world (28). Youth Service Committees have been formed to initiate, organize, fund, and run such weeklong or weekend programs with the same goal: using the natural resources of the site and the season to bring together groups of people living with diabetes to support one another, learn from one another, and have a good time. In Massachusetts, for instance, the American Diabetes Association Youth Services Committee produces approximately eight weekend programs plus two 5 day programs throughout the nonsummer months. Diabetes nurse educators and/or pediatric endocrinologists provide medical support for the program staff, who bring together age-matched families and youth.

Some families may never have taken a vacation because of fears of how diabetes would be managed away from the home. Often this is the first time that fathers can participate in the day-to-day chores of diabetes management and see other fathers doing the same. Sometimes single parents see how other similar parents deal with their unique issues. Some siblings see that there are other families in which the brothers or sisters feel abandoned by parents who must deal with a family member with diabetes or worry that they too might get diabetes, and parents have a chance to see how other parents deal with these stressful situations. Parents can receive support from other parents, and the children in the family see that they are not alone in living with diabetes.

Small group dynamics come into play using ice-breaker sessions on the first evening of the weekend so that participants come to know one another and receive "permission" to discuss feelings often kept submerged at home. Setting the tone for these special and intense weekend experiences is the responsibility of the staff supervising the programs, so that special training in group dynamics and the psychology of group interactions is particularly helpful (29). Immediate bonds can be created. Breakfast the next morning is often shared between families, so that when group activities (in the snow, in the rain, or in the woods) take place shortly afterward, the conversations between and among participants becomes a critical part of the activity. Working to prepare meals or snacks for the other members of the group or having entire families play volleyball or go sledding together in an atmosphere in which diabetes is accepted produces the same feelings of camaraderie as in residential diabetes summer programs and with a speed and intensity that are amazing.

Depending upon the skills and interests of the supervisory medical, nursing, dietary, and activity staff, these staff members can lead discussions about important family issues or research or problem solving, or invited speakers can spend only a few hours with the participants. Some such family weekends focus on age matching the child or teen with diabetes; others merely bring families together. Using role playing for preteenage and teenage participants, as well as adults, is an enjoyable and creative way to deal with such issues as how family members respond to hypoglycemia, not following a meal plan, fears of insulin injections and blood testing, or how health care professionals are viewed by the person with diabetes. Creative drawing (draw a picture of what diabetes would look like "if it were a monster," draw a picture of you having an insulin reactions, or draw a picture of "a cure" for diabetes) sometimes allows feelings to be identified that might otherwise not be stated in school-age children or adolescents, or the adults involved with the drawing session. Adults, teenagers, and young children can all participate and identify with what is placed (safely) on paper in such a fashion,

Table 1 and 2 present youth group themes and parent group themes our multidisciplinary staff has developed for use whenever groups of children, adolescents, or parents are brought together (30).

More recently, grandparent camps have been established, first in Maine by Patricia Stenger, R.N., C.D.E. and Dr. Joan MacCracken and now also in Massachusetts and elsewhere, and serve as a mechanism for safely teaching grandparents how to live with a grandchild who has diabetes and how to do blood glucose testing, administer insulin, and learn about meal planning. Using the same model as the family camping weekends, individual staff are "assigned" to each family unit

Table 1 Youth Group Themes

Fears at diagnosis
Acceptance, denial, anger
Friends who think diabetes is "catching"
Friends who think diabetes is debilitating
Eating snacks at school
Hassles of testing urine or blood
Needle and syringe fears and fantasies
Wearing Medic-Alert identification
Announcing diabetes to the world
Telling your coach, teachers, boyfriend, girlfriend
Guilt
Not being perfect
For teenagers
   Job choices
   Long-term complications

Source: Adapted from New England Diabetes and Endocrinology Cancer (NEDEC), S. J. Brink, M.D., 1994.

Table 2 Parent and Grandparent Group Themes

Fears at diagnosis of devastating Blindness and Amputations
Guilt
Loneliness of going home and coping
Divorced families
Problems of single parents
Mothers versus father's roles
Father "too busy" or never at home
Interference and Sabotage by other family members
School problems
Peer pressures
Sibling rivalry
Oversupervision (nagging) versus undersupervision (laissez-faire)
Normal versus abnormal rebelliousness: when to get counseling
Limit-setting strategies
Causing pain with blood tests, laboratory testing, insulin injections
Expense of diabetes supplies
Trying but not succeeding at blood glucose control
When bad things happen to good people
Holiday and vacation planning

Source: Adapted from New England Diabetes and Endocrinology Center (NEDEC), S. J. Brink, M.D., 1994.

Table 3 Benefits of Diabetes Camping and Youth Support Groups

Increased peer contact and support for child or teen
Increased peer contact and support for parent, sibling, grandparent, others
Identification of youngster or family at risk
Identification of problems needing more treatment or better intervention
Ability to teach in groups
Ability to introduce new concepts in safe fashion
Improved self-esteem and self-confidence
Improved parenting and family relations
Fewer diabetes-related emergencies: severe hypoglycemia and ketoacidosis avoided (?)
Improved compliance and fewer long-term complications (?)

Source: Adapted from New England Diabetes and Endocrinology Center (NEDEC), S.J. Brink. M.D., 1994.

as mentors, but parents specifically are excluded from the weekend. The camper with diabetes and his or her brothers and sisters live with their grandparents for the weekend, and each learns to help the others survive the ordeal. Parents not only get a mini-vacation away from the child with diabetes but find that "experts" teaching their own parents how to take care of diabetes is frequently an easier task than trying to get this accomplished by themselves. The result is a more confident grandparent plus a grandchild proud of grandparents' participation and interest. Parents realize that their own parents are now knowledgeable about diabetes. Grandparents follow meal plans and learn how to decide about food and snack portions. Grandparents receive sham injections with saline, check their own blood glucose levels, and learn how to inject their own grandchildren with insulin, learn about glucagon for emergencies, and learn how to begin interpreting blood glucose results. Universally, grandparents report that their fears were much worse than the reality of needles and lancets and berate themselves for waiting so long to learn how to help.

Other diabetes programs have produced weekend or weeklong retreats designed to have youngsters with diabetes bring a friend who does not have diabetes for the express purpose of teaching that friend how to help them live well with diabetes. Such "wacky weekends" introduce abstract concepts of diabetes care, debunk myths, and help youngsters with diabetes share information with their friends. Table 3 lists the benefits of such youth programs (31).

VIII. NATIONAL YOUTH CONGRESSES AND INTERNATIONAL CAMPS

The idea of bringing teenagers together from different parts of the same country or from different countries around the world who share having diabetes follows the same philosophy of diabetes camping: to help support living well with diabetes and to empower persons with diabetes to take charge of their illness and their lives (32). Combining the experience of travel with the exposure to people from different backgrounds allows young men and women to place their own diabetes management needs and skills into better perspective. Learning from others in a nonthreatening fashion and having to defend (often silently) why one does or does not eat properly, self-monitor, take insulin, or ask for and accept help from health professionals often translate into better decisions about self-management at home. Realizing the benefits or drawbacks of available resources and how these resources are used or ignored allows the possibility for improvement. Teaching leadership skills that make older teenagers and young adults into better counselors at diabetes camps or more active participants in local diabetes associations translates into better self-esteem and perhaps more confidence in living with diabetes. The American Diabetes Association sponsors an annual National Youth Congress each spring. As a training forum for future leaders of the American Diabetes Association and as a "reward" for these young adults' participation in their own states, the National Youth Congress has been invaluable in its efforts to promote improved self-care and improved awareness of the youth efforts of the American Diabetes Association. Programs in Sweden, the United Kingdom, France, Austria, Egypt, Canada, Israel, Chile, Australia, New Zealand, Korea, Japan, and elsewhere have joined those in the United States in sharing such common goals, sharing experiences with diabetes, and bringing back a message of hope in place of frustration, joy instead of sadness, and friendship fostered by diabetes.

IX. FINAL CONSIDERATIONS

It should be pointed out that documentation of benefits of camping and support groups remains anecdotal and without confirmation of any long-term consequences. A substantial improvement in self-esteem associated with the camping experiences has been reported and is expected to be a positive influence on youngsters living with diabetes mellitus, but it is not clear how long such improvements last. Using such outcome measures as glycosylated hemoglobin has also produced varied results, perhaps because of the many other variables involved with improving glycemic control besides what becomes available during any type of camping program. Potential harmful consequences, such as severe hypoglycemia and poorly recognized diabetic ketoacidosis, may occur during camping programs just as they do at other times. One of the great benefits of a diabetes-specific camping experiences comes with the staff training involved with learning to recognize and prevent as well as treat hypoglycemia and ketoacidosis in appropriate fashion so that the severe consequences of each can be minimized. The cost of diabetes camping programs is also extremely variable depending upon support from such organizations as the American Diabetes Association or the Lions International and the fund-raising abilities of each camp staff. Nevertheless, support programs that foster positive approaches to living with a chronic illness like diabetes are an invaluable tool in the armamentarium of the diabetes treatment team.

REFERENCES

1. Wentworth SM. Camping for the child and adolescent with diabetes. In: Brink SJ, ed. Pediatric and Adolescent Diabetes Mellitus, Chicago: Year Book Medical Publishers, 1987:393.
2. Johnson SB. Psychosocial factors in juvenile diabetes: a review. J Behav Med 1980; 3:95–116.
3. Orr DP, Weller SC, Satterwhite MA, Pless IB. Psychosocial implications of chronic illness in adolescence. J Pediatr 1984; 104:152–157.
4. Baker L, Rosman B, Sargent J, Nogueira J, Stanley CA. Family factors predict glycosylated hemoglobin (HbA₁) in juvenile diabetes. Diabetes 1982; 31:15a.
5. Hauenstein EJ, Marvin RS, Snyder AL, Clarke WL. Stress in parents of children with diabetes mellitus. Diabetes Care 1989; 12:18–23.
6. Travis LB, Allen WR. Camps and other similar programs. In: Travis LB, Brouhard H, Schreiner B-J, eds. Diabetes Mellitus in Children and Adolescents. Philadelphia: W. B. Saunders, 1987:226.
7. Travis LB, Allen WR. Camps and other similar programs. In: Travis LB, Brouhard BH, Schreiner B-J, eds. Diabetes Mellitus in Children and Adolescents. Philadelphia: W.B. Saunders, 1987:226–232.
8. Bluebond-Langner M, Perkel D, Goertzel T, Nelson K, McGeary J. Children's knowledge of cancer and its treatment: impact of an oncology camp experience. J Pediatr 1990; 116:207–213.
9. Seeler RA. Disease-specific camping for children. J Pediatr 1990; 116:271–272.
10. Sahler OJZ, Carpenter PJ. Evaluation of a camp program for siblings of children with cancer. Am J Dis Child 1989; 143:690–669.
11. Reavill LK, Wheeler R. Why camp? Diabetes Forecast 1981;27–39.
12. O'Connell KA, Hamera E, Kyner JL. Psychological spread of effects and metabolic control in diabetics. Diabetes 1981; 30:31a.
13. McCraw R, Travis L. Psychological effects of a special summer camp on juvenile diabetes. Diabetes 1973; 22:275–278.
14. Schochet BV. Juvenile diabetes: the adolescent's perspective. Diabetes 1982; 31:79a.
15. American Camping Association, 1993.
16. Brink SJ. Diabetes mellitus in 5- to 9-year old children. In: Brink S, ed. Pediatric and Adolescent Diabetes Mellitus, Chicago: Year Book Medical Publishers, 1987:43–78.
17. Zrebiec JF. Psychosocial commentary on insulin-dependent diabetes in 5- to 9-year old children. In: Brink S, ed. Pediatric and Adolescent Diabetes Mellitus, Chicago: Year Book Medical Publishers, 1987; 79–87.
18. Kurtz SMS, Prus DS. Results of a national survey of diabetes camps. Diabetes 1985; 34:30a.
19. Harkavy J, Johnson SB, Silverstein J, Spillar R, McCallum M Rosenbloom A. Who learns what at diabetes summer camp? J Pediatr Psychol 1982;
20. Travis LB. Care of children with diabetes. In: Moore TD, ed. The Care of Children with Chronic Illness: Report of the 67th Ross Conference on Pediatric Research. Columbus, OH: Ross Laboratories, 1975:57–65.
21. Spevack M, Johnson SB, Silverstein J. The effect of diabetes summer camp on patient adherence, glycemic control and physician behavior. Diabetes 1988; 37:125a.
22. Strickland AL, McFarland KF, Murtiashaw MH, Thorpe SR, Baynes JW. Changes in blood protein glycosylation during a diabetes summer camp. Diabetes Care 1984; 7:183–185.
23. Scharf LS, Leach DC, Adams KM. Diabetes camp as a psychological intervention: some findings. Diabetes 1987; 36:109a.
24. Moffatt M, Pless I. Locus of control in juvenile diabetic campers: changes during camp and relationship to camp assessments. J Pediatr 1984; 103:146–150.
25. Smith KE, Schreiner B-J, Brouhard BH, Travis LB. Impact of a camp experience on choice of coping strategies by adolescents with insulin-dependent diabetes mellitus. Diabetes Ed 1991; 17:49–53.
26. American Diabetes Association. Day Camps for Children with Diabetes, Alexandria, VA, 1990.
27. Kessell M, Resnick MD, Blum RW. Adventure, etc.—a health-promotion program for chronically ill and disabled youth. J Adol Health Care 1985; 6:433–438.
28. Shalom R, Ryan J. Support and education groups for type I diabetics in a college campus. Diabetes 1987; 36:32a.
29. Brink S. Youth and parent groups for patients with juvenile onset type I diabetes mellitus. Pediatr Adol Endocrinol 1982; 10:224–229.
30. Brink SJ. Youth and parent support groups. In: Brink SJ, ed. Pediatric and Adolescent Diabetes Mellitus. Chicago: Year Book Medical Publishers, 1987:359–368.
31. Brink SJ. Youth and parent support groups. In: Brink SJ, ed. Pediatric and Adolescent Diabetes Mellitus. Chicago: Year Book Medical Publishers, 1987:368.
32. Feste C. A practical look at patient empowerment. Diabetes Care 1992; 15:922–925.

48

Hypoglycemia in the Newborn

Richard M. Cowett

Brown University School of Medicine and Women and Infants Hospital of Rhode Island, Providence, Rhode Island

I. INTRODUCTION

Relative to glucose metabolism, the neonate is considered in transition between the complete dependence of the fetus and the complete independence of the adult. The neonate must become independent after birth, balancing between glucose deficiency and excess to maintain euglycemia. The dependence of the conceptus on his or her mother for continuous substrate delivery in utero contrasts with the variable and intermittent exogenous intake orally that is the hallmark of the neonatal period and beyond. Development of carbohydrate homeostasis results from a balance between the specific morbidities to which the neonate is subject, developing hormonal, neural, and enzymatic regulation and substrate availability. Maturation of neonatal homeostasis is influenced by the integrity of the specific pathways of intermediary metabolism important in glucose metabolism. The heterogeneity that is the hallmark of neonatal glucose metabolism is illustrated by the multiplicity of conditions producing or associated with neonatal hypoglycemia and hyperglycemia; however, the latter is not covered in this discussion. The maintenance of euglycemia, especially in the sick or low birth weight neonate, is difficult. This reinforces the concept that the neonate is vulnerable to carbohydrate disequilibrium. This topic has been the subject of a number of recent reviews (1–11).

In this chapter we evaluate the definition of euglycemia (and consider the limits for hypo- and hyperglycemia) and the various methodologies available to measure glucose concentration. Subsequently we evaluate the differential of hypoglycemia and consider its treatment.

II. DEFINITION OF NEONATAL EUGLYCEMIA

A primary example of the heterogeneity that exists in our understanding of neonatal glucose metabolism is that no uniform standards are accepted for specific limits for euglycemia. The definitions of what constitute hypo- and hyperglycemia are quite variable. It is well accepted that glucose is the major substrate for carbohydrate metabolism. At birth, the maternal supply of glucose to the neonate ceases abruptly. Although the neonatal plasma glucose concentration is usually in the normoglycemic range at delivery, its actual concentration depends upon such factors as the last maternal meal, the duration of labor, the route of delivery, and the type of intravenous fluid administered to the mother.

After normal delivery, the plasma glucose concentration declines to approximately 50 mg/dl by 2 h of age but equilibrates at approximately 70 mg/dl at 72 h after birth (10). Cornblath and Reisner have evaluated the blood glucose concentration over time in a classic analysis of both term and low birth weight neonates (12). Their data suggested that concentrations below 40 mg/dl or greater than 125 mg/dl were abnormal after 3 days after birth. Critical adjustments are required by the neonate in the first 72 h after birth to maintain glucose homeostasis.

More recently, Srinivasan et al. evaluated plasma glucose concentrations in normal full-term neonates who weighed between 2500 and 4000 g and were appropriate for age between 37 and 42 completed weeks of gestation (13). The predicted glucose concentrations during the first week of life are noted in Figure 1. All neonates were fed after 3 h. The data indicated that the nadir in plasma glucose concentration is between 1 and 2 h and that a significant rise occurs during hour 3. The authors suggested that a plasma glucose concentration <35 mg/dl should be of concern during the first 3 h of postnatal life. They concluded that a plasma glucose concentration <40 mg/dl between 3 and 24 h and <45 mg/dl after 24 h should be considered in the hypoglycemic range.

Another investigation of this topic was performed by Heck and Erenberg, who evaluated serum glucose concentrations in term neonates during the first 48 h after birth. They concluded that a serum glucose concentration of <30 mg/dl

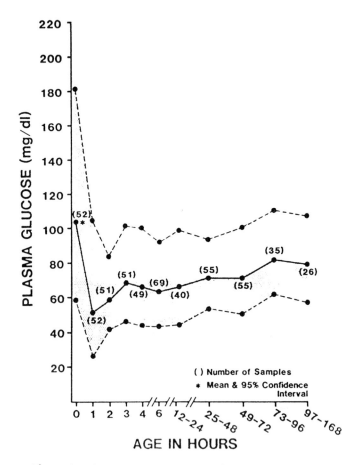

Figure 1 Plasma glucose concentrations in term neonates weighing 2.5–4.0 kg. (From Srinivasan et al., Ref. 13.)

in the first day of life and <40 mg/dl in the second day of life were the limits for the definition of hypoglycemia in the full-term neonate (14).

No similar evaluation of the limits of hypoglycemia have been reported for the preterm neonate. This difficult study is clearly necessary because of the lack of consensus relative to definition. This lack of consensus was studied by Koh et al., who reported a range of hypoglycemia between 18 and 72 mg/dl in the United Kingdom in a survey of health care professionals (15).

The definition of hyperglycemia is equally unsettled (16). However, a consensus may be said to center on concentrations in the range of >125–150 mg/dl (17–19).

What should be apparent from this discussion is the variation not only in the definition of euglycemia but in the "normal" concentration of glucose at any particular point in time. An obvious example of this latter situation is noted in Figure 2. In the four types of neonates commonly cared for in a neonatal unit, the term infant whose size is appropriate for gestational age (AGA), the term infant who is small for gestational age (SGA), the preterm infant who is AGA, and the preterm infant who is SGA, plasma glucose concentration changed constantly and in an apparently random fashion (20).

III. MEASUREMENT OF NEONATAL GLUCOSE CONCENTRATION

The problems involved in the definition of euglycemia are accentuated by the lack of attention given to details of measurement of neonatal glucose concentration. Failure to measure the glucose concentration rapidly enough would allow blood cell oxidation of glucose, resulting in falsely low values. A number of centers use the Dextrostix technique, which was thought to be reliable if directions are followed carefully. However, the company cautions that the reagent strips are not intended for use with neonatal blood. We have suggested that abnormal values, either in the hypoglycemic or hyperglycemic range, should be corroborated with laboratory determination of glucose concentration before correction of the suspected disequilibrium unless the patient is symptomatic (11).

Investigations allow one to question whether the Dextrostix or a like evaluation should be used at all. Several studies have evaluated various means of assessing blood glucose concentration. Frantz et al (21) reported that the Dextrostix test strip was able accurately to identify blood glucose concentrations <50 mg/dl. However, they used fresh heparinized blood from adults to evaluate reliability, which may not be applicable to the neonate. Perelman et al. (22) evaluated rapid glucose determination in the neonate, comparing the Dextrostix Ames Meter, Chemstrip bG test strip, and Stat Tek Meter methods with a glucose analyzer. The authors concluded that there was modest accuracy in estimating whole-blood glucose concentration. They suggested that confirmation by conventional laboratory techniques was necessary before therapeutic intervention. Wilkins and Kaira (23) compared blood glucose test strips for the detection of neonatal hypoglycemia. In 101 blood samples, results of three glucose test strip methods were compared with a laboratory determination of glucose concentration. Two test strips (BM test glycemic 20-800 test strips and the Reflecto-Test hypoglycemia test strips) gave rapid and reliable estimates, but Dextrostix test strips tended to overestimate all blood glucose concentrations.

In another report, Conrad et al. (24) suggested that the Glucostix, the Dextrostix, and the Chemstrip bG test strips were relatively unreliable, with r values of 0.73, 0.74, and 0.83, respectively, compared with the YSI analyzer in tests of 104 neonatal blood samples obtained by heelstick. They tested one glucose reflectance meter (the Glucometer M), which had an r value of 0.73 when correlated with the YSI analyzer. The authors suggested that the YSI analyzer should be used preferentially in the determination of blood glucose concentration in the neonatal intensive care unit.

In a study in our laboratory, we chose four glucose reflectance meters for evaluation (25). The manufacturers claimed that these meters could reliably measure whole-blood glucose concentrations as low as 20 mg/dl. To determine whether the accuracy of the determination would be affected by the technique of obtaining capillary blood by heelstick, we used cord arterial blood from a separate group of neonates for comparison. All blood was sequentially analyzed five different

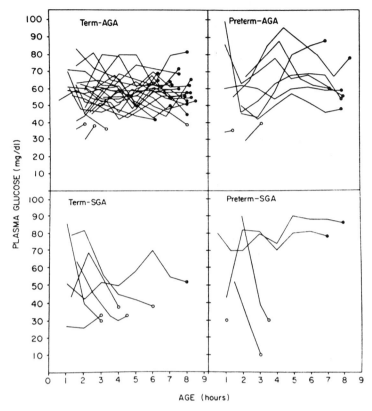

Figure 2 Plasma glucose concentration for the four groups of neonates studied during the first 9 h of life. (From Stanley et al., Ref. 20.)

times on each meter and the YSI analyzer. Evaluation of the data showed that accuracy was limited in heelstick blood whether one evaluated the percentage of difference between the means (Table 1) or the least-squares regression for all the meters tested. The use of cord blood appeared to be associated with greater accuracy than the use of capillary blood obtained by heelstick in the analyses. The reason for the poor correlations with capillary samples and the high variability in the values of blood glucose concentrations remains unclear. There was no relationship between accuracy and reliability of the various glucose reflectance meters (Table 2). The Diascan S meter, which seemed to have accuracy closest to that of the YSI analyzer, was clearly not the most reliable in comparison

Table 1 Accuracy of Reflectance Meters Versus YSI Glucose Analyzer

Reflectance meter	Cord	Heel	p
Difference between means, %			
Glucometer M	− 9.3	−23.2	
Diascan S	0.4	− 0.4	
Accu-Chek II	1.2	16.4	
One Touch	35.2	25.6	
Correlation coefficient r			
Glucometer M	0.88	0.64	<0.05
Diascan S	0.96	0.71	<0.01
Accu-Chek II	0.91	0.71	<0.05
One Touch	0.92	0.86	NS[a]

[a]Not significant

Source: From Reference 25.

Table 2 Reliability of Glucose Analyzer and Reflectance Meters

	Coefficient of variation (%)		
	Cord	Heel	p[a]
YSI analyzer	3.2	3.3	NS
Glucometer M meter	5.6	5.8	NS
Diascan S meter	5.9	7.2	NS
Accu-Chek II meter	5.9	8.0	<0.01
One Touch meter	3.4	3.7	NS

[a]NS, not significant.

Source: From Reference 25.

with the YSI analyzer. On the other hand, the One Touch meter, which had the best reliability among the four glucose reflectance meters tested, was the least accurate. We concluded that, contrary to the manufacturers' claims, glucose reflectance meters should probably not be used for evaluation of capillary blood glucose concentrations in the high-risk neonate. Further work is ongoing in this area in our laboratory and others.

Holtrop et al. evaluated the sensitivity and specificity of glucose oxidase peroxidase chromogen test strips by comparing values of 272 samples of serum glucose concentration with values obtained by Chemstrip bG (26). The diagnostic sensitivity of a test strip $\leq$ 40 mg/dl to predict a serum glucose level $\leq$ 34 mg/dl was 86%, with 78% specificity. The positive predictive value with a 21% prevalence of serum glucose $\leq$ 34 mg/dl was 52%, with a negative predictive value of 95%. Of the serum glucose concentrations 58 were $\leq$ 34 mg/dl, and the strips reported values greater than 40 mg/dl in 8. The authors concluded that more sensitive and specific methods are required for the neonate.

It is important to remember that the blood glucose concentration is usually 10–15% lower than the corresponding plasma glucose value. Finally, care must be taken when the test is performed because erroneously high values can be caused by isopropyl alcohol mixing with the blood on the strip, which is read by reflectance colorimetry (27).

An in vitro model study of 280 glucose samples was recently reported to have reemphasized the general clinical impression of the inability of an umbilical artery catheter sample to measure glucose concentration accurately in the neonate. This is probably because the umbilical artery catheter is usually infused with intravenous glucose as a nutrient supplement for the neonate (28).

In another investigation of differences in glucose concentration related to site of sampling, Cowett and D'Amico evaluated differences in blood glucose concentration between capillary (heelstick) sampling and venous sampling. They were correlated between the two sites ($r^2 = 0.64$). The investigators noted that the heelstick samples provided more variable results than the venous samples, but these differences were probably not significant physiologically (Fig. 3) (29).

IV. CLINICAL HYPOGLYCEMIA IN THE NEONATE

The close relationship between maternal and fetal glucose, the repetitive occurrence of wide swings of neonatal glucose concentration, and the retarded disappearance of an acute glucose load in both term and preterm neonates indicate that the regulation of neonatal carbohydrate metabolism is poorly developed 72 h after birth (30). The birth process brings the necessity of a period of readjustment to allow subsequent control. In the low birth weight neonate especially, this adjustment is delicate and may result in abnormal consequences, such as hypo- or hyperglycemia. We have already discussed the difficulties in the definition of hypo- and hyperglycemia. One of the main clinical difficulties with these definitions is the nonspecific symptomatology, which includes the signs and symptoms listed in Table 3. These

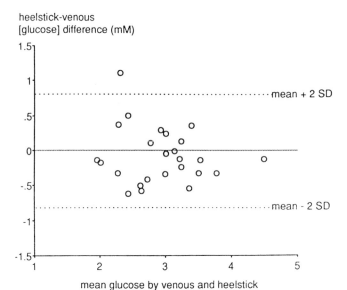

Figure 3   The variability in blood glucose concentration related to the location from which the sample was obtained. SD, standard deviation. (From Cowett and D'Amico, Ref. 29.)

difficulties are compounded by the occurrence of symptoms at different levels of blood glucose in different neonates and the lack of a universal threshold below or above which symptomatology may occur (11). These same conclusions were emphasized by a recent conference on hypoglycemia convened by the CIBA Foundation (31).

A number of different classifications have been employed to categorize the various causes of hypoglycemia seen in the neonatal period. Cornblath and Schwartz (10) and others (32,33) have analyzed the various causes on the basis of clinical course, emphasizing time of presentation, duration, severity, and response to therapy. Another schema considers the biochemical and physiologic parameters and evaluates the relationship between hepatic production and/or uptake in contrast to peripheral utilization (34,35). Differentiation of the various causes of hypoglycemia on the basis of physiologic and biochemical parameters would compare decreased hepatic glucose production as a result of substrate or enzymatic deficiencies to those secondary to increased hormonal insulin concentration. Inadequate glucose production includes those conditions involving decreased availability of substrate

Table 3   Signs and Symptoms of Neonatal Hypoglycemia

Abnormal cry	Hypothermia
Apathy	Hypotonia
Apnea	Jitteriness
Cardiac arrest	Lethargy
Convulsions	Tremors
Cyanosis	Tachypnea

(i.e., glycogen, lactate, glycerol, and amino acids), altered sensitivity to neural or hormonal factors, and/or immature or altered enzymatic pathways (i.e., gluconeogenesis and/or increased peripheral utilization rates).

V. PATHOPHYSIOLOGY OF HYPOGLYCEMIA IN THE NEONATE: IMPRECISE OR DIMINISHED HEPATIC GLUCOSE PRODUCTION

Neonatal hypoglycemia not caused by insulin excess is generally caused by diminished hepatic glucose production. The role of hepatic control of glucose homeostasis and its relationship to its disequilibrium in the neonate has only recently been studied. Conditions in the neonate that produce hypoglycemia relating to either imprecise control of glucose production or diminished substrate availability include prematurely born neonates appropriate for gestational age, small for gestational age neonates, perinatally stressed and asphyxiated neonates, cold-stressed neonates, and neonates with congenital heart disease and/or sepsis. Neonates may also be hypoglycemic because of glucagon deficiency or deficits in intermediary metabolic pathways, such as glycogen storage disease type I or fructose-1,6-diphosphatase deficiency, reflecting a series of hereditary metabolic disorders in which hypoglycemia may be the initial or most obvious presenting feature.

A. Preterm Appropriate for Gestational Age Neonates

Appropriate for gestation age neonates born before term may develop hypoglycemia. Although the first report of this entity concerned small for gestational age neonates (36), subsequent studies documented hypoglycemia in the low birth weight neonate who was appropriate for gestational age. In 1968, Raivio and Hallman reported a frequency of 1.4% of hypoglycemia in these neonates (37). Fluge reported that as many as 14% of AGA neonates evidenced neonatal hypoglycemia (32).

The diminished oral and parenteral intake in the low birth weight neonate in combination with the decreased concentration of substrates may explain the lower plasma glucose seen in these neonates and their propensity to hypoglycemia. Functionally immature gluconeogenic and glycogenolytic enzyme systems present in the neonate potentiate these difficulties. The relatively increased size of the brain (13% of the body mass in the newborn versus 2% in the adult) may be responsible for the greater proportion of glucose consumption during periods of fasting. This effect is magnified in the low birth weight neonate.

B. Small for Gestational Age Infants

Many centers have reported a relatively high frequency of hypoglycemia in SGA neonates ever since Cornblath et al., in 1959, described its occurrence in eight infants born to mothers with toxemia (36). Lubchenco and Bard (38), de-

Leeuw and deVries (39), and others have all substantiated the occurrence of hypoglycemia in these neonates. Toxemia has been repeatedly reported to be associated with hypoglycemia, and its incidence has been shown to be highest (61%) in neonates born to mothers with relatively low urinary estriols, compared with a frequency of 19% in neonates born to mothers with normal estriol levels (39,40). Reduction in energy reserves in the form of decreased glycogen deposition, combined with increased utilization of substrate, may account for the appearance of hypoglycemia.

Recently, a reevaluation of the frequency of hypoglycemia was performed using definitions of euglycemia already noted. Of the SGA infants, 14.7% evidenced hypoglycemia, which occurred at a mean of 6.1 h. Infants evidencing hypoglycemia had a positive history including meconium-stained amniotic fluid and maternal preeclampsia and were predominantly male. The range in the time of occurrence was 0.8–34.2 h after birth (41).

Kliegman studied the effect of maternal nutritional deprivation on fetal and neonatal metabolism in dogs (42). Besides reduced fetal weight at term (251 ± 7 versus 277 ± 7 g), the growth-retarded pups evidenced lower glucose concentrations after 3, 6, and 9 h of fasting, reduced plasma concentrations of free fatty acids at 9 and 24 h and lower ketone bodies at 24 h compared with controls. Although the systemic rates of palmitate and alanine turnover were not affected, systemic glucose production was reduced for 3–9 h after birth, which resulted in the observed hypoglycemia. The author speculated that reduced rates of gluconeogenesis from alanine and reduced oxidation of fuels, such as free fatty acids (FFA), contributed to the hypoglycemia. FFA recycling of triglyceride rather than oxidation contributed to the observed hypoglycemia.

Plasma insulin and blood glucose concentrations were measured in umbilical venous samples from 42 small for gestational age and 68 appropriate for gestational age fetuses by cordocentesis at 17–38 weeks gestation (43). In the AGA fetus, plasma insulin and the insulin-glucose ratio increased exponentially with gestation, suggesting maturation of the pancreas. The major determinant of fetal blood glucose concentration was maternal blood glucose concentration. The insulin-glucose ratio in the SGA fetuses was lower than in the AGA fetuses, suggesting that hypoinsulinemia in the former was the result of hypoglycemia and pancreatic dysfunction. The degree of SGA status did not correlate with plasma insulin or the insulin-glucose ratio, which suggested to the investigators that insulin is not the primary determinant of fetal size.

Following bilateral maternal uterine artery ligation, Bussey et al. studied the sequential changes in plasma glucose, insulin and glucagon concentrations, and hepatic glycogen and phosphoenolpyruvate carboxykinase (PEPCK) during the first 4 h in growth-retarded rat pups (44). Hypoglycemia was noted in the SGA pups compared with control (AGA pups), as was reduced hepatic glycogen stores at birth. Plasma glucagon rose, and plasma insulin fell. PEPCK levels did not rise, either. The investigators concluded that SGA pups developed hypoglycemia because of limited glycogen stores and retarded gluconeogenesis. They speculated that delayed PEPCK induction in these animals may result from inadequate glycogen release at birth or decreased sensitivity to glucagon.

There have been a number of studies evaluating the intermediary metabolism of substrate available postnatally. A functional delay in the development of phosphoenolpyruvate carboxykinase, thought to be the rate-limiting enzyme of gluconeogenesis, in SGA neonates was suggested by Haymond et al. (45). This was substantiated by Williams et al., who studied the effect of oral alanine feeding on glucose homeostasis in the SGA neonate compared with AGA neonates (46). Oral alanine feeding enhanced plasma glucagon in both groups but stimulated hepatic glucose output only in the AGA infants.

The effect of intravenously administered glucagon on plasma amino acids has been evaluated in various types of neonates, including the SGA neonate. SGA neonates in the first hours of life had significantly less total amino acid than a comparable group of AGA neonates, although the response to glucagon in the SGA neonates mimicked that in the control (AGA) group. It was speculated that the inability of the SGA neonate to extract specific gluconeogenic amino acids could account for the susceptibility to hypoglycemia in these stressed neonates (47).

A group of 25 neonates who were small for gestational age received 0.5 mg/day of glucagon to treat hypoglycemia (48). Of the 25, 20 responded within 3 h with a rise in blood glucose to 72 mg/dl; 5 subsequently required hydrocortisone to maintain euglycemia. Rebound hypoglycemia occurred in 9 following discontinuation of the glucagon. The response was poor after maternal β blockade.

The role of glucagon was also evaluated by Mestyan et al. by measuring 17 amino acids before and during glucagon infusion in normoglycemic and hypoglycemia SGA neonates (49). In the normoglycemic group most amino acid concentrations declined significantly, but this did not occur in the SGA neonates who were hypoglycemic. Although the effect was transient, these results reflect the ability of glucagon to produce acute changes in hepatic glucose homeostasis. This was demonstrated in neonatal lambs between 1 and 3 days of age with infusions of somatostatin alone or in lambs that received insulin and glucagon in combination during a 2 h interval. Plasma glucose concentration fell when both insulin and glucagon were suppressed acutely, suggesting that the latter is of importance in maintaining glucose concentration during short-term fasting. It was suggested that the ratio between the two hormones acutely affected glucose homeostasis (50).

The secretion of glucagon and insulin has been evaluated in SGA neonates. Both SGA and AGA neonates, after being fed oral glucose and protein (1 g/kg each after a 4 h fast), had similar secretion of both pancreatic hormones. The investigators speculated that the instability of glucose metabolism in the SGA neonate resulted from the rapid fall in glucose, probably because of a transient deficiency of hepatic gluconeogenic enzymes, but not altered secretory patterns of the hormones (51).

The adequacy of the hormonal response was reinforced in a study of glucose-infused SGA neonates who were evaluated by stable isotope kinetic analysis. Under stimulation of glucose infusion, the SGA neonate and his or her AGA counterpart had similar regulatory responses as well as functional integrity in handling glucose during the second day after birth (52).

Using the newborn piglet model, Fecknell et al. studied the effects of an intravenous glucose infusion on glucose homeostasis in normal and growth retarded piglets using non–steady-state tracer technique (53). Suppression was noted of hepatic glucose output, but hyperglycemia (plasma glucose >180 mg/dl developed in the majority of study subjects. The mechanism of the hyperglycemia was thought to be failure to increase glucose utilization in response to the glucose infusion.

The possibility of hormonal excess producing growth retardation has been emphasized by Ogata et al. (54). The authors adapted methodology to produce maternal hyperinsulinemia in a rat model. This resulted in decreased concentrations of glucose and amino acids in both the mother and fetus, which produced retarded fetal growth, limited hepatic glycogen deposition, and delayed neonatal phosphoenolpyruvate carboxykinase induction.

Sann et al. evaluated the effect of hydrocortisone on intravenous glucose tolerance (1 g/kg) in eight term SGA neonates compared with seven AGA neonates at a mean of 41 h of age (55). The rate of glucose disappearance was decreased in the SGA neonates compared with control neonates. Plasma glucose concentration was similar in both groups, but plasma insulin concentration did not change in the control group. After hydrocortisone administration, plasma insulin concentration increased. The authors concluded that hydrocortisone induced a reduced peripheral uptake of glucose independent of insulin secretion.

Recently, Collins and coworkers measured plasma glucose and insulin concentrations in 27 small for date neonates during the first 48 h after birth. In 10 hypoglycemia was diagnosed, and in half of these neonates, plasma insulin concentrations were elevated. The investigators suggested that hyperinsulinemia is common and may be a mechanism of recurrent hypoglycemia (56).

C. Neonates Experiencing Perinatal Stress or Hypoxia

Neonates who utilize glucose at an increased rate may be prone to hypoglycemia. Because the low birth weight neonate is subject to hypoxia, the combination of decreased substrate availability and increased rate of utilization may result in hypoglycemia. An increased rate of anaerobic glycolysis in combination with an increased rate of glycogenolysis is probably the underlying biochemical mechanism: 2 mol ATP is generated by the Embden-Meyerhof anaerobic pathway, whereas aerobic oxidation results in 36 mol ATP. Thus, 18 times more glucose is required to generate the same amount of ATP. In addition, increased lactate production may result in an associated acidosis. Beard et al. have emphasized the association between hypoxia and hypoglycemia in the low birth weight neonate and noted increased metabolic needs out of proportion to substrate availability (57,58). The difficulties are all accentuated in neonates who are unable to replace substrate from the usual exogenous (oral) sources because of hypoxia or other clinical problems. Metabolic acidosis and lactic acidemia were noted during the first 24 h of life in 4 term and 11 preterm neonates whose Apgar had been 5 at 1 minute after birth and who were fed oral glucose loads (59). Thus, not only may endogenous stores be depleted, but these neonates may be unable to tolerate an exogenous load.

Another complication of perinatal stress is the presence of hyperinsulinism. In another report by Collins and Leonard, hyperinsulinism was noted unequivocally in three small for date neonates and in three who were asphyxiated (60). The etiology of the hyperinsulinism was unclear.

This metabolic derangement was reaffirmed by Schultz and Soltész in three infants who were appropriate for gestational age and asphyxiated at birth. They all recovered spontaneously (61).

A further evaluation of the metabolic effects of neonatal asphyxia was undertaken by Jansen and coworkers (62). Using a rat preparation, they showed that hypoxia drastically altered both metabolic fuel and glucoregulatory hormone availability. They suggested that persistence of the catecholamine surge and tissue hypoxia and acidosis are responsible for the transient surge in glucose and subsequent delay and decrease in insulin and increase in glucagon in the asphyxiated neonatal rat.

D. Cold-Stressed Neonates

Hypoglycemia has been identified in neonates who experience cold injury. Mann and Elliott described 14 neonates who suffered neonatal cold injury following prolonged exposure to environmental temperatures below 90°F (63). Marked hypoglycemia was documented in 3 of 6 neonates in whom it was measured. The hypoglycemia was presumed to be the result of free fatty acid elevation secondary to a cold-induced norepinephrine response (64). Recognition of the potential association of hypoglycemia following cold stress should result in parenteral treatment, if necessary, in conjunction with the warming of the neonate. In addition, this relationship must be considered in the evaluation of blood glucose levels in neonates with either temperature instability or in a suboptimal thermal environment.

Close et al. evaluated the influence of environmental temperature on glucose tolerance and insulin response in the neonatal piglet (65). Temperatures were maintained at 17, 24, and 33°C, during which an intravenous infusion of 1 g glucose/kg body weight was administered. Rectal temperatures were maintained in all piglets subjected to the two higher temperatures, but not the lowest, at which 6 of 18 became hypothermic. A higher glucose disappearance rate was noted KG: 200 and 2.32%/minute was recorded for animals maintaining homeothermic temperatures during 17 and 24°C temperature conditions compared with those kept at thermal neutrality (1.66% minute). The insulin response was comparable. During hypothermia both KG 0.76 ± 0.12%/minute

and the insulin response were decreased. Glucose uptake by skeletal muscle was increased in environmentally cold-exposed homeothermic animals, resulting in an increased metabolic rate.

E. Neonatal Sepsis

Neonatal sepsis has been identified with increased frequency in association with hypoglycemia. Yeung noted the association in 20 of 56 neonates with signs of sepsis (66). He suggested that inadequate caloric intake in these infected neonates may predispose to hypoglycemia. The possibility of an increased metabolic rate was considered because these neonates were infused with 100 kcal/kg/day intravenously. A decreased rate of gluconeogenesis has been documented in laboratory animals following gram-negative bacterial infection (67). The possibility of increased peripheral utilization because of enhanced insulin sensitivity in sepsis has been considered (68). It is likely that one or more of these factors will operate to produce the resultant hypoglycemia.

Neonatal hypoglycemia has been reported in two infants with congenital syphilis who were diagnosed with hypopituitarism. It was recommended that an evaluation for pituitary function should be performed if an infant is diagnosed with congenital syphilis in association with hypoglycemia (69).

Another investigation of neonatal sepsis was recently reported by Fitzgerald et al., who evaluated the effects of sepsis on carbohydrate metabolism in premature neonates weighing ≥1.2 kg and who were appropriate for gestational age. Plasma glucose, lactate, and insulin concentrations were measured repetitively for 48 h after birth in 29 infants, of whom 6 were ultimately found to be septic by culture and countercurrent immunoelectrophoresis. Dextrose was administered to maintain euglycemia. The investigators found significant elevations in plasma lactate and dextrose infusion rates but no change in plasma insulin. They concluded that the alterations in the former parameters may be clinical markers for neonatal sepsis (70).

F. Neonates with Congenital Heart Disease and Congestive Heart Failure

An inverse relationship has been noted between the concentration of cardiac glycogen and the level of maturity of the neonate, exemplified by the low levels in the offspring of mammalian species more mature at birth, that is, human, monkey, sheep, and others. These reserves are rapidly depleted during anoxia (71). Benzing et al. reported a series of 27 patients in whom the simultaneous occurrence of hypoglycemia and acute congestive heart failure was noted in association with congenital heart disease (72). Reduced dietary intake in association with diminished hepatic glycogen resulted in hypoglycemia. This was further substantiated by Amatayakul et al., who noted the association of hypoglycemia with congestive heart failure in neonates without significant heart defects (73). The pathophysiology of hypoglycemia in cyanotic congenital heart disease was studied by Haymond et al. (74). A total of 6 subjects were evaluated between 13 and

67 months of age. Glucose and alanine turnover studies utilizing stable isotope labeling in these neonates were compared with results in controls. A subtle defect in hepatic extraction of gluconeogenic substrates was suspected, possibly secondary to decreased hepatic blood flow. It is apparent that the presence of either hypoglycemia or congestive heart failure should be considered when one or the other appears.

The interrelationship of hypoglycemia and pulmonary edema has been emphasized. Unfortunately, it was unclear whether the pulmonary edema was secondary to the hypoglycemia or caused by treatment of the hypoglycemia because 20% dextrose in water was administered through an umbilical venous catheter into a branch of the left pulmonary vein (75).

A group of 19 neonates with symptomatic ventricular septal defects (VSD) were examined by means of an intravenous (IV) glucose tolerance test and compared with 14 neonates who were healthy (76). The VSD neonates were growth retarded, with lower weight for age and length for age. Glucose tolerance was similar in both groups. Plasma insulin concentration was low in the VSD neonates, but insulin secretion as measured by C peptide concentration was elevated. The authors speculated that increased insulin extraction occurs in the liver, but the mechanism was unknown.

G. Neonates Manifesting Defective Gluconeogenesis or Glycogenolysis

Hypoglycemia has been noted in neonates unable to sustain normal gluconeogenesis. Glucagon is influential in hepatic glucose production because it enhances glycogenolysis and gluconeogenesis. A recent report documented a neonate with isolated glucagon deficiency and neonatal hypoglycemia (77). The diagnosis was based on a low basal glucagon concentration as well as a diminished response to hypoglycemia and alanine infusion, both potent stimulators of glucagon secretion, in a neonate in whom normal insulin secretion was present. Vidnes and Sovik reported three neonates with persistent neonatal hypoglycemia, one of whom evidenced an abnormal subcellular distribution of phosphoenolpyruvate carboxykinase in the extramitochondrial fraction (78,79).

A specific enzymatic deficiency that may affect gluconeogenesis in the neonate is type I glycogen storage disease (glucose-6-phosphatase deficiency). The deficiency is an autosomal recessive genetic defect that may occasionally present in the neonatal period with severe hypoglycemia and hepatomegaly. A second enzymatic defect, fructose-1,6-diphosphatase deficiency, has also been associated with hypoglycemia (80–82).

Galactosemia may present in neonates after birth who are septic and/or have hepatocellular jaundice. Later (1 month) galactosemic infants may present with cataract formation. In some neonates, hypoglycemic symptoms have been reported and a positive reducing test in the urine (to copper or iron) noted. The usual biochemical defect is in galactose-1-phosphate uridyltransferase. The diagnosis involves the demonstration of a low true glucose level (glucose oxidase) in the presence of normal total hexoses, together with the determination of the enzymatic defect, which can be analyzed in both red and white blood cells. Exclusion of milk and milk products (lactose) is the treatment of choice. Because early intervention is preventive, routine neonatal screening has been recommended because the deficiency is inherited as an autosomal recessive condition (83).

Hereditary fructose intolerance may be diagnosed in neonates who are old enough to ingest fruits or juices. The major intolerance is caused by fructose-1-phosphate accumulation secondary to fructose-1-phosphate aldolase deficiency. The hypoglycemia is secondary to an inhibition of hepatic glucose release and absence of a hyperglycemic response to glucagon following ingestion or parenteral administration of fructose.

VI. PATHOPHYSIOLOGY OF HYPOGLYCEMIA IN THE NEONATE: HYPERINSULINISM

Hypoglycemia following increased plasma insulin concentration has now been associated with several discrete disorders of the islets. It may be found in the infant of the diabetic mother, neonates with hemolytic diseases of the newborn, neonates with pancreatic nesidioblastosis, those with discrete or multiple islet cell adenomatosis, and neonates undergoing exchange transfusion. The Beckwith-Wiedemann syndrome should be considered along with other causes of hyperinsulinemic hypoglycemia, β-sympathomimetic treatment to the mother, following high umbilical artery catheter placement, and following maternal ethanol consumption.

In the article cited previously, Holtrop noted that hypoglycemia occurred in large for gestational age (LGA) infants whose mothers were not diabetic with a frequency of 8.1% during the first 48 h after birth. Hypoglycemia occurred at a mean age of 2.9 h (range 0.8–8.5 h). There were no observable differences between LGA neonates and those who were hypoglycemia or euglycemic. The investigator suggested that evaluation for hypoglycemia should continue for 12 h (41).

A. Rh Incompatibility and Hypoglycemia

Hyperinsulinism has been implicated as the cause of the hypoglycemia seen in neonates with severe Rh isoimmunization, although this primary diagnosis is rarely seen currently (84–88). These children are invariably severely affected by their disease, with profound anemia and hepatosplenomegaly at birth. The shock and collapse seen on occasion may be caused primarily by the profound hypoglycemia, and under such circumstances, glucose administration in addition to measures taken to correct the anemia may be critical. The infant of the diabetic mother and severely Rh-affected neonate share several pathologic hallmarks. In addition to the hyperinsulinism and islet cell hyperplasia, both show almost identical edematous placental changes. Both have excessive islands of extramedullary hematopoiesis in both liver and spleen. Although this latter finding may be the result of insulin stimulation, the precise cause of the hyperinsulinism itself in the Rh-affected neonate is uncertain. It has been suggested that an increase in reduced glutathione resulting from massive hemolysis of red blood cells may act as a stimulus to insulin release.

B. Hypoglycemia After Exchange Transfusion

Hypoglycemia, although not often considered, may be a significant problem following exchange transfusion. In this connection, the exchange blood and its preservatives are more critically important in the neonate in whom a double-volume washout is being undertaken than in an adult who is receiving 450 ml blood-preservative mixture to be diluted in a total 5 L or more.

Heparinized blood contains no added glucose. Moreover, the heparin, by raising the free fatty acid levels, contributes to the hypoglycemic potential of the transfusion blood, so that under some circumstances (e.g., severe Rh incompatibility with hyperinsulinism) its use would be contraindicated unless a concomitant IV glucose infusion is administered to prevent and/or treat hypoglycemia (89). With citrated blood, acid citrate dextrose, or citrate phosphate dextrose, the added dextrose yields a blood-preservative mixture containing as much as 300 mg per 100 mg glucose. In this situation, although immediate hypoglycemia is not a problem, the high glucose load may result in a reactive insulin response. This response lags behind the glucose infusion, so that when the glucose "bolus" is suddenly terminated at the end of the exchange procedure, a state of hyperinsulinism ensues. Studies documenting this occurrence have shown a precipitous 2 h postexchange fall in blood glucose to levels below that present before undertaking the exchange procedure (90). Once again, the severely Rh-affected neonate is at greatest risk, but even mildly affected and nonerythroblastotic neonates who undergo an exchange transfusion may respond in such a manner. Recognition of this possibility should lead to its detection and treatment.

C. Beckwith-Wiedemann Syndrome

In 1964, Beckwith and associates described a syndrome characterized by omphalocele, muscular macroglossia, and visceromegaly (91). Wiedemann almost simultaneously described a similar clinical picture in three siblings (92). The etiology of the syndrome remains unclear. Pathologically, islet cell hyperplasia of the pancreas has been demonstrated in these neonates. It was subsequently shown that hypoglycemia may be an associated metabolic component of this syndrome, occurring in approximately 50% of the cases reported, with hyperinsulinism responsible for both the hypoglycemia and the somatic and visceral growth abnormalities. The hypoglycemia is ultimately self-limiting but may be protracted and difficult to control. In a patient with resistant hypoglycemia and hyperinsulinism, Schiff and coworkers (93) were ultimately able to achieve adequate control of glucose levels with a combination of Sus-phrine (epinephrine, aqueous suspension, Cooper Laboratories, Inc.) and diazoxide therapy that suppressed the release of basal and postprandial insulin. The neonate presented at birth with an umbilical hernia, macroglossia, and hepatosplenomegaly, as well as hyperinsulinism and severe, persistent hypoglycemia. Normal glucose control was achieved by 1 month of age. At 6 months, somatic growth was normal and hepatosplenomegaly had receded but the macroglossia was still present. At 2 years of age growth was normal, and the tongue, although still large, could be kept within the mouth without evidence of malocclusion.

D. Nesidioblastosis, Islet Cell Adenomas and Adenomatosis

Although rare, nesidioblastosis (94–96), discrete islet cell adenoma (97,98), or adenomatosis (99,100) has been reported in neonates and successfully treated. Hyperinsulinism without other apparent cause and resistant hypoglycemia should raise these rare but real possibilities. Preoperative confirmation may be sought by means of regular gastrointestinal radiographic studies, peritoneal air insufflation, abdominal angiography, and/or ultrasound examination, but surgical exploration may be necessary as a definitive diagnostic as well as therapeutic measure.

Soltész et al. reported 18 children with hyperinsulinemic hypoglycemia born to nondiabetic mothers (101). Within 3 days of birth, 13 presented, 3 by 20 months, and 2 aged 9 years. The diagnosis was established by an altered insulin-glucose ratio with corresponding low ketone body levels and lactate, alanine, and glycerol concentrations as well. The subjects required increased rates of glucose administration of between 9 and 25 mg/kg/minute and had an increased glucose disappearance rate of KG $7.6 \pm 0.06\%$. The clinical course was quite variable: 4 cases had transient hyperinsulinemia; 2 responded to diazoxide; 2 required both diazoxide and partial pancreatectomy; 2 responded to surgical excision of an isolated adenoma; 5 required total pancreatectomy for nesidioblastosis; and 2 were secondary to drug administration. In this series, a heterogeneity existed in the clinical course of this condition.

Aynsley-Green et al. evaluated plasma proinsulin and C peptide concentrations in 5 children presenting with severe hyperinsulinemic hypoglycemia (102). Data were compared with those from 13 normal neonates; 3 neonates and a 9 year old required partial or total pancreatectomy. All evidenced elevated proinsulin concentrations and had elevated C peptide concentrations as well, given the level of glucose concentration present (normal range for normoglycemia but elevated for hypoglycemia). The authors concluded that the insulin, proinsulin, C peptide concentration profile does not provide a reliable indicator for the pathologic underlying mechanism.

W'uthrich et al. reported two siblings who had persistent neonatal hyperinsulinemic hypoglycemia who were successfully treated with diazoxide at a dose of 10 mg/kg/day for 8 and 1 years, respectively, without the necessity for surgery (103).

Others have suggested that the diagnosis of hypoglycemic hyperinsulinemia may be transmitted as an autosomal recessive disorder with the report of seven pedigrees involving 21 cases (104).

Bruining et al. reported normalization of glucose homeostasis by utilization of a long-acting somatostatin analog, SMS 201-995, in a neonate with nesidioblastosis (105). Because glucose infusions were unable to maintain euglycemia ≥ 36 mg/dl, SMS 201-995 was utilized. Coincident with its use, insulin concentration fell and clinically apparent seizures diminished. As in other cases, a subtotal pancreatectomy was performed for the diagnosis of nesidioblastosis.

Glaser et al. studied six neonates with persistent hypoglycemia secondary to hyperinsulinemia who were treated with the somatostatin analog SMS 201-995 (106). Effective control using the drug alone was achieved in five of six neonates with administration of 10–40 μg/kg/day given by subcutaneous infusion. Most subsequently required subtotal pancreatectomy, but in one case long-term therapy with the drug alone achieved the therapeutic responses necessary to maintain euglycemia.

Nesidioblastosis may be noted in normal tissue and is not the morphologic hallmark of hyperinsulinemic hypoglycemia (107). The authors suggested the term "nesidiodysplasia," which includes in the diagnosis increased, maldistributed, malregulated, or malprogrammed endocrine and cells associated with the endocrine abnormality.

Spitz et al. have emphasized the need for early surgical intervention in infants who demonstrate hyperinsulinemia associated with hypoglycemia unresponsive to vigorous medical management. They suggested this is necessary to avoid the sequela of mental retardation, which may be present by the time the diagnosis is confirmed (108).

E.   β-Sympathomimetic Administration to the Mother in Premature Labor

Reports have described the potential for hypoglycemia after β-sympathomimetic tocolytic therapy, which is being used increasingly to inhibit the premature onset of labor. A possible explanation of the relationship involves increased pancreatic secretion of insulin in response to a specific glucose concentration (109,110). A prospective double-blind study of 35 patients in preterm labor with and without ruptured membranes was conducted. Leake et al. evaluated the neonatal metabolic and cardiovascular effects of maternal ritodrine administration to the mother (111). Patients had either received intravenous and/or oral ritodrine or a placebo. The shortest time from drug administration to delivery was 6 h. No differences were noted in the ritodrine versus the control groups relative to glucose and cardiovascular determinations. The authors concluded that chronic oral administration did not significantly affect the neonate.

These results were confirmed by a review of 30 premature infants whose gestational ages were 27–36 weeks and were compared with results in a matched control group of 37 premature infants whose mothers did not receive either control or ritodrine. However, only a 30 minute postdelivery sample was evaluated (112). In an investigation of the etiology of the clinical situation, a neonatal lamb model was used to evaluate the drug (113). Administration of ritodrine produced both increased insulin secretion from the β cell and glucose production from the liver. It follows that the presence of clinical hypoglycemia depends on the time of administration before delivery.

F.   Hypoglycemia Following Umbilical Artery Catheter Placement

Another cause of relative hyperinsulinism was reported secondary to malposition of an umbilical artery catheter. In a neonate requiring supplemental oxygen because of increasing respiratory distress, hypoglycemia was relieved only when a "high" catheter was repositioned from T11–12 to L4. Following repositioning of the catheter, the child became euglycemic (114). Malik and Wilson reported two neonates who developed hyperinsulinism secondary to malposition of the umbilical arterial catheter. Repositioning resulted in cessation of the hyperinsulinemia (115). Puri et al. reported the association of neonatal hypoglycemia associated with position of an umbilical arterial catheter between thoracic vertebrae 8 and 9, which is the normal position. In this report, the catheter was moved and neonatal hypoglycemia resolved (116). Three neonates were reported whose catheter were placed between thoracic vertebrae 8 and 10. They were noted to have hypoglycemia that responded to catheter withdrawal to lumbar region 3–4. The authors speculated that the cause was a high streaming of glucose to the celiac axis. The mechanism of the hypoglycemia was postulated to be excessive insulin secretion following infusion into the celiac axis (117). This was studied using a neonatal lamb model, and the clinical suspicion was confirmed. The mechanism was thought to be decreased production of hepatic glucose secondary to the presumed increased portal insulin following high catheter placement (118).

Jacob and Davis studied differences in serum glucose concentrations from different extremities in neonates with an umbilical arterial catheter through which dextrose was being infused. Neonates without a catheter had no differences in simultaneous capillary glucose concentrations, obtained from both lower extremities, but neonates with catheters did. Interestingly, neonates with a high catheter did not. As expected, the highest values were in those extremities into which the catheter was placed. This is another study pointing out the heterogeneity possible in glucose determinations depending on the location from which the blood is taken (119).

G.   Hypoglycemia Following Maternal Ethanol Consumption

Finally, the association of neonatal hypoglycemia and maternal ethanol ingestion has been reported. Singh et al. evaluated glucose metabolism in neonatal rats exposed to maternal ethanol ingestion (120). Blood glucose concentration, liver glycogen, and plasma insulin concentrations were decreased in ethanol-treated mothers, as was liter size and average fetal body weight. The pups from ethanol-fed mothers evidenced hypoglycemia and hypoinsulinemia. Within 1 h after birth, an elevation in blood glucose concentration was followed by a decline to hypoglycemic concentrations. Liver glycogen stores were reduced and were quickly mobilized. The hypoglycemic tendency in pups of ethanol-treated mothers disappeared after 4 days.

Witek-Janusek examined the effect of maternal ethanol ingestion on the maternal and neonatal glucose balance in a rat model (121). Controls included an isocaloric liquid pair-fed diet or ad libitum rat chow. Blood for glucose concentration and liver was sampled on days 21 and 22, and pups were studied up to 24 h after birth. Ethanol not only depressed maternal liver glycogen stores but also glycogen in the neonatal liver. Ethanol had no effect on plasma insulin concentrations. Postnatal hypoglycemia could be observed following maternal ethanol ingestion. Singh et al. evaluated the combined effect of chronic ethanol ingestion in pregnant rats and three offspring (122). Fetal body weight and liver weight were reduced in fetuses of alcohol-fed mothers. Blood glucose concentrations were also lower, as was liver glycogen.

H. Other Causes of Hyperinsulinism

Isolated instances have been reported that mimic the problem of insulin excess and resultant hypoglycemia. Zucker and Simon reported symptomatic neonatal hypoglycemia in association with maternal administration of chlorpropamide (123). This resulted in stimulation of the maternal as well as the fetal β cells. Teratogenicity of the drug is a concern, so that its use is limited, especially because it provides poor control of glucose for the management of diabetes in pregnancy. Benzothiazide (thiazide) diuretics have been implicated in producing insulin secretion (124). It has been suggested that these drugs produce elevated maternal blood glucose levels and result in stimulation of the fetal islets with subsequent neonatal hypoglycemia. There is a report of an neonate in whom hypoglycemia may have been caused by an insulin-releasing substance, possibly from the gut (125).

Hypoglycemia has been noted in individuals who are sensitive to leucine. This amino acid, among others, is known to be associated with increased insulin release and may be seen following ingestion of milk (126). Recently, a fourth defect of leucine metabolism, 3-hydroxy-3-methyl glutaryl CoA lyase deficiency, was reported. Hypoglycemia was noted, along with a characteristic excretory pattern of organic acids, but the exact mechanism resulting in the hypoglycemia was not apparent (127).

Neonatal hypoglycemia has followed administration of salicylates, the suggested mechanism being an uncoupling of mitochondrial oxidative phosphorylation (128). The association of congenital adrenal hyperplasia and hypoglycemia has also been recorded (129). Souto et al. studied the effect of equivalent doses of insulin on the adrenal medulla of neonatal and adult rats (130). Glycemia decreased to 33% of the control values in the adult; an equivalent dose of insulin to the neonate decreased glycemia to about 50%. Morphologic evaluation

of the adrenal medulla paralleled the metabolic data. The authors speculated that immaturity of the adrenal chromaffin tissue may be present in the neonate, which is involved in hypoglycemic catecholamine counterregulation.

Actavia-Loria et al. reported a survey of the frequency of hypoglycemia in 165 children who had primary adrenal insufficiency (131). A total of 118 had congenital adrenal hyperplasia, 47% had Addison's disease, and 18% had hypoglycemia. One-half of the episodes were in the neonatal period. The episodes of hypoglycemia were isolated in 13 children, congenital adrenal hyperplasia in 4 neonates, and with 11β-OH deficiency in 1 male. Mechanistically, a significant correlation was noted between plasma glucose concentration and cortisol concentration during the episodes of hypoglycemia.

Hypoglycemia has been noted secondary to indomethacin therapy in premature neonates with patent ductus arteriosus. Unfortunately, the proposed mechanism of indomethacin-mediated lack of prostaglandin inhibition of insulin release was not confirmed because there were no significant changes in plasma insulin concentration (132).

VII. EVALUATION OF THE NEONATE WITH HYPOGLYCEMIA

As noted with other diagnostic dilemmas in neonatology, a detailed maternal history and thorough physical examination are required to determine the probable etiology of neonatal hypoglycemia. Maternal history, including family history of diabetes or other glucose intolerance, drug ingestion (chlorpropamide, benzothiazide diuretics, salicylates, and/or ethanol), blood group incompatibility, preeclampsia or pregnancy-induced hypertension, and the rate of dextrose administered to the mother during labor, should alert the physician to the potential etiology (mechanism) of the observed hypoglycemia.

A thorough physical examination of the neonate indicates whether the neonate is AGA, SGA, or LGA, as well as the gestational age. The appearance of the infant of the well-controlled diabetic mother of classes A, B, and C can usually be differentiated from that of the infant of a class D, E, or F mother (who may be SGA). The neonate with Beckwith-Wiedemann is usually obvious, with evidence of a protuberant tongue, umbilical hernia, and macrosomia. Prolonged jaundice and cataracts are suggestive of galactosemia, as are reducing substances in the urine; unexplained hepatomegaly may indicate glycogen storage disease. Abnormalities that may indicate central defects include abnormal genitalia indicative of pituitary abnormalities and cleft lip and palate.

Appropriate laboratory evaluation should include evaluation of the following: glucose, insulin, growth hormone, cortisol, and thyroid function tests. Evaluation of pH, lactate, pyruvate, and ketones is indicated for glycogen storage disease. Blood is usually drawn when hypoglycemia is present or at a time following a fast of at least 3–4 h. Tolerance tests are reserved for confirmation of a suspected diagnosis, such as a glucagon tolerance test if glycogen storage disease is suspected.

VIII. TREATMENT OF HYPOGLYCEMIA

Treatment of neonatal hypoglycemia begins with identification of its potential in the neonate at risk, documentation of its existence by appropriate laboratory measurement (see earlier), and corrective measures.

Oral administration of nutrients is generally advocated as either 5% dextrose or formula but probably should be used only to maintain a glucose concentration already in the euglycemic range. With 6 mg/kg/minute used as the concentration of glucose required to maintain homeostasis, it is unreasonable to expect that oral feedings alone will provide adequate glucose intake in neonates determined to be hypoglycemic by laboratory evaluation. We advocate parenteral (intravenous) treatment of the hypoglycemic condition with a constant infusion pump to avoid fluctuations in the rate of infusion that would result in irregular rates of endogenous insulin release. Oral feedings should be initiated as tolerated. Repeated documentation of blood or plasma glucose concentration should be an integral part of the treatment of any neonate. The glucose infusions should be gradually reduced rather than abruptly terminated so that sudden reactive hypoglycemia as a result of "uncovered" hyperinsulinism is avoided. Once oral feedings are initiated, evaluation of the glucose concentration just before a subsequent feeding provides an analysis of the neonate's status.

Parenteral therapy should begin with 6 mg/kg/minute, followed by graded increases to achieve euglycemia with the minimal concentration of glucose required. A peripheral vein rather than an umbilical vessel is the preferred route of infusion (118). Other than in an emergency, however, rates greater than 15 mg/kg/minute should be given only when a central venous line is being used. Rates greater than 20 mg/kg/minute are probably contraindicated by either route. Acute administration of 25% glucose by a bolus infusion of up to 4 ml/kg, if required for the relief of acute symptoms (e.g., seizures), must be followed by parenteral infusion until the effect of the bolus infusion on acute pancreatic insulin release is no longer apparent. However, more popular currently is an infusion of 2 ml/kg of 10% dextrose in H_2O (200 mg/dl) given over 1 minute, followed by a continuous dextrose infusion of 8 mg/kg/minute (Fig. 4) (133).

Calculation of parenteral glucose therapy must include the actual concentration of glucose present in the administered fluids. A hydrated form of dextrose ($C_6H_{12}O_6 \cdot H_2O$; molecular weight 198) is used by most manufacturers to prepare the parenteral fluid so that the actual amount of glucose available is approximately 10% less (134). This is of particular concern when very low birth weight or severely hypoglycemic neonates are being treated.

There are increasing reports of the use of lipid infusion to assist in the prevention of hypoglycemia. Sann et al. evaluated the effect of oral lipid supplementation on the prevention of neonatal hypoglycemia in 28 low birth weight neonates whose mean gestational age was 36 ± 1 weeks and whose birth weight was 1778 ± 230 g compared with a

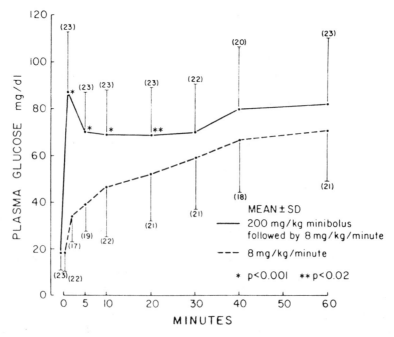

Figure 4 Plasma glucose concentrations in neonates treated with 200 mg/kg minibolus followed by 8 mg/kg/minute constant glucose infusion compared with plasma glucose concentration of neonates treated with constant infusion alone. SD, standard deviation. (From Lilien et al., Ref. 133.)

control group of 23 neonates who had comparable demographic data (135). Hypoglycemia ≤ 31 mg/dl occurred in 8 of 23 neonates in the control group versus 2 of 28 in the supplemented group receiving 2.9 g/day of a solution containing 67% medium-chain triglycerides. Prospectively this study showed that lipid supplementation can prevent the occurrence of hypoglycemia in the low birth weight neonate.

Treatment with a number of specific agents is indicated when parenteral therapy above 15 mg/kg/minute is not effective in maintaining euglycemia. Corticosteroids have been shown to be effective in the therapy of hypoglycemia. Although several glucose-producing reactions are enhanced by the steroids, the major effect is probably that of gluconeogenesis from noncarbohydrate (protein) sources and decreased peripheral glucose utilization. Hydrocortisone is given at a dose of 5 mg/kg/day either intravenously or orally every 12 h, or prednisone is used at a dose of 2 mg/kg/day orally. As with all forms of therapy, gradual diminution of the dosage administered, in concert with decreasing parenteral concentrations of glucose and increasing oral intake of nutrients, should allow success in weaning.

The use of glucagon provides a highly effective method of releasing glycogen from the liver and can indeed be a therapeutic means of assessing whether the liver contains adequate stores. Its failure in some growth-retarded neonates is considered evidence of a lack of hepatic glycogen stores. In the infant of the diabetic mother, there is often a failure to respond to the usual doses (30 μg/kg), despite the presence of more than adequate hepatic glycogen stores. These neonates frequently respond to higher doses (300 μg/kg) with a prolonged and sustained hyperglycemia, so that the higher dose may well be used as initial therapy. Because glucagon may stimulate insulin release, its administration in all probability should be accompanied by a intravenous glucose infusion.

Like glucagon, epinephrine is capable of promoting glycogen to glucose conversion, but in far smaller quantities. For this effect glucagon is the drug of choice. The hyperglycemic potential of epinephrine in blocking glucose uptake by peripheral muscle presupposes an adequate blood level initially and is of little practical benefit in the hypoglycemic state. Epinephrine is a powerful antiinsulin hormone, which explains its success as an effective antihypoglycemic agent in the infant of the diabetic mother as well as in other hyperinsulinemic neonates. The agent most commonly used is a 1:200 epinephrine in aqueous suspension (Sus-Phrine), which can be readily administered subcutaneously (93,136).

Diazoxide at 10–15 mg/kg/day probably exerts its effect by suppressing pancreatic insulin secretion, although some workers have suggested a direct effect on hepatic glucose production (137). The drug should be used only when other methods have failed (138).

Somatostatin, as described earlier, has been utilized to suppress insulin as well as glucagon secretion clinically and experimentally (105,106,139).

Surgical intervention is indicated when an islet cell adenoma or adenomatosis has been confirmed.

IX. SUMMARY

The neonate appears to be in a transitional stage of glucose homeostasis. Maturation of neonatal glucose homeostasis requires coordination of opposing hormonal, neural, and enzymatic controls and hormone receptors and the development of intermediary pathways, along with concerns about substrate availability in the presence of specific clinical morbidities.

The vulnerability of the neonate to carbohydrate disequilibrium has been described by the many examples of neonatal hypoglycemia enumerated. Much information in recent years has increased our understanding of the mechanism of these conditions in the neonate. Continued research on the physiologic and biochemical bases for these alterations in carbohydrate metabolism should further enhance our ability to understand, diagnose, and treat the neonate effectively.

ACKNOWLEDGMENT

We acknowledge the expert secretarial assistance of Ms. Patricia Knight.

REFERENCES

1. Cowett RM. Pathophysiology, diagnosis, and management of glucose homeostasis in the neonate. Curr Probl Pediatr 1985; 15:1–47.
2. Cowett RM. Utilization of glucose during total parenteral nutrition. In: Lebenthal E, ed. Total Parenteral Nutrition in Children: Indications, Complications and Pathophysiological Considerations. New York: Raven Press, 1986:17–27.
3. Ogata ES. Carbohydrate metabolism in the fetus and neonate and altered neonatal glucoregulation. Pediatr Clin North Am 1986; 33:25–45.
4. Pildes RS, Pyati SP. Hypoglycemia and hyperglycemia in tiny infants. Clin Perinatol 1986; 13:2351–2375.
5. Cowett RM, Stern L. Carbohydrate homeostasis in the fetus and newborn. In: Avery G, ed. Neonatology: Pathophysiology and Management of the Newborn, 3rd ed. Philadelphia: Lippincott, 1987:691–709.
6. Cowett RM, Schwartz R. Glucose homeostasis in the newborn. In: Stern L, Vert P, eds. Neonatal Medicine. New York: Masson, 1987:809–831.
7. Cowett RM. Carbohydrate metabolism in the premature and compromised infant. In: Lebenthal E, ed. Textbook of Gastroenterology and Nutrition in Early Childhood, 2nd ed. New York: Raven Press, 1989:311–326.
8. Ogata ES. Problems of glucose metabolism in the extremely-low birth weight infant. In: Cowett RM, Hay WW Jr, eds. The Micropremie: The Next Frontier. Report of the Ninety-Ninth Ross Conference on Pediatric Research. Columbus, OH: Ross Laboratories, 1990:55–63.
9. Cowett RM. Hypo and hyperglycemia in the newborn. In: Polin RA, Fox WW, eds. Neonatal and Fetal Medicine; Physiology and Pathophysiology. Philadelphia: W. B. Saunders, 1992:406–418.
10. Cornblath M, Schwartz R. Disorders of Carbohydrate Metabolism in Infancy, 3rd ed. Philadelphia: 1976.
11. Cowett RM. Neonatal glucose homeostasis. In: Cowett RM, ed. Principles of Perinatal Neonatal Metabolism. New York: Springer-Verlag. 1991:356–389.

12. Cornblath M, Reisner SH. Blood glucose in the neonate and its clinical significance. N Engl J Med. 1965; 273:378–381.

13. Srinivasan G, Pildes RS, Cattamanchi G, Voora S, Lilien L. Plasma glucose values in normal neonates: a new look. J Pediatr 1986; 109:114–117.

14. Heck LJ, Erenberg A. Serum glucose levels in the term neonate during the first 48 hours of life. Pediatr Res 1987; 110:119–122.

15. Koh TH, Aynsley-Green A, Tarbit M, Eyre JA. Neural dysfunction and hypoglycemia. Arch Dis Child. 1988; 63: 1353–1358.

16. Pildes RS. Neonatal hyperglycemia. J Pediatr 1986; 109:905–907.

17. Dweck HS, Cassady G. Glucose intolerance in infants of very low birth weight. I. Incidence of hyperglycemia in infants of birth weights 1,100 grams or less. Pediatrics 1974; 53:189–195.

18. Zarif M, Pildes RS, Vidyasagar D. Insulin and growth hormone responses in neonatal hyperglycemia. Diabetes 1976; 25:428–433.

19. Cowett RM, Oh W, Pollak A, Schwartz R, Stonestreet BS. Glucose disposal of low birth weight infants: steady state hyperglycemia produced by constant intravenous glucose infusion. Pediatrics 1979; 63:389–396.

20. Stanley CA, Anday EK, Baker L, Delivoria-Papdopolous M. Metabolic fuel and hormone response to fasting in newborn infants. Pediatrics 1979; 64:613–619.

21. Frantz ID III, Medina G, Taeusch HW Jr. Correlation of Dextrostix values with true glucose in the range less than 50 mg/dl. J Pediatr 1975; 87:417–420.

22. Perelman RH, Gutcher GR, Engle MJ, MacDonald MJ. Comparative analysis of four methods for rapid glucose determination in neonates. Am J Dis Child 1982; 136:1051–1053.

23. Wilkins BH, Kaira D. Comparison of blood glucose test strips in the detection of neonatal hypoglycemia. Arch Dis Child 1982; 57:948–960.

24. Conrad PD, Sparks JW, Osberg I, Abrams L, Hay WW Jr. Clinical application of a new glucose analyzer in the neonatal intensive care unit: comparison with other methods. J Pediatr 1989; 114:281–287.

25. Lin HC, Maguire C, Oh W, Cowett RM. Accuracy and reliability of glucose reflectance meters in the high risk neonate. J Pediatr 1989; 115:998–1000.

26. Holtrop PC, Madison KA, Kiechle FL, Karcher RE, Batton DG. A comparison of chromagen test strip (Chemstrip bG) and serum glucose values in newborns. Am J Dis Child 1990; 144:183–185.

27. Grazaitis DM, Sexton WR. Erroneously high Dextrostix values caused by isopropyl alcohol. Pediatrics 1980; 66:221–223.

28. Butler LA, Karp T, McCance KL, Ward RM. Neonatal glucose determinations obtained from an umbilical artery catheter: evaluation for accuracy using an in vitro model. Neonatal Netw 1993; 12:31–35.

29. Cowett RM, D'Amico LB. Capillary (heelstick) versus venous blood sampling for the determinations of glucose concentration in the neonate. Biol Neonate 1992; 62:32–36.

30. Shelley HJ, Bassett JM. Control of carbohydrate metabolism in the fetus and newborn. Br Med Bull 1975; 31:37–43.

31. Cornblath M, Schwartz R, Aynsley-Green A, Lloyd JK. Hypoglycemia in infancy: the need for a rationale definition. Pediatrics 1990; 85:834–837.

32. Fluge G. Clinical aspects of neonatal hypoglycemia. Acta Paediatr Scand 1974; 63:826–832.

33. Gutberlet RL, Cornblath M. Neonatal hypoglycemia revisited, 1975. Pediatrics 1976; 58:10–17.

34. Milner RDG. Annotation—neonatal hypoglycemia. A critical appraisal. Arch Dis Child 1972; 47:679–682.

35. Senior B. Current concepts. Neonatal hypoglycemia. N Engl J Med 1973; 289:790–793.

36. Cornblath M, Odell GB, Levin EY. Symptomatic neonatal hypoglycemia associated with toxemia of pregnancy. J Pediatr 1959; 55:545–562.

37. Raivio KO, Hallman N. Neonatal hypoglycemia. Occurrence of hypoglycemia in patients with various neonatal disorders. Acta Paediatr Scand 1968; 57:517–521.

38. Lubchenco LO, Bard H, Incidence of hypoglycemia in newborn infants classified by birth weight and gestational age. Pediatrics 1971; 47:831–838.

39. deLeeuw R, deVries IL. Hypoglycemia in small for dates newborn infants. Pediatrics 1976; 58:18–22.

40. Koivisto M, Jouppila P. Neonatal hypoglycemia and maternal toxaemia. Acta Paediatr Scand 1974; 63:743–749.

41. Holtrop PC. The frequency of hypoglycemia in full term large and small for gestational age newborn. Am J Perinatol 1993; 10:150–154.

42. Kliegman R. Alterations of fasting glucose and fat metabolism in intrauterine growth retarded newborn dogs. Am J Physiol 1989; 256:E380–385.

43. Economides DL, Proudler A, Nicolardes KH. Plasma insulin in appropriate and small for gestational age fetuses. Am J Obstet Gynecol 1989; 160:1091–1094.

44. Bussey ME, Finley S, LaBarbera A, Ogata ES. Hypoglycemia in the newborn growth retarded rat delayed phosphaenol pyruvate carbosy kinase induction despite increased glucagon availability. Pediatr Res 1985; 19:363–367.

45. Haymond MW, Karl IE, Pagliara AS. Increased gluconeogenic substrate in the small gestation age infant. N Engl J Med 1974; 291:322–328.

46. Williams PR, Fiser RH Jr, Sperling MA, Oh W. Effects of oral alanine feeding of blood glucose, plasma glucagon, and insulin concentrations in small for gestational age infants. N Engl J Med 1975; 292:612–614.

47. Reisner SH, Aranda JV, Colle E, et al. The effect of intravenous glucagon on plasma amino acids in the newborn. Pediatr Res 1973; 7:184–191.

48. Carter PE, Lloyd DJ, Duffty P. Glucagon for hypoglycemia in infants small for gestational age. Arch Dis Child 1988; 63:1264–1266.

49. Mestyan MJ, Schultz K, Soltesz G, Horvath M. The metabolic effects of glucagon infusion in normoglycemic and hypoglycemic small for gestational age infants. Changes in plasma amino acids. Acta Paediatr Acad Sci Hung 1976; 17:245–253.

50. Sperling MA, Grajwer L, Leake RD, Fisher DA. Effects of somatostatin (SRIF) infusion on glucose homeostasis in newborn lambs: evidence for a significant role of glucagon. Pediatr Res 1977; 11:962–967.

51. Salle BL, Ruiton-Ugliengo A. Effects of oral glucose and protein load on plasma glucagon and insulin concentrations in small for gestational age infants. Pediatr Res 1977; 11:108–112.

52. Cowett RM, Susa JB, Oh W, Schwartz R. Glucose kinetics in glucose infused small for gestational age infants. Pediatr Res 1984; 18:74–79.

53. Flecknell PA, Wootton R, Royston JP, John M. Glucose homeostasis in the newborn: effects of an intravenous glucose infusion in normal and intrauterine growth retarded neonatal piglets. Biol. Neonate 1987; 52:205–215.

54. Ogata ES, Paul RI, Finley SL. Limited maternal field availability due to hyperinsulinemia retards fetal growth and development in the rat. Pediatr Res 1987; 22:432–437.

55. Sann L, Morel Y, Lasne Y. Effect of hydrocortisone on intravenous glucose tolerance in small for gestational age infants. Helv Paediatr Acta 1983; 38:475–482.

56. Collins JE, Leonard JV, Teale D, et al. Hyperinsulinemic

hypoglycemia in small for dates babies. Arch Dis Child 1990; 65:1118–1120.

57. Beard AG, Panos TC, Marasigan BV. Perinatal stress and the premature neonate. Effect of fluid and caloric deprivation on blood glucose. J Pediatr 1966; 68:329–343.

58. Beard AG. Neonatal hypoglycemia. J Perinat Med 1975; 3:219–225.

59. Tejani N, Lipshitz F, Harper RG. The responses to an oral glucose load during convalescence from hypoxia in newborn infants. J Pediatr 1979; 94:792–796.

60. Collins JE, Leonard JV. Hyperinsulinism in asphyxiated and small for dates infants with hypoglycemia. Lancet 1984; 1:311–313.

61. Schultz K, Soltész G. Transient hyperinsulinemia in asphyxiated newborn infants. Acta Paediatr Hung 1991; 31:47–52.

62. Jansen RD, Hayden MK, Ogata ES. Effects of asphyxia at birth on postnatal glucose regulation in the rat. J Dev Physiol 1984; 6:473–483.

63. Mann TP, Elliott RIK. Neonatal cold injury due to accidental exposure to cold. Lancet 1957; 1:229–234.

64. Schiff D, Stern L, Leduc J. Chemical thermogenesis in newborn infants: catecholamine excretion and the plasma nonesterified fatty acid response to cold exposure. Pediatrics 1966; 37:577–582.

65. Close WH, LeDividish J, Dulee PH. Influence of environmental temperature on glucose tolerance and insulin response in the newborn piglet. Biol Neonate 1985; 47:84–91.

66. Yeung CY. Hypoglycemia in neonatal sepsis. J Pediatr 1970; 77:812–817.

67. LaNaoue KF, Mason AD Jr, Daniels JP. The impairment of glucogenesis by gram negative infection. Metabolism 1968; 17:606–611.

68. Yeung CY, Lee VMY, Yeung CM. Glucose disappearance rate in neonatal infection. J Pediatr 1973; 83:486–489.

69. Daboyl JJ, Kartchmer W, Jones KL. Neonatal hypoglycemia caused by hypopituitarism in infants with congenital syphilis. J Pediatr 1993; 123:983–985.

70. Fitzgerald MJ, Goto M, Myers TF, Zeller WP. Early metabolic effects of sepsis in the preterm infant: lactic acidosis and increased glucose requirement. J Pediatr 1992; 121:951–955.

71. Shelley HJ. Glycogen reserves and their changes at birth and in anoxia. Br Med Bull 1972; 17:137–143.

72. Benzing G, Schubert W, Hug G, Kaplan S. Simultaneous hypoglycemia and acute congestive heart failure. Circulation 1969; 40:209–216.

73. Amatayakul O, Cumming GR, Haworth JC. Association of hypoglycemia with cardiac enlargement and heart failure in newborn infants. Arch Dis Child 1970; 45:717–720.

74. Haymond MW, Strauss AW, Arnold KJ, Bier DM. Glucose homeostasis in children with severe cyanotic congenital heart disease. J Pediatr 1979; 95:220–227.

75. Kerkering KW, Robertson LW, Kodroff MB, Mueller DG, Kirkpatrick BV. Grand round series: hypoglycemia and unilateral pulmonary edema in a newborn. Pediatrics 1980; 65:326–330.

76. Lundell KH, Sabel KG, Eriksson BD, Mellgren G. Glucose metabolism and insulin secretion in infants with symptomatic ventricular septal defect. Acta Paediatr Scand 1989; 78:620–626.

77. Vidnes J, Oyasaeter S. Glucagon deficiency causing severe neonatal hypoglycemia in a patient with normal insulin secretion. Pediatr Res 1977; 11:943–949.

78. Vidnes J, Sovik O. Gluconeogenesis in infancy and childhood. Studies on the glucose production from alanine in three cases of persistent neonatal hypoglycaemia. Acta Paediatr Scand 1976; 65:297–305.

79. Vidnes J, Sovik O. Gluconeogenesis in infancy and childhood. Deficiency of the extramitochondrial form of hepatic phosphoenolpyruvate carboxykinase in a case of persistent neonatal hypoglycemia. Acta Paediatr 1976; 65:307–312.

80. Howell RR, Williams JC. The glycogen storage diseases. In: Stanbury JB, Wyngarden JB, Fredrickson DS, et al., eds. The Metabolic Basis of Inherited Disease. New York: McGraw-Hill, 1983:141.

81. Pagliara AS, Karl IE, Keating JP, Brown BI, Kipnis DM. Hepatic fructose-1,6-diphosphatase deficiency: a cause of lactate acidosis and hypoglycemia in infancy. J Clin Invest 1972; 51:2115–2123.

82. Ralleson ML, Mukle AW, Zigrang WD. Hypoglycemia and lactate acidosis associated with fructos-1,6-diphosphatase deficiency. J Pediatr 1979; 94:933–936.

83. Levy HL, Hammersen G. Newborn screening for galactosemia and other galactose metabolic defects. J Pediatr 1978; 92:871–887.

84. Barrett CT, Oliver TK Jr. Hypoglycemia and hyperinsulinism in infants with erythroblastosis fetalis. N Engl J Med 1968; 278:1260–1263.

85. Molsted-Pedersen L, Trautner H, Jorgensen KR. Plasma insulin and K values during intravenous glucose tolerance test in newborn infants with erythroblastosis foetalis. Acta Paediatr Scand 1973; 62:11–16.

86. Oh W, Yap LL, D'Amodio MD. Hypoglycemia in severely affected Rh erythroblastotic infants (abstract). J Pediatr 1969; 74:813.

87. Schiff D, Lowy C. Hypoglycemia and excretion of insulin in urine in hemolytic disease of the newborn. Pediatr Res 1970; 4:280–285.

88. Katz CM, Taylor PM. Incidence of low birth weight in children with severe mental retardation. Am J Dis Child 1967; 114:80–90.

89. Schiff D, Aranda JV, Chan G, Colle E, Stern L. Metabolic effects of exchange transfusions. Effect of citrated and of heparinized blood on glucose, non-esterified fatty acids, 2-(4-hydroxybenzeneazo)benzoic acid binding and insulin. J Pediatr 1971; 78:603–609.

90. Schiff D, Aranda JC, Colle E, Stern L. Metabolic effects of exchange transfusion. Delayed hypoglycemia following exchange transfusion with citriated blood. J Pediatr 1971; 79:589–593.

91. Beckwith JB, Wang CI, Donel GN. Hyperplastic fetal visceromegaly with macroglossia, omphalocele, cytomegaly of adrenal fetal cortex, postnatal somatic gigantism, and other abnormalities. Newly recognized syndrome (abstract 41). Proc Am Pediatr Soc Seattle, June 16–18, 1964.

92. Wiedemann HR. Complexe malformatif familiale avec hernie ombilicale et macroglossie—un syndrome nouveau? J Genet Hum 1964; 13:223.

93. Schiff D, Colle EC, Wells D, Stern L. Metabolic aspects of the Beckwith-Wiedemann syndrome. J Pediatr 1973; 82:258–267.

94. Heitz PU, Kloppel G, Hacki WH, Polak M, Pearse AG. Nesidioblastosis: the pathologic basis of persistent hyperinsulinemic hypoglycemia in infants. Diabetes 1977; 26:637–642.

95. Schwartz SS, Rich BH, Lucky AW, et al. Familial nesidioblastosis: severe neonatal hypoglycemia in two families. Pediatrics 1979; 95:44–53.

96. Woo D, Scopes JW, Polak JM. Idiopathic hypoglycemia in situ with morphological evidence of nesidioblastosis of the pancreas. Arch Dis Child 1976; 51:528–531.

97. Baerentsen H. Case report: neonatal hypoglycemia due to an islet cell adenoma. Acta Paediatr Scand 1973; 62:207–210.

98. Burst NRM, Campbell JR, Castro A. Congenital islet cell

adenoma causing hypoglycemia in a newborn. Pediatrics 1971; 47:605–610.

99. Habbick BJ, Cram RW, Miller KR. Neonatal hypoglycemia resulting from islet cell adenomatosis. Am J Dis Child 1977; 131:210–212.

100. Gruppuso PA, DeLuca F, O'Shea PA, Schwartz R. Near total pancreatectomy for hyperinsulinism. Spontaneous remission of resultant diabetes. Acta Paediatr Scand 1985; 74:311–315.

101. Soltész G, Jenkins PA, Aynsley-Green A. Hyperinsulinemic hypoglycemia in infancy and childhood: a practical approach to diagnosis and medical treatment based on experience of 18 cases. Acta Paediatr Hung 1984; 25:319–332.

102. Aynsley-Green A, Jenkin P, Tronier B, Heding LG. Plasma proinsulin and C peptide concentrations in children with hyperinsulinemic hypoglycemic. Acta Paediatr Scand 1984; 73:359–363.

103. W'uthrich C, Schubiger G, Zuppinger K. Persistent neonatal hyperinsulinemia hypoglycemia in two siblings successfully treated with diazoxide. Helv Paediatr Acta 1986; 41:455–459.

104. Glaser B, Phillip M, Carml R, Lieberman E, Landau H. Persistent hyperinsulinemic hypoglycemia of infancy ("nesidioblastosis"): autosomal recessive inheritance in 7 pedigrees. Am J Med Genet 1990; 37:511–515.

105. Bruining GJ, Bosschaart AN, Aarsen RRS, Lamberts SW, Sauer PJJ, DelPozo E. Normalization of glucose homeostasis by a long acting somatostatin analog 201-995 in a newborn with nesidioblastosis. Acta Endocrinol Suppl (Copenh) 1986; 279:275–278.

106. Glaser B, Landau H, Smilouici A, Nesher R. Persistent hyperinsulinemic hypoglycemia of infancy: long term treatment with the somatostatin analogue sandostatin. Clin Endocrinol (Oxf) 1989; 31:71–80.

107. Gould UE, Mamoli VA, Dardi LE, Gould NS. Nesidiodysplasia and nesideoblastosis of infancy; structural and functional correlations with the syndrome of hyperinsulinemia hypoglycemia. Pediatr Pathol 1983; 1:7–31.

108. Spitz L, Bhargava RVC, Grant DB, Leonard JV. Surgical treatment of hyperinsulinemic hypoglycaemia in infancy and childhood. Arch Dis Child 1992; 67:201–205.

109. Epstein MF, Nicholls E, Stubblefield PG. Neonatal hypoglycemia after beta-sympathomimetic tocolytic therapy. J Pediatr 1979; 94:449–453.

110. Procianoy RS, Pinheiro CEA. Neonatal hyperinsulinism after short term maternal beta sympathomimetic therapy. J Pediatr 1982; 101:612–614.

111. Leake RD, Hobel CJ, Okada DM, Ross MG, Williams PR. Neonatal metabolic effects of oral ritodrine hypochloride administration. Pediatr Pharm 1983; 3:101–106.

112. Broide E, Bistritzer T, Liune M, Neuman M, Goldberg M, Aladjem M. The effect of prenatal administration of dexamethasone and Ritodrine on cord blood control and glucose concentrations in premature infants with respiratory distress syndrome. J Perinat Med 1992; 20:289–295.

113. Tenenbaum D, Cowett RM. The mechanisms of beta sympathomimetic action on neonatal glucose homeostasis in the lamb. J Pediatr 1985; 107:588–592.

114. Nagel JW, Sims JS, Aplin CE II, Westmark ER. Refractory hypoglycemia associated with a malpositioned umbilical artery catheter. Pediatrics 1979; 64:315–317.

115. Malik M, Wilson DP. Umbilical artery catheterization. A potential cause of refractory hypoglycemia. Clin Pediatr (Phila) 1987; 26:181–182.

116. Puri AR, Alkalay AL, Pomerance JJ, Neufeld ND, Thangavel M. Neonatal hypoglycemia associated with umbilical artery catheter positioned at eighth to ninth thoracic vertebrae. Am J Perinatol 1987; 4:195–197.

117. Carey BE, Zeilinger TC. Hypoglycemia due to high positioning of umbilical artery catheters. J Perinatol 1989; 9:407–410.

118. Cowett RM, Tenenbaum D, Fatoba O, Oh W. The effects of glucose infusion above the celiac axis in the newborn lamb. Biol Neonate 1985; 47:179–185.

119. Jacob J, Davis RF. Differences in serum glucose determinations in infants with umbilical artery catheters. J Perinatol 1988; 8:40–42.

120. Singh SP, Sayder AK, Singh SF. Effects of ethanol ingestion on maternal and fetal glucose homeostasis. J Lab Clin Med 1984; 104:176–184.

121. Wite-Janusek L. Maternal ethanol ingestion: effect on maternal and neonatal glucose balance. Am J Physiol 1986; 251: E178–184.

122. Singh SP, Snyder AK, Pullen GL. Fetal alcohol syndrome—glucose and liver metabolism in term rat fetus and neonate. Alcoholism 1986; 10:54–58.

123. Zucker P, Simon G. Prolonged symptomatic neonatal hypoglycemia associated with maternal chlorpropamide therapy. Pediatrics 1968; 42:824–825.

124. Senior B, Slone D, Shapiro S, Mitchell AA, Heinonen OP. Benzothiadiazides and neonatal hypoglycemia. Lancet 1976; 2:377.

125. Stern C. Idiopathic hypoglycemia. Proc R Soc Med 1973; 66:345–346.

126. Brown RE, Young RB. A possible role for the excrine pancreas in the pathogenesis of neonatal leucine sensitive hypoglycemia. Am J Dig Dis 1970; 15:65–72.

127. Schutgens RBH, Heymans H, Ketel A, et al. Lethal hypoglycemia in a child with a deficiency of 3-hydroxy-3-methyl glutaryl coenzyme A lyase. J Pediatr 1979; 94:89–91.

128. Pickering D. Neonatal hypoglycemia due to salicylate poisoning. Proc R Soc Med 1968; 61:1256.

129. Gemelli M, DeLuca R, Barberio G. Hypoglycemia and congenital adrenal hyperplasia. Acta Pediatr Scand 1979; 68:285–286.

130. Souto M, Piezzi Rs, Bianchi R. Effect of insulin on neonatal and adult adrenal medula in the rat. Acta Anat (Basel) 1985; 122:216–219.

131. Actavia-Loria E, Chaussain JL, Bougneres PF, Job JC. Frequency of hypoglycemia in children with adrenal insufficiency. Acta Endocrinol Suppl (Copen) 1986; 279:275–278.

132. Lilien LD, Srinivasan G, Yeh TF, Pildes RS. Decreased plasma glucose following indomethacin therapy in premature infants with patent ductus arteriosus. Pediatr Pharm 1985; 5:73–77.

133. Lilien LD, Pildes RS, Srinivasan G, Voora S, Yeh TF. Treatment of neonatal hypoglycemia with minibolus and intravenous glucose infusion. J Pediatr 1980; 97:295–298.

134. Cowett RM, Susa JB, Schwartz R, Oh W. Concentration of parenteral glucose solution. Pediatrics 1977; 59:791.

135. Sann L, Mousson B, Rousson M, Maire I, Bethenod M. Prevention of neonatal hypoglycemia by oral lipid supplementation in low birth weight infants. Eur J Pediatr 1988; 147:158–161.

136. McCann ML, Likly B. The role of epinephrine prophylactic therapy in infants of diabetic mothers. Proc Soc Pediatr Res 1967; 3:5.

137. Victorin LH, Thorell JI. Plasma insulin and blood glucose during long-term treatment with diazoxide for infant hypoglycemia. Case report. Acta Paediatr Scand 1974; 63:302–306.

138. Altszular N, Hampshire J, Moraru E. On the mechanism of diazoxide-induced hyperglycemia. Diabetes 1977; 26:931–935.

139. Cowett RM, Tenenbaum D. Hepatic response to insulin in control of glucose homeostasis in the neonatal lamb. Metabolism 1987; 36:1021–1026.

49

Hypoglycemia in the Infant and Child

Mark A. Sperling
University of Pittsburgh and Children's Hospital of Pittsburgh, Pittsburgh, Pennsylvania

I. INTRODUCTION

Glucose plays a central role in mammalian fuel economy. Its carbon serves as a source for energy storage in the form of glycogen, fat, and protein and as an immediate source of energy by providing 38 mol ATP during the aerobic oxidation of each mol glucose. It is particularly important for energy metabolism in brain, where it is usually the preferred substrate whose utilization accounts for all of brain O_2 consumption, 60–80% of hepatic glucose production in the adult, and 80–100% of glucose production in the newborn (1–3). Glucose uptake by the brain occurs via a carrier-mediated, facilitated diffusion process that is glucose concentration dependent (3). The glucose carrier for the brain belongs to a family of glucose transporter molecules whose function is to translocate glucose across the cell membrane (4,5). The molecular basis for these actions and their biochemical regulation have been extensively investigated (4,5). Unlike their counterparts in muscle, glucose transporters in brain cells are not markedly influenced by insulin (Table 1). Therefore, neither glucose entry into brain cells nor its subsequent metabolism is dependent on insulin. To maintain blood glucose concentration and to prevent it from precipitously falling to levels that impair brain function, an elaborate system has evolved.

The defense against hypoglycemia is integrated by the autonomic nervous system and by hormones that, together, act in concert to enhance glucose production via enzymatic modulation of glycogenolysis and gluconeogenesis while limiting peripheral glucose utilization (6–12). In this context, hypoglycemia represents a defect in one or several of the complex interactions that normally integrate glucose homeostasis during feeding and fasting. As discussed in the preceding chapter, understanding of these processes is particularly important for neonates, in whom there is an abrupt transition from intrauterine life, characterized by dependence on transplacental glucose supply, to extrauterine life, characterized ultimately by the autonomous ability to maintain precise glucose balance. Hypoglycemia is an important cause of morbidity in infants and children.

II. DEFINITION

There is no direct correlation between blood glucose concentration and the classic clinical manifestations of hypoglycemia (10). However, the absence of clinical symptoms does not imply that glucose concentration is normal and has not fallen below some optimal level for maintaining brain metabolism. Hypoxemia and ischemia potentiate the role of hypoglycemia in causing brain damage that may permanently impair various aspects of neurologic development (1,10). Any value of blood glucose below 40 mg/dl should be viewed with suspicion and vigorously treated; with serum or plasma, values are generally 10–15% higher. In infants and children, a blood glucose concentration of less than 40 mg/dl (10–15% higher for serum or plasma) is considered to represent significant hypoglycemia (10,12).

III. SIGNIFICANCE AND SEQUELAE

In adults, metabolism by the brain accounts for some 80% of total basal glucose turnover. Studies of cerebral metabolism under in vivo conditions indicate that the brain of infants and children can utilize glucose at a rate in excess of 4–5 mg per 100 g brain weight per minute (13,14). Measurement of endogenous glucose production rate in infants and children using stable isotopes demonstrates values of 5–8 mg/kg body weight per minute (2,15). Thus, almost all endogenous glucose production in infants and young children can be accounted for by brain metabolism. Furthermore, there is a remarkable correlation between glucose production and estimated brain weight at all ages (2). In contrast, the correlation between glucose production and body weight demonstrates a

Table 1 Characterization of Glucose Transporters

| Nomenclature | | | | | |
Name	Numerical	Tissue distribution	Kinetic properties	Location of human gene	Regulation by insulin
HepG2	Glut 1	Many adult and fetal tissues, abundant in human red cells, placenta, brain microvessels	Erythrocyte: asymmetric carrier with exchange acceleration; $K_m \simeq 5{-}30$ mM (variable): V_{max} (influx) $< V_{max}$ (efflux)	$1p35 \to 31.3$	Zero to minimal
Liver	Glut 2	Liver, pancreatic β cells, kidney, intestine	Liver: simple, symmetric carrier; $K_m \simeq 60$ mM; intestine: asymmetric carrier; V_{max} (efflux) $< V_{max}$ (influx)	3q26	Zero to minimal
Fetal muscle, brain	Glut 3	Many adult and fetal tissues, abundant in placenta, brain, kidney	Exchange $K_m \simeq 10$ mM	12p13	Zero
Fat, muscle	Glut 4	White and brown fat, skeletal muscle, heart	Adipocyte: simple, symmetric carrier; $K_m \simeq 2{-}5$ mM	17p13	Dependent on insulin
Intestine	Glut 5	Jejunum, fat, kidney	Incompletely determined	1p31	Zero
Pseudogene (closely related to Glut 3)	Glut 6	Brain, jejunum, placenta, fat, kidney	Fails to encode a functional glucose transporter protein	$5q33 \to 35$	Zero
Liver endoplasmic reticulum type (closely related to Glut 2)	Glut 7	Liver microsomes	Translates into Glut 2 with an added COOH domain that provides endoplasmic reticulum retention	?	Zero to minimal

marked change in slope beyond 40 kg body weight, corresponding to the time when brain growth is completed (2). Because the brain grows most rapidly during the first year of life and the larger proportion of glucose turnover is utilized for brain metabolism, the major impact of hypoglycemia in infants and children is on retarding brain development and function. In the rapidly growing brain, glucose can also be a source of membrane lipids and protein synthesis, that is, structural proteins and myelination, important for normal brain maturation (1). Under conditions of hypoglycemia, these structural substrates may be broken down to a variety of energy-usable intermediates, such as lactate, pyruvate, amino acids, and ketoacids, which can support brain metabolism at the expense of brain growth (1). Although the capacity of the brain of infants and children to take up and oxidize ketone bodies is considerable (13,14,16), the capacity to produce ketone bodies may be especially limited with hyperinsulinemia, which acutely inhibits hepatic glucose output, lipolysis, and ketogenesis, thereby depriving the brain of alternative fuel sources (7,8). The deprivation of the brain's major energy source during hypoglycemia and the limited availability of alternative fuel sources during hyperinsulinemia (7,8,17) have predictable consequences on brain metabolism and growth: decreased brain oxygen consumption, increased breakdown of endogenous structural components to release amino acids and free fatty acid, and destruction of functional membrane integrity (1). All these factors may combine and lead to permanent impairment of brain growth and function (18,19). The potentiating effects of hypoxia may exacerbate brain damage, or indeed be responsible for it, when blood glucose values are not in the classic hypoglycemic range (1).

Thus, the major long-term sequelae of recurrent severe hypoglycemia are neurologic damage with the potential to result in mental retardation, recurrent seizure activity, or both (10,18,19). Subtle effects on personality and intellect are also possible but have not been clearly defined. Permanent neurologic sequelae are present in over one-half of patients with severe recurrent hypoglycemia below the age of 6 months, the period of most rapid brain growth (10). With severe cases, these sequelae may be reflected in pathologic brain changes characterized by atrophic gyri, reduced myelination in cerebral white matter, and atrophy in the cerebral cortex (1,10).

IV. SUBSTRATE, ENZYME, AND HORMONAL INTEGRATION OF GLUCOSE HOMEOSTASIS

In older infants and children, glucose homeostasis is maintained by glycogen breakdown in the immediate postfeeding period and by gluconeogenesis several hours after meals. The liver of a 10 kg child contains approximately 20–25 g glycogen, sufficient to meet glucose requirements of 4–6 mg/kg/minute for only 6–12 h. Beyond this time frame, hepatic gluconeogenesis must be activated. Both glycogenolysis and gluconeogenesis depend upon the metabolic pathway summarized in Figure 1. It should be apparent that defects in gluconeogenesis may not become manifest in infants until the

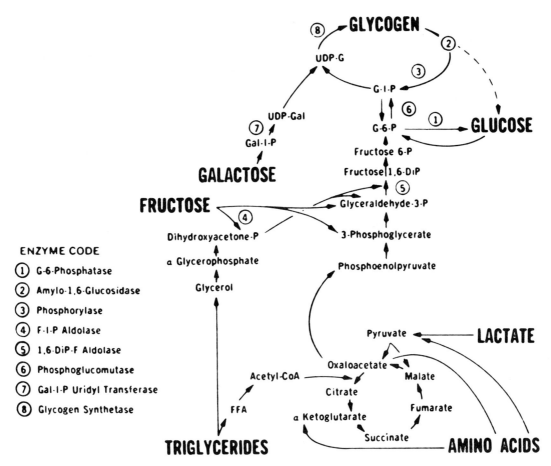

Figure 1 Metabolic pathways involved in glycogen synthesis and degradation and in gluconeogenesis. Key enzymes are designated by number.

practice of frequent feeding at 3–4 h intervals ceases and infants sleep through the night, an event usually accomplished by 3–6 months of age. The source of gluconeogenic precursors is derived primarily from muscle protein. The muscle bulk of infants and small children is substantially smaller relative to body mass than in adults but glucose requirements per unit of body mass are greater in children, so that the ability to compensate for glucose deprivation by gluconeogenesis is more limited in infants and children, as is the ability to withstand fasting for prolonged periods (20). The ability of muscle to generate alanine, the principal gluconeogenic amino acid, may also be limited, particularly in children with inborn errors of amino acid metabolism (21,22). Thus, during fasting in young children, blood glucose falls after 24 h, insulin concentrations fall appropriately to levels of less than 5–10 μU/ml, lipolysis and ketogenesis are activated, and ketones may appear in the urine (20,23).

The switch from glycogen synthesis during and immediately after meals to glycogen breakdown and later gluconeogenesis is governed by hormones, of which insulin is the key (24,25). The control of insulin secretion, its

metabolic effects, and its mechanisms of action are described elsewhere (25). For the present, it is important to emphasize that plasma insulin concentrations increase to peak levels of 50–100 μU/ml after meals, which serves to lower blood glucose through the activation of glycogen synthesis, enhancement of peripheral glucose uptake, and inhibition of gluconeogenesis. In addition, lipogenesis is stimulated whereas lipolysis and ketogenesis are curtailed. During fasting, plasma insulin concentrations fall to 5–10 μU/ml, and together with other hormonal changes, this results in the reversal of metabolic pathways (Fig. 1). Thus, glucose concentrations are maintained through the activation of glycogenolysis and gluconeogenesis, inhibition of glycogen synthesis, and activation of lipolysis and ketogenesis (24–27). It should be emphasized that a plasma insulin concentration of greater than 10 μU/ml, in association with a blood glucose concentration of 40 mg/dl or less, is clearly abnormal, indicating a hyperinsulinemic state and failure of the mechanisms that normally result in suppression of insulin secretion during fasting or hypoglycemia (24,27–29).

The hypoglycemic effects of insulin are opposed by the actions of several hormones whose concentration in plasma increases as blood glucose falls. These counterregulatory hormones are epinephrine, glucagon, growth hormone, and cortisol. Acting in concert, they increase blood glucose concentration by the following mechanisms:

1. Activation of glycogenolytic and gluconeogenic enzymes (glucagon and epinephrine)
2. Induction of gluconcogenic enzymes (glucagon and cortisol)
3. Inhibition of glucose uptake by muscle (epinephrine, growth hormone, and cortisol)
4. Mobilization from muscle of amino acids for gluconeogenesis (cortisol)
5. Activation of lipolysis providing glycerol for gluconeogenesis and fatty acids for ketogenesis (epinephrine, cortisol, growth hormone, and glucagon)
6. Inhibition of insulin release and promotion of growth hormone and glucagon secretion (epinephrine)

There is a hierarchic redundancy in the interaction of these counterregulatory hormones (27). Epinephrine and glucagon act quickly, each signaling its effects via activation of cyclic AMP. Deficiencies of glucagon, as in long-standing type I diabetes mellitus, can be largely compensated by an intact autonomic nervous system with appropriate α- and β-adrenergic signals. Conversely, autonomic failure can be largely compensated if glucagon secretion remains intact. Nevertheless, the defense against insulin-induced hypoglycemia is impaired by deficiency of either glucagon or catecholamine, so that hypoglycemia ensues quite rapidly (Fig. 2). Similarly, growth hormone deficiency can be partly compensated by intact cortisol secretion and vice versa. However, deficiency of either impairs the defense against insulin-induced hypoglycemia, although the decline in blood glucose is more gradual, reflecting the longer time course of the action of these hormones (Fig. 2).

Congenital or acquired deficiencies in these hormones may therefore result in hypoglycemia, which occurs when endogenous glucose production cannot be mobilized to meet energy needs in the postabsorptive state, that is, 8–12 h after meals or during fasting (Fig. 2). Concurrent deficiency of several hormones as in hypopituitarism may result in hypoglycemia that is more severe or appears earlier than with isolated hormone deficiencies.

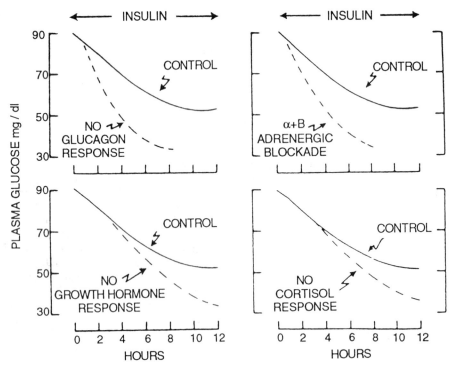

Figure 2 Contribution of counterregulatory hormones to insulin-induced hypoglycemia in healthy young adults. The top two panels illustrate the important roles of glucagon and catecholamines in countering hypoglycemia. Prevention of a glucagon response or a catecholamine response results in a steeper decline in blood glucose and more profound hypoglycemia that occurs within 4 h. The lower two panels illustrate the important roles of growth hormone and cortisol, whose contributions to countering hypoglycemia occurs later, that is, longer than 6 h. (Adapted from Gerich JE. Diabetes 1988; 37:1608–1617. With permission of the author and publisher. See text and references for details.

V. CLINICAL FEATURES

The clinical features of hypoglycemia are generally considered to fall into two categories. The first includes symptoms associated with the activation of the autonomic nervous system and epinephrine release, usually associated with a rapid decline in blood glucose, as illustrated in Table 2. The second category includes symptoms caused by decreased cerebral glucose utilization, usually associated with a slow decline in blood glucose or prolonged hypoglycemia, as also outlined in Table 2. Although these classic symptoms occur in older children, the symptoms of hypoglycemia in infants may be more subtle, as outlined in Table 3. Some of these symptoms may be so mild as to be clinically missed. In childhood, hypoglycemia may present as behavior problems, inattention, ravenous appetite, or seizures, as summarized in Table 4. At any pediatric age level, until proven otherwise, hypoglycemia should always be considered as a cause for an initial episode of convulsions.

Table 2 Symptoms of Spontaneous Hypoglycemia

Symptoms caused in part by activation of autonomic nervous system and epinephrine release (usually associated with rapid decline in blood glucose level)
  Sweating
  Shakiness, trembling
  Tachycardia
  Anxiety, nervousness
  Weakness
  Hunger
  Nausea, vomiting
Symptoms caused by decreased cerebral glucose and oxygen utilization (usually associated with slow decline in blood glucose level and/or severe or prolonged hypoglycemia)
  Headache
  Visual disturbances
  Lethargy, lassitude
  Restlessness, irritability
  Difficulty with speech and thinking, inability to concentrate
  Mental confusion
  Somnolence, stupor, prolonged sleep
  Loss of consciousness, coma
  Hypothermia
  Twitching, convulsions, "epilepsy"
  Bizarre neurologic signs
    Motor
    Sensory
  Loss of intellectual ability
  Personality changes
  Bizarre behavior
    Outburst of temper
    Psychologic disintegration
      Manic behavior
      Depression
      Psychoses
  Permanent mental or neurologic damage

Table 3 Symptoms of Hypoglycemia in Infancy

Cyanotic episodes
Apnea
"Respiratory distress"
Refusal to feed
Brief myoclonic jerks
Wilting spells
Convulsions
Somnolence
Subnormal temperature
Sweating

VI. CLASSIFICATION OF HYPOGLYCEMIA IN INFANTS AND CHILDREN

The classification outlined in Table 5 is based on the knowledge of the control of glucose homeostasis in infants and children as reviewed earlier.

A. Hyperinsulinemia

The majority of children with hyperinsulinemia causing hypoglycemia present in infancy (Chap. 49) (29–34). Like infants born to diabetic mothers, they may be macrosomic at birth, reflecting the anabolic effects of insulin in utero. There is no history, however, and no biochemical evidence of maternal diabetes. Insulin concentrations are inappropriately elevated at the time of documented hypoglycemia. Thus, when blood glucose concentration is less than 40 mg/dl, plasma insulin concentration should be less than 5 μU/ml and no higher than 10 μU/ml. In affected infants, however, plasma insulin concentrations at the time of hypoglycemia are commonly greater than 10 μU/ml. Macrosomic infants present with hypoglycemia from the first days of life (30). Infants with lesser degrees of hyperinsulinemia, however, may manifest hypoglycemia after the first few weeks to months, when the frequency of feedings has been decreased to permit the infant to sleep through the night and hyperinsulinemia prevents the mobilization of endogenous glucose (31,32). The more severe the hyperinsulinemia, the more rapid is the appearance of hypoglycemia after cessation of feeding or during fasting (31). Relatively common presenting symptoms

Table 4 Symptoms of Hypoglycemia in Childhood

Inattention
Staring or strabismus
Lethargy or somnolence
Behavior problems
Ravenous appetite
Convulsions

Table 5 Classification of Hypoglycemia in Infants and Children

Hyperinsulinemic states
  Nesidioblastosis
  B cell hyperplasia
  B cell adenoma
  Beckwith-Wiedemann syndrome
  Leucine sensitivity
Hormone deficiency
  Panhypopituitarism
  Isolated growth hormone deficiency
  ACTH deficiency
  Addison's disease
  Glucagon deficiency
  Epinephrine deficiency
Substrate limited
  Ketotic hypoglycemia
  Branched-chain ketonuria (maple syrup urine disease)
Glycogen storage disease
  Glucose-6-phosphatase deficiency
  Amylo-1,6-glucosidase deficiency
  Liver phosphorylase deficiency
  Glycogen synthetase deficiency
Disorders of gluconeogenesis
  Fructose-1, 6-diphosphatase deficiency
  Pyruvate carboxylase deficiency
  Phosphoenolpyruvate carboxykinase (PEPCK deficiency)
  Acute alcohol intoxication
  Salicylate intoxication
Disorders of fatty acid oxidation
  Carnitine deficiency; medium-chain and long-chain acyl-CoA
    dehydrogenase deficiency
  Valproic acid
Other enzyme defects
  Galactosemia: galactose-1-phosphate uridyltransferase
    deficiency
  Fructose intolerance: fructose-1-phosphate aldolase deficiency
Defects in glucose transporters

and signs include increasing demands for feeding, wilting spells, jitteriness, and frank seizures that occur between feeds or after progressively long period without food as occur at and after weaning. Such symptoms and signs should arouse strong suspicion for the possibility of hypoglycemia caused by some form of organic hyperinsulinism. Provocative tests with tolbutamide or leucine are not necessary in infants; hypoglycemia is invariably provoked through withholding feedings for several vigilant hours, permitting simultaneous measurement of glucose and insulin in the same sample at the time of clinically manifest hypoglycemia (Table 6) (31). Inspection of the data in Table 6 clearly demonstrates that those with hyperinsulinemia tend to present at a younger age, with a mean age at diagnosis of about 7½ months, whereas those with nonhyperinsulinemic causes tend to be diagnosed at much later ages. Similarly, glucose values at the time of

hypoglycemia tend to be significantly lower in those with hyperinsulinemia, although there is considerable overlap. The two striking differences between those with and without hyperinsulinemia are the marked differences in insulin values, mean insulin levels being 22.4 μU/ml in those presenting with hyperinsulinemia as opposed to only 5.8 μU/ml in those without hyperinsulinemia. There is some overlap in the ranges of insulin values observed, but the separation is generally sharp. The most striking difference, however, is the fasting time to hypoglycemia. Infants with hyperinsulinemia tend to develop hypoglycemia within 6 h or so of fasting, generally much more quickly than those without hyperinsulinemia, as evident in Table 6.

Once organic hyperinsulinemia has been established through concurrent measurement of glucose and insulin, the differential diagnosis rests between nesidioblastosis, β cell hyperplasia, and β cell adenoma (35,36). These three entities cannot be distinguished from the plasma levels of insulin alone (33). Although they represent a diffuse or localized abnormality in the pancreas, each is characterized by autonomous insulin secretion that is not appropriately reduced when blood glucose declines spontaneously or in response to provocative maneuvers, such as fasting (33). The autonomous behavior of insulin secretion, with intermittent spikes of release that are unrelated to the ambient glucose concentration, has been shown with islet cell adenomas in vitro. Celiac angiography, which reportedly has a success rate of 60–75% in localizing pancreatic endocrine tumors (adenoma or carcinoma) in adults, has only limited success in infants, in whom the nodules may be small and obscured by the normal rich vascularity. The chances of detecting a tumor "blush" during arteriography must therefore be balanced by the potential risk of vascular trauma in infants under 2 years (34). When present, however, a tumor blush may be helpful in localizing the tumor before surgery. Computed tomography and magnetic resonance imaging may be helpful in localizing a pancreatic adenoma, but the majority of patients have hyperplasia rather than a discrete tumor (24). The term "islet cell dysmaturation syndrome" has been used to encompass the spectrum of localized of diffuse disease (32,33). Thus, with nesidioblastosis, at least four of the cell types of normal islets can be identified within the pancreatic duct walls or scattered in the acinar tissue of single cells, cell clusters, disorganized miniislets, or microadenomas. The pancreatic content of insulin, glucagon, somatostatin, and pancreatic polypeptide is similar in these hypoglycemic infants and normal infants dying from other causes. Thus, secretion, not content, is abnormal (33–36).

Because the definitive diagnosis can be made only by histologic examination of removed tissue, surgical exploration is usually undertaken in *severely* affected neonates (37,38). Nearly total resection of some 85–90% of the pancreas is recommended in severe cases. Further resection of the remaining pancreas may occasionally be necessary if hypoglycemia recurs and cannot be controlled by medical measures, such as the use of long-acting somatostatin or diazoxide with cortisone (39–45). Surgery should be performed by experienced pediatric surgeons in medical centers

Table 6 Hypoglycemia in Infants and Children: Clinical and Laboratory Features

Group	Age at diagnosis (months)	Glucose (mg/dl)	Insulin (μU/ml)	Fasting time to hypoglycemia (h)
Hyperinsulinemia, $N = 12$				
Mean	7.4	23.1	22.4	2.1
SEM[a]	2.0	2.7	3.2	0.6
Nonhyperinsulinemia, $N = 16$				
Mean	41.8	36.1	5.8	18.2
SEM	7.3	2.4	0.9	2.9

[a]Standard error of the mean.
Source: Adapted from Antunes JD, Geffner ME, Lippe BM, et al. J Pediatr 1990; 116:105–108, with permission of the authors and publishers.

equipped to provide the necessary pre- and postoperative support in terms of diagnostic evaluation and management. When the diagnosis is established before 3 months of life, surgery is recommended as the initial approach to treatment. Frequent feedings coupled with pharmacologic agents, such as diazoxide, may, but usually do not, maintain blood glucose concentrations or adequately inhibit insulin release. The result is persistence of hypoglycemia with loss of precious time and the possibility of irreversible brain damage. If hypoglycemia first becomes manifest between 3 and 6 months of life, or later, a therapeutic trial using medical approaches with diazoxide, steroids, and frequent feedings can be attempted for up to 2–4 weeks. Failure to maintain euglycemia without undesirable side effects from the drugs prompts the need for surgery. Some success in suppressing insulin release and correcting hypoglycemia in patients with nesidioblastosis has been reported with the use of long-acting somatostatin, and the long-acting somatostatin analog has also been successful (34,40). Most cases of neonatal nesidioblastosis are sporadic, but occasionally familial forms appear to be inherited in an autosomal recessive manner (44). In these familial forms, recent studies suggest linkage to a gene on chromosome 11.

Before surgery, some patients have been successfully maintained, with a chronic intravenous glucose infusion via the subclavian vein complementing frequent feedings and somatostatin. In occasional patients with diffuse hyperplasia or nesidioblastosis, diazoxide has been effective in suppressing insulin release. The glycemic response is dose related and is reversible on discontinuation of therapy; doses usually range from 5 to 15 mg/kg/day. The side effects of this drug are frequent and include hirsutism, edema, hyperuricemia, electrolyte disturbances, advancement of bone age, IgG deficiency, and, rarely, hypertension (45).

Hypoglycemia associated with hyperinsulinemia is also seen in approximately 50% of patients with Beckwith-Wiedeman syndrome (46). This syndrome is characterized by macrosomia, microcephaly, macroglossia, visceromegaly, and omphalocele. Distinctive lateral or ear lobe fissures are present. Diffuse islet cell hyperplasia and nesidioblastosis both occur in those infants with hypoglycemia. The diagnostic

and therapeutic approach is therefore the same as discussed, although microcephaly and retarded brain development may occur independently of hypoglycemia (42,46). In addition, patients with Beckwith-Wiedeman syndrome have a predilection for eventually developing tumors, including Wilms' tumor, hepatoblastoma, and retinoblastoma.

Leucine-sensitive hypoglycemia does not appear to be diagnosed with the same degree of frequency as in previous years. As originally described, it was considered a subclass of children with idiopathic hypoglycemic in whom protein feeding, specifically leucine, triggered hypoglycemia attacks. Subsequently it was demonstrated that leucine-sensitive hypoglycemia was associated with excessive insulin secretion following leucine and that β cell hyperplasia, adenoma, and nesidioblastosis also demonstrate hyperinsulinemia in response to leucine, tolbutamide, and other provocative tests. Inasmuch as nesidioblastosis may not be diagnosed by a routine histologic examination of islets without employing insulin-specific staining techniques, including immunofluorescent techniques for islet hormones, many of the cases previously diagnosed as leucine sensitive might now be categorized as nesidioblastosis. As awareness of the latter has increased, diagnoses of leucine sensitivity have decreased. Similarly, as the range and precision of diagnostic tools have increased, few patients today are classified as having idiopathic hypoglycemia. Occasionally the diagnosis remains in doubt, because histologic examination of pancreatic tissue is not undertaken as a result of a satisfactory response to a low-leucine diet and diazoxide with or without additional glucocorticoids. In such instances, a functional hyperinsulinemia with leucine sensitivity serves as a descriptive term for patients who eventually outgrow their propensity for hypoglycemia at around 5–7 years of age. Nevertheless, in view of the similarity of excessive insulin response and documented islet cell hyperplasia in previous patients, it is likely that leucine-sensitive hypoglycemia is a variant of the so-called islet cell dysmaturity syndrome (33,35).

Beyond the first 6 months of life, hyperinsulinemic states are uncommon, and a window exists for several years until islet cell adenomas again reappear. Hyperinsulinemia caused by islet cell adenoma should be considered in any child 5 years or older presenting with hypoglycemia and its symptoms, as outlined in Tables 2 and 6. Fasting for 24–36 h usually provokes a hypoglycemic attack; coexistent hyperinsulinemia confirms the diagnosis, providing that factitious administration of insulin by the parents, a form of child abuse also known as Munchausen syndrome by proxy, has been excluded (47,48). Occasionally, the provocative tests may be required. Exogenously administered insulin can be distinguished from endogenous insulin by simultaneous measurement of C peptide concentration. If C peptide levels are elevated, endogenous insulin secretion is responsible for the hypoglycemia; if C peptide levels are low but insulin values are high, exogenous insulin has been administered, perhaps as a form of "child abuse" (49,50). Islet cell adenomas at this age are treated by surgical excision; familial multiple endocrine adenomatosis type I (Wermer syndrome) or type II should be considered possible associations (51). Antibodies to insulin or the insulin receptor may also be associated with hypoglycemia (52,53).

B. Endocrine Deficiency

Hypoglycemia associated with endocrine deficiency is usually a result of adrenal insufficiency with or without associated growth hormone deficiency. In panhypopituitarism, isolated adrenocorticotropic hormone (ACTH) or growth hormone deficiency, or combined ACTH deficiency plus growth hormone deficiency, the incidence of hypoglycemia is up to 20%. In infancy, patients with hypopituitarism may have hypoglycemia as their presenting feature; in males, a microphallus may provide a clue to coexistent deficiency of gonadotropin (54). Congenital hypopituitarism may be associated with a form of "hepatitis" and the syndrome of septooptic dysplasia (55,56). When adrenal disease is severely compromised, as in congenital adrenal hyperplasia caused by enzyme defects (57), adrenal hemorrhage, or congenital absence of the adrenals, disturbances in serum electrolytes with hyponatremia and hyperkalemia or ambiguous genitalia may provide diagnostic clues. In older children, failure of growth raises the possibility of growth hormone deficiency. Hyperpigmentation may provide the clue to Addison's disease with increased ACTH and its inherent MSH activity or adrenal unresponsiveness to ACTH caused by a defect in the adrenal receptor for ACTH (58). The frequent association of Addison's disease in childhood with hypoparathyroidism (hypocalcemia), chronic mucocutaneous moniliasis, and other endocrinopathies should be sought (59). Adrenoleukodystrophy should also be considered in the differential diagnosis of primary Addison's disease in children (60).

The etiology of hypoglycemia in cortisol-growth hormone deficiency may be decreased gluconeogenic enzymes with cortisol deficiency, increased glucose utilization caused by lack of the antagonistic effects of growth hormone on insulin action, and failure to supply endogenous gluconeogenic substrate in the form of alanine and lactate with compensatory breakdown of fat and generation of ketones. Thus, deficiency of these hormones results in reduced gluconeogen-

ic substrate with simulation of ketotic hypoglycemia (see later). Investigation of a child with hypoglycemia therefore requires exclusion of ACTH, cortisol, or growth hormone deficiency and, if diagnosed, its appropriate replacement with cortisol or growth hormone.

Epinephrine deficiency could theoretically be responsible for hypoglycemia (61,62). Urinary excretion of epinephrine has been diminished in some patients with spontaneous or insulin-induced hypoglycemia. Absence of pallor and tachycardia were also noted, suggesting that failure of catecholamine release as a result of a defect anywhere along the hypothalamic-autonomic-adrenomedullary axis is responsible for the hypoglycemia. However, this possibility has been challenged because of the rarity of hypoglycemia in patients with bilateral adrenalectomy, providing they receive adequate glucocorticoid replacement, and because diminished epinephrine excretion is found in normal patients with repeated insulin-induced hypoglycemia. Diminished epinephrine levels with accompanying reduced catecholamine-induced symptoms have been described in patients with type I diabetes who suffer from repeated episodes of insulin-induced hypoglycemia (see later). A reduction in insulin-induced hypoglycemia restores normal catecholamine responses. Consequently, the role of disordered sympathetic activity in childhood hypoglycemia remains unresolved. In addition, many of the patients described as having hypoglycemia with failure of epinephrine excretion fit the criteria for ketotic hypoglycemia.

Glucagon deficiency can also be associated with hypoglycemia, but well-documented cases of in vivo glucagon deficiency have only rarely been described (63).

C. Substrate Deficiency

1. Ketotic Hypoglycemia

Ketotic hypoglycemia is a common form of childhood hypoglycemia (12,24). Usually this condition presents between the ages of 18 months and 5 years and remits spontaneously by the age of 8–9 years. Hypoglycemic episodes typically occur during periods of intercurrent illness when food intake is limited. The classic history is of a child who eats poorly or completely avoids the evening meal, is difficult to rouse from sleep the following morning, and may be observed to have a seizure or to be comatose by the midmorning. At the time of documented hypoglycemia, there is associated ketonuria and ketonemia, and plasma insulin concentrations are appropriately low at 5–10 μU/ml, thereby excluding hyperinsulinemia. A ketogenic provocative diet was formerly used as a diagnostic test, but it is not essential to establish the diagnosis, because fasting alone provokes a hypoglycemic episode, with ketonemia and ketonuria within 12–18 h in susceptible individuals. Normal children of similar age can withstand fasting without developing hypoglycemia during the same time period, although even normal children may develop these features by 36 h of fasting (23). Thus, the provocative nature of a ketogenic diet appears to be more dependent on its hypocaloric nature than its fat content. Therefore, the use of the ketogenic diet as a diagnostic tool has been largely replaced by complete caloric restriction, that is, a 24-h fast (23).

Children with ketotic hypoglycemia have plasma alanine concentrations that are markedly reduced in the basal state after an overnight fast and fall still further with prolonged fasting (21,22). Alanine is the only amino acid that is significantly lower in children with ketotic hypoglycemia, and infusions of alanine (250 mg/kg body weight) produce a rapid rise in plasma glucose without significant changes in blood lactate or pyruvate levels, indicating that the entire gluconeogenic pathway from the level of pyruvate is intact, so that a deficiency of substrate rather than a defect in gluconeogenesis is involved (Fig. 1). The intact nature of the gluconeogenic pathways in affected children is further supported by the normal glycemic response to infusion of fructose and glycerol, and plasma glycerol levels are also normal in these children in both the fed and fasted state. Glycogenolytic pathways are also intact because glucagon induces a normal glycemic response in affected children during the fed state. The metabolic response to infusion of β-hydroxybutyrate does not differ from that of normal children. Finally, the levels of hormones that counter hypoglycemia are appropriately elevated and insulin is appropriately low (21,24).

Alanine is quantitatively the major gluconeogenic amino acid precursor whose formation and release from muscle during periods of caloric restriction is enhanced by the presence of a glucose-alanine cycle, as well as by de novo formation from other substrates within the muscle, principally branched-chain amino acid catabolism. In this way, the release of alanine (and glutamine) for gluconeogenesis by muscle exceeds the content of these amino acids in tissue protein. Thus, the etiology of ketotic hypoglycemia, which is characterized by hypoalaninemia, may be a defect in any of the complex steps involved in protein catabolism, oxidative deamination of amino acids, transamination, alanine synthesis, or alanine efflux from muscle. It was pointed out in the original description of this syndrome that children with ketotic hypoglycemia are frequently smaller than age-matched controls and often have a history of transient neonatal hypoglycemia. Thus, any decrease in muscle mass may compromise the supply of gluconeogenic substrate when glucose demands per unit body weight are already relatively high and thereby predispose to the rapid development of hypoglycemia, ketosis representing the attempt to switch to an alternative fuel supply. Those with ketotic hypoglycemia may represent the low end of the spectrum in the capacity of children to tolerate fasting. A similar relative intolerance to fasting is present in normal children who cannot maintain blood glucose after 30–36 h of fasting compared with the adult's capacity for prolonged fasting. Although the defect may be present at birth, it may not become manifest until the child is stressed by more prolonged periods of caloric restriction. Moreover, the spontaneous remission by age 8–9 years may be explained by the increase in muscle bulk with a resultant increase in the supply of endogenous substrate and the relative decrease in glucose requirement per unit body mass with increasing age.

There is also some evidence to support the contention that impaired epinephrine secretion contributes to ketotic hypoglycemia, perhaps by interacting with the ability to mobilize alanine. However, the rarity of hypoglycemia in glucocorticoid-replaced patients who have undergone bilateral adrenalectomy and therefore lack an adrenal medulla capable of epinephrine production argues strongly against epinephrine deficiency as a major contributing factor for the development of the syndrome of ketotic hypoglycemia. Immaturity of the autonomic nervous system, however, which governs the release of epinephrine, may be involved. This hypothesis of "immaturity" of autonomic innervation may explain the tendency to spontaneous amelioration with increasing age (61).

In anticipation of the spontaneous resolution of this syndrome, treatment of ketotic hypoglycemia consists of frequent feedings of a high-protein, high-carbohydrate diet. During intercurrent illnesses, parents should test the child's urine for the presence of ketones, the appearance of which precedes the hypoglycemia by several hours. In the presence of ketonuria, liquids of high carbohydrate content should be offered to the child. If these cannot be tolerated, the child should be offered a short course of steroids or admitted to the hospital for intravenous glucose administration.

2. Branched-Chain Ketonuria (Maple Syrup Urine Disease)

This autosomal recessive condition is the result of a deficiency of the branched-chain α-ketoacid oxidative decarboxylase(s), resulting in the accumulation of leucine, isoleucine, and valine in plasma and the urinary excretion of ketoacids that imparts the characteristic odor of maple syrup. Manifestations in affected infants include lethargy, vomiting, muscular hypertonia, convulsions, and hypoglycemic episodes. These hypoglycemic episodes were previously attributed to the high levels of leucine, but evidence now indicates interference with the production of alanine. In vitro evidence implicates an important role for branched-chain amino acid catabolism in alanine production. Thus, the hypoglycemia of these patients represents a limitation of the availability of alanine as gluconeogenic substrate during caloric deprivation, akin to the situation in ketotic hypoglycemia (22).

D. Glycogen Storage Disease

A detailed discussion of glycogen synthesis and degradation is beyond the intent of this chapter and can be found elsewhere (64). Consequently, only those glycogen storage diseases associated with hypoglycemia are considered here.

1. Glucose-6-Phosphatase Deficiency (Type I Glycogen Storage Disease)

The deficiency of the enzyme that hydrolyzes glucose-6-phosphate to free glucose, the final step in the glycogenolytic or gluconeogenic pathways (Fig. 1), results in severe hypoglycemia from early infancy. In its classic form, now termed type 1a, affected children develop marked hepatomegaly, resulting in a protuberant abdomen that produces an appearance of exaggerated lordosis. Eruptive xanthomas reflect the hypertriglyceridemia and hypercholesterolemia in the serum, which may be grossly lipemic. Metabolic acidosis is common and is caused by marked ketosis and lactic acidosis. Hyper-uricemia, hypophosphatemia, anomalies in platelet adhesiveness, and severe growth failure are also characteristic features of this form of glycogen storage disease (64–78).

Affected children display a remarkable tolerance to their chronic hypoglycemia; blood glucose values in the range of 20–50 mg/dl are not associated with the classic symptoms of hypoglycemia, possibly reflecting the adaptation of the central nervous system to ketone bodies as an alternative source of fuel. However, the hypoglycemia provokes the appropriate increased secretion of counterregulatory hormones, including growth hormones, glucagon, cortisol, and catecholamines, as well as the suppression of insulin secretion. Thus, whereas insulin concentrations are usually in the low normal range, glucagon and growth hormone are three- to fourfold elevated above their normal fasting concentrations (65). These hormonal changes are responsible for most of the metabolic abnormalities (65). As a result of hypoinsulinemia and the increased concentrations of the counterregulatory hormones, there is increased glycogenolysis and gluconeogenesis to the point of glucose-6-phosphate; the lactic acidosis represents increased formation and decreased utilization of lactate. The hormonal changes also promote exaggerated lipolysis, resulting in the hyperlipidemia and in both the substrate and hormonal setting for accelerated hepatic ketogenesis. Depletion of hepatic ATP and inorganic phosphate as a consequence of ATP consumption during glycogenolysis and the resulting excess glycolysis increase the rate of uric acid production by the degradation of preformed nucleotides (66,67). Endogenous hyperglucagonemia probably contributes substantially to this evolution of hyperuricemia because infusion of exogenous glucagon to patients with type I glycogen storage disease exaggerates the decrease in hepatic ATP and glycogen content while increasing hepatic phosphorylase enzyme activity (66, 67). Hyperuricemia also reflects the decreased renal clearance of urate, which competes with the elevated lactate and ketone concentrations for a common renal tubular secretory site. The defect in platelet adhesiveness and resulting clotting abnormalities may also be the result of ATP depletion (66). Although the liver is laden with glycogen and lipid, liver function tests remain essentially normal, apart from mild elevation in the SGOT.

The kidney and intestinal mucosa also normally contain the enzyme glucose-6-phosphatase. Renal biopsy reveals excessive glycogen deposition, but renal function remains normal except for the occasional development of glycosuria, phosphaturia, and aminoaciduria (Fanconi syndrome). There are no characteristic gastrointestinal symptoms, but diarrhea has occasionally been reported. Liver biopsy with estimation of glucose-6-phosphatase activity remains the classic means for definitive diagnosis.

The hepatic glucose-6-phosphatase system is now known to be a multicomponent system whose enzyme activity is tightly linked to the inner aspect of the endoplasmic reticulum membrane. Three translocase systems that allow entry of glucose-6-phosphate (T_1), exit of phosphate (T_2), and exit of glucose (T_3) from the lumen of the endoplasmic reticulum also participate (71). Whereas classic deficiency of enzyme activity is termed type 1a, deficiency of translocase T_1 is termed type 1b. Type 1a has been described as presenting in adults with hepatomegaly and hypoglycemia (71) and has been implicated in sudden infant death syndrome (72). The human glucose-6-phosphatase cDNA and its gene and expressed protein were recently characterized and reported (73). This achievement has already allowed identification of mutations that inactivate enzyme activity; the molecular basis of this disease, its diagnosis by molecular means, and the potential for gene therapy may now become possible.

Type 1b occurs in children; features are similar to type 1a, with the addition of neutrophil deficiency, oral lesions, perianal abscesses attributed to the neutropenia, and chronic enteritis indistinguishable from Crohn's disease. Treatment with granulocyte-macrophage colony-stimulating factor to increase the neutrophil count ameliorates the Crohn's-like enteritis (74,75). Deficiency of the T_2 transporter as the cause of glycogen storage disease is termed type 1c; T_3 deficiency is termed type 1d, but cases in children have not been reported (71).

Severely affected children manifest growth failure, delayed puberty, mental retardation, and shortened life span unless treated. Recent advances have transformed the prognostic outlook for duration and quality of life and have resulted in reversal of most of the metabolic disturbances. Continuous intragastric feeding or total parenteral nutrition improves the metabolic and clinical findings by reducing the frequency and severity of hypoglycemia, thereby avoiding the secondary hormonal changes that appear to be responsible for the metabolic derangements. Continuous intragastric feeding at night combined with frequent daytime feedings produces equally effective amelioration of the biochemical disturbances (65,68,69). This latter regimen provides a practical long-term solution to the inconvenience of 24 h continuous gastric feeding and avoids the problems associated with long-term parenteral nutrition (69).

The regimen is instituted by daytime feedings given every 3–4 h, consisting of 60–70% of the calories as carbohydrate low in fructose and galactose, 12–15% of the calories as proteins, and 15–25% of the calories as fat. At night, a small nasogastric tube is passed by the patient (or a parent for younger children), and approximately one-third of daily caloric requirements is continuously infused over 8–12 h via a small continuous infusion pump. One commercially available formula for nocturnal infusion (Vivonex, Eaton Laboratories) contains 89% of the calories as glucose and glucose oligosaccharides, 1.8% as safflower oil, and 9.2% as crystalline amino acids. Allopurinol, 100 mg on alternate days, given in addition to this regimen may result in a further fall in uric acid levels to values within the normal range. Acceptance of this regimen, including passage of the nasogastric tube, is reportedly excellent, and the long-term outcome of this innovative approach is promising, although it remains to be determined whether mental retardation or formation of multiple liver nodules is prevented. Possible renal tubular dysfunction also ameliorates with dietary therapy (76). Cornstarch therapy has also been used successfully, and liver transplantation offers promise of long-term cure (69,70,

77,78). Variants of type I glycogen storage disease may present with hypoglycemia.

2. Amylo-1,6-Glucosidase Deficiency (Debrancher Enzyme Deficiency, Type III Glycogen Storage Disease)

Deficiency of this enzyme results in the inability to degrade glycogen beyond the 1:4, 1:6 branch point so that limit dextrin accumulates. The capacity to generate free glucose from glycogen is markedly impaired, although some free glucose results from the action of liver phosphorylase. Moreover, the gluconeogenic pathways are intact (see Fig. 1) so that spontaneous symptomatic hypoglycemia is much less common than in type I glycogen storage disease. During periods of caloric restriction, however, hypoglycemia and ketonuria may appear. Because gluconeogenic pathways are intact, infusions of fructose, galactose, or alanine produce a normal glycemic response, and lactic acidosis is not a feature. Similarly, the lack of persistent hypoglycemia and therefore the lack of a rise in counterregulatory hormones prevents the lipemia, ketonemia, and hyperuricemia. In the fed state, glucagon evokes a normal glycemic response through its activation of phosphorylase enzyme. When liver glycogen reaches the limit dextrin stage through moderate fasting, glucagon no longer elicits a glycemic response because phosphorylase cannot work on limit dextrin.

Children with this disease usually present with hepatomegaly and growth retardation. Liver function tests are normal, with the exception of the SGOT, which may be modestly elevated. In addition to the liver, this enzyme is normally also present in muscle, kidney, and leukocytes. Consequently, muscle weakness and myotonia have occasionally been described. Assay of the enzyme activity in leukocytes has been used to identify affected individuals and presumed heterozygote carriers. Considerable genetic heterogeneity in this enzyme's activity in liver, muscle, or leukocytes among affected individuals and their families precludes the use of leukocytes for the identification of the heterozygous state. Immunoblot analysis of this enzyme using a monoclonal antibody has been reported (79).

Therapy of this condition consists of frequent feedings of a diet high in protein and reduced in carbohydrate, to reduce glycogen deposition and to take advantage of the intact gluconeogenic pathways. Glucose infusions may occasionally be indicated if caloric intake cannot be maintained during intercurrent illness.

3. Liver Phosphorylase Deficiency (Type VI Glycogen Storage Disease)

Normal liver phosphorylase activity involves a complex cascade of events that activate the enzyme capacity to degrade liver glycogen both before and after the debranching step. Consequently, low hepatic phosphorylase activity may result from a defect in any of the steps of activation, and not surprisingly, a variety of defects has been described. In its "classic" form, hepatomegaly, excessive deposition of glycogen in liver, some growth retardation, and occasional symptomatic hypoglycemia occur. A diet high in protein and reduced in carbohydrate usually prevents hypoglycemia. Variants of this condition include a presumed defect in the hormonal activating system for phosphorylase, deficiency of the cAMP-dependent protein kinase that activates phosphorylase, and deficiency of the phosphorylase b kinase that activates phosphorylase a activity (64).

4. Glycogen Synthetase Deficiency

The inability to synthesize glycogen appears to be an extremely rare occurrence, but hepatic glycogen synthetase deficiency has been confirmed through metabolic studies and enzyme assay of liver biopsy material in vivo. The patient, a 9 year old at the time of the study, had symptoms of hypoglycemia since infancy and occasional morning seizures since age 7 years. She had fasting hypoglycemia and hyperketonemia but hyperglycemia with glucosuria after meals. During fasting hypoglycemia, levels of the counterregulatory hormones, including catecholamines, were appropriately elevated or normal and insulin levels were appropriately low. Exogenously administered glucagon produced a glycemic response shortly after meals but no response after a 12 h fast. Gluconeogenic capacity appeared to be intact. The liver was not enlarged. Glycogen synthetase activity was markedly reduced in liver but normal in muscle. Protein-rich feedings at frequent intervals resulted in dramatic clinical improvement, including growth velocity (80). This condition mimics the syndrome of ketotic hypoglycemia and should be considered in the differential diagnosis of that syndrome.

E. Disorders of Gluconeogenesis

1. Fructose-1,6-diphosphatase Deficiency

This disease is inherited as an autosomal recessive trait. From examination of Figure 1, it is apparent that a deficiency of this enzyme results in a block of gluconeogenesis from all possible precursors below the level of fructose-1,6-diphosphate. Infusion of these gluconeogenic precursors results in lactic acidosis without rise in glucose, and acute hypoglycemia may be provoked by acute inhibition of glycogenolysis. Normally, glycogenolysis remains intact, however, and glucagon elicits a normal glycemic response in the fed but not in the fasted state. Accordingly, affected individuals have hypoglycemia only during caloric deprivation, as in fasting or during intercurrent illness. While glycogen stores remain, normal hypoglycemia does not develop. In affected families, several siblings with known hepatomegaly died in infancy with unexplained metabolic acidosis.

Clinical feature simulate those of type I glycogen storage disease. Unlike glycogen storage disease type I, however, hepatomegaly in individuals with fructose-1,6-diphosphatase deficiency is a result of lipid storage rather than glycogen storage. Lactic acidosis, ketosis, hyperlipidemia, and hyperuricemia occur with this enzyme deficiency. As in glycogen storage disease type I, the pathogenesis of these features is related to the severity and duration of hypoglycemia and the resultant low levels of insulin and high levels of counterregulatory hormones. Therapy of these infants in the past consisted of a diet high in carbohydrates (56%), excluding fructose, which cannot be utilized, low in protein (12%), and of normal fat composition (32%). Such a regimen has permitted normal growth and development. The continuous nocturnal provision of calories via the intragastric infusion system described for type I glycogen storage disease is also applicable to children with fructose-1,6-diphosphatase deficiency. During intercurrent illnesses with vomiting, intravenous infusion of glucose is necessary to prevent severe hypoglycemia (81–83).

2. Pyruvate Carboxylase Deficiency

This is predominantly a disease of the central nervous system characterized by a subacute necrotizing encephalomyelopathy and high levels of blood lactate and pyruvate. Deficiency of hepatic pyruvate carboxylase was demonstrated in one case. Hypoglycemia has not been a prominent feature of this syndrome, presumably because gluconeogenesis from precursors other than alanine remains intact: these precursors enter the gluconeogenic pathway at the level of oxaloacetate, thus bypassing the pyruvate carboxylase step. The utilization of alanine as well as that of lactate via pyruvate cannot proceed, however, so that these substrates accumulate in blood and modest hypoglycemia may result during fasting. Affected patients have usually died from progressive central nervous system disease.

3. Phosphoenolpyruvate Carboxykinase (PEPCK) Deficiency

Deficiency of this rate-limiting enzyme, which occupies a key step in gluconeogenesis from various precursors (Fig. 1), is associated with severe fasting hypoglycemia and variable onset after birth. In one well-documented case, onset of hypoglycemia occurred 24 h after birth and defective gluconeogenesis from alanine was documented in vivo. At postmortem, liver, kidney, and myocardium demonstrated fatty infiltration, and there was atrophy of the optic nerve and visual cortex. Although total hepatic PEPCK activity was normal, the extramitochondrial (cytosolic) fraction was completely absent, in contrast to the normal situation, in which one-third of enzyme activity is in cytosol. This cytosolic fraction is believed to be physiologically important for gluconeogenesis. Extensive fatty deposition in liver, kidney, and other tissues has also been reported in two further cases of PEPCK deficiency, but in only one of these was there clinical hepatomegaly. Both patients had electrocardiographic evidence of cardiomegaly with left ventricular hypertrophy. Hypoglycemia was profound, onset being at 3 months of age in one and 19 months in the other. Lactate and pyruvate levels in plasma have been normal in all cases, but a mild metabolic acidosis was present. The fatty infiltration of various organs can be explained on the basis of the diversion of carbon flow as a result of PEPCK deficiency leading to the increased formation of acetyl-CoA, which becomes available for fatty acid synthesis. Diagnosis of this rare entity can be made with certainty only through appropriate enzyme determination of liver biopsy material. Avoidance of periods of fasting through frequent feedings rich in carbohydrate should be helpful because glycogen synthesis and breakdown are intact (84).

4. Acute Alcohol Intoxication

The liver metabolizes alcohol as a preferred fuel, and the generation of reducing equivalents during the oxidation of ethanol alters the NADH/NAD ratio, which is essential for certain gluconeogenic steps. As a result, gluconeogenesis is impaired and hypoglycemia may ensue if glycogen stores are depleted by starvation or by preexisting abnormalities in glycogen metabolism. In children who have been unfed for some time, the consumption of even small quantities of alcohol can precipitate these events. The hypoglycemia responds promptly to intravenous glucose, which should always be given to a child at initial presentation of coma or seizure after taking a blood sample for glucose determination. A careful history allows the diagnosis to be made and may avoid needles and expensive hospitalization and investigation (85, 86).

5. Salicylate Intoxication

Both hyperglycemia and hypoglycemia have been reported to occur in children with salicylate intoxication. Accelerated utilization of glucose caused by augmentation of insulin secretion by salicylates and possible interference with gluconeogenesis may both contribute to hypoglycemia. Infants appear to be more susceptible than older children. Monitoring of blood glucose with appropriate glucose infusion in the event of hypoglycemia should form part of the therapeutic approach to salicylate intoxication in childhood (87,88).

F. Disorders of Fatty Acid Oxidation

The important role of fatty acid oxidation in maintaining gluconeogenesis is underscored by examples of congenital or drug-induced defects in fatty acid metabolism that may be associated with fasting hypoglycemia (Chap. 54) (89–112). The oxidation of fatty acids occurs within mitochondria and requires the transport of fatty acids from plasma to the interior of the mitochondrion (Fig. 3). These complex processes begin by the formation of fatty acid acyl coenzyme A esters, the transfer of the acyl group to carnitine via the enzyme acyl carnitine transferase, and subsequent transfer of the acyl carnitine across the inner mitochondrial membrane. Within the mitochondrion, the carnitine is removed to re-form fatty acid acyl-CoA, which can undergo β oxidation, providing energy for cellular processes, including gluconeogenesis, as well as substrate for ketogenesis. Thus hypoglycemia may result from carnitine deficiency or from any of the required complex enzymatic steps in fatty acid oxidation. In addition, such defects would result in accumulation of acyl-CoA esters and hence lipid storage within affected tissues (Fig. 3).

Systemic carnitine deficiency is a rare, usually fatal syndrome characterized by lipid storage and dysfunction in the skeletal muscle, heart, liver, and kidney (90). Progressive myopathy appearing in late childhood at adolescence is a common presentation, but recurrent episodes of hypoglycemia with hepatic dysfunction also occur. The basic cause for carnitine deficiency remains unknown, but some success in reversing myopathy and other clinical features has been reported through administration of oral carnitine supplements.

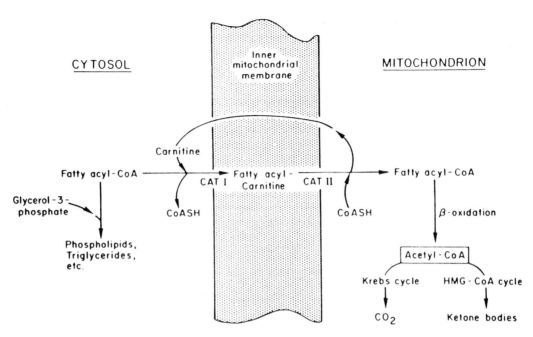

Figure 3   Some major pathways of fatty acid metabolism in liver CAT I is the carnitine acyltransferase located on the outer aspect of the inner mitochondrial membrane, whereas CAT II refers to the same enzyme located on the inner aspect of the inner mitochondrial membrane. (Reproduced from McGarry JD. Diabetes 1979; 28:518, with permission of the American Diabetes Association.)

A muscular form of carnitine deficiency with normal serum and liver carnitine concentrations, not associated with hypoglycemia, has also been described (Tables 7 and 8).

Various congenital enzymatic deficiencies causing defective carnitine or fatty acid metabolism also occur. A severe form of fasting-associated hypoglycemia with hepatomegaly, cardiomyopathy, and hypotonia occurs with long- and medium-chain fatty acid coenzyme A dehydrogenase deficiency (90–97). Plasma carnitine levels are low, ketones are not present in urine, but there is dicarboxylic aciduria. Clinically, patients with acyl-CoA dehydrogenase deficiency present with a Reye-like syndrome, recurrent episodes of severe fasting hypoglycemic, coma, and cardiorespiratory arrest. Severe hypoglycemia and metabolic acidosis without ketosis also occur in patient with multiple acyl-CoA dehydrogenase disorders. Hypotonia, seizures, and acrid odor are other clinical clues. Survival depends on whether the defects are severe or mild; diagnosis is established from studies of enzyme activity in liver biopsy tissue or in cultured fibroblasts from affected patients (96–102).

Recent studies demonstrate that medium-chain acyl co-enzyme A dehydrogenase deficiency (MCAD) has a high prevalence, with an estimated carrier frequency of about 1 in 60, so that the risk of MCAD deficiency in about 1 in 15,000 births (102,105). This high frequency has led to the suggestion for screening for this condition via DNA-based molecular methods in populations known to be at high risk. Avoidance of fasting and supplementation with carnitine may be lifesaving in these patients, who generally present in infancy during the second year of life (104). Lack of ketones in urine in

Table 7   Biochemical Indicators of Disorders of Fatty Acid Metabolism

Increased serum total free fatty acids
Medium-chain dicarboxylic aciduria
Increased acylated and free serum carnitine concentrations

Table 8   Clinical Indicators of Disorders of Fatty Acid Metabolism

I. Primarily muscle manifestations
   A. Chronic weakness and cardiomyopathy:
      primary carnitine deficiency
   B. Episodic rhabdomyolysis:
      carnitine palmityl transferase deficiency
      (muscle type)
II. Primarily systemic manifestations
     A. Medium-chain acyl-CoA dehydrogenase deficiency
     B. Long-chain acyl-CoA dehydrogenase deficiency
     C. Short-chain acyl-CoA dehydrogenase deficiency
     D. Electron transfer flavoprotein deficiency
     E. Electron transfer flavoprotein dehydrogenase
       deficiency
     F. Hydroxymethylglutaryl-CoA lyase deficiency
     G. Carnitine palmityl transferase deficiency (liver type)

association with hypoglycemia should raise the possibility of MCAD deficiency. Hypoglycemia, hypotonia, and cardiomyopathy have been described in long-chain acyl-CoA dehydrogenase deficiency (Tables 7 and 8).

Inference with fatty acid metabolism also underlies the fasting hypoglycemia associated with Jamaican vomiting sickness (110), with atractyloside (111), and with the drug valproate (109,112). In Jamaican vomiting sickness, the unripe akee fruit contains a water-soluble toxic principle, hypoglycin, which produces vomiting, central nervous system depression, and severe hypoglycemia. The hypoglycemic activity of hypoglycin derives from its inhibition of gluconeogenesis secondary to its interference in acyl-CoA and carnitine metabolism, essential for the oxidation of long-chain fatty acids. The disease is almost totally confined to Jamaica, where akee once formed a staple of the diet for the poor. The ripe akee fruit no longer contains this toxic principle. Atractyloside is a reagent that inhibits oxidative phosphorylation in mitochondria by preventing the translocation of adenine nucleotides, such as ATP, across the mitochondrial membrane. Atractyloside is a perhydrophenanthyrenic glycoside from *Atractylis gummifera*. This plant is found in the Mediterranean Basin; ingestion of this "thistle" has been reported to be associated with hypoglycemia and a syndrome similar to that observed in Jamaican vomiting sickness. More commonly, the drug valproate, now used for the treatment of epilepsy, has been associated with side effects that include a Reye-like syndrome, low serum carnitine levels, and the potential for fasting hypoglycemia (109,112). It is important to emphasize that in all these conditions, hypoglycemia is not associated with ketonuria.

G. Other Enzyme Defects

1. Galactosemia (Galactose-1-phosphate Uridyltransferase Deficiency)

The inability to convert galactose-1-phosphate to glucose-1-phosphate via galactose-1-phosphate uridyltransferase and UDP glucose (Fig. 1) results in the intolerance to milk or other products containing lactose or galactose. Affected infants present early in life with failure to thrive and with vomiting, diarrhea, and hypoglycemia following milk feedings. The accumulation of galactose-1-phosphate results in hepatosplenomegaly, impaired liver function, including jaundice, lenticular cataracts, mental retardation, and later renal tubular defects of the Fanconi type (glycosuria, aminoaciduria, and phosphaturia) (113,114). The lenticular cataracts probably reflect the activity of the polyol pathway. The majority of manifestations appear to be caused by a toxic effect of the high levels of galactose-1-phosphate. Hypoglycemia in this condition is a result of an acute impairment of glycogenolysis through the inhibition of the enzyme phosphoglucomutase by galactose-1-phosphate. Galactosemia should be considered in any newborn infant with failure to thrive, hypoglycemia, and the features just described. A presumptive diagnosis can be made by demonstrating a reducing sugar that is not glucose in the urine (urine positive with Clinitest and negative with Clinistix). Definitive diag-

nosis requires the determination of the enzyme activity in red blood cells. The only condition that may simulate some of the clinical findings and have non–glucose-reducing sugars in the urine is hereditary fructose intolerance (113,114).

2. Fructose Intolerance (Fructose-1-phosphate Aldolase Deficiency)

This condition mimics the clinical findings described for galactosemia, including failure to thrive, jaundice, hepatomegaly, and aminoaciduria. Vomiting and hypoglycemia follow the ingestion of foods continuing fructose, which may appear in the urine as a reducing sugar. The acute hypoglycemia is a result of the inhibition by fructose-1-phosphate of glycogenolysis via the phosphorylase system and of gluconeogenesis at the level of fructose-1,6-diphosphate aldolase (Fig. 1). Affected individuals often spontaneously learn to eliminate fructose from the diet (82).

H. Defects in Glucose Transporters

There has been one report of two infants with poorly controlled seizures in whom glucose (and lactate) in the cerebrospinal fluid (CSF) was low and simultaneously measured blood glucose was normal. Whereas the normal ratio of CSF to blood glucose in infants is about 0.8, it was only 0.2–0.4 in the affected infants. The low CSF lactate indicated that the low CSF glucose was not caused by excessive glycolysis as might occur in infection. A defect in the red blood cell glucose transporter was demonstrated, suggesting a similar defect in the related brain glucose transporter (Table 1). Thus, intractable seizures in a child with low CSF, but not blood glucose, should raise the possibility of a glucose transport defect. In the report, the patients were successfully treated with a ketogenic diet that enabled energy utilization by the brain without its customary reliance on glucose (115,116).

VII. DIAGNOSTIC EVALUATION

Table 9 lists the pertinent clinical and biochemical findings in the common childhood disorders associated with hypoglycemia. A careful and detailed history is essential in every suspected or documented case of hypoglycemia. Specific points to be noted include age of onset, temporal relation to meals or caloric deprivation, and a family history of infants known to have hypoglycemia or to have unexplained infant deaths. In the absence of a history and biochemical findings of maternal diabetes, the characteristic large plethoric appearance of an "infant of a diabetic mother" should arouse suspicion of the islet cell dysmaturation syndrome; plasma insulin concentrations above 10–15 μU/ml in the presence of documented hypoglycemia confirm this diagnosis. The presence of hepatomegaly should arouse suspicion of an enzyme deficiency; if non–glucose-reducing sugar is present in the urine, galactosemia is most likely. In males, the presence of a microphallus suggests the possibility of hypopituitarism,

Table 9 Clinical and Differential Diagnoses in Childhood Hypoglycemia[a]

Condition	Hypoglycemia	Urinary ketones (K) or reducing sugars (S)	Hepatomegaly	Serum		Glycemic response to glucagon		Effect of 24–36 h fast on plasma				
				Lipids	Uric acid	Fed	Fasted	Glucose	Insulin	Ketones	Alanine	Lactate
Normal	0	0	0	N	N	↑↑	↑	↓	↓	↑	↓	N
Hyperinsulinemia	Recurrent severe	0	0	N or ↓	N	↑↑	↑↑	↓↓	↑↑	↓↓	N	N
Ketotic hypoglycemia	Severe with missed meals	K+++	0	N	N	↑	0–↑	↓↓	↓	↑↑	↓↓	N
Hypopituitarism	Moderate with missed meals	K++	0	N	N	↑	0–↑	↓↓	↓	↑↑	↓↓	N
Adrenal insufficiency	Severe with missed meals	K++	0	N	N	↑	0–↑	↓↓	↓	↑↑	↓↓	N
Enzyme deficiency												
Glucose-6-phosphatase	Severe constant	K+++	++++	↑↑	↑↑	0	0	↓↓	↓	↑↑	↑↑	↑↑
Debrancher	Moderate with fasting	K++	+	N	N	↑	0	↓↓	↓	↑↑	↓↓	N
Phosphorylase	Mild to moderate	K++	+	N	N	0–↑	0	↓	↓	↑↑	↓↓	N
Fructose-1,6-diphosphatase	Severe with fasting	K++++	++++	↑↑	↑↑	↑	0	↓↓	↓	↑↑	↑↑	↑↑
Galactosemia	After milk or milk products	0–S+++	+++	N	N	↑	0	↓	↓	↑	↓	N
Fructose intolerance	After fructose	0–S+++	+++	N	N	↑	0↑	↓	↓	↑	↓	N
Carnitine deficiency	Moderate to severe with fasting	0	0–+	↓	N	↑	0	↓	↓	↓	N	N–↑

[a]Key: N = normal; 0 = absent; ↑ = low increase; ↑↑ = great increase; ↓ = some decrease; ↓↓ = marked decrease.

which may also be associated with a hepatic jaundice in both sexes.

Beyond the newborn period, clues to the cause of persistent or recurrent hypoglycemia can be obtained through a careful history, physical examination, and the initial laboratory findings (Table 10), which permit a systematic approach using selective and appropriate investigations. The temporal relation of the hypoglycemia to food intake may suggest that the defect is one of gluconeogenesis if symptoms occur 6 h or more after meals. If hypoglycemia occurs shortly after meals, leucine sensitivity, galactosemia, or fructose intolerance is most likely, and the presence of reducing substances in the urine rapidly distinguishes these possibilities. The presence of hepatomegaly suggests one of the enzyme deficiencies in glycogen synthesis or breakdown or of gluconeogenesis as outlined in Table 9. The absence of ketonemia or ketonuria at the time of initial presentation strongly suggests hyperinsulinemia or a defect in fatty acid oxidation (117). As apparent from Table 9, in all other causes of hypoglycemia with the exception of galactosemia and fructose intolerance, ketonemia and ketonuria are present at the time of hypoglycemia provoked by fasting. It cannot be overemphasized that at the time of presentation with hypoglycemia, serum should be obtained for determination of hormones and substrates, followed by repeat measurement after an intramuscular or intravenous injection of glucagon, as outlined in Table 11. The interpretation of the findings is summarized in Table 10. Hypoglycemia with ketonuria presenting between the ages of 18 months and 5 years is most likely to be ketotic hypoglycemia or a hormone deficiency, especially if hepatomegaly is absent. The ingestion of a toxin, including alcohol, can usually be excluded rapidly from the history alone.

When history is suggestive but acute symptoms are not present, a 24–36 h fast can usually provoke hypoglycemia and resolve the question of hyperinsulinema or other conditions (Table 10). Because adrenal insufficiency may mimic ketotic hypoglycemia, plasma cortisol levels should be determined at the time of documented hypoglycemia; increased buccal or skin pigmentation may provide the clue to primary adrenal insufficiency with elevated ACTH (MSH) activity. Short stature or a decrease in the growth rate may provide the clue to pituitary insufficiency involving growth hormone as well as possibly ACTH. Tests of pituitary-adrenal function, such as the arginine-insulin stimulation test for growth hormone and cortisol release, may be necessary.

In the presence of hepatomegaly and hypoglycemia, a presumptive diagnosis of the enzyme defect can often be made through the clinical manifestations, presence of hyperlipidemia, acidosis, hyperuricemia, the response to glucagon in the fed and fasted state, and the response to infusion of various appropriate precursors (Fig. 1 and Table 9). These clinical

Table 10 Diagnosis of Acute Hypoglycemia in Infants and Children

Acute symptoms present	History suggestive: acute symptoms not present
1. Obtain blood sample before and 30 minutes after glucagon.	1. Careful history for relation of symptoms to time and type of food intake bearing in mind age of patient (Table 2–4); exclude possibility of alcohol or drug ingestion; assess possibility of insulin injection; salt craving; growth velocity; intracranial pathology.
2. Obtain urine as soon as possible. Examine for ketones; if not present and hypoglycemia confirmed, suspect hyperinsulinemia or carnitine deficiency; if present, suspect ketotic, hormone deficiency, inborn error of glycogen metabolism, or gluconeogenesis.	2. Examine carefully for hepatomegaly (glycogen storage disease; defect in gluconeogensis); pigmentation (adrenal failure); stature; and neurologic status (pituitary disease).
3. Measure glucose in original blood sample. If hypoglycemia confirmed, proceed with substrate-hormone measurements as in Table 11	3. Admit to hospital for provocative testing:
4. If glycemic increment after glucagon exceeds 40 mg/dl above basal, suspect hyperinsulinemia.	a. 24 h fast under careful observation—when symptom provoked, proceed with steps 1–4 as when acute symptoms present.
5. If insulin level at time of confirmed hypoglycemia is greater than 100 μU/ml, suspect factitious hyperinsulinemia (exogenous insulin injection). Admit to hospital for provocative testing.	b. Pituitary-adrenal function via arginine-insulin stimulation test if indicated.
6. If cortisol less than 10 μg/dl and/or growth hormone less than 5 ng/ml, suspect adrenal insufficiency and/or pituitary disease. Admit to hospital for provocative testing.	4. Liver biopsy for histology and enzyme determination if indicated.
	5. Oral glucose tolerance test (1.75 g/kg; maximum 75 g) if reactive hypoglycemia suspected in an adolescent.

findings and investigative approaches were discussed with each separate condition and are summarized in Table 9. Definitive diagnosis of the glycogen storage disease may require an open-liver biopsy, which should be frozen immediately in liquid nitrogen and maintained at –80°C until determination of glycogen content, enzyme activity, and hepatic ultrastructure. Occasional patients with all the manifestations of glycogen storage disease are found to have normal enzyme activity. Clearly these definitive studies require special expertise available only in certain institutions.

VIII. THERAPEUTIC CONSIDERATIONS

The prevention of hypoglycemia and its resultant effects on central nervous system development is of paramount import-

Table 11 Analysis of Blood Sample Before and 30 Minutes After Glucagon[a]

Substrates	Hormones
Glucose	Insulin
Free fatty acids	Cortisol
Ketones	Growth hormone
Lactate	Thyroxine, thyroid-stimulating hormone[b]
Uric acid	Glucagon

[a]Intravenous or intramuscular Glucagon, 309 μg/kg.

[b]Measure once only before or after glucagon.

ance in the newborn period. With hyperinsulinema in the first 3 months of life, we strongly recommend pancreatectomy, unless hypoglycemia can be readily controlled with diazoxide. The therapeutic approach to specific causes is discussed with the description of each condition. Recent advances in the therapeutic approach to type I glycogen storage disease and fructose-1,6-diphosphatase deficiency represent gratifying examples of the impact of clinical research. As knowledge and understanding of glucose homeostasis has increased, few children are labeled as having idiopathic hypoglycemia and precise rational therapy becomes possible. New investigative tools, such as molecular biology, offer promise for further advances in our understanding and, hence, therapy and possible prevention of neonatal and childhood hypoglycemia.

IX. HYPOGLYCEMIA AND DIABETES

By far the most common type of hypoglycemia in childhood is that in insulin-treated diabetes mellitus. It has been estimated that a typical patient experiences several hundred episodes of severe hypoglycemia in the course of lifelong insulin therapy (118,119). Almost 30% of patient with insulin-dependent diabetes mellitus have experienced hypoglycemic coma at some stage; about 10% of patients experience severe hypoglycemia once annually, and 3–5% experience repeated severe bouts of hypoglycemia (120). Although the pathophysiology of diabetes mellitus in childhood, its treatment, and its complications are dealt with in separate chapters in this book, several important aspects relating to hypoglycemia in diabetes mellitus warrant emphasis.

First and foremost, hypoglycemia in insulin-dependent

diabetes mellitus represents an imbalance between the effects of insulin and those of the counterregulatory hormones. In many instances, this imbalance can be predicted. For example, in the honeymoon phase, recovery of residual endogenous insulin secretion occurs after initial diagnosis, so that the use of additional exogenous insulin frequency results in hypoglycemia. Reducing the dose of exogenous insulin diminishes the episodes of hypoglycemia. This situation represents an example of absolute insulin excess. Absolute insulin excess also occurs with deliberate or inadvertent errors in insulin dosage or when patients are not taking food to cover the effect of the injected insulin. Again, such omissions of food may be inadvertent, but they may be deliberate during attempts to lose weight or as a manifestation of anorexia nervosa. Hypoglycemia may also occur during or after exercise when increased insulin absorption from the injected site results from increased cardiac output and, hence, increased tissue perfusion. As a result of increased insulin absorption from its injection site, serum insulin levels rise during exercise, whereas they normally fall during exercise in a nondiabetic individual. The increase in insulin concentration accentuates the increased glucose consumption by exercising muscle while inhibiting glucose production via the liver. This inhibition of glucose production occurs despite an increase in the counterregulatory hormones that occur with exercise. Normally, the production of counterregulatory hormones in exercise is exquisitely finely tuned to the needs of the exercising muscle, such that the production of glucose and its consumption are equal, resulting in virtually unchanged glucose concentrations during mild to moderate exercise lasting minutes to hours.

Deficiency of counterregulatory hormones may also occur in diabetes. Most patients with insulin-dependent diabetes mellitus lose their ability to secrete glucagon in response to hypoglycemia after 5 years or more of diabetes and then rely almost solely on epinephrine secretion (27,118). The mechanism for the impairment of glucagon secretion is not clear. Epinephrine deficiency may also develop if the patients develop autonomic neuropathy as part of the diabetes complications or if patients are simultaneously using β blockers. As previously mentioned, intensive insulin therapy as instituted in the Diabetes Control and Complications Trial was associated with frequent hypoglycemic episodes that may have resulted in blunted capacity for epinephrine responsiveness (121,122).

Patients with impaired epinephrine response are at risk for "hypoglycemic unawareness." These patients may not experience anxiety, tachycardia, or other manifestations of epinephrine secretion, and the first sign of hypoglycemia may be cerebral dysfunction, including confusion, that may lead to further errors of inappropriate medication or impair the ability to take measures to counter hypoglycemia so that unconsciousness and coma may follow (121–126).

Recent studies have emphasized that for the same hypoglycemic stimulus, children secrete two to five times as much epinephrine as adults (127). This may lead to more intense symptoms of hypoglycemia in such children. Exaggerated epinephrine responses in children relative to adults can also

be demonstrated during oral glucose tolerance testing when the normal nadir of glucose, some 3–4 h after glucose ingestion, results in significantly higher epinephrine secretion in children. In both adults and children, it has now been shown that glycemic thresholds for the activation of glucose counterregulatory systems are higher than the thresholds for symptoms (128–131). Nevertheless, the glycemic threshold for epinephrine release in children is higher than in adults, and modest decrements in plasma glucose concentration may cause early impairment in cognitive function before the activation of counterregulatory mechanisms in the absence of typical hypoglycemic symptoms. Thus, clinicians managing children with diabetes must be alert to the possibility that symptoms consistent with hypoglycemia can occur at blood glucose concentrations not previously considered in the hypoglycemia range and that the definition of hypoglycemia as 40 mg/dl or less for normal children and adults is not applicable to those with diabetes mellitus (132). Strict control of diabetes appears to induce a delayed release of epinephrine so that glucose counterregulation becomes impaired (133, 134). Such mechanisms were probably the basis for the increased incidence and severity of hypoglycemic episodes in the Diabetes Control and Complications trial in which the intensive treatment group experienced approximately a threefold increase in hypoglycemic episodes (135).

There has been considerable debate in the literature that treatment with human insulin, rather than the formerly used beef and pork preparations, results in less awareness of acute hypoglycemic symptoms in insulin-dependent diabetes. However, well-controlled studies demonstrate that the symptomatic and hormonal responses to acute hypoglycemia produced by either pork or human insulin appeared to be indistinguishable, even after carefully selecting patients who complained of hypoglycemia unawareness with human insulin (136–139).

Physicians caring for patients with insulin-dependent diabetes should be aware of a syndrome of cerebral glucopenia with hypoglycemic encephalopathy. In these patients, prolonged severe hypoglycemia that is not recognized or treated may result in seizures and coma that lasts for hours despite correction of blood glucose concentrations. Such patients are often combative and use profane language. Several hours of glucose therapy may be necessary for recovery (133).

REFERENCES

1. Volpe JJ. Hypoglycemia and brain injury. In: Volpe, JJ Neurology of the Newborn. Philadelphia: W.B. Saunders, 1987:364–385.
2. Bier DM, Leake RD, Haymond MW, et al. Measurement of "true" glucose production rates in infancy and childhood with 6,6-dideuteroglucose. Diabetes 1977; 16:1016–1023.
3. Bachelar HS. Glucose transport and phosphorylation in the control of carbohydrate metabolism in the brain. In: Brierly JB, Meldrum BS, eds. Brain Hypoxia. Philadelphia: J.B. Lippincott, 1971:251.
4. Devaskar SU, Mueckler MM. The mammalian glucose transporters. Pediatr Res 1992; 31:1–13.
5. Kahn BB. Facilitative glucose transporters: regulatory mech-

anisms and dysregulation in diabetes. J Clin Invest 1992; 89:1367–1374.

6. Sperling MA, Devaskar S. Insulin action in the fetal-placental unit. In: Draznin B, Melmed S, LeRoith D, eds. Molecular and Cellular Biology of Diabetes Mellitus, Vol. II. Insulin Action. New York: Alan R. Liss, 1989; 203–217.

7. Cryer PE, Gerich JE. Glucose counteregulation, hypoglycemia, and intensive insulin therapy in diabetes mellitus. N Engl J Med 1985; 313:232–241.

8. Cryer PE. Glucose counterregulation in man. Diabetes 1981; 30:261–264.

9. Menon RK, Sperling MA. Carbohydrate metabolism. Semin Perinatol 1988; 12:157–162.

10. Cornblath M, Schwartz R. Disorders of Carbohydrate Metabolism in Infancy, 3rd ed. Boston: Blackwell Scientific, 1991.

11. Sperling MA, DeLamager PV, Phelps D, Fisher R, Oh W, Fisher DA. Spontaneous and amino-acid stimulated glucagon secretion in the immediate newborn period: relation to glucose and insulin. J Clin Invest 1974; 53:1159–1166.

12. Pagliara AS, Karl IE, Haymond M, and Kipnis DM. Hypoglycemia in infancy and childhood. J Pediatr 1973; 82:365–379 (part 1); 558–577 (part 2).

13. Persson B, Settergren G, Dahlquist G. Cerebral arterio-venous difference of acetoacetate and D-hydroxybutyrate in children. Acta Paediatr Scand 1972; 61:273–278.

14. Settergren G, Lindblad BS, Persson B. Cerebral blood flow and exchange of oxygen, glucose, ketone bodies, lactate, pyruvate and amino acids in infants. Acta Pediatr Scand 1976; 65:343–353.

15. Kalhan SC, Savin SM, Adam PAJ. Measurement of glucose turnover in the human newborn with glucose-1-^{13}C. J Clin Endocrinol Metab 1976; 43:704–707.

16. Kraus H, Schlenker S, Schwedesky D. Developmental changes of cerebral ketone body utilization in human infants. Hoppe-Seylers Z Physiol Chem 1974; 355:164–170.

17. Granner D, Andreone T, Sazak K, et al. Inhibition of transcription of the phosphoenol pyruvate carbokinase gene by insulin. Nature 1983; 305:549–551.

18. Chase HP, Marlow RA, Dabiere CS, et al. Hypoglycemia and brain development. Pediatrics 1973; 52:513–520.

19. Lucas A, Morley R, Cole TJ. Adverse neurodevelopmental outcome of moderate neonatal hypoglycemia. BMJ 1988; 297:1304–1308.

20. Chaussain JL. Glycemic response to 24 hour fast in normal children and children with ketotic hypoglycemia. J Pediatr 1973; 82:438-443.

21. Pagliara AS, Karl IE, DeVivo DC, Feigin RD, Kipnis DM. Hypoalaninemia: a concomitant of ketotic hypoglycemia. J Clin Invest 1972; 51:1440–1449.

22. Haymond MW, Ben-Galim E, Strobel KE. Glucose and alanine metabolism in children with maple syrup urine disease. J Clin Invest 1978; 62:398–405.

23. Chaussain JL, Georges P, Olie G, Job JC. Glycemic response to 24-hour fast in normal children and children with ketotic hypoglycemia. II. Hormonal and metabolic changes. J Pediatr 1974; 85:776–781.

24. Haymond MW. Hypoglycemia in infants and children. Endocrinol Metab Clin North Am 1989; 18:211–252.

25. Sperling MA. Diabetes mellitus. In: Kaplan S, ed. Clinical Pediatric Endocrinology. Philadelphia: W.B. Saunders, 1990: 127–164.

26. McGarry JD. New perspectives in the regulation of ketogenesis. Diabetes 1979; 28:517–523.

27. Cryer PE. Glucose homeostasis and hypoglycemia. In: Wilson JD, Foster DW, eds. Williams Textbook of Endocrinology, 8th ed. Philadelphia: W.B. Saunders, 1992:1223–1253.

28. Hill DJ, Milner RDG. Insulin as a growth factor. Pediatr Res 1985; 19:879–886.

29. Stanley CA, Baker L. Hyperinsulinism in infants and children: diagnosis and therapy. Adv Pediatr 1976; 23:315–355.

30. Aynsley-Green A, Polak JM, Bloom SR, et al. Nesidioblastosis of the pancreas: definition of the syndrome and the management of the severe neonatal hyperinsulinemic hypoglycemia. Arch Dis Child 1981; 56:496–508.

31. Atunes JD, Geffner ME, Lippe BM, et al. Childhood hypoglycemia; differentiating hyperinsulinemic from non-hyperinsulinemic causes. J Pediatr 1990; 116:105–108.

32. Gabbay KH, Gang DL. Hypoglycemia in a three-month old girl. N Engl J Med 1978; 299:241–248.

33. Hirsch HJ, Loo SW, Gabbay KH. The development and regulatin of the endocrine pancreas. J Pediatr 1977; 91:518–520.

34. Hirsch HJ, Loo S, Evans N, et al. Hypoglycemia of infancy and nesidioblastosis: studies with somatostatin. N Engl J Med 1977; 296:1323–1326.

35. Jaffe R, Hashida Y, Yunis EJ. Pancreatic pathology in hyperinsulinemic hypoglycemia of infancy. Lab Invest 1980; 42:356–365.

36. Jaffe R, Hashida Y, Yunis EJ. The endocrine pancreas of the neonate and infant. Perspect Pediatr Pathol 1982; 7:137–165.

37. Kramer JL, Bell MJ, DeSchryver K, Bower RJ, Ternberg JL, White NH. Clinical and histologic indications for extensive pancreatic resection in nesidioblastosis. Am J Surg 1982; 143:116–119.

38. Martin LW, Ryckman FC, Sheldon CA. Experience with 95 percent pancreatectomy and splenic salvage for neonatal nesidioblastosis. Ann Surg 1984; 200:355–362.

39. Jackson JA, Hahn HB Jr, Oltorf C, O'Dorisio TM, Vinik AJ. Long-term treatment of refractory neonatal hypoglycemia with long-acting somatostatin analog. J Pediatr 1987; 111:548–551.

40. Thornton PS, Alter CA, Katz LE, Baker L, Stanley CA. Short- and long-term use of octreotide in the treatment of congenital hyperinsulinism. J Pediatr 1993; 123:637–643.

41. Otonkoski T, Anderson S, Simell O. Somatostatin regulation of beta-cell function in the normal human fetuses and in neonates with persistent hyperinsulinemic hypoglycemia. J Clin Endocrinol Metab 1993; 76:184–188.

42. Gerver WJ, Menheere PP, Schaap C, Degraeuwe P. The effects of a somatostatin analogue on the metabolism of an infant with Beckwith-Wiedemann syndrome and hyperinsulinemic hypoglycemia. Eur J Pediatr 1991; 150:634–637.

43. Glaser B, Landaw H. Long-term treatment with the somatostatin analogue SMS 201–995: alternative to pancreatectomy in persistent hyperinsulinemic hypoglycemia of infancy. Digestion 1990; 45(Suppl 1):27–35.

44. Schwartz SS, Rich BH, Lucky AW, et al. Familial nesidioblastosis: severe neonatal hypoglycemia in two families. J Pediatr 1979; 95:44–53.

45. Drash A, Kenny F, Field J, et al. The therapeutic application of diazoxide in pediatric hypoglycemic states. Ann NY Acad Sci 1968; 150:337–355.

46. Roe TF, Kershnar AK, Weitzman JJ, Madrigal LS. Beckwith's syndrome with extreme organ hyperplasia. Pediatrics 1973; 52:372–381.

47. Mayefsky JH, Sarnaik AP, Postellon DC. Factitious hypoglycemia. Pediatrics 1982; 69:804–805.

48. Editorial. Meadow's and Munchausen. Lancet 1983; 1:456.

49. Sperling MA. Insulin biosynthesis and C-peptide: practical applications from basic research. Am J Dis Child 1988; 134:1119–1121.

50. Scarlett JA, Mako ME, Rubenstein AH, et al. Factitious hypoglycemia: diagnosis by measurement of C-peptide im-

munoreactivity and insulin-binding antibodies. N Engl J Med 1977; 297:1029–1032.

51. Jerkins TW, Sacks HS, O'Dorisio TM, Tuttle S, Solomon SS. Medullary carcinoma of the thyroid, pancreatic nesidioblastosis and microadenosis, and pancreatic polypeptide hypersecretion: a new association and clinical and hormonal responses to long-acting somatostatin analog SMS 201–995. J Clin Endocrinol Metab 1987; 64:1313–1319.

52. Walters EW, Tavake JM, Denton RM, Walters W. Hypoglycemia due to an insulin-receptor antibody in Hodgkin's disease. Lancet 1987; 1:241–243.

53. Taylor SI, Barbetti F, Accili D, Roth J, Gorden P. Syndromes of autoimmunity and hypoglycemia: autoantibodies directed against insulin and its receptor. Endocrinol Metab Clin North Am 1989; 18:123–143.

54. Lovinger RD, Kaplan SL, Grumbach MM. Congenital hypopituitarism associated with neonatal hypoglycemia and microphallus: four cases secondary to hypothalamic hormone deficiencies. J Pediatr 1975; 87:1171–1181.

55. Kaufman FR, Costin G, Thomas DW, Sinatra FR, Roe TF, Neustein HB. Neonatal cholestasis and hypopituitarism. Arch Dis Child 1984; 59:787–789.

56. Costin G, Murphree AL. Hypothalamic-pituitary function in children with septo-optic dysplasia. Am J Dis Child 1985; 139:249–254.

57. Miller WL, Levine LS. Molecular and clinical advances in congenital adrenal hyperplasia. J Pediatr 1987; 111:1–17.

58. Geffner ME, Lippe BM, Kaplan SA, et al. Selective ACTH insensitivity, achalasia, and alacrima: a multisystem disorder presenting in childhood. Pediatr Res 1983; 17:532–536.

59. Saenger P, Levine LS, Irvine WJ, et al. Progressive adrenal failure in polyglandular autoimmune disease. J Clin Endocrinol Metab 1982; 54:863–868.

60. Moser HW, Moser AE, Singh I, O'Neill BP. Adrenoleukodystrophy: survey of 303 cases. Biochemistry, diagnosis, and therapy. Ann Neurol 1984; 16:628–641.

61. Dahlquist G, Gentz J, Hagenfeldt L, et al. Ketotic hypoglycemia of childhood—a clinical trial of several unifying etiological hypotheses. Acta Paediatr Scand 1979; 68:649–656.

62. Hanse IL, Levy MM, Kerr DS. The 2-deoxyglucose test as a supplement to fasting for detection of childhood hypoglycemia. Pediatr Res 1984; 18:490–495.

63. Vidnes J, Oyasaeter S. Glucagon deficiency causing severe neonatal hypoglycemia in a patient with normal insulin secretion. Pediatr Res 1977; 11:943–949.

64. Hers HG, Van Hoof F, deBarsy T. Glycogen storage disease. In: Scriver CR, Beaudet AL, Sly WS, Valle D, eds. The Metabolic Basis of Inherited Disease, 6th ed., Vol. 1. New York: McGraw-Hill, 1989: 425–452.

65. Greene HL, Slonim AE, O'Neill JA Jr, Burr IM. Continuous nocturnal intragastric feeding for management of type I glycogen-storage disease. N Engl J Med 1976; 294:423–425.

66. Greene HL, Wilson FA. Hefferan P, et al. ATP depletion, a possible role in the pathogenesis of hyperuricemia in glycogen storage disease type I. J Clin Invest 1978; 62:321–328.

67. Cohen JL, Vinik A, Faller J, Fox IH. Hyperuricemia in glycogen storage disease type I. J Clin Invest 1985; 75:251–257.

68. Schwenk WF, Haymond MW. Optimal rate of enteral glucose administration in children with glycogen storage disease type I. N Engl J Med 1986; 314:682–685.

69. Chen Y-T, Cornblath M, Sidbury JB. Cornstarch therapy in type I glycogen-storage disease. N Engl J Med 1984; 310:171–175.

70. Malatack JJ, Iwatsuki S, Gartner JC, et al. Liver transplantation for type I glycogen storage disease. Lancet 1983; 1:1073–1076.

71. Burchell A, Lang CC, Jung RT, Bennet W, Shepherd AN. Diagnosis of type 1a and type 1c glycogen storage diseases in adults. Lancet 1987; 1:1059–1062.

72. Burchell A, Bell JE, Busuttil A, Hume R. Hepatic microsomal glucose-6-phosphatase system and sudden infant death syndrome. Lancet 1989; 291–294.

73. Lei KJ, Shelly LL, Pan CJ, Sidbury JB, Chou JY. Mutations in the glucose-6-phosphatase gene that cause glycogen storage disease type 1a. Science 1993; 262:580–583.

74. Roe TF, Coates TD, Thomas DW, Miller JH, Gilsanz V. Brief report: treatment of chronic inflammatory bowel disease in glycogen storage disease type 1b with colony-stimulating factors. N Engl J Med 1992; 326:1666–1669.

75. Kirkpatrick L, Garty BZ, Lundquist KF, et al. Impaired metabolic function and signaling defects in phagocytic cells in glycogen storage disease type 1b. J Clin Invest 1990; 86:196–202.

76. Chen Y, Scheinman JI, Park HK, Coleman RA, Roe CR. Amelioration of proximal renal tubular dysfunction in type 1 glycogen storage disease with dietary therapy. N Engl J Med 1990; 323:590–593.

77. Wolfsdorf JI, Keller RJ, Landy H, Crigler JF. Glucose therapy for glycogenosis type 1 in infants: comparison of intermittent uncooked cornstarch and continuous overnight glucose feedings. J Pediatr 1990; 117:384–391.

78. Greene HL, Swift LL, Knapp HR. Hyperlipidemia and fatty acid composition in patients treated for type IA glycogen storage disease. J Pediatr 1991; 119:398–403.

79. Ding J, deBarsy T, Brown BI, Coleman RA, Chen Y. Immunoblot analyses of glycogen debranching enzyme in different subtypes of glycogen storage disease type III. J Pediatr 1990; 116:95–100.

80. Aynsley-Green A, Williamson DH, Gitzelmann R. Hepatic glycogen synthetase deficiency. Arch Dis Child 1977; 52:573–579.

81. Kinugasa A, Kusunoki T, Iwashima A. Deficiency of glucose-6-phosphate dehydrogenase found in a case of hepatic fructose-1,6-diphosphatase deficiency. Pediatr Res 1979; 13:1361–1364.

82. Mock DM, Perman JA, Thaler JM, Morris RC Jr. Chronic fructose intoxication after infancy in children with hereditary fructose intolerance. A cause of growth retardation. N Engl J Med 1983; 309:764–770.

83. Kliegman RM, Sparks JW. Perinatal galactose metabolism. J Pediatr 1985; 107:831–841.

84. Hommes FA, Bendien K, Elema JD, Bremer HJ, Lombeck I. Two cases of phosphoenolpyruvate carboxykinase deficiency. Acta Paediatr Scand 1976; 65:233–240.

85. Lochner A, Wulff J, Madison LL. Ethanol-induced hypoglycemia. I. The acute effects of glucose output and peripheral glucose utilization in fasted dogs. Metabolism 1967; 16:1–18.

86. Arky RA. Hypoglycemia associated with liver disease and ethanol. Endocrinol Metab Clin North Am 1989; 18:75–90.

87. Sperling MA, Ganguli S, Miller J. The role of prostaglandins in glucose homeostasis. In: Chiumello G, Sperling MA, eds. Recent Progress in Pediatric Endocrinology. New York: Raven Press, 1983:115–124.

88. Reye's syndrome and aspirin: epidemiological associations and inborn errors of metabolism. Lancet 1987; 2:429–431.

89. McGarry JD. New perspectives in the regulation of ketogenesis. Diabetes 1979; 28:517–523.

90. Ware AJ, Burton WC, McGarry JD, Marks JF, Weinberg AG. Systemic carnitine deficiency. Report of a fatal case with multisystemic manifestations. J Pediatr 1978; 93:959–964.

91. Turnbull DM, Bartlett K, Stevens DL, et al. Short-chain acyl-CoA dehydrogenase deficiency associated with a lipid-

storage myopathy and secondary carnitine deficiency. N Engl J Med 1984; 311:1232–1236.

92. Coates PM, Hale DE, Stanley CA, Corkey BE, Cortner JA. Genetic deficiency of medium-chain acyl coenzyme A dehydrogenase: studies in cultured skin fibroblasts and peripheral mononuclear leukocytes. Pediatr Res 1985; 19:671–676.

93. Hale DE, Batshaw ML, Coates PM, et al. Long-chain acyl coenzyme A dehydrogenase deficiency: an inherited cause of nonketoic hypoglycemia. Pediatr Res 1985; 19:666–671.

94. Rhead WJ, Wolff JA, Lipson M, et al. Clinical and biochemical variation and family studies in the multiple acyl-CoA dchydrogenation disorders. Pediatr Res 1987; 21:371–376.

95. Corkey BE, Hale DE, Glennon MC, et al. Relationship between unusual hepatic acyl coenzyme A profiles and the pathogenesis of Reye syndrome. J Clin Invest 1988; 82:782–788.

96. Editorial. Carnitine deficiency. Lancet 1990; 335:631–633.

97. Editorial. Sudden infant death and inherited disorders of fat oxidation. Lancet 1986; 2:1073–1076.

98. Ding JH, Roe CR, Iafolla AK, Chen YT. Medium-chain acyl-coenzyme A dehydrogenase deficiency and sudden infant death. N Engl J Med 1991; 325:61.

99. Hug G, Bove KE, Soukup S. Lethal neonatal multiorgan deficiency of carnitine palmitolytransferase II. N Engl J Med 1991; 325:1862–1864.

100. Stanley CA, Hale DE, Berry GT, Deleeuw S, Boxer J, Bonnefont JP. Brief report: a deficiency of carnitine-acylcarnitine translocase in the inner mitochondrial membrane. N Engl J Med 1992; 327:19–23.

101. Scholte HR, van Tol A. Lethal neonatal deficiency of carnitine palmitoyltransferase 2. N Engl J Med 1992; 93:891–892.

102. Mehta J, Singhal S, Revankar R, Walvalkar A, Chablani A, Mehta BC. Frequency of the G985 MCAD mutation in the general population. Lancet 1991; 337:298–299.

103. Morton DH, Kelley RI. Diagnosis of medium-chain acyl-coenzyme A dehydrogenase deficiency in the neonatal period by measurement of medium-chain fatty acids in plasma and filter paper blood samples. J Pediatr 1990; 117:439–442.

104. Medium chain acyl CoA dehydrogenase deficiency. Lancet 1991; 338:544–545.

105. Matsubara Y, Narisawa K, Tada K, et al. Prevalence of K329E mutation in medium-chain acyl-CoA dehydrogenase gene determined from Guthrie cards. Lancet 1991; 338:552–553.

106. Treem WR, Stanley CA, Hale DE, Leopold HB, Hyams JS. Hypoglycemia, hypotonia, and cardiomyopathy: the evolving clinical picture of long-chain acyl-CoA dehydrogenase deficiency. Pediatrics 1991; 87:328–333.

107. Wilcken B, Leung K, Hammond J, Kamath R, Leonard JV. Pregnancy and fetal long-chain 3-hydroxyacl coenzyme A dehydrogenase deficiency. Lancet 1993; 341:407–408.

108. Shapira Y, Gutman A. Muscle carnitine deficiency in patients using valproic acid. J Pediatr 1991; 118:646–649.

109. Kelley RI. The role of carnitine supplementation in valproic acid therapy. Pediatrics 1994; 97:892–893.

110. Bressler R. The unripe akee-forbidden fruit. N Engl J Med 1976; 295:500–501.

111. Chappell JB, Crofts AR. The effect of atractylate and oligomycin on the behavior of mitochondria toward adenine nucleotides. Biochem J 1965; 95:707–716.

112. Nishida N, Sugimoto T, Araki A, Woo M, Sakane Y, Kobayashi Y. Carnitine metabolism in valproate-treated rats: the effect of L-carnitine supplementation. Pediatr Res 1987; 22:500–503.

113. Reichardt JK, Belmont JW, Levy HL, Woo SL. Characterization of two missense mutations in human galactose-1-phosphate uridyltransferase: different molecular mechanisms for galactosemia. Genomics 1992; 12:596–600.

114. Landing BH, Ang SM, Villarreal-Englehardt G, Donnell GN. Galactosemia: clinical and pathologic features, tissue staining patterns with labeled galactose- and galactosamine-binding lectins, and possible loci of nonenzymatic galactosylation. Perspect Pediatr Pathol 1993; 17:99–124.

115. DeVivo DC, Trifiletti RR, Jacobson RI, Ronen GM, Behmand RA, Harik SI. Defective glucose transport across the blood-brain barrier as a cause of persistent hypoglycorrhachia, seizures, and developmental delay. N Engl J Med 1991; 325:703–709.

116. Editorial. The glucose-transporter protein and glucopenic brain injury. N Engl J Med 1991; 325:731–732.

117. Phillip M, Bashan N, Smith CPA, Moses SW. An algorithmic approach to diagnosis of hypoglycemia. J Pediatr 1987; 110:387–390.

118. Gerich JE, Lilly Lecture, 1988. Glucose counterregulation and its impact on diabetes mellitus. Diabetes 1988; 37:1608.

119. Cryer PE, Binder C, Bolli GB, et al. Hypoglycemia in IDDM. Diabetes 1989; 38:1193–1199.

120. Gale EAM. Hypoglycemia and human insulin. Lancet 1989; 2:1264–1266.

121. White NH, Skor DA, Cryer PE, et al. Identification of type I diabetic patients at increased risk for hypoglycemia during intensive therapy. N Engl J Med 1983; 308:485.

122. DCCT Research Group, Bethesda, MD. Epidemiology of severe hypoglycemia in the diabetes control and complications trial. Am J Med 1991; 90:450–459.

123. Amiel SA, Tamborlane WV, Simonson DC, et al. Defective glucose counterregulation after strict glycemic control of insulin-dependent diabetes mellitus. N Engl J Med 1987; 316:1376.

124. Editorial. Awareness of hypoglycemia in diabetes. Lancet 1987; 2:371.

125. Heller SR, MacDonald IA, Herbert M, et al. Influence of sympathetic nervous system on hypoglycemic warning symptoms. Lancet 1987; 2:359.

126. Teuscher A, Berger WG. Hypoglycemic unawareness in diabetics transferred from beef/porcine insulin to human insulin. Lancet 1987; 2:382.

127. Casparie AF, Elving LS. Severe hypoglycemia in diabetic patients: frequency, causes, prevention. Diabetes Care 1985; 8:141.

128. Amiel SA, Simonson DC, Sherwin RS. Exaggerated epinephrine responses to hypoglycemia in normal and insulin-dependent diabetic children. J Pediatr 1987; 110:832.

129. DeFeo P, Gallai V, Mazzota G, et al. Modest decrements in plasma glucose concentration cause early impairment in cognitive function and later activation of glucose counterregulation in the absence of hypoglycemic symptoms in normal man. J Clin Invest 1988; 82:436.

130. Schwartz NS, Clutter WE, Shah SD, et al. Glycemic thresholds for activation of glucose counterregulatory systems are higher than the threshold for symptoms. J Clin Invest 1987; 79:777.

131. Herold KC, Polonsky KS, Cohen RM, et al. Variable deterioration in cortical function during insulin-induced hypoglycemia. Diabetes 1985; 34:677.

132. Gjedde A, Crone C. Blood-brain glucose transfer: repression in chronic hyperglycemia. Science 1981; 214:456.

133. Bergada I, Suissa S, Dufresne J, Schiffrin A. Severe hypoglycemia in IDDM children. Diabetes Care 1989; 12:239–244.

134. Jones TW, Boulware SD, Kraemer DT, Caprio S, Sherwin RS, Tamborlane WV. Independent effects of youth and poor diabetes control on responses to hypoglycemia in children. Diabetes 1991; 40:358–363.

135. Boyle PJ, Schwartz NS, Shah SD, et al. Plasma glucose concentrations at the onset of hypoglycemic symptoms in

patients with poorly controlled diabetes and in nondiabetics. N Engl J Med 1988; 318:1487.

136. Diabetes Control and Complications Trial Research Group. The effect of intensive treatment of diabetes on the development and progression of long-term complications in insulin-dependent diabetes mellitus. N Engl J Med 1993; 329: 977–986.

137. Patrick AW, Bodmer CW, Tieszen KL, White MC, Williams G. Human insulin and awareness of acute hypoglycemic symptoms in insulin-dependent diabetes. Lancet 1991; 338: 528–532.

138. Colagiuri S, Miller JJ, Petocz P. Double-blind crossover comparison of human and porcine insulins in patients reporting lack of hypoglycemia awareness. Lancet 1992; 339:1432–1435.

139. Egger M, Smith GD. Human insulin and hypoglycemia (letter to the editor). Lancet 1992; 340:301.

50

Autoimmune Endocrinopathies

William E. Winter
University of Florida College of Medicine, Gainesville, Florida

Takeshi Chihara
Institute for Comprehensive Medical Science, Fujita Health University, Toyoake, Japan

I. AUTOIMMUNITY AND AUTOIMMUNE DISEASES

Cells of the immune system, including macrophages, T lymphocytes, and B lymphocytes, must recognize one another for proper intercellular communication (Fig. 1) (1). This recognition is afforded by common polymorphic cell surface antigens coded for by genes within the human leukocyte antigen (HLA) complex located on the short arm of chromosome 6. Class I antigens (HLA-A, B, and C) are found on the surfaces of all nucleated cells and are important for cytolytic-T lymphocyte (CD8-positive T lymphocyte) recognition of virus-infected target cells (Fig. 2) (1). CD8-positive killer T cells, via their α/β T cell receptors, recognize target cells, juxtapose cell membranes with the target cell, and then inflict cell membrane damage by the release of perforin, a C9-like protein that forms pores in the target cell membrane (2), and produce nuclear lysis via injection of granzyme and other enzymes into the target cell. The class II antigens (HLA-DR, DP, and DQ) are restricted in their distributions to monocytes, macrophages (and macrophage-derived cells, such as Kupffer cells in the liver and microglia in the brain), B lymphocytes, Langerhans cells in the skin, and dendritic cells in several tissues (3). Via class II molecules, macrophages present antigen to α/β T cell receptors of T helper cells (CD4-positive lymphocytes), facilitating the development of cell-mediated immunity (i.e., cytolytic T cells) and B cell-immunoglobulin (humoral) responses (Fig. 3) (4).

Tolerance toward self antigens is primarily a function of T cells (5,6). Tolerance is acquired by the time of birth and is necessary to ensure that the body does not mount an immune response to self (7,8). Central tolerance results from self-nonself discrimination that occurs in the thymus (9,10). Peripheral tolerance (or anergy) has evolved because not all antigens enter the thymus during T cell ontogeny (Fig. 4) (11). By differentiating self from nonself, a process sustained by thymic T cell education and peripheral tolerance afforded by the multiple polymorphic HLA antigens, the immune system is able to recognize and react to foreign antigens, providing protection from microbiologic invasion and certain cancers that express "new" antigens. The class I antigens are responsible for viral (cytoplasmic) antigen presentation to CD8-positive T killer cells and are responsible for foreign tissue rejection, serving as the classically described transplantation antigens. Class II antigens of macrophages, B lymphocytes, and so on present extracellular peptides to CD-4-positive T helper cells to initiate immune responses. The in vitro mixed lymphocyte reaction results primarily from differences in class II antigens.

When a breakdown in tolerance occurs, the immune system recognizes "self" as "foreign" and mounts a humoral and/or cell-mediated immune response that can result in an autoimmune disease. Loss of tolerance can occur by many theoretical routes; however, loss of peripheral tolerance is the most reasonable explanation based upon the highly selective nature of organ-specific autoimmune responses and diseases (see later). Loss of peripheral tolerance most likely results from molecular mimicry (5). Molecular mimicry occurs, theoretically, when an immune response to a foreign antigen cross-reacts with a self antigen, leading to clinical disease.

The factors that lead to a disruption in self-tolerance, resulting in autoimmunities, have not been fully identified. To a large degree, this phenomenon is genetically programmed because autoimmune diseases are frequently associated with specific immune response gene alleles, that is, specific HLA types. Also, environmental influences, including viral infections and diet, are often implicated in the triggering of autoimmune processes. Molecular mimicry between an environmental antigen and an endogenous antigen could lead to autoimmunity. Whereas eradication of virally infected cells by T cell lysis provides an important defense against viral illnesses, this mechanism may expand beyond its immunologic defense function and lead to an autoimmune disorder.

With refinements in laboratory technique, intracellular

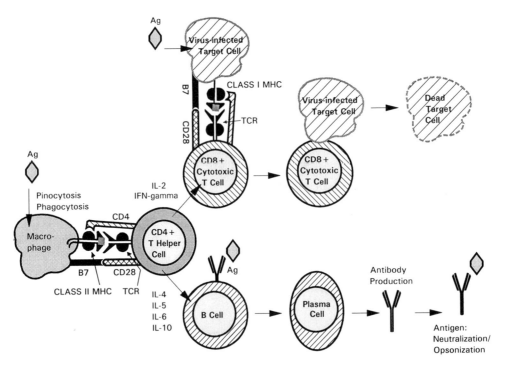

Figure 1   Pathways of the normal immune response.

antigens (i.e., thyroglobulin) can now be found in the circulation of normal subjects. This discovery discredits the earlier "sequestered antigen" theory of autoimmune disease for at least most endocrinopathies. During the aging process, there is a progressive breakdown in self-tolerance and an increased appearance of autoimmune phenomena with self-reactive autoantibodies (6). Clinically apparent autoimmune disease may not be obvious in older persons, however, because of the decreased efficiency of the immune system with advancing age and the limited duration of an autoimmune process that begins in an elderly individual.

Autoimmune diseases can be classified as organ specific, such as autoimmune endocrinopathies (12), or non-organ specific, such as collagen vascular diseases (Table 1). Auto-immune diseases in which an antibody is made to a circulating hormone, including insulin autoantibodies [e.g., autoimmune hypoglycemia), thyroid hormone autoantibodies (13), and autoantibodies against thyroid-stimulating hormone (TSH) (14)], and autoantibodies against adrenocoiticotropic hormone (ACTH) (15), form another group of disorders that lie outside these classifications.

In general, four types of findings support an autoimmune etiology for a disease: (1) evidence of humoral (B cell) and/or cell-mediated (T cell) autoreactivity; (2) ability to transfer disease with either serum or lymphocytes (this is usually performed in animal models of autoimmune disease); (3) disease recurrence in transplanted tissue in the absence of immunosuppression; and (4) ability to prevent or cure disease with immunotherapy, either immunosuppression or induction of tolerance.

Autoantibodies, the hallmark of B cell autoimmunity, can be identified by several methods (Table 2). Their participation in an autoimmune disorder can be assessed by complement fixation and lysis of target cells in tissue culture or by promoting cytolysis of target cells by macrophages in a process of antibody-dependent cell cytolysis. In other diseases, autoantibodies may bind to membrane receptors stimulating target cells, as in Graves' disease, or interfere with receptor functions, as occurs in myasthenia gravis.

The finding of lymphocytic infiltration of a target organ or tissue is evidence of cell-mediated autoimmunity. Cell-mediated autoreactivity can also be shown in vivo by positive delayed-type hypersensitivity reactions during skin testing with specific syngeneic, allogeneic, or xenogeneic "self" antigens. The allogeneic and xenogeneic systems suffer theoretically from the requirement for T killer cell–major histocompatibility complex (MHC) restriction. Ideally, studies of cell-mediated immunity should be performed in syngeneic systems. In vitro, cell-mediated autoimmunity can be assessed by the production of cytokines, such as interleukin-1 (IL-1), IL-2, tumor necrosis factor (TNF), or interferon production. T cell cytolysis of target cells in tissue culture can be measured by ^{51}Cr release or supravital staining.

Cytokines and reactive oxygen intermediates (O_2^-) are being increasingly implicated as mediators or final effectors of autoimmune cell damage (16). Interleukin-1 is often implicated, along with interferon-γ and tumor necrosis factor. In insulin-dependent diabetes mellitus (IDD) in tissue culture, IL-1 is toxic to isolated islets. At low doses, IL-1 inhibits glucose-stimulated insulin release, at higher doses, IL-1 is

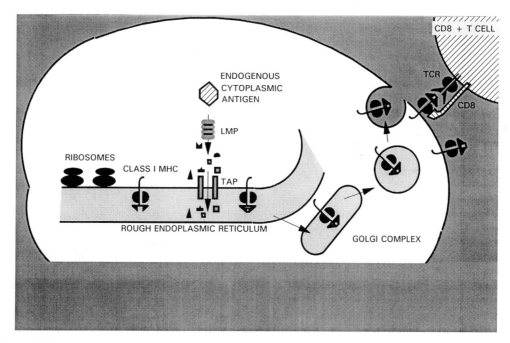

Figure 2 Class I MHC antigen presentation.

directly toxic and leads to islet cell death. Certain lymphokines, such as interferon-γ, may induce high levels of class I MHC expression, as well as low levels of class II MHC expression, that may propagate autoimmune responses once initiated. A marked increase in class I MHC expression on islets during early insulitis in animal models of IDD has been described.

Several other lines of evidence can support an autoimmune etiology for a particular disease: (1) association with known autoimmune diseases; (2) disease association with particular HLA alleles; (3) the ability to induce a similar disease in animals after injection of "self" antigens (often in Freund's adjuvant to exaggerate the response); (4) increased disease frequency in females over males; and (5) increased disease frequency with advancing age. A wide variety of autoimmune mechanisms has been proposed, as outlined in Table 3.

This chapter discusses those endocrinopathies believed to have an autoimmune etiology, with particular reference to genetics and HLA relationships; we classify endocrinopathies into autoimmune polyglandular syndromes and describe their relationship to other nonendocrine autoimmune diseases, discuss available diagnostic tests, and elaborate a clinical approach to the endocrinopathies.

II. AUTOIMMUNITY TO THE PANCREATIC ISLETS, INSULIN RECEPTORS, AND INSULIN

A. Insulin-Dependent Diabetes Mellitus

Insulin-dependent diabetes mellitus is a major clinical problem in both children and adults, and approximately 1:500

children are affected (17). Expected life span from the time of diagnosis is reduced by one-third. Microvascular complications (retinopathy and nephropathy) are major causes of morbidity and mortality in IDD. Premature macrovascular disease (coronary artery, carotid artery, and peripheral vascular disease) and neuropathy are also major contributors to morbidity and mortality.

Although IDD may occur secondarily to pancreatitis, pancreatic malformations (18), poisonings [i.e., the rodenticide Vacor (19)], drug toxicity (20), and viral infections [i.e., coxsackie, B4 (21) and rubella (22)], the majority of cases appear to result from an autoimmune process (23). Multiple lines of evidence support this thesis and are discussed here.

In patients dying within 6 months of diagnosis of IDD, from 60 to ~90% have pancreatic insulitis (24). Insulitis is the histologic description of lymphocytic infiltration of the pancreatic islets, with destruction of the β cells and a depletion in insulin content. With increasing duration of the disease, there is progressive disappearance of pancreatic β cells. According to Gepts and Lecompte (24), some neoislet formation also occurs in the early stages following the clinical diagnosis of IDD, in which islets that contain β cells display renewed evidence of insulitis. Neoislets composed of α cells are not subject to inflammatory changes. Later, the pancreatic islets are populated primarily by glucagon-producing α cells and pancreatic polypeptide (PP) producing cells. The few remaining β cells show degranulation and a pronounced rough endoplasmic reticulum suggestive of increased secretory activity. This evidence suggests that the non-β cells (α, γ, and PP cells) are not the subject of autoimmune targeting or permanent indirect damage. Thus, the β cell most likely carries antigens unique to insulin-producing cells.

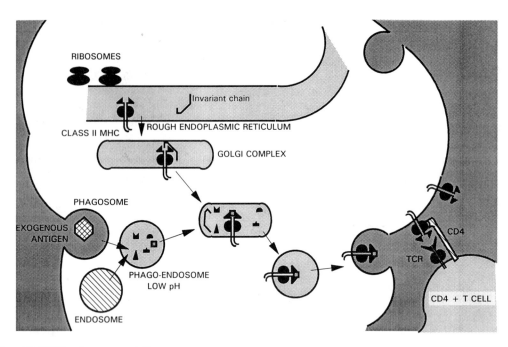

Figure 3   Class III MHC antigen presentation.

Alternatively, if the autoimmune islet attack is not specifically focused on the β cell islet non-β cells may survive, theoretically because of increased resistance to damage, that is, higher activities of superoxide dismutase and increased ability to clear free radicals or a higher reproductive potential than β cells. If β cells have lower endogenous levels of homologous restriction factor, which naturally inhibits the cell membrane pore-forming activity of C9-related protein (C9RP, perforin) that is released by cytotoxic T cells or natural killer cells, they may also be more sensitive to cellular

cytotoxicity. In an animal model of human IDD, the nonobese diabetic (NOD) mouse, there may be an intrinsic fetal defect in islet cell development that could contribute to susceptibility to β cell damage. In the BB (BioBreeding) rat model of human IDD, an islet-venular permeability defect has been demonstrated.

Islet cell cytoplasmic (ICA) and surface (ICSA) autoantibodies have been described in the sera of patients with IDD (25,26). At the time of diagnosis, 70–80% of white children with IDD have ICA; however, the frequency falls

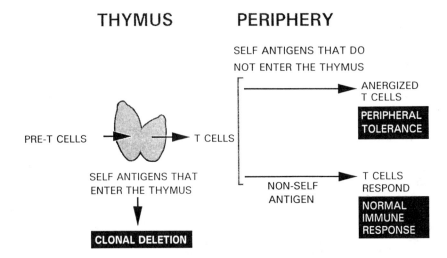

Figure 4   Normal mechanisms that avoid the development of autoimmunity.

Table 1 Autoimmune Disorders

Organ specific
  Antireceptor diseases
    Graves' disease
    Atrophic thyroiditis
    Myasthenia gravis
    Atopic diseases involving β_2-adrenergic receptors
    Insulin-resistant diabetes–acanthosis nigricans syndrome
    Hypoglycemia-insulinomimetic autoantibodies
  Autoimmune endocrinopathies
    Insulin-dependent diabetes mellitus
    Addison's disease
    Hashimoto's thyroiditis
    Autoimmune primary gonadal failure
    Hypophysitis
    Diabetes insipidus with hypothalamic autoantibodies
    Pancreatic α cell autoimmunity
    Hypoparathyroidism
  Miscellaneous
    Lymphocytic gastritis, pernicious anemia
    Chronic active hepatitis
    Primary biliary cirrhosis
    Cryptogenic cirrhosis
    Vitiligo
    Alopecia totalis, areata
    Goodpasture syndrome
    Immune hemolytic anemia
    Immune thrombocytopenic purpura
    Immune leukopenia
    Celiac disease
    Crohn's disease
    Ulcerative colitis
    Multiple sclerosis
    Polymyositis
Non-organ specific
  Systemic lupus erythematosus
  Mixed connective tissue disease
  Progressive systemic sclerosis
  Sjögren syndrome
  Rheumatoid arthritis
  Rheumatic fever
  Reiter syndrome
  Ankylosing spondylitis
  Dermatomyositis
Miscellaneous
  Insulin autoantibodies-hypoglycemia
  Thyroid hormone autoantibodies
  Anti-TSH autoantibodies
  Anti-ACTH autoantibodies

Table 2 Identification of Autoantibodies

Methods
  Cytoplasmic autoantibodies
    Indirect immunofluorescence, Ig, and complement fixing Ig using unfixed human tissue sections as substrates
    Immunohistochemical methods (see above)
    Immunoprecipitation: sera or Ig against cell extracts
    Hemagglutination of tissue antigen-coated red blood cells
    Other methods: radioimmunoassay (RIA), complement fixation assays, ELISA
  Cell surface autoantibody determinations (using isolated xenogeneic or allogeneic target cells) by indirect immunofluorescence, binding of [^{125}I]protein A, antigen precipitation by sera from an affected individual, or as measured by flow cytometry with a fluorescein-labeled second antibody
Determination of autoantibody effects
  Cell metabolism, products: measurement of changes in cell metabolism (i.e., cAMP) or cell products (hormones) after exposure to sera, or purified or partially purified Ig serum fractions; target cells isolated from tissue, tissue culture, or tissue slices
  Cytolysis: measurement of cytolysis by ^{51}Cr release or supravital staining after the addition of sera or purified or partially purified Ig serum fractions
  Transplacental passage: study of the clinical effects of autoantibodies transplacentally passed from mother to fetus or neonate
  Passage to animals: purification of Ig (protein A or $NH_4[SO_4]_2$) and passage to animals

general population is not greater than 1:400 (0.25%). In patients with non–insulin-dependent diabetes, some 5–10% are ICA positive, and with time, these patients tend to progress to insulin dependence (28). Because ICA react with intracellular antigens of all cells of the pancreatic islets, ICA are probably not involved in the pathogenesis of IDD. In vitro, however, sera containing ICSA has been shown to be cytotoxic to rodent islet cells (29) and can inhibit glucose-stimulated insulin release by islets (30). ICSA may also react preferentially with β cells, unlike other islet cell types.

ICA usually predate the clinical presentation of IDD by months or years (31). ICA-positive, nondiabetic patients, evaluated serially by glucose tolerance testing, often show insulinopenia to intravenous glucose injection; later, rises in fasting and stimulated glucose concentrations occur after oral glucose challenge (32,33). According to Bottazzo, ICA are unusual autoantibodies because they are predominantly of the IgG_2 subclass yet still fix complement. To the contrary, work by Schatz et al. concluded that IgG-ICA are polyclonal, including both κ and λ light chains and all four IgG subclasses (34). Bottazzo et al. propose that complement-fixing ICA are more highly associated with progression to IDD than are ICA that do not fix complement. This may simply be the influence of titer, however, because higher titer ICA fix complement

thereafter (27). By 5 years duration of IDD, ICA frequency has declined to approximately 25%, and after 10 years, ICA persists in sera in less than 5% of cases. First-degree relatives of IDD patients have a frequency of IDD similar to their ICA frequency, 3–5%. In our experience, ICA frequency in the

Table 3 Suggested Pathogenic Mechanisms of Autoimmune Endocrinopathies

---

Autoantibody hormone-receptor binding
  Blocking of receptor-hormone activation, e.g., atrophic
    thyroiditis
  Stimulation by autoantibodies with receptor activation, e.g.,
    Graves' disease
Autoantibody-induced target cell destruction, dysfunction
  Formation of local immune complexes with subsequent local
    inflammation
  Complement-dependent cytolysis
  Antibody-dependent cell cytolysis by macrophages, natural
    killer cells, possible role for subsequent IL-1, TNF-
    mediated cytolysis
Autoantibody binding to a circulating protein, with inappropriate
  levels of circulating free hormone producing excessive or
  deficient hormone effects, e.g., autoimmune hypoglycemia
Immune complex formation with distal localization and destruc-
  tion, e.g., immune complex nephritis secondary to auto-
  immune thyroid disease
Cell-mediated (classic $CD8^+$ killing or delayed-type
  hypersensitivity) target cell destruction by T cells without
  participation of autoantibodies
Cytokine and/or free radical destruction of target organ
Combinations of these mechanisms

---

efficiently but lower titer ICA are not able to fix complement efficiently. Furthermore, higher titer ICA would then predict increased risk for the development of IDD. Standardization of ICA testing has been aided by workshops and a proficiency testing program developed by the Immunology of Diabetes Workshops. β Cell destruction is thought to continue during this prodromal period. With greater than 90% β cell destruction, significant insulinopenia results, with consequent hyperglycemia, unrestricted ketogenesis, and clinical "insulin-dependent" diabetes. Using nonhuman pancreas substrates, ICA specific for β cells have been reported (35). This observation requires verification by multiple laboratories. Data from the Pasco County, Florida study indicate that ICA in the general population predicts IDD as well as ICA in nondiabetic first-degree relatives of IDD patients (36), in contrast to the data of Bingley et al. (37). The ability to predict IDD in the general population is most important because 85–90% of IDD patients do not have a first-degree relative with IDD.

Another type of autoantibody found in ~40% of newly diagnosed patients with IDD is the insulin autoantibody (IAA) (38). The enzyme-linked immunosorbent assay (ELISA) for the detection of IAA does not correlate with the development of IDD. However, IAA detected by a serum binding assay when present with ICA are highly predictive of insulinopenia and the eventual development of IDD (38).

Recently, the M_r 64,000 islet immunoprecipable autoantigen (39) was shown to include glutamic acid decarboxylase (GAD) (40). ICA appear to react with GAD, as well as a sialoglycoconjugate target antigen (41). Non-GAD ICA were recently noted by Richter et al. (42). GAD comes in two molecular weights (GAD 65 and GAD 67) that are coded for by separate genes. A primary sequence homology between portions of GAD and the P2-C protein expressed by coxsackie virus has been described (43). GAD cellular autoimmunity has been shown (44). One group of investigators propose that cellular and humoral and GAD reactivity are inversely associated with IDD risk (45). With the isolation and purification of GAD, we expect that commercial assays to detect antibodies to GAD will provide an opportunity for population screening for β cell autoimmunity. Using the older immunoprecipitation assay, Atkinson et al. (46) showed that 64 kD autoantibodies were highly predictive of IDD. GAD autoantibodies in patients with non–insulin-dependent diabetes correlate with insulin deficiency (47).

Besides insulitis, ICA, ICSA, anti-GAD autoantibodies, and IAA, a number of other immunologic abnormalities have been described in IDD: elevated levels of T cells positive for Ia (class II MHC) and TAC (transferrin receptor) (activated T cells), increased K cell levels, perturbed numbers or ratios of T helper/inducer (CD4) and T cytotoxic/suppressor (CD8) cells, lymphocytotoxic autoantibodies, circulating immune complexes, possible decreased IL-2 production by lymphocytes from IDD patients, impaired CD4-positive T lymphocyte function (48), and potentially decreased MHC class I expression (49). Many novel autoantigens and autoantibodies have been described (50): autoantibodies to carboxypeptidase H, islet cell 69 kD (ICA 69) autoantibodies, M_r 38,000 insulin secretory granule protein, rubella-related M_r 52,000 islet autoantigen detected by western blotting, autoantibodies that block uptake of glucose by murine β cells, presumably by binding to GLUT-2, 37/40 kD-derived trypsin-treated 64 kD immunoprecipitating autoantibodies (51), antiproinsulin autoantibodies, and antiinsulin receptor autoantibodies. Antibodies to heat-shock proteins are not related to IDD (52). Many of these immunologic abnormalities are limited to a few weeks or months after the diagnosis of IDD.

In vitro, lymphocytes from IDD patients have been shown to produce migration inhibition factor when exposed to xenogeneic islets or islet homogenates. Lymphocytes in vitro have produced islet adherence and cytolysis and have inhibited insulin release. Serreze and Leiter described an in vitro defect in NOD mouse T cell function in the syngeneic mixed lymphocyte reaction (53). This defect could be corrected with supplementation with IL-2 and could be partially corrected with IL-1 supplementation.

Further evidence of an autoimmune etiology for IDD is found in the association of IDD with other recognized autoimmune diseases (particularly chronic lymphocytic thyroiditis and atrophic gastritis), and with disturbed frequencies of particular HLA-DR and DQ types (54), although IDD does not appear to be inherited as a simple mendelian trait. In contrast to many other autoimmune disorders, IDD is slightly more common in males than females and more commonly presents in childhood than in adult life.

In our studies of over 1000 white patients (of mainly European ancestry) with IDD, ~95% had at least one DR3 and/or DR4. Only 5% lacked either antigen (genotype distribution in white diabetics: 39% DR3/DR4, 25% DR3/non-DR4, and 32% DR4/non-DR3). In African-Americans with IDD, however, only 70% had a DR3 and/or DR4 (only DR4 was significantly increased), suggesting greater heterogeneity of etiology of youth-onset diabetes in African-Americans than in whites (55). Of African-Americans with youth-onset diabetes 30% carried neither DR3 nor DR4 antigens (genotype distribution of HLA-DR antigens in black diabetics: 10% DR3/DR4, 33% DR3/non-DR4, and 31% DR4/non-DR3). ICA frequencies at diabetes onset in African-Americans are also considerably less then in whites (40 versus about 75%), providing further evidence of etiologic heterogeneity. Nondiabetic whites who are heterozygous for DR3 and DR4 are at greater risk for IDD than people with DR3 or DR4 alone. Some authors have proposed that extended haplotypes, including multiple loci (GLO, HLA, A, B, C, complement, DR, and DQ) on chromosome 6, may be more informative for risk of IDD than single-locus typing (56). In individuals with HLA-DR3 or DR4, the second antigen, excluding DR3 and DR4, is most commonly DR1. DR2 and DR5 are usually protective of IDD (57).

Using recombinant DNA methodologies, serologic DR4 has been divided by analysis of DR4-related DQβ genes (DQw3) into IDD-susceptible (DQB1*0302) and IDD-resistant (DQB1*0301 and DQB1*0303) subtypes (58). The susceptibility to IDD is inherited, at least in part, by way of inheritance of DQA1*0501-DQB1*0201 (associated with DR3) and DQA1*0301-DQB1*0302 (associated with DR4) or closely linked alleles. Individuals heterozygous for DQA1*0501-DQB1*0201/DQA1*0301-DQB1*0302 can have a 32-fold increased risk for IDD, which would be a ~6.4% risk based on a general population frequency of IDD of 1 in 500. Dorman et al. proposed that variations in population frequencies of DQB1-β1 nonaspartic acid alleles correlate with the population frequency of IDD (59).

For the DQB1 alleles associated with IDD in whites, at position 57 of the β1 exon, there is a lack of aspartic acid residues (e.g., serine, valine, and alanine), as opposed to IDD resistance alleles, in which aspartic acid is present (60). This amino acid difference is hypothesized (61) to alter the class II MHC antigen binding cleft and thus influence which antigen-peptides are presented. Many studies have associated non-aspartic acid alleles with IDD susceptibility (62,63). Arginine at position 52 in the DQα chain has also been related to IDD susceptibility (64). A combination of these DQA1 and DQB1 alleles (particularly in the trans configuration) further increases risk for IDD (65,66). The DR2- and DR5-associated DQA1-DQB1 haplotypes are DQA1*0102-DQB1*0602 and DQA1*0501-DQB1*0301, respectively (see Ref. 125). As opposed to whites and DQB1, in Japanese DQA1 alleles are the major MHC susceptibility factors (67).

Studies of multiplex families show that the inheritance of IDD is associated with particular parental haplotypes (68). In sibling pairs with IDD, instead of the expected random haplotype distribution (25% HLA identical, 50% haploidentical, and 25% nonidentical), a predominance of like haplotypes is found (60% HLA identical, 25% haploidentical, and

less than 5% nonidentical). There is an apparent transmission bias for IDD: ~7% of children fathered by IDD men develop IDD, as opposed to 2% of the offspring of IDD mothers (69). This is a result of the preferential inheritance of a DR4-bearing haplotype from the affected IDD father (70% transmission to offspring versus expected 50% transmission) (70). In both IDD fathers and mothers, there is transmission bias of DR3 (60% transmission to offspring versus expected 50% transmission).

Polygenic inheritance is almost certain, probably involving insulin gene polymorphisms and possibly involving genes for thyrogastric autoimmunity and gender. In 1984, Bell et al. demonstrated an association between the hypervariable region 5' of the insulin gene and IDD (71). This has been corroborated by data from Van der Auwera et al. (72) and Raffel et al. (73). Insulin gene polymorphisms in noncoding regions appear to have a major impact on IDD susceptibility (74). This influence appears to be independent of DR type (75). C2, C4, and Bf (factor B) alleles of the complement system (class III MHC genes) are most likely associated with IDD: there is linkage disequilibrium between specific class II MHC alleles and class III MHC alleles. GM allotypes of the heavy chain of Ig have no proven influence on susceptibility to IDD. Polymorphisms of T cell receptor genes probably do not affect proclivity to IDD (76).

Because concordance for IDD in identical twins is only 33–50%, environmental factors, such as diet, breast feeding (77), and viral infections, are thought to play some role in the triggering of IDD. There is no unequivocal evidence to suggest that children should avoid cow's milk products to prevent IDD (78). Because of the inherent "plasticity" of the genome, especially with respect to T cell receptor and immunoglobulin gene rearrangements, the supposition that monozygotic twins are immunogenetically identical can be questioned. In persons who develop IDD, the relative contributions of genetic and interacting environmental factors appear to be highly variable. Genetic factors may predominate early in life, and environmental "exposures" may become more important with advancing age. Presumably, once a person is predisposed to IDD by the possession of particular immune response genes (HLA associated and those outside the MHC) and nonimmune response genes, the proper environmental exposure may trigger or foster the initiation of the autoimmune process.

The natural history of IDD can be addressed in five stages: stage 1, genetic susceptibility; stage 2, evidence of humoral and/or cell-mediated autoimmunity without detectable metabolic perturbations; stage 3, declining first-phase insulin response to intravenously administered glucose; stage 4, oral glucose intolerance and potential fasting hyperglycemia; and stage 5, frank clinical IDD.

Immunosuppression of newly diagnosed IDD patients with cyclosporine or azathioprine and glucocorticoids has produced short-lived remissions in newly diagnosed IDD patients (79). Because of the limited success of these trials and the intrinsic toxicities of immunosuppressive agents, researchers recently attempted to induce immunologic tolerance to β cell antigens as a method of preventing IDD. The first β cell antigen to be used in such trials was insulin by subcutaneous injection. Later, oral insulin will probably be used. Presumably, when purified GAD can be isolated in bulk, GAD will be administered in an attempt to prevent IDD. Success in such trials may lead to the routine treatment of prediabetic individuals, enabling one to forestall or actually prevent IDD. Such trials are considered strictly experimental at this time.

B. Insulin-Resistant Diabetes and Acanthosis Nigricans

In this rare syndrome, insulin resistance occurs as a result of autoantibodies directed toward the insulin receptor that interfere with insulin binding (type B insulin resistance and acanthosis nigricans) (80). This condition, which has been described in a few adolescents, is more common in girls and is associated with other autoimmune disorders. In one patient described by Duncan et al., a dramatic remission was induced with steroid therapy (81). Another nonimmunologic form of insulin resistance and acanthosis nigricans (type A) is associated with hypogonadism and/or the Stein-Leventhal syndrome phenotype. In this disorder, there is a decrease in receptor number with normal receptor affinity and no antireceptor autoantibodies.

C. Hypoglycemia Secondary to Insulinomimetic Autoantibodies

Antireceptor autoantibodies usually block insulin action. Patients have been described with antireceptor autoantibodies that displayed insulin-like action, producing hypoglycemia (82). This disorder has been reported in children (83). Hypoglycemia secondary to insulinomimetic autoantibodies has been identified in adults with Hodgkin's disease and lupus.

D. Autoimmune Hypoglycemia

In this disorder, an autoantibody is produced against circulating insulin (84). Whereas insulin antibodies are common in patients who have received exogenous insulin (including human insulin), patients with autoimmune hypoglycemia spontaneously develop such antibodies. Some subjects have developed this syndrome following exposure to antithyroid medications used to treat Graves' disease. The circulating autoantibody-insulin complexes can release insulin inappropriate to metabolic needs, increasing the free insulin concentration. At these times, hypoglycemia results from relative hyperinsulinism. The amount of circulating insulin complexed to autoantibodies may also lead to glucose intolerance or a mild fed diabetic state, as well as hypoglycemia during fasting. This condition is most recognized in Japan but has been reported in studies from Norway. Similar to insulin antibodies resulting from exogenous insulin administration, autoimmune hypoglycemia is associated with HLA-DR4 (85). IAA described in prediabetic individuals do not appear to be

associated with hypoglycemia. In "prediabetes," IAA serve as markers of β cell autoimmunity.

E. Pancreatic α Cell Autoimmunity

Bottazzo and Lendrum in 1976 first described autoantibodies that reacted solely with the cytoplasm of the pancreatic glucagon-producing α cells (86). Another set of autoantibodies reacting with the somatostatin-secreting δ cells was also noted. We have found that the frequency of α cell autoantibodies (ACA) is similar in controls and relatives of IDD patients (0.5 versus 0.6%, respectively) (87). ACA are apparently very rare in IDD patients because ACA were not found in any of 762 ICA-negative IDD patients studied. We also studied 11 ACA-positive patients using arginine infusion and did not find frank glucagon deficiency. Del Prete et al. previously showed normal glucagon responses to arginine infusion in 2 patients with ACA (88). This is a very interesting autoantibody, because as yet there are no clear disease associations with ACA.

III.   AUTOIMMUNE THYROID DISEASE

Autoimmune thyroid disease includes atrophic thyroiditis, Hashimoto's thyroiditis (chronic lymphocytic thyroiditis), and Graves' disease. There is a striking female predominance for all forms of autoimmune thyroid disease.

A.   Chronic Lymphocytic Thyroiditis

Chronic lymphocytic thyroiditis (CLT) is the most common cause of goiter and acquired hypothyroidism in childhood. Patients presenting with a goiter often progress to frank hypothyroidism because of continued gland destruction; other patients may pass through a transient state of hyperthyroidism (hashitoxicosis) (89). In atrophic thyroiditis, an autoantibody to the TSH receptor is present that blocks TSH action (90,91). Goiter is not present in these patients, unlike patients with CLT. Atrophic thyroiditis and Graves' disease often coexist in single pedigrees.

Histologic examination of the thyroid of patients with CLT reveals lymphocytic infiltration with germinal center formation. In the late stages of disease, fibrosis and atrophy are present. Autoantibodies to the thyroid microsomes (TMA), to thyroglobulin (TGA), and to nonthyroglobulin colloid antigen (CA2) can be found in affected patients (92,93). The TMA autoantigen has been shown to be thyroperoxidase (TPO) (94,95). The TMA autoantibody reacts with TPO in its native conformation (96). This may lead to improvements in the TMA assay, but this has yet to be documented (97). A thyroid growth-promoting autoantibody that does not interact with the TSH receptor has been demonstrated (98). In children, TMA correlates best with the presence of CLT, and virtually 100% of children with CLT have TMA, although some also have TGA (94,95). About 2% of the general childhood population have at least one antithyroid autoantibody. Thyroid autoimmunity is also highly associated with gastric autoimmunity: approximately 25%

of TMA-positive patients also have gastric parietal cell autoantibodies (PCA). Similarly, about 25% of PCA-positive patients also have TMA, indicating an underlying genetic predisposition to both thyroid and gastric (thyrogastric) autoimmunities in such patients (99). A target autoantigen in atrophic gastritis is the H^+/Na^+-ATPase pump.

Thyrogastric autoimmunities appear to be frequently inherited as an autosomal dominant trait, with increased expression in female patients. Unlike IDD, thyrogastric autoimmunities are not inherited in association with particular parental HLA haplotypes (100,101). HLA appears to modulate (102) the clinical expression of the disease because DR4 and/or DR5 is associated with CLT and pernicious anemia in population studies and DR3 is associated with Graves' disease.

B. Graves' Disease

Graves' disease is the result of thyroid-stimulating autoantibodies (TSAb) that mimic the action of TSH. These immunoglobulins bind to TSH receptors on the surface of thyroid epithelial follicular cells, stimulate cyclic AMP production, and thus lead to excessive thyroid hormone production and clinical hyperthyroidism. TSAbs were first described in the McKenzie mouse assay system as long-acting thyroid stimulator (LATS) (103). In some patients with low levels of LATS, a substance that blocked LATS absorption by thyroid cells was termed LATS protector (LATS-P) (104). LATS-P corresponds more closely to human specific LATS. Commercial radioimmunoassays to measure thyrotropin binding inhibitory immunoglobulins and thyroid-stimulating immunoglobulins are available (105). TMA/anti-TPO autoantibodies and/or TGA are found in the sera of a large percentage of patients with Graves' disease. As mentioned, Graves' disease is highly associated with HLA-DR3.

Exophthalmos in Graves' disease is also believed to be immunologically mediated (106). Because part of the thyroid's lymphatic drainage traverses the retroorbital space, it is postulated that thyroid antigens, such as thyroglobulin, attach to the eye muscles and cause tissue damage as immune complexes are formed between thyroglobulin and antithyroglobulin autoantibodies. An exophthalmos-stimulating autoantibody has been described. Antibody to a soluble eye muscle antigen has also been demonstrated. A older hypothesis proposes that growth of retroorbital fat in autoimmune exophthalmos may be caused by TSH receptors on fat cells that are affected by thyroid-stimulating immunoglobulins. Clinically euthyroid patients presenting with exophthalmos often have TMA, TGA, and LATS-P (107). Gamblin et al. reported that 68% of patients with Graves' disease without exophthalmos have abnormally increased intraocular pressure on upward gaze (108). As our ability to detect antithyroid autoantibodies improves, it appears more and more likely that exophthalmos and thyroid autoimmunity are tightly linked clinically and etiologically reminiscent of thyrogastric autoimmunity (109–111).

IV. AUTOIMMUNE (NONTUBERCULOUS) ADDISON'S DISEASE

Second only to iatrogenic adrenal suppression by exogenous glucocorticoids, adrenalitis with lymphocytic infiltration of the adrenal cortex is the most common cause of Addison's disease. Similar to ICA for IDD and TMA for CLT, cytoplasmic adrenal autoantibodies precede the clinical manifestations of disease (112,113). Complement-fixing adrenocortical autoantibodies may be more strongly associated with progression to adrenal failure than those that do not fix complement (114). Autoantibodies to the surface of human or murine adrenocortical cells can be detected in some patients by indirect immunofluorescence. Recently, several adrenal enzymes [e.g., 17α-hydroxylase (115), 21-hydroxylase (116), and the side-chain cleavage enzyme] have been shown to be autoantigens in adrenalitis. The side-chain cleavage enzyme autoantibody is identified in sera from patients with autoimmune polyglandular syndrome type I (APS I) but not in patients with isolated idiopathic Addison's disease (117).

Adrenalitis commonly occurs with other autoimmune diseases [autoimmune polyglandular syndrome I and II) (118,119)], and, as discussed later, Addison's disease by itself or as part of autoimmune polyglandular syndrome II is associated with HLA-DR3 and DR4. Therefore, the genetic basis for IDD and Addison's disease is in part similarly linked to an HLA-associated gene or genes.

V. ACQUIRED PRIMARY GONADAL FAILURE

In patients with hypergonadotropic hypogonadism, the presence of serum steroidal cell autoantibodies supports the diagnosis of an autoimmune etiology (120). In patients of either sex, such autoantibodies react with steroid hormone-producing cells in the theca interna/granulosa layer of graafian follicles, cells of the corpus luteum, the placental syncytiotrophoblast, the Leydig cells of the testes, and cells of the normal adrenal cortex. Gonaditis is seen more often in female patients and is usually recognized in association with autoimmune polyglandular syndrome I. Premature menopause, male climacteric, or infertility may be clinically manifest.

VI. "IDIOPATHIC" HYPOPARATHYROIDISM

Autoimmune hypoparathyroidism in children is often seen in association with mucocutaneous candidiasis or Addison's disease (121). Lymphocytic infiltration of the parathyroid glands is observed; however, there is controversy about whether parathyroid autoantibodies can be detected by indirect immunofluorescence (122). In the absence of recognized causes of hypoparathyroidism (i.e., postparathyroidectomy or DiGeorge syndrome) and in the absence of candidiasis and Addison's disease (or adrenal autoantibodies), it is not possible at present to confirm the diagnosis of idiopathic hypoparathyroidism as autoimmune in etiology.

VII. HYPOPHYSITIS AND AUTOIMMUNE DISEASE OF THE PITUITARY

In rare cases of hypopituitarism in which mass lesions of the pituitary were suspected, histologic examination of surgical specimens has revealed hypophysitis (123). In some patients with IDD, as well as their immediate relatives, autoantibodies reactive with prolactin and growth hormone-secreting cells have been visualized by indirect immunofluorescence (124). This study requires confirmation. No associations between such autoantibodies and clinical disease have been recognized. Interestingly, researchers have suggested a stimulatory function for antipituitary antibodies by noting that in some studies, newly diagnosed patients with IDD were taller than their peers (125). Again these data are controversial and may reflect that IDD onset is most common at puberty. Patients who mature sexually earlier are then "able" to develop IDD sooner and are thus relatively taller.

VIII. AUTOIMMUNE DIABETES INSIPIDUS

In some patients with idiopathic diabetes insipidus (DI), autoantibodies to the antidiuretic hormone-producing cells of the hypothalamus have been recognized (126). Problematic is the need for fresh human hypothalamus as a substrate for indirect immunofluorescence. In up to one-third of children with otherwise idiopathic DI, an autoimmune process may be responsible for the condition.

IX. ASSOCIATED NONENDOCRINE AUTOIMMUNE DISEASES

A. Atrophic Gastritis

Atrophic gastritis caused by chronic lymphocytic infiltration of the gastric fundus, as noted previously, is commonly associated with thyroiditis (127). Achlorhydria can be frequently found; however, intrinsic factor secretion is usually preserved except in very long-standing gastric autoimmunity. With prolonged deficiency of intrinsic factor, pernicious anemia and neuropathy may occur during middle to late life. Autoantibodies to the cytoplasm of the gastric parietal cell (PCA) and autoantibodies that block vitamin B_{12} binding to intrinsic factor (IF blocking autoantibodies) or block the absorption of the IF-vitamin B_{12} complex are markers for the disease. In our experience, gastric parietal cell autoantibodies appear early in the course of the disease, are associated with achlorhydria, and are absent in about half the patients by the time pernicious anemia is clinically apparent. Intrinsic factor autoantibodies appear late in the course of disease, often near the onset of pernicious anemia and thereafter.

B. Chronic Active Hepatitis

In the absence of a previous hepatitis B infection, chronic active hepatitis may result from an autoimmune process. The presence of autoantibodies to smooth muscle and mitochondria can serve as markers for this condition (128). Chronic active hepatitis is seen in autoimmune polyglandular syndrome type I.

X. AUTOIMMUNE DISEASE ASSOCIATIONS (TABLE 4)

The concurrence of multiple autoimmune endocrinopathies (with or without other nonendocrine autoimmune diseases) is common. A few consistent associations have been classified into the autoimmune polyglandular syndromes (Table 4) (118). Almost every disease combination has been noted clinically.

A. APS-I

In APS-I, the primary diseases usually present clinically in the order listed in Table 4. If a component disease is "skipped," it usually does not present later. Malabsorption, early-onset pernicious anemia, alopecia, vitiligo, primary hypogonadism, and chronic active hepatitis may frequently accompany APS-I. Curiously, thyroiditis and/or IDD are infrequently encountered. APS-I can be inherited as an autosomal recessive trait, although most cases are sporadic.

B. APS-II

APS-II was first described by Schmidt (Schmidt syndrome: Addison's disease plus chronic lymphocytic thyroiditis) and later as Carpenter syndrome (Schmidt syndrome plus IDD). Unlike APS-I, which presents in childhood, APS-II can occur at any age but occurs more commonly in midlife and shows a female predominance (2:1) similar to that in APS-I (female/male ratio, 4:3). APS-II is strongly associated with HLA-DR3 and DR4 and may share certain common genetic origins with IDD.

Table 4 Autoimmune, Polyglandular Syndromes

Type	Diagnostic criteria
I (Blizzard syndrome)	At least two of the following: Mucocutaneous candidiasis Hypoparathyroidism Addison's disease or adrenal autoantibodies
II	Addison's disease (or adrenal autoantibodies) plus Autoimmune thyroid disease (Schmidt syndrome) Insulin-dependent diabetes Autoimmune thyroid disease and insulin-dependent diabetes (Carpenter syndrome)

C. Other Autoimmune Endocrinopathy Associations (Table 5)

The association of IDD with thyrogastric autoimmunity is of great clinical importance. Approximately 20% of patients with IDD have TMA, and 9% have PCA. These autoantibodies are usually present at the time of diagnosis of IDD. Of IDD patients with TMA, almost one-half eventually manifest thyroid dysfunction. Of these, four-fifths develop primary hypothyroidism, and the remaining 20% manifest Graves' disease. Hyperthyroidism often precedes the clinical onset of IDD (129).

In childhood, frank pernicious anemia is unusual in IDD patients with PCA; however, achlorhydria is commonly associated with the PCA autoantibody. Adrenal autoantibodies are present in 2% of IDD patients and are most commonly associated with TMA and PCA (APS-II). Of children and young adults with IDD and TMA, 6% have adrenal autoantibodies. Approximately one-half of patients with adrenal autoantibodies show evidence of chemical hypoadrenocorticalism (i.e., raised basal renin and ACTH levels); 20% have more overt features of adrenocortical insufficiency when studied (130). At least 1 of 6 such patients ultimately develop clinical Addison's disease, giving an overall prevalence of Addison's disease in IDD patients of 0.33%, or 1 in 300.

In many genetic syndromes, especially those with chromosomal abnormalities (i.e., Down, Turner, and Klinefelter syndromes), increased frequencies of autoimmune endocrinopathies (especially thyrogastric autoimmunity and IDD) are recognized. In patients with congenital infections, such as rubella, the frequencies of autoimmune thyroid disease and IDD are increased.

Table 6 outlines a variety of tests available for autoantibody detection. Those that are in bold print are often of greatest potential value to the clinician.

Table 5 Endocrinopathy Associations

Insulin-dependent diabetes
   Autoimmune thyroid disease
      Hashimoto's thyroiditis
      Graves' disease
   Pernicious anemia
   Adrenal antibodies-Addison's disease
Genetic syndromes
   (Down, Turner, Kleinfelter)
   IDD
   Autoimmune thyroid disease
      Hashimoto's thyroiditis
      Graves' disease
   Pernicious anemia
Congenital infections (rubella)
   IDD
   Hashimoto's thyroiditis

XI. CLINICAL APPROACH TO THE AUTOIMMUNE ENDOCRINOPATHIES AND RELATED DISEASES

In general, whenever one autoimmune disease is suspected or diagnosed, a search for other autoimmune diseases should be launched, guided by knowledge of the common associations noted previously (118,131,132).

Any patient with TMA and anti-TPO autoantibodies should be studied for PCA, and vice versa. Any patient with TMA/anti-TPO autoantibodies and/or PCA should be evaluated for adrenocortical antibodies, especially if IDD is present. Because of the high frequency of chronic lymphocytic thyroiditis and atrophic gastric in patients with IDD, all IDD patients should be screened at the time of diagnosis of IDD for TMA and PCA (133). In patients with serologic evidence of thyroid autoimmunity thyroid-stimulating hormone should be measured yearly to detect incipient hypothyroidism in its earliest stage. PCA-positive patients should have yearly measurements of serum vitamin B_{12} and ferritin levels and be given replacement therapies accordingly. At this time, we do not recommend screening of the general population or first-degree relatives of IDD patients for ICA, IAA, or anti-GAD autoantibodies or HLA typing of these individuals outside the research setting because definitive, safe, and totally efficacious immunotherapy is not currently available. We recommend screening for TMA and PCA in families in which one member has CLT or atrophic gastritis.

Patients with mucocutaneous candidiasis and/or hypoparathyroidism should be tested for adrenal autoantibodies. Patients with adrenal autoantibodies should then have a yearly assessment of adrenal function consisting of morning plasma cortisol and ACTH measurements and peripheral plasma renin activity after the patient has been supine for at least 30 minutes. Patients with APS-I should be tested for steroidal cell autoantibodies and the development of gonadal failure near the time of puberty. They should also be screened for mitochondrial and smooth muscle autoantibodies as indicators of chronic active hepatitis. At that time, serial studies of liver function (e.g., alanine aminotransferase and aspartate aminotransferase) are indicated.

XII. SUMMARY

The majority of endocrine disorders seen in childhood are the result of autoimmune processes. Recognition of the interrelationships among the autoimmune endocrinopathies provides the rationale for autoantibody screening. Identification of autoantibody-positive individuals followed by appropriate endocrine testing allows the clinician to anticipate and treat disease states before their frank clinical presentation.

Table 6 Clinically Useful Tests for the Diagnosis of Autoimmune Endocrinopathies and Related Diseases

Disease	Autoantibody	Technique[a]
Insulin-dependent diabetes	**ICA**: islet cell cytoplasmic auto-antibody	IFL (unfixed type O pancreas)
	IAA: insulin autoantibody	Serum binding RIA
	GAD autoantibody	Radiobinding assay
Chronic lymphocytic thyroiditis	**TMA**: thyroid microsomal auto-antibody	HA, IFL, RIA, CF, latex agglutination
	TGA: thyroglobulin autoantibody	HA, IFL, RIA, CF, latex agglutination
Graves' disease	**TMA, TGA**	See above
	LATS: long-acting thyroid-stimulating immunoglobulin	McKenzie mouse bioassay
	LATS-P: LATS protector	RIA
	TBII: thyrotripin binding inhibitory immunoglobulin	RIA
	TSI: thyroid-stimulating immuno-globulin	RIA
Addison's disease	**AA**: adrenocortical autoantibody	IFL
Primary gonadal failure	**SCA**: steroidal cell autoantibody	IFL
Associated nonendocrine diseases		
Chronic atrophic gastritis, pernicious anemia	**PCA**: gastric parietal cell auto-antibody	IFL
	IFAb: intrinsic factor blocking auto-antibody	RIA
Chronic active hepatitis	**SMA**: smooth muscle autoantibody	IFL
	Mitochondrial autoantibody	IFL
Vitiligo	Melanocyte autoantibody	IFL

[a]IFL, indirect immunofluorescence; CF, complement fixation; HA, hemagglutination; RIA, radioimmunoassay.

REFERENCES

1. Janeway CA. How the immune system recognized invaders. Sci Am 1993; September:73–79.
2. Marx JL. How target cells kill their targets. Science 1986; 231:1367–1369.
3. Korman AJ, Boss JM, Spies T, Sorrentino R, Okada K, Strominger JL. Genetic complexity and expression of human class II histocompatibility antigens. Immunol Rev 1985; 85:45–86.
4. Marrack P. New insights into antigen recognition. Science 1987; 235:1311–1313.
5. Röcken M, Urban JF, Shevach EM. Infection breaks T-cell tolerance. Nature 1992; 359:79–82.
6. Maclaren NK, Riley WJ. Thyroid, gastric, and adrenal autimmunities associated with insulin-dependent diabetes mellitus. Diabetes Care 1985; 8(Suppl. 1):34–38.
7. Nossal GJV. Immunologic tolerance: collaboration between antigen and lymphokines. Science 1989; 245:147–153.
8. Sinha AA, Lopez MT, McDevitt HO. Autoimmune diseases: the failure of self tolerance. Science 1990; 248:1380–1388.
9. Nossal GJV. Life, death and the immune system. Sci Am 1993; September:53–62.
10. Von Boehmer H, Kisielow P. Self-nonself discrimination by T cells. Science 1990; 248:1369–1373.
11. Marrack P, Kappler JW. How the immune system recognizes the body. Sci Am 1993; September:81–89.
12. Maclaren NK, Riley WJ. Autoimmune endocrine diseases and the pediatrician. Pediatr Ann 1982; 11:333–345.
13. Volpe R. Autoimmunity causing thyroid dysfunction. Endocrinol Metab Clin North Am 1991; 20:565–587.
14. Raines KB, Baker JR, Lukes YG, Wartofsky L, Burman KD. Antithyrotropin antibodies in the sera of Graves' disease patients. J Clin Endocrinol Metab 1985; 61:217–222.
15. Carstensen H, Krabbe S, Wulffraat NM, Nielsen MD, Ralfkiaer E, Drexhage HA. Autoimmune involvement in Cushing syndrome due to primary adrenocortical nodular dysplasia. Eur J Pediatr 1989; 149:84–87.
16. Rabinovitch A. Roles of cytokines in IDDM pathogenesis and islet β-cell destruction. Diabetes Rev 1993; 1:215–240.
17. Sperling MA. Diabetes mellitus. Pediatr Clin North Am 1979; 26:149–167.
18. Winter WE, Maclaren NK, Riley WJ, Andres J, Toskes RP, Rosenbloom AL. Congenital pancreatic hypoplasia: a novel diabetes syndrome of exocrine and endocrine pancreatic insufficiency. Pediatrics 1986; 109:465–469.
19. Karam JH, Lewitt PA, Young CW. Insulinopenic diabetes after rodenticide (Vacor) ingestion: a unique model of acquired diabetes in man. Diabetes 1980; 29:971–978.
20. Hauser L, Sheehan P, Simpkins H. Pancreatic pathology in pentamidine-induced diabetes in acquired immunodeficiency syndrome patients. Hum Pathol 1991; 229:926–929.
21. Yoon JW, Austin M, Onodera T, Notkins AL. Virus-induced diabetes mellitus. N Engl J Med 1979; 300:1173–1179.

22. Forrest JM, Menser MA, Burgess JA. High frequency of diabetes mellitus in young adults with congenital rubella. Lancet 1971; 2:332–334.

23. Atkinson MA, Maclaren NK. What causes diabetes? Sci Am 1990; 262:62–71.

24. Gepts W, Lecompte PM. The pancreatic islets in diabetes. Am J Med 1981; 70:105–115.

25. Bottazzo GF, Florin-Christensen A, Doniach D. Islet-cell antibodies in diabetes mellitus with autoimmune polyendocrine deficiencies. Lancet 1974; 2:1279–1283.

26. Maclaren NK, Huang SW, Fogh J. Antibody to cultured human insulinoma cells in insulin-dependent diabetes. Lancet 1975; 1:997–1000.

27. Neufeld M, Maclaren NK, Riley WJ, et al. Islet cell and other organ-specific antibodies in U.S. Caucasians and blacks with insulin-dependent diabetes mellitus. Diabetes 1980; 29:589–592.

28. Niskanen L, Karjalaienen J, Sarlund H, Siitonen O, Uusitupa M. Five year follow-up of islet-cell antibodies in type 2 (non-insulin dependent) diabetes mellitus. Diabetologia 1991; 34:402–408.

29. Dobersen MJ, Scharff JE, Ginsberg-Fellner F, Notkins AL. Cytotoxic autoantibodies to beta cells in the serum of patients with insulin-dependent diabetes mellitus. N Engl J Med 1980; 303:1493–1498.

30. Kanatsuna T, Lernmark A, Rubinstein AH, Steiner DF. Block in insulin release from column-perfused pancreatic beta cells induced by islet cell surface antibodies and complement. Diabetes 1981; 30:231–234.

31. Riley WJ, Maclaren NK, Krischer J, et al. A prospective study of the development of diabetes in relatives of patients with insulin-dependent diabetes. N Engl J Med 1990; 323:1167–1172.

32. Srikanta S, Ganda OP, Eisenbarth GS, Soeldner JS. Islet-cell antibodies and beta cell function in monozygotic triplets and twins initially discordant for type I diabetes mellitus. N Engl J Med 1983; 308:322–325.

33. Palmer JP. Predicting IDDM: use of humoral immune markers. Diabetes Rev 1993; 1:104–115.

34. Schatz DA, Barrett DJ, Maclaren NK, Riley WJ. Polyclonal nature of islet cell antibodies in insulin-dependent diabetes. Autoimmunity 1988; 1:45–50.

35. Gianani R, Pugliese A, Bonner-Weir S, et al. Prognostically significant heterogeneity of cytoplasmic islet cell antibodies in relatives of patients with type I diabetes. Diabetes 1992; 41:347–353.

36. Schatz D, Krischer J, Horne G, et al. Islet cell antibodies predict insulin dependent diabetes in U.S. school age children as powerfully as in unaffected relatives. J Clin Invest 1994; 93:2403–2407.

37. Bingley PJ, Bonifacio E, Gale EAM. Can we really predict IDDM? Diabetes 1993; 42:213–220.

38. Atkinson MA, Maclaren NK, Riley WJ, Winter WE, Fisk DD, Spillar RP. Are insulin autoantibodies markers for insulin-dependent diabetes mellitus? Diabetes 1986; 35:894–898.

39. Baekkeskov S, Nielson JH, Marner B, Bilde T, Ludvigsson J, Lernmark A. Autoantibodies in newly diagnosed diabetic children immunoprecipitate human pancreatic islet cell proteins. Nature 1982; 298:167–169.

40. Baekkeskov S, Aanstoot HJ, Christgau S, et al. Identification of the 64K autoantigen in insulin-dependent diabetes as the GABA-synthesizing enzyme glutamic acid decarboxylase. Nature 1990; 347:151–156.

41. Nayak RC, Omar MAK, Rabizadeh A, Srikanta S, Eisenbarth GS. "Cytoplasmic" islet cell antibodies. Evidence that the target antigen is a sialoglycoconjugate. Diabetes 1985; 34:617–619.

42. Richter W, Seissler J, Northemann W, Wolfahrt S, Meinch H-M, Scherbaum WA. Cytoplasmic islet cell antibodies recognize distinct islet antigens in IDDM but not in stiff man syndrome. Diabetes 1993; 42:1642–1648.

43. Kaufman DL, Erlander MG, Clare-Salzler M, Atkinson MA, Maclaren NK, Tobin AJ. Autoimmunity to two forms of glutamate decarboxylase in insulin-dependent diabetes mellitus. J Clin Invest 1992; 89:283–292.

44. Atkinson MA, Kaufman DL, Campbell L. Response of peripheral blood mononuclear cells to glutamate decarboxylase in insulin-dependent diabetes. Lancet 1992; 339:458–459.

45. Harrison LC, Honeyman MC, DeAizpurua HJ, et al. Inverse relation between humoral and cellular immunity to glutamic acid decarboxylase in subjects at risk of insulin-dependent diabetes. Lancet 1993; 341:1365–1369.

46. Atkinson MA, Maclaren NK, Scharp DW, Lacy PE, Riley WJ. 64 000 M_r autoantibodies as predictors of insulin-dependent diabetes. Lancet 1990; 335:1357–1360.

47. Tuomi T, Groop LC, Zimmet PZ, Rowley MJ, Knowles W, Mackay IR. Antibodies to glutamic acid decarboxylas reveal latent autoimmune diabetes mellitus in adults with a non-insulin-dependent onset of disease. Diabetes 1993; 42:359–362.

48. Schatz DA, Riley WJ, Maclaren NK, Barrett DJ. Defective inducer T-cell function before the onset of insulin-dependent diabetes mellitus. J Autoimmun 1991; 4:125–136.

49. Faustman D, Li X, Lin H, et al. Linkage of faulty major histocompatibility class I to autoimmune disease. Science 1991; 254:1756–1761.

50. Atkinson MA, Maclaren NK. Islet cell autoantigens in insulin-dependent diabetes. J Clin Invest 1993; 92:1608–1616.

51. Bottazzo GF. Banting lecture. On the honey disease. A dialogue with Socrates. Diabetes 1993; 42(5):778–800.

52. Atkinson MA, Holmes LA, Scharp DW, Lacy PE, Maclaren NK. No evidence for serological autoimmunity to islet cell heat shock proteins in insulin dependent diabetes. J Clin Invest 1991; 87:721–724.

53. Serreze D, Leiter EH. Lymphokine deficiencies may underlie immunoregulatory defects in NOD mice. Diabetes 1987; 36(Suppl. 1):68A.

54. Nepom GT. Immunogenetics and IDDM. Diabetes Rev 1993; 1:93–103.

55. Winter WE, Maclaren NK, Riley WJ, Clarke DW, Kappy MS, Spillar RP. Maturity-onset diabetes of youth in black Americans. N Engl J Med 1987; 316:285–291.

56. Segurado OG, Arnaiz-Villena A, Wank R, Schendel DJ. The multifactorial nature of MHC-linked susceptibility to insulin-dependent diabetes. Autoimmunity 1993; 15:85–89.

57. Maclaren N, Riley W, Skordis N, et al. Inherited susceptibility to insulin-dependent diabetes is associated with HLA-DR1, while DR5 is protective. Autoimmunity 1988; 1:197–205.

58. Khalil I, Deschamps I, Lepage V, al-Daccak R, Degos L, Hors J. Dose effect of cis- and trans-encoded HLA-DQ alpha beta heterodimers in IDDM susceptibility. Diabetes 1992; 41:378–384.

59. Dorman JS, LaPorte RE, Stone RA, Trucco M. Worldwide differences in the incidence of type I diabetes are associated with amino acid variation at position 57 of the HLA-DQ β chain. Proc Natl Acad Sci USA 1990; 87:7370–7374.

60. Todd JA, Bell JI, McDevitt HO. HLA-DQβ gene contributes to susceptibility and resistance to insulin-dependent diabetes mellitus. Nature 1987; 329:599–604.

61. Todd JA, Acha-Orbea H, Bell JI, et al. A molecular basis for MHC class II-associated autoimmunity. Science 1990; 240:1003–1008.

62. Morel PA, Dorman JS, Todd JA, McDevitt HO, Turcco M. Aspartic acid at position 57 of the HLA-DQβ chain protects against type I diabetes: a family study. Proc Natl Acad Sci USA 1988; 85:8111–8115.

63. Baisch JM, Weeks T, Giles R, Hoover M, Stastny P, Capra JD. Analysis of HLA-DQ genotypes and susceptibility in insulin-dependent diabetes mellitus. N Engl J Med 1990; 322:1836–1841.

64. Owerbach D, Gunn S, Ty G, Wible L, Gabby KH. Oligonucleotide probes for HLA-DQA and DQB genes define susceptibility to type 1 (insulin-dependent) diabetes mellitus. Diabetologia 1988; 31:751–757.

65. Gutierrez-Lopez MD, Bertera S, Chantres MT, et al. Susceptibility to type 1 (insulin-dependent) diabetes mellitus in Spanish patients correlates quantitatively with expression of HLA-DQ alpha Arg 52 and HLA-DQ beta non-Asp 57 alleles. Diabetologia 1992; 35:583–588.

66. Khalil I, d'Auriol L, Gobet M, et al. Combination of HLA-DQ beta Asp^{57}-negative and HLA DQ alpha Arg^{52} confers susceptibility to insulin-dependent diabetes mellitus. J Clin Invest 1990; 85(4):1315–1319.

67. Ikegami H, Tahara Y, Topyon C, et al. Aspartic acid at position 57 of the HLA-DQβ chain is not protective against insulin-dependent diabetes mellitus in Japanese people. J Autoimm 1990; 3:167–174.

68. Barbosa J, King R, Noreen H, Yunis EJ. The histocompatibility system in juvenile, insulin-dependent diabetic multiplex kindreds. J Clin Invest 1977; 60:989–998.

69. Warram JH, Krolewski AS, Gottlieb MS, Kahn CR. Differences in risk of insulin-dependent diabetes in offspring of diabetic mothers and diabetic fathers. N Engl J Med 1984; 311:149–152.

70. Vadheim CM, Rotter JI, Maclaren NK, Riley WJ, Anderson CE. Preferential transmission of diabetic alleles within the HLA gene complex. N Engl J Med 1986; 315:1314–1318.

71. Bell GI, Horita S, Karam JH. A polymorphic locus near the human insulin gene is associated with insulin-dependent diabetes. Diabetes 1984; 33:176–183.

72. Van Der Auwera BJ, Heimberg H, Schrevens AF, Van Waeyenberge C, Flament J, Schuit FC. 5′ insulin gene polymorphism confers risk to IDDM independently of HLA class II susceptibility. Diabetes 1993; 42:851–854.

73. Raffel LJ, Vadheim CM, Klein R, et al. HLA-DR and the 5′ insulin gene polymorphism in insulin-dependent diabetes. Metabolism 1991; 40:1244–1248.

74. Julier C, Hyer RN, Davies J, et al. Insulin-IGF2 region on chromosome 11p encodes a gene implicated in HLA-DR4-dependent diabetes susceptibility. Nature 1991; 354:155–159.

75. Bain SC, Prins JB, Hearne CM, et al. Insulin gene region-encoded susceptibility to type 1 diabetes is not restricted to HLA-DR4-positive individuals. Nat Genet 1992; 2:212–215.

76. Concannon P, Wright JA, Wright LG, Sylvester DR, Spielman RS. T-cell receptor genes and insulin-dependent diabetes mellitus (IDDM): no evidence for linkage from affected sib pairs. Am J Hum Genet 1990; 47:45–52.

77. Karjalainen J, Martin J, Knip M. A bovine albumin peptide as a possible trigger of insulin-dependent diabetes mellitus. N Engl J Med 1992; 327:302–307.

78. Maclaren NK, Atkinson MA. Is insulin-dependent diabetes mellitus environmentally induced? N Engl J Med 1992; 327:347–349.

79. Silverstein J, Maclaren N, Riley W, Spillar R, Radjenovic D, Johnson S. Immunosuppression with azathioprine and prednisone in recent-onset insulin-dependent diabetes mellitus. N Engl J Med 1988; 319:599–604.

80. Kahn CR, Flier JS, Bar RS, et al. The syndromes of insulin resistance and acanthosis nigricans: insulin-receptor disorders in man. N Engl J Med 1976; 294:739–745.

81. Duncan JA, Shah SC, Shulman DI, Siegel RL, Kappy MS, Malone JI. Type b insulin resistance in a 15-year-old white youth. J Pediatr 1983; 103(3):421–424.

82. Flier JS, Kahn CR, Roth J. Receptors, antireceptor antibodies, and mechanisms of insulin resistence. N Engl J Med 1979; 300:413–419.

83. Elias D, Cohen IR, Schechter Y, Spirer Z, Golander A. Antibodies to insulin receptor followed by anti-idiotype antibodies to insulin in child with hypoglycemia. Diabetes 1987; 36:348–354.

84. Meschi F, Dozio N, Bognetti E, Carra M, Cofano D, Chiumello G. An unusual case of recurrent hypoglycaemia: 10-year follow up of a child with insulin auto-immunity. Eur J Pediatr 1992; 151:32–34.

85. Uchigata Y, Kuwata S, Tokunaga K, et al. Strong association of insulin autoimmune syndrome with HLA-DR4. Lancet 1992; 339:393–394.

86. Bottazzo GF, Lendrum R. Separate autoantibodies to human pancreatic glucagon and somatostatin cells. Lancet 1976; 2:873–876.

87. Winter WE, Maclaren NK, Riley WJ, Unger RH, Ozand P, Neufeld M. Pancreatic alpha cell autoantibodies and glucagon response to arginine. Diabetes 1984; 33:435–437.

88. Del Prete GF, Tiengo A, Nosadini R, Bottazzo GF, Betterle C, Bersani G. Glucagon secretion in two patients with autoantibodies to glucagon producing cells. Horm Metab Res 1987; 10:260–261.

89. Riley WJ, Maclaren NK, Lezotte DC, Spillar RP, Rosenbloom AL. Thyroid autoimmunity in insulin-dependent diabetes mellitus: the case for routine screening. J Pediatr 1981; 98:350–354.

90. Strakosch CR, Wenzel BE, Row VV, Volpe R. Immunology of autoimmune thyroid diseases. N Engl J Med 1982; 307:1499–1507.

91. Editorial. Thyroid autoimmune disease: a broad spectrum. Lancet 1981; 1:874–875.

92. Doniach D, Bottazzo GR, Russell RCG. Goitrous autoimmune thyroiditis. Clin Endocrinol Metab 1979; 8:63–80.

93. Doniach D. Humoral and genetic aspects of thyroid autoimmunity. Clin Endocrinol Metab 1975; 4:267–285.

94. Mariotti S, Caturegli P, Piccolo P, Barbesino G, Pinchera A. Antithyroid peroxidase autoantibodies in thyroid diseases. J Clin Endocrinol Metab 1990; 71:661–669.

95. Banga JP, Barnett PS, McGregor AM. Immunological and molecular characteristics of the thyroid peroxidase autoantigen. Autoimmunity 1991; 8:335–343.

96. Berthold H, Steffens U, Northemann W. Human thyroid peroxidase: autoantibody recognition depends on the natural conformation. J Clin Lab Anal 1993; 7:401–404.

97. Vakeva A, Kontiainen S, Miettinen A, Schlenzka A, Maenpaa J. Thyroid peroxidase antibodies in children with autoimmune thyroiditis. J Clin Pathol 1992; 45:106–109.

98. Valenti WA, Vitti P, Rotella CM, et al. Antibodies that promote thyroid growth, a distinct population of thyroid-stimulating autoantibodies. N Engl J Med 1983; 309:1028–1034.

99. Irvine WJ. The association of atrophic gastritis with autoimmune thyroid disease. Clin Endocrinol Metab 1975; 4:351–377.

100. Phillips D, McLachlan S, Stephenson A, et al. Autosomal dominant transmission of autoantibodies to thyroglobulin and thyroid peroxidase. J Clin Endocrinol Metab 1990; 70:742–746.

101. Roman SH, Greenberg D, Rubinstein P, Wallenstein S, Davies TF. Genetics of autoimmune thyroid disease: lack of evidence

for linkage to HLA within families. J Clin Endocrinol Metab 1992; 74:496–503.

102. Wick G. Concept of a multigenic basis for the pathogenesis of spontaneous autoimmune thyroiditis. Acta Endocrinol Suppl (Copenh) 1987; 281:63–69.

103. McKenzie JM. Humoral factors in the pathogenesis of Graves' disease. Physiol Rev 1968; 48:252–310.

104. Adams DD, Kennedy TH. Evidence to suggest that LATS-protector stimulates human thyroid gland. J Clin Endocrinol Metab 1971; 33:47–51.

105. Fisher DA, Pandian MR, Carlton E. Autoimmune thyroid disease: an expanding spectrum. Pediatr Clin North Am 1987; 34:907–918.

106. Doniach D, Florin-Christensen A. Autoimmunity in the pathogenesis of endocrine exophthalmos. Clin Endocrinol Metab 1975; 4:341–350.

107. Solomon DH, Chopra IJ, Chopra U, Smith FJ. Identification of subgroups of euthyroid Graves' ophthalmopathy. N Engl J Med 1977; 296:181–186.

108. Gamblin GT, Harper DG, Galentine P, Buck DR, Chernow B, Eil C. Prevalence of increased intraocular pressure in Graves' disease—evidence of frequent subclinic opthalmopathy. N Engl J Med 1983; 308:420–424.

109. Salvi M, Zhang ZG, Haegert D, et al. Patients with endocrine ophthalmopathy not associated with overt thyroid disease have multiple thyroid immunological abnormalities. J Clin Endocrinol Metab 1990; 70:89–94.

110. Schifferdecker E, Manfras B, Kuhnl P, Holzberger G, Boehm BO. HLA-DR3 and variations of the T cell receptor beta gene in Graves' disease. Acta Endocrinol (Copenh) 1991; 124:658–660.

111. Weetman AP. Update. Thyroid-associated ophthalmopathy. Autoimmunity 1992; 12:215–222.

112. Riley WJ, Maclaren NK, Neufeld M. Adrenal autoantibodies and Addison's disease in insulin-dependent diabetes mellitus. J Pediatr 1980; 97:191–195.

113. Betterle C, Scalici C, Pedini B, Mantero F. Addison's disease: principal clinical associations and description of natural history of the disease. Ann Ital Med Int 1989; 4:195–206.

114. Betterle C, Zanette F, Zanchetta R, et al. Complement fixing adrenal autoantibodies: a marker for predicting the onset of idiopathic Addison's disease. Lancet 1983; 1:1238–1240.

115. Krohn K, Uibo R, Aavik E, Peterson P, Savilahti K. Identification by molecular cloning of an autoantigen associated with Addison's disease as steroid 17 alpha-hydroxylase. Lancet 1992; 339:770–773.

116. Baumann-Antczak A, Wedlock N, Bednarek J, et al. Autoimmune Addison's disease and 21-hydroxylase. Lancet 1992; 340:429–430.

117. Winqvist O, Gustafsson J, Rorsman F, Karlsson FA, Kämpe O. Two different cytochrome P450 enzymes are the adrenal antigens in autoimmune polyendocrine syndrome type I and Addison's disease. J Clin Invest 1993; 92:2377–2385.

118. Neufeld M, Maclaren NK, Blizzard RM. Two types of autoimmune Addison's disease associated with different polyglandular autoimmune (PGA) syndromes. Medicine (Baltimore) 1981; 60:355–362.

119. Papadopoulos KI, Hallengren B. Polyglandular autoimmune syndrome type II in patients with idiopathic Addison's disease. Acta Endocrinol (Cohenh) 1990; 122:472–478.

120. Elder M, Maclaren N, Riley W. Gonadal autoantibodies in patients with hypogonadism and/or Addison's disease. J Clin Endocrinol Metab 1981; 52:1137–1142.

121. Blizzard RM, Chee P, David W. The incidence of parathyroid and other autoantibodies in the sera of patients with idiopathic hypoparathyroidism. Clin Exp Immunol 1966; 1:19–128.

122. Irvine WJ, Barnes EW. Addison's disease, ovarian failure and hypoparathyroidism. Clin Endocrinol Metab 1975; 4:379–434.

123. Supler M, Mickle JP. Lymphocytic hypophysitis: report of a case in a man with cavernous sinus involvement. Surg Neurol 1992; 37:472–476.

124. Mirakian R, Bottazzo GF, Cudworth AG, Richardson CA, Doniach D. Autoimmunity to anterior pituitary cells and the pathogenesis of insulin-dependent diabetes mellitus. Lancet 1982; 1:775–759.

125. Songer TJ, LaPoerte R, Tajima N, et al. Height at diagnosis of insulin dependent diabetes in patients and their non-diabetic family members. BMJ 1986; 292:1419–1422.

126. Scherbaum WA, Czernichow P, Bottazzo GF, Doniach D. Diabetes insipidus in children. IV. A possible autoimmune type with vasopressin cell antibodies. J Pediatr 107:922–925.

127. Riley WJ, Toskes PP, Maclaren NK, Silverstein JH. Predictive value of gastric parietal cell autoantibodies as a marker for gastric and hematologic abnormalities associated with insulin-dependent diabetes. Diabetes 1982; 31:1051–1055.

128. Meek F, Khoury EL, Doniach D, Baum H. Mitochondrial antibodies in chronic liver diseases and connective tissue disorders: further characterization of the autoantigens. Clin Exp Immunol 1980; 41:43–54.

129. Riley WJ, Winer A, Goldstein D. Coincident presence of thyrogastric autoimmunity at onset of type I diabetes. Diabetologia 1983; 24:418–421.

130. Ketchum C, Riley WJ, Maclaren NK. Adrenal dysfunction in asymptomatic patients with adrenocortical autoantibodies. J Clin Endocrinol Metab 1984; 58:1166–1170.

131. Neufeld M, Maclaren N, Blizzard R. Autoimmune polyglandular syndromes. Pediatr Ann 1980; 9:43–53.

132. Winter WE, Maclaren NK. To what extent is "polyendocrine" serology related to the clinical expression of disease. In: Clinical Immunology and Allergy, Doniach D, Bottazzo GF, eds. Vol. 1. London: Bailliere Tindall, 1987:109–123.

133. Riley W, Maclaren N, Rosenbloom A. Thyroid disease in young diabetics. Lancet 1982; 2:489–490.

51

Disorders of Antidiuretic Hormone Homeostasis
Diabetes Insipidus and SIADH

Hans Henning Bode
School of Pediatrics, University of New South Wales,
Prince of Wales Children's Hospital,
Sydney, New South Wales, Australia

John D. Crawford
Harvard Medical School
and Massachusetts General Hospital, Boston, Massachusetts

Marco Danon
Maimonides Medical Center and State University of New York Health Science Center at Brooklyn,
Brooklyn, New York

I. INTRODUCTION

Neuroendocrinology dates its beginning to simultaneous observations made almost 100 years ago when it was discovered that the posterior pituitary represented the neuronal terminals originating in the brain and that injection of extract of this tissue induced vasoconstriction, uterine contraction, and lactation in appropriately conditioned animals (1–3). Paradoxically, the antidiuretic action of such extracts was not shown until 25 years later.

The recognition that diabetes insipidus represented a hormone deficiency rather than the response to excessive secretion of an unidentified substance followed the independent observations of van den Velden and Farini (who restored urinary concentration ability in affected patients with injection of posterior pituitary extract (4,5).

Nephrogenic diabetes insipidus, the syndrome of target tissue resistance to vasopressin, was first described as an X-linked genetic disease by Waring et al. (6) and Forssman (7) 50 years ago. These investigators established independently that the target resistance was limited to the tissue of the renal medulla and the vasoconstrictive effect of vasopressin was preserved. Elucidation of the molecular genetic basis for nephrogenic diabetes insipidus was only recently accomplished following the characterization by Birnbaumer et al.

(8) and Lolait et al. (9) of the V_2 receptor gene and subsequent documentation of a multiplicity of point mutations of this gene in patients afflicted with nephrogenic diabetes insipidus (10,11).

In contrast to vasopressin deficiency, excessive secretion of this hormone has become a far more frequent problem in modern medicine and is most often related to inappropriate intravenous fluid therapy. This syndrome of inappropriate antidiuretic hormone secretion (SIADH) was first recognized by Schwartz et al. (12) in patients with bronchial carcinoma who received intravenous fluid therapy. Their symptoms and signs were almost identical to those exhibited by volunteers whom Leaf et al. (13) had studied while exposed to constant and excessive amounts of exogenous vasopressin.

In the past decade, many new insights have been gained about vasopressin and its gene structure (14), as well as the diversity of vasopressin receptors and their various different actions (15). Better understanding of the mechanism and control of thirst and its interaction with vasopressin secretion has improved our clinical management of disorders of fluid homeostasis.

Our goal for the future is to elucidate the pathophysiology of disease states associated with chronic hyperosmolality and hypernatremia for which we have at present no unifying concept of etiology or effective therapy.

In this chapter, we review the physiology and pathophysiologic aspects of antidiuretic hormone (ADH) secretion and action as they relate to clinical disease and to the management of children with disorders of fluid and solute homeostasis.

II. ANTIDIURETIC HORMONE PHYSIOLOGY

A. Vasopressin Synthesis

Vasopressin is a nonapeptide with a disulfide bridge between positions 1 and 6. Its synthesis and secretion as related to fluid homeostasis are under the control of the magnocellular neurons located in the supraoptic and paraventricular nuclei of the anterior hypothalamus (Fig. 1).

Vasopressin is initially assembled as a macromolecular precursor, propressophysin, and is packaged within neurocellular granules (16). Subsequently, vasopressin-neurophysin II is cleaved from the latter complex and transported by the cells of the supraoptic and paraventricular nuclei along their axons to the infundibulum and the posterior pituitary (17). It is stored there in microvesicles and released by depolarization of the neurohypophyseal neurons (18). A bundle of shorter axons predominantly originating from the paraventricular nuclei transports vasopressin to the floor of the third ventricle and to the median eminence, where it is secreted into the portal blood supply of the anterior pituitary. Both the synthesis and transport of the microvesicles are stimulated by osmotic and baroreceptor signals.

B. Regulation of Vasopressin Secretion

1. Osmoreceptors

Vasopressin secretion is influenced by a number of variables (Table 1). Under physiologic conditions, the predominant influence on vasopressin release is exerted by the osmoreceptors located near the supraoptic nuclei in the anterolateral hypothalamus (19). These cells are believed to be in direct contact with capillary branches of the anterior cerebral artery and thus to function outside the blood-brain barrier. They are highly sensitive to increases in extracellular tonicity and induce abrupt vasopressin secretion in response to increases in plasma osmolality. The "set point" lies between 275 and 290 mOsmol/kg and varies minimally between individuals and age groups but tends to be slightly higher in mature men than in children or grown women (20). It is also influenced significantly by alterations in blood volume and pressure (Fig. 2) (21). The antidiuretic but not the polydipsic response to increased plasma tonicity remains intact even after surgical separation of the hypothalamus from the rest of the brain (22). An almost linear direct correlation exists between plasma vasopressin concentration and osmolality, the former rising approximately 1 pg/ml for every 1% rise above the set point in plasma osmolality. The slope and the intercept on the x axis of plasma osmolality provide measures of the sensitivity and the threshold of the system.

The differences in plasma vasopressin levels present during fluid overload and fluid restriction are surprisingly small. According to Robertson et al. (23), plasma levels of

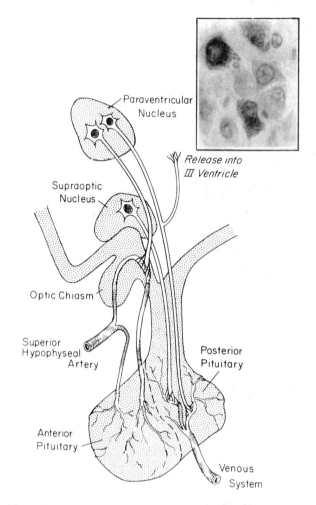

Figure 1 Schematic diagram on the neurohypophyseal system. Vasopressin synthesized in the paired supraoptic and paraventricular nuclei is transported bound to neurophysin along the unmyelinated axons to the posterior pituitary. Separate axons transport vasopressin to the median eminence and the wall of the third ventricle. Interruption of transport from the hypothalamic nuclei within the blood brain barrier does prevent vasopressin release into circulation. The inset depicts a Gomori stain of the large cells in the supraoptic nucleus containing microvesicles with vasopressin granules.

vasopressin average 2.7 ± 1.4 pmol/ml in recumbent subjects whose plasma osmolality is 287 ± 2.1 mOsmol/kg. Vasopressin levels decline to 1.4 ± 0.8 pmol/ml during overhydration and rise to 5.4 ± 3.4 pg/ml after prolonged water deprivation with concurrent increases in plasma osmolality to 292 mOsmol/kg. Rises in plasma vasopressin beyond 8.0 pmol/ml are often observed but do not cause a significant further increase in antidiuretic activity. The sensitivity of the osmoreceptors inducing vasopressin release in response to osmolar challenge is increased during hypoglycemia and hyperglycemia (24). Hyperglycemia stimulates thirst and vasopressin secretion only in insulinopenic diabetes mellitus,

Table 1 Factors Influencing Vasopressin Secretion

Factor	Increased Secretion	Decreased Secretion
Physiologic	Hypovolemia	Hypervolemia
	Hypo-osmolality	Hypo-osmolality
	Upright Position	Recumbent position
	Central hyperthermia	Central hypothermia
Pathologic	Cerebral disease	Diabetes insipidus
	Chest disease	
	Malignancies	
	Adrenal Insufficiency	
Pharmacologic	Carbamazepine, clofibrate	Alcohol
	Nicotine, angiotensin II	Dilantin
	Cholinergic drugs	Anticholinergic agents
	Morphine, barbiturates	

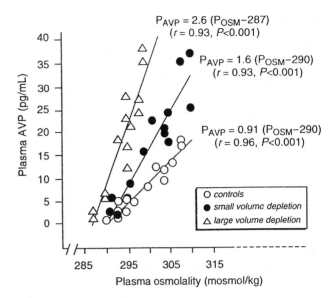

Figure 2 Vasopressin secretion in relation to serum osmolality is amplified by coexisting hypovolemia. In the presence of severe volume depletion vasopressin secretion is augmented even without osmotic stimulus and rises steeply with an osmotic challenge.

suggesting that glucose uptake by the osmoreceptor cells is insulin dependent (25).

2. Baroreceptors

In contrast to the extraordinary sensitivity of the osmoregulatory system, which induces abrupt vasopressin secretion, the vasopressin release mediated by hemodynamic regulatory mechanisms is sluggish when only minor changes in blood pressure and volume take place. Vasopressin release is exponential, however, during more pronounced alterations in blood volume, such as those that occur during acute hemorrhage. With abrupt reduction in effective blood volume, whether by loss or as in syncope or shock, plasma vasopressin rises rapidly to levels far beyond those observed during severe dehydration, reaching concentrations at which its pressor and its action to increase blood coagulation are evident (26). Most but not all baroreceptor signals are mediated through afferent polysynaptic pathways involving the vagal and glossopharyngeal nerves and nucleus tractus solitaris in the brain stem (27). These carry signals from pressure-sensitive receptors in the heart and major arteries. The vasopressin release observed upon assumption of an upright position reflects some of the short-lasting influences of the regulatory system.

Baroreceptors contribute only minimally to the day-to-day maintenance of fluid and electrolyte homeostasis during health, but they influence the set point and slope of vasopressin release controlled by the osmoregulatory mechanism (Fig. 2) (28). Their function becomes clinically significant when "effective" blood volume is diminished as in congestive cardiac failure or nephrosis or in chronically bedridden patients, rendering them susceptible to water intoxication.

A multitude of drugs exert their effect on vasopressin secretion through baroreceptor pathways. Among them are nicotine, morphine, diuretics, prostaglandins, and catecholamines (27).

3. Emesis (29)

Nausea and vomiting, whether occurring spontaneously or drug induced, are extremely potent in releasing vasopressin.

Plasma levels rise to more than 100 times those serving to modulate urine concentration under ordinary circumstances. Effective antiemetic therapy or prophylaxis suppresses the acute rise in plasma vasopressin but does not suppress vasopressin release in response to simultaneous osmolar or hemodynamic stimuli. It is likely that emetic stimuli are at least in part responsible for the vasopressin release observed during cyclophosphalmide infusion, ketoacidosis, or hypoxia.

4. Environmental Factors

Stimulation of vasopressin secretion by regions of the forebrain was documented early by Verney (30), who observed antidiuresis during emotional and physical stress. Pain, physical exercise, and acute exposure to cold have been shown to enhance the release of ADH. Probably more important under these circumstances than the peripheral release of vasopressin and resultant antidiuresis is the release of vasopressin at the median eminence, where it enters the portal vascular system of the anterior pituitary. According to recent observations (31, 32), vasopressin is the major mediator of pituitary adrenocorticotropic hormone (ACTH) release during stress and insulin-induced hypoglycemia; corticotropin-releasing hormone (CRH) plays only a permissive role in the process (33). This may explain the correction of low plasma cortisol concentrations during hypoglycemia or after pyrogen injections in some patients with known anterior pituitary insufficiency (34).

C. Vasopressin Action

The major target organ for arginine vasopressin (AVP) is the kidney. This hormone acts on the collecting ducts and distal tubules and increases their permeability to water. AVP acts on receptor sites of the basal surface of the collecting duct cells and activates adenylate cyclase, thereby stimulating the production of cyclic AMP in the cytoplasm. This makes the cell membranes more permeable, allowing the diffusion of water. More water may also enter because of osmosis. Thus, most of the water is reabsorbed from the tubules, whereas the electrolytes are lost in the urine. As more and more water is retained, there is expansion of the plasma and of the extracellular volume. This corrects the hyperosmolality that stimulated the secretion of AVP.

1. Receptors

The effects of AVP are mediated by two major classes of receptor (35). The V_1 receptor is coupled to phospholipase C and thus increases the turnover of the inositol phosphates and allows the influx of Ca^{2+} to raise intracellular Ca^{2+} concentrations. This receptor is subdivided into V_{1a} and V_{1b} because the binding properties of the pituitary corticotrope (V_{1b}) to a variety of vasopressin agonists and antagonists differ from those of other V_1 receptor tissues. The rat V_{1a} arginine vasopressin receptor was recently cloned in hepatocytes and has seven transmembrane domains (36). The V_2 receptor is coupled via the regulatory G proteins to adenylate cyclase and is found principally in the kidney (37). Both the human and the rat V_2 receptors have been cloned (38,39). The gene, located on the long arm of the X chromosome, encodes a 370 amino acid protein with a transmembrane topography characteristic of G protein-coupled receptors.

2. Control of Diuresis

The ability to dilute and concentrate urine is unique to the mammalian kidney. The formation of dilute urine is achieved by the phylogenetically new architecture of the renal medulla, in which the loops of Henle function as a countercurrent multiplier system.

Approximately 80–90% of the isoosmotic glomerular filtrate is reabsorbed in the proximal tubule. The remaining filtrate enters the descending limb of Henle's loop and equilibrates with the increasingly hypertonic interstitium of the renal medulla through passive reabsorption of water. The osmolar concentration at the tip of the loop in the renal papilla can be as high as 1200 mOsmol/kg. During passage through the ascending limb of Henle's loop, urine osmolality declines and reaches greater dilution than the corresponding interstitial environment through active chloride and sodium removal in the thick section of the limb, which is less permeable to water. Urine delivered to the distal convoluted tubule is therefore always dilute. The active chloride pump in the ascending loop is the source of the concentrating gradient in the renal medulla. Active sodium chloride transport in the medullary portion of the loop is enhanced by vasopressin in several species, but this hormone has no effect on salt transport in the cortical part of the ascending loop (40). The U-shaped vasa recta are in osmotic equilibrium with the interstitial environment. They function as highly efficient countercurrent exchangers and allow the removal of reabsorbed solute and

water. The efficiency of this countercurrent gradient system is dependent on normal urine flow and kidney perfusion.

In the absence of vasopressin, the collecting duct and distal cortical nephron are impermeable and prevent the bulk flow of water into the hypertonic renal medullary interstitium. The dilute urine of the distal convoluted tubule can be changed only minimally in volume and tonicity at the top of the renal papilla, where reabsorption can occur even in the absence of vasopressin. Urine volume in severe diabetes insipidus can be as high as 10% of the total glomerular filtrate. In the presence of vasopressin the collecting duct becomes permeable, allowing the passive bulk flow of water to equilibrate with the surrounding interstitium. Urine volume markedly decreases and osmolality exceeds 1000 mOsmol/kg.

III. REGULATION OF THIRST AND FLUID SATIETY

Under physiologic conditions, water and solute homeostasis is maintained within a very narrow range, even during wide variations in fluid and food intake. This is accompanied by the coordinated control of vasopressin secretion, which acts at the kidney to limit water losses, and drinking behavior and thirst, which modulate water intake. These coordinated functions serve to maintain the essential constancy of systemic tonicity and effective blood volume (Fig. 3).

A. Osmoregulation

Suppression of thirst and vasopressin release occurs during water excess. During water deprivation, thirst is at least as important as vasopressin secretion in maintaining fluid homeostasis, and both share similar neuronal pathways for transmission of osmoregulatory and baroreceptor signals. Strong evidence exists to support the idea that thirst and vasopressin release are both regulated by the osmoreceptors in or near the supraoptic nuclei (28). Inadequate water intake results in systemic hypertonicity. This is "sensed" by the osmoreceptors, which promptly signal for antidiuretic hormone secretion and drinking. Excess water intake, on the other hand, induces less abruptly but reliably a sense of adipsia or water avoidance; the simultaneous suppression of vasopressin release leads to water diuresis and correction of serum hypoosmolality.

Increases in serum osmolality induced by glucose and urea constitute weak stimuli for thirst (41). This suggests that the osmoreceptors are fully permeable to urea and admit glucose freely when insulin is available; when insulin is unavailable, as in diabetes mellitus, glucose becomes a potent stimulus to the osmoreceptors in provoking thirst and polydipsia (25). Nonosmotic control mechanisms of physiologic thirst involve laryngeal and oropharyngeal nerve endings sensitive to temperature changes (42,43). The drinking of ice water markedly reduces thirst during hypertonicity well before the absorption of water and a fall in serum osmolality are demonstrable. Clinicians have taken advantage of this mechanism by offering ice cubes to fluid-restricted patients. Other

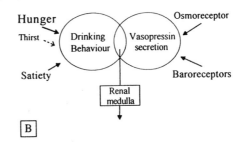

Figure 3 Fluid and osmolar homeostasis is maintained by simultaneous stimulation or suppression of drinking and vasopressin secretion. Both rely on a normally functioning renal medulla which can dilute or concentrate urine over a twentyfold range (A). In infancy (B) hunger is the primary stimulus for drinking and overrides fluid satiety sensation. Therefore vasopressin secretion has to remain suppressed in order to faciliate the excretion of an obligatory dilute urine. Long-acting vasopressin administration in infancy will always lead to dilutional hyponatremia and less frequently to seizures if frequent feeding is maintained.

oropharyngeal neurons prove sensitive to osmotic change. The drinking of hypertonic saline induces thirst and vasopressin secretion before absorption occurs, but neither is stimulated by drinking normal saline (44).

B. Hemodynamic Control

A sudden fall in blood volume or pressure also provokes drinking as well as vasopressin secretion, and both responses may well be mediated by identical baroreceptor pathways (45). Several lines of evidence suggest that angiotensin II plays a physiologic role in the control of thirst, but proof of such a dipsogenic effect has been difficult to establish (46).

A dysfunction of the thirst mechanism and subnormal drinking behavior are the major factors contributing to the syndrome of chronic hypernatremia. The failure of the sense of fluid satiety to override all impulses for water intake is the principal cause of hyponatremia in the ambulatory patient exposed to excess vasopressin. Fluid satiety is regularly overridden by hunger, a phenomenon that disqualifies the use of long-acting vasopressin preparations for the treatment of diabetes insipidus in infants whose diet is provided entirely in liquid form. (Fig. 3B).

IV. INTERRELATIONSHIP OF VASOPRESSIN WITH OTHER HORMONES

The secretion and antidiuretic action of vasopressin are influenced by many other endocrine systems. The amelioration of diabetes insipidus with the onset of hypothyroidism and adrenal insufficiency has been recognized for many years (47). Clinicians have learned from these observations to suspect poor compliance with the prescribed thyroxine replacement whenever their patients with diabetes insipidus and panhypopituitarism claim to have no further need for vasopressin therapy.

Pregnancy is associated with worsening of symptoms from diabetes insipidus. Remarkable polyuria and polydypsia may develop in carriers of the gene for nephrogenic diabetes

insipidus who have hitherto been asymptomatic. These phenomena are attributable primarily by the reduced half-life of vasopressin in blood as a result of increased vasopressinase activity (49). The antidiuretic action of vasopressin is also affected by gender and phase of estrous cycle in animals, but such sexual dimorphism is insignificant in humans (50).

A multifaceted interaction exists between the neurohypophyseal system and the hypothalamic-pituitary-adrenal axis (Fig. 4). AVP augments the ACTH response to CRH stimulus under physiologic conditions and controls ACTH secretion during certain conditions of stress, when CRH plays only a permissive role (31). ACTH and cortisol release during hypoglycemia is thought to be entirely under AVP control (32). A similar mechanism may be involved in the ACTH release observed following pyrogen stimulation in hypopituitary women who underwent pituitary stalk section as part of the treatment of their breast cancer (34). Cortisol and other glucocorticoids, on the other hand, have a negative feedback effect on AVP secretion. Experimentally, dexamethasone reduces the AVP response to nicotine, to CRH, and to insulin-induced hypoglycemia (51). Clinically, glucocorticoid administration induces very rapid correction of SIADH observed in patients with ACTH deficiency (52,53).

Other hormones, such as parathyroid hormone, aldosterone, and catecholamines, exert their influences on fluid homeostasis indirectly by causing renal resistance to AVP during hypercalcemia or hypokalemia or by eliciting baroreceptor stimulation through their vasoactive properties.

V. DIABETES INSIPIDUS

Diabetes insipidus describes all conditions associated with the excretion of copious amounts of dilute urine. The excessive free water turnover may be the result of vasopressin deficiency or resistance, of primary renal disease, or, rarely in childhood, of primary polydipsia. Each of these three conditions exerts a characteristic but different influence on the mechanisms controlling fluid and solute homeostasis. In vasopressin-defi-

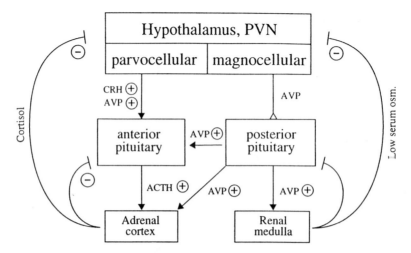

Figure 4 Interaction of the neurohypophyseal system with the hypothalamic-pituitary-adrenal axis. Portal CRH and AVP are important interactive controllers of ACTH secretion. The resulting cortisol secretion from the adrenal cortex exerts negative feedback control over CRH, pituitary ACTH as well as AVP secretion from both the parvocellular and magnocellular neurons of the paraventricular nuclei. In adrenal insufficiency AVP secretion persists regardless of whether hyponatraemia is dilutional in nature and due to anterior pituitary deficiency or due to primary adrenal disease associated with hyperkalemic dehydration. AVP of the posterior pituitary has a minor influence on ACTH secretion and only at very high levels on adrenal cortisol secretion. (33)

cient and nephrogenic diabetes insipidus, the urine-concentrating ability but not the ability to dilute urine is severely reduced. A large water intake is therefore required to prevent plasma hypertonicity; the extent of the obligatory polydipsia is directly proportional to the solute load presenting for renal excretion. In contrast, primary polydipsia causes plasma hypotonicity if the dietary solute intake is insufficient to provide at least 60 mOsmol solute for every liter water requiring excretion. Last, in primary renal disease, both urine dilution and concentration are limited: solute and free water intake therefore must remain more strictly proportional to maintain homeostasis. The emphasis of this chapter is on the discussion of vasopressin-deficient and vasopressin-resistant states.

A. Vasopressin Deficiency Syndrome

1. Etiology

Polyuric states caused by deficient vasopressin delivery to the renal medulla can be caused by defects in the hypothalamic hormone synthesis, packaging, and transport along the neurohypophyseal tract beyond the blood barrier to the posterior pituitary, by abnormalities of the osmoreceptors signaling vasopressin release, or by accelerated inactivation of vasopressin through vasopressinase or circulating antibodies. Clinically, most prominent among these etiologies are disease processes that interfere with vasopressin transport from the hypothalamus beyond the blood-brain barrier and to the posterior pituitary.

   a. Trauma. Accidental head injuries may result in diabetes insipidus within 24 h after injury. In about half of these patients the disease resolves spontaneously. In others, permanent vasopressin deficiency develops after an "interphase" of uncontrolled vasopressin release from the degenerating posterior pituitary (Fig. 5). The antidiuresis of the triphasic pattern usually becomes apparent a few days after trauma, lasts 2–5 days, and rarely persists beyond day 10 after injury (54). The same phenomenon can also be observed after neurosurgical intervention and damage to the hypothalamus or the neurohypophyseal tract. It should be anticipated in all patients developing intra- or early postoperative diabetes insipidus. Appropriate restriction of fluid intake during the interphase effectively prevents symptoms and signs of SIADH. Some children recovering from traumatic stalk section and transient diabetes insipidus form an ectopic posterior pituitary that may be detected on T1-weighted magnetic resonance images (Fig. 6). The ectopic, radiologically "bright" tissue indicates either incomplete descent or prior interruption of the neural pituitary stalk; however, it does not necessarily suggest cessation of the portal blood supply, which governs anterior pituitary hormone release.

   b. Tumor and Infiltrative Diseases. Pituitary and hypothalamic tumors account for diabetes insipidus in at least 30% of affected children (55). Craniopharyngiomas, germinomas, and gliomas are the most frequent types. In patients with craniopharyngiomas, symptoms of vasopressin deficiency are usually preceded by visual disturbances or signs of anterior pituitary deficiency and often are observed only after surgical intervention. In contrast, diabetes insipidus is frequently the first symptom presenting in germinomas. In boys with idiopathic diabetes insipidus, the onset of precocious testosterone secretion should always be considered a sign of human chorionic gonadotropin (hCG) secretion and demands measurement of β-hCG to exclude a dysgerminoma with trophoblasts producing this hormone.

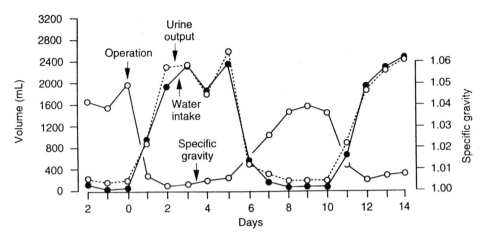

Figure 5 The triphasic response to experimental pituitary stalk section in dogs which mirrors the events after traumatic stalk section in humans. Immediately post-operative a copious excretion of dilute urine indicates onset of diabetes insipidus. This phase is followed by a period of uncontrolled ADH release from the severed posterior pituitary remnant. This so-called "interphase" varies in duration from 1–6 days before either permanent diabetes insipidus ensues as indicated in this figure, or alternatively homeostatic ADH release from a newly formed ectopic pituitary is restored (see also Fig. 6).

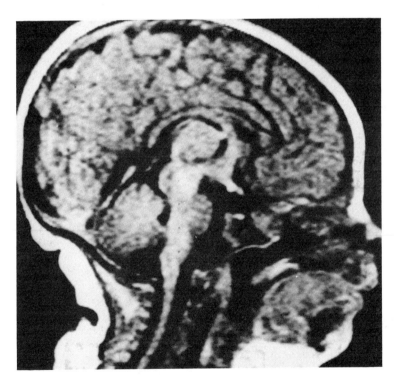

Figure 6 Ectopic posterior pituitary documented on T1 weighted MRI image. In this newborn, incomplete descent of the neurohypophyseal tract during the first trimester prevented connection with the tissue of the Rathke pouch. Increased lipid content of the atrophied adenohypophysis in the sella causes a second area of increased signal intensity. This newborn had secondary anterior pituitary deficiency but not diabetes insipidus as vasopressin is transported normally beyond the blood brain barrier.

Histiocytosis accounts for the majority of the infiltrative diseases of the hypothalamus causing diabetes insipidus. This was formerly considered the most frequent presenting sign of histiocytosis (56) but is now reported to be observed in less than half of the children so affected (57). Sarcoidosis, Wegener's granulomatosis, and tuberculosis are exceedingly rare causes of vasopressin deficiency in childhood (58). In the majority of these children, vasopressin deficiency is permanent, independent of the course of the primary disease. Only occasionally is vasopressin secretion restored after successful medical or radiation therapy of germinomas, granulamatous disease, or histiocytosis (59).

c. Congenital Malformations. Cysts or malformations in the vicinity of the hypothalamus and third ventricle are well known to cause vasopressin deficiency with symptoms presenting in infancy. Septooptic dysplasia is especially prominent among these etiologies. Prolonged hypoxia in the newborn can also cause symptoms and signs of diabetes insipidus. These frequently improve with time. Vascular anomalies, such as aneurysms and thrombosis, have been described in adults as causes of vasopressin deficiency. As in the neonate, diabetes insipidus can be associated with severe hypoxic encephalopathy in older children and usually indicates a poor prognosis for normal neurologic development (60,61).

d. Infection. Infections, including meningitis, encephalitis, and toxoplasmosis, are rare causes of diabetes insipidus (62). Tuberculosis and syphilis, major causes of diabetes insipidus decades ago, are no longer prominent etiologic considerations.

e. Autoimmune Hypophysitis. Approximately one-third of patients with idiopathic diabetes insipidus have circulating antibodies to the vasopressin-producing cells of the hypothalamus. This suggests that in these cases diabetes insipidus may have an autoimmune etiology. However, such antibodies can also be present in patients with diabetes insipidus of other causes. Documentation of such circulating antibodies is therefore not sufficiently reassuring to limit the search for other etiologies (63).

f. Hereditary Vasopressin Deficiency. The familial occurrence of vasopressin-sensitive diabetes insipidus has been known for many years (64). There is variation in severity of the disorders from one pedigree to another, but most affected members do not become symptomatic until after infancy. Recently, normal vasopressin secretion has been documented before the onset of symptoms of deficiency (65). In most families, the disease is inherited as an autosomal dominant trait, but there does not seem to be a uniform mode of inheritance. In several well-studied families, the etiology of the disorder was linked to specific mutations in the arginine vasopressin neurophysin II gene (66-68). These defects do not interfere initially with active vasopressin transport and release but presumably cause secondary degeneration of the neurohypophyseal system resulting in vasopressin deficiency and the paucity of neurosecretory cells discovered at autopsy (69). These observations explain the typical disease-free period in infancy as well as the progressive loss of antidiuretic function with age.

In other affected families, a specific defect in osmoreceptor-mediated vasopressin release has been documented (70). These patients respond to baroreceptor stimuli, and their symptoms are usually milder (Fig. 7). According to at least one study, the vasopressin release to nicotine stimulation is also preserved (71). Affected members of these pedigrees respond well to long-acting vasopressin analogs but also show a dramatic reduction in the daily urine secretion when treated with chlorothiazide or one of its congeners.

Last, there is the autosomal recessively inherited Wolfram syndrome of diabetes insipidus, diabetes mellitus, optic atrophy, and neurosensory deafness (72). Symptoms and disease presentation vary widely. Vasopressin deficiency and progressive deafness are usually late complications of this degenerative disease. The Wolfram syndrome is thought to be a mitochondrially mediated disorder in which defective ATP supply is the unifying etiology for the varying clinical presentation. Recent documentation of a point mutation in mitochondrially encoded tRNA gene as well as of a deletion of mitochondrial DNA provide strong support for this hypothesis (73,74).

g. Idiopathic Diabetes Insipidus. Diabetes insipidus of unknown causes accounted for almost 50% of cases in some of the older published series. This proportion has declined markedly in recent years, and it can be expected that advances in diagnostic technology will lead to a further reduction of cases in this category. As imaging techniques improve and molecular markers become available for clinical use, the etiology of the vasopressin deficiency will be identified in all but a few cases.

2. Clinical Presentation

The symptomatology in children with diabetes insipidus varies widely with age and is influenced not only by the extent of vasopressin deficiency but also by diet, preservation of normal thirst, and anterior pituitary function.

In infants the disease is often masked and may be present with failure to thrive, unexplained fevers, vomiting, and constipation. Poor growth is the likely consequence of chronic hypertonicity as well as of poor nutrition. A history of excessive urine output is often not elicited until laboratory tests reveal hypernatremia.

More than one-third of older children give a history of recent onset of excessive drinking, with nocturia and enuresis developing in a previously toilet-trained child. Practically all children with diabetes insipidus require water during the night and become inconsolable if fluid is withheld. There may be a history indicating preference for ice water because of its superb ability to ameliorate their chronic thirst. These children also tend to avoid diets high in protein and salt, which require them to drink even larger amounts of fluid to provide the water necessary for excretion of the renal solute residue. In children with diabetes insipidus caused by hypothalamic disease, concomitant deficiency of anterior pituitary hormone secretion may cause additional symptoms but has an ameliorating effect on polyuria. Diabetes insipidus associated with headaches and ocular signs, such as visual field restriction,

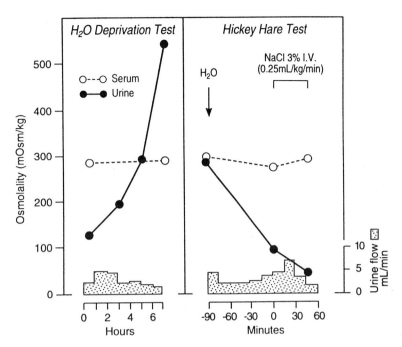

Figure 7 The antidiuretic response to water deprivation and hypovolemia but failure to secrete ADH during normovolemic hypernatremia in a boy with familial diabetes insipidus due to defective osmoregulatory vasopressin release. There is sluggish reduction in urine flow and increased urine concentration during water deprivation suggesting an ADH secretory response. In contrast, hypertonic saline infusion causes further reduction in urine osmolality and increased urine volume pathognomonic for vasopressin deficiency.

optic atrophy, strabismus, and nystagmus, should alert the physician to the presence of an intracranial lesion. In isolated vasopressin deficiency, abnormal physical findings may be limited but a large distended bladder is often easily palpable except when the child is examined soon after voiding.

3. Diagnosis

The diagnosis of diabetes insipidus is confirmed when in the absence of primary or secondary renal disease hypotonic urine is excreted in the presence of serum hypertonicity and hypernatremia. Neurohypophyseal disease is indicated when the symptoms can be relieved by vasopressin administration. The absence of response to vasopressin or desmopressin under these circumstances, especially if the serum vasopressin concentration can be shown to be elevated, is pathognomonic of nephrogenic diabetes insipidus.

The majority of children whose parents seek medical attention for their offspring's polyuria and polydipsia do not have organic disease. Simple screening tests for confirmation of the history should therefore precede detailed diagnostic testing. Usually sufficient are analyses carried out on a fasting urine specimen, the second morning voiding passed after withholding all fluids from midnight on. The urine to be analyzed should be paired with a serum sample taken within a few minutes of the voiding. Determinations in the urine should include osmolality, creatinine, and sodium, in addition to noting the volume, determining the time interval between this and the last prior voiding, and performing a standard urine analysis. The serum sample should be analyzed for

osmolality, sodium, creatinine, calcium, potassium, and vasopressin. Of course, the child's state of comfort, hydration, and weight at the time the blood specimen is drawn should be noted. The outcome of these observations and laboratory analyses guide the pediatrician in deciding what further diagnostic tests are needed. Urine osmolalities consistently approaching isosthenuria (200–400 mOsmol/kg) suggest that primary or secondary renal disease needs to be considered. In children presenting with hypokalemia or hypercalcemia, etiologies other than vasopressin deficiency should be searched for. On the other hand, in those patients excreting consistently dilute urine (<200 mOsmol/kg) while hypertonic and hypernatremic, plasma vasopressin concentration should be determined without delay and the response to exogenous vasopressin measured. For those presenting with less classic signs of diabetes insipidus, a formal water deprivation test must be performed.

a. The Water Deprivation Test. This test is begun in the morning. After a light breakfast the patient is weighed and water, 500 ml/m² body surface, is given by mouth. Thereafter, hourly weights and urine volumes are recorded and the patient is given water in amounts equal to urine volume. Once a steady diuresis is established, initial blood samples are drawn for measurement of serum sodium, osmolality, and vasopressin. Thereafter, fluids are withheld for 6 h. Urine volumes and osmolalities and the patient's weights are recorded hourly. At the termination of the tests, blood and urine samples for sodium, osmolality, and vasopressin determinations are obtained. The persistent excretion of dilute urine with osmolality less than that of plasma, a rise in serum sodium concentration above 145 mmol/L, and serum osmolality above 290 mOsmol/kg coupled with a weight loss of 3–5% suggest the presence of diabetes insipidus. Antidiuretic hormone deficiency is established when the patient responds to vasopressin with a rise in urine tonicity to at least 400 mOsmol/kg beyond the maximum concentration during water deprivation. Hourly weight loss should be compared with urine volumes to exclude surreptitious fluid intake. Urine sodium concentration at the termination of the test should be less than 20 mmol/L despite coexisting hypernatremia. High urine sodium losses suggest the presence of renal disease with loss of sodium conservation ability during hypovolemia. In infants and small children, 6 h of water deprivation is not always necessary or advisable, and this test should therefore be interrupted as soon as the criteria for diagnosis have been reached. In older children, prolongation of the test may be required, but the subjects must be kept under close supervision and the test terminated as soon as possible. Measurement of plasma vasopressin at the end of the test confirms the diagnosis in most patients.

The water deprivation test is designed to measure vasopressin release in response to both osmoreceptor and baroreceptor stimulation. In diabetes insipidus caused by an isolated osmoreceptor defect but with preservation of the normal response to hypovolemia, the water deprivation test provides inconclusive results. In patients with long-standing psychogenic polydipsia, water deprivation does not always lead to a rapid rise in urine osmolality (76). In such patients it may be necessary to examine vasopressin release during a normovolemic, hypernatremic state.

b. Hypertonic Saline Infusion Test (75). Early in the day while fasting, the patient is given 20 ml/kg of 2.5% glucose water intravenously over a period of 1 h. Hydration may be alternatively accomplished with water by mouth, 500 ml/m^2, until steady diuresis is observed. Thereafter, hypertonic sodium chloride solution (2.5%) is infused intravenously at a rate of 0.25 ml/kg/minute over 45 minutes. Urine volume and osmolality are determined every 15 minutes, and serum sodium, osmolality, and plasma vasopressin are measured before and at the end of the hypertonic saline infusion.

Normal subjects show an antidiuresis within 30 minutes after initiation of the saline infusion. Patients with diabetes insipidus show an increase in urine volume and a fall in urine osmolality. Their vasopressin secretion remains subnormal for the degree of serum hypertonicity. In some patients with psychogenic polydipsia, the decrease in urine volume and increase in urine osmolality may be intermediate; however, plasma vasopressin release is linear in proportion to the increase in plasma tonicity, clearly differentiating those with primary polydipsia from those with vasopressin deficiency. This provocative test should never be performed in children unless vasopressin sensitivity has been previously documented because in nephrogenic diabetes insipidus severe hypernatremia will ensue and require large amounts of free water for correction of hyperosmolality.

c. Other Diagnostic Tests. Other diagnostic maneuvers are rarely needed and are only of academic interest. Once the diagnosis of vasopressin-deficient diabetes insipidus is established, the etiology must be carefully investigated. Radiologic procedures should include skull films, which may show distortion of the sella turcica. Supracellar calcification suggests a craniopharyngioma or other tumor; punched out "holes" are typical of histiocytosis. Children with the latter disease may present with a history of loosening of healthy teeth with a bony lesion that can be detected on specific radiologic views. Maculopapular skin rashes are often seen, and a biopsy may serve to establish the diagnosis. Magnetic resonance imaging studies have replaced the computed tomography scan for evaluation of hypothalamic lesions. In the vast majority of healthy children, functioning posterior pituitary tissue can be visualized on the T1-weighted images (Fig. 6). The absence of this bright spot in children with diabetes insipidus suggests interruption of the neurohypophyseal-pituitary communication above or at the blood-brain barrier, or it may support the diagnosis of familial diabetes insipidus (77). The latter etiology demands that screening tests be performed at least in patient's first-degree relatives.

4. Differential Diagnosis

Disorders mimicking the symptoms of vasopressin insufficiency are listed in Table 2. They are divided into two groups: conditions in which polyuria may be a consequence of increased fluid intake while vasopressin secretion is physiologically suppressed and, alternatively, those in which vasopressin is secreted normally but there is a failure of the kidneys to respond appropriately.

Polyuria as a consequence of polydipsia is not infrequently observed in young children. In the vast majority the high fluid intake is a function of the parents' misguided perception that water drinking is beneficial to their children's health and a good preventive measure. Dryness of the mouth either drug induced or caused by mouth breathing can be another cause of polydipsia. Psychogenic polydipsia in adolescence is usually characterized by marked amelioration during sleep. These patients shy away from drinking ice water and often prefer eating a diet high in solutes demanding renal excretion. They can be distinguished from those with partial vasopressin deficiency by their continued fluid intake during exogenous vasopressin infusion, a maneuver that requires close supervision to prevent severe dilutional hyponatremia. The preferred diagnostic maneuver is the infusion of hypertonic saline.

Disease states in which there is an inability of the kidney to elaborate concentrated urine despite vasopressin stimulation vary greatly in etiology. Aside from inherited nephrogenic diabetes insipidus, all these disorders have in common an inability to dilute urine to the same extent as is seen in authentic diabetes insipidus or nephrogenic diabetes insipidus (NDI). Often the polyuria is mild, daily urine volumes not exceeding 2.5L/m^2 body surface. Drug-induced polyuria and that caused by hypercalcemia and hypokalemia usually have a sudden onset and are initially reversible. Hyposthenuria as a result of a secondary hypokalemia is not infrequently

Table 2 Polyuric Conditions Mimicking Vasopressin Deficiency

Physiologic suppression of vasopressin secretion	
Psychogenic polydipsia	
Organic polydipsia (hypothalamic disease)	
Drug-induced polydipsia (thioridazine, tricyclics)	
Reduced renal responsiveness to vasopressin	
Genetics	Nephrogenic diabetes insipidus, Medullary cystic disease
Pharmacologic	Lithium, demeclocycline, penthrane, diuretics
Osmotic diuresis	Diabetes mellitus, reduced nephron population
Electrolyte disturbance	Hypercalcemia, Hypokalaemia
Renal disease	Postobstructive diuresis, Renal tubular acidosis, Pylenonephritis, papillary necrosis, Sickle cell disease
Haemodynamic	Hyperthyroidism

observed in children with cystinosis. Metabolic diseases, such as diabetes mellitus and hyperthyroidism, should not present diagnostic problems.

5. Treatment of Vasopressin Deficiency

Vasopressin deficiency as an isolated defect is not associated with significant morbidity provided that water is always accessible to the patient. During infancy, when the child cannot make its needs known or obtain the water necessary to quench its thirst, it is of particular hazard, as will be evident in considering congenital nephrogenic diabetes insipidus. Once infancy has been survived, the long-term prognosis is good. Untreated diabetes insipidus provides much inconvenience, however, interfering with sleep, interrupting school activities, and reducing the time that can be devoted to leisure (78).

a. Hormone Replacement. The treatment of choice is replacement therapy with the long-acting vasopressin analog

DDAVP (1-desamino-8-D-arginine vasopressin, desmopressin). It is important to keep in mind that this therapy does not restore homeostasis, however: it merely exchanges inconvenient polyuria and polydipsia for a constant antidiuresis. It thus stands to reason that all infants and children dependent upon a high-liquid diet should be disqualified for such treatment because iatrogenically induced SIADH will be the consequence.

DDAVP differs from native vasopressin insofar as the amino terminal in position 1 is absent and L-arginine is replaced by its D isomer in position 8 (Fig. 8). These modifications enhance the ratio of antidiuretic (AD) to vasopressor (VP) activities 200-fold and markedly prolong the biologic half-life (79). As a selective V_2 receptor agonist it is free of the vasoconstrictive side effects that may be prominent with either arginine or lysine vasopressins. Its duration of action is between 6 and 24 h, depending on the dose and state of hydration (80). Nasal insufflation of DDAVP 2.5–10 μg (25–100 μl) will rapidly eliminate polyuria; its

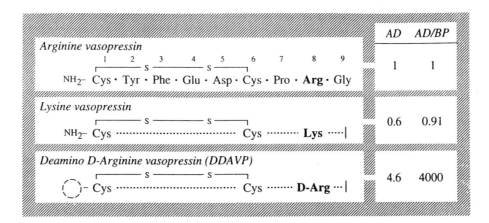

Figure 8 Structure of vasopressin and the synthetic analog DDAVP. Lysine vasopressin, the antidiuretic hormone of the pig family is short acting and available for intranasal application. The antidiuretic potency (AD) and the ratio of antidiuretic/vasopressor activities (AD/BP) are compared with those of arginine vasopressin. The low affinity to V_1 receptors provides DDAVP with a selective antidiuretic action.

action will cease in similarly abrupt fasion. DDAVP is given usually twice daily and the dose titrated for each patient according to needs and effectiveness. Initially a dose between 2.5 and 5.0 $\mu g/m^2$ body surface may be tried. The aim is to provide the child with constant antidiuresis and uninterrupted sleep during the night and allow approximately 1 h of diuresis for correction of a possible water overload before the next evening dose is administered. Excess water intake leading to hyponatremia should be suspected when polyuria develops more than 30 minutes before the expression of thirst. This therapy is enthusiastically accepted and well tolerated, and noncompliance is rare. Reduced and irregular intranasal absorption occurs, especially with upper respiratory infections and allergic rhinitis. Under these conditions doses may be repeated. Other alternatives are the peroral administration of DDAVP, which requires a 20-fold higher dose and is therefore rarely used (81). Given by subcutaneous injection rather than intranasally, the oral DDAVP dose can be reduced by a factor of 10–15; 0.08 μg (0.02 ml/kg) and less in infancy will provoke antidiuresis sustained for 8–15 h. DDAVP is marketed for intranasal administration in a preparation containing 100 $\mu g/ml$. It can be obtained as a nasal spray, the pump-equipped container delivering 0.1 ml or 10 μg per compression. It can also be delivered by rhinal tubes that require the patient to blow a measured dose onto the highly vascular mucosa of the nasal choanal. The rhinal tubes are graduated in 50 ml divisions to facilitate measurement of dose.

DDAVP for parental use is marketed in ampules containing a more dilute solution than that used intranasally. The parental preparation contains 4 $\mu g/ml$ of DDAVP and should always be given by injection to children who are unable to perceive or express thirst, whose fluid intake is restricted, whose management depends on a reliable and predictable antidiuresis, that is, during anesthesia. Short-acting lysine vasopressin (Fig. 8) is commercially available for intranasal use. Its duration of action is limited to a maximum of 4 h. The drug can be used in infants with diabetes insipidus not requiring regular overnight feeding.

b. *Nonhormonal Therapy.* Among the drugs amplifying residual or weak vasopressin secretion or action, chlorpropamide is the most effective and frequently prescribed. It was initially marketed as an oral hypoglycemic drug, and by serendipity it was discovered also to exert vasopressin-enhancing properties. It is a safe drug when administered in moderate doses to patients whose anterior pituitary function is intact; in anterior hypopituitarism the risk of precipitating hypoglycemia is significant. Aside from its ability to potentiate the effect of submaximal amounts of vasopressin, chlorpropamide also stimulates thirst in at least some patients with "essential" hypernatremia and hypodipsia (Fig. 9) (82). Chlorpropamide is administered to responsive patients at a dose of 150 mg/m²/day each morning. Although not as potent an antidiuretic as vasopressin, it restores some degree of fluid homeostasis, providing the patient relief from polyuria as well as the ability to adapt to excess water intake. Other drugs now rarely used for the therapy of diabetes insipidus in childhood are the chlorothiazides and its

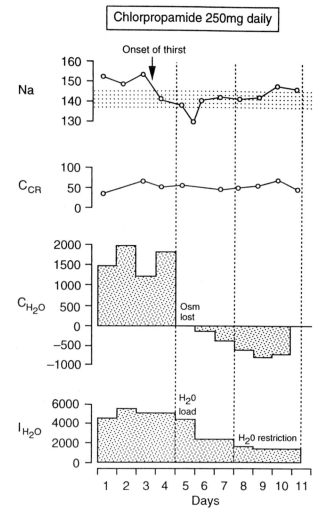

Figure 9 Chlorpropamide-induced restoration of normal drinking behavior and fluid homeostasis in a child with diabetes insipidus, chronic hypernatremia and hypodipsia. Within 36 hours after initiation of chlorpropamide therapy the patient demanded water and later appropriately refused water loading when her serum Na fell to hyponatremic levels. Restriction of fluid intake led to improved antidiuresis and thirst sensation (82).

congeners and the inhibitors of prostaglandin synthesis, especially indomethacin. These drugs are generally reserved for the treatment of nephrogenic diabetes insipidus even though they are equally effective in vasopressin deficiency. This is because their ability to ameliorate polyuria in hormone deficiency is only a fraction of that of vasopressin and its longer acting analogs.

c. *Special Therapeutic Consideration.* The therapy of diabetes insipidus must be adjusted when there is a requirement for a high fluid intake for coverage of caloric needs, that is, in the newborn period and early infancy or when fluid is administered parentally as in the perioperative period.

i. Management of Diabetes Insipidus in Infancy.
Therapy for diabetes insipidus in infancy is especially demanding and difficult. All breast- or formula-fed infants must excrete dilute urine to maintain homeostasis and to eliminate the large amount of free water that derives from their intake. Breast milk and commercial formulas provide only 80–100 mOsmol/L of solute for renal excretion. Vasopressin secretion is therefore chronically suppressed. Exogenous vasopressin administration to infants fed at regular intervals is likely to cause dilutional hyponatremia not infrequently associated with seizures (83). On the other hand, when endogenous vasopressin secretion is severely deficient because of hypothalamic or pituitary damage, the infant requires only dilution of the formula to approximately 30% the strength of the usual preparation or, in breast-fed infants, ad libitum supplementary water intake to remain well hydrated and normonatremic. Also crucial to the therapy of these infants is the frequency of feeding, which should occur every 2 h and may require insertion of a feeding gastrostomy. Therapy can be facilitated by the addition of chlorothiazides as prescribed for patients with nephrogenic diabetes insipidis (see later). In those infants with normal thirst and diabetes insipidus, the addition of a single intranasal application of lysine vasopressin at night further reduces oral fluid needs and allows infants and parents at least a short interval of uninterrupted sleep.

ii. Treatment During Parenteral Fluid Therapy. All patients with diabetes insipidus need adjustment of therapy when intravenous fluid administration is the sole source of water intake. Such adjustment is most often necessary in the perioperative period or during acute gastrointestinal infections. The therapeutic options are again to maintain antidiuresis or to eliminate vasopressin treatment entirely. We prefer therapy designed to produce constant antidiuresis, which can be induced by subcutaneous DDAVP, 0.02 ml (0.08 μg)/kg/body weight administration in 8–12 h intervals, or by intravenous infusion of aqueous vasopressin, 0.03 mμ/kg body weight/minute (0.01 mμ = 25 pg = 2.2 fmol). This dose is within the range required to produce antidiuresis in normal subjects. The volume of intravenous fluid should initially be reduced to approximately 600 ml/m^2/24 h and thereafter be adjusted according to the observed changes in urine and serum sodium concentration and osmolality. With insufficient fluid administration, these patients will complain of thirst. Serum sodium and osmolality will remain normal. At least in the initial phase, their concentrated urine will show a very low sodium concentration, often less than 20 mM. When the patient is thirsty, the urine scant, and the sodium excretion low, the intravenous fluid can be increased by 10–20%. Fluid infusion in excess of needs initially causes very few clinical symptoms, but urine sodium concentrations exceeding 70 mM signal incipient water intoxication unless the rate of intravenous fluid delivery is reduced.

The regimen of constant antidiuresis and restriction of fluid only to those given intravenously is advantageous in unconscious or neurosurgical patients. This regimen eliminates complications associated with unexpected endogenous vasopressin release, such as that during the interphase, and enables the maintenance of serum tonicity and sodium levels within the narrow physiologic range. In neurosurgical patients, surgeons may prefer that the patient be kept "on the dry side" to minimize brain swelling. Paradoxically, this "oliguric" method of management permits much more precise control of fluid balance than the alternative. It is for this reason superior to allowing full diuresis and hourly adjustment of intravenous fluid volumes according to measured urinary and estimated insensible water losses. The latter regimen requires catheterization of the bladder and intensive nursing care and is apt to cause hyperglycemia and hectic fluctuations in serum sodium concentrations and osmolality.

B. Vasopressin-Resistant Syndromes: Nephrogenic Diabetes Insipidus

1. Clinical Presentation and Diagnosis

Nephrogenic diabetes insipidus differs from the disorder caused by vasopressin insufficiency in that there is no renal response to the antidiuretic hormone or any of its analogs. It is a disorder of the hormone receptors analogous to those in testicular feminization of pseudohypoparathyroidism. It is usually familial, the inheritance pattern being that of an X-linked trait (84). Rare instances of apparent autosomal inheritance have been reported; possibly these will be found associated with an anomaly of the gene coding for the water channels (85). The gene coding for these is apparently quite separate from that coding for V$_2$ vasopressin receptor. The renal response to vasopressin depends both upon its binding to and activation of this G protein-coupled receptor as well as the formation and function of the water channels. As in other syndromes of "end organ resistance," hormone levels are normally modulated. Because the receptors are nonfunctional, however, the feedback loop is unsatisfied, and in general, individuals with NDI are chronically hypertonic and dehydrated with high circulating levels of vasopressin.

The "curse" of families in which half of the sons are "drinkers" but never pass on their disability directly but only through their daughters has been chronicled by their own members (86) as well as by physicians. One of the earliest of the latter to describe the disorder and its sex-linked inheritance was McIlraith (87) writing in 1892. Of course, McIlraith (87) was unaware of the hormone unresponsiveness. More relevant to the present consideration, however, was the demonstration by de Lange in 1935 (88) that antidiuretic hormone resistance was a characteristic of some males with congenital diabetes insipidus. However, Forssman (7) in Sweden and Waring, Kadji, and Tappan (6) in the United States, writing in 1945, are generally credited with being the first to associate the sex-linked pattern of inheritance with unresponsiveness to pituitary extract.

In the 60 years since these major features of NDI were first sketched, much detail has been filled in. It has become possible to measure directly the elevated blood levels of arginine vasopressin. Certain of the extrarenal actions of vasopressin have been associated with specific receptors distinct from the renal V$_2$ receptors through which antidiuresis is mediated. In turn, the V$_2$ receptors have been shown to be represented in several extrarenal tissues, where they mediate responses as diverse as release of clotting factors, increase in plasma renin activity, and vasodilation. In NDI, all the functions of the V_2 receptors are absent, whereas the pressor, ACTH release, and glycogenolytic activities mediated through the V_1 receptors are preserved (89). The gene encoding the V_2 receptors has been localized to the distal portion of the long arm of the X chromosome, and lately, the gene structure has been elucidated (8,9). Almost as soon as the structure of the normal gene was known, multiple anomalies associated with absence of function began to be described (10,11). Instead of proving the sturdy gene once imagined, it now became evident that new mutations are relatively frequent, most of which are associated with complete loss of function. These discoveries have "sunk" the "Hopewell hypothesis," whose authors proposed that the anomalous gene had been introduced in North America by Ulster Scot immigrants arriving aboard the ship of that name in Halifax, Nova Scotia in 1761 (84). Even before the precise structure of the V_2 receptor became known, more careful genealogic studies and genetic analyses based on restriction fragment length polymorphisms and variable number tandem repeats had cast doubt on the suggestion that a single family arriving on the Hopewell had been the "founders" of NDI on the North American continent (90).

NDI is a serious condition. Carrier women often become quite uncomfortable during the last trimester. With all pregnancies in these heterozygotes, there is apt to be a mounting polyuria correlated with the rising levels of vasopressinase, a placental aminopeptidase. If the conceptus is an affected male, gestation is complicated by polyhydramnios, increasing the bulk of the uterine contents and compressing the mother's bladder, which is already taxed by increasing urine volume (49).

The affected newborn males, particularly those that are breast fed, may do quite well until solids are added, weaning begun, or an intercurrent infection is superimposed on this normal period of rapid anabolism. With acute infection deterioration may be precipitated but with the gradual introduction of solids and delayed weaning, good progress may give way only gradually to a failure to thrive picture. Commonly the first manifestation of nephrogenic diabetes insipidus is recurrent, unexplained fever. The severity of dehydration may be underestimated by the attending physician because of the continuing abundant urine output. It may not be until it is recommended that the infant be hospitalized and the sodium is discovered to be 160 mmol/L or more that the severity of dehydration is realized. "Adequate" rehydration may be guided by the rules applying to infants with normal renal water conservation ability, tempered by the physician's caution that overrapid correction of hypertonic dehydration can result in seizures. Under such circumstances, valuable time may be lost while it is being discovered that in the face of these measures dehydration has been worsening and hypertonicity increasing. These infants may need such extravagant amounts of "free water" for their intravenous rehydration that the usual concentrations of glucose must be reduced to 2.5% and the highest saline concentration that can be used with benefit is 0.22% (37.5 mmol/L).

Nephrogenic diabetes insipidus is attended by a high mortality and morbidity. In a retrospective study it was found that approximately 20% of patients were lost in childhood or as young adults (55). The analysis suggested that most of the final episodes were aggravated by ill-considered recommendations of physicians. About 80% of affected males showed some degree of mental impairment, in all probability secondary to central nervous system watershed ischemic injury during bouts of dehydration. An equally high percentage of boys showed stunted growth and ended up as short adults. It is to be hoped that this high toll of the disorder has been reduced in recent years with improved knowledge of the special requirements of these patients as well as advances in treatment.

The males who do not succumb as infants often limp through childhood, growing slowly and doing poorly at school. During this period they adapt to the disease by developing bladders of enormous capacity. Megacystis is well tolerated as long as the ureterovesical valves remain competent. Once these give way and the high intravesical pressure begins to be transmitted to the renal parenchyma, the stage is set for development of megaureter and kidney insufficiency. A number of the survivors of the special hazards of infancy are faced by end-stage renal insufficiency as young adults. A few have undergone kidney transplantation and been relieved both of their azotemia and their NDI, inasmuch as the normal kidney is equipped with receptors responsive to the new host's normally modulated vasopressin. This experience provokes the question, should kidney transplantation be considered in infancy for those affected by so devastating a disorder?

Before undertaking a consideration of therapy, note should be taken of the fact that carrier females do not escape with complete impunity. Already the difficulties encountered during pregnancy have been noted. Even when not pregnant, almost all such women show some compromise in their renal water conservation ability. There is a spectrum of disability ranging from women who can concentrate their urine normally (>1000 mOsmol/kg or specific gravity >1.030) to those whose disability is almost as severe as that of the affected male.

2. Treatment

Wastes leaving the body via the kidneys require "packaging" in water. Normally this packaging requirement is so small, under 1 ml/mOsmol of solute, as to be almost negligible. In diabetes insipidus the efficiency of packaging is lost and each milliosmole waste obliges the excretion of 10 ml water. In neurogenic diabetes insipidus, efficiency is restored by administering vasopressin or desmopressin, but in nephrogenic diabetes insipidus there is no response to hormone treatment. Excretion of a solute residue amounting to 600 mOsmol/m^2/day—not an unusual load—requires 6 L water and consumption of at least another L/m^2/day to cover the extra renal water losses. Little wonder that infants and small children with NDI, in whom turnover is so large relative to body water stores, become rapidly dehydrated if they are either unable to drink or denied access to water.

The water requirement of infants and small children can

be markedly reduced by simple dietary measures. Breast milk is the ideal feeding for the neonate with nephrogenic diabetes insipidus. In breast milk the content of minerals, protein, and calories is so closely matched to the infant's needs for growth that the osmotic residue requiring excretion in the urine is minimal, approximately 200 mOsmol/m2/24 h. The water provided in breast milk is abundant even to meet the extravagant needs of diabetes insipidus. Unless the good health of such an infant is interrupted by an illness, extending his water requirement (diarrhea, for example) or reducing his breast milk intake, he may continue to thrive until weaning. At this juncture the substitution of cow milk or initiation of solid foods or both is likely to curtail his water intake and extend the solute load, requiring renal excretion. Dehydration ensues, often first manifest as unexplained episodes of fever. Growth slows and concern increases. Unless a family member familiar with the disorder suggests the diagnosis, it may not be made until a blood sample is obtained, giving insight into the hemoconcentration hitherto unsuspected given the persistent large urine volumes.

The progressive dehydration and failure to thrive syndrome can be greatly relieved by diluting the cow milk with water and adding carbohydrate and fat. The latter provide calories without encumbering the kidneys given that the metabolic by-products of these two food classes are water and carbon dioxide. Alternatively, one of the commercially prepared low renal solute residue formulas can be used in place of the modified cow milk, alternating formula feeds with bottles of plain water or water with 2% glucose. In either case, the frequency of feedings must be increased, otherwise, water intake is limited by the gastric capacity before normotonicity is restored.

a. Thiazides and Other Diuretics. Approximately 30 years ago, it was discovered that the thiazide diuretics had a paradoxic action to improve the water economy of children with nephrogenic diabetes insipidus (91). The list of diuretics having this property has since been extended to include furosemide and amiloride (92). The benefit of these agents appears to lie in a shift of sodium reabsorption to the portions of the nephron proximal to the collecting ducts. In the absence of vasopressin or when, as in nephrogenic diabetes insipidus, there is no response to its normal influence, the epithelium of the collecting ducts is "waterproof," and reabsorption of sodium and other solutes in this distal portion of the nephron generates water from which the dissolved substances have been totally removed—"free water." The same denial substrate for generation of free water can be achieved by strict dietary salt restriction, but the aforementioned diuretics facilitate achievement of this goal.

Amiloride is often coupled with thiazides if the latter drugs are causing hypokalemia or hyperuricemia (93,94). There is evidence that the antidiuretic effects of amiloride are caused by a blockade of sodium reabsorption in the collecting ducts, whereas the thiazides act only to restrict sodium access to this area.

b. Inhibitors of Prostaglandin Synthesis. Fichman et al. (94) were apparently the first to use indomethacin in the treatment of nephrogenic diabetes insipidus. They showed that, when used alone, this inhibitor of prostaglandin synthesis had little effect on the water turnover of two affected brothers. When used in company with a thiazide, however, the reduction in water turnover was approximately twice that achieved with the thiazide alone. It was postulated that the indomethacin reduced the inhibition by prostaglandins of sodium reabsorption in the proximal convoluted tubule, thus further enhancing sodium (and water) reabsorption at this site and denying the passage of sodium to the distal diluting segment. A number of other prostaglandin synthetase inhibitors, including acetylsalicylic acid (95) and tolmetin (96), have been found to share this property with indomethacin. Curiously, ibuprofen, one of the most commonly nonsteroidal antiinflammatory drugs, proved less effective than indomethacin in a controlled trial (97).

VI. CHRONIC HYPERNATREMIA

Neurogenic hypernatremia is a relatively rare syndrome observed primarily in the young and very old. Chronically affected patients have serum sodium concentrations constantly above 145 mEq/L and intermittently show rises to above 180 mEq/L without experiencing the desire to correct the systemic hypertonicity with increased water intake. Unless dehydrated, the children show remarkably few symptoms. They often have coexisting severe neurologic and hypothalamic disease or a history of extensive neurosurgical procedures. Symptomatic diabetes insipidus is present in approximately half of the patients, but all patients show maximal antidiuresis only when very high plasma osmolalities and sodium concentrations have been reached. Plasma vasopressin concentrations are usually measurable but low for the degree of hyperosmolality. It has also been suggested that increased renal sensitivity to vasopressin was present in some of the patients (98).

The primary cause of this disease entity is a defective thirst mechanism and thus loss of an integral part of the regulatory system maintaining fluid homeostasis. Studies of drinking behavior and fluid and electrolyte metabolism have shown a defect in osmoreceptor-mediated thirst and vasopressin secretion in several patients with normal volume receptor function. Several authors have therefore suggested that these patients have reached a new "set point" for serum osmolality at which vasopressin secretion and thirst sensation are initiated (70).

For the clinical management of these patients, we consider it helpful to separate patients with neurogenic hypernatremia into groups according to their defect and adjust therapy accordingly. Clear separation is not always possible, and overlap will occur between the groups. The response to challenges, such as fluid restriction, hypertonic saline infusion, and water loading, should be examined in each patient. Before each test, patients should be well hydrated; elevated plasma renin activity and uric acid concentrations indicate poor renal perfusion and hypovolemia.

The untreated child with nephrogenic diabetes insipdus

is forced to accept a new set point for thirst during infancy, when fluids are not readily available. Serum sodium concentrations in this group of patients vary from 144 to 152 mEq/L. The patients experience normal thirst during water deprivation and systemic hypertonicity. In response to a water load they excrete dilute plasma sodium levels. Their kidneys exhibit normal sodium-conserving mechanisms when overhydrated for a prolonged time. Hyponatremia, therefore, does not occur acutely.

A second group of hypernatremic children are those with abnormal thirst and vasopressin release in response to changes in plasma osmolality. They usually have normal baroreceptor-mediated vasopressin release and are not polyuric. Urine osmolality may reach 1000 mOsmol/kg during prolonged water deprivation when hypovolemia and hypernatremia ensue. Antidiuresis also occurs when a baroreceptor response is elicited pharmacologically by vasodilation or by placing the patient on a tilting table (111, 112). However, deficient vasopressin release can be shown after infusion of hypertonic saline when the hypovolemic stimulus is eliminated. Some of these patients also show abnormal suppression of ADH and develop hyponatremia after a water load is administered. Studies by Dunger et al. (98) suggested that the latter phenomenon may be a consequence of increased renal sensitivity to vasopressin. When their patients were treated with a pure V_2 receptor agonist, such as DDAVP, the condition improved. However, this has not been observed in most of the patients reported by others. Thirst stimulation with chlorpropamide should be tried. The patients will respond to salt restriction and chlorothiazide therapy because this induces mild hypovolemia.

The entity of diabetes insipidus and hypodipsia is seen most often in patients with extensive hypothalamic damage. They experience polyuria and usually concentrate their urine to less than 800 mOsmol/kg during dehydration and severe hyperosmolality. During treatment with long-acting vasopressin preparations, they show wide fluctuations in serum osmolality, even if fluid intake is carefully regulated. Many of these patients respond to chlorpropamide therapy with both antidiuresis and improvement of thirst sensation (82).

Primary hypodipsia is very rarely seen and can be caused by anomalies of the thirst center or by interruption of pathways relating to the limbic system. These patients have normal vasopressin regulation and respond normally to all three challenge tests. Hypernatremia can be avoided by securing an adequate daily fluid intake.

On rare occasions hypernatremia is observed in patients with chronic upper airway obstruction and hypoventilation as a result of obesity. These children have a hypoventilatory response to carbon dioxide stimulation and may have chronic or intermittent hypernatremia. Restoration of normal weight or removal of the upper airway obstruction will cure abnormal ventilation and hypernatremic episodes. It is unclear whether this anomaly is caused by carbon dioxide inhibition, vasopressin secretion, or severe fluid losses from excessive perspiration (99).

VII. THE SYNDROME OF INAPPROPRIATE ADH SECRETION

Any condition associated with continuous fluid intake while exposed to unsuppressed vasopressin will result in dilutional hyponatremia and hypoosmolality. This phenomenon was first observed in human volunteers by Leaf et al. (13). A few years later, Schwartz et al. (12) recognized very similar findings in patients with bronchogenic carcinoma and coined the phrase syndrome of inappropriate ADH secretion.

Under physiologic conditions, fluid and electrolyte homeostasis is maintained by the reciprocal relationship between free water intake and vasopressin secretion. However, when in healthy subjects fluid intake is maintained during chronic exposure to exogenous vasopressin, water retention, weight gain, and dilutional hyponatremia ensue very rapidly, especially in young children, whose fluid turnover per unit body weight is proportionally greater than in adults. During these initial changes, renal blood flow and glomerular filtration rate are excellent, proximal tubular reabsorption of the glomerular filtrate is low, and despite incipient hyponatremia, renin-aldosterone secretion is suppressed but water reabsorption in the distal tubule and final urine osmolality and sodium content are high. With ensuing hyponatremia and loss of the renal medullary concentration gradient, urinary sodium and solute loss decreases, urine volume rises despite continuous vasopressin secretion, and a new equilibrium at lower systemic osmolality is approached. This equilibrium is again very sensitive to any abrupt change in fluid intake or vasopressin activity.

In Fig. 10, the systemic response to this hyponatremic and hypoosmolar challenge is depicted using as an organ example the brain (100). It shows immediate reaction to a fall in the extracellular fluid osmolality, which is a passive shift in water from the extracellular to the more hypertonic intracellular fluid space leading to an expansion of cell volume and brain edema. A solute flow in the reverse direction follows slowly and eventually causes an equilibrium between the extra- and intracellular fluid space and restoration of cell volume. Not depicted are events that occur with very rapid correction of hypoosmolality. During infusion of hypertonic fluids, water flows passively from the intracellular to the extracellular space and causes cells and organ shrinkage before equilibrium is restored. It is during these acute adjustments that cellular damage and permanent complications are most likely to occur. Although stupor and seizures are observed during the acute phase of SIADH development, pontine and extrapontine myelinolysis are associated with overly aggressive correction of the hypoosmolar state (101). It is therefore imperative that correction of hyponatremia and hypernatremia be established slowly and cautiously.

1. Etiology

SIADH is often an iatrogenic disease, found with a frequency of up to 15% among hospitalized patients receiving intravenous fluid therapy. Most patients are only mildly affected by the serum sodium dropping to 130–135 μM, but this asymptomatic SIADH has been shown to amplify manyfold the morbidity and mortality of the underlying disease (102). The

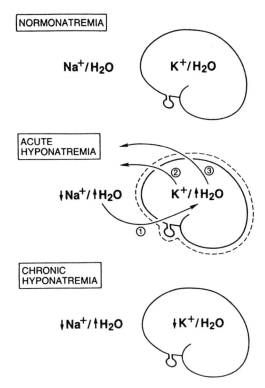

NORMONATREMIA

Na^+/H_2O K^+/H_2O

ACUTE
HYPONATREMIA

$\downarrow Na^+/\uparrow H_2O$ $K^+/\uparrow H_2O$

CHRONIC
HYPONATREMIA

$\downarrow Na^+/\uparrow H_2O$ $\downarrow K^+/H_2O$

Figure 10 Intracerebral fluid and solute shifts during acute and chronic hyponatremia. Acute reduction of extracellular solute (Na^+) leads water to flow along the osmotic gradient into the brain, causing edema (middle panel). Subsequently both water and solute (K^+) rapidly flow back into systemic circulation, a process reducing brain edema and establishing chronic hypotonic equilibrium (lower panel). Moderate corrective measures during acutely developing brain edema may be clinically indicated and will cause rapid improvement. However, very slow correction is required for chronic hyponatremia in order to prevent pontine myelinolysis (100).

etiologies of inappropriate vasopressin secretion are listed in Table 3. Ectopic vasopressin synthesis by malignant tumors is rare in childhood; most children suffering from SIADH have either intracranial or pulmonary disease.

Aside from the narcotics and analgesics, such agents as nicotine, clofibrate, and emetics induce vasopressin release from the pituitary. The prostaglandin inhibitors carbamazepine and chlorpropamide represent drugs that amplify vasopressin action at the level of the kidney (103). Chemotherapeutic agents induce SIADH-like clinical presentations; however, the ADH levels measured under these circumstances are usually only minimally elevated. For several of these agents their mechanism of action is incompletely understood (104), and not infrequently the cause for this syndrome cannot be explained at all.

2. Clinical Presentation

The clinical manifestations of SIADH are largely limited to those symptoms and signs arising from central nervous

Table 3 Etiologies of SIADH

Intrathoracic
   Bronchial carcinoma, mediastinal malignancies
   Pneumonitis: bacterial, viral, mycoplasma etc.
   Acute respiratory failure
   Obstructive lung disease, positive pressure ventilation
Nervous System
   Hydrocephalus, trauma, haemorrhage
   Encephalitis, meningitis, other inflammatory causes
   Demyelinating disease, spinal cord lesions
   Psychosis
Drugs
   ADH amplification (Chlorpropamide)
   Clofibrate, carbamazepine
   Chemotherapeutic agents
   Nicotine, phenothiazides, tricyclics
Others
   Malignancies: intestinal, uterine, urological etc.
   Leukaemia
   Idiopathic

system involvement and dilatation. For the most part they are directly related to the brain swelling described before. Often nausea, headaches, and malaise precede the onset of more severe stages, such as disorientation, confusion, coma, and seizures. The symptomatology is not as much influenced by the severity of hyponatremia as by the velocity with which the changes in systemic osmolality occur. It is not exceedingly rare that a patient with chronic SIADH is still ambulatory and relatively asymptomatic while their serum sodium is 115 mOsmol/kg or below. On the other hand, seizures may occur when serum sodium falls acutely to 130 mOsmol/kg during inappropriately rapid infusion of hypotonic solutions. These observations must be kept in mind when therapeutic interventions are considered (105). Long-standing hyponatremia should be corrected very slowly. On the other hand, acutely presenting neurologic signs often require rapid intervention, which will be very successful if the hyponatremia is only partially corrected and complete restoration is left to occur during periods of no treatment except fluid restriction.

3. Diagnosis

The diagnostic criteria are essentially those established by Schwartz et al. (12) in their original publication. They considered SIADH to be present when a clinically normovolemic patient without renal or adrenal disease exhibits simultaneously low serum sodium and osmolality and excretes an inappropriately concentrated urine of high sodium content. The improvement in this condition with fluid restriction is an additional criterion. However, documentation of persistent vasopressin secretion was not required in their original report and should not be considered because several recent reports have been published of patients who fulfill all diagnostic criteria of SIADH but do not have detectable vasopressin in their serum (106). The nature of this ADH-like antidiuresis is not understood.

4. Differential Diagnosis

All diseases presenting with hyponatremia must be considered in the differential diagnosis of SIADH. The algorithm for clinical evaluation of hyponatremia is outlined in Fig. 11. In the first instance it must be ascertained that the hyponatremia is not spurious and that it is associated with an appropriately suppressed serum osmolality.

Pseudohyponatremia is observed with marked elevation of serum lipids or proteins that artificially suppress plasma water and sodium content but not their proportion to each other or plasma osmolality. Another condition presenting with spuriously suppressed plasma sodium but normal osmolality is induced when another solute replaces sodium in maintaining plasma tonicity. The classic example of this condition is hyperglycemia, especially diabetic ketoacidosis. In this condition the serum sodium rises proportionally with the fall in blood glucose and ketoacids as treatment is initiated.

When considering the differential diagnosis of true hyponatremic, hypoosmolar presentations, it is essential to establish whether the patient's hydration and blood volume status is maintained, excessive, or deficient (Fig. 11). Edema and ascites eliminate excess vasopressin secretion as a primary cause for hyponatremia and should direct the physician to search for anomalies associated with protein deficiency, cirrhosis, renal disease, or cardiac failure. Patients with hypotonic dehydration and hypovolemia, on the other hand, establish that solute depletion is in excess of water loss and indicate the need for isotonic fluid therapy. The history will point to losses from the gastrointestinal tract and excess

sodium loss is aside for extraordinary exposure to dry heat through sweat limited to infants with cystic fibrosis.

In all these conditions, a maximal sodium-conserving effort will be exhibited by the kidney through the excretion of a concentrated urine of low sodium content. Should there be persistent urinary sodium losses during systemic hypovolemia, however, then either adrenal and renal failure or, rarely, excessive diuretic use must be considered. The hyperkalemia will point to adrenal insufficiency, and diuretic use will be eliminated by the history. Renal diseases to be considered are medullary cystic disease, acute interstitial nephritis, and, in newborns, obstructive nephropathy, which may also present with hyperkalemia.

Most patients presenting with hyponatremia and clinically normal kidney function, blood volume, and hydration will have SIADH, but all need to be treated with fluid restriction. In hypothyroidism the hyponatremia is thought to be a consequence of decreased renal blood and tubular urine flow (47). ACTH-deficient patients secrete vasopressin in excess and show rapid correction of their hyponatremia following cortisol administration. Exogenous vasopressin causes SIADH in all children who receive their diet predominantly in liquid form. It is the young children and infants who are less protected against the consequences of drinking excess free water (83). In adults, however, even with severe polydipsia, there will be rarely solute intake sufficiently low to cause hyponatremia.

5. Therapy

Once the diagnosis of SIADH is established and other causes for the hyponatremia have been excluded, therapy must be instituted. In all patients, especially in those who are relatively asymptomatic, fluid restriction alone is the safest and most

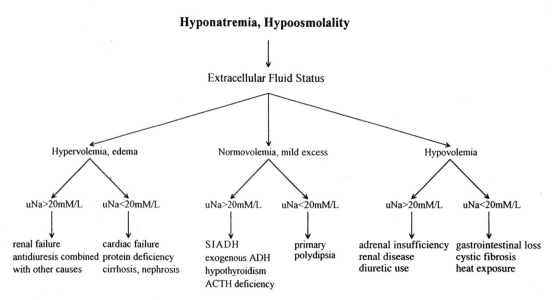

Figure 11 Algorythm for hyponatremia. Circulating blood volume and urinary Na concentration are considered most valuable indicators for deriving at the correct diagnosis.

efficient therapeutic measure to be instituted. In those who show evidence of acute SIADH and present with symptoms of brain swelling, however, immediate but restrained intervention is required. Slow infusion of hypertonic saline, 3–5 ml/kg of 3% NaCl, should be combined with furosemide therapy to maintain diuresis and excretion of dilute urine. This raises serum Na by 5–7 mM and prevents deterioration. As soon as symptoms improve, this therapy should be discontinued and water restriction enforced. The long-term therapeutic goal should be slow correction of hyponatremia over a period extending over at least 48 h (107).

When SIADH is chronic, consistent water restriction often proves insufficient and difficult to enforce. Attempts to compensate for the persistent antidiuresis by providing a diet high in protein, solute, and salt content is equally doomed to fail even when combined with furosemide therapy because it simultaneously stimulates thirst. Until recently, the drug of choice for chronic SIADH was demethylchlortetracycline, which induces a reversible renal tubular resistance to vasopressin (108). This drug becomes effective only after at least 24 h of administration, and the dose requires titration. Its use is clearly preferable to lithium therapy, which has many potential complications. Alcohol is known to suppress ADH release from the posterior pituitary but not ectopic secretion. It is impractical for therapeutic use. Recently, the peroral administration of urea has been advocated as highly successfully in chronic SIADH because it provides solute for renal excretion as well as for formation of dilute urine and seems to have a relative low stimulatory effect on thirst (109). Since the advent of synthetic vasopressin analogs, it has been anticipated that one of these products would be an effective antagonist of ADH, but so far none of these seems to be free of unwanted vasopressor action (110).

Most important in considering SIADH are the aspects of disease prevention. Pediatricians should remain keenly aware that this syndrome is frequently of iatrogenic origin and its occurrence can be limited by more cogent and guarded use of intervenous fluid administration.

REFERENCES

1. Oliver G, Schafer EA. On the physiological action of the extracts of pituitary body and certain other glandular organs. J Physiol (Lond) 1895; 18:277.
2. Dale HH. On some physiological actions of ergot. J Physiol (Lond) 1906; 34:163.
3. Ott I, Scott JC. The action of infundibulin upon the mammary secretion. Proc Soc Exp Biol Med 1910; 8:48.
4. Von den Velden R. Die Nierenwirkung von Hypophysenextrakten beim Menschen. Berl Klin Wochenschr 1913; 50:2083.
5. Farini F. Uber Diabetes Insipidus und Hypophysisterapie. Wien Klin Wochenschr 1913; 26:1867.
6. Waring AG, Kajdi L, Tappan F. A congenital defect of water metabolism. AMA J Dis Child 1945; 69:323.
7. Forssman H. On hereditary diabetes insipidus. Acta Med Scand 1945; 212(Suppl 159): 9–46.
8. Birnbaumer M, Seibold A, Gilbert S, et al. Molecular cloning of the receptor for human antidiuretic hormone. Nature 1992; 357:333–335.
9. Lolait SJ, O'Carroll AM, McBride OW, Konig M, Morel A, Brownstein MJ. Cloning and characterization of a vasopressin V₂ receptor and possible link to nephrogenic diabetes insipidus. Nature 1992; 357:336–336.
10. Davies K. Diabetes defect defined. Nature 1992; 359:434.
11. Holtzman EG, Harris HW Jr, Kolakowski LF Jr, et al. Brief report. A molecular defect in the vasopressin V₂-receptor gene causing nephrogenic diabetes insipidus. N Engl J Med 1993; 328:1534–1537.
12. Schwartz WB, Bennett W, Curelop M, et al. A syndrome of renal sodium loss and hyponatremia, probably resulting from inappropriate secretion of antidiuretic hormone. Am J Med 1957; 23:529.
13. Leaf A, Bartter FC, Santos RF, et al. Evidence in man that urinary electrolyte loss induced by pitressin is a function of water retention. J Clin Invest 1953; 32:868.
14. Mohr E, Richter D. Hypothalamic neuropeptide genes. Aspects of evolution, expression and sub-cellular, mRNA distribution. Ann NY Acad Sci 1993; 689:50–58.
15. Fuhrenholz F, Jurzak M, Gerstberger R, et al. Renal and central vasopressin receptors: immunocytochemical localization. Ann NY Acad Sci 1993; 689:194–206.
16. Russel JT, Brownstein MY, Gainer H. Biosynthesis of vasopressin, oxytocin and neurophysins: isolation and characterization of two common precursors (propressophysin and pro-oxyphysin). Endocrinology 1980; 107:1880.
17. Stopa EG, LeBlanc VK, Hill DH, Anthony ELP. A general overview of the anatomy of the neurohypophysics. Ann NY Acad Sci 1993; 689:6–15.
18. Renaud LP, Bourque CW. Neurophysiology and neuropharmacology of hypothalamic magnocellular neurons secreting vasopressin. Prog Neurobiol 1991; 36: 131–169.
19. Robertson GL, Shelton RL, Athar S. The osmoregulation of vasopressin. Kidney Int 1976; 10:25–37.
20. Zerbe RL, Miller JZ, Robertson GL. Osmoregulation of thirst and vasopressin secretion in human subjects: effects of various solutes. Am J Physiol 1983; 224:E607.
21. Dunn FL, Brennan TJ, Nelson AE, Robertson GL. The role of blood osmolality and volume in regulating vasopressin secretion in the rat. J Clin Invest 1973; 52:3212–3219.
22. Bard P, Woods JW, Bleier R. The locus and functional capacity of the osmoreceptors in the deafferented hypothalamus. Trans Assoc Am Phys 1966; 79:107.
23. Robertson GL, Mahr EA, Athar S, et al. Development and clinical application of a new method for the radioimmunoassay of arginine vasopressin in human plasma. J Clin Invest 1973; 52:2340.
24. Fischer BM, Baylis PH, Frier BM. Plasma oxytocin, arginine vasopressin and atrial natriuretic peptide responses during insulin induced hypoglycemia. Clin Endocrinol (Oxf) 1987; 26:179.
25. Vokes TP, Aycinoma PR, Robertson GL. Effect of insulin on osmoregulation of vasopressin. Am J Physiol 1987; 252:E538.
26. Morris M, Alexander N. Baroreceptor influences on oxytocin and vasopressin secretion. Hypertension 1989; 13:110.
27. Robertson GL. Physiology of vasopressin, oxytocin and thirst. In: Becker KL, ed. Principles and Practice of Endocrinology and Metabolism. Philadelphia: Lippincott, 1990: 222–230.
28. Robertson GL. Physiology of ADH release. Kidney Int 1987; 31:S20.
29. Rowe JW, Shelton RL, Helderman JH, et al. Influence of the emetic reflex on vasopressin release in man. Kidney Int 1979; 16:729.
30. Verney EC. Croonian Lecture. Antidiuretic hormone and factors which determine its release. Proc R Soc Med [B] 1947; 135:25.

31. Plotzky PM, Bruhm TO, Vale W. Evidence for multifactor regulation of the adenocorticotropin secretory response to hemodynamic stimuli. Endocrinology 1985; 116:633.

32. Plotzky PM, Bruhm TO, Vale W. Hypophysiotropic regulation of ACTH secretion in response to insulin-induced hypoglycemia. Endocrinology 1985; 117:323.

33. Raff H. Interactions between neurohypophysial hormones and the ACTH adrenocortical axis. Ann NY Acad Sci 1993; 689:411–425.

34. Van Wyk JJ, Dugger GS, Newsome JF, Thomas PZ. The effect of pituitary stalk section on the adrenal function of women with cancer of the breast. J Clin Endocrinol Metab 1960; 20:157.

35. Guillon G, Couraud P-O, Butlen D, Jard S. Size of vasopressin receptors from rat liver and kidney. Eur J Biochem 1980; 111:287–294.

36. Morel A, O'Carroll A-M, Brownstein MJ, Lolait SJ. Molecular cloning and expression of a rat V_{1a} arginine vasopressin receptor. Nature 1992; 356:523–529.

37. Kokko JP, Rector FC Jr. Countercurrent multiplication system without active transport in inner medulla. Kidney Int 1972; 2:214–223.

38. Birnbaumer M, Seibold A, Gilbert S, et al. Molecular cloning of the receptor for human antidiuretic hormone. Nature 1992; 357:333–335.

39. Lolait SJ, O'Carroll A-M, McBride OW, et al. Cloning and characterization of a vasopressin V_2 receptor and possible link to nephrogenic diabetes insipidus. Nature 1992; 357:336–339.

40. Herbert SC, Reeves WB, Malong DA, Andreoli TE. The medullary thick limb: function and modulation of the single-effect multiplier. Kidney Int 1987; 31:580.

41. Zerbe RL, Robertson GL. Osmoregulation of thirst and vasopressin secretion in human subjects: effects of various solutes. Am J Physiol 1983; 224:E607.

42. Salata RA, Verbalis JG, Robinson AG. Cold water stimulation of oropharyngeal receptors in man inhibits release of vasopressin. J Clin Endocrinol Metab 1987; 64:561.

43. Akaishi T, Homma S. Properties of oropharyngeal/laryngeal afferents regulating vasopressin release. Am NY Acad Sci 1993; 689:455–457.

44. Thompson CJ, Burd JM, Baylis PH. Acute suppression of plasma vasopressin and thirst after drinking in hypernatremic humans. Am J Physiol 1987; 252:R1138.

45. McKinley MJ. Common aspects of the cerebral regulation of thirst and renal sodium excretion. Kidney Int 1992; 37:S102–106.

46. Evered MD. Investigating the role of angiotensin II in thirst: interactions between arterial pressure and the control of drinking. Com J Physiol Pharmacol 1992; 70:791–797.

47. Robinson AG, DeRubertis FR. Disorders of sodium and water balance associated with adrenal, thyroid and pituitary disease. In: Schrier RW, Gottschalk C, eds. Diseases of the Kidney. Boston: Little Brown, 1988:2795–2822.

48. Robson JS, Lambie AT. Cortisone induced polyuria following hypophysectomy. Am J Med 1959; 26:769–782.

49. Iwasaka Y, Osio Y, Kando K, et al. Aggravation of subclinical diabetes insipidus during pregnancy. N Engl J Med 1991; 324:522–526.

50. Rollin C, Hucharczyk J, Lemoine J, et al. Osmoregulation of vasopressin secretion and thirst during the estrous cycle in pigs. Am J Physiol 1989; 256:R270–275.

51. Chiodera P, Coira V. Inhibition by dexamethasone of arginine vasopressin and ACTH responses to insulin induced hypoglycemia and cigarette smoking in normal men. Acta Endocrinol (Coperh) 1990; 123:487–492.

52. Ishikawa S, Fujisawa G, Tsuboi Y, et al. The role of antidiuretic hormone in hyponatremia in patients with isolated ACTH deficiency. Endocrinol Jpn 1991; 38:325–330.

53. Oelkers W. Hyponatremia and inappropriate secretion of vasopressin in patients with hypopituitarism. N Engl J Med 1989; 321:492–496.

54. Hollinshead WH. The interphase of diabetes insipidus. Proc Staff Meet Mayo Clin 1964; 39:92.

55. Crawford JD, Bode HH. Disorders of the posterior pituitary in children. In: Gardner LJ, ed. Endocrine and Genetic Diseases of Childhood. Philadelphia: Saunders, 1975:126.

56. Atkinson FRB. Schuller-Christian's disease. Br J Child Dis 1937; 34:28.

57. Dunger DB, Broadbent V, Yeoman E, et al. The frequency and natural history of diabetes insipidus in children with Langerhans-cell histiocytosis. N Engl J Med 1989; 321:1157–1162; 1994; 40:171–172.

58. Molitch ME, Hedley-Whyte. Case records of the Massachusetts General Hospital, case 5, 1985. N Eng J Med 1985; 312:297–305.

59. Mineham KJ, Cheng MG, Zimmerman D, et al. Radiation therapy for diabetes insipidus caused by Langerhans cell histiocytosis. Int J Radiat Oncol Biol Phys 1992; 23:519–524.

60. Hojo M, Kuno T, Sakamoto K, et al. Central diabetes insipidus: an ominous sign of severe hypoxic encephalopathy. Acta Paediatr Scand 1990; 79:701–703.

61. Arisaka O, Arisaka M, Ikebe A, et al. Central diabetes insipidus in hypoxic brain damage. Childs Central Ner Sys 1992; 8:81–82.

62. Czernichow P, Pomarede R, Brauner R, et al. Neurogenic diabetes insipidus in children. Front Horm Res 1985; 13:190–209.

63. Scherbaum WA, Czernichow P, Bottazzo GF, Doniach D. Diabetes insipidus in children. IV. A possible auto-immune type with vasopressin cell antibodies. J Pediatr 1985; 107:922–925.

64. Weil A. Uber die hereditare Form des Diabetes insipidus. Dtsch Arch Klin Med Leipzig 1908; 93:180.

65. Leod JF, Kovacs L, Gskill MB, et al. Familial neurohypophyseal diabetes insipidus associated with a signal peptide mutation. J Clin Endocrinol Metab 1993; 77:599.

66. Christopher C, Balerioux D, Hanquinet S, et al. The molecular biology of human hereditary central diabetes insipidus. Prog Brain Res 1992; 93:296–306.

67. Ito M, Mori Y, Oiso Y, Saito H. A single base substitution in the region coding for neurophysin II associated with familial central diabetes insipidus. J Clin Invest 1991; 87:725–728.

68. Schmale H, Bahnsen U, Richter D. Structure and expression of the vasopressin precursor gene in central diabetes insipidus. Ann NY Acad Sci 1993; 689:74–82.

69. Bergeron C, Kovacs K, Ezrin C, Mizzen C. Hereditary diabetes insipidus: an immunohistochemical study of the hypothalamus and pituitary gland. Acta Neuropathol (Berl) 1991; 81:345–348.

70. Bode HH. Disorders of the posterior pituitary. In: Kaplan S, ed. Clinical Paediatric Endocrinology. Philadelphia: Saunders, 1990:63–86.

71. Martin FIR. Familial diabetes insipidus. Q J Med N S 1959; 112:573–582.

72. Salih MA, Tuvemo T. Diabetes insipidus, diabetes mellitus, optic atrophy and deafness (DIDMOAD syndrome). Acta Paediatr Scand 1991; 80:567–572.

73. Van den Ouweland JM, Bruining GJ, Lindhout D, et al. Mutation in mitochondrial tRNA genes: non linkage with syndromes of Wolfram and chronic progressive external ophthaloplegia. Nucleic Acids Res 1992; 20:679–682.

74. Rotig A, Cormier U, Chatelain P, et al. Deletion of mitochon-

drial DNA in a case of early-onset diabetes mellitus, optic atrophy and deafness (Wolfram syndrome). J Clin Invest 1993; 91:1095–1098.

75. Hickey RC, Hare K. The renal excretion of chloride and water in diabetes insipidus. J Clin Invest 1944; 23:768.

76. Thompson CJ, Edwards CR, Baylis PH. Osmotic and non-osmotic reputation of thirst and vasopressin secretion in patients with compulsive water drinking. Clin Endocrinol (Oxf) 1991; 35:221–228.

77. Maghnie M, Villa A, Arico M, et al. Correlation between magnetic resonance imaging of posterior pituitary and neurohypophyseal function in children with diabetes insipidus. J Clin Endocrinol Metab 1992; 74:795–800.

78. Hillman DA, Neqzi O, Porter P, et al. Renal (vasopressin resistant) diabetes insipidus: definition of the effects of a homeostatic limitation in capacity to conserve water on the physical, intellectual and emotional development of a child. Pediatrics 1958; 21:430.

79. Pliska V. Pharmacology of deamino D-arginine vasopressin. Front Horm Res 1985; 13:278–291.

80. Harris AS. Clinical experience with desmopressin: efficacy and safety in central diabetes insipidus and other conditions. J Pediatr 1989; 114:711–718.

81. Fjellestad-Paulsen A. Central diabetes insipidus in children: antidiuretic effect and pharmacokinetics of intranasal and peroral DDAVP. Acta Endocrinol (Copenh) 1987; 115:307.

82. Bode HH, Harley BM, Crawford JD. Restoration of normal drinking behavior by chlorpropamide in patients with hypodipsia and diabetes insipidus. Am J Med 1971, 51:304.

83. Crigler JF. Commentary. On the use of pitressin in infants with neurogenic diabetes insipidus. J Pediatr 1976; 88:295.

84. Bode HH, Crawford JD. Nephrogenic diabetes insipidus in North America: the Hopewell hypothesis. N Engl J Med 1969; 280:750.

85. Deen PM, Verdijk MA, Knoers NV, et al. Requirement of human renal water channel aquaporin-2 for vasopressin-dependent concentration of urine. Science 1994; 264:92–95.

86. Rogers GD. Joan at Halfway. New York: GH Doran, 1919.

87. McIlraith CH. Notes on some cases of diabetes insipidus with marked family and hereditary tendencies. Lancet 1892; 2:767–768.

88. De Lange C. Uber erblichen Diabetes insipidus. Jahrbuch Kinderheilk. 1935; 145:1.

89. Bichet DG, Razi M, Lonergan M, et al. Hemodynamic and coagulation responses to 1-desamino (8-D-arginine) vasopressin in patients with congenital nephrogenic diabetes insipidus. N Engl J Med 1988; 318:881–887.

90. Bichet DG, Arthus M-F, Lonergan M, et al. X-linked nephrogenic diabetes insipidus mutations in North America and the Hopewell hypothesis. J Clin Invest 1993; 92:1262–1268.

91. Crawford JD, Kennedy GC, Hill LE. Clinical results of treatment of diabetes insipidus with drugs of the chlorothiazide series. N Engl J Med 1960; 262:737–743.

92. Knoers N, Monnens AH. Amiloride-hydrochlorothiazide versus indomethacin-hydrochlorothiazide in the treatment of nephrogenic diabetes insipidus. J Pediatr 1990; 117:499–502.

93. Gorden P, Robertson GL, Seegmiller JE. Hyperuricemia, a concomitant of congenital vasopressin-resistent diabetes insipidus in the adult. N Engl J Med 1971; 284:1057–1060.

94. Fichman MP, Speckhart P, Zia P, Lee A. Antidiuretic response to prostaglandin inhibition by indomethacin in nephrogenic diabetes insipidus. Clin Res 1976; 24:161A.

95. Monn E. Prostaglandin synthetase inhibitors in the treatment of nephrogenic diabetes insipidus. Acta Pediatr Scand 1981; 70:39–42.

96. Chevalier RL, Rogol AD. Tolmetin-sodium in the management of nephrogenic diabetes insipidus. J Pediatr 1982; 101:787–789.

97. Libber S, Harrison H, Spector D. Treatment of nephrogenic diabetes insipidus with prostaglandin synthesis inhibitors. J Pediatr 1986; 108:305–311.

98. Dunger DB, Seckl JR, Lightman SL. Increased renal sensitivity to vasopressin in two patients with essential hypernatremia. J Clin Endocrinol Metab 1987; 64:185.

99. Schaad U, Vassella F, Zuppinger K, et al. Hypodipsia-hypernatraemia syndrome. Helv Paediatr Acta 1979; 34:63.

100. Verbalis JG. Hyponatremia. Endocrine causes and consequences of therapy. Trends Endocrinol Metab 1992; 3:1–7.

101. Kleinschmidt-DeMasters BK, Norenberg MD. Rapid correction of hyponatremia causes demyelination: relation to central pontine myelinolysis. Science 1981; 211:1068.

102. Anderson RJ, Chuag H, Kluge R, Schrier RW. Hyponatremia: a prospective analysis of its epidemiology and the pathogenic role of vasopressin. Ann Intern Med 1985; 102:164.

103. Crawford JD, Bode HH. Diabetes and the amplifier hypothesis. N Engl J Med 1970; 282:635.

104. Ganong CA, Kappy MS. Cerebral saltwashing in children. The need for recognition and treatment. Am J Dis Child 1993; 147:167–169.

105. Berl T. Treating hyponatremia: damned if we do and damned if we don't. Kidney Int. 1990; 37:1006–1018.

106. Zerbe R, Stropes L, Robertson GL. Vasopressin function in the syndrome of osmoregulation. Am J Med 1982; 72:339.

107. Ayus JC, Krothapalli RK, Arieff AI. Treatment of symptomatic hyponatremia and its relation to brain damage. N Engl J Med 1987; 317:1190–1195.

108. Forrest JN Jr, Cox M, Hong C, et al. Superiority of demeclocycline over lithium in the treatment of chronic syndrome of inappropriate secretion of antidiuretic hormone. N Engl J Med 1978; 298:173.

109. Decaux G, Prospect F, Penninck R, et al. % year treatment of the chronic syndrome of inappropriate secretion of ADH with oral urea. Nephron 1993; 63:460–470.

110. Hofbauer KG, Mah SC. Vasopressin antagonists: present and future. Kidney Int 1987; 31:521.

111. De Ruberbis FR, Michelis MS, Beck N, et al. "Essential" hypernatremia due to ineffective osmolic and intact volume regulation of vasopressin. J Clin Invest 1971; 80:97.

112. Halter BH, Goldberg AP, Robertson GL, et al. Selective osmoreceptor dysfunction in the syndrome of chronic hypernatremia. J Clin Endocrinol Metab 1977; 44:609.

52
Childhood Obesity

Ramin Alemzadeh
University of Tennessee Medical Center at Knoxville, Knoxville, Tennessee

Fima Lifshitz
Maimonides Medical Center and State University of New York Health Science Center at Brooklyn,
Brooklyn, New York

I. INTRODUCTION

Childhood obesity is one of the most complex and poorly understood clinical syndromes in pediatric practice. This is presumably a result of the multiple etiologies and manifestations of this condition, which elude the simple cause-and-effect concept. Nevertheless, obesity is a common nutritional disorder among children and adolescents in the United States, with an estimated prevalence of 25%, compared with 30% in adult population. The percentage of overweight children and adolescents has increased by almost 50% in the past two decades (1). Obesity in childhood is a major public health problem and a well-recognized risk factor for adult obesity, which in turn may lay the foundation for the development of hypertension (1,2), hyperlipidemia (3), respiratory diseases (4), diabetes (5), orthopedic conditions (6,7), psychosocial disorders (8), and important social and economic consequences (9).

The modes of treatment of childhood obesity are difficult to establish, and clinicians continue to face the dilemma of determining how this disease should be treated. It is not known to what extent development of childhood obesity is linked to genetic, congenital, nutritional, metabolic, or behavioral factors. Thus it is difficult to change the natural progression of this disease. It is estimated that 10–20% of obese infants remain overweight as children (10). It has also been observed that about 40% of overweight children continue to be obese during adolescence, and 75–80% of obese adolescents become obese adults (11). It has also been shown that more than a third of obese children eventually become obese adults (12).

This chapter reviews the definition and etiologies of obesity, complications, evaluation of two cases of childhood obesity, differential diagnosis, management, and the prevention of obesity in children at risk.

II. DEFINITIONS AND DIAGNOSTIC CRITERIA

Obesity may be defined as an excessive storage of energy as fat relative to lean body mass. The measurement of body weight, the parameter commonly used to assess adiposity, is not an optimal method to differentiate between being overweight and being obese. Indeed, individuals with larger than average body frames or excess muscle mass (athletes) may be mistakenly considered obese because they have excess body weight. Because they do not have excess body fat, they are not obese, although their relative weight for height may be above 120%, a commonly used criterion of obesity in children.

Age-specific growth charts (13) allow a more precise assessment of a child's nutritional status. These charts help the clinician evaluate a child's weight and its relationship to height. They also provide a view of the previous growth patterns and thus establish the presence of obesity more accurately. However, weight and height nomograms also fail to take into account the frame size and body composition of the patient. The importance of growth charts in the evaluation of childhood obesity is illustrated in the example shown in Figure 1. Julie is a 5-year-old girl with a pattern of morbid obesity. Review of her growth records revealed that Julie's rate of weight gain became excessive after 3 months of age and progressed at an accelerated pace after age 1 year. This coincided with acceleration of linear growth. The final point on Julie's growth chart (weight 50 kg; height 116.5 cm) represents 249% of her ideal body weight for height. In contrast, in Figure 2 the growth chart of Michael, with pattern of constitutional overweight, is shown. In this patient, body weight progression was constant throughout, being two major percentiles above that of the height, with an excess weight for height of 38% throughout his life span. These two types

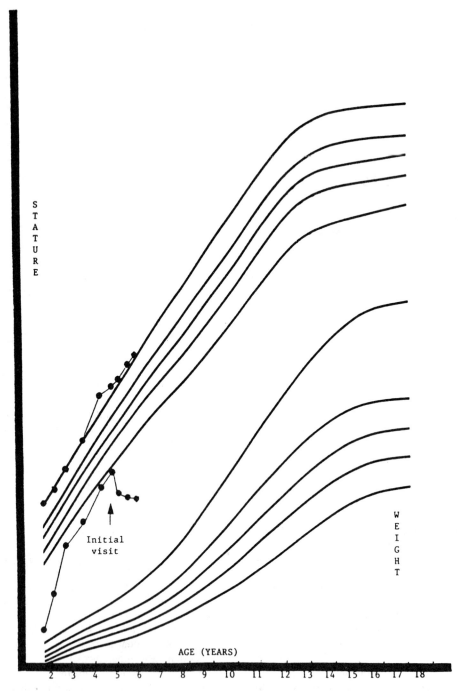

Figure 1 Growth chart illustrating pattern of severe obesity in a 5-year-old girl (Julie). Notice the disproportionate amount of weight gained over time. Height progression also increased, with crossing of percentiles, but to a lesser extent than weight gain.

of growth patterns of the patients shown provide clear evidence of two distinct clinical patterns necessitating different approaches. In Julie's case, all efforts must be made to stop the disproportionate body weight accretion, whereas in Michael's case, caution must be exercised not to interfere with the balance and the adjustment already achieved by the

patient in maintaining body weight. In a survey of high school children, we showed that constitutional patterns of growth are encountered in about 25% of the students with excess body weight for height, remaining proportional throughout the school years (14). The morbid obesity pattern of growth is rare, observed in 0.8% of students. Therefore, the clinical

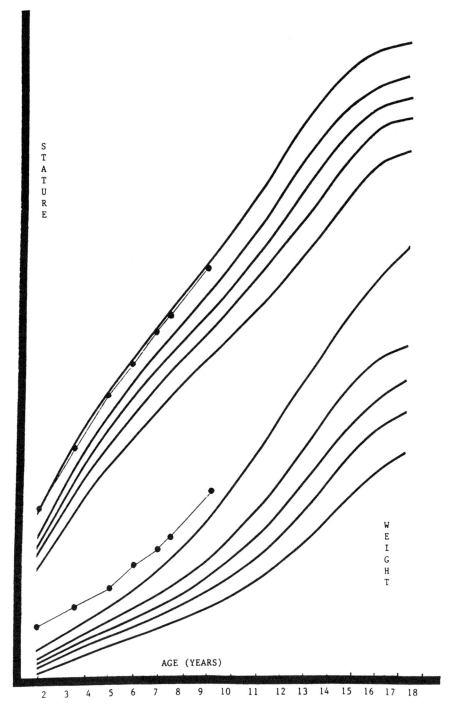

Figure 2 Growth chart illustrating pattern of constitutional overweight in a 9-year-old boy (Michael). Notice the constant body weight progression above the 95th percentile throughout the life of the child. The height progressed on the 90th percentile at a constant rate.

assessment of an obese child must include measurements of height and weight progression for the proper assessment and recommendations for treatment.

Body mass index (BMI) is a widely used method to define the relationship between weight and height (15). BMI is calculated as weight (kg)/height (m²) and provides a practical clinical tool for classification of individuals with normal and those with various degrees of obesity (grades I–III): grade I, BMI 25–29; grade II, BMI 30–40; and grade III, >40 BMI (Table 1). The BMI system of classification of

Table 1 Body Weight (Pounds) in Relation to Height and Body Mass Index

BMI	13	14	15	16	17	18	19	20	21	22	23	24	25	26	27	28	29	30	40
Height (inches)																			
34 (m^2 0.74)	21	23	24	26	28	29	31	32	24	36	37	39	41	42	44	46	47	49	65
35 (m^2 0.79)	22	24	26	28	29	31	33	35	36	38	40	42	43	45	47	49	50	52	70
36 (m^2 0.83)	23	25	27	29	31	33	35	36	38	40	42	44	46	47	49	51	53	55	73
37 (m^2 0.90)	25	27	29	31	33	35	37	39	41	43	45	47	49	51	53	55	57	59	79
38 (m^2 0.93)	27	29	31	33	35	37	39	41	43	45	47	49	51	53	55	57	59	61	82
39 (m^2 0.98)	29	31	33	35	37	39	41	43	45	47	49	51	53	56	58	60	62	64	86
40 (m^2 1.03)	30	32	34	36	38	41	43	45	47	49	51	53	56	59	61	63	65	68	90
41 (m^2 1.08)	31	33	35	38	40	43	45	47	49	53	55	57	59	62	64	66	69	71	95
42 (m^2 1.14)	33	35	37	40	43	45	47	50	52	55	57	59	62	65	67	70	73	75	100
43 (m^2 1.19)	34	37	40	42	45	47	50	53	55	58	61	63	66	68	70	73	76	78	105
44 (m^2 1.25)	36	38	41	44	47	49	52	55	58	60	63	66	69	71	74	77	80	82	110
45 (m^2 1.31)	37	40	43	46	49	52	55	58	60	63	66	69	72	75	78	80	83	86	115
46 (m^2 1.36)	39	42	45	48	51	54	57	60	63	66	69	72	75	78	81	84	87	90	120
47 (m^2 1.42)	41	44	47	50	53	56	59	62	65	69	72	75	78	81	84	87	90	94	125
48 (m^2 1.49)	43	46	49	52	56	59	62	65	69	72	75	78	82	85	88	92	95	98	131
49 (m^2 1.55)	45	48	51	54	58	61	64	67	72	75	78	81	85	88	92	95	99	102	136
50 (m^2 1.61)	47	50	53	56	60	63	66	69	75	78	81	84	88	92	95	99	103	106	142
51 (m^2 1.67)	48	51	55	59	62	66	70	73	77	81	84	88	92	95	99	104	106	110	147
52 (m^2 1.74)	50	53	57	61	65	69	73	76	80	84	88	92	96	99	103	107	111	115	153
53 (m^2 1.81)	52	56	60	64	68	72	76	80	84	88	92	96	100	103	107	111	115	119	159
54 (m^2 1.88)	54	58	62	66	70	74	78	82	86	91	96	100	103	107	111	116	120	124	165
55 (m^2 1.95)	56	60	64	68	73	77	81	86	90	94	99	103	107	111	116	120	124	129	171
56 (m^2 2.02)	58	62	66	71	75	80	84	89	93	98	102	106	111	115	120	124	129	133	178
57 (m^2 2.10)	60	64	69	73	78	83	88	92	97	101	106	111	115	120	124	129	134	138	184
58 (m^2 2.17)	62	67	71	76	81	86	91	95	100	105	110	114	119	124	129	134	138	143	191
59 (m^2 2.24)	64	69	74	79	84	89	94	98	103	108	113	118	123	128	133	138	143	148	197
60 (m^2 2.32)	66	71	76	81	87	92	97	102	107	112	117	112	127	133	138	143	148	153	204
61 (m^2 2.40)	68	74	79	84	90	95	100	105	111	116	121	128	132	137	142	148	153	158	211
62 (m^2 2.50)	71	77	82	88	93	99	104	110	115	121	126	132	137	143	148	154	159	165	220
63 (m^2 2.56)	73	79	84	90	95	101	107	112	118	124	129	135	141	146	152	158	163	169	225
64 (m^2 2.64)	75	81	87	93	99	104	110	116	122	128	133	139	145	151	157	162	168	174	232
65 (m^2 2.72)	78	84	90	96	102	108	114	120	126	132	138	144	150	155	161	167	173	179	239
66 (m^2 2.81)	80	86	93	99	105	111	117	124	130	136	142	148	154	161	167	173	179	185	247
67 (m^2 2.90)	83	89	96	102	108	115	121	128	134	140	147	153	159	166	172	179	185	191	255
68 (m^2 3.00)	86	92	99	106	112	119	125	132	138	145	152	158	165	171	178	185	191	198	264
69 (m^2 3.07)	88	94	101	108	115	121	128	135	142	148	155	162	169	176	182	189	196	203	270
70 (m^2 3.16)	90	97	104	111	118	125	132	139	146	153	160	166	174	181	188	195	202	208	278
71 (m^2 3.25)	93	100	107	114	121	129	136	143	150	157	164	172	179	186	193	200	207	214	286
72 (m^2 3.34)	95	103	110	118	125	132	140	147	154	162	169	176	184	191	198	206	213	220	294
73 (m^2 3.44)	98	106	113	121	129	136	144	151	159	166	174	182	189	197	204	212	219	227	303
74 (m^2 3.53)	101	109	116	124	132	140	148	155	163	171	179	186	194	202	210	217	225	233	311
75 (m^2 3.63)	104	119	120	128	136	144	152	160	168	176	184	192	200	208	216	224	232	240	320

Source: Adapted from Bray GA, Gray DS. Obesity. Part I. Pathogenesis. West J Med 1988; 149:429–441.

obesity is important because it has been found that the risk for medical complications of obese patients increases at BMI levels above 25 (16). According to the National Center for Health Statistics Health and Nutrition Examination Survey (17), individuals with a BMI above 27 have a markedly increased risk for developing hypertension, hypercholesterol-emia, and diabetes mellitus. In contrast, when the BMI index is less than 25, there are no apparent physical effects of obesity on the individual, although there may be social problems and psychologic concerns with body appearance.

Using the BMI classification system, Julie (Fig. 1) would be classified with grade II obesity (BMI 37), whereas Michael represents an example of grade I obesity (BMI 25). The use of BMI has limited applications in the assessment of overweight children, however, because its calculation is based primarily on a stable height, which is not applicable to growing children. Also, the BMI can underestimate the percentage of lean body mass because it does not account for variations in musculature and this could lead to classification of normal children as overweight.

Skinfold thickness from several separate sites, including both trunk and extremities, provides a reliable estimate of obesity and regional fat distribution. The correlation of multiple skinfold measurements with total-body adiposity is in the range of 0.7–0.8. The use of skinfold thickness measurements for the assessment of body adiposity, although appealing, is compounded by methodologic problems. One problem with skinfold measurements is that the equations used must be changed for age, sex, and ethnic background. Body fat increases with age, even through the sum of the skinfolds remains constant. This means that the fat deposition with age occurs in large part at sites other than subcutaneous (18). Also, triceps skinfold (TSF), which is typically the site of measurement, is often difficult to grasp, and measurement reliability can be poor. It has been observed that there is a strong correlation between BMI and TSF among age and sex groups, however, suggesting that these measures are interchangeable for use both in classification of individuals and in the evaluation of secular trends of obesity and superobesity (19).

Several methods are available for the estimation of body fat content. These include methods that measure body density derived from its specific gravity, that is, the weight of the body in and out of the water. This process makes it possible to fractionate the body into its fat and lean components, assuming a density for fat of 0.9168 g/cm^3. The technique remains basically a research method, however.

Other noninvasive methods, such as the use of ultrasound waves applied to the skin, can provide a measure of fat depth. In a group of children, Czinner and Varady demonstrated a significant correlation ($r = 0.969$) between the body adiposity (skinfold thickness) measured with ultrasound and caliper (20). However, the data derived from the ultrasound method were about 15–25% lower than fat obtained by caliper. The authors concluded that the ultrasound-derived body fat estimates represented only the subcutaneous body fat, not the whole-body adiposity (i.e., visceral fat). On the other hand, other studies have shown that sonography is a reliable tool in measuring small variations in quantities of intraabdominal (visceral) fat and is superior to waist-hip ratio in evaluating regional fat distribution and visceral adiposity (21).

Computed tomography (CT) scan and magnetic resonance imaging (MRI) can also be used to quantitate lean and fat tissue. They provide accurate anatomic details and can reliably measure total and regional body adiposity. Numerous studies have shown the feasibility of CT scans to measure human adiposity (22). In a recent study, Ross et al. demonstrated that MRI can provide reliable measure of subcutaneous and visceral adipose tissue in obese subjects (23). A principal benefit of measuring adipose tissue by MRI or CT is the development of mathematic equations from external anthropometry that can predict MRI adipose tissue.

Obesity should also be evaluated in terms of the distribution of body adiposity. Regional body fat patterning has emerged as an independent risk factor predisposing to a variety of metabolic disorders, including hyperinsulinemia, insulin resistance, and non–insulin-dependent diabetes mellitus (NIDDM) (24). In recent years, several studies have revealed major morphologic and metabolic features that distinguish upper from lower body obesity (25–27). In adults, body fat distribution is as or more important than percentage body fat in predicting morbidity. Adults with a preponderance of abdminal fat ("android") have a higher frequency of hypertension, hyperinsulinemia, diabetes, and hyperlipidemia than equally obese individuals with predominantly pelvic ("gynecoid") fat distribution.

The distribution of body fat is assessed using the waist-hip ratio (WHR). Increasing WHR in excess of 0.8 has been accompanied by abnormalities in glucose, insulin, and lipoprotein homeostasis (28,29). Thus, the evaluation of body fat distribution is an essential element in the assessment of obesity. However, it has been observed that WHR cannot predict visceral adiposity in obese individuals (20,23). On the other hand, using CT scan, the visceral-subcutaneous fat tissue ratio (VSR) has been shown to be a better index of regional fat distribution than the WHR (31). Also, the VSR correlates more closely with such metabolic variables serum lipids, isulin, and glucose than the WHR. At present, WHR or VSR standards for children are not available.

III. ETIOLOGY (Table 2)

A. Genetic Factors

It is known that there is strong role of parental fatness in childhood obesity: when both parents are overweight, about 80% of their children will be obese. When one parent is obese, this incidence falls to 40%; and when both parents are lean, obesity prevalence drops to approximately 14% (32). The reasons for these associations are not clear, however: most of the studies fail to separate the genetic and environmental influences in a critical way.

Obesity is a heterogeneous group of disorders that can result from an energy imbalance over an extended period of time in which energy intake exceeds expenditure. It is superficially apparent that obese subjects ingest more food relative to their needs. However, caloric intakes have been reported to be comparable among overweight and normal weight adults (33), therefore suggesting that obese subjects have "increased metabolic efficiency."

The main determinant of basal metabolic rate (BMR) is fat-free mass (FFM), and the main determinant of energy expenditure is physical activity. It is believed that minor alterations in any of these could result in positive energy balance and lead to obesity over prolonged periods of time. For example, obligatory energy expenditure, reflected by a decreased resting metabolic rate, could be the consequence of an increased metabolic efficiency in obese persons. On the

Table 2 Causes of Obesity

Genetic causes
  Polygenetic familial factors
  Monogenetic factors
    Prader-Willi syndrome
    Laurence-Moon-Biedl syndrome
    Alstom syndrome
    Cohen syndrome
    Carpenter syndrome
    Pseudohypoparathyroidism
Environmental causes
  Maternal feeding practices
  Sedentary lifestyle
  Excessive television viewing
Dietary causes
  Excessive food availability
  Gorging practices
  Calorically dense foods (i.e., high fat)
Endocrine causes
  Insulinoma
  Diabetes mellitus
  Mauriac syndrome
  Klinefelter syndrome
  Turner syndrome
  Pituitary dwarfism
  Hypercorticolism (Cushing syndrome; cortico-
    steroid therapy)
  Hypothyroidism
Central nervous system causes
  Frohlich syndrome
  Trauma
  Tumor (i.e., craniophanyngioma)
  Postinfectious (i.e., encephalitis and tuberculosis)
Miscellaneous causes
  Immobilization
  Psychologic or psychiatric disturbances
  Social and cultural pressure

other hand, a reduced level of activity could also lead to an increased energy balance and weight gain. The resting energy expenditure and the baseline activity levels are thought to be genetically determined. In fact, studies among obese Pima have demonstrated low BMR values and, therefore, enhanced metabolic efficiency of energy consumption among some families with obesity (34,35). However, other studies demonstrated that BMR values corrected for FFM among obese subjects were relatively higher than those in nonobese subjects (36,37), suggesting that attainment of energy balance and weight maintenance in obese individuals require a larger energy intake than in nonobese individuals.

The susceptibility to obesity may begin at birth as a consequence of metabolic variations in energy expenditure. Roberts et al. demonstrated that excessive weight gain among a group of infants born to obese mothers was accompanied by reduced level of physical energy expenditure (38). This

was probably because infants mimicking the activity patterns of their moderately inactive parents or siblings.

It is well recognized that children living in a household in which one or both parents are obese have an increased risk of becoming obese. Childhood obesity may be linked to the same physiologic and environmental factors that resulted in parental obesity. Moreover, the tendency for decreased rate of energy expenditure as a cause of excessive weight gain in obese individuals has been found to be prevalent in obese families (34), which is further evidence of the importance of genetic predisposition in the development of obesity.

Ravussin et al. observed decreased levels of energy expenditure in obese compared with nonobese girls (39). In a subsequent study, differences of up to 500 cal per day in energy expended as a result of spontaneous physical activity (i.e., fidgeting) were observed among obese children compared with normal weight children (40). Differences in BMR and physical activity were found in 3- to 5-year-old offspring of obese parents (41). BMR of children with at least one obese parent was 10% lower than that of children with lean parents. Children of lean parents had about a twice greater energy expenditure for physical activities as opposed to children with at least one obese parent, suggesting that children of obese parents are less physically active.

In monogenetic or dysmorphic forms of obesity transmitted by both recessive and dominant modes of inheritance, there are also alterations in energy balance that result in obesity. Patients with Prader-Willi syndrome are characterized by hyperphagia, hypotonia, developmental delay, hypogonadism, and short stature (42). In these children, obesity may start during the first year of life and becomes prominent by the second year, which in the presence of hyperphagia can result in morbid obesity. It was previously suggested that a low metabolic rate caused the obesity in these children (43). However, it has been demonstrated that the lower energy requirement of these children is caused by less fat-free mass, not an unusually low metabolic rate (44).

Translocation or deletion of chromosome 15 has been reported in about 50% of these patients (45). In contrast, Lawrence-Moon-Biedl syndrome is another dysmorphic form of obesity characterized by retinitis pigmentosa, hypogonadism, mental retardation, and polydactyly. It is inherited by an autosomal recessive gene (46). It is believed that excessive weight gain in these children is caused by a disturbance of hypothalamic appetite center(s), which leads to increased food intake. Pseudohypoparathyroidism is also associated with obesity and short stature and is characterized by a short fourth metacarpal, short thick neck, rounded facies, mental retardation, and hypocalcemia (47). It is commonly inherited as a sex-linked dominant trait and may be accompanied by hypothyroidism and gonadal failure. Other genetic syndromes that include obesity are Alstrom, Carpenters, and Cohen. The mechanisms of excess weight in these patients have not yet been elucidated.

The role of genetic factors in obesity was evaluated by Stunkard et al., who demonstrated no relationship between the body fat indices of adoptive parents compared with their adoptive children (48). They showed that body mass index of biologic parents was more closely correlated with the weight status of their offspring, although they did not live together. The importance of the genetic component was also confirmed by a more recent study involving monozygotic twins (49). The BMIs of identical twins reared apart compared with those reared together were essentially the same. Also, the use of skinfold as a genetic marker in twins has been reported (50). With the use of correlation coefficients to estimate the heritability of skinfold thickness, it has been shown that there was a significant environmental component among children under 10 years, whereas heritability estimated in twins over 10 years of age was very high.

B. Environmental Factors

The influence of many environmental factors on the rate of weight gain with or without a genetic susceptibility has been evaluated by some investigators (31). It has long been observed that infants of diabetic mothers have increased body adiposity at birth. It has also been shown that body adiposity and growth of newborns is influenced significantly by maternal weight and rate of weight gain during the antenatal period (51).

Weight gain and adiposity in infancy and early childhood are also influenced by several environmental factors (52,53). For instance, birth weight, duration of feeding, male sex, and age at the introduction of solid foods seem to affect the rate of weight gain during the first year of life significantly, whereas maternal weight becomes a significant determinant for adiposity only during the second year of life. The latter probably reflects the maternal environmental influences, which may contribute significantly to the development of obesity because they determine child's energy intake and expenditure.

It has been demonstrated that vigorous feeding of infants and children may set the ground for the development of obesity (54,55). Overweight children have been observed to eat more rapidly and chew their food less than those with normal weight (54).

The role of physical energy expenditure in the development of obesity is not very clear. Obese individuals have often been described as sluggish or lazy. A study of children and adolescents by Bullen et al. indicated that obese youngsters were less active than their peers (56). However, an earlier study that measured caloric expenditure by measuring oxygen consumption found that obese individuals actually expended more calories through activity compared with normal weight individuals (57). Recently, Maffeis et al. demonstrated that walking and running are energetically more expensive for obese than for nonobese children (58).

It is not clear whether inactivity is a cause or consequence of obesity. However, it is believed that sedentary lifestyle increases the risk of obesity. Physical activity in children has declined over recent decades, implying that children are living an increasingly sedentary lifestyle in Western industrialized countries. The estimates of energy requirements for children were derived at a time when more physical exertion was needed for daily living; therefore, energy requirements for children may be overestimated for today's sedentary lifestyle. Prentice et al. measured energy expenditure in children aged 0–3 years by a doubly labeled water method and found that energy needs were overestimated by 15% (59) as originally recommended by the World Health Organization (WHO) (60). Similarly, Goran et al. showed that energy requirements were 25% overestimated for 4- to 6-year-old children (61). Utilizing a doubly labeled water method, Fontvieille et al. (62) observed that total energy expenditures were overestimated by 24% for 5- to 6-year-old children as previously calculated according to WHO (60). The sedentary lifestyle of today's children may easily account for the consistent overestimates of childhood energy requirements. Indeed, children living a sedentary lifestyle with unlimited access to food consume larger quantities of energy than they expend and are therefore at increased risk of developing obesity.

Child obesity experts have suggested that the relationship between television viewing and obesity may be the consequence of enhanced food consumption, either during viewing or as a result of food advertisement or decreased physical energy expenditure (63). Experimental studies have demonstrated that a causal relationship exists between specific televised messages and children's eating behavior (64,65) and between television viewing and participation in sports (66). Earlier studies among children and adolescents found an association between hours of television viewing and the development of obesity (63,67), but a recent evaluation of body mass index and physical activity among female adolescents over a 2 year period failed to demonstrate meaningful associations with body adiposity, physical activity, or change in either over time (68). It is possible that the way a child watches television and the content of the television programs may be more important than the number of viewing hours. However, it was recently shown that television viewing has a fairly profound lowering effect on metabolic rate in both lean and obese individuals. Thus television viewing may reduce BMR and may thereby serve as an important factor in susceptible children who are at risk for weight gain and may potentially lead to obesity (69). This acute lowering effect of television viewing on basal metabolic rate provides further support for a causal relationship between television viewing and obesity (70).

C. Dietary Factors

The role of dietary intake in obesity remains controversial, although new data have shed more light on this problem. Obese patients often claim that they do not ingest excess food. Some of these patients often seek medical evaluation for failure to lose weight despite a history of severe caloric restriction. They are frequently thought to be hypometabolic and are often treated with thyroid or other hormones, yet they fail to lose weight. Possible explanations for this failure include (1) an energy intake significantly higher than reported and (2) a low total energy expenditure.

A number of studies have demonstrated that obese individuals tend to underreport food intake compared with normal weight subjects (71–73). Indeed, careful metabolic balance studies in some obese adults have shown that failure to lose weight despite a self-reported low caloric intake is a result of substantial misreporting of food intake and physical activity, not an abnormality in thermogenesis (74). However, the problem is often confounded in the clinical setting by the difficulties in assessing food intake and food efficiency.

On the other hand, it has been shown that low total and resting energy expenditure are risk factors for long-term weight gain in infants (38) and adults (35), respectively. However, Dwyer et al. showed that obese children may not eat more than their normal weight peers (75), and they may expend relatively fewer calories to maintain their body weight. This phenomenon has been referred as "adaptation" and results after frequent dieting efforts have taken place. These result in lower energy requirements because of loss of lean body mass (76). Repeated weight reduction attempts result in alterations in body composition and decreased fat free mass. This leads to decreased metabolic demands and thus fewer calories needed to maintain weight (77).

Reduced meal frequency, or "gorging" (i.e., one to two meals daily), has been associated with an increased risk of obesity (78,79). This is also associated with high fasting serum lipid and insulin levels. Insulin stimulates hepatic synthesis of cholesterol and tissue lipogenesis (80,81). Increasing meal frequency, or "nibbling," has been shown to lower serum cholesterol and insulin levels significantly (82). This is thought to have a beneficial effect in decreasing triglycerride synthesis in adipose tissue through a reduction in postprandial glucose and insulin levels. However, this effect may be significantly minimized by a parallel reduction in the postprandial thermogenesis stimulated by insulin and glucose (83).

The high susceptibility to obesity may also be the result of unlimited availability of palatable and high-calorie-density foods. Adult laboratory rats fed a "supermarket diet" consisting of high-carbohydrate and high-fat foods (i.e., chocolate chip cookies, marshmallows, and peanut butter) gained 2.5 times more weight than normal controls (84). In some animals, the weight gain was not reversed after the rat was switched back to chow. It is believed that the supermarket diet not only increases fat cell size but also acts to increase the number of fat cells.

Dietary composition and different rates of nutrient utilization of ingested diet can influence body weight maintenance. Using an indirect calorimetric technique in nonobese males, Flatt et al. demonstrated that under sedentary conditions, ingested carbohydrates are quickly metabolized while the rate of fat oxidation remains unchanged (85). Moreover, it has been suggested that the body tightly regulates carbohydrate balance for up to 36 h after ingestion and is not affected by alterations in the body's fat balance (86). On the other hand, fat balance is believed to be regulated over a varying long term, and it may take several days before the fat balance adjusts to new levels of fat ingestion. Thus, ingesting excess fat calories over a long period of time results in a positive fat balance and weight gain.

Moreover, the medium-chain fatty acids contained in many diets are metabolized in the postprandial period instead of being stored as fat (85). Therefore, fats containing a large proportion of medium-chain fatty acids may provide an alternative to prevent weight gain because of excess fat ingestion. The best way to decrease fat deposition is to reduce fat intake, but incorporation of medium-chain fatty acids into many of the foods that children tend to consume may offer a way to reduce dietary fat that is shunted to body weight gain. Further evaluation of the nutrient utilization of various diets in children will determine whether medium-chain fatty acids can safely substitute for dietary long-chain fatty acids.

Finally, a high carbohydrate content of diets has been demonstrated to increase basal plasma insulin levels in animals and humans (87,88). It has been shown that marked obesity is associated with an elevated basal plasma insulin secretory response to glucose and protein (89,90). The hyperinsulinemia of obesity has been regarded as a compensatory adaptation to the peripheral insulin resistance characteristics of the obese state (91). Because the diets of moderately obese individuals are excessive in both total calories and in the quantity of carbohydrate ingested, the hyperinsulinemia of obesity may also be a consequence of these dietary factors rather than merely a secondary response to insulin resistance. Furthermore, hyperinsulinemia and insulin resistance are thought to cause enhanced insulin-induced lipogenesis and excessive weight gain.

D. Metabolic and Endocrine Alterations (Table 3)

The altered nutritional state in obesity results in many endocrine changes that disappear with weight loss. These include excess insulin secretion, insulin resistance, and alterations at the level of the hypothalamic-pituitary-gonadal and adrenal axes.

On the other hand, endocrine and metabolic disorders are seldom the cause of obesity in children and adolescents. These may include insulinoma, Cushing syndrome, and hypothyroidism.

1. Hyperinsulinemia and Insulin Resistance

Hyperinsulinism and insulin resistance are characteristic features of obesity (92). It has been demonstrated that insulin secretion increases as the severity of obesity increases (93), and this increase in insulin secretion is accompanied by varying degrees of resistance to insulin-mediated glucose uptake (94). Indeed, the observed abnormalities in glucose tolerance in some obese adolescents are consistent with the presence of hyperinsulinemia and insulin resistance. Occasionally, young patients with a strong positive family history of NIDDM develop diabetes. Also, insulin resistance may result in the development of acanthosis nigricans, a hyperpigmentation of skin, which is commonly seen on the back of the neck, axillae, and other flexural areas (95). Hyperinsulinemia is usually accompanied by hyperandrogenism, which leads to hirsutism.

The presence of hyperinsulinemia favors the maintenance of the obese state by stimulating lipogenesis via activation of lipoprotein lipase and by inhibiting lipolysis. The hyperinsulinemia and insulin resistance are believed to cause preferential

Table 3 Endocrine and Metabolic Alterations in Obese Children and Adolescents

Endocrine and metabolic function	Alterations in obese subjects
Pancreatic	Hyperinsululinemia and insulin resistance
	Decreased glucagon release
Reproductive	
Pituitary	Normal or elevated serum FSH and normal LH; early onset of puberty in these with advanced skeletal age
Ovarian	Normal serum (estradiol) but elevated progesterone, decreased SHBG, premature pubarche, hyperandogenism, hirsutism; increased incidence of polycystic ovarian syndrome
Testicular	Decreased total serum testosterone with normal free testosterone caused by decreased SHBG, increased serum estrogen but no clinical feminization; premature pubarche
Adrenal	Normal serum cortisol with increased cortisol production and excretion of its metabolites; normal circadian rhythm, premature adrenarche; elevated serum adrenal androgens and DHEA, normal epinephrine and norepinephrine
Growth factors	Attenuated basal and stimulated growth hormone release following provocative hypothalamic or pituitary stimuli; normal serum somatomedins and normal or accelerated linear growth
Prolactin	Elevated basal serum prolactin but attenuated response to provocative tests
Thyroid	Normal serum thyroxine, triiodothyronine, free thyroxine, and thyroid-stimulating hormone

shunting of substrates to adipose tissue, with conversion of periadipocytes to adipocytes; this is associated with hyperplasia and hypertrophy of fat cells, inducing an unabated lipogenic state and obesity (96). It has also been shown that the lipogenic action of insulin occurs at a lower insulin concentration than its glycoregulatory action (97). Additionally, Le Stunff and Bougnéres recently demonstrated that hyperinsulinemic obese children oxidized more fat and less glucose compared with their lean counterparts (98). This impairment of glucose metabolism may be caused in part by an excessive utilization of fatty substrate (99). This finding supports the concept of decreased glucose utilization and its shunting to fatty acid and triglyceride synthesis.

The hyperinsulinemia of obesity is apparently caused by a combination of increases in pancreatic secretion and a reduction in hepatic extraction (100). The extent of the changes in insulin level is correlated with increasing fat cell size and degree of obesity and is more prominent in individuals with central obesity (100,101). The mechanisms for the enhanced insulin secretion are not well understood, but one explanation is that it is an adaptive response to the diminished insulin binding sites (102). Others, however, have suggested that an islet-stimulating humoral factor may be contributing to the hyperinsulinemia of obesity (103).

The observed metabolic alterations in the insulin-resistant state are predominantly with regard to glucose metabolism, especially with respect to cellular glucose uptake and hepatic glucose production, whereas effects on amino acid metabolism and fat metabolism are less significant. These metabolic changes lead to blood glucose elevation (104) and enhanced fatty acid storage in adipose tissue. Kida et al. demonstrated diminished insulin receptor binding in monocytes of obese children that inversely correlated with their degree of obesity (105). Both receptor and postreceptor binding defects appear to play a role in the insulin resistance of obesity. However, it is not clear whether hyperinsulinemia-induced downregulation of insulin receptors and/or decreased receptor-induced hyperinsulinemia are the mechanisms for the observed alterations. These abnormalities correct toward the normal range with weight loss.

Additionally, other investigators have evaluated the rate of body fat distribution and altered fatty acid metabolism in insulin resistance and hyperinsulinimia of obesity. For instance, obese subjects with an abdominal fat distribution have reduced hepatic insulin binding (106,107). A possible cellular mechanism may be the result of high physiologic free fatty acid (FFA) concentrations. It has been suggested that the inhibitory effect of FFA is energy dependent and does not change the total cellular number of insulin receptors or their binding characteristics, indicating that the receptor internalization or recycling is influenced (108). More recently, Svedberg et al. demonstrated that obesity with high ambient FFA levels influences the internalization and recycling of hepatic insulin receptors, leading to reduced cell surface binding (109). An increased supply of FFAs to muscle have been suggested to restrain glucose transport and disposal through the inhibitory action of the products of FFA oxidation (citrate, acetyl-CoA, and adenosine 5-triphosphate, for example) on key enzymes of glucose metabolism (pyruvate dehydrogenase, phosphofructokinase, and hexokinase) (99). The observed substrate competition is suggested to impede insulin action on glucose metabolism through a derangement of lipid metabolism (110,111). In children, progressive augmentation of fat stores and lipid oxidation during the first years of obesity could therefore induce a progressive reduction in glucose oxidation and decreased insulin action (98). This suggests that the increase in lipid oxidation precedes the changes in glucose oxidation and insulin levels associated with long-duration obesity.

Finally, elevated circulating levels of insulin as a result of insulin-producing tumor (insulinoma) or excessive administration of insulin to an insulin-dependent diabetic patient can lead to obesity. These patients develop obesity, short stature, and hepatomegaly (Mauriac syndrome) (112).

2. Reproductive Function

Puberty may begin early in tall overweight children with advanced skeletal age. Pubertal elevations of follicle-stimulating hormone (FSH) has been observed in 7 to 9-year-old girls without changes in luteinizing hormone (LH) level (113). This is usually complicated by an adiposity-related decrease in circulating concentrations of sex hormone binding globulin (SHBG), which results in a higher fraction of free or unbound serum sex steroids, and thus bioactive, than in lean subjects (114). In general, the sex hormone binding globulin abnormalities correlate with the degree of obesity and are reversed with weight loss (115). Low serum entradiol levels and elevated progesterone levels have been observed in young prepubertal and early pubertal obese girls compared with age-matched lean girls (113).

The emergence of hyperandrogenism in pubertal girls may be associated with rapid weight gain, signs of hirsutism or virilism, and irregular menstrual periods (116). This is usually accompanied by hyperinsulinemia and insulin resistance with or without glucose intolerance. There is strong evidence that insulin exerts a regulatory effect on ovarian androgen synthesis (117). In fact, a positive correlation between the degree of hyperinsulinemia and hyperandrogenism can be found in obese women (118). Because insulin is believed to exert its regulatory action through the effect of luteinizing hormone on ovarian function, some obese patients may also present with polycystic ovaries and abnormally elevated serum LH, low follicle-stimulating hormone, and high free testosterone levels.

Obese adolescent boys appear to have an attenuated testicular response to human chorionic gonadotropin, but this is probably an artifact of decreased sex hormone binding globulin. Indeed, Glass (100) demonstrated that despite a decrease in SHBG levels and increased percentage of free testosterone, the free testosterone levels were normal. The serum dihydrotestosterone level remain normal in obese subjects. Also, aromatization of androgens to estrogens by adipose tissue, in males, appears to be enhanced without evidence of clinical feminization (100). However, free and total testosterone levels may be diminished in morbidly obese males. This is commonly associated with decreased gonadotropin levels, suggesting some degree of hypogonadotropic hypogonadism (119). These alterations in pituitary and gonadal hormones return to the normal range with weight loss (120).

Finally, mild obesity may occur in adolescent patients with Klinefelter (121) and Turner syndrome (122) with primary hypogonadism. It is believed that hypogonadism results in excessive deposition of fat because of the deficiency of anabolic hormones, which are responsible for the growth of muscle. In Klinefelter syndrome, this effect is enhanced by the unopposed influence of estrogen, leading to further fat accumulation in the hips and buttocks to produce the eunuchoid appearance.

3. Adrenal Function

Adrenal glucocorticoid production is enhanced in obese children (112). Obese children tend to maintain normal serum cortisol levels because of increased urinary clearance and in direct proportion to an increase in lean body mass. Increased clearance of cortisol has a stimulatory effect on pituitary adrenocorticotropic hormone (ACTH) release. ACTH stimulates the increased production of adrenal sex steroids, such as dehydroepiandrosterone and testosterone. Increased production of adrenal sex steroids leads to early adrenarche (pubarche) in obese children (123).

The release of cortisol is maintained under a normal circadian rhythm. Further, it is believed that elevated plasma cortisol in some obese individuals is related to the hyperinsulinemnia of obesity and contributes to the characteristic body fat distribution and altered body composition (124). Adrenal hypercorticolism has long been recognized in the differential diagnosis of pediatric obesity. Although some patients have a fat distribution suggestive of Cushing syndrome, the use of corticosteroid therapy for a variety of inflammatory and allergic conditions is also associated with the development of obesity. In most instances, this obesity is transient and resolves once the drug is stopped. This syndrome is a rare cause of obesity. In obese children, serum levels of epinephrine and norepinephrine remain normal.

4. Growth Hormone, Growth Factors, and Prolactin

Obese children are commonly tall for age. This is associated with advanced skeletal maturity and early onset of puberty, as well as premature pubarche (123). The lean body mass is often increased in these children (125). Growth hormone levels are low in overweight subjects, both in the fasted state and following pharmacologic stimulation (126,127). Attenuated growth hormone levels in obese subjects appear to be related to enhanced adipose tissue mass (128).

On the other hand, growth hormone (GH) deficiency or pituitary dwarfism is reported to result in a mild degree of obesity compared with other causes of weight gain. It is believed that weight gain in a growth-deficient child is caused by diminished energy expenditure. Indeed, it has been observed that GH stimulates the growth of muscle tissue and breakdown of fat tissue, therefore affecting body composition (129).

Insulin-like growth factor I (IGF-I) levels are normal to elevated in obese subjects (130). However, overfeeding may cause significant elevations of insulin-like growth factor I (130,131). It has been suggested that the blunted growth hormone response in obese subjects could be secondary to negative feedback inhibition by IGF-I (130). However, other investigators have suggested that the IGF-I level is maintained or even enhanced by the hyperinsulinemia of obesity (132).

Basal prolactin levels are normal or slightly elevated in obese children. However, the prolactin response to provocative stimuli is often diminished (133). Donders et al. suggested that decreased serotonin in the brain was a potential mechanism for the blunted prolactin response. Others have hypothesized that this may be caused by a hypothalamic defect that contributes to the abnormal prolactin response and aberrant appetite regulation, especially when the prolactin response does not return to normal with weight loss in the same obese patients.

5. Thyroid Function

There is no evidence that links thyroid dysfunction to exogenous obesity. Serum levels of thyroxine, free thyroxine, and thyroid-stimulating hormone (TSH) are normal in obese individuals. Hypothyroidism is not a common cause of obesity. Excessive weight gain secondary to an underactive thyroid gland is caused by a combination of decreased metabolic rate and enhanced fluid retention (134). In children, hypothyroidism is associated with poor linear growth. Therefore, a normally growing but overweight child is not likely to be hypothyroid.

E. Neurochemical Factors

The process of feeding is regulated via a complex interplay of central and peripheral brain pathways that include not only hypothalamus but also other brain areas, neurotransmitters, hormones, and circulating metabolites.

Infusion of insulin into the hypothalamic or ventricular cerebrospinal fluid produces satiety and weight loss (135), and insulin is suggested to be a central adiposity signal. Chronically hyperinsulinemic animals, such as obese Zucker rats, are believed to have reduced insulin receptor concentrations in brain capillary endothelium, leading to impaired cerebrospinal fluid insulin uptake (136,137), with consequent reduction of receptor-mediated insulin transport into the brain. These animals display hyperphagia at the time of weaning preceding significant hyperinsulinemia (138).

Experimental infusion of neuropeptide Y in paraventricular nucleus produces severe hyperphagia and leads to the development of obesity (139). Similarly, alterations in dopamine systems and/or abnormalities of monoamines can cause various types of hyperphagia (140). On the other hand, serotonin is believed to act as a satiety factor and an inhibitor of feeding reward in the hypothalamus (141).

The role of other humoral signals in the regulation of appetite and body adiposity has been extensively studied (142,143). For instance, it has been thought that a number of gut hormones (i.e., cholecystokinin) feed back to appetite-controlling areas of central nervous system (CNS) in the regulation of meal size and frequency (143,144). A study by Stromayer et al. (144) demonstrated that administration of a cholecystokinin (CCK) antagonist, L364,718, resulted in increased daily food intake in lean but not obese Zucker rats. This is consistant with other observations that CCK decreases appetite and that a satiety deficit in obese rats contributes to their overeating.

The composition of food has been proposed to affect brain neurotransmitter metabolism in some individuals. For instance, individuals referred to as "carbohydrate cravers" have been described to binge on high-carbohydrate foods during the early evening and night (145). However, most individuals seem to prefer high-fat, low-sugar foods because of the high palatability of such foods. Unfortunately, high-fat meals result in less intense satiety than high-carbohydrate meals of equal caloric value (146).

F. Hypothalamic Obesity

Lesions of the ventromedial area of hypothalamus may result from inflammatory processes, such as encephalitis, arachnoiditis, tuberculosis or trauma, or malignancy (Frohlich syndrome) (147). In children, craniopharyngioma is the most common CNS tumor that leads to hypothalamic and pituitary dysfunction (148,149). It is believed that hypothalamic injury leads to alterations in the appetite center, which can cause hyperphagia and obesity. However, there is increasing evidence that the hyperinsulinemia seen in this disorder plays a role in the development of obesity. Children with hypothalamic obesity may present with history of foraging and stealing of foods. They have a voracious appetite and may display frequent tantrums if food is denied.

IV. MEDICAL COMPLICATIONS

Obesity in children and adolescents affects many organ systems. It is associated with hypertension in about 10–30% of children (1) regardless of age, sex, and duration of obesity. Obese children and adolescents tend to have elevated total serum cholesterol, triglycerides, and low-density lipoprotein levels and decreased high-density lipoproteins (3). They are also at increased risk for developing coronary heart disease as they grow into obese adults with hyperlipidemia (150,151).

Increased cholesterol turnover and its concentration in the bile of obese individuals predispose them to high incidence of steatohepatitis (152) and gallbladder disease (153). Indeed, gallstones (cholelithiasis) have been reported to be three times more common in morbidly obese people than in normal subjects. Gallstones may also result while the obese person is on a hypocaloric diet, probably because of adipose tissue cholesterol mobilization during weight loss (154).

In a more recent study by Must et al., long-term morbidity and mortality of overweight adolescents were examined (155). They demonstrated that overweight in adolescent subjects was associated with an increased risk of mortality from all causes and disease-specific mortality among men, but not among women. On the other hand, the risk of morbidity from coronary heart disease and atherosclerosis was increased in both sexes who had been obese in adolescence. Also, the risk of colorectal cancer and gout was increased among women who had been obese in adolescence. Finally, obesity in adolescence was a more significant predictor of these risks than overweight in adulthood.

Obesity is accompanied by advanced skeletal maturity (bone age) and early menarche (156). Amenorrhea, oligomenorrhea, and/or dysfunctional uterine bleeding are common among obese adolescent females. Some of these patients also develop polycystic ovarian syndrome (157).

The orthopedic complications of obesity are believed to be largely of a mechanical nature. During childhood, a slipped femoral head epiphysis. Legg-Calve-Perthes disease, and genu valgum tend to be more common in obese subjects. Orthopedic disorders, such as Blount disease (tibia vara) and slipped femoral head epiphysis, are frequently seen in obese adolescents (7).

Rapid weight gain or obesity during infancy and childhood tends to be a risk factor for frequent respiratory infections (4). The work of breathing is increased in obese individuals, and the larger body mass places increased demands for oxygen consumption and carbon dioxide elimination. Many obese subjects suffer from chronic hypoxemia secondary to ventilation-perfusion mismatch. This is characterized by increased ventilation of upper lobes and increased perfusion of lower lobes. Insufficient elimination of carbon dioxide in some obese subjects leads to obesity hypoventilation (pickwickian) syndrome (158), which is characterized by chronic hypoxemia and hypercapnia. These subjects have blunted respiratory drive to both hypoxemia and hypercapnia.

Sleep apnea is also seen in severe obesity and is characterized by cessation of airflow for 10 s or longer on 30 occasions during 7 h of sleep. Parents of obese children and adolescents usually report that he or she snores loudly and sometimes appears to stop breathing (159). The apnea may be obstructive, central, or combined. In most patients, there are no anatomic abnormalities of upper airway that can contribute to the development of obstructive sleep apnea (OSA). It has been shown that the occurrence of OSA in obese subjects is related to the size of the region enclosed by the mandible (160) and sites and sizes of fat deposits around the pharynx (161), as well as the weight.

In patients with OSA, alveolar hypoventilation results from the increased oxygen demand during an apneic episode. Cooxistent cardiopulmonary or neuromuscular disease in subjects with OSA can play a role in the development of alveolar hypoventilation. During the apneic episodes, the systemic blood pressure increases, whereas the heart rate and cardiac output decrease. Apnea-associated cardiac arrhythmias have been frequently observed in patients with OSA and increase their risk factor for cardiovascular mortality (162). Relief of respiratory obstruction alleviates obstructive apnea. This may be accomplished by weight loss and continuous positive airway pressure during sleep.

V. PSYCHOSOCIAL COMPLICATIONS

In addition to the medical complications associated with obesity, the juvenile-onset obese subject is also at risk for psychologic morbidity (8). It has also been shown that obesity tends to confer disability greater than that associated with other forms of chronic illness (9). This disability seems to be linked to the public nature of obesity, and peer group discrimination is the factor that prompts parents to seek treatment in their obese child. Even young school-age children have been observed to view their overweight classmates as less desirable playmates (163). Overweight children are frequently teased on the playground and are usually excluded from games. Obese children are under considerable psychologic stress and are generally viewed by society as clumsy, unattractive, and overindulgent.

Lowered self-image, heightened self-consciousness, and impaired social functioning have been noted in some individuals who either become or remain obese during adolescence

(164). Studies of obese adolescents have demonstrated obsession with being overweight, passivity, and withdrawal from social contact (8). Some investigators have found similarities between the behavior of obese subjects and racial minorities expressing prejudice (165). In fact, it has been shown that obese persons were less likely to be admitted to a college than their lean counterparts, although there were no significant differences in their application rates, academic standing, or economic background (166). Moreover, obese individuals more often fail to marry and are of lower income status than normal weight individuals with other chronic medical conditions.

VI. EVALUATION (Table 4)

A child with obesity requires a comprehensive medical and nutritional evaluation during the initial visit. The initial visit focuses on dietary history, family history, review of systems, level of daily physical history, medical history, review of growth records, physical examination, and pertinent laboratory studies.

A. History

This includes an account of duration of excessive weight gain and previous or ongoing attempts to reduce weight gain.

Table 4 Diagnostic and Therapeutic Approach to the Obese Child

Intervention	Components included
Evaluation	Medical, dietary, and family histories
	Assessment of daily exercise
	Review of systems
	Physical examinations including assessment of growth and excess body weight
	Pertinent laboratory studies
Dietary	Special restriction
	Dietary counseling
	Alteration of food availability
Exercise	Development of an exercise program
	Various levels of physical excessive
	Walking, jogging, aerobic exercise, other
Behavioral	Stimulus control procedures: cue control, goal setting, social reinforcement aversion therapy, other
	Managing family problems
	Assertiveness training
Drug therapy	Not recommended
Surgical therapy	Gastric plication procedure (only in selected severely obese adolescents who are refractory to other types of intervention)
Maintenance	Calorie maintenance diet
	Increase exercise
	Weight monitoring
	Reassessment when weight gain occurs

A 3 day food record may help determine estimated caloric intake. However, one should combine a history of usual caloric intake with a history of frequency of high-caloric-density foods. In Julie's case, the reported daily calorie intake was not excessive but consisted of frequent high-carbohydrate and high-fat snacks (i.e., cookies and potato chips). Similarly, Michael's food diary revealed frequent intake of high-fat snacks, but the total daily calories were not excessive.

The family history should focus on overweight members of the family to determine the prevalence of obesity and evaluate the familial health beliefs and attitudes toward the obese child. Family history can also help estimate the risk of obesity-related morbidity. For instance, a strong family history of NIDDM increases the risk of future development of diabetes in the obese patient (167). Additionally, the body fat distribution in family members must be evaluated because of its strong correlation with hyperinsulinism and insulin resistance. Strong family histories of hypertension, hyperlipidemia, and atherosclerotic cardiovascular disease enhance the risk that such diseases will occur later in life if the obese state persists. Julie's family history was significant for obesity and NIDDM in the maternal grandmother, and Michael's extended paternal family was reported to be overweight.

The review of systems should focus on the potential causes or consequences of obesity. For instance, mild mental retardation, learning disability, or congenital syndromes (i.e., Turner and Prader-Willi) identify children at risk for the disease and a family constellation associated with a potentially vulnerable child. Recurrent headaches that have increased in frequency may identify children who must be assessed in the presence of hypothalamic tumor. Previous history of brain injury, infection, or surgery, all of which can lead to hypothalamic dysfunction, must be recorded.

The activity level and capacity of the obese child for physical exercise should be assessed. Both Julie and Michael were reported to be quite sedentary and watched greater than 2 h of television daily. The parents of both children reported that they became easily tired and short of breath after brief periods of walking or running.

History of daytime somnolence may be an important clue to chronic hypercapnia as well as sleep apnea or primary alveolar hypoventilation. Julie snored loudly at night, but this was not associated with daytime somnolence.

Recurrent pain in the ankles or ankle sprain may result from the effect of increased weight bearing. In some adolescents chronic hip pain may indicate imminent fermoral head epiphysis. Julie and Michael did not complain of joint pain.

Psychosocial issues or concerns in obesity must be stressed during the initial evaluation. For instance, Julie complained that other children teased her on the playground and did not want to play with her, whereas Michael was distressed by his parents' frequent remarks about his weight and being lazy.

B. Physical Examination

A review of the growth record of the patient is essential. Rapid weight gain is commonly associated with linear growth acceleration in obese children. Overweight children are frequently taller at all ages than their age- and sex-matched peers, as well as their genetic predisposition. Also, their final adult height is not frequently affected. However, in Julie's case (Fig. 1), excessive weight gain and accelerated growth were accompanied by advanced bone age (BA) of 8 years versus chronologic age (CA) of 5 years. Her height age (HA) was only 6 years, with BA/HA ratio > 1, predicting probable attenuation of her ultimate adult height. On the other hand, Michael's growth chart (Fig. 2) revealed progression of weight gain above and parallel to the 95th percentile and his linear growth proceeded on the 95th percentile. His BA was advanced at 11 years, with CA 9 years and HA 11 years. His BA/HA ratio was 1, which suggested no potential attenuation of final adult height in this child.

In obese children whose heights fall below the 50th percentile or below their genetic potential, causes other than excessive energy intake may be contributing to obesity. Children with Prader-Willi syndrome or pseudohypoparathyroidism commonly present with obesity and short stature.

The physical examination should also include an assessment of fat deposits. A high WHR, greater than 0.8, has been associated with hyperinsulinemia, insulin resistance, and future development of NIDDM in adults. In Julie's case, the WHR was 0.96, with significant upper body adiposity, whereas Michael's WHR was 0.76, with modest subcutaneous adiposity. The presence of upper body obesity in markedly obese children may be associated with the development of acanthosis nigricans (brownish discoloration of skin) along the skin creases of the posterior cervical axilla and other flexural areas. Julie's examination revealed modest pigmentary discoloration in the cervical area. She was found to have growth of pubic hair (Tanner 2) without breast development and/or cliteromegaly. Michael's physical examination revealed a prepubertal male and was basically within normal limits.

C. Laboratory Studies

Pertinent laboratory tests in some obese children help determine associated endocrine and metabolic alterations. These include fasting plasma lipids, glucose, and insulin in morbidly obese children and adolescents with a history of excessive thirst and nocturia. Also, evaluation of pituitary, adrenal, and/or thyroid hormones in some children with the early appearance of secondary sex characteristics or linear growth deceleration helps to identify acquired but rare causes of excessive weight gain, respectively.

In Julie's case, laboratory studies revealed elevated fasting insulin and basal adrenocortical hormones. A dexamethasone suppression test resulted in reduction of adrenocortical DHEA and ruled out androgen-producing adrenal or ovarian tumor. Also, ultrasonographic study of the abdomen and pelvis revealed normally sized adrenal glands and prepubescent uterus and ovaries. These findings were consistent with the diagnosis of hyperinsulinemic morbid obesity complicated by alterations in adrenocortical hormone and the resulting premature pubarche. On the other hand, Michael was assessed to have modest (grade I) obesity with a constitutional pattern of obesity.

VII. MANAGEMENT

Many medical professionals avoid taking care of children with obesity. The patient is usually referred to a dietitian, who reenforces a list of meal plans that has been unsuccessful for the child on several occasions. The physician's approach to the problem of obesity in many instances is biased by the view that a nutritional disorder like obesity is a psychologic problem and that there is not much that can be done to treat or cure the obese individual. Also, some believe that obesity is really the patient's fault. None of this analysis is accurate or valid, and it is the medical professional's responsibility to provide care to patients who are sick.

A number of treatment modalities for childhood obesity exist. However, before institution of any form of therapy, a comprehensive medical evaluation is indicated. This should comprise information on the rate of growth, developmental milestones, and family history. The last is essential to identify those with parental obesity, hypertension, diabetes mellitus, hyperlipidemia, and thyroid dysfunction. Also, the assessment should include nutritional, psychologic, and physical fitness evaluations. It has been reported that a subgroup of obese adolescents and adults (5–43%) engage in binge eating (168). Those who indulge in binge eating are those who are described as rigid dieters and under tremendous psychologic stress. These individuals have a higher dropout rate from weight reduction programs than those who do not binge.

A. Goals of Treatment

The main goal of therapy should be to achieve the objective of lifelong weight control. Therefore, it is important to know the child's pattern of growth and weight gain. In general, any therapeutic approach to childhood obesity is designed to induce decreased energy intake while maintaining normal growth. Intervention to induce weight loss must consider all the factors that are believed to cause obesity and the treatment modalities that have been effective. Because most of our present experience in the treatment of obesity centers on environmental and behavioral factors, these represent the primary areas of intervention. Genetic factors also play a very significant role in obesity and can help identify the child at risk. This allows early intervention in a child predisposed to obesity and is indicated before obesity reaches extreme proportions. Furthermore, any form of treatment for obesity should take into account potential underlying medical conditions (i.e., hypotonia) that may frustrate or render it ineffective. Therefore, the therapeutic plan should be individualized to reach its desired goal.

Eating and exercise behaviors are influenced by a number of physiologic, psychologic, social, and cultural factors. Treatment of childhood obesity must be multifaceted to include sufficiently all the elements necessary for success. Half-hearted attempts to treat obesity can only lead to failure

and frustration and can result in a lifelong struggle with obesity and weight cycling.

1. Weight Cycling

Weight cycling has a profound effect on body composition and its metabolic efficiency (169). Weight loss followed by weight gain results in (1) weight loss from muscle, (2) weight regained as fat, (3) body learns to cope with dieting, (4) increased risk of heart disease, and (5) increased frustration (76,77).

Chronic dieters learn to cope with dieting. They develop a very efficient metabolism and maintain their weight with fewer and fewer calories with each attempt to lose weight. There is loss of muscle mass as a result of body composition changes during weight cycling. The fat mass is increased, which leads to elevation of basal insulin and lipoprotein lipase levels (170), resulting in more fat deposition.

In addition to changes in the body composition, the patient becomes psychologically frustrated as he or she fails to achieve the desired weight loss. The outcome is a patient who ingests very few calories and yet cannot lose weight.

Chronic dieters may also be increasing their risk for heart disease more than if excess weight remained at a stable level. Dieting leads to fat mobilization, and during the regaining phase fat deposition in the arteries occurs. The regained weight is more likely to be distributed in the upper body, where it is potentially more harmful (23) and is associated with a higher incidence of heart disease and more glucose intolerance (28).

Appropriate strategies to avoid weight cycling should be considered at the beginning of a child's weight reduction program. When a child is ready to participate in a weight reduction program, this should represent the serious commitment of all involved.

2. Growth Failure

In the management of childhood obesity, an appropriate balance should exist between the needs of a patient to lose weight and the nutritional requirements for linear growth. A child who loses weight is in a negative energy balance and therefore may not grow in height (171).

To avoid deceleration of linear growth in an obese child, the goals for weight loss should be conservative. In some cases, it may be adequate that a child ceases to gain weight and allows the height to catch up with his or her present weight. Because most obese children are above average for height for their age and demonstrate a more rapid growth rate and earlier sexual maturity than normal weight children, some clinicians may not be concerned with slowing the growth velocity during the management of obesity. However, if a child's height velocity slows, the individual should be reassessed, including an evaluation of daily energy intake. A new dietary regimen should be considered to allow growth to take place. Therefore, accurate assessment of linear growth is essential in the dietary management of childhood obesity. Dietary restriction and weight reduction can only be considered successful if there is a normal growth in height proceeding simultaneously with weight loss. It has been shown that moderate energy restriction does not influence long-term growth (172). The accelerated height of obese children is associated with an earlier growth spurt than in nonobese children (173). Obese children who are taller than expected at baseline experience a deceleration in height velocity during development, which makes their height more similar to parent height.

B. Dietary Intervention

Many special diets and dietary regimens have been used in the management of obesity. Diets are most likely to succeed if they are individualized according to current eating patterns, degree of motivation, intellect, amount of family support, and financial considerations. The best approach is appropriate reduction of energy intake coupled with exercise to increase energy expenditure. A well-balanced diet that provides all the necessary nutrients is the most effective and safest treatment for obesity. The reduction in caloric intake should be based on the weight history of the child in conjunction with the usual calorie intake, body size, rate of growth, degree of adiposity, desired weight, and estimated daily activity level. As a general rule, moderately obese children should be placed on an energy intake and exercise level that slow weight gain or induce a slight weight loss. To accomplish this goal, it can be assumed that for every pound of weight loss 3500 kcal must be used.

For Julie (see Fig. 1), who was 50 kg at 5 years of age, weight loss was considered an important goal of treatment because the workup revealed an underlying hyperinsulinemic state. It was recently demonstrated that hyperinsulinemic obesity is more resistant to weight loss than normoinsulinemic obesity in children (174). Her caloric intake was reported to be 1400–1500 kcal per day. This level of caloric intake was not excessive for maintenance of body weight. However, it contained a high proportion of fats (>35%). Additionally, she was reportedly quiet and sedentary and spent 6–7 h watching television daily, with little or no outdoor physical activities. A realistic goal for Julie was set at 10% of body weight loss and then weight maintenance until her weight caught up with her height and normalized the height-weight ratio. This was a long-term plan that would require a successful attempt of 3 years of body weight maintenance.

Dietary therapy was initiated without reducing calories because her total daily caloric intake did not appear to be excessive; the diet was modified to reduce the fat intake. She was placed on a 1500 kcal meal plan with decreased fat content (27–30%). The parents were counseled about the importance of their supportive role and the need to increase Julie's level of physical activity (i.e., walking and playing outdoors) and decreasing her television viewing to 2 h per day. However, Michael was counseled to decrease or eliminate high-caloric snacks from his diet and increase his level of daily physical activity by walking, biking, and/or participating in sports. This strategy was used to prevent unnecessary weight reduction. Instead, it was aimed to prevent his

rapid rate of weight gain and to maintain his body weight while his growth proceeded at a normal rate.

Overweight children often desire immediate rewards. Severe dietary restriction may lead to loss of lean body mass (175) and many other unphysiologic changes (176), as well as nutritional deficiencies. In a recent study, no long-term advantages were reported among obese patients treated with reduced caloric intake (177). Very low calorie diets may lead to repeated weight loss failures and noncompliance. Supportive counseling and reinforcement can help keep the goals straight between health professionals, patient, and parent for long-lasting results and avoidance of failure and frustration. Refusal to adhere to a weight reduction plan may be the manifestation of lack of family support, insufficient motivation, or other psychologic stresses. For instance, it has been demonstrated that children of married parents lose weight at higher rates than those of divorced parents (178). When a weight reduction plan has been recommended, conflicts frequently arise between the patient and nondieting family members regarding the degree of dietary restriction and who is permitted to eat different foods. Dietary restriction should never be introduced in a punitive fashion. In some cases, the obese child and the entire family may adhere to a diet similar in composition if not quantity. Participation of the entire family should help minimize the feelings of isolation in the obese child.

It should be noted that weight loss may not occur every week, and the overall pattern of weight change for several weeks should be used to assess the child's progress. Obese children and adolescents, especially those who have gone through dieting in the past, may have adjusted to a lower level of dietary consumption while maintaining weight (weight cycling). If weight loss does not occur for 2–3 weeks and there is no obvious noncompliance, then a further reduction in the caloric intake or an increase in energy expenditure may be needed.

The modification of the diet should be based on appropriate nutritional guidelines. This should include the reduction of fat to about one-third of the calories while increasing complex carbohydrates. Our patient, Julie, was managed by increasing vegetables in her diet and eating low-calorie snacks, which substituted for high-fat foods. She was given three meals and three snacks. It is well recognized that frequent meals are more effective for weight control than one large meal (179). Therefore, diets that consist of one or two large meals per day are discouraged.

It should be kept in mind that day-to-day variations in caloric consumption are characteristic of normal eating patterns, and thus they should be allowed as long as they are within an acceptable range. For example, it is appropriate for Julie, on a 1500 kcal meal plan, to have a range of intake from approximately 1200 to 1800 kcal. Although assessment of the rate of weight loss and growth is important, periodic assessment of the nutrient composition of the diet is essential. This is particularly important for such micronutrients as calcium, iron, magnesium, copper, zinc, folacin, and vitamin B_6, because these nutrients are very likely to be deficient on a restricted intake (180).

Figure 1 shows Julie's weight pattern over a 12 month period. She was able to lose 5.0 kg over a period of 8 weeks (1% per week), and her body weight was then maintained. During her most recent evaluation, she weighed 44.5 kg and had maintained excellent growth rate and was 208% of IBW, down from 249% of IBW 12 months earlier.

Several variations of low-calorie diets have become popular in attempts to accelerate the process of weight reduction. These weight loss fixes include total fasting, very low calorie diets, low-carbohydrate diets, protein-sparing diets, and high-protein diets. These aggressive weight loss regimens are not appropriate for obese children because they may cause negative nitrogen balance and loss of lean body mass and may affect proper growth and development. Additionally, they do not have any long-term advantages in weight control (177).

Low-carbohydrate diets are usually high in protein and fat. They encourage the intake of large amounts of meat and restrict carbohydrate-containing foods, such as fruits, vegetables, and grain products. The high intake of fat in such diets can increase the risk of coronary heart disease and other problems, such as gallstones and high cholesterol. The body depends heavily on its fat stores for energy while on a low-carbohydrate diet. This can lead to ketosis. The rapid weight loss on these diets is composed of 60–70% water, and dieters often regain weight rapidly once normal eating is resumed (181,182).

Very low caloric restriction using protein-sparing, modified fast (PSMF) diets (400–800 kcal/day) are designed to produce rapid weight loss, up to 5 pounds (2.3 kg per week), while preserving vital lean body mass. The protein is provided either as food, such as lean meat or fish, or in a milk- or egg-based liquid formula. This is associated with increased risk of medical complications. It has been suggested that these diets spare body protein by decreasing insulin levels and enhancing fat breakdown (183) while inhibiting the release of amino acids from muscle (184). However, in the past, several deaths have been associated with the use of these formulas (185). Moreover, these quick-fix weight loss schemes are unsafe for use in children and do not promote healthy eating behavior for long-lasting weight control.

C. Exercise

Physical activity has a significant influence on energy expenditure, and the energy cost for most activities is generally greater for heavier people. Also, there is some evidence that increased activity in the obese individual may decrease appetite while it increases metabolic rate.

Both obese and lean individuals experience a 19–30% decrease in resting metabolic rate within 24–48 h following caloric restriction (186). Thus caloric restriction without an increase in physical activity may not result in continued weight loss. Regular aerobic exercise combined with energy restriction results in greater reductions in body weight than dieting alone (187).

Dietary management of childhood obesity treatment should always be combined with exercise. However, exercise should be prescribed on an individual basis. An exercise program based upon the initial fitness level with a slow progression of the intensity, frequency, and duration is required to achieve the goal of weight control. For instance, morbidly obese children may achieve maximal energy expenditure during a brisk walk, because prescriptions for more demanding physical activities, such as jogging, are likely to be impossible at the start.

D. Behavioral Modification

Dietary management and physical exercise are essential components for the development of effective treatment, and the area of greatest concern for the psychologist is how to get children to alter food intake and activity behaviors. Because the primary focus is on changing the child's behavior, parenting skills represent an integral component of the intervention.

Stimulus control procedures in the behavioral control of overeating have led to the development of several behavioral techniques for the treatment of obesity, which include (1) self-monitoring of body weight and/or food intake, (2) goal setting, (3) reward and punishment, (4) aversion therapy, (5) social reinforcement, and (6) stimulus control. Several of these modification have been found to be effective with children (188–190).

These interventions are based on the assumption that the obese child is an overeater who is hypersensitive to food stimuli and can be trained to behave like a nonobese person and subsequently lose weight. Moreover, family support has been shown to influence the degree of immediate and long-term weight loss in children and adolescents, parental participation repeatedly showing a positive impact (191).

E. Drug Therapy

Long-term use of medications to suppress appetite or other antiobesity pills are not indicated in the treatment of pediatric obesity. Studies involving the use of anorectic drugs alone and in combination with behavior therapy have demonstrated that weight loss is no greater than when behavior therapy is used alone and that when the drugs are stopped, the weight is regained more rapidly (192). Also, the effectiveness of appetite suppressant drugs (i.e., amphetamines) appears to decrease with time, and there may be side effects.

The addictive potential of amphetamines and the risk of depression associated with fenfluramine have resulted in the minimal use of these agents in children and adolescents. The serotonin agonist fluoxetine has proven useful as an adjunct in weight loss programs for adolescents (193). This drug seems to decrease appetite and carbohydrate craving. Although these drugs are by no means the solution to weight loss, they may help individuals at the beginning of a weight loss program by suppressing appetite, but they must be used with caution and for a very limited time (176).

Bulking agents and nonprescription diet aids, such as methylcellulose and other noncaloric bulk materials, have also been used in experimental and clinical attempts to inhibit food intake. The rational for the use of such agents is that they swell in the stomach and supposedly give a feeling of satiety. However, the use of such agents as appetite suppressants works on a principle that has not proved to be effective in reducing feelings of hunger in patients on weight loss programs. The use of pectin has been shown to reduce gastric emptying and increase satiety, but no long-term trial for obesity treatment has been carried out.

F. Surgery

There are very few applications of surgical procedures in the management of pediatric obesity. Four types of surgical procedures have been used to change eating behavior: jaw wiring, intestinal bypass, gastric bypass procedures, and vagotomy.

Gastric plication is the only procedure that can be recommended for weight loss at the present time. This procedure is considered carefully in a selected group of adolescents with significant medical complications who have been frequently unsuccessful in losing weight (194). Following the gastric plication procedure, patient's food intake is decreased by the sensation of fullness. However, some patients regulate their food intake by nausea, pain, and vomiting. Patients also experience a change in eating patterns by decreasing their intake of fats, sweets, milk, and other dairy products. Patients who have undergone a gastric plication procedure have shown less anxiety, depression, irritability, and preoccupation with food during weight loss compared with their weight reduction attempts before the surgical procedure (195).

VIII. PREVENTION

Early intervention in the management of obesity is critical from a treatment standpoint. Initial calorie excess results in enlarged fat cells ("hypertrophic obesity"). Once the fat cells have their maximum capacity, the actual number of fat cells begins to increase to provide excess fat accretion (triglyceride). This stage of adipose development in a child is termed hyperplastic obesity. The condition tends to be more refractory to treatment than hypertrophic obesity (196).

Children should be encouraged to develop healthy eating habits and exercise patterns that prevent excessive weight gain. This is especially important for children in high-risk groups, for instance, children with obese parents and those who are overweight by the time they enter school (197). In some children who may be genetically susceptible to becoming obese, total calorie intake should be monitored with an emphasis on controlling the percentage of fat calories. Health professionals should inform the parents of the potential risks and provide instructions on preventive measures at an early age.

The introduction of a variety of nutritious foods to children's diet will lead to the development of healthy eating practices in children and adolescents. These foods should include an assortment of fresh or frozen vegetables and legumes; dairy products; fresh fruits; breads (preferably whole grain); and pastas, rice, cereals, and other grain products. Sweets and other nutrient-poor foods should be allowed in limited amounts that do not interfere with the child's consumption of basic foods. With relatively free access to these highly palatable choices, the chances of overeating are increased and may encourage the development of obesity in predisposed children.

Primary public health measures are critical to formulate a sound approach to the prevention of obesity in children. It is the responsibility of schools and government agencies, as well as food industries, to support measures that can improve the food habits and exercise patterns of children and adults. The schools should play an active role in providing healthy food choices in the cafeteria and provide appropriate exercise programs for normal weight and obese children separate from competitive athletics. The government and local authorities can assist schools to implement and promote physical fitness programs and provide affordable exercise facilities in the community. The government should play a more active role in promoting physical activity through the provision of more community facilities for exercise affordable to all residents. The government should also regulate commercial weight loss organizations and provide standards of treatment to reduce deception and fraudulent practices to which obese persons so frequently fall victim. The media should assume a responsible position with regard to idealized concepts of beauty by appropriate programming and feeding messages passed to children and to society at large. Finally, health insurance companies should assume responsibility in paying for obesity treatment before it leads to more costly long-term complications.

REFERENCES

1. Gortmaker SL, Dietz WH Jr, Sobol AM, Wehler CA. Increasing pediatric obesity in the United States. Am J Dis Child 1987; 141:535–540.
2. Ellison RC, Sosenko J, Harper GP, Gibbons L, Pratter FE, Miettinen OS. Obesity, sodium intake, and blood pressure in adolescents. Hypertension 1980; 2:78–82.
3. Williams DP, Going SB, Lohman TG, et al. Body fatness and risk for elevated blood pressure, total cholesterol, and serum lipoprotein ratios in children and adolescents. Am J Public Health 1992; 82:358–363.
4. Tracey VV, De NC, Harper JR. Obesity and respiratory infection in infants and young children. BMJ 1971; 1:16–8.
5. Deschamps I, Desjeux JF, Machinot S, Rolland F, Lestradet H. Effects of diet and weight loss on plasma glucose, insulin, and free fatty acids in obese children. Pediatr Res 1978; 12:757–760.
6. Kelsey JL, Acheson RM, Keggi KJ. The body build of patients with slipped capital femoral epiphysis. Am J Dis Child 1972; 124:276–281.
7. Kling TF Jr. Angular deformities of the lower limbs in children. Orthop Clin North Am 1987; 18:513–527.
8. Wadden TA, Stunkard AJ. Psychopathology and obesity. Ann NY Acad Sci 1987; 499:55–65.
9. Gortmaker SL, Must A, Perrin JM, Sobol AM, Dietz WH. Social and economic consequences of overweight in adolescence and young adulthood. N Engl J Med 1993; 329:1008–1012.
10. Merritt RJ. Obesity. Curr Probl Pediatr 1982; 12:1–58.

11. Stunkard A, Burt V. Obesity and the body image. II. Age at onset of disturbances in body image. Am J Psychiatry 1967; 123:1443–1447.

12. Stark O, Atkins E, Wolff OH, Douglas JWB. Longitudinal study of obesity in the National Survey of Health and Development. BMJ (Clin Res Ed) 1981; 283:13–17.

13. Hamill PV, Drizd TA, Johnson CL, Reed RB, Roache AF, Moore WM. Physical growth: National Center for Health Statistics percentiles. Am J Clin Nutr 1979; 32:607–629.

14. Moses N, Banilivy MM, Lifshitz F. Fear of obesity among adolescent girls. Pediatrics 1989; 83:393–398.

15. Rolland-Cachera MF, Sempe M, Guilloud-Bataille M, Patois E, Pequignot-Guggenbuhl F, Fautrad V. Adiposity indices in children. Am J Clin Nutr 1982; 36:178–184.

16. Pi-Sunyer FX. Obesity. In: Shils ME, Young VR, eds. Modern Nutrition in Health and Disease. Philadelphia: Lea & Febiger 1988:795–816.

17. National Center for Health Statistics, U.S. Department of Health, Education and Welfare. NCHS growth curves for children: birth to 18 years. Series H, No. 165, DHEW Publication No. (PHS)78-1650, 1977.

18. Durnin JV, Womersley J. Body fat assessed from total body density and its estimation from skinfold thickness: measurements on 481 men and women aged from 16 to 72 years. Br J Nutr 1974; 32:77–97.

19. Must A, Dallal GE, Dietz WH. Reference data for obesity: 85th and 95th percentiles of body mass index (wt/ht^2) and triceps skinfold thickness. Am J Clin Nutr 1991; 53:839–846.

20. Czinner A, Varady M. Quantitative determination of fatty tissue on body surface in obese children by ultrasound method. Padiatr Padol 1992; 27:7–10.

21. Armellini F, Zamboni M, Rigo L, et al. Sonography detection of small intra-abdominal fat variations. Int J Obes 1991; 15:847–852.

22. Kvist H, Chowdhury B, Grangard U, Tylen U. Sjostrom L. Total and visceral adipose tissue volumes derived from measurements with computed tomography in adult men and women: predictive equations. Am J Clin Nutr 1988; 48:1351–1361.

23. Ross R, Shaw KD, Martel Y, de Guise J, Avruch L. Adipose tissue distribution measured by magnetic resonance imaging in obese women. Am J Clin Nutr 1993; 57:470–475.

24. Bjorntorp P. Abdominal obesity in the development of non-insulin dependent diabetes mellitus. Diabetes Metab Rev 1988; 4:615–622.

25. Kissebah AH, Vydelingum N, Murray R, et al. Relation of body fat distribution to metabolic complications of obesity. J Clin Endocrinol Metab 1982; 54:254–260.

26. Evans DJ, Hoffmann RG, Kalkhoff RK, Kissebah AH. Relationship of body fat topography to insulin sensitivity and metabolic profiles in premenopausal women. Metabolism 1984; 33:68–75.

27. Kalkhoff RK, Hartz AH, Rupley D, Kissebah AH, Kelber S. Relationship of body fat distribution to blood pressure, carbohydrate tolerance, and plasma lipids in healthy obese women. J Lab Clin Med 1983; 102:621–627.

28. Peiris AN, Hennes MI, Evans DJ, Wilson CR, Lee MB, Kissebah AH. Relationship of anthropometric measurements of body fat distribution to metabolic profile in premenopausal women. Acta Med Scand Suppl 1988; 723:179–188.

29. Peiris AN, Struve MF, Mueller RA, Lee MB, Kissebah AH. Glucose metabolism in obesity: influence of body fat distribution. J Clin Endocrinol Metab 1988; 67:760–767.

30. De Ridder CM, de Boer RW, Seidell JC, et al. Body fat distribution in pubertal girls quantified by magnetic resonance imaging. Int J Obes 1992; 16:443–449.

31. Zamboni M, Armellini F, Milani MP, et al. Evaluation of regional body fat distribution: comparison between W/H ratio and computed tomography in obese women. J Intern Med 1992; 232:341–347.

32. Garn SM, Sullivan TV, Hawthorne VM. Fatness and obesity of the parents of obese individuals. Am J Clin Nutr 1989; 50:1308–1313.

33. Maxfield E, Konishi F. Patterns of food intake and physical activity in obesity. J Am Diet Assoc 1966; 49:406–408.

34. Bogardus C, Lillioja S, Ravussin E, et al. Familial dependence of the resting metabolic rate. N Engl J Med 1986; 315:96–100.

35. Ravussin E, Lillioja S, Knowler WC, et al. Reduced rate of energy expenditure as a risk factor for body weight gain. N Engl J Med 1988; 318:467–472.

36. Felig P, Cunningham J, Levitt M, Hendler R, Nadel E. Energy expenditure in obesity in fasting and postprandial state. Am J Physiol 1983; 244:E45–51.

37. Bandini LG, Schoeller DA, Dietz WH. Energy expenditure in obese and nonobese adolescents. Pediatr Res 1990; 27:198–203.

38. Roberts SB, Savage J, Coward WA, Chew B, Lucas A. Energy expenditure and intake in infants born to lean and overweight mothers. N Engl J Med 1988; 318:461–466.

39. Ravussin E, Burnand B, Schutz Y, Jéquier E. Twenty-four-hour energy expenditure and resting metabolic rate in obese, moderately obese, and control subjects. Am J Clin Nutr 1982; 35:566–573.

40. Ravussin E, Lillioja S, Anderson TE, Christin L, Bogardus C. Determinants of 24-hour energy expenditure in man. Methods and results using a respiratory chamber. J Clin Invest 1986; 78:1568–1578.

41. Griffiths M, Payne PR. Energy expenditure in small children of obese and nonobese parents. Nature 1976; 260:698–700.

42. Bray GA, Dahms WT, Swerdloff RS, Fiser RH, Atkinson RL, Carrel RE. The Prader-Willi syndrome: a study of 40 patients and a review of the literature. Medicine (Baltimore) 1983; 62:59–80.

43. Widhalm K, Veitt V, Irsigler K. Evidence for decreased energy expenditure in the Prader-Labhart-Willi syndrome: assessment by means of the Vienna calorimeter. Proc Int Cong Nutr 1981;

44. Schoeller DA, Levitsky LL, Bandini LG, Dietz WW, Walczak A. Energy expenditure and body composition in Prader-Willi syndrome. Metabolism 1988; 37:115–120.

45. Ledbetter DH, Riccardi VM, Airhart SD, Strobel RJ, Keenan BS, Crawford JD. Deletions of chromosome 15 as a cause of the Prader-Willi syndrome. N Engl J Med 1981; 304:325–329.

46. Bauman ML, Hogan GR. Laurence-Moon-Biedl syndrome. Am J Dis Child 1973; 126:119–126.

47. Spiegel AM. Pseudohypoparathyroidism. In: Scriver, CR, Beadet AL, et al. eds. The Metabolic Basis of Inherited Disease. New York: McGraw-Hill, 1989:2013–2027.

48. Stunkard AJ, Sorensen TI, Hanis C, et al. An adoption study of human obesity. N Engl J Med 1986; 314:193–198.

49. Stunkard AJ, Harris JR, Pedersen NL, McClearn GE. The body-mass index of twins who have been reared apart. N Engl J Med 1990; 322:1483–1487.

50. Bray GA. The inheritance of corpulence. In: Cioffi LA, James WPT, Van Itallie TB, eds. The Body Weight Regulatory System: Normal and Disturbed Mechanisms. New York: Raven Press, 1981:61–64.

51. Udal JN, Harrison GG, Vaucher Y, Walson PD, Morrow G III. Interaction of maternal and neonatal obesity. Pediatrics 1978; 62:17–21.

52. Kramer MS, Barr RG, Leduc DG, Boisjoly C, McVey-White

L, Pless IB. Determinants of weight and adiposity in the first year of life. J Pediatr 1985; 106:10–14.

53. Kramer MS, Barr RG, Leduc DG, Boisjoly C, Pless IB. Infant determinants of childhood weight and adiposity. J Pediatr 1985; 107:104–107.

54. Drabman RS, Cordua GD, Hammer D, Jarvie GJ, Horton W. Developmental trends in eating rates of normal and overweight preschool children. Child Dev 1979; 50:211–216.

55. Agras WS, Kraemer HC, Berkowitz RI, Korner AF, Hammer LD. Does a vigorous feeding style influence early development of adiposity? J Pediatr 1987; 110:799–804.

56. Bullen BA, Reed RB, Mayer J. Physical activity of obese and nonobese adolescent girls appraised by motion picture sampling. Am J Clin Nutr 1964; 14:211–223.

57. Waxman M, Stunkard AJ. Caloric intake and expenditure of obese boys. J Pediatr 1980; 96:187–193.

58. Maffeis C, Schutz Y, Schena F, Zaffanello M, Pinelli L. Energy expenditure during walking and running in obese and nonobese prepubertal children. J Pediatr 1993; 123:193–199.

59. Prentice AM, Lucas A, Vasquez-Velasquez L, Davies PS, Whitehead RG. Are current dietary guidelines for young children a prescription for overfeeding? Lancet 1988; 2:1066–1069.

60. Energy and protein requirements. Report of a joint FAO/WHO ad hoc expert committee. Rome, March 22 to April 2, 1971. FAO Nutr Meet Rep Ser 1973; (52):1–118.

61. Goran MI, Carpenter WH, Poehlman ET. Total energy expenditure in 4-to 6-yr-old children. Am J Physiol 1993; 264:E706–711.

62. Fontvieille AM, Harper IT, Ferraro RT, Spraul M, Ravussin E. Daily energy expenditure by five-year-old children, measured by doubly labeled water. J Pediatr 1993; 123:200–207.

63. Najjar MF, Rowland M. Anthropometric reference data and prevalence of overweight. Vital Health Stat [11] 1987; (238):1–73.

64. Gorn GJ, Goldberg ME. Behavioral evidence for the effects of televised food messages on children. J Consumer Res 1982; 9:200–205.

65. Jeffrey DB, McLellarn RW, Fox DT. The development of children's eating habits: the role of television commercials. Health Ed Q 1982; 9:174–189.

66. Williams TM, Handford AG. Television and other leisure activities. In: Williams TM, ed. The Impact of Television: A Natural Experiment in Three Communities. Orlando, FL: Academic Press, 1986:143–213.

67. Dietz WH Jr, Gortmaker SL. Do we fatten our children at the television set? Obesity and television viewing in children and adolescents. Pediatrics 1985; 75:807–812.

68. Robinson TN, Hammer LD, Killen JD, et al. Does television viewing increase obesity and reduce physical activity? Cross-sectional and longitudinal analyses among adolescent girls. Pediatrics 1993; 91:273–280.

69. Klesges RC, Shelton ML, Klesges LM. Effects of television on metabolic rate: potential implications for childhood obesity. Pediatrics 1993; 91:281–286.

70. Dietz WH, Bandini LG, Gortmaker S. Epidemiologic and metabolic risk factors for childhood obesity. Klin Padiatr 1990; 202:69–72.

71. Schoeller DA. How accurate is self-reported dietary energy intake? Nutr Rev 1990; 48:373–379.

72. Mertz W, Tsui JC, Judd JT, et al. What are people really eating? The relation between energy intake derived from estimated diet records and intake determined to maintain body weight. Am J Clin Nutr 1991; 54:291–295.

73. Bandini LG, Schoeller DA, Cyr HN, Dietz WH. Validity of reported energy intake in obese and nonobese adolescents. Am J Clin Nutr 1990; 52:421–425.

74. Lichtman SW, Pisarska K, Berman ER, et al. Discrepancy between self-reported and actual caloric intake and exercise in obese subjects. N Engl J Med 1992; 327:1893–1898.

75. Dwyer JT, Feldman JJ, Mayer J. Adolescent dieters: who are they? Physical characteristics, attitudes and dieting practices of adolescent girls. Am J Clin Nutr 1967; 20:1045–1056.

76. Rossner S. Weight cycling a "new" risk factor? J Intern Med 1989; 226:209–211.

77. Steen SN, Oppliger RA, Brownell KD. Metabolic effects of repeated weight loss and regain in adolescent wrestlers. JAMA 1988; 260:47–50.

78. Bray GA. Lipogenesis in human adipose tissue: some effects of nibbling and gorging. J Clin Invest 1972; 51:537–548.

79. Fabry P, Tepperman J. Meal frequency a possible factor in human pathology. Am J Clin Nutr 1970; 23:1059–1068.

80. Dietschy JM, Brown MS. Effect of alterations of the specific activity of the intracellarlar acetyl CoA pool on apparent rates of hepatic cholesterogenesis. J Lipid Res 1974; 15:508–516.

81. Lakshmanan MR, Nepokroeff CM, Ness GC, Dugan RE, Porter JW. Stimulation by insulin of rat liver β-hydroxy-β-methylglutaryl coenzyme A reductase and cholesterol-synthesizing activities. Biochem Biophys Res Commun 1973; 50:704–710.

82. Jenkins DJ, Wolever TM, Vuksan V, Brighenti F, Cunnane SC. Nibbling verses gorging: metabolic advantages of increased meal frequency. N Engl J Med 1989; 321:929–934.

83. Acheson K, Jequier E, Wahren J. Influence of β-adrenergic blockade on glucose-induced thermogensis in man. J Clin Invest 1983; 72:981–986.

84. Sclafani A, Springer D. Dietary obesity in adult rats: similarities to hypothalamic and human obesity syndromes. Physiol Behav 1976; 17:461–471.

85. Flatt JP, Ravussin E, Acheson KJ, Jequier E. Effects of dietary fat on postprandial substrate oxidation and on carbohydrate and fat balances. J Clin Invest 1985; 76:1019–1024.

86. Schutz Y, Flatt JP, Jequier E. Failure of dietary fat intake to promote fat oxidation: a factor favoring the development of obesity. Am J Clin Nutr 1989; 50:307–314.

87. Grey NJ, Goldring S, Kipnis DM. The effect of fasting, diet, and actinomycin D on insulin secretion in the rat. J Clin Invest 1970; 49:881–889.

88. Grey NJ, Kipnis DM. Effect of diet composition on the hyperinsulinemia of obesity. N Engl J Med 1971; 285:827–831.

89. Bagdade JD, Bierman EL, Porte D Jr. The significance of basal insulin levels in the evaluation of the insulin response to glucose in diabetic and nondiabetic subjects. J Clin Invest 1967; 46:1549–1557.

90. Floyd JC Jr, Fajans SS, Conn JW, Knopf RF, Rull J. Stimulation of insulin secretion by amino acids. J Clin Invest 1966; 45:1487–1502.

91. Rabinowitz D, Zierler KL. Forearm metabolism in obesity and its response to intra-arterial insulin. Characterization of insulin resistance and evidence for adaptive hyperinsulinism. J Clin Invest 1962; 41:2173–2181.

92. Polonsky KS, Given BD, Van Cauter E. Twenty-four-hour profiles and pulsatile patterns of insulin secretion in normal and obese subjects. J Clin Invest 1988; 81:442–448.

93. Bogardus C, Lillioja S, Mott D, Reaven GR, Kashiwagi A, Foley JE. Relationship between obesity and maximal insulin-stimulated glucose uptake in vivo and in vitro in Pima Indians. J Clin Invest 1984; 73:800–805.

94. Kashiwagi A, Verso MA, Andrews J, Vasquez B, Reaven G, Foley JE. In vitro insulin resistance of human adipocytes isolated from subjects with noninsulin-dependent diabetes mellitus. J Clin Invest 1983; 72:1246–1254.

95. Fier JS. Metabolic importance of acanthosis nigricans. Arch Dermatol 1985; 121:193–194.

96. Caro JF, Dohm LG, Pories WJ, Sinha MK. Cellular alterations in liver, skeletal muscle, and adipose tissue responsible for insulin resistance in obesity and type II diabetes. Diabetes Metab Rev 1989; 5:665–689.

97. Schade DS, Eaton RP. Dose response to insulin in man: differential effects on glucose and ketone body regulation. J Clin Endocrinol Metab 1977; 44:1038–1053.

98. Le Stunff C, Bougnéres PF. Time course of increased lipid and decreased glucose oxidation during early phase of child-hood obesity. Diabetes 1993; 42:1010–1016.

99. Randle PJ, Garland PB, Hales CN, Newsholme EA. The glucose fatty-acid cycle: its role in insulin sensitivity and the metabolic disturbances of diabetes mellitus. Lancet 1963; 1:785–789.

100. Glass AR. Endocrine aspects of obesity. Med Clin North Am 1989; 73:139–160.

101. Rosenbaum M, Leibel RL. Pathophysiology of childhood obesity. Adv Pediatr 1988; 35:73–137.

102. Olefsky JM. Decreased insulin binding to adipocytes and circulating monocytes from obese subjects. J Clin Invest 1976; 57:1165–1172.

103. Lautala P, Akerblom HK, Kouvalainen K, Martin JM. Insulinotropic activity in the serum of obese and nonobese infants and children. Pediatr Res 1986; 20:720–723.

104. DeFronzo RA, Ferrannini E, Simonson DC. Fasting hyperglycemia in non-insulin-dependent diabetes mellitus: contributions of excessive hepatic glucose production and impaired tissue glucose uptake. Metabolism 1989; 38:387–395.

105. Kida K, Watanabe N, Fujisawa Y, Goto Y, Matsuda H. The relation between glucose tolerance and insulin binding to circulating monocytes in obese children. Pediatrics 1982; 70:633–637.

106. Rossell R, Gomis R, Casamitjana R, Segura R, Vilardell E, Rivera F. Reduced hepatic insulin extraction in obesity: relationship with plasma insulin levels. J Clin Endocrinol Metab 1983; 56:608–611.

107. Peiris AN, Mueller RA, Smith GA, Struve MF, Kissebah AH. Splanchnic insulin metabolism in obesity. Influence of body fat distribution. J Clin Invest 1986; 78:1648–1657.

108. Svedberg J, Bjorntorp, Smith U, Lonnroth P. Free-fatty acid inhibition of insulin binding, degradation, and action in isolated rat hepatocytes. Diabetes 1990; 39:570–574.

109. Svedberg J, Bjorntorp P, Smith U, Lonnroth P. Effects of free fatty acids on insulin receptor binding and tyrosine kinase activity in hepatocytes isolated from lean and obese rats. Diabetes 1992; 41:294–298.

110. Felber JP, Ferrannini E, Golay A, et al. Role of lipid oxidation in pathogenesis of insulin resistance of obesity and type II diabetes. Diabetes 1987; 36:1341–1350.

111. Lillioja S, Bogardus C, Mott DM, Kennedy AL, Knowler WC, Howard BV. Relationship between insulin-mediated glucose disposal and lipid metabolism in man. J Clin Invest 1985; 75:1106–1115.

112. Daneman D, Drash AL, Lobes LA, Becker DJ, Baker LM, Travis LB. Progressive retinopathy with improved control in diabetic dwarfism (Mauriac's syndrome). Diabetes Care 1981; 4:360–365.

113. Genazzani AR, Pintor C, Corda R. Plasma levels of gonado-tropins, prolactin, thyroxine, and adrenal and gonadal steroids in obese prepubertal girls. J Clin Endocrinol Metab 1978; 47:974–979.

114. Dunkel L, Sorva R, Voutilainen R. Low levels of sex hormone-binding globulin in obese children. J Pediatri 1985; 107:95–97.

115. Stanik S, Dornfeld LP. Maxwell MH, Viosca SP, Korenman SG. The effect of weight loss on reproductive hormones in obese men. J Clin Endocrinol Metab 1981; 53:828–832.

116. Hartz AJ, Barboriak PN, Wong A, Katayama KP, Rimm AA. The association of obesity with infertility and related menstrual abnormalities in women. Int J Obes 1979; 3:57–73.

117. Poretsky L, Kalin MF. The gonadotropic function of insulin. Endocr Rev 1987; 8:132–141.

118. Pasquali R, Casimirri F, Venturoli S, et al. Insulin resistance in patients with polycystic ovaries: its relationship to body weight and androgen levels. Acta Endocrinol (Copenh) 1983; 104:110–116.

119. Strain GW, Zumoff B, Kream J, et al. Mild hypogonadotropic hypogonadism in obese men. Metabolism 1982; 31:871–875.

120. Strain GW, Zumoff B, Miller LK. The influence of massive weight loss on the hypogonadotropic hypogonadism of obese men. Int J Obes 1987; 11(Suppl. 2):54–59.

121. Ratcliffe SG, Bancroft J, Axworthy D, McLaren W, Klinefelter's syndrome in adolescence. Arch Dis Child 1982; 57:6–12.

122. Polychronakos C, Letarte J, Collu R, Ducharme JR. Carbo-hydrate intolerance in children and adolescents with Turner syndrome. J Pediatr 1980; 96:1009–1014.

123. Jabbar M, Pugliese M, Fort P, Recker B, Lifshitz F. Excess weight and precocious pubarche in children: alterations of the adrenocortical hormones. J Am Coll Nutr 1991; 4:289–296.

124. Freedman DS, Srinivasan SR, Burke GL, et al. Relation of body fat distribution to hyperinsulinemia in children and adolescents: the Bogalusa Heart Study. Am J Clin Nutr 1987; 46:403–410.

125. Forbes GB. Influence of nutrition. In: Forbes GB, ed. Human Body Composition: Growth, Aging, Nutrition and Activity. New York: Springer-Verlag, 1987:209–247.

126. Sims EA, Danforth E Jr, Horton ES, Bray GA, Glennon JA, Salans LB. Endocrine and metabolic effects of experimental obesity in man. Recent Prog Horm Res 1973; 29:457–496.

127. Meistas MT, Foster GV, Margolis S, Kowarski AA. Integrated concentrations of growth hormone, insulin, C-peptide and prolactin in human obesity. Metabolism 1982; 31:1224–1228.

128. Kalkhoff R, Ferrou C. Metabolic differences between obese overweight and muscular overweight men. N Engl J Med 1971; 284:1236–1239.

129. Novak LP, Hayles AB, Cloutier MD. Effect of HGH on body composition of hypopituitary dwarfs. Four-compartment analysis and composite body density. Mayo Clin Proc 1972; 47:241–246.

130. Rosskamp R, Becker M, Soetadji S. Circulating somatomedin-C levels and the effect of growth hormone-releasing factor on plasma levels of growth hormone and somatostation-like immunoreactivity in obese children. Eur J Pediatr 1987; 146:48–50.

131. Forbes GB, Brown MR, Welle SL, Underwood LE. Hormonal response to overfeeding. Am J Clin Nutr 1989; 49:608–611.

132. Kopelman PG, Weaver JV, Noonan K. Abnormal hypothalamic function and altered insulin secretion and IGFBP-1 binding in obesity. Int J Obes 1990; 14(Suppl. 2):75–79.

133. AvRuskin TW, Pillai S, Kasi K, Juan C, Kleinberg DL. Decreased prolactin secretion in childhood obesity. J Pediatr 1985; 106:373–378.

134. Kyle LH, Ball MF, Doolan PD. Effect of thyroid hormone on body composition in myxedema and obesity. N Engl J Med 1966; 275:12–17.

135. Woods SC, Lotter EC, McKay LD, Porte D Jr. Chronic intracerebroventricular infusion of insulin reduces food intake and body weight of baboons. Nature 1979; 282:503–505.

136. Porte D Jr, Woods SC. Regulation of food intake and body weight in insulin. Diabetologia 1981; 20:274–280.

137. Woods SC, Porte D Jr, Bobbioni E, et al. Insulin: its relationship to the central nervous system and to the control of food intake and body weight. Am J Clin Nutr 1985; 42:1063–1071.

138. Stern JS, Johnson PR. Spontaneous activity and adipose cellularity in the genetically obese Zucker rat (fafa). Metabolism 1977; 26:371–380.

139. Sclafani A. Animal models of obesity: classification and characterization. Int J Obes 1984; 8:491–508.

140. Blundell JE. Impact of nutrition on the pharmacology of appetite. Some conceptual issues. Ann NY Acad Sci 1989; 575:163–169; discussion 169–170.

141. Samanin R, Garattini S. Serotonin and the pharmacology of eating disorders. Ann NY Acad Sci 1989; 575:194–207; discussion 207–208.

142. Bray GA. Peptides affect the intake of specific nutrients and the sympathetic nervous system. Am J Clin Nutr 1992; 55(Suppl. 1):265S–271S.

143. Woods SC, West DB, Stein LJ, et al. Peptides and the control of meal size. Diabetologia Suppl 1981; 20:305–313.

144. Stromayer AJ, Greenberg D, Von Heynr, Dornstein L, Balkman C. Blockade of cholecystokinin (CCK) satiety in genetically obese Zucker rats (abstract). Soc Neurosci 1988; 14(2):1196.

145. Wurtman JJ. Disorders of food intake. Excessive carbohydrate snack intake among a class of obese people. Ann NY Acad Sci 1987; 499:197–202.

146. Drewnowski A, Greenwood MR. Cream and sugar: human preferences for high-fat foods. Physiol Behav 1983; 30:629–633.

147. Bray GA, Gallagher TF Jr. Manifestations of hypothalamic obesity in man: a comprehensive investigation of eight patients and a review of the literature. Medicine (Baltimore) 1975; 54:301–330.

148. Banna M, Hoare RD, Stanley P, Till K. Craniopharyngioma in children. J Pediatr 1973; 83:781–785.

149. Thomsett MJ, Conte FA, Kaplan SL, Grumbach MM. Endocrine and neurologic outcome in childhood craniopharyngioma: review of effect of treatment in 42 patients. J Pediatr 1980; 97:728–735.

150. Webber LS, Srinivasan SR, Wattigney WA, Berenson GS. Tracking of serum lipids and lipoproteins from childhood to adulthood: the Bogalusa heart study. Am J Epidemiol 1991; 133:884–899.

151. Webber LS, Cresanta JL, Voors AW, Berenson GS. Tracking of cardiovascular disease risk factor variables in school-age children. J Chron Dis 1983; 36:647–660.

152. Moran JR, Ghishan FK, Halter SA, Greene HL. Steatohepatitis in obese children: a cause of chronic liver dysfunction. Am J Gastroenterol 1983; 78:374–377.

153. Bennion LJ, Knowler WC, Mott DM, Spagnola AM, Bennett PH. Development of lithogenic bile during puberty in Pima indians. N Engl J Med 1979; 300:873–876.

154. Liddle RA, Goldstein RB, Saxton J. Gallstone formation during weight-reduction dieting. Arch Intern Med 1989; 149:1750–1753.

155. Must A, Jacques PF, Dallal GE, Bajema CJ, Dietz WH. Long-term morbidity and mortality of overweight adolescents. A follow-up of the Harvard growth study of 1922 to 1935. N Engl J Med 1992; 327:1350–1355.

156. Dietz WH Jr. Obesity in infants, children and adolescents in the United States. I. Identification, natural history and aftereffects. Nutr Res 1981; 1:117–137.

157. Pasquali R, Casimirri F. The impact of obesity on hyperandrogenism and polycystic ovary syndrome in premenopausal women. Clini Endocrinol (Oxf) 1993; 39:1–16.

158. Mallory GB Jr, Fiser DH, Jackson R. Sleep-associated breathing disorders in morbidly obese children and adolescents. J Pediatr 1989; 115:892–897.

159. Malloy GB Jr, Fiser DH, Jackson R. Sleep-associated breathing disorders in morbidly obese children and adolescents. J Pediatr 1989; 115:892–897.

160. Shelton KE, Gay SB, Hollowell DE, Woodson H, Suratt PM. Mandible enclosure of upper airway and weight in obstructive sleep apnea. Am Rev Respir Dis 1993; 148:195–200.

161. Horner RL, Mohiaddin RH, Lowell DG, et al. Sites and sizes of fat deposits around the pharynx in obese patients with obstructive sleep apnoea and weight matched controls. Eur Respir J 1989; 2:613–622.

162. Shepard JW Jr. Cardiopulmonary consequences of obstructive sleep apnea. Mayo Clin Proc 1990; 65:1250–1259.

163. Staffieri JR. A study of social stereotype of body image in children. J Pers Soc Psychol 1967; 7:101–104.

164. Stunkard A, Mendelson M. Obesity and the body image. I. Characteristics of disturbances in the body image of some obese persons. Am J Psychiatry 1967; 123:1296–300.

165. Monello LF, Mayer J. Obese adolescent girls: an unrecognized "minority" group? Am J Clin Nutr 1963; 13:35–39.

166. Canning H, Mayer J. Obesity: its possible effect on college acceptance. N Engl J Med 1966; 275:1172–1174.

167. Chiumella G, del Guercio MJ, Carnelutti M, Bidone G. Relationship between obesity, chemical diabetes and beta pancreatic function in children. Diabetes 1969; 18:238–243.

168. Lowe MR, Caputo GC. Binge eating in obesity. Toward the specification of predictors. Int J Eating Disorders 1991; 10:49–55.

169. Ravussin E, Burnand B, Schutz Y, Jequier E. Energy expenditure before and during energy restriction in obese patients. Am J Clin Nutr 1985; 41:753–759.

170. Brownell KD, Greenwood MR, Stellar E, Shrager EE. The effects of repeated cycles of weight loss and regain in rats. Physiol Behav 1986; 38:459–464.

171. Dietz WH Jr, Hartung R. Changes in height velocity of obese preadolescents during weight reduction. Am J Dis Child 1985; 139:705–707.

172. Epstein LH, Valoski A, McCurley J. Effect of weight loss by obese children on long-term growth. Am J Dis Child 1993; 147:1076–1080.

173. Garn SM, Clark DC, Guire KE. Levels of fatness and size attainment. Am J Phys Anthropol 1974; 40:447–449.

174. Zannolli R, Rebeggiani A, Chiarelli F, Morgese G. Hyperinsulinism as a marker in obese children. Am J Dis Child 1993; 147:837–841.

175. Hill JO, Sparling PB, Shields TW, Heller PA. Effects of exercise and food restriction on body composition and metabolic rate in obese women. Am J Clin Nutr 1987; 46:622–630.

176. Bray GA, Gray DS. Treatment of obesity: an overview. Diabetes Metab Rev 1988; 4:653–679.

177. Wadden TA. Treatment of obesity by moderate and severe caloric restriction. Results of clinical research trials. Ann Intern Med 1993; 119:688–693.

178. Dietz WH. Nutrition and obesity. In: Grand RJ, Sutphen JL, Dietz WH, eds. Pediatric Nutrition: Theory and Practice. Boston: Butterworths, 1987:525–538.

179. Metzner HL, Lamphiear DE, Wheeler NC, Larkin FA. The relationship between frequency of eating and adiposity in adult men and women in the Tecumseh Community Health Study. Am J Clin Nutr 1977; 30:712–715.

180. Nationwide Food Consumption Survey of Food Intakes by Individuals. Women 19–50 years and their children 1–5 years,

1 day. NCFS, CSFII Report No. 85-1. U.S. Department of Agriculture. Human Nutrition Service, Nutritional Monitoring Division, Washington, D.C., 1985.

181. Andersen T, Backer OG, Stokholm KH, Quaade F. Randomized trial of diet and gastroplasty compared with diet alone in morbid obesity. N Engl J Med 1984; 310:352–356.

182. Wadden TA, Stunkard AJ. Controlled trial of very low calorie diet, behavior therapy, and their combination in the treatment of obesity. J Consult Clin Psychol 1986; 54:482–488.

183. Flatt JP, Blackburn GL. The metabolic fuel regulatory system: implications for protein-sparing therapies during caloric deprivation and disease. Am J Clin Nutr 1974; 27:175–187.

184. Sherwin RS, Hendler RG, Felig P. Effect of ketone infusions on amino acid and nitrogen metabolism in man. J Clin Invest 1975; 55:1382–1390.

185. Sours HE, Frattali VP, Brand CD, et al. Sudden death associated with very low calorie weight reduction regimens. Am J Clin Nutr 1981; 34:453–461.

186. Apfelbaum M, Bostsarron J, Lacatis D. Effect of caloric restriction and excessive caloric intake on energy expenditure. Am J Clin Nutr 1971; 24:1405–1409.

187. Hagan RD, Upton SJ, Wong L, Whittam J. The effects of aerobic conditioning and/or caloric restriction in overweight men and women. Med Sci Sports Exerc 1986; 18:87–94.

188. Brownell KD, Stunkard AJ. Behavioral treatment of obesity in children. Am J Dis Child 1978; 132:403–412.

189. Epstein LH. Review of behavioral treatments for childhood obesity. In: Brownell KD, Foreyt JP, eds. Eating Disorders. New York: Basic Books, 1986:159–179.

190. Epstein LH, Wing RR, Koeske R, Valoski A. Long-term effects of family-based treatment of childhood obesity. J. Consult Clin Psychol 1987; 55:91–95.

191. Epstein LH, Valoski A, Wing RR, McCurley J. Ten-year follow-up of behavioral, family-based treatment for obese children. JAMA 1990; 264:2519–2523.

192. Stunkard AJ, Craighead LW, O'Brien R. Controlled trial of behaviour therapy, pharmacotherapy, and their combination in the treatment of obesity. Lancet 1980; 2:1045–1047.

193. Boeck MA. Safety and efficiency of fluoxetine in morbidly obese adolescent females. Int J Obes 1991; 15(Suppl. 3):60.

194. Soper RT, Mason EE, Printen KJ, Zellweger H. Gastric bypass for morbid obesity in children and adolescents. J Pediatr Surg 1975; 10:51–58.

195. Saltzstein EC, Gutmann MC. Gastric bypass for morbid obesity: preoperative and postoperative psychological evaluation of patients. Arch Surg 1980; 115:21–28.

196. Buckmanster L, Broconell KD. Behavior modification. The state of the art. In: Frankle RT, Yang M, eds. Obesity and Weight Control: The Health Professional's Guide to Understanding and Treatment. Rockville, MD: Aspen Publishers, 1988.

197. Black O, James WPT, Besser GM. A report of the Royal College of Physicians. J Roy Coll Physicians Long 1983; 17:5–65.

53

Low-Renin Hypertension in Childhood

Maria I. New and Christopher Crawford
New York Hospital–Cornell Medical Center, New York, New York

Raffaele Virdis
University of Parma, Parma, Italy

I. INTRODUCTION

Elevated arterial blood pressure, although not generally expected in the child, should never escape notice in even routine pediatric evaluation. The earliest identification and treatment of hypertension will prevent organ damage and minimize the systemic vascular changes that progress into the resistant picture of essential hypertension. Low-renin hypertension in the child or adolescent most often has a clearly definable hormonal cause; thus, although each of its numerous forms is moderately rare, a specific hormonal basis is expected and is sought via complete endocrine evaluation.

First-line endocrine evaluation (after exclusion of the frank pathologies of a cardiologic or great vessel, renovascular, or portal abnormality) is for elevated plasma levels of catecholamines (sympathomedullary neoplasm) or thyroid hormones. In the next phase, the plasma renin activity (PRA) level gives an indication of what further evaluation is appropriate. Hormonal hypertension with high or normal renin conditions is rare. Elevated blood pressure (BP) with high or normal renin levels may in fact be within the normal range in the context of growth at the upper percentile limits, possibly in conjunction with simple obesity. (Obesity, however, is also the leading early manifestation of Cushing's disease or syndrome in the child.) Before the default diagnosis of "essential" hypertension is made, the possibility of a neurogenic basis should be investigated. More often, elevated BP is associated with suppressed PRA, indicating a volume overload and sodium-sensitive form of hypertension. In the greatest number of cases of low-renin hypertension, an underlying hormonal basis may be found. Diagnosis may be made at any age in many of these forms.

The various forms described of childhood hypertension with suppressed renin are listed in Table 1. In all cases with a well-defined genetic basis, the loci concerned are autosomal, and thus both sexes are affected equally. In contrast to the moderate rarity with which these disorders are found to be fully expressed, the pathologic mechanisms represented by each may prove to be operative to a mild degree in the majority of cases of essential hypertension in adult age, for which the genetic bases are currently being sought (1).

II. STEROIDOGENIC ENZYME DEFECTS

The adrenal cortex is divided structurally into zones, with the steroid-producing cells of the zona glomerulosa (the outer zone) and the wide middle zona fasciculata showing distinct histologic features. Clinical data on regulation and secretion support the concept of the zona glomerulosa (ZG) and the zona fasciculata/reticularis (ZF) behaving as two separate glands (2,3). Cortisol is the main product of the ZF, which synthesizes its steroid products under the control of adrenocorticotropin (ACTH). Aldosterone, by contrast, originates exclusively from the ZG, whose activity is modulated principally by angiotensin II and serum potassium concentration (K^+) (Fig. 1) and only secondarily by ACTH.

An adrenal defect in any of the component enzymes of cortisol biosynthesis, because of the feedback relationship between the pituitary and adrenal, induces a secondary increase in plasma ACTH that then drives the ZF to produce cortisol precursors and other steroids in excess, according to the position of the enzymatic block in the adrenal steroidogenic scheme (Fig. 2). These enzymatic defects as a group are termed congenital adrenal hyperplasia (CAH). Each form

Table 1 Forms of Endocrine Hypertension with Suppressed Renin

Signs and symptoms	Hormonal findings	Source	Genetics
A. Steroidogenic enzyme defects			
Steroid 11β-hydroxylase deficiency (hypertensive virilizing congenital adrenal hyperplasia): ambiguous external genitalia in newborn females; precocious isosexual development/virilization and rapid growth in both sexes	Decreased PRA and aldosterone; elevated serum androgens/urine 17-ketosteroids; elevated DOC and 11-deoxycortisol (S)	Glandular: ZF of adrenal cortex	Mutations in gene CYP11B1 (which encodes cytochrome $P_{450}11\beta/18$ of ZF) impair synthesis of cortisol and ZF 17-deoxysteroids
Steroid 17α-hydroxylase/17,20-lyase deficiency (congenital adrenal hyperplasia with male pseudohermaphroditism): female external genital phenotype (internally: blind vagina, no Müllerian derivatives) in males; primary amenorrhea in females	Decreased PRA and aldosterone; low serum/urinary 17-hydroxysteroids; decreased cortisol, increased corticosterone (B) and DOC in plasma; serum androgens and estrogens very low, serum gonadotropins very high	Glandular: ZF of adrenal cortex and interstitial cells of gonads (Leydig cells in testes—ovarian thecal cells)	Mutations in gene CYP17 (which encodes cytochrome P_{450}C17) impair cortisol and sex steroid production
B. Hyperaldosteronism			
Primary aldosteronism associated with aldosterone-producing adenoma (Conn syndrome): muscular weakness; hypokalemia in sodium-replete state	Decreased PRA; elevated plasma aldosterone, 18-hydroxy- and 18-oxocortisol (18-OHF and 18-oxoF); normal 18-OHF/aldo ratio	Adenoma ("clear cell" tumor) (suppression of ipsilateral ZG)	Unknown; very rare in children; sex ratio 2.5 : 1 to 3 : 1 females-males
Adrenocortical hyperplasia (as above)	Plasma findings as above; hormonal source established by radiologic/scan studies	Focal (micro/macronodular) or diffuse adrenal cortical hyperplasia (may be uni- or bilateral)	Unknown
Idiopathic primary aldosteronism (as above)	High plasma aldosterone; elevated 18-OHF/aldo ratio	Hyperactivity of ZG of adrenal cortex	Unknown
Deoxycorticosterone-producing tumor (as above)	High plasma DOC	Adenoma/carcinoma	Unknown
C. Dexamethasone-suppresible hyperaldosteronism (DSH) [glucocorticoid-remediable aldosteronism (GRA)]: Hypokalemia in sodium-replete state	Elevated plasma (and urinary) aldosterone resposive to ACTH and suppressible by dexamethasone within 48 h; Steroids 18-hydroxy-11-deoxycortisol, (18-OHS), 18-OHF, and 18-oxoF elevated in plasma	Abnormal presence of enzymatic activity of adrenal ZF allowing completion of synthesis of aldosterone from 17-deoxy steroids	Hybrid enzyme from chimeric gene that (1) is expressed at high level in ZF (regulated like CYP11B1 gene) and (2) has 18-oxidase activity (functionality of CYP11B2)
D. Apparent mineralocorticoid excess (AME): cardiac conduction changes; + left ventricular hypertrophy (LVH) and vessel remodeling; some Ca ion abnormalities: nephrocalcinosis, rickets	Low plasma ACTH and secretory rates of all corticosteroids; serum F normal because of delayed plasma clearance; extreme hypokalemia and severe hypertension aggravated by any sodium intake—or by hydrocortisone or ACTH—and responding to spironolactone	High F bioactivity in periphery (1) defective oxidase function (F → E) of bidirectional enzyme 11β-hydroxysteroid dehydrogenase or (2) slow clearance by 5α/β reduction to (allo)dihydro-F	Mutations have been identified in type 2 11β-hydroxysteroid dehydrogenase (placental/kidney isoform)

of CAH specifically produces a characteristic plasma and excreted steroid profile and clinical picture (4,5).

The adrenal enzyme defects are all autosomal recessive traits and show a wide range in frequency of occurrence: 21-hydroxylase is most often impaired, and 11β-hydroxylase and 3β-hydroxysteroid dehydrogenase less commonly affected; deficiencies of the 17α-hydroxylase and cholesterol desmolase enzymes are very rare. In two forms of CAH, 11β-hydroxylase deficiency and 17α-hydroxylase deficiency, the steroid precursors that are abnormally elevated exert a net sodium-retaining effect and cause hypertension.

A. Steroid 11β-Hydroxylase Deficiency

Defects in 11β-hydroxylation result in virilizing congenital adrenal hyperplasia that is most often accompanied by hypertension. The abnormal adrenal steroid serum profile exerts a net mineralocorticoid effect, altering renal function and causing sodium retention and volume expansion.

Virilization and hypertension are the salient clinical features of 11β-hydroxylase deficiency. Accumulation of precursors increases substrate availability for ACTH-stimulated 17,20-lyase activity in the unimpeded androgen path-

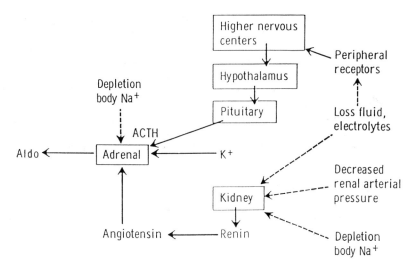

Figure 1 Regulation of aldosterone synthesis.

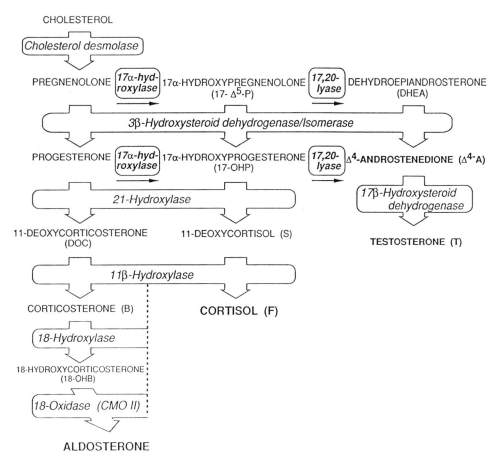

Figure 2 Steroidogenesis.

ways, and adrenal androgen secretion is increased. Development of the female external genitalia is affected in utero by excess fetal adrenal androgens, resulting in ambiguous or frankly masculinized aspect (female pseudohermaphroditism) in all cases. Internal female genital structures are intact. Postnatally, continued excessive adrenal androgen production results in premature and inappropriate somatic development in both boys and girls: progressive penile or clitoral enlargement, appearance of axillary hair, pubic hair, and facial hair, acne, deepening of voice, and rapid skeletal growth. Without treatment, accelerated development is terminated by early epiphyseal closure, resulting in short adult stature.

Hypertension is a less consistent feature than virilization in 11β-hydroxylase deficiency. It is usually not identified until later in childhood or in adolescence, although its appearance in an infant 3 months of age has been documented (6). In addition, hypertension correlates variably with biochemical values (7,8). Potassium depletion develops concomitantly with sodium retention, but hypokalemia is variable (this is also observed in aldosteronism; see later). Renin production is suppressed secondary to steroid-induced sodium retention and volume expansion. Aldosterone production is low secondary to low serum [K$^+$] and low plasma renin. Hyporeninemia, the hallmark serum abnormality, varies widely in degree, and in at least two reported cases has even been absent (9).

Malignant hypertensive changes and considerable mortality are evident in some clinical surveys, yet it also has been observed in steroid 11β-hydroxylase deficiency that the hypertension may in some cases be more amenable to treatment than is usual in hypertension of some years' duration (10). A late-onset form of 11β-hydroxylase deficiency is recognized,

having been identified in several adult patients (11–13). Combined 11β-hydroxylase and 21-hydroxylase deficiencies have also been clinically described (1,2).

Biochemically, 11β-hydroxylase in the ZF is responsible for the conversion of 11-deoxycortisol (compound S) to cortisol in the 17-hydroxy pathway, and, for the conversion in the 17-deoxy pathway, of deoxycorticosterone (DOC) to corticosterone (compound B; Fig. 3). In the ZG, the conversion of DOC to B is one of a number of related conversions that in series yield aldosterone, the regulated product of this zone. As well as being 11β-hydroxylated to B, DOC can instead be 18-hydroxylated to 18-hydroxy-11-deoxycorticosterone (18-OHDOC), which then can be 11β-hydroxylated to 18-hydroxycorticosterone (18-OHB; see Fig. 3). Steroid 18-hydroxylating activity has been termed corticosterone methyloxidase (CMO) type I. The final step of aldosterone synthesis, the 18-oxidation of 18-OHB, an activity that has been termed corticosterone methyloxidase type II, is catalyzed by the enzyme now known as aldosterone synthase (cytochrome P$_{450}$aldo), which is an isoform of 11β-hydroxylase (closely related to but not identical with cytochrome P$_{450}$C11).

Chronic elevation of ACTH in response to low plasma cortisol results in increased synthesis and secretion of steroid intermediates proximal to the 11β-hydroxylase block and their non-11β-hydroxylated products (14). These include 11β-hydroxylase substrates compound S and DOC, the S precursor 17α-hydroxyprogesterone (17-OHP), and, distal to 17-OHP, the androgenic intermediate Δ^4-androstenedione. In female infants with ambiguous genitalia, or male infants with normal genitalia, serum elevations of the S and DOC are characteristic of an 11β-hydroxylase deficiency. Serum 17-OHP and its

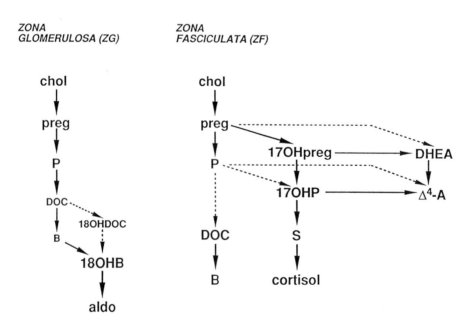

Figure 3   Zona glomerulosa (ZG) and zona fasciculata (ZF) of the adrenal cortex acting as two separate glands.

major urinary metabolite, pregnanetriol, are elevated, but not as greatly as in 21-hydroxylase deficiency CAH.

The significant mineralocorticoid potency of DOC was recognized early in clinical studies in which this steroid was administered as an exogenous agent (15), and the elevation of DOC in the plasma steroid profile is thus presumed to be central to the volume-expanded hypertension induced in 11β-hydroxylase deficiency. Tetrahydro-11-deoxycortisol and tetrahydrodeoxycorticosterone, the principal metabolites of S and DOC, are significantly increased in the urine. Urinary 17-ketosteroids (i.e., 17-oxosteroids) are elevated, reflecting the raised serum levels of adrenal androgens.

Glucocorticoid administration provides cortisol function and normalizes ACTH, which in turn removes the drive for oversecretion of DOC—the adrenal secretion studies of New and Seaman showed that plasma DOC arises largely from the ZF (2)—and in most cases brings about remission of hypertension. Serum DOC is thus the principal steroid index of the 11β-hydroxylase defect and its normalization the indicator of hormonal control of this condition.

In one earlier case report of 11β-hydroxylase deficiency, selective inhibition of 11β-hydroxylation of 17α-hydroxylated steroids with intact 11β-hydroxylation of 17-deoxysteroids was observed (16). Endocrine challenge and suppression studies undertaken to evaluate zonal differences in 11β-hydroxylase deficiency determined that the ZF exhibits reduced 11β-hydroxylation and 18-hydroxylation, but both functions

appear to be spared in the ZG (17). This explains the effect of glucocorticoid treatment, which by diminishing the secretion of DOC and producing natriuresis and diuresis, restores (by contraction) the plasma volume to a normal value, raising plasma renin to levels able to stimulate aldosterone production via the separate 11β-/18-hydroxylating system of the ZG.

The adrenal steroid 11β-hydroxylase is the enzyme cytochrome $P_{450}C11$. Whereas it was for a time thought from biochemical and cell fraction studies that the terminal steps of aldosterone synthesis were also catalyzed by the identical molecular species of cytochrome P_{450} (18), it has now been established that there are two closely related isoforms, cytochrome $P_{450}C11$ and cytochrome $P_{450}aldo$, the products of two homologous genes (19), CYP11B1 (encoding the 11β-hydroxylase isoform) (20) and CYP11B2 (encoding the aldosterone synthase isoform) (21,22). These two genes are located about 30 kb apart on the long arm of chromosome 8.

Steroid 11β-hydroxylase deficiency is the result of mutations affecting the type or expression of the CYP11B1 gene (Fig. 4) (23–26). Mutations also occur affecting the CYP11B2 gene, resulting in a distinct disorder, corticosterone methyloxidase type II deficiency. This disorder was earlier clinically characterized as a disorder of terminal aldosterone synthesis (27). Its genetic basis was sought in DNA studies of affected pedigrees (28), and a mutation in the CYP11B2 gene has now been characterized (29). In contrast with the

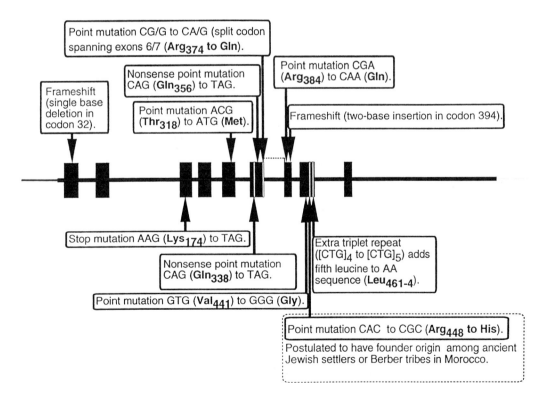

Figure 4 Mutations in the CYP11B1 gene causing steroid 11β-hydroxylase deficiency (CAH).

hypertension of 11β-hydroxylase deficiency CAH, the CMO II disorder causes salt wasting and hypotension.

The homology (Fig. 5) and close location of the two CYP11B genes give rise to a very specific type of gene mutation that produces yet another phenotype. At the DNA level, misalignment of the homologs and crossing over during meiotic reduction result in the creation of a chimeric gene, with regulatory sequence features of CYP11B1 and structural coding features of CYP11B2 (see Fig. 6). Occurring on even one chromosome, such chimeric genes result in the over-expression of a hybrid gene—because the gene is under ACTH (i.e., B1 type) regulation—that has 18-oxidase (i.e., B2 type) capacity (30,31). This is the autosomal dominant disorder dexamethasone-suppressible hyperaldosteronism (DSH), which is discussed in Section IV.

B. Steroid 17α-Hydroxylase Deficiency

A defect in 17α-hydroxylase results in diminished production of cortisol and also of sex steroids, whose production requires the 17,20-lyase function of the same 17α-hydroxylase enzyme. The enzyme defect is shared by adrenals and gonads and reduces the production of all androgens and estrogens; an undifferentiated (i.e., infantile female) sexual phenotype results in both genetic sexes, and puberty fails to occur (32).

Reciprocal elevation of ACTH to low cortisol increases synthesis via the allowed 17-deoxy pathway, notably of the steroids DOC and corticosterone (compound B; see Fig. 3b). As in 11β-hydroxylation, the production of aldosterone, although not enzymatically blocked, is very low secondary to the suppressed renin resulting from the excess DOC.

Since the first description of a female patient with 17α-hydroxylase deficiency by Biglieri et al. (33) and in a male by New (34), reported cases in females and males now number about 120. Most males have been phenotypically female. Males have defective internal genital formation: embryologically, blocked androgen production precludes complete wolffian duct development, and intact testicular Sertoli cell production of antimüllerian hormone inhibits the formation of female structures. Gynecomastia was a notable

feature in the first reported male case, but more often is absent.

Diagnosis is often made with the young female or apparent female presenting at pubertal age with primary amenorrhea or lack of development of secondary sex characteristics. The disorder may be revealed earlier in 46,XY karyotype cases presenting in infancy or childhood with hernia or inguinal mass. These patients are hypokalemic and hypertensive at diagnosis. Alternatively, hypokalemia and hypertension may comprise the primary presentation at any time. In long-standing untreated or undertreated cases, hypertension of considerable severity may develop.

Massive overproduction of corticosterone (compound B) at serum concentrations 30 times normal and higher appears to provide an adequate physiologic response to infection or other stress. Plasma ACTH levels are less elevated than in other conditions of impaired cortisol production, perhaps as a result of limited feedback response to the presence of this marginal glucocorticoid activity. Gonadotropin production is extremely elevated in both sexes because of the absence of any sex steroid feedback.

Treatment consists of glucocorticoid replacement in prepuberty and sex steroid replacement as appropriate for the phenotypic sex starting at pubertal age. In 46,XY patients the testes may be abdominal, inguinal, or labial; if therapy is directed toward phenotypic development as a male, the gonads may be preserved. Estrogen replacement induces the breasts to develop satisfactorily, and menstrual cycles may be established in genetic females.

ACTH stimulation testing evokes steroidogenic responses intermediate between normal and affected values in heterozygotes for 17α-hydroxylase deficiency. The utility of this mode of testing is well known in the clinical study of other adrenal enzyme defects, in particular the commonly occurring steroid 21-hydroxylase deficiency. A study of families has suggested that ACTH testing can identify heterozygotes for 17α-hydroxylase deficiency (35).

It has been established that one protein, cytochrome $P_{450}C17$, functions both as steroid 17α-hydroxylase and as 17,20-lyase (36). The structural gene for cytochrome $P_{450}C17$ has been mapped to chromosome 10 (37), and it has been further localized to subregion 10q24.3 (38).

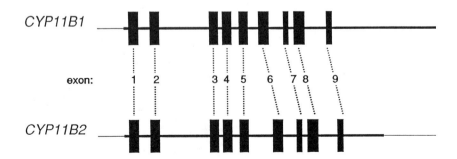

Figure 5   Basic structures of the 11β-hydroxylase genes: CYP11B1 (11β-/18-hydroxylase) and CYP11B2 (aldosterone synthase).

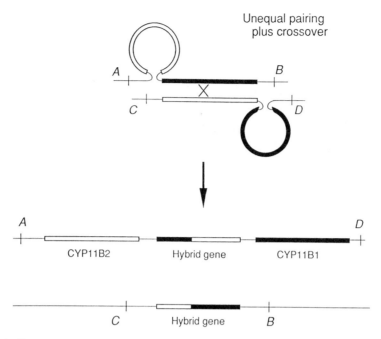

Unequal pairing
plus crossover

Figure 6 Mechanism of misalignment and unequal crossing over.

Homologous or identical mRNA species for $P_{450}C17$ are regulated in the adrenals and gonads by the specific factors controlling steroidogenesis in the respective glands, suggesting that the same gene is active in the expression of the enzyme in each tissue (39). Second and third gene copies have been detected but not mapped.

Mutations in numerous cases of 17α-hydroxylase deficiency (combined 17α-hydroxylase and 17,20-lyase deficiency) have been described (Fig. 7) (40–42). Two patients studied earlier (43) were from Canadian prairie Mennonite families between which there was consanguinity. Determination of the complete exonic sequence for CYP17 revealed a four-base duplication at a corresponding position almost at the carboxyl terminus of the $P_{450}C17$ protein. This shift in reading frame, coupled with the fortuitous appearance of a stop codon near the proper end position, yields a slightly abbreviated sequence in place of the final 29 amino acids of the normal $P_{450}C17$. Of interest for population genetics, the same mutation was identified in DNA from present inhabitants of the Friesland region of the Netherlands, where the first Mennonites originated in the 1500s (44).

The biochemical basis of the differential functions of this enzyme is a topic of continuing interest (45). Changes in the cytochrome $P_{450}C17$ protein, possibly altering the two enzyme functions to different degrees, continue to be sought in site-directed mutagenesis and protein-fusion experiments, as well as in in vivo mutations (40–48).

III. PRIMARY ALDOSTERONISM

The autonomous overproduction of aldosterone with concomitant elevation of serum aldosterone levels produces hypokalemia and mild to moderate hypertension. Primary aldosteronism caused by an aldosterone-producing adenoma (APA), or Conn syndrome, is rare in childhood. Adrenal adenoma is mostly solitary, occurring two to three times more frequently in the left gland; multiple adenomas of clinical significance are observed in 10% of cases, and only one-fifth of these occur bilaterally (49). DOC-producing neoplasms have also been observed, though these are extremely rare, and serum electrolyte and hemodynamic effects comparable to an aldosterone-producing tumor are expected (50).

Primary aldosteronism in childhood is more likely to be caused by bilateral adrenal hyperplasia. The number of reported cases of primary aldosteronism of either cause in childhood is very small, however (51–58). One case has been reported of macronodular adrenal hyperplasia occurring unilaterally (56).

The diagnostic tools used in characterizing primary aldosteronism are adrenal suppression (to assess ACTH sensitivity), bilateral adrenal vein sampling, computed tomographic (CT) scan, scintigraphy (radioiodocholesterol scan), and nuclear magnetic resonance imaging. CT scan is the primary method of identifying the presence of a tumor (59,60). Scintigraphy is of particular value in providing improved preoperative localization of APA in the event of equivocal results on CT scan (61). Surgery is indicated in cases of APA. Surgical treatment of bilateral adrenal hyperplasia by total or subtotal bilateral adrenalectomy in the past has in many cases been unsatisfactory, with recurrence of hypertension. Medical management with the mineralocorticoid antagonist spironolactone is able to achieve a better therapeutic result (62).

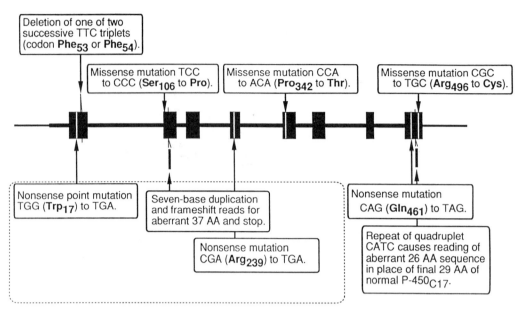

Figure 7 Mutations in the CYP17 gene causing steroid 17α-hydroxylase deficiency.

IV. DEXAMETHASONE-SUPPRESSIBLE HYPERALDOSTERONISM (GLUCOCORTICOID-REMEDIABLE ALDOSTERONISM)

This familial form of hyperaldosteronism, first reported in 1966–1967 (63,64), is known to be transmitted as an autosomal dominant (65). This mendelian genetic pattern and the salient clinical features of DSH have been reported in numerous pedigrees (Fig. 8) (66–72). Certain clinical features are similar to those found in the other types of primary hyperaldosteronism as a result of bilateral adrenal hyperplasia or aldosterone-producing adenoma. However, the unique feature of this familial form is the complete and rapid suppression of aldosterone oversecretion by dexamethasone (or other pure glucocorticoid) administration.

In the young DSH patient, hypertension remits following suppression of aldosterone oversecretion by dexamethasone or other glucocorticoid treatment, whereas in adults diagnosed with DSH, hypertension may persist despite correction of the steroid hormonal abnormalities. This tendency for the hypertension to become resistant to treatment and to require management as essential hypertension underscores the need for early diagnosis.

Circadian measurement of plasma steroids in the untreated state in DSH patients has revealed a characteristic abnormality of aldosterone secretion in DSH, this steroid being produced not only in excess amounts but also following ACTH stimulation, in a manner suggestive of a zona fasciculata rather than zona glomerulosa origin. Further indicating a regulatory dysfunction was the adrenal aldosterone secretory response to exogenous ACTH as shown by the clinical findings on a prolonged (5 day) course of ACTH administration: on monitoring of serum and urinary aldosterone, which

in normal individuals increase and then level off after 3 days, the values in the DSH patients continued to rise unabated through the end of the test (73).

Other factors in addition to elevated aldosterone levels have been considered in the genesis of hypertension in this disorder. In one investigation, whereas ACTH (40 U/day by intravenous infusion) given in the dexamethasone-suppressed state reestablished the hypertension of the untreated state in a DSH patient after 5 days, aldosterone replacement in a large dose [1 mg/day (mean blood production rate of aldosterone in an adult on a normal sodium intake is in the range of 0.1 mg/day)] over 5 days did not (74). Additional replacement of DOC and 18-OHDOC in amounts restoring pretreatment levels of these steroids along with aldosterone also failed to accomplish this. Thus, a significant proportion of the hormonal effect in DSH hypertension may be from (an)other ACTH-stimulable steroid(s) (75,76). [A point underscoring the significance of the cyclic variability of steroid levels: it has been observed that the mineralocorticoid receptor (MR) number on blood lymphocytes in DSH patients is *not* reduced compared to normal values, unlike the case in patients with hyperaldosteronism of other types, in whom the lymphocyte MR number is significantly reduced (77). It may be that downregulation of one or more MR types is in response to the sustained elevation of mineralocorticoid levels, and that with cyclicity and a lower baseline level this downregulation is not induced (other cellular and clinical effects could represent differential sensitivity to this signal).]

Qualitative steroid abnormalities in DSH have in fact been identified, but the summed mineralocorticoid effects of these steroids at their physiologic levels fall far short of the total mineralocorticoid effects observed. The steroids that are apparently specific for DSH and aldosterone-producing adenoma, in contrast with the other types of hyperaldosteronism,

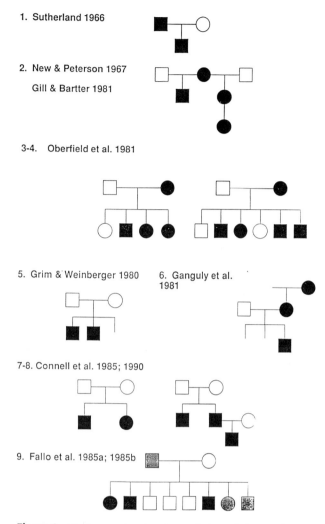

1. Sutherland 1966

2. New & Peterson 1967
   Gill & Bartter 1981

3-4. Oberfield et al. 1981

5. Grim & Weinberger 1980   6. Ganguly et al. 1981

7-8. Connell et al. 1985; 1990

9. Fallo et al. 1985a; 1985b

Figure 8 Pedigrees showing transmission of dexamethasone-suppressible hyperaldosteronism (DSH) as autosomal dominant trait. Solid, affected; open, unaffected; shaded, presumed affected.

An adequate basis for explaining the elevated aldosterone synthesis and its unusual regulation by ACTH has been provided by recent molecular genetic findings. "Chimerism" is a term used to refer to a phenomenon whereby a specific type of gene mutation results, that is, the creation of fusion (chimeric) genes by misalignment of chromatids and unequal crossing over between them during meiotic reduction in gametogenesis.

Chromosomal alignment being directed by similarity of DNA sequences, a predisposing factor in chromatid misalignment is the proximity of homologs, such as is the case for the steroid 11β-hydroxylase and aldosterone synthase genes, CYP11B1 and CYP11B2, occurring in like orientation within a 30 kilobase stretch of the chromosome (see Sec. II.A). Alignment with the homolog and crossing over between strands can approximate complementary parts—the 5' end of a CYP11B1 gene with the 3' end of a CYP11B2 gene—and this results in a gene that (1) is induced by ACTH/ACTH factors (therefore it is inappropriately expressed at high levels under ACTH control in adrenal cells), and (2) directs cellular expression of an enzyme that has catalytic capacity normally encoded only by the CYP11B2 gene (that is, a hybrid 11β-hydroxylase-aldosterone synthase cytochrome P$_{450}$). This model accounts for the molecular genetic findings in all independent pedigrees studied so far. It should be noted, however, that other mechanisms of gene mutation are not excluded. Gene conversion, for instance, could conceivably result in the same phenotype by transferring DNA short sequences, converting either gene to one with characteristics of its homolog. With transfer of part of the regulatory segment of CYP11B1 to CYP11B2, normal-type adrenal aldosterone synthase would be under ACTH induction and overexpressed. With transfer of a part of the CYP11B2 structural sequence critical for specifying the activity of P$_{450}$aldo to the corresponding section of the CYP11B1 gene, there could be a gene induced under a normal adrenal cell ACTH-directed program having abnormal enzymatic activity of the 18-oxidase type.

are 18-hydroxycortisol and 18-oxocortisol (78,79). Apart from the question of hormonal potency (80), these at the least have utility as markers of the conditions (81). That 17α-, 18-dihydroxy- and 17α-hydroxy-18-al C$_{21}$ steroids as a class are synthesized and secreted at such high levels implies a particular type of adrenal abnormality. Normal adrenal cortical cells exposed to ACTH respond with a number of changes in the pattern of steroidogenesis: (1) total steroid secretion increases overall, (2) CYP17 gene and acquisition by the cell induces 17α-hydroxylase activity, and (3) aldosterone synthase activity is involuted. In DSH, when the adrenal corticol cells shift to ACTH regulation, cortisol is produced adequately, but there is an abnormally retained 18-hydroxylating/18-oxidating potential, generating an overabundance of 18-hydroxy/oxo compounds: the signal steroids, from the cortisol pathway, and the aldosterone from 17-deoxy precursors normally present. Models of abnormal adrenal zonation in DSH were proposed (82–84).

V. APPARENT MINERALOCORTICOID EXCESS (AME)

Apparent mineralcorticoid excess (AME) was first defined as a syndrome in 1977 by New and coworkers in their clinical evaluation of a patient with an extremely unusual endocrine profile. In this case (a young female child, a member of the Zuñi tribe of the Southwest), hypertension, significant hypokalemia, metabolic alkalosis, and suppressed renin but undetectable aldosterone and very low secretion rates of all standardly assayable corticosteroids were found, despite no signs of adrenal insufficiency (85). Following observations of possible biochemical defects in the clearance of cortisol and numerous attempts to identify an unknown steroid acting potently as both a glucocorticoid and a mineralocorticoid, it was by 1983 postulated that cortisol itself was the hypertensinogenic agent in this syndrome (86).

Apparent mineralocorticoid excess is difficult to treat

and shows a high degree of morbidity and mortality (87). The hypertension in this disorder is very severe, often leading to early end-organ damage, and with significant mortality. The hypokalemia is extreme. Mineralocorticoid receptor blockade with spironolactone, usually in quite high doses, results in an initial lowering of arterial BP and an increase in serum potassium. Addition of a diuretic may improve management, but patients may unfortunately become refractory to therapy.

The clear indications of excess mineralocorticoid action in the face of levels of serum cortisol in the normal range suggest that numerous systemic responses to cortisol are somehow rendered supersensitive. Such responses included the neuroendocrine feedback loop, because plasma ACTH was very low, and hypothalamic-pituitary-adrenal axis testing by exogenous ACTH produced a sluggish response, both indications of a hypoadrenal state. The levels or characteristics of cortisol binding globulin were normal, ruling out any abnormality of steroid partitioning in the extracellular fluid phases. Delayed metabolic clearance of cortisol was implicated by earlier findings of altered profiles of free cortisol and cortisol metabolites in the urine (88,89).

For many years it has been known that the root of the licorice plant *Glycyrrhizae glabra* can induce sodium retention with elevated blood pressure and potassium wasting. Clinical studies showed that the presence of corticosteroids was necessary for the elaboration of this hypertensinogenic effect because administration of licorice root extracts to Addison's disease patients was without effect. The active principles glycyrrhizic and glycyrrhetinic acid have been isolated from root extracts and further experiments performed.

Also in the intervening years, studies of the type I and type II steroid receptors revealed for the type I receptor, the classic mineralocorticoid receptor, that the isolated receptor (and, later, the recombinant receptor in a cell expression system) had as great an intrinsic affinity for the glucocorticoid corticosterone as for the mineralocorticoid aldosterone. How then, it was asked, could aldosterone, present in the plasma in levels two to three orders of magnitude less than glucocorticoids, access the MR, even allowing for its much lesser protein-bound and increased unbound active fraction?

An answer to this question and explanation of the origin of the excess mineralocorticoid steroid effect in AME came with a new mechanistic postulate, that selectivity of mineralocorticoid action is determined not by the MR ligand binding site, which is in fact nonspecific, but by an intracellular enzyme that systematically inactivates unintended candidate steroids (glucocorticoids) and thereby protects the MR from saturation. The widely distributed enzyme 11β-hydroxy-steroid dehydrogenase (11β-HSD) catalyzes the interconversion of cortisol (F) and cortisone (E) in the opposing steps of 11-oxidation (cortisol to cortisone) and 11β-reduction (cortisone to cortisol) (90) (Fig. 9). In animal species whose principal glucocorticoid is corticosterone, the corresponding conversions are between corticosterone (B) and 11-dehydrocorticosterone (A). The hormonally active 11-hydroxysteroid F (or B) is oxidized by 11β-HSD to the 11-oxo form E (or

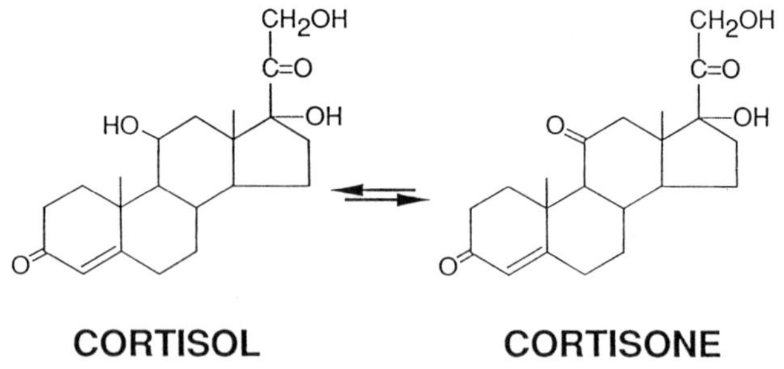

CORTISOL   **CORTISONE**

Figure 9 Cortisol-cortisone shuttle.

A), for which the MR has little affinity, whereas aldosterone (Fig. 10) is not subject to inactivation by the 11β-HSD enzyme and in this way retains full access to the MR. In keeping with the possibility of such a mechanism, immunohistochemical staining has revealed tissue distributions for 11β-HSD activities corresponding with MR distribution patterns.

Altered cortisol metabolism in a pattern like the hallmark pattern of AME—diagnosis of the disorder is made on the basis of an abnormally low serum cortisone-cortisol ratio or low ratio of normally major metabolites tetrahydrocortisone (THE) to tetrahydrocortisol (THF) in the urine—consistent with inhibition of the 11β-hydroxysteroid dehydrogenase enzyme was found also to result correspondingly in sodium retention, in support of the postulate that defective cortisol-cortisone interconversion is the underlying metabolic defect in the syndrome of AME (91,92). Increased availability and binding of cortisol at the mineralocorticoid receptor at the site of the distal collecting tubule of the kidney is the currently accepted pathophysiologic mechanism (Fig. 11).

The human gene first cloned was that for an NADP$^+$/NADPH-dependent 11β-HSD enzyme (93). DNA analysis of AME patients and of subjects with a less well-defined converse defect, 11-oxo-reductase deficiency, revealed no abnormalities in the gene for this bidirectional enzyme (94). The importance of an 11β-hydroxy/11-oxo equilibrium shifted toward oxidation is readily understood for an organ like the kidney (95). Biochemical information on a distinct isoform (96,97)—NAD$^+$-dependent, characteristically unidirectional—was followed by cloning of the human gene (98). The gene nomenclature is HSD11B1 for the type 1, or liver isoform, and HSD11B2 for the type 2, or kidney isoform. Recent DNA analysis of a family with AME-affected members has now identified a mutation in the HSD11B2 gene, confirming that lesions at this site are causative of the disease (99).

Whereas defective steroid 11-oxidation was clearly shown by altered excretory THF + alloTHF/THE ratios initially in all AME patients, a second AME type has been observed in which this ratio is in fact normal. Still consistent with the notion of abnormal bioactivity of cortisol, it has been found in this biochemically distinct group that they have diminished rates of corticosteroid ring A reduction (that is, C_{21} steroid 5α-/5β-reduction). Unlike 11β-oxidoreduction,

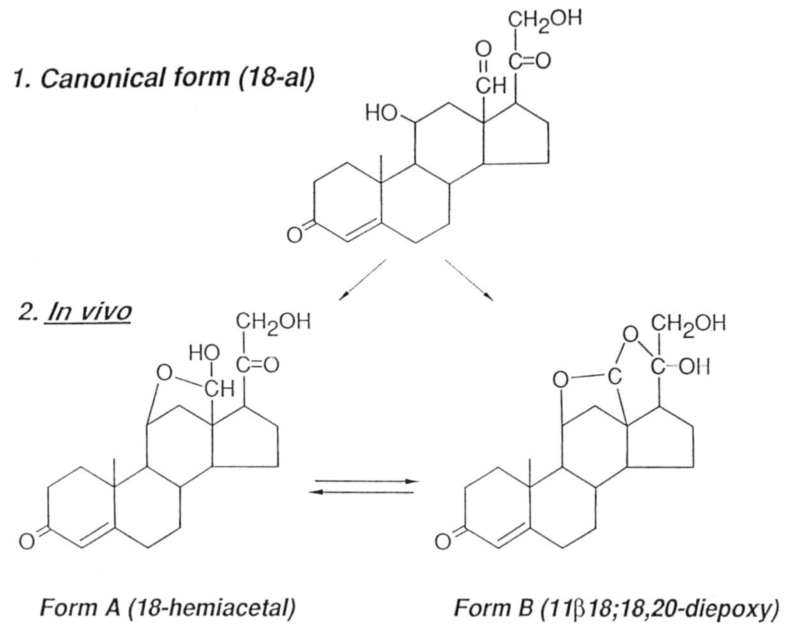

1. Canonical form (18-al)
2. In vivo
Form A (18-hemiacetal)
Form B (11β18;18,20-diepoxy)

Figure 10 Forms of aldosterone.

which as an interconversion of 11β-hydroxy/11-oxo forms within the same metabolic compartment may be shown to be abnormal only by a shift in equilibrium value, ring A reduction is an irreversible transformation, representing a significant pathway in the metabolic clearance of cortisol, and it is argued (1) that a defect of this type of step will always be exhibited in a syndrome of increased cortisol action and (2) that A ring reduction may in fact, like 11β-oxidoreduction, *also* be a significant part of prereceptor mechanisms conferring MR specificity (97).

Just as identification of the rare hypertensive disorder AME (as indeed for the other adrenocortical low-renin disorders earlier discussed) has opened speculation on little understood aspects of steroid hormonal functions, further characterization of this disorder will increase understanding of physiologic processes.

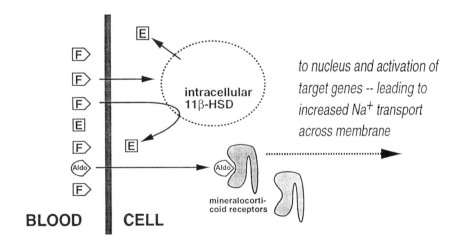

intracellular
11β-HSD
to nucleus and activation of
target genes -- leading to
increased Na+ transport
across membrane
mineralocorti-
coid receptors
BLOOD
CELL
Distal tubule/cortical collecting duct epithelial cell

Figure 11 Mechanism of protection of mineralocorticoid receptors (MR) by the enzyme 11β-hydroxysteroid dehydrogenase (11β-HSD).

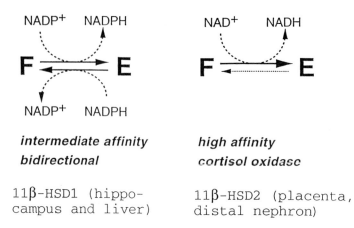

Figure 12   Two forms of the enzyme 11β-hydroxysteroid dehydrogenase (11β-HSD).

VI. SUMMARY

Although oversecretion or altered metabolic handling of specific hormones has been demonstrated in each of the forms of hypertension discussed here, the actions of other steroid compounds found in changed levels in these conditions, and their possible contribution to hypertension, are in many instances not known completely.

The challenge is to identify which hormone is indeed responsible for the hypertension of each case. Excess of DOC (deoxycorticosterone) does not correlate completely with hypertension in 11β-hydroxylase and 17α-hydroxylase deficiencies. Among the forms of primary aldosteronism, hypertension in DSH (dexamethasone-suppressible aldosteronism) has been shown in our studies not to be directly attributable to elevated aldosterone. Cortisol appears to act potently at renal receptor sites in AME (apparent mineralocorticoid excess), but the variability of hypertension in AME and hypercortisolemic states remains unexplained.

Understanding the pathogenesis of childhood hypertension is of the utmost importance because the pharmacologic risks in committing a child to long-term management with antihypertensives are unknown. Specific therapy is best, which means early identification of the underlying cause. For this to be done, these relatively uncommon disorders must be investigated as carefully and completely as possible by study of individual cases. Further elucidation of endocrine origins and course of development of hypertension will improve therapy and benefit affected children.

REFERENCES

1. Williams RR, Hunt SC, Hopkins PN, Hasstedt SJ, Wu LL, Lalouel JM. Tabulations and expectations regarding the genetics of human hypertension. Kidney Int 1994; 45(Suppl. 44):S57–S64.

2. New MI, Seaman MP. Secretion rates of cortisol and aldosterone precursors in various forms of congenital adrenal hyperplasia. J Clin Endocrinol Metab 1970; 30:361.

3. New MI, Levine LS. Hypertension of childhood with suppressed renin. Endocrinol Rev 1980; 1:421–430.

4. New MI, Levine LS. Congenital adrenal hyperplasia. Adv Hum Genet 1973; 4:251–326.

5. New MI, White PC, Pang S, Dupont B, Speiser PW. The adrenal hyperplasias. In: Scriver CR, Beaudet AL, Sly WS, Valle D, eds. The Metabolic Basis of Inherited Disease, 6th ed. New York: McGraw-Hill, 1989; 1771–1817.

6. Mimouni M, Kaufman H, Roitman A, Morag C, Sadan N. Hypertension in a neonate with 11 beta-hydroxylase deficiency. Eur J Pediatr 1985; 143:231–233.

7. Rosler A, Leiberman E, Sack J, et al. Clinical variability of congenital adrenal hyperplasia due to 11β-hydroxylase deficiency. Horm Res 1982; 16:133–141.

8. Rosler A, Leiberman E. Enzymatic defects of steroidogenesis: 11β-hydroxylase deficiency congenital adrenal hyperplasia. Pediatr Adol Endocrinol 1984; 13:47–71.

9. New MI, Nemery RL, Chow DM, et al. Low-renin hypertension of childhood. In: Mantero F, Takeda R, Scoggins BA, et al., eds. The Adrenal and Hypertension: From Cloning to Clinic. New York: Raven Press, 1989; 323–343.

10. Bongiovanni AM. The adrenal and other hormones in human hypertension. In: Giovanelli G, New MI, Gorini S, eds. Hypertension in Children and Adolescents. New York: Raven Press, 1981; 217–222.

11. Dyrenfurth L, Sybulski S, Notchev V, Beck JC, Venning E. Urinary corticosteroid excretion patterns in patients with adrenocortical dysfunction. J Clin Endocrinol Metab 1958; 18:391.

12. Gabrilove JL, Sharma DC, Dorfman RI. Adrenocortical 11β-hydroxylase deficiency and virilism first manifest in the adult woman. N Engl J Med 1965; 272:1189.

13. Cathelineau G, Brerault JL, Fiet J, Julien R, Dreux C, Canivet J. Adrenocortical 11β-hydroxylation defect in adult women with postmenarchial onset of symptoms. J Clin Endocrinol Metab 1980; 51:287–291.

14. Eberlein WR, Bongiovanni AM. Plasma and urinary corticosteroids in the hypertensive form of congenital adrenal hyperplasia. J Biol Chem 1956; 223:85–94.

15. Perera GA, Knowlton AI, Lowell A, Loeb RF. Effect of deoxycorticosterone acetate on the blood pressure of man. JAMA 1944; 125:1030–1035.

16. Zachmann M, Vollmin JA, New MI, Curtius C-C, Prader A. Congenital adrenal hyperplasia due to deficiency of 11β-hydroxylation of 17α-hydroxylated steroids. J Clin Endocrinol Metab 1971; 33:501.

17. Levine LS, Rauh W, Gottesdeiner K, et al. New studies of the 11β-hydroxylase and 18-hydroxylase enzymes in the hypertensive form of congenital adrenal hyperplasia. J Clin Endocrinol Metab 1980; 50:258–263.

18. Yanagibashi K, Haniu M, Shively JE, Shen WH, Hall P. The synthesis of aldosterone by the adrenal cortex. J Biol Chem 1986; 261:3556–3562.

19. Mornet E, Dupont J, Vitek A, White PC. Characterization of 2 genes encoding human steroid 11β-hydroxylase (P450c11). J Biol Chem 1989; 264:20961–20967.

20. Chua SC, Szabo P, Vitek A, Grezeschif K-H, John M, White PC. Cloning of cDNA encoding steroid 11β-hydroxylase (P450c11). Proc Natl Acad Sci USA 1987; 84:7193–7197.

21. Curnow KM, Tusie-Luna M-T, Pascoe L, et al. The product of the CYP11B2 gene is required for aldosterone biosynthesis in the human adrenal cortex. Mol Endocrinol 1991; 5:1513–1522.

22. Kawamoto T, Mitsuuchi Y, Toda K, et al. Role of steroid 11β-hydroxylase and steroid 18-hydroxylase in the biosynthesis of glucocorticoids and mineralocorticoids in humans. Proc Natl Acad Sci USA 1992; 89:1458–1462.

23. White PC, Dupont J, New MI, Leiberman E, Hochberg Z, Rösler A. A mutation in CYP11B1 (Arg[448] → His) associated with steroid 11β-hydroxylase deficiency in Jews of Moroccan origin. J Clin Invest 1991; 87:1664–1667.

24. Curnow KM, Slutsker L, Vitek J, et al. Mutations in the CYP11B1 gene causing congenital adrenal hyperplasia and hypertension cluster in exons 6, 7, and 8. Proc Natl Acad Sci USA 1993; 90:4552–4556.

25. Skinner CA, Rumsby G. Steroid 11β-hydroxylase deficiency caused by a 5-base-pair duplication in the CYP11B1 gene. Hum Mol Genet 1994; 3:377–378.

26. Helmberg A, Ausserer B, Kofler R. Frameshift by insertion of 2 basepairs in codon 394 of CYP11B1 causes congenital adrenal hyperplasia due to steroid 11β-hydroxylase deficiency. J Clin Endocrinol Metab 1992; 75:1278–1281.

27. Rösler A, Rabinowitz D, Theodor R, Ramirez LC, Ulick S. The nature of the defect in a salt-wasting disorder in Jews of Iran. J Clin Endocrinol Metab 1977; 44:279–291.

28. Globerman H, Rosler A, Theodor R, New MI, White PC. An inherited defect in aldosterone biosynthesis is caused by a mutation in or near the gene for steroid 11-hydroxylase. N Engl J Med, 1988; 319:1193–1197.

29. Pascoe L, Curnow KM, Slutsker L, Rösler A, White PC. Mutations in the human CYP11B2 (aldosterone synthase) gene causing corticosterone methyloxidase II deficiency. Proc Natl Acad Sci USA 1992; 89:4996–5000.

30. Lifton RL, Dluhy RG, Powers M, et al. A chimeric 11β-hydroxylase/aldosterone synthase gene causes glucocorticoid-remediable aldosteronism, a mendelian cause of human hypertension. Nature 1992; 355:262–265.

31. Pascoe L, Curnow KC, Slutsker L, et al. Glucocorticoid-suppressible hyperaldosteronism results from hybrid genes created by unequal crossovers between CYP11B1 and CYP11B2. Proc Natl Acad Sci USA 1992; 89:8327–8331.

32. Mantero F, Scaroni C. Enzymatic defects of steroidogenesis: 17α-hydroxylase deficiency. Pediatr Adol Endocrinol 1984; 13:83–94.

33. Biglieri EG, Herron MA, Brust N. 17-Hydroxylation deficiency. J Clin Invest 1966; 45:1946.

34. New MI. Male pseudohermaphroditism due to 17α-hydroxylase deficiency. J Clin Invest 1970; 49:1930.

35. Wit JM, van Roermund HPC, Oostdik W, et al. Heterozygotes for 17α-hydroxylase deficiency can be detected with a short ACTH test. Clin Endocrinol (Oxf) 1988; 28:657–664.

36. Nakajin S, Shinoda M, Haniu M, Shively JE, Hall PF. C21

37. Matteson KJ, Picado-Leonard J, Chung B-C, Mohandas TK, Miller WM. Assignment of the gene for adrenal P450c17 (steroid 17α-hydroxylase/17,20-lyase) to human chromosome 10. J Clin Endocrinol Metab 1986; 63:789.

38. Fan Y-S, Sasi R, Lee C, Winter JSD, Waterman MR, Lin CC. Localization of the human CYP17 gene (cytochrome P450 17α) to 10q24.3 by fluorescence in situ hybridization and simultaneous chromosome banding. Genomics 1992; 14: 1110–1111.

39. Chung BC, Picado J, Haniu M, et al. Cytochrome P450c17 (steroid 17α-hydroxylase/17,20-lyase): cloning of human adrenal and testis cDNAs indicates the same gene is expressed in both tissues. Proc Natl Acad Sci USA 1987; 84:407–411.

40. Yanase T, Simpson ER, Waterman MR. 17α-Hydroxylase/-17,20-lyase deficiency: from clinical investigation to molecular definition. Endocr Rev 1991; 12:91–108.

41. Lin D, Harikrishna JA, Moore CCD, Jones KL, Miller WM. Missense mutation serine[106] → proline causes 17α-hydroxylase deficiency. J Biol Chem. 1991; 266:15992–15998.

42. Rumsby G, Skinner C, Lee HA, Honour JW. Combined 17α-hydroxylase/17,20-lyase deficiency caused by heterozygous stop codons in the cytochrome P450 17α-hydroxylase gene. Clin Endocrinol (Oxf) 1993; 39:483–485.

43. Winter JSD, Couch RM, Muller J, et al. Combined 17-hydroxylase and 17,20-desmolase deficiencies: evidence for synthesis of a defective cytochrome P450c17. J Clin Endocrinol Metab 1989; 68:309–316.

44. Imai T, Yanase T, Waterman MR, Simpson ER, Pratt JJ. Canadian Mennonites and individuals residing in the Friesland region of the Netherlands share the same molecular basis of 17α-hydroxylase deficiency. Hum Genet 1992; 89: 95–96.

45. Kühn-Velten WN, Bunse T, Förster MEC. Enzyme kinetic and inhibition analyses of cytochrome P450XVII, a protein with a bifunctional catalytic site. J Biol Chem 1991; 266:6291–6301.

46. Clark BJ, Waterman MJ. Functional expression of bovine 17α-hydroxylase in COS 1 cells is dependent upon the presence of an amino-terminal signal anchor sequence. J Biol Chem 1992; 267:24568–24574.

47. Imai T, Globerman H, Gertner JM, Kagawa N, Waterman MJ. Expression and purification of functional human 17α-hydroxylase/17,20-lyase (P450c17) in Escherichia coli. J Biol Chem 1993; 268:19681–19680.

48. Koh Y-C, Buczko E, Dufau ML. Requirement of phenylalanine 343 for the preferential Δ[4]-lyase versus Δ[5]-lyase activity of rat CYP17. J Biol Chem 1993; 268:18267–18271.

49. Labhart A. In: Adrenal cortex. Labhart A, ed. Clinical Endocrinology: Theory and Practice. New York: Springer-Verlag, 1974:332–339.

50. Gröndal S, Eriksson B, Hagenäs L, Werner S, Curstedt T. Steroid profile in urine: a useful tool in the diagnosis and follow-up of adrenocortical carcinoma. Acta Endocrinol (Copenh) 1990; 122:656–663.

51. Grim CE, McBryde AC, Glenn JF, Gunnells JC. Childhood primary aldosteronism with bilateral adrenocortical hypertension: plasma renin activity as an aid to diagnosis. J Pediatr 1967; 17:377.

52. New MI, Peterson RE. Aldosterone in childhood. In: Levine SZ, ed. Advances in Pediatrics 1968. Chicago: Yearbook Medical, 1968:111.

53. Baer L, Sommers SC, Krakoff LR, Newton MA, Laragh JH. Pseudoprimary aldosteronism. Circ Res 1970; (Suppl. I) 27:203.

54. George JM, Wright L, Bell NH, Bartter FC. The syndrome of primary aldosteronism. Am J Med 1970; 48:343.

55. Kelch RP, Connors MH, Kaplan SL, Biglieri EG, Grumbach MM. A calcified aldosterone-producing tumor in a hypertensive, normokalemic prepubertal girl. J Pediatr 1973; 83:432.

56. Oberfield SE, Levine LS, Firpo A, et al. Primary hyperaldosteronism in childhood due to unilateral macronodular hyperplasia. Hypertension 1984; 6:75–84.

57. Bryer-Ash M, Wilson D, Tune BM, Rosenfeld RG, Shochat SJ, Luetscher JA. Hypertension caused by an aldosterone-secreting adenoma. Am J Dis Child 1984; 138:673–676.

58. Decsi J, Soltesz G, Harangi F, Nemes J, Szabo M, Pinter A. Severe hypertension in a ten-year-old boy secondary to an aldosterone-producing tumor identified by adrenal sonography. Acta Pediatr Hung 1986; 27:233–238.

59. Prosser PR, Sutherland CM, Scullin DR. Localization of adrenal aldosterone adenoma by computerized tomography. N Engl J Med 1979; 300:1278.

60. Weinberger MH, Grim CE, Hollifield JW, et al. Primary aldosteroneism: diagnosis, localization and treatment. Ann Intern Med 1979; 90:386.

61. Hietakorpi S, Korhonen T, Aro A, et al. The value of scintigraphy and computed tomography for the differential diagnosis of primary hyperaldosteronism. Acta Endocrinol (Copenh) 1986; 113:118–122.

62. Conn JW. Primary aldosteronism and primary reninism. Hosp Pract 1974; 9:131.

63. Sutherland DJA, Ruse JL, Laidlaw JC. Hypertension, increased aldosterone secretion and low plasma renin activity relieved by dexamethasone. Can Med Assoc J 1966; 95:1109.

64. New MI, Peterson RE. A new form of congenital adrenal hyperplasia. J Clin Endocrinol Metab 1967; 27:300.

65. New MI, Oberfield SE, Levine LS, et al. Demonstration of autosomal dominant transmission and absence of HLA linkage in dexamethasone-suppressible hyperaldosteronism. Lancet 1980; 1:550.

66. Miura K, Yoshinaga K, Goto K, et al. A case of glucocorticoid-responsive hyperaldosteronism. J Clin Endocrinol Metab 1968; 28:1807.

67. New MI, Siegal EJ, Peterson RE. Dexamethasone-suppressible hyperaldosteronism. J Clin Endocrinol Metab 1973; 37:93.

68. Giebink GS, Gotlin RW, Biglieri EG, Katz FH. A kindred with familial glucocorticoid-suppressible aldosteronism. J Clin Endocrinol Metab 1973; 36:715.

69. Grim CE, Weinberger MH. Familial dexamethasone-suppressible normokalemic hyperaldosteronism. Pediatrics 1980; 65:597.

70. Oberfield SE, Levine LS, Stoner E, et al. Adrenal glomerulosa function in patients with dexamethasone-suppressible hyperaldosteronism. J Clin Endocrinol Metab 1981; 53:158.

71. Ganguly A, Grim CE, Weinberger MH. Anomalous postural aldosterone response in glucocorticoid-suppressible hyperaldosteronism. N Engl J Med 1981; 305:991.

72. Gill JR Jr, Bartter FC. Overproduction of sodium-retaining steroids by the zona glomerulosa is adrenocorticotropin-dependent and mediates hypertension in dexamethasone-suppressible aldosteronism. J Clin Endocrinol Metab 1981; 53:331.

73. Rauh W, Levine LS, Gottesdiener K, New MI. Mineralocorticoids, salt balance and blood pressure after prolonged ACTH administration in juvenile hypertension. Klin Wochenschr (Suppl I) 1978; 56:161.

74. New MI, Peterson RE, Saenger P, Levine LS. Evidence for an unidentified ACTH-induced steroid hormone causing hypertension. J Clin Endocrinol Metab 1976; 43:1283.

75. Lan NC, Matulich DT, Stockigt JR, et al. Radioreceptor assay of plasma mineralocorticoid activity. Role of aldosterone, cortisol and deoxycorticosterone in various mineralocorticoid-excess states. Circ Res 1980; 46(Suppl. 1):I-94-I-100.

76. Speiser PW, Martin KO, Kao-Lo G, New MI. Excess mineralocorticoid receptor activity in patients with dexamethasone-suppressible hyperaldosteronism is under adrenocorticotropin control. J Clin Endocrinol Metab 1985; 61:297–302.

77. Armanini D, Witzgall H, Wehling M, Kuhnle U, Weber PC. Aldosterone receptors in different types of primary aldosteronism. J Clin Endocrinol Metab 1987; 65:101–104.

78. Ulick S, Chu MD. Hypersecretion of a new cortico-steroid, 18-hydroxycortisol in two types of adrenocortical hypertension. Clin Exp Hypertens 1982; (Suppl. 9/10):1771–1777.

79. Ulick S, Chu MD, Land M. Biosynthesis of 18-oxocortisol by aldosterone-producing adrenal tissue. J Biol Chem 1983; 258:5498–5502.

80. Ulick S, Land M, Chu MD. 18-Oxocortisol, a naturally occurring mineralocorticoid agonist. Endocrinology 1983; 113:2320–2322.

81. Gomez-Sanchez CE, Montgomery M, Ganguly A, et al. Elevated urinary excretion of 18-oxocortisol in glucocorticoid-suppressible aldosteronism. J Clin Endocrinol Metab 1984; 59:1022–1024.

82. Connell JMC, Kenyon CJ, Corrie JET, Fraser R, Watt R, Lever AF. Dexamethasone-suppressible hyperaldosteronism. Adrenal transition cell hyperplasia? Hypertension 1986; 8:669–676.

83. Gomez-Sanchez CE, Gill JR Jr, Ganguly A, Gordon RD. Glucocorticoid-suppressible aldosteronism: a disorder of the adrenal transitional zone. J Clin Endocrinol Metab 1988; 67:444–448.

84. Ulick S, Chan CK, Gill JR Jr, et al. Defective fasciculata zone function as the mechanism of glucocorticoid-remediable aldosteronism. J Clin Endocrinol Metab 1990; 71:1151–1157.

85. New MI, Levine LS, Biglieri EG, Pareira J, Ulick S. Evidence for an unidentified ACTH-induced steroid hormone causing hypertension. J Clin Endocrinol Metab 1977; 44:924–933.

86. New MI, Oberfield SE, Carey RM, Greig F, Ulick S, Levine LS. A genetic defect in cortisol metabolism as the basis for the syndrome of apparent mineralocorticoid excess. In: Mantero F, Biglieri EG, Edwards CRW, eds. Endocrinology of Hypertension, Serono Symposia No. 50. New York: Academic Press, 1982:85–101.

87. Downey MK, Riddick L, New MI. Apparent mineralocorticoid excess: a genetic form of fatal low-renin hypertension. Program and Abstracts, American Society of Hypertension Second World Congress on Biologically Active Atrial Peptides, New York, May 1987.

88. Ulick S, Ramirez LC, New MI. An abnormality in steroid reductive metabolism in a hypertensive syndrome (rapid communication). J Clin Endocrinol Metab 1977; 44:799–802.

89. Ulick S, Levine LS, Gunczler P, et al. A syndrome of apparent mineralocorticoid excess associated with defects in the peripheral metabolism of cortisol. J Clin Endocrinol Metab 1979; 44:757–764.

90. Lakshmi V, Monder C. Evidence for independent 11-oxidase and 11-reductase activities of 11β-hydroxysteroid dehydrogenase: enzyme latency, phase transitions, and lipid requirements. Endocrinology 1985; 116:552–560.

91. Stewart PM, Wallace AM, Valentino R, Burt D, Shackleton CHL, Edwards CRW. Mineralocorticoid activity of liquorice:

11β-hydroxysteroid dehydrogenase deficiency comes of age. Lancet 1987; 2:821–823.

92. Stewart PM, Corrie JET, Shackleton CHL, Edwards CRW. Syndrome of apparent mineralocorticoid excess: a defect in the cortisol-cortisone shuttle. J Clin Invest 1988; 82:340–349.

93. Tannin GM, Agarwal AK, Monder C, New MI, White PC. The human gene for 11beta-hydroxysteroid dehydrogenase. Structure, tissue distribution and chromosomal localization. J Biol Chem 1991; 266:16653–16658.

94. Nikkilä H, Tannin GM, New MI, et al. Defects in the HSD11 gene encoding 11β-hydroxysteroid dehydrogenase are not found in patients with apparent mineralocorticoid excess or 11-oxoreductase deficiency. J Clin Endocrinol Metab 1993; 77:687–691.

95. Whitworth JA, Stewart PM, Burt D, Atherden SM, Edwards CRW. The kidney is the major site of cortisone production in man. Clin Endocrinol (Oxf) 1989; 31:355–361.

96. Brown RW, Chapman KE, Edwards CRW, Seckl JR. Human placental 11beta-hydroxysteroid dehydrogenase. Evidence for and partial purification of a distinct NAD-dependent isoform. Endocrinology 1993; 132:2614–2621.

97. Seckl JR. 11β-Hydroxysteroid dehydrogenase isoforms and their implications for blood pressure regulation. Eur J Clin Invest 1993; 23:589–601.

98. Albiston AL, Obeyesekere VR, Smith RE, Krozowski ZS. Cloning and tissue distribution of the human 11beta-hydroxysteroid dehydrogenase type 2 enzyme. Molec Cell Endocrinol 1994; 105:R11–R17.

99. Wilson RC, Krozowski ZS, Lik, et al. A mutation in the HSD11B2 gene in a family with apparent mineralocorticoid excess. J Clin Endocrinol Metab 1995; 80:2263–2266.

100. Ulick S, Tedde R, Wang JZ. Defective ring A reduction of cortisol as the major metabolic error in the syndrome of apparent mineralocorticoid excess. J Clin Endocrinol Metab 1992; 74:593–599.

54

Emergencies of Inborn Metabolic Diseases

Jose E. Abdenur
*Mount Sinai School of Medicine,
New York, New York*

I. INTRODUCTION

Baby JO was born full term, after an uneventful pregnancy and delivery. He had a normal physical examination and was discharged home at 36 h of age. The mother noted poor sucking and a weak cry 12 h later. He was brought to the hospital and found to be lethargic. A sepsis workup was done, and because a blood gas revealed respiratory alkalosis, an ammonium level was obtained. The value was 1600 μM (normal up to 80). Blood for plasma amino acids was sent, and he was treated with sodium benzoate, sodium phenylacetate, arginine, and a high glucose infusion. Citrulline levels were 2300 μM, and arginine dose was adjusted for treatment of argininosuccinic acid synthetase deficiency. The patient improved and was discharged after 2 weeks on a special diet.

The family history of JO revealed that a brother died at 5 days of age. He also presented with poor suck and lethargy early in life, was admitted into a hospital, and later had seizures and lapsed into coma. The diagnosis was sepsis. This story shows two dramatically different outcomes for two siblings who undoubtedly had the same disease.

Inborn metabolic diseases (IMD) are a group of genetic disorders in which there is a clinically significant block in metabolic pathways. They are usually the product of a single gene defect that affects the activity of an enzyme either directly or through abnormalities in its cofactor or activating protein (1). IMD comprise a variety of disorders affecting the metabolism of small (i.e., amino acids) or large molecules (i.e., sphingolipids). Many patients present with a catastrophic collapse in the neonatal period. However, the age and clinical presentation of IMD are highly variable. Therefore a disease-free period of months or years, or a subacute presentation does not rule out the possibility of an IMD (2). A variable phenotype can even be seen in patients with the same enzyme deficiency (3). Molecular studies suggest that, at least for some IMD, this clinical heterogeneity is the result of a variety of mutations that

affect enzyme activities in different ways (4). When possible, identification of the patient's molecular defect should be done. This information is useful for prenatal diagnosis and may allow one to predict the clinical course of the disease (genotype-phenotype correlation), helping to find the best therapeutic option for each individual.

The availability of newborn screening programs has dramatically changed the outcome of many IMD. Screening programs vary among different states. For example, the IMD screened by New York State are phenylketonuria, galactosemia, biotinidase deficiency, maple syrup urine disease, and homocystinuria.

A complete description of the different IMD can be found in excellent textbooks (5,6). In this chapter, we describe the most common IMD that can present with acute, life-threatening illness, focusing on the diagnosis and treatment of these emergencies.

II. UREA CYCLE DEFECTS (UCD)

A. Pathophysiology

High ammonium levels can be found in a variety of diseases (Table 1). However, the most severe causes of hyperammonemia are the UCD. The urea cycle prevents the accumulation of toxic nitrogen compounds incorporating nitrogen not used for protein synthesis into urea and is also responsible for the biosynthesis of arginine (7). Abnormalities in the urea cycle produce hyperammonemia and elevation of glutamine. The latter produces an intracellular osmotic effect, with secondary swelling of astrocytes and increased intracranial pressure, which is clinically expressed by an acute encephalopathy (7,8). There are five enzymes involved in the urea cycle (Fig. 1): carbamylphosphate synthetase (CPS), ornithine transcarbamylase (OTC), argininosuccinic acid synthetase (AS), argininosuccinic acid lyase (AL), and arginase. Because

Table 1 Causes of Hyperammonemia

Increased ammonium production
    Muscular hyperactivity (seizures, respiratory distress)
    Infections with urease positive bacteria (skin, intestine, urinary tract)
    Asparaginase treatment
Insufficient detoxification
    Urea cycle defects
        N-acetylglutamate synthetase deficiency
        Carbamylphosphate synthetase deficiency
        Ornithine transcarbamylase deficiency
        Argininosuccinic acid synthetase deficiency
        Argininosuccinic acid lyase deficiency
        Arginase deficiency
    Transient hyperammonemia of the newborn
    Transport defects of urea cycle intermediates
        Lysinuric protein intolerance
        Hyperammonemia-hyperornithinemia-homocitrullinuria
    Organic acidemias
    Fatty acid oxidation defects
    Mitochondrial diseases
    Liver insufficiency
        Infections
        Intoxication
    Liver bypass
        Vascular malformations
        Cirrhosis
    Deficient arginine supply in diet

Source: Modified from Reference 9.

N-acetylglutamate (NAG) is required for the activity of CPS, the enzyme responsible for NAG biosynthesis (NAG synthetase) is also considered part of the pathway (9). Except for OTC deficiency, which is X linked, all the UCD are autosomal recessive (7).

B. Clinical and Laboratory Manifestations

Patients with UCD can present with symptoms from birth to adulthood. The neonatal presentation is caused by a complete deficiency of CPS, OTC, AS, or AL, which have almost identical clinical expression (7,9). Although infrequent, NAG synthetase deficiency can also have a similar neonatal course (10). These patients are usually full term and have a normal physical examination at birth. Between the first 24 and 72 h, depending on protein intake, the neonate presents with poor suck, vomiting, and hypotonia, followed by lethargy, seizures, hypothermia, and coma (7). AS deficiency patients may present with hypertonicity (9) and trismus. Hyperventilation and slight liver enlargement are also constant findings. Sepsis, intracranial bleeding, and respiratory distress are the diagnoses considered most often. If hyperammonemia is not detected the patient dies, without the diagnosis of IMD.

Beyond the neonatal period, the clinical expression of the UCD patients varies depending on the degree of enzyme defect, nitrogen intake, and endogenous catabolism. The most common presentation is episodes of vomiting associated with irritability, agitation, ataxia, and/or lethargy, sometimes progressing to coma in a patient with a history of a self-imposed protein restriction. These episodes can be triggered by an exogenous protein load or increased endogenous catabolism (7). This variability also characterizes the presentation in female carriers for OTC deficiency, whose phenotype can range from completely asymptomatic to severe neonatal hyperammonemia because of the different degrees of lyonization in the hepatocytes (11).

The most important biochemical finding in symptomatic patients with OTC, CPS, AS, or AL deficiency is severe hyperammonemia (usually greater than 500 μM), with moderate elevation in liver transaminases and low blood urea nitrogen (BUN). Respiratory alkalosis, as a result of the toxic effect of the ammonia on the brain, is another key to the diagnosis (7). Patients with UCD can also present with metabolic acidosis (9), however, probably secondary to dehydration. Severe hyperammonemia in a sick neonate is strongly suggestive of an IMD. Quantitative plasma amino acids (AAs) and urine organic acid analysis (UOA) should be done as soon as possible, and a urine aliquot should be frozen for determination of orotic acid. An algorithm that combines clinical and biochemical information is a useful aid in the diagnosis of neonatal hyperammonemia (Fig. 2). The most common differential diagnoses are transient hyperammonemia of the newborn (THAN) and organic acidemias (OA; Fig. 2). Patients with THAN are usually preterm babies who present with respiratory distress and severe hyperammonemia (even higher than the UCD) in the first 24 h of life (12). Neonates with OA classically present with metabolic acidosis, high anion gap, and ketonuria. Hyperammonemia can be as severe as in the UCD, and UOA are usually diagnostic (13). Among the different UCD, differential diagnosis depends on the AA pattern. Low or undetected citrulline levels are present in CPS and OTC deficiencies (7). In the latter, the accumulated carbamylphosphate is diverted to the pyrimidine synthetic pathway, producing an increased excretion of orotic acid, which is the basis for the differential diagnosis between these two conditions (Fig. 2) (7). Additionally, uracil, another pyrimidine, may be present in the UOA of patients with OTC deficiency (14). Patients with AS deficiency have markedly increased citrulline levels (usually more than 1000 μM), and patients with AL deficiency have milder elevations in citrulline (100–300 μM) and increased argininosuccinic acid. Other AA abnormalities common to the four enzyme deficiencies are increased glutamine and alanine as a result of nonspecific nitrogen accumulation and decreased arginine and ornithine because of the impaired arginine biosynthesis (7). A liver biopsy for measurement of enzyme activity is seldom necessary for diagnostic purposes.

C. Treatment

1. Supportive Therapy

Treatment of an hyperammonemic episode is an emergency. All nitrogen intake should be discontinued. A central venous line should be placed for intravenous (IV) infusion, and an

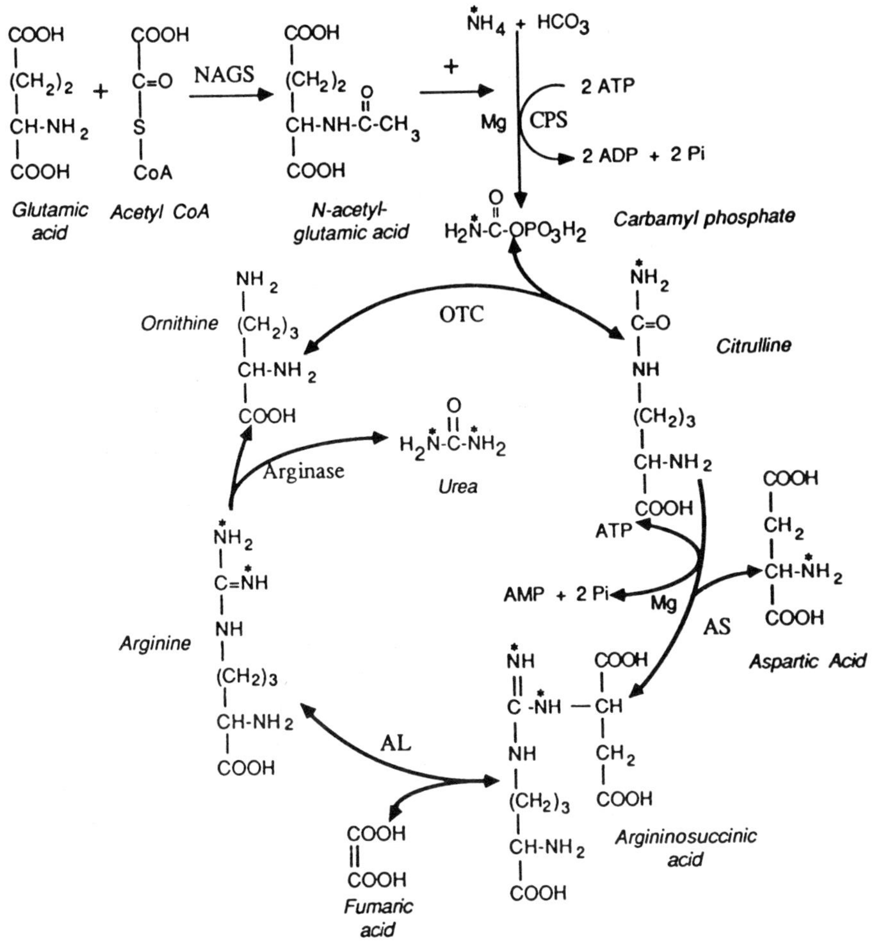

Figure 1 The urea cycle. The asterisks denote waste nitrogen atoms. For abbreviations, see the text. (From Ref. 7.)

arterial line should be available for blood drawing. The hemodialysis team should be alerted. Blood samples for ammonium, blood gas, electrolytes, BUN, glucose, and calcium should be obtained before the beginning of the treatment and every 4 h thereafter. If intracranial pressure is elevated, therapy with mannitol should be started. Corticosteroids should not be used because they produce a negative nitrogen balance (15).

2. Anabolism

To decrease endogenous protein catabolism, calories to cover at least the basal energy expenditure should be provided (60 cal/kg/day in newborns) (16). This requires the use of a high glucose infusion rate (GIR) and. when possible, IV lipids. The different GIR and calories delivered using different concentrations of dextrose can be seen in Tables 2 and 3. In less severely ill patients who can tolerate oral (PO) or nasogastric (NG) feedings, IV calories should be supplemented using one of the protein-free powders available, Pro-Free (Ross Laboratories, Columbus, OH) or Mead-Johnson 80056 (Mead Johnson Laboratories, Evansville, IN).

3. Detoxification

Pharmacologic treatment of the UCD is based on the use of sodium benzoate and sodium phenylacetate (15). The IV preparations of these drugs are still considered investigational and are available only upon application to Dr. Saul Brusilow (17). Both drugs activate alternative pathways for nitrogen excretion. After esterification to their CoA esters, sodium benzoate and sodium phenylacetate produce hippuric acid and phenylacetylglutamine, respectively. These compounds are excreted through the urine, diverting nitrogen from the urea cycle (Fig. 3). According to the protocol (15), both drugs should be given in a priming infusion of 250 mg/kg in 25–35 ml/kg of 10% dextrose over 90 minutes (GIR = 28–39 mg/kg/minute), followed by a sustaining infusion of 250 mg/kg to be given over 24 h in maintenance fluids (Table 4). We have observed hypoglycemia with hyperinsulinism as a result of this sudden change in glucose infusion. To avoid this problem, we delivered the drugs using a separate pump piggybacked to the main IV fluid line, which runs at a constant GIR. Sodium benzoate and sodium phenylacetate provide 6.9 and 6.4 mEq sodium per g, respectively. There-

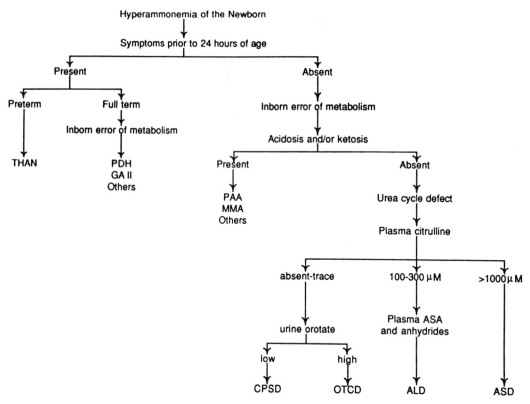

Figure 2   Diagnostic algorithm for neonatal hyperammonemia. See explanation in the text. THAN = transient hyperammonemia of the newborn; PDH = pyruvate dehydrogenase deficiency; GA II = glutaric aciduria type II; PAA = propionic acidemia; MMA = methylmalonic acidemia; ASA = argininosuccinic acid. (From Ref. 7.)

fore, the amount of sodium given to the patient with both drugs in 24 h is approximately 6.7 mEq/kg. These salts can produce potassium loss (15), which in association with the increased potassium uptake secondary to the high GIR may result in hypokalemia. Therefore, serum electrolytes must be followed closely and IV fluids adjusted accordingly. Arginine, which becomes an essential amino acid in UCD, should also be provided. The dose of the IV preparation of arginine HCl (10% solution) varies according to the enzyme defect (Table 4). A side effect of the treatment with arginine HCl is

Table 2   Glucose Infusion Rates (GIR) Calculated from Different Glucose Concentrations (D%) and Fluid Infusion Rates (ml/kg)[a]

ml/kg	D5%	D7.5%	D10%	D12.5%	D15%	D20%
40	1.4	2.1	2.8	3.5	4.2	5.6
50	1.7	2.6	3.5	4.3	5.2	6.9
60	2.1	3.1	4.2	5.2	6.2	8.3
67	2.3	3.5	4.6	5.8	7.0	9.3
75	2.6	3.9	5.2	6.5	7.8	10.4
100	3.5	5.2	6.9	8.7	10.4	13.9
120	4.2	6.2	8.3	10.4	12.5	16.7
150	5.2	7.8	10.4	13.0	15.6	20.8
180	6.2	9.4	12.5	15.6	18.8	25.0

[a]Concentrations of dextrose greater than 12.5% should not be used through a peripheral vein.

Table 3   Calories/kg/Day Provided at Different GIR[a]

Mg/kg/minute	Cal/kg/day
4.0	19.6
5.0	24.5
6.0	29.4
7.0	34.3
8.0	39.2
9.0	44.0
10.0	49.0
11.0	53.9
12.0	58.8

[a]The 3.4 cal provided by 1 g IV glucose was used for the calculations.

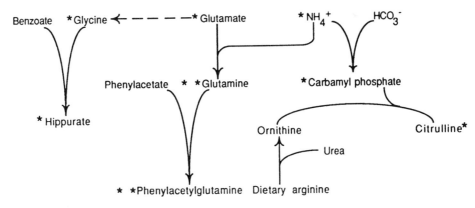

Figure 3 Alternative pathways of nitrogen excretion using sodium benzoate, sodium phenylacetate, and arginine. The asterisks denote nitrogen atoms. (From Ref. 7.)

the development of hyperchloremic metabolic acidosis, which may require treatment with sodium bicarbonate (15). Potassium acetate, rather than KCl, is useful to decrease the hyperchloremia resulting from the arginine administration. If plasma ammonium level does not decrease after 8 h, hemodialysis should be started using the largest catheters allowed by the patient's size (15). Peritoneal dialysis and hemofiltration have only 10% of the efficiency of hemodialysis for ammonium clearance (15).

4. Long-term Management

When ammonium levels are close to normal, protein can be added to the parenteral nutrition at an initial dose of 0.5 g/kg/day. Nasogastric or oral feeds can be started as soon as the clinical condition permits. Protein intake can be increased gradually until reaching 1–2 g/kg/day. The use of essential AAs to provide part of the total protein intake is recommended for OTC and CPS and can also be used in AS and AL deficiencies (18,19). To achieve the desired caloric intake

(120–130 cal/kg for a newborn), the formula should be supplemented with one of the available protein-free powders (see earlier). Enough water should be added to meet the patient's needs and to maintain the caloric density at 20–24 cal/ounce. The diet should be frequently adjusted to ensure growth and development. Protein and calorie requirements per kg body weight decrease with age and vary from patient to patient according to residual enzyme activity (15). Fasting plasma ammonium, branched-chain AAs, arginine, and serum plasma protein should be maintained within normal limits, and plasma glutamine should be below 1000 μM (15). It has been suggested that secondary carnitine deficiency may develop in patients with UCD (20,21). Therefore, carnitine levels should be monitored and therapy should be prescribed only if low levels are present. When PO intake is satisfactory, the appropriate medicines for long-term treatment (sodium phenylbutyrate, citrulline, and/or arginine) can be given PO, mixed with the formula, and the IV can be discontinued. The recommended guidelines for chronic management (15) are outlined in Table 5.

The outcome of patients with AS or AL is better than

Table 4 Pharmacologic Treatment of the Hyperammonemia Caused by the Different Enzyme Deficiencies in the Urea Cycle[a]

	CPS	OTC	AS	AL
Sodium benzoate				
PI	250	250	250	—
SI	250	250	250	—
Sodium phenylacetate				
PI	250	250	250	—
SI	250	250	250	—
Arginine HCl				
PI	210	210	660	660
SI	210	210	660	660

[a]PI = priming infusion, to be given over 90 minutes; SI = sustaining infusion, to be given over 24 h. Doses are in mg/kg.

Table 5 Recommended Management of Patients with Different Enzyme Deficiencies in the Urea Cycle

	CPS or OTC	AS	AL
Diet			
Total protein	1.0 –2.0	1.25–2.0	1.25–2.0
Essential AA	0 –0.7	?	?
Medication			
Sodium phenylbutyrate	0.45–0.60	0.45–0.60	—
Citrulline	0.17	—	—
Arginine (free base)	—	0.4 –0.7	0.4 –0.7

[a]All values are in g/kg/day.

that of those with OTC or CPS deficiencies (7). Neurologic damage may be directly related to the duration and degree of the initial hyperammonemic episode (22). Successful liver transplantation has been reported for OTC deficiency (23). Prospective treatment of children with confirmed prenatal diagnosis or at risk of having UCD has been more effective in patients with AS and AL than in those with OTC or CPS deficiencies (24,25).

III. ORGANIC ACIDURIAS

A. Pathophysiology

The organic acidurias are a group of IMD characterized by an abnormal accumulation of one or more organic acids in body fluids, producing an "intoxication-like" clinical presentation (2). The fatty acid oxidation defects and the primary lactic acidemias, which may also produce abnormal amounts of organic acids, are not included in this section because their pathophysiology differs from that of the classic OA (2). More than 20 different OA have been described (Table 6) (26). They comprise defects in several pathways, are inherited as autosomal recessive conditions, and have a highly variable phenotype. The majority of the OA can present with life-

threatening episodes that require emergency treatment. Iso-valeric aciduria (IVA), propionic aciduria (PA), and methyl-malonic aciduria caused by mutase deficiency (MMA) are the most common. Therefore, we mainly address these conditions. IVA, an IMD of leucine metabolism, results from the deficiency of isovaleryl-CoA dehydrogenase. Patients with IVA accumulate isovaleryl-CoA and excrete its by-products 3-OH-isovaleric acid, isovalerylglycine, and isovalerylcarni-tine (27). PA results from a defect in propionyl-CoA car-boxylase, a biotin-dependent enzyme, and MMA from a deficiency of methylmalonyl-CoA mutase. Activity of the latter could be impaired because of defects in the mutase itself or defects in the synthesis of its cofactor, adenosylcobalamin (28). Both PA and MMA accumulate propionyl-CoA, which derives from the catabolism of valine, isoleucine, threonine, methionine, odd-chain fatty acids, and cholesterol side chain (Fig. 4) (13). Another important source of propionyl-CoA is its endogenous production by the anaerobic gut flora (29,30). In general, patients with OA accumulate acyl-CoA esters and organic acids in the mitochondria. These abnormal metabo-lites inhibit several mitochondrial enzymes, which leads to the secondary biochemical abnormalities frequently seen in OA patients (28). Inhibition of N-acetylglutamate synthetase and carbamylphosphate synthetase are responsible for the hyperammonemia, which usually correlates with the level of

Table 6 Organic Acidurias

Organic aciduria	Enzyme defect
Branched-chain AA metabolism	
Isovaleric aciduria	Isovaleryl-CoA dehydrogenase
3-Methylcrotonylglycinuria	3-Methylcrotonyl-CoA carboxylase
3-Methylglutaconic aciduria	3-Methylglutaconyl CoA hydratase
3-OH-3-methylglutaric aciduria	3-OH-3-methylglutaryl-CoA lyase
Mevalonic aciduria	Mevalonate kinase
—	2-methyl branched-chain acyl-CoA dehydrogenase
2-Methylacetoacetic aciduria	2-methylacetoacetyl-CoA thiolase
3-OH-isobutyric aciduria	3-OH-isobutyryl-CoA dehydrogenase
—	Methylmalonyl/malonyl semialdehyde dehydrogenase
Propionic aciduria	Propionyl-CoA carboxylase
Methylmalonic aciduria	Methylmalonyl-CoA mutase
Methylmalonic aciduria	Cobalamin defects
—	Succynyl-CoA transferase
Malonic aciduria	Malonyl-CoA decarboxylase
Miscellaneous	
Glutaric aciduria type I	Glutaryl-CoA dehydrogenase
2-Ketoadipic aciduria	2-Ketoadipic dehydrogenase
L-2-Hydroxyglutaric aciduria	L-2-hydroxyacid dehydrogenase
4-OH-butyric aciduria	Succinic semialdehide dehydrogenase
Hyperoxaluria type I	Alanine:glyoxylate aminotransferase
Hyperoxaluria type II	D-glyceric dehydrogenase
Glyceroluria	Glycerol kinase
Pyroglutamic aciduria	Glutathione synthetase
Alkaptonuria	Homogentisic acid oxidase

Source: Modified from Reference 26.

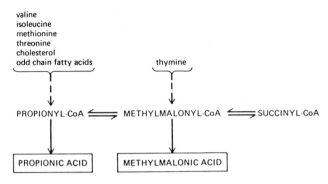

Figure 4 Precursors and schematic pathway of propionate and methylmalonate. Broken arrows indicate the presence of several reactions. (From Ref. 28.)

organic acid accumulation (31,32). Impairment of pyruvate carboxylase and the shunt of malate explain the hypoglycemia and ketosis found in these patients, and inhibition of the glycine cleavage system may be responsible for the hyperglycemia (28). Additionally, decreased ATP synthesis and hyperlactacidemia may result from inhibition of citrate synthase and pyruvic dehydrogenase (13).

B. Clinical and Laboratory Manifestations

The clinical presentation of patients with OA can be divided schematically into a severe neonatal form with metabolic distress, a chronic intermittent late-onset form, and a chronic progressive form (13). Additionally, many asymptomatic patients have been found as a result of screening programs and studies performed in relatives of affected individuals (3).

The severe neonatal form is the most common. The usual presentation is a neonate with a history of normal pregnancy and delivery and a short disease-free period who presents with poor sucking, vomiting, respiratory distress, hypotonia or dystonia, lethargy, and coma (13). Mild dehydration is frequent in MMA and PA, and a strong "sweaty feet" odor in urine and skin is present in IVA. Seizures and a Reye-like syndrome can be present in severely ill patients (2,13). Neutropenia, thrombocytopenia, or pancytopenia is frequent, and other severe complications can worsen the prognosis of this acute crisis (Table 7).

The most characteristic biochemical abnormalities are metabolic acidosis, with elevated anion gap, hyperammonemia, and ketosis. Hypocalcemia and mild hyperlactacidemia are common (13). Blood glucose is usually low but in some patients may be high, even before IV fluids have been started (41,42). This is particularly frequent in patients with ketolysis defects, who present with hyperglycemia and ketosis resembling an episode of diabetic ketoacidosis (43). In contrast, patients with 3-OH-3-methylglutaryl-CoA lyase deficiency present with hypoketotic hypoglycemia (27).

The most important diagnostic test in OA is the UOA performed by gas chromatography and mass spectrometry (GC/MS). The diagnostic possibilities of this test greatly

Table 7 Complications in Patients with OA During Acute Metabolic Decompensation

Pancreatitis (33)
Infections (34)
Generalized staphyloccocal epidermolysis (13,35)
Alopecia (36)
Acute basal ganglion dysfunction[a]

[a]Sudden onset of dystonia and/or movement disorder can be seen caused by involvement of the globus pallidum in patients with MMA and PA (37,38) and changes in the putamen and caudate in patients with glutaric aciduria type I (39,40).

increase if the urine is collected during the acute episode, when the characteristic profile for each OA is most likely to be found (26). In an acutely sick patient, the laboratory performing the test must be alerted, so that the result can be available in less than 24 h. Typical UOA profiles show an elevation in 3-OH-isovaleric and isovalerylglycine in IVA; 3-OH-propionic, methylcitrate, tiglylglycine, and propionylglycine in PA; and a massive increase in methylmalonic acid, with or without slight elevation in propionate metabolites, in MMA because of mutase deficiency (13).

More sophisticated tests, such as analysis of acylcarnitines by fast atom bombardment and tandem mass spectrometry and/or acylglycines by GC/MS stable isotope dilution, are necessary for the diagnosis of some specific OA, especially when a urine sample from the acute episode is not available (26). Quantitative AAs usually show a nonspecific elevation in glycine and glutamine. Total and free carnitine are usually decreased, with elevation in the acylcarnitine/free carnitine ratio (13).

In the intermittent, late-onset form, the disease presents with recurrent attacks of coma or lethargy with ataxia or dystonia. Acute hemiplegia, hemianopsia, and cerebellar hemorrhage have also been described (13). Increased protein intake or endogenous catabolism (caused by an intercurrent illness) may trigger these crisis. The first attack may present at several months or years of age, even in adolescence or adulthood, and has frequently been preceded by episodes of dehydration, anorexia, vomiting, failure to thrive, hypotonia, developmental delay, and/or other symptoms (13,44,45). Between attacks, clinical and laboratory evaluations may appear normal. However, the laboratory profile obtained during the attacks is similar to that described for the severe neonatal form, with the exception of hyperammonemia, which is less frequent (13).

The chronic progressive form is characterized by persistent anorexia, failure to thrive, and vomiting. These symptoms are frequently attributed to gastrointestinal problems. Renal Fanconi syndrome or osteoporosis may develop. Hypotonia with muscle weakness can be present, mimicking congenital or metabolic myopathies. Developmental delay, progressive mental retardation, and seizures can accompany the other symptoms (2,4,13).

C. Treatment

Rapid recognition and treatment of the acute metabolic decompensation in patients with OA can be lifesaving. Treatment should provide supportive therapy, promote anabolism, and remove the offending toxins.

1. Supportive Therapy

The treatment depends on the patient's clinical condition. A central line to assure IV access and an arterial line for blood pressure monitoring and frequent blood drawing should be placed. Assisted ventilation, inotropics, albumin, and/or blood products are frequently needed. After fluid resuscitation is provided, IV hydration should be aimed at correcting dehydration and promoting a good urinary output. If pH is less than 7.25, sodium bicarbonate at an initial dose of 1–3 mEq/kg should be given and repeated as needed. Overcorrection of the metabolic acidosis should be avoided. In severely acidotic patients, sodium overload can be prevented using sodium bicarbonate, instead of sodium chloride, for replacement of the sodium requirements. Blood gases, electrolytes, BUN, glucose, calcium, ammonium, hematocrit, and urine ketones should be monitored every 2–4 h. Liver function tests, amylase, and lipase should be obtained initially and repeated as needed. A sepsis workup should be done and antibiotics started. Staphylococcal and *Candida* infections should be considered in the differential diagnosis, and a complete blood count should be followed daily.

2. Anabolism

It has been shown that endogenous production is an important source of abnormal metabolites in nonacutely ill patients with OA. This production is probably a result of protein turnover (46,47) and is increased by fatty acid breakdown and intestinal production of propionate in patients with PA and MMA (29,30). These endogenous sources of toxic metabolites become even more important in severely ill patients (48). Therefore, to decrease the endogenous production of toxic compounds is mandatory in the treatment of these patients. The first step is to discontinue any oral intake, which must be followed by IV nutrition to promote anabolism. Initially, this goal can be partially achieved by giving a high GIR to provide at least 10 mg/kg/minute (Tables 2 and 3). However, in patients with OA, hyperglycemia and glucosuria are frequently seen, even with low GIR. Insulin has been used empirically in those patients (13,49) and we have found an inadequate insulin response to hyperglycemia during the acute decompensation in OA patients (50).

Insulin requirements vary depending on the severity of the patient's condition and the GIR. In our experience, in a severely ill patient receiving a GIR of 9–11 mg/kg/minute, a dose of 0.05–0.075 U/kg/h is enough to control hyperglycemia. However, it is advisable to start with a lower dose (0.025 U/kg/h) and to adjust it accordingly. Plasma ammonium levels usually decrease in parallel with those of the organic acids (32). When ammonium values are close to normal, total parenteral nutrition (TPN) can be started. TPN has been used successfully in chronic and acutely ill

patients with OA and allows an effective anabolism that cannot be achieved with glucose alone (49,51). Ideally, the initial IV amino acid mixture should be deprived of the AA precursors of the increased organic acid. Such preparations are not available in the majority of medical centers. Therefore, the available amino acid mixture can be used at an initial dose of 0.5 g/kg/day. This dose can be increased gradually to 1 g/kg/day with daily monitoring of AAs, UOA, and ammonium (49,51).

3. Detoxification

In IVA and MMA, the organic acids are effectively excreted through the urine. Therefore, maintaining a good urinary output becomes the initial strategy for toxin removal (13). Hemodialysis or blood exchange transfusions may be necessary in patients who do not improve rapidly. Peritoneal dialysis is an alternative for patients with impaired kidney function. In contrast, urinary excretion of propionic acid is poor. Therefore, in acutely ill patients with PA, hemodialysis or peritoneal dialysis should be considered early in the treatment (48,52). Intravenous carnitine, which should be used in all three conditions, is another resource for toxin removal. This therapy corrects the decreased levels of free carnitine, provides enough substrate for the synthesis of acylcarnitine compounds that can be excreted through the urine, and restores the intramitochondrial levels of CoA (13,27,28).

After obtaining a sample for basal levels, an initial loading dose of 50 mg/kg can be given, followed by a maintenance dose of 50–200 mg/kg/day, divided every 4–6 h. In patients with IVA, treatment with L-glycine increases the conversion of the toxic isovaleryl-CoA to the nontoxic isovalerylglycine, which can be excreted through the urine (27,36). Oral or NG tube supplementation of L-glycine (250–600 mg/kg/day divided in four to eight doses) should be given during the acute episode. Another potential resource for toxin removal is the administration of cofactors, biotin (10 mg/day) in PA and hydroxycobalamin (1 mg/day) in MMA. However, patients with severe neonatal presentation rarely respond to vitamin treatment. Clinical improvement is usually correlated with correction of the metabolic acidosis, hyperammonemia, and ketonuria.

4. Long-term Management

When the patient's condition allows, PO or NG feedings can be started. Chronic management of these patients requires a special diet. Natural protein is restricted to meet the recommended amounts of the AAs involved in the metabolic block. Total protein requirements are achieved by adding special formulas devoid of the offending amino acids. Children with OA require a higher than normal caloric intake. This can be obtained with the use of protein-free powders, fat, or carbohydrate supplements. Oral carnitine (IVA, PA, and MMA) and glycine (IVA) supplementation should be maintained, and vitamin therapy should continue only if a positive response has been documented. Metronidazole has been shown to be effective in decreasing the production of propionate by the gut flora (53). However, experience with chronic treatment is still limited. The long-term prognosis of the patients varies depending upon the particular OA, genotype, response to vitamin therapy, and residual enzyme activity. Family compliance and psychologic adjustment are important factors for the success of the treatment. Despite early diagnosis and intensive treatment, which usually requires NG or gastric tube feedings and/or TPN, OA patients with severe neonatal presentation need frequent hospitalizations and have a shortened life expectancy (13,51). In patients with long survival, several complications may appear (Table 8).

IV. FATTY ACID OXIDATION DEFECTS

A. Pathophysiology

The fatty acid oxidation defects are a relatively new group of IMD. They can present with life-threatening episodes resembling energy deficiency and include several enzymatic defects in different steps of the fatty acid metabolism (2).

Oxidation of free fatty acids is an important source of energy during periods of fasting and/or metabolic stress. Fatty acids of carbon length 20 or less are oxidized in the mitochondria; longer chain fats are metabolized in the peroxisomes (61). Short- and medium-chain fatty acids enter the mitochondrial matrix directly, where they are activated to their corresponding acyl-CoA thioesters by an acyl-CoA synthetase. In contrast, long-chain fatty acids are activated in the cytoplasm and need active transport into the mitochondria (Fig. 5). Transport of long-chain acyl-CoAs is a complex process. Initially, they are conjugated to carnitine by carnitine palmitoyltransferase (CPT) I, located in the outer mitochondrial membrane. Long-chain acylcarnitines are then passed by a translocase to CPT II, located in the inner mitochondrial membrane, which releases carnitine and long-chain acyl-CoAs into the mitochondrial matrix (62). Carnitine itself is transported into the tissues by two transporter proteins, one specific for the liver and the other to the kidney, muscle, and fibroblasts (63). Once in the mitochondrial matrix, acyl-CoAs of all chain lengths undergo a series of cyclic enzymatic reactions (Fig. 5). The first step in the cycle is the dehydrogenation of the acyl-CoA to enoyl-CoA. This reaction is catalyzed by four related enzymes, the acyl-CoA dehydrogenases (ACDs): very long chain, long-, medium-, and short-chain acyl-CoA dehydrogenases (VLCAD, LCAD, MCAD, and SCAD, respectively), which differ in their chain length specificity (61).

Electrons released during these reactions are channeled into the respiratory chain by the electron transfer flavoprotein (ETF) and the ETF dehydrogenase, producing ATP. The enoyl-CoAs produced by the ACDs are then hydrated to the hydroxyacyl-CoAs, which undergo dehydrogenation to ketoacyl-CoAs, followed by cleavage of the thioester bond. This process, which results in the release of acetyl-CoA and a new acyl-CoA molecule that is two carbons shorter, completes one turn of the mitochondrial fatty acid oxidation (FAO) cycle. The exact mechanism of the last three steps varies for substrates of different chain length. For long-chain acyl-CoA substrates the reactions are carried by a trifunctional protein with enoyl-CoA hydratase, hydroxyacyl-CoA dehydrogenase, and acyl-CoA ketothiolase activities (64). In contrast, for shorter chain substrates individual enzymes, each with a single activity, have been identified and purified (65). However, there is overlap in the substrate specificity of these enzymes. The acetyl-CoA moieties produced during the FAO are used as fuel for the tricarboxylic acid cycle or for the production of ketone bodies. The latter can be used as fuel by most tissues, including the brain (61).

Several enzymatic defects in FAO have been found in humans. The majority have been described over the last decade, and our knowledge of these defects is still growing. (Table 9 presents a summary of the known defects.) The multiple acyl-CoA dehydrogenase deficiency (glutaric aciduria type II), which involves defects in the metabolism of fatty acids, branched-chain amino acids, tryptophan, lysine, and sacrosine, is not discussed in this chapter.

B. Clinical and Laboratory Manifestations

The most distinctive features for each FAO defect are outlined in Table 9. However, there is overlapping in the clinical presentation among the different conditions. In general, children present with a hepatic and/or myopathic picture. Growth and development are usually normal until the first acute metabolic decompensation.

The most common FAO defect is MCAD deficiency (MCADD). Its clinical presentation ranges from completely asymptomatic persons to unexplained sudden death during infancy. Most classically, MCADD presents with intermittent episodes of hypoglycemia and lethargy in children 6 months to 2 years of age. A prolonged period of fasting and vomiting usually precedes the episode. An intercurrent illness may be present, as well as hepatomegaly. Ketone bodies are detected in smaller amounts than expected for the degree of hypoglycemia. FFA are increased and the FFA-ketone body ratio is abnormally high (78). Hyperuricemia and metabolic acidosis with mild elevation in lactic acid are nonspecific findings. In more severe cases, hyperammonemia, marked elevation in liver transaminases, and coma may occur. During the acute episode, a liver biopsy under light microscopy shows micro-

Table 8 Chronic Complications in Patients with OA

Poor growth
Malnutrition
Cutaneous lesions (54)
Deficiency of trace elements (55)
Osteoporosis
Mental retardation (56)
Movement disorders
Tubulopathy (57,58)
Chronic renal failure (59)
Cardiomyopathy (60)

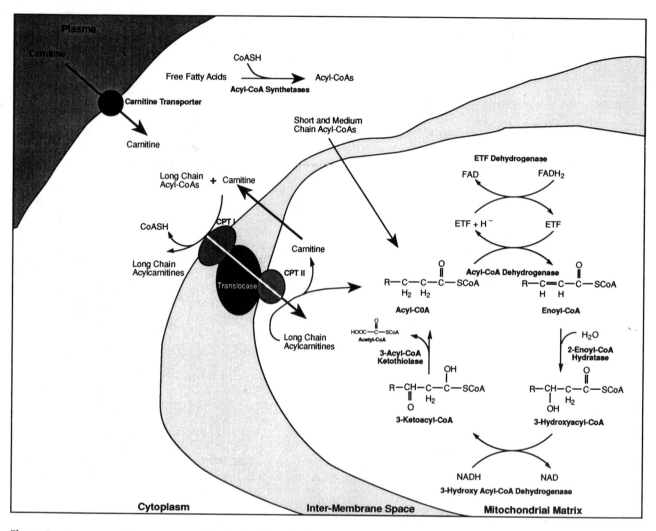

Figure 5   Enzymes and transporter proteins involved in mitochondrial β oxidation. See explanation in the text. CoA = coenzyme A; CoASH = free CoA; CPT = carnitine palmitoyltransferase; ETF = electron transport flavoprotein; FAD = flavin adenine dinucleotide; NAD = nicotinamide-adenine dinucleotide, NADH = reduced form of NAD. (From Ref. 61.)

and macrovesicular steatosis. These abnormalities usually lead to the diagnosis of Reye syndrome. However, electron microscopy does not detect the characteristic mitochondrial changes of Reye syndrome (79). Patients may repeat the metabolic decompensation but remain asymptomatic between episodes. Family history often reveals that a sibling died of sudden infant death syndrome (SIDS) or had a near-death episode. MCADD is inherited as an autosomal recessive disease. Interestingly, several studies have shown that the same mutation, a substitution of a T for an A at nucleotide 985, accounts for more than 90% of mutant alleles in patients with MCADD. The allele frequency of this mutation varies in different populations, however, ranging from 1:40 in Northern Europeans to less than 1:100 in Asians (61). A disease frequency of 1:15,000 persons can be calculated for the white U.S. population (80). This frequency is similar to

or greater than the estimated for phenylketonuria and/or galactosemia, which are screened for in the majority of the states. Additionally, recent data show that MCADD accounts for about 1% of SIDS and 19% of children with MCADD are diagnosed after death, but no affected child died after the diagnosis of MCADD was established (81). This information suggests the need for newborn screening for this condition.

When MCADD or other FAO defects are suspected, blood and urine samples should be obtained immediately for metabolic studies. Total and free carnitine levels are normal or high in CPT I deficiency and extremely low in carnitine transport defect. In all other FAO defects, total and free carnitine are usually decreased and the percentage of acylcarnitines (total − free) is increased (78). The OA profile is typical for some of the FAO defects. However, when samples are collected after the patient has been started on supportive

Table 9 Fatty Acid Oxidation Defects

Enzyme deficiency	Most important features
Carnitine transport	Impaired metabolism of long-chain fatty acids (LCFA), cardiomyopathy, muscle weakness; defect hypoglycemia; severe carnitine deficiency (66)
CPT I	Severe hypoglycemia with hypoketosis; normal or high carnitine levels (67)
Translocase	Hypoketotic hypoglycemia; cardiomyopathy, muscle weakness (68)
CPT II	Classic form in late childhood or early adulthood with episodic myoglobinuria; infantile form with hypoketotic hypoglycemia, hepatomegaly, and cardiomyopathy (69,70)
VLCAD	Impaired LCFA metabolism; hypoketotic hypoglycemia, liver failure, and cardiomyopathy (71)
LCAD	Impaired metabolism of LCFA; hypoketotic hypoglycemia; hypotonia, cardiomyopathy, and myoglobinuria (72)
MCAD	One of the most common inborn errors of metabolism; hypoketotic hypoglycemia; Reye-like episodes; sudden death (61)
SCAD	Failure to thrive, developmental delay, intermittent metabolic acidosis, muscle weakness, and hypotonia (73)
Trifunctional enzyme	Episodes of hypotonia and muscle weakness; high creatine kinase (74)
LCHAD	Marked heterogeneity; Reye-like syndrome; cardiomyopathy, myopathy, neuropathy, retinopathy; some patients may have trifunctional enzyme deficiency (75)
Short chain hydroxy acyl-CoA dehydrogenase (SCHAD)	Hypoketotic hypoglycemia, myoglobinuria, muscle weakness (76)
Dienoyl-CoA reductase	Impaired metabolism of LCFA with even-numbered double bonds; hypotonia and microcephaly (77)

therapy, the abnormal metabolites may not be present in the urine. Therefore, patients with FAO defects can be misdiagnosed if only standard OA analysis is performed (26).

Analysis of plasma acylcarnitines by fast atom bombardment/tandem mass spectrometry and/or acylglycines by GC/MS stable isotope dilution are more sophisticated tests that usually allow diagnosis even when patients are not acutely sick (26). As an exception, patients with SCAD deficiency may show a normal acylcarnitine profile with OA showing the typical increase in ethylmalonic acid. Fasting or loading tests, which are less frequently needed, should be performed only in experienced centers. Enzyme activity can be measured in the majority of these conditions in fibroblasts, liver, and/or muscle. Molecular studies for MCADD are available in several centers.

C. Treatment

Patients with encephalopathy and liver failure should be treated in by experienced pediatric intensive care unit staff. To suppress lipolysis, intravenous fluids should provide a glucose infusion rate of 10 mg/kg/minute or more. Intracranial pressure monitoring should be considered if brain swelling is suspected, and mannitol should be used as needed (82). Patients with long-chain FAO defects who present with coma and severe liver dysfunction may benefit from exchange transfusion (82). Treatment with intravenous carnitine is indicated for the carnitine transport defect (CTD). However, its use for all other FAO defects is controversial (78).

The keys for the chronic treatment of patients with FAO defects are to avoid prolonged periods of fasting and to use a diet restricted in fat (15–20% of total calories). Enough linoleic and linolenic acids should be prescribed to avoid essential fatty acid deficiency (83). Treatment of infants must be aggressive and may require overnight gastric tube feedings (78). Frequent feedings during the day and a high carbohydrate feeding late at night may be enough for older children. The formula to be used depends on the enzymatic defect. Patients with impaired metabolism of long chain fatty acids (LCAD, trifunctional protein, LCHAD, CPT, or CTD) may benefit from the use of formulas rich in medium-chain triglycerides (MCT). In contrast, the use of MCT is contraindicated for patients with MCAD or SCAD deficiencies. After the age of 2 years, the diet can be supplemented with uncooked cornstarch, as used in patients with glycogen storage diseases (78). Chronic treatment with PO carnitine is indicated for the CTD. For all other FAO defects, carnitine levels should be monitored and treatment should probably be considered in patients with low free carnitine levels (61,78). Additionally, glycine supplementation appears to be useful in patients with MCADD (84).

It was initially thought that treated patients with MCADD had a good prognosis. However, recent information revealed several long-term complications, including developmental delay, muscle weakness, failure to thrive, and cerebral palsy (81). There is as yet limited information about the long-term prognosis of patients with other FAO defects.

V. PRIMARY LACTIC ACIDEMIAS

A. Pathophysiology

The primary lactic acidemias (PLA) are a group of IMD with variable clinical presentation, including life-threatening episodes of metabolic acidosis and complex biochemical, enzymatic, and molecular diagnosis. They represent abnormalities in pyruvate metabolism that are recognized biochemically by their primary consequence, hyperlactacidemia, and clinically by symptoms reflecting "energy deficiency" (2). Pyruvic acid produced by the glycolytic pathway can follow different metabolic fates. To produce energy, pyruvate enters the mitochondria and undergoes aerobic catabolism via acetyl-CoA, the Krebs cycle, and the respiratory chain (Fig. 6). Pyruvic acid can also be an intermediary substrate for gluconeogenesis via oxaloacetic acid. A block in any of the many enzymatic steps involved in these pathways can produce an increase in pyruvic acid levels with simultaneous elevation in lactic acid and alanine (Fig. 6).

A detailed description of each enzymatic defect is beyond the scope of this chapter, but in general, the PLA can be divided into four groups: defects in pyruvate oxidation, TCA cycle, respiratory chain, and gluconeogenesis.

Pyruvate oxidation defects are caused by deficiencies in the pyruvic dehydrogenase complex (PDHC). This thiamine-dependent enzymatic complex is responsible for the decarboxylation of pyruvate to acetyl-CoA (Fig. 6). Deficiencies in different components of the PDHC have been reported, and they are one of the most frequent causes of PLA (85–87).

The TCA cycle is responsible for the oxidative decarboxylation of citrate to oxaloacetate (Fig. 6). Several enzymes are involved. However, defects in only two of them have been characterized: α-ketoglutarate dehydrogenase (α-KGD) and fumarase (88–90).

The respiratory chain carries electrons through a series of complex ractions to generate ATP. Our understanding of this system has greatly increased with recent advances in molecular genetics. The respiratory chain is divided into five different complexes. Each complex has several protein components, some of them encoded by nuclear DNA (nDNA) and others by mitochondrial DNA (mtDNA) (91). The only exception is complex II, which has only nDNA-encoded proteins.

Differentiation between abnormalities in the respiratory chain caused by defects in nDNA or mtDNA is important for prenatal diagnosis and genetic counseling: nDNA defects follow a Mendelian inheritance, and mtDNA is maternally transmitted. The mtDNA is a small circular molecule (16.5 kb) that encodes for 13 polypeptide subunits of the respiratory chain, together with ribosomal RNAs and the 22 mitochondrial transfer RNAs necessary for mRNA expression (91). Each cell contains hundreds of mitochondria and thousands of mtDNA. In patients with mtDNA abnormalities, normal and abnormal mtDNA coexist in the same cells (heteroplasmy). During cell division, mitochondria are randomly distributed to the new cells (replicative segregation), and as the cells divide, the relative proportions of normal and abnormal mtDNA change (91). These characteristics of

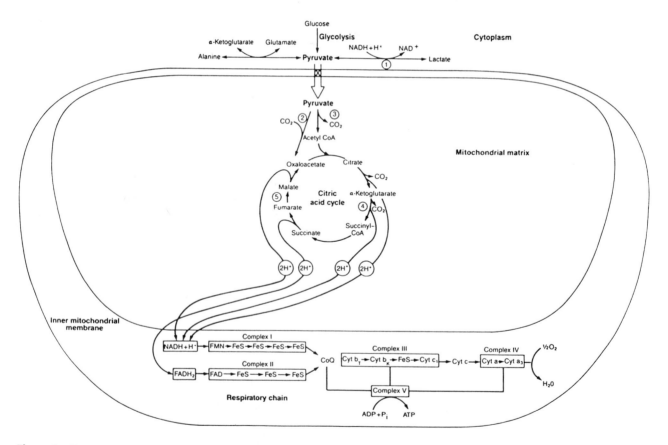

Figure 6 Pyruvate metabolism. See explanation in the text. Enzymes: 1 = lactate dehydrogenase; 2 = pyruvate carboxylase; 3 = pyruvate dehydrogenase complex; 4 = α-ketoglutarate dehydrogenase; 5 = fumarase. (From Ref. 86.)

the mtDNA have clinical implications. In the same patient, some tissues and organs may or may not be affected, depending on their proportion of normal and abnormal mtDNA. Furthermore, tissues that are not affected at one point may become affected when the number of abnormal mitochondria reaches a threshold for phenotypic expression (91). This explains why the same molecular defect can present with different phenotypes, which can also change over time.

Patients with defects of the respiratory chain have been diagnosed based on enzymatic and/or molecular studies. The most common enzyme deficiencies are reported for complex I (NADH-CoQ reductase) (85,86) and IV (cytochrome c oxidase, COX) (92), but deficiencies of complex III and V have also been described (85,86,93). Molecular studies have shown several mutations and deletions of the mtDNA to correlate with more or less well defined syndromes (94,95) (Table 10). Point mutations usually follow maternal inheritance; deletions are usually sporadic (94).

Gluconeogenic defects involve deficiencies in the four regulatory enzymes of this pathway. The most frequent defects are found in pyruvate carboxylase (PC), a biotin-dependent enzyme responsible for the carboxylation of pyruvate to oxaloacetate. Defects in phosphoenolpyruvate carboxykinase and fructose-1,6-diphosphatase are less frequent. The last enzyme in the gluconeogenic pathway, glucose-6-phosphatase, is responsible for glycogen storage disease type I.

Table 10 Clinical Syndromes Associated with mtDNA Defects[a]

Associated with mtDNA mutations
MELAS
MERRF
NARP
LHON
PEO
Cardiomyopathy
Myopathy
Diabetes and deafness (96)
IDDM and NIDM (97)
Diseases associated with mtDNA deletions
Pearson syndrome
Pearson syndrome + nephropathy (98,99)
Kearns-Sayre syndrome/PEO
Wolfram syndrome (DIDMOAD)
Deafness, Fanconi syndrome, and IDDM (100)

[a]MELAS, Mitochondrial encephalomyopathy, lactic acidosis, and stroke-like episodes; MERRF, myoclonic epilepsy and ragged red fibers; NARP, neuropathy, ataxia, and retinitis pigmentosa; LHON, Leber's hereditary optic neuropathy; PEO, progressive external ophthalmoplegia; IDDM, insulin-dependent diabetes mellitus; NIDDM, non–insulin-dependent diabetes mellitus; DIDMOAD, diabetes insipidus, diabetes mellitus, optic atrophy, and deafness.

Table 11 Most Frequent Findings Associated with PLA

Failure to thrive
Episodic vomiting
Developmental delay
Progressive encephalopathy
Structural brain abnormalities (absence of corpus callosum, porencephalic cysts)
Sudden infant death
Leigh's disease
Seizures, myoclonus
Recurrent ataxia
Stroke-like episodes
Cortical blindness
Hypotonia, weakness
Cardiomyopathy, heart block
Ophthalmoplegia
Retinal degeneration
Sensorineural hearing loss
Maternal family history of neurologic disease

B. Clinical and Laboratory Manifestations

Clinical presentation of patients with PLA is highly variable. Correlation between symptoms and enzymatic block is difficult because the same enzymatic defect can present with different phenotypes and different enzyme deficiencies can give a similar clinical presentation.

Patients with neonatal lactic acidemia present a few hours after birth with poor feedings, hypotonia, lethargy, and respiratory distress. Initial laboratory tests disclose severe metabolic acidosis, high anion gap, and markedly elevated lactic acid. Mild hyperammonemia may be present.

The most frequent etiologies for this presentation are PDHC or PC deficiencies. However, a similar course can be seen in the fatal and benign infantile myopathy caused by COX deficiency, as well as in complex I and V deficiencies (85,86,92,93). PLA patients with a subacute or chronic course can have different combinations of symptoms and signs (Table 11) (85,86,95). In general, a respiratory chain defect must be considered when "dealing with an unexplained association of symptoms, with early onset and a rapidly progressive course involving seemingly unrelated organs" (101). Certain combinations are characteristic for specific syndromes (Table 10).

Initial workup for an acute or chronic PLA is similar. Fasting blood levels for lactate (L), pyruvate (P), 3-OH-butyrate (30HB), acetoacetate (AcAc), and AAs and urine for organic acids should be obtained. Accurate measurement of L and P requires rapid and proper handling of the specimens. Arterial samples are preferred, and the use of a tourniquet should be avoided if venous samples are to be obtained. The lactic/pyruvate (L/P) molar ratio should be calculated (normal 10–20). A low to normal value suggests PDHC deficiency. By contrast, PC and respiratory chain defects show elevated

L/P ratios, and a low 30HB/AcAc ratio is seen only in PC deficiency (26). Secondary lactic acidosis as a result of poor perfusion, hypoxia, liver insufficiency, or sepsis also gives elevated L/P ratios and should be ruled out. Some patients with chronic PLA have normal fasting levels of L, P, and ketone bodies. These patients can eventually be diagnosed by measuring the postprandial levels of these metabolites or, in patients with central nervous system (CNS) involvement, by measuring L and P levels in cerebrospinal fluid (CSF) (101). UOA are useful to detect a possible PLA but, with the exception of the TCA cycle defects, cannot determine the site of the metabolic block (26). Usual findings are elevated lactic (pyruvic acid is not well extracted with the standard methods) and 2-hydroxybutyric acids, with or without elevation in TCA cycle intermediates (succinic, fumaric, malic, and 2-ketoglutaric acids). Lactic aciduria together with ketonuria suggests PC deficiency (86). Patients with urinary infections by *Enterobacter cloacae* may show isolated elevation in lactic acid in urine (102). Quantitative plasma AAs have limitations similar to those of UOA. A common finding in all PLA is an elevation in alanine. Elevated citrulline and lysine, together with hyperammonemia, are characteristic of PC deficiency (103) and elevated branched-chain AAs are seen in the E3 subunit deficiency of α-KGD (88). Patients with gluconeogenic defects can also present with hypoglycemia and hepatomegaly. In patients with respiratory chain defects, who are prone to multiorgan involvement, abnormalities in muscle, liver, kidney, pancreas, bone marrow, heart, brain, retina, auditory nerve, and endocrine system should be ruled out (101). In patients with CNS involvement, magnetic resonance imaging (MRI) of the brain usually shows diffuse demyelination, abnormal signaling in the basal ganglia, and variable degrees of cortical atrophy (104). In patients with muscle involvement, a muscle biopsy is indicated. Specimens should be obtained appropriately for light and electron microscopy, immunohistochemistry, and enzyme activity. The presence of ragged red fibers under light microscopy and abnormal mitochondria under electron microscopy are suggestive of a respiratory chain defect (86). Enzymatic diagnosis for defects in pyruvate oxidation, the TCA cycle, and gluconeogenesis can be done in blood or fibroblasts. Enzyme activity for the respiratory chain is best measured in muscle. The assessment is complicated by several factors, however, including different percentages of abnormal mtDNA and different isoforms of the same enzyme in different tissues (92). Additionally,

point mutations in a tRNA of the mtDNA can secondarily affect the enzyme activity of several respiratory chain complexes. Molecular diagnosis of the most common mutations or deletions is available.

C. Treatment

Treatment of acute neonatal lactic acidemia requires an intensive care unit. Sodium bicarbonate in large amounts is usually required to control the metabolic acidosis. If hypernatremic metabolic acidosis develops, it should be treated with peritoneal or hemodialysis. Special solutions with sodium bicarbonate (instead of sodium chloride) and devoid of acetate or lactate should be used in these procedures. A high glucose infusion rate can severely worsen the lactic acidemia in patients with PDHC deficiency. Therefore, initial intravenous fluids should provide a low GIR that can be increased according to clinical and biochemical response.

After the appropriate samples for enzyme diagnosis have been obtained, a vitaminic "cocktail" can be started (105,106) (Table 12). This cocktail contains some of the cofactors involved in the different metabolic pathways, as well as artificial electron acceptors (vitamins C and K$_3$).

Assessment of the response to vitamin therapy is difficult, and well-documented data are rare. When final diagnosis becomes available, an attempt to withdraw those vitamins not involved in the metabolic block should be done, one at the time, with careful monitoring of the clinical and biochemical response. Dichloroacetate stimulates the activity of the PDHC kinase and has been used in the treatment of PLA of unknown origin as well as in PDHC and complex I deficiencies (105,106). However, this drug is still considered experimental and can be used only under the protocol approved by the U.S. Food and Drug Administration. Carnitine supplementation (50–100 mg/kg/day) should be used to maintain normal free carnitine levels. Additionally, treatment with methylene blue, folate, aspartate, vitamin E, succinic acid, corticosteroids, and acetylcarnitine has been advocated for some conditions (105,106). Dietary treatment may have a role in some patients with PLA. A high-fat–low-carbohydrate diet has been useful in some patients with PDHC deficiency, and a low-fat–high-carbohydrate diet with frequent feeds is indicated for the gluconeogenic defects. However, the response to dietary treatment is still controversial (106).

Treatment of subacute and chronic cases also involves vitamin therapy. In these cases it is desired to add one vitamin at the time and to maintain careful monitoring of the patient's response. The long-term prognosis of PLA patients is generally poor, with progressive neurologic and muscle involvement.

Table 12 Vitamin Therapy for PLA

Thiamine, 200–300 mg/day
Lipoic acid, 10–50 mg/kg/day
Biotin, 5–10 mg/day
Riboflavin, 50–300 mg/day
Coenzyme Q, 180–360 mg/day
Vitamin C, 500–3000 mg/day
Vitamin K$_3$ (menadione), 50–500 mg/day
Dichloroacetate, 100–300 mg/kg/day

VI. AMINO ACID DISORDERS

A. Nonketotic Hyperglycinemia (NKH)

1. Pathophysiology

NKH is an autosomal recessive disorder that causes life-threatening illness in newborns. The disease results from defects in the glycine cleavage system (GCS), which consists of four protein components, P, H, T, and L (107). The majority of the patients (87%) have a severe neonatal course and very low enzyme activity in liver. These children have a defect in P protein. The remainder of patients present a milder, late-onset form, have higher enzyme activity, and share a defect in T protein (107). The GCS is present only in liver, kidney, and brain, and its defects produce high levels of glycine in these tissues. Increased levels of glycine in the brain overpotentiates the glutaminergic receptor N-methyl-D-aspartate (NMDA), producing neurologic damage (108).

2. Clinical and Laboratory Manifestations

In the neonatal form, patients present in the first 48 h of age with lethargy, seizures, hypotonia, and hiccups, followed by coma and apnea, which require assisted ventilation. Many neonates die shortly thereafter; others start breathing after few weeks and survive a few months with extremely severe neurologic damage (109). Electroencephalography shows a characteristic burst suppression pattern, which later progresses to hypsarrhythmia (110). Computed tomographic scan or MRI shows atrophy of the brain and hypodensity of the myelin. Organic acids are normal. The diagnosis is confirmed by the presence of an increased glycine level in the CSF with a high CSF/serum glycine ratio (>0.09) in simultaneously obtained samples (110). Differential diagnosis include several nongenetic causes of seizures in the neonatal period (i.e., bleeding), as well as IMD (i.e., molybdenum cofactor deficiency and primary lactic acidemias). Other causes of hyperglycinemias, such as organic acidemias and treatment with valproic acid, should also be ruled out.

The late-onset form of NKH presents with variable degrees of mental retardation in children (109).

The prevalence of NKH is unknown, except in Finland, where there is a high incidence of the disease because of the same mutation affecting the P protein (107).

3. Treatment

Treatment of NKH includes supportive therapy (e.g., assisted ventilation and anticonvulsants) and detoxification with sodium benzoate (250–750 mg/kg/day). Most recently dextromethorphan, a blocker of the NMDA receptor, has been used, with promising results (108,111). However, different responses have been observed at different doses (7.5–20 mg/kg/day), which appears to be secondary to individual variations in dextromethorphan metabolism (112). It is not yet known whether this novel treatment will improve the long-term prognosis of NKH patients.

B. Maple Syrup Urine Disease (MSUD)

1. Pathophysiology

MSUD is an autosomal recessive disease affecting the metabolism of the branched-chain amino acids (BCAA) leucine, isoleucine, and valine. The defect is located in the branched-chain 2-ketoacid dehydrogenase complex (BCKD), which is comprised of four different components: E1-α, E1-β, E2, and E3 (113). BCKD deficiency results in the elevation in the corresponding branched-chain 2-ketoacids (BCKA) 2-ketoisocaproic, 2-keto-3-methylvaleric, and 2-ketoisovaleric. Accumulation of these compounds is responsible for the characteristic odor as well as the clinical course of the disease.

2. Clinical and Laboratory Manifestations

At least three clinical phenotypes have been described, with residual enzyme activity correlating with the severity of the clinical presentation (114). In the most classic form, infants present soon after birth with the characteristic odor, poor feedings, lethargy, seizures, and apnea. This intoxication-like clinical picture resembles that of the OA. Biochemical abnormalities include ketoacidosis, hyperammonemia, and hypoglycemia. Diagnosis can be made by either plasma AAs or UOA. Typical findings in the former are elevated levels of the BCAA, mainly leucine (1000–5000 μM/L), and the presence of L-alloisoleucine, which is a transamination product of the 2-keto-3-methylvaleric acid (26). Routine UOA analysis may show an elevation in branched-chain 2-OH-acids and BCKA. However, the latter are better detected if the sample is previously oximated.

A variant form of MSUD presents in infancy to young adulthood with failure to thrive, ataxia, and less severe ketoacidosis. In these patients, plasma leucine levels range between 400 and 2000 μM/L (114). A milder clinical form presents in children or adults with intermittent ataxia and ketoacidosis triggered by infections or high protein ingestion. Plasma leucine values are usually between 50 and 1000 μM/L (113). A "thiamine-responsive" form of the disease has also been described (115).

MSUD is transmitted as an autosomal recessive condition, and it has been diagnosed in all ethnic groups. The general incidence of the disease is estimated as 1:200,000 (114). This incidence is much higher for some inbred communities (113). Several different mutations have been identified, the majority of them affecting the E2 component. No genotype-phenotype correlation is as yet available. Newborn screening programs are available in many states.

3. Treatment

Acute management of a MSUD patient follows the same principles outlined for the treatment of organic acidemias (see earlier). Although patients with MSUD usually require less bicarbonate than the OA to correct the metabolic acidosis, dialysis should be strongly considered in those patients who present with severe neurologic involvement and/or with leucine levels above 1500 μM/L. If TPN is needed, it should be given with an AA mixture initially devoid of BCAA. Carnitine is not indicated in MSUD patients. Additionally, the administration of thiamine (100–200 mg/day) is indicated for the thiamine-responsive patients. The prognosis of MSUD patients has dramatically improved because of the early diagnosis (newborn screening programs), intensive treatment, and availability of the special formulas. For children treated in specialized centers, survival is 100% (113). However, some degree of psychomotor impairment seems to be present even in patients with early diagnosis (116), and strict dietary treatment appears necessary to avoid CNS involvement (117).

REFERENCES

1. Wappner R. Biochemical diagnosis of genetic diseases. Pediatr Ann 1993; 22:282–297.
2. Saudubray JM, Ogier H. Clinical approach to inherited metabolic disorders. In: Fernandez J, Saudubray JM, Tada K, eds. Inborn Metabolic Diseases. Berlin: Springer-Verlag, 1990:3–25.
3. Haworth JC, Booth FA, Chudley AE, et al. Phenotypic variability in glutaric aciduria type I: Report of fourteen cases in five Canadian Indian kindreds. J Pediatr 1991; 118:52–58.
4. Crane AM, Martin LS, Valle D, Ledley FD. Phenotype of disease in three patients with identical mutations in methylmalonyl CoA mutase. Hum Genet 1992; 89:259–264.
5. Scriver CR, Beaudet AL, Sly WS, Valle D, eds. The Metabolic Basis of Inherited Disease, 6th ed. New York: McGraw-Hill, 1989.
6. Fernandez J, Saudubray JM, Tada K, eds. Inborn Metabolic Diseases. Berlin: Springer-Verlag, 1990.
7. Brusilow SW. Urea cycle enzymes. In: Scriver CR, Beaudet AL, Sly WS, Valle D, eds. The Metabolic Basis of Inherited Disease, 6th ed. New York: McGraw-Hill, 1989: 629–663.
8. Voorhies TM, Ehrlich ME, Duffy TE, Petito CK, Plum F. Acute hyperammonemia in the young primate: physiologic and neuropathologic corelates. Pediatr Res 1983; 17:971–975.
9. Bachmann C. The urea cycle disorders. In: Fernandez J, Saudubray JM, Tada K, eds. Inborn Metabolic Diseases. Berlin: Springer-Verlag, 1990:211–228.
10. Schubiger G, Bachmann C, Barben P, Colombo JP, Tonz O, Schupbach D. N-acetylglutamate synthetase deficiency: diagnosis, management and follow-up of a rare disorder of ammonia detoxification. Eur J Pediatr 1991; 150:353–356.
11. Rowe PC, Newman SL, Brusilow SW. Natural history of symptomatic partial ornithine transcarbamylase deficiency. N Engl J Med 1986; 314:541–547.
12. Hudak ML, Jones D, Brusilow S. Differentiation of transient hyperammonemia of the newborn and urea cycle enzyme defects by clinical presentation. J Pediatr 1985; 107:712–719.
13. Ogier H, Charpntier C, Saudubray JM. Organic acidemias. In: Fernandez J, Saudubray JM, Tada K, eds. Inborn Metabolic Diseases. Berlin: Springer-Verlag, 1990:271–300.
14. Webster DR, Simmonds HA, Barry DMJ, Becroft DMO. Pyrimidine and purine metabolites in ornithine carbamoyl transferase deficiency. J Inherited Metab Dis 1981; 4:27–31.
15. Brusilow SW. Treatment of urea cycle disorders. In: Desnick RJ, ed. Treatment of Genetic Disease. New York: Churchill-Livingston, 1991:79–94.
16. Hendricks KM. Estimation of energy needs. In: Hendricks KM, Walker WA, eds. Manual of Pediatric Nutrition, 2nd ed. Philadelphia: B.C. Decker, 1990:59–71.
17. Brusilow S. Johns Hopkins Hospital, 600 North Wolfe Street, Baltimore, MD 21205. (410) 955-0885.
18. Brusilow SW. Urea cycle disorders. In: Dietary Management of Metabolic Disorders. Evansville, IN: Mead Johnson Laboratories, 1991:40–41.
19. Acosta PB, Yannicelli S. Urea cycle disorders. In: Cameron AM, ed. The Ross Metabolic Formula System. Nutrition Support Protocols. Columbus, OH: Ross Laboratories, 1993: 339–358.
20. Mori T, Tsochiyama A, Nagai K, Nagao M, Oyanagi K, Tsugawa S. A case of carbamylphosphate synthetase-I deficiency associated with secondary carnitine deficiency. L-carnitine treatment of CPSI deficiency. Eur J Pediatr 1990; 149:272–274.
21. Sakuma T. Alteration of urinary carnitine profile induced by benzoate administration. Arch Dis Child 1991; 66:873–875.
22. Batshaw ML, Brusilow S, Waber L, et al. Treatment of inborn errors of urea synthesis. N Engl J Med 1982; 306:1387–1392.
23. Largilliere C, Houssin D, Gottrand F, et al. Liver transplant for ornithine transcarbamylase deficiency in a girl. J Pediatr 1989; 115:415–418.
24. Maestri NE, Hauser ER, Bartholomew D, Brusilow SW. Prospective treatment of urea cycle disorders. J Pediatr 1991; 119:923–928.
25. Melnyk AR, Matalon R, Henry B, Zeler WP, Lange C. Prospective management of a child with neonatal citrullinemia. J Pediatr 1993; 122:96–98.
26. Rinaldo P. Laboratory diagnosis of inborn errors of metabolism. In: Suchy FJ, ed. Liver Disease in Children. St. Louis: Mosby, 1994:295–308.
27. Sweetman L. Branched chain organic acidurias. In: Scriver CR, Beaudet AL, Sly WS, Valle D, eds. The Metabolic Basis of Inherited Disease, 6th ed. New York: McGraw-Hill, 1989:791–819.
28. Rosenberg LE, Fenton WA. Disorders of propionate and methylmalonate metabolism. In: Scriver CR, Beaudet AL, Sly WS, Valle D, eds. The Metabolic Basis of Inherited Disease, 6th ed. New York: McGraw-Hill, 1989:821–844.
29. Bain M, Jones M, Borrielo SP, et al. Contribution of gut bacterial metabolism to human metabolic disease. Lancet 1988; 1:1078–1079.
30. Thompson GN, Walter JH, Bresson JL, et al. Sources of propionate in inborn errors of metabolism. Metabolism, 1990; 11:1133–1137.
31. Coude FX, Sweetman L, Nyhan WL. Inhibition by propionyl-coenzyme A of N-acetyglutamate synthtase in rat liver mitochondria. J Clin Invest 1979; 64:1544–1551.
32. Coude FX, Ogier H, Grimber G, et al. Correlation between blood ammonia concentration and organic acid accumulation in isovaleric and propionic acidemia. Pediatrics 1982; 69:115–117.
33. Khaler SG, Sherwood WG, Woolf D, et al. Pancreatitis inpatients with organic acidemias. J Pediatr 1994; 124:239–243.
34. Berry GT, Yudkoff M, Segal S. Isovaleric acidemia: medical and neurodevelopmental effects of long term therapy. J Pediatr 1988; 113:58–64.
35. Koopman RJJ, Happle R. Cutaneous manifestations of methylmalonic acidemia. Arch Dermatol Res 1990; 282:272–273.
36. Shigematsu Y, Sudo M, Momoi T, Inoue Y, Suzuki Y, Kameyama J, Changing plasma and urinary organic acid levels in a patient with isovaleric acidemia during an attack. Pediatr Res 1982; 16:771–775.
37. Heidenreich R, Natowicz M, Hainline B, et al. Acute extrapyramidal syndrome in methylmalonic acidemia: "Metabolic stroke" involving the globus pallidus. J Pediatr 1988; 113:1022–1027.
38. Andreula CF, DeBlasi R, Carella A. CT and MR studies of methylmalonic acidemia. AJNR 1991; 12:410–412.
39. Bergman I, Finegold D, Gartner C, et al. Acute profound dystonia in infants with glutaric acidemia. Pediatrics 1989; 83:228–234.
40. Chow CW, Haan EA, Goodman SI, et al. Neuropathology in

glutaric acidemia type I. Acta Neuropathol (Berl) 1988; 76:590–594.

41. Boeckx RL, Hicks JM. Methylmalonic acidemia with the unusual complication of severe hyperglycemia. Clin Chem 1982; 28:1801–1803.

42. Williams K, Peden VH, Hillman RE. Isovalercacidemia appearing as diabetic ketoacidosis. Am J Dis Child 1981; 135:1068–1069.

43. Saudubray JM, Specola N. Ketolysis defects. In: Fernandez J, Saudubray JM, Tada K, eds. Inborn Metabolic Diseases. Berlin: Springer-Verlag, 1990:411–420.

44. Shapira SK, Ledley FD, Rosenblatt DS, Levy HL. Ketoacidotic crisis as a presentation of mild methylmalonic acidemia. J Pediatr 1991; 119:80–84.

45. Sethi KD, Ray R, Roesel RA, et al. Adult onset chorea and dementia with propionic acidemia. Neurology 1989; 39:1343–1345.

46. Thompson GN, Chalmers RA. Increased urinary metabolite excretion during fasting in disorders of propionate metabolism. Pediatr Res 1990; 27:413–416.

47. Millington DS, Roe CR, Maltby DA, Inoue F. Endogenous catabolism is the major source of toxic metabolites in isovaleric acidemia. J Pediatr 1987; 110:56–60.

48. Saudubray JM, Ogier H, Charpentier H, et al. Neonatal management of organic acidurias—clinical update. J Inherited Metab Dis 1984; 7:2–9.

49. Kalloghlian A, Gleispach H, Ozand PT. A patient with propionic acidemia managed with continuous insulin infusion and total parenteral nutrition. J Child Neurol (Suppl) 1992; 7:S88–S91.

50. Abdenur J, Greene C. 1992. Unpublished.

51. Khaler SG, Millington DS, Cederbaum SD, et al. Parenteral nutrition in propionic and methylmalonic acidemia. J Pediatr 1989; 115:235–241.

52. Roth B, Younossi A, Skopnik H, Leonard JV, Lehnert W. Haemodialysis for metabolic decompensation in propionic acidemia. J Inherited Metab Dis 1987; 10:147–151.

53. Thompson GN, Chalmers RA, Walter JH, et al. The use of metronidazole in management of methylmalonic and propionic acidemias. Eur J Pediatr 1990; 149:792–796.

54. De Raeve L, Meirleir L, Ramet J, Vandenplas Y, Gerlo E. Acrodermatitis enteropathica-like cutaneous lesions in organic aciduria. J Pediatr 194; 124:416–420.

55. Yannicelli S, Hambidge KM, Picciano MF. Decreased selenium intake and low plasma selenium concentrations leading to clinical symptoms in a child with propionic acidemia. J Inherited Metab Dis 1992; 15:261–268.

56. Surtees RAH, Matthews EE, Leonard JV. Neurologic outcome of propionic acidemia. Pediatr Neurol 1992; 8:333–337.

57. Ohura T, Kikuchi M, Abukawa D, et al. Type 4 renal tubular acidosis (subtype 2) in a patient with methylmalonic acidemia. Eur J Pediatr 1990; 150:115–118.

58. D'Angio CT, Dilon MJ, Leonard JV. Renal tubular dysfunction in methylmalonic acidemia. Eur J Pediatr 1991; 150:259–263.

59. Molteni KH, Oberley TD, Wolff JA, Friedman AL. Progressive renal insufficiency in methylmalonic acidemia. Pediatr Nephrol 1991; 5:323–326.

60. Massoud AF, Leonard JV. Cardiomyopathy in propionic acidaemia. Eur J Pediatr 1993; 152:441–445.

61. Vockley J. The changing face of disorders of fatty oxidation. Mayo Clin Proc 1994; 69:249–257.

62. Murthy MSR, Pande SV. Malonyl-CoA binding site and the overt carnitine palmitoyltransferase activity reside on the opposite sides of the outer mitochondrial membrane. Proc Natl Acad Sci USA 1987; 84:378–382.

63. Treem WR, Stanley CA, Finegold DN, Hale DE, Coates PM. Primary carnitine deficiency due to a failure of carnitine transport in kidney, muscle and fibroblasts. N Engl J Med 1988; 319:1331–1336.

64. Uchida Y, Izai K, Orii T, Hashimoto T. Novel fatty acid B-oxidation enzymes in rat live mitochondria. II. Purification and properties of enoyl-CoA hydratase/3-hydroxyacyl-CoA dehydrogenase/3-keto-acyl-CoA thiolase trifunctional protein. J Biol Chem 1992; 267:1034–1041.

65. Mori M, Amaya Y, Arakawa H, Takiguchi M. Biosynthesis and mitochondrial import of fatty acid oxidation enzymes. Prog Clin Biol Res 1990; 321:663–672.

66. Treem WR, Stanley CA, Finegold DN, Hale DE, Coates PM. Primary carnitine deficiency due to a failure of carnitine transport in kidney, muscle and fibroblasts. N Engl J Med 1988; 319:1331–1336.

67. Demaugre F, Bonnefont JP, Mitchell G, et al. Hepatic and muscular presentations of carnitine palmitoyl transferase deficiency: two distinct entities. Pediatr Res 1988; 24:308–311.

68. Pande SV, Brivet M, Slama A, Demaugre F, Aufrant A, Saudubray JM. Carnitine-acylcarnitine translocase deficiency with severe hypoglycemia and auriculo ventricular block: translocase assay in permeabilized fibroblasts. J Clin Invest 1993; 91:1247–1252.

69. Angelini C, Trevisan C, Isaya G, Pegolo G, Vergani L. Clinical varieties of carnitine and carnitine palmitoyltransferase deficiency. Clin Biochem 1987; 20:1–7.

70. Hug G, Bove KE, Soukup S. Lethal multiorgan deficiency of carnitine palmitoyltransferase II. N Engl J Med 1991; 325:1862–1864.

71. Aoyama T, Uchida Y, Kelley RI, et al. A novel disease with deficiency of mitochondrial very-long-chain acyl-CoA dehydrogenase. Biochem Biophys Res Commun 1993; 191:1369–1372.

72. Treem WR, Stanley CA, Hale DE, Leopold HB, Hyams JS. Hypoglycemia, hypotonia and cardiomyopathy: the evolving clinical picture of long chain acyl-CoA dehydrogenase deficiency. Pediatrics 1991; 87:328–333.

73. Amendt BA, Greene C, Sweetman L, et al. Short-chain-acyl-CoA dehydrogenase deficiency: clinical and biochemical studies in two patients. J Clin Invest 1987; 79:1303–1309.

74. Kamijo T, Wanders R, Saudubray JM, Aoyama T, Komiyama A, Hashimoto T. Mitochondrial trifunctional protein deficiency. J Clin Invest 1994; 93:1740–1747.

75. Wanders RJA, Ijlst L, Duran M, et al. Long-chain 3-hydroxyacyl-CoA dehydrogenase deficiency: different clinical expression in three unrelated patients. J Inherited Metab Dis 1991; 14:325–328.

76. Tein I, De Vivo DC, Hale DE, et al. Short-chain L-3-hydroxyacyl-CoA dehydrogenase deficiency in muscle: a new cause of recurrent myoglobinuria and encephalopathy. Ann Neurol 1991; 30:415–419.

77. Roe CR, Millington DS, Norwood DL, et al. 2,4-Dienoyl-coenzyme A reductase deficiency: a possible new disorder of fatty acid oxidation. J Clin Invest 1990; 85:1703–1707.

78. Treem WR. Inborn defects in mitochondrial fatty acid oxidation. In: Suchy FJ, ed. Liver Disease in Children. St. Louis: Mosby, 1994:852–887.

79. Treem WR, Witzleben CA, Picoli DA, et al. Medium-chain and long-chain acyl CoA dehydrogenase deficiency: clinical, pathologic and ultrastructural differentiation from Reye's syndrome. Hepatology 1986; 6:1270–1278.

80. Matsubara Y, Narisawa K, Tada K, et al. Prevalence of K329E mutation in medium-chain acylCoA dehydrogenase gene determined from Guthrie cards. Lancet 1991; 338:552–553.

81. Iafolla AK, Thompson RJ, Roe CR. Medium-chain acyl-co-

enzyme A dehydrogenase deficiency: clinical course in 120 affected children. J Pediatr 1994; 124:409–415.

82. Partin JC. Reye's syndrome. In: Suchy FJ, ed. Liver Disease in Children. St. Louis: Mosby, 1994:653–671.

83. Acosta PB, Yannicelli S. Mitochondrial fatty acid oxidation defects. In: Cameron AM, ed. The Ross Metabolic Formula System. Nutrition Support Protocols. Columbus, OH: Ross Laboratories. 1993:307–322.

84. Rinaldo P, Schmidt-Sommerfeld E, Posca AP, Heales SJR, Woolf DA, Leonard JV. Effect of treatment with glycine and L-carnitine in medium-chain acyl-CoA dehydrogenase deficiency. J Pediatr 1993; 122:580–584.

85. Robinson BH. Lacticacidemia. Biochim Biophys Acta 1993; 1182:231–244.

86. De Vivo DC, Di Mauro S. Disorders of pyruvate metabolism, the citric acid cycle and the respiratory chain. In: Fernandez J, Saudubray JM, Tada K, eds. Inborn Metabolic Diseases. Berlin: Springer-Verlag, 1990:127–157.

87. Brown GK. Pyruvate dehydrogenase E_1 deficiency. J Inherited Metab Dis 1992; 15:625–633.

88. Yoshida I, Sweetman L, Kulovich S, Nyhan WL, Robinson B. Effect of lipoic acid in a patient with defective activity of pyruvate dehydrogenase, 2-oxoglutarate dehydrogenase and branched-chain keto acid dehydrogenase. Pediatr Res 1990; 27:75–79.

89. Kohlschutter A, Behbehani A, Langenbeck U, et al. A familial progressive neurodegenerative disease with 2-oxo-glutaric aciduria. Eur J Pediatr 1982; 138:32–37.

90. Bourgeron T, Chretien D, Poggi-bach J, et al. Mutation of the fumarase gene in two siblings with progressive encephalopathy and fumarase deficiency. J Clin Invest 1994; 93: 2514–2518.

91. Shoffner JM, Wallace D. Mitochondrial genetics: principles and practice. Am J Hum Genet 1992; 51:1179–1186.

92. DiMauro S, Lombes A, Nakase H, et al. Cytochrome c oxidase deficiency. Pediatr Res 1990; 28:536–541.

93. Pastores GM, Santorelli FM, Shanske S, et al. Leigh syndrome and hypertrophic cardiomyopathy in a patient with a mitochondrial DNA point mutation (T8993G). Am J Med Genet 1994; 50:265–271.

94. De Vivo DC. Mitochondrial DNA defects: clinical features. In: DiMauro S, Wallace D, eds. Mitochondrial DNA in Human Pathology. New York: Raven Press, 1993:39–52.

95. Di Mauro A, Moraes CT. Mitochondrial encephalomyopathies. Arch Neurol 1993; 50:1197–1208.

96. Van den Ouweland JMW, Lemkes HHPJ, Ruitenbeek W, et al. Mutation in mitochondrial tRNA gene in a large pedigree with maternally transmitted type II diabetes mellitus and deafness. Nature Genet 1992; 1:368–371.

97. Kadowaki T, Kadowaki H, Mori Y, et al. A subtype of diabetes mellitus associated with a mutation of mitochondrial DNA. N Engl J Med 1994; 330:962–968.

98. Niaudet P, Heidet L, Munnich A, et al. Deletion of the mitochondrial DNA in a case of Toni-Debre-Fanconi syndrome and Pearson syndrome. Pediatr Nephrol 1994; 8:164–168.

99. Szabolks MJ, Seigle R, Shanske S, Bonilla E, Di Mauro S, D'Agati V. Mitochondrial DNA deletion: a cause of chronic tubulointerstitial nephropathy. Kidney Int 1994; 45:1388–1396.

100. Abdenur JE, Cotter PD, Lieberman K, et al. A new mitochon-

drial DNA deletion disorder presenting with deafness, renal Fanconi syndrome and insulin dependent diabetes mellitus. VI International Congress Inborn Errors of Metabolism. Milan, Abstracts Book 1994:120.

101. Munnich A, Rustin P, Rotig A, et al. Clinical aspects of mitochondrial disorders. J Inherited Metab Dis 1992; 15:448–455.

102. Rogers JG, Wilkinson RG, Skelton I, Danks DM. Tertiary lactic acidosis. J Pediatr 1981; 99:272–273.

103. Coude FX, Ogier H, Marsac D, et al. Secondary citrullinemia with hyperammonemia in four neonatal cases of pyruvate carboxylase deficiency. Pediatrics 1981; 68:914.

104. Kendall BE. Inborn errors and demyelination: MRI and the diagnosis of white matter disease. J Inherited Metab Dis 1993; 16:771–786.

105. Przyrembel H. Therapy of mitochondrial disorders. J Inherited Metab Dis 1987; 10:129–146.

106. Calvani M, Koverech A, Caruso G. Treatment of mitochondrial diseases. In: DiMauro S, Wallace D, eds. Mitochondrial DNA in Human Pathology. New York: Raven Press, 1993: 173–198.

107. Tada K, Kure S. Non-ketotic hyperglycinemia: molecular lesion, diagnosis and pathophysiology. J Inherited Metab Dis 1993; 16:691–703.

108. Schmitt B, Steinmann B, Gitzelmann R, Thun-Hohenstein L, Mascher H, Dumermuth G. Nonketotic hyperglycinemia: clinical and electrophysiologic effects of dextromethorphan, an antagonist of the NMDA receptor. Neurology 1993; 43: 421–424.

109. Nyhan WL. Nonketotic hyperglycinemia. In: Scriver CR, Beaudet AL, Sly WS, Valle D, eds. The Metabolic Basis of Inherited Disease, 6th ed. New York: McGraw-Hill, 1989: 743–753.

110. Tada K. Nonketotic hyperglycinemia. In: Fernandez J, Saudubray JM, Tada K, eds. Inborn Metabolic Diseases. Berlin: Springer-Verlag, 1990:323–330.

111. Hamosh A, McDonald JW, Valle D, Francomano CA, Niedermeyer E, Johnston MV. Dextromethorphan and high dose benzoate therapy for nonketotic hyperglycinemia in an infant. J Pediatr 1992; 121:131–135.

112. Arnold GL, Griebel ML, Valentine JL, Kearns GL. Dextromethorphan metabolism in nonketotic hyperglycinemia. VI International Congress Inborn Errors of Metabolism, Milan, Abstracts Book, 1994:55.

113. Danner DJ, Elsas LJ. Dissorders of branched-chain aminoacid and ketoacid metabolism. In: Scriver CR, Beaudet AL, Sly WS, Valle D, eds. The Metabolic Basis of Inherited Disease, 6th ed. New York: McGraw-Hill, 1989:671–692.

114. Peinemann, Danner DJ. Maple syrup urine disease 1954 to 1993. J Inherited Metab Dis 1994; 17:3–15.

115. Fernhoff P, Lubitz D, Danner DJ, et al. Thiamine responsive maple syrup urine disease. Pediatr Res 1985; 19:1011–1016.

116. Nord A, van Doorninck WJ, Greene C. Developmental profile of patients with maple syrup urine disease. J Inherited Metab Dis 1991; 14:881–889.

117. Treacy E, Clow CL, Reade TR, Chitayat D, Mamera OA, Scriver CR. Maple syrup urine disease: interrelations between branched-chain amino-, oxo- and hydroxyacids; implications for treatment; associations with CNS dysmyelination. J Inherited Metab Dis 1992; 15:121–135.

55

Endocrine Alterations in Human Immunodeficiency Virus Infections

Robert Rapaport

University of Medicine and Dentistry–New Jersey Medical School and Children's Hospital of New Jersey, Newark, New Jersey

I. INTRODUCTION

The first cases of the acquired immunodeficiency syndrome (AIDS) in children were reported in 1983 (1,2). Since that time, more than 3000 cases of AIDS have been reported to the Centers for Disease Control (CDC) in children less than 13 years of age, representing about 2% of all AIDS cases reported (3). Inasmuch as the number of human immunodeficiency virus (HIV)-infected women will continue to increase because of both intravenous drug use and heterosexual transmission, many more cases of AIDS in children are expected to occur (3). HIV-associated disease has been classified by the CDC in three categories: P0 for indeterminate infection, P1 for asymptomatic infection with and without laboratory abnormalities, and P2 for symptomatic infection with or without additional HIV-related infections or neurologic or neoplastic diseases. Reported cases of AIDS, representing only the most severe manifestations of HIV-associated disease, therefore reflect only a small proportion of infants and children with HIV infections (4). Most cases of pediatric HIV infections are a result of perinatal transmission (84%), most mothers acquiring the virus by intravenous drug use and heterosexual contact. Of pediatric HIV cases 7% are caused by infection through blood and blood products in individuals with clotting disorders, such as hemophilia (4). Recent reports have estimated that about 6000 HIV-infected women give birth annually in the United States, with a vertical transmission rate of 30%. It is estimated that 10,000–20,000 HIV-infected children currently live in the United States (4).

Improvement in means of detecting and treating HIV infections has led to improvements in the quality of life and survival of infected children. As these children survive longer, the effects of HIV infections on various organ systems become more apparent. It is therefore imperative to detect and treat HIV-related complications as early and effectively as possible.

The endocrine alterations observed in HIV-infected children may be caused by the direct effects of HIV infections, the severe, often debilitating chronic disease that results from infection with the HIV and/or accompanying opportunistic infections or neoplasms, or the therapeutic agents used to treat HIV-infected children.

Evidence for alterations in the endocrine system by HIV disease derives from pathologic studies of autopsy material as well as from in vitro and clinical studies. In this section I review existing evidence of endocrine system alterations in HIV infections, with special emphasis on studies relating to HIV-infected children.

II. GROWTH

In children with HIV infections, poor growth has been a consistent finding. Of the first 15 children with AIDS reported in 1983, 13 (87%) were described as having "failure to thrive" (FTT) (1,2). A subsequent report described FTT in 14 of 14 infants less than 7 months of age with AIDS (5). This poorly defined term, FTT, has been a frequently reported characteristic of infants and children with AIDS. A dysmorphic syndrome noted in HIV-infected children and named HIV embryopathy by some had as its most commonly found feature FTT, or poor growth (6,7). Reviews of large numbers of HIV-infected children have consistently commented on the occurrence of poor growth in the affected children (8–11).

The cause of the growth failure accompanying HIV infections appears to be postnatal in origin. Johnson et al. (12) studied prospectively 20 children born to HIV-infected mothers for 18 months. All infants had normal birth weights, suggesting no effect of HIV exposure upon intrauterine growth. By the end of the first year of life 12 children had no evidence of HIV infection. None of them was considered to have FTT. Of the 8 infected children, 4 (50%) exhibited FTT, 2 developing a syndrome of growth failure, dermatitis, and early death.

Maas et al. (13) evaluated prospectively the effects of maternal HIV infection on fetal development and neonatal morbidity in 17 neonates and 37 controls, of whom 21 were exposed to opiates. They concluded that prenatal exposure to nicotine and opiates but not HIV infection resulted in fetal growth retardation and neonatal morbidity.

In a group of children with perinatally acquired infection, 10 who had the presence of antigen-induced lymphocyte proliferation were found to grow normally, in contrast to 8 children with absent antigen-induced lymphoproliferation, 7 of whom had failure to thrive (14).

The cause of growth failure in HIV-infected children remains undetermined. We evaluated 31 children with symptomatic HIV infections. We found that as a group they were not smaller than average. When individual patients were evaluated, however, we found that about 1 of 6 of the HIV-infected children was underweight (weight < 3%), and one-third had height and weight velocities less than 3%. Those children who had more opportunistic infections and lower CD4 lymphocyte counts tended to grow most poorly. A substantial number of patients had abnormal thyroid function test results, but most had normal serum growth hormone, somatomedin C, and cortisol levels. Urinary growth hormone excretion was increased in the patients as a group (15).

In a recent retrospective analysis of 198 children enrolled in the Children's Hospital of New Jersey AIDS program, sufficient data for growth analysis were found in 122 subjects. Poor growth, defined as weight or height less than 5% based on National Center for Health Statistics (NCHS) data, was noted in 10 of 22 infants less than 2 years of age, 5 of whom were girls. Of these, 8 had heights and weights less than 5%. Among boys older than 2, 15 of 49 had poor growth, 6 having low weights and heights, 7 only low heights, and 2 only low weights. Of 51 girls, 16 had evidence of poor growth, 6 low heights and weights, 7 low heights, and 2 low weights. These data confirm our earlier finding that height was more affected than weight in HIV-infected children, suggesting that nutritional factors alone could not explain the growth failure. CD4 cell counts were lower and the incidences of opportunistic infections were higher in the poorly growing children. The incidence of progressive encephalopathy was not related to the children's growth patterns (16).

McKinney et al. (17) compared 62 HIV-infected with 108 uninfected children less than 25$^1/_2$ months of age. The weight for length scores through the first 2 years of life were comparable in the two populations, suggesting that the HIV-infected children were not abnormally lean or wasted. However, the uninfected population was significantly longer (higher length for age scores) at 4–24 months of age than the infected children. However, the study did not take into account that 73% of the infected children had received antiretroviral treatment (zidovudine), which has been shown to result in increased weight.

Growth hormone dynamics have been investigated in relatively few children with HIV infections. Jospe and Powell reported an 8-year-old girl with growth hormone deficiency (18). Laue et al. (19) studied 9 children with severe growth failure, with heights between 2 and 5 standard deviations (SD) below the mean. All children had normal levels of insulin-like growth factor I (IGF-I), and 8 of 9 had normal growth hormone responses to stimulation tests with arginine and levodopa. Thyroid and adrenal function tests were by and large normal in these children and could therefore not provide an explanation for their growth failure. Schwartz et al. (20) also found normal growth hormone responses to glucagon stimulation in 12 short children with average heights of 2.23 ± 1.2 SD under the mean. Serum IGF-I levels were low, however. Lepage et al. (21) compared 16 HIV-seropositive children 5–12 years of age with perinatally acquired disease in Kigali, Rwanda with age- and sex-matched seronegative children. Of 16 patients, 12 had short stature, and 7 of 16 had low weight for age. Mean IGF-I concentrations were lower in patients ($n = 11$) than controls, but basal (unstimulated) growth hormone levels were not different between the two groups.

Geffner et al. (22) studied the in vitro colony formation of erythroid progenitor cells derived from HIV-infected children stage P1, stage P2, and short normal children in response to growth hormone, IGF-I, and insulin. They found that P2 subjects had lower erythroid progenitor cell colony formation in response to all stimuli compared with control and P1 subjects. They suggested that it was this resistance to IGF-I that may contribute to the poor growth of HIV-infected children.

Children with hemophilia provide a unique population for the study of the effects of HIV infection upon growth. In one study, 3 of 22 boys had growth failure: 2 had low IGF-I levels and possible neurosecretory dysregulation of growth hormone secretion (23). In another study, Jason et al. (24) noted a decline in weight percentiles in children with hemophilia following the diagnosis of HIV infection. They suggested that the effect of HIV infection on growth may precede both the clinical and laboratory alterations of the immune deficiency. Similarly, Brettler et al. (25) found that growth failure, defined as a decrease of more than 15 percentile points in height or weight for age for 2 consecutive years, was predictive of the development of symptoms in HIV-positive children with hemophilia. The growth failure in many cases predated the lowering in CD4 levels, generally thought to be a prognostic indicator of disease progression. In a multicenter hemophilia growth and development study, entry data revealed that, adjusted for age, HIV-positive subjects were three times as likely as HIV-negative subjects to have height for age decrements (26). In a recent study, Gertner et al. (27) studied a cohort of 300 boys with hemophilia. Those who were HIV infected, 62% of the total, had lower age-adjusted heights and weights compared with the uninfected boys. Despite decrements in growth parameters, the HIV-infected group had no evidence of wasting or malnutrition. The growth failure was postulated to be caused by delays in pubertal maturation, reflected by delays in bone age and caused by differences in testosterone or sex hormone binding globulin secretion.

In adults, severe HIV infections are at times associated with massive, often debilitating involuntary weight loss that has been referred to as cachexia or wasting syndrome. In an analysis of 147,225 individuals with AIDS reported to the Centers for Disease Control between September 1, 1987 and August 31, 1991, it was found that wasting syndrome was the only AIDS indicator condition in 7.1% of subjects. Wasting syndrome was defined as involuntary weight loss of more than 10% of baseline body weight, in addition to either chronic diarrhea (two or more stools/day for more than 30 days) or chronic weakness and documented fever in the absence of other conditions that could explain the symptoms. Patients with wasting syndrome as the only AIDS-defining diagnosis were more likely to be female, black, or Hispanic and to have contracted HIV by drug use, heterosexual contact, or transfusion. The highest proportion of such patients were from Puerto Rico (47%) (28). Although many factors including decreased oral intake, malabsorption and numerous metabolic disturbances may contribute to wasting, its exact cause is yet to be determined. Investigators have compared this wasting syndrome with starvation and with the weight loss associated with cancers, burns, or other severe metabolic illnesses. Hypertriglyceridemia has been described commonly in patients with AIDS, but it was found not to be related to degree of wasting as measured by total-body potassium as an index of body cell mass (29). The role of cytoxines as potential mediators of the wasting syndrome was also investigated. In AIDS, tumor necrosis factor (TNF) and haptoglobin levels were not increased, but interferon-α (IFN-α) and C-reactive protein were. Levels of these cytokines, however, were not related to plasma cholesterol, high-density lipoprotein cholesterol, or free fatty acids. Plasma triglycerides were correlated with IFN-α levels only. The decrease in cholesterol and cholesterol-containing lipoproteins in AIDS precedes the appearance of hypertriglyceridemia and is unrelated to IFN-α or triglyceride levels (30).

Resting energy expenditure (REE) has been found to be increased in stable malnourished HIV-infected patients with both AIDS and AIDS-related complex (ARC) (31). This increased REE was found not to be decreased by decrements in caloric intake, such as during acute infection, leading to more rapid weight loss (32). The many, and sometimes conflicting, metabolic disturbances accompanying the wasting syndrome of AIDS, as well as the role of cytokines, such as TNF, in its etiology were recently elegantly reviewed by Grunfeld and Feingold (33).

Although malnutrition and evidence of carbohydrate malabsorption as detected by lactose hydrogen breath tests and d-xylose absorption studies are common in HIV-infected children, these abnormalities do not seem to be predictive of or correlated with growth failure (34,35).

We have measured serum and cerebrospinal fluid (CSF) levels of TNF in children with HIV infections with and without progressive encephalopathy (PE). We found that neither serum nor CSF levels of TNF were correlated with the degree of cachexia (wasting) in these children. Serum but not CSF TNF levels were increased in the children who had PE (36).

III. ADRENAL FUNCTION

In patients with HIV infections, the adrenal gland has been the most frequently studied of all endocrine organs. Most of the earlier studies concentrated on pathologic evaluations of adrenal gland involvement in autopsy specimens. More recently, in vivo studies of adrenal function have been undertaken, but mostly in adults.

Pathologic studies have demonstrated frequent involvement of the adrenal glands, most commonly by opportunistic infections, such as cytomegalovirus (CMV), mycobacteria, cryptococci, toxoplasma, and pneumocystis. Neoplasms, such as lymphoma and Kaposi sarcoma, have also been shown to affect the adrenal glands. The frequency of adrenal gland involvement on autopsy material varies from 36 to 90% (37–45). The pattern of adrenal gland involvement, the medulla being the site of primary involvement and with areas of focal and generalized hemorrhage affecting both medulla and cortex, initially described by Reichert et al. (37), has been repeatedly reported since. The adrenal gland is the most common extrapulmonary site of CMV infections (39).

Glasgow et al. (42) found CMV adrenalitis in 21 of 41 cases examined and widespread lipid depletion in most cases (a nonspecific finding on autopsies of critically ill patients). The adrenal cortical involvement was limited to 10% of the cortex in most and less than 70% in all cases. In an attempt to establish clinicopathologic correlation, 32 cases were also analyzed for signs and symptoms of adrenal insufficiency. Common findings were hyponatremia (75%), hypotension (34%), hypokalemia (19%), hyperkalemia (16%), vomiting, diarrhea, and fever (percentage not specified). No patient had hyperpigmentation. Morning levels of serum cortisol were normal or elevated in five of five patients. One of two patients tested had a subnormal increase in cortisol after adrenocorticotropic hormone (ACTH) infusion. Despite significant pathologic adrenal abnormalities, no clinical adrenal insufficiency was documented. The degree of adrenal cortical damage seen was considered less than that usually associated with adrenal insufficiency.

Pulakhandam and Dincsoy (46) found CMV infections in half of 74 autopsied cases of AIDS. Of those 37 cases, the adrenal gland was most commonly affected of all organs, 84% compared with the lungs being affected in 55% of cases. CMV inclusions were found in endothelial, cortical, and medullary cells. The CMV adrenalitis was diffuse in 10 cases and focal in 20. Analysis of clinical data in 30 subjects revealed no findings related to the adrenal pathology, with the possible exception of serum sodium-potassium ratio of less than 30 in those with more severe adrenal pathology.

Clinically, adrenal function has been the most commonly studied of all endocrine parameters. Many of the signs and symptoms characteristic of adrenal insufficiency are seen in severely ill patients with HIV infections. However, definite adrenal insufficiency is rare in subjects with AIDS. The results of the many studies of adrenal function in subjects with AIDS vary depending on the nature of the subjects studied, the severity of the disease, the concomitant intercurrent illnesses and medications to which they are exposed, and the means of adrenal testing—baseline or stimulated levels of glucocorticoids and/or ACTH.

Most studies of adrenal function were performed in adults with HIV infections. Early reports documented both normal and diminished cortisol responses to ACTH in patients with AIDS (47–51). Membreno et al. (52) studied 74 randomly selected hospitalized patients with AIDS and 19 patients with AIDS-related complex. Based on subnormal cortisol responses to ACTH stimulation, 4 patients with AIDS were diagnosed as having adrenal insufficiency. Mean basal cortisol levels were higher in patients with AIDS than in normals, but ACTH-stimulated cortisol responses were not different from normal. However, stimulated levels of 17-deoxysteroid levels (corticosterone and 18-OH-deoxycorticosterone, 18-OHDOC) were lower than normal. Patients with ARC responded in a similar manner as those with AIDS. Based on these findings the authors suggested that impaired 17-deoxysteroid levels, especially 18-OHDOC, may be a "harbinger of progressive adrenal disorder." Plasma ACTH levels were not elevated, and plasma renin and aldosterone levels were normal in patients with adrenal insufficiency, suggesting a possible pituitary defect in these patients. Administration of the hypothalamic factor corticotropin-releasing hormone (CRH) resulted in subnormal 18-OHDOC responses in 2 patients. The authors advanced the hypothesis that HIV pituitary infection could lead to selective hypopituitarism and hypoadrenalism, with subsequent HIV adrenal infection leading to complete adrenal insufficiency.

Dobs et al. (53) reported normal cortisol responses to ACTH in 36 of 39 ambulatory patients with AIDS. Merenich et al. (54), although finding no clinical evidence of endocrine disorders, reported lower baseline cortisol and aldosterone and ACTH-stimulated cortisol levels in 40 asymptomatic HIV-infected men compared with 27 HIV-infected age-matched control subjects; 1 patient had low cortisol and also low ACTH-stimulated aldosterone levels.

HIV-infected subjects have been reported to have lower responses in cortisol and/or ACTH to cold stress (55) or tetanus toxoid administration (56).

Several investigators, however, have reported elevated baseline levels (57–59) or 24 h secretion (60) of cortisol and/or ACTH.

Recently, Catania et al. (61) compared propiomelanocortin-derived peptides and cytokines in 80 patients with AIDS and in 80 normal subjects. Average plasma α-melanocyte-stimulating hormone levels were higher in the AIDS patients, but mean levels of cortisol, ACTH, β-endodorphins, interleukin-1 (IL-1), IL-6, and tumor necrosis factor were not different between the two groups.

In a prospective study of 98 HIV-infected patients, Raffi et al. (62) found only 4 patients with low baseline and 7 with low ACTH-stimulated cortisol levels. Only 2 were believed to have adrenal insufficiency.

To explore further the effect of HIV infection on the hypothalamic-pituitary-adrenal (HPA) axis, Azar and Melby (63) administered ovine CRH (oCRH) to 25 non-AIDS ambulatory HIV-infected patients and 10 normal volunteers: 6 patients had diminished cortisol and ACTH responses to CRH, 6 low cortisol and normal ACTH responses, and 13 normal cortisol and ACTH responses. They suggested enhanced hypothalamic CRH production in HIV infections as a possible explanation for their results. Complex interactions between the immune and HPA axis, mediated by cytokines and perhaps lymphocyte-produced ACTH, have been postulated by some to explain the mechanisms by which HIV infections may affect adrenal function (64,65).

Hyponatremia has been reported in 30% to more than 50% of hospitalized patients with AIDS (66). In most patients, however, the hyponatremia has been thought to be caused by renal and/or gastrointestinal losses and the syndrome of inappropriate secretion of antidiuretic hormone (67–69). Hyporeninemic hypoaldosteronism (70) and also mineralocorticoid deficiency have been reported in patients with AIDS (71). However, the adrenal mineralocorticoid pathway has been found to be normal in both the baseline and ACTH-stimulated states in most HIV-infected patients (57,62).

Serum levels of dehydroepiandrosterone have been reported to be decreased in HIV-infected patients, to correlate with CD4 levels, and to be a reliable predictor of the progression of HIV infection to AIDS (72–75).

Norbiato et al. (76) reported nine patients with AIDS and characteristic clinical features of adrenal insufficiency with elevated cortisol levels suggesting resistance to glucocorticoids characterized by abnormal glucocorticoid receptors on lymphocytes.

In children with symptomatic HIV infections, we measured morning serum cortisol levels ($n = 28$) and found that the lowest levels occurred in those with the lowest CD4 levels. ACTH tests performed on the two children with the lowest cortisol levels were normal, sugesting normal adrenal glucocorticoid function. In seven ill children with AIDS suspected of having adrenal insufficiency, we found normal baseline cortisol levels in all. In four subjects ACTH-stimulated cortisol responses were normal, excluding the diagnosis of adrenal insufficiency (15,77).

Oberfield et al. (78) found normal or slightly elevated baseline and ACTH-stimulated cortisol levels, with mildly diminished stimulated serum deoxycorticosterone and corticosterone levels in 12 HIV-infected children, 2 of whom were receiving ketoconazole, a drug known to inhibit adrenal function. Laue et al. (19) reported normal cortisol responses to ACTH in 8 of 9 children with AIDS; the 1 patient with a subnormal response was receiving treatment with ketoconazole. Schwartz et al. (20) found normal cortisol responses to glucagon stimulation in 12 of 12 HIV-infected children.

Although pathologic specimens have been reported to exhibit AIDS- or CMV-related infiltration of adrenal medullary cells, I know of no systematic studies of adrenal medullary function in either adults or children with HIV infections.

IV. THYROID

During the course of HIV infections, the thyroid gland has been reported to be affected by opportunistic infections. In autopsy specimens thyroid pathology has been described in 10–14% of cases analyzed. Cytomegalovirus inclusions, Kaposi sarcoma, and cyptococcal infections in the thyroid have been reported (39–41,79,80). Fine-needle aspiration of an area of decreased thyroid uptake in an individual with biochemical but not clinical evidence of hypothyroidism revealed *Pneumocystis carinii* infection (81). Following antibiotic therapy, the goiter decreased in size and thyroid function tests became normal.

Clinically significant evidence of hypothyroidism in individuals with HIV disease has been extremely rare. However, many reports have attested to altered biochemical parameters of thyroid function in subjects with HIV infections, especially AIDS. The incidence of clinical or subclinical hypothyroidism in studies of larger series of patients has been as low as 1% (82,83). The most consistent abnormalities described have been low levels of triiodothyronine (T_3), especially in the more severely ill patients, and elevated levels of thyrotropin binding globulin (TBG) (54,82–89). The lowering of serum T_3 levels suggested the kind of biochemical thyroid picture noted in ill patients with nonthyroid disease. Some authors have correlated low T_3 levels with severity of the critical illness and mortality among hospitalized patients with AIDS (84,87). In a minority of patients with asymptomatic HIV infections, exaggerated thyroid-stimulating hormone (TSH) responses to thyrotropin-releasing hormone (TRH) administration have been reported, suggesting a "hypothyroid-like" regulation of the hypothalamic-pituitary-thyroid axis in subjects with stable HIV infections (54,88).

In children, studies of thyroid function have been rare. We observed only 1 child with AIDS and evidence of primary hypothyroidism in whom treatment with replacement doses of thyroid hormone resulted in improvement in growth velocity (90). In children with symptomatic HIV infections we noted transiently abnormal thyroid function test results in 3 of 20 patients. Serum levels of T_3 and free thyroxine did correlated with an index of weight retardation, chronologic age minus weight age (15). Hypothyroidism in 1 of 9 short children with AIDS, along with elevated TBG levels in all 9, and evidence of possible central hypothyroidism (based on timed hourly TSH measurements) were reported by Laue et al. (19). Among 12 clinically and biochemically euthyroid children with AIDS, Schwartz et al. (20) reported elevated TSH responses to TRH in 5.

V. GONADS

The vast majority of information regarding gonadal function in HIV-infected individuals is from studies performed on autopsy material derived from adult men. Reports have included normal (37) to atrophic testicular volumes (39–41), as well as evidence of infiltration by CMV (37,39,91), Kaposi sarcoma (37), toxoplasmosis (91,92), tuberculosis (92), retrovirus-like particles (93), and neoplasms (94). Histologically,

the testes exhibited evidence of peritubular fibrosis, arrest of spermatogenesis, germ cell degeneration and loss of tubular and peritubular fibrosis and hyalinization, thickening of seminiferous tubules and basement membranes, epididymal obstruction, prostatic inclusion, and Leydig cell atrophy (37,39–41, 95–99). The presence of focal HIV-associated proteins, such as HIV P17, was documented by anti-HIV P17 monoclonal antibodies in testes and prostate (98). The possibility of immune-mediated gonadal destruction was not substantiated in one study in which immune complex deposits were found not to be increased in the testes of homosexual AIDS patients compared with those of a control group of heterosexual men without AIDS (97).

Studies of the effects of HIV infection upon hypothalamic-pituitary-gonadal function have been performed mostly in adult men. Most have shown some degree of hypogonadism, especially in the most severely affected individuals. Conflicting data exist regarding the etiology of the hypogonadism as primary, gonadal, or hypothalamic pituitary in origin. Clinical evidence of hypogonadism as reflected by a history of decreased libido and impotence was reported in 28 of 42 and 14 of 42 ambulatory patients with AIDS, respectively (53). Of the HIV-infected men, 38% had low serum testosterone levels, the majority having low baseline serum gonadotropin levels. Human chorionic gonadotropin stimulation in 2 men resulted in normal testosterone responses, attesting to a normal testicular ability to produce testosterone. In 7 of 8 men, gonadotropin-releasing hormone (GnRH) stimulation resulted in normal gonadotropin responses, suggesting that the etiology of the gonadal dysfunction was hypothalamic in origin.

In contrast, Croxson et al. (100) described low testosterone levels accompanied by high levels of luteinizing hormone (LH) and follicle-stimulating hormone in patients with AIDS, suggestive of the diagnosis of primary hypogonadism.

Decreased basal and also mean 24 h plasma testosterone have also been reported by others (62,78). One study has documented elevated free testosterone levels and exaggerated LH responses to GnRH (54). Martin et al. (101) recently reported that HIV-positive patients had 39–51% higher levels of sex steroid binding proteins than HIV-negative control subjects.

Isolated LH deficiency (102) and transient gynecomastia (103) have also been described.

Gonadal function has not been investigated in children with HIV infections. The recent report of Gertner et al. (27) documents pubertal delay accompanied by bone age delay in poorly growing boys with hemophilia. More studies are needed to identify and examine gonadal function in children and females of all ages with HIV infections.

VI. PANCREAS

Anatomic evidence for pancreatic involvement by HIV or associated organisms has been more common than clinical evidence of either exocrine or endocrine pancreatic deficiencies (104).

Pancreatic lesions as a result of HIV, CMV toxoplasmosis, Kaposi sarcoma, lymphoma, and pancreatitis have been reported in autopsy material of patients with AIDS (40,41, 105). Clinical correlation in one of these studies (105) revealed no evidence of hyperglycemia. One report described the development of insulin-dependent diabetes mellitus in two HIV-infected, drug-addicted subjects in whom neither antiinsulin nor antiislet cell antibodies were detected (106). In most HIV-infected patients, normal glucose levels were found (53). Hommes et al. (107) used the euglycemic clamp technique to measure insulin sensitivity and clearance in 10 HIV-infected stable patients and 10 healthy control subjects. They found increased rates of insulin clearance and increased peripheral tissue sensitivity in the HIV-infected men.

Clinical evidence of pancreatitis has not generally been reported, although Zazzo et al. (108), in a prospective study of 35 consecutive patients with AIDS admitted to an intensive care unit, found evidence of acute pancreatitis with elevated levels of amylase and lipase in 16. Of these patients, 8 died and had documentation on autopsy of pancreatic infection by CMV, candida, and cryptococci. Because of the lack of sufficient clinical warning signs of pancreatitis, the authors suggested laboratory measurements of amylase and lipase levels in critically ill HIV-infected patients. Pancreatitis has also been reported in one 3-year-old HIV-positive child (109).

VII. PARATHYROID

Lesions of the parathyroid glands have been reported in autopsy studies (39,41), but parathyroid dysfunction has been reported extremely infrequently. Hypercalcemia with low serum levels of parathyroid hormone and calcitriol has been described in two patients with AIDS and disseminated CMV infection (110). The hypercalcemia improved with calcitriol treatment in one patient. It was postulated by the authors that the hypercalcemia may have been caused by increased osteoclast-mediated bone resorbtion resulting from disseminated CMV infection with accompanying renal insufficiency. Six patients with AIDS-associated lymphoma were found to have hypercalcemia ($n = 4$) or hypercalcuria ($n = 2$), presumably because of the deregulated synthesis of a compound like 1,25-dihydroxyvitamin D (111).

VIII. PROLACTIN

Because of the potential immune regulatory property of prolactin, serum prolactin levels were studied in HIV-infected individuals. Compared with HIV-negative homosexual, bisexual, or heterosexual controls, serum prolactin levels were normal in HIV-infected men, including those with AIDS (112,113).

IX. HYPOTHALAMUS AND PITUITARY

The effects of HIV infections on the central nervous system have been the subject of numerous reports (114). Still, specific pathologic documentation of lesions in the hypothalamus or pituitary of affected individuals has been rare. "Panhypopituitarism" secondary to toxoplasmosis (115) and posterior pituitary lesions in HIV-infected children with disseminated CMV (45) have been reported. Evidence of specific hypothalamic-pituitary dysfunctions in endocrine defects was reviewed in previous sections.

X. SECONDARY ENDOCRINE ALTERATIONS

In HIV-infected children and adults, endocrine dysfunction may also be caused by the effects of the various treatment regimens employed. These effects must be separated from endocrine defects caused by HIV and related opportunistic infections.

Hypothyroidism has been reported as a result of drugs that affect cytochrome P_{450} enzyme systems, such as ketoconazole (116,117) and rifampin (118), as well as interferon treatment (119,120).

Hypoadrenalism may result from ketoconazole (121–123) or rifampin (124,125) treatment. Hypogonadism and gynecomastia in men have also been noted during ketoconazole treatment (126,127). Hypoglycemia has been reported in patients with AIDS treated with pentamidine (128–131) and trimethoprim-sulfamethoxazole (132). Hyponatremia has been associated with pentamidine (133) and vidarabine (134) therapy. Hypocalcemic tetany secondary to magnesium loss has been noted during amphotericin B and aminoglycoside treatment (135). Hyperkalemia was reported in a patient with AIDS to be a result of the sodium channel inhibitory effect of trimethoprim (136).

XI. FUTURE HORMONAL THERAPY IN HIV INFECTIONS

Antiretroviral therapy has been the mainstay of therapy of HIV-infected individuals. In children, it has been reported to result in at least short-term improvement in weight gain (137). Treatment of pregnant women may result in growth retardation in a small number of infants (138).

Hormonal therapy in HIV disease is still in the very preliminary stages and awaiting the performance of large, controlled clinical studies. Thymus-derived hormones, such as thymopoietin, have been shown in preliminary reports to lead to an improvement in $CD4^+$ cell counts and CD4/CD8 ratios, thereby, it is hoped, at least slowing the immune deterioration of HIV infections (139,140). Dehydroepiandrosterone was administered in three different doses to subjects with symptomatic HIV disease and CD4 lymphocyte counts of 250–600 cells/ml for 16 weeks. The drug was well tolerated, but it resulted in no sustained improvements in CD4 cell counts or decreases in serum p24 antigens or β_2-microglobulin levels (141).

Considerable attention has focused on the reversal of the weight loss and wasting syndrome accompanying AIDS. Therapeutic strategies have involved the use of appetite stimulants, such as megesterol acetate, anticytokine-directed supplements, such as dietary $N - 3$ fatty acids, anabolic agents, such as anabolic steroids and growth hormone, and metabolic inhibitors, such as hydrazine sulfate (142,143).

The most extensive experience with megesterol acetate in adults was recently summarized (144–146). Initial encouraging results of its effects on improvements in appetite, weight, and quality of life are being studied in multicenter trials in children.

Growth hormone (GH) and insulin-like growth factor I have been utilized in very few HIV-infected patients. In a prospective double-blind clinical trial, 5 patients were assigned randomly to treatment with GH at either 5.0 or 2.5 mg every other day (147). Of the 10, 3 withdrew because of opportunistic infections. In the remaining patients, all of whom were also receiving zidovudine, the higher dose of GH reversed the pretreatment weight loss by increasing lean body mass and total-body water and decreasing total-body fat and urinary nitrogen excretion. Muscle power and endurance also improved. Fasting plasma glucose, insulin, and C peptide increased in all. CD4 cell counts did not change. During treatment 1 patient became p24 antigen positive. The short-term beneficial effects were noted only with the higher GH doses.

In a short-term, carefully conducted clinical trial, Mulligan et al. (148) administered GH, 0.1 mg/kg/day for 7 days, to six HIV-positive men with an average weight loss of 19% and six healthy HIV-negative subjects. Treatment resulted in an increase in body weight, nitrogen retention, increased energy expenditure, lipid oxidation, and glucose flux and decreased protein oxidation in both groups. These short-term effects of increases in protein anabolism and protein-sparing lipid oxidation, should they be sustained during long-term treatment, were postulated to result in increased total-body cell mass.

Recently, Lieberman et al. (149) found that a single injection of growth hormone to 21 patients with AIDS resulted in a smaller increase in IGF-I than in 23 age-matched controls, suggesting partial resistance to growth hormone in AIDS. In 10 subjects low-dose but not high-dose IGF-I administration for 10 days resulted in only a transient anabolic effect as demonstrated by a transient increase in nitrogen retention.

Further studies will undoubtedly be undertaken to study the effects of either GH or IGF-I or the concomitant administration of both agents in larger populations of HIV-infected subjects, including children.

XII. CONCLUSION

In the future, more and more infants and children will be diagnosed with HIV infections. With advances in therapy the survival of HIV-infected children and their quality of life will improve. Pediatric endocrinologists will be called upon more and more to evaluate and treat children suffering from HIV infection-related diseases. It will become increasingly important, therefore, to conduct careful clinical investigations to assess endocrine dysfunction in HIV-infected children, as well as the potential interactions between HIV disease and the endocrine system. Evidence documenting bidirectional communications between the endocrine and immune systems is accumulating at a rapid pace (150).

The evaluation and treatment of endocrine alterations in subjects with HIV infections will continue to become an increasingly important clinical and investigational area of pediatric endocrinology.

REFERENCES

1. Oleske J, Minnefor A, Cooper R Jr, et al. Immune deficiency syndrome in children. JAMA 1983; 249:2345–2349.
2. Rubinstein A, Sicklick M, Gupta A, et al. Acquired immuno-deficiency with reversed T4/T8 ratios in infants born to promiscuous and drug addicted mothers. JAMA 1983; 249: 2350–2356.
3. Rogers MF, Kilbourne BW. Epidemiology of pediatric HIV infection. In: Wormser GP, ed. AIDS and Other Manifestations of HIV Infections, 2d ed. New York: Raven Press, 1992:17–24.
4. Grubman S, Conviser R, Oleske J. HIV infections in infants, children, and adolescents. In: AIDS and Other Manifestations of HIV Infections, 2d ed. New York: Raven Press, 1992:201–216.
5. Scott GB, Buck BE, Leterman JG, Bloom FL, Parks WO. Acquired immunodeficiency syndrome in infants. N Engl J Med 1984; 12(310):76–81.
6. Marion RW, Wiznia AA, Hutcheon RG, Rubinstein A. Human T-cell lympho-tropic virus type III (HTLV-III) embryopathy. Am J Dis Child 1986; 140:638–640.
7. Iosub S, Bamji M, Stone RK, Gromisch DS, Wasserman E. More on human immunodeficiency virus embryopathy. Pediatrics 1987; 80:512–516.
8. Rubinstein A. Pediatric AIDS. Curr Probl Pediatr 1986; 16(7):379–380.
9. Shannon KM, Ammann AJ. Acquired immune deficiency syndrome in children. J Pediatr 1985; 106(332):42.
10. Falloon J, Eddy J, Wiener L, Pizzo PA. Human immunodeficiency virus infection in children. J Pediatr 1989; 114:1–30.
11. Kamani N, Lightman H, Leiderman MS, Krilov LR. Pediatric acquired immunodeficiency syndrome-related complex: clinical and immunologic features. J Pediatr Infect Dis 1988; 7:383–388.
12. Johnson JP, Nair P, Hines SE, et al. Natural history and serologic diagnosis of infants born to human immunodeficiency virus-infected women. Am J Dis Child 1989; 143:1147–1153.
13. Maas U. Kattner E, Koch S, Schafer A, Obladen M. Fetal development and neonatal morbidity in infants of HIV-positive mothers. Monatsschr Kinderheilk 1990; 138:799–802.
14. Blanche S, Le Keist F, Fischer A, et al. Longitudinal study of 18 children with perinatal LAV/HTLV II, infection: attempt at prognostic evaluation. J Pediatr 1986; 109:965–970.
15. Rapaport R, McSherry G, Connor E, et al. Growth and hormonal parameters in symptomatic human immunodeficiency virus (HIV) infected children (abstract). Pediatr Res 1989; 25:187A.
16. Rapaport R, Sills I, Figueroa W, Hoyt I, Mintz M. Growth failure (GF) in HIV infected children (HIV-IC) (abstract). Pediatr Res 1993; 33:82A.
17. McKinney RE, Wesley J, Robertson R. Effect on human immunodeficiency virus infection on the growth of young children. J Pediatr 1993; 123:579–582.
18. Jospe N, Powell KR. Growth hormone deficiency in an

8-year-old girl with human immunodeficiency virus infection. Pediatrics 1990; 86:309–312.

19. Laue L, Pizzo PA, Butler K, Cutler GB Jr. Growth and neuroendocrine dysfunction in children with acquired immunodeficiency syndrome. J Pediatr 1990; 117:541–545.

20. Schwartz LJ, Louis Y, Wu R, Wiznia A, Rubinstein A, Saenger P. Endocrine function in children with human immunodeficiency virus infection. Am J Dis Child 1991; 145: 330–333.

21. Lepage P, Van de Perre P, Van Vliet G, et al. Clinical and endocrinologic manifestations in perinatally human immunodeficiency virus type 1-Infected children aged 5 years or older. Am J Dis Child 1991; 145:1248–1251.

22. Geffner ME, Yeh DY, Landaw EM, et al. In vitro insulin-like growth factor-I, growth hormone, and insulin resistance occurs in symptomatic human immunodeficiency virus-1-infected children. Pediatri Res 1993; 34:66–72.

23. Kaufman FR, Gomperts ED. Growth failure in boys with hemophilia and HIV infection. Am J Pediatr Hematol Oncol 1989; 11:292–294.

24. Jason J, Gomperts E, Lawrence DN, et al. HIV and hemophilic children's growth. J Acquir Immune Defic Syndr 1989; 2:277–282.

25. Brettler DB, Forsberg A, Bolivar E, Brewster F, Sullivan J. Growth failure as a prognostic indicator for progression to acquired immunodeficiency syndrome in children with hemophilia. J Pediatr 1990; 117:584–588.

26. Hilgartner MW, Donfield SM, Willoughby A, et al. Hemophilia growth and development study. Am J Pediatr Hematol Oncol 1993; 15:208–217.

27. Gertner JM, Kaufman FR, Danfield SM, et al. Delayed somatic growth and pubertal development in human immunodeficiency virus-infected hemophiliac boys: hemophilia growth and development study. J Pediatr 1994; 124(6):896–902.

28. Nahlen BL, Chu SY, Nwanyanwu OC, Berkelman RL, Martinez SA, Rullan JV. HIV wasting syndrome in the United States. AIDS 1993; 7:183–188.

29. Grunfeld C, Kotler DP, Hamadeh R, Tierney A, Wang J, Pierson RN. Hypertriglyceridemia in the acquired immunodeficiency syndrome. Am J Med 1989; 86:27–31.

30. Grunfeld C, Pang M, Doerrler W, Shigenaga JK, Jensen P, Feingold KR. Lipids, lipoproteins, triglyceride clearance, and cytokines in human immunodeficiency virus infection and the acquired immuno-deficiency syndrome. J Clin Endocrinol Metab 1992; 74:1045–1052.

31. Melchior C, Salmon D, Rigaud D, et al. Resting energy expenditure is increased in stable, malnourished HIV-infected patients. Am J Clin Nutr 1991; 53:437–441.

32. Grunfeld C, Pang M, Shimizu L, Shigenaga JK, Jensen P, Feingold KR. Resting energy expenditure, caloric intake, and short-term weight change in human immunodeficiency virus infection and the acquired immunodeficiency syndrome. Am J Clin Nutr 1992; 55:455–460.

33. Grunfeld C, Feingold KR. Metabolic disturbances and wasting in the acquired immunodeficiency syndrome. N Eng J Med 1992; 327:329–337.

34. Miller TL, Ovav EJ, Martin SR, Cooper ER, McIntosh K, Winter HS. Malnutrition and carbohydrate malabsorption in children with vertically transmitted human immunodeficiency virus 1 infection. Gastroenterology 1991; 100:1296–1302.

35. Brief critical reviews. Is malabsorption an important cause of growth failure in HIV-infected children? Nutr Rev 1991; 49:341–343.

36. Mintz M, Rapaport R, Oleske JM, et al. Elevated serum levels of tumor necrosis factor are associated with progressive

encephalopathy in children with acquired immunodeficiency syndrome. Am J Dis Child 1989; 143:171–174.

37. Reichert CM, O'Leary TJ, Levens DL, Simrell CR, Macher AM. Autopsy pathology in the acquired immune deficiency syndrome. Am J Pathol 1983; 112:357–382.

38. Tapper ML, Rotterdam HZ, Lerner CW, Al'Khafaji K, Seitzman PM. Adrenal necrosis in the acquired immunodeficiency syndrome. Ann Intern Med 1984; 100:239–241.

39. Welch K, Finkbeiner W, Alpers CE, et al. Autopsy findings in the acquired immune deficiency syndrome. Ann Intern Med 1984; 100:239–240.

40. Mobley K, Rotterdam HZ, Lerner CW, Tapper ML. Autopsy findings in the acquired immune deficiency syndrome. Pathol Ann 1985; 20:45–65.

41. Niedt GW, Schinella RA. Acquired immunodeficiency syndrome. Arch Pathol Lab Med 1985; 109:727–734.

42. Glasgow BJ, Steinsapir KD, Anders K, Layfield LJ. Adrenal pathology in the acquired immune deficiency syndrome. Am J Clin Pathol 1985; 84:594–597.

43. Weiss CD. The human immunodeficiency virus and the adrenal medulla. Ann Intern Med 1986; 105:300.

44. Laulund S, Visfeldt J, Klinken L. Patho-anatomical studies in patients dying of AIDS. Acta Pathol Microbiol Immunol Scand [A] 1986; 94:201–221.

45. Joshi VV, Oleske JM, Saad S, Connor EM, Rapkin RH, Minnefor AB. Pathology of opportunistic infections in children with acquired immune deficiency syndrome. Pediatr Pathol 1986; 6:145–150.

46. Pulakhandam U, Dincsoy HP. Cytomegaloviral adrenalitis and adrenal insufficiency in AIDS. Am J Clin Pathol 1990; 93:651–656.

47. Klein RS, Mann DN, Friedland GH, Surks MI. Adrenocortical function in the acquired immunodeficiency syndrome. Ann Intern Med 1983; 99:566.

48. Greene LW, Cole W, Greene JB, et al. Adrenal insufficiency as a complication of the acquired immunodeficiency syndrome. Ann Intern Med 1984; 101:497–498.

49. Guenthner EE, Rabinowe SL, Van Niel A, Naftilan A, Dluhy RG. Primary Addison's disease in a patient with the acquired immuno-deficiency syndrome. Ann Intern Med 1984; 100: 847–848.

50. Salik JM, Kurtin P. Severe hyponatremia after colonoscopy preparation in a patient with the acquired immune deficiency syndrome. Am J Gastroenterol 1985; 80:177–179.

51. Bleiweiss IJ, Pervez NK, Hammer GS, Dikman SH. Cytomegalovirus-induced adrenal insufficiency and associated renal cell carcinoma in AIDS. Mt Sinai J Med 1986; 53: 676–679.

52. Membreno L, Irony I, Dere W, Klein R, Biglieri EG, Cobb E. Adrenocortical function in acquired immunodeficiency syndrome. J Clin Endocrinol Metab 1987; 65:482–487.

53. Dobs AS, Dempsey MA, Ladenson PW, Polk BP. Endocrine disorders in men infected with human immunodeficiency virus. Am J Med 1988; 84:611–616.

54. Merenich JA, McDermott MT, Asp AA, Harrison SM, Kidd GS. Evidence of endocrine involvement early in the course of human immuno-deficiency virus infection. J Clin Endocrinol Metab 1990; 70:566–571.

55. Kumar M, Kumar AM, Morgan R, Szapocznik J, Eisdorfer C. Abnormal pituitary-adrenocortical response in early HIV-1 infection. J Acquir Immune Defic Syndr 1993; 6:61–65.

56. Catania A, Manfredi MG, Airaghi L, et al. Delayed cortisol response to antigenic challenge in patients with acquired immunodeficiency syndrome. Ann NY Acad Sci 1992; 650: 202–204.

57. Verges B, Chavanet P, Desgres J, et al. Adrenal function in

HIV infected patients. Acta Endocrinol (Copenh) 1989; 121: 633–637.

58. Christeff N, Gharakhanian S, Thobie N, Rozenbaum W, Nuenez EA. Evidence for changes in adrenal and testicular steroids during HIV infection. J Acquir Immune Defic Syndr 1992; 5:841–846.

59. Malone JL, Oldfield EC, Wagner KF, et al. Abnormalities of morning serum cortisol levels and circadian rhythms of CD4 lymphocyte counts in human immunodeficiency virus type 1-infected adult patients. J Infect Dis 1992; 156:185.

60. Villette JM, Dourin P, Doinel C, et al. Circadian variations in plasma levels of hypophyseal adrenocortical and testicular hormones in men infected with human immunodeficiency virus. J Clin Endocrinol Metab 1990; 70:572–577.

61. Catania A, Airaghi L, Manfredi MG, et al. Proopiomelano-cortin-derived peptides and cytokines: relations in patients with acquired immunodeficiency syndrome. Clin Immun Immuno-pathol 1993; 66:73–79.

62. Raffi F, Brisseau JM, Planchon B, Remi JP, Barrier JH, Grolleau JY. Endocrine function in 98 HIV-infected patients: a prospective study. AIDS 1991; 5:729–733.

63. Azar ST, Melby JC. Hypothalamic-pituitary-adrenal function in non-AIDS patients with advanced HIV infection. Am J Med Sci 1993; 305:321–325.

64. Gonovan DS, Dluhy RG. AIDS and its effect on the adrenal gland. Endocrinologist 1991; 1:227–232.

65. Grinspoon SK, Bilezikian JP. HIV disease and the endocrine system. N Engl J Med 1992; 32:1360–1365.

66. Vitting KE, Gardenswartz MH, Zabetakis PM, et al. Frequency of hyponatremia and nonosmolar vasopressin release in the acquired immunodeficiency syndrome. JAMA 1990; 263:973–978.

67. Agarwal A, Soni A, Ciechanowsky M, Chander P, Treser G. Hyponatremia in patients with the acquired immunodeficiency syndrome. Nephron 1989; 53:317–321.

68. Cusano AJ, Thies HL, Siegal FP, Dreisbach AW, Maesaka JK. Hyponatremia in patients with acquired immune deficiency syndrome. J Acquir Immune Defic Syndr 1990; 3:949–953.

69. Tang WW, Kaptein EM, Feinstein EI, Massry SG. Hyponatremia in hospitalized patients with the acquired immunodeficiency syndrome (AIDS) and the AIDS-related complex. Am J Med 1993; 94:169–174.

70. Kalin MF, Poretsky L, Seres DS, Zumoff B. Hyporeninemic hypoaldo-steronism associated with acquired immune deficiency syndrome. Am J Med 1987; 82:1035–1038.

71. Guy RJC, Turberg Y, Davidson RN, Finnerty G, MacGregor GA, Wise PH. Mineralocorticoid deficiency in HIV infection. BMJ 1989; 298:496–497.

72. Merril CR, Harrington MG, Sunderland T. Plasma dehydro-epiandrosterone levels in HIV infection. JAMA 1989; 261: 1149.

73. Jacobson MA, Fusaro RE, Galmarini M, Lang W. Decreased serum dehydroepiandrosterone is associated with an increased progression of human immunodeficiency virus infection in men with CD4 cell counts of 200–499. J Infect Dis 1991; 164:864–868.

74. Mulder JW, Jos Frissen PH, Krijnen P, et al. Dehydroepian-drosterone as predictor for progression to AIDS in asymptomatic human immunodeficiency virus-infected men. J Infect Dis 1992; 165:413–418.

75. Wisniewski TL, Hilton CW, Morse EV, Svec F. The relationship of serum DHEA-S and cortisol levels to measures of immune function in human immunodeficiency virus-related illness. Am J Med Sci 1993; 305:79–83.

76. Norbiato G, Bevilacqua M, Vago T, et al. Cortisol resistance

in acquired immunodeficiency syndrome. J Clin Endocrinol Metab 1992; 74:608–613.

77. Rapaport R, McSherry G, Connor E, Oleske J. Neuroendo-crine function in acquired immunodeficiency syndrome (letter). J Pediatr 1991; 118:828.

78. Oberfield SE, Kairam R, Bakshi S, et al. Steroid response to adrenocorticotropin stimulation in children with human immunodeficiency virus infection. J Clin Endocrinol Metab 1990; 70:578–581.

79. Frank TS, LiVolsi VA, Connor M. Cytomegalovirus infection of the thyroid in immunocompromised adults. Yale J Biol Med 1987; 60:1–8.

80. Machac J, Nejatheim M, Goldsmith SJ. Gallium citrate uptake in cryptococcal thyroiditis in a homosexual male. J Nucl Med Allied Sci 1985; 29:283–285.

81. Battan R, Mariuz P, Raviglione MC, Sabatini MT, Mullen MP, Poretsky L. *Pneumocystis carinii* infection of the thyroid in a hypothyroid patient with AIDS: diagnosis by fine needle aspiration biopsy. J Clin Endocrinol Metab 1991; 72:724–726.

82. Bourdoux PP, DeWit SA, Servais GM, Clumeck N, Bonnyns MA. Biochemical thyroid profile in patients infected with the human immunodeficiency virus. Thyroid 1991; 1:147–149.

83. Tang WW, Kaptein EM. Thyroid hormone levels in the acquired immunodeficiency syndrome (AIDS) or AIDS-related complex. West J Med 1989; 151:627–631.

84. LoPresti JS, Fried JC, Spencer CA, Nicoloff JT. Unique alterations of thyroid hormone indices in the acquired immunodeficiency syndrome (AIDS). Ann Intern Med 1989; 110:970–975.

85. Feldt-Rasmussen U, Sestoft L, Berg H. Thyroid function tests in patients with acquired immune deficiency syndrome and healthy HIV1-positive out-patients. Eur J Clin Invest 1991; 21:59–63.

86. Lambert M, Zech F, DeNayer P, Jamez J, Vandercam B. Elevation of serum thyroxine-binding globulin associated with the progression of human immunodeficiency virus infection. Am J Med 1990; 89:748–751.

87. Fried JC, LoPresti JS, Micon M, Bauer M, Tuchschmidt JA, Nicoloff JT. Serum triiodothyronine values: prognostic indicators of acute mortality due to *pneumocystis carinii* pneumonia associated with the acquired immunodeficiency syndrome. Arch Intern Med 1990; 150:406–409.

88. Hommes MJT, Romijn JA, Endert E, et al. Hypothyroid-like regulation of the pituitary-thyroid axis in stable human immunodeficiency virus infection. Metabolism 1993; 42:556–561.

89. Sato K, Ozawa M, Demura H. Thyroid function in the acquired immunodeficiency syndrome (AIDS). Ann Intern Med 1989; 111:857–858.

90. Rapaport R, McSherry G. Unpublished data. 1993.

91. Chabon AB, Stenger RJ, Grabstald H. Histopathology of testes in acquired immune deficiency syndrome. Urology 1987; 29:658–663.

92. Nistal M, Santana A, Paniagna R, Palacios J. Testicular toxoplasmosis in two men with the acquired immunodeficiency syndrome (AIDS). Arch Pathol Lab Med 1986; 110:744–746.

93. Lecatsas G, Houff S, Macher A, et al. Retrovirus-like particles in salivary glands, prostate and testes of AIDS patients. Proc Soc Exp Biol Med 1985; 178:653–655.

94. Tessler AN, Cantanese A. AIDS and serous cell tumors of the testes. Urology 1987; 30:203–204.

95. Yoshikawa Y, Truong LD, Fraire AE, Kim HS. The spectrum of histopathology of the testis in acquired immunodeficiency syndrome. Mod Pathol 1989; 2:233–238.

96. De Paege ME, Waxman M. Testicular atrophy in AIDS: a study of 57 autopsy cases. Hum Pathol 1989; 20:210–214.

97. De Paege ME, Vuletin JC, Lee MH, Rojas-Corona RR, Waxman M. Testicular atrophy in homosexual AIDS patients. Hum Pathol 1989; 20:572–578.

98. Da Silva M, Shevchuk MM, Cronin WJ, et al. Detection of HIV-related protein in testes and prostates of patients with AIDS. Hum Pathol 1989; 20:572–578.

99. Dalton ADA, Harcout-Webster JN. The histopathology of the testis and epididymis in AIDS—a post-mortem study. J Pathol 1991;

100. Croxson TS, Chapman WE, Miller LK, Levit CD, Senie R, Zumoff B. Changes in the hypothalamic-pituitary-gonadal axis in human immuno-deficiency virus-infected homosexual men. J Clin Endocrinol Metab 1989; 68:317–321.

101. Martin ME, Benassayag C, Amiel C, Canton P, Nunez EA. Alterations in the concentrations and binding properties of sex steroid binding protein and corticosteroid-binding globulin in HIV^+ patients. J Endocrinol Invest 1992; 15:597–603.

102. Garavelli PL, Azzini M, Boccalatte G, Rosti G. Isolated LH deficiency in an AIDS patient (letter). J Acquir Immune Defic Synd 1990; 3:547.

103. Couderc LJ, Clauvel JP. HIV-infection-induced gynecomastia. Ann Intern Med 1987; 107:257.

104. Schwartz MS, Brandt LJ. The spectrum of pancreatic disorders in patients with the acquired immune deficiency syndrome. Am J Gastroenterol 1989; 84:459–462.

105. Brivet F, Coffin B, Bedossa P, et al. Pancreatic lesions in AIDS (letter). Lancet 1987; 2:1212.

106. Vendrell J, Nubiola A, Goday A, et al. HIV and the pancreas (letter). Lancet 1987; 2:1212.

107. Hommes MJ, Romijn JA, Endert E, Eeftinck SchattenkerK JKM, Sauerwein HP. Insulin sensitivity and insulin clearance in human immunodeficiency virus-infected men. Metabolism 1991; 40:651–656.

108. Zazzo JF, Pichon F, Regnier B. HIV and the pancreas (letter). Lancet 1987; 2:1212.

109. Torre D, Montanari M, Fiore GP. HIV and pancreas (letter). Lancet 1987; 2:1212.

110. Zaloga GP, Chernow B, Eil C. Hypercalcemia and disseminated cyto-megalovirus infection in the acquired immunodeficiency syndrome. Ann Intern Med 1985; 102:331–333.

111. Adams JS, Fernandez M, Gacad MA, et al. Vitamin D metabolite-mediated hypercalcemia and hypercalciuria patients with AIDS- and non-AIDS-associated lymphoma. Blood 1989; 73:235–239.

112. Chernow B, Schooley RT, Dracup K, Napolitano LM, Stanford GG, Klibanski A. Serum prolactin concentrations in patients with the acquired immunodeficiency syndrome. Crit Care Med 1990; 18:440–441.

113. Gorman JM, Warne PA, Begg MD, et al. Serum prolactin levels in homosexual and bisexual men with HIV infection. Am J Psychiatry 1992; 149:367–370.

114. Mintz M. Neurologic abnormalities. In: Yogev IR, Connor E, eds. Management of HIV Infection in Infants and Children. Chicago: Mosby Year Book 1992:247–87.

115. Milligan SA, Katz MS, Craven PC, Strandberg DA, Russell IJ, Becker RA. Toxoplasmosis presenting as panhypopituitarism in a patient with acquired immunodeficiency syndrome. Am J Med 1984; 77:760–764.

116. Kitching NH. Hypothyroidism after treatment with ketoconazole. BMJ 1986; 293:993–994.

117. Tanner AR. Hypothyroidism after treatment with ketoconazole. BMJ 1987; 294:125.

118. Isley WL. Effect of rifampin therapy of thyroid function tests in a hypothyroid patient on replacement of E-thyroxine. Ann Intern Med 1987; 107:517–518.

119. Fentiman IS, Thomas BS, Balkwill FR, Rubens RD, Hayward JL. Primary hypothyroidism associated with interferon therapy of breast cancer. Lancet 1985; 1:1166.

120. Burman P, Trotterman TH, Oberg K, Karlsson FA. Thyroid autoimmunity in patients on long-term therapy with leukocyte-derived interferon. J Clin Endocrinol Metab 1986; 63:1086–1090.

121. Sonino N. The use of ketoconazole as an inhibitor of steroid production. N Engl J Med 1987; 317:812–818.

122. Tucker WS Jr, Snell BB, Island DP, Gregg CR. Reversible adrenal insufficiency induced by ketoconazole. JAMA 1985; 253:2413–2414.

123. Best TR, Jenkins JK, Murphy FY, Nicks SA, Bussell KL, Vesely DL. Persistent adrenal insufficiency secondary to low-dose ketoconazole therapy. Am J Med 1987; 82:676–680.

124. Elansary EH, Earis JE. Rifampicin and renal crisis. BMJ 1983; 286:1861–1862.

125. Kryiazopoulou V, Parparadi O, Vagenaskis AG. Rifampicin-induced renal crisis in Addison patients receiving corticosteroid replacement therapy. J Clin Endocrinol Metab 1984; 59:1204–1206.

126. Pont A, Graybill JR, Crayen PC, et al. High dose ketoconazole therapy and renal and testicular function in humans. Arch Intern Med 1984; 144:2150–2153.

127. Pont A, Goldman ES, Sugar AM, Siiteri PK, Stevens DA. Ketoconazole-induced increase in estriol-testosterone ratio. Arch Intern Med 1985; 145:1429–1431.

128. Ganada OP. Pentamidine and hypoglycemia. Ann Intern Med 1984; 100:464.

129. Stahl-Bayliss CM. Pentamidine-induced hypoglycemia in patients with the acquired immune deficiency syndrome. Clin Pharmacol Ther 1986; 39:271–275.

130. Perronne C, Bricaire F, Leport C, Assan D, Vilde JL, Assan R. Hypoglycemia and diabetes mellitus following parenteral pentamidine mesylate treatment in AIDS patients. Diabetic Med 1990; 7:585–589.

131. Hauser L, Sheehan P, Simpkins H. Pancreatic pathology in pentamidine-induced diabetes in acquired immunodeficiency syndrome patients. Hum Pathol 1991; 22:926–929.

132. Gordin FM, Simon GL, Wofsy CB, Mills J. Adverse reactions to trimethoprim-sulfamethoxazole in patients with the acquired immunodeficiency syndrome. Ann Intern Med 1984; 100:495–499.

133. Andersen R, Boedicker M, Ma M, Goldstein EJ. Adverse reactions associated with pentamidine isothionate in AIDS patients: recommendations for monitoring therapy. Drug Intell Clin Pharm 1986; 20:862–868.

134. Semel JD, McNerney JJ Jr. SIADH during disseminated herpes varicella-zoster infections: relationship to vidarabine therapy. Am J Med Sci 1986; 291:115–118.

135. Davies SV, Murray JA. Amphotericin B, aminoglycosides, and hypomagnesemic tetany. BMJ 1986; 292:1395–1396.

136. Choi MJ, Fernandez PC, Coupaye-Gerard B, D'Andrea D, Szerlip H, Kleyman TR. Brief report: Trimethoprim-induced hyperkalemia in a patient with AIDS. N Engl J Med 1993; 328:703–706.

137. Palasanthiran P, Ziegler JB, Kemp AS, et al. Zidovudine (AZT) therapy in children with HIV infection: the Australian experience. J Pediatr Child Health 1990; 26:257–262.

138. Sperling RS, Stratton P, O'Sullivan MJ, et al. A survey of zidovudine use in pregnant women with human immunodeficiency virus infection. N Engl J Med 1992; 326:857–861.

139. Gianotti N, Finazzi R, Uberti Foppa C, Danise A, Migone T, Lazzarin A. The thymic hormones in the treatment of immune deficiency related to HIV infection. Pharmacol Res 1992; 26:62–63.

140. Conant MA, Calabrese LH, Thompson SE, et al. Maintenance

of CD4$^+$ cells by thymopentin in asymptomatic HIV-infected subjects: results of a double-blind, placebo-controlled study. AIDS 1992; 6:135–139.

141. Dyner TS, Lang W, Geaga J, et al. An open-label dose-escalation trial or oral dehydroepiandrosterone tolerance and pharmacokinetics in patients with HIV disease. J Acquir Immune Defic Syndr 1993; 6:459–465.

142. Hellerstein MK, Kahn J, Mudie H, Viteri F. Current approach to the treatment of human immunodeficiency virus-associated weight loss: pathophysiologic considerations and emerging management strategies. Semin Oncol 1990; 17:17–33.

143. Loprinzi CL, Ellison NM, Goldberg RM, Michalak JC, Burch PA. Alleviation of cancer anorexia and cachexia: studies of the Mayo Clinic and the North Central Cancer Treatment Group. Semin Oncol 1990; 17:8–12.

144. Aisner J, Parnes H, Tait N, et al. Appetite stimulation and weight gain with megestrol acetate. Semin Oncol 1990; 17:2–7.

145. Von Roenn JH, Murphy RL, Wegener N. Megestrol acetate for treatment of anorexia and cachexia associated with human immunodeficiency virus infection. Semin Oncol 1990; 17:13–16.

146. Coltman CA, Abrams JS, Aisner J, et al. (panel participants). Therapy to promote weight gain in cancer and acquired immunodeficiency syndrome patients: a panel discussion (Part 1). Semin Oncol 1990; 17:34–37.

147. Krentz AJ, Koster FT, Crist DM, et al. Anthropometric, metabolic, and immunological effects of recombinant human growth hormone in AIDS and AIDS-related complex. J Acquir Immune Defic Syndr 1993; 6:245–251.

148. Mulligan K, Grunfeld C, Hellerstein MK, Nesse RA, Schambelan M. Anabolic effects of recombinant human growth hormone in patients with wasting associated with human immunodeficiency virus infection. J Clin Endocrinol Metab 1993; 77:956–962.

149. Lieberman SA, Butterfield GE, Harrison D, Hoffman AR. Anabolic effects of recombinant insulin-like growth factor-I in cachectic patients with the acquired immunodeficiency syndrome. J Clin Endocrinol Metab 1994; 78:404–410.

150. Rapaport R. Immunomodulation by growth hormone in humans. In: Berczi I, Szelenyi J, eds. Advances in Psychoneuroimmunology. New York and London: Plenum Press, 1994.

56

Endocrine Problems After Cancer Therapy

Raphael Rappaport and Elisabeth Thibaud

Hôpital des Enfants Malades,
Paris, France

I. INTRODUCTION

Advances in the treatment of malignant diseases have resulted in a dramatic fall in mortality rates for most of them, which means that an increasing number of survivors may have to cope with the late effects of cancer treatment. The protocols used include surgery, tumor-targeted radiotherapy, chemotherapy, and, more recently, total-body irradiation and/or intensive chemotherapy followed by bone marrow transplantation. There has now been a sufficient follow-up interval for most conditions and for the current therapeutic regimens, so that most children can be followed with a prospective view of potential complications. Appropriate therapeutic decisions can therefore be taken to avoid or minimize severe complications, such as dwarfism or abnormal pubertal development. Although the primary goal is still to cure the malignant disease, knowledge of the side effects also contributes to the choice of any new therapeutic protocol.

According to the British National Registry of Childhood Tumors, acute leukemias, mostly lymphoblastic leukemias occurring in early childhood, account for one-third of all registrations. Lymphomas, most frequently non-Hodgkin's type, account for a further 10%, with a higher incidence in late childhood. Brain and spinal tumors make up 25% of all tumors, and retinoblastoma, which is often bilateral and familial, is a major condition requiring cranial irradiation in infants. Most of these tumors require high doses of radiation, which severely damage the hypothalamus and pituitary gland. The remaining childhood cancers include gonadal, bone and soft tissue sarcomas, and embryonal tumors, such as Wilms' tumors and neuroblastomas (1).

Because most of the children with malignant diseases are treated according to nationally or internationally driven protocols in pediatric oncology centers, it has now become clear that the most constructive evaluation and follow-up of survivors might be undertaken by a combined endocrinology and oncology clinic. Most treatment protocols combine chemotherapy and irradiation, but chemotherapy is becoming an important and sometimes exclusive form of treatment in many conditions. It is therefore important to consider the detailed structure of a given treatment for each child, focusing on the location of the radiation fields causing direct damage to endocrine glands or to the skeleton and on the use of cytotoxic chemotherapy that could be responsible for direct damage to the gonads (Table 1). In general, the time at which the late endocrine effects may occur is quite variable.

II. GROWTH HORMONE SECRETION

The first case of induced hypopituitarism after cranial radiation for a tumor distant from the hypothalamic-pituitary region was reported in 1966 (2), and growth hormone (GH) deficiency is at present the most common pituitary defect after radiation (Table 2). The hypothalamus is more radiosensitive than the pituitary gland, so that GH deficiency is probably caused by a dysfunction of GH releasing hormone (GHRH)/somatostatin control. This may explain the differences observed between spontaneous and pharmacologically stimulated GH secretion, as well as the persistence of normal GH responses to the GHRH stimulation test (3,4). Experimental studies in monkeys (5) and the changes observed in the other anterior pituitary functions in adult patients (6) support such a hypothesis. The severity and frequency of pituitary defects vary according to the initial disease and its specific therapeutic regimens, but basically the radiation dose effectively delivered to the hypothalamic-pituitary region defines the risk factor. It depends on the total dose, the number of fractions, and the duration of treatment: a given dose delivered in a shorter time period is more likely to cause GH deficiency than one delivered over a long period (Chap. 4) (7,8).

GH deficiency occurs in about 75% of the children treated with cranial doses between 3000 and 4500 cGy. All

Table 1 Endocrine Abnormalities After External Cranial Irradiation in Patients Evaluated at Least 4 Years After Irradiation[a]

| | | Frequency of cases with endocrine abnormality (%) | | | | |
| | | GH deficiency | | | | |
Etiology	Cases (n)	Complete	Partial	Thyroid[b]	ACTH	LHRH[c]
Leukemia, 24 Gy	86	30	22	2	0	3
Face and neck tumors, 25–45 Gy	56	46	22	35	7	16
Medulloblastoma, 25–45 Gy	59	52	24	47	8	20
Optic glioma, 45–55 Gy	39	77	23	46	3	40

[a]Expressed as percentage of affected cases in each patient group. GH deficiency: complete, after stimulation, GH peak < 5 ng/ml; partial, 5–8 ng/ml. ACTH, adrenocorticotropic hormone.

[b]Includes elevated plasma TSH after direct thyroid irradiation.

[c]LH/FSH deficiency or precocious puberty. Evaluated in patients reaching pubertal age. Does not include primary gonadal failure.

Source: From Reference 8.

children irradiated with higher doses are affected and eventually develop panhypopituitarism. The greater the radiation dose, the earlier it is that the GH deficiency develops, with intervals ranging from 1 year in patients irradiated with 4000 cGy for cranial tumors to more than 4 years in leukemic patients (8). The age at time of cranial irradiation is another important risk factor, younger children being more vulnerable (9). It is therefore recommended that cranial irradiation be delayed whenever possible until the child is over 3 years old. Children treated for acute leukemia with radiation doses of 2400 cGy or less do not always develop growth hormone deficiency, and the deficiency may be restricted to the pubertal period (10). Whereas complete GH deficiency is not reversible, the long-term outcome of partial GH deficiency, as observed in patients treated with low-dose cranial irradiation, is not firmly established. This may be partly because of difficulties in quantitatively assessing GH secretion (3). The anterior pituitary function should nevertheless be reevaluated in these patients after adolescence to provide a reference for further follow-up during adulthood.

The reported frequency of GH deficiency after total-body irradiation is quite variable. It occurred after a single dose of 1000 cGy but was also found after fractionated doses (11–14). Generally there seems to be no correlation between GH

secretion and growth, at least during the first few years following irradiation (14). This is not surprising, because many other etiologic factors may play a role.

A. Assessment of GH Secretion

For practical purposes, GH secretion may be first assessed by a pharmacologic GH stimulation test, measuring plasma insulin-like growth factor I (IGF-I) 2 years after therapy (15). If growth is retarded despite normal GH peak responses, the spontaneous GH secretion during a 24 h profile should be measured. Actually, there may be normal GH responses to a pharmacologic stimulus despite subnormal spontaneous GH secretion. This condition, described as a GH neurosecretory dysfunction, may merely reflect a partial GH deficiency. It has generally been reported after 2400 or 1800 cGy cranial irradiation (16). Repeated testing may be necessary in some cases before GH deficiency is diagnosed. Such difficulties arise only in patients treated with low doses of radiation, when pituitary dysfunction appears after an interval of several years. Last, GH secretion and circulating IGF-I values must also be interpreted according to the pubertal status of the patient (Chaps 2 & 4) (8).

B. Growth and Growth Hormone Deficiency

Growth impairment differs from one group of patients to another, and the impact of GH deficiency may be difficult to assess without sufficient follow-up. Growth retardation as a result of GH deficiency following high-dose cranial radiation for brain or facial tumors or retinoblastoma is easy to diagnose because it occurs within a few years in most patients. However, in patients treated with low doses of cranial radiation, there is no clear correlation between growth and growth hormone secretion (8). Prepubertal growth may remain normal in some of these patients despite GH deficiency (17), and early puberty may help to sustain height velocity, sometimes at a cost of excessive bone maturation.

Table 2 Targets Critical to Growth According to Irradiation Protocols

	Cranial	Craniospinal	Total body
Growth hormone[a]	++	++	+
Sex steroids[b]	+	+	+
Thyroid hormone[b]	+	++	++
Skeleton		++	+

[a]Hypothalamic and pituitary defect.

[b]Primary and/or secondary defects according to radiation protocols.

III. PUBERTY

Surprisingly, children who have received cranial irradiation may present with early or true precocious puberty (18,19). This is in contrast with the delayed puberty usually accompanying idiopathic GH deficiency. Early puberty occurred essentially in girls after cranial irradiation for leukemia, and the children who had been irradiated when very young tended to have the earliest puberty (20,21). This is an important consideration because of the risk of excessive bone maturation and early epiphyseal closure (Chap. 13). Puberty not only occurs earlier but it is shortened with early menarche (22), a condition that tends to shorten the time available for human GH (hGH) therapy. The final height loss may even be more severe if full-blown precocious puberty is associated with untreated GH deficiency: in patients with optic glioma presenting with precocious puberty at the time of irradiation, the persistence of a normal growth rate within 1 or 2 years after cranial radiation may be misinterpreted, and excessive progression of bone age will lead to early cessation of growth. GH testing is then necessary 1 year after irradiation to unmask any associated GH deficiency and allow GH therapy to begin (23). Gonadotropin deficiency may develop within a few years after high-dose cranial radiation for tumors, as indicated by arrested puberty, primary amenorrhea in girls, and absence of luteinizing hormone (LH) and follicle-stimulating hormone (FSH) response to an LH-releasing hormone (LHRH) stimulation test (24). Some girls suffer only from menstrual irregularities, and their impact on fertility has not been documented. Gonadotropin deficiency is usually associated with GH deficiency and moderate hyperprolactinemia, a combination indicating multiple hypothalamic pituitary deficiencies.

IV. GONADAL FUNCTION AND FERTILITY

Direct testicular irradiation with 2400 cGy, as performed in some leukemic boys with local relapse, causes permanent testicular atrophy with elevated plasma FSH concentrations. Leydig cell insufficiency is also a frequent complication of irradiation, with a higher risk in boys treated before the age of 5 years (25). It requires androgen replacement therapy (Chap. 18). Because of the high susceptibility of the testicular germinal epithelium, lower doses, such as those delivered during abdominal or low spinal radiation, may damage the testis, with a permanent or transient rise in plasma FSH and later oligospermia or azoospermia (26). Doses of less than 1000 cGy may cause transient damage to the germinal epithelium. In any boy at risk of gonadal failure, the routine follow-up includes checking the progression of testicular volume in relation to age and measuring basal plasma levels of LH, FSH, and testosterone. Semen analyses, if necessary, can only be proposed during adulthood. Ovarian function may also be severely impaired by irradiation because of the susceptibility of a fixed pool of oocytes. Fractionated doses over 1000 cGy are damaging, with complete destruction of the oocytes at 2000 cGy (27). The ovarian risk can therefore be predicted in most radiation protocols if they include the ovaries. Patients at risk are those treated for abdominal, pelvic, or genital tumors and Hodgkin's disease. Primary ovarian dysfunction, resulting in premature menopause, may also occur in patients who received spinal irradiation with scattered irradiation to ovaries. This scattered dose to the ovary may depend on the method of delivering the radiation at a particular treatment center. Ovarian transposition has been shown to protect patients from ovarian failure if performed before puberty (28). After total body irradiation with more than 600 cGy, ovarian failure is almost constant. The follow-up of these girls also focuses on breast development as the best indicator of ovarian activity, on initiation of puberty and menstrual cycles, and on measurement of plasma LH and FSH during puberty.

The impact of cytotoxic chemotherapy on the gonads is variable, depending on several factors, such as the nature and dose regimen of the drugs employed, the association with various other agents, and the age of the patients (29). Boys and girls react differently.

As a rule, drugs causing damage to the gonads include alkylating agents and such drugs as procarbazine, vinblastine, cytarabin, and cisplatin (Table 3). Each regimen used in the management of a given cancer should be evaluated for its potential harm to the gonads. Except for the very aggressive intensive chemotherapy protocols, there are remarkable individual variations that may not be predictable. All boys achieve normal adult sexual characteristics and normal testosterone secretion after chemotherapy. The reproductive function of prepubertal and pubertal boys appears

Table 3 Current Chemotherapy Agents Cytotoxic for the Testis and Ovary

Chemotherapy	Disease
Alkylating agents	
Cyclophosphamide	Lymphoblastic leukemia
	Non-Hodgkin's lymphoma
	Various tumors
Ifosfamide	Soft tissue tumors
	Ewing sarcoma
	Nephroblastoma
Melphalan	Bone marrow transplantation
Busulfan	Bone marrow transplantation
	Chronic myeloid leukemia
Dacarbazine (DTIC)	Soft tissue tumors
Carmustine (BCNU)	Hodgkin's disease
	Brain tumors
Lomustine (CCNU)	Hodgkin's disease
Semustine (methyl-CCNU)	Brain tumors
Other agents	
Cytarabine (cytosinearabinoside)	Lymphoblastic leukemia
Vincristine	Various tumors
Vinblastine (VLB)	Hodgkin's disease
Procarbazine	Hodgkin's disease
Cisplatin (cis-DDP)	Various tumors

to be equally susceptible to chemotherapy. Combined treatments with one or more cytotoxic agents result in elevated plasma FSH concentrations at puberty that are consistent with germ cell damage. For instance, the effects of cyclophosphamide on sperm density are proportional to the dose (30). Although some of these patients may be normally fertile several years after completion of chemotherapy, the prognosis for fertility remains poor for most of them (31). In contrast, ovarian function, including estrogen secretion, and future fertility are less severely impaired by chemotherapy. The plasma FSH concentration may be raised after administration of alkylating agents for leukemia. These changes are most often transient and do not preclude pubertal development or ultimate fertility (32,33). The same trend is observed in girls treated with nitrosureas for brain and spinal tumors. The prospects for normal fertility are therefore rather favorable. Amenorrheic girls with persistently elevated plasma gonadotropins after intensive chemotherapy may even become pregnant. A large survey of patients treated by chemotherapy with alkylating agents showed that fertility was impaired in about 60% of the men but it was normal in women given similar treatment (34). Another study suggested that the pregnancy outcome of leukemia survivors was not adversely affected by treatment with various chemotherapeutic regimens, provided they did not include an alkylating agent or cytarabin (35).

V. GYNECOLOGIC OUTCOME AFTER PELVIC IRRADIATION

Abdominal and pelvic irradiation for Wilms' tumors, Hodgkin's disease, or pelvic and vaginal tumors damages the uterus and its vascularization. When a low radiation dose was delivered to the ovary and fertility was maintained, uterine irradiation may result in a high frequency of miscarriages or premature births. Because of uterine atrophy, as shown by reduced uterine length and endometrial thickness at ultrasound examination, some women are also unlikely to benefit from in vitro fertilization with donor oocytes (36). Breast atrophy may also result from scattered irradiation after whole abdominal or flank irradiation performed before puberty and may require cosmetic surgery (36). Gonadal insufficiency is treated by the usual replacement therapy with sex steroids. Doses should be gradually increased to mimic the normal timing of growth and pubertal development.

VI. THYROID

Hypothalamic failure with defective thyroid-stimulating hormone (TSH) secretion depends on the doses of cranial irradiation. A high dose of external irradiation causes permanent TSH deficiency to develop within 2 years in about half of the treated patients. Its estimated frequency is even higher if a so-called hypothalamic prolonged and elevated plasma TSH response to thyrotropin-releasing hormone (TRH) stimulation is also considered a diagnostic criterion of TSH dysfunction. Low total or free thyroxine with low

TSH is less frequently observed (8). Although mild hypothyroidism does not play a major role in growth retardation, replacement thyroxine therapy should be prescribed. The thyroid function usually remains normal after low-dose prophylactic cranial irradiation in leukemia patients. Direct thyroid irradiation is followed by thyroxine deficiency, elevated plasma TSH being the first detectable abnormality, which is dose dependent in a high proportion of patients. It occurs during the first year following therapy, and its incidence increases for several more years (37,38). Transient hypothyroidism has been reported during induction chemotherapy with L-asparaginase (39).

The risk of developing benign nodules or thyroid cancer in later life is increased after radiation to the neck (Chap. 31). The threshold dose for inducing cancer is as low as 100 cGy. Although most data are derived from patients treated for Hodgkin's disease (37), children given spinal or total-body irradiation should also be followed until adulthood, and any palpable nodule confirmed by ultrasound should be removed. It has been suggested that thyroxine therapy, at doses that suppress TSH secretion, would help avoid the recurrence after surgery of nodules of cancer (6).

VII. OTHER ENDOCRINE COMPLICATIONS

Corticotropin deficiency with clinical symptoms is a rare complication that occurs after high doses of cranial radiation given for brain tumors. If early morning plasma cortisol is low and does not respond to insulin-induced hypoglycemia, hydrocortisone replacement therapy is required. Hyperprolactinemia (plasma prolactin usually remains below 100 ng/ml) can follow high-dose cranial irradiation; it develops during adolescence or adulthood without any clinical significance. As already mentioned, it is an additional indicator of hypothalamic damage (6). Importantly, cranial irradiation is never accompanied by posterior pituitary dysfunction. Calcium homeostasis remains normal, although hyperparathyroidism has been reported to occur after neck irradiation (41). Finally, there is no reported evidence of primary endocrine pancreas or adrenal dysfunction after abdominal irradiation.

VIII. GROWTH

Growth depends on growth hormone secretion and the timing of puberty but also on a number of factors unrelated to pituitary deficiency, such as chemotherapy, associated acute and chronic disease effects, and exposure of cartilage plates to irradiation, as seen in children with spinal or total-body irradiation. Growth after cranial irradiation is shown in Figure 1.

A. After High-Dose Cranial Irradiation

Radiation doses in excess of 3000 cGy reduce final height in most children. The height loss is progressive, reaching about 1 standard deviation (SD) before puberty and 2 SD at final height. Growth retardation develops more rapidly, within 2

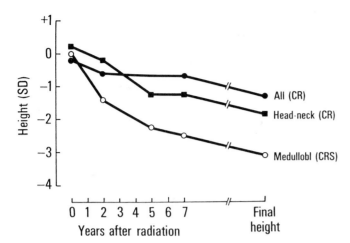

Figure 1 Mean prepubertal height changes after cranial and craniospinal irradiation and final heights in patients treated for leukemia, head and neck tumours, or medulloblastoma. (From Ref. 61.)

years, in patients given 4500 cGy or more. Bone age is delayed, and typical features of GH deficiency may appear in prepubertal patients (8).

B. After Low-Dose Cranial Irradiation

Variable patterns of growth have been reported. Typically, there is a moderate height reduction during the acute phase of the disease and the associated induction chemotherapy. This is followed by a subnormal or normal growth rate until puberty. An additional height loss of 1 SD may occur during puberty (8). A few patients have shown normal growth after irradiation, despite a GH deficiency (17). The overall mean loss in adult height in patients treated with cranial doses of 1800–2400 cGy varies from 0.9 to 1.4 SD (42–44). Final short stature is more likely to occur after intensive induction chemotherapy in children irradiated at a younger age if puberty began earlier and in patients with familial short stature. Because GH deficiency remains the prime candidate as a cause of growth retardation, all children should be tested for GH secretion before and at onset of puberty if they demonstrate a significant decrease in linear growth. This issue is even more critical in patients, most frequently girls, presenting with sexual precocity.

C. After Spinal or Total-Body Irradiation

Some protocols include extensive skeletal irradiation, and these patients are exposed to more severe and early growth retardation. A first group of patients are those given spinal irradiation (generally 2400 cGy) in addition to cranial irradiation for medulloblastoma. They may lose up to 2 SD of height within 2 years following irradiation and have a mean final height loss of 2–3 SD, with a short upper segment largely attributed to the lack of spinal growth (45,46). Children irradiated before age 6 years are more severely affected. Some

degree of reduced spinal growth and disproportion also occurs after whole-abdomen or, more rarely, after flank irradiation, as performed for abdominal malignancies, such as Wilms' tumors (47). Total-body irradiation as conditioning for bone marrow transplantation is another therapy that leads to growth retardation unrelated to GH deficiency. It is increasingly used as the ultimate therapy in leukemia and in some nonmalignant diseases (48,49). The outcome of growth in these patients depends on the radiation dose and its fractionation (14). An immediate growth retardation is observed in patients given a single 1000 cGy dose. The more recent protocols with fractionated doses of 800–1000 cGy have little or no impact on short-term growth. However, adult heights in various groups of patient remain to be documented. Other factors, such as prolonged corticosteroid therapy, renal failure, and chronic graft-versus-host disease, may also contribute to growth retardation. The frequency and severity of GH deficiency depends on the radiation protocols, and GH may not play a major role in the growth disturbance of these patients (14,50–52). Growth retardation may be caused by several factors, the most important being direct skeletal irradiation, so that the contribution of GH deficiency to a decreased growth rate remains difficult to assess. A positive response to hGH treatment is good indicator of GH deficiency.

Primary thyroid insufficiency occurs in most patients given total-body irradiation, elevated plasma TSH appearing within 2 years, but less than 10% of them have overt hypothyroidism. Most of the boys and girls irradiated before puberty develop primary gonadal failure with elevated LH and FSH levels. Delayed or absence of sex steroid secretion then contributes to growth retardation at the age of puberty and requires replacement therapy. Some patients may spontaneously recover ovarian or testicular function.

D. After Chemotherapy

The effect of chemotherapy on growth is difficult to assess because many factors, such as differences between protocols, infection, poor nutrition, and the disease itself, may play a role. These patients do not develop GH deficiency after treatment by chemotherapy alone, but the moderate, early growth retardation, as reported in children also irradiated for leukemia (53) or cranial tumors (46), may be related to the induction chemotherapy and caused by a transient insensitivity to growth hormone (54). However, a recent study showed that the final height of patients treated for leukemia with chemotherapy alone was normal (44). Interestingly, there may even be catch-up growth in immunodeficient growth-retarded children after preparative chemotherapy for bone marrow transplantation (14). Because some data still suggest that chemotherapy has a moderately detrimental effect on growth (43), a follow-up of all patients remains necessary. However, growth is unlikely to be a critical issue in nonirradiated patients.

IX. FOLLOW-UP AND MANAGEMENT

Our experience to date with children surviving childhood malignancies provides guidelines for long-term assessment of growth and endocrine complications. This is part of the regular checkups that are necessary to decide upon replacement treatments. Growth hormone treatment is easy to decide after cranial irradiation for brain and facial tumors because GH deficiency is generally severe. Recombinant growth hormone given at the usual dose of 0.1 u/kg/day (about 0.250 mg/kg/week), (Chapter 5) produces a significant short-term improvement in growth rate. To date, however, the long-term results and final heights achieved have been rather disappointing (55–58). Several factors may have had negative effects compared with patients with idiopathic GH deficiency: (1) these patients have been GH deficient for a shorter period, (2) their bone age was less retarded, and (3) some had early puberty, which accelerated the skeletal maturation faster than the increase in growth rate. Failure to catch up with normal height may also have been related to low hGH dosage in some studies. It is therefore essential to commence hGH therapy as soon as GH deficiency and growth retardation are documented, but preferably not less than 2 years after the primary treatment. This issue is more complex in patients treated for leukemia with low doses of cranial irradiation. In this group GH therapy should be started before puberty only if the height loss exceeds 1 SD, because some of them maintain normal growth rates for several years until puberty despite a GH deficiency, and at time of onset of puberty if short stature and severe GH deficiency predict significant adult height loss. Again, early or precocious puberty is an additional risk factor of short stature. LHRH analog therapy should then be considered in association with the hGH treatment. In this group of patients most authors restrict the use of hGH and/or LHRH analog therapy to the GH-deficient patients most at risk of final short stature because of familial short stature, cranial irradiation at a younger age, and/or early puberty. Whatever the cranial radiation dose, those who have received additional spinal irradiation have a poor response to hGH treatment (58,59). The same suboptimal growth response occurs after high-dose total-body irradiation. Early hGH treatment remains suitable for these patients at high risk of short stature, but it should be started no less than 2 years after the end of intensive chemotherapy and irradiation and maintained only if significant catch-up growth is obtained during the first years of therapy.

One major concern is the potential oncogenic effect of hGH treatment. However, there is at present no evidence that hGH promotes leukemia or tumor relapse or an increased occurrence of a second cancer (60). In the future it will be important to identify better the patients at risk of significant final height loss for an appropriate use of hGH therapy. Because intensive chemotherapy is becoming an alternative to irradiation, it should be required that each protocol be evaluated for its impact on growth, pubertal development, and fertility.

ACKNOWLEDGMENTS

This work was supported by grants from INSERM, University Descartes (Paris V), Assistance-Publique-Hôpitaux de Paris, and Association de recherche contre le cancer.

REFERENCES

1. Stiller CA. Aetiology and epidemiology. In: Plowman PN, Pinkerton CR, eds. Paediatric Oncology. Clinical Practice and Controversies. London: Chapman and Hall Medical, 1992:1–24.
2. Tan BC, Kunaratnam N. Hypopituitary dwarfism following radiotherapy for nasopharyngeal carcinoma. Clin Radiol 1966; 17:302–304.
3. Blatt J, Bercu BB, Gillin JC, Mendelson WB, Poplack DG. Reduced pulsatile growth hormone secretion in children after therapy for acute lymphoblastic leukemia. J Pediatr 1984; 104:182–186.
4. Crosnier H, Brauner R, Rappaport R. Growth hormone response to growth hormone releasing hormone (hp GHRH 1–44) as an index of growth hormone secretory dysfunction after prophylactic cranial irradiation for acute lymphoblastic leukemia (24 grays). Acta Paediatr Scand 1988; 77:681–687.
5. Chrousos GP, Poplack D, Brown T, O'Neill D, Schwade J, Bercu BB. Effects of cranial radiation on hypothalamic-adenohypophyseal function: abnormal growth hormone secretory dynamics. J Clin Endocrinol Metab 1982; 54:1135–1139.
6. Constine LS, Woolf PD, Cann D, et al. Hypothalamic-pituitary dysfunction after radiation for brain tumors. N Engl J Med 1993; 328:87–94.
7. Shalet SM, Beardwell CG, Pearson D, Morris-Jones PH. The effect of varying doses of cerebral irradiation on growth hormone production in childhood. Clin Endocrinol (Oxf) 1976; 5:287–290.
8. Rappaport R, Brauner R. Growth and endocrine disorders secondary to cranial irradiation. Pediatr Res 1989; 25:561–567.
9. Brauner R, Czernichow P, Rappaport R. Greater susceptibility to hypothalamopituitary irradiation in younger children with acute lymphoblastic leukemia. J Pediatr 1986; 108:332.
10. Moell C, Garwicz S, Westgren U, Wiebe T, Albertsson-Wikland K. Suppressed spontaneous secretion of growth hormone in girls after treatment for acute lymphoblastic leukemia. Arch Dis Child 1989; 64:252–258.
11. Sanders JE, Buckner CD, Sullivan KM, et al. Growth and development in children after bone marrow transplantation. Horm Res 1988; 30:92–97.
12. Borgstrom B, Bolme P. Growth and growth hormone in children with bone marrow transplantation. Horm Res 1988; 30:98–100.
13. Ogilvy-Stuart AL, Clark DJ, Wallace WHB, et al. Endocrine deficit following fractionated total body irradiation. Arch Dis Child 1992; 67:1107–1110.
14. Brauner R, Fontoura M, Zucker JM, et al. Growth and growth hormone secretion after bone marrow transplantation. Arch Dis Child 1993; 68:458–463.
15. Rose SR, Ross JL, Uriarte M, Barnes KM, Cassorla FG, Cuttler GB. The advantage of measuring stimulated as compared with spontaneous growth hormone levels in the diagnosis of growth hormone deficiency. N Engl J Med 1988; 319:201–207.
16. Bercu BB, Shulman D, Root AW, Spiliotis BE. Growth hormone (GH) provocative testing frequently does not reflect endogenous GH secretion. J Clin Endocrinol Metab 1986; 63:709–716.
17. Shalet SM, Price DA, Beardwell CG, Morris Jones PH, Pearson D. Normal growth despite abnormalities of growth hormone secretion in children treated for acute leukaemia. J Pediatr 1979; 94:719–722.
18. Brauner R, Czernichow P, Rappaport R. Precocious puberty after hypothalamic and pituitary irradiation in young children. N Engl J Med 1984; 311:920.

19. Pasqualini T, Escobar ME, Domene H, Sackmann-Muriel F, Pavlovsky S, Rivarola MA. Evaluation of gonadal function following long-term treatment for acute leukemia in girls. Am J Pediatr Hematol Oncol 1987; 9:15–22.

20. Leiper AD, Stanhope R, Kitching P, Chessels JM. Precocious and premature puberty associated with the treatment of acute lymphoblastic leukaemia. Arch Dis Child 1987; 62:1107–1112.

21. Uruena M, Stanhope R, Chessels JM, Leiper AD. Impaired pubertal growth in acute lymphoblastic leukaemia. Arch Dis Child 1990; 66:1403–1407.

22. Quigley C, Cowell C, Jimenez M, et al. Normal or early development of puberty despite gonadal damage in children treated for acute lymphoblastic leukaemia. N Engl J Med 1989; 321:143–151.

23. Brauner R, Malandry F, Rappaport R, et al. Growth and endocrine disorders in optic glioma. Eur J Pediatr 1990; 149:825–828.

24. Rappaport R, Brauner R, Czernichow P, et al. Effect of hypothalamic and pituitary irradiation on pubertal development in children with cranial tumors. J Clin Endocrinol Metab 1982; 54:1164–1168.

25. Brauner R, Czernichow P, Cramer P, Schaison G, Rappaport R. Leydig-cell function in children after direct testicular irradiation for acute lymphoblastic leukemia. N Engl J Med 1983; 309:25–28.

26. Shalet SM, Beardwell CG, Jacobs HS, Pearson D. Testicular function following irradiation of the human prepubertal testis. Clin Endocrinol (Oxf) 1978; 9:483–490.

27. Wallace WHB, Shalet SM, Hendry JH, et al. Ovarian failure following abdominal irradiation in childhood: the radio-sensitivity of the human oöcyte. Br J Radiol 1989; 62:995–998.

28. Thibaud E, Ramirez M, Brauner R, et al. Preservation of ovarian function by ovarian transposition performed before pelvic irradiation during childhood. J Pediatr 1992; 121:880–884.

29. Shalet SM. Disorders of gonadal function due to radiation and cytotoxic chemotherapy in children. Adv Intern Med Pediatr 1989; 58:1–21.

30. Lentz AD, Bergstein J, Steffes MW, et al. Postpubertal evaluation of gonadal function following cyclophosphamide therapy before and during puberty. J Pediatr 1977; 91:385–394.

31. Wallace WHB, Shalet SM, Lendon M, Morris Jones PH. Male fertility in long-term survivors of acute lymphoblastic leukaemia in childhood. Int J Androl 1991; 14:312–319.

32. Pasqualini T, Escobar ME, Domené H, et al. Evaluation of gonadal function following long-term treatment for acute lymphoblastic leukaemia in girls. Am J Pediatr Hematol Oncol 1987; 9:15–22.

33. Wallace WHB, Shalet SM, Tetlow LJ, Morris Jones PH. Ovarian function following the treatment of childhood acute lymphoblastic leukaemia. Med Pediatr Oncol 1993; 21:333–339.

34. Byrne J, Mulvihill JJ, Myers MH, et al. Effects of treatment on fertility in long-term survivors of childhood or adolescent cancer. N Engl J Med 1987; 317:1315–1321.

35. Green DM, Hall B, Zevon A. Pregnancy outcome after treatment for acute lymphoblastic leukaemia during childhood or adolescence. Cancer 1989; 64:2335–2339.

36. Critchely HOD, Wallace WHB, Mamtora H, Higginson J, Shalet SM, Anderson DC. Ovarian failure after whole abdominal radiotherapy: the potential for pregnancy. Br J Obstet Gynaecol 1992; 99:392–394.

37. Schimpff SG, Diggs CH, Wiswell JG, et al. Radiation-related thyroid dysfunction: implications for the treatment of Hodgkin's disease. Ann Intern Med 1980; 92:91–98.

38. Barnes ND. Effects of external irradiation on the thyroid gland in childhood. Horm Res 1988; 30:84–89.

39. Ferster A, Glinoër D, Van Vliet G, Otten J. Thyroid function during L-asparaginase therapy in children with acute lymphoblastic leukaemia: difference between induction and late intensification. Am J Pediatr Hematol Oncol 1992; 14:192–196.

40. Murphy ED, Scanlon EF, Garces RM, et al. Thyroid hormone administration in irradiated patients. J Surg Oncol 1986; 31:214–217.

41. Prinz RA, Barbato AL, Braithwaite SS, et al. Simultaneous primary hyperparathyroidism and nodular thyroid disease. Surgery 1982; 92:454–458.

42. Schriock EA, Schell MJ, Carter M, Hustu O, Ochs JJ. Abnormal growth patterns and adult short stature in 115 long-term survivors of childhood leukemia. J Clin Oncol 1991; 9:400–405.

43. Sklar C, Mertens A, Walter A, et al. Final height after treatment for childhood acute lymphoblastic leukemia: comparison of no cranial irradiation with 1800 and 2400 centigrays of cranial irradiation. J Pediatr 1993; 123:59–64.

44. Katz JA, Pollock BH, Jacaruso D, Morad A. Final attained height in patients successfully treated for childhood acute lymphoblastic leukemia. J Pediatr 1993; 123:546–552.

45. Shalet SM, Gibson B, Swindell R, et al. Effect of spinal irradiation on growth. Arch Dis Child 1987; 62:461–464.

46. Brauner R, Rappaport R, Prevot C, et al. A prospective study of the development of GH in children given cranial irradiation, and its relation to statural growth. J Clin Endocrinol Metab 1989; 68:346–351.

47. Wallace WHB, Shalet SM, Morris Jones PH, et al. Effect of abdominal irradiation on growth in boys treated for a Wilms' tumour. Med Pediatr Oncol 1990; 18:441–446.

48. Borton MM, Rimm AA. Increasing utilization of bone marrow transplantation. Transplantation 1986; 42:229–234.

49. Sanders JE, Pritchard S, Mahoney P, et al. Growth and development following marrow transplantation for leukemia. Blood 1986; 68:1129–1135.

50. Borgström B, Bolme P. Growth and growth hormone in children after bone marrow transplantation. Horm Res 1988; 30:98–100.

51. Hovi L, Rajantie J, Perkkio M, Sainio K, Sipilä I, Siimes MA. Growth failure and growth hormone deficiency in children after bone marrow transplantation for leukemia. Bone Marrow Transplant 1990; 5:183–186.

52. Ogilvy-Stuart AL, Clark DJ, Wallace WHB, et al. Endocrine deficit after fractionated total body irradiation. Arch Dis Child 1992; 67:1107–1110.

53. Kirk JA, Raghupathy P, Stevens MM, et al. Growth failure and growth hormone deficiency after treatment for acute lymphoblastic leukaemia. Lancet 1987; 1:190–193.

54. Nivot S, Benelli C, Clot JP, et al. Non parallel changes of GH and IGF-1, IGFBP-3, GHBP, after craniospinal irradiation and chemotherapy. J Clin Endocrinol Metab 1994; 78:597–601.

55. Clayton PE, Shalet SM, Price DA. Growth response to growth hormone therapy following cranial irradiation. Eur J Pediatr 1988; 147:593–596.

56. Clayton PE, Shalet SM, Price DA. Growth response to growth hormone therapy following craniospinal irradiation. Eur J Pediatr 1988; 147:597–601.

57. Lannering B, Albertsson-Wikland K. Improved growth response to GH treatment in irradiated children. Acta Paediatr Scand 1989; 78:562–567.

58. Sulmont V, Brauner R, Fontoura M, et al. Response to growth hormone treatment and final height after cranial or craniospinal irradiation. Acta Paediatr Scand 1990; 79:542–549.

59. Clayton PE, Shalet SM, Price DA. Growth response to growth hormone therapy following craniospinal irradiation. Eur J Pediatr 1988; 147:597–601.

60. Ogilvy-Stuart AL, Ryder WDJ, Gattamaneni HR, Clayton PE, Shalet SM. Growth hormone and tumour recurrence. BMJ 1992; 304:1601–1605.

61. Rappaport R, Brauner R. Endocrine disorders and growth after cranial radiation. Acta Paediatr Jpn (Suppl) 1988; 30:55–60.

57

Endocrine Tumors in Children

Muhammad A. Jabbar

Hurley Medical Center, Michigan State University,
Flint, Michigan

I. INTRODUCTION

Generally speaking, endocrine tumors in children pose a number of fundamental questions: whether the tumor is a nonfunctioning, functioning, or hyperfunctioning entity and whether it is a malignant or a benign process or a hyperplasia responsive to physiologic regulations. Apart from clinical presentations, the answers to these questions often depend on specific hormonal-biochemical, radiologic, and histopathologic findings. Consequently, the optimal assessment and management of these patients remain a challenging task and must include the efforts of endocrinologists, oncologists, surgeons, and other support personnel.

This chapter covers the clinical approach to the children with adrenal, gonadal, and pancreatic tumors. Pituitary, thyroid, and parathyroid tumors are covered in Chapters 2, 29, 30, and 33, respectively.

II. ADRENAL TUMORS

The incidence of adrenal tumors in children is not known (Chap. 22 for adrenal cortex and Chap. 24 for adrenal medulla). Of 58 patients reported by Bertagna and Orth (1), 11 (19%) were between 0.8 and 15 years of age. Adrenal carcinoma represented about 10% of the carcinomas in childhood according to registry-based data from England (2). The age of appearance is usually during the first decade of life (3). Females are more frequently affected than males, with ratio of 2.5:1 (4). Although familial cases are reported (5), the occurrence of adrenal carcinoma in patients with Beckwith syndrome (6), hemihypertrophy (7), and congenital malformations of the genitourinary tract are well known.

Pathologically, corticotropin-independent cortisol overproduction represents a spectrum ranging from benign nodular hyperplasia to malignant adrenal tumors. In the 1960s, Meador et al. (8) described primary adrenocortical nodular dysplasia, characterized by nonmalignant, autonomously secreting le-

sions. In a more recent review (9), a similar condition, predominantly affecting children and young adults, was described with bilateral nodular disease and internodular cortical atrophy and varying degrees of pigmentation. This condition has also been described in association with the Carney complex, which includes myxomas, pigmented skin lesions, peripheral nerve tumors, and various endocrine tumors (10). The etiology of the nodule formation or dysplasia remains to be established. An adrenal-stimulating immunoglobulin has been implicated in the pathogenesis (11). In McCune-Albright syndrome, nodular hyperplasia of the adrenal glands has been reported as the cause of hypercortisolism (Chap. 13) (12). In these patients, somatic mutation of the α subunit of the G protein occurs during fetal development, thus creating a mosaicism of normal and mutant-bearing cells. In the latter, the G protein activation of adenylate cyclase increases cyclic AMP, with formation of multiple nodules and overproduction of cortisol. Inverted diurnal rhythm, subnormal morning cortisol concentration, and low corticotropin in association with gastric inhibitory peptide (GIP) were recently described. Although the causative role of GIP in cortisol overproduction remains undetermined, the data support the hypothesis of abnormal expression of the receptors in the adrenal (13,14).

A. Clinical Features

Adrenal tumors in children are usually functional, giving rise to the constellation of symptoms or signs (Chap. 22). Depending on the duration of the disease and the action of the metabolic, androgenic, and salt-retaining hormones, the clinical spectrum may cover Cushing syndrome and virilization to hypertension. The majority of the tumors secrete cortisol; androgen and aldosterone secretion follow in decreasing frequency. Occasionally, there is alteration of the clinical course with evidence of initial glucocorticoid predominance being overlapped by the androgenic effects, or vice versa, as the disease progresses. An incidental adrenal tumor without clinical manifestation is a distinct entity in adults, but this represents only about 5% of all adrenal tumors in children.

Weight gain, truncal obesity, moon face, and buffalo hump are observed in 40–60% of the children with functional adrenal tumors (Table 1). Obesity and short stature are common presenting features (15–17), although the latter may be the only manifestation of hypercortisolemia in children (18).

Normal or accelerated linear growth may be encountered in children with androgen-producing adrenal tumors. In such cases, acne, hirsutism, hypertrichosis of the face and trunk, deepening of the voice, and, in females, clitoromegaly are the distinguishable physical signs. In prepubertal children, excess androgen leads to virilization, with excess body hair, adrenarche, acne, clitoromegaly or abnormal phallic growth, and rapid skeletal growth, along with excess weight gain (19,20). The disorder tends to be more severe and the clinical findings more flagrant in infants than when the onset occurs in older children (21,22). Premature adrenarche, a common problem in clinical practice, may be the initial presentation, although the severity of the signs and symptoms helps to differentiate the adrenal tumor from benign adrenarche. In postmenarcheal females, rapid weight gain and menstrual irregularity often result from increased androgens (Chaps. 16 and 17). Estrogen-secreting tumors of the adrenals are rare in childhood. In prepubertal boys, these may lead to gynecomastia along with enhancement of growth and skeletal mat-

uration; in girls, sexual precocity characterized by premature thelarche and advanced growth may occur (23). If there is evidence of virilization or elevation in blood pressure, concomitant secretion of androgens or mineralocorticoids should be suspected.

Hypertension, plethora, and fluid retention are also common in children with adrenal tumor, being present in up to 70% of these patients (Chap. 53). In aldosterone-producing tumors, elevated blood pressure is one of the most common manifestations. Both systolic and diastolic blood pressure are abnormally elevated. Muscle weakness, cramping, paresthesia, polydipsia, and polyuria may occur. Despite fluid retention and an increase in the intravascular volume, there is no clinical evidence of edema in these patients. Sodium retention is of only mild to moderate proportion. Hypokalemia is the most reliable laboratory abnormality, with electrocardiographic signs of prolonged ST segment and inverted T wave. Alkalosis is also a frequent finding, causing tetany and Trousseau's sign in untreated patients.

A small percentage of patients are known to have psychiatric symptoms, ranging from acute psychosis and depression to manic depressive behavior. Asymptomatic hypercortisolemia with normal blood pressure has been reported in children. Diffuse osteoporosis, more noticeable in the vertebral column, is also common in these patients. Impaired glucose tolerance is more frequent than overt diabetes, and the incidence of renal stones is higher than that in the general population.

Preoperative differentiation of an adenoma from carcinoma is difficult. Although Cushing syndrome is frequently caused by adenoma and virilization is associated with carcinoma, benign and malignant tumors may be functionally identical and thus clinically inseparable. A normal or exaggerated response to exogenous adrenocorticotropic hormone (ACTH) stimulation is more often encountered in adenoma than carcinoma, but lack of dexamethasone suppression is observed in both (1). The size of the tumor has been noted to be a predictor, tumor size greater than 75 g being more likely to be malignant (16). Histopathologic criteria, such as mitoses, necrosis, and capsular and vascular invasion, were not reliable predictors of a malignant tumor, as demonstrated by the presence of these characteristics in benign adenomas (24,25).

B. Diagnosis

Because of the anatomic location deep in the abdomen as well as nonfunctioning nature of the tumors, adrenal adenoma or carcinoma often remains undiagnosed for a considerable period of time. The size attained by these tumors is therefore enormous in many instances. During evaluation of nonspecific complaints or routine physical examination, an abdominal mass may be detected in such patients.

Hormonal studies are of vital importance in the diagnosis of adrenal tumors. Urinary steroids 17-KS and 17-OHCS are significantly elevated in patients with a functioning adrenal tumor. Plasma cortisol is elevated, along with loss of diurnal rhythm. A complete androgen profile, including DHEA,

Table 1 Clinical Features of Hypercortisolemia in Children and Adults[a]

Symptoms, signs	Children (CS)	Children (CD)	Adult (CD)
General			
Obesity (moon facies)	25	100	85
Growth failure	0	85	NR
Hypertension	13	77	75
Cutaneous			
Plethora	13	77	80
Striae	0	54	50
Acne	88	85	35
Hirsutism	75	85	75
Bruising	0	38	35
Hyperpigmentation	0	38	5
Musculoskeletal			
Osteoporosis	NR	54	80
Weakness	0	46	50
Metabolic			
Glucose intolerance	NR	38	75
Renal stones	NR	15	15
Neuropsychiatric symptoms			
Fatigue, weakness	50	46	85

[a]CS, Cushing syndrome; CD, Cushing's disease; NR, not reported.
Source: Data adapted from Pediatr Clin North Am, 1990; 37(6):1313–1329.

androstenedione, and testosterone levels, should be studied in patients with clinical evidence of virilization (Chap. 17). Differentiation from congenital adrenal hyperplasia is important but difficult. In the hypercortisolemic state, lack of suppression of the plasma cortisol following administration of dexamethasone is characteristic of adrenal tumors. Therefore, performance of a low-dose or high-dose dexamethasone test should be a priority in these patients (Chap. 60). Apart from providing further understanding about the functional relations between the pituitary and the adrenal, a metyrapone test may be useful in differentiating adrenal adenomas from carcinomas. In about 50% of cases, adrenal adenomas are responsive to metyrapone but carcinomas are usually nonresponsive. Because the tumors do not respond and the normal adrenal cortices are atrophic, the ACTH stimulation test has very limited use in the diagnosis of adrenal tumors. Differentiation of central precocious puberty from estrogen-secreting adrenal tumors may be necessary in girls. Urinary estrogens and 17-KS and plasma DHEA, DHEAS, and estrogens are elevated, along with absent gonadotropin response following gonadotropin-releasing hormone stimulation in adrenal tumors.

Measurement of serum and 24 h urinary aldosterone levels, as well as plasma renin activity, is useful for the initial evaluation of suspected aldosterone-producing tumors. To differentiate secondary hyperaldosteronism and avoid false positive results, all medications, particularly the diuretics, should be discontinued before the laboratory studies. In patients with elevated serum aldosterone levels, complete suppression of aldosterone secretion by administration of dexamethasone distinguishes the entity called dexamethasone-suppressible hyperaldosteronism from primary hyperaldosteronism. Elevated aldosterone levels, low renin activity, and high urinary aldosterone with lack of dexamethasone suppression establish the diagnosis of hyperaldosteronism (Chap. 22). Further diagnostic studies, including the imaging studies, should be performed in these patients (Chap. 53).

Radiologic studies are an important component in the diagnosis of adrenal tumors. Computed tomographic (CT) scan and magnetic resonance imaging aim to localize the tumor and define the extent of the disease. Intravenous pyelography is useful to delineate the relationship of the kidney to the tumor mass. Ultrasonography shows an adrenal mass in the majority of cases. The CT scan, however, is the ideal method because it allows visualization of other abdominal organs. Angiography is often required to provide the surgeon with a map of the tumor's blood supply.

C. Treatment

Complete surgical excision with replacement steroid therapy provides the best choice for these patients (17). Preoperative, operative, and postoperative management are of critical importance. For primary pigmented nodular adrenocortical disease, bilateral adrenalectomy with steroid replacement is preferred (24). For adrenal adenoma, the unilateral adrenalectomy or resection of the tumor followed by replacement steroid therapy is the treatment of choice. Replacement

therapy with glucocorticoid is necessary until normal function in the contralateral gland is restored. This is usually for 6–12 months. although suppression from the tumor can persist for up to 2 years.

For adrenal carcinoma, the surgical therapy aims to excise the tumor and local metastasis completely, to enhance the chance of cure. For inoperable or partially resectable carcinoma, combination chemotherapy may offer an alternative management approach (27–29). However, the experience with pediatric patients is largely anecdotal. In addition, medical therapy with metyrapone and aminoglutethimide in combination is useful for control of symptoms. Ketoconazole, an inhibitor of steroid biosynthesis, is the preferred drug to decrease cortisol secretion in selected cases. RU 486, a glucocorticoid antagonist, has also been employed to control the symptoms secondary to hypercortisolism.

D. Prognosis and Follow-up

Early diagnosis and surgery offer the best hope for long-term survival, with adenoma exhibiting an extremely good outcome. Adrenal carcinoma in children, on the other hand, is an extremely progressive disease. Final adult stature is stunted in most of these patients. Replacement therapy with glucocorticoid is required for an indefinite period of time. Careful follow-up at 3–6 month interval is mandatory. Clinical assessment and serum levels of cortisol, DHEA, androstenedione, testosterone, and plasma renin activity are necessary to detect recurrent or metastatic disease. The 24 h urinary 17-KS, 17-OHCS, and free cortisol, along with the other hormones that were initially abnormal, should be measured. Repeat dexamethasone stimulation test should be done to assess the suppressibility of cortisol production.

III. GONADAL TUMORS

A. Testicular Tumors

1. Etiology and Presentation

Constituting about 1% of all cancers in males, testicular tumors occur most commonly during the third and fourth decades of life. Germ cell tumors, accounting for about 90% of all testicular tumors in the pediatric age group, include embryonal carcinoma, endodermal sinus tumor, and teratoma, representing a spectrum of progressive histologic differentiation. In young adults, however, the spectrum includes seminoma, which represent about 30–50% of all germ cell tumors (30,31).

The most well-documented risk factor for the development of germ tumors is cryptorchidism, which is associated with about 10% of germ cell tumors (Chap. 20) (32–34). The degree of maldescent of the testes correlates with the likelihood of tumor formation, with abdominal testes more at risk than those in the inguinal area. Orchidopexy performed before the age of 6, however, reduces this risk significantly. The pathogenesis of the tumors is not clear. The incidence of tumor in the contralateral normally descended testis is higher than that in controls. Although several factors, including higher temperature, higher gonadotropin levels, and congenitally abnormal germ cells, have been proposed, none has provided compelling evidence to attain wide acceptance.

Dysgenetic gonads associated with androgen insensitivity, persistent müllerian syndrome, true hermaphroditism, and Klinefelter syndrome have a higher incidence of germ cell tumors (33–35). Down syndrome and cutaneous icthyosis (35–37) with steroid sulfatase deficiency have also been reported to be associated with the occurrence of testicular tumors. One of the strongest risk factors for the development of a germ cell tumor is a history of contralateral tumor (38–40), although the specific etiologic factor remains undetermined. Familial occurrence of tumor has been reported, with a sixfold increase for a son whose father had a germ cell tumor (41).

Inadequately treated congenital adrenal hyperplasia has been observed to be associated with testicular tumors (42,43). It is presumed that the development and progression of these tumors are enhanced by the chronic stimulatory effect of elevated corticotropin.

A painless mass is the common mode of presentation; however, pain and tenderness are found in half of the cases. Symptoms or signs of metastasis to the retroperitoneal lymph nodes or lungs are the initial findings in a small proportion of patients. Tumor of Leydig cell origin may secrete testosterone, producing signs of sexual development. Unilateral or bilateral gynecomastia may occur as a result of the secretion of estrogen or chorionic gonadotropin by the stromal or germ cell tumors (44).

2. Diagnosis

Careful examination is instrumental to the diagnosis of testicular tumor. An area of hardness, nodularity, or altered consistency should be determined. Localization of the tumor and differentiation of a simple hydrocele from a reactive hydrocele with testicular tumor can be reliably performed by sonographic study. Patients suspected to have germ cell tumor should have radiographic or imaging studies of the chest, abdomen, and skeletal system to detect metastatic disease. The functional and histologic behavior of various testicular tumors is given in Table 2. Preoperatively as well as during the follow-up, measurement of such biomarkers as serum human chorionic gonadotropin (hCG) and α-fetoprotein (AFP) (45) is useful, particularly for monitoring these patients.

3. Treatment

Following the diagnosis of testicular tumor, immediate surgery is indicated. For teratoma, surgery alone is usually sufficient, but localized germ cell tumor requires radical surgery (involving excision of the spermatic cord structures and the testicle). Periodic evaluation of the chest and abdomen and measurement of serum AFP level allows identification of recurrence of the tumor. For malignant tumors with metastatic or recurrent disease, radical surgery and chemotherapy (cisplatin, vinblastine, and bleomycin) offer the best outcome. However, controversy remains about the need for retroperitoneal lymph node resection in pediatric patients.

B. Ovarian Tumors

Ovarian tumors, which represent approximately 1% of childhood malignancies (46), are classified into two categories on the basis of their cells of origin: germ cell tumor and non–germ cell tumor. Germ cell tumors, which are more common than non–germ cell tumors in all age groups, account for 90% of the ovarian tumors in premenarcheal girls (47). The majority of these germ cell tumors are teratomas, having a histologically benign and functionally inactive nature. Non–germ cell tumors, such as granulosa, theca, Sertoli, and Leydig cell tumors, represent a small proportion of the ovarian tumors; however, these tumors are of additional clinical significance because of their secretory activity, the granulosa and theca cell tumors predominantly producing estrogens and the Sertoli and Leydig cell tumors secreting androgens.

Classification, median age, distribution, secretory and histologic characteristics, and the common presentation of the

Table 2 Classification, Median Age, Frequency, and Secretory and Histologic Characteristics of Childhood Testicular Tumors[a]

Classification	Median age (years)	Frequency (%)	Secretory activity	Tumor characteristics
Germ cell tumors				
Endodermal sinus	2	26	AFP	Malignant
Teratoma	3	24	None	Usually benign
Embryonal carcinoma	Late teens	20	AFP, hCG	Both
Teratocarcinoma	Late teens	13	None	Both
Gonadoblastoma	5–10	<1	None	Both
Non–germ cell tumors				
Leydig cell	5	6	Androgen	Benign
Sertoli cell	1	4	Androgen, estrogen	Benign

[a]AFP, α-fetoprotein; hCG, human chorionic gonadotropin.
Source: Data adapted from Reference 45.

ovarian tumors are given in Table 3. Dysgerminoma, the most common germ cell tumor of the ovary, presents with a painless abdominal mass. Endodermal sinus tumor, the most aggressive germ cell tumor, presents as a painful mass with rapid metastasis to distant sites. Teratomas, the most common and benign tumor of germ cell origin, usually remain hormonally inactive. In contrast, embryonal carcinoma, which is typically found as an admixture of dysgerminoma, endodermal sinus tumor, or teratoma, may undergo differentiation, become hormonally active, and manifest with effects of hormone production. Gonadoblastomas are uncommon tumors, yet an important ovarian tumor in girls for two reasons. First, these tumors occur more in phenotypic females with an abnormal karyotype containing components of Y chromosomes (46, XY; 45, X/46, XY; 45, X/46, X fra). Second, these tumors, which occur in dysgenetic gonads in which differentiation into testis or ovary has been absent or incomplete, usually contain both germ cell and stromal cell components and frequently exhibit the tendency of recurrence. Because all the gonadal tissue is potentially involved and carcinoma in situ is always a possibility, removal of the gonads is recommended at an early stage (48).

About 5% of the granulosa cell tumors develop in prepubertal females. In these females, with a median age of 8 years, presenting symptoms are attributed to the hormones produced by these tumors. Precocious sexual development characterized by premature breast development, pubic and axillary hair, white vaginal discharge, or irregular uterine bleeding may be the mode of presentation (48). Excessive weight gain with or without acceleration of linear growth may also occur with advancement in the skeletal age (Chap. 13). On rare occasions, androgen production may lead to virilization with hirsutism and clitoromegaly, along with acceleration

of growth. In postmenarcheal females, unregulated estrogen production may lead to irregular bleeding or amenorrhea. Although hormonally inactive tumors may remain asymptomatic, acute abdominal symptoms may be the presentation in a small proportion of these patients. This is largely the result of torsion or rupture of the tumor. Adequate clinical evaluation of these girls should include pelvic examination, performed under sedation or anesthesia, because a palpable mass is almost always diagnostic of tumor. To complete the endocrine evaluation, pituitary-ovarian axis and estrogen profile should be studied. Estradiol level is usually elevated but luteinizing hormone and follicle-stimulating hormone levels are suppressed, thereby excluding the differential diagnosis of central precocious puberty. Vaginal cytology reveals maturation of squamous cells, reflecting the effect of estrogen. Sonographic study helps to localize the mass in the ovary, although it is not a useful method to exclude adrenal disease. Laparoscopy and biopsy are often necessary. Surgical resection of the lesion, that is, unilateral salpingo-oophorectomy, usually yields a good outcome. Recurrence of the disease is unusual. Compared with adult granulosa cell tumors, juvenile granulosa cell tumors have distinct histologic features characterized by luteinized cells, irregular follicles and fibroblast-like cells and the absence of Call-Exner bodies. The tumors may be cystic, solid, or both. Theca cell tumors are often hormonally active and manifests themselves by causing premature breast development, which is similar to that of granulosa cell tumors. They are usually slowly growing and lack the acuteness often encountered in patients with granucosa cell tumor. Diagnostic studies and management approach are identical in both conditions, however.

As classic virilizing ovarian neoplasms often called arrhenoblastomas, Sertoli-Leydig cell tumors occur most

Table 3 Classification, Median Age, Frequency, Secretory and Histologic Characteristics, and Presentation of Ovarian Tumors in Childhood[a]

Classification	Median age (years)	Frequency (%)	Secretory activity	Tumor and presentation[b]
Germ cell tumors				
Dysgerminoma	16	17	hCG	M, mass
EST	18	11	AFP	H, mass, pain
Embryonal carcinoma	14	4	AFP, hCG	M, sexual precocity
Choriocarcinoma	—	Rare	hCG	M, sexual precocity
Teratoma	10–15	29	None	B, mass
Gonadoblastoma	8–10	Rare	A, hCG	M, virilization
Carcinoid	—	Rare	Serotonin	Nonspecific
Struma ovarii	—	Rare	Thyroxine	Hyperthyroidism
Non–germ cell tumors				
Granulosa-theca cell	8	13	E, P	L, sexual precocity
Sertoli-Leydig cell	8	17	A, P	L, virilization

[a]EST, endodermal sinus tumor; A, androgens; E, estrogens; P, progesterone; AFP, α-fetoprotein; hCG, human chorionic gonadotropin.
[b]Degree of malignant behavior; L, low-grade malignancy; M, moderately malignant; H, highly malignant.
Source: Data adapted from References 53 and 54.

commonly during the teenage or early adult years (49). Because of the effect of androgens, the early symptoms and signs consist of weight gain, amenorrhea, hirsutism, acne, deepening of the voice, and clitoromegaly. Abdominal mass and nonspecific gastrointestinal and urinary symptoms may be concurrently present. Although symptoms and signs are more intense and the progression of the course is more rapid compared with congenital adrenal hyperplasia, androgen-producing adrenal tumor, and polycystic ovarian disease, clinical differentiation may be difficult. ACTH-stimulated adrenal study, GnRH-stimulated gonadotropin profile, and estrogen levels are essential to confirm or exclude these differential diagnoses. Sonographic study of the ovary often provides adequate information to detect cystic lesions. However, CT scan is often required to assess the adrenal disease and noncystic ovarian lesions. Histologically, these tumors show intermediate to poor degrees of differentiation (50). Because of the relatively young age, conservative surgical management with preservation of the uterus and contralateral ovary is the goal of therapy. In advanced or recurrent disease, chemotherapy and irradiation remain the alternative (51,52) although the benefits of such therapy are not proven.

IV. TUMORS OF ENDOCRINE PANCREAS

A. Nesidioblastosis

This is defined, from the pathologist's point of view, as the diffuse proliferation of islet cells budding from the pancreatic duct, leading to the formation of numerous small clusters of B cells (55–57).

Males and females are equally affected, and familial occurrence has been reported. Clinically, the condition is encountered in neonates and infants with persistent symptomic hypoglycemia (Chaps. 48 and 49). Almost exclusively, neonatal hypoglycemia is attributed to impaired hepatic glucose output because of hyperinsulinemia. Severe, persistent hypoglycemia determines the clinical picture (58–60). Seizures, apnea, respiratory distress, listlessness, and cyanosis are the common manifestations (61). Neonates are usually macrosomic, and infants frequently weigh greater than the 97th percentile. Physical examinations are otherwise unremarkable in these patients.

Demonstration of hyperinsulinemia in the face of hypoglycemia and normal liver function, as well as other glucoregulatory hormones, confirms the diagnosis. Medical therapy includes diazoxide, corticosteroids, and epinephrine (61–64). However, partial pancreatectomy is recommended in these patients. Surgery should be performed at the earliest opportunity to minimize episodes of hypoglycemia and consequent brain damage (61).

Such terms as nesidioblastoma, multifocal ductuloinsular proliferation, microadenomatosis, nesidiodysplasia, and islet cell dysmaturation syndrome have been used to describe the morphologic variants of nesidioblastosis (56,65).

Clinical and biochemical means are not helpful to characterize the morphologic patterns in these patients (Table 4). At the functional level, further controversy exists about

Table 4 Distribution (%) of Morphologic Patterns in Nesidioblastosis

Lesions	Reference 61[a]	Reference 69
Hyperplasia	33	29
Nesidioblastosis	17	34
Discrete adenomas	16	29
Normal pancreas	30	8

[a]Report was not available for 4% of the patients.

the relationship between hypoglycemia and nesidioblastosis because pathologic characteristics similar to those of nesidioblastosis are known to exist in patients with normoglycemia and a normal pancreatic morphology has been described in patients with hypoglycemia (66–68).

B. Insulinoma

Functioning β cell tumors have been found from birth to old age, approximately 10% of all cases occurring in individuals below 20 years of age (70,71). There is a slight preponderance in females, adequate reasons for this observation being unclear (72).

Although insulinomas may belong to a spectrum that includes islet cell tumors, nesidioblastosis, and multiple endocrine neoplasia (MEN) type I (73,74), it is important to differentiate this entity from the rest because of the therapeutic implications (Chap. 50). If it is part of MEN type I, long-term follow-up must focus on the detection of other tumors; similarly, nesidioblastosis requires more radical surgical resection than what is necessary for a discrete tumor.

1. Clinical Features

In patients with insulinoma, the hypoglycemia caused by hyperinsulinemia determines the clinical picture. Combinations of adrenergic and neuroglycopenic symptoms, as shown in Table 5, are present in the vast majority of patients

Table 5 Symptoms of Hypoglycemia

Adrenergic	Neuroglycopenic
Anxiety	Headache
Nervousness	Blurred vision
Tremulousness	Paresthesias
Sweating	Weakness
Hunger	Tiredness
Palpitation	Confusion
Irritability	Dizziness
Pallor	Amnesia
Nausea	Incoordination
Flushing	Behavioral change
Angina	Seizures, coma

Source: From Reference 73.

(75,76), although the latter tend to predominate in individuals with organic hyperinsulinism. The time of the day symptoms occur and the relationship of these symptoms to a meal are important. If the symptoms are present in the morning during the fasting state, hyperinsulinemic hypoglycemia remains a strong possibility; if symptoms are reported during the postmeal period, an excessive insulin response because of leucine sensitivity becomes a possibility. Similarly, the presence or absence of other diseases, such as pituitary, adrenal, hepatic, renal, or autoimmune disease, should be ascertained. A family history of MEN type I, possible access to hypoglycemic agents, a history of ethanol ingestion, and the nutritional status of the patient should be specifically determined.

Apart from the symptoms being nonspecific, physical examinations are also noncontributory; thus, the clinical diagnosis of insulin-producing tumor is almost impossible. As shown in Table 6, the initial diagnosis in patients with proven insulinoma is extremely variable, with 50% of patients diagnosed inappropriately. The duration of the symptoms in patients with islet cell tumor is also variable and may be as short as 2 weeks or as long as 20 years. Because they learn to avoid symptoms by eating frequently throughout the day and night, some patients with long-standing disease may present with obesity and increased linear growth, which may also be the direct consequence of the anabolic and growth-promoting effect of insulin.

2. Laboratory Tests

Although normoglycemia and normal serum insulin levels have been documented in a small percentage of patients with insulinoma (77), this condition is usually suspected in nondiabetic individuals with hyperinsulinemic hypoglycemia during the fasting state. Indeed, absolute values of blood glucose and serum insulin, as well as their ratio, normally up to 0.3 in the fasting state, require documentation in these patients before embarking upon more definitive and expensive tests (78). A lack of ketonemia, ketonuria, and acidosis in the presence of fasting hypoglycemia is also strongly supportive of a diagnosis of hyperinsulinemic hypoglycemia.

An amended insulin-glucose ratio, calculated by multiplying the insulin level by 100 and then dividing by the blood glucose minus 30, is considered a better discriminator between normal and abnormal insulin secretions. This ratio, normally 50 or less, measures the degree of suppression of the pancreatic insulin secretion and reduces the false negative results.

Measurement of plasma C peptide and proinsulin levels is also useful in differentiating factitious hypoglycemia from islet cell tumor (79). Normally, the pancreatic insulin secretion parallels the plasma level of the peptides.

In children with concerns of hypoglycemia because of insulinoma, a limited fast of variable duration (6–72 h) is often necessary (80). This is especially the case when hypoglycemia is observed in the absence of inappropriate elevation in insulin levels.

For detection of symptoms of hypoglycemia and measurements of blood glucose, insulin, and urine ketones at the time of the symptoms, hospitalization is necessary.

In patients with insulinoma, the time of development of symptoms during the fast has been variable, ranging from 7 to 60 h. A spontaneous increase in the blood glucose levels has also been reported in such patients.

A provocative test for assessment of insulin secretion is sometimes necessary (81). This is particularly advantageous when the clinical evidence is compelling, yet time limitations do not allow hospitalization for prolonged fasting. Glucagon, leucine, and tolbutamide are β cell stimulatory agents used for this purpose (81–83). Intravenous calcium infusion is also used as a stimulus to insulin secretion (84,85). However, a tolbutamide test should not be used because it may be dangerous.

Depressed glucosylated hemoglobin and fructosamine levels may be present in patients with insulinoma, supporting the presence of hypoglycemia during the preceding 6–8 weeks.

3. Differential Diagnosis

Hypoglycemia caused by various systemic diseases is frequently encountered in clinical practice. Hyperinsulinemia is the primary distinguishing feature between these patients and those with insulinoma. The most difficult differential diagnosis is nesidioblastosis.

4. Localization of the Lesion

Once clinical and biochemical evidence of hyperinsulinemia is established, anatomic localization of the insulin-secreting lesion is indicated. This is accomplished by (1) ultrasonography, (2) CT scan, (3) highly selective arteriography, and (4) percutaneous transhepatic pancreatic venous sampling.

Of all the methods of study, preoperative ultrasonography is the most inexpensive and least invasive technique to localize pancreatic tumors. The accuracy is low, however, with detection of only 25% of pancreatic lesion (86). Using intraoperative ultrasonography by applying the probe to the

Table 6 Initial Diagnosis in 46 of 91 Patients with Proven Insulinoma

Diagnosis	Number of patients
Epilepsy	14
Nervous exhaustion	6
Psychoses	6
Stroke	4
Hysteria	4
Menopause	3
Tetany	2
Brain tumor	2
Diabetes	2
Inebriation	2
Heart attack	1

Source: From Reference 80.

surface of the pancreas, lesions too small to be palpable have been detected. CT scan performed with contrast enhancement can improve the sensitivity of detection up to 40% (87). The detection of the lesion also depends on its size and location: lesions measuring less than 2 cm or located on the head or tail of the pancreas are most likely to be missed. Although ultrasonography and CT scan have low accuracy, these are reasonable first choices for tumor staging and detection of metastasis. Selective arteriography is useful to demonstrate insulinomas, with a success rate ranging from 30 to 90% (88); lesions as small as 0.5 cm in diameter have been detected. This preoperative angiography is utilized to determine the number, size, and location of the tumors. Tumors located in the head or tail of the pancreas are the most likely to be missed.

Transhepatic venous sampling with simultaneous arterial blood sampling has been useful in detecting small tumors that were missed during the preoperative imaging studies (89). Apart from obtaining blood samples from different points in the portal, splenic, and mesenteric venous systems, it is important to draw simultaneous peripheral blood samples to allow change during the course of the procedure. During this study, a venous insulin concentration at least 50% higher than the arterial level is considered diagnostic of insulinoma. There is a considerable risk of complications, such as peritonitis, hemorrhage, or perforation of the gallbladder; consequently, this procedure should be considered if insulinoma is very likely based on the hypoglycemia and hyperinsulinemia and yet ultrasound, CT scan, arteriography have all been negative. Biochemical markers using α-hCG or β-hCG or an immunostaining technique have been found to be helpful in some patients. Differentiation of malignant lesions from benign ones by histologic criteria has been unreliable, because the morphologic characteristics fail to correlate with the metastatic disease (90).

5. Treatment and Prognosis

To avoid irreversible damage to the brain as a result of persistent profound hypoglycemia, intense preoperative management is mandatory. Dietary management should be judicious, particularly ensuring a snack before bedtime. Treatment is particularly difficult in infants and children, however, because of the uncertainty of assuring food intake in a timely manner and the variability of the pathology: diffuse islet cell involvement is more frequent than solitary adenomas, making complete surgical removal of the tumor difficult for the surgeons.

For preoperative patients as well as those with inoperable or undetectable tumor, pharmacologic agents are indicated. Diazoxide, a benzothiadiazine derivative, reduces insulin secretion and increases the epinephrine release and, when administered at a dose of 100–800 mg daily, maintains normoglycemia. Although side effects, such as fluid retention and hypertrichosis, are unacceptable, it is tolerated by most patients. Corticosteroid, used in conjunction with other agents, enhances the effectiveness of maintaining normoglycemia. A long-acting somatostatin analog, SMS 201-995, has shown promise in correcting hypoglycemia (91). Surgical removal of the tumor is the mode of therapy in patients with insulinoma (92) and should be performed at the earliest possible time. Almost 90% of the tumors are benign and carry a favorable prognosis.

C. Glucagonoma

The clinical and diagnostic features of glucagonoma, in comparison with vipoma and somatostatinoma, are presented in Table 7. Apart from insulin, endocrine tumors of the pancreas can produce glucagon, pancreatic polypeptide, and somatostatin, along with peptides that are not normally present, such as vasoactive intestinal peptide (VIP), peptide histidine methionine, growth hormone-releasing factors, gastrin, and calcitonin. Because of cosecretion of these hormones by various tumors, clinical syndromes may overlap and appear to be nonspecific; consequently, it becomes impractical to pursue the diagnosis in all patients who present with these symptoms. However, glucagonoma, vipoma, and so-

Table 7 Characteristic Features of Glucagonoma, Vipoma, and Somatostatinoma

Character	Glucagonoma	Vipoma	Somatostatinoma
Amino acid	29	28	14
Normal source	α Cells of pancreatic islet	Intestinal mucosa, central and peripheral nervous system	D cells of pancreatic islet, hypothalamus-pituitary, intestinal mucosa
Physiologic action	Raise blood glucose	Neurotransmitter; enhances intestinal secretion	Reduces intestinal secretion and motility
Characteristic clinical features	Rash, glossitis, stomatitis	Persistent and profuse diarrhea mimicks cholera	Diabetes, cholestasis, steatorrhea; may have hypoglycemia
Malignancy, %	75	60	60
Incidence in children	Not known, cases reported	Not known	Not known
Diagnosis	Elevated plasma level of glucagon, insulin; CT scan	Elevated plasma level of VIP or PHM; hypokalemia; CT scan; laparotomy	Elevated serum level of somatostatin; CT scan to detect tumor mass

matostatinoma, despite being rare in children, are interesting because of the cause-and-effect relationship between the increased hormone levels and the distinct clinical syndromes (glucagon and hyperglycemia, vasoactive intestinal peptide and diarrhea, and somatostatin and the reduced motility of the gastrintestinal-biliary tract). For a practicing physician, the importance of being familiar with these syndromes is therefore obvious: distinct clinical expression caused by altered biochemical environment, increased availability of precise diagnostic tools, and, most of all, specific therapeutic implications.

The true incidence of glucagonoma is not really known. Postmortem studies in adult patients with neither clinical symptoms nor diabetes have disclosed the presence of glucagonoma (93). However, there are no such data in children.

Glucagon, a 29 amino acid polypeptide, is secreted mostly by the α cells of the pancreatic islets. It stimulates the glycogenolytic process, resulting in elevation in blood glucose.

1. Clinical Features

A characteristic skin rash is the major manifestation in patients with glucagon-secreting islet cell tumor (93–95). Commonly starting in the groin area as erythematous blotches, the lesions migrate to the buttocks, thighs, perineum, and distal extremities. The lesions are necrolytic, with a raised and vesiculopustular appearance, and gradually become confluent. During the acute stage, these lesions are intensely painful and pruritic. After scaling, the lesions heal and become indurated and hyperpigmented. Remission and relapse are typical of these lesions, however, which are caused by the glycogenolytic action of glucagon. Glossitis, angular stomatitis, venous thrombosis, and occasional blackout spells occur in association with these lesions. The most common gastrointestinal symptoms are diarrhea and constipation, which are attributed to the altered motility of the intestine. Other findings include anemia and weight loss, which are primarily a result of the anorexic and catabolic effects of glucagon. Specific biochemical findings include hypoproteinemia, hypoaminoacidemia, and hypocholesterolemia. Mild hyperglycemia caused by the glycogenolytic effect of glucagon is also observed in some patients (97).

2. Diagnosis and Management

In the presence of suggestive clinical findings, the diagnosis is readily confirmed by the finding of elevated serum glucagon concentrations. Plasma insulin is also elevated, which explains the mildness of diabetes. A paradoxic rise in plasma glucagon during an oral glucose tolerance test or an intravenous tolbutamide test provides additional support to the diagnosis of glucagonoma. However, these tests are superfluous in most cases. Preoperatively, a CT scan is necessary to localize the primary and metastatic disease. However, the most valuable technique of tumor localization is selective arteriography: glucagonomas are highly vascular and produce a prominent tumor blush.

Treatment involves surgical resection, which leads to

dramatic improvement in the rash (96,97). Chemotherapy with dacarbazine (98) and streptozotocin (99) has been useful in nonresectable tumors. Somatostatin alleviates the symptoms because of the reduction in glucagon (100,101). Although zinc levels in the blood do not correlate with the presence or absence of the rash, oral zinc administration has been shown to improve the skin lesions (102). Adequate nutritional support and reversal of the negative nitrogen balance stands at the center of the medical and surgical management of these patients. Parenteral infusions of specific amino acids to correct the catabolic hypoaminoacidemia has led to disappearance of the skin lesions (103).

D. Vipoma

Since the first description of this condition in 1957 by Priest and Alexander (104), various investigators have reported manifold clinical features of this condition (105–109). Various synonyms, such as Verner-Morrison syndrome, watery diarrhea hypokalemia-achlorhydria syndrome, and pancreatic cholera syndrome, have represented the same condition (108). In 1973, Bloom, Polak, and Pearse renamed this condition Vipoma syndrome (106).

VIP is a 28 amino acid peptide distributed diffusely in the gastrointestinal submucosa as well as the central nervous system (110). It stimulates water and electrolyte secretion, leading to profuse water loss in the small intestine and colon. Sodium and potassium secretion into the lumen of the bowel also features prominently because of its action. Relaxation of the smooth muscles of gastrointestinal and vascular system, reduction in the gastric acid output, and decrease in the motility of the gallbladder are also caused by the vipoma.

1. Clinical Features

Vipoma is an uncommon disorder in children. Mekhjian and O'Dorisio reported 6 patients (109) of 29 diagnosed cases of this syndrome who were below 5 years of age. Mean age of presentation is 47 years (111), and the incidence has been estimated at 1 per 10 million per year. There is preponderance to females.

Diarrhea, the major manifestation of the vipoma syndrome, is characterized as persistent, secretory, and large in volume, exceeding 700 ml/day. Stool is isotonic with plasma and mimics the description of cholera. Apart from the massive water loss, large amounts of potassium and bicarbonate are lost in the stool. Thus, dehydration, hypokalemia, and acidosis lead to significant morbidity and mortality.

Because of the inhibitory effect of VIP on pentagastrin-mediated acid secretion, gastric acid secretion is frequently decreased in these patients. Differentiation from Zollinger-Ellison syndrome is therefore based on diminished basal acid output. Although serum phosphorus level is normal, hypercalcemia and hypomagnesemia occur in patients with vipoma syndrome. Hypercalcemia is explained on the basis of excessive bone resorption mediated by the VIP. Hyperglycemia, because of the glucagon-like effect of the VIP, is also reported.

2. Diagnosis and Management

Correction of volume deficit, electrolyte abnormalities, hypercalcemia, and hypomagnesemia should be the priority before establishing the diagnosis of vipoma and localization of the tumor.

In the presence of the characteristic clinical syndrome, an elevated plasma VIP concentration is diagnostic. However, normal plasma VIP with increased levels of peptide histidine methionine (PHM), another intestinal secretagogue similar in effect to VIP, has been described in patients with this syndrome. An intestinal perfusion study is useful to document intestinal secretion and confirm the diagnosis of vipoma syndrome. Anatomic localization of the tumor and its metastases is obtained by ultrasound and CT study. However, false negative studies are reported, making exploratory laparotomy the most definitive diagnostic modality.

Surgical resection offers the best chance of cure and provides relief of symptoms. In patients with nonresectable or metastatic disease, chemotherapy with streptozotocin may produce remission of symptoms and normalize the plasma VIP levels. Other drugs, such as corticosteroids and lithium carbonates, have been reported to control the symptoms of diarrhea. Treatment with octreotide, a somatostatin analog, represents a newer method of nonsurgical management of these patients.

E. Somatostatinoma

1. Clinical Features

This is also an unusual disorder in children. Most of the reported cases in the literature involve adult patients. Somatostatin, a 14 amino acid cyclic peptide, is present in the anterior pituitary, hypothalamus, thyroid follicle, D cells of the pancreatic islet, and intestinal mucosa (113–116). As indicated by its name, it inhibits pituitary, pancreatic, gastric, and biliary secretion. Thus, in patients with somatostatinoma and consequent increased serum somatostatin concentration, provocative growth hormone and thyroid-stimulating hormone response is inhibited, insulin and glucagon levels are diminished, and gastrointestinal and biliary secretion is decreased. Additionally, the motility of the gastrointestinal and biliary tract is reduced. Clinically, pancreatic somatostatinoma gives a triad of diabetes, cholelithiasis, and steatorrhea (117,118). Diabetes is usually mild, cholelithiasis is associated with gallbladder stasis, and steatorrhea is caused by insufficient exocrine function of the pancreas. However, cosecretion of the hormones can alter the picture, contributing to various nonspecific symptoms. For instance, diarrhea may be the prominent feature in calcitonin oversecretion. Because of the altered insulin-glucagon balance, hypoglycemia has been reported in some patients with somatostatinoma (119). Extrapancreatic somatostatinoma, usually located in the duodenal mucosa, is more likely to present with biliary obstruction rather than the constellation of the syndrome. Weight loss and anemia are also present in patients with long-standing disease.

2. Diagnosis and Management

In the clinical syndrome, the serum somatostatin level is usually elevated in patients with somatostatinoma. Provocative endocrine studies using a tolbutamide, arginine, or glucose tolerance test may be required in doubtful cases to document the lack of change in the insulin and glucagon (119,120). Detection of tumor mass and metastasis requires a radiologic imaging study, usually by CT scan. Although total surgical resection offers the most favorable outcome, advanced or recurrent disease may require chemotherapy with streptozotocin and 5-fluorouracil (119,121). Prognosis with treatment depends on the extent of the disease at the time of diagnosis.

REFERENCES

1. Bertagna C, Orth DN. Clinical and laboratory findings and results of therapy in 58 patients with adrenocortical tumors admitted to a single medical center (1951 to 1978). Am J Med 1981; 71:855–875.
2. McWhirler WR, Stiller CA, Lennox EL. Carcinoma in childhood. A registry-based study of incidence and survival. Cancer 1989; 63:2242–2246.
3. Kaplan SA. Disorders of the adrenal cortex I. Pediatric Clin North Am 1979; 26:65–76.
4. Luton J, Cedras S, Billard L, et al. Clinical features of adrenocortical carcinoma, prognostic factors and the effect of mitotane therapy. N Engl J Med 1990; 325:1195–1201.
5. Donaldson MDC, Grant DB, O'Hare MJ, Schackleton CHL. Familial congenital Cushing syndrome due to bilateral nodular adrenal hyperplasia. Clin Endocrinol (Oxf) 1981; 14:519–525.
6. Soleto-Avila C, Gonzales-Crussi F, Fowler JW. Complete and incomplete forms of Beckwith-Weidemann syndrome: their oncogenic potential. J Pediatr 1980; 96:47–50.
7. Fraumeni JF Jr, Miller RW. Adrenocortical neoplasms with hemihypertrophy, brain tumors, and other disorders. J Pediatr 1967; 70:129–138.
8. Meador CK, Bowdoin B, Owen WC, Farmer TA. Primary adrenocortical nodular dysplasia: a rare cause of Cushing's syndrome. J Clin Endocrinol Metab 1967; 27:125–163.
9. Larsen JL, Cathey WJ, Odell WD. Primary adrenocortical nodular dysplasia, a distinct subtype of Cushing's syndrome. Case report and review of the literature. Am J Med 1986; 80:976–984.
10. Carney JA, Hruska LS, Beauchamp GD, et al. Dominant inheritance of the complex of myxomas, spotty pigmentation, and endocrine overactivity. Mayo Clin Proc 1986; 61:165–172.
11. Wulffraat NM, Drexhage HA, Wiersinga RD, et al. Immunoglobulins of patients with Cushing's syndrome due to pigmented adrenocortical micronodular dysplasia stimulate in vitro steroidogenesis. J Clin Endocrinol Metab 1988; 66:301.
12. Weinstein LS, Shenker A, Gejman PV, Merino MJ, Friedman E, Spiegel AM. Activating mutations of the stimulatory G-protein in the McCune-Albright syndrome. N Engl J Med 1991; 325:1688–1695.
13. Lacroix A, Bolte E, Tremblay J, et al. Gastric inhibitory polypeptide-dependent cortisol hypersecretion: a new cause of Cushing's syndrome. N Engl J Med 1992; 327:974–980.
14. Reznik Y, Allili-Zerah V, Chayvialle, et al. Food-dependent Cushing's syndrome mediated by aberrant adrenal sensitivity to gastric inhibitory polypeptide. N Engl J Med 1992; 327:981–986.
15. McArthur RG, Cloutier MD, Hayles AB, et al. Cushing's disease in children. Mayo Clin Proc 1972; 47:318–326.

16. Thomas CG Jr, Smith AT, Griffith JM, et al. Hyperadrenalism in childhood and adolescence. Ann Surg 1984; 199:538–548.

17. Tyrell JB. Cushing's disease. N Engl J Med 1978; 298:753–758.

18. Lee PA, Weldon VV, Migeon CJ. Short stature as the only clinical sign of Cushing syndrome. J Pediatr 1975; 86:89–91.

19. Lee PDK, Winter RJ, Green OC. Virilising adrenocortical tumors in childhood. Eight cases and review of literature. Pediatrics 1985; 76:437–444.

20. Lanes R. Adrenocortical carcinoma in a 4 year old. Clin Pediatr (Phila) 1982; 21:164–166.

21. Giombetti R, Hagstrom JW, Landey S, Young MC, New MI. Cushing's syndrome in infancy: a case complicated by *Monilia endocarditis*. Am J Dis Child 1971; 122:264–266.

22. Dahms WT, Gray G, Vrana M, New MI. Adrenocortical adenoma and a ganglineuroblastoma in a child: a case presenting as Cushing's syndrome with virilization. Am J Dis Child 1973; 125:608–611.

23. Comite F, Schiebinger RJ, Albertson BD, et al. Isosexual precocious pseudopuberty secondary to a feminizing adrenal tumor. J Clin Endocrinol Metab 1984; 58:435–440.

24. Cagle PT, Hough AJ, Pysher TJ, et al. Comparison of adrenal cortical tumors in children and adults. Cancer 1986; 57:2235–2237.

25. Moore I, Barker AP, Byard RW, Bourne AJ, Ford WDA. Adrenocortical tumors in childhood—clinicopathological features of six cases. Pathology 1991; 23:94–97.

26. Zeiger MA, Nieman LK, Cutler GB, et al. Primary bilateral adrenocortical causes of Cushing's syndrome. Surgery 1990; 110:1106–1115.

27. Arico M, Bossi G, Livieri C, Raiteri E, Severi F. Partial response after intensive chemotherapy for adrenocortical carcinoma in a child. Med Pediatr Oncol 1992; 20:246–248.

28. Crock PA, Clark ACL. Combination chemotherapy for adrenal carcinoma: response in a 5 and half year old male. 1989; 17:62–65.

29. Schlumberger M, Brugieres L, Gicquel C, Travagli J, Groz J, Parmentier C. 5-Flourouracil, doxorubicin, and cisplatin as treatment for adrenal carcinoma. Cancer 1991; 67:2997–3000.

30. Ulbright TM, Roth LM. Recent developments in the pathology of germ cell tumors. Semin Diagn Pathol 1987; 4:304–319.

31. Jacobson GK, Barlebo H, Oslen J, et al. Testicular germ cell tumors in Denmark 1976–1980: Pathology of 1058 consecutive cases. Acta Radiol Oncol 1984; 23:239–247.

32. Batata MA, Whitmore WFJ, Chu FCH. Cryptorchidism and testicular cancer. J Urol 1980; 124:382–387.

33. Martin DC. Germinal cell tumors of the testis after orchiopexy. J Urol 1979; 121:422–424.

34. Benson RJ, Beard CM, Kelalis PP, et al. Malignant potential of the cryptorchid testis. Mayo Clin Proc 1991; 66:372–378.

35. Cassio A, Cacciari E, D'Errico A, et al. Incidence of intratubular germ cell neoplasia in androgen insensitivity syndrome. Acta Endocrinol (Copenh) 1990; 123:416–422.

36. Dexeus FH, Logothetis CJ, Chong C, et al. Genetic abnormalities in men with germ cell tumors. J Urol 1988; 140:80–84.

37. Lykkesfeldt G, Bennet P, Lykkesfeldt AE, et al. Testis cancer. Icthyosis constitutes a significant risk factor. Cancer 1991; 67:730–734.

38. Aristizabal S, Davis JR, Miller RC, Moore MJ, Boone LM. Bilateral primary germ cell testicular tumors. Report of four cases and review of literature. Cancer 1978; 42:591–597.

39. Thompson J, Williams CJ, Whitehouse JM, Mead GM. Bilateral testicular germ cell tumors: an increasing incidence and prevention by chemotherapy. Br J Urol 1988; 62:374–376.

40. Patel SR, Richardson RL, Kuols L. Synchronous and meta-chronous bilateral testicular tumors. Mayo Clinic experience. Cancer 1990; 65:1–4.

41. Tollerud DJ, Blattner WA, Fraser MC. Familial testicular cancer and urogenital developmental anomalies. Cancer 1985; 55:1849–1854.

42. Radfar N, Bartler FC, Easley R, et al. Evidence for endogenous LH suppression in a man with bilateral testicular tumors and congenital adrenal hyperplasia. J Clin Endocrinol Metab 1977; 45:1194–1203.

43. Srikanth MS, West BR, Ishitani M, et al. Benign testicular tumors in children with congenital adrenal hyperplasia. J Pediatr Surg 1992; 27:639–641.

44. Morrish DW, Venner PM, Siy O, et al. Mechangisms of endocrine dysfunction in patients with testicular cancer. J Natl Cancer Inst 1990; 82:412–418.

45. Castleberry RP, Kelly DR, Joseph DB, Cain WS. Gonadal and extragonadal germ cell tumors. In: Fernbach DJ, Vietti TJ, eds. Clinical Pediatric Oncology, 4th ed. St. Louis: Mosby YearBook, 1991:577–594.

46. Young JL, et al. Cancer, incidence, survival and mortality for children younger than age 15 years. Cancer 1986; 58:598–602.

47. Abell MR, Johnson VJ, Holtz, F. Ovarian neoplasms in childhood and adolescence. Am J Obstet Gynecol 1965; 92:1059–1081.

48. Young RH, Dickerson RG, Scully RE. Juvenile granulosa cell tumor of the ovary. A clinicopathological analysis of 125 cases. Am J Surg Pathol 1984; 8:575–596.

49. Young RH, Scully RE. Ovarian Sertoli-Leydig cell tumors. A clinicopathologic analysis of 207 cases. Am J Surg Pathol 1985; 9:534–569.

50. Roth LM, Anderson MC, Govan ADT, Langley FA, Gowing NFC, Woodcock AS. Sertoli-Leydig cell tumors: a clinico-pathological study of 34 cases. Cancer 1981; 48:187–197.

51. Zaloudek C, Norris HJ. Sertoli-Leydig tumors of the ovary. A clinicopathologic study of 64 intermediate and poorly differentiated neoplasm. Am J Surg Pathol 1984; 8:405–418.

52. Schwartz PE, Smith JP. Treatment of ovarian stromal tumors. Am J Obstet Gynecol 1976; 125:402–411.

53. Carr BR. Disorders of the ovary and female reproductive tract. In: Wilson JD, Foster DW, eds. Williams Textbook of Endocrinology, 8th ed. Philadelphia: W.B. Saunders, 1992: 779.

54. Castleberry RP, Kelly DR, Joseph DB, Cain WS. Gonadal and extragonadal germ cell tumors. In: Fernbach DJ, Vietti T, eds. Clinical Pediatric Oncology, 4th ed. St. Louis: Mosby YearBook, 1991:577–594.

55. Laidlaw G. Nesidioblastoma, the islet tumor of the pancreas. Am J Pathol 1938; 14:12–34.

56. Heitz PV, Kloppel G, Haiki WH, et al. Nesidioblastosis. The pathologic basis of persistent hyperinsulinemic hypoglycemia in infants: morphologic and quantitative analysis of seven cases based on specific immunostaining and electron microscopy. Diabetes 1971; 26:632–642.

57. Nathan DM, Axelrod L, Proppe KH, et al. Nesidioblastosis associated with insulin-mediated hypoglycemia in an adult. Diabetes Care 1981; 4:383–388.

58. Vance JE, Stoll RW, Kitabchi AE, et al. Nesidioblastosis in familial endocrine adenomatosis. JAMA 1969; 207:1679–1682.

59. Schwartz SS, Rich BM, Lucky AW, et al. Familial nesidio-blastosis: severe neonatal hypoglycemia in two families. J Pediatr 1979; 95:44–53.

60. Woo D, Scopes JW, Polak JM. Idiopathic hypoglycemia in sibs with morphological evidence of nesidioblastosis of the pancreas. Arch Dis Child 1976; 51:528–531.

61. Thomas CG Jr, Underwood LE, Carney CN, et al. Neonatal

and infantile hypoglycemia due to insulin excess: new aspects and diagnosis in surgical management. Ann Surg 1977; 185:505–517.

62. Fajans SS, Floyd JC Jr. Diagnosis and medical management of insulinomas. Annu Rev Med 1979; 30:313–329.

63. Fajans SS, Floyd JC Jr, Thiffault CA, et al. Further studies on diazoxide suppression of insulin release from abnormal and normal islet tissue in man. Ann NY Acad Sci 1968; 150:261–280.

64. Field JB, Remer A, Drapanas T. Clinical and physiologic studies using diazoxide in the treatment of hypoglycemia. Ann NY Acad Sci 1968; 150:415–428.

65. Carlson T, Eikhauser ML, DeBoz B, et al. Nesidioblastosis in an adult: an illustrative case and collective review. Am J Gastroenterol 1987; 82:566–571.

66. Rahier J. Relivance of endocrine pancrease nesidioblastosis to hyperinsulinemic hypoglycemia. Diabetes Care 1989; 12:164–166.

67. Karnauchow PN. Nesidioblastosis in adults without insular hyperfunction. Am J Clin Pathol 1982; 78:511–513.

68. Fong T, Warner NE, Kumar D. Pancreatic nesidioblastosis in adults. Diabetes Care 1989; 12:108–114.

69. Field JB. Insulinoma. In: Mazzaferi EL, Samaan NA, eds. Endocrine Tumors. Oxford: Blackwell Scientific, 1993:517–518.

70. Crain EL, Thorn GW. Functioning pancreatic islet cell adenomas: a review of the literature and presentation of two new differential tests. Medicine (Baltimore) 1949; 28:427–447.

71. Stefanini P, Carboni M, Pitrassi N, Bosali A. Beta-islet cell tumors of the pancreas. Results of a study on 1067 cases. Surgery 1989; 75:597–609.

72. Brunelle F, Negre V, Barth MD. Pancreatic venous sampling in infants and children with primary hyperinsulinism. Pediatr Radiol 1989; 19:100–103.

73. Field JB. Hypoglycemia. Definition, clinical presentations, classification, and laboratory tests. Endocrinol Metab Clin North Am 1989; 18:27–43.

75. Turner RC, Oakley NW, Naborro JDN. Control of basal insulin secretion with special reference to the diagnosis of insulinoma. BMJ 1971; 2:132–135.

76. Johnson RG, Bauman WA, Warshaw A, et al. Factitious hypoglycemia due to administration of human synthetic insulin: new diagnostic challenge. Diabetes Care 1987; 10:253–255.

77. Carlett JA, Mako ME, Rubinstein AH, et al. Factitious hypoglycemia: diagnosis by measurement of serum C-peptide immunoreactivity and insulin-binding antibodies. N Engl J Med 1977; 297:1029–1032.

78. Turner RC, Heding LG. Plasma proinsulin, C-peptide and insulin in diagnostic suppression tests for insulinomas. Diabetologia 1977; 13:571–577.

79. Fajans SS, Vinick AI. Insulin-producing islet cell tumors. Endocrinol Metab Clin North Am 1989; 18:45–74.

80. Breidahl HD, Priestly JT, Rynearson EH. Hyperinsulinemia: surgical aspects and results. Ann Surg 1955; 142:698–708.

81. Service FJ, Dale AJ, Elveback R, Jiang NS. Insulinomas: clinical and diagnostic features of 60 consecutive cases. Mayo Clin Proc 1976; 51:417–431.

82. Pun KK, Young RTT, Wang C, et al. The use of glucagon challenge test in the diagnostic evaluation of hypoglycemia due to hepatoma and insulinoma. J Clin Endocrinol Metab 1988; 67:546–550.

83. Kaplan EL, Arganine M, Kong SJ. Diagnosis and treatment of hypoglycemic disorder. Surg Clin North Am 1987; 67:395–410.

84. Kaplan EL, Rubinstein AH, Evans R, et al. Calcium infusion—a new provocative test for insulinoma. Ann Surg 1979; 190:501–507.

85. Roy BK, Abuid J, Wendorff H, et al. Insulin release in response to calcium in the diagnosis of insulinoma. Metabolism 1979; 28:246–252.

86. Gorman B, Charboneau JW, James EM, et al. Benign pancreatic insulinoma. Preoperative and intraoperative sonographic localisation. Am J Roengenol 1986; 147:929–934.

87. Dagget PR, Goodburn EA, Kurtz AB, et al. Is preoperative localization of insulinomas necessary? Lancet 1981; 1:483–486.

88. Galiher AR, Reading CC, Charbonneau JW, et al. Localization of pancreatic insulinoma: comparison of pre- and intraoperative US with CT and arteriography. Radiology 1988; 166:405–408.

89. Cho KJ, Vinik AI, Thompson NW, et al. Localization of the source of hyperinsulinism: percutaneous transhepatic portal and pancreatic vein catheterization with hormone assay. Am J Roentgenol 1982; 139:237–245.

90. Kenny BD, Sloan JM, Hamilton PW, et al. The role of morphometry in predicting prognosis in pancreatic islet cell tumors. Cancer 1989; 64:460–465.

91. Osei K, O'Dorisio TM. Malignant insulinoma: effects of somatostatin analog (compound 201-995) on serum glucose, growth and gastroenteropancreatic hormones. Ann Intern Med 1985; 103:223–225.

92. Koivunen DG, Harrison TS. The hypoglycemic syndrome: endogenous hyperinsulinism. In: Friesen SR, Thompson NW, eds. Surgical Endocrinology: Clinical Syndromes, 2nd ed. Philadelphia: J.B. Lippincott, 1990:221–225.

93. Mallinson CN, Bloom SR, Warin AP, et al. A glucagonoma syndrome. Lancet 1974; 2:1–3.

94. Printz RA, Dorsch TR, Lawrence AM. Clinical aspects of glucagon producing islet cell tumors. Am J Gastroenterol 1981; 76:125–131.

95. Stacpole PW. The glucagonoma syndrome: clinical features, diagnosis and treatment. Endocr Rev 1981; 2:347–361.

96. Higgins GA, Recant L, Fischman AB. The glucagonoma syndrome: surgically curable diabetes. Am J Surg 1979; 137:142–148.

97. Boden G, Owen OE, Rezvani I, et al. An islet cell carcinoma containing glucagon and insulin. Chronic glucagon excess and glucose homeostasis. Diabetes 1977; 26:128–137.

98. Strauss GM, Weitzman SA, Aoki TT. Dimethyltriazionoimidazole carboxamide therapy of malignant glucagonoma. Ann Intern Med 1979; 80:57–58.

99. Danforth DN Jr, Triche T, Doppman JL, Beazley RM, Perrino PV, Recant L. Elevated plasma glucagon-like component with -secreting tumor: effect of streptozotocin. N Engl J Med 1976; 295:242–245.

100. Kahn CR, Bhathena SJ, Recant L, et al. Use of somatostatin and somatostatin analogs in a patient with a glucagonoma. J Clin Endocrinol Metab 1981; 53:543–549.

101. Sohier H, Jeanmougin M, Lombrail P. Rapid improvement of skin lesions in glucagonoma with intravenous somatostatin infusion (letter). Lancet 1980; 1:40.

102. Mallinson C, Bloom SR. The hyperglycemic, cutaneous syndrome: pancreatic glucagonoma. In: Friesen SR, ed. Surgical Endocrinology: Clinical Syndromes. Philadelphia: J.B. Lippincott, 1978:171–202.

103. Norton JA, Kahn CR, Scheibinger R, Gorscboth C, Brennan MF. Amino acid deficiency and the skin rash associated with glucagonoma. Ann Intern Med 1979; 91:213–215.

104. Priest WM, Alexander MK. Islet-cell tumor of the pancreas

with peptic ulceration, diarrhea and hypokalemia. Lancet 1957; 2:1145–1147.

105. Verner JV, Morrison AB. Islet cell-tumor and a syndrome of refractory watery diarrhea and hypokalemia. Am J Med 1958; 25:374–380.

106. Bloom SR, Polak JM, Pearse AGE. Vasoactive intestinal peptide and watery diarrhea syndrome. Lancet 1973; 2:14–16.

107. Murray JS, Paton RR, Pope CE. Pancreatic tumor associated with flushing and diarrhea. Report of a case. N Engl J Med 1961; 264:436–439.

108. Matsumoto KK, Peter JB, Schultze RG, et al. Watery diarrhea and hypokalemia associated with pancreatic islet cell adenoma. Gastroenterology 1966; 50:231–242.

109. Mekhjian HS, O'Dorisio TM. Vipoma syndrome. Semin Oncol 1987; 14:282–291.

110. Pearse AGE. Peptides in brain and intestine. Nature 1976; 262:92–94.

111. Verner JV, Morrison AB. Non-beta islet cell tumors and the syndrome of watery diarrhea, hypokalemia and hypochlorhydria. Clin Gastroenterol 1974; 3:595–608.

112. Gardner JD. Plasma VIP in patients with watery diarrhea syndrome. Am J Dig Dis 1978; 23:370–373.

113. Brazeau P, Vale W, Burgus R, et al. Hypothalamic polypeptide that inhibits the secretion of immunoreactive pituitary growth hormone. Science 1973; 179:77–79.

114. Yamada Y, Ito S, Matsubara Y. Immunohistochemical demonstration of somatostatin-containing cells in the human, dog and rat thyroids. Tohoku J Exp Med 1977; 122:87–92.

115. Sundler F, Alumets J, Hokanson R, et al. Somatostatin immunoreactive cells in medullary carcinoma of thyroid. Am J Pathol 1977; 88:381–386.

116. Reichlin S. Somatostatin, part I. N Engl J Med 1983; 309:1495–1501.

117. Gunther KJ, Orci L, Conlon JM, et al. Somatostatinoma syndrome. Biochemical, morphologic and clinical features. N Engl J Med 1979; 285:285–292.

118. Friesen SR. Tumors of the endocrine pancreas. N Engl J Med 1982; 306:580–590.

119. Pipeleers D, Coutourier E, Gepts W, Reynders J, Somers G. Five cases of somatostatinoma: clinical heterogeneity and diagnostic usefulness of basal and tolbutamide-induced hypersomatostatinoma. J Clin Endocrinol Metab 1983; 56:1236–1242.

120. Boyce EL, Guenter KJ. The inhibitory syndrome: somatostatinoma. In: Friesen FR, Thompson TW, eds. Surgical Endocrinology, 2d ed. Philadelphia: J.B. Lippincott, 1990:249–266.

121. Ganda OP, Weir GC, Soeldner S, et al. Somatostatinoma: a somatostatin-containing tumor of the endocrine pancreas. N Engl J Med 1977; 296:963–967.

58

Nontraditional Inheritance of Endocrine Disorders

Elena Lopez-Rangel and Judith G. Hall
British Columbia Children's Hospital, University of British Columbia,
Vancouver, British Columbia, Canada

I. INTRODUCTION

Over the last few years there have been many new developments in the area of molecular genetics that have uncovered alternative genetic mechanisms leading to human genetic disorders and disease.

Disorders that were previously thought to have a straightforward Mendelian inheritance are now being recognized to have nontraditional forms of inheritance, such as uniparental disomy, mosaicism, mitochondrial disease, imprinting, and somatic recombination. These newly recognized nontraditional forms of inheritance and their importance in endocrine disorders are reviewed in this chapter.

II. UNIPARENTAL DISOMY

Chromosomes are inherited in pairs. The usual "normal" chromosome pair is made up of one chromosome contributed from the father and one from the mother. Studies in mice (1), however, have shown that although this may be the most common inheritance of a chromosome pair, there are instances in which both chromosomes come from only one of the parents. This particular situation has been called uniparental disomy (2).

Uniparental disomy (UPD) has now been described in a number of patients (3–8) involving a number of different chromosomes (9). In UPD, both chromosomes in a pair come from mother or from father. The patients with UPD who have been described so far are usually sporadic but can be expected to be seen occasionally in families with translocations. Uniparental disomy may be associated with abnormalities of growth and behavior, placental abnormalities, and intrauterine death (4,6,7). When two copies of exactly the same chromosome are inherited from one parent, an abnormal gene may be present and thereby both copies of the gene are abnormal. This may lead to an autosomal recessive disease.

This is a very unusual situation for an autosomal recessive disease because only one parent is a carrier. This situation occurs and has been reported in cystic fibrosis, one form of albinism, and several other disorders (3,4).

Uniparental disomy, as mentioned, occurs when the two chromosomes in a pair have been inherited from only one parent. UPD may be uniparental *isodisomy*, in which the two chromosomes originate from the same parental chromosome and are identical, or uniparental *heterodisomy*, in which the two chromosomes originate from the two different parental chromosomes so they are not identical. This difference is important to remember because the phenotype of an individual with UPD for a certain chromosome may vary depending on the sex of the parent who contributed the two chromosomes and on whether there is isodisomy or heterodisomy for the particular chromosome. In some situations involving chromosomes that have been involved in crossing over during meiosis, partial isodisomy and partial heterodisomy can exist.

The classic examples of UPD are Prader-Willi syndrome (PWS) and Angelman syndrome. Prader-Willi syndrome is a disorder that may present to the endocrinologist. The affected individuals have a round face, obesity, mental retardation, and hypogonadism. In the newborn period they are usually markedly hypotonic. PWS is associated with absence of paternal contribution of chromosome 15 because of a deletion or because of maternal UPD for chromosome 15 (6). Angelman, on the other hand, presents with a very long face, mental retardation, uncontrolled bouts of laughter, and seizures and is associated with absence of a maternal contribution of chromosome 15 because of a deletion or paternal UPD for chromosome 15 (7).

Maternal UPD for chromosome 7 has been reported in two patients with cystic fibrosis (3,4). Another case of maternal UPD for chromosome 7 was reported by Spotila et al. (5). All patients reported so far with maternal UPD for chromosome 7 have had intrauterine and postbirth growth and mental retardation.

UPD for other chromosomes, however, is not always associated with an abnormal phenotype. Several reports have shown that UPD for chromosome 22, for example, has no phenotypic abnormalities (10,11).

In summary, it is important to keep in mind that UPD for certain chromosomes or chromosome regions must be considered a possible mechanism producing disease, particularly related to disorders of growth, such as sporadic autosomal disorders and abnormal associations of two recessive disorders.

III. MOSAICISM

"Mosaicism" is the term used to describe an individual who has two different cell lines derived from a single zygote. Studies of placental tissue from chorionic villus sampling have shown that at least 2% of all conceptions are mosaic for chromosomal anomalies at or before 10 weeks of pregnancy (12). This suggests that mosaicism may be quite frequent in human. Among early abortuses, 50% have a chromosomal anomaly, the most common being trisomy and triploidy. Complete trisomies are usually nonviable and, in most cases, aborted. However, the development of a normal cell line may rescue or allow a trisomic conception to come to term and be viable. In trisomies 13 and 18, Kalousek (12) has shown that all pregnancies that survive to birth have some normal cells in the placenta.

Depending upon the point at which the new cell line arises during early embryogenesis, a patient may have a variety of clinical presentations. In some situations, the trisomic cell line may be lost or overgrown. Mosaicism may be present in some tissues but not in others. Mosaicism may lead to a patchy or asymmetric distribution for abnormal tissue. There are many conditions that are asymmetric or patchy, such as Ollier, multiple exostosis, and McCune-Albright syndrome (MAS), that are best explained on the basis of mosaicism.

McCune-Albright was first described in 1924 (13) as a sporadic disorder characterized by polyostotic fibrous dysplasia, café au lait pigmentation, sexual precocity, and hyperfunction of multiple endocrine glands (Chap. 13). Because MAS is usually sporadic and has a characteristic lateralized pattern of cutaneous hyperpigmentation, it has been thought for some time to be likely caused by a somatic mutation occurring early in development, with some cells affected but others not affected. The occurrence and severity of the disease in bone, skin, and endocrine abnormalities in a patient depend on the number of cells carrying the mutated gene in the specific tissue.

Recent research has shown that MAS is a result of a specific mutation in the stimulatory G protein of adenyl cyclase (14,15). This mutation leads to constitutive activation of the G_s protein, inducing proliferation and hyperfunction of cells responsive to hormones. This mutation is not the same in all patients, and different patients have different specific mutations and different distributions of tissue involvement.

Studies of specific patients have shown that the mutated gene has a mosaic distribution and in general is present in low levels in blood and high levels in skin (16). These findings support the suggestion and the segmental distribution and variable expression of the skeletal, cutaneous, and endocrine abnormalities in MAS are caused by underlying somatic mosaicism (17).

IV. GERMLINE MOSAICISM

Germline mosaicism refers to germ cells (eggs and sperm) only and occurs when some germ cells are normal and others carry a genetic abnormality, such as a mutation. Because this situation is exclusive to the germ cells, it does not become apparent until a couple has children. In this case parents can have two or more children with the same new mutation but who appear to be and test perfectly normal themselves. Germline and somatic mosaicism have been documented on a bichemical and DNA level in some cases of osteogenesis imperfecta (18,19).

V. IMPRINTING

"Imprinting" is a term used to refer to the differences in the phenotype of a disorder depending on the parent of origin (20,21). Most of the information on imprinting comes from studies done in mice and, more recently, from specific clinical findings in humans.

One of the first indications that male and female genetic contributions were different came from pronuclear transplantation experiments. Pronuclear transplantation allows the pronuclei of the oocyte and the sperm to be manipulated before fertilization. This technique was used in mice to produce zygotes that have two female pronuclei (gynogenetic) or two male (androgenetic) pronuclei. These studies showed that the zygote with two maternal contributions developed embryos, but the placentas were very small. Embryos with only a paternal contribution, on the other hand, had normal placentas but the embryos were very small. These studies clearly showed both maternal and paternal genetic information is necessary to form a healthy embryo that grows to be born. The maternal and the paternal genetic contributions are different, complementary, and necessary (20).

More evidence for imprinting comes from mice and human uniparental disomies, from differences in mouse transgene expression, and from certain types of cancer studies (21).

Mouse and human chromosomes have homologous regions. This has prompted the suggestion that several genes known to be imprinted in mice may also be imprinted in homologous chromosomal regions in humans. Several genes known to be imprinted in mice have been associated with disorders of growth in humans and consequently have been suggested to be "at risk" of being imprinted (Table 1) (23–25).

Insulin-like growth factor type II and the H19 genes, for example, are located in the mouse chromosome 7 (26). In humans these genes map to 11p15, which is the area

Table 1 Endocrine Disorders "at Risk" to Be Imprinted[a]

Chromosome	Endocrine Disorder
6	Insulin-dependent diabetes
	H-Y antigen
	Prolactin
	21-OH
	Paget's disease of bone
	Estrogen receptor
	MEN I
11	Hypoparathyroidism
	Adrenocortical cancer
	MODY
19	Insulin receptor
	Infertility (LH)
	Chorionic gonadotrophic cluster
20	Diabetes insipidus
	Albright hereditary osteodystrophy
	Growth hormone-releasing factor
22	Thyroid-stimulating hormone
	MEN II

[a]MEN, multiple endocrine neoplasia; LH, luteinizing hormone.

associated with Beckwith-Wiedemann syndrome, a fetal overgrowth disorder characterized by a predisposition to tumours and hyperinsulinism (Chap. 12).

Because disorders that are imprinted in humans show a difference in the phenotype depending on the parent transmitting the gene, endocrine and other disorders should be suspected to be imprinted if varying phenotypes are seen in a pedigree (Figs. 1 and 2). Two examples of disorders suspected to be imprinted on the basis of varying phenotype in the pedigrees are Albright's hereditary osteodystrophy and paragangliomas.

Albright's hereditary osteodystrophy (AHO), also known as pseudo-pseudohypoparathyroidism, is characterized by short stature, mental retardation, round face, obesity, brachydactyly, and subcutaneous calcifications in the presence of

PATERNAL

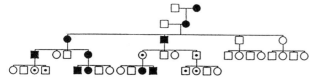

Figure 1 Pedigree suggestive of paternal imprinting. Phenotypic effects occur only when the gene is transmitted from the mother but not when transmitted from the father. An equal number of males or females are affected or unaffected phenotypically in each generation. A nonmanifesting transmitter gives a clue to the sex of the parent who passes the expressed genetic information; in other words, in paternal imprinting there are "skipped" female nonmanifesting individuals.

MATERNAL

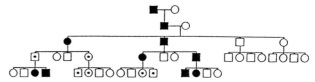

Figure 2 In pedigrees suggestive of maternal imprinting, phenotypic effects occur only when the gene is transmitted from the father but not when transmitted from the mother. Equal numbers of males or females are affected or unaffected phenotypically in each generation. A nonmanifesting transmitter gives a clue to the sex of the parent who passes the expressed genetic information; in other words, in paternal imprinting there are "skipped" female nonmanifesting individuals.

hypocalcemia and parathyroid hormone resistance. A family reported by Schuster et al. (15) supports the suggestion that AHO may be imprinted. In this report, the mildly affected members of the family had inherited the disorder from their father but the severely affected index case had inherited it from his mother.

A recent review of reported cases of AHO has shown that in fact there is a marked difference in the phenotype of AHO depending on the parent transmitting the disorder. Davies and Hughes (23) collected data on 36 AHO-transmitting parents. They found that in 92% of the affected cases the allele was inherited from the mother and the phenotype was fully expressed (AHO + hormone resistance + pseudohypoparathyroidism). The remaining 8% were paternally inherited and the phenotype was only partially expressed (AHO alone).

Mutations of the G_s protein have been observed in patients with AHO, but in contrast to MAS patients these mutations cause deficient expression of the G_s protein (27). The gene for G_s protein has been mapped to chromosome 20q13.11, which is homologous to the mouse area 2H, which is known to be imprinted (28). This evidence points to the differential expression of the phenotype and supports the suggestion that AHO is indeed imprinted.

VI. MITOCHONDRIAL INHERITANCE

Diabetes mellitus (DM) is another disorder often encountered by endocrinologists. DM is a heterogeneous disorder that may be inherited in various forms. It has been associated with imprinting (29), and there have been suggestions that it is also associated with segregation distortion and/or mitochondrial involvement (30,31). Immunologic predisposition as a result of specific inherited HLA markers has been documented to play an important role in the etiology of DM (32).

VII. SUMMARY

It is clear that nontraditional mechanisms of inheritance may be playing an major role in a number of endocrine disorders, and it is important to look for parent of origin effects in all disorders. This will allow better understanding of some of the genetic mechanisms causing disease, which could lead to better diagnosis and counseling of patients and their families.

REFERENCES

1. Cattanach BM, Kirk M. Differential activity of maternally and paternally derived chromosome regions in mice. Nature 1989; 315:496–498.
2. Engel F. A new genetic concept: uniparental disomy and its potential effect. Am J Med Genet 1980; 6:137–143.
3. Spence JE, Perciaccante RG, Greig GM, et al. Uniparental disomy as a mechanism for human genetic disease. Am J Hum Genet 1988; 42:217–226.
4. Voss R, Ben-Simon E, Vital A, et al. Isodisomy of chromosome 7 in a patient with cystic fibrosis: could uniparental disomy be common in humans? Am J Hum Genet 1989; 45:373–380.
5. Spotila LD, Sereda L, Prockop DJ. Uniparental disomy as a mechanism for human genetic disease. Am J Hum Genet 1988; 42:217–226.
6. Knoll JHM, Nicholls RD, Magenis RE, Graham JM Jr, Lalande M, Latt SA. Angelman and Prader-Willi syndrome share a common chromosome 15 deletion but differ in paternal origin of the deletion. Am J Med Genet 1989; 32:285–290.
7. Nicholls RD, Knoll JHM, Butler MG, Karam S, Lalande M. Genetic imprinting suggested by maternal heterodisomy in non-deletion Prader-Willi syndrome. Nature 1989; 324:281–285.
8. Henry I, Priech A, Riesewijk A, Ahnine L, Mannens M, Beldjord C, Bitoun P, Tournade MF, Landrieu P, Imieu C. Somatic mosaicism for partial paternal isodisomy in Wiedemann-Beckwith syndrome: a postfertilization event. EJHG 1993; 1:19–29.
9. Engel E, Delozier-Blanchet D. Uniparental disomy, isodisomy and imprinting: probable effects in man and strategies for their detection. Am J Hum Genet 1991; 40:432–439.
10. Schinzel AA, Basaran S, Bernasconi F, Karaman B, Yuksel-Apak M, Robinson WF. Maternal uniparental disomy for chromosome 22 has no impact on the phenotype. Am J Hum Genet 1994; 54:21–24.
11. Kirkels VG, Hustinx TW, Scheres JM. Habitual abortion and translocation (22q;22q): unexpected transmission from mother to her phenotypically normal daughter. Clin Genet 1980; 18:456–461.
12. Kalousek DK. The role of confined placental mosaicism in placental function and human development. GGH 1988; 4:1–3.
13. Albright F, Burnett CH, Smith PH, Parson W. Pseudohypoparathyroidism—an example of Seabright bantam syndrome. Endocrinology 1942; 30:922–932.
14. Weinstein LE, Shenker A, Gejman P, Merino MJ, Friedman E, Spiegel AM. Activating mutation of the stimulatory G protein in the McCune-Albright syndrome. N Engl J Med 1991; 325:1688–1695.
15. Schuster V, Eschenhagen T, Kruse K, Gierschlik P, Kreth HW. Endocrine and molecular biological studies in a German family with Albright hereditary osteodystrophy. Eur J Pediatr 1993; 152:185–189.
16. Schuwindinger WF, Francomano CA, Levine ME. Identification of a mutation in the gene encoding the alpha subunit of the stimulatory G protein of adenylyl cyclase in McCune-Albright syndrome. Proc Natl Acad Sci USA 1992; 89:5152–5156.
17. Happle R. Mosaicism in human skin. Understanding the patterns and mechanisms. Arch Dermatol 1993; 129:1460–1470.
18. Cohn DH, Starman BJ, Blumberg B, Byers PH. Recurrence of lethal osteogenesis imperfecta due to parental mosaicism for a dominant mutation in a human type I collagen gene (COL1A1). Am J Hum Genet 1990; 46:591–601.
19. Wallis GA, Starman BJ, Zinn AB, Byers PH. Variable expression of osteogenesis imperfecta in a nuclear family is explained by somatic mosaicism for a lethal point mutation in the alpha 1(I) gene (COL1A1) of type I collagen in a parent. Am J Hum Genet 1990; 46:1034–1040.
20. Solter D. Differential imprinting and expression of maternal and paternal genomes. Annu Rev Genet 1988; 22:127–226.
21. Surani MA, Reik W, Allen ND. Transgenes as molecular probes for genomic imprinting. Trends Genet 1988; 4:59–62.
22. Surani MA, Kothary R, Allen ND, et al. Genome imprinting and development in the mouse. Development 1990; 108:203–211.
23. Davies SJ, Hughes HE. Imprinting in Albright's hereditary osteodystrophy. J Med Genet 1992; 30:101–103.
24. Ohlsson R, Nystrom A, Pfeifer-Ohlsson S, et al. IGF2 is parentally imprinted during human embryogenesis and in the Beckwith-Wiedemann sundrome. Nat Genet 1993; 4:94–97.
25. Giannoukakis N, Deal C, Paquette J, Gooyer CG, Polychronakos C. Parental imprinting of the human IGF2 gene. Nat Genet 1993; 4:98–101.
26. Ekstrand J, Ehrenborg E, Sten I, Stellan B, Zech L, Luthman H. The gene for insulin-like growth factor-binding protein is localized to human chromosome region 7p14-p12. Genomics 1990; 6:413–418.
27. Levine MA. The McCune-Albright syndrome. The whys and wherefores of abnormal signal transduction. N Engl J Med 1991; 24:1688–1694.
28. Gopal Rao VVN, Schnittger S, Hansmann I., G protein (GNAS1), the probable candidate gene for Albright herediatry osteodystrophy, is assigned to hyman chromosome 20q12-q13.2. Genomics 1991; 10:257–261.
29. McCarthy BJ, Dorman JS, Aston CE. Investigating genomic imprinting and susceptibility to insulin dependent diabetes mellitus: an epidemiologic approach. Genet Epidemiol 1991; 8:77–86.
30. Alcolado JC. Mitochondrial DNA defects in diabetes mellitus. Diabetologia. 1993; 36:578–579.
31. Reardon W, Ross RJ, Sweeney MG, et al. Diabetes mellitus associated with a pathogenic mutation in mitochondrial DNA. Lancet 1992; 340:1376–1379.
32. Julier C, Hyer RN, Davies J, et al. Insulin-IGF2 region on chromosome lip encodes a gene implicated in HLA-DR dependent diabetes susceptibility. Nature 1991; 354:155–159.

59

Eating Disorders

Eric A. Lifshitz

UCLA Neuropsychiatric Institute,
Los Angeles, California

I. INTRODUCTION

With both biologic and psychologic factors at play, eating disorders can be perplexing to understand and treat. The primary aims of treatment are relatively straightforward: normalize eating patterns and maintain weight within a normal range. These seemingly simple goals are often met with a great deal of resistance, and this difficulty points to our need for a fuller understanding of the underlying determinants that make treatment challenging. As described in this chapter, eating disorders (ED) represent an attempt at mastery and self-control in individuals who have often felt unable to achieve this otherwise. Because of the often central role of eating disorders in the individual's sense of self-evaluation, they are relinquished reluctantly. Identifying patients with eating disorders and prescribing a course of treatment is likely to be ineffective unless the clinician is able to develop a therapeutic alliance by being open, truthful, patient, tolerant, and able to relate well to eating-disordered patients and their families (1).

ED typically begin in the late teens, and the female-male ratio is at least 10:1 (1). ED have potentially profound physiologic effects, such as stunted growth, delayed sexual development, and increased risk of death. ED also have profound psychologic consequences. Normal adolescents have many developmental obstacles to overcome, and the burden of eating disorders hampers this process and robs them of the opportunity to grow and develop normally. The self-preoccupative, obsessive nature characteristic of these disorders can have long-lasting effects on self-esteem and peer relations (2). These disorders also exist in a social milieu in which thinness and perfect bodies are idealized. In fact, ED are typically found in more developed affluent cultures. These messages affect young women. As we shall see, not infrequently, more serious ED first begin with attempts at dieting. Early successes in controlling their bodies may lay the template for a much more serious disorder (1). Obviously,

not all women who diet develop ED, and the differences between those who do and those who do not progress to disordered eating are also addressed in this chapter.

The diagnosis of eating disorders is also complicated by the fact that outwardly many of these women may lead successful lives and are, by and large, high-achieving perfectionists (3). Moreover, there is often a great deal of shame surrounding the disorder. Secrecy is not uncommon, and unless the clinician is familiar with the signs and symptoms of eating disorders, they may go undetected and undiagnosed (4).

This chapter focuses on anorexia nervosa and bulimia nervosa, because these are the two most common forms of eating disorders. A review of the diagnostic parameters and epidemiology of these severe eating disorders and their physiologic complications, underlying psychologic determinants, and, finally, treatment strategies is presented.

II. DIAGNOSIS

Several questions are usually asked in the initial evaluation of a patient with a possible eating disorder (5). Inquiring about what the patient views as the highest and lowest weight with which he or she would be comfortable can give the clinician a sense of the degree of body image distortion that may be present. If the patient mentions specific periods of weight fluctuations, asking about possible concurrent life events helps to introduce the patient to think psychologically about the relationship between food, weight and shape, and life events. Patients are asked how much emphasis is placed on thinness and appearance by family members and friends. Patients are also asked to describe daily eating patterns, dieting behaviors, frequency of binging and purging, possible events or emotional states that trigger binge-eating episodes, and about how important it is for them to purge (5).

Anorexia nervosa (AN), which means "nervous loss of

appetite," and bulimia nervosa, which means "hunger of the ox," share in common the primary symptom of extreme weight preoccupation and behaviors designed to control the weight and body shape (6).

AN is one of the few childhood psychiatric disorders that can cause death; it has a 6% mortality rate, the highest of any psychiatric disorder (7,8). In particular, children with AN are more likely to have diminished fluid intake and become dehydrated than older patients. Children have less total-body fat than either adolescents or adults and may become emaciated more quickly. Starvation in prepubertal girls can delay menarche and permanently minimize stature and breast development (7). DSM-IV, the latest *Diagnostic and Statistical Manual of Mental Disorders*, lists the following diagnostic criteria for AN (9).

1. Refusal to maintain body weight at or above a minimally normal weight for age and height (e.g., weight loss leading to maintenance of body weight less than 85% of that expected or failure to make expected weight gain during period of growth, leading to body weight less than 85% of that expected)
2. Intense fear of gaining weight or becoming fat, even though underweight
3. Disturbance in the way in which one's body weight or shape is experienced, undue influence of body weight or shape on self-evaluation, or denial of the seriousness of the current low body weight
4. In postmenarcheal females, amenorrhea, that is, the absence of at least three consecutive menstrual cycles (a woman is considered to have amenorrhea if her periods occur only following hormone, e.g., estrogen administration)

There are two types of AN that must be specified:

1. Restricting type: during the current episode of anorexia nervosa, the person has not regularly engaged in binge-eating or purging behavior, that is, self-induced vomiting or the misuse of laxatives, diuretics, or enemas
2. Binge-eating/purging type: during the current episode of anorexia nervosa, the person has regularly engaged in binge-eating or purging behavior (i.e., self-induced vomiting or the misuse of laxatives, diuretics, or enemas)

DSM-IV diagnostic criteria differ from those previously listed in DSM-III-R by the further specification of two subtypes of AN. As described later, this distinction is important because of the differing psychologic features associated with each.

The anorectic's intense fear of gaining weight or becoming fat manifests itself as an obsessive preoccupation and is usually not alleviated by weight loss. In fact, concern about weight gain often increases even as actual weight continues to decrease (9). It is difficult to appreciate the extent to which a patient will go to maintain an abnormally low weight. When monitoring their weight, clinicians should be aware that anorectic patients often "pad" their weight by wearing several layers of clothing, placing heavy objects in their pockets, or withholding urine and stool to increase body weight before measurements.

One frequently used reference is the Metropolitan Table of Height and Weight (10). The weights in this table reflect women in light clothing and 2 inch heels. Another useful rule of thumb for estimating expected weight for height for female patients is the Hamwi formula (5 feet = 100 pounds and 5 pounds is added for each additional inch) (11). This calculated weight, give or take 10%, gives an acceptable weight range for most patients. The inclusion of the DSM-IV of failure to make expected weight gain during period of growth is useful in assessing younger patients who are still growing (9). For these younger patients, it is best to refer to the growth charts and to monitor weight and height and their progression over time (see Chaps. 1 and 8). The morbid fear of fat present in anorectics is a feature that helps differentiate anorexia nervosa from other psychiatric disorders (12). In addition to the body image disturbance criteria found in DSM-III-R, DSM-IV has further emphasized the central concern of weight and shape in the person's self-evaluation and incorporated the denial of the serious consequences of low body weight seen in patients with anorexia nervosa (1,9): for example, a 5 foot 6 inch patient can weigh 80 pounds and still believe she is too fat.

Bulimia nervosa (BN) has been recognized as an official diagnosis since 1980. The DSM-IV diagnostic criteria for bulimia nervosa are as follows:

1. Recurrent episodes of binge eating. An episode of binge eating is characterized by both of the following:
   a. Eating, in a discrete period of time (e.g., within any 2 h period), an amount of food that is definitely larger than most people would eat during a similar period of time and under similar circumstances
   b. A sense of lack of control over eating during the episode (e.g., a feeling that one cannot stop eating or control what or how much one is eating)
2. Recurrent inappropriate compensatory behavior to prevent weight gain, such as self-induced vomiting; misuse of laxatives, diuretics, enemas, or other medications; fasting; or excessive exercise.
3. The binge eating and inappropriate compensatory behaviors both occur, on average, at least twice a week for 3 months.
4. Self-evaluation is unduly influenced by body shape and weight.
5. The disturbance does not occur exclusively during episodes of anorexia nervosa.

As in AN, bulimia nervosa also presents in two subtypes:

1. Purging type: during the current episode of bulimia nervosa, the person has regularly engaged in self-induced vomiting or the misuse of laxatives, diuretics, or enemas

2. Nonpurging type: during the current episode of bulimia nervosa, the person has used other inappropriate compensatory behaviors, such as fasting or excessive exercise, but has not regularly engaged in self-induced vomiting or the misuse of laxatives, diuretics, or enemas.

Although there has been no current consensus on what constitutes a binge, DSM-IV has defined binges as episodes in which the person consumes an amount of food that is out of proportion to what most would eat in the same setting. Binges can involve the consumption of as many as 3000–20,000 cal at a time (13). For example, a binge may consist of two boxes of cereal, 2 pints of ice cream, and a pizza. An important characteristic of binges is the subjective sense of loss of control experienced by the patient. Patients tend to feel helpless both in preventing the onset of a binge and in terminating it once it has begun. Individuals also describe a dissociative quality during or following binge episodes. An individual may be in a frenzied state while binging but can stop when a roommate walks in. Typically binges are preceded by a dysphoric or unpleasant emotional state, interpersonal stressors, intense hunger following dietary restraint, or feelings related to body weight, body shape, and food. Binges are often characterized by rapid consumption and continue until the individual is uncomfortably or even painfully full (9). Binges often have the immediate effect of providing relief from the negative mood or stressor that triggered them, but this is soon followed by physical discomfort secondary to the binge, as well as guilt feelings about the amount of food eaten. This then triggers a fear of gaining weight, and in response to this, bulimic patients resort to various purging techniques, including vomiting, laxative, thyroxine, and diuretic abuse, and vigorous exercise for several hours daily (14,15). Vomiting frequency can occur 20 times or more in a single day. Also, bulimic patients with diabetes mellitus have been known to omit insulin to induce glycosuria to promote weight loss (16–18). In DSM-IV, the presence of these compensatory behaviors has been included as part of the diagnostic criteria for bulimia nervosa. Moreover, DSM-IV has refocused the overconcern with body weight and shape to the influence of these on the person's self-evaluation. With the addition of the two subtypes of AN, bulimic patients who fall below 85% of their expected weight are now considered to have AN, binge-eating/purging type. Shape and weight concerns, which are commonly found among the general female population, differ from BN and AN in intensity and by the central role they play in influencing the person's self-evaluation and self-esteem (see later) (12).

Although anorexia nervosa and bulimia nervosa have different diagnostic criteria, many people view these disorders as occurring along the same continuum. Many patients demonstrate both anorectic and bulimic behaviors, either concurrently or at different times. Up to 50% of AN patients develop bulimic symptoms, and a significant number of patients who are initially bulimic develop anorectic symptoms. Moreover, both subtypes of AN may coexist in the same patient (19).

Both AN restrictors and AN bulimics share characteristics of high academic achievement and perfectionism (20). Compared with AN restrictors, AN bulimics generally weigh more before the illness and more commonly have been obese. They also come from families in which obesity is more common. They are more likely to induce vomiting and misuse laxatives while attempting to control their weight and, on the whole, tend to be more impulsive and display more depression and mood lability (12). They are more often raised in homes with disturbed family interaction patterns and have a higher prevalence of family history of affective disorders. They also have higher rates of substance abuse, suicide attempts, and stealing (21). All these characteristics are also true of patients with bulimia nervosa (12). Interestingly, the psychologic issues seen in the bulimic subtype of AN appear to be state dependent; that is, while the patient is underweight the issues are similar to AN restrictors, but with weight gain they begin to resemble those seen in bulimia nervosa (22). Bulimic AN are similar in personality to bulimics but differ by the loss of large amounts of weight.

AN restrictors, on the other hand, tend to be more steady, deliberate, and conscientious. They frequently display avoidant personality traits. From a nutritional standpoint, they can limit their energy intake to several hundred kilocalories per day and tend to eat irregularly and to skip meals. A large majority of them fast and eat nutrient-poor diets, avoiding certain food items, such as red meat, sweets, and carbohydrates, and can display peculiar food rituals (13).

DSM-IV diagnostic criteria also include the category of eating disorder not otherwise specified, which is used for disorders of eating that do not meet the criteria for a specific eating disorder. Examples include, for females, that all the criteria for AN are met except that the individual has regular menses; all the criteria for BN are met except for the frequency of binging and purging; and nonpurging bulimics (9). Bulimics who do not purge or engage in other compensatory mechanisms to maintain their weight tend to be obese and tend to represent small sample of patients seen in eating disorder clinics, approximately 6% (12). On the other hand, among obese women seeking treatment for weight loss, 23–46% engage in binge eating (23).

Other types of disordered eating have been reported in middle childhood or early adolescence. These "atypical" eating disorders include the syndromes of fear of obesity (24) and fear of hypercholesterolemia (25). These children do not meet the criteria for an ED according to DSM-IV but display abnormal eating patterns that can lead to nutritional dwarfing and other physiologic abnormalities, such as delayed puberty (13). These individuals restrict their dietary intake by avoiding "junk foods," dairy products, meat, and eggs in an attempt to comply with a specific fear or health belief. They typically ingest an insufficient amount of calories for age, usually about two-thirds of their normal daily caloric requirements. Additionally, the low-calorie, low-fat diets preferred by these patients lead to intakes of iron and zinc of below 30 and 40%, respectively, of the recommended dietary allowance. This in turn can also cause growth failure and delayed puberty (13). In contrast to the

ED described in DSM-IV, these atypical eating disorders are not associated with any obvious signs of psychiatric disorders or disturbed behavioral functioning. A study by Sandberg et al. found no difference in an eating disorders screening questionnaire between patients with nutritional dwarfing and a matched control group (26).

Other eating disorders seen in children and infants, described in DSM-IV, include pica, rumination disorder of infancy, and feeding disorder of infancy or early childhood (9). Pica is characterized by the persistent eating for more than 1 month of nonnutritive substances, which is inappropriate to the developmental level and is not part of a culturally sanctioned practice (in some cultures, the eating of dirt is believed to be of value). Pica is more commonly seen in young children and occasionally in pregnant women. Rumination disorder describes the repeated regurgitation and re-chewing of food that develops in infants or children after a period of normal functioning and lasts for at least 1 month. This behavior is not caused by an associated gastrointestinal or other medical condition. Rumination is most commonly seen in infants but may occur in older individuals, particularly those with mental retardation. Infants with the disorder display a characteristic position of straining and arching the back with the head held back, making sucking movements with their tongues and giving the impression of gaining satisfaction from the activity. The criterion requiring weight loss, described in DSM-III-R, was omitted in DSM-IV (9).

Feeding disorder of infancy or early childhood is a new category that was added to DSM-IV to provide diagnostic coverage for infants and children, before age 6, who fail to eat adequately and who then have problems in gaining or maintaining weight. This condition is not caused by an associated medical disorder and may encompass up to half the 1–5% of all pediatric hospital admissions for failure to gain adequate weight (9,27). This category also includes the syndrome of infantile anorexia nervosa, previously described by Chatoor (28).

The EAT (eating attitudes test) is a commonly used questionnaire to screen for attitudes and behaviors suggestive of the diagnosis of an eating disorder (see Table 1) (29). For children age 8–13, a modified version, the ChEAT (children's eating attitude test), is used. Despite its wide usage, criticisms of the EAT include that it may have a relatively low predictive value (low specificity). Also, because it is a self-report questionnaire and anorectics tend to deny their illness, responses may not always be reliable (2).

III. EPIDEMIOLOGY

The prevalence of bulimia nervosa is approximately 1–3% among adolescent and young adult females; in males it is one-tenth of this (7,9). Anorexia nervosa primarily affects young females, with a bimodal peak incidence at age 14 and 18. There has also been an increased incidence reported in recent years among women age 15–24. Eating disorders are more prevalent among young white (of mainly European ancestry) females from middle to upper social classes in Western cultures, affecting 1–4% of adolescent and young adult women in these groups, and appears to be increasing in incidence (1). The prevalence among nonwhites in Western societies is not known, but the incidence is lower than that in whites (30).

It has also been suggested that the incidence of AN may be increasing in developed countries and that immigrants from other cultures tend to develop abnormal eating attitudes and behaviors as they become acculturated. Clearly, a relationship exists between the social norms and attitudes toward food, weight, and body shape and the development of eating disorders among people in those populations most concerned about dieting weight and shape. (1). In Western societies and developed countries, dieting and body shape concerns are ubiquitous. Garner et al., in a study looking at weight and shape measurements of *Playboy* centerfolds and Miss America pageant winners over a 20 year period, found a trend toward a thinner and more tubular standard in the context of increasing population weight norms (31). Approximately two-thirds of adolescent girls at any age are dissatisfied with their weight. Adolescents often know what their ideal weight should be but often prefer to be 10% less than the ideal weight for height (32,33). More than one-half of all girls are also dissatisfied with the shape of their bodies, and this positively correlates with their weight. More than 55% of high school students frequently use bathroom scales to monitor their weight (33). A history of dieting has been reported in 44–72% of adolescent girls, and one study found 60% of 12-year-old girls had tried to lose weight (34). A high prevalence of dieting attempts has also been found in children as young as the third grade (35). Interestingly, dieting is more common among girls with below-average body fat compared with those of average weight or who are overweight. One study found that 46% of girls with below-average body fat had dieted; another study showed that 31% of girls of average weight had dieted (34). At all ages, both black and white females tend to be fatter than males. Females also tend to gain fat and males to lose fat during adolescence.

Dieting is less common in boys but may be increasing in prevalence. Boys are more likely to use physical activity for weight loss; however, it is unusual for any boy not overweight to want to lose weight. In one study, almost all the boys stated they wanted to be taller (1).

Vomiting has been reported in an unselected population of adolescent girls at a rate of 9–11%. In another study, Phelps et al. looked at the prevalence of purging in female adolescents. They sampled middle and high school students three times over a 7 year period. These students were 99% white, of middle socioeconomic status. A significant decrease in the use of appetite suppressants was found in high school students, but an increase was noted among middle school students. An increase in vomiting among middle school students was also noted (36). Another study by Pugliese et al. reviewed the growth records of 1017 high school students of middle socioeconomic status and found that over 25% of these students were below 90% of the ideal body weight for height. Also, 1.8% exhibited linear growth retardation associated with poor weight gain (37).

Table 1 Eating Attitudes Test.*

Please place an (X) under the column which applies best to each of the numbered statements. All of the results will be *strictly* confidential. Most of the questions directly relate to food or eating, although other types of questions have been included. Please answer each question carefully. Thank you.

	ALWAYS	VERY OFTEN	OFTEN	SOMETIMES	RARELY	NEVER
1. Am terrified about being overweight.	( )	( )	( )	( )	( )	( )
2. Avoid eating when I am hungry.	( )	( )	( )	( )	( )	( )
3. Find myself preoccupied with food.	( )	( )	( )	( )	( )	( )
4. Have gone on eating binges where I feel that I may not be able to stop.	( )	( )	( )	( )	( )	( )
5. Cut my food into small pieces.	( )	( )	( )	( )	( )	( )
6. Aware of the calorie content of foods I eat.	( )	( )	( )	( )	( )	( )
7. Particularly avoid foods with high carbohydrate content (e.g., bread, potatoes, rice, etc.).	( )	( )	( )	( )	( )	( )
8. Feel that others would prefer if I ate more.	( )	( )	( )	( )	( )	( )
9. Vomit after I have eaten.	( )	( )	( )	( )	( )	( )
10. Feel extremely guilty after eating.	( )	( )	( )	( )	( )	( )
11. Am preoccupied with a desire to be thinner.	( )	( )	( )	( )	( )	( )
12. Think about burning up calories when I exercise.	( )	( )	( )	( )	( )	( )
13. Other people think that I am too thin.	( )	( )	( )	( )	( )	( )
14. Am preoccupied with the thought of having fat on my body.	( )	( )	( )	( )	( )	( )
15. Take longer than others to eat my meals.	( )	( )	( )	( )	( )	( )
16. Avoid foods with sugar in them.	( )	( )	( )	( )	( )	( )
17. Eat diet foods.	( )	( )	( )	( )	( )	( )
18. Feel that food controls my life.	( )	( )	( )	( )	( )	( )
19. Display self-control around food.	( )	( )	( )	( )	( )	( )
20. Feel that others pressure me to eat.	( )	( )	( )	( )	( )	( )
21. Give too much time and thought to food.	( )	( )	( )	( )	( )	( )
22. Feel uncomfortable after eating sweets.	( )	( )	( )	( )	( )	( )
23. Engage in dieting behavior.	( )	( )	( )	( )	( )	( )
24. Like my stomach to be empty.	( )	( )	( )	( )	( )	( )
25. Enjoy trying new rich foods.	( )	( )	( )	( )	( )	( )
26. Have the impulse to vomit after meals.	( )	( )	( )	( )	( )	( )

*Scores are derived as follows: A mark on "always" yields 3 points, "very often" 2 points, "often" 1 point; and others 0 points. The only exception is No. 25, which is reversed scoring. Any patient scoring above 20 may have a severe eating disorder.

From Garner DM, Olmstead MP, Bohr Y, Garfinkel PE. The Eating Attitudes Test: Psychometric features & clinical correlates. Psychol Med 1982; 12:871–878. Reprinted by permission of Cambridge University Press.

Although a large number of children and adolescents may not meet the strict criteria for the more serious ED, the clinician must inquire about possible inappropriate eating behaviors in any child or adolescent who is failing to gain sufficient weight and growth along the same channels in the growth chart. Parents in particular can set the stage for these innapropriate eating behaviors by using pressure to get their children to eat or by depriving them of a variety of foods. Parents who go to extremes in keeping their children from snacks may set the stage for food obsessions and hoarding (13,38).

The relationship between childhood eating pathology and the development of eating disorders later in life is unclear, and proposed entry mechanisms for ED are discussed in the etiology section. Patients with AN and BN have reported more control by external forces, being less able to display self-assertion and experience decreased self-esteem and higher levels of self-directed hostility in terms of guilt and self-criticism compared with obese dieters, nonobese dieters, and normal controls (39).

In assessing at-risk populations, adolescent and young adult women athletes have shown prevalences of disordered eating (not strict definition of ED) as high as 62%. In the general population it has been reported that 2–5% of women have amenorrhea. The observed prevalence is higher in athletes, ranging from 3.4 to 66%. The characteristics that apparently increase an athlete's risk of developing these conditions include a pressure to excel, as well as constant attention given to achieving or maintaining an ideal body weight and/or optimal body fat (40).

There has been some evidence of a higher concordance rate of AN in monozygotic twins than in dizygotic twins, and there is an increased risk of AN among first-degree biologic relatives. An increased risk of mood disorders has also been found in family members of patients with eating disorders, particularly those who exhibit binge-eating and purging behaviors (9,41).

IV. PATHOPHYSIOLOGY

Many of the detrimental effects of the eating disorders are a result of the physiologic consequences of starvation and malnutrition common to these disorders, as well as the deleterious consequences of the various purging or weight-eliminating techniques employed.

Anorexia nervosa is typified by malnutrition and its sequelae. Patients complain of constipation, cold intolerance, lethargy, and abdominal pain (9). Physical signs include emaciation, hypotension, hypothermia, and dry skin. Additionally, one may see lanugo, a fine babylike hair, over the patient's body. Anorexia nervosa can lead to compromised cardiovascular status, arrested sexual maturation, delayed or stunted growth, bradycardia, drop in orthostatic blood pressure, and increase in pulse rate, as well as sudden death (18,19). Prolonged amenorrhea (more than 6 months) is associated with potentially irreversible osteopenia and a higher rate of pathologic fractures. Patients may suffer from

dehydration, electrolyte imbalances, gastrointestinal motility disturbances, infertility, hypothermia, and other signs of hypometabolism. Abnormal computed tomographic scans of the brain may be found in more than half of patients with AN, as a consequence of malnutrition (19). Interestingly, laboratory findings may be normal despite profound malnutrition. Abnormalities that may be seen are listed in Table 2. Changes in endocrine functioning can also occur and are discussed here.

Many of the physical complications seen in bulimia nervosa result from purging behaviors. In patients who vomit, one can see a hypokalemic, hypochloremic alkalosis, mineral and fluid imbalances, hypomagnesemia, gastric and esophageal irritation, and bleeding. Mallory-Weiss esophageal tears occur rarely. Abraded knuckles (Russell's sign), caused by the use of the hand to induce vomiting, and erosion of dental enamel secondary to the effects of gastric acid on the teeth are also common. Frequent vomiting can also cause parotid enlargement and accompanying hyperamylasemia. Abuse of ipecac to induce vomiting may cause cardiomyopathies (with sudden death) or peripheral muscle weakness. Laxative abuse can lead to large bowel abnormalities, including cessation of function. Resting bradycardia, hypotension, and decreased metabolic rates are observed in some bulimic patients and may reflect decreased activity in the sympathetic nervous system and the thyroid axis (18,19).

A number of neuroendocrine and neurotransmitter changes are seen in anorexia nervosa. These changes also occur in states of starvation and malnutrition, however, and tend to normalize with weight restoration (42,43). Growth hormone (GH) levels have been found to be increased in AN, as well as in most severely malnourished children. Glucose does not suppress GH in either population (44). Insulin-like growth factor I, which mediates the anabolic effects of GH, has been found to be decreased in severe, chronic childhood malnutrition, as well as in AN (45). Thyroid hormone changes in AN are also seen in other states of malnutrition and likely reflect an adaptation to starvation. These changes include a low-normal thyroxine level, a decreased triiodothyronine (T_3) level, increased reverse T_3, and normal thyrotropin (thyroid-stimulating hormone) levels (46). Total circulating thyroxine

Table 2 Laboratory Abnormalities in Anorexia Nervosa

Leukopenia and mild anemia
Hypercholesterolemia
Abnormal liver function
Hypoglycemia
Hypercortisolemia
Hypokalemia
Hypophosphatemia
Hypomagnesemia
Hypozincemia
Hypercarotenemia

Source: From Reference 19.

concentrations appear to depend more on the concentrations of serum binding proteins than on glandular secretions. Because of this, measurements of free thyroxine by analog radioimmunoassay may be decreased but the free fraction measured using equilibrium dialysis may be increased (44).

The hypothalamic-pituitary-adrenal (HPA) axis has also been implicated (47). Similarities have been found to exist in the functional status of the HPA in patients with AN and those with depressive illness. They both have elevated 24 h urinary free cortisol excretion and inadequate suppression of plasma cortisol after dexamethasone. Corticotropin-releasing hormone causes a blunted adrenocorticotropic hormone response but an increased cortisol response. Cortisol production returns to normal with weight restoration, but complete recovery may take a long time (44).

Such sophisticated studies have not been performed in malnourished children; however, other groups of malnourished patients also show elevated levels of plasma cortisol, slowed rates of cortisol metabolism, and inadequate suppression of plasma cortisol (Chap. 8). In contrast, bulimic patients of normal weight appear to show normal plasma cortisol levels (44,46). Amenorrhea is a hallmark of AN; however, not all amenorrhea is secondary to weight loss. Approximately 25% of AN patients develop amenorrhea before severe weight loss. The amenorrhea of AN and BN is mitigated by abnormal pituitary gonadotropin secretion, which is likely caused by abnormal secretion of gonadotropin-releasing hormones (48).

Neurotransmitter changes in AN include decreased levels of cerebrospinal fluid norepinephrine and possible alterations in the serotonin system. It has been hypothesized that endogenous opioids play a role in the denial of hunger seen in AN patients. Preliminary studies have reported dramatic weight gains in some patients administered opiate antagonists (41).

Cholecystokinin (CCK) is known to regulate satiety in animals and humans, and some evidence has suggested that glucagon and gastrin-releasing peptide also act as physiologic signals for satiety (49). One study by Pirke et al. looked at CCK plasma levels in patients with anorexia and bulimia nervosa. They measured CCK-8-S levels in the pre- and postmeal plasma of patients with anorexia nervosa and bulimia nervosa and age-matched controls. The basal CCK-8-S levels in plasma were similar among the three groups, but the increase after the test meal was significantly lower in patients with bulimia nervosa than in either the anorectic or control group, suggesting that impaired feelings of satiety in bulimic patients was accompanied by low CCK-8-S secretion (50). CCK, glucagon, and gastrin-releasing peptide appear to act peripherally and may offer new treatments in the future for overeating in obesity and BN.

V. DIFFERENTIAL DIAGNOSIS

Anorexia nervosa can be confused with depression, gastrointestinal (GI) disorders, and certain brain tumors. Depression also causes loss of appetite and weight loss. However, the other eating disorder criteria are seldom present. One of the

GI diseases that most mimics an eating disorder is inflammatory bowel disease, especially Crohn's disease (8). Crohn's disease can present with weight loss, anorexia, nausea, vomiting, and diarrhea. Irritable bowel syndrome, which classically presents between 15 and 35 years of age, has an age of onset very similar to that of eating disorders. Additionally, both groups of patients tend to be compulsive and high achievers (8). Again, the importance of low weight in the person's self-evaluation is a useful distinguishing feature. Serum cholesterol is usually normal or elevated in eating disorder patients and has also been reported as a helpful test in differentiating eating disorders from inflammatory bowel disease or malabsorptive problems. The serum albumin concentration is also usually normal, even in severely malnourished patients with AN (in contrast to GI inflammatory states, such as Crohn's, ulcerative colitis, pancreatitis, or hepatitis). Cu deficiency is rare in humans, however, and Casper et al. found low serum Cu concentrations in AN patients (8).

Parotid enlargement associated with hyperamylasemia can be found in BN. A serum lipase or salivary isoamylase test can help distinguish this from pancreatitis. The most common electrolyte abnormality seen in BN is an elevated serum bicarbonate. An isolated hypokalemia in an otherwise healthy young female with complaints of nonspecific GI problems can be a sign of an eating disorder.

Clinicians should inquire about nutritional intake, a history of eating disorders, and weight-reducing behaviors as part of the routine assessment of patients with disorders of reproductive function, including failure to ovulate, oligomenorrhea, amenorrhea, reduced sex drive, infertility, hyperemesis gravidarum, small babies for gestational age, low birth weight infants, increased neonatal morbidity, and problems in infant feeding (51).

VI. ETIOLOGY AND PSYCHOLOGIC FACTORS

The etiology of eating disorders has been conceptualized as multifactorial, with psychologic, biologic and social components. The social pressures and norms regarding weight and shape have been discussed. As women respond to these pressures for "ideal" bodies, they diet. Adolescents are perhaps more vulnerable to these forces because, as Hsu has postulated, "adolescent dieting provides an entree into an eating disorder if such dieting is intensified by adolescent turmoil, low self and body concept, and poor identity formation" (1).

Important psychologic tasks of adolescent girls are viewed as including separation and individuation, identity formation, development of intimacy, and acquiring understanding and control of their impulses (52). AN has also been conceptualized as an attempt to return to an earlier developmental age, when these impulses were not as threatening. Anorectics are often horrified by the development of breasts and puberty and try to return their bodies to a prepubertal state (1).

Early psychoanalytic theories saw the anorectic's behavior as a means of warding off unconscious oral or sexual wishes. In a later interpersonal model, Bruch (53) proposed that, early in development, the child's needs were not adequately addressed, nor were the expression of these needs encouraged or validated. The effect of this ultimately is to leave the child at a loss as to how to "decode" his or her emotional needs or how to respond adequately to external pressures and demands. This view is summarized by Casper (22):

> These deficits in self-awareness and initiative became manifest only when the person was confronted with having to adapt to new situations such as puberty . . . the anorectic patient, Bruch believed, tried to compensate for this lack of inner structure and control by rigid discipline and control over her body size and food intake to attain a sense of structure and personal identity.

Anorectics also deal harshly with their bodies and view them as "rebellious, willful objects in need of control" (22). Zerbe (54) believes this intense body hatred results from a highly pathologic relationship, early in life, with the child's primary caretaker. Even in infancy, future anorectics learn they are responsible for their mother's emotional needs rather than vice versa. Their mothers were likely unable to allow them to develop personal autonomy, and starvation of her body is a way for the anorectic to kill off the internal mother from whom she wishes to be freed (54).

The anorectic somehow merges aspects that are unacceptable to her, such as low self-esteem, with body fat. The body becomes split into good and bad parts, and weight gain is linked to losing one's sense of self (22).

During adolescence, individuals normally turn away from their parents and become immersed in peer relationships. Patients prone to develop AN likely feel helpless and ineffective in relationships and turn to controlling their bodies as the only way of feeling some sense of mastery. Moreover, these patients tend to be especially sensitive to traumatic events, and disappointments in relationships cause them to question the value of close relationships and contribute to maintaining a detached stance (22). The discovery of making herself feel better by controlling her body shape becomes a powerful reinforcer of the anorectic's behavior.

Strober (55) studied personality variables in anorexia and found that patients with AN exhibit particular traits, including an extreme tendency toward harm avoidance, lessened reward dependence, and decreased novelty seeking. This withdrawn posture is believed to leave the anorectic with a defective sense of self and unready to handle the pressures and demands of separation and independence. Earlier theories focused on the fears of sexual development, but more recent thought conceives of anorexia nervosa as a way to compensate for and counterbalance a poor self-concept. Because of their profound sense of internal emptiness and the inability of anorectics to handle developmental demands adequately, they become "dependent" on controlling their bodies. Anorectics deal with anxiety by the development of an ideal body image that is maintained at any cost, including death (22).

Patients cling to their bony bodies as a way to maintain an identity. The symptom of mirror gazing, in which patients admire their bony structure and caved-in abdomen in the privacy of their bedrooms, suggests that patients are able to perceive their figures visually but somehow are unable to integrate this information and remain unaware of the life-threatening implications of the emaciation. Prepubertal patients seem not to display this pathologic body attachment (22).

Many of the psychologic sequelae of AN are also seen in starvation. A study conducted in 950 by Keys et al. (56) evaluated the effect of restricting caloric intake in 36 young, healthy, psychologically normal men. Food was restricted over a 6 month period, and the men lost an average of 25% of their original body weight. A dramatic increase in food preoccupation developed.

Concentration was decreased as the men were plagued by persistent thoughts of food and eating. The men spent much more time planning how they would eat their food and would often eat in silence, devoting total attention to consumption. Some of the men also developed binge-eating behaviors and, even after a 3 month rehabilitation period, complained of experiencing increased hunger immediately following a large meal. There was an overall lowering of the threshold for depression, with an increase in anxiety and irritability. The men became progressively more withdrawn and isolated, and sexual interest was drastically reduced. Of interest were changes in body fat and muscle composition. Weight decreased by an average of 25%, body fat fell almost 20%, and muscle decreased by 40% during the restricting phase. Upon refeeding, a greater proportion of the regained weight was fat. After 8 months of rehabilitation, volunteers were 110% of their original body weight but 140% of their original body fat. The men became more fearful of weight gain and reported feeling fat and being worried about developing distended stomachs. The changes in fat percentage returned to normal levels after 1 year (20).

AN patients show features of interpersonal withdrawal, like those seen in starvation, but with even more profound emotional disengagement from relationships. Lack of food leads to preoccupation with food, decreased interest in people and outside activities, and a personal investment in body weight loss. Unlike normal people with starvation who experience lethargy and fatigue, many patients with AN actually report an energizing effect with starvation. The anorectic patient also operates according to new values: being hungry is good, and eating is bad (22).

Most cases of bulimia nervosa result from unsuccessful dieting attempts motivated by a wish for a fashionable body shape (22,57). Excessive dieting leads to hunger, which can precipitate episodes of binge eating. Women learn that by vomiting or employing other purging techniques not only can they rid themselves of these calories, but it provides relief from the concomitant feelings of guilt and depression induced by binging. Vomiting eliminates unwanted food, but it does not help to deal with the mounting hunger. Although the aim of purging is to compensate for a binge, it actually tends to make it more likely, not less likely, that the person will binge again. It is not difficult to see, then, how a binge-purge cycle can escalate as the patient more desperately attempts to regain control of her eating. In this way, a binge-purge cycle can lead to weight gain rather than weight loss. This is an important psychoeducational principle that should be conveyed to patients. This phenomenon also occurs with other purging methods and this is discussed further in the treatment section.

Bulimics tend to feel internally chaotic, and this tends to be reflected by the turbulent nature of their eating behavior. This level of disorganization is further highlighted by the fact that many bulimic patients have dissociative symptoms, sexual conflicts, and a variety of impulsive behaviors that frequently involve overspending, shoplifting, promiscuity, and self-mutilation (19). Genetic predisposition, personality factors, family transactional patterns, and early upbringing experiences all may exert an influence and determine whether a pathologic dieter goes on to develop AN or BN (1).

The issue of childhood sexual abuse as a risk factor for the development of BN has been a matter of considerable debate. The majority of studies investigating this issue have not found statistically significant differences for BN patients compared to controls. A study by Rorty et al., however, found that women with BN have reported significantly higher levels of childhood physical, psychologic and multiple abuse. Sexual abuse was not a discriminating factor between women with BN and control groups, except in combination with other forms of abuse (58).

VII. TREATMENT

Unless one has a clear understanding of the psychologic underpinnings of ED, the treatment process is likely to fail. Because of the shame and secrecy surrounding these disorders, an insensitive clinican can easily alienate an already wary patient. An appreciation of the value a patient places on weight and shape can help the clinician to develop more effectively a sense of trust and rapport with the patient.

ED have in common that they are an attempt by the patient's self to maintain control and handle overwhelming conflicting demands. They are a final common pathway. Because this control is so vital and central to the patient's world view, he or she may view treatment as a threat. In the absence of a strong therapeutic alliance, the clinician and the treatment process are invariably perceived by the patient as further intrusions and attempts to wrest away what little control he or she has been able to achieve, and the patient actively resists treatment. This is particularly true in AN, in which treatment means refeeding and thus changing her body shape against her will. Insistence on weight gain recreates an interaction reminiscent of her early interpersonal experiences, and these patients can become depressed and suicidal. The risk of refeeding can be minimized by taking a personal interest in the patient. "Patients with AN are deeply distrustful and highly sensitive. They are excellent observers . . . and the patient needs to sense that we are not merely interested in her physical survival but equally interested in her personal suffering (22).

There are differences in the treatment of patients with AN and BN, and these relate to the more profound disturbances of weight and shape often seen in AN patients. Practice guidelines for the treatment of AN and BN have been established by the American Psychiatric Association, and the following includes a brief synopsis of these (19).

A. Anorexia Nervosa

The foundation of treatment of AN is weight restoration accompanied by individual and family psychotherapies. Target weights should reflect the resumption of menses and reversal of bone demineralization. The use of body mass index as a standard of nutritional status may be employed in adults—body mass index = weight (kg)/height (m) squared—and appropriate tables should be consulted. For children, the growth charts are more appropriate (see Chap. 8). Inpatient hospitalization is often required, particularly when the patient is 70% or less of ideal body weight or in patients with rapidly falling weight or metabolic instability. For those patients who are less than 20% below average weight for height, successful outpatient treatment requires a highly motivated patient, cooperative family, and history of brief symptom duration. A goal of 0.5–2 pounds/week of weight gain is appropriate in an outpatient setting. If after several weeks of treatment there is no progress, inpatient hospitalization should be considered. In hospitalized patients, a goal of 1–3 pounds/week of weight gain should be expected. During the weight restoration phase of treatment, particularly in severely malnourished individuals, one must pay attention to the development of edema, rapid weight gain as a result of fluid overload, and the risk of congestive heart failure. As stated previously, patients may attempt to pad their weight and should be weighed in the morning after voiding, wearing only a gown. Excess physical activity aimed at weight loss should be curbed.

Nutritional rehabilitation is best started at about 500 cal/day over that necessary for weight maintenance and gradually increased. Patients may require up to 70–100 kcal/kg per day during the weight gain phase and 40–60 kcal/kg/day during weight maintenance. If patients require more than this, it may be an indication that they are exercising frequently, vomiting, or discarding food. Another approach is to aim for a 10–20% increase above the amount of calories needed to maintain weight. Because of their malnourished states, a decline in basal energy requirements has taken place, and the use of calculated basal caloric requirments from tables derived from normal populations overestimates the needs of the undernourished patient (13). Using liquid supplements initially can help coax a patient back into eating more calories. The use of nasogastric feeding should be reserved for life-endangering conditions rather than solely for weight restoration, although some believe that early renourishment in severely malnourished patients is more easily accepted as passive feeding than active eating. Giving the patient explicit information about refeeding or food to be consumed also helps to introduce cognitive control.

Patients should preferably be hospitalized in a setting

in which the staff is knowledgeable about eating disorders. If the staff does not have this knowledge, the clinician or a psychiatric consultant should spend some time educating the staff. Staff should be able to help the patient deal with her concerns about weight gain and body image changes. "Lenient" treatment settings, in which initial bed rest and threat of returning the patient to bed if weight gain does not occur may be as effective as "stricter" approaches utilizing meal-by-meal caloric measurements and punishment. Using a more lenient approach also reduces the staff's policing functions and encourages more cooperation. Any program, though, should include such routine monitoring as accompanying the patient to the bathroom after meals to restrict purging.

Eliciting family cooperation should be an integral part of the treatment plan. One should generally anticipate resistance on the part of patients at the onset of treatment, and repeated wishes to leave the hospital during the first few weeks of treatment are not uncommon. Families should be educated about the nature of the patient's condition and the relationship between semi-starvation and symptoms of AN. Particularly for children and adolescents, family therapy should be initiated on or before admission. Individual psychotherapy is also important, not only for support and empathy to help the patient adjust to her changing body shape but also to address the psychopathologic and personality disturbance features underlying the disorder.

Inpatient discharge criteria are determined by weight gain, motivation, and family dynamics. Speed of weight gain provides no assurance of long-term outcome (19). In fact, too vigorous a weight gain may induce a patient to begin or intensify purging behavior, such as vomiting. In the absence of psychotherapeutic support, the patient may also deteriorate psychologically.

It must also be remembered that these patients usually have had a chronic malnourished state to which they have adapted. Too rapid a weight gain has been associated with fatal reactions and biochemical changes, such as severe drops in serum phosphorous levels or zinc concentrations. In general, the best approach to nutritional rehabilitation has been described as the least restrictive one that leads to weight gain. The ultimate target weight should be one at which normal reproductive function resumes and bone demineralization is reversed, but it should be kept in mind that normal physiologic function can be achieved even when mild malnutrition persists and body weight is not at an ideal level (13,19). Normal menstruation may not occur even when body weight deficits are fully restored. For those patients without adequate psychologic support to help them tolerate the weight gain, the aim should be a slower rate of weight gain and, in some cases, a lower target weight (13).

Psychotropic medications have a limited role in the treatment of AN. Because depression often improves with weight restoration, it is advisable to wait for this to occur and use antidepressants if the depression persists. Serotonin is thought to be involved in hunger and satiety, and the serotonin antagonist cyproheptadine has had some use for weight restoration. Some beneficial effects have been noted in patients with the restricting subtype of AN, but negative effects have occurred in those with the bulimic subtype.

Malnourished depressed patients may be more prone to side effects and less responsive to antidepressant medications. Tricyclic antidepressants may also add to the risk of hypotension and arrythmias in patients with AN. Uncontrolled studies have suggested that fluoxetine has been helpful with weight restoration. The weight loss and impaired appetite seen in normal-weight and obese patients taking fluoxetine (60 mg/day) has not been reported in AN patients taking lower dose. Low-dose neuroleptics may have a role in patients with marked obsessionality. Antianxiety agents may also be used selectively before meals to reduce anticipatory anxiety. Bupropion is contraindicated in patients with AN and BN because of the increased rate of seizures in these populations.

Estrogen replacement is sometimes used in older AN patients; however, experts recommend waiting 1 year before initiating estrogen replacement for adolescent patients (19).

B. Bulimia Nervosa

BN can usually be managed on an outpatient basis, unless there is unremitting purging or laxative abuse, concomitant substance abuse, major personality disorders, or suicidality. Brief or group psychotherapy, cognitive-behavioral therapy, interpersonal, and psychodynamic therapies have all been shown to be effective. Simple behavioral techniques, such as planned meals and keeping of food diaries, can be quite helpful for initial symptom management (19).

Cognitive-behavioral therapy (CBT) has been found to be more effective than interpersonal or behavioral therapy in changing patient's disturbed attitudes to shape and weight, as well as extreme dieting attempts. The three treatments have not differed, however, in their effect on reduction of bulimic episodes at the end of treatment. Cognitive-behavioral therapy has also been found to be marginally superior to psychodynamic therapy in reducing purging.

Interpersonal psychotherapy may actually have the best long-term outcome. The combination of nutritional and cognitive treatments has been found to be especially effective in decreasing bulimic behaviors and inducing remission. In patients who also have personality disorders or complicating factors, a more interpersonal, psychodynamic approach is warranted (59).

The most effective method of treatment in uncomplicated cases has been found to be cognitive-behavioral therapy. The goals of this therapy are based on the hypothesis that bulimia results from a disturbance in body image. The cognitive distortion is addressed, and the patient learns healthier ways to eat. The binge-purge cycle is disrupted by focusing on decreasing purge behavior. It is thought that, with the introduction of nutritionally balanced meals and snacks, the urge to binge is decreased.

Cognitive-behavioral therapy is divided into three stages and typically consists of 19 sessions of individual treatment over a 20 week period (60). The first stage involves education about BN and a general orientation to this method of treatment. The patient is taught how proper nutrition and weight regulation are essential to the elimination of the ED. The patient learns how to begin self-tracking food intake and eating habits and to assess situations that trigger binge eating and purging. The goal of this stage is to return the patient to eating three meals a day, with healthy snacks between meals. The second stage of CBT helps the patient to develop a more focused means of evaluating dysfunctional attitudes regarding shape, weight, and eating. Procedures and coping skills are introduced to help cut down on dietary restraint and to resist binge eating. This is achieved by encouraging patients to try behavioral experiments in eating that directly challenge some of their misconceptions. For example, patients' fears of loss of control and increased binge eating if they abandon dietary restraint and subtitute three regular meals per day can be effectively disconfirmed when they make these behavioral changes. The third stage of CBT shifts the focus to relapse prevention strategies (60,61). Some helpful dietary principles for bulimic patients are provided in Table 3. The following are some psychoeducational principles that are useful when treating ED patients (20):

1. Patient's weights are predetermined within a certain range, and the body operates according to a "set-point" principle. Below a certain weight the body hypometabolizes food, and above a certain weight it hypermetabolizes it. Thus, the patient's body resists being at too high or too low a weight..

2. Severe dietary restraint causes binging. The way to reduce binging is to eat three regular meals per day with healthy snacks between meals.

3. Vomiting, laxatives, and diuretics are ineffective in controlling weight because they lead to increased binging. Laxatives primarily affect emptying of the large intestine, occuring after calories have been absorbed in the small bowel. Diuretics have absolutely no effect on calories or body fat.

In contrast to AN, there is a greater role for the use of medication in treating BN. A review of controlled trials of pharmacotherapy by Mitchell et al. found 13 studies to date that have examined the use of antidepressants in the treatment of BN. In studies comparing the use of the tricyclic antidepressants imipramine (150–200 mg) and desipramine (150–300 mg) to placebo groups, a significant reduction was seen in the frequency of binging and vomiting. Binge-eating frequency was reduced between 47 and 91% in these studies. Abstinence from bulimic symptoms was found to have a mean of 24%, although this figure may be inflated because of one study. Overall, most studies looking solely at the use of antidepressants found poor abstinence rates. This is important because long-term prognosis may be predicted by abstinence rates at the end of treatment (59).

Two controlled trials using the monoamine oxidase inhibitors (MAOIs) phenelzine and isocarboxide had reductions in bulimic symptoms, comparable to those seen with the tricyclic antidepressants. Because of side effects encountered, as well as the additional dietray restraints required (tyramine-free diets), MAOIs are not often used as first-line agents. Trazodone (400–650 mg) led to a reduction in binge-eating frequency of 50% and an abstinence rate of 10%. Bupropion was effective in reducing binge-eating behavior; however, the higher than expected rate of clonic-tonic seizures in these patients has made this medication contraindicated in ED populations (59,62). The Fluoxetine Bulimia Nervosa Collaborative Study group (63) reported a multicenter trial of fluoxetine, comparing doses of 20 and 60 mg/day with placebo in a total of 382 BN patients. Both doses led to more improvement than placebo; however, the 60 mg/day dose led to markedly better results than the 20 mg/day dose.

BN has been thought of by some as a variant of affective disorders. Responsiveness to antidepressant medication, high incidence of depression in these patients, and higher than expected frequency of affective disorders in their relatives supports this hypothesis. The effect of antidepressant medication in the treatment of BN, though, appears equally in depressed and nondepressed bulimic patients, and the evidence indicates that the therapeutic effect is a result of more than an antidepressant effect alone. Of note, however, is that studies that have looked at the use of medication in the absence of psychotherapy have shown poor efficacy. Thus it is the combination of the two that appears to be most effective (14,59).

VIII. PROGNOSIS

More than 40 outcome studies of AN have been published in the last 30 years, and the rates of recovery found are 17–77% after follow-up of 4–20 years (64). Overall, about 44% of AN patients have a good outcome at least 4 years after onset of illness. Predictors of poorer prognosis include initial lower minimum weight, the presence of vomiting, prior treatment

Table 3 Diet Recommendations to Aid the Bulimic Patient

Avoid finger foods; eat foods requiring the use of utensils

Include warm foods, rather than cold or room-temperature foods, to increase meal satiety

Include vegetables, salad, and/or fruit at a meal to prolong the mealtime; choose whole-grain and high-fiber breads and cereals

Diet and meals should be well balanced to increase satiety and to increase variety of foods consumed

Use foods that are naturally divided into portions, such as potatoes (rather than rice or pasta); rolls or bagels (instead of bread); 4 and 8 ounce containers of yogurt, ice cream, or cottage cheese; precut steaks or chicken parts; and frozen dinners and entrees

Include adequate fat to enhance meal satiety by slowing gastric emptying

Include generous portions of carbohydrate-containing foods

Eat meals and snacks sitting down

Plan meals and snacks; keep a food diary by recording food before eating

Source: From Reference 48.

failures, premorbidly disturbed family relationships, and being married. Mortality, primarily from suicide or cardiac arrest, reached about 20% among patients followed for more than 20 years. Predictors of positive outcome may include early onset of illness (19,64).

There are fewer outcome studies for BN. Short-term treatment studies have reported 50–90% reductions in binge eating and purging. Follow-up studies of longer duration, however, have found recovery rates ranging from 13 to 69% (19,64). Negative prognostic predictors for BN include alcohol abuse, suicide attempts, and increased binging and vomiting at baseline (64). Stable weight and having good friendships have been found to be positive predictors of recovery (11).

A study by Rorty et al. evaluated the subjective appraisals of 40 women recovered from BN for a year or more. They found that empathic and caring relationships with others were highlighted as essential by recovered subjects. Lack of understanding by important persons or treating personnel was seen as hampering the recovery process (11).

Eating disorders are multifactorial in etiology and a challenge to treat. It is the hope of this author that this chapter has been able to shed some light on the complexities of these disorders and of the importance of a strong therapeutic alliance in the treatment of patients with eating disorders.

REFERENCES

1. Hsu LK. Eating Disorders. New York: Guilford Press. 1990: 14–58, 77–103.
2. Lask B, Bryant-Waugh R. Early onset anorexia nervosa and related eating disorders. J Child Psychiatry 1992; 33:281–300.
3. Revised diagnostic subgroupings for anorexia nervosa. Nut Rev 1994; 52:213–215.
4. Zerbe K. Selves that starve and suffocate: the continuum of eating disorders and dissociative phenomena. Bull Meninger Clin 1993; 57:319–327.
5. Johnson C. Initial consultation for patients with bulimia and anorexia Nervosa. In: Garner DM, Garfinkel PE, eds. Handbook of Psychotherapy for Anorexia Nervosa and Bulimia. New York: Brunner/Mazel, 1988:56–79.
6. Garner DM, Fairburn C. Relationship between anorexia nervosa and bulimia nervosa: diagnostic implications. In: Garner DM, Garfinkel PE, eds. Diagnostic Issues in Anorexia Nervosa and Bulimia Nervosa. New York: Brunner/Mazel, 1988: 56–79.
7. Childress A, Brewerton T, Hodges E, Jarrell M. The kids' eating disorders survey (KEDS): a study of middle school students. J Am Acad Child Adol Psychiatry 1993; 32:843–850.
8. McClain C, Humphries L, Hill K, Nicki N. Gastrointestinal and nutritional aspects of eating disorders. J Am Coll Nutr 1993; 12:466–474.
9. American Psychiatric Association, Diagnostic and Statistical Manual of Mental Disorders, 4th ed. Washington, D.C., 1994.
10. 1983 Metropolitan height and weight table. Stat Bull Metrop Life Found 1983; 64:3–9.
11. Rorty M, Yager J, Rossotto E. Why and how do women recover from bulimia nervosa? The subjective appraisals of forty women recovered for a year or more. Int J Eating Dis 1993; 14:249–260.
12. Garfinkel PE. Classification and diagnosis. In: Halmi K, ed. Psychobiology and Treatment of Anorexia Nervosa and Bulimia Nervosa. Washington, D.C.: APA Press, 1992:37–60.
13. Lifshitz F. Eating disorders: nutrition for special needs. In: Lifshitz F, Finch NM, Lifshitz JZ, eds. Children's Nutrition. Boston: Jones and Bartlett, 1991:271–294.
14. Walsh T, Devlin M. The pharmacologic treatment of eating disorders. Psychiatr Clin North Am March 1992; 15:149–160.
15. Mitchell J. Bulimia Nervosa. Minneapolis: University of Minnesota Press, 1990:16–23.
16. Hudson J, Wentworth SM, Hudson MS, et al. Prevalence of anorexia nervosa and bulimia among young diabetic women. J Clin Psychiatry 1985; 46:88–89.
17. Hudson JI, Hudson MS, Wentworth SM. Self-induced glycosuria: a novel method of purging in bulimia. JAMA 1983; 249:2501.
18. Mitchell J, Seim H, Colon E, Pomeroy C. Medical complications and medical management of bulimia. Ann Intern Med 1987; 107:71–77.
19. American Psychiatric Association. Practice guideline for eating disorders. Am J Psychiatry February 1993; 150:213–228.
20. Garner DM, Rockert W, Olmsted MP, Johnson C, Coscina D. Psychoeducational principles in the treatment of bulimia and anorexia nervosa. In: Garner DM, Garfinkel PE, eds. Handbook of Psychotherapy for Anorexia Nervosa and Bulimia. New York: Guilford Press, 1985:513–572.
21. DaCosta M, Halmi K. Classifications of anorexia nervosa: question of subtypes. Int J Eating Dis 1992; 11:305–313.
22. Casper R. Integration of psychodynamic concepts into psychotherapy. In: Halmi K, ed. Psychobiology and Treatment of Anorexia Nervosa and Bulimia Nervosa. Washington, D.C.: APA Press, 1992:287–306.
23. Zwaan M, Mitchell J. Binge eating in the obese. Ann Med 1992; 24:303–308.
24. Pugliese MT, Lifshitz, F, Grad G, et al. Fear of obesity: a cause of short stature and delayed puberty. N Engl J Med 1983; 309:513–518.
25. Lifshitz F, Moses N. Growth failure—a complication of hypercholesterolemia treatment. Am J Dis Child 1989; 143: 537–542.
26. Sandberg D, Smith MM, Fornari V, Goldberg T, Lifshitz F. Nutritional dwarfing: is it a consequence of disturbed psychosocial functioning? Pediatrics 1991; 88:926–933.
27. Powell GF, Low JF, Speers MA. Behavior as a diagnostic aid in failure to thrive. J Dev Behav Pediatr 1987; 8:18–24.
28. Chatoor I. Infantile anorexia nervosa: a developmental disorder of separation and individuation. J Am Acad Psychoanal 1989; 17:43–64.
29. Garner DM, Olmstead MP, Bohr Y, Garfinkel PE. The eating attitudes test: psychometric features and clinical correlates. Psychol Med 1982; 12:871–878.
30. Dolan B. Cross-cultural aspects of anorexia nervosa and bulimia: a review. Int J Eating Dis 1991; 10:67–78.
31. Garner DM, Garfinkel PE, Schwartz D, Thompson M. Cultural expectations of thinness in women. Psychol Rep 1980; 47:483–491.
32. Lifshitz F. Fear of obesity in childhood. Ann NY Acad Sci 1993; 699:230–236.
33. Moses N, Banilvy M, Lifshitz F. Fear of obesity among adolescent girls. Pediatrics 1989; 83:393–398.
34. Moore D. Body image and eating behavior in adolescents. J Am Coll Nutr 1993; 12:505–510.
35. Maloney MJ, McGuire J, Daniels DR, Specker B. Dieting behavior and eating attitudes in children. Pediatrics 1989; 84:482–487.
36. Phelps L, Andrea R, Rizzo F, et al. Prevalence of self-induced vomiting and laxative/medication abuse among female adoles-

cents: a longitudinal study. Int. J Eating Dis 1993; 14:375–378.

37. Pugliese MT, Recker B, Lifshitz F. A survey to determine the prevalence of abnormal growth patterns in adolescence. J Adol Health Care 1988; 9:181–187.

38. Pugliese MT, WeYman-Daum M, Moses N, Lifshitz F. Parental health beliefs as a cause of non-organic failure to thrive. Pediatrics 1987; 80:175–182.

39. Williams GJ, Power KG, Millar HR, et al. Comparison of eating disorders and other dietary/weight groups on measures of perceived control, assertiveness, self-esteem, and self-directed hostility. Int J Eating Dis 1993; 14:27–32.

40. Yeager K, Agostini R, Nattiv A, Drinkwater B. The female athlete triad: disordered eating, amenorrhea, osteoporosis. Med Sci Sports Exerc April 1993; 25:775–777.

41. Kaplan H, Sadock B. Synopsis of Psychiatry, 6th ed. Baltimore: Williams & Wilkins, 1991:740–749.

42. Fichter M. Starvation-related endocrine changes. In: Halmi K, ed. Psychobiology and Treatment of Anorexia Nervosa and Bulimia Nervosa. Washington, D.C., APA Press, 1992:193–220.

43. Winterer J, Gwirtsman H, George D, et al. Adrenocorticotropin-stimulated adrenal androgen secretion in anorexia nervosa: impaired secretion at low weight with normalization after long-term weight recovery. J Clin Endocrinol Metab 1985; 61:693–697.

44. Lifshitz F, Brasel J. Nutrition and endocrine disease. In: Kappy MS, Blizzard RM, Migeon CJ, eds. Wilkins Diagnosis and Treatment of Endocrine Disorders in Childhood and Adolescence, 4th ed. Springfield, IL: Charles C. Thomas, 1994:535–571.

45. Hill K, Hill D, McClain M, et al. Serum insulin-like growth factor-I concentrations in the recovery of patients with anorexia nervosa. J Am Coll Nutr 1993; 12:475–478.

46. Danforth EJ, Burger AG. The impact of nutrition on thyroid hormone physiology and action. Ann Res Nutr 1989; 9:201–210.

47. Gold P, Gwirtsman H, Avgerinos P, Nieman L, et al. Abnormal hypothalamic-pituitary-adrenal function in anorexia nervosa. N Engl J Med 1986; 314:1335–1342.

48. Fornari V. Eating disorders. In: Lifshitz F, ed. Pediatric Endocrinology, 2nd ed. New York: Marcel Dekker, 1991:905–920.

49. Gibbs J. The physiological control of food intake. Contemp Nutr 1994; 19(3).

50. Pirke K, Philipp E, Schweriger U, Broocks A, Wilckens T. Neuroendocrine and reproductive function. In: Halmi K, ed. Psychobiology and Treatment of Anorexia Nervosa and Bulimia Nervosa. Washington, D.C.: APA Press, 1992:151–167.

51. Stewart D. Reproductive functions in eating disorders. Ann Med 1992; 24:287–291.

52. Ponton L. Issues unique to psychotherapy with adolescent girls. Am J Psychother 1993; 47:353–372.

53. Bruch H. Preconditions for the development of anorexia nervosa. Am J Psychoanal 1980; 40:169–172.

54. Zerbe K. Whose body is it anyway? Understanding and treating psychosomatic aspects of eating disorders. Bull Menninger Clin 1993; 57:161–177.

55. Strober M. Disorders of the self in anorexia nervosa: an organismic-developmental paradigm. In: Johnson C, ed. Psychodynamic Theory and Treatment for Eating Disorders. New York: Guilford, 1990:354–373.

56. Keys A, Brozek J, Henschel A, Mickelsen O, Taylor HL. The biology of human starvation. Minneapolis: University of Minnesota Press, 1950.

57. Patton G. Eating disorders: antecedents, evolution and course. Ann Med 1992; 24:281–285.

58. Rorty M, Yager J, Rossotto E. Childhood sexual, physical, and psychological abuse in bulimia nervosa. Am J Psychiatry 1994; 151:1122–1126.

59. Mitchell J, Raymond N, Specker S. A review of the controlled trials of pharmacotherapy and psychotherapy in the treatment of bulimia nervosa. Int J Eating Dis 1993; 14:229–247.

60. Wilson GT, Fairburn C. Cognitive treatments for eating disorders. J Consult Clin Psychol 1993; 6:261–269.

61. Fairburn C, Hay P. The treatment of bulimia nervosa. Ann Med 1992; 24:297–302.

62. Medical Economics Data Production Company. Physician's Desk Reference. Montvale, NJ, 1994.

63. Fluoxetine Bulimia Nervosa Collaborative Study Group. Fluoxetine in the treatment of bulimia nervosa. Arch Gen Psychiatry 1992; 49:139–147.

64. Herzog D, Sacks N, Keller M, et al. Patterns and predictors of recovery in anorexia nervosa and bulimia nervosa. J Am Acad Child Adol Psychiatry 1993; 32:835–842.

60

Laboratory Aids and Tolerance Testing in Pediatric Endocrinology: A Practical Approach

Fred I. Chasalow
Maimonides Medical Center, Brooklyn, New York

Lori J. Ginsberg
North Shore University Hospital, Manhasset, New York

I. INTRODUCTION

This chapter consists of three basic sections. The first section is a discussion of laboratory operation and understanding laboratory results. The second section includes general considerations of tolerance testing. The third section includes detailed instructions for the performance and interpretation of specific tolerance tests. This chapter can assist the reader in making the testing procedure as understandable and painless as possible for patients.

II. ROLE OF THE LABORATORY

Many endocrine disorders can only be distinguished by laboratory tests. The clinical symptoms of an inherited biosynthetic disorder frequently cannot be distinguished from an inherited receptor defect. For example, a child (46, XY) with ambiguous genitalia could have a biosynthetic defect in 17-keto-steroid reductase or 17-hydroxylase/lyase or a defect in the androgen receptor (androgen insensitivity syndrome; Chap. 18). These disorders cannot be distinguished by the clinical presentation but only by differences in laboratory parameters. Testosterone replacement therapy may be useful for either enzyme defect, but in contrast, replacement hormone therapy is not useful therapy for a child with androgen insensitivity. Thus, laboratory results are absolutely required for distinguishing the pathophysiologic basis of related disorders and for planning therapy.

The most striking fact in endocrinology today is that virtually all hormones are assayed with antibody-based technology. Endocrinology, as we know it, would not exist if not for the development of radioimmunoassay. The use of antibody-based technology has some specific consequences: (1) the specificity of an assay is limited by the specificity of the antibody; (2) the presence of a large amount of a closely related substance can interfere with the assay; and (3) different assay formats have precision in different portions of the standard curves. Each of these points affects the utility of a laboratory result.

A. General Considerations in Interpreting Tolerance Test Results (1–4)

For many disorders, evaluation of basal hormone levels is sufficient for diagnosis. However, some hormones are secreted episodically and others are secreted only as part of the response to particular stimuli. Thus, tolerance testing attempts to evaluate either a transient process or the "reserve" of an ongoing process.

The first consideration in understanding the result of a tolerance test is to consider the units used by a reference laboratory. Many laboratories do not report results with the same units as are used in publications. The units reported can be divided into two types: (1) mass-based units, usually used for small molecules, such as steroids and thyroid hormones, and (2) standard preparation-based units, usually used for proteins. Each of the types has specific problems.

Most small molecules are generally reported in mass units (e.g., ng/dl). The pure materials are readily available and inexpensive; solutions of known concentration can be readily compared from laboratory to laboratory. Some laboratories report results as ng/dl however, and others use ng/ml. Thus, one laboratory's 100 might be another laboratories 1.

(Is 210 a normal value for 17-hydroxyprogesterone? Yes, if it is ng/dl; no, if it is ng/ml.) To avoid this problem, perhaps under pressure from journals, small molecules are now being reported in SI units (moles per liter).

For peptide hormones, when these assays were first established, pure materials were not readily available and each laboratory generated its own standard. For example, the first standard unit for somatomedin C assay was a pool of adult serum prepared in the investigator's laboratory. Each investigator's pool was different, however. As a consequence, results could not be readily compared from laboratory to laboratory. To solve this problem, groups with international support (National Institutes of Health and/or the World Health Organization) made large standard preparations and defined the amount of active hormone present as an International Unit (IU). As needed, a vial of the standard, with a defined concentration in IU/L would be reconstituted. Over time, the original international standards were depleted and new standards were collected, but the new standards did not have exactly the same amount of hormone as the old. Thus, depending on when a particular laboratory established its assay, the normal values in International Units will be different but each is properly called an International Unit. Hence, knowing that a hormone is reported as IU/L does not specify the normal or expected values. Another source of differences in laboratory results is microheterogeneity. Many peptide hormones are glycoproteins with variable amounts of carbohydrate groups, perhaps a partial cause of inactive or hyperactive molecules. Because the epitopes frequently overlap with the glycosyl groups, specific antibodies may be more (or less) immunoreactive with the active hormone or with metabolites or fragments and the different standards may also be more or less contaminated with metabolites or fragments. Thus, as a consequence of the microvariation, immunoreactivity and bioactivity correlate to a variable extent. For example, assays of human chorionic gonadotropin (hCG) are frequently used to determine whether a woman is pregnant. However, hCG is a heterodimer consisting of an α subunit shared with thyroid-stimulating hormone (TSH), luteinizing hormone (LH), and follicle-stimulating hormone (FSH) and a specific β subunit. Some assays measure only the β subunit, others measure the amount of intact hormone, and still others detect specific glycosylated isoforms. As a consequence, the range of expected values indicative of pregnancy varies from 25 to 50 IU/L. In this case, if needed, a repeat sample a few days later will resolve an initial ambiguous result. In summary, it is not sufficient to report results as IU/L because different IUs are in use. This problem becomes more important if an endocrinologist is using several different laboratories, perhaps because of insurance company or health maintenance organization requirements.

B. Assay Format and Design

The most commonly used format for antibody-based assays is displacement analysis. With this format, (1) a limited amount of antibody is allowed to bind to a limited amount of specific tracer for the hormone, (2) the antibody-bound tracer is separated from the free tracer, and finally, (3) the antibody-bound tracer is quantitated. If the tracer is a radioactive hormone, then the assay is classified as a radioimmunoassay (RIA); if the tracer is a hormone coupled to an enzyme, then the assay is classified as an enzyme immunoassay. If the tracer is a fluorescent compound, then the assay might be classified as fluorescent immunoassay. In each format, a standard curve is generated by adding known amounts of unlabeled hormone and determining the decrease (displacement) in tracer bound to the antibody. For determination of the serum concentration of a hormone, the observed displacement is compared to the standard curve. The important point here is that if (1) additional amounts of antibody (or binding proteins) are present in the serum or (2) there are closely related forms of the hormone in the serum, then the assay result is unreliable. The forms can be (1) closely related steroids for a steroid assay, (2) glycoproteins with differences in glycosyl groups, (3) closely related hormones, such as the activin-inhibin or LH-hCG pairs, or (4) isoforms, such as the 20 K and 22 K isoforms of growth hormone. In each of these formats, the least analytic precision occurs at the lowest concentration of analyte. Thus, alternative methodology must be used if the clinically important analyte concentration is at the lowest range of ligand concentration. Examples of ligands that usually require an alternative format are hCG (one cannot be a little bit pregnant) and TSH assays when used to evaluate hyperthyroidism.

In the ELISA (enzyme-linked immunosorbent assay) format, a small amount of hormone is prebound to each well of a 96-well plate (alternatively to a plastic or glass tube); then, the standards and unknowns are added. The hormone-specific antibody is added and allowed to react with both the prebound and free hormone. More is bound if there is less free hormone added. The amount of antibody bound is then quantitated by a suitable technique, typically by eliminating all unbound proteins and adding a second antibody that is specific for the first antibody and to which an active enzyme is bound. Finally, the amount of active enzyme is specifically determined in each well and compared to the known amount of hormone added and a standard curve generated for comparison with the unknowns. This format is best used for assays to detect the presence of important compounds. Perhaps the best example of this is the presence of disease-specific antibodies for specific infectious agents, for example, antibodies specific for human immunodeficiency virus for risk of the acquired immunodeficiency syndrome.

In the IRMA (immunoradiometric assay) format, one hormone-specific antibody is attached to the solid support. The standards and unknowns are added, and a second hormone-specific antibody is added. Note that the second antibody used in IRMA is ligand specific rather than specific for the first antibody, as would be the case in RIA or ELISA. The second antibody is labeled with (1) radioactive tracer, (2) fluorescent or other non-radioactive tracer, or (3) an enzyme. After a suitable incubation period, all unbound materials are washed away. Only when the desired analyte forms a bridge between (1) the (first) antibody bound to the solid support and (2) the soluble (second) antibody is the tracer or enzyme bound to the solid support and available for detection. It should be noted that if a pair of epitopes are very closely spaced on a ligand of interest, then the combination of antibodies cannot be used in an IRMA. As a consequence of the format, the amount of tracer bound to the bridge is approximately proportional to the amount of ligand present. At high ligand concentrations, the amount of ligand can exceed the amount of either one of the antibodies. This leads to a "high-dose hook effect" and results in low estimations of ligand concentration. IRMA reagents are generally more expensive than reagents suitable for displacement analysis because of the requirement for two matched specific antibodies. As a compensating advantage, however, in contrast to displacement analysis, the IRMA format has its greatest analytic precision at the lowest analyte concentrations. The improved sensitivity at low concentrations and the improved specificity inherent in the method has led to widespread replacement of kits for displacement analysis (including RIA) for all analytes large enough for the generation of suitable antibodies.

C. Assay Specificity

The specificity of an assay is limited by two factors: (1) the amount and nature of sample preparation and (2) the specificity of the antibody. The necessity for a chromatographic step (an example of a type 1 step) in an assay for a steroid adds a significant amount to the cost of an individual determination. Thus, most laboratories minimize type 1 factor steps and rely on type 2 as much as possible. The difference between an alcohol and a ketone (such as between androstenedione and testosterone) generally permits a 10- to 50-fold difference in sensitivity based on a suitable antibody (a type 2 factor). Thus, for steroids present in similar concentrations, an antibody can usually provide sufficient specificity. In patients with biosynthetic defects, however, specific intermediates may be present to 10,000-fold excess. For example, an assay kit for testosterone would not be specifically tested or approved for use in children with congenital adrenal hyperplasia. At the time of diagnosis of the non–salt-losing form (typically a boy 4–6 years of age), 17-hydroxyprogesterone levels might exceed 50,000 ng/dl. Even if the testosterone antibody had only 1% cross-reactivity with 17-hydroxyprogesterone, then the contribution of 17-hydroxyprogesterone to the apparent testosterone concentration would be 500 ng/dl, a level much greater than the normal range for a 4- to 6-year-old boy. The large amount of 17-hydroxyprogesterone would also serve as a substrate for synthesis of testosterone. Thus, both large amounts of testosterone and a cross-reacting steroid may be contributing to the apparent hormone levels. Type 1 procedures would be necessary to evaluate the actual testosterone level in such a case, but most laboratories are not equipped or experienced in appropriate techniques. Thus, when one hormone concentration is present to large excess, it may carry over to other closely related hormones and cause a lack of specificity.

In addition to factors in the assay, there are biologic factors that lead to loss of inherent specificity. Lack of

specificity can also be compounded because of age-specific differences in secretion. Dehydroepiandrosterone (DHEA) kits are usually tested on adult serum and would not be specifically approved for use in serum from newborns, even though DHEA assay might be requested to evaluate 3β-hydroxysteroid dehydrogenase function in a newborn. A comparison of three approved kits for the assay of DHEA is shown in Figure 1. Reagent kits B and C showed substantial equivalence, but both detected more DHEA in cord serum than kit A. Studies of possible cross-reacting steroids showed that kits B and C both detected 16-hydroxy-DHEA as DHEA, but kit A did not. In adults, this compound is not present in significant amounts, but newborns produce more of it than of DHEA itself. Thus, apparent levels of DHEA would be elevated if the laboratory used kit B or C, and a faulty diagnosis of 3β-hydroxysteroid dehydrogenase deficiency might be suggested. These problems require good rapport between a physician and the director of the clinical laboratory service.

The combination of reliance on type 2 steps and differences in age specificity can easily lead to delays in proper diagnosis. For example, apparently high levels of DHEA sulfate were associated with a clinical history of severe salt wasting and ambiguous genitalia and with facial features suggestive of Smith-Lemli-Opitz syndrome. The high levels of DHEA sulfate suggested a diagnosis of congenital adrenal hyperplasia caused by 3β-hydroxysteroid dehydrogenase deficiency. However, when type 1 steps (chromatography) were added to the assay method, large amounts of DHEA sulfate and 16-hydroxy-DHEA sulfate but no 15-hydroxy-DHEA sulfate or 15,16-dihydroxy-DHEA sulfate was found, in contrast to normal infants of the same age, in whom all four compounds are present. Thus, the infants had a defect in 15-hydroxylase activity not in 3β-hydroxysteroid dehydrogenase activity. In summary, complete reliance on type 2 specificity for hormone assays in infants must be carefully considered.

There are two different mechanisms by which binding proteins can also contribute to the lack of clinical utility of a particular assay. First, if the affinity constant of the binding protein is comparable to the affinity constant of the antibody, then it may interfere with the assay by providing additional binding sites. This would probably lead to inappropriately low hormone levels. Second, because the definition of a hormone includes passage through the blood and control of the function of a second organ, serum binding proteins (BPs) can interfere with or supplement the activity of the parent hormone. For example, some binding proteins increase the half-life of a short-lived hormone (for example, insulin-like growth factor, IGF, BP-3); others increase the amount present in the serum by increasing the solubility of a lipophilic compound (testosterone-estradiol binding globulin); others seem to have hormonal functions of their own (corticosteroid binding globulin). The function of thyroid binding globulin is unclear because individuals with TBG deficiency seem to have no clinical problems. Whatever functional role is fulfilled by a particular binding protein, however, it becomes possible to evaluate an additional parameter, the free hormone

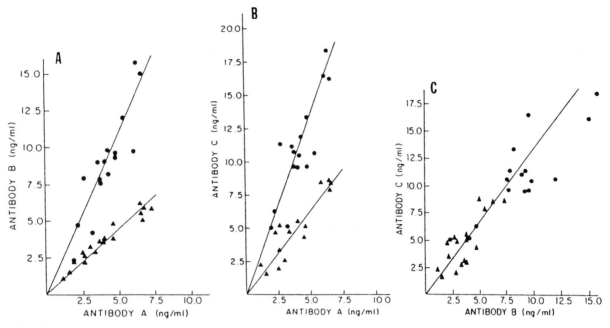

Figure 1 Comparison of results obtained with three antibodies to DHEA in serum from adults (triangles) and cord serum (circles). Antibody A was prepared by immunization with DHEA-3-hemisuccinate-BSA (bovine serum albumin) conjugate. Antibody B was prepared by immunization with DHEA-7-oxo- CMO-BSA conjugate. Antibody C was prepared by immunization with DHEA-15-oxo-CMO-BSA conjugate. Kits using similar antibodies with similar cross-reactivities have been approved by the FDA. Note the discordant results obtained with cord serum when antibody A is compared with either antibody B or C. (By permission from Steroids 1985; 45:187–193.)

concentration, and identify an additional basis for a pathophysiologic disorder, binding protein deficiency, or excess. Changes in binding protein concentrations can lead to large changes in total hormone levels without corresponding changes in free levels, which are presumably the active form. To date, however, no common disorders are associated with any binding protein deficiency (with the possible exception of Laron syndrome). The best known example of this phenomenon is thyroid binding globulin deficiency. Individuals with this deficiency have low total thyroxine levels and normal free thyroxine levels, but to date there are no known pathophysiologic consequences.

Although there is no mysticism in immunoassay there are many places for error, and no single laboratory value should be considered diagnostic without confirmation. In general, because of the "one disease to a customer" rule in pediatrics, until all laboratory results suggest a single disorder, the clinician should not consider the diagnostic process complete. This discussion should suggest alternatives for a clinician to consider when a laboratory result is not consistent with the clinical index of suspicion.

D. Impact of the Regulatory Environment on Laboratory Operation (5–7)

Clinical laboratories have come under close regulatory scrutiny with a new set of regulations, collectively called CLIA-88

(Clinical Laboratory Improvement Act of 1988). Because these regulations limit the operation of a laboratory, one must understand their application. Smaller clinical laboratories purchase reagents (kits) for all analytes they evaluate. Their list of analytes is limited, by the availability of approved kits, to the more frequently ordered analytes. Larger laboratories purchase some reagents from commercial manufacturers and have developed their own (in-house) reagents for some of the newer, less common analytes. Thus, larger clinical laboratories both establish normal pediatric results and introduce new analytes of interest to pediatric endocrinologists. It is not clear whether they will all seek U.S. Food and Drug Administration (FDA) approval under the CLIA-88 regulations for their in-house reagents. This point is important because under CLIA-88 regulations, laboratories may be allowed to use reagents only with FDA approval. Thus, the regulations may serve to stifle innovation.

As defined by CLIA88, almost all endocrine testing is classified as high-complexity testing. To perform high-complexity testing, CLIA88 describes three types of personnel: (1) directors, (2) consultants, and (3) technologists and supervisors. The director of the laboratory must have completed a doctoral-level training program, but it may include an M.D. (or D.O.), a Ph.D. (or Sc.D.), or both. The organizational structure for the laboratory requires both a technical consultant (who provides advice on reagent and kit selection, as well as troubleshooting when results fail quality control parameters) and a clinical consultant (who aids physicians in making diagnosis and must be an M.D. or D.O.). If the director has an M.D., he or she may serve as the clinical consultant and/or technical consultant; however, if the director has a Ph.D. degree and serves as the technical consultant, then the laboratory must also have clinical consultants. Patient diagnosis may only be made by an M.D. (or D.O.), but the distinction between reporting normal levels and/or levels expected in specific disorders and actual diagnosis may become small. In most cases, the actual testing is performed by a technologist, not a technician. Technicians are not required to have a college degree and may work only under direct supervision. In contrast, a technologist must have a college degree in chemistry, biology, or medical technology and at least 1 year of experience and be capable of working without direct supervision. *Note*: calling a technologist a technician is not a good way to foster a relationship. Once one understands the functions of the people who work in the laboratory and may be available to speak to you on the phone, one can begin to receive proper advice. Thus, in addition to the name of the answerer, it is absolutely appropriate to inquire about their function in the laboratory.

Basically, for common analytes, manufacturers can gain FDA approval to market reagent kits by showing general equivalence to a test already marketed for clinical diagnostic use. For pediatrics, however, this procedure is often inappropriate. In general, the FDA approves reagents for clinical diagnostic uses based on adult normal samples and adult disease populations. Hormone levels and interfering substances are frequently different in children, especially in infants. A pediatrician might order DHEA (see Fig. 1) or DHEA-S as part of the diagnosis of ambiguous genitalia or congenital adrenal hyperplasia. Figure 2 shows results with nine different assays for DHEA-S on cord serum. Although each of the nine reagents was quite capable of assaying DHEA-S in adult serum samples and seven of the nine had FDA approval (reagents 1 and 2 were not specifically approved at the time of the study), results on cord serum were discordant. In cord sera from normal infants, some of the kits detected 3–10 times more DHEA-S than the others. This was caused by the detection of 16-hydroxy-DHEA-S and other androstene sulfates that are not present in corresponding concentrations in adults. The original FDA-approved kits for the assay of digoxin also cross-reacted with this same class of compounds. During the period when the fetal adrenal zone was functional, these interfered with the monitoring of digoxin therapy because there were apparent high levels of digoxin, which was detected by RIA, present before the initiation of therapy. Thus, FDA approval is no guarantee of a suitable kit for pediatrics.

Reagent kits for novel analytes can be marketed, at present, as *For Research Use Only*. Each laboratory using reagents marked in this way is obligated to establish normal ranges and clinical utility by itself. Of course, most laboratories do not perform these studies, nor do they have the capability of doing the required studies. Under the guidelines in CLIA-88, laboratories are only allowed to use kits specifically approved for diagnostic use. As a consequence of this

rule, widespread evaluation of new analytes cannot proceed through this intermediate mechanism and introduction of new diagnostic markers to clinical practice will probably be delayed.

In summary, the changing regulatory environment will standardize clinical laboratory services. The high cost of kits and equipment may lead to a decrease in the number of hospital laboratories offering service, and at the same time, laboratories may become more price conscious in the selection of kits. Fewer novel analytes will be available for the diagnosis of rare disorders. Insurance reimbursement will also prevent an endocrinologist from relying on a single laboratory. Thus, a knowledge of kits and reagents used for different laboratories will become more necessary for clinicians.

III. PRACTICAL CONSIDERATIONS

Meticulous attention to detail, both in the selection of laboratory tests and in the tolerance test room, are the keys to a successful procedure. In particular, the most important details to evaluate are the sample size requirements, the type of tubes (e.g., serum, EDTA, or heparin) used to collect the blood, and the specific sample-processing requirements, including whether serum samples should be separated and if they could, should, or must be frozen. In consultation with the laboratory, one should determine the amount of serum required for each analyte and prepare a table listing the exact time of sampling, the analytes for that time point, and the

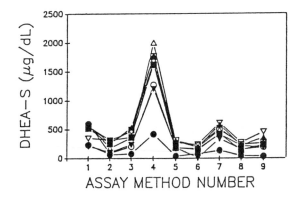

Figure 2 DHEA-S levels as determined with nine different methods. Methods 1 and 2 utilized published methods based on commercially available antibodies and tracers. Methods 3–9 were complete kits approved by the FDA (3 = Diagnostic Products; 4 = Nuclear Medical Sciences; 5 = Diagnostic Systems Laboratories; 6 = Cambridge Medical Diagnostics; 7 = Wien Laboratories; 8 = ICN (RSL); 9 = Pantex). In experiments not shown, each method adequately assayed "spiked" samples, both on charcoal-treated and on whole serum. Serum from normal adults and children yielded essentially equivalent results with each method. The DHEA-S level detected in cord serum obtained at birth from eight infants. Note the large variation in apparent concentration. (By permission from Steroids 1989; 54:373–383.)

amount of blood required by the laboratory. The proper number and type of blood collection tubes should be collected. Recall that if a mistake is made and inappropriate or inadequate blood samples are obtained, the protocol will probably have to be repeated. Finally, arrangements must be made to transport samples to the laboratory in a manner that does not lead to degradation.

A. Mechanics

Successful testing is accomplished primarily through organization. A tray should be prepared to hold completed laboratory slips, the correct number and types of tubes, labels, syringes, alcohol, arm board, and tape. This allows methodical sampling throughout the test, without having to look for necessities while the test is in progress. Medications should also be ordered the day before the test. These advance preparations ensure that, on the day of the test, everything proceeds smoothly, with the least discomfort to the patient.

A heparin lock is extremely useful because it permits an indwelling line for both withdrawal of blood samples and delivery of medication with minimal discomfort to the patient. The standard solution for the heparin lock is a mixture of 9 ml normal saline and 1 ml of 1:1000 sodium heparin. Withdraw and discard 0.5–1.0 ml from the line before sampling; after sampling, the line may be cleared by injection of an equal volume of the heparin solution. An intravenous setup is a suitable alternative but leaves the patient somewhat less comfortable during the protocol. In a child younger than 4 years of age, it is appropriate to maintain a separate intravenous line with 0.25 normal saline, in addition to the heparin lock, for emergencies during potentially hazardous testing, such as insulin tolerance protocols. Although this may cause some added discomfort to the patient, loss of a line is common in young children and a patent line is essential to address any untoward events.

The size of the heparin lock needle must be selected on the basis of its intended use. A 24 gauge angiocatheter needle in a scalp vein may be adequate for infusion for an infant or young child; however, it is futile to attempt to obtain multiple blood samples from such a small needle or vein. Generally, a 22 or 23 gauge angiocatheter is adequate for both infusion and sampling. Infants and children with poor venous access may require various measures to obtain access. Choice of site should be made after careful assessment of the child and the necessity of the test. It is strongly suggested that when a complex protocol is performed on an infant, a colleague is present who can respond to a compromising situation and provide help during an emergency.

Many of the protocols for tolerance tests include an overnight fast. Because the nothing by mouth order is usually written for after midnight, a snack should be given just before midnight, if the child is awake at that time. Otherwise, the snack should be given at bedtime. For infants and very young children, however, an overnight fast may be too long. Therefore, the fast should conform to the child's eating patterns (i.e., an infant may be on a 3–4 h feeding schedule).

In general, to avoid unnecessary fasting by young children, most tolerance tests should be started as early in the morning as possible. If the test must be postponed, the child should be fed and refasted. However, it should be noted that if a protocol is delayed, diurnal variation must be considered in the interpretation of the results.

In most cases, patient medications that might interfere with the test should be discontinued for at least 1 week. If this is not possible, the effects of the medication on the tolerance test must be considered when interpreting the results. Other factors, such as extreme agitation or exercise, can also affect the results and should be noted.

A critical factor when conducting a tolerance test is the total amount of blood that must be obtained if, as is usually the case, multiple samples are required. The amount of blood that can be safely withdrawn without compromise to the patient must be considered. The usual guideline is a maximum, within a 2 week period, of 5% of the total blood volume, which is calculated by multiplying the body weight (kg) by 80 ml/kg. Remember to include any other testing planned for the same time or within 2 weeks of the tolerance test. If the amount required is more than 5% of the patient's total blood volume, the protocol must be modified.

B. Person-to-Person Considerations

One of the greatest challenges is informing the parents and the child about the purposes and mechanics of the test; this is an important point because an informed patient is calmer and more cooperative. While explaining the procedure to the patient and the parents, the greatest fear is often expressed when you describe the necessity for repeated blood samples. The terror of repeated venipuncture and its inevitable pain can often be alleviated by a description of the indwelling line that will be placed. Some of the fear may be relaxed if the apparatus to be used can be shown (i.e, the heparin lock) and its use demonstrated for obtaining blood samples without additional discomfort. It may be useful to emphasize that only one "stick" is needed, although blood may be drawn many times. You may have greater cooperation from the child and the parents if they are convinced that the child will not suffer more pain than absolutely necessary.

Of greatest importance is the explanation of the significance of the test. This must be done in terms understandable both to the parents and to the child. Allow sufficient time for questions and answers. A simplified drawing of the specific hormonal system is valuable as an aid to understanding the test protocol. While you are describing the test, judge whether the parents should stay in the room with the child during the test. Most parents respond to a clear, logical, and honest estimation of what will happen during the test and frequently remain more in control than you estimate. On the other hand, a parent's anxiety may be unconsciously relayed to the child and may make the situation more difficult. In deciding whether to allow the parents to stay, exercise discretion on an individual basis.

C. Time-of-Day Considerations

The largest single diagnostic group of tolerance tests is evaluation of short stature and possible growth hormone deficiency. Almost all of these tests must be performed on fasting subjects. Hence, in most offices, they are scheduled for the first appointment in the morning in preestablished time blocks. Protocols not requiring fasting are usually scheduled for the same time blocks because those blocks are already established as tolerance test time blocks. Hence, most protocols are usually performed in the morning, whether or not there is any physiologic purpose for this restriction. As a consequence, normal and expected values are all based on testing in the morning. It should be noted that there are circadian rhythms in many hormonal secretion patterns that can be superimposed on other patterns. For example, LH and FSH are both secreted episodically with 90 minute cycles but the amplitude of the cycle is increased in the morning. As a consequence, (1) pituitary responses to gonadotropin-releasing hormone (GnRH) may be different and (2) basal testosterone levels are higher in the morning and one cannot measure an acute response to hCG. Adrenocorticotropic hormone (ACTH) is also secreted episodically with a 90 minute cycle, but episodes of secretion occur more frequently in the morning and the ratio of cortisol to adrenal androgen secretion also changes with time of day. Hence, if testing is or must be performed at times other than morning, care must be used in comparing observed values to expected values. The exception to this requirement is in young infants, in whom circadian patterns have not yet been established.

IV. PRACTICAL PROTOCOLS FOR TOLERANCE TESTING IN CHILDREN

The concept of a tolerance test is to provide a means to evaluate a physiologic pathway that may function only episodically or in response to a specific metabolic event. The physiologic response may require only one organ or several organs to generate the specific response. In many cases, the metabolic state must be controlled at the start of the test. The factors that must be controlled can include access to food, access to fluids, time of day, or even prior treatment with metabolites, substrates, or even other hormones. The physiology of a tolerance test can be as simple as a decrease in serum glucose levels after insulin infusion (which would direct glucose uptake by the liver) or as multistepped as an increase in serum cortisol levels after insulin infusion (which requires functioning of the complete hypothalamus-pituitary-adrenal cortex axis). Typically, the end point of a tolerance test is (1) the secretion of a hormone that controls other processes or (2) a change in serum glucose levels. Hence, the interpretation of test results almost always depends on the evaluation of specific serum hormone or metabolite levels.

A. Tolerance Tests for Growth Hormone (GH) Deficiency

1. Screening Tests for GH Deficiency (8)

a. Background. Growth hormone deficiency is only one of many causes of growth failure. The overall incidence of GH deficiency is approximately 1 in 5000 children. This is equivalent to only 1 to 250 children in the shortest five percentiles. In view of the high cost and effort for evaluating GH secretory dynamics, screening tests have been developed to increase the success rate in identifying children with GH deficiency. The proper control group for evaluation of a screening test is children with short stature rather than children of normal stature.

The most widely used screening test for GH deficiency is evaluation of serum IGF-I levels. IGF-I (somatomedin C or sulfation factor) is a 3000 dalton peptide that is secreted in response to GH. Its various names are based on specific aspects of its physiologic function. (Remember the story of the blind men and the elephant?) Most, but not all, of the physiology of GH action requires IGF-I as a mediator. Serum levels are age and sex dependent in normal children, with a sharp increase at the time of puberty. Low levels of IGF-I also occur in children with (1) GH receptor and/or postreceptor defects, (2) thyroid disorders, and (3) delayed puberty. Thus, low IGF-I levels are a good indicator of a defect in the physiology of growth but do not specifically implicate GH deficiency.

In serum, the IGFs are mostly bound to specific binding proteins. The most important binding protein is designated BP-3 and is GH dependent. BP-3 has less age and sex dependence than IGF-I levels. In 1990, Blum pioneered BP-3 as a specific screening test for GH deficiency.

There are four possible outcomes to screening tests. A negative result implies that the test was within the normal range and that definitive testing confirmed the absence of GH deficiency. A positive result implies that the test result was out of the normal range and that definitive testing confirmed the diagnosis of GH deficiency. In contrast, a false negative result implies a level within the normal range but definitive testing suggested a diagnosis of GH deficiency, and a false positive result implies a level below the normal range but definitive testing eliminated a diagnosis of GH deficiency. In view of the low expected frequency of GH deficiency in the population, the most important parameter is a very low false negative result. If there were higher false negative results, then there would be a need to evaluate GH secretion in individuals with negative results and the utility of the screening test fails.

b. Indications. Children at increased risk for GH deficiency should be screened, including (1) children in the lowest five height, growth, or bone age percentiles, when proper consideration is made for family history; (2) children with syndromes associated with short stature; (3) children who have acute changes in their growth charts; and (4) children who have had possible insults to the pituitary, such as chemotherapy, radiotherapy, or physical injury to the head.

c. Preparation and Medication. None are needed.

d. Sampling. A single sample is obtained at the time of a routine patient visit. There is no time of day or diet restriction. *Note*: Some laboratories require plasma, rather than serum, for IGF-I assays. Check with the laboratory before collecting a sample. BP-3 levels are determined on serum. Thus, both serum and plasma may be needed.

e. Normal and Expected Values (IGF-I Levels). Normal levels were determined by collecting samples from children of normal height. However, the desired test comparison is between children with short stature without GH deficiency and children with short stature with GH deficiency. Tables 1 and 2 show the results of IGF-I screening tests from our laboratory. Samples were obtained from 109 healthy normal children (age 0.5–18 years); from 151 healthy children with heights less than the fifth percentile (all children had at least one GH over 10 ng/ml after pharmacologic testing, and none had any recognized syndrome associated with short stature); and from 50 children with short stature and GH deficiency, defined as having no serum GH level above 10 ng/ml on two pharmacologic tests (we thank Diagnostic Systems Laboratory [DSL, Webster, TX] for providing reagents for the assay of IGF-I).

Although some investigators have suggested the use of levels that change every year, our experience suggests a simpler algorithm: GH deficiency should be considered in (1) children less than 9 years of age with IGF-I below 50 ng/ml and (2) children over 9 years of age with IGF-I levels below 100 ng/ml and testosterone levels below 200 ng/dl. Boys with testosterone levels over 200 ng/dl have already started puberty and may have limited remaining growth potential. In our experience, criteria including lower IGF-I levels lead to a higher incidence of false negative results.

f. Normal and Expected Values (BP-3 Levels). The normal range is from 2.5 to 10 mg/dl, with a small dependence, compared with the normal variation in RIA or IRMA assays, on differences in age and sex. Serum levels

Table 1 IGF-I Levels in Children[a]

	Normal stature	Short stature	GH deficiency
Age range, years	0.5–5 (37 children)		
Number	25	5	7
IGF-I, ng/ml	80 ± 52	92 ± 63	17 ± 15
Age range, years	5–9 (61 children)		
Number	21	39	11
IGF-I, ng/ml	158 ± 52	100 ± 71	25 ± 17
Age range, years	9–13 (109 children)		
Number	29	63	17
IGF-I, ng/ml	249 ± 77	149 ± 97	51 ± 32
Age range, years	>13 (93 children)		
Number	34	44	15
IGF-I, ng/ml	312 ± 150	197 ± 125	64 ± 45

[a]Mean ± standard deviation).

Table 2 IGF-I Levels as a Screening Test for GH Deficiency in Children

	Normal stature	Short stature
Age range, years	0.5–9 (62 children)	
IGF-I levels, ng/ml	<50	>50
Short stature	13	31
GH deficiency	18	0
Age range, years	9–15 (139 children)	
IGF-I levels, ng/ml	<100	>100
Short stature	20	82
GH deficiency	27	5[a]

[a]These five subjects were boys over 13 years of age with testosterone levels in excess of 200 ng/ml.

less than 2.4 mg/dl are associated with GH deficiency. Slightly higher values occur at the time of puberty.

g. General Considerations. About 50% of the positive results are not associated with GH deficiency but with receptor and postreceptor defects. In addition, a positive screening test with normal GH secretory dynamics is an indication to consider other nonorganic disorders associated with growth failure, such as (1) nutritional inadequacies, (2) inadequate spontaneous GH secretion, and (3) psychosocial growth failure.

h. Basic Physiology of Growth Hormone Secretion (9–13). For most short children (less than the fifth percentile in height), the final diagnosis is constitutional short stature or constitutional growth delay and there is no specific therapy other than to maintain adequate nutrition (Chap. 1). A few individuals (1 in 5000 or 1 in 250 short children) have GH deficiency, and replacement therapy with biosynthetic hormone may be effective, but at a cost of $5000–20,000 per year (Chap. 5). Present understanding suggests that only individuals with inadequate growth hormone secretion have improved final height when treated with growth hormone; others only reach their final height sooner and then stop growing. Thus, the problem is to identify the individuals who will benefit and to exclude those who will not benefit.

GH is secreted episodically, most episodes occurring during rapid eye movement sleep (Chap. 4). Most random serum samples (at least 90%) do not contain GH and cannot be used to evaluate GH deficiency. Isolated random samples are only of use to rule out the diagnosis of acromegaly. Over the years, many pharmacologic agents have been identified that induce GH secretion, and suitable tolerance test procedures have been developed. There are two factors necessary for the evaluation of the response to pharmacologic stimuli for GH secretion: first, knowledge of normal and inadequate responses to the particular protocol and, second, laboratory selection of methods and reagents for the evaluation of serum GH levels.

Assays for serum GH levels are complicated by the molecular nature of GH in serum. There are multiple isoforms, a binding protein, and specific metabolites that all can interfere or be detected differentially by the particular assay. On the favorable side, first, GH has a short serum half-life, reducing the amount of metabolites that can accumulate, and second, GH is not a glycoprotein, which eliminates one major source of molecular variation. Finally, the GH binding protein has less affinity than most antibodies and, as a consequence, does not generally interfere with the assay. Several laboratories have investigated the response of different assays on the same samples. Although each of the kits nominally uses the same standard, specific kits produce widely different estimates for the serum GH level. The most striking differences are observed with the Hybritech IRMA kit. With this kit, for GH to be detected, each GH molecule must have two specific intact epitopes. The most common isoform, with 191 amino acids (22K), but not the isoform with 176 amino acid residues (20K), has both epitopes used in the IRMA. Thus, in children with normal growth rates, partially because of the presence of 20K, this kit reports about 30% lower GH levels than many other kits. It is in widespread use by clinical laboratories but is less commonly used than several other kits. Expected values must account for this difference in apparent GH concentration. Throughout the remainder of this section, for ease of explanation, quantitative discussions assume that the physician is not using a laboratory that relies on Hybritech reagents. If the laboratory relies on these reagents, then the quantitative values to identify children with growth hormone deficiency should be decreased by about 30%.

At the present time, the generally recognized criteria for GH deficiency is a response of less than 10 ng/ml (or 10 μg/l) to two different pharmacologic stimuli for GH secretion. The stimuli can have their effects at the level of the hypothalamus, the pituitary, or both. High serum glucose levels inhibit GH secretion. Thus, each protocol must also include a significant period of fasting before the test.

i. Normal Values. With most assay reagents, serum GH concentration over 10 ng/ml indicates adequate GH response to pharmacologic stimulation. (As noted earlier, if the laboratory uses Hybritech assay kits, then levels above 7 ng/ml probably indicate adequate GH response.) If peak serum levels do not exceed the nominal normal values, the test is considered consistent with GH deficiency.

The pharmacodynamics of GH secretion and metabolism determine the design of the serum-sampling protocol. Episodes of active GH secretion by the pituitary last about 5–10 minutes, and the half-life of GH is about 20–30 minutes. Thus, the specific protocol for a tolerance test must collect serum every 20–30 minutes to detect an episode of secretion. With each of the tolerance tests, first a single value over 10 ng/ml is sufficient to evaluate the response, and second, there will usually not be a second serum sample with a concentration over 10 ng/ml because GH concentration will decrease by half (one half-life) before obtaining the next sample.

j. Expected Frequency of Inadequate GH Secretion in Response to a Tolerance Test. Children with (1) Prader-Willi syndrome, Russell-Silver syndrome, Down syndrome, or other syndromes associated with short stature, (2) Turner syndrome (in girls), or (3) a history of cranial irradiation or of treatments for leukemia have a very high frequency, perhaps up to 100%, of inadequate GH secretion (Chap. 56). Thus, there should be a high index of suspicion for a diagnosis of GH deficiency if a child also has one of these syndromes. However, in the absence of a specific syndrome associated with GH deficiency, about 1 child in 5000 has idiopathic GH deficiency. This corresponds to an incidence of 1 in 250 children who are less than the fifth percentile for height. Hence, most short children do not have GH deficiency. Children with GH deficiency frequently continue to cross growth lines on growth charts and have increasing amounts of bone age delay. Over time, the clinical symptoms of GH deficiency become more pronounced and more easily recognized. However, children with exaggerated bone age delay do not completely "catch up" to their genetic potential when therapy is started (Chap. 5). Hence, it is important to make the diagnosis as soon as possible, and thus, if a physician notes that most of his or her patients fail GH testing, he or she is probably not testing soon enough or frequently enough. In my laboratory, about one-fifth of all children tested actually had GH deficiency. Thus, the clinical judgment, screening tests, and experience of the clinical endocrinologists increased the incidence of GH deficiency from 1 in 250 short children to 1 in 5 for those children actually tested.

k. General Considerations. The following sections describe protocols for tolerance tests to evaluate the adequacy of GH secretion. Most physicians develop their own favorites and tend to use the same tests for most patients.

Near the time of puberty, for adequate GH secretion to occur, there must be adequate androgen levels. However, many short boys have delayed puberty or constitutional delay. To evaluate GH secretion in boys near puberty, testosterone priming should be added to the GH stimulation test. One protocol for androgen priming is the administration of 100 mg depot testosterone between 1 week and 10 days before the actual GH tolerance test. The same priming protocol could be used for any of the protocols. For girls, some endocrinologists prime with estrogens, but this does not seem to be as widely utilized.

2. Arginine and Combined Arginine-L-Dopa Test for GH Secretion (14–16)

a. Indications. The arginine stimulant apparently works by inducing insulin secretion and by blocking somatostatin secretion. The combined test thus stimulates GH secretion by two separate mechanisms. Perhaps as a consequence, the combined protocol has fewer false positive results then when either agent is administered alone. The test is used primarily when a second pharmacologic test for GH secretion is required.

b. Preparation. Indicate nothing by mouth after midnight or bedtime snack. Arrange with pharmacy to have arginine and to prepare it for administration. Plan ahead: not all pharmacies have stocks of arginine, and it may have to be specially ordered.

c. Medications. After the baseline serum sample is obtained, arginine HCl (0.5 g/kg to a maximum of 30 g) is administered intravenously over a 30 minute period.

If the combined arginine-L-Dopa protocol is used, L-Dopa is administered orally (PO) immediately after the baseline blood sample is obtained. Then administer arginine. The dose of L-Dopa should be as follows: (1) 125 mg for children less than 13.5 kg; 250 mg for children between 13.5 and 31.5 kg; and (3) 500 mg for children over 31.5 kg.

d. Sampling. Blood for GH assay should be sampled at 0, 30, 60, 90, and 120 minutes.

e. Special Considerations. As with the L-Dopa protocol, nausea and vomiting frequently occur in toddlers. Be prepared. Do not stop taking blood samples. Children should be recumbent and may be given water throughout the test.

3. Clonidine Stimulation Test for GH Secretion (17–20)

a. Specific Indications. This agent is probably the best choice for avoiding false positive results. Children who fail to secrete GH in response to pharmacologic doses of clonidine seldom secrete GH in response to any other test.

b. Preparation. The patient should receive nothing by mouth for at least 4–6 h before the test and should be off all other medications.

c. Medications. Administer clonidine, 5 μg/kg, after baseline sample is drawn, to a maximum of 250 μg.

d. Sampling. Blood for GH assay should be drawn at 0, 60, and 90 minutes and blood for cortisol assay at 0 and 90 minutes. Usually, the 60 minute sample has the highest amount of GH, the 90 minute sample being about 30% lower.

e. Special Considerations. Clonidine is an agent that lowers blood pressure. Blood pressure should be monitored at 0, 30, 60, and 90 minutes. In young children, clonidine frequently causes drowsiness, which lasts for several hours. Parents should be aware of this possible, benign side effect. Patients should have a place to lie down and may sleep or lie quietly throughout the procedure. Water may be given freely throughout the test period.

4. Dexamethasone Response Test (21–24)

a. Indications. Dexamethasone can be used to induce growth hormone secretion with the same time course as glucagon. When used in this way, dexamethasone administration has no reported side effects.

b. Preparation. Patients should fast after midnight.

c. Medications. After collection of the baseline serum sample, dexamethasone (2 mg/m^2) is administered intravenously as a bolus.

d. Sampling. After bolus administration of dexamethasone, serum samples should be obtained every 30 minutes for 2 h, every 15 minutes for 2 h, and then every 30 minutes for the fifth hour. The serum samples may be withdrawn from a heparin lock.

e. Normal Values. A peak of GH secretion should occur between 2 and 4 h after dexamethasone administration.

The peak GH concentration should exceed 5 ng/ml in normal individuals. In patients with GH deficiency, the peak response does not exceed 5 ng/ml. Patients with obesity may also respond poorly.

f. General Considerations. Patients can drink water as desired throughout the test. At the conclusion of the protocol, patients should be fed.

Like the galanin test, this protocol has not been widely utilized. Additional study is necessary to improve the response pattern.

5. Exercise-Induced GH Secretion (25,26)

a. Indications. This test is frequently used as a screening test to evaluate the need for more formal testing for GH secretion. This is a suggested protocol to take advantage of an active (hyperactive) child. Use caution with exercise-challenged children.

b. Preparation. The patient should have fasted for 3–4 hours before the test.

c. Medications. None are needed.

d. Sampling. The stimulus is 20 minutes of mild exercise: (1) up and down stairs, (2) run up and down corridor, and (3) 20 minutes on exercise cycle or bicycle; final heart beat should exceed 120 beats per minute.

Obtain blood samples at the end of exercise and at 20 and 40 minutes after completion of exercise or severe crying episode.

e. General Considerations. Water should be provided freely, as requested. As soon as the first serum sample is obtained at the conclusion of the exercise period, the child may eat and drink as desired.

Most offices do not have the equipment for an exercise test. The usual occasion to use this protocol is chance recognition of exercise, inadvertently performed by an active young boy.

6. Galanin Response Test (23,27,28)

a. Indications. Galanin is a neuropeptide that participates in the regulation of GH secretion, apparently in the hypothalamus. Thus, the response to galanin should test the hypothalamus-pituitary secretory pathway.

b. Preparation. As with most of the pharmacologic tests to evaluate GH secretion, the test should be performed in the morning after an overnight fast.

c. Medication. Galanin (*p*-galanin 1–29; Clinalfa AG, Switzerland) is administered over 1 h as an intravenous infusion at a total dose of 15 μg/kg body weight.

d. Sampling. After a baseline sample is obtained, galanin infusion is started and additional serum samples are obtained every 15 minutes for 2 h.

e. Normal Values. The peak response occurs between 1 and 2 h after the start of the infusion. The expected peak response is a peak level greater than 5 ng/ml. Note that the expected response is lower than with many other pharmacologic tests for GH secretion. Obese children respond poorly or do not respond at all.

f. General Considerations. Patients can drink water, if desired, during the test. At the conclusion of the serum-sampling protocol, patients should be allowed to eat. The only side effect reported is a temporary bad taste when the infusion is started.

Galanin infusion has fewer side effects than either clonidine or insulin administration. This may be caused by the fact that galanin is a natural part of the GH secretion mechanism. However, galanin is not yet approved by the FDA as a pharmaceutical agent in the United States and must be obtained as part of a research protocol at this time. The protocol described here is the first reported attempt at using galanin as an inducer for GH secretion. Additional studies are needed to establish a protocol with a better response pattern. The change required might be the same dose of galanin administered over a shorter time period.

7. GH Releasing Hormone (GHRH) Test for Pituitary Reserve for GH Secretion (29–33)

a. Indications. Administration of GHRH evaluates the ability of the pituitary to secrete GH. If a patient secretes GH in response to GHRH but not to pharmacologic stimuli that function in the hypothalamus, then a defect in the hypothalamus is indicated. This distinction may be of importance if the FDA approves either a GHRH substitute or a hexarelin analog to increase GH secretion.

b. Preparation. The test should be performed in a fasting child in the morning.

c. Medication. Inject intravenous human pituitary GHRH at a dose of 1 μg/kg over a period of 1 minute. The patient may experience some flushing immediately after the infusion.

d. Sampling. Serum samples for evaluation of GH should be obtained at 0, 15, 30, 45, and 60 minutes. Earlier protocols also collected a late sample at 90 minutes, but this does not seem to be needed because the peak generally occurs within the first hour after administration of GHRH.

e. Normal Values. Children with pituitary defects fail to secrete GH to a peak of 10 ng/ml. The peak serum level usually occurs in the 15 or 30 minute sample.

f. General Considerations. Most individuals with idiopathic GH secretion have a defect in hypothalamic regulation of pituitary secretion of GH. Hence, most patients secrete GH in response to GHRH but do not secrete GH in response to normal physiologic processes.

High endogenous (or exogenous) levels of somatostatin block the effect of GHRH.

8. Glucagon Test for GH Secretion (34,35)

a. Indications. This test is frequently a good choice in young children or infants. Because the test induces GH secretion by inducing endogenous insulin secretion to compensate for elevated serum glucose levels, it is a good substitute for the insulin tolerance test.

b. Preparation. Indicate nothing by mouth after midnight. Patients must have normal glucose reserves at the start of the test.

c. Medications. After baseline sample is drawn, glucagon is administered intramuscularly (IM) or subcutaneously (SC) at a dose of 0.03 mg/kg to a maximum of 1 mg.

d. Sampling. For evaluation of GH secretion, serum samples should be obtained at 0, 1, 2, 2$^{1}/_{2}$, and 3 h after administration of glucagon. For other indications for the glucagon tolerance test, different sampling protocols are required.

e. Normal Values. At least one sample with a GH concentration over 10 ng/ml of GH secretion usually occurs between 2 and 3 h after glucagon administration. Be sure to collect the last samples.

f. Specific Considerations. The administration of glucagon causes a temporary increase in serum glucose levels. As part of the rebound process, insulin is oversecreted and serum glucose levels decrease, in turn directing other counterregulatory mechanisms, including GH secretion. Hence, a glucagon tolerance test cannot be used as a stimulus for GH secretion in individuals with a limited ability to secrete insulin.

Young children frequently develop nausea and vomit during the course of this test. Be prepared.

9. IGF-I (Somatomedin C) Generation Test (36–38)

a. Indications. IGF-I is a GH-dependent polypeptide that mediates growth. This procedure evaluates GH function by evaluating its ability to increase serum IGF-I levels. This test is useful for identifying patients with GH resistance.

b. Preparation. No specific preparation is necessary, but an adequate diet must be maintained.

c. Medications. Daily doses (four) of GH (0.1 mg/kg per day) are given IM or SQ. Parents or guardians can administer the additional GH.

d. Sampling. A baseline sample should be obtained before the first GH injection. Additional samples should be obtained 8–16 h after the last injection. Samples on intermediate days are often helpful but are not required.

e. Normal Values. Basal levels consistent with GH deficiency are as follows: (1) less than 50 ng/ml for children less than 5 years of age; (2) less than 100 ng/ml for older children until puberty; (3) less than 100 ng/ml in premenstrual girls or boys with testosterone levels less than 100 ng/ml; and (4) less than 150 ng/ml in girls after the start of menses or in boys with testosterone levels over 100 ng/ml. These levels elimination false negative results but have a high incidence of false positives. Lower levels reduce the false positive incidence at the expense of false negative results.

In response to GH administration, serum levels of IGF-I should triple or increase to more than 250 ng/ml (1 U/ml).

f. General Considerations. The GH should be administered at the same time each day, either in the morning or in the evening. The dose administered is equivalent to the normal daily secretion. There are no reported side effects.

Children who do not respond to GH administration with

an increase in IGF-I levels are not good candidates for GH therapy. When GH was scarce, this test was used to assure that a particular patient would benefit from therapy. Now, this test is not as widely used as in the past, because when the diagnosis of GH deficiency leads to uninterpretable results, children are frequently given a 6 month trial period of GH therapy. However, with the expanding concern for cost containment, this test may be requested more often.

10. Insulin Stimulation Test for GH Secretion (39–41)

a. Specific Indications. This test is generally considered the "gold standard." The mechanism of stimulation is the counterregulatory response to insulin-induced hypoglycemia. Although there are few children with responses classified as false negatives, however, there are many children who have responses classified as false positive. A false positive response is a patient who fails to secrete GH in response to insulin but secretes GH in response to other pharmacologic stimuli. In contrast, a false negative response occurs if a patient secretes GH in response to insulin but does not secrete GH in response to other pharmacologic or physiologic stimuli. False positive responses may be caused by insulin insensitivity, which leads to inadequate hypoglycemia.

The reserve of the adrenal cortex for cortisol secretion can also be confirmed during this protocol. If cortisol reserve is adequate, then at least one sample will have a cortisol level over 20 μg/dl. Thus, the same samples assayed for GH can also be assayed for cortisol to verify the function of the pituitary-adrenal cortex axis.

b. Preparation. Indicate nothing by mouth after midnight. Calibrate and prepare for use a bedside device for rapid serum glucose measurement. Prepare a 50% glucose solution, and fill a 25 ml syringe. (Fill two syringes if the patient is larger than 25 kg.) An intravenous line with 0.25 N saline should be established in small children.

c. Medications. In children over 4 years of age, to start the protocol, 0.1 U/kg of regular insulin should be administered. For younger children, a dose of 0.05 U/kg is usually sufficient.

d. Sampling. Serum samples should be obtained before insulin administration and then 15, 30, 45, and 60 minutes later. Serum glucose levels must be evaluated at the bedside at each time point during the protocol. The pharmacologic stimulus for GH secretion is mediated by serum glucose levels. Hence, glucose levels must decrease by 50% of the initial value or to less than 40 mg/dl. However, more severe hypoglycemia must be avoided because it can lead to seizures, coma, or death.

e. Monitoring and Dangers of Hypoglycemia. At the bedside, each blood sample must be immediately evaluated for serum glucose levels, as you would for a child with diabetes. It is not sufficient to send the sample to the hospital laboratory. If a child develops symptoms of hypoglycemia (blood glucose level less than 40 mg/dl, rapid pulse, sweating, hot, and lethargy) and the signs do not improve by the next scheduled blood sampling, the 50% glucose should be administered (1 ml/kg) from the previously prepared syringes. If this occurs, do not stop collecting serum samples according to the protocol. After the test protocol is complete, either administered the glucose solution (0.5–1.0 g/kg) or require the patient to eat. The patient must be monitored until serum glucose levels return to normal. Water should be provided as requested.

f. Normal and Expected Values. About 20 minutes after the glucose nadir, there should be an episode of GH secretion. The peak level should be above 10 ng/ml. In some patients the response is delayed. Children with GH deficiency have a response of less than 10 ng/ml. In about 20% of children with short stature and severe bone age delay, the pituitary does not secrete GH during this test but secretes GH in response to other tests. The complete physiologic basis for this false positive response is unknown.

g. Special Considerations. Secretion of GH occurs as part of the counterregulatory system for hypoglycemia. For the test to be valid, serum glucose levels must decrease more than 50% from the baseline or to less than 40 mg/dl. If signs of severe hypoglycemia occur, administer glucose but continue to collect serum for GH assay.

Children with GH deficiency frequently have enhanced response to insulin, thus making them more likely to have an episode of severe hypoglycemia. Hence, this test requires the presence of either an experienced nurse or a physician.

Shah et al. (39) recently reported three cases of iatrogenic illness as a result of tolerance tests for GH deficiency (two with insulin and one with glucagon). Two of the three children died as a result of hyperglycemic hyperosmolar coma, perhaps as a result of inappropriate management after the test. Both children who died were shown to have GH deficiency when the serum obtained during the test was analyzed. Examination of the case reports suggests that the coma may have been avoided had immediate, appropriate action (not overreaction) been taken by an attending physician. In each case, analysis of serum samples showed severe hyperglycemia as a consequence of excessive administration of glucose to treat hypoglycemia or rebound hypoglycemia induced by the tolerance test.

11. L-Dopa Stimulation Test for GH Secretion (42)

a. Indications. For the diagnosis of GH deficiency by evaluating a response to pharmacologic stimulation, this test is frequently used as the second test necessary to confirm the diagnosis of GH deficiency.

b. Preparation. Indicate nothing by mouth after midnight on the night before the test.

c. Medications. L-Dopa is given PO immediately after the baseline blood sample is obtained. The dose is as follows: (1) 125 mg for children less than 13.5 kg; (2) 250 mg for children between 13.5 and 31.5 kg; and (3) 500 mg for children over 31.5 kg.

d. Sampling. Draw blood for GH assay at 0, 30, 60, 90, and 120 minutes.

e. Normal Values. At least one serum value should

be above 10 ng/ml. Usually, the samples with high levels of GH are the last samples collected during the protocol.

f. Expected Values. If there is no sample with a concentration of GH greater than 10 ng/ml, then the test is diagnostic for GH deficiency.

g. Special Concerns. Nausea and vomiting frequently occur in toddlers. Be prepared. Do not stop taking blood samples. Children should be recumbent and may be given water throughout the test.

12. Overnight Test for Spontaneous GH Secretion (43,44)

a. Indications. This procedure is used to evaluate spontaneous GH secretion rather than secretion in response to pharmacologic stimulation. This is the diagnostic test necessary for documentation of inadequate spontaneous GH secretion or a neurosecretory defect in GH secretion.

b. Preparation. Patients can be tested in the hospital or at home with the aid of a home care service. In either case, patients should go to bed at the usual time but not later than 11 P.M. A heparin lock can be used to cause the least disturbance in sleep pattern.

c. Medication. No medication needed as part of the tolerance test.

d. Sampling. Serum samples should be obtained every 20 minutes from 8 P.M. to 8 A.M., a total of 37 samples over 12 h.

e. Normal Values. There are two criteria for evaluating the adequacy of overnight GH secretion: (1) mean levels and (2) number and height of episodes of secretion. The mean level is the simple average of the 37 samples collected. This is a representation of the total amount of GH secreted during the 12 h period. The evaluation of normal values is confounded by practical and ethical considerations: IRBs do not permit testing truly normal individuals. With this caveat, most reports suggest a normal lower limit of the mean about 3 ng/ml. Means below this limit probably indicate inadequate physiologic secretion.

The second method of evaluating results is after deconvolution analysis using the Veldhuis and Johnson cluster analysis program. The program permits the evaluation of the number of episodes of secretion and the half-life of serum GH. There should be 6–10 episodes of secretion, with at least four peaks over 10 ng/ml. Fewer peaks of less peak height are consistent with the diagnosis of inadequate spontaneous secretion or neurosecretory defect.

f. Special Concerns. In view of the large number of samples collected and the general limitation of using no more than 5% of total blood volume for laboratory testing in any 2 week period, it is frequently necessary to limit the amount of serum obtained in each sample. Hence, it is necessary to discuss with your laboratory the absolute minimum amounts of blood necessary for each sample. For example, if your laboratory requests 1 ml serum for a GH assay, then each sample collected must have 2 ml whole blood and the total volume collected is about 75 ml. If the patient weighs 10 kg, then total blood volume is only approximately 800 ml and

the amount necessary would represent almost 10% of the total, an unacceptable proportion.

B. Tests for Thyroid Function

1. Calcium-Pentagastrin Test (45,46)

a. Indications. Generally used for the detection of thyroid medullary carcinoma as part of the workup for multiple endocrine neoplasia (MEN) syndrome, in patients with MEN who are at high risk for the disorder, this test should be repeated on a yearly basis to confirm the absence of a new thyroid medullary carcinoma.

b. Preparation. Patients should be fasted after midnight or bedtime snack; water is permitted as desired. The test should be performed in a supine position.

c. Medications. Elemental calcium (2 mg/kg) is infused intravenously over a 1 minute period; pentagastrin (0.5 μg/kg) is administered as a bolus immediately thereafter. The elemental calcium content of some common calcium salts is (1) calcium gluconate, 10%; (2) calcium lactate, 13%; and (3) calcium chloride, 27%.

d. Sampling. Serum samples for calcitonin are obtained at 0, 1, 2, 3, 5, and 10 minutes after administration of both stimulants.

e. Normal Values. Normal values should be established in conjunction with the laboratory.

f. Expected Values. An increase of five times over the baseline level during the test is diagnostic of medullary thyroid carcinoma.

g. General Considerations. The test protocol leads to some minor discomfort. (1) Infusion of calcium may be accompanied by a mild generalized flush or feeling of warmth, the urge to urinate, and a sensation of gastric fullness. These symptoms are self-limited and usually do not last longer than 5 minutes. (2) Pentagastrin may cause some discomfort in the pharynx and substernal and retrosternal areas, a sense of gastric fullness, abdominal cramping and nausea, and dyspepsia. These symptoms also last less than 2 minutes.

It is extremely important to maintain patent, noninfiltrated intravenous access during the calcium infusion; infiltration of calcium into subcutaneous tissue can cause tissue necrosis.

2. Thyroid Suppression Test (47,48)

a. Indications. This test is used in the diagnosis of thyrotoxicosis. Radioiodine uptake by the thyroid gland should be decreased by exogenous thyroid hormone in a properly functioning gland. If uptake continues after treatment with thyroid hormone, then the gland is autonomous and the patient is at risk for thyrotoxicosis.

b. Preparation. Medications that affect thyroid function should be discontinued at least 1 week before the test.

c. Medications. Triiodothyronine (75 μg; Cytomel) PO every day (25 μg PO three times per day) for 7–10 days.

d. Sample. Radioactive iodine uptake studies should be performed before and after treatment.

e. Normal Values. Radioactive iodine uptake in the thyroid should decrease by ≥50% of the initial value. Failure to suppress is indicative of an autonomous gland.

f. General Considerations. No side effects of this test have been reported. However, the test is contraindicated during pregnancy.

3. TRH Test (49,50)

a. Indications. The first generation of assays could only quantitate TSH levels greater than 1 mIU/l. In many cases, however, a TSH test could not discriminate between hyperthyroidism and euthyroidism. In response to thyrotropin-releasing hormone (TRH) TSH is secreted, reaching a maximal level about 5–10 times the basal TSH level. Thus, during a TRH tolerance test in euthyroid individuals, the serum TSH increased into the range that could be detected by the assay methodology even though the basal level could not be detected. In contrast, the TSH levels in individuals with hyperthyroidism remained undetectable or very nearly so. With the new third- and fourth-generation TSH tests, it is possible to evaluate very low levels of TSH, and TRH is not widely used to evaluate hyperthyroidism. At the present time, TRH tolerance tests are used primarily for evaluation of prolactin secretion.

b. Preparation. The patient should be off all thyroid medication and chronic aspirin therapy for at least 1 week before the test.

c. Medication. TRH (7 μg/kg up to a maximum of 400 μg) should be administered intravenously over a 90 s period.

d. Sampling. Samples should be collected before the administration of TRH and at 15 minute intervals for 1 h after treatment. Baseline samples should be assayed for triiodothyronine and thyroxine. All the samples should be assayed for TSH and prolactin.

e. Normal Results. TSH should increase to 5–10 times higher than the basal level. Prolactin levels should increase to 3–5 times over basal levels, with the peak secretion 15–30 minutes after TRH administration.

f. Expected Values. Individuals with hyperthyroidism do not raise their TSH levels into the normal range. High basal prolactin levels without an increase during the tolerance test are suggestive, but not diagnostic, of prolactinoma.

g. General Considerations. TRH may cause an increase in blood pressure and is contraindicated in patients with hypertension or cardiovascular disease.

Because during the infusion of TRH subjects may feel a strong urge to urinate, it is useful to suggest urination before the start of the protocol. Other side effects of TRH infusion are nausea, vomiting, and facial flushing. These effects last only for 30–90 s. Because of the nausea, although not directly required for the test, an overnight fast or omission of the last meal should be considered.

C. Tests for Parathyroid Function

The following protocols were used to evaluate parathyroid function before the availability of RIA tests for parathyroid hormone (PTH). At present, these protocols are occasionally used to detect and evaluate minimal degrees of dysfunction, perhaps associated with partial resistance to PTH or partial protein S deficiency.

1. Ethylenediaminetetraacetic Acid (EDTA) Infusion Test (51,52)

a. Indications. This test is a direct method for detecting disorders of the parathyroid gland, including both hypoparathyroidism and pseudohypoparathyroidism in its different forms. EDTA is a calcium-specific chelating agent. It is metabolized by excretion in urine with its chelated cations, mostly calcium. Thus, the infusion of EDTA leads to a decrease in serum calcium levels, and it is the response to this stimulus that comprises the test. Under the regulation of hormones secreted by the parathyroid gland, normal individuals respond to this stimulus by mobilization of calcium stores and restoration of serum calcium levels within 12 h.

b. Preparation. Patient should fast overnight before the test. Patients should be recumbent for the duration of the test.

c. Medication. Intravenous infusion of 50 mg/kg of trisodium EDTA in 300 ml of 5% dextrose over a 1 h period. To reduce discomfort at the site of infusion, procaine hydrochloride, 1 or 2%, or lidocaine (Xylocaine) should be added to the infusion. Care should be taken to assure that the tubing is primed with the anesthetic before the administration of EDTA.

d. Sampling. Draw blood for calcium immediately before EDTA infusion, immediately after infusion, and at 4, 8, and 12 h after start of the infusion. Serum samples can also be assayed directly for parathyroid hormone and calcitonin to differentiate the basis for the disorder.

e. Normal Values. Preinfusion values of calcium values should be within the normal range for the laboratory. Postinfusion levels should fall immediately by 2–3 mg/dl. The failure of calcium levels to return to preinfusion levels within 12 h after the EDTA infusion is indicative of the lack of proper function of the parathyroid hormone. Further tests may be necessary to identify the exact nature of the disorder.

f. General Considerations. Patients in whom calcium stores may be challenged should be monitored carefully until normal serum calcium levels are restored. Paresthesias of the face and extremities may occur, and patients should be forewarned. Positive Chvostek's and/or Trousseau's signs may be seen at any time in the 24 h period. Patients should be observed carefully for signs of tetany; appropriate measures should be taken should tetany or seizures ensue.

2. Ellsworth-Howard Test (53–55)

a. Indications. The test is used to differentiate between hypoparathyroidism and pseudohypoparathyroidism.

b. Preparation. All supplemental medications used to treat hypoparathyroidism and pseudohypoparathyroidism, such as calcium or vitamin D, should be withheld for 8–12 h before the testing period. Patients should be fasted over the same period.

c. Medications. Over a 15 minute period, PTH, 200–300 IU, is administered intravenously in 50 ml normal saline with 0.5% human serum albumin.

d. Sampling. Collect urine 1 h before PTH infusion and afterward for 5 h. Assay for cyclic AMP.

e. Expected Values. Expected values are listed in Table 3.

D. Tests for Prolactin Secretion

1. *Dopamine Inhibition of Prolactin Secretion (56)*

a. Indications. Dopamine normally inhibits prolactin secretion. Thus, this test is used when hypersecretion of prolactin is suspected.

b. Preparation. On the night before the test, indicate nothing by mouth from midnight or after the bedtime snack.

c. Medication. L-Dopa is given PO immediately after the baseline blood sample is obtained. The dose is as follows: (1) 125 mg for children less than 13.5 kg; (2) 250 mg for children between 13.5 and 31.5 kg; and (3) 500 mg for children over 31.5 kg.

d. Sampling. Draw blood for prolactin assay at 0, 40, 60, 90, 120, and 180 minutes after administration of L-Dopa. In view of the method of evaluation of the result, two baseline samples should be obtained, one 15 minutes before and the second just before the administration of L-Dopa.

e. Normal Values. Prolactin levels should decrease to less than 50% of the baseline value within 1–3 h. Lack of suppression suggests autonomous or hypersecretion of prolactin.

f. General Considerations. Nausea and vomiting frequently occur in toddlers. Be prepared. Do not stop taking blood samples. Children should be recumbent and may be given water throughout the test.

Table 3 Expected cAMP Values After PTH Infusion

Diagnosis	Cyclic AMP after PTH infusion (μmol)
Normal adults	3.90 ± 0.35
Pseudohypoparathyroidism	0.63 ± 0.12
Idiopathic hypoparathyroidism	4.43 ± 0.54
Pseudo-pseudohypoparathyroidism	2.98 ± 0.49

2. *TRH-Induced Prolactin Secretion (57)*

a. Indications. This test is often used for the confirmation of abnormalities of prolactin secretion. Although the mechanism is unknown, TRH stimulates prolactin secretion.

b. Preparation. The patient should be off all thyroid medication and chronic aspirin therapy for at least 1 week before the test. For their own comfort, patients should be requested to urinate before the start of the test.

c. Medication. After collection of a baseline sample, TRH (7 μg/kg up to a maximum of 400 μg) should be administered intravenously over a 90 s period.

d. Sampling. Serum should be collected every 15 minutes for 1 h after administration of TRH. The samples should be assayed for prolactin.

e. Normal Values. In children, prolactin levels should increase three- to fivefold during the test. The peak usually occurs at 15 or 30 minutes. Men have a similar response. In women, the increase can be somewhat larger.

f. General Considerations. TRH may cause an increase in blood pressure and is contraindicated in patients with hypertension or cardiovascular disease.

Because during the infusion of TRH subjects may feel a strong urge to urinate, it is useful to suggest urination before the start of the protocol. Other side effects of TRH infusion are nausea, vomiting, and facial flushing. These effects last only for 30–90 s. Because of the nausea, although not directly required for the test, an overnight fast or omission of the last meal should be considered.

E. Tolerance Tests for Adrenal Cortex Function

1. *Basic Physiology of Adrenal Cortex Function*

ACTH has two major effects on the adrenal cortex: (1) it serves as a growth factor, and (2) it stimulates the secretion of steroids. Within 15 minutes of an endogenous or exogenous episode of ACTH secretion, the adrenal cortex secretes cortisol in large amounts and smaller amounts of androgens and intermediates. Within the adrenal, the blood flow pattern is from the cortex through the medulla. In the medulla, the high levels of cortisol stimulate the conversion of norepinephrine to epinephrine. The cortex is divided into three intertwined layers: (1) the outermost layer, the glomerulosa, secretes mineralocorticoids primarily under the regulatory influence of angiotensin; (2) the middle layer, the fasciculata, secretes cortisol; and (3) the inner layer, the reticularis, secretes androgens. At the time of biochemical adrenarche, the reticularis increases the production of DHEA, but the serum level of DHEA-S is not increased during an ACTH stimulatory episode. Tolerance testing for the adrenal cortex primarily involves testing for the adequacy of cortisol production and for excessive production of either (1) intermediates of cortisol production or (2) adrenal androgens other than DHEA-S.

Despite that evaluating the adequacy of cortisol production is one of the main purposes of ACTH tolerance testing, direct assay of cortisol is often not sufficient. Typically, as part of an attempt to rule out glucocorticoid insufficiency, perhaps caused by a steroid biosynthetic defect, a physician requests serum cortisol levels, but every cortisol assay that I have tested does not completely discriminate 21-deoxycortisol from cortisol. Individuals with 21-hydroxylase deficiency produce excessive amounts of 21-deoxycortisol, thus often contributing to apparently normal levels of cortisol. Only by the simultaneous evaluation of 17-hydroxyprogesterone levels can the diagnosis of 21-hydroxylase deficiency be eliminated or confirmed.

Following are specific protocols to evaluate different aspects of adrenal function.

2. *Dexamethasone Suppression Test (Overnight) (58)*

a. Indications. This test is a screening test for Cushing syndrome or excessive cortisol and/or androgen production. In women or girls with hirsutism, it can also be used to differentiate between the ovary and the adrenal as the source of excess androgen production. If the source of excess androgen production is the ovary or autonomous adrenal function, then androgen levels are not suppressed by overnight dexamethasone.

b. Preparation. No specific preparation is needed. The test need not be performed in the hospital. Dexamethasone can be provided to the parent and administered at the proper time at home and the child brought for serum collection the following morning.

c. Medication. For children larger than 25 kg, prescribe 1 mg dexamethasone at bedtime. For children smaller than 25 kg, administer 0.5 mg dexamethasone at bedtime.

d. Samples. A single serum sample is obtained between 8 and 9 A.M.

e. Normal Values. The morning serum cortisol level should be less than 2 μg/dl. In our experience, of almost 200 tests evaluated in our laboratory, only 5 had serum levels between 2 and 3 μg/dl: a boy who was highly stressed because of a car accident on the way to the hospital and 4 women who were taking oral contraceptives.

f. Expected Values. In the absence of extenuating circumstances, serum cortisol levels in excess of 2 μg/dl are abnormal and a physiologic basis should be explored. Children with Cushing syndrome may have cortisol levels after dexamethasone suppression of as little as 4 μg/dl in the early course, and this level should slowly increase under the continuing ACTH-induced hyperplasia.

g. General Considerations. Most texts and review articles suggest cutoff values of 5–10 μg/dl. However, these values were obtained with chemical tests for cortisol that were less specific then the RIAs now used. The use of 2 μg/dl (more than 2.5 standard deviations above the mean) might result in a few more false positive results, but it leads to fewer false negatives, which is the real purpose of a screening test.

Dexamethasone suppresses ACTH secretion and therefore prevents its function as a growth factor for the adrenal cortex. Repeated administration leads to inadequate adrenal reserves.

3. *Dexamethasone Suppression Test (High Dose) (59,60)*

a. Indications. This test is used to define further the control of cortisol secretion for individuals who do not have adequate suppression with the overnight dexamethasone test.

b. Preparation for Part 1. No specific preparation is needed.

c. Medication for Part 1. Dexamethasone, 20 μg/kg per day, to a maximum of 0.5 mg/dose, is given PO every 6 h for 2 days beginning on day 3 of the test. Older children and adults may be given 0.5 mg every 6 h for eight doses.

d. Sampling for Part 1. The 24 h urine collections are started on day 1. Each urine sample should be assayed for 17-ketogenic steroids, urinary free cortisol, and creatinine. Serum should be collected each morning and assayed for DHEA-S and cortisol.

e. Normal Values for Part 1. The 17-ketogenic steroids should fall to $\leq$7 mg/day ($\leq$3 mg/g creatinine) by the day of the test. Urinary free cortisol should suppress by more than 50% in normal subjects.

f. General Considerations for Part 1. Food and water should be available as desired throughout the test period. The test can be done on an outpatient basis. Patients who do not suppress the urinary free cortisol levels should be tested with high doses of dexamethasone, part 2 of the protocol. In general, if the results have not been returned from the laboratory or are ambiguous, part 2 of the protocol should be performed immediately.

g. Preparation for Part 2. Part 2 should be performed immediately after completion of part 1 as days 5 and 6 of the combined protocol.

h. Medication for Part 2. Dexamethasone, 2 mg/dose, is given PO every 6 h for 2 days beginning on day 5 of test.

i. Sampling for Part 2. The 24 h urine samples are collected on days 5 and 6. Each urine sample should be assayed for 17-ketogenic steroids, urinary free cortisol, and creatinine. Serum should be collected each morning and assayed for DHEA-S and cortisol.

j. Normal Values for Part 2. The 17-ketogenic steroids and urinary free cortisol should suppress by more than 50% even in subjects with adrenal hyperplasia or Cushing syndrome. In patients in whom they are not suppressed during part 2 of the protocol, the presence of an independent, steroid-producing tumor must be explored.

4. *ACTH Stimulation Test (61–64)*

a. Indications. This protocol is used to evaluate the adequacy of cortisol secretion and adrenal reserve, primarily to eliminate a diagnosis of Addison's disease or congenital ACTH unresponsiveness.

b. Preparation. The patient should be off medications that interfere with ACTH secretion, especially high-dose glucocorticoids or other steroids. High-dose steroids must be discontinued for at least 1 week to permit restoration of the normal biosynthetic reserve. *Be aware*: a dose considered a low dose by an immunologist or neonatologist is considered a high dose by an endocrinologist.

c. Medications. In the morning, after collection of baseline serum samples, a single intravenous bolus of 0.25 mg Cortrosyn is administered.

d. Sampling. Before the administration of Cortrosyn, a baseline sample is obtained. An additional sample is collected 30 minutes after administration of Cortrosyn. Each sample is assayed for cortisol, 17-hydroxyprogesterone, progesterone, and 17-hydroxypregnenolone. The exact interval between the administration of ACTH and the second sample must be noted.

e. Normal and Expected Values. Cortisol levels should exceed 16 μg/dl in either the baseline or post-ACTH sample; levels of less than 4 μg/dl are indicative of inadequate secretion. Cortisol levels may not be decreased in individuals with 21-hydroxylase deficiency.

For evaluation of 21-hydroxylase deficiency, the sum of the increase in progesterone and 17-hydroxyprogesterone concentration is divided by the time between the samples. If the increase is more than 7 ng/ml/h, then the test is considered indicative of 21-hydroxylase deficiency; increases above 4 ng/ml/h are typical of heterozygotes for 21-hydroxylase deficiency. However, endogenous episodes of ACTH secretion can confound the interpretation.

For evaluation of 3β-hydroxysteroid dehydrogenase deficiency, the ratio of 17-hydroxypregnenolone to 17-hydroxyprogesterone levels is considered. Normal individuals have a ratio of less than 10, and higher ratios are considered diagnostic.

f. General Considerations. However, because of (1) the variable timing of the morning endogenous ACTH secretory episodes and (2) the secretion of ACTH when a child is frightened, the baseline values are often already stimulated.

5. Dexamethasone-Suppressed ACTH Stimulation Test (65–67)

a. Indications. This protocol differs from the simple ACTH stimulation test by the administration of a single dose of dexamethasone at bedtime before the test. This step serves to block the normal morning episodes of ACTH secretion and eliminates the ongoing secretion of cortisol and its intermediates. As a consequence, before the administration of ACTH, the adrenal cortex synthesizes and secretes only small amounts of steroids. Without the dexamethasone treatment, the fear of doctors experienced by many children leads to immediate ACTH secretion and thus to high levels of steroids in the baseline samples. In fact, on many occasions, the baseline samples have higher levels of steroids than the samples obtained after ACTH administration. In contrast, after dexamethasone pretreatment, the presence of steroids in the baseline samples can be attributed either to gonadal secretion or to ACTH-independent pathways. The protocol is used to confirm a suspected diagnosis of complete or partial steroid biosynthetic defects. The phenotype

characteristic of heterozygote carriers for 21-hydroxylase deficiency can also be identified. The dexamethasone-pretreated protocol was specifically developed to overcome the variation in baseline steroid intermediate levels caused by uncontrolled endogenous episodes of ACTH secretion.

b. Preparation. A single dose of dexamethasone (0.5 mg/m^2) is administered just before the subject goes to bed, usually between 10 and 11 P.M. Patients should be fasted from the time of dexamethasone treatment until the completion of the test. Water may be consumed as desired. Menstruating women should be tested in the follicular phase of the cycle.

c. Medications. In the morning, after collection of baseline serum samples, a single intravenous bolus of 0.25 mg Cortrosyn is administered.

d. Sampling. Before the administration of Cortrosyn, two baseline samples are obtained 15 minutes apart. Additional samples are collected 30, 45, and 60 minutes after the administration of Cortrosyn.

e. Normal and Expected Values. The test is evaluated by considering the difference in steroid levels between the baseline and stimulated samples. The baseline level is obtained by averaging the two baseline samples; the stimulated level is the average of the two highest samples obtained after Cortrosyn administration. It should be noted that as a consequence of the continued function of the long-acting synthetic glucocorticoid, the morning episodes of ACTH secretion do not occur. Thus, baseline levels of steroid intermediates are not elevated.

Expected values are listed in Table 4.

f. General Considerations. Girls (but not boys) with idiopathic, premature adrenarche frequently have response phenotypes similar to those of carriers for 21-hydroxylase deficiency. It is not clear whether the genotype is also similar to that in carriers for 21-hydroxylase deficiency. About 15% of girls with features of hyperandrogenism have steroid secretory patterns typical of nonclassic 21-hydroxylase or 3β-hydroxysteroid dehydrogenase deficiency. When older populations are tested, the frequency of deficiency syndromes decreases, perhaps because of prior identification of severely affected individuals.

After dexamethasone suppression, there are four common causes of elevated baseline levels of cortisol, androgens, or steroid intermediates: (1) the subject did not take the dexamethasone, (2) breakthrough ACTH secretion, (3) gonadal secretion of steroids, and (4) lack of regulatory control, perhaps caused by Cushing syndrome. If the subject does not take the dexamethasone, the baseline samples are frequently similar to stimulated values. Breakthrough ACTH secretion was recognized in 1 of 200 tests. In this case, the subject had driven himself to the hospital for the test and had been involved in a significant traffic accident. Ovarian secretion of 17-hydroxyprogesterone, DHEA, and androstenedione is most common in patients with polycystic ovarian disorder or during the luteal phase of the menstrual cycle. The source of excess steroids in the baseline samples can be attributed to the ovary if the cortisol level is less than 2 μg/dl or less than 5 μg/dl if a woman is taking birth control pills. Finally, with

Table 4 Expected Steroid Values

Steroid	Baseline levels	Stimulated levels
Normal individuals		
Cortisol, μg/dl	≤2	12– 24
17-Hydroxyprogesterone, ng/dl	≤50	50– 150
Androstenedione, ng/dl	≤50	50– 200
Dehydroepiandrosterone, ng/dl	≤200	400– 800
Heterozygote (carriers) for 21-hydroxylase deficiency		
Cortisol, μg/dl	≤2	12– 24
17-Hydroxyprogesterone, ng/dl	≤50	150– 500
Androstenedione, ng/dl	≤50	50– 200
Dehydroepiandrosterone, ng/dl	≤200	900–1300
Individuals with 21-hydroxylase deficiency		
Cortisol, μg/dl	≤2	12– 24
17-Hydroxyprogesterone, ng/dl		≥2000
Androstenedione, ng/dl	≤50	50– 200
Dehydroepiandrosterone, ng/dl	≤200	900–1300
Individuals with 3β-hydroxysteroid dehydrogenase deficiency		
Cortisol, μg/dl	≤2	12– 24
17-Hydroxyprogesterone, ng/dl	≤50	150– 500
Androstenedione, ng/dl	≤50	50– 200
Dehydroepiandrosterone, ng/dl	≤400	1600–8000

the exceptions noted, baseline cortisol levels in excess of 2 μg/dl are suggestive of Cushing syndrome. Thus, the addition of dexamethasone pretreatment the night before the administration of ACTH increases the discrimination of the entire Cortrosyn tolerance test procedure.

6. Metyrapone Test (68–70)

a. Indications. Metyrapone blocks the conversion of compound S (11-desoxycortisol or cortexolone) to cortisol. The test is used to assess: (1) pituitary ACTH reserve, (2) adrenal insufficiency, and (3) the extent of adrenal suppression for patients on prolonged glucocorticoid therapy for any reason.

b. Warning. With patients in whom adrenal insufficiency (Addison's disease) is suspected, an appropriate steroid medication should be kept at bedside in case of an adverse reaction. Addison's disease was first recognized in a patient with tuberculosis, and with the current epidemic of drug-resistant tuberculosis, this may become a more common problem.

c. Preparation. The patient should be off all medications that interfere with ACTH production, including (1) glucocorticoids, (2) drugs that accelerate the action of metyrapone, such as diphenylhydantoin, and (3) drugs that alter the concentration of 17-ketogenic steroids, such as penicillin and its variants.

d. Medication and Sampling: 24 h Test. Metyrapone, 300 mg/m^2 in children or 750 mg in adults, is orally administered every 4 h for six doses. Basal 24 h urine should be collected before the administration of metyrapone and for the next 3 days. The urine is assayed for creatinine and for 17-ketogenic steroids. Serum should be obtained 4 h after the last dose of metyrapone and assayed for ACTH, cortisol, and compound S.

e. Normal Values: 24 h Test. In normal individuals, 17-ketogenic steroids should double during the metyrapone treatment. Plasma cortisol levels should be less than 8 μg/dl, and compound S levels should exceed 10 μg/dl.

f. Medication and Sampling: Single-Dose Test. Metyrapone, 30 mg/kg to a maximum of 1 g, is administered as a single oral dose at midnight. Serum should be obtained at 8 A.M. and assayed for ACTH, cortisol, and compound S.

g. Normal Values: Single-Dose Test. The results of the test should be considered in the following order: (1) ACTH levels should be elevated. Inadequate ACTH secretion suggests inadequate pituitary reserve for secretion of ACTH. (2) Cortisol levels should be less than 8 μg/dl. Higher levels suggest inadequate therapy (rapid metabolism) or excessive production of cortisol, perhaps caused by Cushing syndrome. (3) Compound S levels should exceed 10 μg/dl. Lower levels suggest adrenal insufficiency, caused by either lack of recovery from high-dose therapy or Addison's disease.

h. General Considerations. Hypotension and vomiting may occur during the administration of metyrapone. Transient vertigo may be avoided by administering the drug with milk or a meal. Activity should be mild throughout the day of drug treatment.

F. Tests for Pheochromocytoma

This diagnosis is frequently suspected but is actually very rare in children. In this disorder, catecholamine secretion from the adrenal medulla no longer responds to proper hormonal regulation.

1. Clonidine Suppression Test (71,72)

a. Indications. Clonidine suppresses catecholamines arising from the sympathetic neuroendocrine system but not from a pheochromocytoma.

b. Preparation. Indicate nothing by mouth after midnight or for 10–12 h before the test. β-Adrenergic blocking drugs should be discontinued 48 h before the test; concomitant administration of these drugs can lead to severe bradycardia and decreased cardiac output. Adequate hydration must be maintained (or restored) before the test because of the possibility of potentiation of hypovolemia.

c. Medication. Clonidine, 0.005 mg/kg to a maximum of 0.25 mg, is administered as a single oral dose.

d. Sampling. Draw blood for free catecholamines (epinephrine and norepinephrine) at 0, 1, 2, and 3 h after clonidine administration.

e. Normal Values. By 3 h after clonidine treatment,

circulating catecholamines should decrease to less than 500 pg/ml. Failure to suppress the circulating levels is usually diagnostic of pheochromocytoma.

f. General Considerations. Because of the hypotensive effects of clonidine, blood pressure should be monitored during the protocol and the patient should be in a supine position. Patients may become very drowsy about 30–45 minutes after clonidine administration. Various clinical laboratories have different instructions for the handling of blood plasma for catecholamine assay. Hence it is necessary to identify the specific laboratory you intend to use and their specific protocol.

2. Glucagon Test (73)

a. Preparation. The patient should rest quietly in a supine position without environmental stress or distraction. A heparin lock should be established at least 30 minutes before the start of the test.

b. Medication. After collection of baseline blood pressure data and serum, the test is started by the intravenous administration of 0.5 mg glucagon.

c. Sampling. Blood pressure should be determined at –10, –5, 0, 5, 10, 20, 25, and 30 minutes after glucagon treatment. Plasma should be collected for catecholamine levels at 0, 5, and 10 minutes after glucagon administration.

d. Normal Values. In normal patients, there should not be a rise in blood pressure. If a 0.5 mg dose of glucagon does not produce a rise in blood pressure, the test can be repeated with 1 mg glucagon administered as an intravenous bolus. A significant elevation in blood pressure and catecholamines for 5–15 minutes after glucagon administration is indicative of pheochromocytoma.

e. General Considerations. Patients must be supine throughout the test period. A darkened room without disturbance is often helpful. Various clinical laboratories have different instructions for the handling of blood plasma for catecholamine assay. Hence it is necessary to identify the specific laboratory you intend to use and their specific protocol.

G. Test for Acromegaly: Glucose Test for Suppression of GH Secretion (74)

a. Indications. GH is normally secreted episodically, only a few episodes occurring during the day. However, some individuals develop autonomous continuous secretion from the pituitary, either from an adenoma or from a GHRH-secreting tumor in some other location. In normal individuals, high serum glucose levels block GH secretion. Thus, the administration of glucose should cause a decrease in serum GH levels and confirm that GH secretion is not autonomous. The inability of GH levels to be suppressed by high serum glucose levels is indicative of GH excess, including acromegaly. It should be noted that young infants and diabetics in poor control often have paradoxic GH secretion.

b. Preparation. Overnight fast is prescribed before the test.

c. Medication. After collection of a baseline serum sample, glucose, 1.75 g/kg body weight to a maximum of 75 g, is given by mouth (Glucola, Trutol, or Dextol Cola is commonly used).

d. Sampling. Serum should be obtained for glucose and GH at the time of glucose administration and every 30 minutes for 2 h.

e. Normal Values. GH levels should decrease to less than 5 ng/ml. GH levels above 10 ng/ml confirm a diagnosis of GH excess. Values between 5 and 10 ng/ml are inconclusive.

f. General Considerations. As desired, patients can drink water and walk during the protocol.

H. Tests for Regulation of Serum Glucose Levels

1. Glucose Tolerance Tests (75,76)

a. Indications. This test is useful for the evaluation of impaired glucose tolerance and insulin resistance or hypersensitivity. The test must include insulin levels to make an accurate diagnosis. Fasting blood sugars must be less than 140 mg/dl. The intravenous protocol should be used in patients who have gastrointestinal disturbances and cannot tolerate an oral glucose load. The intravenous protocol may also be preferred when assessing insulin secretion because the direct stimulus is not dependent on the absorption of glucose in the gastrointestinal tract.

b. Preparation. For 3 days before the test, patients should be on a high-carbohydrate diet with at least 60% of calories as carbohydrates. Patients should be fasted after midnight or after a bedtime snack the night before the test. Medications that may act as hyper- or hypoglycemic agents should be discontinued.

c. Medication: Oral Protocol. After the baseline serum sample is obtained, glucose solution, 1.75 g/kg body weight to a maximum of 75 g, is administered as an oral solution. Trutol, Glucola, and Dextol Cola are commonly used commercial solutions.

d. Sampling: Oral Protocol. Draw blood for glucose and insulin at 0, 1/2, 1, 1 1/2, 2, 3, and 4 h after glucose administration. Urine is measured for sugar and acetone at each void throughout the protocol.

e. Normal Values: Oral Protocol. Peak response should not exceed 200 mg/dl (Table 5). Higher levels suggest

Table 5 Normal Peak Glucose Response

Time (h)	Glucose (mg/dl)	Insulin 2–6 years	(μU/ml) 6–11 years
0	≤110	8	15
1	≤160	40	60
2	≤140	35	55
3	≤130	18	20

impaired glucose tolerance. Serum glucose levels within the normal range but glucose present in the urine suggests a low renal threshold for glucose.

f. Expected Values: Oral Protocol. In 1979, the National Diabetes Data Group (NDDG) established criteria to evaluate the results of oral glucose tolerance tests in children and adults suspected of having diabetes. The NDDG criteria for normal glucose tolerance are as follows (all three criteria must be satisfied):

1. Fasting plasma glucose < 115 mg/dl
2. A 2 h plasma glucose < 140 mg/dl
3. $1/2$, 1, and $1^1/2$ h plasma glucose < 200 mg/dl

The glucose tolerance results diagnostic for diabetes are as follows:

1. Symptoms and unequivocal hyperglycemia (>200 mg/dl) on 2 separate days
2. Fasting plasma glucose > 140 mg/dl
3. A 2 h plasma glucose over 200 mg/dl and $1/2$, 1, or $1^1/2$ plasma glucose < 200 mg/dl

Any one one of these three criteria must be satisfied. Impaired glucose tolerance by NDDG criteria is as follows (all three criteria must be satisfied):

1. Fasting plasma glucose < 140 mg/dl
2. The 2 h plasma glucose between 140 and 200 mg/dl
3. A $1/2$, 1, or $1^1/2$ h plasma glucose > 200 mg/dl

Indeterminate glucose tolerance by NDDG criteria is any pattern not fulfilling any of the other criteria.

g. Medication: Intravenous Protocol. After the baseline serum sample is obtained, glucose, 0.5 g/kg body weight, is given as an intravenous bolus over a 3–4 minute period. It is preferable to have two separate intravenous lines, one for infusion of glucose and one for obtaining blood samples. The first line may be discontinued after the infusion is complete.

h. Sampling: Intravenous Protocol. Draw blood for glucose and insulin at 0, 1, 3, 5, 10, 20, 30, 45, and 60 minutes after the start of the glucose infusion.

i. Normal Values: Intravenous Protocol. For quantitative evaluation of the first-phase insulin response (FPIR), the parameter used is the sum of plasma insulin values for 1 and 3 minutes [designated insulin $\Sigma(1' + 3')$]. Normal values for individuals over 8 years of age are insulin $\Sigma(1' + 3') > 100$ μU/ml. Normal values for individuals between 3 and 8 years of age are insulin $\Sigma(1' + 3') > 60$ μU/ml. Individuals at high risk for developing diabetes have a low FPIR.

The disappearance curve of glucose is plotted as a function of time on semilogarithmic paper and the K value (glucose disappearance rate) determined.

$$K = \frac{0.693 \times 100}{T_{1/2}}$$

where $T_{1/2}$ is time in minutes for the glucose to fall to half of its initial value.

A K value of less than 1.4 indicates impaired glucose

tolerance in persons less than 50 years of age. Insulin levels should reach their peak within 10 minutes of the start of the infusion.

j. General Considerations. Patients may drink water and move about freely during the test. The test should be postponed until 2 weeks after any acute illness. There is a risk of hyperosmolality in patients with elevated baseline blood glucose levels.

2. *Hypoglycemia Workup (77–79)*

a. Indications. The following plan is valuable when evaluating hypoglycemia in children. Hyperinsulinemia, glycogen storage disease, factitious hypoglycemia, carnitine deficiency, fatty acid oxidation disturbance, and inborn errors of metabolism are indications for the use of this workup. The protocol evaluates metabolic changes that occur during a fast.

b. Preparation. The test should be conducted under close supervision. For younger children, maintain a separate intravenous line with 0.25 N saline, in addition to the heparin lock, both for hydration, if necessary, and to ensure a patent venous line other than the heparin lock.

The patient should be on a high-carbohydrate diet (60% of calories from carbohydrates) for 3 days. The diet should include frequent feedings.

No high-fat foods should be allowed on the evening before the start of the test, and the patient should be fasted after midnight or bedtime snack.

Test and prepare for use a device to measure glucose (Dextrostix, Chemstrip bG, or equivalent).

In anticipation of hypoglycemia, have at hand syringes prepared with (1) glucagon, 30 μg/kg, and (2) 50% glucose, 1 ml/kg body weight.

c. Medications. Administer glucagon, 30 μg/kg to a maximum of 1 mg, for two individual glucagon tolerance measurements. Glucagon is administered by slow intravenous push after baseline samples are drawn.

d. Sampling: Part 1. Approximately 4 h after fast is begun, collect baseline blood sample and administer the first glucagon challenge. The baseline serum should be assayed for glucose at bedside and the hypoglycemia panel (insulin, GH, cortisol, venous blood gases, phosphorus, uric acid, lactate, alanine, ketones, β-hydroxybutyrate, free fatty acids, carnitine, and glucagon).

At 5, 15, 30, and 60 minutes after glucagon administration, draw blood for glucose and insulin.

e. Sampling: Part 2. All urine is collected and evaluated for ketones and specific gravity. Every 2 h blood should be collected and assayed for glucose at bedside. Every 4 h blood should be collected and assayed for glucose at bedside and hypoglycemia panel.

f. Sampling: Part 3. If blood glucose at any time is less than 40 mg/dl in whole blood (or less than 45 mg/dl in serum or plasma) with or without symptoms, then confirm with laboratory glucose measurement and assay for the hypoglycemia panel. Repeat the glucagon tolerance test as described in part 1. Terminate the test with a 50% glucose solution, 1 ml/kg as an intravenous push.

If severe symptomatic hypoglycemia and/or convulsions occur at any point, collect the serum sample and terminate the fast at once by administering the 50% glucose solution, 1 ml/kg. The serum should be assayed for the hypoglycemia panel and electrolytes.

If no hypoglycemia occurs within 24 h of the first glucagon test, perform a second glucagon tolerance test and terminate the protocol.

If no hypoglycemia occurs but the patient develops metabolic acidosis (HCO_3 less than 15 mEq/L, with or without normal pH), repeat the glucagon tolerance test and terminate immediately.

g. Sampling: Part 4. After the fast, you may consider the following additional tolerance tests needed for further evaluation of defective gluconeogenesis: 0.5 g/kg of alanine, 1.0 g/kg of glycerol, and 1.0 g/kg of fructose. In each case blood should be collected at 0, 15, 30, 45, 60, and 120 minutes after administration and assayed for glucose, serum ketones, lactic acid, and β-hydroxybutyrate.

h. Normal Values. Glucose levels should remain above 40 mg/dl throughout the 24 h fast. Episodes of hypoglycemia are considered abnormal at any time throughout the test, whether or not there are symptoms.

Episodes of GH secretion greater than 10 ng/ml should follow about 20 minutes after any hypoglycemic episodes.

Cortisol levels of 8–20 μg/dl are normal under nonstressful conditions. Under the conditions of this fast, levels should increase by 10 μg/dl or exceed 20 μg/dl.

In samples obtained during hypoglycemic episodes, low glucose-insulin ratios (ratio of 3 versus ratio of 6 as observed in normal individuals) are indicative of hyperinsulinism. The concentration of metabolites must be considered to evaluate the pathophysiology of hypoglycemia in other patients.

i. General Consideration. Only children over 4 years of age should be submitted to the full 24 h fast protocol. Patients must remain quiet but can sit in a chair or lie down as they desire. They can drink water and use the bathroom freely. The intravenous infusion rate should be adjusted according to water intake. Parents should be encouraged to remain with the child, if this will lower stress.

Glucagon may cause some mild abdominal discomfort and/or nausea. Hence, it should be administered by slow intravenous push. Patient should be checked frequently for vital signs and symptoms of hypoglycemia, including convulsions, stupor, tremors, coma, decreased blood pressure, or thready pulse. A flow sheet should be maintained and all data recorded as rapidly as possible.

I. Tests for Gonadal Function

1. Acute Response to hCG Administration (80,81)

a. Indications. This protocol is useful to confirm the diagnosis of nonclassic 17-ketosteroid reductase deficiency, typically in a teenage boy with severe gynecomastia.

b. Preparation. The test should be performed in the morning. Patients should eat a normal breakfast and can continue to eat and drink as desired and as appropriate.

c. Medications. At bedtime at home, the patient should take 1 mg dexamethasone. In the morning (about 9 A.M.), the patient should receive 4000 IU hCG as an intramuscular injection.

d. Samples. Serum samples should be obtained before the administration of hCG and 2, 4, 6, 24, and 48 h later.

e. Normal Values. In normal males, the testosterone-androstenedione ratio increases in response to hCG. The final testosterone levels should exceed 300 ng/dl, which are adult normal levels. In patients with partial 17-ketosteroid reductase deficiency, the sum of testosterone and androstenedione concentrations equals the adult normal levels, but the ratio is about equal rather than in excess of 4:1.

f. General Considerations. The two major sources of androstenedione are the adrenal and the testis. Administration of dexamethasone serves to eliminate secretion from the adrenal and thus permits monitoring of testicular synthesis.

Compared with testosterone, androstenedione is the preferred substrate for aromatization. Thus, the excess production of androstenedione leads to excess production of estrogens and the development of gynecomastia. Many boys at puberty develop mild gynecomastia that disappears as testosterone production increases. In normal individuals, the 17-ketosteroid dehydrogenase is substrate (androstenedione) and product (testosterone) activated, thus leading to complete conversion of androstenedione to testosterone. However, the enzyme of some individuals does not have the proper kinetic properties and does not fully convert all androstenedione to testosterone. The incomplete deficiency disorder is inherited as an autosomal recessive trait. This test helps to identify these patients.

2. Tonic Response to hCG Administration (82,83)

a. Indications. This test is used to aid in the diagnosis of vanishing testis syndrome, disorders of steroidogenesis, micropenis, ambiguous genitalia, or other circumstances in which there is a question about normal testicular function.

b. Preparation. No specific preparation is needed.

c. Medication. Four daily doses of hCG (5000 IU/m^2 per dose) are administered as IM injections. Alternative protocols use only 3000 IU/m^2 every day or every other day.

d. Samples. A baseline serum sample and a stimulated sample obtained 24 h after the last dose of hCG should be assayed for testosterone and androstenedione.

e. Normal Values. Testosterone should increase to normal adult levels or greater than 300 ng/dl. Androstenedione should not exceed one-quarter of the observed testosterone level.

f. General Considerations. Prolonged administration of hCG can lead to bone age advancement. Progesterone or other intermediates can be assayed if the testosterone response is inadequate.

3.   Gonadotropin Sleep Study (84,85)

a. Indications. This test is useful in suspected polycystic ovarian disease and in suspected precocious puberty.

b. Preparation and Medication. None are needed.

c. Sampling. Sample serum for LH and FSH from the heparin lock every 20 minutes, overnight for up to 12 h. In small children for whom the amount of blood drawn may be a critical factor, the test may be modified by limiting the period of sample collection and increasing the interval to 30 minutes.

d. Normal Values. Normal, prepubertal children have no nocturnal episodes of gonadotropin secretion.

e. General Considerations. There are no side effects of this protocol.

4.   GnRH (Factrel) Response Test (86–90)

a. Indications. The response to the administration of gonadotropin-releasing hormone is useful for evaluating the role of pituitary dysfunction in children with premature or delayed puberty. Tolerance test responses can be used to distinguish central nervous system dysfunction from peripheral dysfunction in both premature and delayed puberty. In children with premature puberty, peripheral dysfunction (testotoxicosis, McCune-Albright syndrome, and ovarian follicular cysts) is frequently associated with hypogonadotropinism, whereas hypergonadotropinism can be caused by central nervous system dysfunction (hamartoma or craniopharyngioma). In contrast, in children with delayed puberty, peripheral dysfunction is associated with hypergonadotropinism (Turner syndrome) and hypogonadotropinism suggests dysfunction in the central nervous system (Kalmann syndrome, Prader-Willi syndrome, and constitutional delay). The test is also useful in evaluating the extent of damage caused by radiation or chemotherapy in children with leukemia or brain tumors. In this group, the results can indicate the need for endocrine replacement therapy.

b. Preparation. Although not required, many physicians request that (1) the patient should be fasted overnight before the test and (2) the test should be performed in the morning. Certainly, there is time-of-day variation in the secretory pattern for LH and FSH, and most of the normal data have been collected in this manner. Thus, using the same protocol eases comparison of results to previous studies.

c. Medications. Administer an intravenous bolus dose of 10 μg GnRH (Factrel, Ayerst Laboratories, New York, NY).

d. Sampling. Baseline samples ($n = 2$) should be obtained 15 minutes apart before the administration of the GnRH. Stimulated samples should be obtained 15, 30, 45, 60, and 90 minutes after treatment. For comparison with published values, the baseline samples and the three highest stimulated samples should be averaged. This protocol minimizes slight variations in secretory pattern and in laboratory values.

e. Normal Values. The response pattern changes with age, sex, and development. After 6 months of age and before puberty, basal levels for both LH and FSH are frequently less than 2 IU/L. Stimulated levels less than 5 IU/L are indicative of hypogonadotropinism, and levels in excess of 50 IU/L are indicative of hypergonadotropinism. With a few exceptions, the increase in both gonadotropins should be similar in magnitude. Girls within a year of menarche often have FSH levels about twice those of LH. Individuals with mild or partial steroid biosynthetic defects often have higher LH than FSH levels.

FSH and LH are both glycoproteins and thus are very subject to microheterogeneity; as a consequence, there is significant intermethod variability. Microbioassay methods have been developed to attempt to determine the amount of functional hormone present, but these methods are expensive and time consuming. Although bioassay results are useful in studying the mechanisms and regulation of pubertal development, generally they do not yet aid diagnosis because of an inadequate understanding of expected results for normal children.

f. General Considerations. Patients need not remain seated but can walk about during the test. There are many units for LH and FSH. Be sure to check that the units reported by the laboratory are the same units used for reporting normal values.

J.   Test for Diabetes Insipidus: Water Deprivation Test (91–93)

a. Indications. This protocol is most useful in the diagnosis of diabetes insipidus and in differentiating between neurogenic (hypothalamic central) diabetes insipidus, nephrogenic (renal) diabetes insipidus, and primary polydipsia (inappropriate thirst mechanism or psychogenic diabetes insipidus).

b. Preparation. No special preparation is necessary. Treatment for diabetes insipidus with vasopressin, desmopressin (DDAVP), or analogs should be discontinued 48–72 h before the protocol.

c. Medication. After obtaining the first pair of urine and plasma samples, water and food are restricted for 3 h. At the end of the period of restriction, a second pair of urine and plasma samples are obtained. No food or drink may be consumed during the protocol.

d. Sampling. Paired samples are evaluated for Uosm (urine osmolality) and Posm (plasma osmolality).

e. Normal Values. At any time during the protocol, baseline Uosm in excess of 400 mOsm/kg with normal Posm (between 275 and 300 mOsm/kg) eliminates a diagnosis of diabetes insipidus. Baseline Uosm less than 300 mOsm/kg with normal Posm is consistent either with overhydration or with diabetes insipidus.

After the 3 h water deprivation period, individuals with overhydration or with diabetes insipidus may still have Uosm less than 30 mOsm/kg. However, individuals with overhydration have Posm between 275 and 290 mOsm/kg but Posm remains above 290 mOsm/kg in individuals with diabetes insipidus.

f. General Considerations. Some physicians have extended the period of water deprivation to 7 h.

REFERENCES

1. Blum WF, Horn N, Kratzsch J, et al. Clinical studies of IGF-BP-3 by radioimmunoassay. Growth Regul 1993; 3:100–104.
2. Martin JL, Baxter RC. Insulin-like growth factor binding protein-3: biochemistry and physiology. Growth Regul 1992; 2:88–99.
3. Chasalow FI, Blethen SL. Dehydroepiandrosterone (DHEA) measurements in cord blood. Steroids 1985; 45:187–193.
4. Chasalow FI, Blethen SL, Taysi K. Possible abnormalities of steroid secretion in children with Smith-Lemli-Opitz syndrome and their parents. Steroids 1985; 46:827–843.
5. Chasalow FI, Blethen SL, Duckett D, Zeitlin S, Greenfield J. Serum levels of dehydroepiandrosterone sulfate as determined by commercial kits and reagents. Steroids 1989; 54:373–383.
6. Smith TW, Butler VP, Haber E. Determination of therapeutic and toxic digoxin concentrations by radioimmunoassay. N Engl J Med 1969; 281:1212–1216.
7. Chasalow FI, Blethen SL. Characterization of digoxin-like materials in human cord serum. In: Castegnetta L, D'Aquino S, Bradlow HL, Labrie F, eds. Steroid Formation, Degradation and Action in Peripheral Normal and Neoplastic Tissues. Ann NY Acad Sci 1990; 595:212–221.
8. Blethen SL, Chasalow FI, Davis MJ. Screening for GH deficiency with IGF-1 assays: a revisit. J Endocrinol Invest 1992; 15(Suppl 4):93.
9. Blethen SL, Chasalow FI. Use of a 2-site immunoradiometric assay for growth hormone in identifying children with growth hormone dependent growth failure. J Clin Endocrinol Metab 1993; 57:1031–1035.
10. Reiter EO, Morris AH, MacGillivray MH, Weber D. Variable estimates of serum growth hormone concentrations by different radioassay systems. J Clin Endocrinol Metab 1988; 66:68–71.
11. Celniker AC, Chen AB, Wert RM, Sherman BM. Variability in the quantitation of circulating growth hormone using commercial immunoassays. J Clin Endocrinol Metab 1989; 68:469–476.
12. Martin LG, Clark JW, Conner TB. Growth hormone secretion enhanced by androgens. J Clin Endocrinol Metab 1968; 28:425–431.
13. Rosenfield RL, Furlanetto RW. Physiologic testosterone or estradiol induction of puberty increases plasma somatomedin C. J Pediatr 1985; 107:415–417.
14. Weldon VV, Gupta SK, Klingensmith G, et al. Evaluation of growth hormone release in children using arginine and L-dopa in combination. J Pediatr 1975; 87:540–544.
15. Alba-Roth J, Muller OA, Schopohl J, Von Werder K. Arginine stimulates growth hormone secretion by suppressing endogenous somatostatin secretion. J Clin Endocrinol Metab 1988; 67:1186–1189.
16. Merimee TJ, Lillicrap DA, Rabinowitz D. Effect of arginine on serum levels of growth hormone. Lancet 1965; 2:688–680.
17. Lanes R, Recker B, Fort P, Lifshitz F. Low dose oral clonidine—a simple and reliable growth hormone screening test. Am J Dis Child 1985; 139:87–88.
18. Fraser NC, Seth J, Brown S. Clonidine is a better test for

19. growth hormone deficiency than insulin hypoglycemia. Arch Dis Child 1983; 58:355–358.
Gil-Ad I, Topper E, Laron Z. Oral clonidine as a growth hormone stimulation test. Lancet 1979; 2:278–280.
20. Nussbaum M, Blethen SL, Chasalow FI, Jacobson M, Shenker R, Feldman J. Blunted growth hormone responses to clonidine in adolescent girls with early anorexia nervosa. J Adol Health Care 1990; 11:145–148.
21. Martul P, Pineda J, Dieguez C, Casanueva FF. Corticoid induced growth hormone (GH) secretion in GH-deficient and normal children. J Clin Endocrinol Metab 1992; 75:536–539.
22. Pineda J, Dieguez C, Casanueva FF, Martul P. Decreased growth hormone response to dexamethasone stimulation test in obese children. Acta Paediatr 1994; 83:103–105.
23. Martul P, Pineda J, Pombo M, Penalva A, Bokser L, Dieguez C. New diagnostic tests of GH reserve. J Pediatr Endocrinol 1993; 6:317–323.
24. Casanueva FF, Burguera B, Alvarez CV, Zugaza JL, Pombo M, Dieguez. Corticoids as a new stimulus of growth hormone secretion in man. J Pediatr Endocrinol 1992; 5:85–90.
25. Eisenstein E, Plotnick L, Lanes R, Lee P, Migeon C, Kowarski AA. Evaluation of the growth hormone exercise test in normal and growth hormone deficient children. Pediatrics 1978; 62:526.
26. Buckler JMH. Plasma growth hormone response to exercise as a diagnostic aid. Arch Dis Child 1973; 48:565–567.
27. Loche S, Cella SG, Puggione R, Stabilini L, Pintor C, Muller EE. The effects of galanin secretion on growth hormone secretion in children of normal and short stature. Pediatr Res 1989; 26:316–319.
28. Bauer FE, Rokaeus A, Jornvall H, McDonald TJ, Mutt V. Growth hormone release in man induced by galanin, a new hypothalamic peptide. Lancet 1986; 2:192–195.
29. Takano K, Hizuka N, Shizume L, et al. Plasma growth hormone (GH) response to GH-releasing factor in normal children with short stature and patients with primary dwarfism. J Clin Endocrinol Metab 1984; 58:236–41.
30. Butenandt O. Diagnostic value of growth hormone-releasing hormone tests in short children. Acta Paediatr Scand (Suppl) 1989; 349:93–99.
31. Martha PM, Blizzard RM, McDonald JA, Thorner MO, Rogol AD. A persistent pattern of varying pituitary responsiveness to exogenous growth hormone (GH) releasing hormone in GH deficient children: evidence supporting periodic somatostatin secretion. J Clin Endocrinol Metab 1988; 67:449–454.
32. Gelato MC, Malozowski S, Caruso-Nicoletti M, et al. Growth hormone (GH) responses to GH-releasing hormone during pubertal development in normal boys and girls: comparison to idiopathic short stature and GH deficiency. J Clin Endocrinol Metab 1986; 63:174–179.
33. Williams T, Berelowitz M, Joffe SN. Impaired growth hormone responses to growth hormone-releasing factor in obesity. A primary defect reversed by weight reduction. N Engl J Med 1984; 311:1403–1407.
34. Mitchell ML, Suvunrungsi P, Sawin CT. Effects of propranolol on the response of serum growth hormone to glucagon. J Clin Endocrinol Metab 1971; 32:470–475.
35. Mitchell ML, Savin CT. Growth hormone responses to glucagon in diabetic and non-diabetic persons. Isr J Med Sci 1972; 8:867.
36. Furlanetto RW, Underwood LE, VanWyk JJ, D'Ercole AJ. Estimation of somatomedin C levels in normals and patients with pituitary disease by radioimmunoassay. J Clin Invest 1977; 50:648–657.
37. Plotnick LP, Van Meter QL, Kowarski AA. Human growth hormone treatment of children with growth failure and normal

growth hormone level by radioimmunoassay: lack of correlation with somatomedin generation. Pediatrics 1983; 71:324–327.

38. Jorgensen JOL, Blum WF, Moller N, Ranke MB, Christiansen JS. Short-term changes in serum insulin-like growth factors (IGF) and IGF binding protein 3 after different modes of intravenous growth hormone (GH) exposure in GH-deficient patients. J Clin Endocrinol Metab 1991; 72:582–587.

39. Shah A, Stanhope R, Mathew D. Hazards of pharmacological tests of growth hormone secretion in childhood. BMJ 1992; 304:173–174.

40. Greenwood FC, Landon J, Stamp TCB. The plasma sugar, free fatty acid cortisol and growth hormone response to insulin in control subjects. J Clin Invest 1966; 45:429–436.

41. Brauman H, Gregoire F. The growth hormone response to insulin induced hypoglycemia in anorexia nervosa and control underweight or normal subjects. Eur J Clin Invest 1975; 5:289–295.

42. Weldon VV, Gupta SK, Haymond MW, et al. The use of L-dopa in the diagnosis of hyposomatropinism in children. J Clin Endocrinol Metab 1973; 36:42–46.

43. Veldhuis JD, Johnson ML. A novel general biophysical model for simulating episodic endocrine gland signaling. Am J Physiol 1988; 255:E740–E759.

44. Tapanainen P, Rantala H, Leppaluoto J, Lautala P, Kaar M-L, Knip M. Nocturnal release of immunoreactive growth-hormone releasing hormone and growth hormone in normal children. Pediatr Res 1989; 26:404–409.

45. Gharib H, Kao PC, Heath H. Determination of silica-purified plasma calcitonin for the detection and management of medullary thyroid carcinoma: comparison of two provocative tests. Mayo Clin Proc 1987; 62:373–378.

46. Leshin M. Multiple endocrine neoplasia. In: Wilson JD, Foster DW, eds. Williams Textbook of Endocrinology. Philadelphia: W.B. Saunders, 1981:1274–1289.

47. Burke G. The triidothyronine suppression test. Am J Med 1967; 42:600–608.

48. Wallack MS, Adelberg HM, Nicoleff JT. A thyroid suppression test using a single dose of L-thyroxine. N Engl J Med 1970; 283:402–405.

49. Whitley RJ. Thyrotropin-releasing hormone (TRH) stimulation test. Am Assoc Clin Chem Endocr In-Service Training Contin Educ 1993; 11:207–209.

50. Spencer CA, Schwarzbein D, Guttler RB, et al. Thyrotropin (TSH)-releasing hormone stimulation test responses employing third and fourth generation TSH assays. J Clin Endocrinol Metab 1993; 76:494–498.

51. Dillon RS. Handbook of Endocrinology, 2nd ed. Philadelphia: Lea & Febiger, 1980:416.

52. Jones KH, Fourman P. Edetic acid test of parathyroid insufficiency. Lancet 1963; 2:119–121.

53. Ellsworth R, Howard JE. Studies on the physiology of the parathyroid glands. VII. Some responses of normal human kidneys and blood to intravenous parathyroid extracts. Bull Johns Hopkins Hosp 1934; 55:296.

54. Chase LR, Melson GL, Aurbach GD. Pseudohypoparathyroidism: Defective excretion of 3′,5′-AMP in response to parathyroid hormone. J Clin Invest 1969; 48:1832–1844.

55. Mikati MA, Melham RE, Najjar SS. The syndrome of hyperostosis and hyperphosphatemia. J Pediatr 1981; 99:900–904.

56. Buckman M, Kaminsky N, Conway M, et al. Utility of L-dopa and water loading in evaluating hyperprolactinemia. J Clin Endocrinol Metab 1973; 36:911–919.

57. Foley TP, Jacobs LS, Hoffman W, et al. Human prolactin and thyrotropin concentrations in normal and hypopituitary children before and after administration of synthetic TRH. J Clin Invest 1972; 51:2143–2150.

58. Blethen SL, Chasalow FI. Overnight dexamethasone suppression test: normal responses and the diagnosis of Cushing's syndrome. Steroids 1989; 54:185–193.

59. Liddle GW. Test of pituitary-adrenal suppressibility in the diagnosis of Cushing's syndrome. J Clin Endocrinol 1960; 20:1539.

60. Pavlatos FC, Smilo RP, Forsham PH. A rapid screening test for Cushing's syndrome. JAMA 1965; 193:720.

61. Temeck JW, Pang S, Nelson C, New MI. Genetic defects of steroidogenesis in premature adrenarche. J Clin Endocrinol Metab 1987; 64:609–617.

62. Childs DF, Bu'lock DE, Anderson DC. Heterogeneity in adrenal steroidogensis in normal men and women. Clin Endocrinol (Oxf) 1979; 11:383–389.

63. Childs DF, Bu'lock DE, Anderson DC. Adrenal steroidogensis in heterozygotes for 21-hydroxylase deficiency. Clin Endocrinol (Oxf) 1979; 11:391–398.

64. Gutai JP, Kowarski AA, Migeon CJ. The detection of heterozygote carrier for congenital virilizing adrenal hyperplasia. J Pediatr 1977; 90:924–929.

65. Granoff AB, Chasalow FI, Blethen SL. 17-Hydroxyprogesterone responses to adrenocorticotrophin in children with premature adrenarche. J Clin Endocrinol Metab 1985; 60:409–415.

66. Rich BH, Rosenfield RL, Lucky AW, Helke JC, Otto P. Adrenarche: changing adrenal response to adrenocorticotropin. J Clin Endocrinol Metab 1981; 52:1129–1136.

67. Hawkins LA, Chasalow FI, Blethen SL. The role of adrenocorticotrophin testing in evaluating girls with premature adrenarche and hirsutism/oligomenorrhea. J Clin Endocrinol Metab 1992; 74:248–253.

68. Liddle GW, Estep HL, Kendall KW, et al. Clinical application of a new test of pituitary reserve. J Clin Endocrinol 1959; 19:875.

69. Gold EM, Kent JR, Forsham PH. Clinical use of a new diagnostic agent methoapyrapone (SU-4885), in pituitary and adrenocortical disorders. Ann Intern Med 1961; 54:175.

70. Sparks LL, Smilo RP, Pavlotos FC, Forsham PH. Experience with a rapid oral metrapone test and the plasma ACTH content in determining the cause of Cushing's syndrome. Metabolism 1969; 18:175–192.

71. Schulman D, Zamanillo J, Lowitt S, et al. Effect of clonidine upon anterior pituitary function and plasma catecholamine concentrations in short children and adolescents. J Pediatr Endocrinol 1985; 1:211–216.

72. Bravo EL, Tarazi RC, Fouad FM, Vidt DG, Gifford RW. Clonidine suppression test: a useful aid in the diagnosis of pheochromocytoma. N Engl J Med 1981; 305:623–626.

73. LeFebvre PJ, Cession-Fossion A, Luyckx AS. Glucagon test for phaeochromocytoma. Lancet 1966; 2:1366.

74. Beck P, Parker ML, Daughaday WH. Paradoxical hypersecretion of growth hormone in response to glucose. J Clin Endocrinol Metab 1966; 26:463–469.

75. Rosenbloom AL, Wheller L, Bianchi R, Chin FT, Tiwary CM, Grgic A. Age-adjusted analysis of insulin responses during normal and glucose tolerance tests in children and adults. Diabetes 1975; 24:820–828.

76. Kahn CB, Soeldner JS, Gleason RE, Rojas L, Camerini-Davalos RA, Marble A. Clinical and chemical diabetes in offspring of diabetic couples. N Engl J Med 1969; 281:343–347.

77. Cornblath M, Schwartz R. Disorders of Carbohydrate Metabolism in Infancy. Philadelphia: W.B. Saunders, 1976:355–361.

78. Cornblath M, Poth M. Hypoglycemia. In: Kaplan S, ed. Clinical Pediatric and Adolescent Endocrinology. Philadelphia: W.B. Saunders, 1982:157–170.

79. Stanley CA, Baker L. Hyperinsulinism in infants and children: diagnosis and therapy. Adv Pediatr 1976; 23:324–325.

80. Rogers DG, Chasalow FI, Blethen SL. Partial deficiency in 17-ketosteroid reductase deficiency presenting as gynecomastia. Steroids 1985; 45:195–200.

81. Saez JM, Bertand J. Studies on testicular function in children: plasma concentrations of testosterone, dehydroepiandrosterone and its sulfate before and after stimulation with human chorionic gonadotropin. Steroids 1968; 12:749–761.

82. Chasalow FI, Blethen SL, Marr HB, French FS. An improved method for evaluating testosterone biosynthetic defects. Pediatr Res 1984; 18:759–763.

83. Zachmann M. Evaluation of gonadal function in childhood and adolescence. Helv Pediatr Acta (Suppl) 1974; 34:53–62.

84. Matthews MJ, Parker DC, Rebar RW, et al. Sleep associated gonadotropin and oestradiol patterns in girls with precocious sexual development. Clin Endocrinol (Oxf) 1982; 17:601–607.

85. Beck W, Stubbe P. Pulsatile secretion of luteinizing hormone and sleep-related gonadotropin rhythms in girls with premature thelarche. Eur J Pediatr 1984; 141:168–170.

86. Roth JC, Kelch SL, Kaplan Sl, Grumbach MM. FSH and LH responses to luteinizing hormone releasing factor in prepubertal and pubertal children, adult males, and patients with hypogonadotropic and hypergonadotropic hypogonadism. J Clin Endocrinol Metab 1972; 35:926–930.

87. Partsch CJ, Hummelink R, Lorenzen F, Sippell WG. Significance of the LHRH test in diagnosis of premature sexual development in girls: the stimulated LH/FSH ratio differentiates between central precocious puberty and premature thelarche. Monatsschr Kinderheilkd 1989; 137:284–288.

88. Job JC, Garnier PE, Chaussain JL, Milhaud G. Elevation of serum gonadotropins (LF and FSH) after releasing hormone (LH-RH) in normal children and patients with disorders of puberty. J Clin Endocrinol Metab 1972; 35:473–476.

89. Chasalow FI, Granoff AB, Tse TF, Blethen SL. Adrenal steroid secretion in girls with pseudoprecocious puberty due to autonomous ovarian cysts. J Clin Endocrinol Metab 1986; 63:828–834.

90. Zipf WB, Kelch RP, Hopwood NJ, Spencer ML, Bacon GE. Suppressed responsiveness to gonadotropin releasing hormone in girls with unsustained isosexual precocity. J Pediatr 1979; 95:38–43.

91. Richman RA, Post EM, Notman DD, Hochberg Z, Moses AM. Simplifying the diagnosis of diabetes insipidus in children. Am J Dis Child 1981; 135:839–841.

92. Frasier SD, Kutnik LA, Schmidt RT, Smith FG. A water deprivation test for the diagnosis of diabetes insipidus in children. Am J Dis Child 1967; 114:157–160.

93. Robertson GL. Diagnosis of diabetes insipidus. Horm Res 1985; 13:176–189.

61

Reference Charts Used Frequently by Endocrinologists in Assessing the Growth and Development of Youth

Bridget F. Recker
Maimonides Medical Center, Brooklyn, New York

III.   STANDARD GROWTH CHARTS FOR CHILDREN WITH GENETIC OR PATHOLOGICAL CONDITIONS

I. STANDARDS OF GROWTH AND DEVELOPMENT

A. Neonates: Figures 1–7

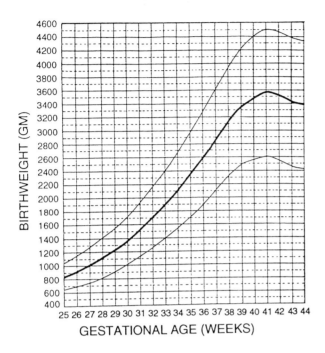

Figure 1 Smoothed curve values for the mean ± 2 SD of birth weight against gestational age. (From Usher R, McLean F. Intrauterine growth of live-born Caucasian infants at sea level: Standards obtained from measurements in 7 dimensions of infants born between 25 and 44 weeks of gestation. J Pediatr 1969; 74(6):901–910.)

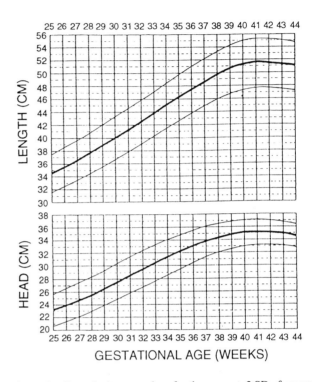

Figure 2 Smoothed curve values for the mean ± 2 SD of crown heel length and head circumference against gestational age (From Usher R, McLean F. Intrauterine growth of live-born Caucasian infants at sea level: Standards obtained from measurements in 7 dimenstions of infants born between 25 and 44 weeks of gestation. J Pediatr 1969; 74(6):901–910.)

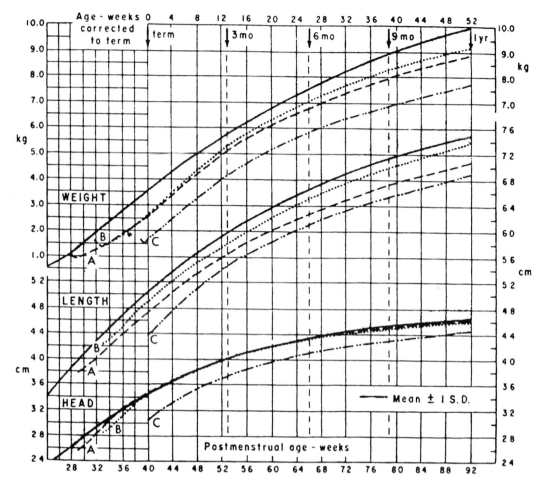

Figure 3   Mean growth curves of three groups of low-birth-weight infants. (A) Very premature and appropriate in size; (B) moderately premature and appropriate in size; (C) full-term but severely undergrown. These curves are plotted against the gestational age for that group. (From Babson SG. Growth of low birth weight infants. J. Pediatr 1970; 77(1):11–18.)

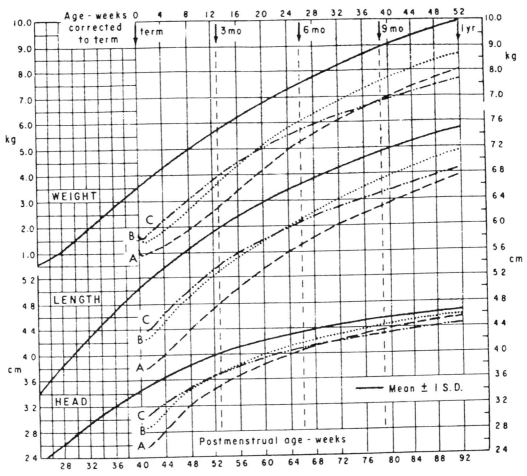

Figure 4 Growth curves of three groups of low-birth-weight infants plotted without correction for gestational age. (From Babson SG. Growth of low-birth-weight infants. J Pediatr 1970; 77(1):11–18.)

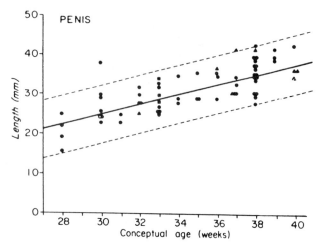

Figure 5 Phallic length of premature and full-term infants. Stretched phallic length of 63 normal premature and full-term male infants (●), showing lines of mean ± 2 SD. Correlation coefficient is 0.80. Superimposed are data for two small-for-gestational-age infants (△), seven large-for-gestational-age infants (▲), and four twins (■), all of which are in the normal range. (From Feldman KW, Smith DW. Fetal phallic growth and penile standards for newborn male infants. J Pediatr 1975; 86(3):395–398.)

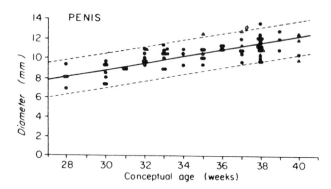

Figure 6 Phallic diameter of premature and full-term infants. Phallic diameter of 63 normal premature and full-term male infants (●), showing lines of mean ± 2 SD. Correlation coefficient is 0.82. Superimposed are data for two small-for-gestational-age infants (△), seven large-for-gestational-age infants (▲), and four twins (■), all of which are in the normal range. (From Feldman KW, Smith DW. Fetal phallic growth and penile standards for newborn male infants. J Pediatr 1975; 86(3):395–398.)

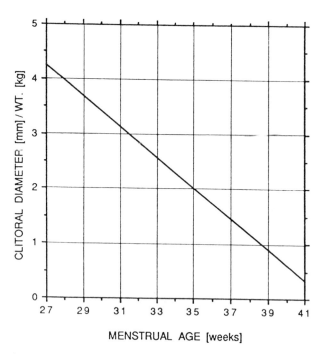

Figure 7 Ratio of clitoral diameter to infant's weight plotted against menstrual age. Measurements were made with calipers on 69 premature and 90 term infants in the first 3 days of life. There was no difference in measurements between black infants and white infants. Clitoral diameter had reached term size by 27 weeks' menstrual age. Clitoral diameter varied from 2 to 6 mm, but did not change with menstrual age. The ratio clitoral diameter to body showed a significant negative correlation to menstrual age. (From Riley WS, et al. J Pediatr 1980; 96:918.)

B. Females: Figures 8–15

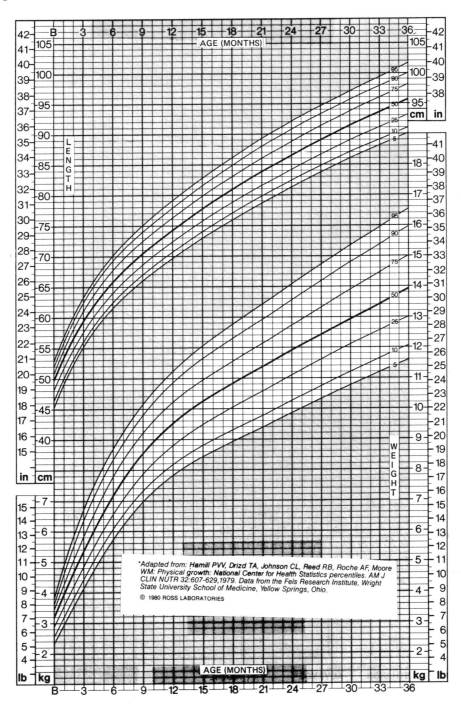

Figure 8 Female: length and weight (birth to 36 months.) (Reproduced with permission from Ross Laboratories, Columbus, Ohio 43216. © 1980, Ross Laboratories.)

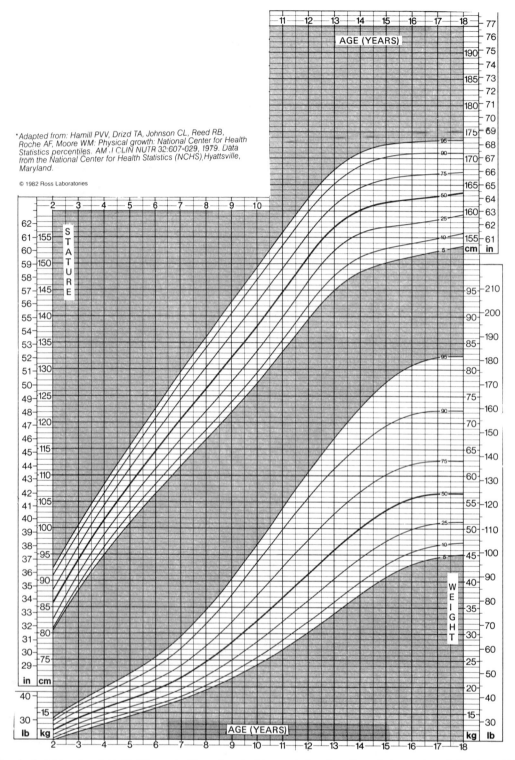

Figure 9 Female: height and weight (2–18 years). (Reproduced with permission from Ross Laboratories, Columbus, Ohio 43216. © Ross Laboratories.)

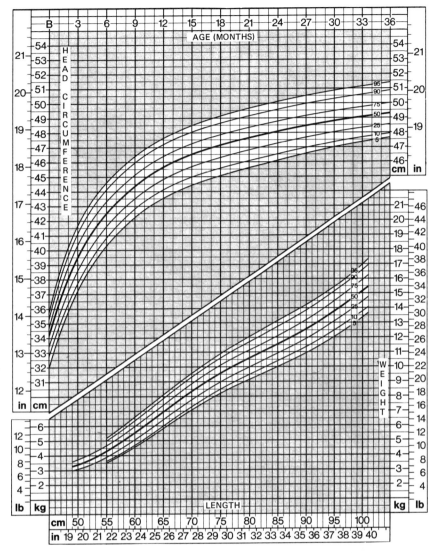

Figure 10 Female: head circumference and length/weight percentiles (birth to 36 months). (Reproduced with permission from Ross Laboratories, Columbus, Ohio 43216. © 1982, Ross Laboratories.)

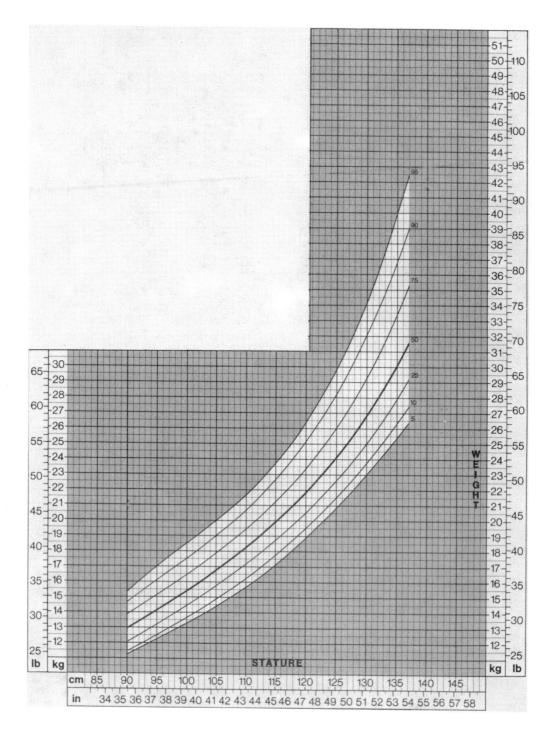

Figure 11 Height/weight percentiles. (From Ross Laboratories, Columbus, Ohio 43216. © 1982, Ross Laboratories.)

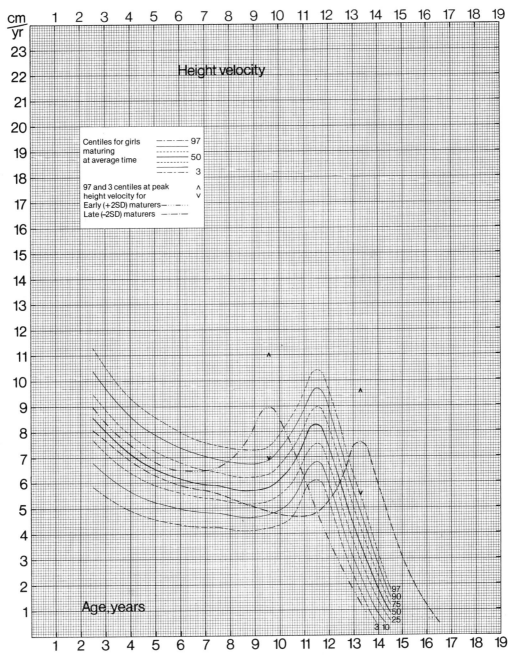

Figure 12 Female: height velocity. (© 1985, Castlemead Publications, Hertford, England. From Tanner JM, Davis PSW. J Pediatr 1985; 107.)

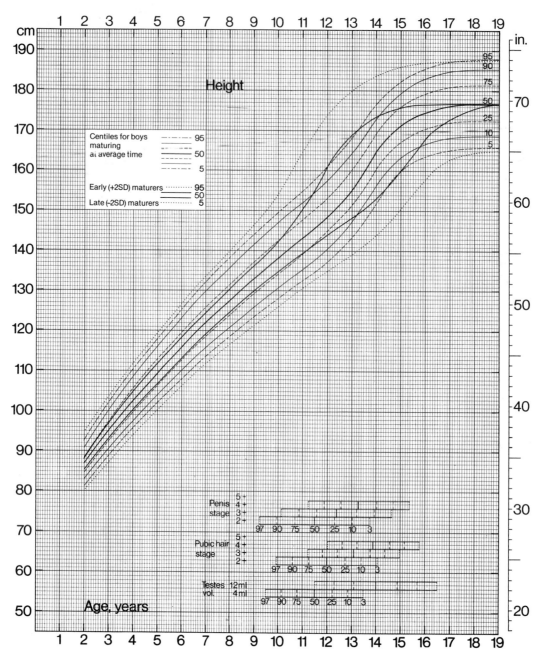

Figure 13 Female: height and pubertal development. (© 1985, Castlemead Publications, Hertford, England. From Tanner JM, Davis PSW. J Pediatr 1985; 107.)

Typical Progression of Female Pubertal Development

Pubertal development in size of female breasts.

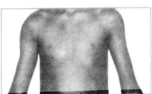
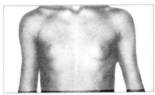

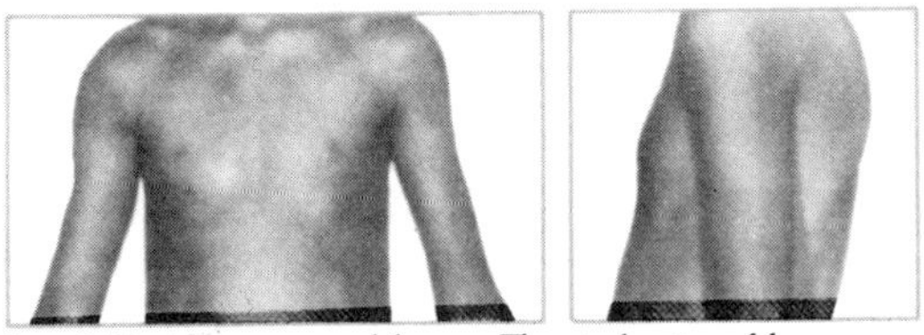

Stage 1. The breasts are preadolescent. There is elevation of the papilla only.

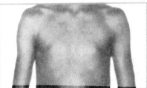
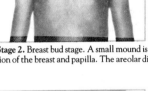
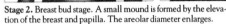
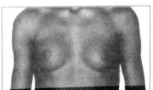

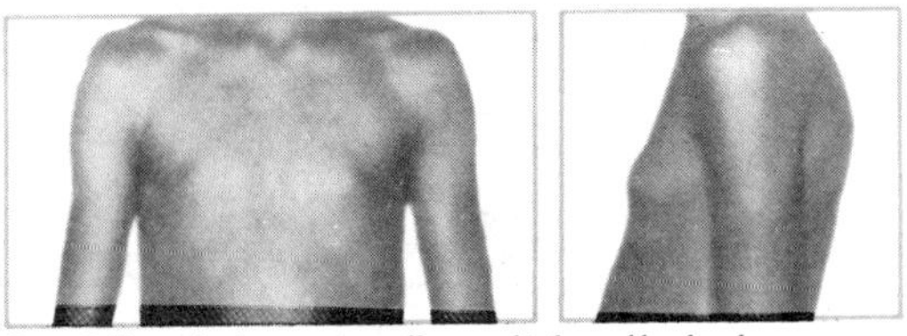

Stage 2. Breast bud stage. A small mound is formed by the elevation of the breast and papilla. The areolar diameter enlarges.

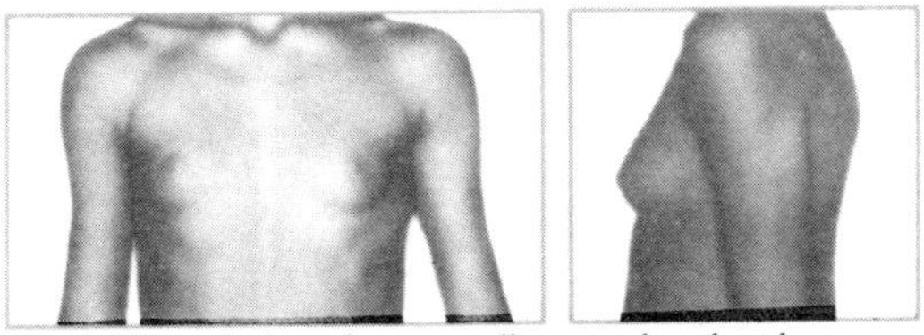

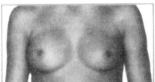

Stage 3. There is further enlargement of breasts and areola with no separation of their contours.

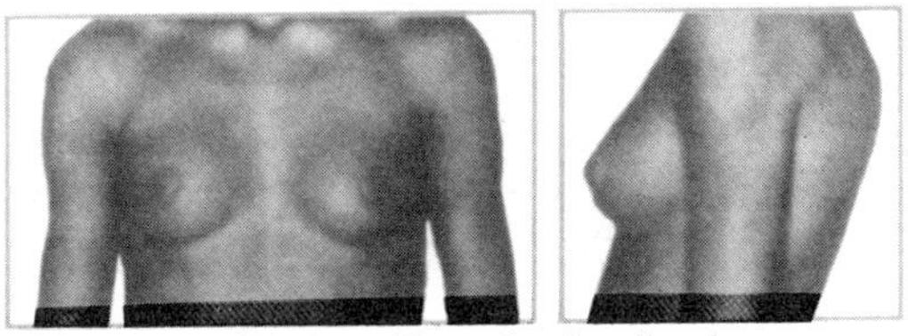

Stage 4. There is a projection of the areola and papilla to form a secondary mound above the level of the breast.

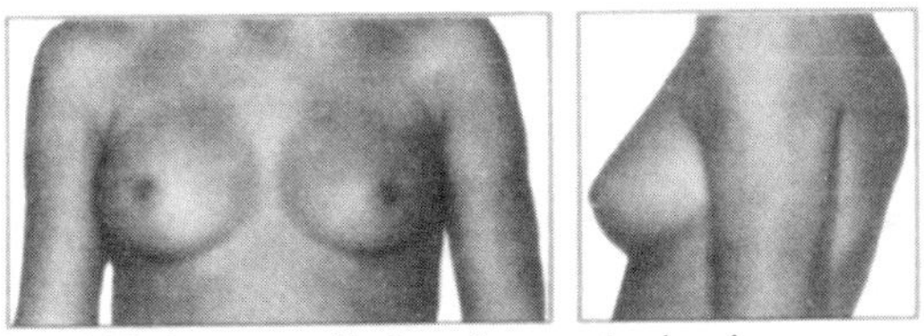

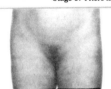

Stage 5. The breasts resemble those of a mature female as the areola has recessed to the general contour of the breast.

Pubertal development of female pubic hair.
Stage 1. There is no pubic hair.

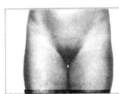
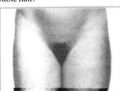
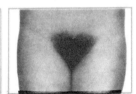

Stage 2. There is sparse growth of long, slightly pigmented, downy hair, straight or only slightly curled, primarily along the labia.

Stage 3. The hair is considerably darker, coarser, and more curled. The hair spreads sparsely over the junction of the pubes.

Stage 4. The hair, now adult in type, covers a smaller area than in the adult and does not extend onto the thighs.

Stage 5. The hair is adult in quantity and type, with extension onto the thighs.

Figure 14 Female: typical progression of pubertal development. (Reproduced with permission from Ross Laboratories, Columbus, Ohio 43216. © Ross Laboratories.)

Age	Height	s.d.	Age	Height	s.d.	Age	Height	s.d.	Age	Height	s.d.
2.0	86.80	3.16	7.0	120.60	5.35	12.0	151.50	7.11	17.0	163.10	6.32
2.1	87.39	3.18	7.1	121.19	5.39	12.1	152.15	7.13	17.1	163.17	6.30
2.2	87.99	3.20	7.2	121.77	5.42	12.2	152.79	7.16	17.2	163.23	6.28
2.3	88.62	3.22	7.3	122.35	5.45	12.3	153.41	7.18	17.3	163.29	6.25
2.4	89.28	3.25	7.4	122.92	5.49	12.4	154.02	7.21	17.4	163.34	6.22
2.5	90.00	3.28	7.5	123.50	5.53	12.5	154.60	7.23	17.5	163.40	6.20
2.6	90.77	3.32	7.6	124.08	5.58	12.6	155.15	7.24	17.6	163.46	6.18
2.7	91.59	3.37	7.7	124.66	5.63	12.7	155.68	7.25	17.7	163.52	6.17
2.8	92.43	3.42	7.8	125.24	5.68	12.8	156.18	7.25	17.8	163.58	6.16
2.9	93.27	3.48	7.9	125.82	5.73	12.9	156.65	7.24	17.9	163.64	6.15
3.0	94.10	3.53	8.0	126.40	5.78	13.0	157.10	7.23	18.0	163.70	6.14
3.1	94.90	3.58	8.1	126.98	5.82	13.1	157.52	7.22			
3.2	95.67	3.63	8.2	127.56	5.86	13.2	157.92	7.21			
3.3	96.42	3.68	8.3	128.14	5.89	13.3	158.30	7.19			
3.4	97.16	3.72	8.4	128.72	5.93	13.4	158.66	7.18			
3.5	97.90	3.77	8.5	129.30	5.96	13.5	159.00	7.17			
3.6	98.65	3.82	8.6	129.88	6.00	13.6	159.32	7.16			
3.7	99.40	3.87	8.7	130.45	6.03	13.7	159.63	7.15			
3.8	100.14	3.92	8.8	131.03	6.07	13.8	159.91	7.14			
3.9	100.88	3.97	8.9	131.61	6.10	13.9	160.17	7.13			
4.0	101.60	4.01	9.0	132.20	6.14	14.0	160.40	7.11			
4.1	102.30	4.05	9.1	132.79	6.17	14.1	160.60	7.09			
4.2	102.98	4.08	9.2	133.39	6.21	14.2	160.77	7.07			
4.3	103.66	4.12	9.3	133.99	6.24	14.3	160.92	7.04			
4.4	104.33	4.15	9.4	134.59	6.28	14.4	161.06	7.01			
4.5	105.00	4.19	9.5	135.20	6.32	14.5	161.20	6.99			
4.6	105.68	4.23	9.6	135.81	6.37	14.6	161.33	6.97			
4.7	106.36	4.28	9.7	136.43	6.42	14.7	161.47	6.95			
4.8	107.05	4.33	9.8	137.05	6.47	14.8	161.59	6.92			
4.9	107.73	4.39	9.9	137.67	6.52	14.9	161.70	6.90			
5.0	108.40	4.44	10.0	138.30	6.57	15.0	161.80	6.87			
5.1	109.06	4.49	10.1	138.93	6.61	15.1	161.88	6.84			
5.2	109.71	4.54	10.2	139.57	6.66	15.2	161.94	6.80			
5.3	110.35	4.59	10.3	140.21	6.69	15.3	162.00	6.76			
5.4	110.98	4.64	10.4	140.85	6.72	15.4	162.05	6.72			
5.5	111.60	4.68	10.5	141.50	6.75	15.5	162.10	6.69			
5.6	112.21	4.72	10.6	142.15	6.77	15.6	162.16	6.66			
5.7	112.81	4.75	10.7	142.81	6.79	15.7	162.22	6.64			
5.8	113.41	4.79	10.8	143.46	6.82	15.8	162.28	6.62			
5.9	114.01	4.82	10.9	144.13	6.84	15.9	162.34	6.60			
6.0	114.60	4.86	11.0	144.80	6.87	16.0	162.40	6.57			
6.1	115.20	4.90	11.1	145.48	6.91	16.1	162.46	6.53			
6.2	115.80	4.95	11.2	146.16	6.95	16.2	162.51	6.49			
6.3	116.40	5.00	11.3	146.84	6.99	16.3	162.57	6.45			
6.4	117.00	5.06	11.4	147.52	7.02	16.4	162.63	6.41			
6.5	117.60	5.11	11.5	148.20	7.05	16.5	162.70	6.38			
6.6	118.20	5.16	11.6	148.87	7.07	16.6	162.78	6.36			
6.7	118.81	5.21	11.7	149.54	7.08	16.7	162.86	6.35			
6.8	119.41	5.26	11.8	150.19	7.09	16.8	162.94	6.34			
6.9	120.01	5.31	11.9	150.85	7.10	16.9	163.02	6.33			

Figure 15 Mean height and SD for females. (From Hamill PVV, Dzird TA, Johnson CL, Reed RR, Roche AF. NCHS growth curves for children from birth to 18 years: United States. DHEW publication (PHS) 78-1650. Washington DC: US government Printing Office; Vital Health Stat 1977; (11) 165: 1-74.)

C. Males: Figures 15–25

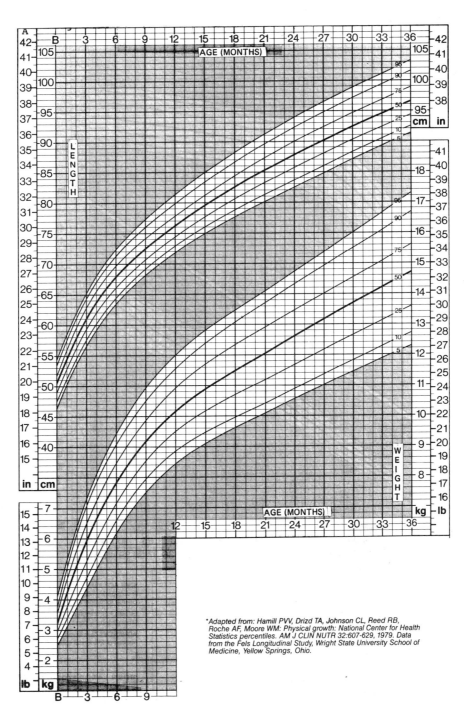

Figure 16 Male: length and weight (birth to 36 months). (Reproduced with permission from Ross Laboratories, Columbus, Ohio 43216. © 1982, Ross Laboratories.)

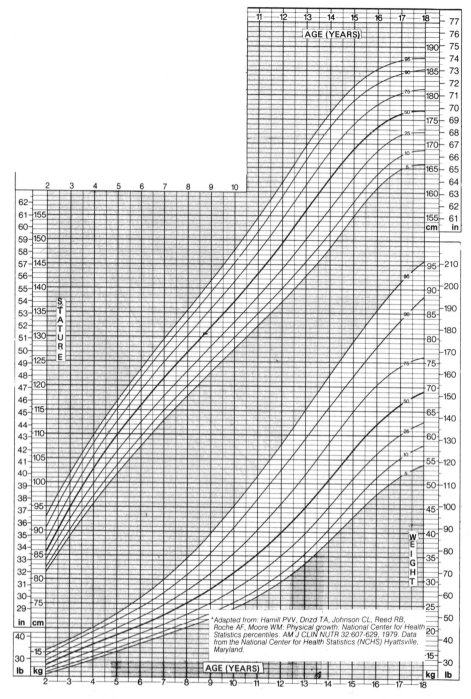

Figure 17 Male: height and weight (2–18 years). (Reproduced with permission from Ross Laboratories, Columbus, Ohio 43216. © 1982, Ross Laboratories.)

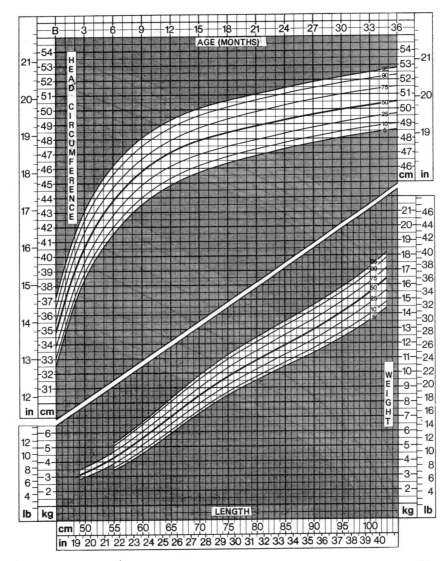

Figure 18 Male: head circumference and length/weight percentiles (birth to 36 months). (Reproduced with permission from Ross Laboratories, Columbus, Ohio 43216. © 1982, Ross Laboratories.)

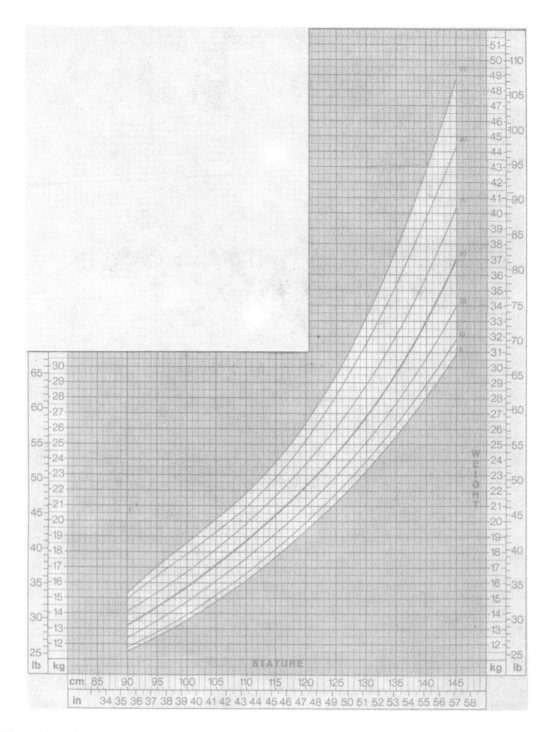

Figure 19 Height/weight percentiles. (From Ross Laboratories, Columbus, Ohio 43216. © 1982, Ross Laboratories.)

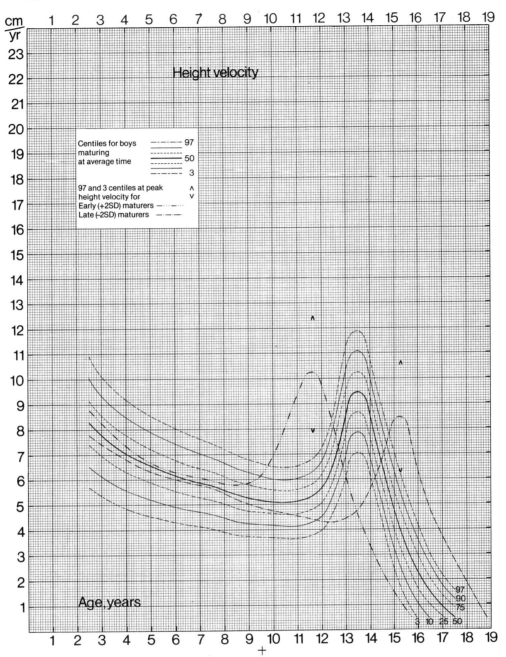

Figure 20 Male: height velocity. (© 1985, Castlemead Publications, Hertford, England. Tanner JM, Davis PSW. J Pediatr 1985; 107.)

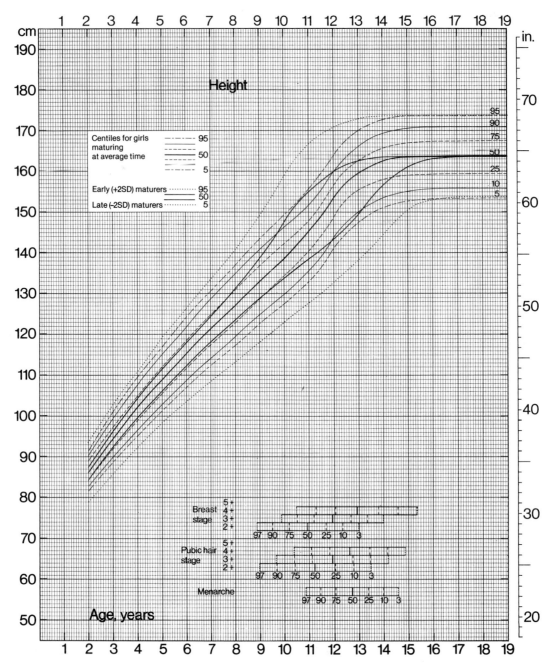

Figure 21   Male: height and pubertal development. (© 1985, Castlemead Publications, Hertford, England. Tanner JM, Davis PSW. J Pediatr 1985; 107.)

Typical Progression of Male Pubertal Development

Pubertal development in size of male genitalia.

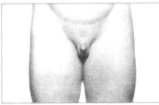

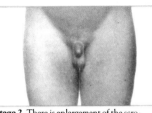

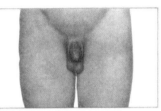

Stage 1. The penis, testes, and scrotum are of childhood size.

Stage 2. There is enlargement of the scrotum and testes, but the penis usually does not enlarge. The scrotal skin reddens.

Stage 3. There is further growth of the testes and scotum and enlargement of the penis, mainly in length.

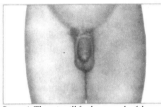

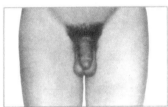

Stage 4. There is still further growth of the testes and scrotum and increased size of the penis, especially in breadth.

Stage 5. The genitalia are adult in size and shape.

Pubertal development of male pubic hair.

Stage 1. There is no pubic hair.

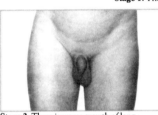

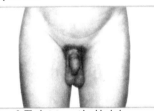

Stage 2. There is sparse growth of long, slightly pigmented, downy hair, straight or only slightly curled, primarily at the base of the penis.

Stage 3. The hair is considerably darker, coarser, and more curled. The hair spreads sparsely over the junction of the pubes.

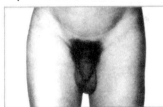

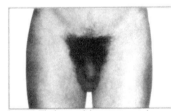

Stage 4. The hair, now adult in type, covers a smaller area than in the adult and does not extend onto the thighs.

Stage 5. The hair is adult in quantity and type, with extension onto the thighs.

Figure 22 Male: typical progression of pubertal development. (Reproduced with permission from Ross Laboratories, Columbus, Ohio 43216. © Ross Laboratories.)

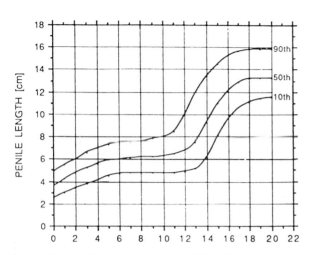

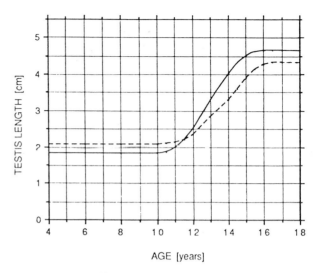

Figure 23 Penile growth in stretched length from the pubic ramus to the tip of the glans; from infancy into adolescence. (From Schonfield WA. Am J Dis Child 1943; 65:535.)

Figure 24 Testicular growth in length, adapted from normal standards of testicular volume. (Solid line from data in Zurich; broken line from data of Laron A, Zilka E. J Clin Endocrinol Metab 1969; 29;1409; adapted from data of Praeder A. Recognizable Patterns of Human Malformation, 3rd ed. Philadelphia: WB Saunders, 1982.)

Age	Height	s.d.	Age	Height	s.d.	Age	Height	s.d.	Age	Height	s.d.
2.0	86.80	2.61	7.0	121.70	5.29	12.0	149.70	7.36	17.0	176.20	6.87
2.1	87.47	2.50	7.1	122.24	5.30	12.1	150.34	7.44	17.1	176.33	6.83
2.2	88.15	2.40	7.2	122.78	5.31	12.2	150.97	7.52	17.2	176.45	6.80
2.3	88.86	2.34	7.3	123.33	5.33	12.3	151.61	7.60	17.3	176.55	6.78
2.4	89.61	2.35	7.4	123.87	5.34	12.4	152.28	7.69	17.4	176.64	6.76
2.5	90.40	2.43	7.5	124.40	5.35	12.5	153.00	7.78	17.5	176.70	6.75
2.6	91.25	2.60	7.6	124.93	5.36	12.6	153.77	7.88	17.6	176.74	6.74
2.7	92.14	2.84	7.7	125.45	5.37	12.7	154.57	7.97	17.7	176.77	6.74
2.8	93.06	3.10	7.8	125.97	5.38	12.8	155.38	8.07	17.8	176.79	6.74
2.9	93.99	3.37	7.9	126.48	5.39	12.9	156.16	8.17	17.9	176.80	6.75
3.0	94.90	3.59	8.0	127.00	5.41	13.0	156.90	8.27	18.0	176.80	6.75
3.1	95.79	3.75	8.1	127.52	5.43	13.1	157.57	8.36			
3.2	96.65	3.86	8.2	128.04	5.45	13.2	158.18	8.45			
3.3	97.49	3.93	8.3	128.56	5.48	13.3	158.75	8.52			
3.4	98.30	3.97	8.4	129.08	5.50	13.4	159.32	8.58			
3.5	99.10	4.01	8.5	129.60	5.53	13.5	159.90	8.63			
3.6	99.88	4.06	8.6	130.12	5.56	13.6	160.51	8.66			
3.7	100.64	4.11	8.7	130.64	5.58	13.7	161.14	8.68			
3.8	101.40	4.17	8.8	131.16	5.60	13.8	161.79	8.69			
3.9	102.15	4.24	8.9	131.68	5.63	13.9	162.45	8.69			
4.0	102.90	4.32	9.0	132.20	5.65	14.0	163.10	8.69			
4.1	103.65	4.40	9.1	132.72	5.67	14.1	163.74	8.69			
4.2	104.41	4.48	9.2	133.23	5.70	14.2	164.38	8.68			
4.3	105.15	4.56	9.3	133.75	5.72	14.3	165.00	8.67			
4.4	105.89	4.63	9.4	134.27	5.75	14.4	165.60	8.65			
4.5	106.60	4.68	9.5	134.80	5.78	14.5	166.20	8.63			
4.6	107.29	4.72	9.6	135.33	5.81	14.6	166.78	8.60			
4.7	107.96	4.74	9.7	135.87	5.84	14.7	167.35	8.55			
4.8	108.61	4.76	9.8	136.41	5.88	14.8	167.91	8.51			
4.9	109.26	4.78	9.9	136.95	5.92	14.9	168.46	8.45			
5.0	109.90	4.80	10.0	137.50	5.96	15.0	169.00	8.39			
5.1	110.55	4.83	10.1	138.05	6.00	15.1	169.53	8.33			
5.2	111.19	4.86	10.2	138.60	6.05	15.2	170.05	8.26			
5.3	111.84	4.90	10.3	139.16	6.10	15.3	170.56	8.19			
5.4	112.47	4.94	10.4	139.72	6.15	15.4	171.04	8.11			
5.5	113.10	4.98	10.5	140.30	6.20	15.5	171.50	8.02			
5.6	113.72	5.01	10.6	140.89	6.25	15.6	171.93	7.93			
5.7	114.32	5.04	10.7	141.48	6.31	15.7	172.35	7.83			
5.8	114.92	5.06	10.8	142.09	6.37	15.8	172.74	7.73			
5.9	115.51	5.09	10.9	142.69	6.43	15.9	173.12	7.63			
6.0	116.10	5.11	11.0	143.30	6.50	16.0	173.50	7.54			
6.1	116.69	5.14	11.1	143.91	6.58	16.1	173.87	7.46			
6.2	117.28	5.16	11.2	144.52	6.66	16.2	174.24	7.38			
6.3	117.86	5.19	11.3	145.13	6.75	16.3	174.58	7.31			
6.4	118.44	5.21	11.4	145.76	6.84	16.4	174.91	7.24			
6.5	119.00	5.23	11.5	146.40	6.93	16.5	175.20	7.17			
6.6	119.55	5.25	11.6	147.05	7.02	16.6	175.46	7.10			
6.7	120.09	5.26	11.7	147.72	7.11	16.7	175.68	7.04			
6.8	120.63	5.27	11.8	148.39	7.19	16.8	175.88	6.98			
6.9	121.16	5.28	11.9	149.05	7.28	16.9	176.05	6.92			

Figure 25 Mean height and SD for males. (From Hamill PVV, Dzird TA, Johnson CL, Reed RR, Roche AF. NCHS growth curves for children from birth to 18 years: United States. DHEW publication (PHS) 78-1650. Washington DC: US government Printing Office; Vital Health Stat 1977; (11) 165: 1-74.)

II. MISCELLANEOUS STANDARDS: FIGURES 26–34

| AGE | HEIGHT (In.) | | SPAN | | | | AGE | HEIGHT (In.) | | SPAN | | | |
| | | | Absolute | | Relative | | | | | Absolute | | Relative | |
	M	F	M	F	M	F		M	F	M	F	M	F
Birth	20.2	19.9	19.3	18.9	95.7	95.2	7½ Yrs.	48.2	47.9	47.6	47.0	98.7	98.1
1 Mo.	21.9	21.5	21.0	20.5	95.7	95.2	8 Yrs.	49.2	48.9	48.8	48.1	99.1	98.3
2 Mos.	23.1	22.7	22.1	21.6	95.7	95.2	8½ Yrs.	50.2	49.9	50.0	49.2	99.6	98.6
3 Mos.	24.1	23.7	23.1	22.6	95.8	95.3	9 Yrs.	51.2	50.9	51.2	50.3	100.0	98.8
4 Mos.	25.0	24.6	24.0	3.4	95.8	95.3	9½ Yrs.	52.2	51.9	52.4	51.4	100.4	99.0
5 Mos.	25.7	25.3	24.6	24.1	95.8	95.3	10 Yrs.	53.2	53.0	53.6	52.6	100.7	99.2
6 Mos.	26.4	26.0	25.3	24.8	95.8	95.3	10½ Yrs.	54.2	54.1	54.7	53.8	100.9	99.4
7 Mos.	27.1	26.6	26.0	25.4	95.9	95.4	11 Yrs.	55.2	55.3	55.8	55.1	101.2	99.6
8 Mos.	27.6	27.1	26.5	25.9	95.9	95.4	11½ Yrs.	56.2	56.5	56.9	56.3	101.4	99.8
9 Mos.	28.1	27.6	26.9	26.3	95.9	95.4	12 Yrs.	57.1	57.6	58.0	57.6	101.6	100.0
10 Mos.	28.6	28.1	27.4	26.8	95.9	95.9	12½ Yrs.	58.0	58.7	59.1	58.7	101.8	100.1
11 Mos.	29.1	28.6	27.9	27.3	96.0	95.5	13 Yrs.	58.9	59.7	60.1	59.9	102.0	100.3
12 Mos.	29.5	29.0	28.3	27.7	96.0	95.5	13½ Yrs.	59.8	60.6	61.1	60.9	102.2	100.4
15 Mos.	30.7	30.2	29.5	28.9	96.1	95.6	14 Yrs.	60.7	61.4	62.1	61.7	102.3	100.6
18 Mos.	31.9	31.4	30.7	30.0	96.2	95.7	14½ Yrs.	61.6	62.0	63.1	62.4	102.5	100.7
21 Mos.	32.9	32.4	31.7	31.0	96.3	95.7	15 Yrs.	62.4	62.5	64.0	63.0	102.6	100.8
24 Mos.	33.9	33.4	32.6	32.0	96.3	96.8	15½ Yrs.	63.2	62.9	64.9	63.5	102.7	100.9
30 Mos.	35.7	32.1	34.4	33.7	96.4	96.0	16 Yrs.	64.0	63.2	65.8	63.0	102.8	101.0
36 Mos.	37.3	30.7	30.0	35.0	96.6	96.2	16½ Yrs.	64.7	63.5	66.6	64.2	102.9	101.0
42 Mos.	38.8	38.2	37.5	36.5	96.8	96.4	17 Yrs.	65.4	63.7	67.4	64.4	103.0	101.2
48 Mos.	40.2	39.6	39.0	38.2	97.0	96.6	17½ Yrs.	66.0	63.9	68.1	64.6	103.1	101.2
54 Mos.	41.5	40.9	40.3	39.6	97.2	96.8	18 Yrs.	66.6	64.0	68.7	64.8	103.2	101.3
60 Mos.	42.7	42.2	41.6	40.9	97.4	97.0	18½ Yrs.	67.1	64.0	69.3	64.8	103.3	101.3
5½ Yrs.	43.9	43.4	42.8	42.2	97.6	97.2	19 Yrs.	67.5	64.0	69.8	64.8	103.4	101.3
6 Yrs.	45.0	44.6	44.0	43.4	97.8	97.4	19½ Yrs.	67.8	64.0	70.1	64.8	103.4	101.3
6½ Yrs.	46.1	45.7	45.2	44.6	98.1	97.6	20 Yrs.	68.0	64.0	70.4	64.8	103.5	101.3
7 Yrs.	47.2	46.8	46.4	48.9	98.4	97.8							

Figure 26   Span in relation to age and standing height. (From Engelbach W Endocrine Medicine. Courtesy of Charles C Thomas, Publisher, Springfield, Illinois, 1932.)

AGE:	STANDING HEIGHT (In.)		SITTING HEIGHT, ABSOLUTE		SITTING HEIGHT, RELATIVE	
	M	F	M	F	M	F
Birth	20.2	19.9	13.6	13.4	67.3	67.3
1 Month	21.9	21.5	14.6	14.4	66.7	66.8
2 Months	23.1	22.7	15.3	15.1	66.2	66.3
3 Months	24.1	23.7	15.8	15.6	65.6	65.7
4 Months	25.0	24.6	16.3	16.1	65.1	65.2
5 Months	25.7	25.3	16.6	16.4	64.6	64.7
6 Months	26.4	26.0	16.9	16.7	64.1	64.2
7 Months	27.1	26.6	17.3	17.0	63.8	63.9
8 Months	27.6	27.1	17.5	17.2	63.4	63.5
9 Months	28.1	27.6	17.7	17.4	63.1	63.2
10 Months	28.6	28.1	18.0	17.7	62.8	62.9
11 Months	29.1	28.6	18.2	17.9	62.6	62.7
12 Months (1 yr)	29.5	29.0	18.4	18.1	62.3	62.4
15 Months	30.7	30.2	18.9	18.6	61.6	61.7
18 Months	31.9	31.4	19.4	19.1	60.9	61.0
21 Months	32.9	32.4	19.8	19.5	60.3	60.4
24 Months (2 yrs)	33.9	33.4	20.3	20.0	59.8	59.9
30 Months	35.7	35.1	21.0	20.7	58.9	59.0
36 Months (3 yrs)	37.3	36.7	21.7	21.4	58.2	58.3
42 Months	38.8	38.2	22.3	22.0	57.6	57.6
48 Months (4 yrs)	40.2	39.6	22.9	22.5	57.0	56.9
54 Months	41.5	40.9	23.4	23.1	56.5	56.4
60 Months (5 yrs)	42.7	42.2	23.9	23.6	56.0	55.9
5½ Years	43.9	43.4	24.4	24.1	55.6	55.5
6 Years	45.0	44.6	24.9	24.6	55.2	55.2
6½ Years	46.1	45.7	25.3	25.1	54.9	54.9
7 Years	47.2	46.8	25.8	25.5	54.6	54.5
7½ Years	48.2	47.9	26.2	26.0	54.3	54.2
8 Years	49.2	48.9	26.6	26.4	54.1	54.0
8½ Years	50.2	49.9	27.1	26.9	53.9	53.8
9 Years	51.2	50.9	27.5	27.3	53.7	53.6
9½ Years	52.2	51.9	27.9	27.7	53.4	53.3
10 Years	53.2	53.0	28.3	28.1	53.2	53.0
10½ Years	54.2	54.1	28.8	28.6	53.0	52.8
11 Years	55.2	55.3	29.2	29.1	52.9	52.6
11½ Years	56.2	56.5	29.6	29.7	52.7	52.6
12 Years	57.1	57.6	30.0	30.3	52.6	52.6
12½ Years	58.0	58.7	30.4	30.9	52.5	52.7
13 Years	58.9	59.7	30.9	31.5	52.4	52.8
13½ Years	59.8	60.6	31.3	32.0	52.3	52.8
14 Years	60.7	61.4	31.7	32.5	52.3	52.9
14½ Years	61.6	62.0	32.2	32.8	52.4	52.9
15 Years	62.4	62.5	32.8	33.0	52.5	52.9
15½ Years	63.2	62.9	33.3	33.2	52.6	52.9
16 Years	64.0	63.2	33.7	33.4	52.7	52.9
16½ Years	64.7	63.5	34.1	33.5	52.8	52.9
17 Years	65.4	63.7	34.5	33.6	52.8	52.8
17½ Years	66.0	63.9	34.8	33.7	52.8	52.8
18 Years	66.6	64.0	35.1	33.8	52.7	52.8
18½ Years	67.1	64.0	35.3	33.8	52.6	52.8
19 Years	67.5	64.0	35.5	33.8	52.6	52.8
19½ Years	67.8	64.0	35.6	33.8	52.5	52.8
20 Years	68.0	64.0	35.7	33.8	52.5	52.8

Figure 27 Sitting height in relation to age and standing height. (From Engelbach W. Endocrine Medicine. Courtesy of Charles C Thomas, Publisher, Springfield, Illinois, 1932).

Age Yrs.	Boys Height cm	annual incr.	Weight kg	Lower Segment cm	Ratio U/L	Girls Height cm	annual incr.	Weight kg	Lower Segment cm	Ratio U/L	Both Sexes Head cm	Chest cm	Span Difference Span minus Height Male cm	Female cm
Birth	50.8		8.4	18.8	1.70	50.8		3.2	18.8	1.70	35	35	−2.5	−2.5
½	67.8		8.5	25.7	1.62	65.8		7.7	25.3	1.60	43.4	44	−2.5	−3.0
1	76.1	25.3	10.8	30.0	1.54	74.2	23.4	9.9	20.4	1.52	46.5	47	−2.5	−3.3
1½	81.9		12.2	32.8	1.50	80.0		11.3	32.5	1.46	48.0	48	−2.7	−3.3
2	87.4	11.4	13.2	36.1	1.42	86.1	11.9	12.5	36.7	1.41	49.0	50	−3.0	−3.5
2½	92.2		14.8	38.9	1.37	91.1		13.6	38.9	1.34			−3.0	−3.8
3	96.4	9.0	15.8	41.0	1.35	95.4	9.3	14.7	41.5	1.30	50.0	52	−2.7	−4.0
3½	100.2		16.3	43.6	1.30	99.5		15.9	43.8	1.27			−2.7	−4.0
4	104.0	7.6	17.3	46.4	1.24	103.3	7.9	16.9	46.5	1.22	50.5	53	−3.0	−3.8
4½	107.6		18.4	48.5	1.22	107.2		18.1	49.0	1.19			−3.0	−3.5
5	110.7	6.7	19.4	50.6	1.19	110.6	7.3	10.2	51.4	1.15	50.8	55	−3.3	−3.5
6	117.7	7.0	21.9	55.5	1.12	117.6	7.0	21.9	56.0	1.10	51.2	56	−2.5	−3.3
7	123.8	6.1	21.6	60.0	1.07	123.8	6.2	21.7	60.1	1.06	51.6	57	−2.5	−2.0
8	120.9	6.1	27.6	61.0	1.03	120.8	6.0	28.1	64.2	1.02	52.0	50	−1.8	−1.8
9	135.4	5.5	31.0	67.0	1.02	135.4	5.6	31.6	67.3	1.01		60	0	−1.2
10	141.0	5.0	34.8	70.8	0.99	141.0	5.6	35.4	70.5	1.00	58.0	61	0	−1.0
11	145.9	4.9	38.8	73.7	0.95	147.7	6.7	40.1	74.2	0.90			0	0
12	151.4	5.5	43.2	76.4	0.98	154.2	0.5	45.5	77.5	0.99	53.2	66	+8.0	0
13	157.5	6.1	47.9	80.0	0.97	150.5	5.3	50.1	79.7	1.00			+3.3	0
14	161.8	7.3	54.0	83.6	0.97	102.9	3.4	54.5	80.6	1.01	54.0	72*	+3.3	0
15	171.1	6.3	60.0	86.3	0.95	104.8	1.9	57.4	81.5	1.01			+4.3	+1.2
16	175.2	4.1	64.4	88.0	0.99	165.5	0.7	59.2	81.9	1.01	55.0	77*	+4.6	+1.2
17	176.6	1.4	66.9	88.8	0.99	165.5	0	60.5	81.9	1.01	55.4	82*	+5.8	+1.2

*Males only.

Figure 28   Average anthropometric measurements. (From Wilkins, Lawson. The Diagnosis and Treatment of Endocrine Disorders in Childhood and Adolescence. Courtesy of Charles C. Thomas, Publisher, Springfield, Illinois, 1966.)

Site	Grade	Definition
1. Upper lip	1	A few hairs at outer margin.
	2	A small moustache at outer margin.
	3	A moustache extending halfway from outer margin.
	4	A moustache extending to midline.
2. Chin	1	A few scattered hairs.
	2	Scattered hairs with small concentrations.
	3 & 4	Complete cover, light and heavy.
3. Chest	1	Circumareolar hairs.
	2	With midline hair in addition.
	3	Fusion of these areas, with three-quarter cover.
	4	Complete cover.
4. Upper back	1	A few scattered hairs.
	2	Rather more, still scattered.
	3 & 4	Complete cover, light and heavy.
5. Lower back	1	A sacral tuft of hair.
	2	With some lateral extension.
	3	Three-quarter cover.
	4	Complete cover.
6. Upper abdomen	1	A few midline hairs.
	2	Rather more, still midline.
	3 & 4	Half and full cover.
7. Lower abdomen	1	A few midline hairs.
	2	A midline streak of hair.
	3	A midline band of hair.
	4	An inverted V-shaped growth.
8. Arm	1	Sparse growth affecting not more than a quarter of the limb surface.
	2	More than this: cover still incomplete.
	3 & 4	Complete cover, light and heavy.
9. Forearm	1, 2, 3, 4	Complete cover of dorsal surface; 2 grades of light and 2 of heavy growth.
10. Thigh	1, 2, 3, 4	As for arm.
11. Leg	1, 2, 3, 4	As for arm.

Figure 29 Hair-grading system. (From Ferriman D, Gallwey JD. J Clin Endocrinol Metab 1961; 21:1440–1447.

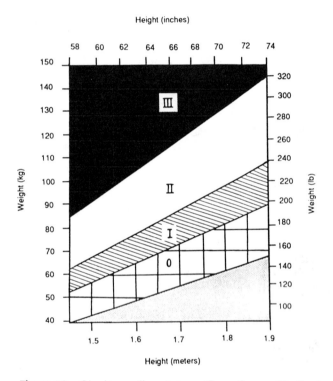

Figure 30 Obesity grading system. (From Garrow JS. Treat Obesity Seriously. New York: Churchill Livingstone, 1981:3.)

PRIMARY (DECIDUOUS) TEETH

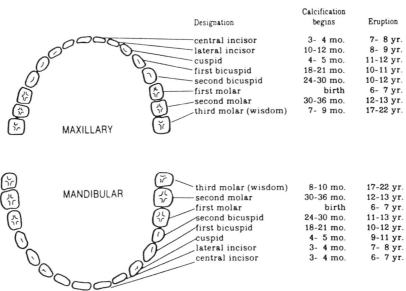

Designation	Calcification (fetal month)	Eruption (months)	Shedding (years)
MAXILLARY			
central incisor	5	6- 8	7- 8
lateral incisor	5	8-11	8- 9
cuspid	6	16-20	11-12
first primary molar	5	10-16	10-11
second primary molar	6	20-30	10-12
MANDIBULAR			
second primary molar	6	20-30	11-13
first primary molar	5	10-16	10-12
cuspid	6	16-20	9-11
lateral incisor	5	7-10	7- 8
central incisor	5	5- 7	6- 7

DESIGNATION OF TEETH

$$\frac{211111 \mid 101112}{211110 \mid 11111}$$

Deciduous teeth designated by 1; permanent teeth by 2, missing teeth by O. Upper row indicates maxillary teeth, lower row of numbers indicates mandibular teeth. Vertical line locates the midline.

SECONDARY (PERMANENT) TEETH

Designation	Calcification begins	Eruption
MAXILLARY		
central incisor	3- 4 mo.	7- 8 yr.
lateral incisor	10-12 mo.	8- 9 yr.
cuspid	4- 5 mo.	11-12 yr.
first bicuspid	18-21 mo.	10-11 yr.
second bicuspid	24-30 mo.	10-12 yr.
first molar	birth	6- 7 yr.
second molar	30-36 mo.	12-13 yr.
third molar (wisdom)	7- 9 mo.	17-22 yr.
MANDIBULAR		
third molar (wisdom)	8-10 mo.	17-22 yr.
second molar	30-36 mo.	12-13 yr.
first molar	birth	6- 7 yr.
second bicuspid	24-30 mo.	11-13 yr.
first bicuspid	18-21 mo.	10-12 yr.
cuspid	4- 5 mo.	9-11 yr.
lateral incisor	3- 4 mo.	7- 8 yr.
central incisor	3- 4 mo.	6- 7 yr.

Figure 31 Development of dentition. (From Simon FA, Stevenson RE. Pediatric Patient Care. University of Texas Press, 1975.)

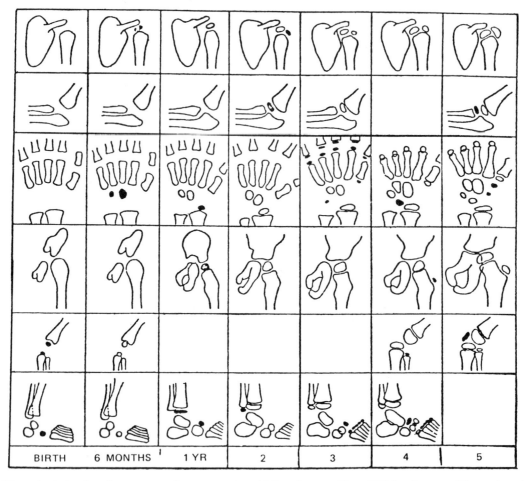

Figure 32 Chronological order of appearance of osseous centers, birth to 5 years. (From Wilkins, Lawson. Diagnosis and Treatment of Endocrine Disorders in Childhood and Adolescence. Courtesy of Charles C Thomas, Publisher, Springfield, Illinois, 1966.)

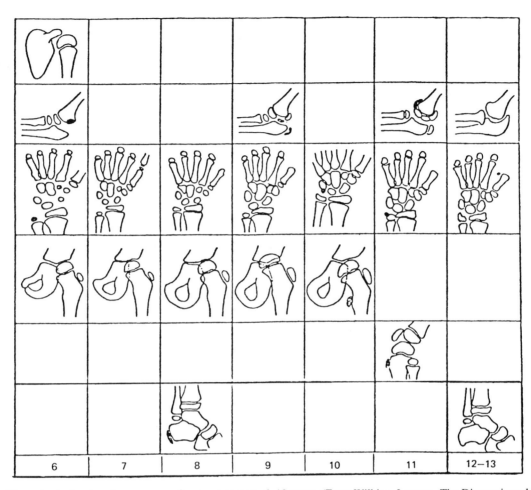

Figure 33 Chronological order of appearance of osseous centers, 6–13 years. (From Wilkins, Lawson. The Diagnosis and Treatment of Endocrine Disorders in Childhood and Adolescence. Courtesy of Charles C Thomas, Publisher, Springfield, Illinois, 1966.)

	12 Yrs.	13 Yrs.	14 Yrs.	15 Yrs.	16 Yrs.	17 Yrs.	18 Yrs.
Shoulder							Head of humerus Great tuberosity
Elbow	Trochlen & capitelium	Olecranon	Ext. epicondyle Head of radius				
Hand		Styloid of ulna		Ep. metacarpals & phalanges			Ep. radius & ulna
Hip				Head of femur Trochanters			
Knee							Ep. femur, tibia & fibula
Foot	Ep. os raleis			Ep. metatarsals & phalanges		Ep. tibia & fibula	

Figure 34   Chronological order of union of epiphysis with diaphysis. (From Wilkins, Lawson. The Diagnosis and Treatment of Endocrine Disorders in Childhood and Adolescence. Courtesy of Charles C Thomas, Publisher, Springfield, Illinois, 1966.)

III. STANDARD GROWTH CHARTS FOR CHILDREN WITH GENETIC OR PATHOLOGICAL CONDITIONS: FIGURES 35–57

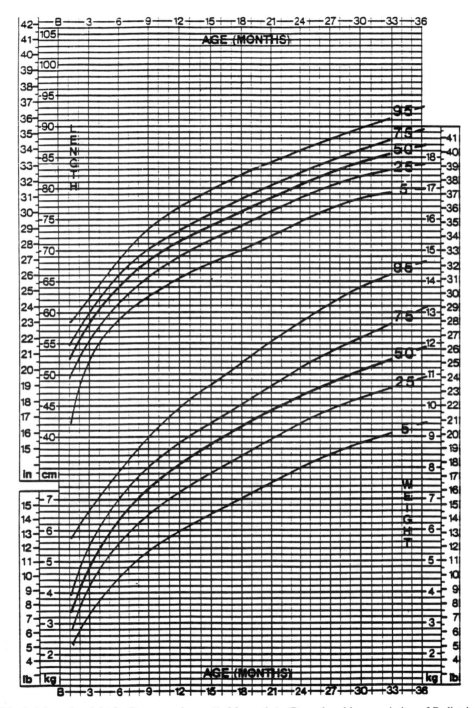

Figure 35 Male: height and weight for Down syndrome (1–36 months). (Reproduced by permission of Pediatrics 1988; 81:102.)

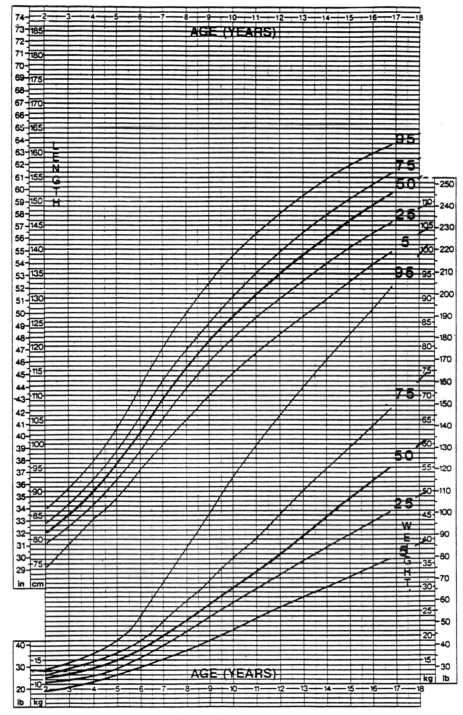

Figure 36 Male: height and weight for Down syndrome (2–18 years). (Reproduced by permission of Pediatrics 1988; 81:102.)

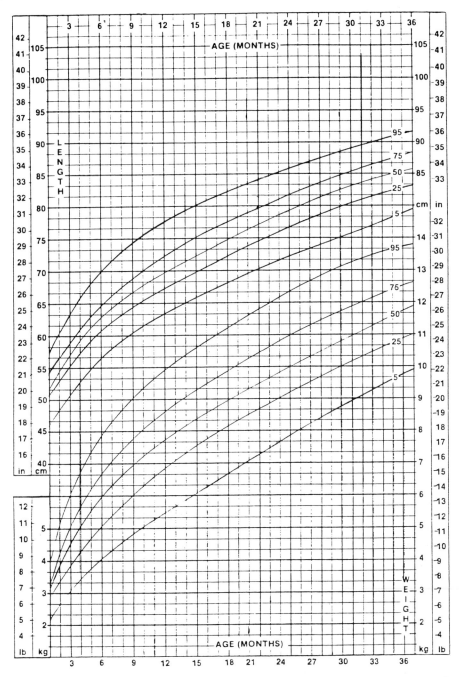

Figure 37 Female: height and weight for Down syndrome (1–36 months). (Reproduced by permission from Pediatrics 1988; 81:102.)

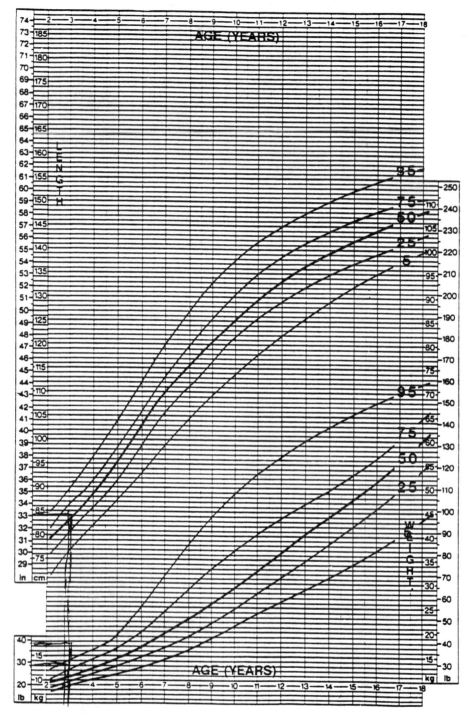

Figure 38 Female: height and weight for Down syndrome (2–18 years). (Reproduced by permission from Pediatrics 1988; 81:102.)

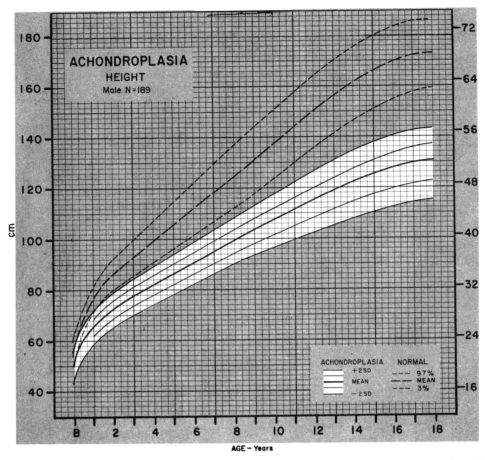

Figure 39   Male: height curve for achondroplasia compared to normal height curve. (From J Pediatr 1978; 93(3):435–438.)

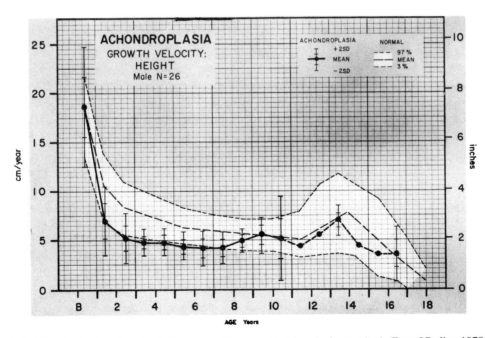

Figure 40   Male: height velocity for achondroplasia compared to normal height velocity standard. (From J Pediatr 1978; 93(3):435–438.)

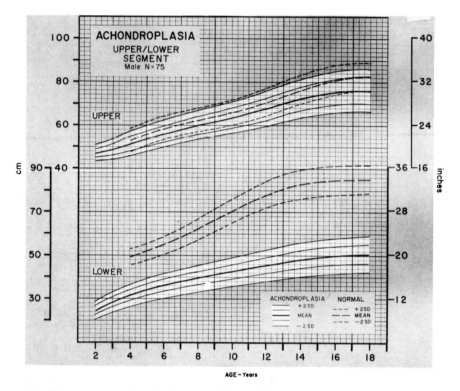

Figure 41   Male: upper and lower segment lengths for achondroplasia compared to normal segment lengths. (From J Pediatr 1978; 93(3):435–438.)

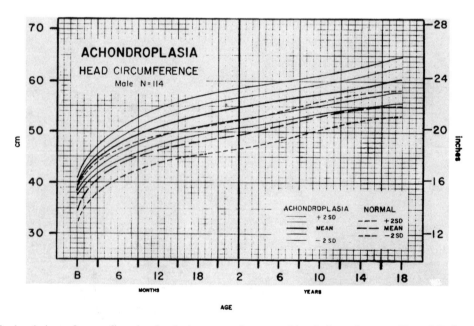

Figure 42   Male: head circumference for achondroplasia compared to normal head circumference. (From J Pediatr 1978; 93(3):435–438.)

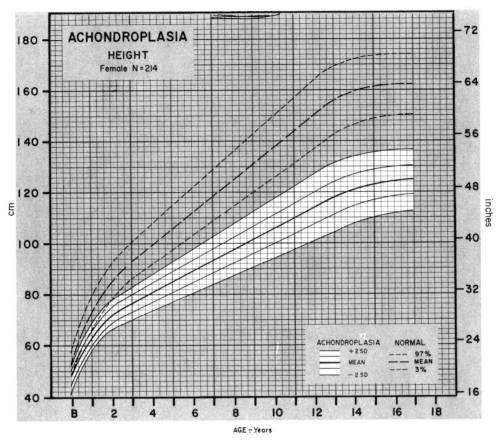

Figure 43 Female: height curve for achondroplasia compared to normal standard curve. (From J Pediatr 1978; 93(3):435–438.)

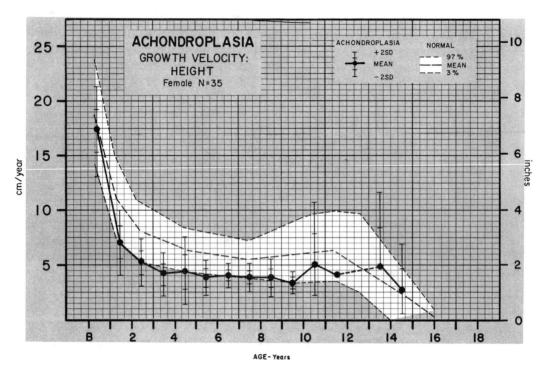

Figure 44 Female: height velocity for achondroplasia compared to normal height velocity standard. (From J Pediatr 1978; 93(3):435–438.)

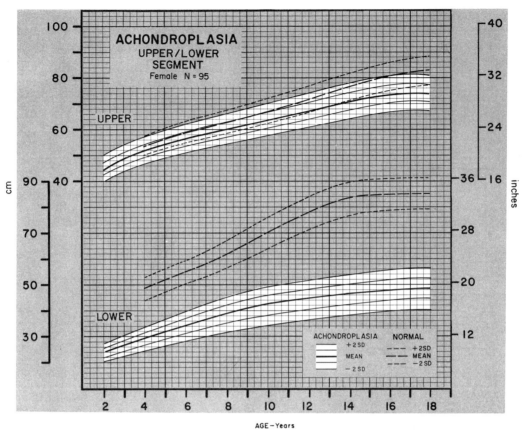

Figure 45 Female: upper and lower segment lengths for achondroplasia compared to normal segment lengths. (From J Pediatr 1978; 93(3):435–438.)

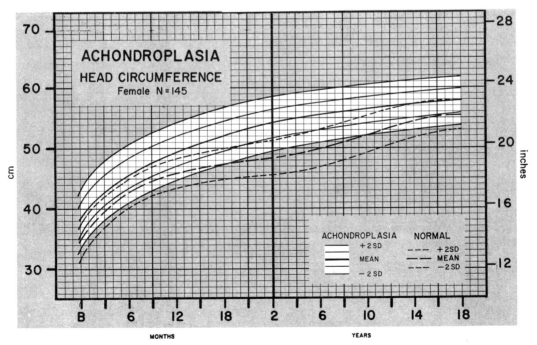

Figure 46 Female: head circumference for achondroplasia compared to normal head circumference. (From J Pediatr 1978; 93(3):435–438.)

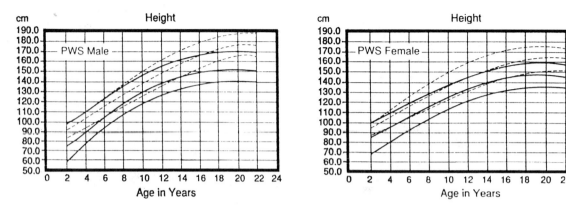

Figure 47 Curves for height of males and females with Prader-Willi syndrome (solid lines) and healthy individuals (broken lines). (From Pediatrics 1991; 88:853.)

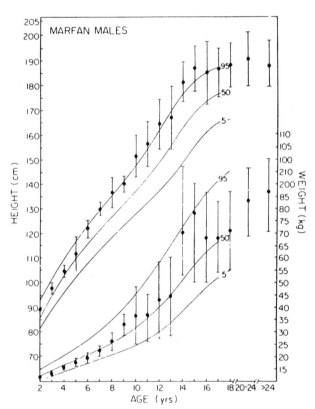

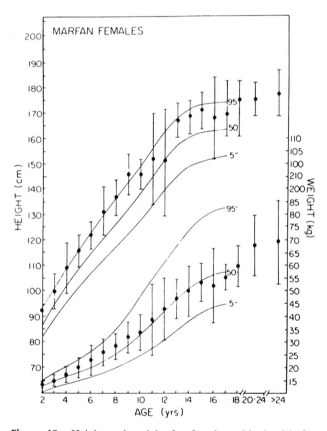

Figure 48 Height and weight for males with the Marfan syndrome, superimposed on normal growth curves (5th, 50th, and 95th percentiles). Cross-sectional and longitudinal data from 200 Caucasian patients with Marfan syndrome were used. Patients were not treated with hormones. Bars shown ± one standard deviation. (From Pyeritz RE. Marfan syndrome. In: Principles and Practice of Medical Genetics. New York: Churchill Livingstone, 1983.)

Figure 49 Height and weight for females with the Marfan syndrome, superimposed on normal growth curves (5th, 50th, and 95th percentiles). Cross-sectional and longitudinal data from 200 Caucasian patients with Marfan syndrome were used. Patients were not treated with hormones. Bars shown ± one standard deviation. (From Pyeritz RE. Marfan syndrome. In: Principles and Practice of Medical Genetics. New York: Churchill Livingstone, 1983.)

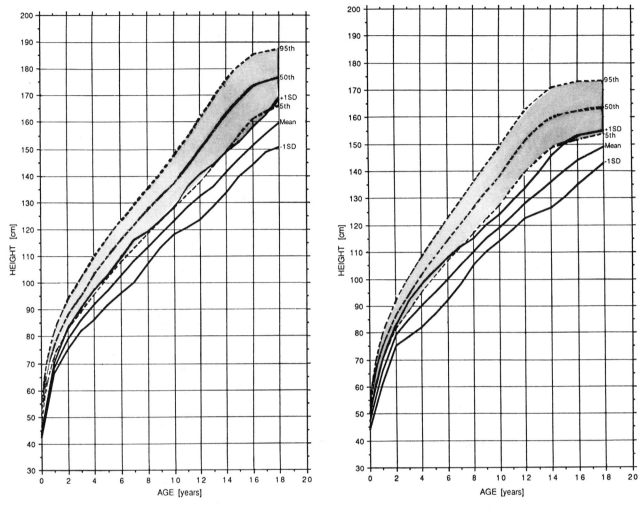

Figure 50 Growth curve for height in males with Noonan syndrome (solid lines) compared to normal values (dashed lines). Data obtained in 64 Noonan syndrome males from a collaborative retrospective review. (From Witt DR, et al. Clin Genet 1986; 30:150.)

Figure 51 Growth curve for height in females with Noonan syndrome (solid lines) compared to normal values (dashed lines). Data obtained in 48 Noonan syndrome females from a collaborative retrospective review. (From Witt DR, et al. Clin Genet 1986; 30:150.)

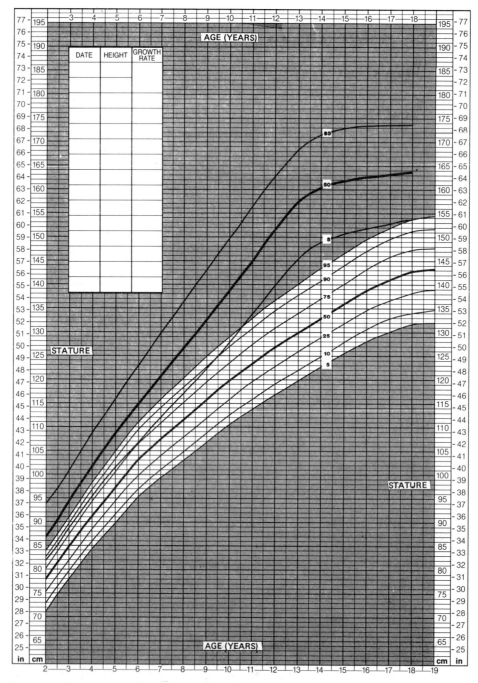

Figure 52 Growth chart for Turner syndrome compared to normal female growth. The solid line shows growth in normal girls; percentiles derived from the National Center for Health Statistics. The broken line shows growth in untreated Turner syndrome girls; percentiles derived from Lyon AJ, Preece MA, Grant DB. Arch Dis Child 1985; 60:932–935. (© Genetech, Inc., 1987. All rights reserved.)

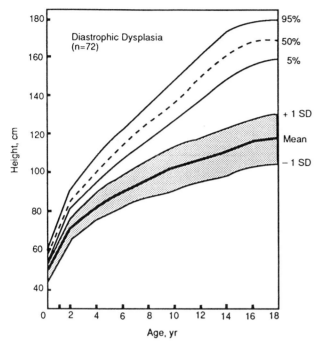

Figure 53 No gender specified: growth curve for diastrophic dysplasia. (From Am J Dis Child 1983; 136:316–319. © AMA.)

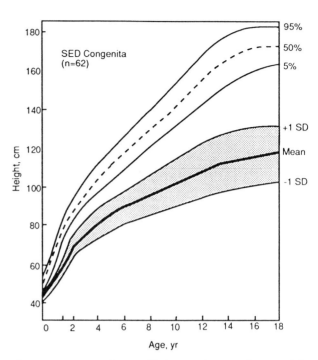

Figure 54 No gender specified: growth curve for spondylo-epiphyseal dysplasia congenita. (From Am J Dis Child 1983; 136:316–319. © AMA.)

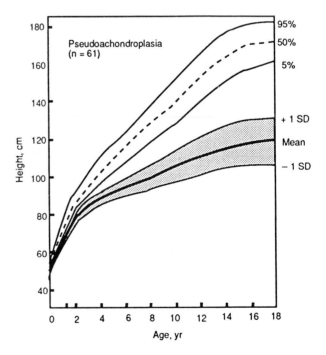

Figure 55 No gender specified: growth curve for pseudoachondroplasia. (From Am J Dis Child 1983; 136:316–319. © AMA.)

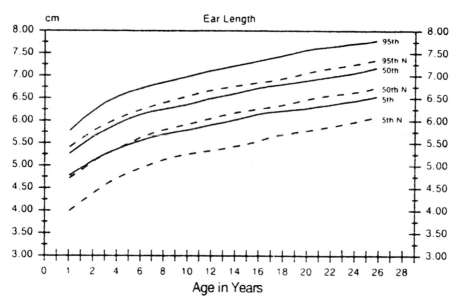

Figure 56 Curves for ear length of males with fragile X syndrome (solid lines) and normal individuals (dotted lines). (From Butler MG, Brunschwig A, Miller, LK, et al. Pediatrics 1992; 89:1059–1062.)

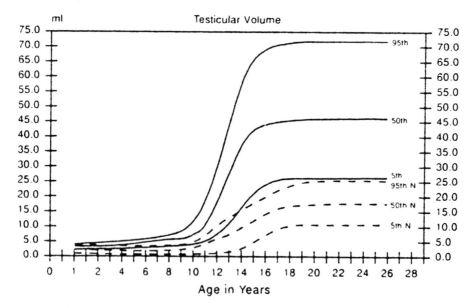

Figure 57 Curves for testicular volume of males with fragile X syndrome—birth to 28 years. (From Butler MG, Brunschwig A, Miller, LK, et al. Pediatrics 1992; 89:1059–1062.)

Index